Second Edition

Clinical Procedures in

Emergency Medicine

JAMES R. ROBERTS, M.D., F.A.C.E.P.

Professor of Emergency Medicine and
Director, Division of Toxicology,
The Medical College of Pennsylvania,
Philadelphia, Pennsylvania

Chairman, Department of Emergency Medicine,
Mercy Catholic Medical Center,
Philadelphia, Pennsylvania

JERRIS R. HEDGES, M.D., M.S., F.A.C.E.P.

Associate Professor of Emergency Medicine and
Director, Emergency Medicine Research Programs,
Oregon Health Sciences University,
Portland, Oregon

Attending Physician, University Hospital and
Veterans Affairs Medical Center Hospital,
Portland, Oregon

President, Society for Academic Emergency Medicine (1990–1991)

W.B. SAUNDERS COMPANY
Harcourt Brace Jovanovich, Inc.
Philadelphia ▪ London ▪ Toronto ▪ Montreal ▪ Sydney ▪ Tokyo

W. B. SAUNDERS COMPANY
Harcourt Brace Jovanovich, Inc.

The Curtis Center
Independence Square West
Philadelphia, PA 19106

Library of Congress Cataloging-in-Publication Data

Clinical procedures in emergency medicine /
[edited by] James R. Roberts, Jerris R. Hedges.—2nd ed.

p. cm.

Includes bibliographical references.
Includes index.

ISBN 0-7216-7611-1

1. Emergency medicine.   I. Roberts, James R.
   II. Hedges, Jerris R.   [DNLM: 1. Emergencies.
   2. Emergency Medicine—Methods.   WB 105 C641]

RC86.7.C55 1991

616.02′5—dc20

DNLM/DLC   90–9244

Listed here is the latest translated edition of this book, together with the language of translation and the publisher.

1st ed. Spanish. Editorial Medica Panamericana, Buenos Aires, Argentina.

Editor: Darlene Pedersen
Developmental Editor: Hazel Hacker
Designer: W. B. Saunders Staff
Production Manager: Bill Preston
Manuscript Editors: Lee Ann Draud, Phyllis Skomorowsky, Amy Eckenthal, and Jessie H. Raymond
New Illustrations: Karen Giacomucci and Elizabeth Strausburg
Illustration Coordinator: Peg Shaw
Indexer: Linda Van Pelt
Cover Designer: Michelle Maloney

Clinical Procedures in Emergency Medicine, Second Edition   ISBN 0–7216–7611–1

Printed in the United States of America.

Last digit is the print number: 9   8   7   6   5   4   3   2

To
George Roberts, George H. Roberts,
and Albert J. Forte
three exceptional self-made men who have given
guidance, inspiration, and support,
often in ways they will never know.

JAMES R. ROBERTS

While second editions of textbooks should be less difficult than the original effort, this edition was decidedly more time-consuming and challenging than the first. This edition is dedicated to my children, Andrew Ryan and Emily Roseanne, who have seen considerably less of their father than I would have preferred during the preparation of this second edition. Someday they will understand my commitment to this project when they observe the effect of my efforts and their sacrifice upon future generations of emergency physicians who will use this textbook to advance the clinical practice of emergency medicine.

JERRIS R. HEDGES

Contributors

Tom I. Abelson, M.D.

Assistant Clinical Professor of Otolaryngology, Case Western Reserve University School of Medicine, Cleveland, Ohio; Assistant Otolaryngologist, University Hospitals of Cleveland, Cleveland, Ohio; Staff Otolaryngologist, Mt. Sinai Medical Center and Hillcrest Hospital, Cleveland, Ohio; Consulting Staff, Veterans Administration Hospital of Cleveland, Cleveland, Ohio; Adjunct Staff, Department of Otolaryngology and Communicative Disorders, The Cleveland Clinic Foundation, Cleveland, Ohio.

James T. Amsterdam, D.M.D., M.D., F.A.C.E.P.

Associate Professor of Emergency Medicine, Northeastern Ohio Universities College of Medicine, Rootstown, Ohio; Visiting Associate Professor of Medicine (Dental Medicine), Medical College of Pennsylvania, Philadelphia, Pennsylvania; Chairman, Department of Emergency Medicine, Western Reserve Care Systems, Youngstown, Ohio.

Paul B. Baker, M.D.

Staff Physician, Emergency Department, Holy Cross Hospital, Silver Spring, Maryland.

William J. Barker, M.D., F.A.C.E.P.

Assistant Clinical Professor of Emergency Medicine, George Washington University, Washington, D.C.; Chairman, Department of Emergency Services, Fair Oaks Hospital, Fairfax, Virginia.

Richard C. Barnett, M.D.

Associate Clinical Professor of Family and Community Medicine, University of California, San Francisco, Medical School, San Francisco, California; Former Director, Family Practice Program, Community Hospital of Sonoma County, Santa Rosa, California.

David H. Barr, M.D.

Attending Ophthalmologist, Northwest Hospital, Ballard Hospital, and Stevens Hospital, Seattle, Washington.

Robert L. Bartlett, M.D., F.A.C.E.P.

Associate Educational Director and Director of Research, Department of Emergency Medicine; Richland Memorial Hospital, Columbia, South Carolina; Clinical Instructor of Surgery, Medical University of South Carolina, Charleston, South Carolina.

Calvin Bell, M.D.

Faculty, Joint Military Medical Command—San Antonio, Emergency Medicine Residency Program, Department of Emergency Medicine, Brooke Army Medical Center, Fort Sam Houston, Texas.

Georges C. Benjamin, M.D., F.A.C.P., F.A.C.E.P.

Clinical Instructor, Department of Emergency Medicine, Georgetown University, Washington, D.C.; Chairman, Department of Community Health and Ambulatory Care, District of Columbia General Hospital, Washington, D.C.

Richard E. Berger, M.D.

Associate Professor, Department of Urology, University of Washington, Seattle, Washington; Attending Urologist, University Hospital, Seattle, Washington; Chief of Urology, Harborview Medical Center, Seattle, Washington; Attending Urologist, Seattle Veterans Administration, Seattle, Washington; Children's Orthopedic Hospital and Medical Center, Seattle, Washington.

Garrett E. Bergman, M.D., M.B.A.

Clinical Professor, Department of Pediatrics, Medical College of Pennsylvania, Philadelphia, Pennsylvania; Attending Pediatrician, St. Christopher's Hospital for Children, Philadelphia, Pennsylvania; Director, Medical and Scientific Affairs, Armour Pharmaceutical Company, Blue Bell, Pennsylvania.

Courtney A. Bethel, M.D., M.P.H.

Resident, Department of Emergency Medicine, Medical College of Pennsylvania, Philadelphia, Pennsylvania.

G. Richard Braen, M.D., F.A.C.E.P.

Professor and Chairman, Department of Emergency Medicine, State University of New York at Buffalo, School of Medicine, Buffalo, New York; Head, Emergency Department, Buffalo General Hospital, Buffalo, New York.

Frank P. Brancato, Ph.D.

Former Affiliate Professor, University of Washington, Department of Microbiology, Seattle, Washington; Former Director, Microbiology Service, USPHS Hospital, Seattle, Washington.

Michael L. Callaham, M.D.

Professor of Medicine, University of California, San Francisco, San Francisco, California; Chief, Division of Emergency Medicine, University of California, San Francisco Medical Center, San Francisco, California.

Carl R. Chudnofsky, M.D.

Clinical Instructor, Department of Medicine, Division of Emergency Medicine; Associate Research Director, Division of Emergency Medicine, University of Massachusetts Medical Center, Worcester, Massachusetts.

Joseph E. Clinton, M.D.

Senior Physician, Hennepin Faculty Association, Minneapolis, Minnesota; Assistant Chief, Emergency Medicine, Hennepin County Medical Center, Minneapolis, Minnesota.

Samuel Timothy Coleridge, D.O., F.A.C.E.P.

Clinical Assistant Professor of Emergency Medical Services, The University of Texas Health Science Center at San Antonio, Texas; Clinical Assistant Professor of Military Medicine, Uniformed Services University of The Health Sciences, F. Edward Hébert School of Medicine, Bethesda, Maryland; Clinical Associate Professor, Division of Emergency Medicine Department of General and Family Practice, Texas College of Osteopathic Medicine, Fort Worth, Texas; Chief, Department of Emergency Medicine, Brooke Army Medical Center, Fort Sam Houston, Texas; Medical Staff, Bexar County Hospital District, San Antonio, Texas.

William C. Dalsey, M.D.

Chairman, Department of Emergency Medicine, Albert Einstein Medical Center, Philadelphia, Pennsylvania.

Scott M. Davis, M.D., F.A.C.E.P.

Associate Professor of Emergency Medicine, Northeastern Ohio Universities College of Medicine, Rootstown, Ohio; Attending Emergency Physician, Akron City Hospital, Akron, Ohio.

Richard Davison, M.D.

Associate Professor of Medicine and Chief, Divisions of Cardiology and Critical Care, Northwestern University Medical School, Chicago, Illinois; Director, Medical Intensive Care Area, Northwestern Memorial Hospital, Chicago, Illinois.

Mohamud R. Daya, M.D., F.A.C.E.P.

Assistant Professor, University of Toronto, Toronto Hospital, Toronto, Ontario, Canada.

Edwin Dean, M.D.

Assistant Professor of Clinical Emergency Medicine, University of Southern California; Attending Staff, Emergency Department, Los Angeles County and University of Southern California Medical Center, Los Angeles, California.

Thom Dick, EMT-P

Lecturer, University of California, San Diego, San Diego, California; Paramedic, Hartson Ambulance Service, San Diego, California; Associate Editor, Journal of Emergency Medical Services.

Lynnette Doan-Wiggins, M.D., F.A.C.E.P.

Assistant Professor of Medicine, Loyola University of Chicago Stritch School of Medicine, Maywood, Illinois; Associate Director, Emergency Department, Loyola University Medical Center, Maywood, Illinois.

David Doezema, M.D., F.A.C.E.P.

Assistant Professor, Division of Emergency Medicine, University of New Mexico School of Medicine, Albuquerque, New Mexico; Emergency Medicine Physician, University of New Mexico Hospital, Albuquerque, New Mexico.

Alice M. Donahue, R.N., M.S.N.

Saint Mary Hospital, Langhorne, Pennsylvania.

Steven C. Dronen, M.D.

Associate Professor of Emergency Medicine, University of Cincinnati College of Medicine, Cincinnati, Ohio; Staff Physician, Department of Emergency Medicine, University Hospital, Cincinnati, Ohio.

David J. Dula, M.D., F.A.C.E.P.

Associate in Emergency Medicine, Geisinger Medical Center, Danville, Pennsylvania.

Susan M. Dunmire, M.D., F.A.C.E.P.

Assistant Professor of Medicine, University of Pittsburgh School of Medicine, Division of Emergency Medicine, Pittsburgh, Pennsylvania; Attending Physician, Presbyterian University Hospital, and Academic Coordinator, Emergency Department, Presbyterian University Hospital, Pittsburgh, Pennsylvania.

William Durston, M.D.

Assistant Clinical Professor of Medicine, University of California, Davis, Davis, California; Staff Emergency Physician, Kaiser Foundation Hospital, Sacramento, California.

William A. Engle, M.D.

Assistant Professor of Pediatrics, James Whitcomb Riley Hospital for Children, Indiana University School of Medicine, Indianapolis, Indiana; Indiana University Hospital, Indianapolis, Indiana; Wishard Memorial Hospital, Indianapolis, Indiana.

Michael E. Ervin, M.D.

Associate Clinical Professor of Emergency Medicine, Wright State University School of Medicine, Dayton, Ohio.

Sandra L. Ezell, M.D.

Assistant Professor, Department of Surgery, Howard University College of Medicine, Washington, D.C.; Director of Trauma Service, District of Columbia General Hospital, Washington, D.C.

Roy G. Farrell, M.D.

Emergency Physician, Seattle, Washington.

Carol S. Federiuk, M.D., Ph.D.

Assistant Professor, Division of Emergency Medicine, Oregon Health Sciences University, Portland, Oregon; Attending Physician, University Hospital, Oregon Health Sciences University, Portland, Oregon.

Dan L. Field, M.D.

Teaching Faculty, Department of Emergency Medicine, University of California, Sacramento, California; Staff Physician, Kaiser Foundation Hospital, Sacramento, California.

Mark W. Fourré, M.D.

Clinical Assistant Professor of Surgery, University of Vermont College of Medicine, Burlington, Vermont; Attending Physician, Department of Emergency Medicine, Maine Medical Center, Portland, Maine.

Thomas G. Frohlich, M.D.

Assistant Professor of Clinical Medicine, Northwestern University Medical School, Chicago, Illinois; Associate Director, Cardiac Catheterization Laboratory, Evanston Hospital Corporation, Evanston, Illinois.

Kenneth Frumkin, M.D., Ph.D.

Emergency Physician and Chief, Department of Emergency Services, Humana Hospital—Sunrise, Las Vegas, Nevada.

Stephen Gazak, M.D.

Staff Physician, Department of Emergency Medicine, Methodist Hospital, Philadelphia, Pennsylvania.

Jonathan M. Glauser, M.D.

Director, Department of Emergency Medicine and Residency Training Program in Emergency Medicine, Mt. Sinai Medical Center, Cleveland, Ohio.

Morton G. Glickman, M.D.

Professor of Diagnostic Radiology and Surgery/Urology, Yale University School of Medicine, New Haven, Connecticut; Chief of Genitourinary Radiology, Yale–New Haven Hospital, New Haven, Connecticut.

Michael I. Greenberg, M.D.

Clinical Associate Professor of Emergency Medicine, Medical College of Pennsylvania, Philadelphia, Pennsylvania; Chief, Department of Emergency Medicine, Sacred Heart Hospital, Norristown, Pennsylvania.

Edith L. Hambrick, M.D., F.A.C.E.P.

Associate Professor, Program Director, Emergency Medicine, Howard University, Washington, D.C.; Vice-Chairman, Emergency Department, Howard University Hospital, Washington, D.C.

Dwight E. Helmrich, M.D.

Staff, Department of Emergency Service, Wilford Hall USAF Medical Center, San Antonio, Texas.

Geoffrey E. Herter, M.D.

Clinical Instructor of Surgery, University of Connecticut, Farmington, Connecticut; Clinical Instructor of Surgery, Yale New Haven Hospital, New Haven, Connecticut; Senior Attending Physician, Middlesex Memorial Hospital, Middletown, Connecticut.

John M. Howell, M.D., F.A.C.E.P.

Instructor in Emergency Medicine, Northeastern Ohio Universities College of Medicine; Faculty, Akron City Emergency Medicine Residency Program; Staff, Emergency Department, St. Thomas Medical Center, Akron, Ohio.

Mary Ann Howland, Pharm.D., A.B.A.T.

Clinical Professor of Pharmacy, St. John's University College of Pharmacy, Jamaica, New York; Consultant, New York City Poison Control Center; Consultant, Bellevue Hospital, Emergency Medical Services, New York, New York.

J. Stephen Huff, M.D., F.A.C.E.P.

Associate Residency Director, Division of Emergency Medicine, Eastern Virginia Graduate School of Medicine, Norfolk, Virginia; Staff Physician, Emergency Physicians of Tidewater, Norfolk, Virginia.

Kenneth V. Iserson, M.D., M.B.A., F.A.C.E.P.

Associate Professor of Surgery, Residency Director in Emergency Medicine, University of Arizona College of Medicine,

Tucson, Arizona; Staff Emergency Physician, University Medical Center, Tucson, Arizona.

Steven M. Joyce, M.D.

Associate Professor, Division of Emergency Medicine, Department of Surgery, University of Utah School of Medicine, Salt Lake City, Utah; Emergency Physician, University of Utah Hospital, Salt Lake City, Utah.

Jon Jui, M.D., F.A.C.E.P.

Assistant Professor, Division of Emergency Medicine, Oregon Health Sciences University, Portland, Oregon.

Robert L. Katz, M.D., F.A.C.S.

Associate Clinical Professor of Otolaryngology, Case Western Reserve University, Cleveland, Ohio; Otolaryngologist, University Hospitals of Cleveland, Cleveland, Ohio.

Seung K. Kim, M.D.

Assistant Clinical Professor of Surgery, Division of Plastic Surgery, Stanford University School of Medicine, Stanford, California; Attending Plastic Surgeon, Stanford University Medical Center, Stanford, California.

Robert Knopp, M.D.

Associate Clinical Professor of Medicine, University of California, San Francisco, San Francisco, California; Associate Chief, Emergency Medicine, Valley Medical Center, Fresno, California.

Marc E. Kobernick, M.D.

San Diego, California.

Jon C. Kooiker, M.D.

Clinical Assistant Professor of Medicine (Neurology), University of Washington School of Medicine, Seattle, Washington; Attending Neurologist, St. Peter Hospital and Black Hills Community Hospital, Olympia, Washington.

Thomas J. Krisanda, M.D.

Attending Physician, Department of Emergency Medicine, York Hospital, York, Pennsylvania.

Richard L. Lammers, M.D.

Assistant Clinical Professor of Family and Community Medicine, University of California School of Medicine, San Francisco, California; Assistant Chief of Emergency Medicine, Valley Medical Center, Fresno, California.

Robert G. R. Lang, M.D., F.R.C.S.(C)

Attending Neurosurgeon and Chairman, Department of Surgery, St. Peter Hospital, Olympia, Washington; Attending Neurosurgeon, Capital Medical Center, Olympia, Washington.

Jody Riva Lewinter, M.D.

Attending Physician, Department of Emergency Medical Services/Trauma, Hartford Hospital, Hartford, Connecticut.

John L. Lyman, M.D., F.A.C.E.P.

Assistant Director, Emergency Department, Bay Medical Center, Panama City, Florida.

Sharon E. Mace, M.D., F.A.C.E.P., F.A.A.P.

Clinical Assistant Professor, Emergency Medicine, University of Rochester Medical Center, Rochester, New York; Faculty and Former Emergency Medicine Residency Director, Department of Emergency Medicine, Mt. Sinai Medical Center, Cleveland, Ohio; Director, Emergency Department, St. Mary's Hospital, Rochester, New York; Faculty, Emergency Medicine Residency Program, Department of Emergency Medicine, Mt. Sinai Medical Center, Cleveland, Ohio.

A. Roy Magnusson, M.D., F.A.C.E.P.

Assistant Professor, Associate Residency Director, Division of Emergency Medicine, Oregon Health Sciences Center, Portland, Oregon.

Lancing P. Malusky, D.P.M.

Volunteer Instructor, Department of Surgery, University Hospital, Cincinnati, Ohio; Director, Department of Podiatry, Divison of Department of Surgery, University Hospital, Cincinnati, Ohio.

Ronald J. Mariani, EMT-P

Clinical Instructor, Oregon Health Sciences University; Instructor, Portland Community College, Portland, Oregon; Instructor II, Fire Standards Accreditation Board, Portland, Oregon; Firefighter/Paramedic, Portland Fire Bureau, and Flight/Paramedic, Emanuel Hospital LifeFlight, Portland, Oregon.

David H. Neustadt, M.D., F.A.C.P.

Clinical Professor of Medicine, Division of Rheumatology, University of Louisville, School of Medicine, Louisville, Kentucky; Attending Physician, Humana Hospital–University, Louisville, Kentucky; Attending Physician, Jewish Hospital, Louisville, Kentucky; Consultant, Veterans Administration Hospital, Louisville, Kentucky.

William L. Newmeyer, M.D.

Associate Clinical Professor of Surgery, University of California, San Francisco, San Francisco, California; Active Staff, Chief of Surgery, St. Francis Memorial Hospital, San Francisco, California; Active Staff, Children's Hospital of San Francisco, San Francisco, California; Courtesy Staff, St. Mary's Hospital, Seton Medical Center, Daly, California; Consultant Staff, Martinez Veterans Administration Hospital, University of California Hospitals, Martinez, California.

Robert Norton, M.D.

Assistant Professor of Emergency Medicine, Division of Emergency Medicine, Oregon Health Sciences University, Portland, Oregon; Emergency Physician, University Hospital, Portland, Oregon.

Michael Orlinsky, M.D.

Assistant Professor of Clinical Emergency Medicine, University of Southern California, Los Angeles, California; Area Director, Emergency Trauma, Los Angeles County and University of Southern California Medical Center, Los Angeles, California.

Edward J. Otten, M.C.

Director, Division of Toxicology, Associate Professor, Department of Emergency Medicine, University of Cincinnati, Cincinnati, Ohio; University Hospital and St. Luke Hospital, Florence, Kentucky.

Steven A. Pace, M.D.

Faculty Physician, Emergency Medicine Residency Program, Madigan Army Medical Center, Fort Lewis, Washington.

Paul M. Paris, M.D.

Associate Professor and Chief, Division of Emergency Medicine, Department of Medicine, University of Pittsburgh School of Medicine, Pittsburgh, Pennsylvania; Presbyterian University Hospital, Pittsburgh, Pennsylvania; Montefiore University Hospital, Pittsburgh, Pennsylvania.

Douglas A. Propp, M.D., F.A.C.E.P.

Assistant Professor of Clinical Emergency Medicine, University of Illinois College of Medicine, Chicago, Illinois; Education Director, Department of Emergency Medicine, and Director, Employee Health Center and Outpatient Department, Lutheran General Hospital, Park Ridge, Illinois.

Thomas B. Purcell, M.D.

Adjunct Assistant Professor, Department of Medicine, University of California, Los Angeles, Los Angeles, California; Residency Director, Department of Emergency Medicine, Kern Medical Center, Bakersfield, California.

Elaena Quattrocchi, Pharm.D.

Associate Professor of Clinical Pharmacy, Arnold and Marie Schwartz College of Pharmacy and Health Sciences, New York, New York; Clinical Coordinator of Pharmacy, Staten Island University Hospital, Staten Island, New York.

Frederick J. Rescorla, M.D.

Assistant Professor of Surgery, Indiana University School of Medicine, Indianapolis, Indiana; Attending Physician, James Whitcomb Riley Hospital for Children, Indiana University Hospital, and Wishard Memorial Hospital, Indianapolis, Indiana.

David S. Ross, M.D.

Associate Professor of Clinical Emergency Medicine, University of Cincinnati College of Medicine, Cincinnati, Ohio; Medical Director, Emergency Department, St. Luke Hospital West, Florence, Kentucky.

Ernest Ruiz, M.D.

Assistant Professor of Surgery, University of Minnesota Medical School, Minneapolis, Minnesota; Chief of Emergency Medicine, Hennepin County Medical Center, Minneapolis, Minnesota.

Alfred D. Sacchetti, M.D., F.A.C.E.P.

Clinical Assistant Professor, Section of Emergency Medicine, Thomas Jefferson University School of Medicine, Philadelphia, Pennsylvania; Research Director, Department of Emergency Medicine, Our Lady Of Lourdes Medical Center, Camden, New Jersey; Staff Emergency Physician, Jersey Shore Medical Center, Neptune, New Jersey.

John R. Samples, M.D.

Associate Professor, Glaucoma Service, Department of Ophthalmology, Oregon Health Sciences University, Portland, Oregon.

Leonard Samuels, M.D., F.A.C.E.P.

Attending Physician, Mt. Sinai Medical Center, Cleveland, Ohio.

Arthur B. Sanders, M.D., F.A.C.E.P., F.A.C.P.

Professor, Section of Emergency Medicine, Department of Surgery, University of Arizona College of Medicine, Tucson, Arizona; Attending Physician, University Medical Center, Tucson, Arizona.

Martin Schiff, Jr., M.D.

Clinical Professor of Surgery/Urology, University of Arizona College of Medicine, Tucson, Arizona; Attending Physician, University Medical Center, Tucson, Arizona; Consultant, Tucson Veterans Administration Hospital, Tucson, Arizona; Consultant, Tucson Medical Center, Tucson, Arizona.

David P. Sklar, M.D., F.A.C.E.P.

Associate Professor, Department of Family, Community, and Emergency Medicine, Division of Emergency Medicine, University of New Mexico School of Medicine, Albuquerque, New Mexico; Attending Physician, University of New Mexico Hospital, Albuquerque, New Mexico.

Anders E. Sola, M.D.

Clinical Assistant Professor of Anesthesiology and Consultant Algologist, Multidisciplinary Pain Center, University of Washington, Seattle, Washington.

William H. Spivey, M.D.

Associate Professor of Emergency Medicine, and Chief, Division of Research, Department of Emergency Medicine, Medical College of Pennsylvania, Philadelphia, Pennsylvania; Associate Director of the Emergency Department, and Director of Fellowships, Department of Emergency Medicine, Medical College of Pennsylvania, Philadelphia, Pennsylvania.

Thomas Stair, M.D.

Associate Professor and Chairman, Department of Emergency Medicine, Georgetown University Hospital, Washington, D.C.

Scott A. Syverud, M.D., F.A.C.E.P.

Assistant Professor, Department of Emergency Medicine, University of Cincinnati Medical Center, Cincinnati, Ohio; Attending Physician, Emergency Department, St. Luke Hospital West, Florence, Kentucky; Attending Physician, University Hospital, Cincinnati, Ohio.

Dan Tandberg, M.D.

Associate Professor, Division of Emergency Medicine, University of New Mexico School of Medicine, Albuquerque, New Mexico; Attending Physician, University of New Mexico Hospital, Albuquerque, New Mexico; Medical Director, New Mexico Poison and Drug Information Center, Albuquerque, New Mexico.

Thomas E. Terndrup, M.D., F.A.C.E.P.

Assistant Professor, Critical Care and Emergency Medicine and Pediatrics, SUNY Health Science Center at Syracuse, Syracuse, New York; Attending Physician, Emergency Department, University Hospital, Syracuse, New York.

Alexander Trott, M.D.

Associate Professor of Clinical Emergency Medicine, University of Cincinnati School of Medicine; Director, Clinical Affairs, University Hospital Center for Emergency Care, Cincinnati, Ohio.

William G. Troutman, Pharm.D.

Regent's Professor of Pharmacy, College of Pharmacy, University of New Mexico, Albuquerque, New Mexico; Director, New Mexico Poison and Drug Information Center, University of New Mexico, Albuquerque, New Mexico.

David E. Van Ryn, M.D., F.A.C.E.P.

Director, Department of Emergency Medicine, Elkhart General Hospital, Elkhart, Indiana; Director, Pre-Hospital Medical Services, Goshen General Hospital, Goshen, Indiana.

Lars M. Vistnes, M.D.

Professor and Chairman, Department of Functional Restoration, Stanford University School of Medicine, Stanford, California; Chief of Functional Restoration Service, Stanford University Hospital, Stanford, California.

J. Thomas Ward, Jr., M.D.

Clinical Instructor, Department of Internal Medicine, University of Texas Southwestern Medical Center at Dallas, Dallas, Texas; Emergency Department Staff Physician, HCA Medical Center, Plano, Texas; Consulting Medical Staff, Parkland Memorial Hospital, Dallas, Texas; EMS Medical Director, City of Plano, Plano, Texas.

Todd M. Warden, M.D.

Chairman, Department of Emergency Medicine, Our Lady of Lourdes Medical Center, Camden, New Jersey.

Terry M. Williams, M.D., F.A.C.E.P.

Assistant Chief, Emergency Medicine, South Sacramento Kaiser Hospital, Sacramento, California.

William J. Witt, M.D.

Assistant Clinical Professor of Otolaryngology, Case Western Reserve University School of Medicine, Cleveland, Ohio; Otolaryngologist, University Hospitals and Mt. Sinai Medical Center, Cleveland, Ohio.

Seth W. Wright, M.D.

Assistant Professor of Surgery and Medicine, Vanderbilt University Medical Center, Nashville, Tennessee.

Donald M. Yealy, M.D.

Assistant Professor, Division of Emergency Medicine, Texas A & M University College of Medicine, College Station, Texas; Adjunct Assistant Professor, Division of Emergency Medicine, University of Pittsburgh School of Medicine, Pittsburgh, Pennsylvania.

Gary P. Young, M.D.

Chief, Emergency Medicine, Portland Veterans Affairs Medical Center, Portland, Oregon; Assistant Professor of Emergency Medicine and Internal Medicine, Oregon Health Sciences University, Portland, Oregon.

Ivan Zbaraschuk, M.D.

Chief of Surgery, Good Samaritan Hospital, Puyallup, Washington.

Foreword

The emergency physician has the unique responsibility to offer his or her skills at all times to all people (young and old, friendly and hostile, rich and poor). No other health providers are always there. In emergency medicine, our responsibilities have grown and our horizons as emergency physicians have been expanded because of our commitment to people. We have built a system that creates a caring environment from the home to the street and on to the hospital; we have built a system that integrates fire fighters, police officers, paramedics, nurses, clerks, students, pharmacists, and physicians into the caring service. Roberts and Hedges' text, *Clinical Procedures in Emergency Medicine*, takes another step in the pursuit of excellence in the provision of that care. If we are prepared with the basic skills and the rationale for their use, as defined by Roberts and Hedges, we will all have the potential to provide the type of care that our patients seek and deserve.

The last 15 to 20 years in the history of emergency medicine have seen a remarkably rapid evolution in care. Organized medicine has often been criticized for its inability to change thought patterns and approaches to care, but emergency physicians cannot be criticized in this area. We have undertaken our responsibilities in a new area, created new relationships, and developed new perspectives on clinical medicine. In the past, medical providers have also been criticized for not looking at their techniques and technology effectively. This text exemplifies and describes the tremendous progress in thought and technology that marks the success of emergency medicine in America today.

The rapid growth of prehospital care, the ever-increasing access to emergency care, and the evident clinical issues and research dilemmas in emergency medicine have led to the development of a new type of physician in the emergency department. This text defines the true extent of academic emergency medicine and the enormous task to which each clinician must be dedicated.

In emergency medicine, as in many other fields, physicians have felt a need to specialize in a particular aspect of care. These chapters are written by individuals with highly specialized knowledge. All of the chapters in this second edition have been rewritten. A reevaluation of the clinical and academic roles of the emergency physician has led to the expansion, redirection, and refinement of this second edition. As the basic science and clinical practice of emergency medicine have been further developed, this book has grown to represent our speciality. In this edition the editors have placed a special emphasis on filling clinical gaps noted in the first edition. They have included many basic procedures such as the determination of vital signs and approaches to the patient who is hyperthermic. The detailed elucidation of the principles of intubation, anesthesia, and fluid resuscitation reemphasizes the emergency physician's vital role in the evolution of these areas. Special additional emphasis is also placed on life-threatening gynecologic and obstetric procedures. New chapters on wound care (splints, burns, dressings), esophageal foreign body removal, and expanded efforts in microbiologic procedures give a better balance to the emergency and urgent interventions offered in the emergency department.

The first edition of this text filled a void in medical practice. We all believe in the principles of correct diagnosis, appropriate patient advice and reassurance, and effective treatment. However, procedural interventions in the emergency department had previously been largely undefined. The emergency physician who is trained in these techniques can develop the requisite technical skills and combine them with the warmth and humanity essential to rendering concerned, committed, and compassionate emergency care. Knowledge of these skills and their indications, as well as of the risks and benefits of practice, will allow emergency physicians to achieve a high level of service and to initiate quality research.

Understanding this remarkable spectrum of responsibility as emergency physicians is our essential task. We shall succeed as providers if we understand our patients and their needs, the pathophysiology of emergency medicine and its therapeutics, and our procedures and their pitfalls. Roberts and Hedges' *Clinical Procedures in Emergency Medicine* goes a long way toward providing the emergency physician enough thoughtful information to be prepared to care for the emergency department patient in an intellectually sound manner while retaining a humane approach to medical technology.

Although there are few physicians other than emergency physicians who will use all the technology detailed in the text, there are many others who can and will profit immensely from this book. The techniques are well defined, well illustrated, and well referenced by clinicians who obviously use them daily. This effort was unique with respect to its depth and breadth in its first edition, and this edition reinforces the importance and potential value of Roberts and Hedges's work while defining areas for future direction and improvement.

The understanding and application of the principles defined in this edition should be considered essential for each emergency physician in his or her attempt to improve continuously the delivery of our patients' health care.

LEWIS GOLDFRANK, M.D.

Director, Emergency Medical Services,
Bellevue Hospital Center and
New York University Medical Center;
Associate Professor of Clinical Medicine,
New York University School of Medicine;
Medical Director, New York City Poison
Control Center

Preface

Emergency medicine is a procedure-oriented specialty. Indeed, the decision-making process that goes into the performance of a procedure represents a major aspect of clinical emergency medicine. Most standard textbooks discuss procedures only briefly and provide little information regarding the rationale or thought process involved in the decision to use a given method. Technique manuals are often more like cookbooks, replete with assumptions and complemented by only sparse text and inadequate illustrations. Dogma is often espoused, unsubstantiated statements are made, and alternative techniques may be overlooked in favor of each particular author's preferred method. This textbook offers the reader the well referenced clinical rationale for procedures, alternative methods where appropriate, and potential complications with advice on how to avoid them. Tricks of the trade and personal experience are incorporated throughout the text.

The concept for this book originated over 15 years ago, when the editors began to practice the new specialty of emergency medicine and attempted to teach residents the basic procedures of the discipline. It was obvious that emergency physicians often faced problems or circumstances that were different from the traditionalist when performing well established or newer procedures. Often, problems encountered in the emergency department required their own unique solutions. For example, availability of makeshift equipment became paramount, and the time element was always present. Older techniques had to be modified and new ones had to be created to meet the needs of a rapidly expanding specialty. No longer did the otolaryngology text suffice for an emergency physician's approach to epistaxis, nor did the urology text suffice for evaluation of acute genitourinary trauma at 3 A.M. when a urologist could not be found.

A number of experts from a variety of specialties have contributed to this book. The experience and opinions of the contributing authors have been collated by the editors into a presentation that encompasses the majority of procedures performed in clinical emergency medicine. The second edition has 18 new, additional chapters, on such common procedures as the outpatient management of burns, splinting techniques, and the seemingly simple concept of measuring vital signs. The chapter on local anesthesia has been completely rewritten, and includes newer concepts regarding the use of topical anesthesia and buffered lidocaine. The chapter on pharmacologic adjuncts to tracheal intubation contains material difficult to find elsewhere and is especially relevant to emergency medicine. Depending on one's practice, some procedures, such as central venous access, may be performed frequently, while others, such as emergency burn escharotomy and the amobarbital interview, may seldom be encountered by even the busiest emergency physician. Some of the procedures are uncommon and may be previously unknown to the reader; others may be totally familiar. In the latter circumstances, one will find objective data upon which to base clinical decisions and helpful suggestions for modification of even the most familiar techniques.

This book was written to satisfy the needs of physicians with varied backgrounds and training and can be adapted to a number of practice situations. Specialists in emergency medicine will undoubtedly consider this text an essential ingredient in their practice. Family physicians, pediatricians, general internists, general surgeons, and other specialists will find the text of value for review of infrequently used procedures. Physicians involved in the education of residents and medical students will find the book a valuable source of didactic information. Finally, the physician in training will value this text as a ready authoritative source in those lonely hours when a procedure must be performed but on-site consultation is unavailable.

Although the editors had hoped that the text would be all-inclusive, such a goal is not practical. In both editions of this textbook, the editors have avoided the cookbook presentation of procedures by protocol as presented in Basic Cardiac Life Support, Advanced Cardiac Life Support, Advanced Trauma Life Support, and other similar courses. While emergency physicians must be familiar with the general approach to patient care taught in those courses, the purpose of this textbook is to emphasize the procedures themselves.

Many emergency procedures are learned by a "see one, do one, teach one" format, and techniques are handed down from resident to intern to medical student. Often critical details or basic concepts are lost or distorted in the transmission. The editors have attempted to present a clear and straightforward discussion without assuming that the reader has had previous experience with the technique. Some points, therefore, may seem obvious, unnecessary, or superfluous to the experienced physician, but they have been provided for thoroughness.

While no textbook can equal the bedside guidance of a skilled clinician's tutorial, the availability of fully referenced and detailed procedural descriptions, written by a practicing physician with personal experience, should aid the seasoned practitioner and novice house staff alike.

An area that will require further discussion in future editions is the protection of both the practitioner and the patient from exposure to contagion during the performance of clinical procedures. Of paramount concern are those infections for which medical science has no cure. In addition to the human immunodeficiency virus (which may be present in the blood of up to 10 per cent of patients bleeding because of penetrating trauma), hepatitis B virus and other viral agents pose real risks every day to the clinician. Although this textbook encourages "universal precautions" (i.e., treating all body substances as potentially infectious), the most practical application of such precautions is uncertain. Furthermore, the setting in which a practitioner with AIDS may perform procedures with no appreciable risk to the patient remains to be established. Until further data become available, we advise that the practitioner at risk of contact with body substances always be appropriately protected. The use of latex gloves, a face mask with an eye shield, and a gown is recommended for high-risk settings. Sharp objects (e.g., sutures, staples, scalpels, needles, and trocars) should be promptly placed in puncture-proof containers. Needles should *not* be recapped, but disposed of in the puncture-proof containers. When possible, injections should be administered through intravenous extension tubing side ports so that direct contact with patient blood is avoided should a subsequent needle stick occur. Irrigation shields to minimize side spray during wound irrigation should be used. *All health care providers should be immunized against hepatitis B.* During all invasive procedures, extreme caution is warranted and urged.

James R. Roberts
Jerris R. Hedges

Contents

Section IX
Genitourinary Procedures

Section X
Obstetric and Gynecologic Procedures

Section XI
Neurologic Procedures

Respiratory Procedures

Chapter 1

Emergency Airway Management Procedures

Joseph E. Clinton and Ernest Ruiz

INTRODUCTION

Airway management is widely preached as the first priority in the management of any seriously ill or injured patient. However, in spite of the lip service given to the importance of airway management, it is often overlooked and, consequently, can be a source of error in the care of the critically ill or injured patient. Although appropriate airway management is evident in all smooth resuscitations, inappropriate management often presages a cycle of patient deterioration and misguided therapeutic intervention.

Unfortunately, recognition of the need for airway management is only the first part of the problem in emergency resuscitation. Managing the airway may be one of the most difficult aspects of the entire resuscitation. Because of the sheer variety of airway obstructions possible, even the most skilled resuscitator can find the task challenging. Blood, loose teeth, vomitus, swollen or distorted landmarks—all of these present formidable barriers to successful management. When obstruction occurs in conjunction with reflex clenching of the jaws and possible cervical spine injury, conventional airway management tools may be rendered useless. Time pressures imposed by the need to avoid cerebral anoxia force one to make difficult decisions concerning the use of risky maneuvers such as moving the neck, administering paralyzing agents, or using invasive procedures. Tools must be at hand, skills must be well practiced, and decision making must be sharp if optimal emergency airway management is to occur.

Some solutions to the dilemmas faced in emergency airway management are presented in this chapter. Nonsurgical and minimally invasive approaches to airway establishment and ventilatory control are described. Detailed description of procedures is not meant to imply that the procedure can be performed in only one fashion. Rather, the descriptions are intended to offer an acceptable answer to those "obvious" procedural questions that are often left unanswered.

Decision algorithms are presented to assemble the pieces of the airway management puzzle into a logical scheme. Study of the algorithms will serve to clarify and facilitate decision making in times of stress. The reader is urged to spend time with the algorithms and apply them to hypothetical cases. Coupling of manipulative skills with sound decisions should lead to appropriate airway management as a prelude to successful resuscitation.

ESTABLISHMENT OF AIRWAY PATENCY

The first concern in the management of a patient in critical condition is adequacy of the airway. Partial or complete airway obstruction must be overcome quickly. In some cases, such as an airway obstructed by a tongue, simple maneuvers will suffice. In other cases, particularly those in which a myriad of obstructing agents are conspiring to block the airway, the task will be formidable. The tongue, dentures, swollen or distorted tissues, blood, and vomitus are common obstructing agents that make intubation difficult. Clearing or bypassing these agents may be made more difficult by reflex clenching of the jaws. Moreover, the neck motion required for suction and intubation may be imprudent in certain patients with acute injuries because of the possibility of cervical spine injury.

Airway Maneuvers

Partial or complete airway obstruction resulting from *lax musculature* and *tongue occlusion* of the posterior pharynx may be overcome by a variety of maneuvers. The relative benefits of various airway-opening maneuvers have been examined. In a study of 120 anesthetized patients whose airways were obstructed by their tongues, Guildner compared the ease of performance of the neck-lift and head-tilt method, the jaw-thrust method, and the chin-lift method. He concluded that the chin lift was the easiest to perform and produced the greatest airway patency of the three methods tested.[1] Besides offering greater patency, the chin-lift method has the additional advantage that neck extension is unnecessary (Fig. 1–1, Tables 1–1 and 1–2).

Partial airway obstruction in the patient with a decreased level of consciousness is commonly due to posterior displacement of the tongue. This may be recognized readily in the presence of snoring or stridor, but an apneic patient or one who is moving minimal air may not exhibit any audible evidence of airway obstruction. Some type of jaw-thrust or chin-lift maneuver should be performed on every unconscious patient to ensure airway patency. When uncertain about cervical spine status, the neck must be maintained in the neutral position. If the patient was found with a flexed or extended neck, the neck should first be restored to neutral position with gentle longitudinal traction. The chin-lift or jaw-thrust method is then performed. A combination of these maneuvers will usually clear airways obstructed as a result of the position of the neck itself. The neck-lift and head-tilt maneuver, as described in cardiac life support courses, should not be used when cervical spine injury is suspected, because the extension of the spine produced during the maneuver endangers the spinal cord.

Clearing the airway of foreign material requires more than a simple jaw thrust. The occasional patient who presents with complete airway obstruction secondary to food aspira-

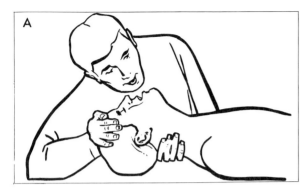

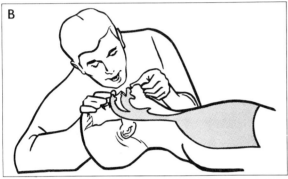

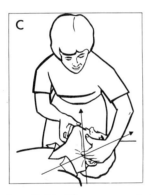

Figure 1–1. Illustration of chin-lift maneuver. *A,* Neck lift. *B,* Chin lift. *C,* Jaw thrust. (From Guildner CW: Resuscitation—opening the airway: A comparative study of techniques for opening an airway obstructed by the tongue. JACEP 5:588, 1976. Reproduced by permission.)

tion may be treated with abdominal thrusts as described in basic cardiac life support.[2]

Partial or complete airway obstruction can be the result of upper airway hemorrhage, accumulation of the patient's own secretions, vomitus, or fractured dentition. When deciding on airway-clearing maneuvers, one must take these circumstances into account. Neck extension is clearly contraindicated if the probability of a cervical spine injury is high. When stability of the spine is a concern, application of the abdominal thrust should be limited to the supine method described for unconscious victims. The abdominal thrust carries a significant risk of complication, compelling the rescuer to weigh the benefits of its application.

The Chin-Lift Maneuver. The rescuer places the tips of the fingers, volar surface superiorly, beneath the patient's chin. The jaw is lifted gently forward. The patient's mouth is opened by drawing down on the lower lip with the thumb of the same hand. Mouth-to-mouth or other means of positive-pressure ventilation is provided if the patient is not ventilating spontaneously.

The Jaw-Thrust Maneuver. The jaw-thrust maneuver

Effectiveness	Neck Lift		Chin Lift		Jaw Thrust	
	No.	%	No.	%	No.	%
Total obstruction						
Unable to ventilate	7	5.8	—	—	1	0.8
Partial obstruction						
Inadequate ventilation	8	6.7	2	1.7	2	1.7
Partial obstruction						
Adequate ventilation but with difficulty	58	48.3	9	7.5	23	19
Good airway						
Easy ventilation	47	39.2	109	90.8	94	78

(From Guildner CW: Resuscitation—opening the airway: A comparative study of techniques for opening an airway obstructed by the tongue. JACEP 5:588, 1976. Reproduced by permission.)

is the second choice, again because neck extension is not necessary. Forward traction on the mandible is achieved by using two hands to grasp the mandibular rami and pull them forward.

The Abdominal Thrust. The abdominal thrust is a method to relieve a completely obstructed airway. The technique was popularized by Dr. Henry Heimlich and is commonly referred to as the *Heimlich maneuver.*[3]

The conscious patient with an obstructed airway is characterized by increased respiratory effort, anxiety, aphonia, and occasionally cyanosis. In the conscious patient, the maneuver is performed with the rescuer positioned behind the upright patient. The rescuer's arms are circled about the patient's midsection with the radial side of the clenched fist placed in the epigastrium of the patient. Care is exercised to position the fist midway between the umbilicus and the xiphoid of the patient. After proper positioning, the rescuer grasps the fist with the opposite hand and delivers an inward and upward thrust to the abdomen. A successful maneuver will cause the obstructing agent to be expelled from the patient's airway by the force of air exiting the lungs.

An unconscious, supine patient must be handled differently: the rescuer kneels next to the patient's pelvis facing cephalad. The palmar bases of the hands are placed in an overlapping fashion on the epigastrium at the same spot as that used in the upright patient. Inward, upward thrusts are delivered in this fashion with the same objective.

Abdominal thrusts are relatively contraindicated in pregnant patients and others with protuberant abdomens. A chest thrust similar to that delivered in closed chest massage may be used instead. The upright patient may be delivered a chest thrust by placing the fist over the sternum. Primate studies that model infant airway obstruction show

Effectiveness (Tidal Volume)	Neck Lift		Chin Lift		Jaw Thrust	
	No.	%	No.	%	No.	%
0–50 ml	13	43.3	—	—	1	3.4
50–250 ml	9	30	2	6.7	3	10
250–400 ml	6	20	7	23.3	7	23.3
Over 400 ml	2	6.7	21	70	19	63.3

(From Guildner CW: Resuscitation—opening the airway: A comparative study of techniques for opening an airway obstructed by the tongue. JACEP 5:588, 1976. Reproduced by permission.)

higher peak airway pressures with chest thrusts than with abdominal thrusts; a combined (simultaneous) chest and abdominal thrust produces even higher peak airway pressures.[4] Hence, a combined maneuver should be considered in the case of total airway obstruction that is unresponsive to simple abdominal thrusts.

Visceral injury can occur with the Heimlich maneuver.[5-7] Excessive force may be responsible in such cases. In others, incorrect placement of the hands may play a role. Nonetheless, the technique can be life saving and should be used when needed. Attention to proper execution may limit mistakes.

Positioning

Positioning the patient who has sustained multiple trauma can be a problem. Spinal injury and airway access priorities dictate that the patient should be kept in the supine position while immobilized on a backboard. Turning the patient on the side will allow upper airway hemorrhage, secretions, and vomitus to drain externally rather than collect in the patient's mouth, which can lead to aspiration and airway obstruction.

Guidelines for patient positioning must take into account the status of the patient's spine and the use of gravity to enable secretions to drain rather than accumulate in the airway. A judicious approach to airway management in a patient *with spontaneous respiration* is the following:

1. Initial airway maintenance accomplished by the chin-lift maneuver and the application of cervical stabilization.
2. Immobilization of the patient on a spinal backboard.
3. With the position of the neck controlled, transportation of the patient on the side to facilitate airway drainage.

Suctioning

Patient positioning and airway opening and clearing maneuvers are often inadequate to achieve the degree of airway patency desired. Ongoing hemorrhage, vomitus, and particulate debris often require suction to clear and maintain the respiratory passage. Three basic types of suctioning devices are available, each suited to different types of airway obstruction problems. Figure 1–2 illustrates the three types of devices that are useful in the management of the traumatized patient's airway.

Dental tip suction is most useful for clearing particulate debris from the upper airway. Vomitus is most readily cleared with this tip because it is least likely to become obstructed itself by particulate matter. The *tonsil* tip (Yankauer) suction device is used most effectively to clear upper airway hemorrhage and secretions. Its design is intended to prevent the obstruction of its tip by tissue and clot. The rounded tip is also less traumatic to soft tissues.

Unfortunately, the *catheter* tip suction device is the one most readily available in many hospitals. Often it is the only type of suction available. This device is virtually useless before the patient has been intubated, at which time it is used for suctioning the trachea and bronchi through the tracheal tube. The dental tip device should be used during the resuscitation period and should be kept ready at the bedside. The dental tip allows rapid clearing of both particulate matter and hemorrhage, thereby expediting airway control.

Optimally, stabilization of the patient with multiple injuries will involve all three types of suction tips. The tonsil or dental tip should be attached to the suction source during

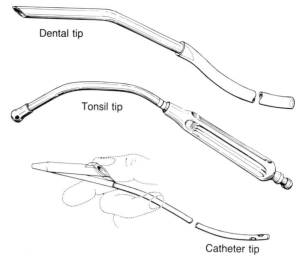

Figure 1–2. Three types of suction tips: dental, tonsil, and catheter tips. (From Clinton, JE, Ruiz E: Trauma Life Support Manual, 1982.)

the interval between patients because it will most likely be the one needed on short notice. Both the tonsil tip and catheter tip should be stored next to the suction source so they can be attached when needed. It is essential that all physicians and nurses know the location of suction equipment and *know how to turn it on* during an emergency. In the resuscitation rooms, the equipment should be connected and ready to operate and not kept in cabinets or wrapped in difficult-to-open packaging material. Latex suction tubing allows the three tips to be interchanged easily. Interposition of a suction trap at the base of the dental tip suction device prevents clogging of the latex tubing with particulate debris. A trap that fits directly onto a tracheal tube has been described; use of this device will allow effective suctioning during intubation (Fig. 1–3).[8]

Although no specific contraindications to airway suctioning exist, complications of incorrectly performed suctioning may be significant. Nasal suction is seldom required to improve oxygenation (except in infants), because most adult airway obstruction occurs in the mouth and oropharynx. Vigorous nasal suction can induce epistaxis and further complicate an already difficult situation. Suctioning that is prolonged may not be recognized during an emergency, but it should be avoided because it may lead to significant hypoxia, especially in children. *Suctioning should not exceed 15-second intervals,* and the provision of supplemental oxygen should be routine. Basilar skull fractures can allow the inadvertent placement of nasal suction tubes in the brain (Fig. 1–4). Extreme care should be exercised when a basilar skull or facial fracture is suspected because communication between nasal and intracranial cavities may exist.

Generally, it is best to perform suctioning *under direct visual inspection* or with the aid of the laryngoscope. Forcing a suction tip blindly into the posterior pharynx can injure tissue or convert a partial obstruction to a complete obstruction.

Complications may be avoided by anticipating problems and providing appropriate care during suctioning maneuvers. Epistaxis may be avoided by limiting the force applied during suctioning. Vasoconstrictor drops, such as 0.25 per cent phenylephrine, will constrict the nasal mucosa and reduce the injury potential in patients who require repeated nasopharyngeal suctioning. The operator must be aware that the occasional patient may develop transient pupillary dilation following use of the drops if the vasoconstrictor solution drips into the conjunctival space. Naigow and Powasner found that suctioning induced hypoxia in dogs consistently and that it was best avoided by hyperventilating the animals before and after suctioning.[9]

Artificial Airways

INDICATIONS AND CONTRAINDICATIONS

Once the airway has been established through various maneuvers and suctioning, the patient may require further temporary support to maintain airway patency. The semiconscious patient who is breathing with an adequate rate and tidal volume at the time of the chin-lift maneuver may develop hypoxia because of recurrent obstruction if the maneuver is discontinued. Oxygen supplementation and an artificial airway may be all the support that is necessary. The use of an artificial airway will also allow more efficient use of rescuer skills and relief from fatigue that is caused by the continuous application of chin-lift or jaw-thrust maneuvers.

Positive-pressure ventilation with a bag-valve-mask (BVM) device may be necessary to bolster the patient's inadequate ventilatory effort or to provide total ventilation in cases of apnea. By maintaining airway patency, artificial airways facilitate spontaneous and bag-mask ventilation. Specialized airways, including the esophageal obturator airway (EOA), the esophageal gastric tube airway (EGTA), the pharyngeal-tracheal lumen airway, and the esophageal combitube airway, are designed for use in the unconscious patient who requires positive-pressure ventilation. The esophageal occluding cuff built into these devices provides the added advantage of reducing gastric regurgitation.

AIRWAY PLACEMENT

The simplest artificial airways are the oropharyngeal and nasopharyngeal airways (Fig. 1–5). Both are intended to prevent the tongue from obstructing the airway by falling back against the posterior pharyngeal wall. The oral airway may also prevent teeth clenching. The oropharyngeal airway may be inserted by either of two procedures. In the first procedure, the airway is inserted in an inverted position along the patient's hard palate. When it is well into the patient's mouth, the airway is rotated 180 degrees and advanced to its final position along the patient's tongue, with the distal end of the airway lying in the hypopharynx. The second procedure involves the performance of a jaw-thrust maneuver, either manually or with a tongue blade, and the simple advancement of the airway into the mouth to its final position. No rotation is performed when the airway is placed in this manner. Once inserted, the oral airway may have to be taped in place to prevent expulsion by the patient's tongue.

The nasopharyngeal airway is placed by gently advancing the airway into a nostril, directing the tip along the floor of the nose toward the nasopharynx. When in final position, the flared external end of the airway should rest at the nasal orifice. Either of these two airways will provide airway patency similar to a correctly performed chin-lift maneuver, but the nasal airway may be better tolerated by the semiconscious patient.

COMPLICATIONS

Few complications are encountered in the use of these airways. The oropharyngeal airway may obstruct the airway if during its placement the tongue is pushed against the posterior pharyngeal wall. Care in placement will prevent this occurrence. In the patient whose reflexes are intact, the gag reflex may stimulate retching and emesis, and the semiconscious patient may not tolerate the oropharyngeal airway. If gagging is a persistent problem, the airway should be removed and a nasal airway or a tracheal intubation should be considered. If the patient is comatose and lacks a gag reflex, the oropharyngeal airway *should not be used* as a definitive airway; tracheal intubation should be used instead. The oropharyngeal airway will keep the mouth partially open if an orogastric tube is placed for gastric lavage or suction, and it will prevent clenching of the teeth, which can obstruct an orotracheal tube.

The nasopharyngeal airway may offer an advantage over the oropharyngeal airway in that the nasopharyngeal airway is less likely to induce gagging. The same considerations that apply to nasal suctioning apply to placement of the nasopharyngeal airway, that is, care must be exercised not to induce epistaxis, and extreme caution is indicated in patients with a suspected basilar skull fracture or facial injury. All patients with oral or nasal pharyngeal airways should be observed constantly, because these devices are temporary measures and cannot substitute for tracheal intubation.

BAG-VALVE-MASK VENTILATION

Indications and Contraindications

Correctly performed, the BVM method of ventilation appears to be simple and effective. Still, it is fraught with difficulty and therefore deserves special mention.

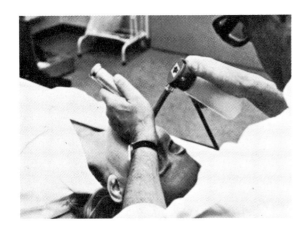

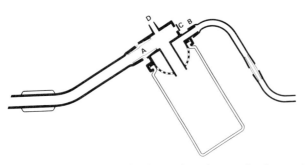

Figure 1–3. Suction booster of Ruben. The Ruben suction booster is designed to allow high-capacity suctioning through the endotracheal tube during intubation. Schematic diagram: *A,* Tracheal tube connection. *B,* Connection to suction. *C,* Introducer opening in the closed position. *D,* Opening that is kept closed when suction is needed through the tracheal tube. Note: All suction should be done under direct vision. (From Ruben H, Hansen E, MacNaughton FI: High capacity suction technique. Anesthesia 34:349, 1979. Reproduced by permission.)

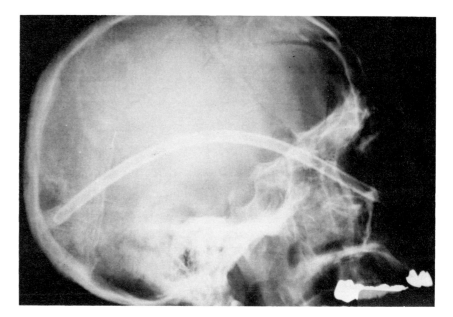

Figure 1–4. Intracranial intubation. Lateral skull x-ray showing nasogastric tube placed into brain through skull fracture. (From Clinton JE, Ruiz E: Trauma Life Support Manual, 1982.)

Bag-valve-mask ventilation should be used by experienced individuals who are able to ensure a tight mask seal in situations requiring positive-pressure ventilation. The BVM is often used with an oropharyngeal or nasopharyngeal airway in place.[2]

Inexperience is a relative contraindication to the use of a BVM. A rescuer who is not skilled with the BVM will achieve much better ventilation with mouth-to-mouth or mouth-to-mask breathing than with a BVM. Although BVM ventilation may provide excellent respiratory support in the anesthetized, paralyzed patient in the operating room, the device frequently is of marginal value during cardiopulmonary resuscitation (CPR), during an ambulance run, or in the combative patient. A tight mask seal is mandatory to prevent loss of air volume during ventilation. Another hazard of BVM ventilation occurs when vomitus, blood, or other debris is present in the mouth or pharynx. The foreign material may be insufflated down the trachea if it is not cleared before ventilation. The three major problems encountered with BVM ventilation are inadequate tidal volumes, inadequate oxygen delivery, and gastric distention.

Ventilation Technique

Achieving adequate tidal volume with BVM ventilation requires a tight mask seal and adequate compression of the

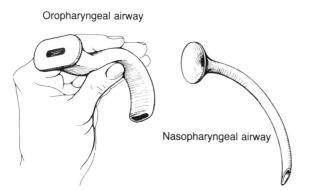

Oropharyngeal airway

Nasopharyngeal airway

Figure 1–5. Simple artificial airways: oropharyngeal and nasopharyngeal. (From Clinton JE, Ruiz E: Trauma Life Support Manual, 1982.)

bag. Even trained paramedics practicing on mannikins have difficulty delivering tidal volumes above 650 ml, which is well below the 800 ml recommended by the American Heart Association. A variety of mask configurations are available to facilitate a tight seal, but none substitutes for the practiced skill of the rescuer. For the single rescuer, only one hand can be used to achieve the seal because the other must squeeze the bag. The rescuer's hand must be large enough to apply pressure anteriorly while simultaneously lifting the jaw forward. The thumb and index finger provide anterior pressure while the fifth and fourth fingers lift the jaw. Care must be exercised to deliver an adequate tidal volume by full compression of the bag. Dentures generally should be left in place to help ensure a better seal with the mask.

It has been suggested that effective BVM ventilation during CPR requires two hands and therefore, two rescuers.[10] When practical, we suggest using the two-rescuer technique (Fig. 1–6A and B). The presence on the device of a pop-off valve may further frustrate ventilation efforts in the patient with reduced compliance. When using pediatric BVM devices such as the Hope II (Ohio Medical Products), the rescuer must recognize the presence of a pressure release valve.[11] The valve may need to be occluded with a digit to ventilate when dealing with high airway pressures.

All BVM devices should be attached to a supplemental oxygen source (with a flow rate of 15 L/min) to avoid hypoxia. A significant problem with the BVM method is the low oxygen saturation achieved with various reservoirs. The amount of delivered oxygen is dependent on the ventilatory rate, the volumes delivered during each breath, the oxygen flow rate into the ventilating bag, the "filling time" for reservoir bags, and the type of reservoir used. The commonly used corrugated tube reservoir is the least effective of those examined by Campbell and colleagues.[12] It is too sensitive to ventilatory technique and does not alert the clinician to changes in oxygen flow. A 2.5-L bag reservoir and a demand valve are the preferred supplementation technique during BVM ventilation.[12]

Complications

Hypoventilation often occurs because of the difficulty of carrying out the technique properly. Three mechanisms can result in complications: poor mask seal, failure to achieve

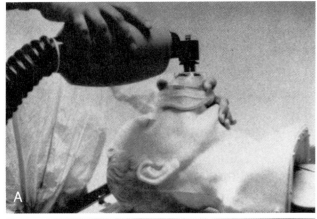

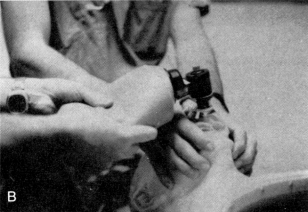

Figure 1–6. Bag-valve-mask ventilation is very difficult for one person to do *(A)*, and it frequently fails to deliver adequate tidal volumes, especially during cardiopulmonary resuscitation. With the two-person method *(B)*, one person uses both hands to hold the mask firmly against the face and extend the head. The other person uses both hands to squeeze the bag. (From Jesudian MC, Harrison RR, Keenan RL, Maull KI: Bag-valve-mask ventilation: Two rescuers are better than one. Crit Care Med 13:122, 1985. © Williams & Wilkins, 1985.)

airway patency, and low tidal volume. Practiced skill development is necessary to avoid these errors. Gastric distention can also result from poor airway patency. Air is insufflated down the esophagus, which inflates the stomach. Consequently, the risk of regurgitation and aspiration increases. When assistance is available, the application of firm posterior pressure on the cricoid ring will help reduce gastric inflation during BVM ventilation.[13] The technique must be used carefully in infants, whose airway is more pliable and subject to obstruction with excessive cricoid pressure. Even with proper BVM technique, aspiration can occur. The rescuer must be vigilant to recognize complications early and take corrective action.

INTERMEDIATE AIRWAYS

Intermediate airways are those interventions that go beyond the maintenance of a patent airway. They represent a midpoint between airway establishment and true airway control. Airway control is secured by maneuvers such as tracheal intubation and tracheotomy, in which an endotracheal cuff isolates the trachea. The devices described in this section occlude the esophagus and allow ventilation across the larynx. Two are designed to occlude only the esophagus, and two offer versatility of use whether placed into the esophagus or the trachea.

Esophageal Obturator Airway and Esophageal Gastric Tube Airway

The EOA and the EGTA maintain airway patency in ways similar to the oral and nasal airways, but they also protect the airway by occluding the esophagus to reduce gastric distention and regurgitation. The face mask permits use of these airways as positive-pressure ventilating devices. Air insufflated through the airway traverses the upper airway before crossing the larynx and entering the trachea. Ventilation from the EOA exits the airway through numerous ports in its hypopharyngeal portion (Fig. 1–7A and B). Ventilation from the EGTA is identical to mask ventilation, with the addition of esophageal occlusion. A port is available on the EGTA to vent the stomach. The attractiveness of the EOA and the EGTA for use in the apneic patient stems from their retention of much of the simplicity of the artificial airway with the addition of an important feature of more complicated airways—some protection against regurgitation and reduction of gastric distention.

INDICATIONS AND CONTRAINDICATIONS

A significant advantage of the esophageal airway is the speed with which airway control can be achieved. Trained individuals can successfully place an esophageal airway in an average of 5 seconds, whereas the same individuals need 20 seconds to perform a tracheal intubation.[14, 15] In one prehospital system, failure to intubate was much higher with the endotracheal tube (19.4 per cent) than with the EOA (1.7 per cent).[16] Neck motion is not as necessary with the esophageal airway as it is with tracheal intubation. For these reasons, the EOA may be an effective adjunct in the management of the unconscious injured patient who requires respiratory assistance. Hypercarbia may occur more commonly with EOA ventilation as compared with endotracheal ventilation.[17, 18] The most difficult aspect of this form of ventilation is securing a tight fit with the mask. Dentures should be left in place to give support to the lips. Adequate tidal volume must be delivered to ventilate the lungs.[19]

There are various contraindications to the use of the EOA and the EGTA. Because the airway is not protected from pharyngeal secretions, the presence of active oropharyngeal bleeding and excessive secretions represents a relative contraindication to EOA and EGTA use. Because of attendant discomfort, the devices cannot be used in the awake patient. Size specifications preclude its use in the pediatric patient; sixteen is the age usually cited as the lower limit for EOA and EGTA use. The actual limiting factors are the size of the esophagus and the face; an adult-sized 14 year old would certainly tolerate an EOA or EGTA if necessary. However, a small adult may not receive an appropriate fit. Other contraindications include esophageal injury or conditions predisposing to perforation. A patient who has ingested a caustic agent or one with a known esophageal stricture should not undergo esophageal intubation. As a precaution against pressure-related complications, it is recommended that the device not be left in place for longer than 2 hours. It must be recognized that the EOA and the EGTA are *temporary* forms of airway control. This form of airway control has been used most in prehospital care.

PROCEDURE

Placement of the EOA and the EGTA is accomplished with the head in the neutral position. Neck motion is unnecessary. The jaw is grasped by the rescuer and pulled forward. At this point, the assembled airway, with the mask attached, is introduced. The obturator tip is directed into

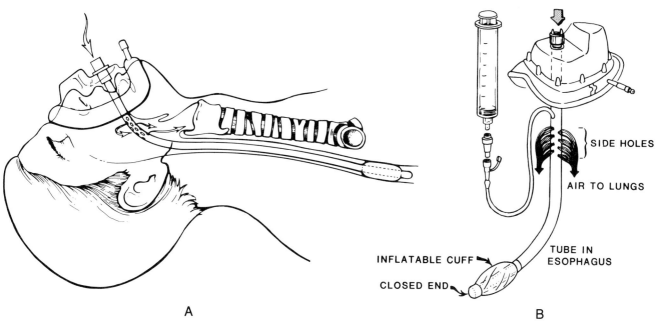

Figure 1–7. *A*, Esophageal obturator airway. Correct placement of the esophageal airway with the cuff inflated in the esophagus caudad to the bifurcation of the trachea. (From Clinton JE, Ruiz E: Trauma Life Support Manual, 1982.) *B*, Esophageal obturator airway. (From Jacobs LM: The importance of airway management in trauma. J Natl Med Assoc 80:873, 1988.)

the patient's posterior pharynx with gentle, steady pressure. The obturator is advanced down the esophagus until the mask rests flush against the face of the patient. Figure 1–7*A* illustrates the correct position at placement. The cuff should lie in the esophagus just distal to the carina of the trachea. Inflation of the balloon is postponed until proper position is confirmed. The patient is ventilated with a tight mask seal on the face, and the lungs are auscultated. For effective ventilation, the mask seal must be tight. Breath sounds should be audible bilaterally. Unilateral breath sounds or failure of auscultation should lead the rescuer to reassess the airway placement. Pneumothorax or hemothorax may explain unilateral sounds, as may inadvertent main stem bronchus intubation. Tracheal intubation will result in the absence of breath sounds. The possibility of bronchial or tracheal intubation requires removal and replacement of the airway. Once satisfactorily placed, the esophageal balloon is inflated to 20 to 25 ml.

COMPLICATIONS

A 5 per cent incidence of inadvertent tracheal intubation has been reported by Don Michael in experience with 29,000 placements.[15] In a subsequent smaller sample, a 2.9 per cent (5 of 170) incidence was reported with a 100 per cent mortality among the five patients.[20] One study comparing prehospital EOA placement with endotracheal tube placement found that the occurrence rate for complications of the EOA that prevented resuscitation (tracheal placement, tube kinking) was nearly three times higher for the EOA (8.7 versus 2.6 per cent).[21] If not quickly rectified, tracheal intubation with the EOA or tube kinking are disastrous complications that produce occlusion of the patient's airway. Disciplined examination for bilateral breath sounds is critical.

Esophageal lacerations of undetermined depth were found in 8.5 per cent of autopsies of patients in whom the EOA was used.[16] Esophageal rupture has been found and reported in case histories.[22, 23] Since Scholl and Tsai first reported esophageal ruptures in 1977, recommended balloon inflation volume was reduced from 35 to 20 ml. No further ruptures or leakage around the cuff have been

reported. However, factors other than balloon inflation volume that theoretically can contribute to rupture include careless balloon removal without deflation and forceful attempts at placement when obstruction is met.

Tracheal intubation must be performed *before* removal of the EOA, because vomiting often occurs following deflation of the balloon and EOA removal. If the EOA cuff has been overinflated, it may partially occlude the trachea and make intubation difficult. In such cases, the balloon is partially deflated to facilitate tracheal intubation.

The Pharyngeal-Tracheal Lumen Airway and the Esophageal-Tracheal Combitube

The pharyngeal-tracheal lumen airway (PTLA) and the esophageal-tracheal combitube (ETC) are two variations on the concept of the modified esophageal airway. Both of these airways do away with the EOA-EGTA face mask, and both allow for effective ventilation, whether the esophagus or the trachea is intubated. Both can be introduced with limited movement of the patient's neck.

The PTLA (Respironics, Inc., Monroeville, Pa.) has two

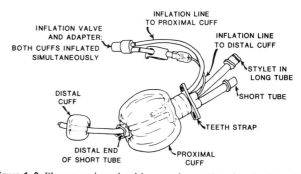

Figure 1–8. Pharyngeal-tracheal lumen airway (Respironics Inc., 530 Seco Road, Monroeville, PA 15146; Tel. [412] 373-8114, FAX [412] 373-1183.) (From Jacobs LM: The importance of airway management in trauma. J Natl Med Assoc 80:873, 1988.)

lumina (Fig. 1–8). The proximal lumen is designed to reside in the patient's hypopharyngeal area. The length of the distal lumen allows the tip to rest in either the trachea or the proximal esophagus. Two cuffs seal the airway. The large proximal cuff occludes the upper oral and nasal pharynx. The distal cuff is similar to the cuff on an endotracheal tube. It seals either the esophagus or the trachea. Both cuffs are inflated simultaneously as the rescuer blows into the single port. Once inflated, each cuff can be sealed with a separate clamp. Fixation straps are connected to the airway to be fastened around the head after balloon inflation.[24]

The ETC airway (Fig. 1–9; Sheridan Catheter Corp., Argyle, NY) differs slightly from the PTLA. The proximal cuff on the ETC is smaller. It is designed to occlude the nasopharynx proximal to the hard palate. The palate then acts as a barrier to external migration of the tube. The proximal lumen consists of numerous fenestrations in the tube at the hypopharyngeal level. The distal lumen and cuff are reminiscent of an endotracheal tube.[25]

INDICATIONS AND CONTRAINDICATIONS

The ETC and the PTLA are designed for use by emergency personnel not trained in endotracheal intubation. They also appear promising for use in patients who have failed initial endotracheal intubation or whose cervical spine is considered unstable. Tube placement with the PTLA and the ETC has been found to be more rapid than with endotracheal intubation.[26, 27] Furthermore, the small increase in expiratory pressure with the ETC provides arterial oxygenation as good as or better than that provided by endotracheal intubation.[28, 29]

These devices may not avert aspiration if the cuffed tube is placed in the esophagus and extensive upper airway secretions or hemorrhage are present. These devices are not for use in patients under 16 years of age or under 5 feet in height, individuals with an intact gag reflex, or persons with known or suspected proximal esophageal disorders (e.g., following a caustic ingestion).

PROCEDURE

Reported clinical experience with the PTLA and the ETC is limited.[24-29] To ensure placement location, both tubes require auscultation during ventilation through each of the

two lumina. The use of a lighted stylet[30] or a CO_2 detection device[31] (e.g., FEF, FENEM, Inc., New York, NY) may facilitate documentation of endotracheal placement. If the distal lumen is in the esophagus, then ventilation is carried out through the proximal lumen. If it is in the trachea, the distal lumen is used as an endotracheal tube. The proximal balloon eliminates the need for a face mask and thereby facilitates ventilation.

COMPLICATIONS

Preliminary experience with the PTLA has shown that external migration of this tube is a potential hazard. This problem does not seem to occur with the ETC.[27] More clinical experience is necessary to determine the usefulness of these devices.

TRACHEAL INTUBATION

General Indications and Contraindications

The critically ill patient must be well oxygenated with a protected airway. If the airway is not obstructed and respiration is spontaneous and adequate, oxygen supplementation and artificial airway placement may suffice. When these conditions are absent, as in the patient with a head injury who is hypoventilating or the patient with a flail chest, the airway must be protected and ventilation assisted. Breathing is a dynamic function that must be monitored constantly. In general, the significantly injured patient with a tidal volume of less than 500 ml or the patient with a respiratory rate of less than 10 or more than 24 breaths per minute is a candidate for airway control and assisted ventilation.

Patients who are unconscious from head trauma should be tracheally intubated and hyperventilated. Borderline cases should receive airway control if blood gases indicate hypoxia or acidosis or if clinical deterioration occurs. A decreased level of consciousness secondary to head injury is considered an indication for hyperventilation to an arterial P_{CO_2} of 25 to 30 mm Hg.[32] In the trauma victim, failure of the patient's spontaneous respiratory effort to achieve this level of hyperventilation often indicates the need for airway control. The patient with hypovolemic shock that does not respond rapidly to oxygen supplementation and volume replacement will soon display clear indications for airway control, such as decreasing level of consciousness, acidosis, hypoxia, or hypoventilation. All unconscious patients who lack the gag reflex must be intubated to protect against aspiration and to provide ventilation if their condition deteriorates.

Definitive control of the airway by nonsurgical means is, for practical purposes, synonymous with tracheal intubation. Tracheal intubation may be accomplished by various means, each with its own advantages and disadvantages. The existence of several differing approaches attests to the difficulty of the problem of nonsurgical airway control. Nowhere is the problem more difficult or the variety of approaches more necessary than in the patient with multiple injuries. This chapter describes the various means of passing a tracheal tube through either the mouth or the nose. The skills to be described are listed in Table 1–3.

Special Considerations

Cervical Spine Injury. Any patient who has sustained a significant injury has the potential for cervical spine injury. Approximately 3 per cent of initial survivors of all types of

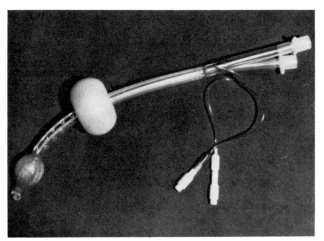

Figure 1–9. Esophageal-tracheal combitube airway. (From Frass M, Frenzer R, Zdrahal F, et al: The esophageal tracheal combitube: Preliminary results with a new airway for CPR. Ann Emerg Med 16:770, 1987.)

Table 1–3. Tracheal Intubation Skills
Direct laryngoscopy
Orotracheal intubation
with laryngoscope
around esophageal airway
Nasotracheal intubation
under direct vision
blind
with bronchoscope
Retrograde tracheal intubation

major trauma seen in emergency departments will have significant cervical spine injury; interestingly, this prevalence is not increased in the setting of significant head injury.[33] Falls from heights and motor vehicle crashes are common causes of spinal instability. Any patient sustaining a fall should be considered as potentially having spinal injury, even if the initial injury is an isolated penetrating injury.

In patients with multiple injuries, the possibility of cervical spine injury warrants caution when considering tracheal intubation involving the use of the laryngoscope. Until adequate radiographs of the cervical spine are obtained, the patient's ventilation is best maintained by means that provide adequate oxygenation yet limit neck extension. However, if the patient is severely hypoxic or apneic, immediate tracheal intubation may be necessary.

Methods of positive-pressure ventilation that can be accomplished with limited neck motion are listed in Table 1–4. Mouth-to-mouth and bag-mask ventilation can be done with minimal neck motion, but these frequently require some degree of neck extension to open the airway. Therefore, they are the least desirable of the methods listed in Table 1–4.

Many institutions and some prehospital systems use pharmacologic adjuncts, in-line cervical stabilization, and orotracheal intubation before cervical spine films are initiated. In the patient who is comatose, combative, or in severe respiratory distress without definite evidence of spinal cord injury, this approach may be life saving. Although this approach has been practiced successfully by a number of emergency medical services (EMS) systems[34, 35] and trauma centers,[36–38] a risk is taken in such situations that must be justified by the overall risk to the patient's life posed by failure to secure airway control.

Jaw Clenching. Hypertonus induced by neurologic dysfunction is a common complicating factor of airway management, especially in the patient with multiple injuries, the drug overdose patient, and those with seizures. Jaw clenching may be a lethal complication when it prevents clearing of blood, vomitus, or foreign bodies in the airway. No more difficult airway problem exists than occlusion of the nasal and oral passages by vomitus while the patient's teeth are tightly clenched. Respiratory efforts may lead to severe aspiration, and although the hypertonus will gradually give way as the brain stem becomes progressively hypoxic, the cerebrocortical hypoxic insult sustained in the process may be irreversible. Various disease states can lead to a similar scenario, in which the jaws are clenched during airway hemorrhage or the accumulation of secretions.

Jaw clenching and cervical spine injury can, of course, occur together. Fortunately, the nasotracheal routes of intubation may be adequate for airway management while minimizing the risk of further spine injury. However, at least a small degree of spontaneous air movement should be present for the blind nasotracheal approach to be successful. Although a serendipitous success may occur in the apneic patient, it is recommended that time not be wasted on this approach in the completely apneic patient. A tube stylet

technique that permits the nasotracheal tube to be passed blindly over a "nasogastric" tube passed into the *trachea* during cricoid pressure (Sellick maneuver) appears promising but requires clinical validation.[39] For either the stylet or bronchoscopic nasotracheal approach to succeed, the airway must be nearly free of foreign debris or blood. The patient with complete airway obstruction and clenched teeth fails to meet the prerequisite for each of these approaches. In this most difficult case, it is first necessary to find a way of opening the mouth to clear the airway.

Neuromuscular blocking agents are the ideal way to overcome jaw clenching. Both neuromuscular depolarizing and nondepolarizing agents may be administered intravenously to the injured patient to induce paralysis to allow orotracheal intubation. Neuromuscular blocking agents are discussed in Chapter 2.

Time Constraints. Prolonged efforts to intubate may result not only in hypoxia but also in cardiac decompensation. Pharyngeal stimulation can produce profound bradycardia or asystole; when it is feasible, an assistant should view the cardiac monitor during intubation of a patient who has not suffered cardiac arrest. Atropine should be available to reverse vagal-induced bradycardia that often occurs secondary to suctioning or laryngoscopy. Prolonged pharyngeal stimulation may also result in laryngospasm, bronchospasm, and apnea.

Selection of the airway management approach must always reflect a consideration of the degree of hypoxic insult imposed before and during the maneuver. Thirty seconds is the maximum interval allowable for routine intubation of the apneic patient. As a guide, one should limit the time of an intubation attempt to the amount of time a single deep breath can be held. This is especially important in a child because the functional residual capacity of a child's lungs is less than that of an adult. Failure to achieve control within this time frame demands an interval of BVM ventilation before intubation is attempted again. The use of preoxygenation to minimize hypoxia is strongly recommended. An oxygen saturation monitor can also be used to monitor explicitly for hypoxia. Assuming optimal preoxygenation of the patient to greater than 98 per cent O_2 saturation, attempts at intubation should be halted until the patient is reoxygenated whenever the O_2 saturation drops below 95 per cent, equal to a P_{O_2} of about 70 to 75 mm Hg.

When ventilation is not achievable, irreversible brain damage can result within minutes. Therefore, the maximum interval allowable for conservative airway management maneuvers is about 3 minutes; one must then choose alternative methods. The algorithms at the end of this chapter (see Figs. 1–21 and 1–22) reflect the relevant considerations and the many maneuvers discussed in a logical scheme for management of the airway.

Priorities in Cardiac Arrest Airway Management. Mouth-to-mouth and bag-mask ventilation may suffice for prehospital care with short transport times or for the initial few minutes of ventilation in cardiac arrest. However, optimal bag-mask ventilation during CPR is impossible. Mouth-

Table 1–4. Nonsurgical Airway Management Methods That Require Minimal Neck Motion
Mouth-to-mouth ventilation
Bag-valve-mask ventilation
Esophageal obturator airway
Esophageal gastric tube airway
Pharyngeal-tracheal lumen airway
Esophageal-tracheal combitube airway
Blind nasotracheal intubation
Bronchoscopic nasotracheal intubation

1. An assistant should be in the room, watching the cardiac monitor and blood pressure and observing the patient for signs of decompensation. The assistant should be instructed to inform the intubator if more than 30 sec have elasped without ventilation.

2. An intravenous infusion should be running properly. Oxygen should be administered to the patient.

3. Draw the necessary drugs (e.g., atropine, lidocaine, succinylcholine, and a barbiturate or a benzodiazepine).

4. Attach the bag-valve-mask to an oxygen source (rate of 15 L/min).

5. If used, a stylet should be inserted properly into the tracheal tube.

6. Check the integrity of the balloon on the tracheal tube.

7. Have tape or commercial tube stabilizer available.

8. Check the light source of the laryngoscope. Have a second light source, a selection of blades, and additional endotracheal tubes available.

A

9. Turn on the oral suction device and place the suction tip under the mattress to the left of the patient's head. Prepare the catheter suction for postintubation use.

10. Place the syringe to inflate the endotracheal tube balloon on the stretcher to the right of the patient's head. An option is to attach a syringe to the pilot balloon of the endotracheal tube.

11. Elevate the stretcher so the patient's head is at the level of the intubator's lower sternum. A towel or sheet may be placed under the patient's occiput to raise it 10 cm.

12. If the patient is awake, restrain the hands.

13. Remove the patient's dentures.

14. Check the cardiac monitor leads and the rhythm strip immediately before the intubation attempt.

15. Radiology should be alerted in case a postintubation chest radiograph is needed.

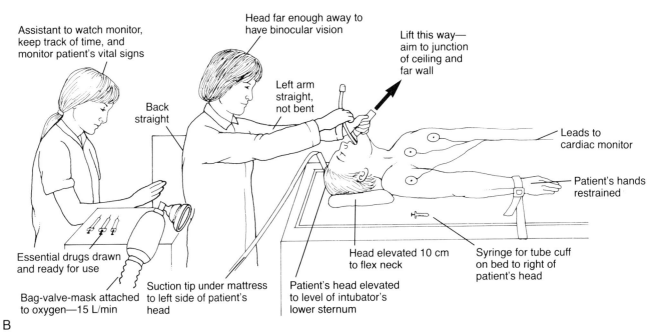

B

Figure 1–10. A, Suggested preintubation checklist. *B,* Essentials for a smooth intubation.

to-mouth and bag-mask ventilation are adequate and effective in the anesthetized or paralyzed patient with an empty stomach in the absence of chest compression, but they are *inadequate* for prolonged ventilation in the patient in cardiac arrest. Proper bag-mask ventilation is probably harder to master than tracheal intubation, and prolonged attempts during CPR usually only distend the stomach and give the uninitiated a false sense of security. *Patients in cardiac arrest should be orotracheally intubated.* Most cardiopulmonary arrests will not be associated with cervical spine injury. Although a high index of suspicion should be maintained, the fear of a cervical spine injury should not preclude tracheal intubation in nontrauma patients in cardiac arrest or in trauma patients with injuries unlikely to produce cervical spine injuries.

Preparing for Intubation

Before beginning intubation, a number of issues should be addressed. It is a common error to fail to position the patient properly or to proceed with the procedure before the proper equipment is assembled or checked. Such simple omissions as failing to restrain the patient's hands or misplacing the suction device can seriously hamper the proper performance of the procedure. A suggested preintubation check list and scheme are presented in Figure 1–10*A* and *B*.

It may be possible to predict most patients who will be particularly difficult to intubate and thereby alert the physician to change the approach to increase the chances for success. It should be stressed, however, that even individuals who appear to be perfectly normal and without any medical history that would predict a complicated intubation may quite unexpectedly be difficult to intubate.

Previous operations in or around the airway may make intubation difficult by changing anatomic landmarks, producing edema or scar tissue, or otherwise hampering the view of the vocal cords. Recent intubation, caustic ingestions, thermal or chemical burns, cancer, infection of the oral cavity, inflammation of the larynx or epiglottis, or trauma may distort normal anatomy. Facial or skull fractures may preclude using the nasal route for intubation. Thermal or chemical burns to the neck, radiation, severe arthritis, and developmental abnormalities (such as a small mandible or large tongue, noted with Down syndrome) may limit the motion of the jaw and neck and may complicate intubation.

In addition to the historical parameters and obvious developmental abnormalities, a short muscular neck poses the greatest problem for oral intubation. In the individual with a short neck, the larynx is anatomically higher than in other individuals. This means that the larynx, now approximately opposite the fourth cervical vertebra, is harder to visualize with the laryngoscope, the so-called anterior larynx. In such situations it is prudent to opt for the straight blade and have an assistant apply cricoid pressure. In the patient with a hypoplastic mandible, there is less room to displace the tongue, and forward movement of the epiglottis is also hampered. Potential difficulty in such cases may be predicted by measuring the chin to hyoid distance as suggested in Figure 1–11.

Direct Laryngoscopy

INDICATIONS AND CONTRAINDICATIONS

Any clinical situation in which visualization of the vocal cords is necessary and neck motion is permissible is an indication for use of the laryngoscope. Direct laryngoscopy is useful in the trauma patient who requires tracheal intubation or suctioning of the hypopharynx. The most expeditious method of tracheal intubation is the orotracheal route

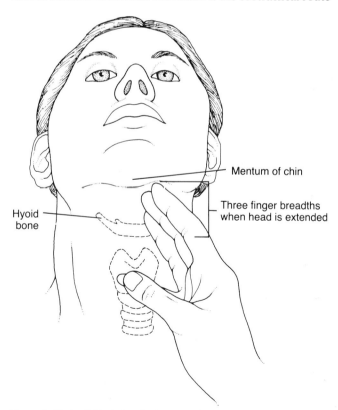

Figure 1–11. A difficult intubation may be expected if the distance from the mentum of the chin to the hyoid bone in an adult is less than three finger breadths when the head is extended. Patients with a shortened distance often have a hypoplastic or poorly developed mandible or a short fat neck, producing an anterior larynx that may best be approached with the straight blade and cricoid pressure.

using the laryngoscope. Cervical spine injury or the potential for such an injury is a *relative* contraindication to direct laryngoscopy.

EQUIPMENT

Facility in the use of the direct laryngoscope is a prerequisite to orotracheal intubation. Various adult and pediatric blade sizes are available. Two basic blade designs—curved (MacIntosh) and straight (Miller, Wisconsin)—are available. Slight variations in laryngoscopic technique follow from one's choice of blade design, a choice that is often a matter of personal preference. The tip of the straight blade lifts the epiglottis directly, whereas the curved blade fits into the vallecula and lifts the epiglottis passively by moving the larynx. The straight blade is usually a better choice in children, in patients with a very anterior larynx, or in the individuals whose larynx is fixed by scar tissue. In adults, however, the straight blade is more likely to damage the teeth. A straight blade may inadvertently be advanced into the esophagus and initially present one with unfamiliar anatomy until it is withdrawn. The straight blade has a light bulb at the tip that may hamper vision slightly. The wider curved blades are helpful in keeping the tongue retracted from the field of vision and are generally preferred in uncomplicated adult intubations.

PROCEDURE

Adults. The use of the curved and straight laryngoscope blades is illustrated in Figure 1–12. The laryngoscopist is stationed at the patient's head. To maintain the best mechanical advantage, the intubator keeps his or her back straight and does not hunch over the patient. The patient's head should be at the level of the intubator's lower sternum. While the patient is generally supine, sitting direct laryngoscopy can be performed with the laryngoscopist on a step stool behind the patient.[40] The sitting position may be helpful for intubating the severely dyspneic patient. The patient's head is placed in the "sniffing" position, with the head extended on the neck and the neck slightly flexed in relation to the trunk. Figure 1–13 illustrates how this position facilitates intubation by aligning the larynx with the intubator's field of vision. A small towel under the occiput (to raise it 10 cm) may facilitate this positioning. It is a common mistake to position the patient improperly or to fail to restrain the hands. Any dentures or partial plates are removed before laryngoscopy.

The laryngoscope is grasped in the rescuer's *left* hand with the blade directed toward the patient from the hypothenar aspect of the rescuer's hand. The patient's lower lip is drawn down by the rescuer's right thumb, and the tip of the laryngoscope is introduced into the *right* side of the patient's mouth. The blade is slid axially along the right side of the patient's tongue, gradually displacing the tongue toward the patient's left as the blade is moved to the center of the patient's mouth. If the blade is placed in the middle of the tongue, the tongue will fold over the edge of the blade and obscure the airway (Fig. 1–14). *Placing the blade in the middle of the tongue and failure to move the tongue to the left are the two most common errors that prevent visualization of the cords.* The rescuer exerts force anteriorly along the line of the laryngoscope handle, being careful not to pry the blade on the patient's upper teeth. It is important to keep the left arm straight. Do not bend at the elbow, as this tends to place the teeth as a fulcrum for the blade. If the left arm is kept straight, the jaw is lifted rather than pried open—the head is virtually suspended from the laryngoscope blade. If needed, suctioning is performed at this point. The epiglottis

Labels on figure:
Mentum of chin
Three finger breadths when head is extended
Hyoid bone

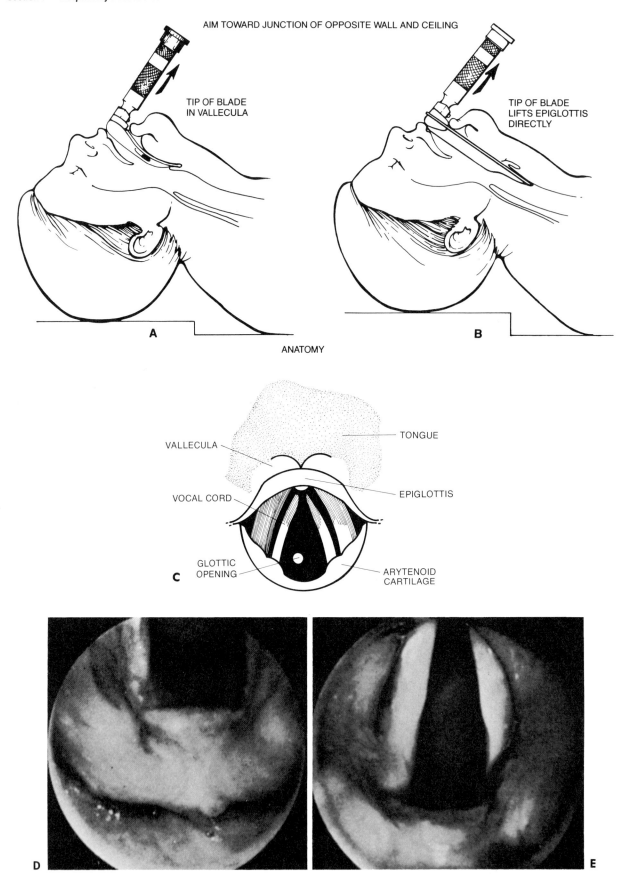

Figure 1–12. Direct laryngoscopy. *A,* Use of curved laryngoscope blade. *B,* Use of straight laryngoscope blade. (From Clinton JE, Ruiz E: Trauma Life Support Manual, 1982.) *C,* Diagram of anatomy of larynx entrance exposed by direct laryngoscopy. (From AHA Advanced Life Support Slide Series, 1976.) *D,* Direct laryngoscopic view during tracheal intubation: exposure of arytenoids. *E,* Direct laryngoscopic view during tracheal intubation: exposure of glottis. The anterior commissure is not fully seen. The posterior commissure is below. (From Holinger PH, Anison GC, Johnston KC: Bronchoscopic and esophagoscopic cinematography. J Thorac Surg 17:178, 1948.)

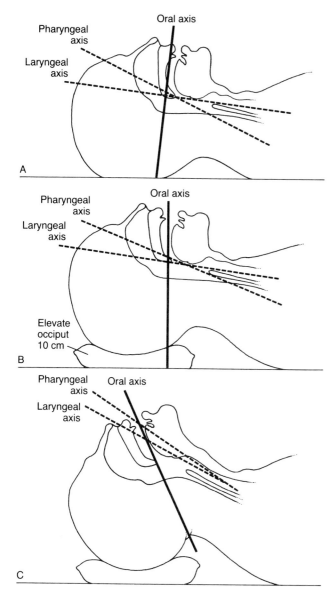

can directly elevate the epiglottis (Fig. 1–15). An infant has a small "omega"-shaped epiglottis that is firmer than that of the older child and generally does not require direct elevation. The child's proportionately larger head generally places the child naturally in the sniffing position, so a towel is not used under the occiput. If the larynx is too low to permit an adequate view of the vocal cords, a small towel can be put under the child's shoulders. One can also have an assistant lightly apply cricoid pressure, or the laryngoscopist can use the little finger of the hand holding the laryngoscope blade for this purpose. If no laryngeal structures are visible after cricoid pressure, the laryngoscopist should retract the blade gently, because a common error is to advance the blade initially into the esophagus (Table 1–5).

COMPLICATIONS

One should check for loose or missing teeth in children before and after the procedure. Any newly missing teeth

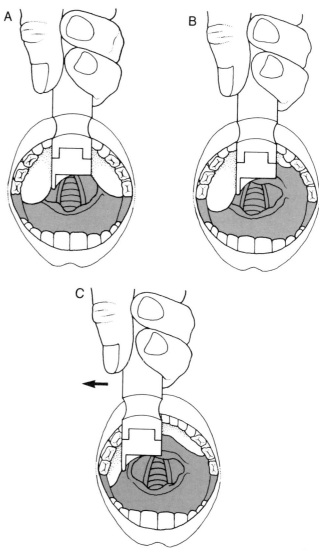

Figure 1–13. Head positioning for tracheal intubation. *A,* Neutral position. *B,* Head elevated. *C,* "Sniffing" position, flexed neck, extended head. Note how flexing the neck and extending the head to line up the various axes allows for intubation. Position *C* creates the shortest distance and straightest line between the teeth and the vocal cords.

is best visualized when the intubator keeps the back straight and uses both eyes to view the cords rather than hunching over close to the patient's mouth. When using a straight blade, the epiglottis is lifted with the tip of the blade. When using a curved blade, the tip of the blade is placed anterior to the epiglottis into the vallecula. Continued anterior elevation of the base of the tongue and epiglottis will expose the vocal cords. Proper neck positioning and pressure on the larynx by an assistant will facilitate visualization and intubation of an anterior larynx.

Infants and Children. Direct laryngoscopy in the child (up to the age of 8 to 9 years) generally requires a straight blade (Miller size 0 for premature infants, size 1 for normal-sized infants, and size 2 for older children). The child's large tongue to oral pharynx diameter ratio, floppy epiglottis and shorter neck hinder forward displacement of the tongue and associated structures. Subsequently children are most easily intubated by the smaller diameter straight blade that

Figure 1–14. Placing the laryngoscope blade in the center of the tongue *(A)* allows the tongue to fold over the sides, obscures the cords and blocks the path of the tracheal tube. This is a common mistake. Placing the laryngoscope in the right side of the mouth is necessary to move the tongue to the left, but if the laryngoscope stays in the midline, the tongue is still in the way *(B),* and the laryngoscope may block passage of the tracheal tube. The proper position for the laryngoscope is slightly to the left of midline, pushing the tongue totally out of the way and allowing space for the tracheal tube to be inserted *(C).*

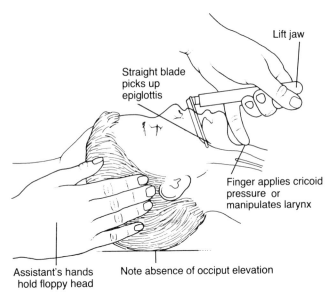

Lift jaw

Straight blade picks up epiglottis

Finger applies cricoid pressure or manipulates larynx

Assistant's hands hold floppy head

Note absence of occiput elevation

Figure 1–15. Oral intubation in a child, using a straight blade. The proportionately large, floppy head of the child may present some difficulty, and an assistant may be required to hold the head straight.

warrant a postlaryngoscopy chest film to rule out aspiration of a tooth. Swallowed teeth are of no consequence. In a study of 366 patients, McGovern and coworkers found broken teeth to be the most common complication of laryngoscopy.[41] Laceration of the mucosa of the lips, especially the lower lip, may be easily produced if adequate care is not taken. Failure to visualize the larynx may lead to complications to be discussed under tracheal intubation.

Tracheal Tubes

Sizing of endotracheal tubes can be a source of confusion because three different sizing systems have been employed. The most common system is the measure, in millimeters, of the tube's internal lumen diameter. French size is roughly equivalent to the tube's external circumference. Because circumference is given by π times the tube diameter, and π equals 3.14, the external diameter in millimeters of a French size tube can be calculated by dividing the French size by 3. Magill sizes are rarely used but consist of a gradation of diameters ranging from 0 for infants to 10 for adults.

Internal diameter sizing, the most descriptive of the three systems described previously, is the preferred tube sizing system. The internal diameter is 2 to 4 mm less than the external diameter, depending on the thickness of the walls of the tube.[42] Internal diameter sizes that are commonly used are listed in Table 1–6.

It is a common error to underestimate the proper tube size initially. A tube that is as large as possible without damaging the airway should be chosen to minimize airway resistance. Excessive airway resistance is a significant problem in attempting to wean a patient with chronic respiratory disease from the respirator. Because resistance to airflow varies to the fourth power of the tube diameter, even a 0.5 mm difference in tube size may be important.

Most adult females can be orally intubated with a 7.5- to 8.0-mm tube. Adult males can usually accept an 8.0- to 9.0-mm tube. One can estimate the size for a tube in a child by comparing the diameter of the tube with the diameter of the child's little finger. For nasal intubation, a slightly smaller tube (by 0.5 to 1.0 mm) is usually chosen. If one foresees

the need for bronchoscopy, at least an 8.0-mm tube should be used.

Adult tubes will accept a standard adaptor to which the ventilator tubing will fit. Pediatric tubes require a special adaptor with a distal end small enough to accommodate the small tube size. Most tubes with an internal diameter of less than 7 mm do not have inflatable cuffs. They are used in children younger than 8 years old. In an emergency, one might be tempted to select a smaller than adequate tube, thinking that the smaller tube will pass more easily. In children, however, choosing a smaller tube presents a problem, because a tight seal between the uncuffed tube and the soft trachea is required to prevent aspiration. The current use of cuffed tubes in children younger than 8 years of age is primarily limited to patients requiring mechanical ventilation and having reduced lung compliance. The use of cuffed tubes does not appear to increase the risk of postextubation stridor in such patients.[43]

Although cuff inflation can compensate for choosing a small tube size in an adult, the proper-sized tube should be chosen for the first intubation in children. In a child, the smallest airway diameter is at the cricoid ring rather than at the vocal cords as for adults. Hence, a tube may pass the cords but go no farther in the child. Should this occur, the next smaller sized tube should be passed after reoxygenation. An uncuffed tube will manifest an air leak at a ventilation pressure of 15 to 20 mm Hg but should provide a good seal at lower inflation pressures.

The introduction of high-volume, low-pressure cuffs has greatly reduced the incidence of tracheal injury from intubation. Initially, the proper amount of air required to produce a seal is estimated by slowly filling the balloon until the air leak with positive-pressure ventilation stops and all vocal sounds are eliminated. This occurs with 5 to 8 ml of air if the proper-sized tracheal tube has been selected. For long-term use, cuff pressure should be measured and maintained at 20 to 25 mm Hg. Capillary blood flow is compromised in the tracheal mucosa when the cuff pressure exceeds 30 mm Hg.

The cuff should be ascertained to be functional before beginning the intubation procedure. A persistent air leak during ventilation usually means one of three things: (1) the cuff is leaking because of damage to the balloon, (2) the pilot balloon is leaking, or (3) the cuff is positioned above the vocal cords and cannot maintain a proper seal.

Orotracheal Intubation

Indications for orotracheal intubation are the same as for airway control in general. The only relative contraindication is potential cervical spine injury.

Procedure

The most difficult steps in orotracheal intubation technique have been described: clearing the airway and visualizing the vocal cords by laryngoscopy. Once the vocal cords have been visualized with the laryngoscope, all that remains is to pass an endotracheal tube of the appropriate size between the vocal cords and, under direct vision, into the trachea. With the laryngoscope in place and the vocal cords visualized, orotracheal intubation is achieved.

The tube is held in the rescuer's right hand while the vocal cords are visualized. The concavity of the tube should be oriented toward the tongue during placement. A wire stylet may be placed in the lumen of the tube to assist in the placement by increasing the tube's stiffness. The angle of the curve is most acute in the distal one third to allow easier

Table 1–5. Comparison of the Airway in the Adult and Child

Comparison	Child	Adult	Clinical Consequences or Adjustments for Child
Head	Proportionately larger (up to about age 10)	Proportionately smaller	Child normally in a sniffing position when supine; do not place towel or sheet under occiput; may benefit from elevation of shoulders; large head in child may be "floppy"; have assistant hold head straight during intubation attempt.
Teeth	Easily knocked out	Stable unless decay or trauma is a factor	Teeth may be knocked out and aspirated or forced into trachea
Tonsils or adenoids	Large and friable	Generally not a problem	Nasal intubation in child may cause excessive bleeding; vision may be obscured by mass; adenoid or tonsil tissue may plug endotracheal or nasotracheal tube or be aspirated into lungs
Tongue	Relatively large	Relatively smaller	Difficult to displace tongue in child; should consider the straight blade
Larynx	Opposite C-2, C-3	Opposite C4–C6	In child curved blade may fold epiglottis down; structures are more "anterior" and harder to displace; consider straight blade
Epiglottis	U-shaped, shorter, stiffer	Flatter, more flexible	Epiglottis more difficult to manipulate in child; more accurate placement of straight blade required
Vocal cords	Concave upward. Anterior attachment of cords lower than posterior, creating a slant	Horizontal	Concave shape does not affect intubation, but it may affect ventilation efforts; for partial airway obstruction or to break laryngospasm in a child, combine positive-pressure ventilation with chin thrust to open arytenoids; slant to vocal cords may cause endotracheal tube to hang up on anterior commissure as it passes into larynx; rotate tube if it gets hung up
Length of trachea	Relatively short	Relatively longer	Straight blade may be advanced too far into esophagus, past the epiglottis; slowly withdraw under direct vision to visualize structures; with short trachea, main stem bronchus intubation likely to occur. FORMULA: in child advance endotracheal tube to a cm depth of ($\frac{1}{2}$ age + 12) measured at the corner of the mouth.
Airway diameter	Relatively smaller; smallest diameter is at the cricoid ring	Relatively larger; smallest diameter is between vocal cords	Laryngoscope-induced trauma, edema, foreign matter will significantly alter airway diameter in child; be gentle; extremes of flexion or extension may kink airway; if trouble with bag-valve-mask ventilation, reassess the degree of head flexion or extension; cricoid pressure may also cause complete airway obstruction; small diameter at cricoid ring allows wedging of endotracheal tube to obtain seal without use of balloon on tube, allowing for maximum-diameter endotracheal tube to be used.
Residual lung capacity	Relatively smaller	Relatively larger	Child may become hypoxic more quickly than adult; do not allow prolonged periods without ventilation; child's metabolic rate significantly higher than adult's; an option is to attach oxygen tubing to laryngoscope blade to add supplemental oxygen if respirations are spontaneous (e.g., epiglottitis or croup)

Table 1–6. Tracheal Tube Sizes for Average Patients*

Age	French Size	Internal Diameter (mm)	Equivalent Tracheotomy Tube Size
Premature			00
newborn	12	2.5	00–0
6 months	16	3.5	0–1
1 year	20	4.5	1–2
2 years	22	5.0	2
4 years	24	5.5	3
6 years	26	6.0	4
8 years	28	6.5	4
10 years	30	7.0	4
12 years	32	7.5	5
14 years	34	8.0	5
Adult			
Female	34–36	7.5–8.5	5
Male	36–40	8.0–9.0	6
Special cases			8–10

(Modified from Applebaum EL, Bruce DL: Tracheal Intubation. Philadelphia, WB Saunders Co, 1976.)

*A slightly smaller size may be required for nasotracheal intubation.

direction toward the larynx. The stylet should not extend past the tip of the tube.

The tube is advanced toward the patient's larynx from an angle and not down the slot of the laryngoscope blade. This way, the operator's view of the larynx is not obstructed by the hand or the tube until the last possible moment before the tube enters the larynx.

The tube is advanced into the larynx until the proximal aspect of the cuff is observed to pass between the vocal cords and out of view. The tube is advanced 2 to 3 cm beyond this point. The tube should be passed during inspiration when the vocal cords are open. The cuff is inflated with 5 to 10 ml of air to the point of minimal air leak on positive-pressure inspiration. In emergency intubation, 10 ml of air is placed in the cuff, and inflation volume is adjusted after the patient is stabilized. Both lungs are auscultated under positive-pressure ventilation. Care is taken to auscultate laterally in the lung periphery, because midline auscultation may lead to an erroneous impression of tracheal placement when the tube is actually in the esophagus. When the tube is correctly placed and the cuff is inflated, the tube is secured in place with umbilical (nonadhesive cloth) tape by tying the tape securely around the tube and the patient's head. The tube should be positioned in the corner of the mouth where the tongue cannot expel it. This position is also more comfortable for the patient and allows for suctioning. Other methods of securing the tube, including commercial ties with adhesive, adhesive tape, or clamp-on devices, are also useful (Fig. 1–16A and B). Adhesive tape should not be placed over the lips. A bite block or oral airway to prevent endotracheal tube crimping or damage from biting is commonly incorporated into the system used to secure the tube.

COMPLICATIONS

Complications of orotracheal intubation include those that have been described for laryngoscopy. The most severe complications are related to tube placement. The best "test" for proper placement is for the intubator to see the tube pass through the vocal cords (Table 1–7). Placement of the endotracheal tube into the esophagus, if unrecognized, is a disastrous complication. *Esophageal placement is not always immediately obvious.* One may hear "normal" breath sounds if only the midline is auscultated. One way to check for tracheal placement after a ventilation or during spontaneous respiration is to note whether air is felt or heard to exit through

the tube following cuff inflation. If the lungs are ventilated, the exit of air should be obvious. Importantly, if the tube is in the trachea, the patient cannot groan, moan, or speak, and any verbalization should suggest esophageal placement.

A chest radiograph should be taken shortly after the intubation to confirm one's clinical impression of tube location. The assessment of tube position should also be the first step in the emergency department evaluation of a patient who has been intubated in the field by paramedics.

Asymmetric breath sounds indicate probable main stem bronchus intubation. When asymmetric sounds are heard, the cuff should be deflated and the tube withdrawn until equal breath sounds are present. Bloch and colleagues report accurate supracarinal placement if the tube is withdrawn a certain distance beyond the point at which equal breath sounds are first heard—2 cm in children under 5 years of age and 3 cm in older children.[44] An estimate of the proper depth to which the tube should be passed can be derived from the following formulae, in which the length represents the distance from the tube tip to the upper incisors or gum line in children[45, 46] and from the tube tip to the corner of the mouth in adults[47, 48]:

Children:
Airway length (cm) = age (years)/2 + 12
           = height (cm)/10 + 5
           = weight (kg)/15 + 12

Adults:
Airway length (cm) = 21 cm (women)
           = 23 cm (men)

Bissinger and coworkers noted that endobronchial intubation was clinically unrecognized without a chest film in 7 per cent of reviewed cases.[49] Delayed tube repositioning can lead to unilateral pulmonary edema.[50] Persistent asymmetry of breath sounds after appropriate tube positioning indicates probable unilateral pulmonary pathology (e.g., main stem bronchus obstruction, pneumothorax, or hemothorax).

Absent or diminished breath sounds, increased abdominal size, or gurgling sounds during ventilation suggest esophageal placement. Exhaled carbon dioxide measurement has become an important indicator of proper tube placement. Measurement devices are available that detect CO_2 and indicate levels digitally, graphically, or colorimetrically. Tracheal placement of the tube in a perfusing patient produces the expected high CO_2 reading during exhalation. An esophageal placement will show a low or decreasing reading. Some devices demonstrate the fluctuation of CO_2 between lung inflation and deflation. Little difference is seen in these capnographic tracings with esophageal placement of the tube. One simple device (FEF, Fenem, Inc., New York, NY) for detecting exhaled CO_2 changes color when it is placed over the tracheal tube if the exhaled CO_2 level is appropriate for tracheal intubation. Unfortunately, when lung perfusion is poor during CPR, even tracheal intubation may not show sufficient CO_2 excretion to produce the desired color change.[31]

If an endotracheal tube is removed from the esophagus, vomiting frequently occurs, probably from a combination of vagal stimulation and air exiting from a distended stomach. Vomiting should be anticipated and suction readied. Cricoid pressure should be applied immediately after tube removal and maintained until intubation is successful.

When stimulated, the vocal cords may close (laryngospasm) and prevent passage of the tube. Much of the spasm responsible for this closure can be eliminated through the use of local topical anesthetics before intubation. Two or 4

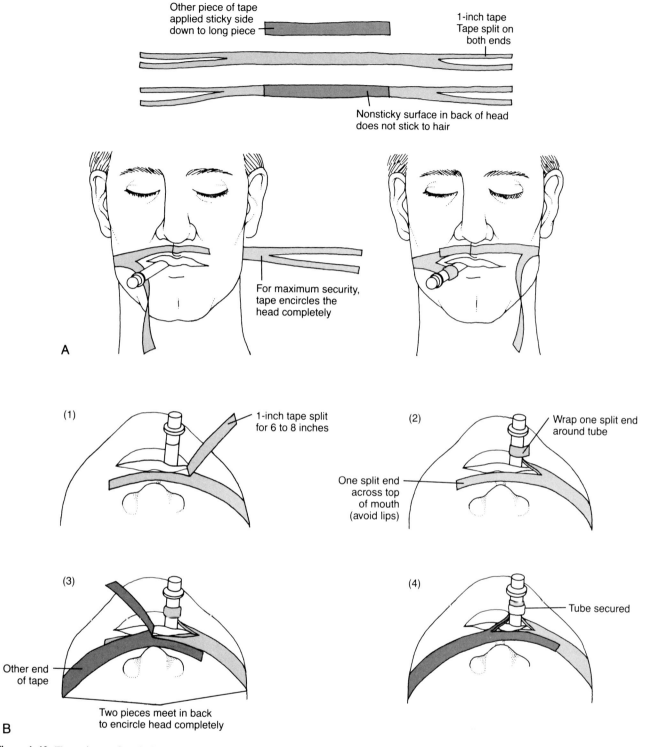

Figure 1-16. Two views of technique for taping the tracheal tube. It is important to secure the tracheal tube properly. The method illustrated can be replaced by using a commercial holder or less tape when the patient is stabilized. Avoid taping the lips.

per cent lidocaine may be sprayed directly on the cords or introduced via a puncture of the cricothyroid membrane with the spray directed cephalad. Occasionally, prolonged spasm is a significant problem. Spasm is best overcome through the application of gentle, sustained pressure with the tip of the tracheal tube. At no time should the tube be forced, because permanent damage to the vocal cords may result. In cases of life-threatening need for intubation, intense spasm may be overcome with diazepam (Valium) or succinylcholine. If vocal cord spasm prevents passage in a

child, a chest thrust maneuver may momentarily open the passage.[51]

In the past, tracheal stricture as a result of intubation has been a serious complication of long-term intubation. In recent years, high-volume, low-pressure cuffs have replaced low-volume, high-pressure cuffs on tracheal tubes. The principle behind this change has been that the high-volume cuffs distribute a lower pressure over a wider area of the trachea. Most investigators believe that this innovation has lessened the degree of tracheal injury associated with long-

Table 1–7. *Assessing Proper Tube Placement*

Test	Interpretation
Observe tube pass through the vocal cords	Accurate way to ensure placement; if in doubt, look again after intubation
Auscultation of breath sounds over the chest	May be misleading, especially if only midline is examined; listen in both axillae
Auscultation over the stomach	Gurgling indicates esophageal placement
Condensation (fog) forms inside tube with each breath	Quite reliable
Observe chest rise with positive pressure and fall with release	Generally reliable but may be absent in patients with small tidal volume or severe bronchospasm
Feel air exiting from end of tube following inflation	Reliable
Air remains in lung after end of tube is occluded and exits when occlusion is removed	Reliable but one may "ventilate" a closed area of the esophagus
Ask patient to speak; listen for moaning or other sounds	If tube is in proper place, no sound is possible
Chest radiograph	Generally reliable but can be misleading
End-tidal carbon dioxide measurements	Carbon dioxide not persistently detected if esophagus is intubated

term intubation.[51–56] Nonetheless, tracheal mucosal pressure even with low-pressure cuffs can still be excessive when high inspiratory pressures are used to overcome poor lung compliance.[57] Tubes with high-pressure cuffs are obsolete and should be avoided. If they are inserted, they should be replaced as soon as possible.

OROTRACHEAL INTUBATION WITH EOA OR EGTA IN PLACE

The unconscious patient who requires ventilatory assistance may benefit from the temporary use of the EOA or similar device as described earlier. Although this may be an effective means of ventilation, it is at best a temporary measure. The patient experiencing upper airway hemorrhage with the EOA in place may have oropharyngeal blood insufflated into the trachea. Also, an endotracheal tube is the preferable airway because of its convenience of ventilation. Although the EOA may allow rapid airway support until cervical spine injury can be ruled out, it is recommended that the EOA not be left in place for more than 2 hours.

Replacement of the EOA with an orotracheal tube requires appropriate care. Removal of the esophageal cuff before placement of the endotracheal tube is fraught with danger. Spontaneous gastric regurgitation often occurs on EOA removal. The rescuer must therefore learn to perform endotracheal intubation around the esophageal obturator to protect the patient from aspiration.

The patient is hyperventilated through the EOA before intubation is attempted around it. The EOA mask is then removed, and the EOA tube is moved to the *left* side of the patient's mouth. Laryngoscopy and intubation are then performed in the usual fashion. If resistance to passage of the tracheal tube is met, the volume of the EOA balloon should be reduced, because the balloon may be producing distortion of the larynx. Next, the operator deflates the EOA balloon completely and slides it out of the patient's esophagus. If resistance is met, the operator must be sure the esophageal cuff has been deflated completely.

OROTRACHEAL INTUBATION WITH THE PTLA OR ECT IN PLACE

The pharyngeal balloon prevents tracheal intubation around these tubes. First, the airways must be removed, a maneuver that represents an added risk over the EOA and EGTA but one that may be justified on the grounds of the improved ventilation these airways provide. The exercise of appropriate caution will prevent regurgitation during the procedure; also, the stomach should be emptied before device removal via a gastric tube placed through the esophageal port of the airway. Deflation of the cuffs and device removal follow. On removal of the tube, the rescuer must then intubate quickly.

Nasotracheal Intubation

INDICATIONS AND CONTRAINDICATIONS

Nasotracheal intubation is technically more difficult than oral intubation, but it may be advantageous in certain patients. When in place the tracheal tube traverses the nasal cavity, the nasal hypopharynx, and the larynx with the tip resting in the trachea. The patient cannot bite the tube or manipulate it with the tongue. Oral injuries may be cared for without interference by the tube. A nasotracheal tube is more easily stabilized and generally easier to care for than an orotracheal tube; also, it is better tolerated by the patient, allows easier movement in bed, and produces less reflex salivation than do the oral tubes. For acute epiglottitis, nasotracheal intubation is the method of intubation preferred by many clinicians.

The tube may be placed with the aid of the laryngoscope, but placement by blind technique or with the aid of the bronchoscope offers the additional advantages of minimizing neck motion and avoiding having to open the mouth. Patients with a clenched jaw or suspected cervical spine injury may be intubated with a minimum of preparation. The need for cervical spine films, jaw spreading, or paralyzing agents as preliminaries to airway control may be avoided with this technique.

Nasotracheal intubation may be relatively advantageous in patients who have short, fat necks or other anatomic or pathologic characteristics that would make orotracheal intubation difficult. The drug overdose patient with a decreased level of consciousness can often benefit from nasotracheal intubation. Such patients are often intubated before gastric lavage. They may be sufficiently awake to make orotracheal intubation without paralyzing agents difficult, but they are breathing enough to facilitate nasotracheal intubation by the blind technique. However, one study found that orotracheal intubation after use of paralyzing agents was more successful than nasotracheal intubation in the obtunded overdose patient.[58]

Blind nasotracheal intubation is possible with the patient in the sitting position, a distinct advantage in elective intubation of the patient with congestive heart failure, who will not tolerate the supine position. In fact, patients in respiratory distress are often more easily intubated by the nasal route because their air hunger facilitates entry into the trachea.

Nasal intubation should be avoided in patients with severe nasal or midface trauma. In the presence of a skull fracture, a nasal tube may inadvertently enter the brain through a fracture in the base of the skull or an ethmoid sinus. Nasal intubation is relatively contraindicated if the patient is taking anticoagulants or known to have a coagulopathy.

In addition to the obvious time delay encountered in

difficult nasotracheal intubations, the major immediate disadvantage of the nasal route is that it often precipitates bleeding. Although hemorrhage itself is usually not life-threatening, bleeding into the pharynx may precipitate vomiting and aspiration. In the presence of a clenched jaw or an obtundent patient, this complication is serious. Although a nasal tube is generally better tolerated than an oral tube, in the long-term patient the nasal tube has been associated with serious sinus infections, edema, and inflammation of the nasopharynx.

PLACEMENT UNDER DIRECT VISION

This technique is nearly equivalent to orotracheal intubation. The indications and precautions are similar, and the importance of considering cervical spine injury before performance is identical. Likewise, the need for jaw opening by physical or pharmacologic means is unchanged. The primary indication for preferring this method over orotracheal intubation is when the presence of an orotracheal tube would be a nuisance and would interfere with surgical repair in the management of an oral injury.

Before intubation the operator may choose to anesthetize the area with lidocaine spray (10 per cent) and constrict the nasal mucosa with 0.25 per cent phenylephrine, oxymetazoline spray (Afrin), or 4 per cent cocaine spray. If available, cocaine is ideal because it is both a vasoconstrictor and an anesthetic. Caution is necessary in hypertensive patients. The most patent nostril should be chosen for passage of the tube. The most patent nostril can be identified by direct vision, assessing air flow with the opposite side pinched off, or by gently inserting the lubricated gloved finger into the nostril. The tube is lubricated with viscous lidocaine or K-Y jelly. Viscous lidocaine may also be placed directly in the nostril.

Although the ideal lubricating agent is unknown, we prefer a water-soluble, gel-like substance over an ointment. Lubrifax may be used, but many physicians prefer viscous lidocaine, 2 per cent gel. The addition of an anesthetic agent over a plain lubricant is of theoretic advantage, but to be of benefit the anesthetic agent should be placed directly in the nostril rather than only as a coating on the tube. An effective method to dilate the nasal passage is to pass a lubricated soft nasopharyngeal airway (nasal trumpet) into the selected nostril first. This airway is left in place for 1 to 5 minutes, and progressively larger trumpets may be used if time permits. An alternative method is to insert the gloved index finger gently into the nose and advance it the full length. Although distasteful for the patient, this is an excellent way to dilate the passage and determine the most patent nostril.

The well-lubricated tube is inserted into the nostril directly posteriorly along the floor of the nasal cavity until the tip of the tube is in the hypopharynx. This is usually the most traumatic portion of the procedure, and it must be done gently. Twisting the tube may help bypass soft tissue obstruction.

Laryngoscopy is performed as described earlier to visualize the vocal cords and the tip of the endotracheal tube. The endotracheal tube should be grasped proximal to the cuff with the Magill forceps and directed toward the larynx (Fig. 1–17). An assistant advances the tube gently while the operator directs the tip into the larynx and trachea. Cricoid pressure may facilitate the passage. Often the larynx can be manipulated sufficiently with the laryngoscope so that the physician can advance the tube with the right hand and guide it between the cords without using the Magill forceps. Occasionally, the natural curve of the tracheal tube guides it through the cords without any manipulation. The cuff is

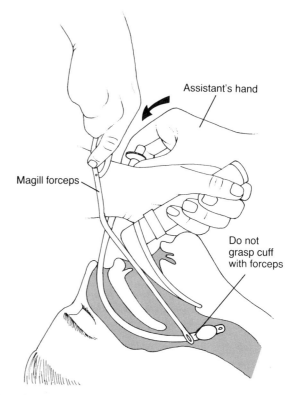

Figure 1–17. Nasotracheal intubation with the aid of a laryngoscope and Magill forceps. Note that the forceps do not pull the tube but only guide it through the vocal cords while an assistant advances it. The cuff is frequently damaged if it is grasped.

inflated, and both lungs are auscultated to ensure ventilation. When placement is satisfactory, the tube is secured.

BLIND PLACEMENT

Blind nasotracheal intubation is a useful airway control maneuver in the multiply injured or critically ill patient who exhibits some degree of spontaneous respiration. It is often successful in the air-hungry patient who seems literally to inhale the tube. The patient's breath sounds are used to guide the tube into the trachea. It is unnecessary for the operator to visualize the larynx, or to open the jaws or extend the neck. The technique, therefore, circumvents two of the most frustrating obstacles in airway management: potential cervical spine injury and hypertonus.

Any patient requiring airway control who has some spontaneous ventilation is a candidate for blind nasotracheal intubation. Specific indications that favor this approach over others are (1) inability to open the mouth, (2) inability to move the neck, (3) dental injuries, (4) gagging or resisting the use of the laryngoscope, and (5) short stocky neck.

Some would argue that the inability to open the mouth is a relative contraindication because emesis may be induced that could not be cleared. The operator must exercise judgment in the individual case and be prepared to use neuromuscular blocking agents or to bypass the upper airway with a surgical technique if such a complication develops.

Apnea is the major contraindication to blind nasotracheal intubation. Attempts to place the tube without respiration as a guide are futile. Relative contraindications include anterior fossa fracture and nasal injury.[59, 60] Furthermore, significant bleeding may occur if the patient is anticoagulated or has a coagulopathy. Patient combativeness also represents a strong contraindication.

The technique of blind nasotracheal intubation was first described by Magill in 1928.[61] Little change in technique has occurred since. Modifications have been described to increase the success rate and limit complications.

The nasal mucosa is constricted with 0.25 to 1.0 per cent phenylephrine drops. Topical anesthesia with cocaine or lidocaine spray (10 per cent) may be used if the patient is responding to pain. A well-lubricated endotracheal tube with a 7.0, 7.5, or 8.0 internal diameter is inserted along the floor of the nasal cavity, using breath sounds transmitted through the tube to guide advancement. The tube is *not* directed toward the frontal sinus. The tube is advanced into the hypopharynx, and usually one feels a "give" as it turns the corner into the posterior pharynx. Once in the nasopharynx, the tube is used as a nasopharyngeal airway to ensure that ventilation is occurring through the tube and that it is not obstructed. As the tube approaches the vocal cords, fogging of the inside may be noted, and breath sounds are heard in the tube. The tube is most easily advanced into the trachea during an inspiratory effort. If the patient can cooperate, success is enhanced by maintaining the "sniffing" position. Often the patient will cough or wheeze during this maneuver, ensuring the intubator of success. Continued air passage through the tube indicates that the tube is in the trachea rather than the esophagus. Once the tube is in the trachea, moaning and groaning noises should disappear. If they continue, esophageal passage is likely. Use of cricoid pressure may help avert esophageal passage. Reflex swallowing during blind nasotracheal intubation may direct the tube posteriorly and away from the larynx. If passage is difficult, the conscious patient should be directed to stick out the tongue to inhibit swallowing and secure the larynx to facilitate intubation.

Following intubation, both lungs are auscultated while applying positive-pressure ventilation. If only one lung is being ventilated, the tube is withdrawn until both lungs are ventilated. The cuff is inflated, and the tube is secured.

Most of the time the endotracheal tube will pass into the trachea when it is advanced gently and swiftly during inspiration. Jacoby[62] has described five possible locations of the misplaced tube:

1. Left piriform sinus
2. Right piriform sinus
3. Anterior to the epiglottis
4. In the esophagus
5. Above the vocal cords but unable to pass

Observation of the soft tissues of the neck during attempted passage of the nasotracheal tube will often allow the operator to determine the location of the misplaced tube. Maneuvers to correct the misplacement may be made on the second attempt. Bulging of the neck laterally and superior to the larynx indicates the presence of the tube in the piriform sinus on either side. A midline bulge at the same level suggests positioning anterior to the epiglottis. Esophageal placement is detected by passage of the tube to a greater depth with loss of breath sounds. In addition, attempted ventilation while auscultating the stomach leaves no doubt as to an esophageal placement. If the tube is advanced beyond the larynx level into the esophagus, it should be withdrawn back into the hypopharynx. The tube should not be removed from the nose because this will create additional trauma to the nasal soft tissues. Resistance to passage at the level of the larynx without anterior bulging suggests a location above the vocal cords. Methods of achieving success when facing one of the misplacements are listed in the following discussions.

Piriform Sinus. The tube should be rotated away from the side of the misplacement, and placement should be reattempted. An alternate method is to abduct the patient's head toward the side of the misplacement and reattempt placement. For example, a tube placed in the *right* nostril tends to advance diagonally toward the *left* piriform sinus. Abducting or cocking the patient's head toward the left tends to straighten the tube's course toward the larynx, away from the sinus.[62]

Anterior to the Epiglottis. Extension of the head on the neck is decreased by forward flexion. A tube with a lesser degree of curvature may produce the same positive effect.

Esophageal Placement. The tube should be withdrawn to the hypopharynx (not out of the nose) and passage reattempted while applying cricoid pressure. Increased extension of the head on the neck during placement may help.

Placement above the Cords (as in Laryngospasm). Intubation may be reattempted with a smaller tube. Laryngeal anesthesia should be reassessed, and transcricothyroid anesthesia with 2 ml of 4 per cent lidocaine should be considered before further attempts are made.[63] The potenial presence of cervical spine injury must be kept in mind constantly when considering these corrective maneuvers. Any maneuver that moves the neck significantly should not be used when alternatives that do not jeopardize the spinal cord exist.

COMPLICATIONS

Epistaxis is a common complication of nasotracheal intubation in the emergency situation. Severe epistaxis was encountered in five of 300 cases reported by Danzl and Thomas.[64] Tintinalli and Claffey encountered severe bleeding in one of 71 cases and less serious bleeding in 12 others.[65] Bleeding is usually not a problem unless it provokes vomiting or aspiration, a serious potential problem in obtunded patients with a clenched jaw or a decreased gag reflex. Other complications that have been reported include turbinate fracture, nasal necrosis, intracranial placement through basilar skull fracture, retropharyngeal laceration or dissection, and delayed or unsuccessful placement.[58, 59, 66, 67] Unsuccessful placement may be minimized by selection of a smaller tube and by gentle technique. Sinusitis in patients with nasotracheal tubes is common and can be an unrecognized cause of sepsis.[68–70]

Delayed placement deserves special discussion. Manipulation of the endotracheal tube through the nose and with the Magill forceps during the direct vision technique involves additional steps that require time. Because time is of the essence in the resuscitation of the critically ill patient, orotracheal intubation may be preferable. A stylet is rarely used during nasotracheal intubation. If the tube is not easily passed through the nose, orotracheal intubation is performed.

Complications with blind tube placement are similar to those described for nasotracheal intubation under direct vision. Retropharyngeal laceration and esophageal intubation are more of a threat in blind placement techniques because they are more likely to go unrecognized.[65] One unique problem associated with nasotracheal intubation is damage of the tube cuff with the Magill forceps.

Guided Intubation

Laryngoscopy is notoriously difficult in the patient with a short or an immobile neck. Although blind nasotracheal intubation is the most widely used alternative in this setting, other techniques are described in the sections that follow.

DIGITAL INTUBATION

Digital intubation uses the index and middle fingers to guide the tube blindly through the larynx. The technique is indicated in comatose patients when the larynx cannot be visualized by other means. Failure to visualize the larynx may be due to the presence of blood, secretions, or other debris in the airway. In addition, anatomic constraints may prevent laryngeal visualization, or neck motion may be contraindicated because of cervical spine injury.

Minimal neck motion is necessary during digital intubation. The tracheal tube is prepared with a stylet in its lumen that is formed to the shape of a "J" with a gentle curve distally. The intubator stands at the patient's right side facing the patient. The intubator's left index and ring fingers are introduced into the right angle of the patient's mouth and slid along the surface of the tongue until the epiglottis is palpated. The tube is then introduced from the patient's left between the tongue and the rescuer's fingers. The tip of the tube is guided to pass beneath the epiglottis, and gentle anterior pressure directs the tube into the larynx. After the tip of the tube is securely in the larynx, the stylet is withdrawn, and the tube is advanced simultaneously (Fig. 1–18).[71]

Preliminary experience with the technique has demonstrated an 89 per cent success rate in the hands of paramedics.[72] Digital intubation is particularly advantageous in prehospital situations with trapped victims when positioning for intubation is compromised.

Complications of the technique have not been addressed specifically but appear to be rare. The greatest risk seems to be to the intubator, whose fingers may be bitten. Use of a bite block, gauze teeth guards, and gloves have been recommended during the procedure.

LIGHTED STYLET INTUBATION

Prehospital airway management has stimulated innovation in the form of a lighted stylet for airway placement. A bright light placed in the larynx can be seen to illuminate the overlying skin in darkened surroundings. This principle

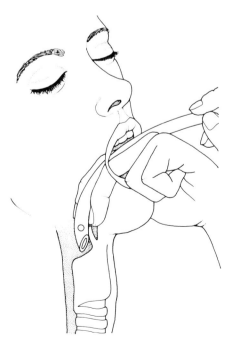

Figure 1–18. Tactile intubation.

was used to devise a flexible lighting system to be used as a stylet in both blind oral and tracheal intubation.[73–75]

This technique is indicated in situations in which the larynx cannot be visualized or the neck moved. It is relatively contraindicated in situations in which lighting is bright and cannot be dimmed. The bright lighting can prevent perception of the illumination.

The technique as described by Ellis and colleagues[73] is as follows: The intubator approaches the patient from the patient's right side. A lighted stylet is formed with an angle at the tip. The site of stylet angulation is estimated by measuring the distance from the submental area of the mandible to the hyoid bone, using the intubators fingers to estimate the distance. Stylet angulation is then formed at that distance from the base of the lamp on the stylet (Fig. 1–19). After angulation the stylet is introduced into the tracheal tube. The tube is held in a pencil-type of grip and advanced along the surface of the tongue. Successful entry into the larynx is indicated by the illumination of the overlying skin. The tube is then advanced off the stylet into the trachea.[73] Auscultation of both lungs and the epigastrium should be carried out to ensure correct placement at this point.

The reported success rate for the procedure on first attempt has varied from 70 to 88 per cent, and the success rate after several attempts has ranged from 88 to 100 per cent.[73–75] Measurement of mandibular-hyoid distance increased the success rate on the first attempt from 54 to 85 per cent. The average time to intubation with the technique ranged from 20 to 38 seconds.[73]

Complications have been minimal. Breakage with dislodgement of the stylet bulb in early reports was corrected by redesign of the bulb stylet linkage.

PLACEMENT OVER FIBEROPTIC BRONCHOSCOPE

Flexible fiberoptic scopes allow placement of endotracheal tubes under direct vision in circumstances in which other techniques are not applicable.[76–78] The recent development of small-caliber (4 mm) intubating fiberoptic scopes (such as the Olympus) with both a suction and an oxygen delivery port has greatly simplified this procedure. Two approaches to placement using the fiberoptic scope are possible; one is a nasotracheal method, and the other is an orotracheal approach.

Although blind nasotracheal intubation is commonly used in the patient with potential cervical spine injury who is breathing spontaneously, it is occasionally unsuccessful in spite of corrective maneuvers, and it is not feasible in the apneic patient. Failure of blind nasotracheal intubation and apnea are potential indications for use of the fiberoptic bronchoscope. Jaw clenching and potential cervical spine injury remain significant factors in the decision to use this maneuver. Contraindications to fiberoptic placement of a nasotracheal tube are similar to those of other forms of nasotracheal intubation. An impediment to the success of this technique is the presence of significant airway hemorrhage, secretions, or foreign material. The degree of obstruction may be significant enough to contraindicate an attempt at fiberoptic placement. Two means of handling mild hemorrhage and secretions exist. The first is to use the suction port of the bronchoscope, which may be effective in cases with limited bleeding or secretions. Another less cumbersome technique is to attach oxygen tubing to the suction port for insufflation of oxygen during intubation. The insufflation serves to keep debris away from the tip of the bronchoscope while providing the patient with some supplemental oxygen.

Fiberoptic-Assisted Nasotracheal Intubation. The en-

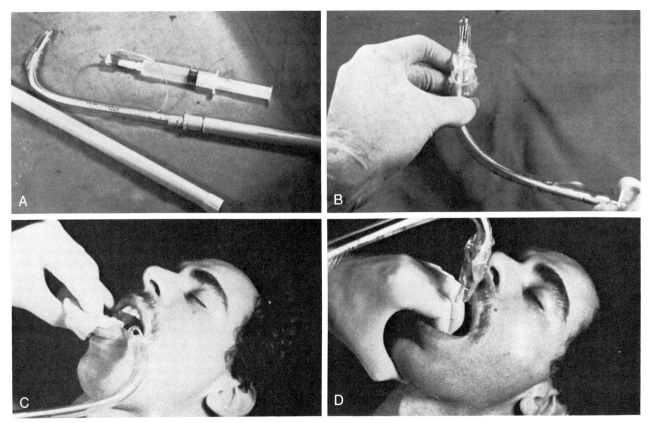

Figure 1–19. Lighted stylet intubation. *A,* Flexilum surgical light used as a stylet. *B,* Tube/stylet bent to slightly greater than 90 degrees when patient is in a neutral position. *C,* Tongue is gently pulled out, lifting the epiglottis and allowing the tube to pass. *D,* Alternate technique: pulling the jaw forward. (From Vollmer TP, Stewart RD, Paris PM, et al: Use of a lighted stylet for guided orotracheal intubation in the prehospital care setting. Ann Emerg Med 14:324, 1985.)

dotracheal tube is inserted *without* the fiberoptic scope along the floor of the patient's nasal cavity into the nasopharynx or hypopharynx. The lubricated bronchoscope is inserted through the endotracheal tube to a premeasured distance corresponding to the point at which the bronchoscope tip is at the tip of the endotracheal tube. The vocal cords are visualized through the fiberoptic scope, and the scope is advanced through the endotracheal tube toward the cords without moving the endotracheal tube. The bronchoscope is advanced past the vocal cords into the trachea. The endotracheal tube is then slid over the bronchoscope into the trachea. Thereafter the bronchoscope is removed, the cuff inflated, and the patient ventilated. Both lungs are auscultated to ensure adequate ventilation. As always, the tube must be repositioned if asymmetrical ventilation exists. When confident of adequate placement, the tube is secured.

The complications of this technique are identical to those of blind nasotracheal intubation. Delayed intubation during attempts is a much greater hazard with the fiberoptic intubation technique. The manipulation is much more complicated, and the operator may become intrigued with the procedure and lose awareness of the passage of time. One must be particularly disciplined in timing these attempts to avoid unnecessary hypoxic insult. Alternatively, an O_2 saturation monitor can be used by an assistant to monitor for the development of hypoxia and direct further ventilation and oxygenation.

Fiberoptic-Assisted Orotracheal Intubation. Inability to visualize the vocal cords with a laryngoscope because of anatomic variation may necessitate the orotracheal use of the fiberoptic scope as an adjunct for intubation. The patient with a short "bull" neck or one with a spinal deformity may be particularly refractory to direct laryngoscopy with the

laryngoscope. Failure to visualize the vocal cords or anticipation of such a difficulty may lead the operator to choose the fiberoptic scope as an adjunct for *orotracheal* intubation in the patient *without* a cervical spine injury.

Contraindications and complications of this technique are identical to those for orotracheal intubation with a laryngoscope. Again, excessive time consumption is a greater hazard when using the fiberoptic scope. Two operators are necessary to apply this technique.

The lubricated fiberoptic scope and endotracheal tube are assembled by inserting the scope through the tube lumen until the fiberoptic tip is protruding from the distal end of the tube. The first operator retracts the tongue with the laryngoscope in a manner similar to that in laryngoscopy. The first operator grasps the assembled fiberoptic scope and endotracheal tube and slowly advances the combination in the direction of the larynx. The second operator visualizes the vocal cords through the fiberoptic scope as it is advanced toward the larynx. The tip is manipulated with the controls to pass between the vocal cords. The tube is advanced to its final position in the trachea. The fiberoptic scope is removed, and the cuff is inflated. The lungs are auscultated to ensure good ventilation. When the position is adequate, the tube is secured.

Retrograde Orotracheal Intubation

The technique of retrograde intubation represents a more invasive procedure than those described thus far. The technique requires puncturing the cricothyroid membrane to place a guide up through the mouth, over which an endotracheal tube may be slid into the trachea (Fig. 1–20).

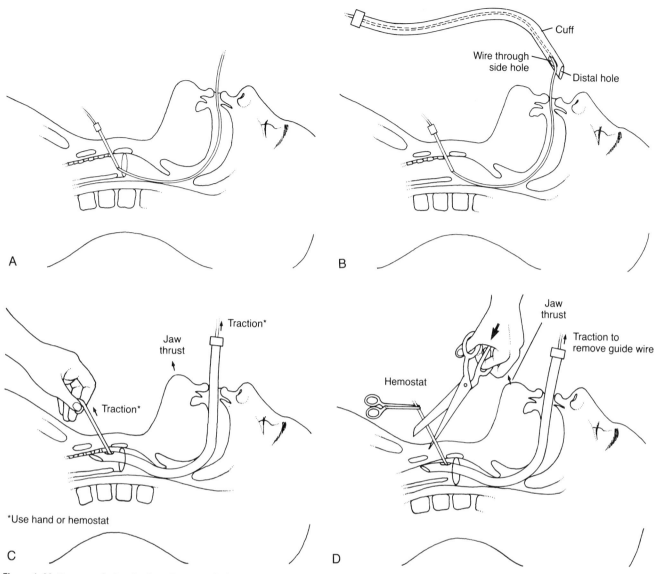

Figure 1–20. Retrograde intubation. Retrograde intubation using a catheter threaded from the larynx by cricothyroid membrane puncture. (*A* redrawn from Clinton JE, Ruiz E: Trauma Life Support Manual, 1982.)

The technique combines elements of both nonsurgical airway control maneuvers already described and an invasive maneuver (i.e., cricothyroid membrane puncture).

The technique was originally described in 1960 as a means of intubating patients with a tracheostomy in place.[79] Subsequent modifications of the technique have been applied in conjunction with puncture of the larynx, allowing the technique to be used in any patient in need of airway control.[80–85]

INDICATIONS AND CONTRAINDICATIONS

Because retrograde intubation is a relatively invasive technique, it should be reserved for patients in whom more conservative approaches to management of the airway have failed. It may be particularly useful when too much airway debris prevents fiberoptic scope intubation and neck motion is limited. When it can be performed rapidly (after failure of any of the more conservative nonsurgical approaches), retrograde intubation may be a reasonable alternative to emergency surgical airway techniques.[85]

Contraindications to this procedure include the ability to secure airway control by less invasive means. Clenched teeth preclude grasping the retrograde-passed guide. Cervical spine injury does not pose a problem because neck motion is unnecessary for retrograde intubation.

Although nasotracheal retrograde intubation has been described, it is too complicated and time consuming to be of significant benefit to the acutely ill or injured patient.[79, 80] The technique described here is the retrograde orotracheal approach.[81, 82, 84]

EQUIPMENT

1. 60-cm intravenous catheter-needle combination or 80-cm (0.88 mm diameter) spring guide wire (J tip preferred)
2. Tracheal tube of appropriate size
3. Long forceps (e.g., Magill) for grasping catheter in pharynx
4. Materials for securing endotracheal tube
5. Syringe for tube cuff
6. 2 hemostats
7. Local anesthetic and skin preparation materials

PROCEDURE (see also Chapters 3 and 7)

Three anatomic landmarks must be located by palpation: the cricoid cartilage, thyroid cartilage, and hyoid bone. The prepared skin over the cricothyroid membrane is anesthetized. Next, the lower half of the cricothyroid membrane is punctured with a needle directed slightly cephalad. The bevel should also face cephalad. Air must be aspirated to ensure that the needle tip is in the lumen of the larynx. The catheter is threaded through the needle until the tip is visible in the patient's mouth. The forceps are then used to grasp the catheter and draw it out through the mouth. The catheter must be long enough to be held at the puncture site and extend through the oropharynx (and subsequently endotracheal tube) to be grasped at the other end.

The tube is slid over the catheter by introducing the catheter through the endotracheal tube side port into the lumen and out the proximal end of the tube. A common error is to insert the guide wire through the distal opening of the tracheal tube. Tension is applied over the catheter by pulling on both ends of the catheter. This is most easily done by securing both ends of the catheter with hemostats. The endotracheal tube is advanced into the larynx over the catheter until resistance is felt at the cricothyroid puncture site. This is the most crucial point in the procedure. Because it is a blind technique, one may mistake abutment of the tip of the tracheal tube against the piriform sinus or vallecula as indicating the tube tip is distal to the vocal cords. The catheter is cut at the puncture site while the endotracheal tube is simultaneously advanced into the trachea. The distal end of the catheter is withdrawn out of the patient's mouth. The lungs are ventilated and auscultated to verify correct position. The tube may then be secured in the standard fashion.

An attractive alternative technique is to introduce a vascular guide wire.[85] The technique differs in that the guide wire is used instead of the catheter. Use of a J-tipped wire permits rotation of the wire for easy grasping of the curved tip in the oropharynx. As before, after passage of the wire, the guide wire is introduced first into the tracheal tube side port until the distal end of the guide wire can be grasped. The wire is held taut at both ends during tube advancement. After tube advancement past the vocal cords, the guide wire is withdrawn through the tube, and the tube is advanced simultaneously.

COMPLICATIONS

Complications of the technique are largely related to cricothyroid membrane puncture. They are (1) failure to achieve intubation, (2) hemorrhage, (3) subcutaneous emphysema, and (4) soft tissue infection. Investigators have stressed two points to minimize failure. The first is to keep the catheter taut during passage of the tracheal tube to prevent kinking and obstruction. Second, the technique for threading the catheter up the tracheal tube has received considerable attention. Figure 1–20*B* illustrates the recommended method, in which the catheter is threaded up the side hole of the tube rather than up the end hole. This method *allows the maximum length of the tube to be advanced into the larynx before the catheter is cut.* There also is less chance of the tube being displaced out of the larynx into the esophagus when it is threaded in this manner.[81] Hemorrhage is minimized by taking care to puncture the cricothyroid membrane in its lower half to avoid the cricothyroid artery. Subcutaneous emphysema may be unavoidable but usually is of little significance because no air is insufflated during this technique. A small incidence of soft tissue infection is reported with translaryngeal needle procedures (see Chapters 3 and 7) and can be expected to occur with this technique as well.

Intubation in Acute Epiglottitis

A problem that deserves special consideration is the management of suspected acute epiglottitis. A cautious approach is necessary to avoid stimulation that may convert borderline airway patency to complete obstruction.

Epiglottitis is often considered a disease of children between the ages of 2 and 8 years, but it is being recognized in adults with increasing frequency.[86] The most common pathogen in children and a frequent pathogen in adults is *Haemophilus influenzae* type B. The typical presenting picture is that of an adult or child sitting upright, drooling, or spitting up oral secretions rather than swallowing. The voice may sound muffled. There is a history of a relatively abrupt onset of a "sore throat" that rapidly becomes more painful. Children commonly present with a high temperature, but adults usually are only mildly febrile.[86] The disease is especially treacherous in children because of their small airways and their tendency to panic when an oral examination or an intravenous intubation is attempted. Small children are most calm when allowed to sit on a parent's lap. An oxygen mask with oxygen flowing at 10 L/min can be held by the parent several centimeters from the child's face. If the child is using accessory muscles to breathe, every attempt should be made to keep the child calm. If a lateral radiograph of the neck taken on inspiration can be obtained without disturbing the child, it will often establish the diagnosis.[87] On radiography, the inflamed epiglottis will often appear thickened and rounded. The hypopharynx will be dilated above the obstruction.

In cases of respiratory compromise, an epiglottitis protocol should be implemented rapidly. This protocol can save many minutes of time otherwise spent trying to reach all of the personnel needed to manage this critical emergency. When a child is suspected of having epiglottitis because of the history and clinical presentation, the safest course of action is to call immediately for the most experienced pediatric intubator available to meet the child in the operating room. The emergency physician should accompany the child to the operating room, remain until the airway is safely secured, and be prepared to intervene if needed. Otolaryngologist notification should be included in the protocol because a tracheostomy may be necessary.[88] When operating room space or personnel are not available immediately, emergency department personnel must be prepared to manage the airway.

If the child lapses into a coma or stops making ventilatory efforts, the first step is to attempt to force oxygen past the obstruction by using mouth-to-mouth respiration or a BVM apparatus. Because the obstruction is edematous supraglottic tissue and epiglottis, positive-pressure ventilation often can displace the edema enough to allow adequate ventilation. If this effort is unsuccessful, the emergency physician should attempt oral intubation. However, a normal larynx will not be visible because of the edema. The intubator should attempt to pass an endotracheal tube through the slit-like opening that remains for the supraglottic airway. An assistant can compress the chest to force bubbles through the airway, as a means of locating the airway.[89] The assistant can also palpate the larynx and the trachea to detect the tube's entry into the trachea. If orotracheal intubation fails, the intubator should go directly to transtracheal needle ventilation (TTNV) (see Chapter 3). The obstruction of epiglottitis is mainly inspiratory, so there should be no difficulty with chest hyperinflation with intermittent TTNV. This method should facilitate subsequent orotracheal intubation, because the path of the airway should be readily apparent as exhaled gases pass through it.

It is recommended that all children with acute epiglottitis be intubated endotracheally.[87] If the child is not in distress, an intravenous line can be established before intubation for appropriate drug administration (see Chapter 2).

Adults with suspected epiglottitis can be examined directly. It is good practice to visualize the epiglottis and the vocal cords of any adult patient complaining of difficulty swallowing. A mirror, fiberoptic scope, or a right-angle scope can be used to do this. The pharynx and tonsils usually do not appear inflamed, a finding that would explain the symptoms. Adults with epiglottitis do not always need to be intubated if rigorous monitoring can be accomplished, a skilled intubator is immediately available, and the patient is not in distress.[86] Orotracheal intubation for epiglottitis is not as difficult in adults as it is in small children. Transtracheal needle ventilation can also be used in adults who are difficult to intubate.

Intravenous ampicillin and chloramphenicol or a third-generation cephalosporin (e.g., ceftriaxone) is recommended after the airway has been secured in children or on making the diagnosis in adults, pending results of throat and blood cultures.[90]

Changing Tracheal Tubes

The tracheal tube whose cuff develops a leak is a vexing problem, especially if the original intubation was difficult. A method of replacement of the tube without losing control of the tracheal lumen is preferred. This can be achieved using a guide to remove the tracheal tube over which the new tube can be introduced.

A simple guide can be made using a standard nasogastric tube. A copper wire placed inside the tube gives it the proper stiffness for the task, although the standard 18 French Salem sump tube is generally stiff enough by itself. The TTX tracheal tube exchanger (Sheridan Catheter Corporation, Argyle, NY) is a similar commercially available device.

The patient is hyperventilated before placing the introducer through the tube. The guide is advanced so that its tip is well within the tracheal lumen. While cricoid pressure (Sellick maneuver) is applied, the tracheal tube is withdrawn over the guide. The replacement tube is then slid over the guide and gently advanced into the trachea. The guide is withdrawn. The cuff is inflated, and the lungs are auscultated. After correct placement has been verified, the new tube can be secured.

Many of the technical problems of this procedure are eliminated if a commercially available endotracheal tube changer is used. However, if a Salem sump nasogastric tube is used, a few caveats should be emphasized (Table 1–8). The proximal end of this nasogastric tube flares, and the proximal 6 to 8 cm must be cut off. The plastic of the tracheal tube and the plastic of the nasogastric tube create considerable friction. Therefore, it is necessary to lubricate the guiding catheter with K-Y jelly before use. (This makes the tube quite slippery, so gloves are required for handling it.) It is best to remove the standard adapter from the new tracheal tube because the guiding stylet occasionally gets hung up at this point. Finally, it may be necessary to use a large hemostat to force the guide back through the new tracheal tube.

Complications are related to the time required to change the tube. A successfully performed procedure should be accomplished within 30 seconds. Injury to the patient from forcing the guide or the tube is a possibility to consider when placing the tube.

Table 1–8. Procedure for Changing an Orotracheal Tube Using a Salem Sump Nasogastric Tube as a Guide

1. Cut off the proximal 6 to 8-cm flared end of an 18 French Salem sump nasogastric tube.
2. Test the balloon or cuff of the new tracheal tube. An 8.0-mm tracheal tube should be used. Remove the proximal adapter from the new tracheal tube.
3. Sedate the patient and restrain the hands as necessary. Preoxygenate as much as possible.
4. Lubricate the entire length of the nasogastric tube with water soluble (K-Y, Lubrifax) lubricant.
5. Advance the nasogastric tube as far as possible into the trachea through the existing tracheal tube.
6. Deflate the balloon of the existing tracheal tube and remove it. *Now only the nasogastric tube remains in the trachea, to be used as a guiding stylet.*
7. Thread the proximal end of the nasogastric tube through the distal end of the new tracheal tube. This is facilitated by the use of a hemostat.
8. Advance the new tracheal tube over the guide until the nasogastric tube exits through the proximal opening in the new tracheal tube.
9. Grasp the exiting nasogastric tube, have an assistant *lift the patient's jaw*, and advance the tracheal tube over the guide into the trachea.
10. Remove the guide.
11. Replace the adapter on the new tracheal tube, inflate the cuff, and ventilate the patient. Confirm proper placement of the new tube.

ROLE OF SURGICAL AIRWAY PROCEDURES

We have described several techniques for dealing with many different scenarios of airway compromise in the emergency situation. We have discussed variable degrees of airway obstruction, clenching of teeth, and coexistence of cervical spine injury. As yet we have offered no solution to the situation when time is not available to implement some of the more complex techniques even though they are otherwise indicated. Moreover, no solution has been offered for the patient who is apneic with airway obstruction and clenched teeth following trauma.

Surgical techniques come into play when time is not available to accomplish more conservative airway management. These surgical techniques are discussed in Chapter 3.

DECISION MAKING IN AIRWAY MANAGEMENT

The physician must have many tools at hand to deal with the acutely compromised airway. Even though the physician may be proficient in the performance of all the previously described maneuvers, the choice of which maneuver to use often must be made when no time is available for contemplation. It is critical that consideration of potential scenarios take place before airway management must be carried out in the clinical situation. Failure to do so will lead to unnecessarily aggressive management in some situations and, worse, to irreversible hypoxic injury as a result of delays due to indecisiveness.

Several parameters must be assessed quickly before an airway management choice can be made. The parameters to be considered are the following:

1. Adequacy of current ventilation
2. Time of hypoxia
3. Patency of airway
4. Malleability of jaws (teeth clenching)
5. Cervical spine stability
6. Safety of technique

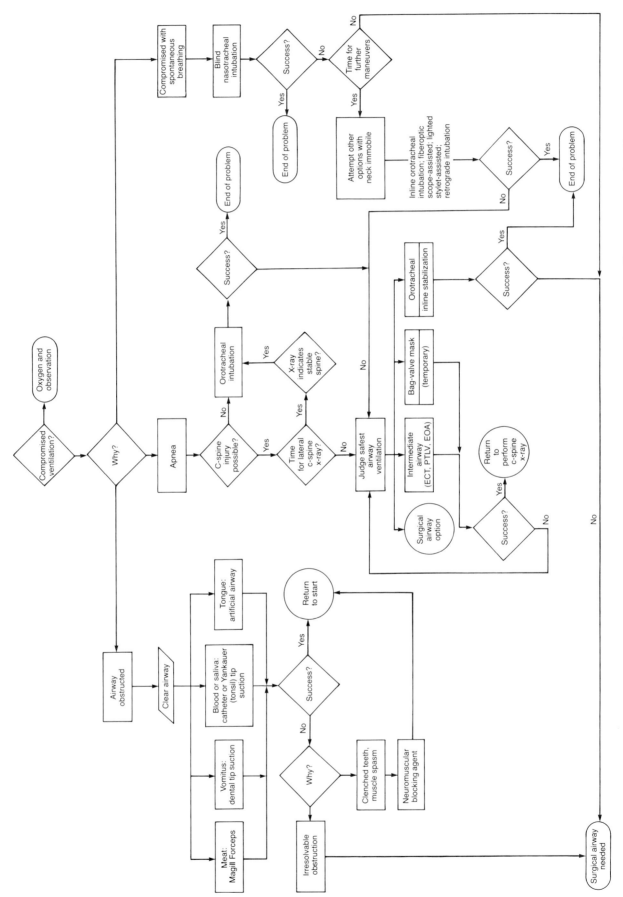

Figure 1-21. Nonsurgical airway management algorithm. (A redrawn from Clinton JE, Ruiz E: Trauma Life Support Manual, 1982.)

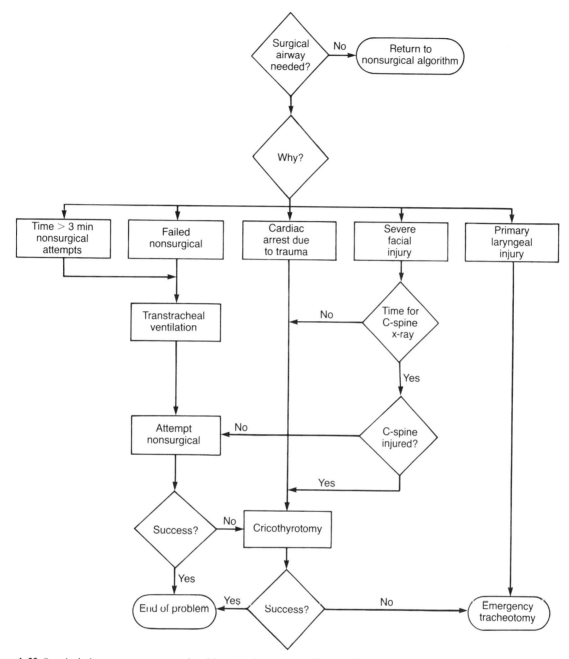

Figure 1–22. Surgical airway management algorithm. (Redrawn from Clinton JE, Ruiz E: Trauma Life Support Manual, 1982.)

Consideration of these factors will allow a choice to be made of the optimal procedure among those described. This initial choice is relatively straightforward. Real difficulty is encountered when the initial choice is unsuccessful. Time becomes more of a factor and safety of technique becomes less important as the risk of irreversible hypoxic injury is approached. Anxiety increases in such a clinical situation, and the potential for error is compounded. No substitute exists for forethought and practice in making these decisions.

Schemata are offered in Figures 1–21 and 1–22 that outline the logic behind the airway choices. The first diagram is the most complicated. It represents the choices among nonsurgical approaches to airway management that we have described. The end point of this diagram is either success or the decision to pursue surgical management. Note that the overriding time-oriented diagram in the upper right corner of the first diagram forces a judgment in favor of

surgical airway management when time is running out. The second diagram in Figure 1–22 is much simpler. Now that the decision to manage the airway surgically has been made, one need only choose among three available options. Consideration of patient condition, definitiveness of the airway approach, and degree of invasiveness are factors to be weighed in the final decision.

CONCLUSION

Airway management in the critically ill or injured patient with acute airway compromise is a most demanding task for the emergency physician. Mastery of several nonsurgical and three surgical techniques of airway control is necessary to meet any emergency situation that might occur. Preparation involving mastery of technique, preparation of equipment, and experience in decision making is essential. Scenario visualization is a means of practicing making the difficult decisions that will afford the patient the most expeditious and safest means of airway control available under the circumstances. In this chapter we have described the techniques and offered a logical schema for their use in the patient with an acutely compromised airway.

REFERENCES

1. Guildner CW: Resuscitation—opening the airway: A comparative study of techniques for opening an airway obstructed by the tongue. JACEP 5:588, 1976.
2. Standards and guidelines for cardiopulmonary resuscitation (CPR) and emergency cardiac care (ECC). JAMA 255:2905, 1986.
3. Guildner CW, Williams D: Airway obstructed by foreign material: The Heimlich maneuver. JACEP 5:675, 1976.
4. Straugh FK, Pryor RW, Matson JR, et al: Comparison of three methods to clear the totally obstructed airway. Crit Care Med 17:S124, 1989.
5. Cowan M, Bardole J, Dlesk A: Perforated stomach following the Heimlich maneuver. Am J Emerg Med 5:121, 1987.
6. Valero V: Mesenteric laceration complicating a Heimlich maneuver. Ann Emerg Med 15:105, 1986.
7. Razabini RM, Brathwaite CEM, Dwyer W: Ruptured jejunum following Heimlich maneuver. J Emerg Med 4:95, 1986.
8. Ruben H, Hansen E, MacNaughton FI: High capacity suction technique. Anaesthesia 34:349, 1979.
9. Naigow D, Powasner MD: The effect of different endotracheal suction procedures on arterial blood gases in a controlled experimental model. Heart Lung 6:808, 1977.
10. Jesudian MC, Harrison RR, Keenan RL, Maull KI: Bag-valve-mask ventilation: Two rescuers are better than one. Crit Care Med 13:122, 1985.
11. Hirschman AM, Kravath RE: Venting vs ventilating: A danger of manual resuscitation bags. Chest 82:369, 1982.
12. Campbell TP, Stewart RD, Kaplan RM, et al: Oxygen enrichment of bag-valve mask units during positive-pressure ventilation: A comparison of various techniques. Ann Emerg Med 17:232, 1988.
13. Betito SP, Russell WJ: The prevention of gastric inflation: A neglected benefit of cricoid pressure. Anaesth Intensive Care 16:139, 1988.
14. Schofferman J, Oill P, Lewis AJ: The esophageal obturator airway: A clinical evaluation. Chest 69:67, 1976.
15. Don Michael TA: Esophageal obturator airway. Med Instrum 11:231, 1977.
16. Goldenberg IF, Campion BC, Siebold CM, et al: Morbidity and mortality in patients receiving the esophageal obturator airway and endotracheal tube in prehospital cardiopulmonary arrest. Minn Med 69:707, 1986.
17. Auerbach PS, Geehr EC: Inadequate oxygenation and ventilation using the esophageal gastric tube airway in the prehospital setting. JAMA 255:3067, 1983.
18. Meislin HW: The esophageal obturator airway: A study of respiratory effectiveness. Ann Emerg Med 9:54, 1980.
19. Hammargren Y, Clinton JE, Ruiz E: A standard comparison of the esophageal obturator airway and endotracheal tube ventilation in cardiac arrest. Ann Emerg Med 14:953, 1985.
20. Gertler JP, Cameron DE, Shea K, et al: The esophageal obturator airway: Obturator or obtundator? J Trauma 25:424, 1985.
21. Hankins D, Carruthers N, Frascone RJ, et al: Prehospital complications of esophageal obturator airway (EOA) and endotracheal tube (ET) placement. Prehosp Disaster Med 4:77, 1989.
22. Johnson KR, Genovesi MG, Lassar KH: Esophageal obturator airway: Use and complications. JACEP 5:36, 1976.
23. Scholl DG, Tsai SH: Esophageal perforation following the use of the esophageal obturator airway. Radiology 122:315, 1977.
24. McCabe CJ, Browne BJ: Esophageal obturator airway, ET tube, and pharyngeal-tracheal lumen airway. Am J Emerg Med 4:64, 1986.
25. Frass M, Frenzer R, Zdrahal F, et al: The esophageal tracheal combitube: Preliminary results with a new airway for CPR. Ann Emerg Med 16:768, 1987.
26. McMahon JM, Bartlett R, Martin S, et al: Comparison of the pharyngeal tracheal lumen airway to the endotracheal tube: An EMS field trial. Prehosp Disaster Med 4:77, 1989.
27. Frass M, Johnson JC, Atherton GL, et al: Esophageal tracheal combitube (ETC) for emergency intubation: Anatomical evaluation for ETC placement by radiology. Resuscitation 18:95, 1989.
28. Frass M, Frenzer R, Rauscha F, et al: Ventilation with the esophageal tracheal combitube in cardiopulmonary resuscitation: Promptness and effectiveness. Chest 93:781, 1988.
29. Frass M, Rodler S, Frenzer R, et al: Esophageal tracheal combitube, endotracheal airway and mask: Comparison of ventilatory pressure curves. J Trauma 29:1476, 1989.
30. Stewart RD, LaRosee A, Stoy WA, et al: Use of a lighted stylet to confirm correct endotracheal tube placement. Chest 92:900, 1987.
31. MacLeod GJ, Heller MB, Yealy DM: Verification of endotracheal intubation using a disposable end-tidal CO_2 detector. Prehosp Disaster Med 4:74, 1989.
32. Crockard HA, Coppel DL, Morrow WFK: Evaluation of hyperventilation in treatment of head injuries. Br Med J 4:634, 1973.
33. O'Malley KF, Ross SE: The incidence of injury to the cervical spine in patients with craniocerebral injury. J Trauma 28:1476, 1988.
34. Hedges JR, Dronen SC, Feero S, et al: Succinylcholine-assisted intubations in prehospital care. Ann Emerg Med 17:469, 1988.
35. Syverud SA, Borron SW, Storer DL, et al: Prehospital use of neuromuscular blocking agents in a helicopter ambulance program. Ann Emerg Med 17:236, 1988.
36. Holley JE, Jorden RC: Airway management in patients with unstable cervical spine fractures. Ann Emerg Med 18:1237, 1989.
37. Rhee KJ, Green W, Holcroft JW, et al: Oral intubation in the multiply injured patient: The risk of exacerbating spinal cord damage. Ann Emerg Med 19:511, 1990.
38. Stellin GP, Barker S, Murdock M, et al: Oral-tracheal intubation in trauma patients with cervical fractures. Crit Care Med 17:S37, 1989.
39. Nakhgevany KB, McCloskey DS, Sariego J, et al: A new technique for emergency endotracheal intubation in trauma patients. Am J Emerg Med 7:664, 1989.
40. Fontanarosa PB, Goldman GE, Polsky SS, et al: Sitting oral-tracheal intubation. Ann Emerg Med 17:336, 1988.
41. McGovern FH, Fitz-Hugh GS, Edzeman LJ: The hazards of endotracheal intubation. Ann Otol Rhinol Laryngol 80:556, 1971.
42. Applebaum EL, Bruce DL: Tracheal Intubation. Philadelphia, WB Saunders Co, 1976, pp 35–37.
43. Reynolds GE, Deakers TW, Clemens D, et al: Cuffed endotracheal tube intubation in children. Crit Care Med 17:S109, 1989.
44. Bloch EC, Ossey K, Ginsberg B: Tracheal intubation in children: A new method for assuring correct depth of tube placement. Anesth Analg 67:590, 1988.
45. Cole F: Pediatric formulas for the anesthesiologist. Am J Dis Child 94:472, 1957.
46. Morgan GAR, Steward DJ: Linear airway dimensions in children: Including those with cleft palate. Can Anaesth Soc J 29:1, 1982.
47. Spadafora MP, Roberts JR: Technique for determining proper depth of orotracheal tube placement in the critically ill adult patient. (Abstract.) Ann Emerg Med 15:657, 1986.
48. Owen RL, Cheney FW: Endobronchial intubation: A preventable complication. Anesthesiology 67:255, 1987.
49. Bissinger U, Lenz G, Werner K: Unrecognized endobronchial intubation of emergency patients. Ann Emerg Med 18:853, 1989.
50. Kramer MR, Melzer E, Sprung CL: Unilateral pulmonary edema after intubation of the right mainstem bronchus. Crit Care Med 17:472, 1989.
51. Milstein JM, Goetzman BW: The Heimlich maneuver as an aid in endotracheal intubation of neonates. Pediatrics 60:749, 1977.
52. Lewis FR, Schlobohm RM, Thomas AN: Prevention of complications from prolonged tracheal intubation. Am J Surg 135:452, 1978.
53. Black AMS, Seegobin RD: Pressures on endotracheal tube cuffs. Anaesthesia 36:498, 1981.
54. Grillo HC, Cooper JD, Geffin B, et al: A low pressure cuff for tracheostomy tubes to minimize tracheal injury: A comparative clinical trial. J Thorac Cardiovasc Surg 62:898, 1971.
55. Vogelhut MM, Downs JB: Prolonged endotracheal intubation. Chest 76:110, 1979.
56. Loeser EA, Hodges M, Gliedman J, et al: Tracheal pathology following short-term intubation with low- and high-pressure endotracheal tube cuffs. Anesth Analg 57:577, 1979.
57. Guyton DC, Banner MJ, Kirby RR: High-volume, low pressure cuffs: Are they really low-pressure? Crit Care Med 17:S24, 1989.
58. Dronen SC, Merigian KS, Hedges JR, et al: A comparison of blind nasotracheal and succinylcholine-assisted intubation in the poisoned patient. Ann Emerg Med 16:650, 1987.
59. Horellou MF, Mathe D, Feiss P: A hazard of naso-tracheal intubation. Anaesthesia 33:73, 1978.
60. Zwillnick C, Pierson DJ: Nasal necrosis: A common complication of nasotracheal intubation. Chest 64:376, 1973.
61. Magill IW: Endotracheal anaesthesia. Proc R Soc Med 22:4, 1928.
62. Jacoby J: Nasal endotracheal intubation by an external visual technique. Anesth Analg 49:731, 1970.
63. Iserson KV: Blind nasotracheal intubation. Ann Emerg Med 10:468, 1981.
64. Danzl DF, Thomas DM: Nasotracheal intubation in the emergency department. Crit Care Med 8:677, 1980.
65. Tintinalli JE, Claffey J: Complications of nasotracheal intubation. Ann Emerg Med 10:142, 1981.
66. Taryle DA, Chandler JG, Good JT, et al: Emergency room intubations—complications and survival. Chest 75:541, 1979.
67. Blanc VF, Tremblay NA: The complications of tracheal intubation: A new classification with a review of the literature. Anesth Analg 53:202, 1974.
68. Grindlinger GA, Niehoff J, Hughes L, et al: Acute paranasal sinusitis related to nasotracheal intubation of head-injured patients. Crit Care Med 15:214, 1987.
69. Deutschman CS, Wilton P, Sinow J, et al: Paranasal sinusitis associated with nasotracheal intubation: A frequently unrecognized and treatable source of sepsis. Crit Care Med 14:111, 1986.
70. Knodel AR, Beekman JF: Unexplained fevers in patients with nasotracheal intubation. JAMA 248:868, 1982.

71. Stewart RD: Tactile orotracheal intubation. Ann Emerg Med 13:175, 1984.
72. Hardwick WC, Bluhm D: Digital intubation. J Emerg Med 1:317, 1984.
73. Ellis DG, Steward RD, Kaplan RM, et al: Success rates of blind orotracheal intubation using a transillumination technique with a lighted stylet. Ann Emerg Med 15:138, 1986.
74. Vollmer TP, Steward RD, Paris PM, et al: Use of a lighted stylet for guided orotracheal intubation in the prehospital setting. Ann Emerg Med 14:324, 1985.
75. Fox DJ, Castro T, Rastrelli AJ: Comparison of intubation techniques in the awake patient: The Flexi-lum^R surgical light (lightwand) versus blind nasal approach. Anesthesiology 66:69, 1987.
76. Taylor PA, Towey RM: The bronchofiberscope as an aid to endotracheal intubation. Br J Anaesth 44:611, 1976.
77. Lindholm CE, Grenvik A: Flexible fiberoptic bronchoscopy and intubation in intensive care. In Ledingham IM (ed): Recent Advances in Intensive Therapy. Edinburgh, Churchill Livingstone, 1977, pp 47–66.
78. Rucker RW, Silva WJ, Worchester CC: Fiberoptic bronchoscopic nasotracheal intubation in children. Chest 76:56, 1979.
79. Butler FS, Cirillo AA: Retrograde tracheal intubation. Anesth Analg 39:333, 1960.
80. Waters DJ: Guided endotracheal intubation for patients with deformities of the upper airway. Anesthesia 18:158, 1963.
81. Powell WF, Ozdel T: A translaryngeal guide for tracheal intubation. Anesth Analg 46:231, 1967.
82. Bourke D, Levesque P: Modification of retrograde guide for endotracheal intubation. Anesth Analg 53:1013, 1974.
83. McNamara RM: Retrograde intubation of the trachea. Ann Emerg Med 16:680, 1987.
84. King H, Wang L, Khan AK, et al: Translaryngeal guided intubation for difficult intubation. Crit Care Med 15:869, 1987.
85. Barriot P, Riou B: Retrograde technique for tracheal intubation in trauma patients. Crit Care Med 16:712, 1988.
86. Stair TO, Hirsch BE: Adult supraglottitis. Am J Emerg Med 3:512, 1985.
87. Vernon DD, Sarnaik AP: Acute epiglottitis in children: A conservative approach to diagnosis and management. Crit Care Med 14:23, 1986.
88. Robb PJ: Failure of intubation in acute inflammatory airway obstruction in childhood. J Laryngol Otol 99:993, 1985.
89. Rosen P, Barkin RM: Respiratory distress in the child. J Emerg Med 3:157, 1985.
90. Grodin MA: Epiglottitis. J Emerg Med 1:13, 1983.

Chapter **2**

Pharmacologic Adjuncts to Intubation

Steven C. Dronen

INTRODUCTION

Endotracheal intubation in the acute care setting presents a challenge distinct from that associated with intubation of the fasted, premedicated patient in the operating room. The emergency department patient is frequently uncooperative, unstable, and completely unknown to the treating physician. Often within a matter of minutes, the physician is expected to assess and control the airway as well as to diagnose and manage other life-threatening problems.

In 1979, Taryle and colleagues reported that complications occurred in 24 of 43 patients intubated in a university hospital emergency department. They called for improved house officer training in endotracheal intubation as well as "more liberal use of the procedures used in the operating room, such as sedation and muscle relaxation."[1] In the past decade, training programs in both critical care and emergency medicine have been greatly expanded, resulting in a significant improvement in the expertise of physicians who provide acute airway management. Simultaneously, the use of established pharmacologic adjuncts to intubation previously available only in the operating room has increased.[2-8] In addition, new drugs have been developed that are potent, rapid acting, and relatively safe, giving the physician greater ability to tailor therapy to specific clinical problems.[9, 10] Because of these developments, physicians may now concentrate not only on the manual skill of intubation but also on the pharmacology of intubation. Specific pharmacotherapeutic goals include provision of analgesia and sedation, muscle relaxation, and avoidance of the complications of intubation, including systemic and intracranial hypertension. This chapter reviews the pharmacology and use of the drugs currently available to facilitate intubation in the acute care setting.

ANALGESIA AND SEDATION

Overview

Laryngoscopy in the awake patient has been likened to the "mouth being held open with a wrench."[11] The upper airway is richly innervated by sensory branches of the fifth, seventh, ninth, and tenth cranial nerves. In addition to pain fibers, there are stretch receptors that stimulate coughing and gagging reflexes with even minor airway manipulation. It is therefore essential that adequate analgesia be provided before intubation in all but the most critical circumstances. Treatment options include topical application of anesthetic agents to the pharyngeal and tracheal mucosa and intravenous infusion of analgesic or sedative agents.

Local Anesthesia

Local or topical anesthesia techniques may be used in patients who are awake, either in place of or as a supplement to intravenous analgesia or sedation. They are particularly useful as adjuncts to nasotracheal intubation but do not generally provide the degree of analgesia or relaxation desirable for orotracheal intubation. In addition, it is time consuming to achieve good topical anesthesia, which may limit the usefulness of these techniques in emergency situations.

Topical anesthesia may be achieved by direct spraying under laryngoscopy, by cricothyroid membrane puncture, or by inhalation of a nebulized anesthetic.

DIRECT APPLICATION USING LARYNGOSCOPY

Achieving anesthesia of the oral and pharyngeal mucosa is a relatively simple procedure using commonly available agents such as a 4 per cent lidocaine or benzocaine-tetracaine (Cetacaine). Achieving anesthesia of the hypopharynx is more difficult because optimal results require application of the anesthetic under direct vision to the epiglottis and vocal cords.

This procedure is begun by spraying the tongue and pharynx with a topical agent. After allowing at least 2 to 3 minutes to permit numbing of the tongue and pharynx, the epiglottis and vocal cords are visualized using a laryngoscope and are sprayed directly with the anesthetic agent. Even if laryngoscopy is not used to facilitate this procedure, it is at best an unpleasant experience. It is also time consuming because of the inherent delay associated with mucosal absorption of an anesthetic agent. An alternative is the percutaneous injection of an anesthetic agent into the trachea at the level of the cricothyroid membrane.[12-13]

CRICOTHYROID MEMBRANE PUNCTURE

The cricothyroid membrane is identified in the trapezoidal space between the cricoid and thyroid cartilages. After appropriate skin preparation with an alcohol or a povidone-iodine swab, the overlying tissue and membrane are punctured with a 22-gauge needle in the midline and just above the superior border of the cricoid cartilage. Care should be taken to maintain the needle in the midline at all times to avoid injury to the recurrent laryngeal nerves. The needle should be advanced until air can be aspirated, indicating placement of the tip in the trachea. A volume of 2 ml of 4 per cent lidocaine is then injected rapidly. Alternatively, 1 or 2 per cent lidocaine (3 to 4 ml) that is used for local anesthesia may be injected if the 4 per cent concentration is not available. Typically this will precipitate a cough, which adequately distributes the anesthetic over the upper trachea, vocal cords, and epiglottis. (See also Chapters 3 and 7.)

NEBULIZED ANESTHESIA

This simple and painless technique can be used to facilitate awake intubation when the patient's condition is stable enough to permit a several-minute delay.[14] The anesthetic is delivered using a standard nebulizer and face mask connected to an oxygen source that delivers 4 to 8 L/min. A volume of 4 ml of a 4 per cent solution is nebulized over about 5 minutes. Bourke and colleagues reported achieving consistently good anesthesia using this technique, although their patients were often premedicated with narcotics, sedatives, or both.[15]

Intravenous Analgesia or Sedation

OVERVIEW

The intravenous infusion of analgesic, anesthetic, or sedative agents either alone or in combination is an excellent means of facilitating relatively painless intubation. In recent years a number of drugs have been released that are characterized by high potency, rapid onset of action, short half-life, and minimal potential for cardiorespiratory depression. Properly used, these agents provide rapid, safe, and effective anesthesia.

NARCOTICS (FENTANYL)

Pharmacology. A number of useful agents exist, including morphine, meperidine, and fentanyl. Only the last-mentioned drug will be discussed because it possesses significant advantages over the other agents.

Fentanyl is a synthetic opiate related to the phenylpiperidine family. Since its introduction in 1968, fentanyl has been used widely in a variety of settings, often replacing meperidine as the agent of choice for rapid short-term analgesia.[16-20] Its pharmacologic properties that are responsible for this preference include a highly lipophilic nature, rapid serum clearance, high potency, and minimal histamine release.[21-24] Fentanyl crosses the blood-brain barrier rapidly, producing analgesia in as little as 1.5 minutes. Serum levels decline rapidly from peak concentrations because of extensive tissue uptake.[25, 26] Unlike morphine, the brain concentration of the drug falls in conjunction with the serum level. The duration of analgesic action is 30 to 40 minutes, although at high doses a second peak of activity may be seen several hours later because of the release of the bound drug from tissue stores. Fentanyl is about 50 to 100 times as potent as morphine sulfate.[27] This unique combination of potency and short half-life permits the administration of numerous small doses that can be titrated to the desired clinical effect.

Dose. The relative safety of fentanyl permits considerable latitude in dosing. When used as a primary anesthetic agent for major surgical procedures, doses ranging from 50 to 100 μg/kg produce minimal side effects.[28] Comparatively tiny doses provide good analgesia for intubation, and 3 to 5 μg/kg, given at a rate of 1 to 2 μg/kg/min, is generally an effective analgesic dose. More rapid administration will cause greater depression of the level of consciousness. Mostert and coworkers reported successful awake intubation in 99 of 103 patients who were administered an average dose of 3.7 μg/kg.[21] Most of these patients were able to follow commands, and many recalled the events surrounding the intubation. A small percentage could not be intubated even after receiving 500 μg of fentanyl.

Larger doses, perhaps up to 25 μg/kg, may be needed to produce ideal intubating conditions, although if given rapidly, 10 μg/kg is usually adequate. Administering large doses is generally impractical for an emergency intubation because it is time consuming and produces a longer period of unresponsiveness than may be desirable. It is preferable to combine a low dose of fentanyl (2 to 3 μg/kg) for analgesia with a paralytic agent, such as succinylcholine, to produce adequate muscle relaxation and a sedative, such as midazolam, to reduce anxiety and produce amnesia for the event.

Complications. Unlike other narcotics, fentanyl causes little or no histamine release, and its use is seldom associated with hypotension. It is probably the safest narcotic to use in the hypovolemic patient. Fentanyl also has less emetic effects than other narcotics. Complications that have been reported with fentanyl are few and primarily follow the rapid intravenous infusion of very large doses. Like other narcotics, fentanyl may cause rigidity of the skeletal musculature including the chest wall and diaphragm. Typically this occurs with doses in excess of 15 μg/kg, but it has been reported with doses as low as 10 μg/kg.[21, 29] The muscular rigidity may be prevented or treated with standard doses of succinylcholine or naloxone.[30] Grand mal seizures have also been reported, but they are very uncommon.[31-33] Chudnofsky and colleagues[7] reported a complication rate of less than 1 per cent in 841 emergency department patients treated with fentanyl. The most common complication was respiratory depression, and it generally occurred when fentanyl was given in combination with other central nervous system depressants.

BENZODIAZEPINES (MIDAZOLAM)

Pharmacology. The benzodiazepines are a widely used class of drugs characterized by anxiolytic, hypnotic, sedative, anticonvulsant, muscle relaxant, and amnestic effects. Several of these properties make the benzodiazepines ideal adjuvant agents for intubation, particularly when used in combination with narcotics. It is important to remember that benzodiazepines do not have analgesic effects. Although they may produce excellent sedation and impair the patient's memory of an unpleasant experience, they will not prevent the pain associated with intubation.

Diazepam has been used widely to facilitate intubation, but its use has been supplanted in recent years. Diazepam has a variable onset of action and a long elimination half-life, and it causes significant infusion site pain and frequently phlebitis when given intravenously.

Midazolam is a recently introduced benzodiazepine that has to a great extent replaced diazepam as a preoperative sedative agent.[34, 35] Midazolam is also used widely as an anesthesia induction agent even in high-risk elderly and cardiac patients.[36-38] Compared with diazepam, the primary advantages of midazolam include a twofold increase in potency, a shorter half-life, and a lessened potential for cardiorespiratory depression. Midazolam possesses a unique imidazole ring that is stable and water soluble in an acid medium but highly lipophilic at physiologic pH.

Because it does not require suspension in propylene glycol, midazolam is not a tissue irritant. It causes minimal pain on injection, is rarely associated with phlebitis, and can be given intramuscularly when a very rapid onset of action is not required. The highly lipophilic character of the drug permits rapid accumulation in the central nervous system with an onset of sedation in as little as 1 to 2 minutes. Rapid penetration into fatty tissue coupled with extensive binding to plasma proteins causes a prompt fall in serum levels after intravenous administration. This may account for the paucity of side effects outside the central nervous system. The half-life of elimination is 1 to 4 hours and is dependent on release of the drug from adipose tissue and protein-binding sites. The period of sedation following a single intravenous dose is considerably shorter. Emergence from a 0.15 mg/kg dose occurs in 15 to 20 minutes.[39]

Clinical experience using midazolam for conscious sedation before the performance of surgical and dental procedures or as an adjunctive agent for the induction of anesthesia is considerable. Baker and Gordon reported the use of midazolam to achieve conscious sedation in 400 ambulatory surgery patients.[35] Used in combination with either fentanyl or ketamine, midazolam was felt to be both effective and safe.

Dose. The recommended dose for conscious sedation with midazolam is 0.02 to 0.04 mg/kg given in 1 mg boluses and not exceeding 2.5 mg over 2 minutes. Doses up to 0.1 mg/kg may be needed to produce good conditions for intubation. All patients receiving midazolam should be monitored closely, and personnel skilled and prepared to manage the airway should be present.

Complications. Although initially touted to be free of cardiorespiratory side effects, recent experience suggests that the potential complications of midazolam are quite similar to those of other benzodiazepines. A small increase in heart rate is seen frequently, as is a small decrease in systolic blood pressure.[40] The change in blood pressure may be exaggerated in the presence of hypovolemia.[41] Cardiac index and coronary artery blood flow are generally not affected. Respiratory depression may occur even at standard doses but most often follows rapid administration of an excessive dose. Respiratory depression is also more likely to occur in debilitated or elderly patients and in those simultaneously receiving narcotics. Reports of fatalities soon after midazolam's introduction in the United States prompted changes in the recommendations for its use. These included lowering of the dosage schedule, reduction of the speed of administration, and careful patient monitoring during administration.[42]

Limited information is available on the use of midazolam to facilitate emergency department intubation. Wright and colleagues reported its use in 289 emergency department patients, of whom 20 were undergoing intubation.[43] The overall complication rate was 1.4 per cent, including 2 cases of hypotension and 2 cases of respiratory depression. In every case, patients had received other drugs in combination with midazolam that may have been responsible for the observed adverse effects. Seventy-one per cent of the patients in this study also received fentanyl. The midazolam-fentanyl combination has been reported to provide an excellent level of conscious sedation that is also of rapid onset and short duration.[44, 45]

BARBITURATES (THIOPENTAL AND METHOHEXITAL)

Pharmacology. Although they are the most popular agents used to induce preoperative anesthesia, barbiturates are used infrequently to facilitate intubation outside the operating room. This is most likely because of their reputation as cardiorespiratory depressants. Although it is true that barbiturate use may be associated with significant complications, these can usually be avoided by careful attention to proper dosing and patient selection. Used appropriately, barbiturates provide the practitioner with a highly effective tool to facilitate intubation. Both thiopental (Pentothal) and methohexital (Brevital) may be used, depending on the period of sedation desired.

Following intravenous injection, barbiturates bind rapidly to plasma proteins, particularly albumin. Unbound barbiturate quickly accumulates in highly vascular organs, reaching peak brain levels in as short a time as 50 seconds. The drug then diffuses from the brain, ultimately reaching equilibrium between the intracerebral and plasma concentrations. Degradation occurs primarily in the liver, producing inactive metabolites that are excreted in the urine or gut depending on the drug used. Single-pass hepatic clearance is substantially higher for methohexital than for thiopental, which accounts for the former drug's shorter duration of action. The period of anesthesia following a single intravenous dose of methohexital is 4 to 6 minutes compared with 5 to 10 minutes for thiopental.[46, 47]

The barbiturates are central nervous system depressants that are capable of producing mild sedation to deep coma. They do not block afferent sensory impulses to a significant extent and therefore should be used in conjunction with an analgesic agent such as fentanyl if a painful procedure is to be performed. It is, however, common practice to intubate patients who have received only barbiturates.[47]

Advantages of barbiturates as adjuncts to intubation include their high potency, rapid onset, and short duration of action, traits they share with fentanyl and midazolam. The barbiturates are also known to reduce cerebral metabolism and oxygen consumption and, secondarily, cerebral blood flow and intracranial pressure.[48, 49] For this reason, thiopental is considered the agent of choice for anesthesia induction and maintenance in patients with elevated intracranial pressure. Some have stated that thiopental is the drug of choice to temporarily anesthetize the patient with a head injury before intubation. It has not been proved, however, that barbiturates exert a protective effect on the central nervous system when used for a short period of time during rapid-sequence intubation. Moreover, their use in trauma patients may lead to systemic hypotension and impaired cerebral perfusion pressure that may offset the theoretic advantages of barbiturate therapy.

Dose. The recommended dose of thiopental is 3 to 5 mg/kg administered as a 2.5 per cent solution at a rate not to exceed 2 mg/kg/min. Normal saline should be used as a diluent. Methohexital is given at 1 to 2 mg/kg over 30 to 60 seconds.

Complications. It has been stated that barbiturates are "fatally easy" to use.[47] This is an overstatement that reflects improper use of the drugs more than an inherent danger associated with their use. The most significant complication of barbiturate therapy is depression of the vasomotor center and myocardial contractility leading to significant hypotension. This may be particularly pronounced in the presence of hypovolemia or cardiovascular disease.

Barbiturates also depress the brain stem respiratory centers when given rapidly or in large doses. This effect may be accelerated by simultaneous treatment with narcotics. Patients with asthma or chronic bronchitis may experience bronchospasm. Laryngospasm may occur in patients who were anesthetized lightly with barbiturates during manipulation of the upper airway. Laryngospasm usually responds to positive-pressure ventilation or paralysis with succinylcholine. In addition, the high pH of the barbiturate solution may cause tissue necrosis following extravascular administration and severe pain, vessel spasm, and thrombosis following intra-arterial infusion.[47]

KETAMINE

Pharmacology. Unique among anesthetic agents currently in use, ketamine produces a dissociative anesthesia, characterized by excellent analgesia and amnesia despite the appearance of wakefulness. As a drug that is potent and relatively safe and possesses a rapid onset and brief duration of action, ketamine fits the profile of a drug that could be used effectively to facilitate intubation. It does, however, possess a number of pharmacologic properties that limit its use to very select circumstances.

Ketamine is a water- and lipid-soluble drug with rapid penetration into the central nervous system. Like the barbiturates, ketamine accumulates rapidly in highly vascular organs and then undergoes redistribution. The half-life of redistribution from the plasma to the peripheral tissues is 7 to 11 minutes, and the half life of elimination is 2 to 3 hours. Degradation occurs primarily in the liver.[50]

Unlike other anesthetic agents that depress the reticular activating system, ketamine acts by interrupting association pathways between the thalamoneocortical and limbic systems. Characteristically the eyes remain open, and patients exhibit spontaneous, although not purposeful, movements. Increases in blood pressure, heart rate, cardiac output, and myocardial oxygen consumption are seen—effects that are most likely mediated through the central nervous system. In vitro studies indicate that ketamine is a myocardial depressant, but the central nervous system–mediated pressor effects generally mask the direct cardiac effects.[51, 52] Respirations are initially rapid and shallow after ketamine administration, but they soon return to normal.

Other features of ketamine anesthesia include increase in skeletal muscle tone, preservation of laryngeal and pharyngeal reflexes, hypersalivation, and relaxation of bronchial smooth muscle. Intracranial pressure is increased most likely as a consequence of increased cerebral blood flow.[50]

Ketamine has been recommended for anesthesia induction in children because of its relative safety and the infrequency of postanesthesia emergence reactions in this group. There is no evidence, however, that it offers any advantage over agents such as fentanyl or midazolam. Ketamine has also been recommended for the unstable critically ill patient because it does not depress the cardiovascular system.[53, 54] This recommendation is too vague to be useful to the clinician, and it ignores the fact that ketamine is potentially harmful in patients with cardiac ischemia (because it increases myocardial oxygen consumption) or acute intracranial pathology (because it increases intracranial pressure). Ketamine may be useful during hemorrhagic shock because of its cardiostimulatory effect. Its administration to patients in shock has been reported to cause a fall in blood pressure only when the shock state was prolonged.[55, 56]

The most promising use of ketamine to facilitate intubation has been in acute bronchospastic disease. Ketamine relaxes bronchial smooth muscle either directly, through the enhancement of sympathomimetic effects, or through the inhibition of vagal effects. Ketamine also increases bronchial secretions, which may decrease the incidence of mucous plugging commonly reported in autopsies of asthmatic patients.[57] Clinical studies have demonstrated a reduction in airway resistance and an increase in pulmonary compliance that occurs within minutes of ketamine administration.[58, 59] L'Hommedieu and Arens[8] reported prompt improvement in respiratory acidosis in 5 asthmatics intubated with ketamine and succinylcholine. Although this is a small study,

their report suggests that ketamine may be a helpful agent when intubation of the asthmatic patient is indicated.

Dose. The recommended dose of ketamine before intubation is 1 to 2 mg/kg administered intravenously over 1 minute. Anesthesia occurs within 1 minute of completing the infusion and lasts approximately 5 minutes. A smaller dose (0.5 to 1.5 mg/kg) may be given 5 minutes after the initial dose if there is a need to maintain anesthesia. The simultaneous administration of succinylcholine and midazolam is recommended to provide adequate muscle relaxation and to decrease the incidence of postanesthesia emergence reactions.

Complications. A side effect that has greatly limited the use of ketamine is its tendency to produce post-anesthesia emergence reactions, a characteristic that it has in common with the structurally similar drug phencyclidine. The reactions typically include floating sensations, dizziness, blurred vision, out-of-body experiences, and vivid dreams or nightmares. The reported incidence of these reactions varies from 5 to 30 per cent.[60, 61] They are less common in children than in adults.

Of the drugs that have been evaluated for their ability to suppress postanesthesia emergence reactions, the benzodiazepines show the most promise. Both diazepam and lorazepam are useful, but the latter is more effective, most likely owing to its enhanced amnestic effect.[62–65] Midazolam has not been evaluated as thoroughly as have the other benzodiazepines, but it has potent amnestic effects and offers the advantage of a short duration of action. White[66] reported a 55 per cent incidence of postemergence dreaming in patients receiving ketamine and complete suppression of dreaming with the addition of midazolam. Evidence also suggests that midazolam may inhibit the cardiostimulatory effects of ketamine.

Although ketamine produces excellent analgesia and is relatively safe, its use as an agent to facilitate intubation is somewhat limited. The widely held belief that aspiration does not occur with ketamine because of preservation of pharyngeal and laryngeal reflexes is incorrect.[67, 68] Moreover, ketamine does not relax skeletal muscle. The production of desired intubating conditions requires the simultaneous administration of a paralytic agent, thereby removing any upper airway reflexes.

MUSCLE RELAXATION

Overview

For many years the neuromuscular blocking agents (NMBs) have been used to facilitate intubations in the operating room, but only recently has their use spread to acute care settings. This practice reflects in large part a lack of physician familiarity and in some cases hospital administrative policies restricting the use of NMBs to anesthesiologists. Some have stated that muscle relaxation may be achieved by other means (e.g., intravenous sedation) or that alternatives to orotracheal intubation (e.g., nasotracheal intubation) should be used. Undoubtedly, these techniques also have a place in the armamentarium of the well-trained acute care physician, but they should not be used to the exclusion of NMBs. Any physician involved in airway management on a regular basis should be thoroughly familiar and comfortable with the use of NMBs. To maximize safety, it is recommended that the use of these agents be guided by a departmentally approved protocol (Table 2–1).

Neuromuscular blocking agents are classified as either depolarizing or nondepolarizing. The recommended dose, onset, and duration of action of the commonly used agents are listed in Table 2–2.

Table 2–1. Representative Departmental Protocol for Endotracheal Intubation Using Succinylcholine

1. Assemble required equipment:
   Bag-valve-mask connected to functioning oxygen
      delivery system
   Working suction with Yankauer suction tip attached
   Endotracheal tube(s) with stylette and intact cuff
   Laryngoscope with blades and bright light
   Cricothyrotomy tray

2. Check to be sure that a functioning, secure intravenous line is in place.

3. Connect patient to a cardiac monitor.

4. Preoxygenate (denitrogenate)) the lungs by providing 100% oxygen by mask (if ventilatory assistance is necessary, bag gently while applying cricoid pressure).

5. Monitor oxygen saturation with pulse oximeter. If oxygen saturation falls below 95% *during* intubation attempt(s), stop the intubation attempt and ventilate the patient. (If pulse oximeter is not available, proceed as for item 10 below.)

6. Premedicate as appropriate:
   Midazolam—0.02 to 0.04 mg/kg IV in l-mg boluses,
      for sedation of awake patients
   Fentanyl—2 to 3 µg/kg given at a rate of 1 to 2 µg/
      kg/min IV for analgesia in awake patients
   Atropine—0.01 mg/kg IV push for children or
      adolescents (miminum dose of 0.1 mg recommended)
   *Lidocaine—1.5 to 2.0 mg/kg intravenously over 30 to 60
      seconds

7. Apply cricoid pressure to occlude the esophagus until intubation is completed successfully and the endotracheal tube cuff is inflated.

8. Give succinylcholine 1.5 mg/kg IV push (use 2.0 mg/kg for infants and small children).

9. Apnea, jaw relaxation, and decreased resistance to bag-mask ventilations indicate that the patient is sufficiently relaxed to proceed with intubation.

10. Perform endotracheal intubation. If unable to intubate during the first 20-second attempt, stop and ventilate the patient with the bag-mask for 30 to 60 seconds. If the patient is insufficiently relaxed, give a second dose of succinylcholine (1.0 to 1.5 times the initial dose). If repeated intubation attempts fail, ventilate the patient with the bag-mask until spontaneous ventilations return. If endotracheal intubation fails and the patient cannot be ventilated with the bag-mask, perform cricothyrotomy (emergency equipment for a surgical airway should be on hand before initiating an intubation attempt).

11. Treat bradycardia occurring during intubation with atropine, 0.5 mg IV push (smaller dose for children; see item 6). Halt the intubation attempt temporarily and ventilate the patient with the bag-mask and 100% oxygen.

12. Once intubation is completed, inflate the cuff and confirm the endotracheal tube placement by auscultating for bilateral breath sounds.

13. Release cricoid pressure and secure endotracheal tube.

*Lidocaine is given to suppress the cough reflex and intracranial hypertension in patients with head trauma. Its use is controversial.
   IV, intravenously.

Indications and Contraindications

The primary indication for the use of NMBs is the need for additional muscle relaxation. Orotracheal intubation is markedly easier to perform when the musculature of the oropharynx is completely relaxed. This is especially true when intubation must be performed quickly under less than ideal circumstances. Sedatives may in some cases provide adequate muscle relaxation, but they generally cannot be given in a high enough dose or quickly enough to provide good relaxation without risking cardiac depression. The combination of an NMB and a sedative or an analgesic agent is generally superior to the use of either agent alone. Also, NMBs are indicated to facilitate intubation of the patient with a head injury because they prevent bucking and gagging that may cause an acute rise in intracranial pressure.

The only absolute contraindication to the use of NMBs is the inability to manage the airway once the patient becomes apneic. Although not absolutely contraindicated, it is relatively inhumane to paralyze and intubate an alert patient. A sedative or analgesic agent should be administered simultaneously if the patient is able to perceive pain.

Controversy surrounds the use of neuromuscular blocking agents to facilitate intubation in the patient who may have a cervical spine injury. Despite claims to the contrary, there is no evidence that orotracheal intubation performed during inline stabilization, with or without paralysis, is dangerous. Cadaver studies[69–71] purporting to demonstrate the dangers inherent in this practice simply do not simulate the condition of a living patient accurately.[72] Conversely, no studies prove conclusively that orotracheal intubation following the use of NMBs is a safe practice, but it has been performed for a number of years in operating rooms without reported detrimental effects even in patients with unstable cervical spine fractures.[73, 74]

Depolarizing Agents

Pharmacology. The standard depolarizing agent in use today is succinylcholine, which was introduced in 1952. It has a chemical structure similar to that of acetylcholine and is therefore able to depolarize the postjunctional neuromuscular membrane. Administration is followed by a brief period of muscle fasciculation that corresponds to the initial membrane depolarization. Unlike acetylcholine, which is released in minute amounts and hydrolyzed in milliseconds, succinylcholine requires several minutes for significant hydrolysis to occur. During this time, the neuromuscular membrane remains depolarized, but the muscles relax and will not contract until the neuromuscular end plate and adjacent sarcoplasmic reticulum return to the resting state and are again depolarized. Relaxation proceeds from the small, distal, rapidly moving muscles to the proximal, slower-moving muscles. The diaphragm is one of the last muscles to relax.[75]

Succinylcholine is rapidly hydrolyzed in the serum by the enzyme pseudocholinesterase. Only a small amount ever reaches the neuromuscular junction, and that portion is quickly drawn back into the serum by a concentration gradient produced by serum clearance. The duration of action of a single dose is 3 to 5 minutes. Relaxation may be maintained by repeated intravenous injections or a constant infusion. Prolonged or repeated use of the drug may, however, enhance its effects at either the vagal or sympathetic ganglia. Vagal stimulation may result in bradycardia and hypotension as well as other muscarinic effects. These effects may be seen even at normal doses, particularly in children.[76] For this reason atropine pretreatment is recommended in all children and in adults receiving multiple doses.[77]

Repeat dosing may also produce desensitization blockade in which the neuromuscular membrane returns to the resting state and becomes resistant to further depolarization with succinylcholine.[78, 79] Clinically this is indicated by an unsustained contraction in response to a tetanic stimulus and response to a test dose of edrophonium.[80] In general, there is little need for repeated doses of succinylcholine. If

Table 2-2. Commonly Used Neuromuscular Blocking Agents				
	Succinylcholine*	Pancuronium†	Vecuronium‡ (Lower Dose)	Vecuronium‡ (Higher Dose)
Dose	1.5 mg/kg	0.1 mg/kg	0.1 mg/kg	0.25 mg/kg
Onset	1 min	2–5 min	3 min	1 min
Duration	3–5 min	40–60 min	30–35 min	60–120 min

*Anectine™: 20 mg/ml.
†Pavulon™: 1 or 2 mg/ml.
‡Norcuron™: 1 mg/ml (supplied as a powder that must be reconstituted).

paralysis in excess of 3 to 5 minutes is desired, agents such as vecuronium or pancuronium should be used.

Dose. The recommended dose of succinylcholine is 1.0 to 1.5 mg/kg given intravenously. It is better to err on the side of too large a dose, thereby guaranteeing complete relaxation and avoiding the need for repeat dosing.

Complications. There are a number of potential complications of succinylcholine use. These include muscle fasciculations and their side effects, hyperkalemia, stimulation of autonomic ganglia, malignant hyperthermia, prolonged apnea, histamine release, and elevation of intracranial pressure.

As noted previously, muscle fasciculations accompany the initial depolarization of the neuromuscular membrane. They may be prevented by preadministration of a subparalytic dose (0.01 mg/kg) of pancuronium. Fasciculations are most prominent in muscular adolescents but are uncommon in children. Their most frequent side effect is deep aching muscle pain that may last for several days.[81] Fasciculations of the abdominal wall may elevate intragastric pressure and cause regurgitation of stomach contents. This is an uncommon complication that most often follows overzealous bag-mask ventilation before intubation. Distention of the stomach with air and failure to perform the Sellick maneuver (firm cricoid pressure to occlude the esophagus during airway management procedures) are more likely to cause vomiting than are muscle fasciculations alone. It is also important to note that oropharyngeal manipulation of the nonparalyzed patient is far more likely to cause vomiting than are succinylcholine-induced fasciculations.

Other reported but distinctly uncommon side effects of muscle fasciculations include elevations of intraocular pressure and skeletal fractures or dislocations. The clinical significance of a transient rise in intraocular pressure in a patient with a penetrating eye injury is unknown. There has never been a reported case of vitreous expulsion occurring during a rapid-sequence intubation with succinylcholine despite its widespread use in open eye surgery.[82] It is certain, however, that paralysis will prevent spontaneous patient motor activity such as coughing or gagging that is associated with a greater risk of vitreous expulsion. Although it may be prudent to use a nondepolarizing agent in patients with penetrating eye injuries, a necessary intubation using succinylcholine should never be delayed or avoided because of this theoretic concern.[83]

The precise mechanism by which succinylcholine causes hyperkalemia is unknown, but it is thought to occur secondary to the asynchronous depolarization of muscle cells and resultant cellular injury. The elevation is typically less than 0.5 mEq/L.[84] In certain pathologic states the hyperkalemic response may be as much as 5.0 mEq/L. These conditions include severe burns,[85] major muscle trauma,[86] and upper motor neuron disease.[87, 88] These large elevations occur only in patients who have had significant tissue injury or muscle denervation for several days or weeks before succinylcholine use. Succinylcholine is not contraindicated in the acute initial management of these patients.

Malignant hyperthermia is a very uncommon complication with an autosomal dominant inheritance pattern. It occurs in approximately one in 15,000 children and one in 50,000 adults.[89] The clinical syndrome consists of high fever, tachypnea, tachycardia, cardiac arrhythmias, hypoxia, acidosis, myoglobinuria, and impaired coagulation. Muscle spasm rather than relaxation is frequently seen.[90] Treatment includes aggressive cooling measures, volume replacement, and correction of hypoxia and acid-base and electrolyte abnormalities. Dantrolene sodium, a direct-acting skeletal muscle relaxant, has been shown to be effective in reducing muscle hypermetabolism that causes the fever.[91]

An associated abnormal response to succinylcholine is isolated masseter spasm.[92] Barlow and Isaacs reported two cases in which masseter spasm was the first abnormality noted in fatal episodes of malignant hyperthermia.[93] Masseter spasm may be more common in patients with neuromuscular disorders such as myotonia congenita.

Prolonged apnea may occur because of decreased cholinesterase levels (e.g., in hepatic disease, anemia, renal failure, pregnancy, advanced age, bronchogenic carcinoma, connective tissue disorders) or, more commonly, because of the inheritance of an atypical cholinesterase present in about 0.03 per cent of the population. This atypical enzyme has both a decreased affinity for the succinylcholine molecule and a decreased ability to hydrolyze it. The period of apnea is therefore increased from 3 to 5 minutes up to several hours. Patients with markedly decreased levels of a normal cholinesterase experience only a two- to threefold increase in the duration of apnea.[94] Patients with cocaine intoxication may experience prolonged muscle relaxation if given succinylcholine because cocaine is also metabolized by cholinesterases.

The magnitude and significance of the increase in intracranial pressure that occurs with succinylcholine use remain controversial.[95–97] Increases in the range of 5 to 10 mm Hg have been reported by several investigators, but other researchers have shown no increase. Nor is there evidence of neurologic deterioration associated with these transient elevations in intracranial pressure. A mechanism that has been proposed to explain this rise is an increase in cortical electrical activity with a resultant increase in cerebral blood flow, blood volume, and intracranial pressure. Minton and colleagues have demonstrated that pretreatment with vecuronium (0.14 mg/kg) reduces the rise in intracranial pressure following succinylcholine administration from mean values of 5 to 1 mm Hg.[98] It has been postulated that nondepolarizing blockade prevents muscle spindle firing and the increase in cortical activity that may lead to increased intracranial pressure. Pretreatment with a nondepolarizing agent may not be practical when intubation must be performed rapidly; furthermore, the dose that has been shown to be effective is itself a paralyzing dose and would obviate the need for succinylcholine.

At the present time, questions concerning the safety of succinylcholine use in the setting of acute intracranial pathology do not have clear answers. The drug has been used widely and successfully in this setting, and its continued use seems reasonable. The eminent risk of airway compromise without the use of a depolarizing agent must always be weighed against the rare harmful effects mentioned.

Nondepolarizing Agents

OVERVIEW

Nondepolarizing agents act in a competitive manner to block the effects of acetylcholine at the neuromuscular junction. These agents have a significant theoretic advantage over succinylcholine in that they do not cause fasciculations and their undesirable side effects. Drugs in this class include d-tubocurarine, pancuronium, atracurium, and vecuronium. Of these, pancuronium has been used the most widely, but its comparatively slow onset of action and long half-life make it less than ideal. The recently introduced agent vecuronium is preferable in most instances, although it too has an onset of action that may be too long to be consistently useful before intubation.

PANCURONIUM (PAVULON)

Pharmacology. Pancuronium is classified as a long-acting NMB with an onset of action of 2 to 5 minutes and a duration of action of 40 to 60 minutes. Ninety per cent of a single intravenous dose is excreted unchanged in the urine within the first hour.[99]

Dose. The recommended dose is 0.1 mg/kg delivered intravenously. Paralysis may be maintained safely by repeating this dose, but because the effects of the drug are cumulative, repeated dosing significantly lengthens the duration of paralysis.

Reversal. Because nondepolarizing agents act competitively, their effects may be reversed by increasing the concentration of acetylcholine. Cholinesterase inhibitors such as neostigmine or edrophonium may be used but not until some spontaneous signs of reversal are seen. Thus the concept of reversal is of limited clinical importance. When reversal is required, neostigmine 0.02 to 0.04 mg/kg is given by slow intravenous push. Additional doses of 0.01 to 0.02 mg/kg may be given in 5 minutes if reversal is incomplete, but the total dose should not exceed 5 mg in the adult. Atropine 0.01 mg/kg (with a minimum dose of 0.1 mg for children and a maximum dose of 1.0 mg for adults) should be given concurrently with neostigmine to block its cholinergic effects.[100, 102]

Complications. There are few complications associated with the use of pancuronium. Many patients experience an increase in heart rate, blood pressure, and cardiac output because of a vagolytic effect of the drug. This may be undesirable in patients with underlying cardiac disease. Ventricular tachycardia and severe hypertension have been reported but are quite rare.[103, 104] Pancuronium may cause histamine release that results in bronchospasm or anaphylactic reactions.[105] Prolonged paralysis may also occur, primarily in patients with myasthenia gravis or those with significant impairment of renal function.

VECURONIUM (NORCURON)

Pharmacology. Vecuronium was introduced in 1984 as the end product of a search for the "ideal" NMB. The desired pharmacologic properties included a rapid onset and short duration of action, absence of cardiovascular side effects or histamine release, minimal activity at sites other than the neuromuscular junction, reversibility, and lack of cumulative effects. Vecuronium closely approximates this ideal profile. Compared with pancuronium, vecuronium offers the advantages of a shorter onset and duration of action and an absence of cumulative effects with repeated doses.[106] Perhaps more important, vecuronium does not have vagolytic activity and does not cause hypertension or tachycardia. Compared with succinylcholine, vecuronium does not cause fasciculations or their side effects. The primary factor limiting its use as the only muscle relaxant needed for intubation is its onset and duration of action, both of which are excessive for many intubations. Vecuronium may be used safely in conjunction with succinylcholine if continued neuromuscular blockade is desired after intubation.[10]

Dose. Vecuronium is classified as an intermediate-acting NMB with an onset of action of about 3 minutes and a duration of action of 30 to 35 minutes at the recommended dose of 0.1 mg/kg, given intravenously. Paralysis may occur in as little as 1 minute at a dose of 0.25 mg/kg, but the period of paralysis will last 1 to 2 hours. This may be the ideal method of obtaining muscle relaxation when a long period of paralysis is desired. Some would object to the use of an intermediate or long-acting agent before intubation because of the risk of failed intubation. This argument is understandable, but in fact, even the 5 minutes of apnea commonly seen with succinylcholine is excessive if an adequate airway cannot be established.

An alternative technique that results in paralysis that is of rapid onset and short duration makes use of the priming principle. It has been observed previously with other nondepolarizing agents that administration of a subparalytic dose several minutes before a smaller than normal "intubating" dose results in a more rapid onset of paralysis. Because a smaller total dose of the drug is used, motor functions return sooner. In a study by Schwarz and colleagues,[107] the administration of 0.015 mg/kg followed 6 minutes later by 0.05 mg/kg resulted in paralysis in about 60 seconds with a duration of 21 minutes. Similarly, Kunjappan and colleagues,[108] using a priming dose of 0.015 mg/kg followed 4 minutes later by 0.085 mg/kg, reported an onset time of 82 seconds and a duration of 28 ± 4 minutes. Because of the 4- to 6-minute interval between the priming and intubating doses, this technique is not practical for emergency intubations but could be used in patients whose condition permits a brief delay in establishing an airway.

With vecuronium, unlike both pancuronium and succinylcholine, there are no side effects specifically related to repeated dosing. A repeat dose of 0.01 to 0.02 mg/kg will extend the period of paralysis 12 to 15 minutes.

PREVENTION OF COMPLICATIONS OF INTUBATION

The Pressor Response

OVERVIEW

The pressor response to stimulation of the pharynx, larynx, and trachea was first described by King and coworkers in 1951.[109] It is a reflex mediated by the sympathetic nervous system consisting of a transient increase in the blood pressure and pulse rate. Stretching of the hypopharynx that occurs with laryngoscopy is the most common precipitant of the pressor response, but any manipulation of the upper airway, including nasotracheal intubation or suction, may elicit a potent response.[110–112]

Considerable variation exists in the magnitude and duration of the pressor response. Studies of young healthy normotensive subjects have shown that an average increase of 20 to 25 mm Hg in mean arterial pressure occurs with laryngoscopy and intubation.[113–117] The magnitude of the response increases as the duration of the stimulus increases, reaching a peak at 45 seconds. Data from controls in several studies of patients with a broad spectrum of medical problems reveal a range of blood pressure increases from 14 to 48 mm Hg, with an average of about 30 mm Hg. Similarly, the increase in heart rates ranges from 8 to 45 beats per minute, with an average of approximately 30. Typically these elevations last less than 5 minutes. The magnitude of the pressor response may be increased in hypertensive patients and those with cardiovascular disease even if the hypertension is adequately controlled before intubation.

In addition to sinus tachycardia, a number of dysrhythmias have been reported following intubation. These are primarily ventricular in origin, including ectopic beats, bigeminy, and, occasionally, short runs of ventricular tachycardia. Bradyarrhythmias have been reported uncommonly. Electrocardiographic changes suggestive of ischemia have been reported, particularly in patients with dramatic increases in blood pressure.[118, 119]

Since the discovery of the pressor response, numerous clinical studies have been conducted that have investigated methods to prevent or blunt it. The drugs studied include lidocaine, atropine, fentanyl, thiopental, nitroprusside, hydralazine, phentolamine, practolol, and midazolam.[120–125] The results of these studies are confusing and contradictory. The differences among their results can be attributed to differences in study design, patient selection, mode of drug delivery, concomitant use of other drugs, and, in some cases, major design flaws. Among studies that have demonstrated pharmacologic blunting of the pressor response, the differences in blood pressure and pulse rate between treated and untreated patients have averaged about 10 to 15 mm Hg and 20 beats per minute. Although the results of these studies were often statistically significant, their clinical significance is unproven. It is also important to note that these studies have produced very limited information supporting claims that the pressor response is harmful.

In 1977[126] Fox reported two patients, both of whom deteriorated after induction of anesthesia and orotracheal intubation. This report has been widely quoted as evidence that the pressor response should be prevented. There are however, no studies reporting comparative data and none establishing a relationship between the response and clinical deterioration in a large patient population. It is also not well documented that attenuation of the pressor response will prevent dysrhythmias or electrocardiographic evidence of ischemia. Although it is prudent to avoid sudden increases in blood pressure in unstable patients with acute cardiac or atherosclerotic vascular disease, it is likely that the pressor response is of little clinical significance in the majority of patients intubated in the emergency department.

PREVENTION

Of the drugs that have demonstrated some ability to attenuate the pressor response, most are impractical for emergency intubations because they either induce deep levels of anesthesia or lead to hemodynamic instability. Drugs that may be useful include lidocaine and fentanyl. Lidocaine, administered either topically or intravenously, has been studied the most extensively but with equivocal results. Lidocaine may work by producing anesthesia of the upper airway or by a direct myocardial depressant effect. Topical lidocaine is generally given in doses sufficient to raise systemic concentration to levels comparable with those seen in intravenous administration, thereby making it difficult to differentiate local and systemic effects. It is clear that topical lidocaine administration by laryngoscopy is not effective because laryngoscopy itself induces the pressor response. Unfortunately, several of the clinical studies were conducted in precisely this manner.[127, 128] Studies by Venus and colleagues[113] and Abou-Madi and coworkers[129] have shown attenuation of the pressor response following inhalation of nebulized 4 per cent lidocaine over a 5-minute period before anesthesia induction. Hartigan and colleagues[110] demonstrated that 60 mg of a 10 per cent lidocaine spray blunted the response when administered more than 5 minutes before nasotracheal intubation. These techniques are too time consuming to be of value in most emergency intubations. Furthermore, they have not been shown to be uniformly effective.[130]

The response to intravenous lidocaine has also been variable, but two well-designed studies have failed to demonstrate any effect. Chraemmer-Jorgensen and coworkers[115] showed no effect on the pressor response in a randomized double-blind comparison of intravenous lidocaine (1.5 mg/kg) and placebo. Similarly, Laurito and colleagues[117] demonstrated in a randomized double-blind and placebo-controlled study no salutary effects of lidocaine given by either topical or intravenous routes.

Perhaps the drug that may be the most useful for suppression of the pressor response in the emergency situation is fentanyl citrate. This drug appears to be at least as effective as lidocaine and simultaneously provides analgesia and sedation. Although not as widely studied as lidocaine, fentanyl is known to prevent the pressor response completely at an anesthetic dose of 50 μg/kg.[131] This is considerably larger than standard sedating doses, but it appears that substantially smaller doses may also be effective. Dahlgren and Messeter[114] showed that patients treated with 5 μg/kg of fentanyl 3 minutes before laryngoscopy exhibited only small elevations in mean arterial pressure and pulse rate—increases that were significantly less than those of controls (12 mm Hg versus 44 mm Hg and 12 beats per minute versus 36 beats per minute). Kautto[116] compared fentanyl in doses of 2 and 6 μg/kg with placebo and demonstrated attenuation of the response of the lower dose and nearly complete suppression at 6 μg/kg. It is important to note that patients in both of these studies also received 5 mg/kg of intravenous thiopental. Although thiopental alone does not affect the pressor response at this dose, a synergistic effect cannot be excluded.

Intracranial Hypertension

Physical stimulation of the respiratory tract by maneuvers such as laryngoscopy, tracheal intubation, and endotracheal suctioning is commonly associated with an acute rise in intracranial pressure. The exact significance of a transient increase in intracranial pressure in the setting of acute intracranial pathology is unknown, but it is probably best avoided. This response is thought to be caused by coughing and subsequent transmission of intrathoracic pressure to the cerebral circulation. Therefore, cough suppression may be the best measure of a drug's ability to prevent this response.

Several drugs, including fentanyl, lidocaine, thiopental, nitrous oxide, and succinylcholine, have been studied to evaluate their ability to prevent the rise in intracranial pressure that is associated with stimulation of the upper respiratory tract. Intravenous lidocaine (1.5 mg/kg) has been shown to suppress coughing induced by citric acid inhalation.[132] Yukioka and colleagues[133] demonstrated dose-dependent suppression of coughing during intubation with maximum suppression at a lidocaine dose of 2 mg/kg, given intravenously. Studies by Hamill and coworkers[134] and Donegan and Bedford[135] indicated that both lidocaine and thiopental effectively suppress the rise in intracranial pressure that is associated with orotracheal intubation, but these studies were conducted on paralyzed patients who could not cough. Intravenous lidocaine (1.5 mg/kg) does not suppress the rise in intracranial pressure that follows tracheal suctioning in nonparalyzed patients. Lidocaine administered intratracheally does suppress this response, but the instillation of lidocaine into the trachea itself produced a cough response. A study by White and colleagues[136] in which several drugs were compared demonstrated that only succinylcholine was effective. Because it completely blocks the motor responses thought to cause acute rises in intracranial pressure, paralysis may be the only sure mechanism by which this side effect may be prevented. Alternatively, intravenous lidocaine at

2 mg/kg may be effective, although this has not been clearly demonstrated.

It is logical to assume that significant elevations in blood pressure, pulse rate, and intracranial pressure are detrimental to patients with head trauma or intracranial hypertension who undergo tracheal intubation in the emergency department. The exact clinical consequences of intubation-induced physiologic changes in such patients have not been studied extensively nor has the exact role of drugs to ameliorate these changes been defined at the present time. Despite a lack of data, one should attempt to protect patients at theoretic risk. The approach outlined in Table 2–3 is recommended.

RAPID-SEQUENCE INDUCTION FOR INTUBATION

The previous discussion has focused on a number of drugs that facilitate the process of intubation, including those that provide analgesia and sedation. These same drugs given rapidly and in higher doses may be used to induce general anesthesia. In the critically ill patient, it is frequently necessary to gain immediate control of the airway while at the same time avoiding the risk of regurgitation and aspiration of stomach contents. Traditionally, this has been accomplished by the process of rapid-sequence induction. As described by Stept and Safar,[137] the sequence includes the following steps: (1) establish an intravenous line, (2) assemble and check necessary equipment, (3) insert a nasogastric tube, (4) clear the mouth of foreign material, (5) denitrogenate the lungs with 100 per cent oxygen for at least 2 minutes, (6) elevate the trunk approximately 30 degrees to decrease the risk of aspiration and place the head in the sniffing position, (7) monitor the cardiac rhythm, (8) give a subparalytic dose of a nondepolarizing NMB and wait 2 minutes, (9) give thiopental 3 to 5 mg/kg intravenously, (10) as the patient loses consciousness, tilt the head back and apply cricoid pressure continuously until the endotracheal tube is in place and the cuff is inflated, (11) give succinylcholine 1.5 mg/kg intravenously, (12) do not stimulate the oropharynx until respirations have ceased completely, and (13) place the endotracheal tube, inflate the cuff, and release the cricoid pressure.

The steps outlined here have been used successfully in the operating room for a number of years, but they have

Table 2–3. Suggested Protocol for Intubation of the Patient with a Head Injury

1. Preoxygenate with 100% O$_2$ for 2 minutes.
2. *Optional:* Administer 1.5 to 2 mg/kg lidocaine (see text).
3. *Optional:* If succinylcholine will be used, 1 mg pancuronium can be given to prevent fasciculations (see text).
4. *Optional:* If patient is *not* hypotensive, administer thiopental, 3 to 5 mg/kg (see text).
5. If thiopental is not administered, sedate with 3 to 5 μg/kg fentanyl
   or 0.1 mg/kg midazolam
   or 2 to 3 μg/kg fentanyl *and* 0.02 mg/kg midazolam.
   (Alternatively, sedative agents may be given *immediately* after administration of paralytic agents.)
6. Paralyze with 1.5 mg/kg of succinylcholine
   or 0.1 to 0.25 mg/kg vecuronium
   or 1.5 mg/kg succinylcholine *and* 0.1 mg/kg vecuronium.
7. Apply cricoid pressure; perform intubation.
8. Maintain postintubation analgesia or sedation to prevent bucking and gagging.
9. Maintain paralysis if indicated (vecuronium or pancuronium).

Table 2–4. Recommended Anesthetic Doses for Rapid-Sequence Induction

Drug	Dose
Thiopental	3–5 mg/kg IV push
Midazolam	0.1 mg/kg IV push
Fentanyl	10 μg/kg IV push *or*
	5 μg/kg and midazolam 0.05 mg/kg IV push
Ketamine	1–2 mg/kg IV push *or*
	0.75 mg/kg and midazolam 0.05 mg/kg IV push

Any one of the six options can be used before the administration of a neuromuscular blocking agent to induce anesthesia; see text.

IV, intravenous.

some limitations that may require modification in the emergency department setting. Insertion of a nasogastric tube is time consuming; it may provoke rather than avoid vomiting, and it may render an agitated or confused patient totally uncooperative. Furthermore, the gagging associated with passage of a nasogastric tube is potentially harmful in the presence of acute intracranial pathology and cervical spine injury.

Pretreatment with a subparalytic dose of a nondepolarizing NMB is another step that is best eliminated when intubation must be performed rapidly. Not only is this therapy time consuming, but it is of questionable value. The risk of regurgitation associated with succinylcholine-induced fasciculations is greatly overstated. It has not been observed in several studies in which succinylcholine was given without pretreatment.[2, 4, 6, 138] Careful use of the Sellick maneuver and avoidance of overdistention of the stomach with bag-mask ventilation play a much more significant role in the prevention of regurgitation than does the use of a nondepolarizing NMB.

Finally, the use of thiopental to induce anesthesia deserves mention. This agent has been favored because it is rapid acting, highly effective, and relatively safe.[139] In addition, it reduces cerebral blood flow and, secondarily, intracranial pressure. As noted previously, thiopental has potential deleterious effects, including myocardial depression, lack of analgesic effect, potential to induce spasm of the larynx and bronchi, and potential to cause tissue necrosis if extravasation occurs. Given these possible problems, it may be appropriate to use agents that have fewer potential side effects, such as midazolam and fentanyl, particularly in patients who have underlying cardiac disease or are potentially hypovolemic. White has shown that midazolam is as effective as thiopental for the rapid induction of anesthesia, although the onset of unconsciousness was slightly delayed.[140] Fentanyl is also highly effective and provides analgesia that the other drugs do not. The choice of an agent for rapid-sequence induction should be tailored to the specific medical problems of the patient and founded on thorough physician familiarity with its potential side effects.

Drugs intended to induce rapid anesthesia should generally be given by intravenous push infusion. The protocol for rapid-sequence induction follows that described in Table 2–1 with the exception of higher doses and more rapid administration. Recommended doses for rapid-sequence induction are listed in Table 2–4.

CONCLUSION

This chapter has described a number of pharmacologic adjuncts that permit a much more sophisticated approach to intubation of the critically ill patient. As the expertise of physicians practicing in acute care settings increases, it is appropriate that they incorporate these adjuncts into their airway management protocols. The agents discussed in this chapter are representative of drugs currently used to facilitate intubation in United States emergency departments. Other agents in these drug classes may also prove of value in the future. For example, etomidate (Hypnomidate) is a short-acting induction agent found advantageous for prehospital intubation in Germany and now receiving increasing attention in the United States.

References

1. Taryle DA, Chandler JE, Good JT, et al: Emergency room intubations—complications and survival. Chest 75:541, 1979.
2. Hedges JR, Dronen SC, Feero S, et al: Succinylcholine-assisted intubations in prehospital care. Ann Emerg Med 17:469, 1988.
3. Roberts DJ, Clinton JE, Ruiz E: Neuromuscular blockade for critical patients in the emergency department. Ann Emerg Med 15:152, 1986.
4. Dronen SC, Merigian KS, Hedges JR, et al: A comparison of blind nasotracheal and succinylcholine-assisted intubation in the poisoned patient. Ann Emerg Med 16:650, 1987.
5. Thompson JD, Fish S, Ruiz E: Succinylcholine for endotracheal intubation. Ann Emerg Med 11:526, 1982.
6. Syverud SA, Borron SW, Storer DL, et al: Prehospital use of neuromuscular blocking agents in a helicopter ambulance program. Ann Emerg Med 17:236, 1988.
7. Chudnofsky CR, Wright SW, Dronen SC, et al: Safety of fentanyl use in the emergency department. Ann Emerg Med 17:881, 1988.
8. L'Hommedieu CS, Arens JJ: The use of ketamine for the emergency intubation of patients with status asthmaticus. Ann Emerg Med 16:568, 1987.
9. Kanto JH: Midazolam: The first water-soluble benzodiazepine. Pharmacotherapy 5:138, 1985.
10. Fahey MR, Morris RB, Miller RD, et al: Clinical pharmacology of ORG NC 45 (Norcuron): A new non-depolarizing muscle relaxant. Anesthesiology 55:6, 1981.
11. Thomas JL: Awake intubation. Anaesthesia 24:28, 1969.
12. Danzl DF, Thomas DM: Nasotracheal intubations in the emergency department. Crit Care Med 8:677, 1980.
13. Boster SR, Danzl DF, Madden RJ, et al: Translaryngeal absorption of lidocaine. Ann Emerg Med 11:461, 1982.
14. Sutherland AD, Sale JP: Fibreoptic awake intubation—a method of topical anaesthesia and orotracheal intubation. Can Anaesth Soc J 33:502, 1986.
15. Bourke DL, Katz J, Tonneson A: Nebulized anesthesia for awake endotracheal intubation. Anesthesiology 63:690, 1985.
16. Billmire DA, Neale HW, Gregory RO: Use of IV fentanyl in the outpatient treatment of pediatric facial trauma. J Trauma 25:1079, 1985.
17. Colon GA, Gubert N: Lorazepam (Ativan) and fentanyl (Sublimaze) for outpatient office plastic surgical anesthesia. Plast Reconstr Surg 78:486, 1986.
18. Michelson LN, Lindenthal JJ, Peck GC, et al: Diazepam and fentanyl as adjuncts to local anesthesia. Aesthetic Plast Surg 11:207, 1987.
19. Stephens MJ, Gibson PR, Jakobovits AW, et al: Fentanyl and diazepam in endoscopy of the upper gastrointestinal tract. Med J Aust 1:419, 1982.
20. Miller DL, Wall RT: Fentanyl and diazepam for analgesia and sedation during radiologic special procedures. Radiology 162:195, 1987.
21. Mostert JW, Trudnowski RJ, Seniff AM, et al: Clinical comparison of fentanyl with meperidine. J Clin Pharmacol 8:382, 1968.
22. Rosow CE, Philbin DM, Keegan CR, et al: Hemodynamics and histamine release during induction with sufentanil or fentanyl. Anesthesiology 60:489, 1984.
23. Rosow CE, Moss J, Philbin DM, et al: Histamine release during morphine and fentanyl anesthesia. Anesthesiology 56:93, 1982.
24. Flacke JW, Flacke WE, Bloor BC, et al: Histamine release by four narcotics: A double-blind study in humans. Anesth Analg 66:723, 1987.
25. Schleimer R, Benjamini E, Eisele J: Pharmacokinetics of fentanyl as determined by radioimmunoassay. Clin Pharmacol Ther 23:188, 1978.
26. McClain DA, Hug CC: Intravenous fentanyl kinetics. Clin Pharmacol Ther 28(1):106, 1980.
27. Finch JS, DeKornfeld TJ: Clinical investigation of the analgesic potency and respiratory depressant activity of fentanyl, a new narcotic analgesic. J Clin Pharmacol 46:1967.
28. Stanley TH, Webster LR: Anesthetic requirements and cardiovascular effects of fentanyl-oxygen and fentanyl-diazepam-oxygen anesthesia in man. Anesth Analg 57:411, 1978.
29. Comstock MK, Carter JG, Moyers JR: Letters to the editor. Anesth Analg 60:362, 1981.
30. Hill AB, Nahrwold ML, De Rosayro AM: Prevention of rigidity during fentanyl-oxygen induction of anesthesia. Anesthesiology 55:451, 1981.
31. Goroszenuik T, Albin M, Jones RM: Generalized grand mal seizure after recovery from uncomplicated fentanyl-etomidate anesthesia. Anesth Analg 64:979, 1986.
32. Safwat AM, Daniel D: Grand mal seizure after fentanyl administration. Anesthesiology 59:78, 1983.
33. Hoien A: Another case of grand mal seizure after fentanyl administration. Anesthesiology 60:387, 1984.
34. Whitwam JG, Al-Khudhairi D, McCloy RF: Comparison of midazolam and diazepam in doses of comparable potency during gastroscopy. J Anaesth 55:773, 1983.
35. Baker TJ, Gordon HL: Midazolam (Versed) in ambulatory surgery. Plast Reconstr Surg 82:244, 1987.
36. Kanto J, Analtonen L, Himberg JJ, et al: Midazolam as an intravenous induction agent in the elderly: A clinical and pharmacokinetic study. Anesth Analg 65:15, 1986.
37. Westphal LM, Cheng EY, White PF, et al: Use of midazolam infusion for sedation following cardiac surgery. Anesthesiology 67:257, 1987.
38. Marty J, Nitenberg J, Blanchet S, et al: Effects of midazolam on the coronary circulation in patients with coronary artery disease. Anesthesiology 64:206, 1986.
39. Reves JG, Fragen RJ, Vinik HR, et al: Midazolam: Pharmacology and uses. Anesthesiology 62:310, 1985.
40. Kawar P, Carson W, Clarke SJ, et al: Haemodynamic changes during induction of anaesthesia with midazolam and diazepam (Valium) in patients undergoing coronary artery bypass surgery. Anaesthesia 40:767, 1985.
41. Adams P, Gelman S, Reves JG, et al: Midazolam pharmacodynamics and pharmacokinetics during acute hypovolemia. Anesthesiology 63:140, 1985.
42. Roche Laboratory Communication: Important new information on the administration of Versed (midazolam hydrochloride) injection for conscious sedation. Nutley, NJ.
43. Wright S, Chudnofsky C, Dronen SC: Midazolam use in the emergency department. Am J Emerg Med March 8:97, 1990.
44. Ayre-Smith G: Fentanyl and midazolam: An alternative to diazepam. Radiology 164:285, 1987.
45. Miller RI, Bullard DE, Patrissi GA: Duration of amnesia associated with midazolam/fentanyl intravenous sedation. J Oral Maxillofac Surg 47:155, 1989.
46. Harvey SC: Hypnotics and sedatives. In Gillman AG, Goodman LS, Rall TW, Murad F (eds.): The Pharmacologic Basis of Therapeutics. New York, Macmillan, 1985.
47. Dripps RD, Eckenhoff JE, Vandam LD: Intravenous anesthetics. In Dripps RD, Eckenhoff JE, Vandam LD (eds.): Introduction to Anesthesia. 7th ed. Philadelphia, WB Saunders Co, 1988.
48. Bedford RF, Persing JA, Pobereskin L, et al: Lidocaine or thiopental for rapid control of intracranial hypertension? Anesth Analg 59:435, 1980.
49. Shapiro HM, Wyte SR, Loeser J: Barbiturate-augmented hypothermia for reduction of persistent intracranial hypertension. J Neurosurg 40:90, 1974.
50. White PF, Way WL, Trevor AJ: Ketamine—its pharmacology and therapeutic uses. Anesthesiology 56:119, 1982.
51. Wong DHW, Jenkins LC: An experimental study of the mechanism of action of ketamine on the central nervous system. Can Anaesth Soc J 21:57, 1974.
52. Schwartz DA, Horwitz LD: Effects of ketamine on left ventricular performance. J Pharmacol Exp Ther 194:410, 1975.
53. Barson P, Arens JF: Ketamine as an induction anesthetic for poor-risk patients. South Med J 67:1398, 1974.
54. Lorhan PH, Lippman M: A clinical appraisal of the use of ketamine hydrochloride in the aged. Anesth Analg 50:448, 1971.
55. Bond Ac, Davies CK: Ketamine and pancuronium for the shocked patient. Anaesthesia 29:59, 1974.
56. Chasapakis G, Kekis N, Sakkalis C, Kolios D: Use of ketamine and pancuronium for anesthesia for patients in hemorrhagic shock. Anesth Analg 52:282, 1973.
57. Lundy PA, Gowdey CW, Calhoun EH: Tracheal smooth muscle relaxant effect of ketamine. Br J Anaesth 46:333, 1974.
58. Fisher M: Ketamine hydrochloride in severe bronchospasm. Anaesthesia 32:771, 1977.
59. Betts EK, Parkin CE: Use of ketamine in an asthmatic child: A case report. Anesth Analg 50:420, 1971.
60. Oduntan SA, Gool RY: Clinical trial of ketamine (CI-581). Can Anaesth Soc J 17:411, 1970.
61. Krestow M: The effect of post-anaesthetic dreaming on patient acceptance of ketamine anaesthesia: A comparison with thiopentone-nitrous oxide anaesthesia. Can Anaesth Soc J 21:385, 1974.
62. Dundee JW, Lilburn JK: Ketamine-lorazepam: Attenuation of the psychic sequelae of ketamine by lorazepam. Anaesthesia 37:312, 1977.
63. Lilburn JK, Dundee JW, Nair SG, et al: Ketamine sequelae—evaluation of the ability of various premedicants to attenuate its psychic actions. Anaesthesia 33:307, 1978.
64. Dundee JW, McGowan AW, Lilburn JK, et al: Comparison of the actions of diazepam and lorazepam. Br J Anaesth 51:439, 1979.
65. Kothary SP, Pandit SK: Orally administered diazepam and lorazepam—sedative and amnesic effects. Anesthesiology 53:S18, 1980.
66. White PF: Pharmacologic interactions of midazolam and ketamine in surgical patients. Clin Pharm Ther 31:280, 1982.

67. Taylor PA, Towey RM: Depression of laryngeal reflexes during ketamine anesthesia. Br Med J 2:688, 1971.

68. Penrose BH: Aspiration pneumonitis following ketamine induction for a general anesthetic. Anesth Analg 51:41, 1972.

69. Bivins HG, Ford S, Bezmalinovic Z, et al: The effect of axial traction during orotracheal intubation of the trauma victim with an unstable cervical spine. Ann Emerg Med 17:25, 1988.

70. Aprahamian C, Thompson BM, Finger WA, et al: Experimental cervical spine injury model: Evaluation of airway management and splinting techniques. Ann Emerg Med 13:584, 1984.

71. Majernick TG, Bieniek R, Houston JB, et al: Cervical spine movement during orotracheal intubation. Ann Emerg Med 15:417, 1986.

72. Dronen SC, Syverud S: Answering the airway management question. Ann Emerg Med 17:1132, 1988.

73. Holley J, Jordon R: Airway management in patients with unstable cervical spine fractures. Ann Emerg Med 18:1237, 1989.

74. Fraser A, Edmonds-Seal J: Spinal cord injuries. A review of the problems facing the anesthetist. Anaesthesia 37:1084, 1984.

75. Taylor P: Neuromuscular blocking agents. In Gillman AG, Goodman LS, Rall TW, Murad F (eds.): The Pharmacologic Basis of Therapeutics. New York, Macmillan, 1985.

76. Leigh MD, McCoy DD, Belton MK, et al: Bradycardia following intravenous administration of succinylcholine chloride to infants and children. Anesthesiology 18:699, 1957.

77. Nugent SK, Laravuso R, Rogers MC: Pharmacology and use of muscle relaxants in infants and children. J Pediatr 94:481, 1979.

78. Katz RL, Ryan JF: The neuromuscular effects of suxamethonium in man. Br J Anaesth 41:381, 1969.

79. Galindo A: Depolarizing neuromuscular block. J Pharmacol Exp Ther 178:339, 1971.

80. Miller RD: Antagonism of neuromuscular blockade. Anesthesiology 44:318, 1976.

81. Bennike KA, Neilson E: Muscle pain following suxamethonium. Dan Med Bull 11:122, 1964.

82. Libonati MM, Leahy JJ, Ellison N: The use of succinylcholine in open eye surgery. Anesthesiology 62:637, 1985.

83. Bourke DL: Open eye injuries. Anesthesiology 63:727, 1985.

84. Bourke DL, Rosenberg M: Changes in total serum Ca^{++}, Na^+, and K^+ with administration of succinylcholine. Anesthesiology 49:361, 1978.

85. Tolmie JD, Joyce TH, Mitchell GD: Succinylcholine danger in the burned patient. Anesthesiology 28:467, 1967.

86. Mazze RI, Escue HM, Houston JB: Hyperkalemia and cardiovascular collapse following administration of succinylcholine to the traumatized patient. Anesthesiology 31:540, 1969.

87. Smith RB, Grenvik A: Cardiac arrest following succinylcholine in patients with central nervous system injuries. Anesthesiology 33:558, 1970.

88. Gronert GA, Theye RA: Pathophysiology of hyperkalemia induced by succinylcholine. Anesthesiology 43:89, 1975.

89. Donlon JV, Newfield P, Sreter F, Ryan JF: Implications of masseter spasm after succinylcholine. Anesthesiology 49:298, 1978.

90. Tsang HS, Frederick GS: Malignant hyperthermia. Illinois Med J 149:471, 1976.

91. May DC, Morris SW, Stewart RM, et al: Neuroleptic malignant syndrome: Response to dantrolene sodium. Ann Intern Med 98:183, 1983.

92. Barnes PK: Masseter spasm following intravenous suxamethonium. Br J Anaesth 45:759, 1973.

93. Barlow M, Isaacs H: Malignant hyperpyrexia deaths in a family. Br J Anaesth 45:1072, 1970.

94. McStravog LJ: Dangers of succinylcholine in anesthesia. Laryngoscope 84.929, 1974.

95. Halldin M, Wahlin H: Effect of succinylcholine on intraspinal fluid pressure. Acta Anaesthesiol Scand 38:155, 1959.

96. Burney R, Winn HR: Increased cerebrospinal fluid pressure during laryngoscopy and intubation for induction of anesthesia. Anesth Anal 54:687, 1975.

97. Shapiro HM, Wyte S, Harris A, Galindo A: Acute intraoperative intracranial hypertension in neurosurgical patients: Mechanical and pharmacological factors. Anesthesiology 37:399, 1972.

98. Minton MD, Grosslight K, Stirt JA, Bedford RF: Increases in intracranial pressure from succinylcholine: Prevention by prior nondepolarizing blockade. Anesthesiology 65:165, 1986.

99. Roizen MF, Feeley TW: Pancuronium bromide. Ann Intern Med 88:64, 1978.

100. Foldes FF: The rational use of neuromuscular blocking agents: The role of pancuronium. Drugs 4:153, 1972.

101. Rupp SM, McChristian JW, Miller RD, et al: Neostigmine and edrophonium antagonism of varying intensity. Neuromuscular blockade induced by atracurium, pancuronium, or vecuronium. Anesthesiology 64:711, 1986.

102. Breen PJ, Doherty WG, Donati F, et al: The potencies of edrophonium and neostigmine as antagonists of pancuronium. Anaesthesia 40:844, 1985.

103. Anderson EF, Rosenthal MH: Pancuronium bromide and tachyarrhythmias. Crit Care Med 3:13, 1975.

104. Fraley DS, Lemoncelli GL, Coleman A: Severe hypertension associated with pancuronium bromide. Anesth Analg 57:265, 1978.

105. Bodman RI: Pancuronium and histamine release. Can Anaesth Soc J 25:40, 1978.

106. Sohn YJ, Bencini AF, Scaf AHJ, et al: Comparative pharmacokinetics and dynamics of vecuronium and pancuronium in anesthetized patients. Anesth Analg 65:233, 1986.

107. Schwarz S, Ilias W, Lackner F, et al: Rapid tracheal intubation with vecuronium: The priming principle. Anesthesiology 62:388, 1985.

108. Kunjappan VE, Brown EM, Alexander GD: Rapid sequence induction using vecuronium. Anesth Analg 65:503, 1986.

109. King BD, Harris LC, Greifenstein FE, et al: Reflex circulatory responses to direct laryngoscopy and tracheal intubation performed during general anesthesia. Anesthesiology 12:556, 1951.

110. Hartigan M, Cleary J, Schaffer DW: A comparison of pre-treatment regimens for minimizing the haemodynamic response to blind nasotracheal intubation. Can Anaesth Soc J 31:497, 1984.

111. Wycoff C: Endotracheal intubation: Effects on blood pressure and pulse rate. Anesthesiology 21:153, 1960.

112. Takeshima K, Noda K, Higaki M: Cardiovascular response to rapid anesthesia induction and endotracheal intubation. Anesth Analg 43:201, 1964.

113. Venus B, Polassani V, Pham CG: Effects of aerosolized lidocaine on circulatory responses to laryngoscopy and tracheal intubation. Crit Care Med 391, 1984.

114. Dahlgren N, Messeter K: Treatment of stress response to laryngoscopy and intubation with fentanyl. Anaesthesia 36:1022, 1981.

115. Chraemmer-Jorgensen B, Hoilund-Carlsen PF, Marving J, Christensen V, et al: Lack of effect of intravenous lidocaine on hemodynamic responses to rapid sequence induction of general anesthesia: A double-blind controlled clinical trial. Anesth Analg 65:1037, 1986.

116. Kautto UM: Attenuation of the circulatory response to laryngoscopy and intubation by fentanyl. Acta Anaesth Scand 26:217, 1982.

117. Laurito CE, Baughman VL, Becker GL, et al: Effects of aerosolized and/or intravenous lidocaine on hemodynamic responses to laryngoscopy and intubation in outpatients. Anesth Analg 67:389, 1988.

118. Prys-Roberts C, Meloche R, Foex P: Studies of anaesthesia in relation to hypertension I: Cardiovascular responses of treated and untreated patients. Br J Anaesth 43:122, 1971.

119. Prys-Roberts C, Greene LT, Meloche R, Foex P: Studies of anaesthesia in relation to hypertension II: Haemodynamic consequences of induction and endotracheal intubation. Br J Anaesth 43:531, 1971.

120. Lehtinen AM, Hovorka J, Widholm O: Modification of aspects of the endocrine response to tracheal intubation by lignocaine, halothane and thiopentone. Br J Anaesth 56:239, 1984.

121. Davies MJ, Cronin KD, Cowie RW: The prevention of hypertension at intubation. Anaesthesia 36:147, 1981.

122. Forbes AM, Dally FG: Acute hypertension during induction of anaesthesia and endotracheal intubation in normotensive man. Br J Anaesth 42:618, 1970.

123. Fassoulaki A, Kaniaris P: Does atropine premedication affect the cardiovascular response to laryngoscopy and intubation? Br J Anaesth 54:1065, 1982.

124. Martin DE, Rosenberg H, Aukburg SJ, et al: Low-dose fentanyl blunts circulatory responses to tracheal intubation. Anesth Analg 61:680, 1982.

125. Boralessa H, Senior DF, Whitwam JG: Cardiovascular response to intubation. Anaesthesia 38:623, 1983.

126. Fox EJ, Sklar GS, Hill CH, et al: Complications related to the pressor response to endotracheal intubation. Anesthesiology 47:524, 1977.

127. Denlinger JK, Ellison N, Ominsky AJ: Effects of intratracheal lidocaine on circulatory responses to tracheal intubation. Anesthesiology 41:409, 1974.

128. Derbyshire DR, Smith G, Achola KJ: Effect of topical lignocaine on the sympathodrenal responses to tracheal intubation. Br J Anaesth 59:300, 1987.

129. Abou-Madi MN, Keszler H, Yacoub JM: Cardiovascular reactions to laryngoscopy and tracheal intubation following small and large intravenous doses of lidocaine. Can Anaesth Soc J 24:12,1977.

130. Youngberg JA, Graybar G, Hutchings D: Comparison of intravenous and topical lidocaine in attenuating the cardiovascular responses to endotracheal intubation. South Med J 76:1122, 1983.

131. Lunn JK, Stanley TH, Webster L, et al: High dose fentanyl anesthesia for coronary artery surgery: Plasma fentanyl concentrations and influence of nitrous oxide on cardiovascular responses. Anesth Analg 58:390, 1979.

132. Poulton TJ, James FM: Cough suppression by lidocaine. Anesthesiology 50:470, 1979.

133. Yukioka H, Yoshimoto N, Nishimura K, et al: Intravenous lidocaine as a suppressor of coughing during tracheal intubation. Anesth Analg 64:1189, 1985.

134. Hamill JF, Bedford RF, Weaver DC, et al: Lidocaine before endotracheal intubation: Intravenous or laryngotracheal? Anesthesiology 35:578, 1981.

135. Donegan MF, Bedford RF: Intravenously administered lidocaine prevents intracranial hypertension during endotracheal suctioning. Anesthesiology 52:516, 1980.

136. White PF, Schlobohm RM, Pitts LH, et al: A randomized study of drugs for preventing increases in intracranial pressure during endotracheal suctioning. Anesthesiology 57:242, 1982.

137. Stept WJ, Safar P: Rapid induction/intubation for prevention of gastric-content aspiration. Anesth Analg 49:633, 1970.

138. Talucci RC, Shaikh KA, Schwab CW: Rapid sequence induction with oral endotracheal intubation in the multiply injured patient. Am Surg 54:185, 1988.
139. Barr AM, Thornley BA: Thiopentone and suxamethonium crash induction. Anaesthesia 31:23, 1976.

140. White PF: Comparative evaluation of intravenous agents for rapid sequence induction—thiopental, ketamine, and midazolam. Anesthesiology 57:279, 1982.

Chapter 3

Cricothyrotomy

Sharon E. Mace

INTRODUCTION

The primary consideration in the management of any seriously ill patient is establishment of the airway. Simple maneuvers and treatment including head tilt with chin lift or jaw thrust in the noninjured patient; modified jaw thrust in the trauma patient; and supplemental oxygen via mouth to mouth, pocket mask, nasal cannula, nonrebreather mask, or bag-valve-mask ventilation can be critical parts of the initial management of a seriously ill patient.[1-8] Definitive airway control, however, may be needed. The usual method for obtaining definitive airway control is by oral or nasal intubation.[1-9] There are clinical situations in which intubation is difficult, impossible, or even contraindicated.[9-13] Under these circumstances, cricothyrotomy may be the quickest, easiest, safest, and most effective way to obtain an airway and is the procedure of choice in such critically ill patients in whom intubation is difficult or absolutely contraindicated.[9-13]

The cricothyroid membrane is a thin membrane lying between the thyroid and cricoid cartilages in the area of the anatomic larynx (Fig. 3–1).[14-18] Cricothyrotomy is the procedure by which an opening is made in the cricothyroid membrane to establish an airway. Cricothyrotomy is also known as a laryngostomy, laryngotomy, cricothyroidotomy, or coniotomy.[19, 20]

There are two methods for performing a cricothyrotomy: surgical or needle cricothyrotomy.[21, 22] A surgical cricothyrotomy indicates the use of a surgical technique with a blade to create the opening in the cricothyroid membrane; a needle cricothyrotomy implies the use of a percutaneous technique with a needle or cannula to puncture the cricothyroid membrane.[21, 22] Once access to the airway is created, whether by the surgical or needle method, oxygen is administered through the opening in the cricothyroid membrane.[21, 22] Thus, an emergency cricothyrotomy allows oxygenation of the lungs and prevents hypoxemia and all of its complications, including anoxic encephalopathy and death.[9-13, 21-22]

BACKGROUND

Obtaining an airway is the first priority, or the *A* in the ABC's (airway, breathing, and circulation) of patient care.[1-8] Because the physician has only 3 to 5 minutes in which to obtain an airway and achieve effective ventilation to prevent the complications of hypoxemia, management of the airway is of paramount importance.[23-25]

Indeed, the importance of securing an airway has been recognized since ancient times. Egyptian tablets dating from 3600 B.C. depict a surgical tracheostomy.[12] Historical records from ancient times give credit for the first tracheostomy to Asclepiades of Prusa in 124 B.C.[26] In the second century A.D., the writings of Galen suggested tracheostomy as the treatment for emergency management of airway obstruction,[27] and Antyllus is recorded as performing a tracheostomy with an incision between the third and fourth tracheal rings.[28]

In the United States, tracheostomies were being performed long before the twentieth century. Even in colonial times, tracheostomies were a known procedure. In 1796 Herholdt and Rohn advocated tracheostomies as a possible treatment for drowning victims.[29] George Washington's physician contemplated performing a tracheostomy on him in 1799 "as a means of prolonging life and of affording time for the removal of the obstruction to respiration in the larynx which manifestly threatened immediate dissolution" but his medical colleagues vetoed a tracheostomy, and the patient died.[30] During the nineteenth century, a Frenchman, Bretonneau, advocated tracheostomies for the treatment of diphtheria.[27] In 1886 Colles reported a tracheostomy mortality rate of about 50 per cent and a high complication rate with frequent resultant airway stenosis, which was itself usually fatal.[31]

Although tracheostomies and cricothyrotomies were successful (and lifesaving) on occasion, they were generally done only on already severely hypoxic, terminally ill patients, thus contributing to the high morbidity and mortality of the surgical procedure. Unfortunately, the fear of complications of the surgical procedure often led to a reluctance on the part of the physician to intervene actively until the patient was near death. This clinical situation was depicted by Hupp in 1914, who stated "certainly the delay due to this great dread of tracheostomy was itself largely accountable for the fatality attending its performance."[32]

Perhaps the first recorded "successful" case of a surgical *cricothyrotomy* was in 1852. Interestingly, the procedure was a suicide attempt performed by a patient. The cricothyrotomy was successful, but the patient died later from airway stenosis, a complication of the procedure.[33]

In his landmark paper in 1909, Jackson described the surgical technique for tracheostomy and detailed the factors that are critical for both successful tracheostomy or cricothyrotomy surgery.[34] These factors, which are still important today, include (1) obtaining the best airway control possible before surgery; (2) using local anesthesia initially rather than sedation or general anesthesia, which can lead to respiratory arrest in patients with an already compromised airway (although sedation and general anesthesia may be acceptable if the patient is already intubated); (3) emphasizing careful, precise surgical technique with good exposure; (4) using an inert, appropriately sized and shaped tracheostomy tube; and (5) ensuring meticulous postoperative care, which helps avoid contamination or infection and other complications. Jackson noted a surgical mortality of approximately 3 per cent, which is similar to that reported in current series.

Because of his classic work, Jackson achieved worldwide recognition and patient referrals regarding cricothyrotomy complications. In 1921, a second classic study by Jackson was published, an investigation of 200 patients referred to him with tracheal stenosis.[35] The study was biased in that patients who did well and had no surgical complications (e.g., no laryngeal stenosis) were not referred to Jackson. In addition, many of the patients had stenosis because of their underlying medical condition or disease and not because of the procedure. Furthermore, other factors relating to surgical technique and postoperative care were not controlled, including factors such as aseptic technique, location of the opening in the larynx, and size and type of the tracheostomy tube. In this paper, Jackson condemned cricothyrotomy because of the complication of chronic subglottic stenosis. Thus although the study's patient population was biased and surgical procedures were performed under uncontrolled conditions by surgeons with various and often questionable technical skills, Jackson's opinion that cricothyrotomy was to be avoided was accepted universally because of his worldwide reputation.

Years later Jackson's negative opinion of cricothyrotomy was challenged. In their landmark study published in 1976, Brantigan and Grow reported the results of cricothyrotomy on 655 patients.[36] In their series, only eight patients (8 out of 655 = 0.01 per cent) developed airway stenosis, and none of the patients developed

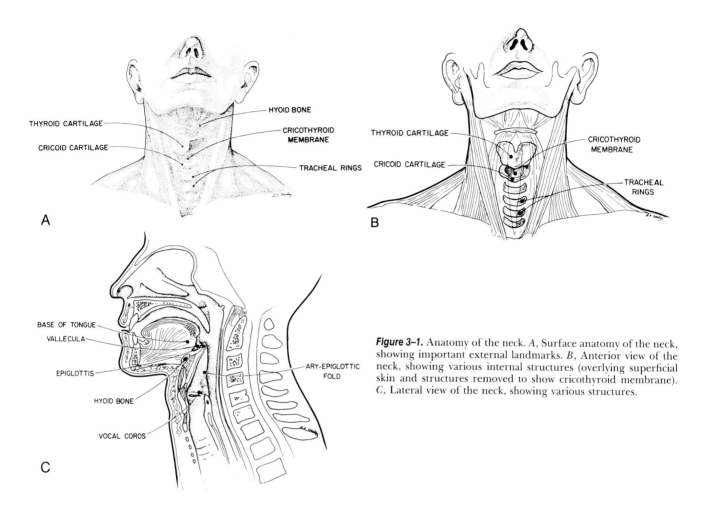

A

B

C

Figure 3–1. Anatomy of the neck. *A,* Surface anatomy of the neck, showing important external landmarks. *B,* Anterior view of the neck, showing various internal structures (overlying superficial skin and structures removed to show cricothyroid membrane). *C,* Lateral view of the neck, showing various structures.

chronic subglottic stenosis. Furthermore, major vessel hemorrhage and operative misadventures were absent, and the complication rate, which included minor problems, was only 6.1 per cent.

A review of the literature in recent years supports the conclusions of Brantigan and Grow that cricothyrotomy is a valid procedure for airway management with relatively few complications.[36–44] In Habel's series of 30 patients[44] and in Morain's series of 16 patients,[40] there were no cases of subglottic stenosis, and there were no significant complications in either series, even though one patient was intubated for 14 months. Another series by Greissy and colleagues of 61 patients undergoing cricothyrotomies at the bedside in an intensive care unit reported no cases of subglottic stenosis and complications in only 8 per cent of the patients.[43]

Clinical reviews of patients with cricothyrotomy have found no signs of laryngeal stenosis or damage when examined at bronchoscopy.[42] Similarly, animal studies of cricothyrotomy have documented a normal larynx after the cricothyrotomy, with no evidence of laryngeal stenosis or damage.[45] Indeed, all the current objective data confirm Brantigan and Grow's conclusion that cricothyrotomy is a safe and effective procedure with relatively few complications.[36–45]

ANATOMY

Cricothyrotomy, whether by needle or surgical technique, is accomplished by creating an opening in the cricothyroid membrane. Knowledge of the anatomy of the neck and the upper airway is essential when performing a cricothyrotomy. The airway lies anterior to the esophagus and the cervical spine and is usually located in the midline of the neck. The surface anatomy of the neck is usually easily recognizable. In the anterior part of the neck, the anatomic

landmarks include the hyoid bone, the thyroid cartilage, the cricoid cartilage, and the tracheal rings (see Fig. 3–1A).[14–20]

The hyoid bone is located midway between the mental protuberance of the mandible and the third cervical vertebra (see Fig. 3–1).[14–20] The hyoid bone is a U-shaped structure that is deficient posteriorly. It functions as a movable base for the tongue. The hyoid bone is held in position by many muscles that connect it to various bones and cartilage, including muscle attachments from the hyoid bone to the mandible, skull, sternum, scapula, and thyroid cartilage. Because the airway is suspended from the mandible and from the base of the skull via the hyoid bone, the hyoid bone can serve as an important landmark. The midpoint of the body of the hyoid is also the transverse midpoint of the neck and can function as an anchor for stabilizing the airway in an edematous neck.

The thyroid cartilage and the cricoid cartilage are both part of the larynx, and the tracheal rings are the major supporting structures of the trachea. The larynx is a hollow tube supported by cartilaginous rings of the tubular part of the airway. Anatomically, the larynx consists of the thyroid and cricoid cartilages with muscle and ligament attachments. In the adult, the larynx lies anterior to the fourth, fifth, and sixth cervical vertebrae. The functions of the larynx include (1) serving as the conduit for the airway located between the pharynx and the trachea and (2) the production of the voice.

The trachea is the downward continuation of the larynx and is the conduit for the airway. The trachea is supported by cartilaginous rings that are deficient posteriorly. The trachea is continuous from the larynx cephalad (inferior cricoid cartilage) to its caudal bifurcation, the right and left main stem bronchi. Thus the upper part of the trachea is in the neck, and the lower part of the trachea is in the chest. Posteriorly, the trachea lies against the esophagus.

The thyroid cartilage is the most rostral of the cartilages in the neck. The thyroid cartilage is located directly inferior and midline to the mandible and is also caudal to the hyoid bone. The thyroid cartilage consists of two approximately quadrilateral-shaped laminae of hyaline cartilage that fuse anteriorly to form the laryngeal prominence. Above the laryngeal prominence is the superior thyroid notch where the two laminae are separated (see Fig. 3–1). The anterior superior edge of the thyroid cartilage, the laryngeal prominence, is known as the "Adam's apple" and is usually easily seen in men. Except in the infant, the markedly obese patient, or the patient with massive neck edema, the laryngeal prominence of the thyroid cartilage is usually easily recognized and palpable (see Fig. 3–1*A* and *B*). It is probably the most important landmark in the neck when performing a cricothyrotomy.

Proceeding caudally in the neck, the next cartilaginous structure is the cricoid ring or cricoid cartilage. The cricoid cartilage is the only circumferential ring in the larynx. It is shaped like a signet ring with the shield located posteriorly. The cricoid cartilage helps to maintain the laryngeal lumen. The cricoid cartilage forms the inferior border of the cricothyroid membrane, and the thyroid cartilage forms the superior border of the cricothyroid membrane.

The highly vascular thyroid gland lies over the trachea at the level of the second and third tracheal rings. If the tracheal rings or the thyroid gland is encountered when performing a cricothyrotomy, then the clinician is too low in the neck and must redirect the incision superiorly toward the cricoid and thyroid cartilages. It is desirable to avoid the thyroid gland, which when injured may cause marked bleeding.

The cricothyroid membrane is a dense fibroelastic membrane located between the thyroid cartilage superiorly and the cricoid cartilage inferiorly and bounded laterally by the cricothyroideus muscles. The cricothyroid membrane covers an area between the thyroid and cricoid cartilages that is roughly trapezoidal in shape. The average size of the cricothyroid membrane in the adult is approximately 22 to 30 mm wide and 9 to 10 mm high.[46–50] The cricothyroid membrane can be identified by palpating a notch, a slight indentation or "dip" in the skin inferior to the laryngeal prominence (see Fig. 3–1). The cricothyroid membrane is located approximately 2 to 3 cm below the laryngeal prominence in an adult.

There are several anatomic and physiologic features that make the cricothyroid membrane an excellent choice for gaining access to the airway. The membrane is immediately subcutaneous in location. It does not calcify with age. It has no overlying muscles or facial layers. No major arteries, veins, or nerves are in the region. Although the right and left cricothyroid arteries, branches of the right and left superior thyroid arteries, respectively, transverse the superior part of the cricothyroid membrane (i.e., nearer the thyroid than the cricoid cartilage) and anastomose in the midline (Fig. 3–2*A*), these vessels generally have not been found to be of clinical significance or to cause problems when performing a cricothyrotomy.

ANATOMIC VARIATIONS

The larynx has a few anatomic features that vary according to age and sex. In children, the larynx is much higher than it is in the adult. The larynx descends from approximately the level of the second cervical vertebra at

birth to the level of the fifth or sixth cervical vertebra in the adult.[19, 51]

The laryngeal prominence, where the two approximately quadrilateral-shaped laminae of the thyroid cartilage fuse anteriorly, also varies according to age and sex. The angle at which these two laminae of the thyroid cartilage meet anteriorly varies from 90 to 120 degrees. This angle is smaller in the male, which makes the laryngeal prominence meet at a more acute angle or a sharper, more prominent point than that in the female.

In infants, the prominent structures in the anterior neck are the hyoid bone and the cricoid cartilage. The laryngeal prominence does not develop until adolescence and young adulthood.[19, 51, 52]

A few vascular anomalies in the neck result in a major artery crossing the midline of the neck. However, this is usually not a problem because these vascular anomalies are almost always located lower in the neck.[19, 53, 54]

SURGICAL CRICOTHYROTOMY

Indications

There are several indications for cricothyrotomy (Table 3–1). The most common reason is inability to perform endotracheal intubation because intubation is either contraindicated or cannot be easily and quickly performed because of various clinical conditions or circumstances.[8, 9, 52, 55–61]

Clinical conditions in which endotracheal intubation is difficult at best and often impossible include significant bleeding of any of the structures in the upper airway (e.g., massive oral, nasal, or pharyngeal hemorrhage), massive emesis or regurgitation, masseter spasm, clenched teeth, spasm of the larynx or pharynx or both, laryngeal stenosis, and structural deformities of the upper airway (e.g., congenital or acquired abnormalities or deformities of the oronasopharynx).[62–64] Whenever several unsuccessful attempts at endotracheal intubation cause an inordinate delay in airway control and oxygenation, cricothyrotomy is indicated to prevent cerebral anoxic damage.[10, 52, 56–61, 65]

Obstruction of the upper airway is yet another indication for cricothyrotomy.[60, 61, 66–70] Both traumatic injuries and nontraumatic lesions can cause airway obstruction.[61] Indeed, it has been stated that "patients who are completely obstructed or in extremis are best managed by establishing an airway via the cricothyroid membrane."[60] When simple airway clearing procedures are unsuccessful, cricothyrotomy should be undertaken without delay.

When maxillofacial, cervical spine, head, or soft tissue neck injuries are present, several factors may inhibit intubation. These factors include (1) gross distortion of structures, (2) airway obstruction, (3) disruption of upper airway structures, (4) massive emesis, (5) significant hemorrhage of upper airway structures, (6) patient discomfort, and (7) the possibility of aggravating existing or suspected injuries that would result in additional damage. In such patients, cricothyrotomy is an excellent alternative for obtaining definitive control of the airway.[9, 10]

Historically, cricothyrotomy has been recommended for (1) patients with a known cervical spine injury or a high probability of cervical spine injury in whom definitive airway control is needed before the cervical spine can be assessed and (2) patients with certain head injuries, especially those who have basilar skull fractures or cribriform plate fractures.[9, 71–74] In trauma patients with known or anticipated cervical spine injury, movement of the neck while positioning the patient for intubation is to be minimized because of the possibility of causing additional cervical spine injury.[9, 52, 62, 75–79]

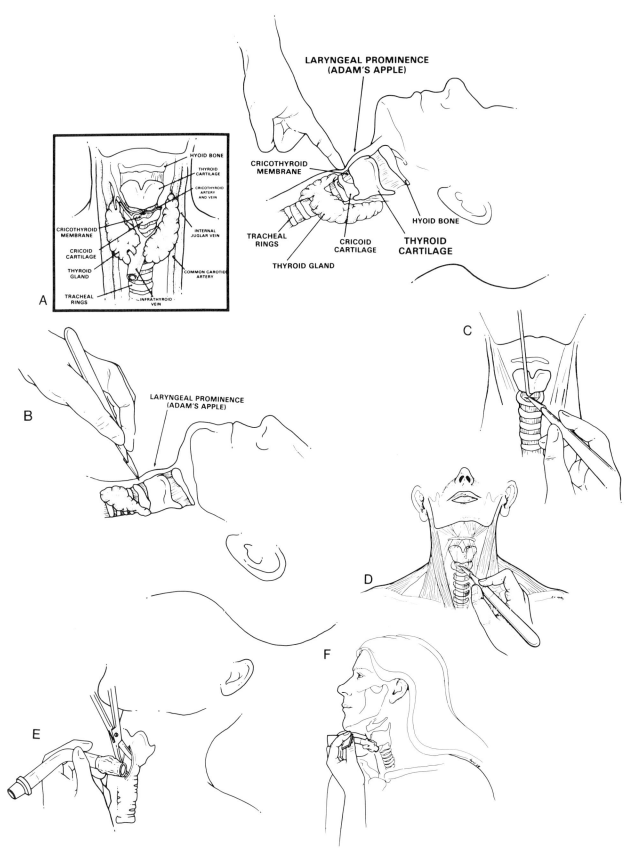

Figure 3–2. The procedure for surgical cricothyrotomy. *A,* Locate the cricothyroid membrane. The insert shows further anatomic details of the region. *B,* A vertical skin incision is made over the cricothyroid membrane. *C,* The larynx is stabilized with a tracheal hook (held in the nondominant hand) while an incision is made in the cricothyroid membrane. *D,* The surrounding anatomy of the neck is shown with the incision being made in the cricothyroid membrane. *E,* After the incision in the cricothyroid membrane is widened using hemostats, curved Mayo scissors, or the blunt end of the scalpel, the tracheostomy tube is inserted between the curved hemostats or tracheal dilator. *F,* Lateral view, showing insertion of the tracheostomy tube.

I. Failure of oral or nasal endotracheal intubation
   A. Massive oral, nasal, or pharyngeal hemorrhage
   B. Massive regurgitation or emesis
   C. Masseter spasm
   D. Clenched teeth
   E. Structural deformities of oronasopharynx, congenital or acquired
   F. Stenosis of upper airway (pharynx or larynx)
   G. Laryngospasm
   H. "Mass" effect (cancer, tumor, polyp, web, or other mass)
II. Airway obstruction (partial or complete)
   A. Nontraumatic
      1. Oropharyngeal edema
      2. Laryngospasm
      3. "Mass" effect (cancer, tumor, polyp, web, or other mass)
   B. Traumatic
      1. Oropharyngeal edema
      2. Foreign body obstruction
      3. Laryngospasm
      4. Obstruction secondary to a mass effect or displacement
      5. Stenosis
III. Traumatic injuries making oral or nasal endotracheal intubation difficult or potentially hazardous
   A. Maxillofacial injuries
   B. Cervical spine instability
IV. Need for prolonged intubation
V. Need for definitive airway during procedures on face, neck, or upper airway
   A. Laryngeal surgery
   B. Oral surgery
   C. Maxillofacial surgery
   D. Laser surgery
   E. Bronchoscopy

Under these circumstances, cricothyrotomy has been recommended, although the extent of cervical motion during cricothyrotomy in the unstable cervical spine is unknown.

Cricothyrotomy has been recommended when prolonged tracheal intubation is needed.[36, 80–82] There are several advantages of cricothyrotomy over tracheostomy in patients requiring prolonged intubation.[40, 82–84]

An additional indication for cricothyrotomy has been for definitive airway control before elective surgery of the face, head, and neck.[85–89] Cricothyrotomy, especially needle cricothyrotomy, has become a routine method of ventilation during procedures (both endoscopy and surgery) on the upper airway.[85–89] The use of cricothyrotomy during procedures on the upper airway has gained popularity because it allows better access to and visualization of the upper airway for the surgeon or endoscopist than is possible with intubation from above the larynx, which often obscures and limits the surgical field. Cricothyrotomy is less likely to damage the mucosa of the upper airway, especially structures that have just been operated on. It decreases the chance of "flames" or a mini "explosion" that may occur during laser surgery or other procedures that require flammable anesthetics or other gases.[89]

Cricothyrotomy versus Tracheostomy

The numerous advantages of cricothyrotomy over tracheostomy suggest that cricothyrotomy is the procedure of choice for airway control in patients needing prolonged intubation[36, 80–84] (Table 3–2).

The decreased incidence of complications with cricothyrotomy compared with that of tracheostomy is due at least partly to anatomy. Anatomic considerations make tracheos-

tomy a relatively complicated and difficult procedure. Many delicate complex structures in the neck lie in close proximity to the trachea, including the carotid arteries, jugular veins, recurrent laryngeal nerves, thyroid gland, dome of the pleura, and esophagus. There is less encroachment on the mediastinum with a cricothyrotomy than with a tracheostomy because the cricothyroid membrane is higher up and further away than the trachea from the mediastinum and other critical structures.[12, 36, 40, 69, 70, 80–84] Therefore, early complications including pneumothorax, pneumomediastinum, and mediastinal perforation occur less often with cricothyrotomy. Because the tracheal cartilage, unlike the cricoid and thyroid cartilage, is deficient posteriorly, there is a greater chance of damage with a tracheostomy to the posterior structures lying immediately behind the airway. Specifically, the esophagus is more likely to be injured during a tracheostomy than during a cricothyrotomy. The incidence of late complications, including fistulas, erosion of the innominate vessels, swallowing problems, and voice disturbances, decreases also.

In general, cricothyrotomy is preferred over tracheostomy for definitive emergency management of the airway when intubation is impossible or contraindicated.[12, 59, 90] The few exceptions to this recommendation are for the infant (although some recommend needle cricothyrotomy rather than tracheostomy), for severe edema of the neck with loss of landmarks (although a modification of cricothyrotomy for patients with massive neck edema now makes surgical cricothyrotomy an acceptable alternative in these patients), and for transection of the trachea with retraction of the distal trachea into the mediastinum[12, 59]

Contraindications

Cricothyrotomy has relatively few contraindications (Table 3–3).[12, 13, 59] Cricothyrotomy should not be done in patients who can be quickly, easily, and safely intubated orally or nasally and in those for whom there are no contraindications to endotracheal intubation. Transection of the trachea with retraction of the distal end is a contraindication to cricothyrotomy. A fractured larynx or other significant damage to the larynx or cricoid cartilage is another contraindication.[59]

I. Advantages due to anatomic considerations
   Immediate subcutaneous location (versus deep dissection)
   Absence of critical structures overlying cricothyroid membrane
   Easily seen landmarks, recognizable from the surface anatomy
   Less chance of esophageal injury (circumferential cricoid cartilage versus deficient tracheal cartilage posteriorly)
   Further away from mediastinum, dome of pleura (less encroachment on thoracic structures)
II. Overall advantages
   Easier to do, faster, safer
   Does not need to be done in an operating room
   Less need for hyperextension of the neck
   Better cosmetic appearance of scar (shorter, less adherent)
   Decreased incidence of late complications (e.g., swallowing problems, voice disturbances, fistulas, erosion of innominate artery)
   Decreased incidence of early complications (e.g., pneumothorax, pneumomediastinum, mediastinal perforation, esophageal injury) because there is less encroachment on the mediastinum and other critical structures
   Can be done quickly by nonsurgeons
   Requires a minimum of instruments

Table 3–3. *Contraindications to Surgical Cricothyrotomy*

Table 3–3. *Contraindications to Surgical Cricothyrotomy*

I. Absolute contraindications
   A. Endotracheal intubation can be accomplished easily and quickly, and no contraindications to endotracheal intubation are present
   B. Transection of trachea with retraction of distal end into the mediastinum
   C. Fractured larynx or significant damage to the cricoid cartilage or larynx
II. Relative contraindications*
   A. Infants and toddlers (for those less than 5 years of age, transtracheal ventilation may be preferred over surgical cricothyrotomy)
   B. Bleeding diathesis
   C. Patients with massive neck edema (may use modified technique for these patients)
   D. Acute laryngeal disease

*Relative contraindications may be overlooked in the true emergency situation because it is more important to obtain an airway and to avoid hypoxemia.

To avoid the now rare but potential complication of subglottic stenosis, some have recommended limiting cricothyrotomy to certain clinical conditions, if possible.[91] In the past, the factors associated with subglottic stenosis have been prolonged intubation, underlying laryngeal disease, and younger age (e.g., infants and small children).[91–103] Thus some believe that these three conditions are relative contraindications to cricothyrotomy.[91] However, more current studies indicate that subglottic stenosis is not as common a complication of cricothyrotomy as in the past[36–44] and that patients can have a cricothyrotomy for months without having subglottic stenosis.[36, 40, 43] Thus, these considerations (i.e., prolonged intubation and underlying laryngeal disease) may no longer be valid contraindications, and the notion that a cricothyrotomy should be converted immediately to a surgical tracheostomy is incorrect.[36]

Acute laryngeal disease has been a relative contraindication to cricothyrotomy in the past.[91] However, current findings suggest that subglottic stenosis is a rare event even in the presence of laryngeal pathology.[36, 44] A bleeding diathesis is not an *absolute* contraindication for an *emergency* cricothyrotomy because it is easier to obtain hemostasis with a cricothyrotomy than with a tracheostomy.[13] Loss of cervical landmarks with massive neck edema makes the procedure more difficult, although one approach using a measured estimation of the cricothyroid membrane location in this setting is promising.[90] These relative contraindications may be overlooked in a true emergency because it is more important to obtain an airway than to suffer the consequences of hypoxemia.

Equipment

In the emergency department, the instruments needed for a surgical cricothyrotomy should be easily accessible. Ideally, a sterile tray containing all the necessary instruments in an organized fashion should be part of the standard equipment stocked in the major resuscitation area (Table 3–4). Prepacked percutaneous kits (e.g., Pertrach, Inc.) have been introduced that greatly simplify the procedure and are recommended for those who perform cricothyrotomies only occasionally.

In an emergency, the only essential instrument is a sharp blade.[55] Any hollow tube may be used to maintain the airway. Under more controlled conditions, an appropriate-sized tracheostomy tube should be selected (Table 3–5). A

small tube becomes obstructed more easily by secretions, whereas a large tube may damage the surrounding cartilage and even lead to a fractured larynx. In an adult, a tracheostomy tube with an 8-mm internal diameter, such as a number 5 Portex or Shiley tube, is usually an appropriate size (see Table 3–5).

If an appropriately sized tracheostomy tube is not available immediately, an endotracheal tube can be modified easily for use as a tracheostomy tube (Fig. 3–3).[56] The uncuffed (proximal) end of the endotracheal tube is cut to an appropriate length (see Fig. 3–3A). The adapter is then attached to the cut end (see Fig. 3–3B), and the modified endotracheal tube is inserted like any tracheostomy tube (see Fig. 3–2D). A flexible endotracheal tube stylet can be used to aid insertion. Caution is required to keep the stylet from protruding beyond the shortened endotracheal tube. After insertion, the cuff of the endotracheal tube should be inflated, if possible. The adapter is reattached to the cut end of the endotracheal tube for ventilation (see Fig. 3–3).[56]

The essential equipment for airway management, specifically supplemental oxygen, suction, and a bag-valve device, also should be readily available.

Procedure

The procedure for surgical cricothyrotomy varies somewhat depending on whether it is done as an emergency or an elective procedure. In the elective situation, the best possible airway control should be obtained before the procedure. Usually, this means endotracheal intubation. In an emergency situation in which endotracheal intubation is contraindicated or impossible, the best airway control may consist of using basic airway techniques such as a modified jaw-thrust maneuver, supplemental oxygen, and bag-valve-mask ventilation.

The instruments and the equipment needed for the procedure should be readily available. Sedation and general anesthesia are usually possible for elective cricothyrotomy. In a truly emergency situation, time is critical, and there may not be enough time even for local anesthesia. Furthermore, because of the dangers of respiratory depression in a patient who may have a compromised airway already, sedation and general anesthesia may be contraindicated.

The patient is positioned to expose the neck and its landmarks. Suction equipment and adequate lighting are essential. If there are no contraindications, such as known or suspected cervical spine injury, the patient's head may be hyperextended, a frequently forgotten maneuver that can greatly enhance the landmarks.

The cricothyroid membrane is located by identifying

Table 3–4. *Equipment for Surgical Cricothyrotomy Tray*

Scalpel with number 15 blade and scalpel with number 11 blade
Tracheal dilator (Trousseau dilator) or spreader
Two hemostats
Scissors
Tracheal hook
Needle holder
Tracheostomy tube (appropriate-size Portex or Shiley tube—number 5–6 in an adult)
25-gauge needle and syringe containing lidocaine with epinephrine (for local anesthesia)
Preparation solution
Sterile gauze pads
Sterile tracheal suction catheter
Suture or circumferential "tie" (to secure tracheostomy tube in place)

the dip or notch in the neck below the laryngeal prominence. The cricothyroid membrane is bounded by the thyroid cartilage superiorly and the cricoid cartilage inferiorly. If time permits, local anesthesia and skin preparation with povidone-iodine may be used, The skin and subcutaneous tissue immediately above the cricothyroid membrane may be infiltrated using lidocaine *with epinephrine* via the usual sterile technique.

A skin incision is made over the cricoid membrane. If time permits, aseptic technique should be used. In an emergency situation, however, this is not always possible. A midline vertical skin incision about 3 to 4 cm long is made for an emergency cricothyrotomy.[13, 20, 56–58] Alternatively, for an elective cricothyrotomy, a 2-cm horizontal skin incision can be made.[19, 52] A vertical skin incision is preferred during an emergency, because if the skin incision is too high or too low, a vertical skin incision merely needs to be extended, thus saving time and avoiding a second incision.[13, 56–58] As an option, one can insert a 20- to 25-gauge needle through the cricothyroid membrane and confirm intratracheal positioning by aspirating air. The needle is *left in place to serve as a guide* for the surgical procedure and removed before insertion of the tracheostomy tube.

The larynx is stabilized by using a tracheal hook (see Fig. 3–2) or by holding it between the nondominant thumb and middle finger. A short horizontal stabbing incision about 1 cm long is made in the lower part of the cricothyroid membrane (i.e., nearer the cricoid cartilage than the thyroid cartilage to avoid the cricothyroid arteries, if possible). The stabbing incision is made in such a way that only the tip of the scalpel blade enters the trachea (see Fig. 3–2).

Curved Mayo scissors are inserted beside the scalpel blade and then spread horizontally to widen the space. An alternative method advocated by some is to widen the opening by using a scalpel handle and turning the scalpel 90 degrees or vertically instead of using curved Mayo scissors. The scalpel handle then is removed and a tracheal (Trousseau) dilator or curved hemostat is inserted into the incision site in the cricothyroid membrane. The dilator is then opened to enlarge the opening in the cricothyroid membrane.

When attempting to insert the tracheostomy tube, the larynx may be displaced posteriorly. Posterior displacement of the larynx may make it difficult or impossible to insert the tracheostomy tube. Stabilization of the larynx is important to lift and hold the larynx anteriorly in proper anatomic position so that this potential problem can be avoided. The

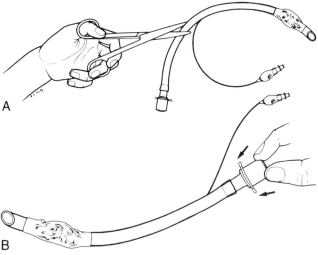

Figure 3–3. Modification of an endotracheal tube for use as a tracheostomy tube. *A,* An appropriate-sized endotracheal tube is cut to an appropriate length. *B,* An adapter is attached to the cut end before the modified endotracheal tube is inserted into the larynx via the opening in the cricothyroid membrane.

tracheostomy tube is inserted between the tracheal dilator or curved hemostat blades (see Fig. 3–2*D*). The dilator or hemostat is then removed. The cuff of the tracheostomy tube is inflated.

For "routine" cricothyrotomy, the following tracheostomy tube sizes are recommended.[12, 55] McGill and colleagues[57] recommend a number 4 Shiley tube in an emergency cricothyrotomy to avoid the potential complication of a fractured larynx. In an adult, a number 5 or 6 Shiley tracheostomy tube is usually an appropriate size (number 5 is an adult female and number 6 in an adult male).[35, 58] Other tube size guidelines are provided in Table 3–5.

If a tracheostomy tube is not available immediately, then a modified endotracheal tube can be used as a temporary airway device, as discussed in the section on equipment.[56] The modified endotracheal tube can be replaced later when an appropriate-sized tracheostomy tube is available.

The lungs are ventilated, and proper tube placement should be ensured. The tracheostomy tube is secured in

Table 3–5. Tracheostomy Tube Sizes			
Age	Internal Diameter of Tracheostomy Tube (mm)	Holinger or Magil Tube Size	Internal Diameter of Endotracheal Tube (mm)
Premature (less than 4 pounds)		000	2.5
Premature (less than 4 pounds)		00	2.5
Newborn	2.5	00 or 0	3.0
0–6 months	3.5	0	3.5
6–12 months	4.0–4.5	1	4.0
1 year	4.5–5.0	1 or 2	4.5
2 years	5.0	2	5.0
4 years	5.5	3	5.5
6 years	6.0	4	6.0
8 years	6.5	4	6.5
10 years	7.0	4	7.0
12 years	7.5	5	7.5
14 years	8.0	5	7.5
Adult female	8.0–8.5	5	7.5–8.5
Adult male	8.5–9.5	6	8.0–9.0

place via a circumferential tie around the neck or by suturing. After confirming proper tube placement, the tracheostomy tube may be attached to a ventilator or a bag-valve device. Flexible connector tubing is recommended to avoid excessive forces on the tracheal wall during mechanical ventilation.

Precautions

Several precautions should be remembered during a cricothyrotomy. The skin incision and the incision in the cricothyroid membrane should not be made too far laterally (see Figs. 3–1 and 3–3A). A central incision will decrease the chance of hemorrhage due to accidental laceration of the carotid arteries, jugular veins, or various laryngotracheal vessels. The skin incision should not be made too far caudally in the neck, thus avoiding hemorrhage from and damage to the highly vascular thyroid gland (see Figs. 3–1 and 3–2A).

If possible, the stabbing incision should be made in the lower half of the cricothyroid membrane (i.e., nearer the cricoid cartilage instead of the thyroid cartilage) in an attempt to avoid bleeding from the cricothyroid arteries, which course superiorly across the cricothyroid membrane near the lower edge of the thyroid cartilage (see Figs. 3–1 and 3–3A).

Transection of the cricoid cartilage or tracheal rings should be avoided (see Fig. 3–1). These structures help maintain the stability of the laryngeal lumen. Injury to these structures may predispose to late complications, including subglottic stenosis.

The scalpel should not be directed in a cephalad direction, so that hitting and injuring the vocal cords is avoided (see Fig. 3–1). The vocal cords are located above the cricothyroid membrane and are protected by the thyroid cartilage on three sides. When a "surgical" cricothyrotomy is being done, the scalpel should be directed posteriorly at a 90-degree angle to the cricothyroid membrane (see Fig. 3–2).

The physician should avoid making a "blind stab" with the scalpel in the region. Controlled, anatomically placed incisions will minimize hemorrhage and injury to any of the adjacent structures, including the thyroid gland, thyroid cartilage, cricoid cartilage, trachea rings, vocal cords, laryngotracheal vessels and nerves. Anatomic perspective is facilitated if one first identifies the cricothyroid membrane and trachea with an aspirating needle and leaves the needle in place during the surgical procedure.

The handle of the scalpel should be held in such a way that only the tip of the scalpel blade can enter the trachea during the initial stab incision through the cricothyroid membrane. For control, the physician should place the thumb and index finger lower down on the handle of the scalpel (just above the scalpel blade). Following this procedure should help avoid injury to the posterior wall of the trachea, esophagus, and other posterior structures by limiting the depth of insertion of the scalpel.

Placement of too large a tracheostomy tube through the cricothyroid membrane should be avoided. Placement of an oversized tracheostomy tube can lead to a fractured larynx.[57] In the adult, the average size of the cricothyroid membrane is about 2 to 3 cm wide and 1 cm high. Thus the appropriate tracheostomy tube in an adult is one with an 8- to 9-mm internal diameter, or a number 5 (in an adult female) and a number 6 (in an adult male) tracheostomy tube size.

Infants and Children

There are several differences in anatomy of the upper airway when infants and children are compared with adults.[14–18] Because of these and other differences, cricothyrotomy may be technically more difficult (as with tracheostomy) in infants and children than in adults and may have a higher rate of problems or complications.

The smaller size of the structures in the infant's or child's neck; the closer proximity of major vessels and other structures to the larynx; the shorter length of the larynx; the higher position of the larynx in the neck, making it less easily accessible; and the lack of the laryngeal prominence in the infant and child[14–18] make it more difficult to palpate and identify the landmarks in the neck and perform a cricothyrotomy.

Because the laryngeal prominence is not well developed until adolescence and young adulthood, the most prominent structures in the anterior neck of the infant or child are the hyoid bone and the cricoid cartilage.[17, 51, 52] In children younger than 5 years of age, the cricoid is the narrowest part of the airway, and the cricothyroid membrane is quite small. Furthermore, the larynx is higher, relatively less accessible, and smaller in the child than in the adult.

Some have advocated tracheostomy rather than cricothyrotomy in infants and children (when endotracheal intubation is contraindicated or impossible) because of the difficulty in palpating and identifying the important landmarks of the neck, including the cricothyroid membrane, and because of the small diameter of the cricoid cartilage.[91] However, others note that emergency surgical cricothyrotomy has fewer complications than emergency tracheostomy in infants and children. To avoid the complications of tracheostomy and surgical cricothyrotomy in infants and children, some have recommended needle cricothyrotomy as the procedure of choice. It has also been suggested that a surgical cricothyrotomy be converted to a tracheostomy when the infant or child is stabilized to reduce the possibility of subglottic stenosis.

The Patient with Massive Neck Swelling

One method of surgical cricothyrotomy uses the hyoid bone as a landmark and an anchor or framework to stabilize the mobile airway in a patient with massive neck edema.[90, 105–107] The horizontal midpoint of the body of the hyoid is also the midpoint of the neck. The key measurement in this technique is distance from the angle of the mandible to the mental protuberance (or mentum) of the chin (line A′ on Fig. 3–4). Distances can be measured using a piece of suture or a string. This distance from the angle of the mandible to the mentum is divided in half.

Next, a point is identified on the anterior midline of the neck below the chin (point C), which equals line B′ or one half the length of the line A′ (see Fig. 3–4). A needle is placed at a point C and directed toward the midline so that it will reach an imaginary line connecting both angles of the mandible. The tip of the needle should hit the hyoid bone. A large-bore (e.g., 18 gauge) spinal needle should be used because the needle must be long enough to pass through massive neck swelling and hit the hyoid bone. If the hyoid bone is not found, the angle of the needle should be adjusted.

When the hyoid bone is found, the needle is left in position, and a number 11 blade is inserted along the needle tract until the hyoid bone is reached. A skin hook is placed alongside the scalpel's tract and under the hyoid bone to retract the hyoid superiorly and anteriorly. A vertical skin incision is made inferiorly from the skin hook with care to stay in the midline. The hyoid bone acts as a fulcrum, holding and stabilizing the larynx in position, so that the incision will stay in the midline despite massive swelling of

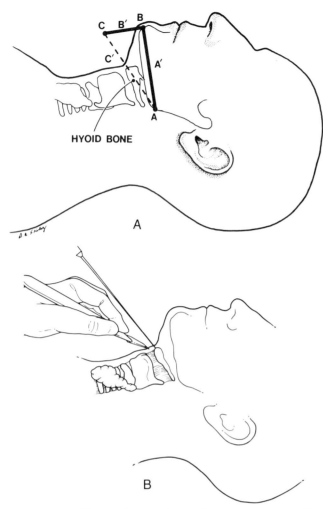

HYOID BONE

A

B

Figure 3–4. Modification for a patient with a massive neck swelling. *A,* Landmarks in the neck. *B,* The procedure for a patient with a massive neck swelling uses a spinal needle to find and identify the hyoid bone and then make the skin incision in the midline going inferiorly from the midpoint of the hyoid bone over the thyroid cartilage until the cricothyroid membrane is exposed.

the neck. The incision is extended caudad over the thyroid cartilage until the cricothyroid membrane is exposed. The remainder of the procedure follows the routine steps for cricothyrotomy.

The only additional supplies needed for this modification of cricothyrotomy in patients with massive neck edema are the suture (or string) to measure the distance from the angle of the mandible to the mentum of the chin and an 18-gauge spinal needle to find the hyoid bone.

Complications

The incidence of complications for an "elective" surgical cricothyrotomy is approximately 6 to 8 per cent.[36, 42, 80] The complication rate for an emergency cricothyrotomy ranges from 10 to 40 per cent.[52, 57] Thus the complication rate for emergency cricothyrotomy compares favorably with that for tracheostomy, which has an average complication rate of approximately 45 per cent.[13, 103, 108, 109] Similarly, the mortality rate for cricothyrotomy of 0.15 per cent is less than that for tracheostomy, which is 1.6 to 5.0 per cent and as high as 16.0 per cent in recent series.[12, 13, 109–112] In general, there has been a higher incidence of complications with cricothyrot-

omy in infants and children than in adults.[91] However, this is also true for tracheostomy. Tumor, inflammation, other masses, certain congenital anomalies, and significant trauma may distort the anatomic features of the neck and airway, creating additional difficulty in performing a cricothyrotomy and increasing the complication rate for this procedure.

Minor complications are more common than serious complications (Table 3–6).[52, 57] Likewise, early complications are more frequent than late complications.[52, 57, 113, 114] In one series of patients who had emergency cricothyrotomies, the overall incidence of complications was 39 per cent, with only 2 per cent long-term complications.

The most common complications are bleeding, incorrect site of tube placement, unsuccessful tube placement, and prolonged procedure time (see Table 3–6). The overall procedure time for cricothyrotomy should be less than 3 minutes.[62] It is not unusual for surgical cricothyrotomy to be completed in 30 to 60 seconds.[115, 116]

Bleeding from the procedure is usually minor and occurs early. Such bleeding can usually be controlled by packing the cricothyrotomy site with gauze. It is unusual for bleeding vessels to require ligation. When present, persistent hemorrhage is usually attributable to vessels located at the edges of a horizontal skin incision. Thus this complication is minimized if a vertical skin incision is made.[57, 117] Potential bleeding may also be minimized by making the stab incision in the lower part of the cricothyroid membrane nearer the cricoid cartilage to avoid the cricothyroid arteries.[52] Although major bleeding generally has not been a problem in most clinical studies,[40, 81, 87] with a few notable exceptions,[41, 46, 57] one cadaver study noted a high number of vessels in the region of the cricothyroid membrane that are at risk during a cricothyrotomy. Thus according to this study, significant hemorrhage could be a problem even if the technique of cricothyrotomy is done correctly and all the guidelines for the procedure are followed.[118] Furthermore, even a small amount of bleeding could be life-threatening if it occurs endotracheally and leads to pneumonitis or suffocation.[112, 119–122] The mortality from acute bleeding during a tracheostomy has been attributed to airway obstruction from

Table 3–6. **Complications of Surgical Cricothyrotomy**

I. Immediate or early complications
  A. Common
    1. Bleeding, hematoma
    2. Incorrect tube placement
    3. Unsuccessful tube placement
    4. Prolonged procedure time
    5. Subcutaneous emphysema
    6. Obstruction
  B. Infrequent
    1. Esophageal perforation
    2. Mediastinal perforation
    3. Pneumothorax, pneumomediastinum
    4. Vocal cord injury
    5. Laryngeal fracture or disruption of laryngeal cartilage
    6. Aspiration
II. Late complications
  A. Most common
    1. Obstructive problems
    2. Voice changes or dysphonia
    3. Infections
    4. Late bleeding
    5. Persistent stoma
    6. Subjective feeling of "lump in the throat"
  B. Infrequent complications
    1. Subglottic or glottic stenosis
    2. Tracheosophageal fistula
    3. Tracheomalacia

the blood and not from volume loss.[36, 118] In the management of postcricothyrotomy or posttracheostomy bleeding, the airway is protected if the tracheostomy tube is in place and the cuff is inflated. If the airway is protected, then the pressure on the bleeding vessels and the usual surgical procedures of locating and then tying off bleeding vessels can be done in a controlled fashion.

Late bleeding is fortunately a rare complication and may result from erosion of vessels by the tracheostomy tube.[123] Significant hemorrhage has not been reported following cricothyrotomy.[36] The cuff of the tracheostomy tube with a cricothyrotomy is located a safe distance away from the brachiocephalic artery.[124] Theoretically, however, the use of an improperly modified endotracheal tube poses the risk of erosion into the brachiocephalic artery.

An incorrectly placed horizontal skin incision (i.e., an incision located above or below the correct location over the cricothyroid membrane) may lead to bleeding, incorrect or unsuccessful tube placement, or both.[57] For example, too low a skin incision may lead to tube placement between the tracheal rings. In an emergency, a vertical skin incision is preferred because a misplaced vertical skin incision, whether too high or too low, can be extended easily.[57]

Other less common early and late complications include infection and airway obstruction.[36, 113, 114, 125] An indwelling tube, whether an endotracheal tube or a tracheostomy tube, will become colonized by bacteria even if meticulous care is given. Infection can result from this colonization. Infection can occur in the structures or tissues of the neck, in the tracheobronchial tree, or in both. Potential infections include cellulitis, perichondritis, abscess in the incision site, and laryngotracheitis.[12, 36]

Acute airway obstruction can occur with tracheostomy or cricothyrotomy.[36, 113, 114] The most common cause of acute airway obstruction is a mucus plug. A mucus plug that causes obstruction, whether partial or complete, should be cleared from the airway by careful suctioning, using a sterile technique. If this cannot be accomplished, then the entire tracheostomy tube may need to be changed. Less frequently, acute airway obstruction can be caused by overinflation of the tracheostomy balloon with herniation of the balloon over the tip of the tracheostomy tube. Finally, the tracheostomy tube can be passed into a subcutaneous fascial or tissue plane instead of into the trachea. This complication can occur during insertion of the tracheostomy tube or more commonly during a tube change, especially during the immediate postoperative period.

Long-term complications following cricothyrotomy are unusual.[52, 57] The major long-term complication is a change in voice or dysphonia.[126] Laryngeal damage may occur secondary to a laryngeal fracture caused by using a tracheostomy tube that is too large for the size of the cricothyroid membrane.[57] Dysphonia can also be caused by direct injury to the vocal cords.

Other late and rare complications include a suture sinus, a subjective feeling of a "lump in the throat," a persistent stoma, and subglottic or glottic stenosis.[12, 36] Swallowing problems have been reported in tracheostomy patients[127] but not in cricothyrotomy patients.

Airway stenosis is a potential complication whenever a tube is placed in the airway. Airway stenosis can occur with oral or nasal intubation, cricothyrotomy, or tracheostomy. At present, the most common cause of subglottic stenosis is endotracheal intubation and not cricothyrotomy or tracheostomy.[100–102, 128–130] The pathophysiology of subglottic stenosis involves mucosal ulceration and damage secondary to a tube eroding the mucosal surface, laryngeal disease along with bacterial colonization of the region or both.[131] Excessive cuff pressures, frequent tube motion, and rigid tubes that

are anatomically incorrect, also contribute to mucosal damage. The use of flexible, anatomically correct tubes with low-pressure cuffs and flexible tubing between the tube and the ventilator will minimize mucosal damage.

Prolonged endotracheal intubation followed by tracheostomy or cricothyrotomy is associated with a higher incidence of subglottic stenosis than either the endotracheal intubation or the surgical procedure (tracheostomy or cricothyrotomy) alone.[97, 98] The airway stenosis produced by an indwelling tube is generally located at the cuff site of the tube. If airway stenosis occurs with a standard tracheostomy, the stenosis occurs quite distal in the trachea, thus making it difficult to reach during surgical repair.

Early aggressive surgical management of granulation tissue associated with mucosal injury has been successful in limiting the number of cases of chronic airway stenosis.[132, 133] In one study of subglottic stenosis after endotracheal intubation, early aggressive therapy that included antibiotics, steroids, and dilations of the obstructions was successful in maintaining an airway in the majority of the patients.[133] Laser endoscopic resection of granulation tissue is one therapy that has been especially useful in the treatment of subglottic stenosis.[133, 134] In recent studies of cricothyrotomy, subglottic or glottic stenosis is rarely encountered if at all.[36, 37, 39, 42–44, 135]

There are other theoretic complications of cricothyrotomy. These include pneumothorax, pneumomediastinum, major vessel hemorrhage (e.g., bleeding secondary to erosion into the brachiocephalic artery), tracheoesophageal fistula, and esophageal perforation. These complications are seen with tracheostomy but have not yet been reported as complications of cricothyrotomy.[65, 136, 137]

The complications of asphyxia including dysrhythmias and cardiac arrest during the performance of tracheostomy or cricothyrotomy are generally due to the lack of adequate oxygenation and not to the procedure itself or to a vagal reaction. Because cricothyrotomy is one of the easiest, quickest, and safest ways to achieve definitive airway control and oxygenation, the complications of hypoxemia should be less than those seen when a tracheostomy is performed in critically ill patients.

PERCUTANEOUS TRANSLARYNGEAL VENTILATION (NEEDLE CRICOTHYROTOMY)

Overview

During needle cricothyrotomy an opening is made in the cricothyroid membrane with a needle to establish an airway.[19, 20] Thus needle cricothyrotomy consists of two parts: needle puncture of the cricothyroid membrane followed by administration of oxygen through the puncture wound or opening in the cricothyroid membrane.

The technique of puncture of the cricothyroid membrane is relatively simple and has many widely accepted uses, ranging from obtaining sputum samples (see Chapter 7) to giving local anesthesia before intubation (see Chapter 2) to ventilating the patient.[138–143] Whether the lungs can be ventilated adequately via a needle or cannula in the cricothyroid membrane has been debated in the past.[5, 144] We now know that percutaneous transtracheal ventilation can be an effective and relatively safe procedure for obtaining and maintaining an airway for extended periods of time provided that appropriate equipment and techniques of ventilation are used.[5, 144]

Needle cricothyrotomy has also been referred to as transtracheal or translaryngeal oxygenation and percutaneous transtracheal or translaryngeal ventilation.[5, 144] Because needle cricothyrotomy involves placing a needle through the skin, then through the subcutaneous tissue, and finally through the cricothyroid membrane without using a formal incision, it is a percutaneous technique.

Historically, oxygen was simply passed through the needle or cannula in the cricothyroid membrane. In this way, hypoxia was treated and generally oxygenation was adequate. However, clinical studies and animal experiments noted that although the P_{O_2} was adequate, CO_2 was retained, and the elevated P_{CO_2} led to a respiratory acidosis.[145–147] Thus the patient could be maintained for only about 30 minutes because of the severe hypercapnia and resultant respiratory acidosis even when the hypoxia was treated successfully.[145–147] This procedure whereby oxygen is run continuously through a needle or cannula in the cricothyroid membrane is referred to as *translaryngeal oxygenation.*

The solution to avoiding a rise in P_{CO_2} and respiratory acidosis is to "ventilate" the patient, allowing time for both inhalation and exhalation, thus simulating normal respiration.[148–150] Intermittent bursts of oxygen provide time for both inhalation and exhalation thus avoiding hypercapnia and respiratory acidosis. *Translaryngeal (jet) ventilation,* then, is the ventilation of the lungs by intermittent bursts of oxygen through a needle or cannula in the cricothyroid membrane with time for exhalation as well as inhalation.

Therefore, *percutaneous translaryngeal ventilation* is the desired procedure, not percutaneous translaryngeal oxygenation. Percutaneous translaryngeal ventilation also is a better term than *needle cricothyrotomy,* which only implies that a needle is in the cricothyroid membrane but does not specify whether the patient is being oxygenated passively or ventilated actively with intermittent bursts of oxygen or air. Percutaneous transtracheal ventilation is the same procedure except that the needle or cannula is placed in the trachea.

Background

Although the idea of gas insufflation via an opening in the trachea was described in the early seventeenth century by Hooke[151] and in animal experiments years ago,[152] the current usage of the technique has only become popular in the last 20 years. Moreover, a lack of understanding of the basic definitions and the differences between transtracheal oxygenation and ventilation as well as a failure to standardize the technique itself (with regard to such factors as pressure, volume, intermittent versus continuous administration of air versus oxygen, size of opening in the membrane, and location of opening in the airway [e.g., trachea versus cricothyroid membrane]) has led to conflicting studies or reports in the literature[9, 144] and to many misconceptions about the technique.[9, 13, 59, 78]

Studies as early as 1909 showed that animals could survive for approximately 30 minutes when oxygen was given via a needle placed in the cricothyroid membrane. Reed and colleagues in 1954 showed that animals could be kept alive for a longer period of time and with a normal pH if the animals were ventilated with intermittent bursts of compressed air instead of a continuous flow of oxygen.[145] The key to avoiding respiratory acidosis and thus maintaining a normal pH was the use of a method allowing for "ventilation" or the simulation of an inspiratory cycle, not just a continuous inflow of oxygen or air that created a respiratory acidosis.[148–150]

A popular misconception is that percutaneous transtracheal ventilation is a temporizing procedure good for only 30 minutes at best.[5, 144] This misconception, which has been almost universally accepted and stated even in standard textbooks,[9, 13, 59] needs to be corrected.[5, 144] Animal experiments and clinical studies have demonstrated that proper transtracheal ventilation is an effective, quick, fairly simple, and safe way to obtain and maintain an airway for a prolonged period of time.[148–159, 153–154] Percutaneous transtracheal ventilation with sufficient time allowed for inhalation and exhalation via an adequate-sized opening with appropriate pressures and sufficient volumes is an acceptable method of maintaining an airway and has been used for extended periods, even for weeks.[148–150, 153–154]

Clinical transtracheal oxygenation was performed as early as 1951 when Jacoby and coworkers used a 14-gauge needle to puncture the tracheas of five patients and then insufflated the lungs with oxygen via the needle.[147] Although the procedure of ventilation using a high-pressure source of oxygen through a small cannula was popularized by Sanders in 1967 when he administered oxygen through a bronchoscope,[155] percutaneous transtracheal ventilation using a small catheter to administer intermittent bursts of oxygen was first performed in 1969 by Toye and Weinstein[156] and then in 1971 by Spoerel and associates during anesthesia.[148] The first use of percutaneous transtracheal ventilation for resuscitation was by Ja-

cobs in 1972.[157, 158] This was followed by a report of transtracheal ventilation before tracheostomy by Smith in 1974.[159]

In 1978, Dunlap's animal experiments and clinical studies again demonstrated that adequate oxygenation, normal pH, and avoidance of respiratory acidosis could be achieved by using intermittent bursts of oxygen via a 14-gauge catheter inserted into the cricothyroid membrane.[150] Furthermore, Dunlap's studies showed that percutaneous transtracheal ventilation could be used quickly and easily during resuscitation in the emergency department and that percutaneous transtracheal ventilation could correct abnormal blood gases and eliminate hypoxia, hypercapnia, and respiratory acidosis.[150]

Transtracheal ventilation has been used extensively as a means of ventilation during head and neck surgery, bronchoscopy, and oral surgery.[37, 89, 154] More recently, percutaneous transtracheal ventilation has also been used during laser microsurgery of the larynx and other structures of the upper airway.[160–162] Percutaneous transtracheal ventilation has several major advantages, and some advocate its use as the airway of choice during these surgical procedures. Thus percutaneous translaryngeal and transtracheal ventilation is a rapid procedure for obtaining airway control in both elective and emergency situations in patients of all ages and in many clinical situations.[163–177]

Special Considerations

Anatomy. The anatomic considerations (see Fig. 3–1) are essentially the same for needle cricothyrotomy as for surgical cricothyrotomy (see the earlier section on surgical cricothyrotomy).

Advantages Over Endotracheal Intubation. The advantages of percutaneous translaryngeal ventilation over standard endotracheal intubation, especially during surgical procedures on the upper airway and during bronchoscopy,[85–89, 154, 177] include the following:

1. Elimination of the endotracheal tube—hence better visualization and access to the larynx and other upper airway structures during surgery.[85, 89, 154]
2. Decreased mucosal damage to the upper airway.[85, 89, 154]
3. No mucosal pressure with resultant granulation or scarring of tissue, especially tissue in the upper airway, which may have been operated on recently.
4. No requirement for sedation—patients may eat, cough, and speak during ventilation.[153]
5. Greatly decreased risk of catheter ignition during laser surgery in this region.[178]

Advantages Over Surgical Cricothyrotomy. The advantages of needle cricothyrotomy over surgical cricothyrotomy include (Table 3–7) faster performance (may take only 10 seconds), easier performance, less equipment and surgical set-up required, no need for an assistant, smaller scar, less bleeding, expulsion of oropharyngeal secretions and other particles or small objects out of the proximal trachea, less

Table 3–7. **Advantages of Percutaneous Translaryngeal Ventilation versus Surgical Cricothyrotomy**

Faster (may take as little as 10 seconds versus 30 seconds to 3 minutes for surgical cricothyrotomy)
Less bleeding (due to smaller opening, smaller incision)
Simpler technique, easier to perform
Does not need an assistant, can be done by nonsurgeons
Requires fewer instruments
Lesser need for extensive surgical set-up (lighting, equipment, and preparation)
Smaller scar (stoma is only as large as the size of the tube)
Less tracheal erosion
Less subglottic or glottic stenosis
Forces oropharyngeal secretions out of the proximal trachea
May force foreign body out of proximal trachea with a partial airway obstruction

tracheal erosion, and lesser incidence of subglottic or glottic stenosis (see Table 3–1).[85] Some of the advantages are because of the smaller size of the opening and the percutaneous technique (e.g., needle insertion versus surgical incision).

Advantages Over Tracheostomy. The advantages of needle cricothyrotomy over tracheostomy are similar to those given for a surgical cricothyrotomy (see Table 3–2).[36, 40, 80, 81-84] In addition, the procedure can be done by nonsurgeons, requires fewer instruments, does not require an operating suite, and produces fewer early and late complications.[36, 40, 80-84, 153] In patients who require prolonged intubation, needle cricothyrotomy has been used successfully and has several advantages over tracheostomy. These advantages include less bleeding, a smaller scar, a lower infection rate, and a lesser incidence of tracheal erosion.[36, 83, 84, 153]

The advantages of needle cricothyrotomy over tracheostomy can be attributed to less encroachment on the mediastinum with needle cricothyrotomy, the smaller opening with a needle puncture versus a surgical incision,[73-79] and the ease of performance without requiring a surgical set-up or skills.

Disadvantages. The disadvantages of percutaneous transtracheal ventilation are that (1) the catheter does not allow for "complete" control of the airway or prevent aspiration (unlike an endotracheal tube with intubation or a trachostomy tube with surgical cricothyrotomy), (2) barotrauma (subcutaneous emphysema or pneumothorax) is likely if exhalation is inadequate and airway pressure is elevated, and (3) adequate suctioning cannot be done through a percutaneous catheter set-up.[179] Although there may not be complete control of the airway, airway protection during transtracheal ventilation is attained by positioning the patient to allow drainage of secretions or blood away from the larynx (when possible); also, during expiration, gas flow is upward through the larynx, causing debris (secretions, blood, etc.) to be blown away from the larynx.[154]

High-Frequency Jet Ventilation. High-frequency jet ventilation is a variation of translaryngeal ventilation that has gained increasing popularity in the last few years.[180-185] High-frequency jet ventilation, also referred to as high-frequency positive-pressure ventilation, is a means of artificial ventilation that uses low tidal volumes and high respiratory rates. The technique can maintain adequate gas exchange at respiratory rates of up to 500 per minute at low tidal volumes, which approaches or is less than the dead space volume. The technique of high-frequency jet ventilation has been suggested as an alternative to conventional artificial ventilation and as an alternative method of positive end-expiratory pressure (PEEP).[180-185] High-frequency jet ventilation has a major advangage over PEEP because at the levels of peak airway pressure commonly used, high-frequency jet ventilation causes no alterations of hemodynamic function. It commonly generates a mean airway pressure of 2.9 to 10.0. mm Hg without any circulatory compromise. High-frequency jet ventilation has been used successfully in all types and all ages of patients, even in premature newborns, without complications.[180-182, 186-191] Because a special ventilator device is needed to produce high-frequency jet ventilations, this technique is not commonly used in the emergency department. Further discussion in this text will be limited to low-frequency translaryngeal ventilation.

Indications

Indications for percutaneous translaryngeal ventilation are similar to that for surgical cricothyrotomy. Cricothyrotomy, whether needle or surgical, is indicated in any situation in which orotracheal or nasotracheal intubation is contraindicated or cannot be performed (see Table 3–1).[5, 9, 46, 59, 60, 184]

Failure to achieve endotracheal intubation in a timely fashion and thus causing an inordinate delay in definitive airway control and oxygenation, is an indication for needle or surgical cricothyrotomy to prevent hypoxemia.[5, 9, 46, 59, 60, 184] Whenever intubation is contraindicated, cricothyrotomy is usually the procedure of choice for airway management.

Percutaneous translaryngeal ventilation can be used in a patient with airway obstruction, but it requires an adequate-sized catheter or catheters.[192-194]

Transtracheal ventilation has been recommended as the procedure of choice for airway control and oxygenation during various surgical procedures, including head and neck surgery, oral surgery, bronchoscopy, and laser microsurgery of the larynx and other upper airway structures.[85, 89, 154, 160-162, 186, 187]

Thus percutaneous translaryngeal ventilation has numerous indications, both as an emergency and as an elective procedure, and has been used successfully in patients of all ages, even in premature infants,[188, 189] for extended periods of time.[5, 9, 11, 12, 46, 60, 61, 144, 184-191]

Contraindications

The absolute contraindications to surgical or needle cricothyrotomy are when endotracheal intubation is not contraindicated and can be accomplished easily and rapidly; when the trachea has been transected and the distal end has retracted into the mediastinum, and when known significant direct damage to the cricoid cartilage or larynx has occurred (see Table 3–3).[5, 12, 195-198]

Known complete airway obstruction requires an adequate-sized catheter or catheters to avoid barotrauma and hypercarbia.[5, 12, 91, 149] Barotrauma with high pressures occurring in the trachea can lead to complications such as a pneumothorax, pneumomediastinum or both during percutaneous transtracheal ventilation with intermittent ventilatory bursts at 50 psi.[5, 12, 13] If intratracheal pressures less than or equal to 20 cm H_2O are maintained, the complication rate of percutaneous transtracheal ventilation is low. If complete upper airway obstruction is present, surgical cricothyrotomy is generally preferred over percutaneous translaryngeal ventilation,[5, 12] although percutaneous translaryngeal ventilation could be used with partial or complete airway obstruction provided appropriate-sized catheters are used.[192-194]

Other relative contraindications to percutaneous translaryngeal ventilation are different from those for surgical cricothyrotomy.[5, 12, 59, 62, 63, 195] Although age less than 5 years has been mentioned as a relative contraindication to surgical cricothyrotomy,[80, 91, 199, 200] age is not a factor in deciding to perform percutaneous translaryngeal ventilation. Because percutaneous translaryngeal ventilation involves a "needle stick" or puncture wound through the cricothyroid membrane rather than a surgical incision, percutaneous translaryngeal ventilation has been recommended by some as the procedure of choice in infants and young children as a means of obtaining an airway, especially in an emergency, rather than tracheostomy or surgical cricothyrotomy.[201, 202]

Equipment

Translaryngeal jet ventilation requires three components: an oxygen supply at 50 psi, a manual in-line valve (e.g., Y-connector or side port cut in the tubing) to allow for the intermittent administration of oxygen, and a needle or cannula with a bore larger than or equal to 13 or 14 gauge in the cricothyroid membrane (Table 3–8).

OXYGEN SUPPLY

The oxygen supply must be at a pressure of 50 psi to deliver enough volume to ventilate the lungs rapidly between periods of exhalation through the glottic opening. An oxygen source of 50 psi can be obtained by attaching a connector to the piped oxygen line found in any emergency department, attaching the tubing to the flush valve of an anesthetic machine, or attaching the oxygen tubing directly into an oxygen tank line (regulator) but not to the flow valve of the oxygen cylinder. The oxygen tanks in ambulances or other patient transport vehicles for prehospital care should have two components: (1) an outlet that leads directly into the cylinder line, and (2) a simple, easy to connect, device that allows the oxygen hose to be quickly attached to the outlet.

Stewart recommends unscrewing the demand valve connection from the oxygen regulator of the tank and rapidly connecting the oxygen hose that has a nipple in place for fitting into the outlet.[144] He further suggests leaving a small wrench fastened to the oxygen hose to allow a rapid transfer.

Two additional key points should be remembered: (1) high-pressure tubing should be used throughout the system, and (2) all connections and attachments should be well secured to avoid any disconnection under high pressure. Ligatures or other fasteners may be helpful in securing the attachments.

VALVE (MANUAL VENTILATION) APPARATUS

It is essential to have the proper attachment or hookup of oxygen to the cannula or needle. Whatever the device or valve apparatus selected, it is critical to have all the equipment ready, all the connections available, and everything easily accessible. The apparatus can be gathered together and placed in one bag or kit and should be stored with the other airway management equipment. The equipment for translaryngeal jet ventilation should be maintained as any other critical equipment found in the emergency department to ensure that it will work when needed.

The valve principle is the same no matter what the specific device (Fig. 3–5). First, high-pressure tubing goes from the oxygen source at 50 psi to a manually controlled device or area of the tubing that allows for the intermittent flow of oxygen, which is then connected via high-pressure tubing to the cannula or needle in the cricothyroid membrane.

There are several simple set-ups for bag-valve–driven system described in the literature (Fig. 3–6). These systems represent temporizing measures at best. A 50-psi oxygen

source is needed for optimal ventilation. There are also several manual valves available commercially. Stewart recommends the manual valve by Instrumentation Industries (Bethel Park, Pa.), although others such as the "Manujet" by VBM (Germany) are also available.[144] The advantages of the commercial manual valve devices are that the intermittent flow of oxygen conserves oxygen and the valve is easy to use, durable, and reusable (after sterilization).

CANNULA OR NEEDLE

The third piece of equipment required is the cannula. A 13- or 14-gauge needle catheter with a length of about 2 cm (or 1¼ inches) or a 3-mm internal diameter cannula is preferred for percutaneous translaryngeal ventilation. The size of the needle or cannula is critical. Too small a needle or cannula will not allow for sufficient ventilation, causing hypercapnia and even hypoxia to develop.

Several modifications for the needle catheter or cannula have been suggested: side holes, a slight curve, and a plate or flange. The advantage of side holes is that they will help keep the end or point of the cannula away from the tracheal wall. Thus the full force of the 50 psi oxygen source is not directed at just one area of the laryngeal wall or larynx but is centered in the larynx. A curve in the cannula facilitates its initial placement. A fixation plate, flange, or side "handle" helps secure the cannula into place. A snug fit of the cannula will help prevent subcutaneous emphysema from ventilation of overlying soft tissue.

COMMERCIAL DEVICES

Several cannulas designed for percutaneous translaryngeal ventilation are available commercially. These include NU-TRAKE and PEDIA-TRAKE (International Medical Devices, Inc., Northridge, Calif.), Abelson cricothyrotomy cannula (Gilbert Surgical Instruments, Inc., Bellmawr, NJ), Pertrach (Long Beach, Calif.), and the Trans-Cricothyrotomy device (VBM, Sulz am Neckar, Germany) (Table 3–9). The use of an 8 French vascular introducer via the Seldinger technique is another technique.[203–205] The Seldinger technique using prepackaged kits is a relatively new development. Experience is limited, but this procedure is easily accomplished and is recommended as an option for those who have limited surgical expertise or who perform the procedure only occasionally (Fig. 3–7). The use of a self-contained, specially designed instrument kit following the procedure outlined later has been described by Schachner and colleagues.[206]

It should be remembered that the indications, contraindications, and complications are generally independent of the device used. For example, bleeding or subcutaneous emphysema may occur as a result of the procedure,[207] and its occurrence is not eliminated by the use of any one specific device.[208–211]

Procedure

The actual technique of needle cricothyrotomy is fairly simple (Fig. 3–8). The anatomy, landmarks, and several of the steps in the technique are identical to that for surgical cricothyrotomy (see Figs. 3–1 and 3–2).

The patient can be positioned for the procedure. If there are no contraindications, such as known or suspected cervical spine injury, the head of the patient should be extended. However, cricothyrotomy may be done without

---

Table 3–8. *Equipment for Needle Cricothyrotomy*

I. Oxygen source
   High-pressure oxygen source at 50 psi
   Deliver 100% oxygen at 20 bursts/minute with I:E = 1:2

II. Manual jet ventilator device
   A. High-pressure tubing (to be attached to cannula or catheter and oxygen at other end with the manual jet ventilator device in the middle)
   B. Manual jet ventilator device (Y-connector or push-button device) to allow for "ventilation" with inhalation and exhalation

III. Cannula
   Large bore (gauge less than or equal to 13- or 14-gauge needle) with a Teflon or plastic cannula or, alternatively, one of the commercial cricothyrotomy devices

I, inhalation; E, exhalation.

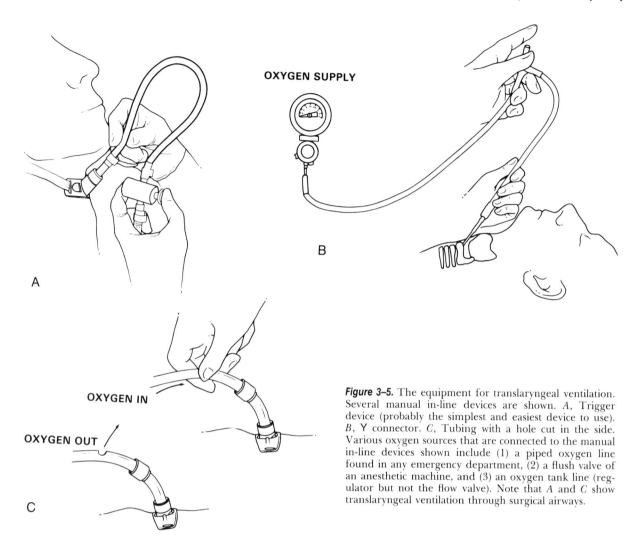

OXYGEN SUPPLY

A

B

OXYGEN IN

OXYGEN OUT

C

Figure 3–5. The equipment for translaryngeal ventilation. Several manual in-line devices are shown. *A*, Trigger device (probably the simplest and easiest device to use). *B*, Y connector. *C*, Tubing with a hole cut in the side. Various oxygen sources that are connected to the manual in-line devices shown include (1) a piped oxygen line found in any emergency department, (2) a flush valve of an anesthetic machine, and (3) an oxygen tank line (regulator but not the flow valve). Note that *A* and *C* show translaryngeal ventilation through surgical airways.

cervical hyperextension. A towel may also be placed under the shoulders.

The cricothyroid membrane is located by identifying the notch in the neck below the laryngeal prominence. The area immediately above the cricothyroid membrane may be prepared with povidone-iodine solution and anesthetized with lidocaine (preferably with epinephrine) if the patient is conscious and if time permits. If the patient is responsive, 1 to 2 ml of lidocaine may be injected into the larynx to prevent reflex coughing when the needle or cannula enters the larynx.

A small 3- to 5-ml syringe containing 1 to 2 ml of sterile normal saline or water is attached to a large-bore needle (≤ 13 or 14 gauge). Alternatively, if lidocaine will be injected, the 1 to 2 ml of 1 per cent lidocaine without epinephrine should be in the syringe.

While the dominant hand (usually the right) holds the syringe, with the needle directed caudally at less than a 45-degree angle to the skin, the other hand (nondominant) holds and stabilizes the larynx. The thumb and middle fingers of the nondominant hand stabilize the cricoid cartilage, and the index finger palpates the cricothyroid membrane.

The needle is inserted through soft tissues and the cricothyroid membrane (see Fig. 3–8). While negative pressure is exerted on the barrel of the syringe, the needle is inserted through the cricothyroid membrane into the larynx. Air bubbles in the saline-filled syringe signify entry into the larynx. After entering the larynx, the cannula is advanced

into the larynx, and then the needle is removed. The cricothyroid membrane should be punctured in the inferior aspect (i.e., nearer the cricoid cartilage than the thyroid cartilage) to avoid the cricothyroid arteries (see Fig. 3–2A).

If there is much resistance to the needle's or catheter's passage through the skin, subcutaneous tissue, or cricothyroid membrane, then kinking or bending of the catheter may occur unless a stiffer catheter is used. A small skin nick may be needed to facilitate passage through the dermis into the subcutaneous tissue.

Next, the cannula is secured by suturing it to the skin or by placing a circumferential tie around the neck. Then the oxygen source is connected to the cannula. It is critical that the proximal end of the cannula be snug or tightly fitting and securely held around the puncture wound opening. If not securely held in place, subcutaneous emphysema will certainly result, or the cannula may be dislodged out of the larynx, or both may occur. A trial of several bursts of oxygen flow is recommended to make certain that the cannula is correctly placed and the set-up is working and ventilating properly.

The hypoxic patient should receive 100 per cent oxygen in intermittent bursts at approximated 50 psi at a rate of 20 bursts per minute. The percentage of inspired oxygen concentration can then be adjusted depending on blood gas results. For children, 30 psi has been recommended. The inspiratory phase or insufflation with the burst of oxygen should last approximately 1 second, and exhalation or the expiratory phase approximately 2 seconds.

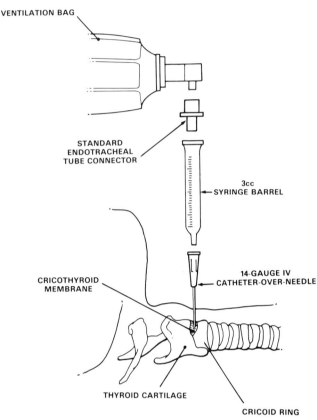

Figure 3–6. A simple set-up for translaryngeal ventilation using standard equipment found in any emergency department. This set-up is temporizing at best. High pressure (50 psi) ventilation systems (see Fig. 3–5) are optimal.

Table 3–9. Commercial Devices

I. *Commercial Cricothyroidotomy Devices*
   There are many commercial cricothyrotomy devices. A few of them are listed below. Mention is not intended to imply endorsement of these devices.
   1. NU-TRAKE and PEDIA-TRAKE are distributed by International Medical Devices, Inc., P.O. Box 408 Canoga Park, 19355 Business Center Drive, Suite 8, Northridge, CA 91324, or P.O. Box 408 Canoga Park, CA 91305; phone (818) 701-5433 or (800) 522-LIFE (outside California)
   2. Pertrach: Pertrach, Inc., 900 Davisson Run Road, Suite 301, Clarksburg, WV 26301, phone (304) 624-7122 or (800) 736-3194.
   3. Abelson cricothyrotomy cannula: Gilbert Surgical Instruments, 115 Harding Avenue, P.O. Box 458, Bellmawr, NJ 08031, phone (609) 933-2770.
   4. Quick Trach emergency cricothyrotomy device for adults and infants: VBM Medizintechnik GMBH, D-7247 Sulz am Neckar, Germany, phone (07454)6211; telefax (07454)4953
   5. Portex Mini Trach Kit
II. *Commercial Transtracheal Puncture Devices*
   Also designed for transtracheal puncture, the Trans-Cricothyrotomy device is distributed by VBM Medizintechnik (same address and phone as above).
III. *Commercial Manual Ventilator Devices*
   1. Manual valve that allows for the flow of oxygen when the control button is pushed. Manual Valve, by Instrumentation Industries, Bethel Park, PA
   2. Manujet: a manual jetting device by VBM Medizintechnik GmbH, Bruhlstrasse 10, 0-727 Sulz am Neckar, Germany

Precautions

Several precautions are useful during needle cricothyrotomy. The location of the needle puncture (or incision) in the skin and cricothyroid membrane is critical. The preferred location is near the midline in the inferior aspect of the cricothyroid membrane just above the cricoid cartilage. The needle (or scalpel) is directed at an approximately 45-degree angle to the skin in a caudal direction. The key landmarks in the neck should be identified before inserting the needle-cannula combination into the cricothyroid membrane.

Too small an opening in the cricothyroid membrane will lead to hypoxia, hypercapnia, and respiratory acidosis.[90, 149, 164, 212–215] In an adult, a 13- or 14-gauge needle or larger bore with a 3-mm internal diameter is needed to provide an adequate-sized opening.[90, 149, 164, 212–215]

Likewise, use of a bag-valve device or a demand valve resuscitator apparatus to ventilate a patient through a translaryngeal cannula is generally inadequate. Using a 50 psi oxygen source, up to 1300 ml per minute can be delivered through a 13-gauge cannula, and up to 1200 ml per minute can be delivered through a 14-gauge cannula. Additional side holes or ports in the cannula to allow for the additional egress of oxygen into the trachea and to limit the obstruction of the cannula by mucus plugs are desirable.

During the insufflation phase of percutaneous translaryngeal ventilation, secretions in the upper airway are blown out of the mouth and nose. Thus it is recommended that personnel stand clear of the patient's face during insufflation to avoid being sprayed with secretions when oxygen exits through the patient's glottis and pushes oropharyngeal se-

---

Table 3–10. Complications of Percutaneous Translaryngeal Ventilation

I. Common
   Subcutaneous emphysema—most common (less occurrence if there is a "secure" fit at the skin)
   Kinking of the catheter
   Blockage or obstruction of the catheter
   Coughing (in a conscious patient)
II. Infrequent
   Bleeding (minor), hematoma
   Infections
   Aspiration
   Incorrect or unsuccessful catheter placement
   Prolonged procedure time
   Persistent stoma
   Subjective feeling of a "lump in the throat"
   Pneumatocyst
III. Serious, rare complications
   Barotrauma (secondary to high airway pressures, more common with complete airway obstruction)
   Pneumothorax
   Pneumomediastinum (less occurrence if high airway pressures are avoided, and not performed with complete airway obstruction)
   Mediastinal perforation
   Esophageal perforation
   Dysphonia or voice changes (secondary to vocal cord injury, laryngeal fracture, or disruption of laryngeal cartilage)
IV. Potential or theoretic complications (not yet commonly associated with percutaneous translaryngeal ventilation although reported with tracheostomy and other airway procedures)
   Subglottic/glottic stenosis
   Trachesophageal fistula
   Damage to laryngotracheal mucosa (such as tracheobronchitis)
   Swallowing problems

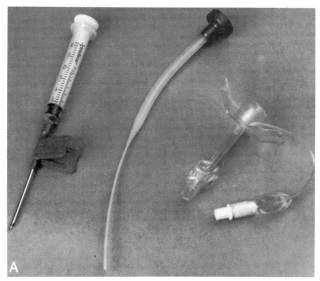

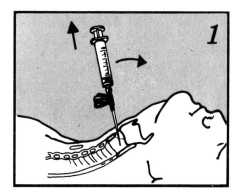

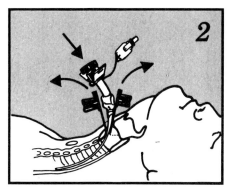

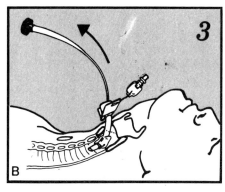

Figure 3–7. *A,* Commerical device used in performing a cricothyrotomy with a modified Seldinger technique. The adult Pertrach percutaneous emergency airway provides a means of rapidly and safely inserting a tube into a patient's trachea (through either cricothyroid membrane or trachea) in certain clinical situations. It provides an adequate airway that can, by its standard 15-mm adapter, be used to allow the patient to breathe. The unit allows full control of the airway with inflation of the cuff. The pediatric device is provided uncuffed in three sizes for infants and children of various sizes. The 15-mm adapter is part of each unit. (Tracheostomy *only* is recommended in children and infants.) *B,* Method of establishing an airway with the Pertrach cricothyrotomy kit. (1) The number 14 needle is inserted into the trachea through a cricothyroid membrane or upper trachea. Placement in the airway is verified by drawing air. The syringe is removed. (2) The leader of the dilator is inserted into the trachea through the needle, which is then split and removed. The dilator and trachea tube are inserted into the trachea. Note that a small skin incision at the puncture site is needed to facilitate passage of the trachea tube. (3) The dilator is removed. The cuff can then be inflated and a respirator applied. Thus a needle puncture becomes an airway. In the child, only tracheostomy is done. (Courtesy of Pertrach, Inc., Clarksburg, WV 26301.)

cretions out the glottis and then out the nose and mouth. This may be a useful side effect if partial upper airway obstruction is present, as with a foreign body such as a bolus of meat or a peanut, because some of the delivered volume of air exiting through the patient's glottis might dislodge such a foreign body. The risk of aspiration is decreased or eliminated by lowering the head.[216] Another key point is that the proximal end of the cannula should be snug against the puncture wound to minimize localized subcutaneous emphysema and should be secured in place to prevent the cannula from being dislodged.[5, 149, 150]

Complications

The exact incidence of complications[217–219] with percutaneous translaryngeal ventilation is not known but is thought to be low,[220] considering that the complication rate of translaryngeal puncture alone is in the range of 0.03 to 0.8 per cent (Table 3–10).[141, 143]

Bleeding can occur at the site of the needle puncture, but this is usually not a major problem.[5, 49, 118, 149, 150] Hemoptysis following cricothyrotomy, either surgical or needle, may occur but is infrequent.[150] Fatal hemorrhage secondary to transtracheal aspiration for sputum cultures has been reported,[121, 122] although no bleeding fatalities secondary to percutaneous transtracheal ventilation have been reported.[5, 82, 177] Again, as with surgical cricothyrotomy, knowing the anatomy of the region and puncturing the cricothyroid membrane in the area near the cricoid cartilage may result in less chance of significant bleeding.[56, 57, 118]

Although minor bleeding is one of the most common complications of a surgical cricothyrotomy, subcutaneous emphysema is the most frequent complication of a percutaneous translaryngeal ventilation.[5, 149, 150] With percutaneous translaryngeal ventilation, subcutaneous emphysema will occur if egress of gas is prevented by inadequate exhalation (e.g., with occlusion of the mouth and nose or with inadequate cannula size).[5, 149] The development of subcutaneous emphysema with percutaneous transtracheal ventilation is often immediate and dramatic.[5, 143, 149] If this complication does occur, the subcutaneous emphysema may be gently squeezed away from the midline and the trachea often recannulated and successfully ventilated.[5, 150] Subcutaneous emphysema can be decreased or avoided by making sure that the flange or hub of the cannula fits securely against the skin.

Barotrauma secondary to high airway pressures may occur if percutaneous translaryngeal ventilation is used when complete airway obstruction is present. Such barotrauma could lead to serious complications including pneumothorax

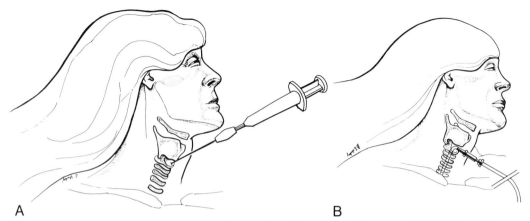

Figure 3–8. The procedure for transtracheal ventilation. *A,* The cricothyroid membrane is punctured with the needle or catheter aimed caudally at approximately a 45 degree angle. *B,* The inner needle has been removed, and the catheter is hooked up to a manual in-line device and then to a source of oxygen. A valve device or tubing modification as shown in Figure 3–5 is also required.

and pneumomediastinum as well as subcutaneous emphysema.

Another side effect that can occur with percutaneous transtracheal ventilation but not with surgical cricothyrotomy is coughing with each burst of oxygen in the conscious patient.[5] A few milliliters of 1 or 2 per cent lidocaine may be injected into the larynx to help prevent coughing when the cannula enters the larynx. Because the patient undergoing cricothyrotomy in the emergency department is almost always critically ill and is rarely conscious, this is usually not a problem.[52, 57]

Percutaneous translaryngeal ventilation for an extended period of time can dry the membranes of the airway unless appropriate humidification is obtained.[122] Techniques or devices for humidification are available.[221]

One complication that may occur with needle cricothyrotomy but not surgical cricothyrotomy is kinking of the catheter as it enters the neck.[90, 177, 222] This problem can be overcome if a stiffer catheter is used. A 14-gauge (1¼ inch) catheter[150] or any device approximately 2 cm long from the hub or flange of the cannula[223] has been recommended as the best length because it puts the tip of the catheter in the middle or midstream of the airway.

Infection, ranging from cellulitis, perichondritis, or laryngotracheitis, is a possible complication of percutaneous translaryngeal ventilation but has not been reported in most series.[57, 65, 136, 137, 224] Careful technique and follow-up care should help prevent these complications of infection and obstruction by blockage of the tube.

Damage to the laryngotracheal mucosa including necrotizing tracheobronchitis from percutaneous translaryngeal ventilation is a theoretic complication that has not been reported.[57, 65, 136, 137] Indeed, most studies[148, 183] have concluded that percutaneous translaryngeal ventilation or high-frequency jet ventilation may be "performed" without undue risk of tracheobronchial injury.[189]

Blockage or obstruction of the tube from bleeding[225] or from a mucus plug occurs infrequently, although such blockage can cause acute airway obstruction. Additional small holes near the tip of the catheter may help to prevent this problem.

A pneumatocyst caused by incorrect needle placement is a rare and benign complication and can be treated by aspiration with a needle.[226] Misplacement of the cannula can lead to tracheal, mediastinal, or esophageal perforation if the needle is advanced too far.[5, 149, 150] Other complications that occur with surgical cricothyrotomy could also occur with needle cricothyrotomy, such as damage to the laryngeal cartilage, which may cause dysphonia or voice changes.[126, 127]

CONCLUSION

Cricothyrotomy, whether surgical or needle, is a simple, reliable, rapid, and effective means of achieving airway control and ventilation. It has relatively few complications. The value of cricothyrotomy as a life-saving procedure in emergency situations has been clearly demonstrated and its usefulness has been well established in emergency care. It has also been well documented that both surgical cricothyrotomy and needle cricothyrotomy can be used for an extended period of time if ventilation factors are appropriately maintained. Likewise, cricothyrotomy has gained acceptance as an "elective" procedure for surgical access to the airway. In many instances, cricothyrotomy is the airway procedure of choice.

REFERENCES

1. Jackson RE: Basic cardiopulmonary resuscitation. In Tintinalli JE, Rothstein RJ, Krome RL (eds): Emergency Medicine—A Comprehensive Study Guide. New York, McGraw-Hill Book Co, 1985, pp 3–13.
2. Kettrick RG, Ludwig S. Resuscitation—pediatric basic and advanced life support. In Fleisher GR, Ludwig S (eds): Textbook of Pediatric Emergency Medicine. Baltimore, Williams & Wilkins, 1983, pp 1–30.
3. McIntyre KM: Standards for cardiopulmonary resuscitation and emergency cardiac care. JAMA 5:453, 1987.
4. Albarran-Sotelo R, Flint LS, Kelly KJ (eds): Introduction to the performance of CPR. In Healthcare Providers' Manual for Basic Life Support. Dallas, American Heart Association, 1988, pp 33–34.
5. Stewart RD: Field airway control for the trauma patient. In Campbell JE(ed): Basic Trauma Life Support. Englewood Cliffs, NJ, Prentice-Hall, Inc, 1988, pp 42–90.
6. Donegan J, Albarran-Soteto R, Jaffee AS, Paraskos JA (eds): Adjuncts for airway control, ventilation, and supplemental oxygen. Textbook of Advanced Cardiac Life Support. Dallas, American Heart Association, 1987, pp 27–44.
7. Karren KJ, Hafen BQ: Airway care and pulmonary resuscitation in first responder. Englewood, Colo, Morton Publishing Co, 1986, pp 56–57.
8. Yealy DM, Paris PM: Recent advances in airway management. Emerg Med Clin North Am 7:83, 1989.
9. Collicott PA, Aprahamian C, Carrico CJ, et al: Upper airway management. In Advanced Trauma Life Support Course. Chicago, American College of Surgeons, 1984, pp 155–161.
10. Weymuller EA Jr, Partlow RC: Emergencies of the ear, facial structures, and upper airway. In Wilkins EW, Dineen JJ, Moncure AC (eds): MGH Textbook of Emergency Medicine. Baltimore, Williams & Wilkins, 1981, pp 625–657.
11. Edgerton MT: Emergency care of maxillofacial injuries. In Zuidema GD, Rutherford RB, Ballinger WF (eds): The Management of Trauma. Philadelphia, WB Saunders Co, 1979, pp 285–292.
12. Kastendieck J: Airway management. In Rosen P, Baker FJ, Braen GR, et al (eds): Emergency Medicine: Concepts and Clinical Practice. St. Louis, CV Mosby Co., 1983, pp 26–53.
13. Danzl DF: Advanced airway support. In Tintinalli JE, Rothstein RJ, Krome RL (eds): Emergency Medicine—A Comprehensive Study Guide. New York, McGraw-Hill Book Co, 1985, pp 20–31.
14. McVay CB: Anterior regions of the neck. In Surgical Anatomy. Philadelphia, WB Saunders Co, 1984, pp 253–272.
15. Romanes GJ: The larynx. In Cunningham's Manual of Practical Anatomy: Head and Neck and Brain. Vol. 3. London, Oxford University Press, 1972, pp 168–171.

16. Grant JCB: Head and neck—larynx. In An Atlas of Anatomy. Baltimore, Williams & Wilkins, 1972, p 621.
17. Gray H: Surface and topographical anatomy—the neck, and the respiratory system—the larynx. In Gross CM (ed): Anatomy of the Human Body. Philadelphia, Lea & Febiger, 1963, pp 69 and 1176.
18. DeWeese DD, Saunders WH: The larynx—anatomy, physiology, paralysis. In Textbook of Otolaryngology. St. Louis, CV Mosby Co, 1973, pp 91–99.
19. Stillman, RM, Sawyer PN: Cricothyroidotomy. In Surgical Resident's Manual. New York, Appleton-Century-Crofts, 1982, pp 102–104.
20. Wright D: Tracheostomy and laryngotomy. In Ballantyne J (ed): Operative Surgery—Fundamental Techniques: Nose and Throat. London, Butterworths, 1981, pp 246–248.
21. Clinton JE, Ruis E: Emergency airway management procedures. In Roberts JR, Hedges J (eds): Clinical Procedures in Emergency Medicine. WB Saunders Co, 1985, pp 2–29.
22. Yearly DM: Surgical methods of emergency airway control. Emergency Care Quart 3:11, 1987.
23. Albarran-Sotelo R, Flint LS, Kelly KJ (eds): Techniques of CPR—airway. In Health Care Providers Manual for Basic Life Support. Dallas, American Heart Association, 1988, pp 35–38.
24. Hafen BQ, Karren KJ: Respiratory emergencies. In Prehospital Emergency Care and Crisis Intervention. Engelwood, Colo, Morton Publishing Co, 1986, p 88.
25. Eisenberg MS, Bergner L, Hallstrom A: Cardiac resuscitation in the community. Importance of rapid provision and implications from program planning. JAMA 241:1905, 1979.
26. Mitchell SA: Cricothyroidostomy revisited. Ear Nose Throat 58:214, 1979.
27. Hudson GC: Handbook on Tracheostomy Care. Kent, England, Portex Ltd, 1972, pp 1–32.
28. Brady M: History of tracheostomy. Nursing Times 1548, 1966.
29. Herholdt JD, Rohn CG: Lifesaving Measures for Drowning Person. Copenhagen, H Tikiob, 1796.
30. Marx R: A medical profile of George Washington. American Heritage, August 1955, p 43.
31. Colles CJ: On stenosis of the trachea after tracheostomy for croup, diptheria. Ann Surg 3:499, 1886.
32. Hupp FL: Tracheotomy: A new retractor and tube pilot for the emergency operation. Surg Gynecol Obstet 19:67, 1914.
33. Upham JB: Report of a case of an incised wound of the throat resulting in closure of the larynx by cicatrix. New Hampshire J Med 2:206,1852.
34. Jackson C: Tracheotomy. Laryngoscope 18:285, 1909.
35. Jackson C: High tracheotomy and other errors the chief causes of chronic laryngeal stenosis. Surg Gynecol Obstet 32:392, 1921.
36. Brantigan CO, Grow JB: Cricothyroidotomy: Elective use in respiratory problems requiring tracheotomy. J Thorac Cardiovasc Surg 71:72, 1976.
37. Toye FJ, Weinsten JD: Clinical experience with percutaneous tracheostomy and cricothyrotomy in 100 patients. J Trauma 26:1034, 1986.
38. Brantigan CO: Emergency cricothyrotomy. In Roberts JR, Hedges J (eds): Clinical Procedures in Emergency Medicine. Philadelphia, WB Saunders, 1985, pp 123–132.
39. Schechter WP, Wilson RS: Management of airway obstruction in the intensive care unit. Crit Care Med 9:577, 1981.
40. Morain WD: Cricothyrotomy in head and neck surgery. Plast Reconstr Surg 65:424, 1980.
41. Boyd AD, Conlan AA: Emergency cricothyrotomy: Is its use justified? Surg Rounds 2;19, 1979.
42. Boyd AD, Ronita MC, Conlan AA: A clinical evaluation of cricothyrotomy. Surg Gynecol Obstet 149:365, 1979.
43. Greissy H, Quarntromo, Willen R: Elective cricothyrotomy: A clinical and histopathological study. Crit Care Med 10:387, 1982.
44. Habel DW: Cricothyroidostomy as a site for elective tracheostomy. Trans Pacific Coast Otolaryngol Soc Annual Meeting 58:181, 1977.
45. Romita MC, Colvin SB, Boyd AD: Cricothyroidotomy: Its healing and complications. Surg Forum 28:174, 1977.
46. Caparosa RJ, Zavatsky AR: Practical aspects of the cricothyroid space. Laryngoscope 67:577, 1957.
47. Carter DR, Meyers AD: The anatomy of the subglottic larynx. Otolaryngology (Rochester) 86:279, 1979.
48. Kirchner JA: Cricothyroidotomy and subglottic stenosis. Plast Reconstr Surg 68:828, 1979.
49. Safar P, Penninckx J: Cricothyroid membrane puncture with a special cannula. Anesthesiology 28:943, 1967.
50. Gold MI, Buechel DR: Translaryngeal anesthesia: A review. Anesthesiology 20:181, 1959.
51. Love JT: Embryology and anatomy. In Bluestone CD, Stool SE (eds): Pediatric Otolaryngology. Philadelphia, WB Saunders Co, 1983, p 59.
52. Kress TD, Balasubramaniam S: Cricothyroidotomy. Ann Emerg Med 11:197, 1982.
53. Snell RS: Atlas of Clinical Anatomy. Boston, Little, Brown & Co, 1978, p 390.
54. Clemente CD: Anatomy—A Region Atlas of the Human Body. 2nd ed. Baltimore, Urban and Schwarsenberg, Inc, 1981.
55. Mitchell SA: Airway obstruction: Surgical intervention. Hospital Medicine, April 1988, pp 49–68.
56. Mace SE: Cricothyrotomy. J Emerg Med 6:309, 1988.
57. McGill J, Clinton JE, Ruiz E: Cricothyrotomy in the emergency department. Ann Emerg Med 11:197, 1982.
58. Narrod JA, Moore EE, Rosen P: Emergency cricothyrostomy—technique and anatomical considerations. J Emerg Med 2:443, 1985.
59. Simon RR, Brenner BE: Airway procedures. In Procedures and Techniques in Emergency Medicine. Baltimore, Williams & Wilkins, 1982, pp 30–82.
60. Roven AN, Clapham MC: Cricothyroidotomy. Ear Nose Throat J 62:68, 1983.
61. Jacobson S.: Upper airway obstruction. Emerg Med Clin North Am 7: 205, 1989.
62. Tintinalli JE, Claffey J: Complication of nasotracheal intubation. Ann Emerg Med 10:142, 1981.
63. Salem MR, Mathrubhutham M, Bennett EJ: Difficult intubation. New Engl J Med 293:879, 1976.
64. Guiffrida JG, Levowitz BS, Boyd AD, Jacobson S: Four ways to open an airway. Emerg Med January 15, 1980, pp 27–36.
65. Miklus RM, Elliott C, Snow N: Surgical cricothyrotomy in the field: Experience of a helicopter transport team. J Trauma 29:506, 1989.
66. Dailey RH: Acute upper airway obstruction. Emerg Med Clin North Am 1:261, 1983.
67. Smith RG, Parker TJ, Anderson TA: Noninfectious acute upper airway obstruction. J Oral Maxillofac Surg 45:701, 1987.
68. DeWeese D, Saunders WA: Tracheotomy. In Textbook of Otolaryngology. St. Louis, CV Mosby Co, 1982.
69. Barratt GE, Coulthard SW: Acute upper airway obstruction—diagnosis and management options. Contemp Anesth Pract 9:73, 1987.
70. Sarant G: Acute epiglottitis in adults. Ann Emerg Med 10:1, 1981.
71. Danzl DF, Thomas DM: Nasotracheal intubations in the emergency department. Crit Care Med 8:677, 1980.
72. Iverson KV: Blind nasotracheal intubation. Ann Emerg Med 10:468, 1981.
73. Ignelsji RJ, Vander Ark GD: Analysis of the treatment of basilar skull fractures with and without antibiotics. Neurosurg 43:819, 1975.
74. Bouzarth WF: Intracranial nasogastric tube insertion (editorial). Trauma 18:819, 1978.
75. Hockberger RS, Doris PE: Spinal injury. In Rosen P, Baker FJ, Braen GR, et al (eds): Emergency Medicine Concepts and Clinical Practice. St. Louis, CV Mosby Co, 1983, pp 289–330.
76. Cloward RB: Acute cervical spine injuries. Clin Symp 32:1, 1980.
77. Sarant G, Chipman C: Early management of cervical spine injuries. Postgrad Med J 71:164, 1982.
78. Thal ER, Ramenofsky ML, Aprahamian C, Brown R, et al: Initial assessment and management. In Advanced Trauma Life Support. Chicago, American College of Surgeons, 1989, p 13.
79. Dula DJ: Cervical spine injuries. In Kravis TC, Warner CG (eds). Emergency Medicine: A Comprehensive Review. Rockville, M, Aspen Systems Corp, 1983, p 625.
80. Sise MJ, Shackford SR, Cruickshank JC, et al. Cricothyroidostomy for long term tracheal access. Ann Surg 200:13, 1984.
81. Brantigan CO, Grow JB: Cricothyroidotomy revised again. Ear Nose Throat J 59:26, 1980.
82. McDowell DE: Cricothyroidostomy for airway access. South Med J 75:282, 1982.
83. Weymuller EA: Cricothyroidotomy (letter). Ann Otol Rhinol Laryngol 91:670, 1982.
84. Najarian JS, Delaney JP: Emergency Surgery. Chicago, Year Book Medical Publishers Inc, 1984, p 260.
85. Layman PR: Transtracheal ventilation in oral surgery. Annals of Surgery (England) 65:318, 1983.
86. Ravissin P, Freeman J: A new transtracheal catheter for ventilation and resuscitation. Can Anaesth Soc J 32:60, 1985.
87. Layman PR: Bypassing an airway problem. Anaesthesia 38:478, 1983.
88. Barham CJ: Difficult intubation. Bolliere's Clin Anesthesiol 1:779, 1987.
89. Monnier PH, Ravussin P, Savary M, Freeman J: Percutaneous transtracheal ventilation for laser endoscopic treatment of laryngeal and subglottic lesions. Clin Otolaryngol 13:209, 1988.
90. Behrendt RE, Kidwell KG, Rund DA: Surgical and needle airways. Am J Emerg Med 2:474, 1984.
91. Esses BA, Jofek BW: Cricothyroidotomy: A decade of experience in Denver. Ann Otol Rhinol Laryngol 96:519, 1987.
92. Kennedy TL: Epiglottic reconstruction of laryngeal stenosis secondary to cricothyroidostomy. Laryngoscope 90:1130, 1980.
93. Montagano J, Passy V: Letter to the editor. Plast Reconstr Surg 67:98, 1981.
94. Donkle SK, Schuller DE, McClead RE: Risk factors for neonatal acquired subglottic stenosis. Ann Otol Rhinol Laryngol 95:626, 1986.
95. Hawkins DB: Pathogenesis of subglottic stenosis from endotracheal intubation. Ann Otol Rhinol Laryngol 96:116, 1987.
96. Marcovich M, et al: Subglottic stenosis in newborns after mechanical ventilation. Prog Pediatr Surg 21:8, 1987.
97. Lesser TH, et al: Laryngeal trauma vs. length of intubation. J Laryngol Otol 101:1165, 1987.
98. Weymuller EA Jr: Laryngeal injury from prolonged intubation. Laryngoscope 98(8, Pt 2, Suppl 45):1, 1988.
99. Brantigan CO: Cricothyroidotomy (letter to the editor). Laryngoscope 90:1980.

100. Orringer MB: Endotracheal intubation and tracheostomy indications, techniques, and complications. Surg Clin North Am 60:1447, 1980.
101. Deane RS, Shinosaki T, Morgan J: An evaluation of the cuff characteristics and laryngeal complications using a nasotracheal tube in prolonged intubations. J Trauma 17:311, 1977.
102. Volpi D, Lin PT, Kuriloff DB, et al: Risk factors for intubation injury of the larynx. Ann Otol Rhinol Laryngol 96:684, 1987.
103. Stauffer JL, Olsen DE, Petty TL: Complications of endotracheal intubation and tracheotomy. Am J Med 70:65, 1981.
104. Gillespie RW, Collicott PA: Airway management. Emerg Med 12(19):39, 1980.
105. Simon RR, Brenner BE: Emergency cricothyrotomy in the patient with massive neck swelling: Part I: Anatomical aspects. Crit Care Med 11:114, 1983.
106. Simon RR, Brenner BE, Rosen MA: Emergency cricothyrotomy in the patient with massive neck swelling. Part II: Clinical aspects. Crit Care Med 11:119, 1983.
107. Simon RR: Emergency tracheostomy in patients with massive neck swelling. Emerg Med Clin North Am 7:95, 1989.
108. Head JM: Tracheostomy in the management of respiratory problems. New Engl J Med 264:587, 1961.
109. Meade JW: Tracheotomy — its complications and their management. New Engl J Med 265:519, 1962.
110. Mulder D, Rubesh J: Complications of tracheostomy. J Trauma 9:389, 1983.
111. Chew J, Cantrell R: Tracheostomy, complications and their management. Arch Otolaryngol 96:538, 1972.
112. Miller JD, Kopp JP: Complications of tracheostomy in neurosurgical patients. Surg Neurol 22:186, 1984.
113. Abelson L: Cricothryoidotomy vs. tracheotomy. Laryngoscope 98:1358, 1988.
114. Cole RR, Aguilar EA: Cricothyroidotomy vs. tracheotomy: An otolaryngologist's perspective. Largyngoscope 98:131, 1988.
115. Menn SJ: Airway management. In Kravis TC, Warner CG (eds): Emergency Medicine. A Comprehensive Review. Rockville, Md, Aspen Systems Corp, 1983, pp 821–830.
116. Montgomery WW, Fabian RL, et al: Fundamental otolaryngologic procedures. In Schwartz GR, Safar P Stone JH, et al (eds): Principles and Practice of Emergency Medicine. Philadelphia, WB Saunders Co, l978, pp 419–425.
117. Little CM, Parker MG, Tarnopolsky R: Modification of cricothyroidostomy. Ann Emerg Med 15:1254, 1986.
118. Little CM, Parker MG, Tarnopolsky R: The incidence of vasculature at risk during cricothyroidostomy. Ann Emerg Med 15:805, 1986.
119. Caroline NL: Emergency Care in the Streets. 2nd ed. Boston, Little, Brown & Co, 1983, p 227.
120. Donald PJ, Bernstein L: Subglottic hemorrhage following translaryngeal needle aspiration. Arch Otolaryngol 101:395, 1975.
121. Schillaci RF, Jacovoni VE, Conte RS: Transtracheal aspiration complicated by fatal endotracheal hemorrhage. N Engl J Med 295: 488, 1976.
122. Holt GR, Davis WE, Ailor EI, et al: Massive airway hemorrhage after transtracheal aspiration. South Med J 71:325, 1978.
123. Brantigan CO: Delayed major vessel hemorrhage following tracheostomy. J Trauma 13: 235, 1973.
124. Oshinsky AE, Rubin JS, Gwozdz CS: The anatomical basis for post tracheotomy innominate artery rupture. Laryngoscope 98:1061, 1988.
125. Stock MC. et al: Perioperative complications of elective tracheostomy in critically ill patients. Crit Care Med 14:861, 1986.
126. Gleeson MJ, Pearson RC, Armistead S, et al: Voice changes following cricothyrotomy. J Laryngol Otol 98:1015, 1984.
127. Nash M: Swallowing problems in the tracheotomised patient. Otolaryngol Clin North Am 21:701, 1988.
128. Astrachan DL, Kirchner JC, Goodwin WJ, Jr: Prolonged intubation vs tracheotomy: Complications practical and psychological considerations. Laryngoscope 98:1165, 1988.
129. Kuriloff DB, et al: Laryngotracheal injury following cricothyroidotomy. Laryngoscope 99:125, 1989.
130. Joshi VV, Mandavia SG, Stern L, et al: Acute lesions induced by endotracheal intubation. Am J Dis Child 124:632, 1972.
131. Koopman CF Jr, Feld RA, Coulthard SW: The effects of cricoid cartilage injury and antibiotics in cricothyrotomy. Am J Otolaryngol 2:282, 1981.
132. Brantigan CO, Grow JB Sr: Subglottic stenosis after cricothyroidotomy. Surgery 91: 217, 1982.
133. Hawkins DB: Glottic and subglottic stenosis from endotracheal intubation. Laryngoscope 87:339, 1977
134. Lofgren LA: Treatment of severe subglottic stenosis in children with the CO_2 laser—a preliminary report on a few successful cases. Acta Otolaryngol Suppl (Stockh) 449:101, 1988.
135. O'Connor JV, Reddy K, Ergen MA, Griepp RB. Cricothyroidotomy for prolonged ventilatory support after cardiac operations. Ann Thorac Surg 39:353, 1985.
136. Erlandson MJ, Clinton JE, Ruis E, Cohen J: Cricothyrotomy in the emergency department revisited. J Emerg Med 7:115, 1989.
137. vanHassett EJ, Bruining HA, Hoeve LJ: Elective cricothyrotomy. Intensive Care Med 11:207, 1985.
138. Kalinske RW, Parker RH, Brandt D, et al: Diagnostic usefulness and safety of transtracheal aspiration. New Engl Med 276:604, 1967.
139. Pecora DV: A comparison of transtracheal aspiration with other methods of determining the bacterial flora of the lower respiratory tract. New Engl J Med 269:664, 1963.
140. Ries K, Levison ME, Kaye D: Transtracheal aspiration in pulmonary infection. Arch Intern Med 133:453, 1974.
141. Gold MI, Buechal DR: Translaryngeal anesthesia: A review. Anesthesiology 20:181, 1959.
142. Matthews HR, Hopkinson RB: Treatment of sputum retention by minitracheotomy. Br J Surg 71:147, 1984.
143. Lyons CD, Garrett ME, Fourrier DG: Complications of percutaneous transtracheal procedures. Ann Otol Rhinol Laryngol 86:633, 1977.
144. Stewart RD: Manual translaryngeal jet ventilation. Emerg Med Clin North Am 7:155, 1989.
145. Reed JP, Kemph JP, Hamelberg HA, et al: Studies with transtracheal artificial respiration. Anesthesiology 15:28, 1954.
146. Jacoby JJ, Hamelberg W, Reed JP, et al. Simple method of artificial respiration. Am J Physiol 167:798, 1951.
147. Jacoby JJ, Hamelberg W, Ziegler CH, et al: Transtracheal resuscitation. JAMA 162:625, 1956.
148. Spoerel WE, Narayanana PS, Singh NP: Transtracheal ventilation. Br J Anaesth 43:932, 1971.
149. Neff CC, Pfister RC, Van Sonnenberg E: Percutaneous transtracheal ventilation: Experimental and practical aspects. J Trauma 23:84, 1983.
150. Dunlap LB: A modified simple device for the emergency administration of percutaneous transtracheal ventilation. JACEP 7:42, 1978.
151. Hooke R: Account of an experiment made by R. Hooke, of preserving animals alive by blowing through their lungs with bellows. Philos Trans R Soc Lond 2:539, 1667.
152. Meltzer SJ, Auer J: Continuous respiration without respiratory movement. J Exp Med 11:622, 1909.
153. Matthews HR, Fischer BJ, Smith BE, Hopkinson RB; Minitracheotomy, a new delivery system for jet ventilation. J Thorac Cardiovasc Surg 92:673, 1986.
154. Norton ML, Strong MS, Vaughan CW: Endotracheal intubation, venturi (jet) ventilation for laser microsurgery of the larynx. Ann Otol Rhinol Laryngol 85:656, 1976.
155. Sanders RD: Two ventilating attachments for bronchoscopies. Del Med J 39:170, 1967.
156. Toye FJ, Weinstein JD: A percutaneous tracheostomy device. Surgery 65:384, 1969.
157. Jacobs HB: Needle catheter brings oxygen to the trachea. JAMA: 222:1231, 1972.
158. Jacobs HB: Emergency percutaneous transtracheal catheter and ventilator. J Trauma 12:50, 1972.
159. Smith RB: Transtracheal ventilation during anesthesia. Anesth Analg 53:225, 1974.
160. Carden E, Becker G, Hamood H: An improved percutaneous jetting system for use during microlaryngeal operations. Am Anaesth Soc J 24:118, 1977.
161. Carden E, Ferguson GB: A new technique for microlaryngeal surgery in infants. Laryngoscopy 83:691, 1973.
162. Smith RB, MacMillan BB, Petroseak J, Pfaeffle IM: Transtracheal ventilation for laryngoscopy. Ann Otol Rhinol Laryngol 82:347, 1973.
163. Smith RB, Myers EN, Sherman H: Transtracheal ventilation in pediatric patients. Br J Anaesth 46:313, 1974.
164. Attia RR, et al: Transtracheal ventilation. JAMA 234:1152, 1975.
165. Smith RB, Schaer WB, Pfaeffle H: Percutaneous transtracheal ventilation for anesthesia: A review and report of complications. Can Anaesth Soc J 22:607, 1975.
166. Spoerel WE, Greenway RE: Technique of ventilation during endolaryngeal surgery under general anesthesia. Can Anaesth Soc J 20:369, 1973.
167. Carden E, Vest HR: Further advances in anesthetic techniques for microlaryngeal surgery. Anesth Analg 53:584, 1974.
168. Smith RB, Babinski M, Klain M, Pfaeffle H: Percutaneous transtracheal ventilation. JACEP 5:765, 1976.
169. Chakravarty K, Narayanan PS, Spoerel WE: Further studies on transtracheal ventilation. Br J Anaesth 45:733, 1973.
170. Hughes RK: Needle tracheostomy. Arch Surg 93:83, 1966.
171. Patel R: Systems for transtracheal ventilation (letter). Anesthesiology 59:165, 1983.
172. Delisser EA, Muravchick S: Emergency transtracheal ventilation (letter). Anesthesiology 55:606, 1981.
173. Gildar JS: A simple system for transtracheal ventilation (letter). Anesthesiology 58:106, 1983.
174. Scuderi PE, McLeskey CH, Comer PB: Emergency percutaneous transtracheal ventilation during anesthesia using readily available equipment. Anesth Analg 61:867, 1982.
175. Aye LS: Percutaneous transtracheal ventilation. Anesth Analg 62:619, 1983.
176. Smith RB, Cutaia F, Hoff BH, et al: Long term transtracheal high frequency ventilation in dogs. Crit Care Med 9:311, 1981.
177. Weymuller EA, et al: Management of difficult airway problems with percutaneous transtracheal ventilation. Ann Otol Rhinol Laryngol 96:34, 1987.
178. Patel KF, Hicks JN: Prevention of fire hazards associated with use of carbon dioxide laser. Anesth Analg 60:885, 1981.

179. Carden E, Becker G, Hamood H: Percutaneous transtracheal ventilation for anesthesia: A review and report of complications. Can Anaesth Soc J 22:607, 1975.
180. Klain M, Smith RB: High frequency percutaneous transtracheal jet ventilation. Crit Care Med 5:280, 1977.
181. Klain M, Miller M: High frequency ventilators, and methods of their use. Presented at Critical Care Medicine 20th Annual Symposium, Las Vegas, Nevada, 1982.
182. Klain M, Miller J, Kalla R: Emergency use of high frequency jet ventilation. Crit Care Med 9:160, 1981.
183. Rock JJ, Pfaeffle H, Smith RB, et al: High pressure jet insufflation used to prevent aspiration and its effect on the tracheal mucosal wall (abstract). Crit Care Med 4:135, 1976.
184. McLellan I, Gordon P, Khawaja S, et al: Percutaneous transtracheal high frequency jet ventilation as an aid to difficult intubation. Can J Anaesth 35:404, 1988.
185. Squires SJ, Frampton MC: The use of minitracheostomy and high frequency jet ventilation in the management of acute airway obstruction. J Laryngol Otol 100:1199, 1986.
186. Carden E, Crutchfield W: Anesthesia for microsurgery of the larynx (a new method). Can Anaesth Soc J 20:378, 1973.
187. Watanabe Y, Murakami S: The clinical value of high frequency jet ventilation in major airway reconstructive surgery. Scand J Thor Cardiovasc Surg 22:227, 1988.
188. Schur MS, Maccioli GA, Azizkhan RG, et al: High frequency jet ventilation in the management of congenital tracheal stenosis. Anesthesiology 68:952, 1988.
189. Kercsmar CM, Martin RJ, Chatburn RL, Carlow A: Bronchoscopic findings in infants treated with high frequency jet ventilation versus conventional ventilation. Pediatrics 82:884, 1988.
190. Yealy DM, Stewart RD, Kaptan RM: Myths and pitfalls in emergency translaryngeal ventilation: Correcting misimpressions. Ann Emerg Med 17:690, 1988.
191. Lewis GA, Hopkinson RB, Mathews HR: Minitracheostomy: A report of its use in intensive therapy. Anaesthesia 41:931, 1986.
192. Campbell CT, Harris RC, Cook MH, et al: A new device for emergency percutaneous transtracheal ventilation in partial and complete airway obstruction. Ann Emerg Med 17:927, 1988.
193. Frame SB, Timberlake GA, Kerstein MD, et al: Transtracheal needle catheter ventilation (TNCV) in complete airway obstruction—an animal model. Ann Emerg Med 18:127, 1989.
194. Frame SB, Simon JM, Kerstein MD, McSwain NE: Percutaneous transtracheal catheter ventilation (PTCV) in complete airway obstruction—a canine model. J Trauma 29(6):774, 1989.
195. Schaefer SD, et al: Acute management of laryngeal trauma update. Ann Otol Rhinol Laryngol 98:98, 1989.
196. Fitz Hugh GS, Wallenborn WA, McGavern F: Injuries of the larynx and cervical trauma. Ann Otol Rhinol Laryngol 71: 419, 1962.
197. Mace SE: Blunt laryngotracheal trauma: The recognition and management of the acute laryngeal fracture. Ann Emerg Med 15:836, 1986.
198. Trone TH, Schaefer SD, Carder HM: Trauma: A 13-year review. Otolaryngol Head Neck Surg 88:259, 1980.
199. Arcand P, Granger J: Pediatric tracheostomies: Changing trends. J Otolaryngol 17:121, 1988.
200. Balkany TJ, Rutherford RB, Narrod I, et al: The management of neck injuries. In Zuidema GD, Rutherford RB, Ballinger WF (eds): The Management of Trauma. Philadelphia, WB Saunders Co, 1978,pp 419–425.
201. Linscott MD, Horton WC: Management of upper airway obstruction. Otolaryngol Clin North Am 12:351, 1979.
202. Gordon B: Cricothyroidotomy. Emerg Digest, July 1980, p 1.
203. Corke C, Cransurck P: A Seldinger technique for minitracheostomy insertion. Anaesth Intensive Care 16:206, 1988.
204. Hart AM, Cashman JN, Baldock GJ, Dick JA: Minitracheostomy in the treatment of sputum retention. Intensive Care Med 13:81, 1987.
205. Ciaglia P, Firsching R, Syniec C: Elective percutaneous dilational tracheostomy: A new simple bedside procedure; preliminary report. Chest 87:715, 1985.
206. Schachner A, Ovil Y, Sidi J, et al: Percutaneous tracheostomy–a new method. Crit Care Med 17:1052, 1989.
207. Tran Y, Hedley R: Misplacement of a minitracheotomy tube (letter). Anaesthesia 42:783, 1987.
208. Weiss S. Evaluation of nu-trake (letter). Crit Care Med 15:1830, 1987.
209. Ravlo O, et al: A comparison between two emergency cricothyroidotomy instruments. Acta Anaesthesiol Scand 31:317, 1987.
210. Bjoraker DG, Kumar NB, Brown AC: Evaluation of an emergency cricothyrotomy instrument. Crit Care Med 15:157, 1987.
211. Ruhe DS, Williams GV, Proud GO: Emergency airway by cricothyroid puncture or tracheostomy. A comparative study of methods and instruments. Trans Am Acad Ophthalmol Otolaryngol 64:182, 1960.
212. Rone CA, et al: Studies in transtracheal ventilation catheter. Laryngoscope 92:1259, 1982.
213. Bougus TP, Cook CD: Pressure-flow characteristics of needles suggested for transtracheal resuscitation. New Engl J Med 262:311, 1960.
214. Jorden RC, Moore EE, Marx JA, et al: Percutaneous transtracheal ventilation in a canine model with an open thorax. Ann Emerg Med, 13:22, 1984.
215. Jorden RD, Moore EE, Marx JA, et al: A comparison of PTV and endotracheal ventilation in an acute trauma model. J Trauma 25:978, 1985.
216. Yealy DM, Plewa MC, JJ, et al: Aspiration during manual low frequency jet ventilation (abstract). Ann Emerg Med 18:458, 1985.
217. Spencer DC, Beaty HN: Complications of transtracheal aspiration. New Engl J Med 286:304, 1972.
218. Levinson MM, Scuderi PE, Gibson RL, et al: Emergency percutaneous transtracheal ventilation (PTV). JACEP 8:396, 1979.
219. Rosen P: A cautionary note about percutaneous translaryngeal ventilation (editorial). JACEP 5:812, 1976.
220. Jordan RC: Percutaneous transtracheal ventilation. Emerg Med Clin North Am 6:745, 1988.
221. Smith BE: The Penlon Bromsgrove high frequency jet ventilator for adult and paediatric use. A solution to the problem of humidification. Anaesthesia 40:790, 1985.
222. Dobbinson TL, Whalen J, Pelson DA, et al: Needle tracheostomy: A laboratory study. Anaesth Intensive Care 8:72, 1980.
223. Carlton DM, Zide MF: An easily constructed cricothyroidotomy device for emergency airway management. J Oral Surg 38:623, 1980.
224. Adriani J: Complications following transtracheal anesthesia. Am J Surg 84:11, 1952.
225. Letter: Complications of transtracheal aspiration. New Engl J Med 289:1094, 1973.
226. Carden E, Calcoterra TC, Lechtman A: Pneumatocele of the larynx: A complication of percutaneous translaryngeal ventilation. Anesth Analg 55:600, 1976.

Chapter **4**

Tracheotomy Care

Robert L. Katz

INTRODUCTION

Historically, tracheotomies have been performed since ancient times. The exact origin, though often attributed to Hippocrates, is uncertain. Throughout modern medicine, tracheotomy has proved to be a life-saving operation. It is primarily indicated to relieve upper airway obstruction, to provide mechanical access to the trachea and lower airway for respiratory assistance, and to assist with lower respiratory toilet. Appelbaum has categorized the conditions that may require tracheotomy into skeletal, neuromuscular, central nervous system, upper respiratory tract, pulmonary, and cardiovascular.[1]

Care of the tracheotomy begins before the surgical procedure. Judgments made by the operative surgeon before surgery contribute significantly to the ease or difficulty of tracheotomy care. The position and size of the incision, the amount of deep dissection, and the method of entering the trachea itself may either increase or decrease the extent of direct wound care required. The size and type of tracheotomy tube used, as well as the method of its attachment to the neck, are also significant factors.

Tracheotomy tubes are made of many materials, including metal, Silastic, Teflon, polyethylene, and rubber. They may be cuffed or uncuffed (Fig. 4–1). They may have a single lumen or an inner cannula (Fig. 4–2). It is important that the emergency physician recognize these options; however, the basic care of the tracheotomy itself is relatively independent of the type of tube used.

The key to optimal care is cleanliness, specifically, keeping the tracheotomy free of obstruction.

IMMEDIATE POSTOPERATIVE CARE

In the immediate postoperative period, high humidity must be provided. Humidity may be provided through a neck collar attached to a nebulizer or vaporizer or through a controlled environment, such as in a tent or steam room. *High humidity* is critical in maintaining liquefaction of the patient's mucus for adequate suctioning.

Suctioning of the tracheotomy tube should be done routinely, approximately every 1 to 2 hours in the immediate postoperative period, but it is gradually reduced according to each patient's needs. When suctioning, relatively sterile techniques should be used. The suction catheter should be introduced into the tracheotomy lumen by a gloved hand.

The size of the catheter used is dictated by the size of the tracheotomy tube; the largest size that can be passed without difficulty is best. When the catheter has been introduced into the trachea itself (it need not be introduced further), continual suction is applied and the catheter is slowly removed, aspirating the produced mucus (Fig. 4–3). When the catheter touches the tracheal mucosa, coughing may result. Unless excessive, or in the presence of increased intracranial pressure, coughing is desirable, because it not only brings mucus into the trachea for aspiration but also expands the distal alveoli, which may collapse in the absence of laryngeal resistance. Excessive stimulation, however, may abuse the tracheal mucosa as the catheter rubs against the tracheal wall during the coughing effort. Coughing can be suppressed by the instillation of a topical mucosal anesthetic such as 1 to 5 ml of 1 per cent lidocaine instilled with a 3-ml syringe. The suctioning should be repeated until the trachea has been cleared of secretions and as often as necessary to keep the airway clear. Prolonged suctioning may produce significant hypoxia, and short periods of suctioning (5 to 8 seconds) with oxygen supplementation in between are preferred.

In the infant with limited respiratory reserve, active support of respiration by Ambu bag or mechanical ventilator with supplemental oxygen is encouraged, particularly before and between suctioning efforts. A suction catheter (Neo-Cath, Pulmonary Medical Devices, Atlanta, Ga.) that can alternately provide oxygen or suctioning has been found helpful for reducing hypoxia and hyperoxia in neonates.[2]

Mucus plugs can often be softened for aspiration by the instillation of saline or acetylcysteine (Mucomyst) drops before suctioning. In individuals with bradycardic responses to suctioning, intravenous or nebulized atropine (0.05 mg/kg ideal body weight) may be helpful.[3] Further discussion of tracheal suctioning techniques is provided in Chapter 7.

The neck wound should be kept clean with hydrogen peroxide as needed. Antibiotic ointments can also be used.

During the first 24 to 48 hours following tracheotomy, careful and constant observation is required. It is during this period of time that the tracheotomy tube can most easily become dislodged or malpositioned. Early recognition of these abnormalities may be life saving to the patient. Cardiac and respiratory monitors should be used, and constant, attentive nursing care is mandatory.

CHANGING A TRACHEOTOMY TUBE [4]

When long-term tracheotomy care is required, the previously discussed philosophies hold true but are modified according to need. The degree of humidity required gradually lessens. Suctioning, though needed periodically, is often replaced by an effective cough, and long-term monitoring is rarely required except in children.

Once the tracheotomy wound has matured, generally at about 5 days, routine changing of the tracheotomy tubes (Fig. 4–4) can be carried out safely and *must* be done to clean them satisfactorily. Before changing the tracheotomy tube, the new tube should be carefully checked. One must be certain that all component parts fit together comfortably and that if a cuffed tube is being used, the integrity of the cuff under pressure is checked. Once this has been accomplished, the patient is placed in a controlled, comfortable position with the *neck hyperextended*, when possible. Adults may sit or lie down; however, children should be lying down and held firmly in the controlled position. Some patients may require soft hand restraints during the changing procedure.

The patient's tracheotomy tube should be removed in a single sweeping motion, and the new tube, which has been readied with the *obturator in position*, should be gently and immediately inserted into the stoma with the same sweeping circular motion. This is most easily accomplished by wetting or lubricating the tube slightly and inserting it during inspiration. There should be no force exerted, because creating false passages is deceptively easy and may prove to be disastrous.

Once the tracheotomy tube is in position, the obturator is removed and the inner cannula (if needed) is placed. Once inserted, the tracheotomy tube should be tied snugly around the patient's neck while the head is held in flexion. The physician should be certain that the tape is in direct approximation to the skin all around the neck and that nothing is intervening that when removed would result in loose tape

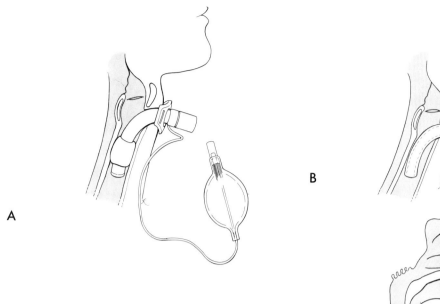

Figure 4–1. Tracheotomy tubes in place. *A,* Cuffed tracheotomy tube with the cuff inflated. *B,* A relatively large uncuffed tube. *C,* This smaller uncuffed tracheotomy tube permits the passage of air up through the vocal cords. If, during expiration, the patient's finger is placed over the tube, all expired air will pass through the vocal cords, permitting vocalization. (From Alperin K, Levine H, Grover M: Tracheostomy Care Manual. New York, Thieme-Stratton, Inc, 1982. Reproduced by permission.)

and possible extubation. The tape should be tied with a square knot and double checked when it is in place. If an inner cannula is being used, it should be removed and cleaned, usually with hydrogen peroxide, pipe cleaners, and small wire brushes, as often as necessary to keep it mucus free.

Note that the removable inner cannula is that portion of the tracheotomy tube that provides the actual airway. The advantage is that *only the inner cannula need be removed for periodic cleaning,* leaving the tube proper in place (see Fig. 4–2). The cleaning schedule will vary. In general the entire tube should be changed approximately every 1 to 2 weeks, and the inner cannula should be cleaned twice daily. If the tubes need to be changed and cleaned more often, this should be done to keep them mucus free and functioning optimally. The adult patient should actively participate in the home cleaning of the tracheotomy tube whenever possible to prevent obstruction. The physician should ascertain the patient's understanding of the cleaning procedure (using pad and pencil for communication if needed).

OBSTRUCTED TRACHEOTOMY TUBE

A tracheotomy patient who presents to the emergency physician with respiratory distress should be *assumed to have a plugged tracheotomy tube.* Such patients should immediately be placed on high-flow humidified oxygen, with the flow directed either at the tracheotomy tube or over the mouth, if appropriate. *The usual cause of obstruction is inspissated mucus,* which is commonly a problem in the winter because of the low humidity of inspired air. Obstruction usually occurs in the tracheotomy tube itself, although more distal tracheal plugging can also occur.

Immediate suctioning is appropriate in an attempt to clear the tracheotomy tube (see Fig. 4–3). Thin mucus may be suctioned easily but dried plugs in the trachea may be stubborn. If suctioning is not successful, 2 to 4 ml of sterile saline should be injected into the trachea and suctioning repeated. This loosens mucus and stimulates coughing, often enough to dislodge a large obstructing plug. If an inner cannula is present, it should be removed so it can be cleaned and obstructing plugs removed. If suctioning and removal of the inner cannula do not immediately clear the airway obstruction, the entire tracheotomy tube should be removed and replaced with a new tube. Hesitancy at total removal and changing of tubes may be a fatal mistake. In an emergency, *one should not hesitate to remove a tracheotomy tube,* because most patients are able to breathe easier through a stoma than through a partially blocked tube.

Occasionally a tracheotomized patient will present with severe shortness of breath that has no relationship to the tracheotomy tube or underlying *upper* respiratory tract disease. When the tube has been changed and the patient remains significantly short of breath, attention must be turned to an evaluation of cardiopulmonary status. A chest film, electrocardiogram, and arterial blood gases must be obtained immediately in search of the unexpected cardiac dysrhythmia, myocardial infarction, pulmonary embolism, pneumothorax, atelectasis, or pneumonia. Appropriate therapy should then be directed at the underlying cause. Recurrent cancer is an *uncommon* cause of acute dyspnea because the tip of the tracheotomy tube is usually well below the operative site (i.e., the larynx).

A tracheotomy patient may present with the tracheotomy tube in hand, stating that the tube came out, either during cleaning or coughing, and could not be replaced because the stoma was closing. It is important to note that

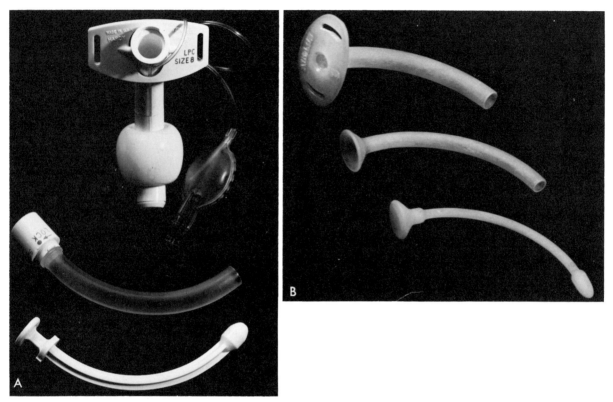

Figure 4–2. *A,* Cuffed tracheotomy tube with the cuff inflated. The tube has a translucent plastic inner cannula that can be removed for cleaning. An obturator, which is used only during insertion of the tracheotomy tube, is also illustrated. *B,* A plastic uncuffed tracheotomy tube with inner cannula and obturator. Some uncuffed tracheotomy tubes such as those designed by Jackson are made of metal. (From Alperin K, Levine H, Grover M: Tracheostomy Care Manual. New York, Thieme-Stratton, Inc, 1982. Reproduced by permission.)

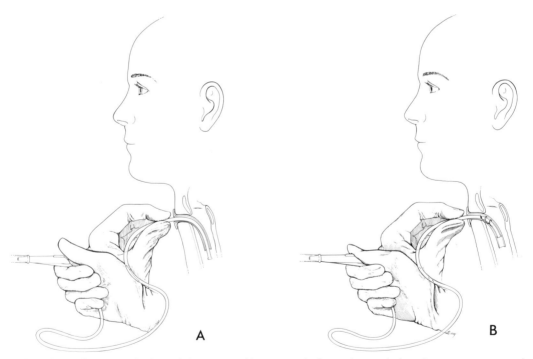

Figure 4–3. Suctioning of a tracheotomy tube is carried out as an aid to removal of secretions or is done in an emergency setting to evaluate the patency of a tracheotomy tube. *A,* The suction catheter is inserted only a short distance past the end of the tracheotomy tube. The thumb is kept off the hole in the suction catheter during placement. Suction is applied only during withdrawal. *B,* The suction catheter can be twisted during removal. Short periods of suctioning (5 to 8 seconds) with respiratory support and supplemental oxygen are necessary in infants and hypoxic adults. Instilling a few milliliters of sterile saline may loosen dried or thick mucus and facilitate suctioning significantly. *Note:* The leading cause of dyspnea in a patient with a tracheotomy tube is blockage of the tube with mucus. (From Alperin K, Levine H, Grover M: Tracheostomy Care Manual. New York, Thieme-Stratton, Inc, 1982. Reproduced by permission.)

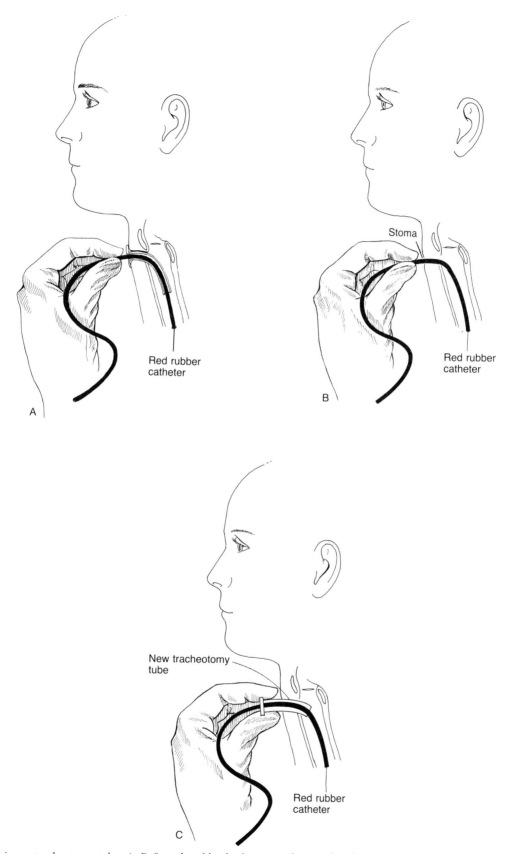

Figure 4–4. Changing a tracheotomy tube. *A,* Before the old tube is removed, a small red rubber catheter is passed into the proximal trachea. *B,* The tracheotomy tube has been removed over the catheter, and only the rubber catheter remains in the trachea. The catheter serves as a guide for easy and atraumatic insertion of a new tube. Note that the neck should be slightly hyperextended. *C,* A new tracheotomy tube is threaded over the guide catheter; once the tube is in place, the catheter is removed. Similarly, if the tracheotomy tube has already been removed, the catheter may be passed through the stoma before a new tube is advanced.

the stoma may close quite quickly, and even if the tube has been out for *only a few hours*, compromise of the stoma may have already begun. It is appropriate to accept the patient's judgment that the old tube will not fit. Forceful attempts to insert the tube may create false passages, bleeding, and traumatic edema, making reintubation almost impossible. The physician should resist the temptation to forcibly dilate the stoma with a hemostat. Although this may occasionally be successful, it often precipitates bleeding and compounds edema. The patient's tube should be inspected to identify its size, which can usually be found on the flange of the outer cannula. The sizes of tubes are designated by numbers progressing sequentially from 00 to 10, from smallest to largest. When the size of the patient's tube has been determined, a new tracheotomy tube one or two sizes smaller can generally be inserted with relative ease. *Care should be taken to avoid false passages.* The tube should be inserted with ease, not forced. Once the smaller tube has been inserted to maintain the trachea stoma, it may gradually be enlarged on a daily basis until the appropriate-sized maintenance tube can again be worn. In the emergency department, it is better to accept a patent airway with a smaller tube that can be enlarged on an elective basic than to cause problems with forceful attempts to insert an identical-sized tube.

A stressful situation can develop when a blocked tracheotomy tube has been removed and the proper passage for easy insertion of a new tube cannot be found. Often, simple extension of the neck will line up tissue planes and facilitate passage. If time permits, it is safer and certainly less stressful for the inexperienced physician to insert a small red rubber catheter into the tracheotomy tube for a short distance down the trachea before the old tracheotomy tube is removed (see Fig. 4–4). When the old tracheotomy tube is withdrawn, the catheter remains in the passage to serve as a guide for atraumatic insertion of a new tube. Once the new tube is in place, the catheter can be removed easily. If the tracheostomy tube has already been removed, as a safety precaution a catheter may also be placed in the stoma prior to advancing a new tube.

A flexible pediatric laryngoscope can, on occasion, be used to identify the lumen and the entrance into the trachea. In difficult situations, a tracheotomy tube can be introduced over the flexible laryngoscope. The appropriate-sized tracheotomy tube should be threaded over the laryngoscope before insertion of the scope into the stoma. The stenosed stoma should be carefully suctioned free of mucus. The laryngoscope can then be introduced into the stoma, and under direct observation, the tracheal lumen can be identified. Once the laryngoscope is comfortably in place within the trachea, the tracheotomy tube can be advanced over the laryngoscope, which functions as a lumen guide.

Bleeding at a tracheotomy site can be an annoying or a life-threatening problem. Minor bleeding is usually secondary to skin irritation or minor trauma. If the tube erodes into a blood vessel, bleeding is often from an arterial source and can be massive. Hemorrhage, can quickly produce hypovolemia or aspirated blood can asphyxiate the patient. Treatment includes volume replacement and control of the bleeding. Do not immediately remove the tracheotomy tube because it may be the best way to ensure a patent airway. Under good lighting and suction, the site is examined. Direct pressure may suffice or occasionally a vessel may be ligated or clamped. Bleeding may be tamponaded if the balloon of the tracheotomy tube is overinflated and traction is applied, the object being to compress the bleeding area from under the skin.

REFERENCES

1. Applebaum EL, Bruce DL: Tracheal Intubation. Philadelphia, WB Saunders Co, 1976.
2. Graff M, France, J, Hiatt, M, et al: Prevention of hypoxia and hyperoxia during endotracheal suctioning. Crit Care Med 15:1133, 1987.
3. Winston, SJ, Gravelyn, TR, Sitrin RG: Prevention of bradycardic responses to endotracheal suctioning by prior administration of nebulized atropine. Crit Care Med 15:1009, 1987.
4. Alperin K, Levine H, Grover M: Tracheostomy Care Manual. New York, Thieme-Stratton, Inc, 1982.

Chapter 5

Noninvasive Assessment and Delivery of Oxygen and Inhaled Medications

*Dan L. Field
and Jerris R. Hedges*

OVERVIEW

Ensuring delivery of oxygen to the cell is the primary critical action in emergency medicine. Without oxygen fueling cellular energy production, the cells ultimately falter and the organism dies. Except during cardiopulmonary bypass, tissue perfusion is dependent on an adequate inspired oxygen content, ventilatory effort, alveolar gas exchange, blood oxygen carrying capacity, and cardiac output. This chapter covers emergency department assessment of spontaneous ventilation and oxygen delivery, noninvasive means of improving inspired oxygen concentration, and delivery of inhalant medications for the treatment of reactive airway disease.

Respiratory illness has been poorly understood until recent times. The Talmud, the ancient lawbook of the Israelites, blames the etiology of asthma-like illness on a malignant spirit.[1] Later, Celsus (A.D. 25), an encyclopedist of the late Roman period, noted a favorable prognosis for a respiratory illness if the "expectoration is white as if mucus from the nose, but unfavorable if sputum is purulent, and accompanied by fever," descriptions that are consistent with chronic bronchitis and pneumonia. Celsus recommended bleeding, purgatives, emetics, and diuretics; this therapy was less preferable perhaps to his prescription for phthisis (tuberculosis), for which he recommended a leisurely sojourn down the Nile, drinking tea and honey.[1]

The Greek word ασθμα signified panting and was applied generally to difficult breathing and respiratory illness; the term eventually gave rise to the word *asthma*. The earliest comprehensive distinction between asthma and other respiratory diseases came from Aretaeus of Cappadocia, who first recognized and recorded the chronic recurrent nature of the disease.[9]

In 1698, Sir John Floyer wrote the first book devoted entirely to asthma and recorded the first description of pulsus paradoxus. Atropine therapy began in England in 1802, and in 1830 John Eberle deduced that "it is highly probable, therefore, that asthma

Table 5–1. Causes of Respiratory Failure*	
Neurologic	**Lower Airway**
Drug overdose	Tracheobronchitis
Stroke	Tracheal stenosis
Central hypoventilation	Bronchospasm
Guillain-Barré syndrome	
Head trauma	**Lung Parenchyma**
Poliomyelitis	Adult respiratory distress
Botulism	syndrome
	Emphysema
Muscles and Chest Wall	Pneumonia
Myopathy	Interstitial pneumonitis
Myasthenia gravis	
Kyphoscoliosis	**Heart**
Flail chest	Pulmonary edema
	Mitral stenosis
Oropharynx	
Foreign body	
Laryngospasm	
Tonsillar hypertrophy	

*Disease at any level of the respiratory system, central or peripheral nervous system, bellows mechanism, or heart may cause respiratory failure.

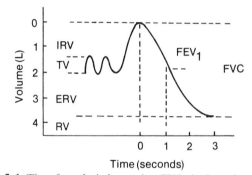

Figure 5–1. Time-forced vital capacity (FVC) is the volume of gas forcibly expelled following a maximal inspiration. Forced expiratory volume in 1 second (FEV_1) is the volume of gas expelled during the first second of the forced expiration. The other lung volumes obtainable are the tidal volume (TV), which is the volume of gas moved during quiet respiration; the inspiratory reserve volume (IRV), which is the volume of gas that can be inspired in addition to the tidal gas volume; and the expiratory reserve volume (ERV), which is the volume of gas that can be forcibly expired at the end of a tidal expiration. Some gas cannot be expired and remains in the chest. This is known as the residual volume (RV).

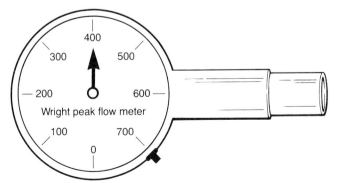

Figure 5–2. Wright peak flow meter. After resetting the dial to zero, the patient inhales fully and exhales forcefully through the disposable paper mouthpiece. The best of three attempts is recorded. A tight seal of the lips around the mouthpiece is required.

consists essentially in a peculiar irritation of the pneumo-gastric nerves (vagus), in consequence of which the smaller bronchial tubes and air-cells are thrown into a state of spasmodic constriction."[3] The American Thoracic Society statement on asthma in 1962 is an often-quoted definition of the disease: asthma is a disease characterized by an increased responsiveness of the trachea and bronchi to various stimuli and manifested by a widespread narrowing of the airways that changes in severity either spontaneously or as a result of therapy. The term *asthma* is not appropriate for bronchial narrowing, which results solely from widespread bronchial infection; from destructive diseases of the lung, as in pulmonary emphysema, or from cardiovascular disorders.

A national study carried out in 1975 reported that asthma was the most common chronic disease of childhood and among the most frequent complaints of adults, resulting in 2 million outpatient visits; it was also the most common cause of absence from school and work.[4] Although asthma is said to affect 3 to 4 per cent of the United States population, chronic obstructive pulmonary diseases afflict up to 15 per cent of adults, with similar economic consequences.[5] Although many investigators and studies distinguish between asthma (pure reactive airway disease) and chronic obstructive pulmonary diseases, which include chronic bronchitis (airway inflammation with increased mucus secretion) and emphysema (airway destruction and loss of airway elasticity), clinically the distinction is blurred by the similarities in emergency department management. In fact, the current literature cites studies that can document little to distinguish the response of either entity to bronchodilators.[6] These diseases must, however, be separated from other causes of dyspnea and respiratory distress (Table 5–1), many of which are associated with wheezing.

PULMONARY FUNCTION TESTING

Introduction

Airway maintenance and breathing are given primacy in the ABC's of emergency medicine. Clinical assessment always begins with the patient's ventilatory function. The physician notes quickly the patient's mental status, level of distress, skin color, character of effort, use of accessory muscles, presence of diaphoresis, lung sounds, and vital signs. In conjunction with this clinical overview, a brief clinical history provides the physician with sufficient information on which to initiate therapy. Unfortunately, the physician's initial clinical impression of the patient's ventilatory status is based on imprecise subjective findings that may not detect all seriously ill patients. For instance, one study reported that in patients with reactive airway disease, the ability of experienced physicians to detect compromised pulmonary function when compared with that of pulmonary function testing was only moderately better than chance alone.[7] The sensitivity of clinical impression did not improve when the clinicians underwent a training period that provided instruction on common and more subtle signs of respiratory distress. Patients were superior to physicians in predicting their own pulmonary function, with a correlation coefficient of 0.86 compared with a predicted physician correlation coefficient of 0.66. Patients were also better at assessing day-to-day variation in disease, using pulmonary function testing as the "gold standard."[8]

Regardless of the initial clinical presentation, a subjectively asymptomatic patient with reactive airway disease will attain after treatment at best only 40 to 50 per cent of predicted normal pulmonary function and 60 to 70 per cent when all abnormal physical signs have resolved.[9,10] This potentially undetected degree of dysfunction may contribute to recrudescence. Objective measures of pulmonary dysfunction are desirable both to quantify results of therapy and as possible predictors of admission.

Spirometry has been used for decades by pulmonary specialists to assess airway limitation. The spirometric measurements were originally validated based on comparisons with clinical and body plethysmographic data. The terminology of pulmonary function testing was derived from the various measured subsegments of spirometry (Fig. 5–1). More recently electronic meters, which are hand-held, less expensive, and much easier to use, have replaced formal spirometry in many clinical settings.[11,12] These relatively inexpensive devices frequently measure or calculate the peak expiratory flow rate (PEFR), forced expiratory volume in 1 second

(FEV₁), forced vital capacity (FVC), and per cent FEV₁/FVC. The Wright peak flow meter (Fig. 5–2) was originally designed by Wright and McKerrow for use in their pneumoconiosis unit in 1959. Subsequently, development of the mini-Wright peak flow meter (Fig. 5–3), both a less complex and less expensive plastic device, allowed for widespread use in acute care settings.[13] In the acute clinical situation, PEFR meter readings correlate well with formal spirometry, offer simplicity, and reduce the need for patient cooperation.[14]

Indications and Contraindications

In the emergency department, acute respiratory diseases such as asthma and chronic lung diseases that have been exacerbated make up the bulk of the situations requiring the objective assessment of ventilatory status. Because of the insensitivity of the physical examination, emergency department pulmonary function testing with either the peak flow meter or spirometer has become commonplace for assessing pulmonary status and patient response to therapy.[10, 15, 16] These tests may facilitate patient transfer at the time of admission by providing an objective and reproducible measure of the patient's failure to improve. Studies have found excellent correlation between PEFR and FEV₁[16] as well as between Wright and mini-Wright meters.[17] Although opportunities will be infrequent, physicians evaluating neuromuscular diseases that affect ventilatory function, such as the Guillain-Barré syndrome, may find these techniques useful in both initial and ongoing assessment. Near respiratory arrest may be the only true contraindication to seeking the measurements discussed earlier because of the limited patient cooperation and the incumbent time delay.

Equipment

A *spirometer* is a tube connected to a bellows-type device having communication with a recording device. The subject breathes in and out through an orifice, causing expansion and contraction of the bellows, which in turn activates the recorder that traces a curve corresponding to the lung volume. This traditional volume method is complex and cumbersome.[12] Hand-held electronic spirometers now available use sensing devices either to translate the pressure of exhalation (e.g., Respiradyne, Fig. 5–4) or to detect the number of rotations of a small turbine (e.g., Pocket Spirometer, Micro Medical Instruments, Rochester, NY) by an optical system. Both systems are self-calibrating, take little practice to use, and can calculate PEFR, FEV₁, and FVC. Some systems, such as the transducer-based Respiradyne, may also give additional calculated information such as per cent FEV₁/FVC and forced midexpiratory flow rate (FEF₂₅₋₇₅%). Results are displayed digitally and maintained in memory until cleared.

Peak flow meters are simple mechanical devices that use the force of exhalation to rotate or push a membrane-

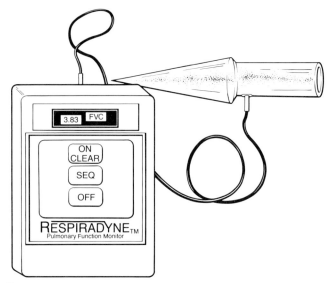

Figure 5–4. The Respiradyne portable spirometer. The device is turned on or "cleared" from the last effort. The patient exhales forcefully into the hand-held mouthpiece following maximal inhalation. The "sequence" button permits selection of the desired spirometry measurements. The best of several tries should be recorded.

coupled measuring arm to statically record a position of maximum flow. Low-flow units designed for children exist for both the Wright and mini-Wright instruments.

Procedure

The operation of peak flow meters and electronic spirometers is similar in many ways. Disposable mouthpieces are inserted or attached. The electronic devices must be switched on for a 30-second self-calibration period. Both the hand-held spirometers and the peak flow meters can be operated with the same respiratory maneuver—a maximal inhalation followed by a maximum forced expiration into the mouthpiece. Three attempts are standard, and the highest value is recorded. Children as young as 3 years of age have consistently achieved the level of cooperation necessary to perform PEFR testing.[13]

Interpretation

One adult study investigating the use of PEFR measurements to predict the need for admission early in the emergency department treatment found that in patients previously noted to be severely compromised, with initial PEFRs less than 16 per cent of the predicted value, an improvement of less than 16 per cent of predicted value (or improvement in PEFR less than 60 liters per minute) after the first epinephrine treatment indicated the need for admission.[18] Nowak and colleagues similarly found an initial FEV₁ ≤ 0.6 liter and a posttreatment FEV₁ ≤ 1.6 liters to be predictive of the need for inpatient therapy.[19] Nowak and coworkers found similar FEV₁ values and PEFR values of less than 100 liters per minute initially and less than 300 liters per minute after treatment as predictive of the need for inpatient therapy in a follow-up study.[16] These studies have been criticized because the admitting physician was not blinded to the results of the pulmonary function tests. A subsequent study found that neither the initial PEFR reading nor the percentage response to the first bronchodilator treatment

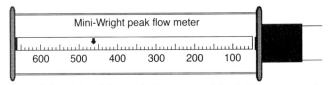

Figure 5–3. Mini-Wright peak flow meter. The indicator arrow is moved back to zero. The patient inhales fully and then exhales forcefully through the disposable paper mouthpiece. The best of three attempts is recorded. Patient cooperation and a tight seal of the lips around the mouthpiece are required.

was helpful in predicting admission.[20] In fact, in this double-blind study, with strict admission criteria and with the additional use of nebulized bronchodilators, less than 50 per cent of those requiring admission were detected by initial measurements. However, measurements performed later in therapy, just before release, were more accurate in predicting relapse.[20]

An examination of pediatric asthmatic patients using initial spirometric and clinical values found that although the initial spirometric values correlated with admission, there were many false positives.[21] Furthermore, the initial spirometric values were unable to identify from among a group of children released from the emergency department who would relapse. Another pediatric study found that PEFR correlated with admission but also had a poor predictive value.[22]

These studies indicate that when initial flow rates are very poor, admission is likely. In patients with decreased flow rates, the response to therapy (which is dependent in part on the therapy and the duration of the therapy chosen) is more important. Prediction of the need for admission based on PEFR and FEV_1 values obtained shortly after presentation is largely unsuccessful because of patient variability in response to bronchodilator therapy.[10, 16] Also previous studies used treatment protocols based on multidose subcutaneous epinephrine and failed to account for delayed clinical improvement found with the prolonged polydrug approach common today. Studies correlating current post-therapeutic pulmonary function with clinical outcome are needed to guide admission decisions more accurately.

Nonetheless, initially low flow rates (PEFR <100 liters per minute) and spirometry values (FEV_1 < 1.0 liter) identify sick patients with the potential need for admission or close follow-up. In the setting of upper airway obstruction, severe airway impairment is suggested when a patient has a PEFR less than 100 liters per minute and the lack of response may indicate the need for intubation or a surgical airway. The chief value of these measurements in the emergency department appears to be for monitoring and documenting response to bronchodilator therapy. In particular, these measurements aid in the transfer of clinical information to the care team at the point of admission to the hospital. Furthermore, one can reserve blood gas analysis for patients with poor initial flow measurements or lack of improvement in pulmonary function and hence reduce the expense and morbidity of evaluation for reactive airway disease.[23, 24]

There has been some disagreement over which test is best for assessment of pulmonary function, but most investigators believe that PEFR measurements are functionally equivalent to the newer hand-held forms of spirometric evaluation.[11, 12, 14] Table 5–2 lists approximate peak flow and spirometry values for various degrees of obstruction.

Table 5–2. Approximate Values for Spirometry and Peak Flow for Various Degrees of Obstruction in Adults

	FEV_1 (L)	FEV_1/FVC (%)	Peak Flow (L/min)
Normal	4.0–6.0	80–90	550–650 males 400–500 females
Mild	3.0	70	300–400
Moderate	1.6	50	200–300
Severe	0.6	40	100

Peak flow and spirometry values vary with height, sex, and distance above sea level; men and taller persons in general have larger flow rates. The reduced barometric pressures found at higher elevations also increase airflow.

ASSESSMENT OF OXYGENATION

Introduction

Adequate tissue perfusion with oxygen-enriched blood is the primary goal of resuscitation. There are several objective means of assessing blood oxygenation in the emergency department. The familiar arterial blood gases (ABG) analysis (see Chapters 6 and 19) is the standard to which other methods are compared. Recent technical advances have made noninvasive techniques promising alternatives (Table 5–3).

Transcutaneous and Transconjunctival Oxygen Monitoring

BACKGROUND

The partial pressure of oxygen tension in blood that perfuses the skin was first linked to levels at the body surface in 1851.[25] A century later, Baumberger and Goodfriend estimated arterial oxygen tension by measuring the oxygen tension in a buffer solution surrounding an immersed finger.[26] Modern measurement of oxygen tension by blood gas machines and noninvasive oxygen monitors uses a modification of Clark's membrane-covered electrode.[27] The electrodes are created by layering a thin film of potassium chloride over a silver chloride anode set between a polyethylene membrane and a platinum cathode disk. An external power source provides a negative potential to the platinum electrode, thus reducing all oxygen molecules diffusing through the polyethylene membrane. While varying the potential of the electrode, the current is measured to determine the oxygen content of a test sample. Refinements of the electrode principle for measuring oxygen tension have permitted the development of similar electrodes for the measurement of blood carbon dioxide tension and pH. Both transcutaneous ($P_{tc}O_2$) and transconjunctival ($P_{cj}O_2$) oxygen monitoring use modified versions of the Clark electrode to measure oxygen diffusing through tissue.[27]

$P_{tc}O_2$ was originally developed by the National Aeronautics and Space Administration to monitor the tissue oxygenation of astronauts who may become ill or injured in an environment in which conventional invasive assessment may be difficult or unavailable. The technique requires heating the skin site to 45° C to liquefy the underlying stratum corneum, permitting the diffusion of oxygen to the sensor, followed by 5 to 10 minutes for device stabilization. The electrode can be used on most keratinized skin surfaces; the anterior chest and arms are common sites. Heating induces variations in local oxygen metabolism, a rightward shift of the oxyhemoglobin dissociation curve, and local perfusion changes. $P_{tc}O_2$ reflects local tissue oxygen tension and hence is sensitive to tissue perfusion. When perfusion is inadequate, additional oxygen consumption will occur in the underlying tissue, and less oxygen will be available for diffusion to the skin surface. In the patient with adequate cardiac output and no vascular insufficiency, the readings will parallel the arterial oxygen tension (Pa_{O_2}).

$P_{cj}O_2$ avoids the problems of tissue heating by the application of the electrode to the thin *non*keratinized conjunctival tissue. The electrode is incorporated into a polymethylacrylate ring formed to sit within the conjunctival fornices with the sensor over the lateral aspect of the superior palpebral conjunctiva. The tissue depth between the underlying capillary bed and the electrode has been estimated as 30 μm. Perfusion of the underlying capillary bed is from the ophthalmic branch of the carotid artery. Readings can be obtained in 1 minute, and because heating is unnecessary, the device does not affect capillary blood flow or tissue metabolism. However, $P_{cj}O_2$ is also affected by local tissue perfusion and will not necessarily reflect cerebral oxygen levels during low-flow states and in the presence of vasoactive drugs. Although not currently in common emergency department use, transconjunctival monitors have been developed with both oxygen and carbon dioxide sensors in the same eyepiece.[28, 29]

INDICATIONS

An important point raised by the proponents of these measurements is that commonly accepted measures of the

Table 5–3. *Oxygen Monitoring*

	Technique	Performance Time	Advantages	Disadvantages	Comments
Arterial blood gas (ABG)	See Chapter 19	5–15 minutes	Offers pH, Pa_{O_2}, P_{CO_2}, Sa_{O_2} Reliable when arterial sample Physician familiarity	Time consuming, delayed results Costly Possibility of venous sampling Painful Single-point sampling Serious complications possible Fastidious handling of sample needed	The "gold standard"
Transcutaneous ($P_{tc}O_2$)	Clean and dry site Apply adhesive electrode Set electrode temperature Calibrate Allow for 5–10 minutes stabilization Draw baseline ABG	10–20 minutes for initial value	Easily performed Correlates well with Pa_{O_2} in normovolemic patients Continuous readings	Heating skin site risks burns and changes local metabolism Recalibration after moving site Measures tissue P_{O_2} Value dependent on perfusion	Can act as a vital sign with greater utility than blood pressure or pulse
Transconjunctival ($P_{cj}O_2$)	Calibrate device Anesthetize conjunctiva Insert sensor Allow for 1–2 minutes stabilization Draw baseline ABG	<5 minutes	Easily performed Correlates well with Pa_{O_2} in normovolemic patients Continuous readings No heating required	Measures tissue P_{O_2} Value dependent on perfusion	In addition to the above comment, this method shares the same arterial blood supply as the brain
Pulse oximetry (Sa_{O_2})	Clip sensor to any extremity Self-calibrating	1 minute	Extremely simple, rapid Correlates well with Pa_{O_2} Continuous data capability Many easily accessible sites	Requires adequate perfusion Only Sa_{O_2} measured	Large cost savings available when used to reduce number of ABG determinations Could be performed routinely as a "vital sign" during triage

adequacy of resuscitation may not adequately reflect tissue oxygen delivery. The reliance of $P_{cj}O_2$ and $P_{tc}O_2$ measurements on local tissue perfusion has been cited as both an advantage and a disadvantage of these techniques. Because oxygen delivery is dependent on both the arterial oxygen content and the cardiac index, a fall in $P_{tc}O_2$ with a satisfactory Pa_{O_2} indicates a low perfusion state.[30] Conversely, when perfusion is adequate, a fall in $P_{tc}O_2$ or $P_{cj}O_2$ indicates inadequate oxygenation. Hence, these measures appear useful for monitoring volume resuscitation when oxygenation is adequate. Animal and human studies suggest that these techniques are more sensitive than standard vital sign parameters for determining the end point of adequate volume resuscitation.[30–34]

Similarly, these measures may be helpful as early warning monitors for low perfusion. Clinical case reports have shown precipitous declines in $P_{cj}O_2$ before the development of ventricular tachycardia, fibrillation, asystole, and pericardial tamponade.[35–37] $P_{tc}O_2$ monitoring may also be used to assess isolated limb perfusion in the setting of presumed regional ischemia that is due to either vascular insufficiency or trauma.[38] $P_{cj}O_2$ monitoring can assess unilateral carotid perfusion and can monitor intraoperatively carotid and cerebral perfusion.[39] In the setting of adequate volume status and perfusion, these measures are helpful for monitoring systemic oxygenation. Patients with a wide range of respiratory disorders are amenable to such monitoring. $P_{tc}O_2$ is especially useful for monitoring neonates to minimize the morbidity of arterial blood draws and the associated red blood cell and plasma loss with repeated phlebotomy. These techniques also are helpful during transport of a critically ill patient when noise interferes with blood pressure auscultation and vibrations complicate cardiac monitoring. In one study of patients transported by helicopter, 36 per cent were found to have compromise of their ventilatory or circulatory status that was undetected by conventional measurements.[40]

CONTRAINDICATIONS

Contraindications to the use of transcutaneous or transconjunctival monitoring are seldom mentioned in the medical literature. Given the dependence of $P_{tc}O_2$ on a properly functioning integument, the transcutaneous sensor should not be placed on injured (e.g., burned or crushed) or infected skin. Because 20 minutes may be required for calibration and stabilization of the monitor, this technique should not be used for making therapeutic decisions until electrode stabilization has occurred. $P_{tc}O_2$ monitoring has not been evaluated in the setting of hypothermia. Current practice favors the use of blood gas results uncorrected for patient core temperature during resuscitation of hypothermic patients (see Chapter 91); hence the effect of tissue warming by the technique on measured $P_{tc}O_2$ values is unknown. Furthermore, the intense vasoconstriction seen clinically during hypothermia, coupled with local heating of the skin to 45° C, is likely to produce injury at the electrode site. For this reason, $P_{tc}O_2$ monitoring should be avoided during resuscitation of the profoundly hypothermic patient.

$P_{cj}O_2$ monitoring is contraindicated in the setting of ocular trauma and conjunctival foreign material. $P_{cj}O_2$ monitoring has not been reported in the setting of conjunctivitis. The presence of the $P_{cj}O_2$ electrode device as a conjunctival foreign body is likely to inhibit adequate clearance of the infectious agent even with supplemental antibiotic use, and the underlying infection-induced hyperemia may produce misleading estimates of systemic oxygenation. Thus we recommend avoidance of $P_{cj}O_2$ monitoring in the setting of conjunctivitis. Because tears may contain viable viruses (e.g., hepatitis B virus and human immunodeficiency virus), the electrode must be sterilized before reuse, if used for more than one patient. Additionally, the $P_{cj}O_2$ electrode does not function if the conjunctival temperature is below 33° C; hence this technique is not effective in profound hypothermia.[41]

EQUIPMENT

$P_{tc}O_2$ monitors evaluated in clinical studies include the TCM-2 (Radiometer America, Westlake, Ohio),[30] TCOM (Novametrix Medical Systems, Inc., Wallingford, Conn.),[34] and Transcend (Sensor Medics, Anaheim, Calif.).[42] Additional supplies include adhesive-backed O-rings to apply the electrode to the skin.

$P_{cj}O_2$ monitors evaluated in clinical studies include the COS (Orange Medical Instruments, Costa Mesa, Calif.)[32, 43, 44] and the NCC Insight (Mallinckrodt, St. Louis, Mo.).[45] Additional supplies include a polymethylacrylate ophthalmic conformer and topical anesthesia.

PROCEDURE

For $P_{tc}O_2$ monitoring, excessive hair is shaved, and the skin is prepared with alcohol to ensure a clean adherent surface for the adhesive-backed O-ring that secures the electrode. The sensor temperature is set at 45° C and after warming is calibrated to room oxygen tension (percentage of oxygen in inspired air × barometric pressure). Contact gel is placed in the O-ring followed by the electrode. The unit is placed on the chosen site (e.g., shoulder, hip, chest, arm, leg) and allowed to heat the skin between 5 and 10 minutes until the measured values stabilize. At this time, a baseline ABG should be drawn to compare the $P_{tc}O_2$ reading and the Pa_{O_2}. The ABG can be repeated each time the $P_{tc}O_2$ reading significantly changes. If the Pa_{O_2} is adequate and the $P_{tc}O_2$ reading is low, a low perfusion state should be suspected. If the Pa_{O_2} is low, the low $P_{tc}O_2$ reading is likely due to inadequate oxygenation. The sensor is moved every 4 hours (2 hours in neonates) to avoid burns and to prevent a time-dependent, site-related decrease in $P_{tc}O_2$ readings. With each change in site, a recalibration is performed.

For $P_{cj}O_2$ monitoring, the machine is calibrated to room oxygen tension (percentage of oxygen in inspired air × barometric pressure). Stabilization and calibration take less than 1 minute for the $P_{cj}O_2$ monitor rather than the several minutes required for heating and stabilization of the $P_{tc}O_2$ monitor before calibration. In conscious patients, a drop of local anesthetic solution is instilled before insertion of the ophthalmic conformer. The miniaturized oxygen electrode contained in the ophthalmic conformer is placed onto the lateral palpebral conjunctiva. After 1 minute for stabilization, measurements are begun, and a baseline ABG is drawn for a comparison Pa_{O_2} value.

INTERPRETATION

It is important to remember that both $P_{tc}O_2$ and $P_{cj}O_2$ monitoring techniques assess tissue oxygen levels and not Pa_{O_2}. $P_{tc}O_2$ values are linearly related to Pa_{O_2} when perfusion is adequate, but during shock or other low-perfusion situations, $P_{tc}O_2$ values will instead parallel perfusion. $P_{tc}O_2$ values reflect low perfusion even in the setting of vasopressor-induced normotension during hemorrhagic shock.[46] $P_{tc}O_2$ to Pa_{O_2} ratios of less than 0.5 suggest the need to initiate aggressive resuscitation measures, although higher levels may also be associated with inadequate perfusion or oxygenation.

With adequate perfusion, the $P_{tc}O_2$ to Pa_{O_2} ratio is approximately 0.79, with a correlation coefficient of 0.89.[47] The infusion of sodium nitroprusside does not affect $P_{tc}O_2$ values or the $P_{tc}O_2$ to Pa_{O_2} ratio.[48] Stokes and coworkers suggest that the Pa_{O_2} can be estimated from the $P_{tc}O_2$ in normodynamic or hyperdynamic patients by the following equation:

$$Pa_{O_2} = 1.1 \times P_{tc}O_2 - 0.28 \times Fi_{O_2} + 45.5,$$

where the Fi_{O_2} is the percentage of inspired oxygen content.[42] Comparison of $P_{tc}O_2$ values from different body regions can indicate regional perfusion abnormalities. A limb to chest $P_{tc}O_2$ level ratio markedly less than 1.0 represents severe extremity perfusion insufficiency. Restoration of flow to the limb should increase this ratio, although small vessel disease, as seen with diabetes, will also produce a low ratio.[48a]

$P_{cj}O_2$ values are similarly related to both perfusion and oxygenation. Animal studies of controlled hemorrhage indicate that a decrease in $P_{cj}O_2$ value is seen before a decrease in the $P_{tc}O_2$ value and that $P_{cj}O_2$ provides a better estimate of volume resuscitation than $P_{tc}O_2$.[49] In hemodynamically stable patients, the $P_{cj}O_2$ to Pa_{O_2} ratio is 0.6 to 0.7.[45, 50–52] Abraham and colleagues suggest that a $P_{cj}O_2$ to Pa_{O_2} ratio of 0.5 or less has strong predictive value for a significant blood volume deficit[51] and that the $P_{cj}O_2$ to Pa_{O_2} ratio does not exceed 0.50 until the volume replacement exceeds 90 per cent of the volume loss. The volume loss at which $P_{cj}O_2$ changes first occur remains to be determined. One study of five healthy adults was unable to show a change in either the absolute $P_{cj}O_2$ value or the $P_{cj}O_2$ to Pa_{O_2} ratio after a phlebotomy of 450 ml.[45]

Baseline $P_{cj}O_2$ values decrease with increasing age,[53] and the baseline $P_{cj}O_2$ to Pa_{O_2} ratio can show considerable variability.[43] The $P_{cj}O_2$ value changes seen with age may be related to underlying carotid pathology. Carotid insufficiency or occlusion can be detected by a low $P_{cj}O_2$ value.[39] Hyperventilation with hypocapnia-induced ophthalmic artery vasospasm will reduce $P_{cj}O_2$ levels.[44] One animal study suggests that in the presence of epinephrine, $P_{cj}O_2$ values do not parallel cerebral oxygen levels.[54]

Although threshold values for $P_{tc}O_2$ and $P_{cj}O_2$ provide useful warnings for hypoxia, low perfusion states, or both, the use of these monitoring techniques is most effective when trends are sought. When therapy fails to produce an improvement in the monitored values, the clinician should reevaluate the situation clinically, troubleshoot the device, and consider a blood gas for determination of actual oxygenation.

COMPLICATIONS

$P_{tc}O_2$ monitoring has been associated with local burns when the electrode is left in one site for prolonged periods (>6 hours for adults, >4 hours for neonates).[55] Periodic electrode site changes will avert this complication. $P_{cj}O_2$ monitoring may be associated with corneal or conjunctival abrasions if foreign material is not removed before ocular placement. Prolonged sensor placement in one eye (>6 hours), especially in the setting of globe exposure, may lead to a punctate keratopathy or chemosis.[41] The use of artificial tear solution and lid closure will minimize this complication. The keratopathy is treated as a minor corneal defect (see Chapter 85).[40]

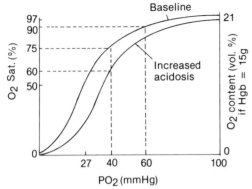

Figure 5–5. Oxyhemoglobin dissociation curve.

Although the spread of infection has not been reported with the use of $P_{cj}O_2$ electrode conformers, the device needs sterilization before reuse. Guidelines have not been formalized for conformer sterilization, but application of a viricidal solution, thorough rinsing of the device to remove any residual viricidal solution, and subsequent air drying should be effective.

Pulse Oximetry

BACKGROUND

Pulse oximetry is a simple, easy-to-use technology that can provide significant information quickly and cheaply. Oximetry was first developed in 1932 by Nicolai and was applied during World War II to measure pilot hemoglobin desaturation and guide automatic adjustment of the oxygen supply to the aviator's mask. It was not until 1980 that the pulse oximeter reached modern form with fiberoptic cables and an onboard computer.[56] Acceptance in clinical practice was initially slow, but now the devices are used in numerous settings.

INDICATIONS

After an extensive review of the history of pulse oximetry, Severinghaus (the "father of respiratory physiology") concluded that pulse oximetry is " . . . the most significant technological advance ever made in monitoring the well-being and safety of patients during anesthesia, recovery and critical care. Its use in patients who are unconscious or unable to maintain adequate ventilation and gas exchange without assistance may become mandatory."[56] Oxygen saturation of hemoglobin (Sa_{O_2}) as measured by pulse oximetry

Table 5–4. *Factors Affecting Pulse Oximetry Readings*

1. Severe anemia: satisfactory readings obtained down to Hgb level of 5 mg/dl
2. Motion-artifact: greatly reduced with new, lightweight, disposable sensors
3. Dyes: transient effect
4. Light-artifact: greatly reduced with new, lightweight, disposable sensors
5. Hypoperfusion: readings can be obtained during *effective* cardiopulmonary resuscitation
6. Electrocautery
7. Deep pigmentation: use fifth finger, earlobe, or other area of lighter pigmentation
8. Dark nail polish: remove with acetone
9. Dyshemoglobin states (such as carboxyhemoglobin, methemoglobin): falsely elevate saturation reading
10. Elevated bilirubin: able to read for bilirubin up to 20 mg/dl in adults: no problem reported for jaundiced children

has even been suggested as a fifth "vital sign."[57] Pulse oximetry offers the physician an arguably more physiologic means of assessing the adequacy of oxygenation than the ABG by providing either continuous or frequent intermittent Sa_{O_2} measurements.[58–60]

The Sa_{O_2} correlates well with Pa_{O_2}, but the relationship is nonlinear and is described by the oxyhemoglobin dissociation curve (Fig. 5–5). For the hypoxic patient, small changes in Sa_{O_2} represent large changes in Pa_{O_2} because these Sa_{O_2} values fall on the steep portion of the curve.[61] In one study, Sa_{O_2} had 100 per cent sensitivity for identifying hypoxemia; an Sa_{O_2} of less than 95 per cent correlated with a Pa_{O_2} of less than 70 mm Hg.[62] Furthermore, Sa_{O_2} measures the large reservoir of oxygen carried by hemoglobin, 20 ml O_2/100 ml blood, compared with Pa_{O_2}, which only measures the relatively small amount of oxygen dissolved in the plasma, approximately 0.3 ml O_2/100 ml blood.[63]

Blood gas samples must be drawn from an arterial source and quickly transported under specific conditions to a machine that is often distant from the patient's bedside. With pulse oximetry, test results are available at the bedside without an invasive arterial procedure. Also eliminated are complicated and time-consuming calibration steps, electrode placement, and "arterialization" of the site (with the possibility of burns), as seen with transcutaneous oxygen monitoring. Furthermore, transcutaneous and transconjunctival methods give a mixed arterial-venous determination contrasted with pulse oximetry's pure arterial value.[58] Pulse oximetry has advantages over PEFR and spirometry as an objective measure of patient condition and response to therapy in that it provides non-effort-dependent continuous values and requires no patient education.[64] Its advantage in children, in lieu of arterial sampling, is obvious. Hypothermia to a low of 26.5° C,[65] hypotension (as long as a pulse is present), skin pigmentation, and pressor infusions do not reduce the accuracy of the pulse oximeter.[61]

As physicians readjust to using Sa_{O_2} rather than Pa_{O_2} in assessment of oxygenation, they may find it interesting to know that this approach is a return to respiratory physiology before the invention of the Clark electrode, when oxygen saturation was the key variable monitored.[56]

Contraindications

The disadvantages of pulse oximetry fall into two groups. First, in comparison with ABG determination, pulse oximetry gives no information on pH, or Pa_{CO_2} levels. Second, the mechanics of the sampling technique may be subject to light and motion interference or may fail to give any reading at all in circumstances of extreme anemia, hypoperfusion, or jaundice. Both ABG determination and pulse oximetry are not as useful for dyshemoglobin states, such as those found in carbon monoxide poisoning and methemoglobinemia. Other conditions affect readings as well (Table 5–4).

Differences between device readings must be taken into account. The pulse oximeter calculates oxygen saturation using empiric algorithms that are based on a sampling of small human populations (five Olympic athletes in one case). Furthermore, each manufacturer may have calibrated its device using a different cooximeter. Some manufacturers have chosen to base the oxygen saturation calculation on what is sometimes called the *fractional* Sa_{O_2}, in which

the percentage of Hb_{O_2} =
$$100 \times (Hb_{O_2}/[Hb + Hb_{O_2} + Hb_{CO} + MetHb])$$

instead of the more traditional calculation of what is now called the *functional* Sa_{O_2}, in which

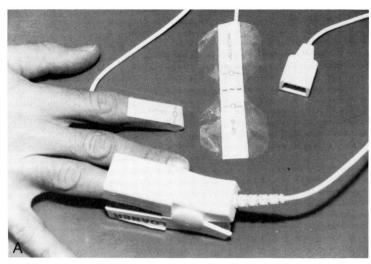 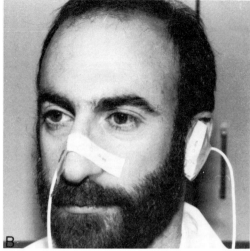

Figure 5–6. *A*, Pulse oximeter sensors attached to digits. *B*, Pulse oximeter sensors attached to the dorsum of the nose and the earlobe. Only one site is measured at a time.

the percentage of $Hb_{O_2} = 100 \times (Hb_{O_2})/(Hb + Hb_{O_2})$.

Hence, as much as a 3 per cent variation in oxygen saturation may be seen among different pulse oximeters.[66]

Despite the potential for mechanical problems, paramedic crews in a prehospital study have successfully used an off-the-shelf model with relative ease and an extremely low failure rate.[59]

EQUIPMENT

Pulse oximetry applies Beer's law: The absorption of light by a solution is a function of the concentration of the solute and the absorption depth of the solution. Light-emitting diodes (in the red and infrared wavelengths) set into a reusable clip or disposable patch are simply placed across an oxygen-rich arterial bed such as a finger tip. The device spectrophotometrically measures the difference in absorption between reduced hemoglobin and oxyhemoglobin to calculate Sa_{O_2}. Additionally, the pulse oximeter eliminates interference from light transmitted through constituents other than arterial blood by using the differences between the light absorption of the pulsating arterial blood at its greatest and least volumes. Using only the changes in absorption measured during peak changes in blood volume, the oxygen saturation of *arterial* blood is calculated selectively.[67] The data are frequently displayed as a plethysmograph of the pulse strength within a few seconds and then as a beat-to-beat recording of the Sa_{O_2}. Because the pulse oximeter generally uses only two wavelengths, the machine is unable to differentiate oxyhemoglobin from hemoglobin saturated with carbon monoxide or from methemoglobin. In each case, oxygen saturation is overestimated.[61]

Pulse oximetry monitors documented in emergency department studies include the Biox 3700 (Ohmeda, Boulder, Colo.),[61] the Biox III (Ohmeda, Boulder, Colo.),[64] and the Nellcor (Nellcor, Inc., Hayward, Calif.).[59, 67a] Short and colleagues recently evaluated pulse oximeters for aeromedical use.[67b] The reader is referred to their article for further product information.

PROCEDURE

The location for the probe is determined by the clinical situation and the probes available. A reusable clip-on probe makes the digits easily accessible. Motion interference can result with digital probes, but this phenomenon is transient and seldom influences assessment. Little is needed in the way of preparation, and even nail polish may generally remain. Other sites (Fig. 5–6) include the ear lobe, the nasal bridge or septum, the temporal artery, and the foot or palm of an infant. Some machines are more susceptible to interference from heavy pigmentation; in this situation the fifth digit has been suggested as the optimal site. Tape and splints can be used to secure the digit probe and to minimize motion.

After placement of the probe, the machine is turned on. The computer analyzes the incoming data to identify the arteriolar pulsation and displays this in beats per minute; newer devices also display a pulse plethysmograph. Simultaneously, oxygen saturation is displayed on a beat-to-beat basis. Some machines have hard copy capability and can provide paper documentation of the patient's status. If the oximeter fails to detect pulsatile flow, either the reading will not be displayed or the Sa_{O_2} value is given with a poor signal quality warning, depending on the machine.

INTERPRETATION

Patients with good gas exchange have oxygen saturations between 97 and 100 per cent. When the Sa_{O_2} falls below 95 per cent, hypoxia is present, although patients with chronic lung disease may live in this range. Oxygen saturations below 90 per cent represent relatively severe hypoxia. In the final analysis, as with PEFR and spirometry, attempts to correlate isolated early measurements of Pa_{O_2} or Sa_{O_2} with the need for admission often fail because of the wide variability of response to therapy;[64, 67a] however, as pieces of the clinical puzzle, these values provide the physician with objective information on which to base decisions.

As noted in Chapters 1 and 2, the Sa_{O_2} monitor can be a useful device for monitoring oxygenation during airway procedures. Undoubtably this technique will be applied in other procedural settings as a means of monitoring the patient's oxygenation. When used during intubation, the monitor provides objective evidence of preoxygenation ($Sa_{O_2} \geq 99$ per cent) and potential hypoxia during the procedure (Sa_{O_2} is less than 95 per cent). In the presence of potential hypoxia, the procedure should be halted until further oxygenation can be provided. The monitor can also be used to detect hypoxia during weaning from a ventilator.[62]

Table 5–5. *Arterial Oxygen Tension at Increasing Altitudes*

Altitude (ft)	Barometric Pressure (mm Hg)	Pa_{O_2} (Expected)
0 (sea level)	760	96
1000	733	91
2000	707	87
3000	687	83
4000	656	79
5000	631	75
6000	604	71
8000	564	63

OXYGEN THERAPY

Introduction and Background

Earlier sections have dealt with ventilation and assessment of oxygenation. Delivery of oxygen is impaired in many clinical situations. Neurologic dysfunction is an early sign of hypoxemia. Otherwise healthy individuals begin to experience short-term memory loss, euphoria, and impaired judgment when approaching a Pa_{O_2} of 55 mm Hg. Progressive loss of cognitive and motor function, increasing tachycardia, and other physical signs occur between 30 and 55 mm Hg. Below 30 mm Hg the patient loses consciousness. Pa_{O_2} is a function of the fraction of inspired oxygen tension (FI_{O_2}), the alveolar ventilation, and the relative distribution of both ventilation and perfusion in the lung. Supplemental oxygen can increase the amount of oxygen dissolved in blood enough to deliver one third of the body's resting metabolic requirements. This section reviews the noninvasive delivery of supplemental oxygen.

Indications

Oxygen therapy is generally indicated when hypoxia is present (Pa_{O_2} is less than 60 mm Hg, Sa_{O_2} is less than 90 to 95 per cent). Clinical situations that are commonly associated with hypoxia and generally benefit from supplemental oxygen include pulmonary disease, cerebral vascular accidents, gastrointestinal bleeding, shock, and trauma. Supplemental oxygen is also indicated when hypoxia is anticipated from a procedure such as intubation or before a procedure in which intravenous analgesics may cause respiratory depression.

High altitude also results in hypoxia; the effect of increasing altitude on Pa_{O_2} is shown in Table 5–5. Commercial airlines maintain cabin pressures at levels equivalent to 8500 feet or less. Patients with chronic hypoxia may require supplemental oxygen and before flying must contact the airline to make appropriate arrangements. Oxygen is specifically indicated for carboxyhemoglobinemia; 100 per cent oxygen reduces the half-life of carboxyhemoglobin from 4 hours to 1 hour; hyperbaric (more than 1.0 atmosphere) oxygen can lessen this time by half again. Hyperbaric oxygen may also enhance the release of carbon monoxide from cytochrome oxidase sites.[68]

Contraindications

Paraquat turns oxygen into free radicals, thus making oxygen a substrate of the poison. Similar toxins in this group

Table 5–6. *Oxygen Cylinders (approximate values)*

Cylinder Type	Volume (L)	Cylinder Factor	Hours O_2 at 2 L/min
D	450	0.20	3.5
E	650	0.28	5.0
G	5600	2.41	44.0
H, K	6900	3.14	58.0

include bleomycin, doxorubicin, ozone, and nitrous dioxide.[69, 70] Hence, oxygen therapy in the absence of documented hypoxia is contraindicated for this group of toxins.

Fears of ventilatory shutdown in the presence of CO_2 retention have made physicians hesitant to give supplemental oxygen in amounts greater than 2 liters per minute. However, if hypoxia remains after low-flow O_2 is initiated, the oxygen delivery must be increased. Continuous monitoring of spontaneous respiration is required in this setting, and preparations to perform intubation should be made to assist the patient's ventilation if indicated. Note that inspired oxygen levels may actually rise with low-flow oxygen therapy as respiratory effort wanes because there is less room air entrained with shallow breaths. A high CO_2 level is not a contraindication to appropriate oxygen therapy.

Equipment

The two most common sources of oxygen for the patient in the hospital are wall outlets linked to a large reservoir of liquid oxygen and oxygen tanks (green by convention) of various sizes, listed in Table 5–6. Both provide outlet pressures in the range of 30–50 psi. An oxygen-concentrating system capable of delivering greater than 90 per cent oxygen has been developed as a central supply source and is used in some hospitals.[70] Oxygen cylinders are used to service the home population as well, and, by means of transfilling procedures, allow portable systems to be recharged for ambulatory use. An approximation of the amount of time left in a given tank at a given flow rate may be calculated using the following formula:

minutes of O_2 = gauge pressure (psi)
$\times$ cylinder factor/flow rate (liters per minute)

Cylinder factors are shown in Table 5–6. Reservoirs of liquid oxygen exist for domicile use as well; these systems store enough to last between 4 and 7 days at 2 liters per minute. The numerous methods available to deliver oxygen from the source to the patient are listed in Table 5–7.

Procedure

The amount of O_2 prescribed should be sufficient to correct the hypoxia. Supplemental oxygen should be given to increase the Pa_{O_2} to between 60 and 80 mm Hg or greater than 90 to 95 per cent Sa_{O_2}. Bedside pulse oximetry can provide prompt monitoring of changes in Sa_{O_2}, allowing adjustments to be made without repeated ABG determination. Evidence of CO_2 retention such as decreasing mental status and failing respiratory drive indicate the need for an ABG determination to document the Pa_{CO_2}; however, the decision to intubate generally should be made on clinical grounds. The need to humidify bedside low-flow oxygen is unproven. One small clinical study found no subjective differences when hospitalized patients receiving 1 to 4 liters per minute of oxygen were treated with or without humidification.[71] This conclusion also was reached during one national consensus conference.[70] Providing oxygen from cylinders involves several steps that are outlined in Table 5–8.[24]

Complications

Three distinct areas of risk accompany supplemental oxygen use: (1) respiratory dysfunction, (2) cytotoxic injury, and (3) physical hazards. Respiratory dysfunction results

Table 5–7. Oxygen Delivery Systems

System	Flow Rate L/min	FI_{O_2} (% Oxygen)	Advantages	Disadvantages
Nasal cannulas	1	25	Simple, comfortable, inexpensive, allow eating and drinking	Can cause local irritation and drying of mucous membranes (primarily for flow rates > 4 L/min)
	2	29		
	3	33		
	4	37		
	5	41		
	6	45		
Simple oxygen masks	>5 L/min	35–50	Deliver higher flow rates than nasal prongs	Must be removed for airway care, eating, and drinking
Masks with reservoir bag	Up to 15 L/min	60	Higher FI_{O_2} at lower flow rates	Risk of atelectasis and oxygen toxicity (with prolonged use)
Venturi masks	4	24–28	More precise control of final oxygen concentration	Same as above
	6	31		
	8	35–40		
	10	50		
Reservoir nebulizers, includes CPAP, T tubes	40 L/min plus:	60–90	Can deliver increased humidity, positive pressure	Risk of barotrauma

from CO_2 retention and atelectasis. Variations in CO_2 level provide the main stimulus to breathe in normal subjects. Patients with chronic obstructive pulmonary disease have a decreased sensitivity to CO_2 levels secondary to chronic exposure to higher CO_2 levels, and hypoxia provides backup support for the respiratory drive. Oxygen given in sufficient amounts can remove the remaining chemical stimulus to respiration and has the potential to cause respiratory shutdown.

The complete abolition of the hypoxic drive has been reported to require a Pa_{O_2} of 200 mm Hg.[72] However, administration of 100 per cent oxygen to 22 patients with chronic obstructive pulmonary disease in acute respiratory distress (mean baseline blood gas values Pa_{CO_2} = 65 mm Hg, Pa_{O_2} = 38 mm Hg) for 15 minutes resulted in only a transient decrease in minute ventilation.[73] The lowest values for minute ventilation were reached between 20 and 180 seconds from onset of inhalation, followed by a slow rise over the next 12 minutes to within 93 per cent of the control value. The decrease was the result of falls in both tidal volume and respiratory rate; however, after 15 minutes, these parameters had returned to baseline levels. Despite little difference in these parameters at the 15 minute point, Pa_{CO_2} had risen a mean of 23 mm Hg, and Pa_{O_2} had risen a mean of 225 mm Hg.[73] The mechanism leading to atelectasis is less clear. Elevated oxygen levels may affect under-perfused or under-ventilated pulmonary segments by decreasing hypoxic vasoconstriction. The increased perfusion could lead to greater absorption of the remaining gas, destabilizing the alveolar units and bringing on collapse.[74]

Cytotoxic damage, theoretically secondary to free radical production, leads to tracheobronchitis and adult respiratory distress syndrome manifested by pulmonary edema and focal lung collapse with pulmonary fibrosis as a long-term consequence. The mechanism of damage has been shown experimentally to include oxidation of carbohydrates with disruption of cell surface receptors, DNA-RNA alterations, lipid peroxidation, and protein denaturation. The previously mentioned consequences of the administration of an inappropriately high level of oxygen are not usually seen within the time frame of the emergency department visit. The risk of oxygen toxicity depends on several factors, including oxygen tolerance (the state of biologic resistance to oxygen-induced damage, which is itself dependent on antioxidant defenses, age, and nutritional and hormonal factors), concentration of oxygen delivered, and duration of treatment. In general, delivering the minimal amount of oxygen to achieve adequate tissue levels is the goal. During resuscitation and most emergency care, 100 per cent oxygen can be delivered safely to most patients without fear of cytotoxic injury. Healthy adult volunteers have received 100 per cent oxygen for up to 6 hours without evidence of pulmonary injury. Except in special circumstances, such as paraquat poisoning, oxygen at concentrations of 50 per cent or less is safe for 2 to 7 days.[70]

Physical risks associated with oxygen therapy include trauma associated with tank explosions, fire hazard, local irritation, and drying of mucous membranes.

Continuous Positive Airway Pressure

Continuous positive airway pressure (CPAP) has been used successfully on alert patients who might otherwise succumb to respiratory failure. The technique involves placing a tight, well-fitting mask over the patient's mouth and nose. Oxygen is delivered under a variable amount of pressure to the airway with the desirable effect of increasing the end-expiratory pressure in the lungs and thus maintaining the patency of alveoli with an effect similar to that of positive end-expiratory pressure (PEEP) on ventilator-bound patients. Clinically, CPAP results in decreased work of breathing. It is indicated in traumatized individuals with

Table 5–8. Operation of Oxygen Cylinders

1. Secure the tank in an upright position so that it will not move or fall while being manipulated.
2. Remove the cylinder seal ("E" tank) or cylinder cap ("G," "H" tank).
3. Turn the cylinder valve on and off quickly to clear ("crack") the valve. On the "E" tank, this is done with a wrench; on the "G" or "H" tank, it is done with the cylinder handle.
4. Check the yoke to ensure that it is compatible for use with oxygen, and place it on the cylinder, being sure that the fittings are compatible.
5. Tighten the yoke, making certain that any necessary gasket is in place.
6. Close the needle valve.
7. Slowly open the cylinder valve until the pressure maximizes.
8. Observe that the cylinder contains an adequate supply of gas.
9. Connect the desired secondary delivery system (e.g., nasal cannula).
10. Open the needle valve so that the desired oxygen flow registers on the flow meters.

early signs of respiratory failure such as tachypnea, hypocarbia, and hypoxia.[75] Other conditions such as cardiogenic pulmonary edema and postextubation hypoxia have also been treated with this method.[76, 77] A nasogastric tube may be required to prevent passive esophageal and gastric dilation in conjunction with CPAP when higher pressures (8 to 10 cm H_2O) are delivered. Contraindications include severe maxillofacial trauma and high esophageal or tracheal injuries. Patients with basilar skull fractures may be at risk for pneumocephalus.

Conclusions

With rare exceptions, most patients seen in the emergency department with respiratory problems and various other complaints benefit from at least low-flow oxygen by nasal cannulas. Patients with known or suspected CO_2 retention are no exception. Such patients require close monitoring and occasionally ventilatory support. Use of pulse oximetry or other oxygen monitoring techniques can help pinpoint patient needs and fine tune delivery of oxygen therapy.

DELIVERY SYSTEMS FOR INHALED MEDICATIONS

Introduction

Inhaled substances have been used for medicinal (and social) purposes since the beginnings of recorded history. Among the earliest such records of the treatment of respiratory disease comes from a monograph written in 2737 B.C. by the Chinese emperor Shen Nung on the use of inhaled cannabis for the treatment of asthma.[80] Later in the fifteenth century B.C. the Chinese *Pharmacopeia* refers to cannabis[81] and to Ma Huang,[78] a medicinal that contained ephedrine, as therapy for asthma.

Through the 1900s, atropinic effects were obtained from ingestion and inhalation of medicinals such as *Atropa belladonna* and *Datura stramonium.* Thus long before the era of modern medicine, β-adrenergic and antimuscarinic stimulation by inhalation were established in the physician's armamentarium.

When compared with oral or parenteral delivery, the aerosolized delivery of certain medications to patients suffering from bronchospasm has been found to be particularly effective. With fewer side effects and better patient acceptance, aerosolization has become the route of choice in contemporary clinical practice.[78] Aerosolized medications are easily delivered using portable self-contained sprays called metered-dose inhalers (MDI) and by nebulizer devices propelled by air compressors or wall oxygen. Either method can be used in the home, outpatient department, or inhospital setting. Nebulized treatment can also be delivered in-line with ventilation equipment for intubated patients and by mask for young or weak patients.[79] Intermittent positive-pressure breathing (IPPB) as a means of assisting simple nebulizer therapy has received much criticism and has been deemphasized (see subsequent discussion). Delivery systems using inhaled dry medication have recently been introduced in the United States. These systems appear promising, although their efficacy for acute bronchospasm is unknown. Hence, these systems will not be mentioned further.

Indications and Contraindications

Nebulizers and MDIs are used in the delivery of medications absorbed by the pulmonary route for the treatment of bronchospasm. Metered-dose inhalers are also used to deliver steroids, mucolytics, and ergotamine tartrate for migraine headache.[82] Gentamicin and other antibiotic solutions have been nebulized for antimicrobial therapy. Aerosolized pentamidine has been developed for the treatment of pneumocystis pneumonia. Spacer devices permit effective drug delivery with MDIs even in patients with poor hand-inhalation coordination.[83] In the setting of effective pulmonary drug delivery, inhalant therapy is preferred over the intravenous or subcutaneous routes for reasons of convenience, safety, and patient comfort.[84]

The MDI is used primarily in the home and nebulizers primarily in the inpatient and outpatient clinical settings; however, this division is becoming less distinct as more patients obtain compressor-driven devices for home nebulizer use and the MDI is restudied for use in the hospital setting. In fact, the MDI is now being offered as a cost-effective replacement for the nebulizer in the hospital.[85, 86] The benefits of replacing nebulizers in the hospital setting include decreased costs, quicker treatments, and better patient education in anticipation of later home use. Less nursing and respiratory technician time are required with MDI therapy.[87] A study comparing the use of an MDI plus spacer with a greater dose of medication delivered by nebulizer detected no clinical difference in either moderate or severe asthmatics.[88]

Nebulizers have two advantages over the MDI: (1) more than one medication can be given simultaneously; and (2) the system can be used in a hands-off fashion for the young, critically ill, or intubated patient. Spacers are indicated for patients who cannot adequately coordinate activation of the MDI with inhalation and for prevention of oral candidiasis in the case of inhaled steroids.

There are few contraindications to these devices. The MDI may be difficult for the very young, elderly, or critically ill to use, either because of inability to cooperate, weakness, or difficulty coordinating breathing with activation of the MDI. Spacer devices make the coordination of MDI use with inspiration less critical. Oxygen-powered nebulization may be contraindicated in the case of CO_2-retaining patients.[89]

Use of Metered-Dose Inhalers

EQUIPMENT AND PARTICLE DELIVERY

Metered-dose inhalers consist of small canisters of highly pressurized liquid with a freon propellant. An activator valve allows the delivery of consistent doses of medication in an aerosolized form. Particles of 1 to 5 μm in diameter are the most desirable size to achieve efficient peripheral airway deposition.[90] Ideally, the MDI output will have up to 13 per cent of particles in this range as opposed to only 1 to 5 per cent for the nebulizer. The deposition of aerosol in the lower respiratory tract is a function of inertia and gravitational sedimentation.

Inertia limits the quantity of drug delivered to the therapeutic site because particles in motion, such as the drug suspended in nebulized liquid, have a tendency to move in a straight line, resulting in the majority of the drug bombarding the posterior pharynx. The open-mouth technique (as opposed to lips closed around the inhaler) with the inhaler held a few centimeters from the mouth has been found to reduce this pharyngeal deposition.[91] By slowing the velocity of the particle, the airflow into the respiratory tract can have proportionately more time to effect transport or "entrain" the drug.

Spacer devices (see the following section) similarly allow for deeper penetration by reducing particle velocity, which in turn reduces droplet size both through the evaporation of the propellant that coats the drug crystal and the sedimentation of the larger particles. More central deposition occurs in patients with severe bronchial asthma and chronic bronchitis because of the underlying airway obstruction. In this situation, fewer particles remain to be deposited further downstream because of early gravitational sedimentation. Centrally deposited particles are carried by mucociliary transport to the larynx and swallowed, increasing the systemic absorption. Breath-holding enhances absorption by allowing the deposition of the smaller particles (less than 5 μm) that require up to 2 seconds to settle onto the walls of the terminal bronchioles.[91]

PROCEDURE

The most important factor in determining the successful use of the MDI is the patient. Up to 75 per cent of patients use the inhaler incorrectly,[92] and even after careful instruction 14 per cent still fail to perform efficiently. Frequent follow-up checks of MDI technique have been recommended.[78] Furthermore, when house staff and attending staff were evaluated, half the physicians could not assemble the device correctly, and only four out of 55 performed all seven steps correctly; three out of these four were asthmatics.[93]

Lower temperatures decrease the internal pressure and result in an increase in the size of the particles; therefore, the canister should be kept at room temperature. Lack of use can result in abnormally low doses, up to 50 per cent less than expected. If the device has not been used for several days, it should be activated once or twice before actual use.[82] In the past, patients have been told to activate the inhaler at the beginning of inhalation, immediately after full expiration. Studies of patients with diseased small airways suggest that beginning activation somewhat later in the inspiration period may result in a greater bronchodilator effect by overcoming the requirement for a higher opening pressure,[94, 95] but this finding remains controversial.[96, 97] Spacer devices and inspiration-triggered inhalers exist for the patient who has difficulty coordinating these tasks.

To optimize *maintenance* use of the MDI, the canister is shaken first and held in the inverted position. The patient exhales as much as possible. The mouthpiece of the nebulizer is placed approximately 2 to 4 cm from the open mouth, or, if a spacer device is used, the lips are placed around the spacer mouthpiece. The patient activates the device at or shortly after inspiration and inhales *slowly*, with the tongue and teeth as removed as possible to decrease oropharyngeal deposition. Inhalation is continued as long as possible and held 10 seconds if possible. The inhalation is repeated in 1 to 5 minutes to allow the medication's preliminary effects to enhance the penetration of the second treatment. One pediatric study in which full exhalation and breath-holding subsequent to inhalation were omitted found improved outcome in this group, probably because of enhanced compliance with the easier instructions.[98]

In the *acute* exacerbation setting, in which the physician elects to use the MDI over nebulizer therapy, the following approach is suggested. A fresh canister (or the patient's MDI if adequate medication remains; see the "float test" in Fig. 5–7) is obtained. A spacer device can be used to maximize the therapeutic effect. The patient is instructed carefully on the correct technique as described previously. (Demonstration of the technique in front of a family member is very helpful, and often family members are quite eager to ensure optimal care.) When treating bronchospasm, the patient should take four consecutive puffs of a β-adrenergic drug, such as albuterol, and then one to two puffs per minute until benefit is obtained or side effects such as tremor or dysrhythmia intervene.[99] Alternatively, the physician can hold the inhaler 10 cm from the patient's mouth and activate the inhaler for up to six consecutive breaths. As with nebulizer therapy discussed below, this *multidose* procedure can be repeated every 20 to 30 minutes for several treatments.

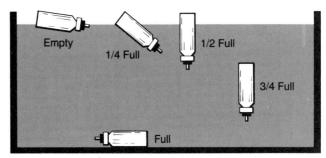

Figure 5–7. Testing a metered-dose inhaler for the quantity of medication remaining. The quantity of medication remaining in the metered-dose inhaler can be approximated by placing the canister in water and comparing the canister's position with that of those in the diagram.

Failure of home therapy with the same medication does not preclude successful emergency department therapy for at least three reasons: (1) inadequate patient compliance, (2) use of a canister empty of drug, and (3) inadequate dosing. Several studies comparing the efficacy of the MDI and the nebulizer support the use of the MDI in the emergency setting.[87, 100–103] The previous apparent superiority of the nebulizer in clinical studies stems from the reliance of patients and physicians on using the two-puff maintenance regimen for the MDI, which has been shown to produce a subtherapeutic dose for the patient during an acute exacerbation of reactive airway disease. Furthermore, the two-puff regimen may not be sufficient for maintenance in some patients.

Patients are often strongly cautioned against overuse of the MDI and may develop a fear of taking more than the ordered two puffs. Both physicians and patients should be comforted to know that double the current recommended dose, much less the occasional extra puff, is quite safe when it is realized that the patient will have a dose of 2.5 mg (a typical dose of albuterol) delivered to the upper airway by nebulizer, whereas less than 0.2 mg is delivered per puff of the corresponding MDI—less than one tenth the dose. In addition, the nebulizer is frequently given three or more times over the course of several hours of treatment. Nonetheless, the patient and family should be cautioned that increased inhaler requirement indicates an exacerbation of the underlying disease, frequently from infection, and that medical evaluation is advised.

SPACER DEVICES

Spacer devices serve as adjuncts to successful use of the MDI for the large subgroup of inhaler users using suboptimal technique. One study demonstrated a ninefold reduction in oropharyngeal deposition and a greater than double increase in deposition over the whole lung with one of these instruments.[90] Additionally, spacers reduce the incidence of oral candidiasis for steroid inhalers by decreasing oropharyngeal deposition.[83]

Essentially, there are two types of spacers: the tube and the airbag type. The simple toilet roll tube, the plastic cola bottle, or the commercially available Aerochamber (Monaghan Medical Corp., Plattsburgh, N.Y.) are basically *fixed tubes* of various lengths and shapes (Fig. 5–8). The inhaler is placed at one end and the patient's mouth at the other. The patient activates the inhaler and breathes in slowly, exhales to the air, and takes a second slow breath from the tube. Other adjuncts fall into the *airbag* group, wherein the inhaler is either attached to or placed within an air-filled bag. The canister is activated, and the patient subsequently breaths in and out of the bag. The commercial InspirEase

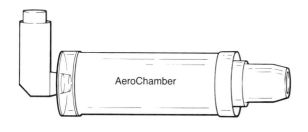

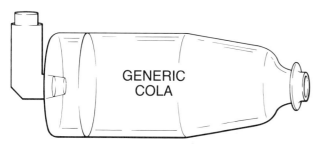

Figure 5–8. Fixed tube spacers. *A*, A commercial device. A mask may be attached to the proximal end to facilitate the treatment of children. *B*, A homemade device fashioned from a plastic 1-liter bottle. See text for details of spacer use.

(Schering Laboratories; Fig. 5–9) and the homemade freezer bag set-up are examples of this approach. In early 1990, Schering Laboratories recalled InspirEase devices manufactured after October 1989 because of a mechanical malfunction. The reader is advised to check with his or her pharmacist regarding the availability of this device.

One version of the airbag we have found particularly useful is achieved by cutting a hole in the permanently sealed end of a Ziplock-type quart bag, placing the inhaler shell orifice in the small hole, and taping the plastic tightly around the shell. The canister is removed; the bag is inflated with air; and the canister is replaced, activated, and promptly removed. The shell than acts as a mouthpiece, and the patient breathes in and out of the bag four to five times.[104] These adjuncts have been used successfully in children as young as 3 years of age.[105] Reeds producing horn-like sounds are frequently incorporated into commercial versions of spacers to facilitate achievement of the proper flow rates.

COMPLICATIONS

In the 1960s MDIs were blamed for excessive deaths in the asthmatic population. Subsequent studies have placed the blame on inadequate and untimely systemic steroid therapy during asthmatic exacerbations.[106] Current opinion is that there is no inherent danger in MDI use.[106, 107]

Many treatment failures can also be attributed to untimely exhaustion of the drug contained in the inhaler that catches the patient unaware. A simple method to assess drug quantity by placing the canister in a bowl of water is shown in Figure 5–7. Oral candidiasis is a complication of inhaled steroids and can be controlled or eliminated by the use of spacers or by activating the MDI at a distance, as discussed previously.

Hand-Held Nebulizer

EQUIPMENT

Nebulizers work on two principles. One type, based on the Bernoulli effect, uses oxygen or air at a flow rate of 5

to 10 liters per minute to aerosolize a liquid from a reservoir and carry the particles of medication through a tube and into the patient's upper respiratory tract. A second type of nebulizer produces an aerosol using the ultrasonic action of piezoelectric crystals to create the medicated mist.

PROCEDURE

As with the MDI, patient compliance with correct nebulizer technique is poor. In the 1000-patient IPPB Trial Group study, which compared IPPB and the simple nebulizer, compliance with the assigned regimen was approximately 55 per cent. This degree of noncompliance occurred despite an intensive effort to obtain maximum compliance, wherein "patients were asked, told and exhorted," with repeated instruction and monthly visits by nurse practitioners over the 3 years of the study.[108]

For the procedure, a reservoir is filled with the medication or medications, along with normal saline as a liquid carrier. The reservoir is then connected to the piezoelectric generator or to a source of propellant gas, either air or oxygen at 5 to 10 liters per minute. The aerosol is delivered via a mouthpiece or a ventilation mask to the patient's upper respiratory tract. The patient inhales slowly and deeply until the chamber is empty or until intolerable side effects intervene. In the absence of nausea, tremors, or palpitations, several treatments 20–30 minutes apart may be given for an acute attack of bronchospasm.[108a]

Hand-held nebulizers have been found to have less nasopharyngeal effect than the face-mask type. A reduction in aerosol losses secondary to striking the baffles of the nebulizer can be achieved by increasing the amount of the normal saline diluent used to fill the nebulizer. Doubling the diluent reportedly increases the drug delivered by a factor of three.[106, 107] Tapping the sides of the reservoir releases droplets of medication that are trapped on the baffles. Further, enhanced deposition in the peripheral airways can be achieved using an increased flow rate to raise the fraction of appropriate-sized particles.[90]

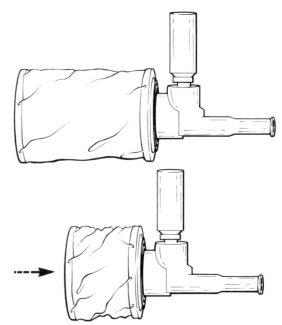

Figure 5–9. A commercial bag-type spacer. *A*, A metered-dose inhaler is activated when the bag is expanded. *B*, The bag collapses during inhalation. See text for details of spacer use.

COMPLICATIONS

Oxygen-powered nebulizers were felt to be the cause of death in five out of six patients who developed hypercarbia after receiving oxygen-powered nebulized salbutamol for severe respiratory distress. Two died despite intubation.[89] Transient severe decreases in Pa_{O_2} with nebulizer use[109, 110] have been found to be of significance only for the most severely compromised patient and can be overcome by exercising the proper vigilance due such a critical patient.[111] Cautious administration of supplemental oxygen during nebulizer therapy appears to minimize this effect.[112]

Intermittent Positive-Pressure Breathing Therapy

For a 40-year period, from the 1930s to the late 1970s, IPPB enjoyed popularity as a means of overcoming severe bronchoconstriction and delivering bronchodilator drugs to those with asthma and other obstructive lung diseases. However, from nearly its inception, IPPB was a controversial method.[113] A major assumption underlying the therapeutic use of IPPB was the capacity to attain deep penetration with aerosolized medications. In 1977, researchers using radioactive tracers showed deeper penetration with quiet breathing than with IPPB. IPPB was found to deliver 32 per cent less aerosolized medication to the lungs.[114] By 1984, a review of 15 studies comparing IPPB with nebulizer or MDI therapy, or both, found equivalence in 12, superiority of IPPB in three, and inferiority in one of the studies to that date.[115]

Although IPPB has been labeled as a potential cause of cardiac toxicity, pulmonary infection, pneumothorax, and pneumomediastinum,[115] its reputation seems to be anecdotal in origin. The implied linkage of increased nosocomial pulmonary infection with IPPB decried in one editorial[116] was found to be a function of the presence of a mainstream reservoir of nebulizer fluid; IPPB machines without such reservoirs had no greater infection rate than that of free air.[117] Nonetheless, the lack of proven efficacy, combined with the great economic costs associated with IPPB—rather than the frequently mentioned but basically undocumented risks—brought this once popular technique into disfavor.

Conclusions

There appears to be little controversy in the current literature as to the safety, efficacy, and superiority of the inhalant route of therapy for acute bronchospasm. The choice of MDI versus nebulizer in various settings has become much less clear cut. The nebulizer requires no significant instruction or effort once the various components have been assembled and presented to the patient. The MDI, when used correctly, is cheaper, less prone to contamination, and far more convenient for patients both in and out of the hospital.

The appearance of a patient suffering from an exacerbation of reactive airway disease should be viewed as an opportunity for medical personnel to observe and correct the patient's use of the MDI—a powerful therapeutic method when used correctly. Failure of the patient to demonstrate correct use of the MDI suggests the need to implement a spacer device. The spacer is a low-cost, highly efficient device that could pay for itself many times over in reduced future visits. Correction of poor technique and treatment of the acute process with the MDI will reduce the impression that there is some magical property inherent in nebulizer use, simplify home therapy for many, and decrease medical costs.

MEDICATIONS

Introduction

The lung parenchyma is innervated by two well-known pathways: the sympathetic (adrenergic) and the parasympathetic (cholinergic) systems. Additionally, a third, poorly understood, pathway called the *peptidergic* (nonadrenergic, purinergic) inhibitory system is currently being investigated, but it will not be covered here.[118] The parasympathetic system stimulates contraction of the bronchial smooth muscle and is responsible for the resting tone of the airways. A major difference in the vigor and reactivity of this system can be seen when comparing patients with reactive airway disease, either from chronic obstructive pulmonary disease or asthma, and controls without respiratory disease. Normal subjects have little or no resting motor tone, but patients with reactive airway disease have a more intense tone that can be antagonized by atropine.[119]

The adrenergic mechanism is less clear. It is known that sympathetic terminals on the airway smooth muscle are rare or nonexistent. Adrenergic neurons cause bronchodilation by inhibition of the cholinergic system at parasympathetic preganglionic sites. Factors such as secretion of mucus, mast cell degranulation, and α-adrenergic neuronal activity are significant effectors in dictating the severity of the disease and are more subject to adrenergic effects in asthma than chronic obstructive pulmonary disease. The rapid response of airways to β_2 agonists in asthma strongly supports their direct role on bronchial smooth muscle tone in addition to the previously mentioned factors. This may explain the greater effect of β_2 agonists compared with anticholinergics.[119]

Formerly, the anticholinergics were thought to affect mainly the larger airways, with the β_2 agonists causing bronchodilation of the peripheral airways.[120] Current evidence suggests the route of drug delivery determines the site of greatest activity. When given intravenously, anticholinergic agents have uniform action throughout the respiratory tract.[119] Despite studies demonstrating greater initial efficacy of parenteral β_2-agonist drugs in the case of severe airway obstruction or bronchospasm, the use of the inhaled route is well accepted. In addition to decreased side effects and increased patient acceptance, the clinical outcome is generally equivalent.

Clonidine, an α_2 agonist, has been studied as a bronchodilator. Its proposed mechanisms of action are direct bronchodilation; central stimulation of the α_2 adrenoreceptors, which may serve presynaptically to inhibit the vagal reflex; and inhibition of allergen-induced histamine release. Because high concentrations of clonidine have been required in vitro to obtain relaxation, the first mechanism is doubtful. Alpha$_2$ adrenoreceptors may be involved in the integration of feedback control of vagal tone. One study demonstrated a 42 to 65 per cent reduction in allergen-evoked bronchospasm after pretreatment with clonidine.[121]

Calcium channel blocking agents would seem to have a rational basis for bronchodilation because smooth muscle contraction is mediated by intracellular calcium. However, in one study, inhaled verapamil was unsuccessful in increasing bronchodilation and in blocking bronchospasm in response to allergens.[122] Beclomethasone treatment of β_2-agonist resistance (see "Complications," discussed later) in acute exacerbations of asthma is well reported.[123]

Background

The use of inhaled medications in Western medicine can be divided into three phases. The period from prerecorded history to the 1800s was covered briefly in the previous section on inhaled drug delivery mechanisms. Atropine was isolated by Vaquelin in 1809 and recognized as an alkaloid by Brandes in 1819.[124] However, the *Datura* genus of plants has supplied indigenous practitioners in many parts of the world with anticholinergic compounds for several thousand years. References can be found to use of these plants by the Chinese, Assyrians, and native Americans. The ancient Siddha and Ayurvedic systems on the Indian subcontinent used specific *Datura* preparations. In 1800, British physicians in India adopted the use of these plants, with the first recorded application in Britain in 1802.[125] Shortly thereafter anticholinergics became a mainstay of treatment for respiratory disease in Great Britain.[118]

Although early atropinic compounds were produced from plants, observers termed the effects crude, unpredictable, malodorous to inhale, and potentially addicting. The synthesis of the first highly efficacious catecholamines in the early part of this century led to the decline in the use of anticholinergics.[125] Of note is that the use of cannabis for respiratory disease underwent a historical course parallel to that of the early atropinic agents; however, despite ongoing research, there has been no significant revival in the therapeutic use of cannabis.

Beginning in 1903 with the advent of adrenaline (epinephrine), the use of anticholinergics (and cannabis) gave way to the catecholamines in the management of bronchospasm. By the mid-1930s, adrenaline 1:100 administered by bulb syringe was available. One investigator wrote that "it was so effective, and the medical profession so opposed to it, that most patients knew enough not to admit to their doctors that they were taking it."[125] Epinephrine remained the standard therapy until the discovery of isoprenaline (isoproterenol) in 1940 led to the concept of α- and β-receptors and the search for ever more β-selective drugs.[126]

In 1964, isoetharine (Bronkosol) promised longer duration and slightly greater β_2 specificity. The drug replaced isoproterenol (Isuprel, Medihaler-Iso) and in turn has given way to the more specific agents such as terbutaline (Bricanyl, Brethine), metaproterenol (Metaprel, Alupent), and salbutamol (albuterol, Ventolin, Proventil).[127] Equally specific but longer-lasting drugs such as formoterol[128] and fenoterol (Berotec)[129] are under investigation.

Meanwhile, a resurgence in the use of anticholinergics has been fueled by the development of quaternary ammonium compounds such as ipratropium bromide (Atrovent) and glycopyrrolate (Rubinol). These charged molecules have bronchodilator properties similar to atropine and have a longer duration of action than the current β_2 agonists. Because of minimal lung membrane penetration, these inhaled anticholinergic drugs have almost no systemic side effects.[130] Atropine sulfate has been administered intravenously and has been nebulized with benefit, but it has also produced a number of side effects. Ipratropium bromide delivered by MDI is superior to atropine as a bronchodilator and has minimal systemic effects, but a nebulizable solution is not available in the United States. Glycopyrrolate is an anticholinergic drug known to anesthesiologists for years and is a nebulizable bronchodilating compound two to four times more potent than atropine. Glycopyrrolate has a duration of action greater than ipratropium bromide—approximately 8 to 12 hours[131] compared with 6 to 8 hours for ipratropium bromide. Glycopyrrolate has a low side effect profile similar to ipratropium bromide; approval by the United States Food and Drug Administration for use as a bronchodilator has not been sought.

Indications

REACTIVE AIRWAY DISEASE

Overview. Studies that directly compare anticholinergics with β_2 agonists have identified specific areas in which each is superior and a few instances in which a specific agent is indicated (Table 5–9). β_2 agonists are superior for treating extrinsic asthma caused by antigens, irritants, or exercise and for treating cold air-induced asthma. They have a relatively quick onset of action when compared with anticholinergics (5 minutes versus 30 minutes) and are therefore the mandatory first-line drug in severe acute respiratory distress due to reactive airway disease. Anticholinergics are the agents of choice in cholinergic toxicity; psychogenic asthma; β-adrenergic blockade from coincidental use of β-blocking agents for other therapeutic indications; and adjunctive therapy in acute reactive airway disease, including β-blocker–induced asthma. Some patients may present with severe bronchospasm and coincidentally may be suffering from systemic β-adrenergic effects, in which case the slower onset of the anticholinergics may be more tolerable than increased β-receptor stimulation.

Maintenance Therapy. For maintenance of patients with chronic obstructive pulmonary disease, anticholinergics appear to be more efficacious; ipratropium bromide is the leading drug prescribed for these conditions outside of the United States.[132] Furthermore, Vakil and colleagues suggest

Table 5–9. Indications for Bronchodilating Medications

Anticholinergic (ipratropium bromide, glycopyrrolate)
Infant, neonate
    Acute asthma
Children
    Asthma maintenance
General
    Maintenance therapy
        Chronic obstructive pulmonary disease
        Chronic bronchitis
        Asthma
    Acute care
        Adjunctively for asthma
        Adjunctively for chronic obstructive pulmonary disease
        Cholinergic toxicity
        Psychogenic asthma
        β-adrenergic blockade incidentally present from therapeutic use of β-blocking agent during bronchospasm
        Bronchospasm specifically due to β-blocking agents
        Organophosphate poisoning

Sympathomimetics (albuterol, metaproterenol)
Children
    Asthma maintenance
    Acute asthma
General
    Exercise and cold air–induced asthma
    Minor and major exacerbations
        Chronic obstructive pulmonary disease
        Chronic bronchitis
        Asthma
    β-adrenergic blockade incidentally present from therapeutic use of β-blocking agent during bronchospasm
    Bronchospasm specifically due to β-blocking agents

that a number of asthmatics might benefit from the use of ipratropium bromide as a maintenance drug as well.[133] A large, multicenter, double-blind, randomized study comparing ipratropium bromide with metaproterenol for 90 days found no significant difference in efficacy. However, responsiveness to the β_2 agonist fell over time, whereas no change was noted for the anticholinergic.[134] A second, longer study[133] placed 20 stable asthmatics on ipratropium bromide for a year and found this agent to be an efficacious and safe maintenance therapy. There was a fall in the "rescue" use of the β_2 agonist over time. One blind study that compared albuterol, ipratropium, and placebo (delivered by MDI) in patients with stable chronic obstructive pulmonary disease found ipratropium superior to albuterol at each measured time interval from 30 minutes to 6 hours.[135] That study also noted that although 40 per cent of the patients had less than a 15 per cent response to β-adrenergics, no patient treated with ipratropium failed to improve by this baseline amount.[135]

Acute Therapy. One study of patients with chronic obstructive pulmonary disease receiving supramaximal doses of atropine methonitrate (a drug functionally similar to ipratropium bromide) before or after administration of a supramaximal dose of salbutamol suggests that anticholinergic therapy is superior to β_2-agonist therapy.[119] When the drugs were given in combination, the greatest improvement achieved equaled that of the anticholinergic drug alone. When the β_2 agonist was given first, subsequent anticholinergic therapy led to clinical improvement. When the order was switched, no additional benefit occurred.

Numerous studies have found additive effects when the medications are used in submaximal doses;[136] submaximal therapy studies of asthmatics show a β_2-agonist–sparing role for the anticholinergics. Most studies in this field were done on stable patients and used small sample sizes. Rebuck and associates[137] examined 199 patients with acute airway obstruction using ipratropium and fenoterol (a long-acting β_2 agonist) alone and in combination and found that although both were effective as bronchodilators for patients in the group defined as "asthmatic," there were significant additive effects. In the "chronic obstructive pulmonary disease" group, combination therapy was no more effective than either therapy alone. This study also confirmed that those with the greatest need (FEV_1 less than 1 liter at presentation) received the greatest benefit from bronchodilator therapy.

Children. Sympathomimetics remain the first line in the treatment of children older than 18 months with acute respiratory distress from reactive airway disease. Before 18 months, children have rarely been responsive to β_2 agonists or aminophylline, although anticholinergic agents have been found useful in some patients. A study using ipratropium bromide in children with acute reactive airway disease found that 40 per cent of premature neonates, infants, and young children obtained benefit. The maximum dose per treatment for preterm patients is 20 μg. For patients up to 3 years of age the dose is 20 to 125 μg; and for those over the age of 3, 250 μg is considered optimal.[138] Other studies have shown that older children can benefit from ipratropium bromide but indicate the need for higher-than-prescribed doses to obtain benefit and caution against the use of an anticholinergic as a single-drug therapy in acute disease.[120, 139]

OTHER ACUTE CARE INDICATIONS

Bronchospasm secondary to allergic reactions, pulmonary infections, cystic fibrosis, and tumors all benefit from the use of aerosolized bronchodilators.[140] Ipratropium bromide may be particularly useful in patients with cystic fibrosis. Investigators using radioactively labeled erythrocytes found (despite the fear that atropinic compounds might increase mucous plugging) that ipratropium bromide doubled mucociliary clearance in patients with chronic bronchitis.[141] Additionally, bronchodilators may relieve some of the dyspnea associated with so-called cardiogenic wheezing from heart failure; here a parasympathetic agent would be preferable to avoid excess β stimulation. Pulmonary atropine has been used to mitigate the poisoning effect of organophosphate toxins on acetylcholine receptors.[142]

In two similar circumstances, unrelated to asthma or chronic obstructive pulmonary disease, patients may benefit from the use of an anticholinergic agent. First, nonasthmatic patients may suffer an anaphylactic reaction to a β-blocking drug. Attacks are characterized by profound hypotension; bradycardia, with or without atrioventricular nodal block; severe sustained bronchospasm; urticaria; or angioedema and are typically very resistant to treatment. These attacks occur independently of the presence of hyperreactive airways. Because of the β-blockade present, epinephrine, the current first-line therapy, has the risk of introducing unopposed α stimulation. Anticholinergics are useful for offering an alternative mechanism for attacking the bronchospasm present.[143] Second, a patient may suffer an anaphylactic reaction to an antigen (e.g., food, contrast material, insect stings, antibiotics, drugs, or allergy antigen injections) with the concurrent presence of therapeutic β-blockade as noted previously. Psychogenic asthma is vagally mediated, and anticholinergic agents offer excellent protection against this type of reactive airway disease.[118]

Contraindications

Inhaled atropine can cause voiding difficulties in men with prostatic hypertrophy, flushing of the skin, tachycardia, blurred vision, and gastrointestinal disturbances. Inhaled ipratropium bromide causes none of these. Atropine is contraindicated in glaucoma, but again ipratropium bromide, even in large doses, is not. Narrow-angle glaucoma is listed under precautions, and patients should avoid medication spray in their eyes. Tremor, a frequent side effect of β_2-agonist therapy is not seen with anticholinergics. The only contraindication to ipratropium bromide and other similar quaternary ammonium compounds is known hypersensitivity to these agents. No adverse drug reactions have been reported.

Sympathomimetics are contraindicated in the presence of tachydysrhythmias and in cases of known hypersensitivity. Life-threatening cases of paradoxical bronchospasm and fatalities from excessive use have been reported. Caution is advised in patients with coronary artery disease, hypertension, hyperthyroidism, and diabetes mellitus according to the manufacturer. The use of β-selective agents such as albuterol (salbutamol) and terbutaline reduces the potential for adverse drug reactions and side effects.

Dosage and Availability (Table 5–10)

Previous recommendations for MDI spray use (e.g., salbutamol and other β_2 agonists) were "two puffs taken four times daily," in part because of concerns generated by asthma-related deaths in the United Kingdom and other countries. The deaths were initially believed to be linked to the increased sale of β-sympathomimetic bronchodilators,[144, 145] but this theory has been discarded.[90] Cumulative dose response curves with isoproterenol indicate that between 8 and 10 puffs per treatment period are required for maximum bronchodilation.[146] Salbutamol requires 4 to 8 puffs per treatment period. Similar work on ipratropium bromide suggests that significantly greater use than the standard two puffs is both safe and therapeutically desirable.[139, 147]

A reasonable recommendation for *maintenance* MDI is 2 to 4 puffs four to six times per day as needed to control symptoms. Because of the low level of side effects, ipratropium bromide is the logical first-choice maintenance drug, with albuterol or another β_2-selective drug reserved for "rescue." As noted previously in the section on drug delivery systems, *more aggressive MDI use is warranted during acute exacerbations* of reactive airway disease. The patient should be cautioned that increased requirements for medication may signal the presence of infection and should prompt the patient to seek medical evaluation for a course of antibiotics, steroids, or both.

Complications

Few complications are associated with the use of the bronchodilators discussed in this chapter. Package inserts for the current β_2 agonists warn of fatalities following excessive use of sympathomimetics; however, this caution probably reflects more on past events such as the unexpected increase in the death rate due to respiratory disease that occurred in Great Britain during the 1960s. The "excess mortality" in the United Kingdom was initially linked to the over-the-counter sales of the MDI, 87 per cent of which were for isoproterenol (much of the sales were for "forte" or double-strength isoproterenol). After a series of published warnings beginning in 1965 through 1968, the respiratory mortality declined, but it did so at a faster rate proportionally than did bronchodilator sales. The United States did not experience a concurrent mortality increase; many factors may explain the variance. Etiologic factors for the United

Table 5–10. Aerosolized Bronchodilators

Agent	Brand Names	Dosage*	Onset of Action	Duration of Action‡
Sympathomimetics†				
Isoetharine	Bronkosol	2.5–5.0 mg (adults) (0.25–0.5 ml 1% solution)	1–2 minutes	1 hour
Metaproterenol	Alupent } Metaprel	10–15 mg (adults) (0.2–0.3 ml 5% solution)	2 minutes	2–4 hours
Salbutamol (albuterol)	Proventil } Ventolin	2.5–5.0 mg (adults) 2.5 mg (children <5 years)	2 minutes	4–6 hours
Terbutaline	Bricanyl } Brethine	2.5–5.0 mg (adults) 0.2 mg/kg (children, max 5.0 mg)	2 minutes	4–6 hours
Anticholinergics				
Atropine		0.05 mg/kg (children) 0.025 mg/kg (adults)	30–60 minutes	4–5 hours
Glycopyrrolate	Robinul	0.2–1.0 mg (adults)	30–60 minutes	6–8 hours

*The amount of nebulizer diluent, usually about 2.5 ml normal saline, may be varied to provide a longer, more complete nebulization of the medication, up to the total amount the reservoir contains. See text for details.

†Epinephrine and isoproterenol are not included in this chart for reasons of short duration and lack of β_2 selectivity; isoetharine remains because, although clearly not a first-choice drug, it is still widely used.

‡Dosing interval should reflect patient need and be balanced against the severity of the side effects present.

Kingdom respiratory deaths probably include poor patient compliance; overuse of powerful, unrestricted drugs; and failure to begin systemic steroids because of patient overreliance on home treatment.[148] Current pharmacy-dispensed formulations are considered to have a greater therapeutic index. Interestingly, several potent and potentially dangerous bronchodilator preparations containing epinephrine are still marketed over the counter. Of note is a single case of myocardial infarction, reported in 1975, said to be associated with the inhalation of 675 mg of aerosolized isoproterenol over less than 3 days—18 times the maximum prescribed dose.[149]

Oxygen desaturation after sympathomimetic therapy has been attributed to increased ventilation-perfusion mismatch. One postulated mechanism is that the bronchodilator has relatively greater deposition within the most well-ventilated portions of the lung, resulting in a relative increase in ventilation of underperfused segments of the lung.[150] Additionally, because β_2 agonists are potent pulmonary vasodilators, there is an increased perfusion of underventilated lung.[151] Oxygen desaturation can be blunted with supplemental oxygen.[112]

The development of resistance to sympathomimetic agents (tachyphylaxis, subsensitivity, or refractoriness) has been called a myth by some[152] but is still being investigated by others.[123] Although tachyphylaxis appears in vitro as a progressive and often prompt loss of the excitability of the cell from repeated exposure to a β_2-agonist catecholamine, its clinical significance is questionable.[127] A progressive loss of response to increasing doses of intravenous β_2 agonist has been found in normal subjects but not in asthmatic patients.[153] Another study found a transient decrease in β_2-agonist receptors but no decrease in airway response to bronchodilators.[154] One group used terbutaline for a year without any loss of response.[155] Inhaled beclomethasone was found to have a salutary effect on β-receptor function within 1 hour of inhalation.[123] Factors such as seasonal variation in climate and air-borne pollutants may influence receptor function in a significant way. Previous unsuccessful use of sympathomimetics (self-administered or otherwise) does not imply a refractory state or preclude a successful outcome when the same drug or another sympathomimetic is administered in the emergency department.[85]

The dose of ipratropium bromide needed to reduce salivary secretions is 300 times that found to inhibit cholinergic-mediated bronchoconstriction.[156] Hence, there is a large therapeutic index. Because the drug is poorly absorbed through both the lung and the gastrointestinal tract, ipratropium bromide is so safe that no instructions for overdose are included on the package insert.

Conclusions

Anticholinergics have been criticized as being less effective bronchodilating agents than β_2 agonists. The criticism is frequently based on studies in which large doses of the β_2 agonists have an overriding effect. Yet careful tailoring of drugs with different mechanisms to the individual's needs will frequently allow the patient to receive better coverage with less risk from toxic side effects. In addition, conclusions drawn from studies treating stable patients are frequently extrapolated widely, overlooking the variability in the disease state. Increased responsiveness to anticholinergics has been found in some patients with acute exacerbations of reactive airway disease. Inter- and intrapatient variability and the variety of study methods reported prevent conclusive statements about the relative role of adrenergic versus anticholinergic drugs in reactive airway disease.

REFERENCES

1. Castiglioni A: A History of Medicine. 2nd ed. New York, Alfred A. Knopf, 1947, p 76.
2. Adams F: The Extant Works of Aretaeus the Cappadocian. London, Sydenham Society, 1856, pp 316–319.
3. McFadden ER Jr, Ingram HR: Asthma: Perspectives, definition and classification. In Pulmonary Diseases and Disorders. New York, McGraw-Hill Book Co, 1980, pp 562–564.
4. Gershwin M: Bronchial Asthma, Principles of Diagnosis and Treatment. New York, Harcourt Brace Jovanovich, 1986, pp 3–4.
5. National Center for Health Statistics: Monthly vital statistics report, annual summary for the U.S., vol.22, no.13, 1973.
6. Gross NJ: COPD: A disease of reversible air-flow obstruction. Am Rev Resp Dis 133:725, 1986.
7. Godfrey S, Edward RHT, Campbell EJM: Repeatability of physical signs in airways obstruction. Thorax 24:4, 1969.
8. Shim CS, Williams MH: Evaluation of the severity of asthma: Patients versus physicians. Am J Med 68:11, 1980.
9. Godfrey S, et al: Spirometry, lung volumes and airway resistance in normal children aged 5–18 years. Br J Dis Chest 64:15, 1970.
10. Kelsen SG, Kelsen DP, Fleegler BF, et al: Emergency room assessment and treatment of patients with acute asthma: Adequacy of the conventional approach. Am J Med 64:622, 1978.

11. Hosie HE, Nimmo WS: Measurement of FEV_1 and FVC%—comparison of a pocket spirometer with the Vitalograph. Anaesthesia 43:233, 1988.
12. Gunawardena KA, Houston K, Smith AP: Evaluation of the turbine pocket spirometer. Thorax 42:689, 1987.
13. Milnar AD, Ingram D: Peak expiratory flow rates in children under 5 years of age. Arch Dis Child 45:780, 1970.
14. Jain SK, Singh V, Sharma DA: The correlation of peak expiratory flow rate and spirometry in normal healthy subjects. J Appl Physiol 31:297, 1983.
15. McFadden ER Jr, Kiser R, deGroot WJ: Acute bronchial asthma: Relations between clinical and physiological manifestations. N Engl J Med 288:221, 1973.
16. Nowak RM, Pensler M I., Sankar DD, et al: Comparison of peak expiratory flow and FEV_1 admission criteria for acute bronchial asthma. Ann Emerg Med 11:64, 1982.
17. Brown LA, Sly RM: Comparison of mini-Wright and standard Wright peak flow meters. Ann Allergy 45:72, 1980.
18. Banner AS, Shah RS, Addington WW: Rapid prediction of need for hospitalization in acute asthma. JAMA 235:1337, 1976.
19. Nowak RM, Gordon KR, Wroblewski DA, et al: Spirometric evaluation of acute bronchial asthma. JACEP 8:9, 1979.
20. Martin TG, Elenbaas RM, Pingleton SH: Failure of peak expiratory flow rates to predict hospital admission in acute asthma. Ann Emerg Med 11:466, 1982.
21. Silver RB, Ginsburg CM: Early prediction of the need for hospitalization in children with acute asthma. Clin Pediatr 23:81, 1984.
22. Ownby DR, Abarzua J, Anderson JA: Attempting to predict hospital admission in acute asthma. Am J Dis Child 138:1062, 1984.
23. Martin TG, Elenbass RM, Pingleton SH: Use of peak expiratory flow rates to eliminate unnecessary arterial blood gases in acute asthma. Ann Emerg Med 11:70, 1982.
24. Nowak RM, Tomlanovich MC, Sankar DD, et al: Arterial blood gases and pulmonary function testing in acute bronchial asthma: Predicting patient outcomes. JAMA 249:2043, 1983.
25. Gerlach JV: Uber das Hautahmen. Arch Anat Physiol (Leipzig) 431:455, 1981.
26. Baumberger JP, Goodfriend RB: Determination of arterial oxygen tension in man by equilibration through intact skin. Fed Proc 10:10, 1951.
27. Severinghaus JW, Astrup PB: History of blood gas analysis. V. Oxygen measurement. J Clin Monit 2:174, 1986.
28. Mahutte CK, Michiels TM, Hassell KT: Evaluation of a single transcutaneous P_{O_2}-P_{CO_2} sensor in adult patients. Crit Care Med 12:1063, 1984.
29. Whitehead MD, Lee BVD, Reynolds EOR: Estimation of arterial oxygen and carbon dioxide tensions by a single transcutaneous sensor. Arch Dis Child 60:356, 1985.
30. Reed RL, et al: Correlation of hemodynamic variables with transcutaneous P_{O_2} measurements in critically ill adult patients. J Trauma 145:1045, 1985.
31. Smith M, Abraham E: Conjunctival oxygen tension monitoring during hemorrhage. J Trauma 26:217, 1986.
32. Abraham E, Fink S: Cardiorespiratory and conjunctival oxygen tension monitoring during resuscitation from hemorrhage. Crit Care Med 14:1004, 1986.
33. Dronen SC, Maningas PA, Foutch R: Transcutaneous oxygen tension measurements during graded hemorrhage and reinfusion. Ann Emerg Med 14:534, 1985.
34. Waxman K, Sadler R, Eisner ME, et al: Transcutaneous oxygen monitoring of emergency department patients. Am J Surg 146:35, 1983.
35. Harding SM, Podolsky S, Wertheimer JH: Conjunctival oxygen monitoring: Relationship to ventricular arrhythmia. Am J Emerg Med 6:244, 1988.
36. Waxman K, Wong DH, O'Neal K: Early diagnosis of shock due to pericardial tamponade using transcutaneous oxygen monitoring. Crit Care Med 15:1156, 1987.
37. Abraham E, Smith M, Silver L: Conjunctival and transcutaneous oxygen monitoring during cardiac arrest and cardiopulmonary resuscitation. Crit Care Med 12:419, 1984.
38. Kram HB, Shoemaker WC: Diagnosis of major peripheral arterial trauma by transcutaneous oxygen monitoring. Am J Surg 147:780, 1984.
39. Shoemaker WC; Lawner PM: Method for continuous conjunctival oxygen monitoring during carotid artery surgery. Crit Care Med 11:946, 1983.
40. Abraham E, Lee G, Morgan MT: Conjunctival oxygen tension monitoring during helicopter transport of critically ill patients. Ann Emerg Med 15:782, 1986.
41. Isenberg SJ, Shoemaker WC: The transconjunctival oxygen monitor. Am J Ophthalmol 64:622, 1983.
42. Stokes CD, Blevins S, Siegel JH, et al: Prediction of arterial blood gases by transcutaneous O_2 and CO_2 in critically ill hyperdynamic trauma patients. J Trauma 27:1240, 1987.
43. Podolsky S, Wertheimer J, Harding S: The relationship of conjunctival and arterial blood gas oxygen measurements. Resuscitation 18:31, 1989.
44. Nisam M, Albertson TE, Panacek E, et al: Effects of hyperventilation on conjunctival oxygen tension in humans. Crit Care Med 14:12, 1986.
45. Klein M, Hess D, Eitel D, et al: Conjunctival oxygen tension monitoring during a controlled phlebotomy. Am J Emerg Med 6:11, 1988.

46. Tremper KK, Barker SJ, Hufstedler SM, et al: Transcutaneous and liver surface PO_2 during hemorrhagic hypotension and treatment with phenylephrine. Crit Care Med 17:537, 1989.
47. Tremper KK, Shoemaker WC: Transcutaneous oxygen monitoring of critically ill adults with and without low flow shock. Crit Care Med 9:706, 1981.
48. Tremper KK, Waxman KS, Applebaum RA, et al: Transcutaneous P_{O_2} monitoring during sodium nitroprusside infusion. Crit Care Med 13:65, 1985.
48a. Rooke TW, Osmundson PJ: The influence of age, sex, smoking, and diabetes on lower limb transcutaneous oxygen tension in patients with arterial occlusive disease. Arch Intern Med 150:129, 1990.
49. Gottrup F, Gellet S, Kirkegaard L, et al: Effect of hemorrhage and resuscitation on subcutaneous, conjunctival, and transcutaneous oxygen tension in relation to hemodynamic variables. Crit Care Med 17:904, 1989.
50. Abraham E, Oye RK, Smith M: Detection of blood volume deficits through conjunctival oxygen tension monitoring. Crit Care Med 12:931, 1985.
51. Abraham E, Smith M, Silver L: Continuous monitoring of critically ill patients with transcutaneous oxygen and carbon dioxide and conjunctival oxygen sensors. Ann Emerg Med 13:1021, 1984.
52. Shoemaker WC, Vidyasagar D: Physiologic and clinical significance of $PtcO_2$ and $PcjO_2$ measurements. Crit Care Med 9:689, 1981.
53. Isenberg SJ, Green BF: Changes in conjunctival oxygen tension and temperature with advancing age. Crit Care Med 13:683, 1985.
54. Guerci AD, Thomas K, Hess D, et al: Correlation of transconjunctival P_{O_2} with cerebral oxygen delivery during cardiopulmonary resuscitation in dogs. Crit Care Med 16:612, 1988.
55. Peabody JL, Gregory GA, Willis MM, et al: Transcutaneous oxygen tension in sick infants. Am Rev Respir Dis 118:83, 1978.
56. Severinghaus JW, Astrup PB: History of blood gas analysis. VI. Oximetry. J Clin Monit 2:270, 1986.
57. Neff TA: Routine oximetry—a fifth vital sign? Chest 94:227, 1988.
58. New W: Pulse oximetry versus measurement of transcutaneous oxygen. J Clin Monit 1:126, 1985.
59. McGuire TJ, Pointer JE: Evaluation of a pulse oximetry in the prehospital setting. Ann Emerg Med 17:1058, 1988.
60. Yelderman M, New W: Evaluation of pulse oximetry. Anesthesiology 59:349, 1983.
61. Jones J, Heiselman D, Cannon L, et al: Continuous emergency department monitoring of arterial saturation in adult patients with respiratory distress. Ann Emerg Med 17:463, 1988.
62. Niehoff J, DelGuercio C, LaMorte W, et al: Efficacy of pulse oximetry and capnometry in postoperative ventilatory weaning. Crit Care Med 16:701, 1988.
63. Gilbert R: Spirometry and blood gases. In Henry JB (ed): Clinical Diagnosis and Management by Laboratory Methods. 16th ed. Philadelphia, WB Saunders Co, 1979, p 113.
64. Hedges JR, Amsterdam JR, Cionni DJ, et al: Oxygen saturation as a marker for admission or relapse with acute bronchospasm. Am J Emerg Med 5:196, 1987.
65. Palve H, Vuori A: Pulse oximetry during low cardiac output and hypothermia states immediately after open heart surgery. Crit Care 17:66, 1989.
66. Choe H, Tashiro C, Fukumitso K: Comparison of recorded values from six pulse oximeters. Crit Care Med 17:678, 1989.
67. Gussack SG, Tacchi EJ: Pulse oximetry in the management of pediatric airway disorders. South Med J 80:1381, 1987.
67a. Rosen LM, Yamamoto LG, Wiebe RA: Pulse oximetry to identify a high-risk group of children with wheezing. Am J Emerg Med 7:567, 1989.
67b. Short L, Hecker RB, Middaugh RE, et al: A comparison of pulse oximeters during helicopter flight. J Emerg Med 7:639, 1989.
68. Myers RA, Linberg SE, Cowley RA: Carbon monoxide poisoning: The injury and its treatment. JACEP 8:479, 1979.
69. Friedman PA: Poisoning and its management. In Petersdorf RG, Adams RD, Braunwald E, et al (eds): Harrison's Principles and Practice of Internal Medicine. New York, McGraw-Hill Book Co, 1983, p 1271.
70. Fulmer JD, Snider GL: American College of Chest Physicians (ACCP)—National Heart, Lung, and Blood Institute (NHLBI) Conference on Oxygen Therapy. Arch Intern Med 144:1645, 1984.
71. Estey W: Subjective effects of dry versus humidified low flow oxygen. Respir Care 25:1143, 1980.
72. Koslawski S, Rasmussen B, Wilkoff WG: The effect of high oxygen tensions on ventilation during severe exercise. Acta Physiol Scand 81:385, 1971.
73. Aubier M, Murciano D, Milic-Emili J, et al: Effects of the administration of oxygen on ventilation and blood gases in patients with chronic obstructive pulmonary disease during acute respiratory failure. Am Rev Respir Dis 122:747, 1980.
74. Dantzker DR, Wagner PD, West JB, et al: Instability of lung units with low VA/Q ratios during breathing. J Appl Physiol 38:886, 1975.
75. Hurst JM, DeHaven CB, Branson RD: Use of CPAP mask as the sole mode of ventilatory support in trauma patients with mild to moderate respiratory insufficiency. J Trauma 25:1065, 1985.
76. Rasanen J, Heikkila J, Downs J, et al: Continuous positive airway

pressure by face mask in acute cardiogenic pulmonary edema. Am J Cardiol 55:296, 1985.

77. DeHaven CB, Hurst JM, Branson RD: Postextubation hypoxemia treated with continuous positive airway pressure. Crit Care Med 13:46, 1985.

78. Paterson IC, Crompton GK: Use of pressurized aerosols by asthmatic patients. Br Med J 1:76, 1976.

79. MacIntyre NR, et al: Aerosol delivery in intubated, mechanically ventilated patients. Crit Care Med 13:81, 1985.

80. Grinspoon L: Marijuana. Sci Am 221:17, 1969.

81. Cohen S: Therapeutic aspects of marijuana. National Institute on Drug Abuse Research Monograph Series. New York, 1980, p 196.

82. Hayton WL: Propellant powered nebulizers. J Am Pharm Assoc 16:201, 1976.

83. Newman SP, Woodman M, Clarke SW, et al: Effect of InspirEase on the deposition of metered-dose aerosols in the human respiratory tract. Chest 89:551, 1986.

84. Jenkins D: Use of nebulizer for acute asthma. J Royal Col Gen Pract 33:725, 1983.

85. McFadden ER: Critical appraisal of the therapy of asthma—an idea whose time has come. Am Rev Respir Dis 133:723, 1986.

86. Summer W, Elston R, Tahrpe L, et al: Aerosol bronchodilator delivery methods—relative impact on pulmonary function and cost of respiratory care. Arch Intern Med 149:618, 1989.

87. Berenberg MJ, Cupples LA, Baigelman W: Comparison of metered-dose inhaler attached to an Aerochamber with an updraft nebulizer for the administration of metaproterenol in hospitalized patients. J Asthma 22:87, 1985.

88. Salzman GA, Steele MT, Pribble JT, et al: Aerosolized metaproterenol in the treatment of asthmatics with severe airflow obstruction. Chest 95:1017, 1989.

89. Lim TK, Tan WC: Acute carbon dioxide narcosis during inhalational therapy with oxygen powered nebulizers in patients with chronic airflow limitation. Ann Acad Med Singapore 14:439, 1985.

90. Laurenco RV, Contromanes E: Clinical aerosols I. Characterization of aerosols and their diagnostic uses. Arch Intern Med 142:2163, 1982; II. Therapeutic aerosols. Arch Intern Med 142:2299, 1982.

91. Connolly CH: Method of using pressurized aerosols. Br Med J 3:21, 1975.

92. Orehek J, Gayrard P, Grimaud CH, et al: Patient error in the use of bronchodilator metered aerosols. Br Med J 1:76, 1976.

93. Kelling JS, et al: Physician knowledge in the use of canister nebulizers. Chest 83:612, 1983.

94. Newman SP, Pavia D, Bateman JRM, et al: Bronchodilator response after administration of pressurized aerosols at different lung volumes in patients with airways obstruction. Clin Sci 56: 10P, 1979.

95. Riley DJ, Weitz BW, Edelman WH: The responses of asthmatic subjects to isoproterenol inhaled at differing lung volumes. Am Rev Respir Dis 114:509, 1976.

96. Dolovich M, Ruffin RE, Roberts R: Optimal delivery of aerosols from metered dose inhalers. Chest 80:911, 1981.

97. Sackner MA, Kim CS: Auxillary MDI aerosol delivery systems. Chest 88:161, 1985.

98. Pedersen S, Steffensen G: Simplification of inhalation therapy in asthmatic children. Allergy 41:296, 1986.

99. Newhouse MT, Dolovich MB: Aerosols therapy: Nebulizer vs MDI. Chest 91:799, 1987.

100. Jenkins SC, et al: Comparison of domiciliary nebulized salbutamol and salbutamol from a MDI in stable chronic airflow obstruction. Chest 91:804, 1987.

101. Tarala RA, et al: Comparative efficacy of salbutamol by pressurized aerosol and wet nebulizer in acute asthma. Br J Clin Pharmacol 10:393, 1980.

102. Gunawardena KA, Smith AP, Shankleman J, et al: A comparison of MDIs with nebulizers for the delivery of ipratropium bromide in domiciliary practice. Br J Dis Chest 80:170, 1986.

103. Turner JR, Corkery KJ, Eckman D, et al: Equivalence of continuous flow nebulizer and MDI with reservoir bag for the treatment of acute airflow obstruction. Chest 93:476, 1988.

104. Feisal AE: "Aerosol-in-bag" administration of inhaled bronchodilators. Eur J Respir Dis 70:234, 1987.

105. Haeseon L, Evans HE: Aerosol bag for administration of bronchodilators to young asthmatic children. Pediatrics 73:230, 1984.

106. Tobin MJ: Use of bronchodilator aerosols. Arch Intern Med 145:1659, 1985.

107. Newhouse MT, Dolovich MB: Control of asthma by aerosols. N Engl J Med 315:870, 1986.

108. IPPB Trial Group: IPPB in COPD (editorial). Chest 86:341, 1984.

108a. Nelson MS, Hofstadter A, Parker J, et al: Frequency of inhaled metaproterenol in the treatment of acute asthma exacerbation. Ann Emerg Med 19:21, 1990.

109. Taguchi JT: Effect of ultrasonic nebulization on blood gas tensions in chronic obstructive pulmonary disease. Chest 60:356, 1971.

110. Phlug AE, Cheney FW, Butler J: The effects of ultrasonic aerosol on pulmonary mechanics and arterial blood gases in patients with chronic bronchitis. Am Rev Respir Dis 101:710, 1970.

111. Flick MR, Moody LR, Block AJ: Effect of ultrasonic nebulization on arterial oxygen saturation in chronic obstructive pulmonary disease. Chest 71:366, 1977.

112. Hedges JR, Cionni DJ, Amsterdam JT, et al: Oxygen desaturation in adults following inhaled metaproterenol therapy. J Emerg Med 4:77, 1987.

113. Noehren TH: IPPB therapy—where do we go from here? Chest 67:471, 1975.

114. Dolvich MB, Killian D, Wolff RK, et al: Pulmonary aerosol deposition in chronic bronchitis: IPPB versus quiet breathing. Am Rev Respir Dis 115:397, 1977.

115. Gonzalez ER, Burke TG: Review of the status of IPPB therapy. Drug Intell Clin Pharm 18:974, 1984.

116. Petty TL: A critical look at IPPB. Chest 66:1, 1974.

117. Reinarz JA, et al: Potential role of inhalant therapeutic equipment in nosocomial pulmonary infection. J Clin Invest 44:831, 1965.

118. Gross NJ, Skorodin MS: Anticholinergic, antimuscarinic bronchodilators. Am Rev Respir Dis 129:856, 1984.

119. Gross NJ, Skorodin MS: Role of the parasympathetic system in airway obstruction due to emphysema. N Engl J Med 311:421, 1984.

120. Lin MT, Lee-Hong E, Collins-Williams C: A clinical trial of the bronchodilator effect of SCH 1000 aerosol in asthmatic children. Ann Allergy 40:326, 1978.

121. Lingren BR, Ekstrom T, Andersson RG: The effect of clonidine in patients with asthma. Am Rev Respir Dis 134:266, 1986.

122. Fish JE, Norman PS: Effects of calcium channel blocker, verapamil, on asthmatic airway responses to muscarinic, histaminergic, and allergenic stimuli. Am Rev Respir Dis 133:730, 1986.

123. Pansegrouw DF, Weich DJV, le Roux FPJ: The treatment of acute resistant asthma with a combination of beclomethasone and fenoterol inhalations (abstract). Am Rev Respir Dis 139 (Suppl): A435, 1989.

124. Shutt LE, Bowes JB: Atropine and hyoscine. Anaesthesia 34:476, 1979.

125. Gandevia B: Historical review of parasympatholytic agents in the treatment of respiratory disorders. Postgrad Med J 51(Suppl 7):13, 1975.

126. Ahlquist RP: A study of the adrenotropic receptors. Am J Physiol 153:586, 1948.

127. Seale JP: Whither β-adrenoceptor agonists in the treatment of asthma. Progr Clin Biol Res 263:367, 1988.

128. Larsson S, Löfdahl GC, Arvidsson P: Formoterol, a new long-acting β₂-agonist for inhalation in a 12 month comparison with salbutamol (abstract). Am Rev Respir Dis 139 (Suppl):A432, 1989.

129. Owens GR: New concepts in bronchodilator therapy. American Family Practice 33:218, 1986.

130. Atsmon J: Topics in clinical pharmacology: Ipratropium bromide in COPD and asthma. Am J Med Sci 296:140, 1988.

131. Schroeckenstein DC, Bush RK, Chervinsky P, et al: Twelve hour bronchodilation in asthma with a single dose of the anticholinergic compound glycopyrrolate. J Allergy Clin Immunol 82:115, 1988.

132. Gross NJ, Petty TL, Freidman M, et al: Dose response to ipratropium bromide as a nebulized solution in patients with chronic obstructive pulmonary disease. A three-center study. Am Rev Respir Dis 139:1188, 1989.

133. Vakil DV, Ayiomanitis A, Nizami RM, et al: Use of ipratropium bromide in long-term management of asthma. J Asthma 22:165, 1985.

134. Storms WW, Bodman SF, Nathan RA, et al: Use of ipratropium bromide in asthma. Am J Med 81 (Suppl 5A) :61, 1986.

135. Braun SR, McKenzie WN, Copeland C: A comparison of the effect of ipratropium and albuterol in the treatment of chronic obstructive airway disease. Arch Intern Med 149:544, 1989.

136. Bruderman I, Cohen-Aronovski R, Smorzik J: A comparative study of various combinations of ipratropium bromide and metaproterenol in allergic asthmatic patients. Chest 83:208, 1983.

137. Rebuck AS, Chapman KR, Abboud R, et al: Nebulized anticholinergic and sympathomimetic treatment of asthma and chronic obstructive airways disease in the emergency room. Am J Med 82:59, 1987.

138. Milner AD: Ipratropium bromide and airways obstruction in childhood. Postgrad Med J 63:53, 1987.

139. Friberg S, Graff-Lonnevig V: Ipratropium bromide (Atrovent) in childhood asthma: A cumulative dose-response study. Ann Allergy 62:131, 1989.

140. Shwachman H: Cystic fibrosis. In Petersdorf RG, Adams RD, Braunwald E, et al (eds): Harrison's Principles and Practice of Internal Medicine. New York, McGraw-Hill Book Co, 1983, p 1544.

141. Matthys H, et al: Influence of 0.2 mg of ipratropium bromide on mucociliary clearance in patients with chronic bronchitis. Respiration 48:329, 1985.

142. Kanto J, Klotz U: Pharmacokinetic implications for the clinical use of atropine, scopalamine and glycopyrrolate. Acta Anaesth Scand 32:69, 1988.

143. Toogood JH: Risk of anaphylaxis in patients receiving beta-blocker drugs. J Allergy Clin Immunol 81:1, 1988.

144. Inman WH, Adelstein AM: Rise and fall of asthma mortality in England and Wales in relation to the use of pressurized aerosols. Lancet 2:279, 1969.

145. Inman WH: Recognition of unwanted drug effects with special reference to pressurized bronchodilators aerosol. In Burley DM (ed): Evaluation of Bronchodilator Drugs. London, Trust for Education and Research in Therapeutics. London, 1974, pp 191–206.

146. Cohen AA, Hale SC: Comparative effects of isoproterenol on airway resistance in obstruction pulmonary disease. Am J Med Sci 249:309, 1965.

147. Hockley B, Johnson NM: A comparison of three high doses of ipratropium bromide in chronic asthma. Br J Dis Chest 79:379, 1985.
148. Paterson JW, Woolcock AJ, Shenfield GM: Bronchodilator drugs. Am Rev Respir Dis 120:1149, 1979.
149. Aelony J, Laks MM, Beall G: An electrocardiographic pattern of acute myocardial infarction associated with excessive use of aerosolized isoproterenol. Chest 68:107, 1975.
150. Knudson RJ, Constantine HP: An effect of isoproterenol on ventilation perfusion in asthmatic versus normal subjects. J Appl Physiol 22:402, 1967.
151. Field GB: The effects of posture, oxygen, isoproterenol, and atropine on ventilation-perfusion relationships in the lung in asthma. Clin Sci 32:279, 1967.
152. Salzman GA, Pyszczynski DR: Drug therapy in asthma. Emerg Decisions 1:36, 1985.
153. Holgate ST, Baldwin CJ, Tattersfield AE: β-adrenergic agonist resistance in normal human airways. Lancet 2:375, 1977.
154. Busse WW, Sharpe G, Smith A, et al: The effect of procaterol treatment on beta-adrenergic bronchodilation and polymorphonuclear leukocyte responsiveness. Am Rev Respir Dis 132:1194, 1985.
155. Herjavecz I, Böszörményi-Nagy G, Szeitz A, et al: Development of drug tachyphylaxis in asthmatic patients treated with beta-adrenergic drugs. Acta Physiol Hungarica 70:329, 1987.
156. Bryant DH: Anti-cholinergic agents and their use in asthma. In Armour CL, Black JL (eds): Mechanisms in Asthma: Pharmacology, Physiology, and Management. New York, Alan R. Liss, Inc, 1988, pp 367–377.

Chapter **6**

Mechanical Ventilation

William Durston

Mechanical ventilation is truly a form of life support. All physicians who treat critically ill patients need to be thoroughly familiar with this mode of therapy. As in many other areas of medicine, there has been a proliferation of information and technology in the field of mechanical ventilation. The purpose of this chapter is to provide the reader with a practical yet complete review of the subject, including discussions of indications for mechanical ventilation, ventilator settings, characteristics of modern ventilators, potential complications of mechanical ventilation, and weaning techniques. Sections on the choice of a ventilator and on the set-up of representative modern pediatric and adult ventilators are also included.

HISTORICAL BACKGROUND

The notion that a person who is not breathing independently can be resuscitated by someone or something to help with the breathing dates back at least to 850 B.C., when it was recorded in the Bible that the prophet Elisha resuscitated a Shunammite boy: "And he put his mouth on his mouth and the flesh of the child waxed warm."[1] Not until the Industrial Revolution many centuries later was the first mechanical device for artificial ventilation described. In 1864, Alfred E. Jones of Lexington, Kentucky, was issued the first patent for a mechanical ventilator, a negative-pressure device that he claimed "cured paralysis, neuralgia, rheumatism, seminal weakness, asthma, bronchitis, and dyspepsia" (Fig. 6–1A).[2] In 1929, Drinker and Shaw patented the first practical iron lung, designed for the treatment of respiratory failure.[3] With this ventilator, the patient lay on a sliding bed with the head outside the apparatus, a rubber collar around the neck, and the remainder of the body inside the metal tank, which was evacuated and recompressed by an electrical pump (Fig. 6–1B). Although it was extremely cumbersome, the Drinker-Shaw iron lung, with few modifications, was used extensively for three decades and contributed to the survival of many polio victims with respiratory insufficiency.[4]

Techniques for positive-pressure ventilation during general anesthesia were developed during the 1920s but were not applied to patients outside of the operating room until the Scandinavian polio epidemic of 1952–1953, when the Danish anesthesiologist Bjorn Ibsen showed that survival was improved in patients ventilated through a cuffed endotracheal tube as compared with patients ventilated in iron lungs.[5] The positive pressure for Ibsen's patients was supplied by teams of nurses, medical students, and interns squeezing rubber anesthesia bags. By 1955, when a polio epidemic struck New England, a positive-pressure ventilator was available commercially, and once again the superiority of positive-pressure ventilation was demonstrated.[6] Respiratory intensive care units soon proliferated, and as the incidence of polio declined, positive-pressure mechanical ventilation came to be used not only in patients with respiratory failure due to neuromuscular disease but also in patients with a variety of other pulmonary and cardiac disorders. The explosive growth in the application of mechanical ventilation is illustrated in the records of Massachusetts General Hospital, where the number of patients treated on ventilators increased from 66 in 1958 to approximately 1500 in 1971.[7] In addition to the development of more reliable ventilators, the invention of the clinical blood gas electrode in the early 1960s contributed to the more widespread application of mechanical ventilation.[8]

Almost all patients who require mechanical ventilation today are treated with positive-pressure ventilation by means of an endotracheal tube or a tracheostomy tube. In a few select cases, however, negative-pressure ventilation is the method of choice. Patients with chronic respiratory insufficiency resulting from neuromuscular diseases have been managed successfully out of the hospital for prolonged periods with cuirass or tank-type negative-pressure ventilators.[9, 10] For the most part, however, negative-pressure ventilators are of historical interest only. In the remainder of this chapter, only positive-pressure ventilation is discussed. The abbreviations that will be used in this chapter are listed in Table 6–1.

INDICATIONS FOR MECHANICAL VENTILATION

The principal indication for mechanical ventilation is respiratory failure. Respiratory failure can be defined in terms of arterial blood gases, although criteria based on pulmonary mechanics have also been proposed. The indications for mechanical ventilation are summarized in Table 6–2.

Respiratory failure in adults is usually defined as a Pa_{O_2} less than 60 mm Hg while the patient is breathing the maximum oxygen concentration achievable by mask or a Pa_{CO_2} greater than 50 mm Hg with a pH less than 7.30. These criteria must sometimes be modified by the clinical situation. For example, a patient with chronic obstructive pulmonary disease (COPD) who is a CO_2 retainer but who has an acute loss of bicarbonate due to a diarrheal illness might have blood gases with a Pa_{O_2} of 55 mm Hg, a Pa_{CO_2} of 50 mm Hg, and a pH of 7.32 and be stable from the pulmonary standpoint. A young asthmatic with the same blood gases might be in need of immediate intubation and mechanical ventilation.[11]

In addition to arterial blood gases, other indices of pulmonary function may be helpful in determining whether a patient needs mechanical ventilation. In adults, a respiratory rate of greater than 35 to 40 breaths per minute usually cannot be sustained for prolonged periods, and if this rate is required to maintain a normal pH or Pa_{CO_2}, tachypnea

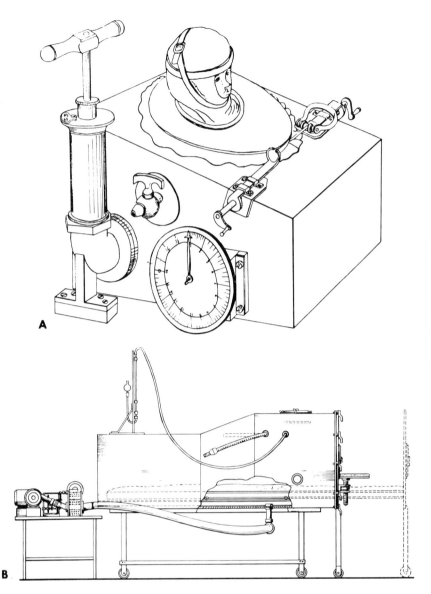

Figure 6–1. *A*, The first mechanical ventilator, patented by Alfred Jones of Lexington, Kentucky, in 1864. (From Crit Care Med 6:310, 1978. © by Williams & Wilkins, 1978. Reproduced by permission.) *B*, The Drinker-Shaw iron lung, patented in 1929, was the standard ventilator for polio victims during the early 1950s. (From Crit Care Med 7:226, 1979. © by Williams & Wilkins, 1978. Reproduced by permission.)

may be an indication for mechanical ventilation. A forced expiratory volume in 1 second (FEV_1) of less than 1000 ml or less than 10 ml/kg indicates severe airway obstruction and, if not readily reversible, predicts that the patient may need ventilatory assistance. A vital capacity (VC) less than 10 ml/kg and a maximum inspiratory force (MIF) less than 25 cm H_2O are other indications that the patient will not be able to maintain adequate ventilation independently. Similarly, a dead space to tidal volume ratio (V_D/V_T) of greater than 0.6 implies a high minute volume requirement and a need for ventilatory assistance in most patients.

Respiratory failure in adults is usually caused by primary pulmonary disease, cardiac disease, neuromuscular disease, drug overdose, or a combination of these conditions. In neonates, respiratory failure usually results from hyaline membrane disease, meconium aspiration, sepsis, or congenital cardiopulmonary anomalies. Respiratory failure in children beyond the neonatal period is most often due to respiratory infections, asthma, or accidents such as near-drowning or chemical aspiration. Indications for mechanical ventilation based on pulmonary mechanics are difficult to apply in infants and children because the patients are usually unable to cooperate in measuring VC, FEV_1, and MIF. Respiratory rates of 35 to 40 breaths per minute are normal in neonates and common in febrile children, and tachypnea

alone is not an indication for mechanical ventilation. The blood gas criteria for respiratory failure in infants are similar to those in adults, except that more deviation from the physiologic norm may be allowed before mechanical ventilation is instituted. Typical blood gas criteria for respiratory failure in infants cited in the literature include a pH less than 7.25, a Pa_{CO_2} greater than 60 mm Hg, and a Pa_{O_2} less than 55 to 60 mm Hg. Infants who are hypoxemic but not hypercapnic may first be tried on continuous positive airway pressure (CPAP) with high inspired oxygen concentrations before mechanical ventilation is instituted.[12-14] As with adults, other clinical factors must be weighed in deciding whether to institute mechanical ventilation. Apneic or bradycardiac periods may warrant ventilatory support, and low-birth-weight or premature infants are more likely to require mechanical ventilation.

In the absence of respiratory failure, there are few other indications for mechanical ventilation. Flail chest was formerly considered one of these. The concept of "alkalotic apnea for internal pneumatic stabilization of the critically crushed chest" was proposed in 1956 by Avery and colleagues, who found that positive-pressure ventilation was more effective and humane in the treatment of flail chest than were the older methods of external stabilization with Hudson traction and towel clips.[15] For two decades following

Table 6–1. Abbreviations Used in This Chapter

A–a D_{O_2}	Alveolar-arterial oxygen difference
ARDS	Adult respiratory distress syndrome
C_a	Oxygen content of systemic arterial blood
C_c	Oxygen content of pulmonary capillary blood
C_v	Oxygen content of mixed venous blood
COPD	Chronic obstructive pulmonary disease
CPAP	Continuous positive airway pressure
f	Respiratory rate or frequency
FEV_1	Forced expiratory volume in 1 second
FI_{O_2}	Per cent oxygen content of inspired gas
HFV	High-frequency ventilation
IMV	Intermittent mandatory ventilation
IRV	Inverse ratio ventilation (I:E ratio >1)
MIF	Maximum inspiratory force
MVV	Maximum voluntary minute volume
PA_{CO_2}	Alveolar carbon dioxide tension
Pa_{CO_2}	Arterial carbon dioxide tension
PA_{O_2}	Alveolar oxygen tension
Pa_{O_2}	Arterial oxygen tension
PE_{CO_2}	Tension of carbon dioxide in mixed expired air
PEEP	Positive end-expiratory pressure
Q_s/Q_t	Shunt fraction (ratio of right-to-left shunt to total pulmonary blood flow)
R	Respiratory quotient (ratio of carbon dioxide produced by the body to oxygen consumed)
SIMV	Synchronized intermittent mandatory ventilation
VA	Alveolar ventilation
$\dot{V}A$	Alveolar minute ventilation
VC	Vital capacity
$\dot{V}_{CO_2}$	Carbon dioxide production per minute
VD	Dead space volume
$\dot{V}E$	Expired minute volume
VT	Tidal volume

Avery's report, it was largely accepted that most patients with flail chest segments should be treated with mechanical ventilation to minimize chest wall motion caused by spontaneous respiratory effort and to allow the fractured ribs to heal. More recently, it has been recognized that patients who have flail segments but who do not meet usual blood gas criteria for respiratory failure do better if treated only with pain control, including epidural and intercostal blocks, than if treated with mechanical ventilation.[16]

Mechanical ventilation may be instituted in the absence of respiratory failure in patients who require hyperventilation. In patients with increased intracranial pressure, hyperventilation to a Pa_{CO_2} of 25 to 30 mm Hg has been advocated to rapidly reduce cerebral blood flow and brain swelling.[17] Hyperventilation has also been proposed to produce a respiratory alkalosis as a means of preventing seizures and ventricular dysrhythmias in patients suffering from tricyclic antidepressant overdose.[18]

In severely hypothermic patients, the administration of warm nebulized air is an effective means of core rewarming.[19] Although such patients usually require mechanical ventilation for other reasons, the need for rewarming might be considered an additional indication. Postoperative mechanical ventilation is also used "prophylactically" in certain surgical patients who are at high risk for the development of respiratory failure, atelectasis, or pneumonia. Conditions that may place a patient in a high-risk category include shock, morbid obesity, COPD, neuromuscular disease, or other debilitating illnesses. Patients also are at increased risk for the development of respiratory complications following cardiothoracic surgery.[7]

There are no absolute contraindications to mechanical ventilation. Some consider COPD with chronic carbon dioxide retention to be a relative contraindication, because patients with this condition are notoriously difficult to wean back to spontaneous breathing. When the COPD patient presents with respiratory failure, however, the condition has usually been precipitated by an acute process, such as a pulmonary infection, which can be reversed while the patient receives ventilatory assistance. The complication rate is unusually high in patients with asthma during mechanical ventilation as a result of the high pressures required to ventilate these patients.[20] Although barotrauma should be anticipated in treating severe asthmatics with mechanical ventilation, mechanical ventilation nonetheless may be life saving. In some patients with terminal illness or chronic debilitating disease, a decision not to initiate mechanical ventilation may be made on moral grounds.

TYPES OF VENTILATORS

Mechanical ventilators manufactured by more than a dozen companies are currently available in the United States; most manufacturers offer several different models. Despite the diversity of these machines, they may be grouped and classified according to a few basic characteristics that describe their operation.

Inspiratory Flow

There are basically two types of inspiratory flow patterns built into modern ventilators. The inspiratory flow either is constant during the inspiratory cycle or varies from the start to the end of the cycle. In general, ventilators with constant flow are called *flow generators*, whereas ventilators with variable flow are classified as *pressure generators*.[21] In a constant-*flow* generator, a high-pressure gradient is established between the ventilator and the patient. The machine is built with a high internal resistance so that changes in the resistance and compliance of the patient's airways make relatively little contribution to the total resistance of the system. The result is a constant, or square wave, flow pattern (Fig. 6–2A). In a constant-*pressure* generator, the machine develops a constant pressure that is only slightly above the pressure in the patient's airways. An exponential flow pattern results, with flow approaching zero as the patient's airway pressure approaches the pressure from the ventilator (Fig. 6–2B).

Table 6–2. Indications for Mechanical Ventilation

Blood gas criteria
    Pa_{O_2} less than 55 to 60 mm Hg on maximum FI_{O_2} by mask
    Pa_{CO_2} greater than 50 mm Hg and pH less than 7.30
Blood gas criteria in neonates
    Patient on CPAP of 5 to 8 cm H_2O and FI_{O_2} up to 0.80
    Pa_{O_2} less than 55 to 60 mm Hg
    Pa_{CO_2} greater than 60 mm Hg
    pH less than 7.25
Criteria based on pulmonary mechanics
    Vital capacity less than 10 ml/kg
    FEV_1 less than 10 ml/kg
    MIF less than 25 cm H_2O
    VD/VT greater than 0.6
Indications other than respiratory failure
    Need for hyperventilation
        Increased intracranial pressure
        Tricyclic antidepressant overdose
    Hypothermia
        Mechanical ventilation used as means of core rewarming
    Prophylactic postoperative mechanical ventilation
        In postoperative patients with shock, morbid obesity, COPD, neuromuscular disease, or other debilitating illness or following cardiothoracic surgery

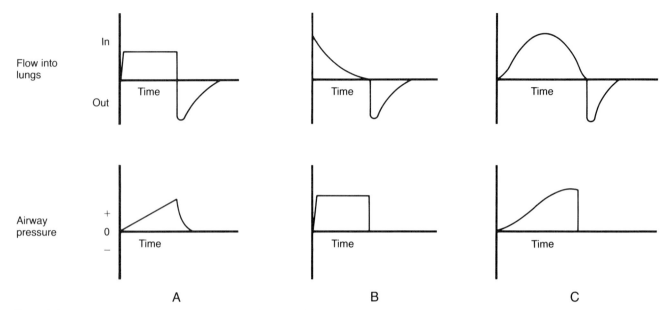

Figure 6–2. Flow and pressure waveforms generated by ventilators. *A,* The constant flow generator produces a square inspiratory flow wave. *B,* The constant pressure generator produces a decelerating inspiratory flow wave. *C,* A sine wave flow pattern is produced by a piston on an eccentric cam. (From Kirby RR, Desautels DA, Modell JH, Smith RA: Mechanical ventilation. In Burton GG, Gee EN, Hodgkin JE: Respiratory Care. Philadelphia, JB Lippincott Co, 1977. Reproduced by permisssion.)

It is apparent that constant-flow generators and constant-pressure generators are not conceptually different but rather are the opposite ends of a spectrum. By reducing internal resistance and machine pressure, one can convert a constant-flow generator into a constant-pressure generator. A sine wave flow pattern is also available on some ventilators (Fig. 6–2C). Such a flow pattern is produced by gas being driven by a piston on an eccentric cam.

The flow patterns of ventilators are of more interest to bioengineers than to clinicians, except that some modern ventilators have controls that allow the operator to switch from one flow pattern to another. As discussed in the section on ventilator settings, by changing the flow pattern, one may sometimes effect small but significant improvements in ventilation of the patient.

Cycling

In addition to being classified according to their inspiratory flow characteristics, ventilators are classified according to the factor that determines when the ventilator cycles from the inspiratory phase to the expiratory phase. Basically, there are three different types: pressure-cycled, volume-cycled, and time-cycled.

Pressure-Cycled. In pressure-cycled ventilators, the inspiratory phase is terminated, and expiration begins when a preset pressure limit is reached. The tidal volume received by the patient is not set directly but depends on the set pressure limit and the patient's chest and lung compliance and airway resistance. As long as the patient's compliance and resistance do not change, the tidal volume will be the same with each breath. If the patient's compliance falls or resistance increases, the tidal volume will also fall, and hypoventilation may result.

Because of the problem of a changing tidal volume caused by changing patient compliance, pressure-cycled ventilators have been largely replaced by volume- or time-cycled ventilators for mechanical ventilation in adults. Pressure-cycled ventilators still have certain advantages, however. They are less expensive than volume- and time-cycled ma-

chines. They are more compact and can be run off compressed gas sources without the need for an electrical source, making them well suited for ambulance transport. For reasons discussed later, pressure-cycled machines also remain popular for ventilating infants and neonates.

Volume-Cycled. In volume-cycled ventilators, inspiration is terminated and expiration begins when a preset tidal volume is delivered. The gas is usually delivered from a compressible bellows. Since the introduction of the Puritan-Bennett MA-1 volume ventilator in 1968, volume ventilators have become the standard for mechanical ventilation in adults. They have an important advantage over pressure-cycled ventilators: delivery of a relatively constant tidal volume despite changes in the patient's compliance. Even with volume-cycled machines, however, the delivered tidal volume will fall slightly if the patient's compliance falls. This is because although a constant volume is delivered from the ventilator bellows, as the patient's lungs become stiffer, more of this gas is lost to expansion of the ventilator tubing. This phenomenon becomes very important in infants. The compliance of the child's chest and lungs may be less than the compliance of the ventilator tubing, and more gas will go to expansion of the tubing than to ventilation of the patient.

Most modern volume ventilators have adjustable secondary pressure limits such that when the airway pressure exceeds the set limit, inspiration is terminated. Thus volume-cycled ventilators may function as pressure-cycled ventilators when the pressure limit is set low enough.

Time-Cycled. In time-cycled ventilators, inspiration is terminated and expiration begins after a preset time has elapsed. The tidal volume that is delivered is determined by the integral of the inspiration flow–inspiratory time curve. Time-cycled ventilators resemble volume-cycled machines in that they deliver a relatively constant tidal volume despite changes in the patient's compliance. They may also function as pressure-limited ventilators when the secondary pressure-limits are adjusted. Time-cycled ventilators are becoming increasingly popular. They allow great flexibility in adjustment of the inspiratory to expiratory ratio, and their internal circuitry is such that they can be manufactured at a lower cost than most volume-cycled machines.

CHOOSING VENTILATOR SETTINGS

To optimize ventilator therapy, the physician must understand the capabilities of the ventilator, the pathophysiology of the patient, and how to match the ventilator settings to the patient's condition to achieve the desired results. In this section, the rational choice of ventilator settings is discussed. Not all of the settings described in this section are available on every ventilator. To learn the capabilities of a given ventilator, the physician should consult the operating manual supplied with that particular machine. A summary of recommended initial ventilator settings is provided in Table 6–3.

Rate and Tidal Volume

The two most important settings on a volume-cycled ventilator (and those that are usually set first) are the rate and tidal volume. To provide an understanding of the way in which the rate and tidal volume determine alveolar ventilation and the arterial carbon dioxide tension (Pa_{CO_2}), it is necessary to review briefly some aspects of pulmonary physiology.

Minute Volume and Alveolar Ventilation. The volume of air (or any other gas mixture) that moves in and out of a patient's lungs per minute is termed the minute volume ($\dot{V}_E$). Minute volume is the product of V_T and respiratory frequency or rate (f):

$$\dot{V}_E = V_T \times f \tag{1}$$

Tidal volume can be further broken down into alveolar ventilation (V_A) and dead space ventilation (V_D):

$$V_T = V_A + V_D \tag{2}$$

In healthy young persons, the anatomic dead space can be accounted for by the trachea and the larger airways and is approximately 1 ml per pound of lean body weight. In disease states, in addition to the anatomic dead space, there is also a variable amount of "pathologic" dead space corresponding to ventilated alveoli and respiratory bronchioles that are not adequately perfused. The sum of the anatomic and pathologic dead spaces is often referred to as the physiologic dead space.

Alveolar minute ventilation ($\dot{V}_A$) is the product of rate times tidal volume minus dead space:

$$\dot{V}_A = (V_T - V_D) \times f \tag{3}$$

Alveolar minute ventilation and the rate of carbon dioxide production by the body ($\dot{V}_{CO_2}$) determine the partial pressure of carbon dioxide in the alveoli (PA_{CO_2}), which is approximately equal to the systemic arterial carbon dioxide tension (Pa_{CO_2}). This relationship is shown in equation 4:

$$Pa_{CO_2} \simeq PA_{CO_2} = k \times (\dot{V}_{CO_2}/\dot{V}_A) \tag{4}$$

Where the value of the constant is 0.863 when the partial pressure of carbon dioxide is measured in mm Hg at 37° C saturated with water vapor, $\dot{V}_{CO_2}$ is measured in milliliters per minute, and $\dot{V}_A$ is measured in liters per minute.

Using equations 3 and 4, one can work through the example of an average 150-pound man with a typical spontaneous tidal volume of 500 ml, respiratory rate of 12 breaths per minute, carbon dioxide production of 200 ml per minute, and dead space of 150 ml and see that a normal Pa_{CO_2} results:

$$\dot{V}_A = (0.500 - 0.150) \times 12$$
$$= 4.2 \text{ liters/minute}$$

and

$$Pa_{CO_2} = 0.863 \times (200/4.2)$$
$$= 41.0 \text{ mm Hg}$$

If this same 150-pound man were to develop respiratory failure purely on a neurologic basis without any change in his dead space or carbon dioxide production, one might

Table 6–3. *Recommended Initial Ventilator Settings*

Parameter	Recommended Setting	Comment
Tidal volume	10 to 15 ml/kg	8 to 12 ml/kg in infants (see section on rate and tidal volume).
Rate	12 to 14 breaths per minute	Starting rates of 25 to 30 per minute used in infants. Rates of 18 per minute or greater used in adults when hyperventilation is indicated or when V_D/V_T is very high (see section on rate and tidal volume).
FI_{O_2}	0.5 to 1.0	To avoid oxygen toxicity, reduce FI_{O_2} to below 0.5 as soon as possible, guided by blood gas results.
Ventilator mode	Assist control, IMV, or SIMV	(See section on ventilator mode.)
PEEP	None	Start with PEEP of 5 cm H_2O and increase in 5–cm H_2O increments if Pa_{O_2} less than 60 mm Hg with FI_{O_2} greater than or equal to 0.50 (see section on PEEP and CPAP).
Inspiratory waveform	Square wave	(See section in inspiratory flow.)
Inspiratory flow	50 L/min	8 to 15 L/min in infants (see section on inspiratory flow rate.)
Inspiratory pause	None	(See section on inspiratory pause.)
I:E ratio	1:2	(See section on I:E ratio.)
Peak pressure	50 cm H_2O	With pressure-cycled ventilators, starting pressures of 20 to 30 cm H_2O should be used in infants and in adults with normal compliance (see section on peak pressure).
Expiratory retard	None	(See section on expiratory retard.)
Sighs	None	(See section on sighs.)
Humidifier temperature	35° C	Use higher temperature (40° C) for rewarming hypothermic patients, lower temperature for cooling febrile patients.

assume that the appropriate ventilator settings would be a tidal volume of 500 ml and a rate of 12 breaths per minute. It has been found empirically, however, that *when patients are ventilated with tidal volumes that are in the normal range for spontaneous breathing, atelectasis and hypoxemia develop.*[7] One can prevent this by ventilating patients at higher tidal volumes, in the range of 10 to 15 ml/kg. Also, mechanical ventilation alters the normal ventilation-perfusion relationships in the lungs, causing relatively greater ventilation of the less well perfused upper lung regions, which in turn results in an increase in physiologic dead space.[22] The magnitude of this effect is roughly to double the predicted dead space when a patient converts from spontaneous breathing to mechanical ventilation.[23]

Returning to the case of our 150-pound man, assuming a physiologic dead space on the ventilator of 300 ml, a desired tidal volume of 12 ml/kg (850 ml), and a desired Pa_{CO_2} of 40 mm Hg, one can use equations 3 and 4 to solve for the desired ventilator rate:

$$Pa_{CO_2} = 0.863 \ (\dot{V}_{CO_2}/\dot{V}_A)$$
$$40 = 0.863 \ \times \ (200/\dot{V}_A)$$

Solving for $\dot{V}_A$:

$$\dot{V}_A = (0.863 \times 200)/40$$
$$= 4.3 \text{ liters per minute}$$

Putting this value for $\dot{V}_A$ into equation 3 and solving for f:

$$\dot{V}_A = (V_T \ - \ V_D) \times f$$
$$4.3 = (0.850 \ - \ 0.300) \times f$$
$$f = 4.3 \ \div \ (0.850 \ - \ 0.300)$$
$$= 7.8 \text{ breaths per minute}$$
$$\cong 8 \text{ breaths per minute}$$

In practice, such a low rate is rarely prescribed as the initial ventilator setting. Most patients requiring mechanical ventilation have more than normal dead space, and it is usually safer to risk mild hyperventilation than hypoventilation. Starting rates of 12 to 14 breaths per minute are recommended for most adult patients.

Changes in Pa_{CO_2} as a Result of Changes in Rate and Tidal Volume. Once a patient has been placed on a ventilator at a rate and tidal volume that are deemed appropriate, it is necessary to check arterial blood gases to be sure that the patient is being adequately ventilated and oxygenated. *Arterial blood gases are customarily drawn 15 minutes after the initiation of mechanical ventilation or after changes in ventilator settings.* This interval is supported by indirect evidence suggesting that blood gases reach equilibrium within 15 minutes after ventilator changes in most patients with severe pulmonary disease and much sooner in patients with normal lungs.[24, 25] In most patients, achieving a normal Pa_{CO_2} (36 to 44 mm Hg) is the goal. In some cases, however, a higher or lower Pa_{CO_2} is desired. For example, most experts warn against rapid reduction of Pa_{CO_2} to normal in patients with chronic carbon dioxide retention. The resultant alkalemia may have many undesirable consequences, including diminished cardiac output, diminished cerebral blood flow, hypokalemia, hypocalcemia with associated seizures, increased airway resistance, and a shift in the hemoglobin-oxygen dissociation curve to the left with impaired release of oxygen to the tissues.[22] However, in patients with increased intracranial pressure due to trauma, infection, or cerebrovascular accident, a lower than normal Pa_{CO_2} may be desired to lower intracranial pressure.

Whatever the desired Pa_{CO_2}, if the measured Pa_{CO_2} differs from the desired level, the ventilator rate or tidal volume must be adjusted accordingly. One can easily calculate the amount of change in ventilator settings needed to produce the desired change in Pa_{CO_2} using the relationship

$$\dot{V}_{E_2} = (Pa_{CO_2}{}^1/Pa_{CO_2}{}^2) \times \dot{V}_{E_1} \qquad (5)$$

where $\dot{V}_{E_2}$ is the desired minute volume, $\dot{V}_{E_1}$ is the present minute volume, $Pa_{CO_2}{}^2$ is the desired Pa_{CO_2}, and $Pa_{CO_2}{}^1$ is the present Pa_{CO_2}. (Strictly speaking, Pa_{CO_2} varies inversely with alveolar minute ventilation and not with total minute ventilation, which includes both alveolar ventilation and wasted, dead space ventilation. It has been observed empirically, however, that the ratio of V_D/V_T remains relatively constant despite changes in tidal volume.[26] Thus equation 5 holds whether rate or tidal volume or both are altered. As an example, suppose that a 70-kg patient is being ventilated at a rate of 10 breaths per minute with a tidal volume of 900 ml. The observed Pa_{CO_2} is 50 mm Hg, and the desired Pa_{CO_2} is 30 mm Hg. The desired minute volume is calculated as:

$$\dot{V}_{E_2} = (50/30) \times 9.0 \text{ liters per minute}$$
$$= 15 \text{ liters per minute}$$

To obtain a Pa_{CO_2} of 30, the rate could be increased to 16 and the tidal volume to 940 ml, giving a new minute volume of approximately 15 liters per minute.

Adding Dead Space. Some patients who are placed on ventilators and who are allowed to trigger the machine themselves, as in the assist control mode, will spontaneously hyperventilate. If the Pa_{CO_2} drops as low as 25 to 30 mm Hg in a patient who is used to a normal Pa_{CO_2}, the same complications may develop as described previously for rapidly lowering the carbon dioxide to normal in a chronically hypercapnic patient. An approach that may be useful in dealing with patients who spontaneously hyperventilate is to add dead space to the ventilator tubing so that the patient rebreathes some of the expired air. A formula has been developed that predicts the amount of dead space that must be added to give a desired increase in Pa_{CO_2}.[27] This formula is somewhat complicated, though, and requires determination of the concentration of carbon dioxide in the expired air. Empirically, it has been found that the addition of 50 ml of dead space will lead to an increase in Pa_{CO_2} of approximately 5 mm Hg in most patients.[27]

Another approach to raising the Pa_{CO_2} in a patient who spontaneously hyperventilates is to add carbon dioxide to the inspired air. A rise of 1 per cent in the inspired carbon dioxide concentration leads to a rise in Pa_{CO_2} of approximately 5 mm Hg.[28] The disadvantage of using this method rather than adding dead space is that it requires an expensive piece of additional equipment, the carbon dioxide mixer. Paradoxically, it has been found that increasing the Pa_{CO_2} by either method leads to a rise, rather than a decline, in Pa_{O_2}.[27, 28] This seems to be a result of the increased cardiac output that occurs with normalization of the Pa_{CO_2}. The problem with adding either dead space or inspired carbon dioxide is that the patient may hyperventilate even more, returning the Pa_{CO_2} to harmfully low levels. If this occurs, the patient should be sedated or changed to a different ventilator mode, as will be discussed subsequently.

The Dead Space to Tidal Volume Ratio (V_D/V_T). As noted earlier, in addition to their anatomic dead space, patients with pulmonary disease have variable amounts of pathologic dead space. The ratio V_D/V_T is useful to follow as an index of the severity of a patient's pulmonary disease. The normal V_D/V_T ratio is 0.20 to 0.35.[29] Patients with

V_D/V_T ratios of 0.6 or greater usually need ventilatory assistance, because they require large minute volumes to maintain adequate alveolar ventilation. The V_D/V_T ratio may be calculated using the Bohr equation:

$$V_D/V_T = (P_{A_{CO_2}} - P_{E_{CO_2}})/P_{A_{CO_2}} \qquad (6)$$

where $P_{E_{CO_2}}$ is the partial pressure of carbon dioxide in mixed expired air and $P_{A_{CO_2}}$ is the partial pressure of carbon dioxide in alveolar air, which is assumed to be the same as $P_{a_{CO_2}}$. To use this equation, one must have access to a carbon dioxide analyzer. Although these analyzers are commercially available, they are not standard equipment in all emergency departments or intensive care units. For this reason, a graph has been constructed from which V_D/V_T can be determined if one knows the patient's minute ventilation and $P_{a_{CO_2}}$ (Fig. 6–3).[30] The graph assumes a normal carbon dioxide production of 200 ml per minute. Although critically ill patients tend to have higher rates of carbon dioxide production, it has been found empirically that V_D/V_T ratios determined by the graph correlate well with V_D/V_T ratios measured directly in patients in intensive care units.[30] The graph can also be used to predict the necessary minute ventilation to produce a desired $P_{a_{CO_2}}$ in a patient with a known V_D/V_T ratio.

Compliance. Measurement of pulmonary compliance is useful in following the progression of a patient's pulmonary disease as well as in determining the optimal tidal volume and level of positive end-expiratory pressure (PEEP—see the following discussion). Compliance is defined as change in volume over change in pressure:

$$\text{Compliance} = \Delta V/\Delta P \qquad (7)$$

Total pulmonary compliance can be subdivided into the compliance of the lung and the compliance of the chest wall.

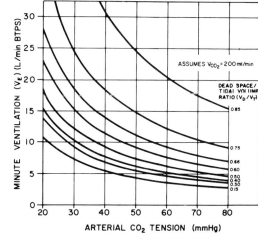

Figure 6–3. The relationship of $\dot{V}_E$ to $P_{a_{CO_2}}$ is shown graphically for various V_D/V_T ratios. Once $\dot{V}_E$ is determined from the ventilator settings and $P_{a_{CO_2}}$ is determined by blood gas analysis, the V_D/V_T ratio can be read from the graph. Conversely, once the V_D/V_T ratio is known, the change needed in $\dot{V}_E$ to produce a desired change in $P_{a_{CO_2}}$ can be predicted from the graph (see text). Assumptions made in constructing this graph are that $\dot{V}_{CO_2}$ is 200 ml/min (the basal metabolic rate for a 70-kg man) and that V_D/V_T remains constant whether rate or tidal volume is changed. (From Selecky PA, Wasserman K, Klein M, and Ziment I: A graphic approach to assessing interrelationships among minute ventilation, arterial carbon dioxide tension, and ratio of physiologic dead space to tidal volume in patients on respirators. Am Rev Respir Dis 117:181, 1978. Reproduced by permission.)

For practical purposes in managing most ventilator patients, only the total compliance need be considered. Total compliance in a ventilator patient may be measured as either static compliance, which is the tidal volume delivered divided by the plateau airway pressure after the patient has been held in full inspiration for 1 second, or as dynamic compliance, which is the tidal volume divided by the peak airway pressure. (When measuring compliance in a patient on PEEP, one considers the change in pressure to be the difference between the peak or plateau inspiratory pressure and the positive end-expiratory pressure level.)

In monitoring ventilator therapy, measurements of static compliance are usually preferred, because dynamic compliance is affected not only by the elastic recoil properties of the patient's chest wall and lungs but also by the patient's airway resistance. Normal static compliance in a healthy young adult undergoing general anesthesia is approximately 50 ml per cm H_2O.[31] It is believed that the tidal volume that leads to the greatest total compliance is that which results in maximal recruitment of alveoli without overdistention. In most patients, the best compliance is found with tidal volumes of 12 to 15 ml/kg.[32] In addition to being affected by tidal volume, compliance is also affected by PEEP and characteristics of inspiratory flow, as will be discussed later.

Set Tidal Volume versus Delivered Tidal Volume. As was mentioned in the discussion of the different types of ventilators, an advantage of volume- and time-cycled ventilators is that they deliver a relatively constant volume despite changes in the patient's compliance. One must remember that even with volume- and time-cycled ventilators, delivered tidal volume will drop slightly if the patient's compliance goes down. This drop in delivered volume occurs because the ventilator tubing has compliance of its own. Although most of the gas mixture delivered by the ventilator bellows goes to expansion of the patient's lungs, a certain amount is lost to expansion of the ventilator tubing.

The compliance of the tubing varies from ventilator to ventilator. For a typical modern volume ventilator, such as the Bear-2, the compliance of the inflow circuit is 3 ml per cm H_2O.[33] To calculate the difference between the set tidal volume and that actually received by the patient, one can multiply the pressure read from the inspiratory pressure gauge at the end of inspiration by the tubing compliance. For example, if the set tidal volume is 850 ml and the peak inspiratory pressure is 30 cm H_2O, then the volume delivered to the patient is:

$$
\begin{aligned}
\text{delivered volume} &= \text{set volume} - (\text{tubing compliance} \times \\
&\qquad \text{peak pressure}) \\
&= 850 - (30 \times 3) \\
&= 760 \text{ ml}
\end{aligned}
$$

The lower the patient's compliance, the higher the peak inspiratory pressure will be and the more gas mixture will be captured in the ventilator tubing.

Tidal Volume and Rate in Infants. Some controversy remains concerning the appropriate rate and tidal volume for mechanical ventilation of infants. Some researchers recommend lower tidal volumes, in the range of 8 to 12 ml/kg, and correspondingly rapid rates of 25 to 30 breaths per minute.[12] In neonates with hyaline membrane disease, rates as high as 60 to 100 breaths per minute may be used in an attempt to synchronize the ventilator with the infant's own breathing pattern.[34] Other investigators recommend higher tidal volumes (15 to 20 ml/kg) and lower respiratory rates (16 to 22 breaths per minute).[35] Most ventilators used for adults and larger children are not capable of delivering the small tidal volumes required in infants and neonates. (An exception is the Siemens-Elema Servo Ventilator.[36]) Therefore, special ventilators have been developed for neonatal intensive care. The compliance and dead space of the ventilator tubing and the valves have special importance in neonates. The total pulmonary compliance of a newborn with hyaline membrane disease may be 1 ml per cm H_2O, which is the same as the compliance of some ventilators designed especially for use in neonates. Thus with each breath delivered by the machine, one half of the volume goes to expand the patient's lungs and the other half goes to expand the ventilator tubing. This technical problem has to some extent hampered the development of volume ventilators for infants.[37] Another problem in infants and children is that leaks around uncuffed endotracheal tubes prevent accurate determinations of volumes delivered to the lungs. Adequacy of ventilation must be ensured by clinical observation of chest excursions, auscultation of breath sounds, and blood gas determinations.[38]

Inspired Oxygen Concentration (FI_{O_2})

After rate and tidal volume have been set, the next variable that the physician usually fixes is the FI_{O_2}. The goal should be to deliver the lowest oxygen concentration that provides adequate arterial oxygenation. Adequate arterial oxygenation is difficult to define and may vary from patient to patient. Most experts recommend maintaining a Pa_{O_2} of 60 mm Hg or greater, because a Pa_{O_2} of 60 corresponds to the shoulder on the normal hemoglobin-oxygen dissociation curve at which hemoglobin is 90 per cent saturated with oxygen. Beyond this point, increases in Pa_{O_2} lead to relatively little rise in hemoglobin saturation, whereas below this point, small decrements in Pa_{O_2} cause large drops in hemoglobin saturation. Conditions such as acidemia, fever, hypercarbia, and certain hemoglobinopathies result in a shift in the curve to the right so that at a Pa_{O_2} of 60, the hemoglobin will be less than 90 per cent saturated. Thus a Pa_{O_2} of 60 mm Hg may not be adequate in such patients.[39]

Oxygen Toxicity. When one is initiating mechanical ventilation, it is better to err on the side of a higher than necessary FI_{O_2} than to risk making a patient hypoxemic. FI_{O_2}'s in the range of 0.50 to 1.00 are commonly prescribed as initial settings. With long-term ventilator support, however, a higher than necessary FI_{O_2} may have serious adverse effects. The phenomenon of pulmonary oxygen toxicity has been recognized since the turn of the century, although the pathophysiology is still not completely understood.[40] The syndrome begins with tracheal irritation, cough, and chest pain, followed by diminished vital capacity and dyspnea. In the later stages, hypoxemia develops with associated alveolar edema and infiltrates on chest radiographs. Finally, as the process becomes irreversible, alveoli become replaced by fibrosis.

Although the exact dose-time relationship of pulmonary oxygen toxicity has not been established, it is known that at atmospheric pressure an FI_{O_2} of 0.40 is well tolerated for 30 days or more, an FI_{O_2} of 0.70 will lead to signs and symptoms of toxicity by 2 days, and an FI_{O_2} of 1.00 leads to toxicity within 30 hours.[40] In general, an FI_{O_2} of 0.50 or greater should be considered potentially toxic if used for more than a few days.

In neonates, two other manifestations of oxygen toxicity may occur: retrolental fibroplasia and bronchopulmonary dysplasia.[41, 42] The dose-time relationship of oxygen administration to the development of these two conditions is even less well established than oxygen toxicity in adults. A multicenter cooperative study designed to develop guidelines for the safe administration of oxygen in neonates was unable to yield any firm recommendations.[43]

The Alveolar-Arterial Oxygen Difference. After the patient has been on a given FI_{O_2} for 15 minutes, arterial blood gases should be checked. Besides confirming the adequacy of arterial oxygenation, blood gas results can be used to measure the efficiency of the lungs in oxygenating venous blood. One way to quantify how well the lungs are doing their job is to compare the oxygen concentration delivered to the alveoli with the oxygen tension in arterial blood. The difference between these two values is known as the alveolar-arterial oxygen difference (A–a D_{O_2}). The arterial oxygen tension (Pa_{O_2}) is easily obtained by blood gas analysis, and the alveolar oxygen tension PA_{O_2} is calculated using the alveolar air equation:

$$PA_{O_2} = [FI_{O_2} \times (P_B - P_{H_2O})] - PA_{CO_2}$$
$$\times \left[FI_{O_2} + \frac{1 - FI_{O_2}}{R} \right] \qquad (8)$$

where P_B is barometric pressure (760 mm Hg at sea level), P_{H_2O} is the pressure of water vapor in the patient's lungs (47 mm Hg at 37° C), and R is the respiratory quotient (assumed to be 0.8 unless it has been directly measured). The alveolar carbon dioxide partial pressure, PA_{CO_2}, is assumed to be the same as the arterial carbon dioxide tension, Pa_{CO_2}. When the patient is breathing 100 per cent oxygen, this equation simplifies to

$$PA_{O_2} = 713 - PA_{CO_2} \qquad (9)$$

At room air, an approximation that is easy to remember (for sea level calculations) is:

$$PA_{O_2} = 150 - 1.2 \times Pa_{CO_2} \qquad (10)$$

The normal A–a D_{O_2} is approximately 8 mm Hg in healthy young adults and 16 mm Hg in healthy 60 year olds with the subjects breathing room air at atmospheric pressure. With increasing inspired oxygen concentrations, the normal value for A–a D_{O_2} increases, although not in a strictly linear fashion. The normal A–a D_{O_2} for a healthy young adult breathing 100 per cent oxygen is 30 to 50 mm Hg.[44]

Right-to-Left Shunts and Ventilation-Perfusion Mismatch. The alveolar-arterial oxygen gradient reflects the amount of ventilation-perfusion mismatch and right-to-left shunting that occurs in the lungs. To quantitate further the amount of right-to-left shunting and ventilation perfusion mismatch, known collectively as venous admixture, the so-called shunt equation can be used. This equation states:

$$Q_s/Q_t = (C_c - C_a)/(C_c - C_v) \qquad (11)$$

where Q_s is the pulmonary blood flow that does not become oxygenated, Q_t is the total pulmonary blood flow, C_c is the oxygen content of pulmonary capillary blood (which is calculated based on the assumption that the oxygen tension in the pulmonary capillaries equals the partial pressure of oxygen in the alveoli), C_a is the oxygen content of systemic arterial blood, and C_v is the oxygen content of mixed venous blood (ideally obtained from the distal port of a pulmonary artery catheter). The oxygen content C (expressed in milliliters of O_2 per 100 ml of blood) equals the product:

$$0.003 \times P_{O_2} + 1.34 \times S_{O_2} \times Hgb \qquad (12)$$

Here S_{O_2} is the oxygen saturation estimated for a given P_{O_2}, and Hgb is the patient's hemoglobin level. Cane and coworkers[45] have shown empirically that in the absence of a mixed venous blood sample, equation 11 can be approximated by

$$Q_s/Q_t = [C_c - C_a]/[(C_c - C_a) + 3.5 \text{ ml/dl}] \qquad (13)$$

This equation assumes a fixed arterial–mixed venous oxygen content difference of 3.5 ml O_2 per 100 ml of blood.

With the patient breathing 100 per cent oxygen, the effect of ventilation-perfusion mismatching is eliminated, and calculation of Q_s/Q_t reflects only the true right-to-left shunting. The normal Q_s/Q_t ratio in healthy young adults is 2 to 3 per cent.[44] A Q_s/Q_t ratio of greater than 50 per cent results in severe hypoxemia, even at 100 per cent inspired oxygen. In Figure 6–4, the relationship of Pa_{O_2} to PA_{O_2} is shown for various Q_s/Q_t ratios. It can be seen from this figure that when Q_s/Q_t is small, large increases in PA_{O_2} lead to similarly large increases in Pa_{O_2}. With high Q_s/Q_t ratios, however, large increases in PA_{O_2} lead to only slight increases in Pa_{O_2}. The clinical application of this observation is that in diseases characterized mainly by ventilation-perfusion mismatching, such as COPD, hypoxemia responds well to oxygen supplementation, whereas in conditions marked by large degrees of right-to-left shunting, such as intracardiac shunts, pneumonia, pulmonary edema, and the adult respiratory distress syndrome (ARDS) large increases in FI_{O_2} may lead to relatively little improvement in arterial oxygenation.

Ventilator Mode

After rate, tidal volume, and FI_{O_2} have been set, the next priority is to set the mode of ventilation. Although not all the modes discussed in this section are available on all ventilators, most modern machines allow the operator to choose more than one mode. The airway pressure and flow characteristics of the different modes are shown diagrammatically in Figure 6–5.

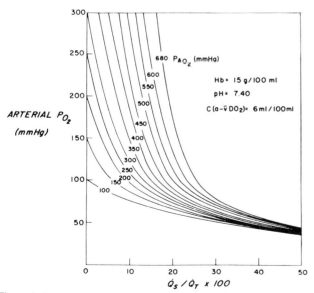

Figure 6–4. The relationship between Pa_{O_2} and Q_s/Q_t for various levels of PA_{O_2}. This graph is constructed from the shunt equation, assuming normal values for hemoglobin, arterial-mixed venous oxygen difference, and hemoglobin-oxygen dissociation curve. (From Pontoppidan H, Geffin B, Lowenstein E: Acute respiratory failure in the adult. N Engl J Med 287:744, 1982. Reproduced by permission.)

Controlled Ventilation. In this mode, the patient is ventilated at the rate set by the operator. The patient cannot breathe between machine breaths. This mode may be used in an unconscious patient with depressed respiratory drive, in a heavily sedated patient, in a patient who has been paralyzed with drugs, or in a patient who is being deliberately hyperventilated. Other patients may attempt to inhale against the closed inspiratory valve, resulting in apprehension, asynchronous chest movement, increased oxygen consumption and carbon dioxide production, and high peak pressures.

Assist Control. In this mode, the operator sets the minimum rate for the patient to be ventilated. If the patient makes no respiratory effort, the prescribed number of breaths will be delivered and no more. If the patient does try to breathe, the machine will deliver an extra breath with the same tidal volume as the others, when the patient generates a sufficient inspiratory effort. The amount of negative inspiratory pressure that the patient must generate to trigger the machine is controlled by the operator. The sensitivity is set so that it is neither too difficult for the patient to initiate a breath (in which case the ventilator would actually be functioning in the control mode) nor too easy (in which case small movements by the patient might trigger the machine). The advantage of assist control over the control mode is that it allows the patient to regulate the minute volume in part. This mode is usually preferred in conscious patients. A disadvantage of assist control is that some patients spontaneously hyperventilate to an undesirable degree in this mode.

IMV and SIMV. Intermittent mandatory ventilation (IMV) was introduced in the early 1970s.[46] As in the assist control mode, the patient may breathe at a rate faster than the set ventilator frequency. With IMV, however, when the patient initiates a spontaneous breath, the machine offers no assistance, and the patient receives only the tidal volume that is self-generated. This is usually smaller than the tidal volume delivered by the ventilator. As in the assist control mode, the patient may determine the minute volume in part. An advantage of IMV is that there is less tendency for the patient to hyperventilate spontaneously. Also, because the patient must work harder to generate a spontaneous breath, it is believed that IMV may help maintain the tone of the respiratory muscles. An additional potential advantage of IMV over assist control and controlled ventilation is that mean airway pressures tend to be lower in the IMV mode, resulting in less impedance to return of blood to the right side of the heart.[22] (See the section on complications of mechanical ventilation.) The IMV mode is particularly well suited for weaning a patient from mechanical ventilation. Over a period of hours to days, the IMV rate can be turned down gradually, so that the patient makes a smooth transition from depending mainly on the ventilator to breathing entirely independently. Some researchers have claimed that the use of IMV facilitates weaning in difficult patients,[46] although others have questioned the assertion that it speeds the weaning process.[47]

Older ventilators, such as the Puritan-Bennett MA-1, do not have IMV circuits built into them but may be converted to the IMV mode through the use of additional tubing and an independent oxygen source. This system wastes oxygen, because the patient may breathe only a small fraction of the air-oxygen mixture that is continuously flowing through the IMV circuit. Newer ventilators have IMV circuits built into them so that gas flows through the IMV circuit only when the patient initiates a breath. Another problem that occurred with older IMV systems was that the ventilator sometimes delivered a tidal volume just as the patient had completed a spontaneous inspiration. This so-called stacking of a machine

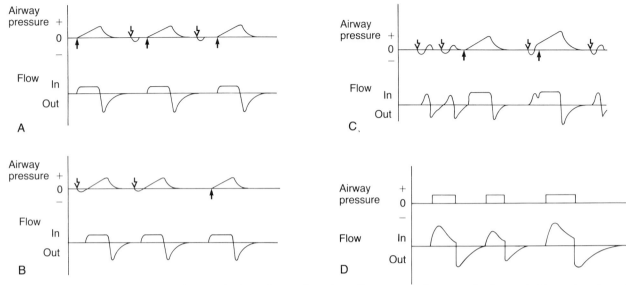

Figure 6–5. Ventilator modes. *A,* Controlled ventilation. The ventilator is cycling at a regular rate *(closed arrows)*. The patient is making inspiratory efforts *(open arrows)* but does not receive any breaths at these times. *B,* Assist control. Each time the patient makes a sufficient inspiratory effort *(open arrows)*, the ventilator delivers a full tidal volume. If the patient's spontaneous rate drops below the set ventilator rate, then the ventilator cycles on its own *(closed arrow)*. *C,* IMV. The patient is breathing at a rate faster than the ventilator is set *(open arrows)*. The ventilator does not assist the patient but cycles at an independent rate *(closed arrows)*. The second ventilator breath falls coincidentally on top of a spontaneous breath (so-called stacking), leading to a high peak pressure. In the SIMV mode, the ventilator is designed to avoid stacking by timing ventilator breaths either to coincide with the initiation of a spontaneous breath or to fall in between spontaneous breaths. *D,* Pressure support. The ventilator provides flow at a constant pressure each time the patient initiates a spontaneous breath *(open arrows)*. The ventilator cycles into expiration when inspiratory flow drops to 25 per cent of peak level. Note that tidal volume (the area under the flow curve) may vary from breath to breath.

breath on top of a spontaneous breath could lead to overdistention of the lungs and dangerously high peak pressures. This problem has been overcome by the development of synchronized IMV (SIMV). This mode is the same as IMV except that the ventilator times the machine breaths to fall in a pause in the patient's spontaneous respiratory cycle or to coincide with the initiation of a spontaneous breath.

Pressure Support. This mode of ventilation, which was the basic mode on the old intermittent positive-pressure breathing machines, has been reintroduced, with some refinements, on some of the newer ventilators such as the Servo 900C. When the patient initiates a breath, the ventilator provides a constant inspiratory pressure, until inspiratory flow drops to 25 per cent of the peak level. The patient determines the rate, and tidal volume depends on the patient's compliance and the inspiratory pressure set by the operator. If the patient's compliance goes down, the tidal volume will go down. The pressure support mode is obviously not desirable in patients with fluctuating ventilatory drive or pulmonary mechanics. It has been found useful, however, in patients with stable pulmonary disease and patients being weaned from mechanical ventilation. In such patients, pressure support results in better patient comfort, slower spontaneous ventilatory rates, less patient work, and lower peak airway pressures than the SIMV mode. Pressure support may also be used in combination with SIMV.[48]

Peep and CPAP

Positive end-expiratory pressure and CPAP were introduced in the late 1960s and early 1970s as means of improving oxygenation in hypoxemic patients. Originally PEEP was used in patients with ARDS,[49] and CPAP was first used in infants with hyaline membrane disease,[50] but both techniques have since been applied to patients of all ages with hypoxemia from various causes.

The term *PEEP* is used to denote positive end-expiratory pressure in a patient who is receiving assisted ventilation. In this mode, airway pressure is positive not only at end expiration but also throughout the respiratory cycle. The term *CPAP* is used to denote continuous positive-airway pressure in a patient who is breathing spontaneously. The CPAP circuits are designed so that airway pressure drops slightly during inspiration but remains above ambient pressure because of a continuous flow of gas through the inspiratory circuit.

When using PEEP, the ventilator can be in the control, assist control, IMV, SIMV, or pressure support modes. In older ventilators, application of PEEP involved cumbersome extra circuitry. In newer machines, the capability for PEEP is built in, and one sets the level merely by turning a knob. Although CPAP is usually applied by way of an endotracheal tube with a ventilator supplying the positive pressure, it can also be applied by means of a tight-fitting mask or a head-enclosing box.[51, 52]

Theoretically, PEEP and CPAP improve oxygenation by keeping alveoli open during expiration. Whether they actually work by this mechanism is a moot point.[53] What is known is that they lead to improved oxygenation and narrowing of the A–a D_{O_2} in most patients.

The number of indications for PEEP and CPAP is currently increasing as more experience is being gained with these modes of ventilator therapy. A generally accepted indication for PEEP is failure to achieve adequate oxygenation (e.g., Pa_{O_2} less than 60 mm Hg) with safe levels of inspired oxygen (e.g., FI_{O_2} less than or equal to 0.50). Other indications are more controversial. There is a prevalent philosophy in the surgical literature that PEEP has prophylactic value in preventing the respiratory distress syndrome or that it hastens its resolution.[54] One basis for this belief is that PEEP alters the appearance of infiltrates on chest films, making them appear less dense. In one study, skilled radiologists interpreted pre- and post-PEEP chest films differently in 25 per cent of cases after patients had been on 10 to 20 cm PEEP for only 15 minutes.[55] Thus some surgical intensive care units routinely use low levels of PEEP (5 to 8 cm H_2O) in patients who require postoperative ventilation but who are not hypoxemic on safe levels of $F_{I_{O_2}}$. The prophylactic and therapeutic value of PEEP has been questioned in the medical literature, however.[56] In one large retrospective study, use of PEEP did not seem to improve survival in critically ill patients.[57] Animal studies designed to assess the influence of PEEP on pulmonary edema have shown either no change or an increase in lung water after institution of PEEP.[58]

Determination of the optimal level of PEEP is also controversial. A conservative approach is to use a level of PEEP that is just enough to provide adequate arterial oxygenation with an inspired oxygen concentration under 50 per cent. In patients requiring higher $F_{I_{O_2}}$'s, PEEP may be started at 5 cm H_2O and may be increased in increments of 3 to 5 cm H_2O at 15-minutes intervals. At each new level, one should measure and record pulse and blood pressure, static compliance, peak airway pressure, arterial blood gas tension, and cardiac output. The pulmonary artery wedge pressure should probably also be measured, although it may not accurately reflect left ventricular filling pressure in patients on PEEP.[56] The $F_{I_{O_2}}$ can usually be gradually turned down as PEEP is increased and the A–a D_{O_2} narrows.[59]

Most patients exhibit a fall in cardiac output at levels of PEEP above 12 to 15 cm H_2O. This drop is due in part to decreased venous return and can be at least partially overcome by expansion of intravascular volume.[60] Diminished myocardial blood flow at higher levels of PEEP may also contribute to diminished cardiac output.[60] A useful method of determining when a fall in cardiac output negates the effect of a rise in Pa_{O_2} is to calculate the peripheral oxygen delivery at different levels of PEEP.[59, 62] One can calculate the peripheral oxygen delivery by multiplying the cardiac output by the arterial oxygen content:

$$O_2 \text{ delivery to periphery} = \text{cardiac output} \times \text{arterial } O_2 \text{ content} \quad (14)$$

One calculates the arterial oxygen content by using equation 12.

Measurement of static compliance also has been advocated as a means of determining the optimal level of PEEP. One small study found that the best PEEP from the point of view of oxygen delivery to the periphery coincided with the level at which static compliance was highest, usually in the range of 6 to 12 cm H_2O.[63] Other researchers have questioned the reproducibility of this association.

The most extensive use of CPAP has been in infants with hyaline membrane disease. In this setting, CPAP is usually initiated at levels of 2 to 8 cm H_2O before mechanical ventilation is begun.[12] In some cases, CPAP leads to enough improvement in the A–a D_{O_2} that assisted ventilation can be avoided. Recently, CPAP has also been advocated for adults with a variety of pulmonary diseases who are hypoxemic on high inspired oxygen concentrations but who are able to maintain normal arterial carbon dioxide tensions. Some have also claimed that CPAP has been of benefit in weaning difficult patients from mechanical ventilation.[64] This indication is discussed further in the section on weaning.

Dual Synchronous Ventilation

In some patients with severe unilateral lung disease, adequate oxygenation, ventilation, or both cannot be maintained with safe levels of $F_{I_{O_2}}$ and reasonable pressures. In such patients, PEEP may actually worsen ventilation perfu-sion mismatch by causing overdistention of the more normal lung and shunting of blood flow to the more diseased lung. A novel approach to ventilating such patients is to use a different ventilator, with different tidal volumes and pressures, for each lung. Dual-lumen endotracheal tubes are available for this purpose, and some ventilators, such as the Servo 900C, are specifically designed to be used synchronously with another twin ventilator. Patients with unilateral lung disease due to pneumonia and bronchopleural fistulas have been ventilated successfully with this technique.[65]

Characteristics of Inspiratory and Expiratory Flow

On modern ventilators, many variables of inspiratory and expiratory flow can be altered by the operator. These include inspiratory flow wave form, inspiratory flow rate, inspiratory time, inspiratory-expiratory (I:E) ratio, peak inspiratory pressure, and expiratory resistance. These variables, along with rate and tidal volume, are interrelated, so that a change in one affects the others. Which variable is set by the operator and which variable is secondarily determined depends on the ventilator design. For example, in a pressure-cycled ventilator, flow and pressure are set and tidal volume is determined, whereas in a volume-cycled ventilator, flow and tidal volume are set and pressure is determined. With a time-cycled ventilator, the I:E ratio is set, whereas with pressure- and volume-cycle ventilators, the I:E ratio is determined. Although changes in the characteristics of inspiratory and expiratory flow tend to result in relatively small changes in the final measures of oxygenation and carbon dioxide elimination, by adjusting these variables appropriately, one can fine-tune the ventilator to optimize the therapy of critically ill patients.

Inspiratory Flow. The basic flow pattern built into most ventilators is a constant flow (square wave). In many modern ventilators, this basic pattern can be altered by the operator to produce an accelerating (tapered wave) pattern. In most cases, a square wave is chosen as the initial setting, since this leads to lower peak pressures for a given inspiratory time and tidal volume. In some patients with very uneven ventilation of different regions of the lungs, however, use of a tapered inspiratory waveform may result in more even ventilation by allowing more time for the inspired gas to pass through airways with increased resistance to flow.[66]

Inspiratory Flow Rate. In volume- and pressure-cycled ventilators, the inspiratory flow rate is initially set in the range of 40 to 50 liters per minute in adults and 8 to 15 liters per minute in infants. In time-cycled ventilators, one may secondarily determine the inspiratory flow by setting the tidal volume and inspiratory time. An inspiratory flow rate that is too rapid may lead to dangerously high peak pressures or unequal ventilation of lung units with different time constants, whereas an inspiratory flow rate that is too slow may lead to an undesirably long inspiratory time with inadequate time for exhalation.

Inspiratory Pause. Some ventilators allow the operator to add a pause to the end of inspiration, during which time airway pressure is held constant and the patient cannot exhale. Like other maneuvers that prolong the inspiratory phase, an inspiratory pause leads to more even ventilation.[66] The pause may also lead to air trapping. An inspiratory pause is also analogous to PEEP in that by increasing mean airway pressure, it may lead to decreased venous return and decreased cardiac output. An inspiratory pause is usually not initially prescribed but may be added when hypoxemia due to uneven ventilation is a problem.

I:E Ratio. To allow complete exhalation, the expiratory

phase of the ventricular cycle should usually be at least twice the length of the inspiratory phase. Higher I:E ratios may lead to air trapping, overdistention, and high peak pressures. It was found in the late 1970s, however, that in infants with hyaline membrane diseases, so-called inverse ratio ventilation (IRV) with I:E ratios of 2:1 improved oxygenation and reduced the time infants had to be on high inspired oxygen concentrations and PEEP.[67] Inverse I:E ratios as great as 4:1 have also been used in adults with severe hypoxemia due to ARDS, pneumonia, and cardiogenic pulmonary edema.[68, 69] Inverse ratio ventilation is similar to PEEP in that it improves oxygenation, increases mean airway pressure, reduces V_D/V_T and Q_s/Q_t, and may reduce cardiac output. It leads to lower peak pressures than PEEP, however, with less risk of barotrauma. The mechanism by which IRV achieves its beneficial effects is not known for certain, but it is theorized that the long inspiratory time may lead to more even ventilation, and the short expiration time may prevent collapse of diseased alveoli.

Peak Pressure. With pressure-cycled ventilators, peak pressure is a set variable and determines tidal volume. Starting pressures of 20 to 25 cm H_2O are commonly used in adults with normal compliance, although pressures of 40 cm H_2O and above are usually required in patients with a pathologic pulmonary condition.

With time- and volume-cycled ventilators, peak pressure is determined mainly by tidal volume. Typical peak pressures for patients with respiratory failure are in the range of 40 to 50 cm H_2O. Peak pressures greater than 60 cm H_2O are not uncommon but are associated with a high incidence of barotrauma. In exceptional cases, peak pressures of 100 cm H_2O and above are required. Modern volume- and time-cycled ventilators have adjustable peak pressure limits such that when the airway pressure exceeds the set limit, inspiration is terminated. The limit is usually set at 10 cm H_2O above the peak pressure that is observed when the patient is initially placed on the ventilator. If the peak pressure alarm sounds later, it is a sign that the patient's compliance has dropped or resistance has increased, and a cause must be sought. (Typical causes of acute increases in peak pressure include attempts by the patient to override, or "buck," the ventilator, development of pneumothorax, migration of the tip of the endotracheal tube into the right main stem bronchus, kinking of the tube, or plugging of the tube or a major airway.)

Expiratory Retard. Many ventilators have an adjustable expiratory resistance, or retard. The development of such a mechanism was inspired by the observation of COPD patients who breathe through pursed lips, apparently in an effort to increase their own expiratory resistance. Theoretically, this resistance to expiration may prevent the premature collapse of small airways and may paradoxically lead to more complete exhalation. Whether this is actually the reason for pursed-lip breathing and whether expiratory retard is a useful setting on a ventilator remain controversial.[21, 70]

Sighs. In the early 1960s, it was shown that patients who were being mechanically ventilated during anesthesia showed a progressive decline in compliance and widening of their A–a D_{O_2}.[71] These changes were thought to be caused by atelectasis and were reversed by intermittent deep breaths. Based on this work, "sigh" functions have been built into mechanical ventilators, allowing the operator to introduce a breath 1½ to 2 times the usual tidal volume at regular intervals. A problem with the original study that demonstrated the benefit of "sighs," however, was that patients were ventilated with low tidal volumes. With tidal volumes in the range of 10 to 15 ml per kg that are used today, it has not been demonstrated that progressive atelectasis occurs. The optimal rate and volume of sighs are unknown,

as is whether sighs are beneficial at all. Indeed, it has been argued that incorporation of a sigh function into a ventilator adds only needless extra expense.[72]

Humidification

Normally, inspired air is humidified and warmed in the oropharynx and the nasopharynx before reaching the lower airway. In an intubated patient, inspired air bypasses the nasopharynx and the oropharynx and is injected directly into the trachea. To prevent drying of the mucosa of the lower airways, all modern ventilators are equipped with systems for humidifying and warming inspired air. The set-up of these systems varies from ventilator to ventilator and is described in the operating manuals supplied by the manufacturers. A commonly overlooked setting, however, is the temperature of the inspired air. Normally, the air temperature should be 35° C at the point at which the gas enters the endotracheal tube. One should remember that in patients who are hypothermic, heating the inspired air is an effective means of core rewarming.[19] Likewise, cooling the inspired air will lower the body temperature in febrile patients.

Medication Nebulizers

Most modern ventilators have in-line medication nebulizers for the administration of bronchodilator drugs. The dosages are the same as for medication nebulizers for patients who are breathing spontaneously. Special mention should be made of ribavirin, a synthetic nucleoside analogue approved for aerosol treatments of infants and young children with severe respiratory syncytial virus infections. Ribavirin has been reported to cause malfunction of ventilators because of precipitation of the drug on the valves and in the ventilator tubing. Special filters must be used when this drug is delivered via the nebulizer on a mechanical ventilator.[73]

VENTILATOR USE

Choosing a Ventilator

With the large variety of commercial ventilators available today, choosing the best ventilator for one's hospital or hospital department can be a difficult decision. One factor in deciding which ventilator is best is the setting in which the ventilator will be used. In an emergency department in which mechanical ventilation is done infrequently and for short periods, a relatively simple ventilator that is easy to set up and operate may be preferable to a more complex machine that offers more controls and monitors. Although some ventilators such as the Servo 900C can be used for both infants and adults, ventilators designed specifically for infants are usually preferred in pediatric and neonatal intensive care units. Safety and reliability are major concerns in choosing a ventilator. Fortunately, most modern ventilators have both features. Cost is another factor to be considered. The improvements in ventilator technology over the past decade have not come cheaply. Many ventilators today cost more than $20,000. Table 6–4 lists some features that are most desirable in a ventilator and some other features that may add significantly to the cost but may not be as necessary.

Table 6–4. Desirable Features in a Ventilator

Desirable Features
Operational Characteristics
Volume- or time-cycled
VT 10–200 ml in infants, 50–500 in children, and 200–2000 in adults
Variable inspiratory flow rate (up to 150 L/min in adults)
Variable I:E ratio
Peak inspiratory pressure limit of 60 mm Hg in infants, 100 mm Hg in children and adults
Assist control and IMV or SIMV modes
PEEP or CPAP to 50 cm H_2O
Frequency 0–60
Internal air compressor

Alarms
Self-resetting alarms (operator cannot turn off alarm for more than 1–2 minutes before alarm reactivates)
Minimum and maximum airway pressures
O_2 concentration
Low minute volume
Electrical or pneumatic power failure

Monitors
Airway pressure
Frequency
Tidal volume or minute volume
Inspired gas temperature
Actual FI_{O_2}

Other Less Necessary Features That May Add to Cost
Microprocessor-driven controls, alarms, and monitors
Sigh, inspiratory pause, expiratory retard
Variable inspiratory waveform
Capability of high-frequency ventilation

(From Kirby RR, Smith RA, Desautels DA: Mechanical ventilation. In Burton GG, Hodgkin JE (eds): Respiratory Care. 2nd ed. Philadelphia, JB Lippincott Co, 1984. Modified with permission.)

Ventilator Set-up

The actual set-up of a ventilator is usually done by a respiratory therapist under the direction of a physician. In some cases, a respiratory therapist or other knowledgeable nonphysician may not be available immediately, and the physician may need to do the actual ventilator set-up. Unfortunately, it is not practical to describe in this chapter the step-by-step set-up of every ventilator in use currently. Instead, the set-up of a "state of the art" infant ventilator, the Infant Star, and the set-up of the versatile Servo 900C, which can be used in both infants and adults, are described. The descriptions of ventilator set-up that follow are not intended to provide everything one needs to know to operate either of these ventilators safely. Rather, these descriptions are intended to serve as examples of the typical steps in the set-up of modern ventilators. For complete instructions regarding the set-up of these or other ventilators, the operator should consult the operating manuals supplied by the manufacturers. Copies of these manuals should be available in any departments in which the ventilators are in use.

If at any point during ventilator set-up, the patient appears to have inadequate ventilation, the patient should be taken off the ventilator and should be bag ventilated. Trouble shooting of ventilator set-ups should *not* occur while the patient is dependent on the ventilator.

SET-UP OF THE INFANT STAR

The Infant Star is a time-cycled ventilator, designed especially for mechanical ventilation of infants and children. The actual ventilator is shown in Figure 6–6, and the control and display panels are depicted schematically in Figure 6–

7. The ventilator is controlled by two microprocessors that allow precise tailoring of ventilator settings and provide alarms and monitors not found on most other pediatric ventilators. The ventilator may be connected by a standard computer cable to an IBM-compatible personal computer for making printouts of monitored parameters and trends. The ventilator software is updatable, and high-frequency ventilation is an enhancement that is currently available.

There are basically two modes available on the Infant Star—CPAP and intermittent mandatory ventilation (IMV). With either mode, continuous or demand flow is possible. Demand flow conserves the hospital oxygen supply, with minimal, if any, increase in the work of breathing as a result of the rapid response time of the microprocessor-controlled inspiratory flow valves. Set-up in the IMV mode with demand flow is described here.

Step-by-Step Set-up

1. Air, oxygen, and electrical power hookups at the back of the ventilator are connected to hospital sources.
2. Inspiratory and expiratory arms of patient breathing tubes are connected to the ports labeled TO PATIENT and FROM PATIENT on the compressor front panel. (Note that a separate humidifier must be used.) Special 1/8-inch tubing is connected from the patient wye to the PROXIMAL AIRWAY PRESSURE port.
3. The power switch at the back of the ventilator is turned on, and the operator checks that all digital displays are illuminated and bright, that an audible alarm sounds momentarily, and that all light-emitting diode indicators are illuminated, except POWER LOSS, VENT INOP, and INTERNAL BATTERY.
4. Ventilator settings are made by turning the appropriate knobs on the control panel and compressor. Although the appropriate settings will be determined by the clinical situation, typical settings for an infant would be FLOW RATE 20 liters per minute, RATE 30 breaths per minute, PEAK INSPIRATORY PRESSURE 50 cm H_2O, INSPIRATORY TIME 1 second, and LOW INSPIRATORY PRESSURE 10 cm H_2O.
5. Connect the patient wye to a test lung to check inflation and deflation at the appropriate rate.
6. Disconnect the patient wye from the test lung and check that the LOW INSPIRATORY PRESSURE ALARM is activated. Obstruct the tube at the patient wye to be sure that the OBSTRUCTED TUBE alarm is activated. Partially obstruct the patient wye and rotate the pop-off valve on the front of the compressor until gas is felt to escape from the valve at a pressure of about 60 cm H_2O as read off the analogue pressure gauge. Reconnect the patient wye to the test lung and push the ALARM SILENCE and VISUAL RESET buttons.
7. Set the desired FI_{O_2} on the front of the ventilator compressor.
8. Connect the ventilator to the patient and observe for rise and fall of the patient's chest and appropriate pressures, I:E ratio, and expiration time. Readjust the PEAK INSPIRATORY PRESSURE to 5 to 10 cm H_2O above the observed peak inspiratory pressure and the LOW INSPIRATORY PRESSURE to 5 to 10 cm H_2O below the observed peak inspiratory pressure. Readjust the pop-off valve to 13 cm H_2O above the set peak inspiratory pressure limit.

Alarms and Monitors on the Infant Star. The Infant Star has nine alarm systems, plus an indicator to signal that the ventilator is running on its internal battery if the outside power source fails. All alarms are both audible and visual, except for a portion of the OBSTRUCTED TUBE alarm. Alarm lights are located on the lower right-hand corner of the ventilator control panel (see Fig. 6–7). Audible alarms can

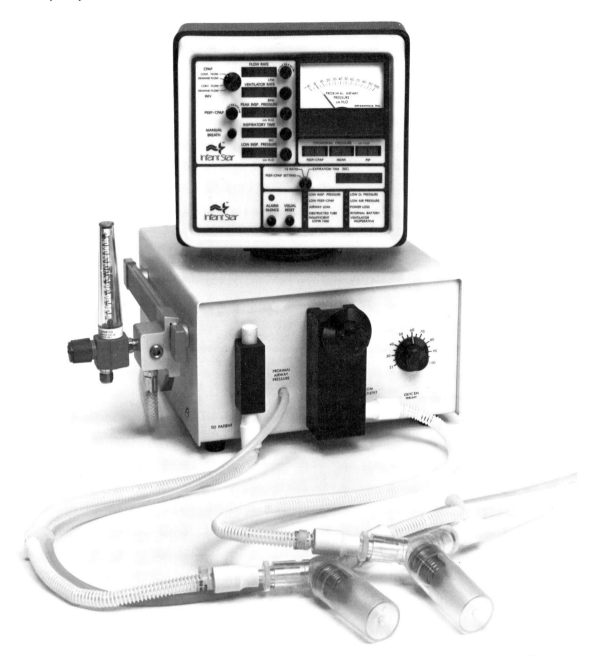

Figure 6–6. The Infant Star ventilator. (Reproduced with permission from Infrasonics, Inc., San Diego, Calif.)

be silenced for 60 seconds by pushing the ALARM SILENCE button, with the exception of the VENTILATOR INOPERATIVE and POWER LOSS alarms, which cannot be silenced.

1. LOW INSPIRATORY PRESSURE. This alarm is activated when the peak inspiratory pressure of a given breath does not reach the set alarm limit. By setting the alarm limit within 5 to 10 cm H_2O of the observed peak inspiratory pressure, the alarm will detect any significant leaks in the inspiratory circuit. Setting the alarm limit closer to the observed peak inspiratory pressure will lead to frequent false alarms.

2. LOW PEEP/CPAP. The microprocessor automatically sets the low PEEP and CPAP limits to 2 to 5 cm H_2O below the set PEEP and CPAP levels. The alarm is activated if PEEP or CPAP falls below the automatic limits.

3. AIRWAY LEAK. This alarm is activated when demand flow exceeds background flow for 4 seconds. It supplements the low inspiratory pressure and low PEEP/CPAP alarms.

4. OBSTRUCTED TUBE. This alarm is activated when peak inspiratory pressure or PEEP or CPAP significantly exceeds the set levels, usually indicating an obstructed breathing tube. The alarm is actually sensitive to five different specific violations, and the exact violation is displayed in coded form in the window above the alarm lights. Explanations of the five different codes and the most likely malfunction associated with each alarm code are described in detail in the operating instructions provided with the ventilator.

5. INSUFFICIENT EXPIRATORY TIME. This alarm is activated when exhalation time for mandatory breaths is less than 0.3 seconds.

6 and 7. LOW O_2 PRESSURE and LOW AIR PRESSURE. These alarms are activated when the pressure of gases into the ventilator drops below 45 psi. Below this pressure, the blender may be affected, and inaccurate $F_{I_{O_2}}$ settings may result.

8 and 9. POWER LOSS and INTERNAL BATTERY. The internal battery light comes on whenever outside power fails and the ventilator is running on its internal battery. Five to

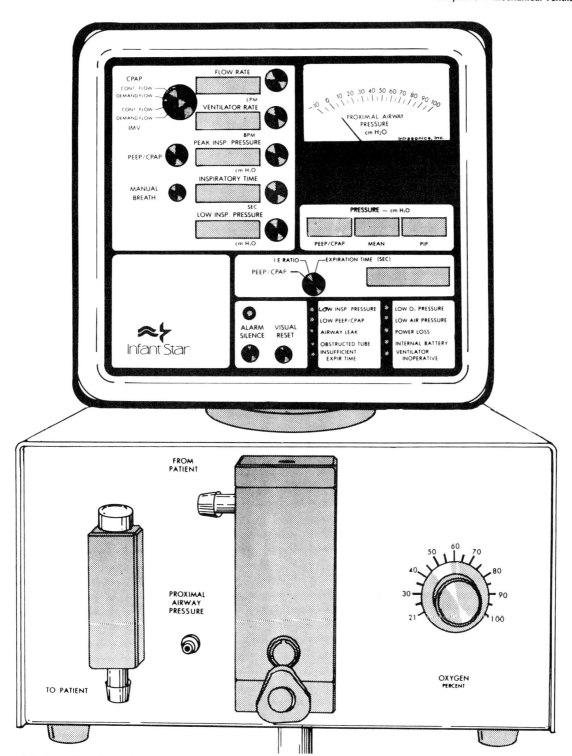

Figure 6–7. Controls and monitors on the Infant Star. (Reproduced with permission from Infrasonics, Inc., San Diego, Calif.)

10 minutes before the internal battery is exhausted, the internal battery and power loss lights alternately flash. When fully charged, the internal battery provides up to 30 minutes of operation.

10. VENTILATOR INOPERATIVE. This alarm signals a major malfunction, which makes the ventilator unsafe. When this alarm activates, the ventilator shuts down and all valves open, allowing the patient to breathe ambient air. Possible causes of ventilator malfunction are detailed in the operating instructions.

Monitors on the Infant Star include an analogue proximal airway pressure manometer; digital displays for PEEP and CPAP, mean airway pressure, and peak inspiratory pressure; and a digital display with a three-way switch that may be turned to read PEEP/CPAP, I:E RATIO, or EXPIRATION TIME. The monitors are for the most part self-explanatory. The MEAN AIRWAY PRESSURE monitor is a particularly useful feature of the Infant Star, because mean airway pressure has a direct bearing on the risk of barotrauma and on oxygenation and cardiac output.

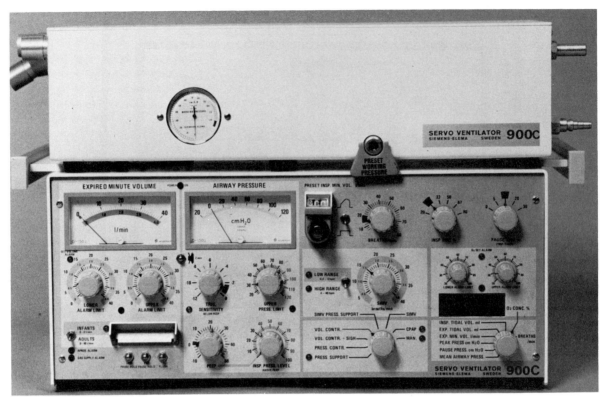

Figure 6–8. Siemens Servo Ventilator 900C time-cycled ventilator. (Courtesy of Siemens Life Support Systems, Schaumburg, Ill.)

SET-UP OF THE SIEMENS SERVO VENTILATOR 900C

The Servo Ventilator 900C is a compact yet versatile and dependable modern ventilator, which operates almost silently. With its many accessories, it can be used as a ventilator for infants, children, or adults; as an anesthesia machine; or as a diagnostic instrument. Although it is basically a time-cycled ventilator, volume and pressure limits can be set to make it function like either a volume-cycled or a pressure-controlled machine.

The modes available on the Servo 900C deserve special mention, because they are somewhat different from those available on most other ventilators. In the VOLUME CONTROL mode, the ventilator functions much like a typical volume-cycled ventilator, except that the operator sets the desired minute volume rather than the desired tidal volume. The operator then sets the desired respiratory rate and I:E ratio, and through its internal electronic circuitry, the ventilator determines the inspiratory flow necessary to deliver the set minute volume. A VOLUME CONTROL PLUS SIGH mode, in which every hundredth breath is delivered with double the basic tidal volume, is also available. By adjusting the TRIGGER SENSITIVITY appropriately, the VOLUME CONTROL mode becomes analogous to "assist control" in a volume-cycled ventilator. In the PRESSURE CONTROL mode, the ventilator delivers a constant pressure, with a decelerating flow pattern, during a set inspiratory time. The inspiratory pressure, respiratory rate, and inspiratory time determine the tidal volume received by the patient. PRESSURE SUPPORT is a unique mode in which the patient must initiate all breaths independently but is assisted by positive pressure from the ventilator each time a sufficient inspiratory effort is made. The tidal volume of each breath depends in part on the set inspiratory pressure and in part on the amount of effort made by the patient. This mode is suggested by the manufacturer for

weaning patients from anesthesia or from mechanical ventilation.

The synchronized intermittent mandatory ventilation (SIMV) mode is the same as that in a volume-cycled ventilator, except as for the VOLUME CONTROL mode, minute volume rather than tidal volume is set. SIMV PLUS PRESSURE SUPPORT combines these two modes, providing the patient with a set minute volume at a set rate but allowing the patient to breathe spontaneously in between machine breaths with the ventilator applying positive pressure during the spontaneous inhalations. The CPAP mode is the same as that in a volume ventilator. A MANUAL mode is also available for providing manual ventilation during the administration of anesthesia or while a patient is being suctioned.

The external appearance of the Servo 900C is shown in Figure 6–8. The assembly of the ventilator to this point as well as the attachment of the humidifier, the oxygen-air mixer, and the patient tubing are discussed in detail in the manufacturer's instruction manual. The power supply cord (which must be plugged into a standard 110-volt AC outlet) and the on/off switch are located at the rear of the electronic unit. The further set-up of the ventilator is illustrated in Figure 6–9 and is discussed here. Set-up is described for the ASSIST CONTROL mode, because this is the mode that is most appropriate for initial ventilation of most adult patients in the emergency department or the critical care unit. The set-up in other modes varies slightly and is covered in the manufacturer's manual.

Step-by-Step Set-up

1. The WORKING PRESSURE adjustment on the pneumatic unit, which is mounted above the electronic unit, determines the maximum pressure that the ventilator will deliver and provides a secondary safeguard against the inadvertent exposure of the patient to dangerously high pressures. (The primary safeguard is the UPPER PRESSURE

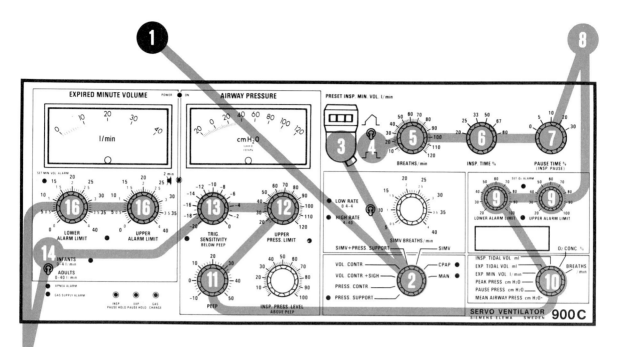

15 Connect the patient.

12 To protect the patient against high pressures, always start from a low value.

1
Set the WORKING PRESSURE.

2
Set the mode selector at VOL. CONTR. or VOL. CONTR.+SIGH.

3
Set the desired minute volume (e.g. by means of a Radford nomogram).

4
Select the curve shape for the inspiration flow.

5
Set the respiratory rate, BREATHS/min.

6
Set the INSP. TIME %.

7
Set the PAUSE TIME %.

8
Set the mixer.

9
Set the LOWER ALARM LIMIT and UPPER ALARM LIMIT for O₂ CONC. %.

10
Set the parameter selector.

11
Set the PEEP-level.

12
Set the UPPER PRESS. LIMIT for AIRWAY PRESSURE to approximately 10 cm H₂O above the patient's airway pressure.

13
Set the TRIG. SENSITIVITY.

14
Set the scale INFANTS/ADULTS.

15
Connect the ventilator to the patient and check:
– that the patient's chest rises and falls in time with the preset respiratory rate.
– the tidal volumes on the digital display and the reading on the EXPIRED MINUTE VOLUME meter.
– that the AIRWAY PRESSURE meter gives a reading during inspiration, and that the reading falls to 0 cm H₂O, or alternatively, to PEEP-level, during expiration.

16
Set the LOWER ALARM LIMIT and UPPER ALARM LIMIT for EXPIRED MINUTE VOLUME.

If the VOL. CONTR.+SIGH mode is selected, it may be necessary to increase the UPPER ALARM LIMIT for EXPIRED MINUTE VOLUME, as well as the UPPER PRESS. LIMIT for AIRWAY PRESSURE. This is done in order to avoid activating the alarms when the sigh occurs.

In VOL. CONTR. or VOL. CONTR.+ SIGH mode with respiratory rate above 80 breaths/min, INSP. TIME % should be set at 33 or 50%. Otherwise the ventilator may give incorrect minute volumes and incorrect EXPIRED MINUTE VOLUME meter readings.

Figure 6–9. Set-up of the Servo Ventilator 900C in the assist control mode. (Courtesy of Siemens Life Support Systems, Schaumburg, Ill.)

LIMIT setting on the ventilator control panel, described in step 12.) The recommended working pressure for most adult patients is 60 cm H₂O. Higher pressures, up to 120 cm H₂O, may be required in rare cases.

2. The mode selector switch may be turned to either VOLUME CONTROL or VOLUME CONTROL PLUS SIGH. As discussed previously, the sigh function is not recommended.

3. The PRESET INSPIRATORY MINUTE VOLUME control determines the minute volume that the ventilator will deliver if the patient initiates no breaths independently. As discussed in the section on set tidal volume versus delivered tidal volume, not all of the volume delivered by the ventilator actually reaches the patient, because some is lost to compression within the humidifier and the patient tubing. The

difference between the preset inspiratory minute volume and the minute volume that the patient actually receives is on the order of 400 to 600 ml per minute for a typical adult patient. A method of calculating the exact difference is given in the operating manual.

4. Either a square wave or an accelerating inspiratory flow pattern may be selected. In most cases, a square wave is the appropriate initial setting (see discussion in the section on inspiratory flow).

5. The BREATHS/MINUTE knob determines the minimum number of breaths that the patient will receive. One determines the tidal volume of each breath by dividing the preset inspiratory minute volume by the breaths per minute. The patient may trigger the ventilator at a faster rate than the breaths/minute setting, in which case the patient will receive more than the preset inspiratory minute volume. The tidal volume of the ventilator breaths will not change, however.

6 and 7. The INSPIRATORY TIME PER CENT setting determines the fraction of each respiratory cycle that is spent in inspiration. The PAUSE TIME PER CENT setting may be used to provide a pause at the end of inspiration that is up to 20 per cent of the respiratory cycle. In combination, the inspiratory time per cent and pause time per cent settings determine the I:E ratio, which may be set anywhere from 1:4 to 4:1. The recommended initial setting is an inspiratory time of 33 per cent with no pause, resulting in an I:E ratio of 1:2. (See the sections on inspiratory pause and I:E ratio for a discussion of the use of an inspiratory pause and different I:E ratios.)

8. The inspired oxygen concentration is set by a control on the air-oxygen mixer attached to the right side of the ventilator.

9. The UPPER and LOWER ALARM LIMIT controls should be set approximately 6 per cent above and below the desired oxygen concentration. When the $F_{I_{O_2}}$ varies outside the set limits, as detected by the internal oxygen analyzer on the ventilator, visible and audible alarms are activated.

10. The PARAMETER SELECTOR knob determines which parameter is displayed in the digital readout window on the control panel above the knob. The available parameters include breathing rate (sum of spontaneous and mechanical), actual $F_{I_{O_2}}$, inspiratory tidal volume, expiratory tidal volume, expired minute volume, peak pressure, pause pressure, and mean airway pressure.

11. If PEEP is required, one sets the desired level by turning the PEEP knob.

12. The UPPER PRESSURE LIMIT knob allows the operator to set a ceiling for airway pressure above which inspiration is terminated and visible and audible alarms are activated. The limit should be set at approximately 50 cm H_2O initially and should be readjusted with the patient on the ventilator to 10 to 15 cm H_2O above the observed peak pressure. If the upper pressure limit is set above the working pressure (see step 1), inspiration will end when the working pressure is reached, but no alarms will be activated.

13. The TRIGGER SENSITIVITY control determines how much inspiratory effort the patient must make to trigger an assisted ventilator breath. The sensitivity is usually set so that an inspiratory effort of -1 to -3 cm H_2O is required.

14. The EXPIRED MINUTE VOLUME meter at the top left corner of the ventilator control panel has dual scales: from 0 to 40 liters per minute for adults and from 0 to 4 liters per minute for children. The proper scale is selected with the INFANTS/ADULTS switch at the lower left corner of the control panel. This switch also sets the scale for the UPPER and LOWER ALARM LIMIT controls (see step 16).

15. The ventilator is now connected to the patient. In addition to observing the clinical response of the patient, one should use the PARAMETER SELECTOR control and EX-PIRED MINUTE VOLUME and AIRWAY PRESSURE meters to be sure that the rate, tidal volume, minute volume, $F_{I_{O_2}}$, and airway pressures are in the desired range.

16. After the patient has been on the ventilator for a few minutes and it has been determined that the patient is receiving an appropriate minute volume, the UPPER and LOWER ALARM LIMIT controls should be set approximately 20 per cent above and below the desired minute volume. When the expired minute volume deviates from this range, visible and audible alarms are activated.

Alarms on the Servo 900C. The alarms that are included for patient safety are depicted in Figure 6–10. Alarms are given in the form of audible signals as well as flashing red lights. One can switch off most of the audible alarms for 2 minutes by depressing the ALARM SILENCE button on the control panel.

In addition to the features discussed previously, available options on the Servo 900C include a carbon dioxide monitor, which analyzes end-tidal carbon dioxide and has alarms for levels of carbon dioxide above or below set limits, a lung mechanics calculator, which calculates airway resistance and compliance, and a paper strip recorder, which can print pressure-flow curves or graphically present the digital displays from the ventilator control panel.

SEDATION AND PARALYSIS

Whereas many patients adapt readily to mechanical ventilation and synchronize their own breathing with the ventilator breaths, other patients "fight the machine." By coughing, bucking, and breathing out of phase with the ventilator, they generate high peak airway pressures and increase their oxygen consumption and carbon dioxide production. When their airway pressures exceed the peak pressure limits, they receive less than the prescribed tidal volume, and hypoventilation results. In such cases, *a complication or a mechanical problem must first be ruled out.* One should check the inspired oxygen concentration with an oxygen analyzer to be sure that the set $F_{I_{O_2}}$ is really being delivered. While the patient is being "bagged" by hand, increased resistance to inflow of air, suggesting a plugged or kinked endotracheal tube, can be sensed. Malposition of the endotracheal tube and pneumothorax should be ruled out by auscultation and a chest film. The patient should be suctioned to remove any large airway obstruction due to mucus, blood, or other debris. Other causes for agitation, such as hypotension or pain, should be considered. If coherent, the patient should be reassured.

When all of these measures have been taken, no complication or malfunction has been found, and the patient continues to fight the ventilator, sedation should be considered. Diazepam is a useful drug in this setting. Diazepam acts rapidly and provides excellent relaxation, sedation, and amnesia. The usual starting dose in adults is 2.5 to 5.0 mg intravenously, given at a rate of 2.5 mg per minute. Because the main side effect is respiratory depression, much larger doses, up to 1 mg/kg, can be given in a mechanically ventilated patient, although some cardiac depression occurs at very high doses (greater than 3 mg/kg).[74]

An alternative to diazepam is morphine sulfate. Morphine is usually given in 2- to 4-mg increments intravenously and titrated to effect. As with diazepam, the main side effect of morphine is respiratory depression, which is not a problem in the mechanically ventilated patient with a secure airway. The drug also causes a small drop in blood pressure, probably a result of peripheral vasodilation rather than a direct cardiac depressant effect.[75] Morphine is also known to cause histamine release, which could theoretically lead to increased bronchospasm.[75] Whether this effect is of clinical significance is unknown. Advantages of morphine over di-

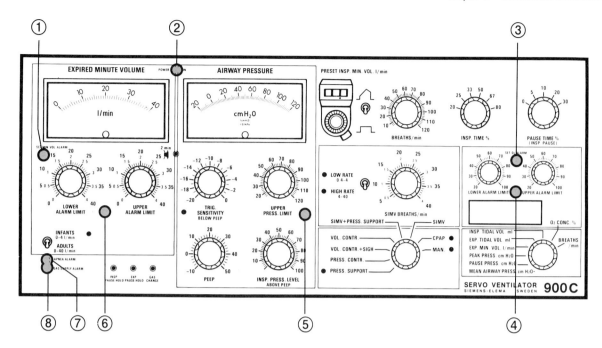

❶

Set minute volume alarm

Indicates that the alarm limits for expired minute volume have not been set.

❷

Power supply failure

The green lamp for POWER ON goes out. Slow audible signals which stop after 5–10 minutes.

❸

Set O₂ alarm

Indicates that the alarm limits for O_2 concentration have not been set.

❹

Alarm limit, O₂ concentration

Upper or lower alarm limit has been passed.

If the O_2 cell is not mounted, neither digital displays nor alarm is given.

A deterioration in the linearity and/or a rapid fall in the values of O_2 concentration, despite adequte O_2 supply, indicates that the O_2 cell is exhausted.

❺

Upper pressure limit, airway pressure

The airway pressure exceeds the preset upper pressure limit. When the alarm is activated, inspiration and/or pause in progress is immediately terminated and changed to expiration. The alarm is given as a single audible signal and a visual flashing signal.

❻

Alarm limit, expired minute volume

Upper or lower alarm limit has been passed. There are two alarm limit settings:
UPPER ALARM LIMIT 3–43 l/min (adults)
　　　　　　　　　0–4.3 l/min (infants)
LOWER ALARM LIMIT 0–37 l/min (adults)
　　　　　　　　　0–3.7 l/min (infants)

❼

Apnea alarm

The APNEA ALARM is activated with audible signals and flashing light if the time between any two consecutive breaths, spontaneous or mandatory or a combination of the two, is greater than approximatively 15 seconds (4 breaths per minute or less). The APNEA ALARM is not intended to and will not monitor for disconnections. The APNEA ALARM is operative in CPAP, PRESS, SUPPORT, SIMV and SIMV + PRESS. SUPPORT.

❽

Gas supply alarm

This alarm is inoperative if the respiratory rate exceeds 80 breaths/min (with inspiration time 20 or 25%).

In the CPAP and PRESS. SUPPORT modes, a patient trig is required to activate the alarm.

Figure. 6–10. Alarms on the Servo Ventilator 900C. (Courtesy of Siemens Life Support Systems, Schaumburg, Ill.)

azepam are that it is a potent analgesic and its effect is readily reversible with naloxone.

When sedation and analgesia are ineffective in preventing the patient from fighting the ventilator, a paralyzing drug may be used. Pancuronium bromide is the drug of choice for inducing paralysis in ventilator patients. Pancuronium is a nondepolarizing blocker of neuromuscular transmission. The main side effects of the drug are a mild increase in pulse and blood pressure, although it has also been reported to cause severe hypertension, ventricular dysrhythmias, and anaphylactic reactions on rare occasions.

Pancuronium is preferred over *d*-tubocurarine, which commonly causes hypotension, and the depolarizing agent succinylcholine, which is short acting and causes fasciculations and cholinergic side effects.[76] The dose of pancuronium is 0.02 to 0.06 mg/kg intravenously. Paralysis occurs within 1 to 3 minutes and lasts 1 to 2 hours, after which time repeat doses may be given. Paralysis induced by pancuronium can be reversed by neostigmine, 0.06 to 0.08 mg/ kg intravenously up to a total of 2.5 mg. Physostigmine should *not* be used for reversal, because it crosses the blood-brain barrier and may induce seizures. Atropine, 0.01 to 0.02 mg/kg up to a total of 1 mg, should be given in the same syringe to block the cholinergic side effects of neostigmine. Paralysis with pancuronium has been reported to be particularly effective in asthmatics.[77] This agent is also used frequently in neonates with hyaline membrane disease, in whom it has been shown to increase compliance and Pa_{O_2}.[78]

It is important to remember that although a patient who is paralyzed with pancuronium may appear asleep and calm, the drug has no sedative or analgesic properties. A paralyzed patient must be given liberal doses of sedatives and analgesics at regular intervals. Hospital personnel should treat the patient as if fully awake, talking to the patient in a reassuring manner and avoiding bedside discussion of the case. Finally, the patient must be continually observed and ventilator function and alarms must be checked frequently, because the patient will be entirely unable to breathe independently should the ventilator fail.

WEANING FROM MECHANICAL VENTILATION

Deciding when a patient can be safely weaned from mechanical ventilation may be more difficult than deciding when mechanical ventilation should be initiated. The patient who is being considered for weaning is often just recovering from a life-threatening illness, and the physician is usually reluctant to do anything that might further cause stress and disturb a precarious equilibrium. However, the longer the patient remains on a ventilator, the more likely complications are to develop. To help the physician in this dilemma, objective criteria have been developed to determine when a patient may be safely weaned.[79–82] These criteria are summarized in Table 6–5. It should be noted that weaning from mechanical ventilation is not necessarily equivalent to extubation. Patients with altered mental status caused by conditions such as stroke, head injury, or drug ingestion may be able to breathe adequately on their own but may not be able to clear their secretions or protect their airways and may therefore require continued intubation after they have been weaned from mechanical ventilation.

The simplest and most reliable predictors of successful weaning are a vital capacity of greater than 10 ml/kg and a maximum inspiratory force of -20 cm H_2O or greater. These parameters are measured easily at the bedside but require cooperation of the patient. In patients with COPD or asthma, either FEV_1 of less than 10 ml per kg or peak flow of less than 25 to 30 per cent of the predicted rate indicates moderately severe airway obstruction and a low likelihood of successful weaning. In patients with high carbon dioxide production and oxygen demands, it is useful to measure the resting minute volume. The patient with a resting minute volume of greater than 10 liters per minute is unlikely to be weaned successfully, because this minute volume could probably not be maintained during spontaneous breathing. Also, the patient should have a maximum

Table 6–5. Weaning Criteria

Measured indices of pulmonary mechanics
  VC greater than 10 ml/kg
  MIF greater than or equal to -20 cm H_2O
  FEV_1 greater than 10 ml/kg
  Peak flow greater than 25 per cent predicted
  Resting $\dot{V}E$ less than 10 L /minute
  MVV greater than two times resting $\dot{V}E$
  Static compliance greater than or equal to 30 ml/cm H_2O

Calculated indices of efficiency of gas exchange
  A–a D_{O_2} on 100 per cent oxygen less than 350 mm Hg
  Q_s/Q_t less than 15 per cent
  V_D/V_T less than 0.6

Clinical indices at the end of 30-minute T-piece trial with $F_{I_{O_2}}$ of 0.40
  Pa_{O_2} greater than or equal to 60 mm Hg
  Pa_{CO_2} and pH normal (An elevated Pa_{CO_2} may be accepted in a patient with chronic carbon dioxide retention provided that the pH is normal.)
  Blood pressure change (up or down) less than 20 mm Hg
  Pulse less than 110
  Respirations less than 30

voluntary ventilation that is at least twice the resting minute volume to provide a margin of safety during time of stress. A static compliance of greater than 30 ml/cm H_2O has also been suggested as a useful weaning parameter. The work of breathing may be too great for a patient with a lower compliance.

Calculated indices of the efficiency of gas exchange may be helpful in predicting successful weaning. A patient with an alveolar-arterial oxygen gradient of greater than 300 to 350 mm Hg on 100 per cent O_2 would be hypoxemic on inspired oxygen concentrations that can be readily administered by mask. Likewise, a shunt fraction of greater than 15 per cent is predictive of hypoxemia following extubation. A V_D/V_T ratio of greater than 0.6 corresponds to a high minute volume requirement and predicts the need for continued ventilatory assistance in most patients.

Once the patient has satisfied criteria for weaning, there are several alternative ways to proceed toward spontaneous breathing. Some physicians use a "sink-or-swim" approach, extubating the patient directly from the assist control or control mode. A more cautious approach is to discontinue mechanical ventilation and allow the patient to breathe spontaneously for a period of approximately 30 minutes while still intubated. An oxygen-enriched mixture (usually 40 per cent) is supplied by a T piece from a wall source or from the ventilator. The patient is observed for signs of anxiety or respiratory distress, vital signs are monitored, and at the end of 30 minutes, arterial blood gases are drawn. If the patient appears clinically stable and arterial blood gases are good, extubation can be carried out. If not, mechanical ventilation is reinstituted.

A third approach, and the one most commonly used today, is to wean patients from the IMV mode. Even before patients satisfy weaning criteria, they may be placed on an IMV rate that provides adequate ventilation but encourages them to take a few breaths on their own. As the patient's pulmonary status improves, the IMV rate is gradually turned down, until finally the patient is breathing entirely independently. Although it has not been proved that this approach hastens weaning, it certainly provides a smooth transition from assisted ventilation to spontaneous breathing.

Some researchers have advocated that patients be weaned to CPAP rather than to breathing at atmospheric pressure.[64] It has been observed that patients breathing spontaneously through an endotracheal tube have a lower

Pa_{O_2}, a lower functional residual capacity, and a higher shunt fraction than when they are breathing the same oxygen mixture after extubation. The improvement in Pa_{O_2} after extubation is on the order of 10 mm Hg while the patient is breathing 40 per cent oxygen. If the same patients breathe spontaneously with a CPAP of 5 cm H_2O, their Pa_{O_2}, functional residual capacity, and shunt fraction are the same before and after extubation. Their Pa_{CO_2} is approximately 2 mm Hg higher while they are on CPAP as compared with spontaneous breathing with or without an endotracheal tube. Thus borderline patients who fail a trial of spontaneous breathing at atmospheric pressure because of hypoxemia may succeed at a CPAP of 5 cm H_2O and go on to be safely extubated.

In addition to the weaning criteria described previously, one should consider other clinical parameters in deciding when a patient may be weaned safely. Weaning should be deferred in patients with unstable, life-threatening cardiac dysrhythmias, because the stress of weaning may exacerbate the dysrhythmias. Also, a cardiac arrest is easier to manage in an intubated patient. Patients with marked anemia may be difficult to wean despite meeting usual weaning criteria, because their oxygen delivery to the periphery is impaired by their low hemoglobin levels. Patients who require heavy doses of sedatives or narcotics may be weanable between doses but lose their respiratory drive when their drugs peak. An example would be a burn patient who receives high doses of narcotics for debridement of wounds. A patient with a metabolic acidosis may be difficult to wean, because hyperventilation is necessary to maintain a normal pH. In contrast, a metabolic alkalosis may be an impediment to weaning in a COPD patient, because it may allow the Pa_{CO_2} to rise to narcotizing levels before the development of acidemia stimulates an attempt to breathe.

COMPLICATIONS OF MECHANICAL VENTILATION

In a prospective study of 354 episodes of mechanical ventilation at the University of Colorado from 1972 to 1973, there were 400 complications.[83] Although most were minor, some were associated with increased patient mortality. It is probably not surprising that there is a high incidence of complications with mechanical ventilation, because it is an invasive form of therapy using complex equipment in critically ill patients for prolonged periods. To some extent, however, the complications are preventable. Others that are not preventable at present should at least be anticipated so that when they occur, they can be recognized and dealt with promptly.

The potential complications of ventilator therapy are listed in Table 6–6. Complications related to intubation and the presence of an endotracheal tube are dealt with in more detail elsewhere in this text but deserve mention here. Intubation of the right main stem bronchus was one of the most common complications in the University of Colorado study and was associated with other problems, including pneumothorax and atelectasis, as well as with decreased survival. Complications related to pressure from the endotracheal tube cuff have declined since the introduction of high-volume, low-pressure cuffs, which require less than 25 mm Hg to produce a seal. Whereas it was recommended in the older literature that a tracheostomy be performed in patients requiring mechanical ventilation for more than 1 to 2 weeks, more recent studies have reported fewer complications with soft cuff endotracheal tubes in place for up to 3 weeks than with tracheostomies.[84] There has been one report of orotracheal intubation for 2 months without com-

Table 6–6. Potential Complications of Mechanical Ventilation

Complications related to endotracheal or tracheostomy tube
 Tube malfunction (leaking cuff, kinked tube, obstruction caused by herniation of balloon over end of tube)
 Pressure phenomena (nasal and tongue necrosis due to pressure from the tube, laryngeal ulceration and polyps, tracheal stenosis and malacia, fistulas into esophagus and innominate artery)
Complications resulting from machine malfunction and operator error
 Failure of ventilator to deliver set tidal volume, rate, Fi_{O_2}, and so forth
 Inappropriate settings ordered
 Settings not fixed as ordered (commonly includes wrong rate, tidal volume, and Fi_{O_2}; assist control sensitivity too high or too low)
 Alarm failure
 Alarm turned off and left off
 Inadequate humidification
 Over- or underheating of inspired air
 Patient accidentally disconnected from ventilator
Direct effects of positive-pressure ventilation
 Barotrauma (pneumothorax, tension pneumothorax, pulmonary interstitial emphysema, subcutaneous emphysema, pneumomediastinum, pneumoperitoneum, air embolism)
 Decreased venous return and cardiac output
Other complications
 Ventilator-associated pneumonia
 Oxygen toxicity and retrolental fibroplasia
 Bronchopulmonary dysplasia

plications.[85] The safety of orotracheal versus nasotracheal intubation has not been studied systematically. In general, nasotracheal intubation is better tolerated by the patient, is more secure, and allows better mouth care. On the other hand, it leads to a higher incidence of sinusitis and necrosis of the nasal mucosa and cartilage.

The incidence of complications related to ventilator malfunction has declined as ventilators have become more reliable, but operator errors remain a significant problem. One of the most common yet potentially serious errors is to turn off a ventilator alarm and forget to turn it back on. This happens most frequently when the patient is disconnected briefly from the ventilator for suctioning. With many older ventilators, such as the Puritan-Bennett MA-1, one can permanently silence the alarm that signals when the patient has failed to receive a full tidal volume by turning off a single switch. If this alarm is not turned back on after the patient has been suctioned, the patient later may, in turning the head, cause the ventilator tubing to become disconnected from the endotracheal tube. The next indication that something is wrong may be the development of a ventricular dysrhythmia on the cardiac monitor. To prevent this occurrence, many modern ventilators have been designed with alarms that can be turned off by the operator only for 1 to 2 minutes before they reactivate themselves.

Barotrauma remains a relatively common complication of ventilator therapy. Pneumothorax is the most common form of barotrauma and may be preceded or accompanied by pulmonary interstitial emphysema, pneumomediastinum, subcutaneous emphysema, and pneumoperitoneum. In patients receiving ventilatory assistance, pneumothorax is more often than not of the tension type. The reported incidence of pneumothorax in mechanically ventilated patients varies in the literature from 0.5 to 14 per cent.[86–88] The highest incidence of barotrauma occurs with the use of levels of PEEP greater than 24 cm H_2O,[89] whereas levels of PEEP of 5 cm H_2O and below do not seem to be associated with increased risk.[88] The incidence of pneumothorax is also particularly high in patients with asthma.[20]

It has been reported that the incidence of barotrauma is lower with pressure-cycled than with volume-cycled ventilators.[87] This is not surprising when it is considered that higher pressures are commonly used with volume-cycled ventilators, because it is generally believed that it is safer to risk barotrauma but maintain an adequate tidal volume than to risk hypoventilation by limiting peak pressure. Judicious use of sedation and paralysis may help reduce pressures and thereby lower the risk of barotrauma. It has been argued that it is safer to allow patients with asthma to remain hypercapnic for periods of hours to days rather than to use peak pressures above 50 cm H_2O.[90]

In patients who are on high levels of PEEP or who require high peak pressures, the development of barotrauma should be anticipated. A pneumothorax should be suspected whenever there is a sudden deterioration in compliance and blood gases. Pneumothorax should be confirmed by auscultation, palpation of the position of the trachea, and, if time permits, a chest film. In the patient who is deteriorating rapidly, needle thoracostomy is both diagnostic and therapeutic (see Chapter 8).

Pneumoperitoneum is a form of barotrauma that deserves special mention. The incidence of pneumoperitoneum and pneumoretroperitoneum has been reported to be as high as 4 per cent in patients on PEEP.[91] Pneumoperitoneum is typically preceded by pulmonary interstitial emphysema, subcutaneous emphysema, and pneumomediastinum and is usually, but not always, accompanied by pneumothorax. Patients with ventilator-induced pneumoperitoneum have been subjected to needless laparotomies in a search for the cause of the free air in their abdomens.[92] Another unusual form of barotrauma is fatal arterial and venous air embolism, which has been reported in association with tension pneumothorax in premature infants receiving mechanical ventilation.[93]

Another potential problem that is a direct effect of positive-pressure ventilation is diminished cardiac output. As discussed in the section on PEEP and CPAP, a clinically significant fall in cardiac output usually occurs at levels of PEEP of 12 to 15 cm H_2O and above. A drop in cardiac output has also been shown to be a result of positive-pressure ventilation without PEEP.[26] The fall in cardiac output seen with mechanical ventilation is thought to be caused by decreased venous return as a result of increased intrathoracic pressure. This effect is greatest when mean airway pressures are highest, as in controlled ventilation with PEEP, and is negligible when low mean airway pressures are used, as in the IMV mode with a low mechanical breathing frequency.[22] It has been shown in the case of PEEP that the fall in cardiac output is at least partly reversible with blood volume expansion.[60] The influence of positive-pressure ventilation on venous return also depends on the extent to which airway pressure is transmitted to the pleural space. When lung compliance is high and chest wall compliance is low, as in COPD, much of the airway pressure is transmitted to the pleural space, and venous return is impaired more than in conditions such as ARDS, in which lung compliance is low.

It should not be assumed that the effect of positive-pressure ventilation on cardiac function is always detrimental. It has been shown that patients with respiratory distress may generate highly negative intrathoracic pressures during spontaneous breathing and that this negative pressure acts as increased afterload on the heart.[94] Although venous return into the thorax is enhanced by negative intrathoracic pressure, ejection of blood out of the thorax is impeded, and the more negative the intrathoracic pressure, the harder the left heart must pump to reach a given systemic arterial pressure.[95] Mechanical ventilation substitutes positive for negative intrathoracic pressure, thereby decreasing afterload on the left heart. In most cases, the effect of positive-pressure ventilation in decreasing venous return to the heart outweighs its effect in decreasing afterload, and decreased cardiac output results. In patients breathing spontaneously on PEEP as compared with those breathing spontaneously without PEEP, however, an increased cardiac output has been demonstrated.[96] Positive-pressure ventilation would be expected to be particularly beneficial in the treatment of patients with cardiogenic pulmonary edema, because it would decrease both the increased preload and the increased afterload which are involved in the pathogenesis of this condition.

Pneumonia is one of the more common complications of intubation and mechanical ventilation. In a review of infections related to medical devices, it was found that ventilator-associated pneumonia was second in frequency only to catheter-related cystitis, and it was estimated that 75,000 ventilator patients a year acquire a nosocomial pneumonia with a fatality rate of 40 per cent.[97] In another large-scale retrospective study, the incidence of nosocomial pneumonia was 0.3 per cent in patients not on ventilators, 1.3 per cent in patients ventilated by endotracheal tube, and a surprising 66 per cent in patients ventilated by tracheostomy.[98] No pneumonias developed in patients ventilated less than 24 hours, whereas there was an abrupt rise in risk for patients ventilated more than 5 days.

Most cases of ventilator-associated pneumonia resulted from enteric gram-negative organisms. Ventilator-associated pneumonias may be preventable in part by strict adherence to sterile technique during suctioning and by avoidance of prolonged ventilation or tracheostomy whenever possible. Ventilator humidification systems are a potential source of bacterial contamination, and it is the policy at many hospitals to change the ventilator tubing and humidification system every 24 hours. With the cascade humidifiers used on most modern ventilators, however, there is probably little risk of introducing bacteria into the inspired gas mixture, and it has been shown that the system need not be changed more often than every 48 hours.[99]

Oxygen toxicity was discussed as a potential complication of mechanical ventilation in the section on inspired oxygen concentration. Although the exact dose-time relationship of oxygen toxicity has not been worked out, it should be assumed that an FI_{O_2} of 0.50 or greater is potentially toxic. One can avoid oxygen toxicity in many cases by using measures such as PEEP, which improve the A–a D_{O_2} and allow one to use lower inspired oxygen concentrations.

A final condition that should be included as a potential complication of mechanical ventilation is bronchopulmonary dysplasia. Bronchopulmonary dysplasia is a form of chronic lung disease that occurs in infants who have been mechanically ventilated for severe hyaline membrane disease. It is characterized radiographically by cystic enlargement of the airways with intermingled dense, strand-like infiltrates. The incidence of bronchopulmonary dysplasia is 6 to 11 per cent in survivors of hyaline membrane disease.[42] It is not known whether bronchopulmonary dysplasia results from high inspired oxygen concentrations, high airway pressures, or the evolution of hyaline membrane disease itself. One small study has suggested that intramuscular administration of vitamin E may modify the development of bronchopulmonary dysplasia.[100] Until more is known about the actual cause of this condition, however, it cannot be considered preventable.

HIGH-FREQUENCY VENTILATION

A chapter on mechanical ventilation would not be complete without at least some mention of high-frequency ventilation (HFV). More than 800 articles have been published on this topic since the technique was introduced in Sweden in 1967, and it has been the subject of several recent reviews.[101–103] High-frequency ventilation differs radically from the traditional approach of using tidal volumes and frequencies in the physiologic range. Instead, tidal volumes of a few milliliters per kilogram are used at rates from 60 to 3000 breaths per minute. The chest does not rise and fall in patients on HFV unless they breathe spontaneously around the ventilator. One might expect that only the dead space gas would be exchanged and that no alveolar ventilation would occur at all. In fact, however, it is found that adequate ventilation and oxygen exchange do occur by mechanisms that are still not completely understood but that include facilitated diffusion of gases along the vibrating column of air.

High-frequency ventilation has found practical application in laryngeal surgery, in which it allows the surgeon a clear view of a motionless larynx. It has also been used successfully to ventilate patients with large bronchopleural fistulas in whom conventional mechanical ventilation has failed because of massive air leaks. High-frequency ventilation has been tried in adults with ARDS and in infants with hyaline membrane disease in hopes that adequate oxygenation and ventilation could be achieved with lower airway pressures than with conventional mechanical ventilation and PEEP. Conflicting results have been reported in these situations, and whether HFV offers a definite advantage remains to be established.

Problems that have been encountered with high-frequency ventilation include difficulties in humidifying the inspired air adequately. Mucosal injury and increased pulmonary secretions have been encountered. Conventional alarm systems for detecting apnea, inadequate tidal volume, and excess airway pressure are not applicable in HFV. Although there are now ventilators available commercially that are capable of delivering HFV, there are still no well-established guidelines to aid the clinician in deciding which of the several different ventilator types to choose from or what tidal volume or rate is best for a given patient.

High-frequency ventilation will undoubtedly remain an area of intense research over the next several years. At this point, it seems unlikely that HFV will replace conventional mechanical ventilation in the majority of patients. With further refinements in technology and greater understanding of the physiology involved, however, it is probable that the number of indications for HFV will expand and that ventilator designs and settings will become more standardized.

REFERENCES

1. Brewer LA: Respiration and respiratory treatment. A historical overview. Am J Surg 138:342, 1979.
2. Crit Care Med 6:310, 1978.
3. Crit Care Med 7:226, 1979.
4. Comroe JH: Man-cans. Am Rev Respir Dis 116:945, 1977.
5. Shapiro BA, Harrison RA, Trout CA: Clinical Application of Respiratory Care. 2nd ed. Chicago, Year Book Medical Publishers, 1979, p 326.
6. Pontoppidan H, Wilson RS, Rie MA, Schneider RC: Respiratory intensive care. Anesthesiology 47:96, 1977.
7. Pontoppidan H, Geffin B, Lowenstein E: Acute respiratory failure in the adult (3 parts). N Engl J Med 287:690, 743, 799, 1972.
8. Laver MB, Safen A: Measurement of blood oxygen tension in anesthesia. Anesthesiology 26:73, 1965.
9. Downer DH, Hoffman LG: Bedside construction of a custom cuirass for respiratory failure in kyphoscoliosis. Chest 74:469, 1978.
10. Man GCW, Jones RL, MacDonald GF, King EG: Primary alveolar hypoventilation managed by negative-pressure ventilators. Chest 76:219, 1979.
11. McFadden ER, Lyons HA: Arterial blood gas tension in asthma. N Engl J Med 278:1027, 1968.
12. Krauss AN: Assisted ventilation: A critical review. Clin Perinatol 7:61, 1980.
13. Spahr RC, Klein AM, Brown DR, MacDonald HM, and Holzman IR: Hyaline membrane disease. A controlled study of inspiratory to expiratory ratio and its management by ventilator. Am J Dis Child 134:373, 1980.
14. Krauss AN, Auld PAM: Evaluation of methods of assisted ventilation in hyaline membrane disease. Arch Dis Child 53:878, 1978.
15. Avery EE, Morch ET, Benson DW: Critically crushed chests. A new method of treatment with continuous mechanical hyperventilation to produce alkalotic apnea and internal pneumatic stabilization. J Thorac Cardiovasc Surg 32:291, 1956.
16. Shackford SR, Virgilia RW, Peters RM: Selective use of ventilator therapy in flail chest injury. J Thorac Cardiovasc Surg 81:194, 1981.
17. Gordon G: Controlled respiration in the management of patients with traumatic brain injury. Acta Anaesthesiol Scand 15:193, 1971.
18. Callaham M: Tricyclic antidepressant overdose. JACEP 8:413, 1979.
19. Reuler JB: Hypothermia: Pathophysiology, clinical settings, and management. Ann Intern Med 89:519, 1978.
20. Scoggin CH, Sahn SA, Petty TL: Status asthmaticus. A nine-year experience. JAMA 238:1158, 1977.
21. Kirby RR, Smith RA, Desautels DA: Mechanical ventilation. In Burton GG, Hodgkin JE (eds): Respiratory Care. 2nd ed. Philadelphia, JB Lippincott Co, 1984, pp 556–647.
22. Douglas ME, Downs JB: Cardiopulmonary effects of intermittent mandatory ventilation. Int Anesthesiol Clin 18:97, 1980.
23. Downs JB, Mitchell LA: Pulmonary effects of ventilatory pattern following cardiopulmonary bypass. Crit Care Med 4:295, 1976.
24. Ayres SM: Analysis of ventilation and perfusion abnormalities by washout in alveolar air and arterial blood and continuous measurement of inert gas. Crit Care Med 4:261, 1976.
25. Smith LL, Walton DM, Wilson DR, Jackson CL, Hinshaw DB: Continuous blood gas and pH monitoring during cardiovascular surgery. Am J Surg 120:249, 1970.
26. Hedley-Whyte J, Pontoppidan H, Morris MJ: The response of patients with respiratory failure and cardiopulmonary disease to different levels of constant volume ventilation. J Clin Invest 45:1543, 1966.
27. Suwa K, Bendixen HH: Change in Pa_{CO_2} with mechanical dead space during artificial ventilation. J Appl Physiol 24:556, 1968.
28. Breivik H, Grenvik A, Millen E, Safar P: Normalizing low arterial CO_2 tension during mechanical ventilation. Chest 63:525, 1973.
29. West JB: Respiratory Physiology. 3rd ed. Baltimore, Williams & Wilkins, 1985, p 19.
30. Selecky PA, Wasserman K, Klein M, Ziment I: A graphic approach to assessing interrelationships among minute ventilation, arterial carbon dioxide tension, and ratio of physiologic dead space to tidal volume in patients on respirators. Am Rev Respir Dis 117:181, 1978.
31. Grimby G, Hedenstierna G, Lofstrom B: Chest wall mechanics during artificial ventilation. J Appl Physiol 38:576, 1975.
32. Suter PM, Fairley HB, Isenberg MD: Effect of tidal volume and positive end-expiratory pressure on compliance during mechanical ventilation. Chest 73:158, 1978.
33. Bear Medical Systems, Inc: Bear-2 Adult Volume Ventilator Instruction Manual. Riverside, Calif, Bear Medical Systems, Inc.
34. Ramsden CA, Reynolds EOR: Ventilator settings for newborn infants. Arch Dis Child 62:529, 1987.
35. Frankel LR, Lewiston NJ, Smith DW, Stevenson DK: Clinical observations on mechanical ventilation for respiratory failure in bronchiolitis. Pediatr Pulmonol 2:307, 1986.
36. Rawlings DJ, McComb RC, Williams TA, Thompson TR: The Siemens Elema Servo ventilator 900B for the management of newborn infants with severe respiratory distress syndrome. A 22 month trial. Crit Care Med 8:307, 1980.
37. Bazaral MG: Volume ventilation systems for infants. Anesthesiology 54:240, 1981.
38. Kanter RK, Blatt SD, Zimmerman JJ: Initial mechanical ventilator settings for pediatric patients: Clinical judgement in selection of tidal volume. Am J Emerg Med 5:113, 1987.
39. Shapiro BA, Harrison RA, Walton JR: Clinical Application of Blood Gases. 2nd ed. Chicago, Year Book Medical Publishers, 1977, pp 85–86.
40. Menn SJ, Tisi GM: Oxygen as a drug. In Burton G, Gee GN, Hodgkin JE (eds): Respiratory Care. Philadelphia, JB Lippincott Co, 1977, pp 386–399.
41. Weiter JJ: Retrolental fibroplasia: An unsolved problem. N Engl J Med 305:1404, 1981.
42. Northway WH: Bronchopulmonary dysplasia and vitamin E. N Engl J Med 299:599, 1978.
43. Kinsey VE, et al: Pa_{O_2} levels and retrolental fibroplasia: A report of the cooperative study. Pediatrics 60:655, 1977.
44. Murray JF: The Normal Lung. 2nd ed. Philadelphia, WB Saunders Co, 1986, pp 196–197.
45. Cane RD, Shapiro BA, Templin R, et al.: Unreliability of oxygen tension-based indices in reflecting intrapulmonary shunting in critically ill patients. Crit Care Med 16:1243, 1988.
46. Downs JB, Klein EF, Desautel SD, et al: Intermittent mandatory ventilation: A new approach to weaning patients from mechanical ventilators. Chest 64:331, 1973.

47. Schacter EN, Tucked D, Beck GJ: Does intermittent mandatory ventilation accelerate weaning? JAMA 246:1210, 1981.

48. MacIntyre NR: Respiratory function during pressure support ventilation. Chest 89:677, 1986.

49. Ashbaugh DG, Bigelow DB, Petty TL, Levine BE: Acute respiratory distress in adults. Lancet 2:319, 1967.

50. Gregory GA, Kitterman JA, Phibbs RH, et al: Treatment of the idiopathic respiratory distress syndrome with continuous positive airway pressure. N Engl J Med 284:1333, 1971.

51. Greenbaum DM, Milien JE, Eross B, et al: Continuous positive airway pressure without tracheal intubation in spontaneously breathing patients. Chest 69:615, 1976.

52. Hoff BN, Flemming DC, Sasse F: Use of positive airway pressure without endotracheal intubation. Crit Care Med 7:559, 1979.

53. Dantzker DR, Brook CJ, Dehart P, et al: Ventilation perfusion distribution in the adult respiratory distress syndrome. Am Rev Respir Dis 120:1039, 1979.

54. Schmidt GB, O'Neill WW, Kotb K, et al: Continuous positive airway pressure in the prophylaxis of the adult respiratory distress syndrome. Surg Gynecol Obstet 143:613, 1976.

55. Zimmerman JE, Glodman LR, Shaituari MBG: Effect of mechanical ventilation and PEEP on chest radiograph. Am J Radiol 133:811, 1979.

56. Weisman IM, Rinaldo JE, Rogers RM: Positive end-expiratory pressure in adult respiratory failure. N Engl J Med 307:1381, 1982.

57. Springer RR, Stevens PM: The influence of PEEP on survival of patients in respiratory failure. A retrospective analysis. Am J Med 66:196, 1979.

58. Rizk NW, Murray JF: PEEP and pulmonary edema. Am J Med 72:381, 1982.

59. Lutch JS, Murray JF: Continuous positive-pressure ventilation: Effects on systemic oxygen transport and tissue oxygenation. Ann Intern Med 76:193, 1972.

60. Jardin F, Farcot J, Boisaute L, et al: Influence of positive end-expiratory pressure on left ventricular performance. N Engl J Med 304:387, 1981.

61. Venus M, Jacobs K: Alterations in regional myocardial blood flows during different levels of positive end-expiratory pressure. Crit Care Med 12:96, 1984.

62. Powers SR, Mannal R, Neclerio M, et al: Physiologic consequences of positive end-expiratory pressure ventilation. Ann Surg 178:265, 1973.

63. Suter PM, Fairley B, Isenberg MD: Optimum end-expiratory airway pressure in patients with acute pulmonary failure. N Engl J Med 292:284, 1975.

64. Annest SJ, Gottlieb M, Paloski WH, et al: Detrimental effects of removing end-expiratory pressure prior to endotracheal extubation. Ann Surg 191:539, 1980.

65. Parish JM, Gracey DR, Southorn PA, et al: Differential mechanical ventilation in respiratory failure due to severe unilateral lung disease. Mayo Clin Proc 59:822, 1984.

66. Dammann JF, McAslan TC, Maffeo CJ: Optimal flow pattern for mechanical ventilation of the lungs. Crit Care Med 6:293, 1978.

67. Spar RC, Klein AM, Brown DR, et al: Hyaline membrane disease. A controlled study of inspiratory to expiratory ratio in its management by ventilator. Am J Dis Child 134:373, 1980.

68. Cole AGH, Weller SF, Sykes MK: Inverse ratio ventilation compared with PEEP in adult respiratory failure. Intensive Care Med 10:227, 1984.

69. Gurevitch MJ, Van Duke J, Young ES, Jackson K: Improved oxygenation and lower peak airway pressure in severe adult respiratory distress syndrome: Treatment with inverse ratio ventilation. Chest 89:211, 1986.

70. Shapiro BA, Harrison RA, Trout CA: Clinical Application of Respiratory Care. 2nd ed. Chicago, Year Book Medical Publishers, 1979, pp 349–363.

71. Bendixen HH, Hedley-Whyte J, Chir B, Laver MB: Impaired oxygenation in surgical patients during general anesthesia with controlled ventilation. N Engl J Med 269:991, 1963.

72. Kirby RR: Mechanical ventilation in acute ventilatory failure: Facts, fiction, and fallacies. Curr Probl Anesth Crit Care Med 3:5, 1977.

73. Hall CB, McBride JT: Vapors, viruses, and views. Am J Dis Child 140:331, 1986.

74. Clarke RSJ, Lyons SM: Diazepam and flunitrazepam as induction agents for cardiac surgical operations. Acta Anaesthesiol Scand 21:282, 1977.

75. Jaffe JH, Martin WR: Narcotic analgesics and antagonists. In Goodman LS, Gilman H (eds): The Pharmacological Basis of Therapeutics. 5th ed. New York, Macmillan Inc, 1975, pp 245–283.

76. DeGarmo BH, Dronen S: Pharmacology and clinical use of neuromuscular blocking agents. Ann Emerg Med 12:48, 1983.

77. Levin N, Dillow JB: Status asthmaticus and pancuronium bromide. JAMA 222:1265, 1972.

78. Stark AR, Frantz ID: Muscle relaxation in mechanically ventilated infants. J Pediatr 94:439, 1979.

79. Freely TW, Hedley-Whyte J: Weaning from controlled ventilation and supplemental oxygen. N Engl J Med 292:903, 1975.

80. Sahn SA, Lakshminarayan S, Petty TL: Weaning from mechanical ventilation. JAMA 235:2208, 1976.

81. Sahn SA, Lakshminarayan S: Bedside criteria for discontinuation of mechanical ventilation. Chest 63:1002, 1973.

82. Bowser MA, Hodgkin JE, Burton GG: Techniques of ventilator weaning. In Burton G, Gee GN, Hodgkin JE (eds): Respiratory Care. Philadelphia, JB Lippincott Co, 1977, pp 664–671.

83. Zwilich CW, Pierson DJ, Creagh CE, et al: Complications of assisted ventilation. A prospective study of 354 consecutive episodes. Am J Med 57:161, 1974.

84. Stauffer JL, Olson DE, Petty TL: Complications and consequences of endotracheal intubation and tracheostomy. A prospective study of 105 critically ill patients. Am J Med 70:65, 1981.

85. Vogelhut MM, Downs JB: Prolonged endotracheal intubation. Chest 76:110, 1979.

86. Kumar A, Pontoppidan H, Falke KJ, et al: Pulmonary barotrauma during mechanical ventilation. Crit Care Med 1:181, 1973.

87. DeLatorre FJ, Tomasa A, Klamburg J, et al: Incidence of pneumothorax and pneumomediastinum in patients with aspiration pneumonia requiring ventilatory support. Chest 72:141, 1977.

88. Cullen DJ, Caldera DL: The incidence of ventilator-induced pulmonary barotrauma in critically ill patients. Anesthesiology 50:185, 1979.

89. Kirby RR, Downs JB, Civetta JM, et al: High level positive end-expiratory pressure in acute respiratory insufficiency. Chest 67:156, 1975.

90. Darioli R, Perret C: Mechanical controlled hypoventilation in status asthmaticus. Am Rev Respir Dis 128:385, 1984.

91. Altman AR, Johnson TH: Pneumoperitoneum and pneumoretroperitoneum. Consequences of positive end-expiratory pressure therapy. Arch Surg 114:208, 1979.

92. Summers B: Pneumoperitoneum associated with artificial ventilation. Br Med J 1:1528, 1979.

93. Banagale RC: Massive intracranial air embolism: A complication of mechanical ventilation. Am J Dis Child 134:799, 1980.

94. Buda AJ, Pinsky MR, Ingels NB, et al: Effect of intrathoracic pressure on left ventricular performance. N Engl J Med 301:453, 1979.

95. McGregor M: Pulsus paradoxicus. N Engl J Med 301:480, 1979.

96. Sturgeon CL, Douglas ME, Downs JB, Dannemiller FJ: PEEP and CPAP: Cardiopulmonary effects during spontaneous ventilation. Anesth Analg 56:633, 1977.

97. Stamm WE: Infections related to medical devices. Ann Intern Med 89:764, 1978.

98. Cross AS, Roup B: Role of respiratory assistance devices in endemic nosocomial pneumonia. Am J Med 70:681, 1981.

99. Craven DE, Connolly MG, Lichtenberg DA, et al: Contamination of mechanical ventilators with tubing changes every 24 or 48 hours. N Engl J Med 306:1505, 1982.

100. Ehrenkranz RA, Bonta BW, Ablow RC, Warshaw JB: Amelioration of bronchopulmonary dysplasia after vitamin E administration. N Engl J Med 299:564, 1978.

101. Froese AB, Bryan CA: High frequency ventilation. Am Rev Respir Dis 135:1363, 1987.

102. Gallagher TJ: High frequency ventilation. Med Clin North Am 67:633, 1983.

103. Wetzell R, Gioia FR: High frequency ventilation. Pediatr Clin North Am 34:15, 1987.

Chapter *7*

Tracheal Suctioning and Transtracheal Needle Aspiration

Steven M. Joyce

Tracheal Suctioning

INTRODUCTION

Tracheal suctioning removes secretions, aspirated material, or both from the airways of patients whose cough reflex has failed or is bypassed by an artificial airway. Removal of secretions prevents atelectasis, improves gas exchange, and helps eliminate infected material. Secretions obtained by suctioning may also be useful in diagnosis of pulmonary infections. With minimal training, the procedure may be performed by respiratory therapists, nurses, or physicians. Although tracheal suctioning may be performed easily at the bedside, there is a potential for serious complications, so the proper precautions must always be taken.

Tracheal suctioning has been practiced since the introduction of positive-pressure ventilation in the 1950s as a method of removing tracheobronchial secretions. The technique remains vitally important for the maintenance of proper gas exchange in endotracheally intubated patients and in selected patients whose cough reflex is otherwise impaired. The development of new materials has resulted in the availability of suction catheters of various diameters and tip designs to minimize mucosal injury and allow selective bronchial catheterization. Other features such as concomitant oxygen delivery with in-line systems optimize secretion removal while minimizing hypoxemia. Substantial clinical research has been devoted to evaluating methods for minimizing complications of tracheal suctioning.

INDICATIONS AND CONTRAINDICATIONS

The following discussion refers principally to tracheal suctioning through an endotracheal tube. Nasotracheal suctioning is discussed separately.

The basic indications for tracheal suctioning are the need to perform bronchopulmonary toilet in intubated or obtunded patients and to sample lower respiratory tract secretions for diagnostic tests (when coughed specimens are inadequate or cannot be obtained). In an emergency setting, prompt tracheal suctioning is usually performed immediately after endotracheal intubation to clear the airways of aspirated materials or accumulated secretions.

Bronchopulmonary toilet is indicated when secretions are visible at the endotracheal tube orifice; auscultation of the lungs reveals coarse rales, rhonchi, or tubular breath sounds; or the sudden onset of dyspnea or arterial oxygen desaturation occurs in patients at risk for airway occlusion. Those at risk include all patients with artificial airways (which prevent coughing), especially those patients with bronchopulmonary infections and excess secretions.

Most authors agree that routine suctioning is unwarranted and potentially dangerous and that the procedure need only be performed on an as-needed basis when the previously mentioned indications exist.[1-3] The only relative contraindication to tracheal suctioning is cardiovascular instability, which is exacerbated by the procedure, as in the patient with cardiogenic pulmonary edema and hypoxemia. However, even in such cases, when treatment of the underlying disorder is not sufficient to maintain adequate gas exchange, tracheal suctioning should be undertaken carefully.

EQUIPMENT

Appropriate vacuum settings for optimal secretion removal and minimal mucosal trauma have been proposed by Wilkins.[2] Settings of 60 to 80 mm Hg for infants, 80 to 120 mm Hg for children, and 120 to 150 mm Hg for adults are recommended. Higher settings cause turbulent flow through the catheter, which actually reduces the efficacy of secretion removal and may increase tracheal mucosal injury.

Catheters made of polyvinylchloride are most commonly used. They are flexible, require no lubrication, and are translucent, allowing visualization of secretions.[1]

The external diameter of the suction catheter should be approximately one half the internal diameter of the endotracheal tube.[3] Larger catheters may prevent adequate air flow into the airways during suctioning, and the resultant evacuation of gases may result in atelectasis and hypoxemia. However, the largest catheter that will fit the airway should be used for life-threatening airway obstruction. Smaller-diameter catheters may not remove secretions effectively.

Catheter tip designs vary, depending on the intended use. Conventional catheters with an end hole and several side holes are most commonly available in an emergency department setting. Tips designed for specialized uses do exist but offer no great advantages for uncomplicated tracheal suctioning. Catheters designed for selective bronchial suctioning are seldom used in an emergency situation. An in-line system that does not require interruption of the ventilator circuit has been developed for use in ventilated patients who have unstable cardiovascular conditions or are dependent on positive end-expiratory pressure (PEEP).[3]

PROCEDURE

Assemble all equipment and ensure that it is functioning properly, including the suction source (of appropriate setting), catheters, tubing, manual resuscitation bag-valve assembly (or ventilator), cardiac monitor, oxygen source, and 10-ml syringe of sterile nonbacteriostatic saline. Standard resuscitation drugs and equipment should be immediately available.

Aseptic technique should be used as much as possible. Hands are washed with antimicrobial soap, and a sterile glove is used to manipulate the suction catheter. In emergencies, asepsis may not be practical, but one should try to minimize contamination of the airways.

Preoxygenate the patient by delivering 6 to 7 breaths of 100 per cent oxygen either by hand-held bag or ventilator. Be aware that many ventilators will not deliver an FI_{O_2} of 1.0 for up to 2 minutes after the setting is changed.[2]

Immediately after preoxygenation, introduce the sterile catheter into the endotracheal tube with the gloved hand, taking care *not* to occlude the vacuum vent during insertion. Pass the catheter tip past the distal end of the artificial airway until resistance is met (usually at the carina). Pull the catheter back slightly before applying suction. Then occlude the vent to apply suction and rotate the catheter in a circular motion around the tube lumen while slowly withdrawing it from the airway.

This entire procedure should interrupt the patient's ventilation for only approximately 20 seconds, with the catheter actually in the airway for less than 15 seconds, to minimize hypoxemia and atelectasis.[3]

Immediately following the procedure, the patient should be reoxygenated using a combination of hyperoxygenation, hyperventilation, and hyperinflation. Hyperoxygenation is achieved by delivering an $F_{I_{O_2}}$ higher than the patient's maintenance value (usually 100 per cent). Hyperinflation is achieved by delivering up to one and one-half times the usual tidal volume, again as estimated either by bag ventilation or by using the ventilator sigh function. A clinical study by Baun as well as an exhaustive review by Barnes and Kirchoff supports the combination of these techniques to minimize postsuctioning hypoxemia and its attendant complications.[4, 5]

Thick secretions may be difficult to remove. In these cases, 5 to 10 ml of sterile normal saline should be injected into the artificial airway, after which several deep breaths should be delivered by bag or ventilator just before suctioning. Following the procedure, $F_{I_{O_2}}$ and other ventilator settings should be returned to presuctioning values. Clotted blood or other thick secretions not removed by suctioning may be retrievable by extraction with number 6 Fogarty catheters.[5a, 5b] The catheter is passed beyond the occluding material and then inflated. The material is pulled ahead of the catheter during its withdrawal.

Secretions for microbiologic studies may be obtained using a sterile mucus trap. The specimen is transported in the sealed trap for prompt processing, as described under "Transtracheal Needle Aspiration."

COMPLICATIONS

As with most invasive procedures, tracheal suctioning is not without the potential for serious complications. Fortunately, most can be prevented or minimized.

Difficulty in passing a suction catheter may be due to the patient's biting the endotracheal tube, airway kinking, inspissated secretions, herniation or rupture of the cuff balloon, tube malalignment, or placement of the tube outside the trachea. Solutions to these problems include placement of a bite block; removal of redundant endotracheal tube to prevent kinking; injection of saline to loosen secretions; and prompt replacement of blocked, malfunctioning, or malpositioned tubes.

Hypoxemia, although transient, is perhaps the most serious complication of tracheal suctioning, as it can lead to life-threatening cardiac dysrhythmias. Inadequate oxygenation before or after suctioning, prolonged (more than 15 seconds) suctioning, and excessive catheter size are the most common causes. Hypoxemia may be presumed when dysrhythmias develop during or just after the procedure. Dynamic oxygen saturation measurement with a transcutaneous oximeter may prove helpful. Fortunately, hypoxemia may be prevented or minimized by proper oxygenation techniques (as described in the section on procedure).

Dysrhythmias may be caused by hypoxemia, as discussed previously, as well as by tracheal irritation. When the mucosa is irritated by the suction catheter, both vagal and sympathetic afferents may be stimulated. Vagal stimulation may produce bradycardia with resultant hypotension, whereas sympathetic stimulation can precipitate tachydysrhythmias or even ventricular fibrillation, especially when hypoxemia is present. The incidence of dangerous dysrhythmias during suctioning is unknown but is probably not rare. Shim and

coworkers described significant dysrhythmias (some persisting for 2 minutes) that occurred in 6 of 17 patients undergoing suctioning while breathing air; all dysrhythmias were abolished when the patients breathed 100 per cent O_2 for 5 minutes before undergoing the procedure.[6] Attention to the cardiac monitor during and after suctioning is thus very important. Suctioning should be terminated immediately when dysrhythmias (other than preexisting dysrhythmias or sinus tachycardia) are observed, and oxygenation should be provided as previously described.

Intracranial pressure (ICP) may increase transiently during tracheal suctioning, which leads to theoretic concerns in patients whose cerebral perfusion pressure is already marginal. Rudy and colleagues reviewed a number of studies examining this transient ICP elevation; none were found to demonstrate a clinically significant deleterious effect in the patients studied.[7] They also reviewed studies that examined the efficacy of pretreatment with various drugs to prevent increases in ICP with tracheal suctioning. A significant effect of lidocaine, fentanyl, thiopental, or succinylcholine in abating the ICP increase with suctioning was not demonstrated, with the exception of intravenous lidocaine (1.5 mg/kg) in patients receiving concurrent pentobarbital therapy. Studies by Yano and colleagues[8] and White and coworkers[9] on patients with head injuries who had baseline elevations of ICP suggest that the cough reflex is the predominant cause of ICP rise with suctioning in the unanesthetized and unparalyzed patient. Cautious spraying of the trachea with lidocaine before suctioning[8, 9] or temporary paralyzation[9] may be helpful in the patient with a severe head injury. Using appropriate technique and vacuum settings should further minimize tracheal irritation during suctioning. However, for most patients, routine pretreatment with drugs to prevent transient ICP increases cannot be recommended at this time.

Tracheal mucosal injury is a frequent complication of tracheal suctioning. Some degree of irritation accompanies even properly performed suctioning, but it can be minimized. Catheters of soft polyvinylchloride should be chosen, and appropriate suction settings should be used. Suctioning should be performed no more frequently than indicated, because mucosal damage occurs more often in the absence of secretions. Tracheitis may occur as the result of frequent or improperly performed suctioning; it can be recognized by a persistent hacking cough and blood-streaked secretions. Tracheitis may be treated by instillation of 1 ml of 1 per cent lidocaine every 2 to 4 hours as needed and by reducing the frequency of endotracheal suctioning.[3]

Atelectasis has been reported as a complication of suctioning and is thought to be related to the diameter of the suctioning catheter, the suction setting, and the duration of suctioning. Atelectasis can best be avoided by proper selection and use of materials for suctioning and can be treated by postprocedural hyperinflation, as described. Prevention and prompt treatment of atelectasis will reduce the chances of suction-induced hypoxemia.

Bronchoconstriction may result from mechanical airway irritation. Cessation of the procedure, positive-pressure ventilation, and bronchodilators as needed should allow a resolution of this complication.

Sudden death has been reported during tracheal suctioning and is probably due to one or more of the complications discussed earlier. For this reason, provisions for cardiopulmonary resuscitation and resuscitative drugs should always be close at hand before the procedure is begun.

INTERPRETATION

Successful tracheal suctioning is evidenced by clearing of rhonchi or rales, relief of dyspnea, improvement of oxygenation (when monitored), and removal of visible secretions. The procedure should be repeated only if indications remain.

The analysis of respiratory secretions obtained by tracheal suctioning is discussed briefly at the end of this chapter and in more detail in the chapters in Section 11, "Microbiologic Procedures."

NASOTRACHEAL SUCTIONING

Nasotracheal suctioning is an infrequently used procedure that is technically more difficult to perform than suctioning through an endotracheal tube and potentially more hazardous.[1–3] Nasotracheal suctioning is reserved for patients who require assistance in clearing secretions due to partial airway obstruction, impaired cough reflex, or excess secretions. Many would argue correctly that these are sufficient indications for endotracheal intubation. However, rare instances may occur in which nonintubated patients require tracheal suctioning. An example is the patient with chronic emphysema who refuses intubation but whose cough is insufficient to clear the excess secretions produced by an intercurrent bacterial bronchitis.

The indications and contraindications for nasotracheal suctioning are the same as those discussed previously for endotracheal suctioning. Secretions may be visualized in the oropharynx rather than in the endotracheal tube. Materials are the same, with the addition of a water-soluble lubricant for easier passage of the catheter through the nose. Airflow sounds are heard through the unattached proximal catheter opening when the distal tip approaches the glottis. Gentle, rapid advancement during inspiration should allow the tip to pass into the trachea. Successful tracheal placement is signified by a vigorous cough and the inability of the patient to phonate much above a whisper. If the catheter instead enters the esophagus or valleculae, airflow sounds are lost, no cough is produced, and the gag reflex may be stimulated. After successful tracheal placement, reoxygenate the patient by allowing several deep breaths of 100 per cent oxygen before suctioning. Then attach the catheter to the suction source at the appropriate setting, advance the tip to about the level of the carina, and occlude the suction port and suction as discussed earlier, taking care to ensure reoxygenation following the procedure.

All of the complications discussed for endotracheal tube suctioning can occur during nasotracheal suctioning. In addition, nosebleeds, gagging, aspiration, and laryngospasm may occur, or the operator may simply be unable to direct the catheter tip into the trachea. Because of these drawbacks, nasotracheal suctioning is seldom the procedure of choice for clearance of airway secretions, nor is it an ideal method for obtaining specimens for microbiologic study, because contamination by nasopharyngeal flora is inevitable.

CONCLUSION

Tracheal suctioning is an important adjunct to bronchopulmonary toilet in patients whose cough reflex is impaired, whether by an endotracheal tube or otherwise. Although easily taught, the procedure is not without the potential for serious morbidity or even mortality. Tracheal suctioning should be undertaken only when indications exist and should be performed by trained individuals with a full appreciation of its potential complications.

Transtracheal Needle Aspiration

INTRODUCTION

Patients with signs and symptoms of acute bronchopulmonary infection require expeditious diagnosis and treatment. Examination and culture of lower respiratory tract secretions are desirable in these patients and are mandatory in those who are critically ill. Although expectorated sputum is always contaminated somewhat with oropharyngeal flora, properly screened expectorated sputum is a sufficient specimen in most cases. Occasionally, results of sputum examination and culture are equivocal or an adequate specimen simply cannot be obtained. In selected cases, the emergency physician may wish to use the technique of transtracheal aspiration to obtain a specimen of tracheobronchial secretions before initiation of antibiotic treatment.

Since the introduction of antibiotics, examination of the Gram stain and culture of expectorated sputum has been a safe and simple method of identifying pathogens in lower respiratory tract infections. In patients who are unable to generate a sputum specimen, tracheal suctioning has been used to collect tracheobronchial secretions. Tracheal suctioning may be performed via a catheter through the nose or through an artifical airway, as well as via a bronchoscope. Specimens obtained by the aforementioned methods are subject to contamination by oropharyngeal or skin flora, which can mean that culture results will be inaccurate. Pecora and Yegian[10] found a poor correlation between cultures of expectorated sputum and those of lower respiratory tract secretions obtained by open lung biopsy. Recognizing the need for uncontaminated culture specimens, Pecora[11] introduced transtracheal needle aspiration, a modification of the technique commonly used for translaryngeal anesthesia.

Cultures of lower respiratory tract secretions obtained by transtracheal needle aspiration are more predictive of pulmonary infection than are those obtained from expectorated washed sputa[12] or bronchoscopic aspirates.[13, 14] Bartlett[15] found that in a series of 488 patients, cultures of transtracheal aspirates agreed 100 per cent with blood cultures from those patients with bacteremic pneumonias. In that same series, the overall diagnostic accuracy of transtracheal aspirate bacteriologic studies was greater than 90 per cent, with 1 per cent false-negative and 21 per cent false-positive incidences. (False-positive results usually reflected an exacerbation of chronic bronchitis.) Transtracheal aspiration specimens have been shown to be especially useful in the diagnosis of unusual pulmonary infections, including those caused by anaerobic bacteria,[16] tuberculosis bacilli,[17] *Aspergillus*,[18] and *Pneumocystis carinii*.[18] The technique has also been suggested as an aid to bacteriologic diagnosis in hospital-acquired and partially treated pneumonias.[19]

INDICATIONS

Failure to obtain adequate expectorated sputum is the primary reason for performing transtracheal needle aspiration. Many patients with pneumonia are obtunded and are unable to produce a coughed sputum specimen. Several investigators have suggested that expectorated sputum containing less than 25 squamous epithelial cells per $100\times$ microscopic field and greater than 25 leukocytes per $100\times$ field generally is representative of lower respiratory tract secretions.[12] These criteria can be checked by quick microscopic screening of a coughed sputum sample. Furthermore, when no predominant organism is found or when multiple organisms are seen on the Gram stain of the screened sputum, transtracheal aspiration should be considered (see also Chapter 88).

Patients with complicated or unusual pulmonary infections may benefit from transtracheal aspiration. This is especially true in anaerobic infections. When putrid sputum or necrotizing roentgenographic lesions suggest anaerobic pneumonia or abscess, secretions obtained by transtracheal aspiration are *preferred* over those obtained by expectoration, because contamination of a sputum specimen by oral anaerobic flora may alter the results of anaerobic cultures.

In addition, transtracheal aspiration has been shown to be useful in obtaining specimens of fastidious organisms, such as *Aspergillus, Pneumocystis carinii, Nocardia,* and tubercle bacilli.[20] Patients with hospital-acquired pneumonia or with partially treated but poorly responding infections may also benefit from transtracheal aspiration performed to establish the correct pathogen.

CONTRAINDICATIONS

Absolute contraindications involve patient safety. Uncooperative patients are most likely to suffer tracheal damage and bleeding. Patients with bleeding diatheses should not be considered for the procedure.

A bleeding diathesis is suggested by documentation of a prothrombin time greater than twice normal, a platelet count less than 100,000, or a prolonged bleeding time.[21] Hypoxia may predispose patients to potentially dangerous cardiac dysrhythmias. Supplemental oxygen should be administered, and an arterial P_{O_2} of greater than 70 mm Hg should be documented before beginning the procedure.[21] In addition, the inability to identify the proper anatomic landmarks for cricothyroid puncture should preclude use of this technique.

A relative contraindication to the use of transtracheal needle aspiration is the presence of chronic respiratory disease. The transtracheal aspirate from the patient with chronic bronchitis may yield false-positive culture results. A severe paroxysmal cough increases the likelihood of subsequent subcutaneous emphysema and hence is also a relative contraindication.

Finally, transtracheal aspiration should never be used when an adequate expectorated sputum specimen can be obtained and is suitable for proper diagnosis.

EQUIPMENT

The equipment needed for transtracheal needle aspiration is minimal and is usually readily available. Material for sterile preparation of the neck includes gloves, drapes, and a povidone-iodine or isopropyl alcohol solution. One per cent or 2 per cent lidocaine (with or without epinephrine) and a syringe for administration of local anesthetic should be available. Commercially available intravenous catheter sets consisting of either a 14- or a 16-gauge needle with a 6- to 8-inch through-the-needle polyethylene catheter are commonly used. A large (10 to 50 ml) syringe should be used to collect the sample. Two to 5 ml of *nonbacteriostatic* normal saline in a syringe should be available. Cardiac monitoring is desirable, and resuscitative drugs should be available.

PROCEDURE

Transtracheal needle aspiration can be performed safely when precautions are taken. The patient or family should be counseled regarding the procedure, and informed consent should be obtained. The patient's ability to suppress a cough on command should be assessed, because coughing while the needle is being inserted may result in tracheal laceration. Supplemental oxygen should be applied well in advance of the procedure (e.g., 100 per cent O_2 for 5 minutes).

When time permits, results of clotting studies and an arterial blood gas or transcutaneous oximeter reading should be obtained and confirmed to be within the acceptable limits discussed previously. An intravenous line and cardiac monitor are desirable, should dysrhythmias requiring treatment occur. Premedication with atropine, 0.4 mg intramuscularly, 20 to 30 minutes before the procedure may minimize the incidence of bradycardia.

The patient is positioned as shown in Figure 7–1A, with a pillow or rolled towel between the shoulder blades to allow full extension of the neck. The neck is sterilized and draped. The operator then palpates the cricothyroid membrane, and a small intradermal wheal is raised with local anesthetic directly over the membrane (Fig. 7–1B).

Next, the 14- or 16-gauge needle is introduced in the midline through the lower portion of the cricothyroid membrane while the larynx is stabilized (with the application of bilateral support) by the operator or an assistant. The tip of the needle should be angulated approximately 45 degrees caudad to avoid injury to laryngeal structures. A "pop" or a sudden give will be felt as the needle enters the tracheal lumen, and air will be aspirated easily into a syringe attached to the needle. As soon as tracheal entry is confirmed, the needle should be advanced *only a few millimeters* to ensure that the entire needle tip is within the lumen. The needle should then be stabilized and advanced *no further* (to avoid injury to the posterior tracheal wall or adjacent structures).

The polyethylene catheter is then inserted quickly through the needle to its full length, and the needle tip is immediately withdrawn through the skin surface. A vigorous cough will almost always be produced when the catheter is introduced, so the needle should be withdrawn as soon as possible to minimize the chance of laryngeal injury. Once inserted, *the catheter must never be withdrawn through the needle*—catheter fragments are easily sheared off by the needle bevel and may become lodged in the trachea. Alternatively, over-the-needle catheter systems can be used. These catheters are generally less desirable because of their limited length.

As soon as the catheter is in place, a 10- to 50-ml syringe

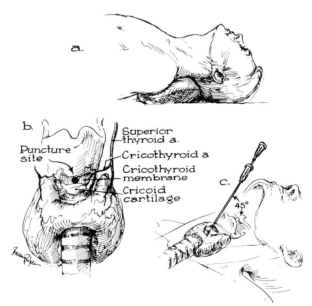

Figure 7–1. Transtracheal aspiration: *a,* position of patient; *b,* anatomic landmarks; *c,* technique of puncture. The Intracath needle is inserted just above the cricoid cartilage through the cricothyroid membrane with its bevel up at a 45-degree angle to the skin. (From Eknoyen G: Medical Procedures Manual. Chicago, Year Book Medical Publishers, 1981. Reproduced by permission.)

is attached to the catheter hub, and suction is applied. Usually, it is easy to obtain a specimen of secretions. Enough fluid to fill the catheter hub is sufficient for analysis.

If a specimen is not forthcoming, 2 to 5 ml of sterile, nonbacteriostatic saline may be injected rapidly through the catheter; suction should be reapplied immediately. Saline will dilute the sample, however, and may decrease the yield of positive cultures. In addition, small volumes of saline may temporarily depress arterial oxygen tension.

As soon as a suitable amount of sample is obtained, the catheter is withdrawn and direct pressure is applied to the puncture site. The patient is instructed to avoid coughing as much as possible in the next 24 hours and should not receive intermittent positive-pressure breathing (IPPB) treatments or other forms of therapy that stimulate coughing during this period.

Proper handling and screening of the aspirate is essential. The catheter and syringe assembly should be transported promptly to the bacteriology laboratory for processing. A smear for Gram stain is made, and cultures are plated as soon as possible, including anaerobic cultures. One may inspect the Gram stain under 100× dry magnification to ascertain that the specimen meets criteria for lower respiratory tract secretions (less than 25 squamous epithelial cells; more than 25 leukocytes per field).[22] Oil immersion magnification should reveal a predominant organism in bacterial infections (see Section XIII, "Microbiologic Procedures"). Antibiotic therapy may be started immediately, based on organism morphology, epidemiology, and roentgenographic appearance of the infiltrate(s). Subsequent culture results should confirm the diagnosis and, as mentioned, are highly accurate when specimens are obtained by transtracheal aspiration.

COMPLICATIONS

When proper precautions are taken and patients are selected appropriately, the complication rate of transtracheal needle aspiration is very low. The overall mortality in more than 1500 cases reviewed is less than 0.1 per cent. Complications are discussed from most to least common.

Subcutaneous emphysema may be observed in up to 20 per cent of patients. It is usually confined to the anterior neck and is self-limiting without specific treatment. One may minimize the incidence of subcutaneous emphysema following transtracheal aspiration by instructing the patient to avoid strenuous coughing, by forgoing (for 24 hours) IPPB and other treatments that stimulate coughing, and by avoiding positive-pressure ventilation when possible. Mediastinal emphysema is very rare and is likewise self-limited.

Some minimal hemoptysis may occur for 1 to 2 minutes following the procedure, but sustained hemoptysis is rare (1 to 2 per cent of cases). Careful assessment of the patient's coagulation studies and caution in needle placement (with prompt needle withdrawal as soon as the catheter is placed) will minimize the risk of injury to the cricothyroid arteries. Digital pressure over the cricothyroid puncture site for 5 minutes will prevent prolonged intratracheal or paratracheal hemorrhage in most instances. Persistent intratracheal hemorrhage has caused death from asphyxia in at least one case.[23] Prompt recognition of intratracheal hemorrhage, placement of a cuffed endotracheal tube, and correction of any coagulopathies will prevent aspiration and serious complications.

Cardiac dysrhythmias are probably secondary to vagal stimulation during tracheal suctioning and occur with an unknown frequency. Cardiac monitoring is recommended. Hypoxia most certainly enhances dysrhythmias and is easily

prevented by administration of supplemental oxygen and monitoring of the arterial P_{O_2} by pulse oximetry. One case of bronchospasm, bradycardia, and hypercarbia that developed during transtracheal needle aspiration and resulted in myocardial ischemia has been reported.[24] Premedication with atropine as described should offer some protection against vagally mediated bradycardia. Atropine as well as other cardioresuscitative drugs and equipment should be immediately available during the procedure.[25]

Anterior cervical infections following transtracheal aspiration have been reported (0.4 to 0.8 per cent of cases).[20] The pathogen is usually the same as that isolated from the transtracheal aspirate. Treatment consists of appropriate antibiotic therapy and incision and drainage of abscesses. Mediastinitis from inadvertent esophageal puncture has not been reported.

Catheter fragments may be sheared free when the catheter of a through-the-needle catheter system is withdrawn without concurrent needle removal. Fragments can be located radiographically and removed by bronchoscopy. Other rare complications, such as pneumothorax, are treated by observation or tube thoracostomy as indicated.

INTERPRETATION

When properly obtained, screened, and processed, cultures of transtracheal aspirate are highly predictive of the pathogen responsible for pulmonary infection. Careful screening by Gram stain minimizes the likelihood of oral contaminants and gives preliminary information as to the identity of the pathogen.[22]

Gram-stained slides of aspirated material that contain fewer than 25 squamous epithelial cells and more than 25 leukocytes per 100× field may be considered to represent lower respiratory tract specimens (approximately 66 per cent accuracy).[12] Antibiotic treatment may be instituted immediately, based on the morphology of stained organisms and the patient's history, clinical presentation, and roentgenographic and laboratory tests. Special staining, as for acid-fast bacilli, should be done when clinically indicated.

Specimens containing more than 25 squamous epithelial cells per 100× field should be considered to be contaminated by oral secretions. In these instances, repeat transtracheal aspiration may be attempted, or the physician may proceed with treatment with the understanding that the culture of such material is likely to contain oral flora, which may obscure or suppress growth of the actual pathogen.[12]

The accuracy of culture results from properly handled specimens is very high in most studies. Bartlett[15] found an incidence of 1 per cent false-negative and 21 per cent false-positive cultures in 488 samples obtained by transtracheal aspiration. A negative culture was found to indicate an alternative diagnosis in 60 per cent of cases and a suppression of growth by prior antibiotic treatment in 37 per cent of cases. Of the false-positive cultures, 25 per cent were considered to reflect exacerbated chronic bronchitis, whereas 75 per cent of the false-positive cultures were presumed to be caused by oral flora contamination. When correctly processed, materials from transtracheal aspiration are highly predictive even of fastidious pathogens or unusual infections, including anaerobic pulmonary infections.[16, 17] However, Berger and Arango[26] found poor correlation between cultures and secretions obtained by endotracheal suction or by transtracheal aspiration with presumed true pathogens in 19 patients with *nosocomial* pneumonias.

CONCLUSION

In the infrequent instances in which tracheobronchial secretions are not obtainable from expectorated sputum and accurate bacteriologic diagnosis is essential to care of the patient with suspected pulmonary infection, transtracheal needle aspiration is a safe, practical method for obtaining such a sample. When one adheres to the precautions and guidelines presented herein, the procedure has low morbidity, high yield, and high diagnostic accuracy.

REFERENCES

1. Imle PC, Klemic N: Methods of airway clearance: Coughing and suctioning. In Mackenzie CF (ed): Chest Physiotherapy in the Intensive Care Unit. Baltimore, Williams & Wilkins, 1981, pp 91–107.
2. Wilkins RL: Suctioning and airway care. In Kacmarek RM, Stoller JK (eds): Current Respiratory Care. Toronto, Canada, BC Decker, 1988, pp 90–95.
3. Caldwell SL, Sullivan KN: Artificial airway care techniques. Suctioning protocol. In Burton SG, Hodgkin JE (eds): Respiratory Care; A Guide to Clinical Practice. 2nd ed. Philadelphia, JB Lippincott, 1984, pp 513–520, 1028–1029.
4. Baun MM: Physiological determinants of a clinically successful method of endotracheal suction. West J Nurs Res 6:213, 1984.
5. Barnes CA, Kirchoff KT: Minimizing hypoxemia due to endotracheal suctioning: A review of the literature. Heart Lung 15:164, 1986.
5a. Allen RP, Siefkin AD: Emergency airway clot removal in acute hemorrhagic respiratory failure. Crit Care Med 15:985, 1987.
5b. Lieman BC, Hall ID, Stanley TH: Extirpation of endotracheal tube secretions with a Fogarty arterial embolectomy catheter. Anesthesiology 62:847, 1985.
6. Shim C, Fine N, Fernandez R, Williams MH: Cardiac arrhythmias resulting from tracheal suctioning. Ann Int Med 71:1149, 1969.
7. Rudy EB, Baun MM, Stone K, Turner B: The relationship between endotracheal suctioning and changes in intracranial pressure: A review of the literature. Heart Lung 15:488, 1986.
8. Yano M, Nishiyama H, Yokota H, et al: Effect of lidocaine on ICP response to endotracheal suctioning. Anesthesiology 64:651, 1986.
9. White PF, Schlobohm RM, Pitts LH, Lindauer JM: A randomized study of drugs for preventing increases in intracranial pressure during endotracheal suctioning. Anesthesiology 57:242, 1982.
10. Pecora DV, Yegian D: Bacteriology of the lower respiratory tract in health and chronic diseases. N Engl J Med 258:71, 1958.
11. Pecora DV: A method of securing uncontaminated tracheal secretions for bacterial examination. J Thorac Surg 37:653, 1959.
12. Geckler RW, Gremillion DH, AcAllister CK, Ellenbogen C: Microscopic and bacteriologic comparison of paired sputa and transtracheal aspirates. J Clin Microbiol 6:396, 1977.
13. Jordon GW, Wong GA, Hoeprich PD: Bacteriology of the lower respiratory tract as determined by fiberoptic bronchoscopy and transtracheal aspiration. J Infect Dis 134:428, 1976.
14. Pecora DV: A comparison of transtracheal aspiration with other methods of determining the bacterial flora of the lower respiratory tract. N Engl J Med 269:664, 1963.
15. Bartlett JG: Diagnostic accuracy of transtracheal aspiration bacteriologic studies. Am Rev Respir Dis 115:777, 1977.
16. Bartlett JG, Rosenblatt JE, Finegold SM: Percutaneous transtracheal aspiration in the diagnosis of anaerobic pulmonary infection. Ann Intern Med 79:535, 1973.
17. Schouteus E, Dekoster JP, Vereerstraeten J, et al: Use of transtracheal aspiration in the bacteriological diagnosis of bronchopulmonary infection. Biomedicine 19:160, 1973.
18. Lau WK, Young LS, Remington JS: *Pneumocystis carinii* pneumonia: Diagnosis by examination of pulmonary secretions. JAMA 236:2399, 1976.
19. Jay SJ, Stonehill RD (eds): Manual of Pulmonary Procedures. Philadelphia, WB Saunders Co, 1980, pp 170–179.
20. Eknoyan G: Medical Procedures Manual. Chicago, Year Book Medical Publishers, 1981.
21. Pratter MR, Irwin RS: Transtracheal aspiration, guidelines for safety. Chest 76:518, 1979.
22. Joyce SM: Sputum analysis and culture. Ann Emerg Med 15(3):325, 1986.
23. Schillaci RR, Iacovoni VE, Conte RS: Transtracheal aspiration complicated by fatal endotracheal hemorrhage. N Engl J Med 295:488, 1976.
24. Pitts JC, Brantigan COK, Hoperman AR: Myocardial ischemia associated with transtracheal aspiration. JAMA, 237:2527, 1977.
25. Shim C, Fine N, Fernandez R, et al: Cardiac arrhythmias resulting from tracheal suctioning. Ann Intern Med 71:1149, 1969.
26. Berger R, Arango L: Etiologic diagnosis of bacterial nosocomial pneumonia in seriously ill patients. Crit Care Med 13:833, 1985.

Chapter **8**

Thoracentesis

David S. Ross

INTRODUCTION

The term *thoracentesis* is derived from the Greek *thorakos* (chest) and *kentesis* (to pierce). Although a broad definition could include the introduction of any object into the chest, including thoracostomy tubes, common usage is confined to the temporary insertion of a needle or small catheter into the pleural space. Traditionally, thoracentesis is considered to be the method of removing a pleural effusion for diagnostic or therapeutic purposes. In the emergency situation, the removal of air from the pleural space (e.g., from a tension pneumothorax) may also be referred to as thoracentesis. In this chapter, both aspects are discussed. (Tube thoracostomy and the use of catheter drainage for longer periods of time are discussed in Chapter 9.)

Thoracentesis may be performed whenever the appropriate indications are present and suitable equipment is available. Because a tension pneumothorax may quickly cause death, all physicians should be familiar with its clinical appearance and the appropriate indications and techniques for relief of this life-threatening complication. In many communities, paramedical and nursing personnel are also trained in needle or catheter thoracentesis for treatment of tension pneumothorax. Removal of pleural fluid by thoracentesis may be performed by any physician experienced with its indications, precautions, and techniques. It may be performed in the emergency department or on medical and surgical floors.

The pleural space is a potential space between the visceral and parietal pleura that contains a thin physiologic layer of pleural fluid. With normal inspiration, a negative pressure is developed within the thorax and is transmitted through the pleural space to the pulmonary parenchyma, allowing a normal influx of air. During normal expiration, the elasticity of the pulmonary parenchyma and chest wall allows exhalation.

If fluid, blood, or air accumulates in the pleural space, normal ventilatory mechanisms may be affected. If the volume of fluid or air is large, respiratory compromise may be the result. If the accumulation is rapid and progressive (e.g., tension pneumothorax), there may be cardiovascular compromise in addition to severe respiratory effects. The underlying etiology of an effusion will also affect the severity of symptoms.

BACKGROUND

Thoracentesis (originally called *paracentesis thoracis*) was first described by Hippocrates for relief of empyema.[1] Various operative approaches using trocars or open drainage were advocated during the ensuing centuries. Professional wound suckers who assisted with drainage were replaced by the aspiration syringe, described in 1674. Anel reported the first successful evacuation of a pneumothorax in 1707.[2] Laennec used thoracentesis for the relief of an apparent pneumomediastinum with a possible associated tension pneumothorax.[3]

In the nineteenth century, more interest developed in thoracentesis. Boerhaave advocated the use of a flexible tube for evacuation of a hemothorax.[2] Bowditch provided the first description of thoracentesis in the American literature in 1851.[4] Hunter adapted the newly developed hypodermic needle into a modern instrument for thoracentesis in 1859. An underwater seal was later designed by Playfair.[2] Hewett described continuous pleural drainage for empyema in 1876.[5]

Antiseptics and improved sterile technique enabled widespread successful use of thoracentesis in the twentieth century. In World War II, thoracentesis and chest drainage replaced routine thoracotomy for most chest injuries, and during the Korean conflict, repeated thoracentesis was advocated for penetrating chest wounds.[3, 6] At the time of the war in Vietnam, the improvement in thoracostomy tubes made them more effective, and tube thoracostomy came to be preferred to simple or repeated thoracentesis.[7]

INDICATIONS

In the emergency setting, thoracentesis is most often indicated as a life-saving intervention in cases of suspected tension pneumothorax. It is usually done as a temporizing measure before thoracostomy tube placement. Occasionally, a pleural effusion may require emergency evacuation for therapeutic reasons in the compromised patient. More often, thoracentesis will be done semielectively for diagnostic purposes. Thoracentesis has also been performed for evacuation of a small, stable pneumothorax.

There are two general approaches to performing thoracentesis. The anterior approach is most often recommended for removal of air. The posterior approach is chosen most commonly for removal of pleural fluid. Each is discussed separately with further detail regarding clinical indications. The current indications for each approach are summarized in Table 8–1.

Anterior Approach for Evacuation of Air

STABLE PNEUMOTHORAX

Etiology. Pneumothorax is defined as air within the pleural space. It usually enters from a rent in the airway but may also enter through the chest wall or from a perforated hollow viscus. Many pneumothoraces occur spontaneously in patients predisposed by the presence of such conditions as chronic obstructive lung disease, asthma, aspiration pneumonia, or malignancy. Others occur without evidence of preexisting lung disease. These idiopathic spontaneous pneumothoraces typically occur in young tall males and may be recurrent.[8, 9] They occur more frequently in smokers.[10] Catamenial pneumothorax may occur in women at the time of menses but is rare.[11] Bilateral spontaneous pneumothoraces have been reported.[12] In the emergency department, most pneumothoraces occur secondary to trauma, either blunt or penetrating, and may be associated with a hemothorax. Pneumothorax may also occur iatrogenically secondary to central venous catheterization; cardiopulmonary resuscitation; intubation; mechanical ventilation; positive end-expiratory pressure (PEEP); and any needle insertion into the chest wall, such as thoracentesis, electromyography, and breast or node biopsy.[13–17] Drug abusers may induce a

Table 8–1. Indications for Thoracentesis

Evacuation of Air: Anterior Approach
Emergency diagnosis and treatment of suspected tension
    pneumothorax (temporary treatment before tube
    thoracostomy)
Evacuation of simple stable pneumothorax

Evacuation of Fluid: Posterior Approach
Diagnostic analysis of pleural effusion
Acute treatment of large symptomatic pleural effusion and
    tension hydrothorax

pneumothorax from "pocket shooting" drugs into the internal jugular veins as well as from a Valsalva maneuver performed to enhance a "high" while smoking marijuana or cocaine.[18, 19]

Diagnosis. Patients with a pneumothorax typically experience dyspnea and pleuritic pain that is localized to the involved hemithorax. Cough may also be present. Symptoms vary greatly depending on the size of the pneumothorax and its etiology, as well as any underlying lung disease. Physical findings also vary and may include tachypnea, tachycardia, diminished breath sounds, and increased hyperresonance to percussion.[9] Subcutaneous emphysema may occur. Increased resonance to percussion of the ipsilateral clavicle has been reported.[20]

Radiographic diagnosis of a pneumothorax is made by noting the presence of a visceral pleural line and the absence of pulmonary markings peripheral to that line. An upright expiratory chest film or a lateral decubitus view with the involved side up may enhance the visibility of a small pneumothorax. In the absence of pleural adhesions, the pleural air is free flowing, so a pneumothorax will assume the apical-lateral position on an upright chest radiograph. Pneumothorax must be differentiated from bullae in patients with chronic obstructive pulmonary disease.[8]

In the supine patient, a small pneumothorax may collect in several recesses. The most common is an anteromedial collection in which a radiolucent band is seen parallel to and enhancing the heart border. Another common location is subpulmonic, in which a radiolucent band is seen superior and parallel to the diaphragm, outlined by the visceral pleura.[21, 22] Other locations include the costophrenic sulcus and the posteromedial recess. In the former, the sulcus appears deepened, often with an oblique radiolucent band projected across the upper abdomen. In the latter, retrocardiac air is seen outlining a collapsed lower lobe and adjacent structures. Other signs of pneumothorax on the supine chest film include hyperlucency of the hemithorax, depressed diaphragm, double diaphragmatic contour, increased delineation along with the inferior cardiac border, and visualization of lobulated pericardial fat at the cardiac apex.[21]

Any of these small pneumothoraces may proceed to a tension pneumothorax.[22] Several additional views may help with their diagnosis, including cross-table lateral, abdominal, and oblique views of the chest. If the patient can be repositioned, the free pleural air will rise, as can be demonstrated on a semirecumbent, upright, or lateral decubitus film. Computed tomography (CT) of the abdomen may demonstrate the pneumothorax.[23] Some suggest performing a limited CT of the lower chest of the major trauma patient, particularly when the patient is having a CT for evaluation of other trauma.[24]

The size of a pneumothorax is often underestimated because volume is a cubic measurement and not always appreciated by viewing its linear dimensions. An accurate nomogram (see Chapter 9) has been designed for determining pneumothorax size.[25] However, in the emergency department, from a practical standpoint, categorization of pneumothorax size may be adequate. Pneumothoraces may be functionally categorized as small (marginal), moderate, and large (massive).[26]

Treatment. The usual treatment for a pneumothorax is tube thoracostomy, as discussed in Chapter 9. Conservative management has been advocated in selected cases.[27] Stable spontaneous pneumothoraces (less than 20 per cent) are commonly absorbed gradually at the rate of 1.25 per cent daily.[28] This absorption will be enhanced by the administration of oxygen. Small or marginal, stable spontaneous pneumothoraces may be observed for resolution,[8] although some advocate thoracentesis to hasten the resorption and increase patient comfort.[29] In a Detroit study, patients with simple pneumothoraces of varying sizes were treated successfully with catheter aspiration, followed by a 6-hour observation period, and then were discharged from the emergency department successfully in 76 per cent of cases.[30] Similar catheter aspiration and outpatient management proved successful in self-inflicted pneumothoraces among "pocket shooters".[18] Small pigtail catheters and small-bore thoracostomy tubes have also been used successfully to treat pneumothoraces, with the use of the Seldinger (guide wire) technique.[31–34] (For further discussion of the Seldinger technique for vascular access see Chapter 23.)

TENSION PNEUMOTHORAX

Mechanism. A tension pneumothorax is marked by the progressive collection of air in the pleural space through a rent in the airway, with subsequent increasing pleural pressures and often a shift of the mediastinum away from the side of the pneumothorax. During inspiration, negative intrapleural pressure facilitates flow into the pleural space. During expiration, air is less able to exit the pleural space in the patient with a tension pneumothorax, because there is a relative compression of the bronchioli and alveoli and subsequent collapse of the rent in the airway owing to positive intrathoracic pressure. This creates a one-way valve mechanism, which favors collection and trapping of additional air in the pleural space.

As the volume of intrapleural air continues to expand, the intrapleural pressure rises. This pressure is transmitted against the lungs, causing a continued decrease in functioning lung volume. First the ipsilateral and then the contralateral lung become compressed. Resultant parenchymal collapse leads to respiratory compromise as ventilation-perfusion mismatching develops and hypoxia and acidosis ensue. In addition, the increase in the volume of the intrapleural air causes a shift of the mediastinum away from the side of the tension pneumothorax. There may be some decrease in the systemic venous return because of a combination of increased intrathoracic pressure and mechanical collapse of the vena cavae. Originally, it was felt that compromised venous return was the primary cause of diminished cardiac output that led to cardiovascular collapse. Animal studies, however, suggest that progressive hypoxia and CO_2 retention may be the primary mediators of cardiovascular depression and collapse.[35, 36] The rapidity with which these events occur is variable. They can proceed quickly and lead to death in a matter of minutes. Therapeutic intervention may often be necessary before full diagnostic evaluation can be carried out.

Etiology. A tension pneumothorax may develop as a result of any of the usual causes of pneumothorax described earlier (see also Chapter 9). It may develop either primarily as a complication of a previously stable pneumothorax or as a result of positive-pressure ventilation. Although occasionally occurring in the patient with spontaneous pneumothorax, it is seen more often in patients following trauma and may occur following instrumentation of the chest, such as during central line insertion. It has been reported following incorrect placement of a nasogastric tube in an elderly patient.[37] Certain factors may predispose to the development of a tension pneumothorax in a patient with an otherwise stable pneumothorax. A major predisposing factor is the use of positive-pressure ventilation, either by bag-valve devices or by mechanical ventilators.[38] The addition of PEEP may further increase the risk of developing a tension pneumothorax.[39] Likewise, cardiopulmonary resuscitation may predispose to the development of a tension pneumothorax.[8]

Clinical Diagnosis. Tension pneumothorax should always be suspected in any patient when there is sudden respiratory or cardiac deterioration. Development of sudden difficulty ventilating a patient should alert the clinician to the possibility of tension pneumothorax.[8] The clinical presentation in the patient who is awake includes the sudden development of dyspnea, agitation, or diminished consciousness. Tachypnea, tachycardia, hypotension, cyanosis, and diaphoresis may be present and may progress to cardiac or respiratory arrest. The following classic constellation of findings may be seen, although they are not necessarily uniformly present. These include tympany to percussion, decreased breath sounds over the involved hemithorax, tracheal deviation toward the contralateral side, and the presence of an overinflated, immobile, ipsilateral hemithorax. Jugular venous distention may also be seen. Other signs of chest trauma or respiratory distress should prompt one to consider the possibility of an underlying pneumothorax with potential tension.

In the patient who suddenly deteriorates, other diagnostic considerations should include massive pulmonary embolus, pericardial tamponade, pneumomediastinum, respiratory failure from reactive airway disease, and myocardial infarction. Traumatic diaphragmatic hernia has also been reported to simulate a tension pneumothorax.[40] The patient with a tension pneumothorax who is being ventilated mechanically will show signs of increased airway resistance, evidenced by increased ventilatory pressures, prolonged inspiratory times, elevated central venous pressure, and elevated pulmonary artery pressure.[39]

When the patient is in extremis, the diagnosis should be made by needle or catheter thoracentesis. The patient will show clinical improvement following thoracentesis. The successful relief of a tension pneumothorax is also marked by the rapid efflux of air through the thoracentesis needle during both inspiration and expiration. If a syringe (ideally premoistened) is attached to the thoracentesis needle, the plunger may be driven outward if sufficient pressure has developed. Likewise any drainage apparatus that directs the efflux of air through a water seal will reveal vigorous bubbling of air in inspiration as well as expiration until the high-pressure air has been released. In a similar manner, a flutter-valve apparatus attached to the needle may continue to show evidence of massive air efflux. If an intubated patient is being ventilated, *diagnostic tube thoracostomy is preferred* to thoracentesis when time permits. There is a theoretic risk of creating a tension pneumothorax by indiscriminate thoracentesis in a patient who is receiving positive-pressure ventilation.

Radiologic Diagnosis. Withholding treatment of a tension pneumothorax until radiographic confirmation is made is not advised except in the following circumstances: patients who are stable with only moderate respiratory compromise; patients in whom tension pneumothorax is suspected but physical evidence is lacking; patients in whom other likely conditions are being considered such as a ruptured diaphragm, in which needle decompression may be relatively contraindicated; and patients in whom portable chest radiographs may be completed immediately.

A patient who has even the most remote possibility of a tension pneumothorax should *never be sent to the radiology suite unless accompanied by a physician* who is prepared to perform immediate thoracentesis or tube thoracostomy. Despite an increased awareness of the possibility of a tension pneumothorax on clinical grounds, the diagnosis is often not recognized until a chest film has been taken.[41]

Radiographic diagnosis is made by noting the presence of the usual signs of pneumothorax described previously, combined with a flattening of the diaphragm and a shift of the mediastinum away from the side of the pneumothorax.[8]

In most cases, even in the supine patient, tension pneumothorax is easily diagnosed. Several exceptions exist. In the case of bilateral pneumothoraces, no mediastinal shift may be seen. In these cases, tension pneumothorax may be diagnosed clinically on decompression of the chest. Localized areas of tension pneumothorax may occur secondary to adhesions. In patients with adult respiratory distress syndrome (ARDS) on PEEP, localized subpulmonic or paracardiac tension pneumothoraces have been reported despite the presence of thoracostomy tubes.[42] These cases will be suspected clinically because of the presence of increased respiratory pressures and diagnostic criteria for localized pneumothorax discussed earlier, with flattening of the cardiac border and a depression or contour change of the diaphragm.

Treatment. Treatment of a tension pneumothorax should begin as soon as it is recognized clinically. It should be emphasized that although *the preferred and definitive treatment of a tension pneumothorax is immediate tube thoracostomy,*[43] this may not be possible in many clinical settings. If a patient deteriorates suddenly and rapid tube thoracostomy is not possible immediately, thoracentesis is an appropriate temporary treatment and may be life saving. Thoracentesis is most commonly and safely performed by simple needle or catheter aspiration in the midclavicular line, second or third intercostal space. Once a tension pneumothorax is confirmed by this method, a thoracostomy tube should be placed as soon as possible (see Chapter 9). This is particularly important in the patient on positive-pressure ventilation.

Thoracentesis may also be used in the prehospital care setting, when a patient in extremis is suspected of having a tension pneumothorax. To facilitate the continued drainage of the pneumothorax, an expedient flutter valve, underwater seal, or commercially available one-way valve may be attached.[44]

McSwain has developed a self-retaining catheter and trocar (McSwain Dart, from Medical Dynamics, Inc.), which can be placed in the chest and attached to a drainage system.[45] Although this apparatus has been suggested as an alternative to needle or catheter placement, it may be associated with increased risk of pulmonary injury, particularly if placed incorrectly when a pneumothorax is not present[46] (see Chapter 9). Use of a guide wire–directed minicatheter is currently preferred to use of a minitrocar system.[32–34]

Contraindications

In clinical situations in which a tension pneumothorax is suspected, several relative contraindications to the use of thoracentesis are important to remember. If tube thoracostomy is readily available, it may be the preferred procedure, and thoracentesis may only serve to delay the more definitive treatment. In patients who are being ventilated manually or by respirator, extreme caution should be exercised when performing thoracentesis. If the presumptive diagnosis of a tension pneumothorax is incorrect, the insertion of a thoracentesis needle may actually create a pneumothorax, which may be converted into a tension pneumothorax by the positive-pressure ventilation.

An absolute contraindication to thoracentesis is the insertion of a needle through an area of infection.[8] In such cases, an alternate insertion site should be selected. In patients who have bleeding diatheses or who are on anticoagulants, thoracentesis for evacuation of a stable, small pneumothorax may be relatively contraindicated, with observation being the preferred treatment.

Equipment

The equipment needed to perform rapid thoracentesis for tension pneumothorax or aspiration of a spontaneous pneumothorax is listed in Table 8–2. Because several techniques are described, the necessary equipment for all techniques is included in this list. Evacuation of a tension pneumothorax can be accomplished by insertion of a needle only, a through-the-needle catheter, or an over-the-needle catheter. Although the needle insertion technique can be performed most rapidly, the catheter insertion techniques may theoretically be safer, allowing continued drainage of the relieved tension pneumothorax without the presence of a rigid needle in the thorax. The drawbacks to the use of a catheter are the possibility of the catheter crimping or collapsing as well as the increased resistance to drainage caused by the catheter's length. The catheter technique is recommended in relief of tension pneumothorax in the prehospital setting.[47] Likewise, when evacuating a simple, stable pneumothorax, the catheter techniques may be preferred because they are less likely to pierce the expanding lung. Small thoracostomy tubes and pigtail catheters may be used for the stable pneumothorax and are placed using the Seldinger technique (see also Chapter 23).

Procedure

The anterior thoracentesis approach is used primarily for relief of a tension pneumothorax and evacuation of a simple pneumothorax. Because treatment is urgently required in the first case, the procedure chosen should be performed in an appropriately expedient manner. Likewise, the amount of preparation and equipment needed is dictated by each particular clinical situation. Informed consent is likely to be impossible to obtain in cases of tension pneumothorax, but an attempt to secure it may be considered in patients with a stable pneumothorax.

Table 8–2. Equipment Needed for Thoracentesis Evacuation of Air

Tension Pneumothorax
Antiseptic solution and sterile gauze sponges (if condition allows)
Catheter or needle (either)
   Over-the-needle catheter (14- to 16-gauge needle)
   Through-the-needle catheter (14-gauge needle)
   Hypodermic needle (14 to 20 gauge)
Drainage equipment (either)
   5- to 10-ml syringe (premoistened if condition allows)
   Flutter value (commercial or fashioned from sterile glove fingertip)
   Sterile intravenous tubing with water-filled basin

Stable Pneumothorax
Antiseptic solution and sterile basin
Sterile gauze sponges
Sterile towels
Syringes (5 to 10 ml) for anesthetic infiltration
Needles (22 and 25 gauge) for anesthetic infiltration
Catheter (either)
   Over-the-needle catheter (16- to 18-gauge needle)
   Through-the-needle catheter (14- to 16-gauge needle)
   Pigtail catheter (6.0 to 8.5 French)*
   Small chest tube (8 French)*
Drainage equipment (either)
   Flutter valve (commercial or fashioned from sterile glove fingertip)
   Sterile intravenous tubing with water-filled basin
   Syringe (30 to 50 ml) with three-way stopcock

*Requires additional equipment for Seldinger technique (see Chapter 23).

INSERTION SITE AND PATIENT POSITION

The conventional approach has been to evacuate tension pneumothoraces by using the anterior approach, with the patient in a supine position and the head of the stretcher elevated 30 degrees. The recommended insertion site is the second intercostal space in the midclavicular line (Fig. 8–1). The rationale for this approach is that free pleural air will rise to the anterior upper chest. With a tension pneumothorax, however, the collapsed lung is moved away from the entire ipsilateral chest wall, making a lateral approach also possible. If the patient is in a supine position and if the anterior chest is obscured (e.g., subclavian vein catheter bandage, chest monitoring leads, subcutaneous emphysema) or if a chest wall infection is present, a lateral approach may be more practical. The lateral approach is accomplished by inserting the needle into the fourth or fifth intercostal space in the midaxillary or anterior axillary line. This location can be identified quickly in males by extending the horizontal nipple line laterally into the axilla. In females who have large breasts, reliable approximation can be made by extending an imaginary horizontal line between the inferior tips of the scapulae laterally into the axilla.

There are two major problems when the lateral approach is chosen. The first is the greater risk of parenchymal injury if neither a tension nor a large pneumothorax is present. The second problem is the danger of adhesions. Previous empyema, hemothorax, tuberculosis, and other inflammatory processes may cause pleural adhesions, which frequently occur in dependent portions of the thorax. Therefore, the anterior approach is theoretically safer and is recommended for most cases in which relief of tension pneumothorax is required. Likewise, for the evacuation of a simple, stable pneumothorax, the anterior approach is recommended unless a loculated pneumothorax dictates an alternate approach.

NEEDLE OR CATHETER INSERTION FOR EVACUATION OF AIR

Patient Preparation. The patient is positioned as previously discussed. An explanation of the procedure is appropriate if the patient is awake, but it should not delay the procedure. Because the patient is usually in extremis, sedation is contraindicated. Restraining the patient may be necessary if the patient is hypoxic and confused. Oxygen should be administered. The insertion site is swabbed rapidly with povidone-iodine or another suitable antiseptic, when time permits. If a stable pneumothorax is being evacuated, an appropriate explanation and a careful preparation of the sterile field is indicated.

Anesthesia. Local anesthesia is usually inappropriate in the case of relieving a tension pneumothorax and will only delay the procedure. If the patient has a slowly progressive tension pneumothorax or a stable pneumothorax and is not in extremis, local anesthesia with 1 per cent lidocaine or its equivalent may be used. It is administered through a 5- to 10-ml syringe with a 25- to 27-gauge needle. An intradermal wheal is raised over the upper edge of the third or fourth rib after localization with palpation. Anesthetic is infiltrated down to the periosteum. The needle is then withdrawn.

Insertion Techniques. A 14- to 20-gauge needle is selected and attached to a 5- to 10-ml syringe premoistened with saline, if time allows. The third rib is again identified by palpation. The needle is inserted perpendicularly in the midclavicular line over the upper edge of the rib. As the rib is encountered, the needle is "walked" over the superior aspect of the rib and into the lower portion of the second intercostal space. This approach should avoid the intercostal vessels positioned near the lower border of each rib, as

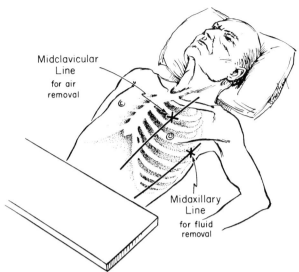

Figure 8–1. For relief of a tension pneumothorax, the second intercostal space in the midclavicular line is preferred. The head of the stretcher is elevated 30 degrees. The midaxillary line, fourth or fifth intercostal space site, has been used for thoracentesis of pleural fluid (see text). (From Fishman NH: Thoracic Drainage: A Manual of Procedures. Chicago, Year Book Medical Publishers, Inc, 1983, p 26. Reproduced by permission.)

indicated in Figure 8–2. The syringe is gently aspirated as the needle is advanced. A "pop" may be felt as the pleural space is entered and air is encountered. A pneumothorax under tension may create enough pressure to drive the plunger of a premoistened syringe the length of the barrel without manually withdrawing it. If the needle has been inserted without a syringe attached, a rush of air exiting the chest may be heard in inspiration as well as during expiration. Either of these findings will confirm the presence of a tension pneumothorax. Inserting a needle without an attached syringe or other drainage device invites the possibility of creating a pneumothorax if none is already present. If

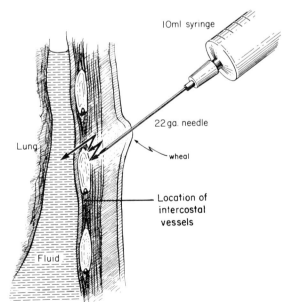

Figure 8–2. Walking the anesthetic needle over the superior aspect of the rib. (From Fishman NH: Thoracic Drainage: A Manual of Procedures. Chicago, Year Book Medical Publishers, Inc, 1983, p 28. Reproduced by permission.)

any pneumothorax is confirmed, a one-way drainage device should be attached as soon as possible.

Alternate methods of relief of a tension or stable pneumothorax include the use of standard intravenous needle and catheter insertion sets (Fig. 8–3). This can be accomplished by attaching the syringe to the hub of an *over-the-needle catheter* (with a 14- to 18-gauge needle). Larger sizes should be chosen for a tension pneumothorax. A small scalpel blade may be used to pierce the skin at the entry site to facilitate catheter entry. The pleura is entered through the second or third intercostal space, as previously described, and the catheter is advanced over the needle into the pleural space. The needle is then removed, and the syringe or another drainage device is attached to the hub of the catheter. A tension pneumothorax is confirmed by the same findings as those discussed earlier. The catheter may be secured with sutures. A drainage system is then attached.

A *through-the-needle catheter* (with a 14- to 16-gauge needle) of the shortest available length may also be used. The larger diameter should be chosen for a tension pneumothorax. Once the needle has entered the pleural space, the catheter is advanced fully into the thorax through the needle. The needle is then withdrawn, and a drainage device is attached to the catheter hub. The "needle guard" should be attached to prevent a laceration of the catheter by the surrounding needle. The catheter may be secured by suturing it to the chest wall. A one-way drainage system should be attached.

For evacuation of a *stable, simple pneumothorax*, either the over-the-needle or through-the-needle technique may be used. In these cases, it is important to attach a one-way drainage system before piercing the chest because the pneumothorax will not be under pressure, and an exposed catheter lumen may enlarge the pneumothorax. Commercial thoracentesis kits and specialized equipment may also be used (see "Needle or Catheter Insertion for Evacuation of Fluid").

The Seldinger technique may also be used to insert a pigtail catheter (6.5 to 8.5 French) or a small chest tube (approximately 8 French) for evacuating a stable pneumothorax. A 16- to 18-gauge needle is attached to a syringe and inserted into the pleural space until air is encountered as described previously. While holding the needle securely, the syringe is removed, and the hub of the needle is covered with a gloved finger. A fine, flexible-tipped guide wire is inserted through the needle and advanced into the pleural space. The needle is withdrawn, leaving the wire in place. A small scalpel blade is used to pierce the skin adjacent to the guide wire. As an option, a dilator may be threaded over the wire and then removed after enlarging the opening. A pigtail catheter or small chest tube is threaded over the exposed guide wire and gently advanced into the pleura to an adequate depth such that all side openings are well within the chest. The wire is then removed, and the catheter should be secured to the chest wall. The catheter should be attached to a drainage device as soon as possible.

Initially air may be evacuated with a 60-ml syringe and a 3-way stopcock. If expansion is incomplete, continuous suction may be used (see Chapter 9). The expanding lung may kink the catheter, requiring placement of a larger catheter. The physician may also instruct the patient to change position (e.g., supine to sitting) or cough to help free the catheter and permit complete lung expansion.

Drainage. After the diagnosis of a pneumothorax has been made, drainage should be instituted. In the case of a tension pneumothorax, drainage should be continued until a thoracostomy tube can be placed. Continuous drainage can be accomplished by attaching the distal end of an intravenous tubing set without one-way valves to the needle

or catheter hub. The proximal end of the intravenous tubing is placed under water in a basin to create an underwater seal. This prevents air from entering the pleural space. An alternative is to attach a commercial flutter valve such as the Heimlich valve. An expedient drainage device may also be made using a premoistened finger cut from a sterile examination glove (Fig. 8–4). The cut edge of the glove finger will act as a one-way flutter-valve.

Any of the previously mentioned techniques may be used for drainage of a stable pneumothorax. Evacuation by attaching a three-way valve to a large (30 to 50 ml) syringe may facilitate the removal of air without creating a danger of increasing the pneumothorax size. Care must be taken to exert gentle negative pressure when aspirating air because greater negative pressure may cause postexpansion pulmonary edema (see "Complications"). If a pigtail catheter or small chest tube has been placed, a standard pleural drainage system may be used (see Chapter 9).

If a tension pneumothorax is found and confirmed by any of the aforementioned methods, a thoracostomy tube should be placed as soon as possible. A chest film is also indicated following thoracentesis or tube thoracostomy to confirm the successful relief of the pneumothorax, absence of hemothorax or other complications, and (if performed) thoracostomy tube placement. This confirmation is best obtained with an upright expiratory chest film.

Posterior Approach for Evacuation of Fluid

PLEURAL EFFUSION

Physiology. Pleural fluid is normally created as a result of several physiologic mechanisms, including hydrostatic pressure, colloid oncotic pressure, and intrapleural pressure.[8, 48] With normal pleural homeostasis, the hydrostatic pressure generated by the systemic capillaries across the parietal pleura is greater than the hydrostatic pressure generated by the pulmonary capillaries across the visceral pleura. Because the colloid oncotic and intrapleural pressures exert symmetric forces, a gradient is created that allows for the formation of normal fluid at the parietal pleura and absorption by the visceral pleura. Lymphatic flow also facilitates absorption. A summary of the homeostatic forces involved is shown in Figure 8–5.

The integrity of this system can be disrupted by changes in hydrostatic pressure, colloid oncotic pressure, intrapleural pressure, lymphatic flow, capillary permeability, and pleural fluid surfactant composition.[48, 49] Fluid can accumulate because of two processes, transudation and exudation. Transudation may occur from increased pulmonary capillary pressure, as in left ventricular failure, or from decreased colloid oncotic pressure secondary to hypoalbuminemic states, as in the nephrotic syndrome and cirrhosis. Structural abnormalities such as peritoneal-pleural communications in cirrhotic patients with ascites have been reported.[50]

The exudation of fluid into the pleural space may occur as the result of abnormalities, such as changes in surfactant or altered capillary permeability seen with inflammatory disease, infection, pulmonary infarction, respiratory distress syndrome, and neoplasm.[8, 48, 49] Lymphatic malignancy may decrease fluid resorption. Likewise, trauma to the lymphatic duct, esophagus, or vascular structures leads to the direct flow of the contents of these structures into the pleural space.

Etiology. Numerous etiologies may account for the formation of abnormal pleural fluid. Rapid or relatively acute accumulations may be seen with hemothorax, esophageal rupture, pulmonary infarction, infection, empyema, obstructive uropathy, thoracic duct injury, or iatrogenic causes (such as intrapleural placement of a subclavian vein catheter). Chronic effusions are also commonly seen in many disease states. The most common atraumatic causes of effusion are congestive heart failure, infection, and neoplasm.[8] Effusions due to pneumonia are referred to as parapneumonic. Massive effusions causing mediastinal shift (tension hydrothorax) due to malignancy, dialysis, and following iatrogenic intrapleural infusion of parenteral hyperalimentation solution have been reported.[51–53] Traditionally, effusions have been classified as transudates or exudates. Transudates typically have a low specific gravity and protein concentration. Exudates usually have an increased specific gravity and high protein concentration (see "Pleural Fluid Analysis"). Common causes of effusions are listed in Table 8–3.

Clinical Diagnosis. A pleural effusion may be asymptomatic or may produce varying degrees of dyspnea or pleuritic pain. Other symptoms such as cough, fever, weight loss, or edema may be present and may be related to the underlying cause of the effusion.

The physical signs of pleural effusion vary according to its size. Small effusions do not usually produce physical findings. Moderate-sized effusions may produce physical findings over the area of the effusion. A pleural friction rub may be present. Breath sounds may be diminished, there may be dullness to percussion, and tactile fremitus may be decreased. Occasionally, decreased chest excursions are evident. In very large effusions, breath sounds may change from vesicular to bronchovesicular, gradually becoming absent as compression of the underlying lung occurs. A tension hydrothorax may produce mediastinal shift, with tracheal

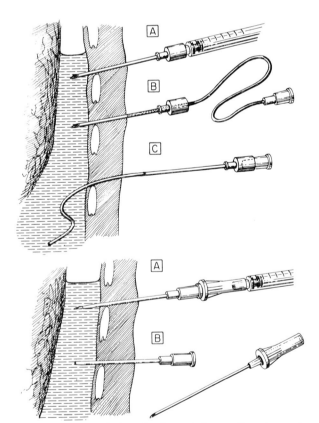

Figure 8–3. Insertion technique for through-the-needle and over-the-needle catheters. Separate intercostal spaces depict the steps *(A, B, C)* that occur at a single intercostal space. (From Fishman NH: Thoracic Drainage: A Manual of Procedures. Chicago, Year Book Medical Publishers, Inc, 1983, p 30. Reproduced by permission.)

deviation, displacement of the cardiac impulse, and bulging of the intercostal spaces.[52, 53]

Radiographic Diagnosis. The radiographic findings of pleural effusions vary with the location and amount of fluid present. Slight elevation of the hemidiaphragm or lateral displacement of the diaphragmatic dome on the posteroanterior chest film suggests a small subpulmonic effusion. Blunting of the costophrenic angle may be seen on an upright chest film and represents at least 175 ml of fluid.[54] A fluid level with an upwardly concave meniscus indicates a considerably larger effusion. The higher level of the meniscus laterally is due partly to the fact that the lung exerts pressure outwardly from the hilum, pushing the fluid toward the periphery.[55] In addition, the increased density of the fluid viewed tangentially at the edge of the chest renders it visible, whereas the fluid located medially may not be of sufficient depth to be visualized. A fluid level without a meniscus is indicative of a coexisting pneumothorax. A massive pleural effusion with contralateral shifting of the mediastinum and diaphragmatic inversion indicates a tension hydrothorax.[53]

Lateral decubitus views of the chest with the involved side down may help to identify small amounts of pleural fluid.[56] Comparison of bilateral decubitus views may help to differentiate fluid from other densities as well as enable viewing underlying lung previously obscured by pleural fluid.[57]

On a supine anteroposterior film, a generalized increased density over the lung field(s), costophrenic blunting, apical capping, widening of the minor fissure, and obscuring of the hemidiaphragm may be suggestive of a pleural effusion.[58] A pleural effusion may be differentiated from an infiltrate by the lack of air bronchograms and the absence of a "silhouette sign" obscuring the heart border.[8] A lateral decubitus or upright chest film helps to confirm this diagnosis.

Other findings may be seen in various views, including thickening of the pleural fissures. A "middle lobe step" has been described on the upright lateral film in which the major and minor fissures outline the middle lobe while the lower lobe is compressed.[8] Loculated effusions along the pleural border due to adhesions from previous hemothorax or empyema may be seen occasionally. Elliptic thickening of the fissures is suggestive of loculated effusions. Ultrasonic examination of the chest may help differentiate loculated effusions from solid tumors, as well as help localize fluid for thoracentesis.[59] A CT of the chest may help evaluate underlying pathologic findings in the presence of an effusion.[60] It may also help identify subpulmonic effusion, atelectasis, and subphrenic fluid.[61, 62]

Treatment. Management of pleural effusions must be directed toward treatment of the underlying condition. In most cases, thoracentesis is indicated for diagnostic purposes. Exceptions to the need for diagnostic thoracentesis may be made for congestive heart failure or for the stable, previously diagnosed effusion in which the cause is clear. Thoracentesis may be withheld in these situations if the effusion responds to medical management.[63] In cases in which tuberculosis or malignancy are suspected, pleural biopsy may also be indicated. The timing of the thoracentesis and biopsy should be coordinated.

Repeated thoracentesis has been recommended by some to monitor the pH of a parapneumonic effusion; a decreasing pH may indicate progression to a complicated parapneumonic effusion that requires thoracostomy tube drainage.[64] Other conditions such as empyema or hemothorax diagnosed by thoracentesis usually require thoracostomy tube insertion to facilitate more thorough evacuation. Likewise, chylothorax due to thoracic duct trauma is often

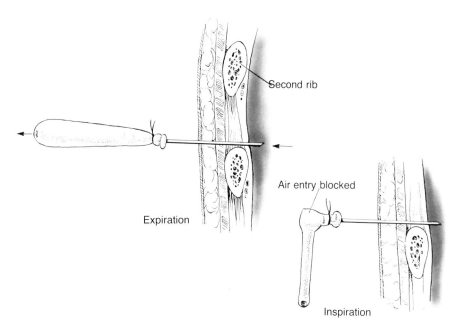

Figure 8–4. Use of a needle and a sterile finger cot or a finger from a sterile glove to fashion a one-way (flutter) valve for emergency evacuation of a tension pneumothorax. (Redrawn from Cosgriff JH: An Atlas of Diagnostic and Therapeutic Procedures for Emergency Personnel, Philadelphia. JB Lippincott Co, 1978, p 243.)

managed by thoracostomy drainage and total parenteral hyperalimentation.[65] A ruptured esophagus usually requires thoracotomy and surgical repair.

Another major indication for thoracentesis is evacuation of a large symptomatic pleural effusion. If the effusion is quite large, has accumulated rapidly, or causes inversion of the diaphragm, the effusion itself may seriously impair respiratory function by decreasing lung volume and increasing shunting.[66] Tension hydrothorax likewise causes significant respiratory compromise and may impair venous return.[67]

In the conditions mentioned previously, removing a large amount of pleural fluid may provide significant therapeutic benefit by improving oxygen saturation, improving the alveolar-arterial oxygen gradient, decreasing shunting, and improving vital capacity.[68, 69] Although removing a maximum of 1000 to 1500 ml has been a general rule of thumb,

as it was thought to prevent postevacuation pulmonary edema, larger amounts may be removed safely by monitoring the pleural pressures and maintaining gentle negative pressure (see "Complications"). In cases of intractable malignant effusions, placement of a pleuroperitoneal shunt may be useful.[70]

HEMOTHORAX

Historically, repeated thoracentesis was used initially to evacuate hemothoraces. With the advent of effective tube thoracostomy, however, this method has become nearly obsolete. There are several major arguments for the decline in this practice. Repeated violation of the pleura and persistence of the hematoma may increase the risk of infection. The effectiveness of evacuation is inferior to that of tube thoracostomy with continuous suction. Likewise, thoracostomy tube drainage allows better monitoring of the rate of bleeding. Failure of complete resorption of a hemothorax may create a fibrous "peel," or fibrothorax, which can lead to restricted ventilation and may subsequently require open thoracotomy and decortication. Finally, tamponade of the bleeding source may theoretically be enhanced by complete expansion of the lung.

Nevertheless, some investigators suggest that thoracentesis may be used safely in select cases such as a small, stable traumatic hemothorax.[71] In one series, thoracentesis was used in traumatic hemothorax for 104 of 502 patients with only one patient requiring subsequent thoracotomy for fibrinothorax.[72] In a second series of 130 patients, thoracentesis was used for hemothorax evacuation in 48 patients, with 10 per cent developing fibrinothorax.[73] The results were poorest in patients with hemopneumothorax. Other isolated successful uses of thoracentesis in cases of nontraumatic hemothorax have been reported, including in Osler-Weber-Rendu disease and spontaneous hemothorax in the newborn.[74, 75] (Traumatic hemothorax is discussed in Chapter 9.)

Contraindications

The removal of pleural fluid by thoracentesis should be avoided in patients with a bleeding diathesis and in those on anticoagulants before correction of the clotting deficits.[8]

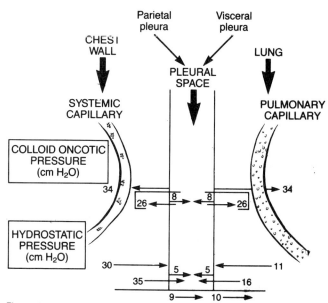

Figure 8–5. Diagrammatic representation of the pressures involved in the formation and absorption of pleural fluid. (From Fraser RG, Paré JAP: Diagnosis of Diseases of the Chest. Philadelphia. WB Saunders Co, 1970, p 65. Reproduced by permission.)

Table 8–3. Causes of Pleural Effusion

Transudates
Congestive heart failure
Cirrhosis with ascites
Nephrotic syndrome
Hypoproteinemia
Acute glomerulonephritis
Peritoneal dialysis
Urinary obstruction (urinothorax)
Superior vena caval obstruction
Acute atelectasis
Myxedema

Exudates
Neoplasm
Pulmonary infarction (embolus)
Bacterial pneumonia (parapneumonic effusion)
Empyema
Lung abscess
Other pneumonias
  Viral
  Tuberculous
  Fungal
  Rickettsial
  Parasitic
Collagen vascular disease (lupus erythematosus, dermatomyositis,
  rheumatoid pleuritis)
Pancreatitis
Drug reactions (nitrofurantoin, methysergide, practolol)
Asbestosis
Meigs syndrome
Dressler syndrome
Lymphatic disease (chylothorax)
Trapped lung (fibrothorax)
Subphrenic and hepatic abscess
Sarcoidosis
Chronic atelectasis
Uremia
Urinary obstruction (urinothorax)
Pulmonary or vascular disruption (hemothorax)
Esophageal rupture

Thoracentesis is also contraindicated unless performed under ultrasound or fluoroscopic guidance if the patient has an ipsilateral ruptured diaphragm. Extreme caution should be used when thoracentesis is being performed in a patient who has pleural adhesions, such as from previous tuberculosis, hemopneumothorax, or empyema, because of the danger of piercing the closely approximated visceral pleura and lung. Should there be an infection of the chest wall, thoracentesis is contraindicated unless an alternate puncture site without soft-tissue infection can be selected. In patients who require removal of large quantities of fluid, needle insertion techniques may be relatively contraindicated because of an increased risk of parenchymal damage.[8]

Equipment

For removal of fluids, more equipment is necessary than that required for aspiration of a pneumothorax. The additional equipment permits thorough patient preparation, more adequate anesthesia, controlled evacuation of fluid, and careful collection of specimens. In Table 8–4, the basic and alternative equipment is listed. The simple needle method has the potential risk of perforating the visceral pleura as the fluid is withdrawn, whereas the catheter of narrow diameter and long length may limit the removal of thick, tenacious fluids. Catheters also have the drawback of crimping if not handled carefully.

Either needle insertion or catheter insertion techniques

may be used for diagnostic thoracentesis when only a relatively small amount of fluid is being withdrawn. Needle insertion techniques may increase the risk of parenchymal injury when large quantities of fluid are removed for therapeutic purposes.[8] Likewise, catheter insertion techniques may be preferable when only a small amount of fluid is available and the risk of contact with the lung is greater.

Pigtail catheters also have been used successfully to remove effusions.[32, 33, 76] The Seldinger technique is used to aid in their insertion.

Procedure

Thoracentesis is generally an elective procedure and should be performed after an adequate number of diagnostic radiographic studies have been obtained. The procedure should be carried out with sufficient preparation, after all available equipment has been tested and under properly controlled circumstances. Informed consent should usually be obtained and documented, according to hospital policy.

The posterior approach is most often recommended when performing thoracentesis for removal of pleural effusions for either diagnostic or therapeutic purposes. A lateral approach may be used in certain circumstances that are described later.

INSERTION SITE AND PATIENT POSITION

The choice of insertion site for removal of pleural fluid depends on many clinical factors. If the fluid collection is large and if the patient is able to sit upright for a prolonged period of time, the following approach is recommended. The patient is seated, leaning forward slightly, supported by the back of a chair or a table. Some physicians recommend that the patient's back be vertical to keep the fluid in the dependent posterior chest (Fig. 8–6).[8] The site chosen for aspiration is the midscapular line or the posterior axillary line at a level below the top of the fluid. This level is best determined clinically at the time of the procedure by the height of dullness to percussion and the decrease in tactile fremitus.[77] A single interspace below this level should be selected.[8]

A chest film of the patient in an upright position should be taken to diagnose and locate the general position of the effusion, but reliance on the film is less precise than clinical assessment. Radiographic determination of fluid levels may

Table 8–4. Equipment Needed for Removal of Fluid

Basin for preparation solution
Antiseptic solution (povidone-iodine)
Sterile gauze sponges
Sterile towels
Syringes (5 to 10 ml) for anesthetic
Needles (22 and 25 gauge) for infiltration
Local anesthetic (e.g., 1% lidocaine)—10 ml
Syringe (50 ml) for aspiration
Catheter or needle (either)
  Hypodermic needle (18 to 22 gauge, 1½ to 2 inch)
  Over-the-needle catheter (16- to 20-gauge needle)
  Through-the-needle catheter (14- to 18-gauge needle)
  *Pigtail catheter (6.0 to 8.5 French)
Two curved hemostats
Three-way stopcock
Sterile intravenous extension tubing
Specimen bowl (may be calibrated for volume measurement) or
  sterile vacuum bottle with intravenous tubing
Sterile dressing and adhesive tape

*Requires additional equipment for Seldinger technique (see chapter 23).

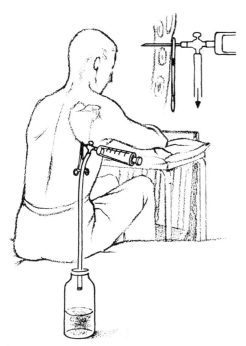

Figure 8–6. Upright positioning of patient for drainage of pleural fluid. Note the use of the hemostat to limit the depth of penetration of the thoracentesis needle. (From Nealon TF Jr: Fundamental Skills in Surgery. 3rd ed. Philadelphia, WB Saunders Co, 1979, p 291. Reproduced by permission.)

occasionally be misleading, because the position of the fluid changes with respiration and patient position. In addition, one should be reminded that the fluid level seen on a chest film of a patient in an upright position is actually higher than the bottom of the fluid meniscus.[55] The raised lateral edge of the fluid level represents the height of fluid available at the periphery. An exception to this distribution of pleural fluid occurs when a combined pneumothorax and pleural effusion produces a flat air-fluid level. In all cases, the lowest level recommended for thoracentesis is the eighth intercostal space. The highest level clinically indicated is generally chosen to minimize inadvertent abdominal insertion of the needle. If a catheter has been inserted and insufficient fluid is obtained, the patient can subsequently be repositioned to make the insertion site more dependent.[77]

The following alternative approaches have been described. If the patient is unable to remain seated, a catheter (through-the-needle, over-the-needle, or pigtail) may be inserted into the midaxillary or posterior axillary line in the fourth or fifth intercostal space while the patient is in a supine position (see Fig. 8–1).[55] It may be prudent to evaluate the height of the fluid both clinically and radiographically in this position before attempting this approach. If the patient can tolerate some elevation, it has been suggested that the patient recline against the raised head of the bed for support while the needle is inserted in the midaxillary or posterior axillary line at the appropriate level.[8] A lower interspace also may be used in these cases. Another suggestion is that the patient lie in a lateral decubitus position with a posterior site chosen for insertion.[8] If the amount of fluid is small and the need for diagnostic analysis is considerable, fluid can be aspirated from beneath the patient in the midaxillary line with the patient in the lateral decubitus position.[78] This technique requires that the patient be placed across an open space between stretchers in such a way that the physician can aspirate from below the patient and between the supporting structures.

For small or loculated effusions, ultrasound-guided thoracentesis may be preferable.[8,79] Fluoroscopic and CT-scan guidance have also been used successfully.[80]

NEEDLE OR CATHETER INSERTION FOR EVACUATION OF FLUID

Patient Preparation. The patient should be placed in the appropriate position, as described previously. Proper explanation of the procedure is essential when there is adequate time. If the patient is comfortable and cooperative, sedation is not needed. When the patient is uncooperative and in extremis, restraint may be necessary. If the patient is restrained, access to the insertion site must be clear, and one's ability to manage the patient and the airway must not be compromised. Sedation should be avoided if possible. In cases in which some sedation is essential, extreme caution and careful monitoring must be done; a rapid-acting or reversible sedative agent should be used. Supplementary oxygen by nasal prongs or mask should be given if it is clinically indicated and may minimize postevacuation hypoxia (see "Complications"). A wide area around the thoracentesis site should be prepared, using povidone-iodine or another suitable antiseptic to allow selection of several intercostal spaces. Sterile towels should be draped around the site. A patent intravenous line should be established, and atropine sulfate for intravenous administration should be available if the patient becomes vasovagal.

Anesthesia and Pleural Fluid Localization. Local anesthesia should be used before removal of pleural fluid. A 1 per cent solution of lidocaine or equivalent anesthetic is usually chosen. The anesthetic (5 to 10 ml) is drawn into a syringe, and a 25- or 27-gauge needle is attached. The previously selected insertion site is relocated by palpation. A small skin wheal is raised at the upper edge of the rib. The syringe is withdrawn, and a 3.75-cm, 22-gauge needle is attached and then inserted through the wheal toward the upper border of the rib. The subcutaneous tissue and muscle are alternately aspirated and infiltrated as the needle is advanced down to the periosteum of the rib. At this point, the needle is "walked" above the superior edge of the rib. It is then held perpendicularly to the chest and advanced while the aspiration-infiltration process is continued through the intercostal space until the pleura is entered (see Fig. 8–2). A pop may be felt, and fluid should be aspirated to ensure that the pleural space has been reached. If no fluid is encountered, the chosen intercostal space may be too low, and a higher site may be indicated. If air bubbles are encountered, the lung parenchyma may have been entered; the chosen intercostal space may be too high, and a lower site may be indicated. Once fluid is aspirated, a curved hemostat may be applied to the needle at the skin surface, or the needle may be grasped with the thumb and index finger to indicate the proper depth of penetration.[77] The needle and hemostat or fingers should be removed together.

Needle Insertion Techniques. The following technique is used for diagnostic thoracentesis when a moderate to large amount of fluid is present. A 3.75- to 5-cm, 18- to 22-gauge needle is selected. The smaller-diameter needles may decrease the risk of hemothorax and are usually adequate to remove pleural fluid.[8] The needle and a 50-ml syringe are attached to a three-way stopcock. The syringe and needle may be premoistened with heparin. A drainage tube is attached to the stopcock. The lever of the stopcock is set to allow passage of fluid between the needle and the syringe. The depth of the pleural space as determined from the anesthetic needle is now marked on the larger aspiration needle by gently placing a second hemostat or grasping the needle with the index finger and thumb. The pleural space is again entered through the previous anesthetic site while gentle negative pressure is applied. Attention to the indicated depth will prevent insertion of the needle farther than necessary, thus decreasing the chance of lacerating the underlying lung. Fluid is first aspirated with the syringe. The stopcock lever is then turned, and the fluid is expelled through the drainage tube into a sterile container or sterile vacuum bottle or into open specimen tubes. An assistant is needed to handle the specimen tubes. The process of aspirating and ejecting the fluid through the drainage tubing is repeated until an adequate amount of fluid to accommodate all needed specimens has been drained.

Thoracentesis performed for diagnostic purposes requires removal of 50 to 100 ml. The specimens obtained are listed in Table 8–5. It is suggested that the appropriate laboratories be contacted to ensure the optimal collection technique for a specific analysis. It may, for example, be best to collect fluid for cytology in the morning to ensure examination of freshly obtained cells. Once the desired amount of fluid has been removed, the needle is withdrawn. A sterile dressing is applied over the insertion site. An upright expiratory chest film is taken to ensure that an iatrogenic pneumothorax was not created.

Catheter Insertion Techniques. An alternative method of removing the pleural fluid can be accomplished by either of the following techniques. Catheter insertion techniques (see Fig. 8–3) may be preferable when either small amounts of fluid are present and needed for diagnostic analysis or when large quantities are to be removed for therapeutic relief.[8] An *over-the-needle catheter* (16-to 20-gauge needle) is attached to the 50-ml syringe. The syringe may be premoistened with heparin. A small scalpel blade to pierce the skin at the selected insertion site may ease entry of the catheter through the skin. The proper depth of the pleural space is indicated on the catheter by grasping it between a gloved index finger and thumb. The needle and catheter are inserted into the pleural space, as previously described. As

fluid is encountered, the needle and the catheter are angled slightly caudally. The catheter is advanced into the pleural space, and the needle is withdrawn. The exposed lumen of the catheter hub is covered with a gloved finger to prevent the entry of air. A three-way stopcock with an attached 50-ml syringe and a drainage tube are again attached to the catheter hub. Fluid is removed following the same process for the needle insertion technique. For diagnostic purposes, 50 to 100 ml of fluid should be adequate. If the purpose of the thoracentesis is therapeutic drainage, the fluid is removed in 50-ml aliquots until the respiratory distress appears to be relieved. Although it has usually been recommended that no more than 1000 to 1500 ml of pleural fluid be removed because of the potential for excessive loss of protein or the risk of postevacuation pulmonary edema,[8, 77] more fluid may be removed with gentle negative pressure. Measuring the pleural pressure frequently using a manometer may be appropriate if larger quantities are removed[8, 81] (see "Complications"). Aftercare is the same for catheter drainage as for needle drainage.

A second alternative method involves the use of a *through-the-needle catheter* (14- to 18-gauge needle). The catheter is withdrawn from the needle before the procedure. A three-way stopcock is attached to the catheter hub and adjusted to close the catheter to the passage of air or fluid. The catheter and stopcock are temporarily set aside with sterile technique. The empty outer needle is attached to a 50-ml syringe. The syringe may be premoistened with heparin. The depth is again marked on the needle with a hemostat or index finger and thumb, as previously described, to indicate the depth of the pleural fluid as determined from the anesthetic needle. The needle is inserted into the pleural space through the anesthetized area while constant, gentle, negative pressure is applied. Once fluid is encountered, the needle is held securely as the syringe is detached. Again, it is essential to cover the needle hub with a gloved finger. The needle is then held securely and angled caudally as the catheter is inserted through the needle into the pleural space and advanced its full distance. The needle is withdrawn, leaving the catheter within the chest wall. The "needle guard" is then attached to the needle tip to prevent shearing off of the catheter. The catheter *must not be drawn back through* the needle, because such action may lacerate the catheter and allow its free entry into the pleural space. The catheter is then held securely within the chest wall without bending or kinking. The syringe is reattached to the stopcock, and the stopcock lever is turned to allow passage of fluid into the syringe. Fluid is withdrawn according to the guidelines described for the previous over-the-needle catheter technique. Should repositioning be needed, care must be taken to avoid crimping the catheter. After an adequate amount of fluid has been withdrawn, the catheter is removed and the entry site is covered with a sterile bandage. A follow-up chest film is again indicated.

Commercial Thoracentesis Kits and Miscellaneous Equipment. Commercial prepackaged kits have been developed that provide the general equipment needed to perform thoracentesis for the removal of pleural effusion. Most include the basic equipment previously described. Use of a kit saves time. Some kits include equipment such as drainage bags or applicators for the preparation solution. Others may provide unique equipment such as automatic two-way valves, self-sealing diaphragms, or collection apparatus.[82] In general, their drawbacks may include increased cost and limited options for equipment. Some may provide brief instructions on technique. It is suggested that each manufacturer's description of thoracentesis technique be consulted and that the equipment be reviewed to allow assembly of any additional equipment before beginning the procedure. The tech-

---

Table 8–5. Diagnostic Pleural Fluid Specimens

In all cases:
6.5-ml plain (red-top) specimen tube
  Lactate dehydrogenase (LDH)
  Glucose
  Protein
5-ml EDTA (lavendar-top) specimen tube
  Appearance
  Color
  Specific gravity
  Cell counts
  Differential counts
  Crystals

If exudate or clinically indicated:
6.5-ml plain (red-top) specimen tubes
  Amylase
  Triglycerides, cholesterol (lipoprotein electrophoresis)
  Complement levels
  Rheumatoid factor
  Countercurrent immunoelectrophoresis (CIE)
  Carcinoembryonic antigen (CEA)
10-ml sterile container
  Gram stain
  Aerobic cultures
  Anaerobic cultures
  Acid-fast bacilli culture and stain
  Fungal culture and stain
10- to 50-ml plain bottle or (red-top) specimen tubes
  Cytology 5-ml heparinized (green-top) specimen tube
  Lupus erythematosus cells
2-ml iced heparinized syringe with air expelled pH

Table 8–6. *Diagnostic Features of Pleural Fluid*[8, 84, 86]

Pleural Fluid	Description	WBC Count	Predominant Leukocyte	Glucose	pH	Comments
Exudates						
Parapneumonic	Turbid	Elevated	P	Low	>7.3	If pH < 7.2 may need thoracostomy tube; CIE may identify some aerobic bacteria[64]
Empyema	Turbid, purulent	Elevated	P	Low	<7.3	Positive gram stain, culture; CIE may identify some aerobic bacteria
Tuberculosis	Straw color, serosanguinous	<10,000	M or P	Low	<7.4	Positive AFB stain, culture or pleural biopsy
Malignancy	Turbid, bloody	<10,000	M	Low	<7.3	Positive cytology, pleural biopsy, CEA
Pulmonary embolism or infarction	Straw color, bloody	Elevated	M or P	Serum	7.4	Hypoxia; positive lung scan
Collagen vascular disease	Turbid	Variable	M or P			Positive serum ANA, pleural complement
Rheumatoid arthritis	Green	Variable	M or P	Very low	<7.3	Elevated pleural rheumatoid factor
Systemic lupus erythematosus	Yellow	Variable	M or P	Serum	>7.3	Positive pleural LE cells
Hemothorax	Bloody	Variable	P	Serum	<7.3	Hematocrit > 50% peripheral level
Chylothorax	White, cloudy	Variable	M			Elevated pleural triglycerides; chylomicrons present; positive Sudan III stain
Pancreatitis	Turbid, serosanguinous	Elevated	P	Serum	>7.3	Pleural amylase > serum
Esophageal rupture	Turbid, bloody	Elevated	P		<<7.3	Pleural amylase elevated
Transudates						
Congestive heart failure	Clear, straw color	<1000	M	Serum	7.4	Clinical features
Cirrhosis	Clear, straw color	<500	M	Serum	7.4	Clinical features
Nephrotic syndrome or hypoproteinemia	Clear, straw color	<1000	M	Serum	7.4	Clinical features
Transudate or Exudate						
Urinothorax	Straw color to bloody			Low		Obstructive uropathy; pleural creatinine > serum[92]

P, polymorphonuclear cells; M, mononuclear cells (e.g., lymphocytes, macrophages, mesothelial and plasma cells); WBC, white blood cell; CIE, counterimmunoelectrophoresis; AFB, acid-fast bacilli; CEA, carcinoembryonic antigen; ANA, Antinuclear antibody; LE, lupus erythematosus.

(From Ross DS: Pleural effusion. In Harwood-Nuss AL, Linden CH, Luten RC, et al (eds): The Clinical Practice of Emergency Medicine. JB Lippincott Co, Philadelphia, 1990. Reproduced by permission.)

niques used should follow the guidelines described earlier, depending on the general type of needle or catheter included in the kits.

Occasionally, specialized equipment that has been developed for other purposes can be used for thoracentesis. An example is an on-off "flow switch" produced in England (Viggo) that has been incorporated into a 13-cm over-the-needle catheter for central venous cannulation. The flow through this catheter may be turned off while removing the introducing needle and attaching a syringe.[83] If the catheter is used for thoracentesis, the flow switch may serve to prevent the inadvertent creation of a pneumothorax.

Pigtail Catheter Insertion. A new method of catheter insertion using the Seldinger technique allows the insertion of small pigtail catheters (6.0 to 8.5 French) to evacuate fluid. A 16- to 18-gauge needle is attached to a syringe and inserted through the appropriate interspace into the pleural space until fluid is encountered. The needle is held securely as the syringe is removed and the exposed hub of the needle is covered. A small flexible guide wire is then threaded through the needle, which is angled caudally. The needle is removed with the wire remaining within the chest. A puncture is made through the skin next to the guide wire with a small scalpel blade. An optional dilator may be threaded over the wire and then removed to enlarge the opening.

The pigtail catheter is inserted over the wire and advanced gently into the chest so that all side openings are well within the pleura. The wire is removed and a stopcock and drainage system are attached to the catheter. The catheter should be attached to the chest wall.

Pleural Fluid Analysis

Whether fluid is removed for diagnostic or for therapeutic purposes, certain specimens should be sent for laboratory analysis based on clinical indications.[84] Of diagnostic thoracenteses, 92 per cent provide clinically useful information.[85]

Whenever thoracentesis is performed, visual inspection of the fluid should be performed. Bloody or blood-tinged fluid most commonly indicates hemothorax, malignancy, pulmonary infarction, or tuberculosis. White or milky fluid suggests a chylothorax or chyliform effusion as described later. A thick purulent fluid, often with a foul odor, indicates an empyema. Other effusions may range from clear, straw colored to turbid (Table 8–6).

Establishing whether an effusion is a transudate or an exudate provides useful information. If a transudate is diagnosed, it has been suggested that minimal additional testing will be needed.[86] Typically, transudates have protein levels below 3 gm/100 ml and a specific gravity of less than 1.016. Exudates have values above these levels. Additional criteria have been advocated that provide a more accurate differentiation. These include (1) a ratio of pleural fluid protein to serum protein of ≤ 0.5, (2) a pleural lactate dehydrogenase (LDH) level of ≤ 200 IU/ml, and (3) a ratio of pleural fluid LDH to serum LDH of ≤ 0.6. Transudates have values below these levels, and exudates have at least one finding above these levels (Table 8–7).[87] These recommendations should be tempered by clinical suspicion. In all cases, fluid should be held for possible additional analysis in the appropriate specimen container (see Table 8–5).

Cytology is an extremely important diagnostic test. If abnormal cellular components of pleural fluid are found, it is highly significant. Cytology may identify malignancies in more than 60 per cent of cases.[88, 89] Many specimens may be needed if the suspicion is high. White blood cell (WBC), differential, and red blood cell (RBC) counts on pleural fluid, however, may provide some general information, but their usefulness in differentiating the etiology of effusions is limited.[88, 89] The highest WBC levels are usually seen with empyema, with values often greater than 50,000 per mm³.[64] Differential cell counts may be grouped by the predominant cell, usually reported as polymorphonuclear cells or mononuclear cells (which include lymphocytes).[8] Typical WBC and differential findings in pleural fluid are summarized in Table 8–6.

Other patterns may include eosinophilia counts above 10 per cent seen with blood or air within the pleural space as well as with parasitic and fungal disease.[8] An RBC count above 100,000 per mm³ suggests trauma, malignancy, or pulmonary infarction.[87] A pleural fluid hematocrit may be performed on bloody effusions. Values greater than half the peripheral hematocrit should indicate a hemothorax.[8]

Numerous chemical analyses of pleural fluid are available and may help differentiate the causes of effusions. Glucose levels are usually low (less than 60 mg%) in malignancy, rheumatoid pleuritis, empyema, or, occasionally, tuberculosis.[8] Amylase levels above 160 Somogyi units suggest pancreatitis, pancreatic malignancy, esophageal rupture, or occasionally lung cancer.[90] Creatinine levels elevated above the serum level may be found in those pleural effusions due to obstructive uropathy.[91, 92] Pleural fluid lactate greater than or equal to 10 mmol per liter above blood lactate suggests a pyogenic pleural effusion.[93] The pH of the pleural fluid may be decreased below 7.30 in cases of malignancy, rheumatoid disease, and occasionally tuberculosis. This is also particularly helpful in delineating empyemas and those complicated parapneumonic effusions that may need thoracostomy tube drainage. pH levels below 7.2 to 7.3 are considered significant.[8, 64]

Table 8–7. Classification of Pleural Effusions

	Transudates	Exudates
Ratio of pleural fluid protein to serum protein	<0.5	>0.5
Pleural fluid lactate dehydrogenase	<200 IU/ml	>200 IU/ml
Ratio of pleural fluid lactate dehydrogenase to serum lactate dehydrogenase	<0.6	>0.6
Specific gravity	<1.016	>1.016
Pleural fluid protein	<3 gm/dl	>3 gm/dl

(From Ross DS: Pleural effusion. In Harwood-Nuss AL, Linden CH, Luten RC et al (eds): The Clinical Practice of Emergency Medicine. Philadelphia, JB Lippincott Co, 1990. Reproduced by permission.)

Milky fluids due to thoracic duct disruption from trauma or lymphoma are known as chylous effusions and may be differentiated from chyliform effusions seen in tuberculosis, rheumatoid disease, and trapped lung.[87] This is most important because chylothorax may require tube thoracostomy. Triglyceride levels above 110 mg% and chylomicrons, which stain with Sudan III stain, are seen in chylous effusions. Chyliform effusions have elevated cholesterol levels, may demonstrate cholesterol crystals on microscopic examination, and do not stain with Sudan III stain. The previously mentioned lipid values may also be obtained by lipoprotein electrophoresis. It has also been suggested that cholesterol levels above 60 mg% may help define an exudate.[94]

If the clinical suspicion warrants, further laboratory tests of pleural fluid may provide useful information. Reduced complement levels may be found in pleural effusions due to rheumatoid arthritis and systemic lupus erythematosis. Lupus erythematosis cells may be seen on a Wright stain. Rheumatoid factor titers greater than 1:320 suggest a rheumatoid pleural effusion. Elevated carcinoembryonic antigen may be suggestive of adenocarcinoma.[8]

The presence of bacteria may be identified in Gram stains and anaerobic and aerobic cultures of empyema and parapneumonic effusions. Countercurrent immunoelectrophoresis may also detect the presence of bacterial antigens in parapneumonic effusions.[8] Stains for acid-fast bacillus and tuberculosis cultures may identify tuberculous pleural effusions. Fungal and mycoplasma cultures may also be obtained.

THORACENTESIS IN PEDIATRIC PATIENTS

Indications

The indications for performing thoracentesis are much the same in children as in adults: relief of a suspected tension pneumothorax, diagnostic tap of a pleural effusion, and therapeutic drainage of a large symptomatic pleural effusion.

Pneumothorax and tension pneumothorax may develop in children for similar reasons as in adults. In all ages, mechanical ventilation and PEEP increase the risk of developing pneumothorax. During the neonatal period, however, the incidence of pneumothorax seems to increase.[95] It occurs with increasing frequency with fetal distress, difficult deliveries, meconium aspiration, cardiopulmonary resuscitation, hyaline membrane disease (respiratory distress syndrome), pulmonary interstitial emphysema, and phenobarbital sedation of low-birth-weight infants.[96] A second contralateral pneumothorax may occur in neonates on positive-pressure ventilation.[97] In the older child, trauma is a common cause of pneumothorax. Spontaneous pneumothorax also occurs and may be associated with asthma, bronchiolitis, cystic fibrosis, staphylococcal pneumonia, empyema, metastatic carcinoma, dermatomyositis, Ehlers-Danlos disease, and Marfan syndrome.[98] Cystic fibrosis has an increased incidence of tension pneumothorax that may occasionally occur bilaterally.[99] In children at any age, pneumothorax can progress to tension pneumothorax, particularly in those being mechanically ventilated and those on PEEP.

Pleural effusions may be encountered in the pediatric age group for most of the same reasons as they occur in adults. Juvenile rheumatoid arthritis and systemic lupus erythematosus may also be causes.[100] Parapneumonic effusions are common causes of pleural effusions and are most often due to pneumococcal infection. Empyema usually occurs because of a staphylococcal infection.[98, 101] In the neonate, spontaneous hemothorax may be due to hemorrhagic disease of the newborn, disseminated intravascular coagulation, arteriovenous malformations, and pleural vascular rupture.[75]

DIAGNOSIS OF TENSION PNEUMOTHORAX

The newborn child with a tension pneumothorax may present with increasing respiratory difficulty marked by irritability, grunting, tachypnea, intercostal and supraclavicular retractions, and nasal flaring. Cervical crepitus may be present. Cyanosis and cardiovascular collapse and decreased mental status may occur. The findings of a tracheal shift and ipsilateral tympany to percussion may be found but are often not appreciated in the newborn. A hyperinflated, relatively immobile hemithorax and decreased breath sounds may be seen occasionally but are frequently absent. This absence may be due in part to the ease with which breath sounds are transmitted from the uninvolved side in the neonate. A shift in the apical pulse may be a more reliable sign.[8]

In the older child, a pneumothorax usually causes dyspnea and pleuretic chest pain. A tension pneumothorax may reveal decreased breath sounds, tympany to percussion, and tracheal shift. Tachycardia, tachypnea, agitation, use of accessory muscles, nasal flaring, and cyanosis may be seen. Subcutaneous emphysema and cardiovascular collapse should suggest the progression of a tension pneumothorax.

A pneumothorax is best seen on an upright chest film. In the neonate, a cross-table lateral radiograph may be more useful than a supine chest film.[102] Tension pneumothorax is easily recognized on an upright posteroanterior chest film by the presence of absent pulmonary markings, shift of the mediastinum, and flattening of the diaphragm. Pneumomediastinum and subcutaneous emphysema may be seen. However, it is appropriate to relieve a tension pneumothorax by needle or catheter aspiration when it is recognized clinically. Awaiting radiographic diagnosis is only indicated when the patient's cardiopulmonary status is relatively stable or when the diagnosis of tension pneumothorax is in doubt. The diagnosis may be confirmed by a rush of air and clinical improvement with decompression.

A bilateral tension pneumothorax may be difficult to diagnose clinically. On a chest film, microcardia, flattened diaphragms, and the bilateral absence of lung markings are seen. In such a case, bilateral chest decompression confirms the diagnosis.

DIAGNOSIS OF PLEURAL EFFUSION

In the pediatric population, pleural effusions may be asymptomatic or may appear with respiratory compromise, pleuritic chest pain, cough, dyspnea, or signs and symptoms of underlying systemic illness such as fever or weight loss. A pleural friction rub may be heard. Bronchial breath sounds may be heard in the infant.[98] A moderate to large pleural effusion may be recognized on physical examination by the presence of decreased breath sounds, dullness to percussion, and decreased excursions of the ipsilateral hemithorax.

Large pleural effusions may be seen on a standard upright chest film displaying the same findings as in the adult. For small effusions, lateral decubitus films may be necessary. Bilateral decubitus views may help assess the underlying lungs as well as whether the effusion is loculated.

TREATMENT

Treatment is directed toward the underlying etiology. Supplemental oxygen may be beneficial. The indications for thoracentesis in children include relief of a tension pneumothorax and diagnostic or therapeutic drainage of a pleural effusion. In cases of parapneumonic effusion from lobar pneumococcal pneumonia, thoracentesis may be withheld.[98]

Position

Immobilization of the child may pose a significant problem because of the child's size as well as the inability of the frightened child to comprehend the explanation for the procedure. Gentle and simple explanations are appropriate for older children. Sedation may be helpful when respiratory distress is minimal. Oxygen saturation (see Chapter 5) should be monitored if sedation is used. Children should be held securely by an assistant. It is important to position the child as described for adults to provide the proper access to the insertion site and reliable landmarks. To relieve a tension pneumothorax, a child may be positioned supinely on a stretcher. The head may be elevated 30 degrees. For removal of pleural fluid, the child should be seated, leaning against the back of a chair or table in the same manner as indicated for adults. If pillows are used, care must be taken to ensure an adequate airway. For the child unable to sit up, the lateral decubitus position may be used. A neonate may be held in the "burping" position by an assistant.[103]

Insertion Site and Procedure

The insertion sites for relieving tension pneumothorax and removing pleural fluid are much the same as those recommended for adults. The second or third intercostal space in the midaxillary line is usually recommended for relief of a tension pneumothorax. The fourth or fifth intercostal space in the anterior axillary line is also suggested.[103] A needle or catheter may be inserted using the smaller suggested gauge as recommended for adults. The procedure follows the same technique as in adults.

Pleural fluid is best removed from the seventh or eighth intercostal space in the posterior axillary line. In children, the seventh intercostal space, located at the tip of the scapula when the arm is slightly elevated, is a reliable landmark.[104] Confirmation by physical examination and chest film is appropriate. A standard needle, a butterfly "scalp vein" needle, over-the-needle catheter, or a through-the-needle catheter may all be used. Again, the smaller gauge needle suggested for adults is recommended. The techniques for needle or catheter insertion are the same as those described for adults. Pigtail catheters have been used successfully in children to drain both pneumothoraces and effusions.[33, 34] The Seldinger technique as described earlier for adults is used for inserting the catheters.

Once a tension pneumothorax is diagnosed, a thoracostomy tube is indicated and should be inserted, even if the patient has experienced temporary relief from needle decompression. A thoracostomy tube should also follow thoracentesis if a hemothorax or empyema is found.

COMPLICATIONS

The most frequent complication caused by inserting a thoracentesis needle or catheter into the thorax from any approach is the *creation* of a pneumothorax. Although many patients already have a small pneumothorax, it may become larger or even become a tension pneumothorax during the procedure. The mechanisms for this complication are a laceration of the underlying lung, an inadequate coverage of the hub of the needle or catheter after the pleural space is entered, an inadequate drainage system, or an air leak in the drainage system or thoracentesis apparatus. The risk of pneumothorax or tension pneumothorax secondary to lung puncture may be increased with patients who are intubated and on positive-pressure ventilation. Iatrogenic pneumothorax also appears to occur more often when performing therapeutic thoracentesis and when malignancy is present.[85] If a pneumothorax is found on a follow-up chest film, tube thoracostomy may also be indicated, according to the criteria in Chapter 9. Approximately one third of pneumothoraces induced during thoracentesis require a thoracostomy tube.[85]

Cough is another frequently (9 per cent) encountered complication.[85] Although seemingly only a symptomatic problem, it may be associated with the creation of an iatrogenic pneumothorax. It has been suggested that on encountering coughing, one should consider terminating the procedure.

Although rare, unilateral pulmonary edema may occur following thoracentesis. It was initially reported following the use of excessive negative pressures in the evacuation of a pneumothorax.[105, 106] Unilateral pulmonary edema has, likewise, been seen following evacuation of a pleural effusion.[107] The pulmonary dysfunction may be the consequence of local hypoxia in the atelectatic lung, with resultant changes in the basement membrane or loss of surfactant, as well as from excessive pleural negative suction pressure. When performing thoracentesis for evacuation of air, one can minimize these changes by applying a passive underwater seal. Any negative suction pressure should be applied gently and may best be accomplished via controlled pressure drainage systems and tube thoracostomy. When removing large pleural effusions, the incidence of postexpansion pulmonary edema may also be decreased by applying gentle evacuation pressures and by frequent measuring of pleural pressures, using a column manometer held below the entry site. It is recommended to cease the evacuation if pressures go below -18 cm H_2O.[81] Once pulmonary edema develops, administering oxygen is appropriate for relief of hypoxia. Rarely, PEEP may be needed to correct this complication. A case has been reported in which the hypoxia associated with reexpansion pulmonary edema actually improved following the inadvertant redevelopment of the pneumothorax.[108]

Reexpansion hypotension has also been reported following rapid evacuation of persistant unilateral pneumothoraces of at least 1-week duration. The hypotension occurred in association with unilateral reexpansion pulmonary edema, a rising hematocrit level, and anuria despite relatively normal pulmonary capillary wedge pressures. Intravascular volume depletion and myocardial depression are the suggested mechanisms.[109, 110]

Transient hypoxia has been noted as a consistent finding after thoracentesis.[111] There may be a ventilation-perfusion mismatch with perfusion of atelectatic lung or areas of localized pulmonary edema. Although the hypoxia usually is not significant clinically, oxygen administration may be indicated, particularly in the patient with minimal respiratory reserve. Oxygen saturation monitoring (see Chapter 5) may be useful in such patients.

Although hemothorax and hemoperitoneum are uncommon, they represent significant potential complications of thoracentesis. Hemothorax may be due to laceration of the lung and diaphragmatic, intercostal, or internal mammary vessels. Cardiac perforation has been reported following thoracentesis in a pneumonectomized patient.[112] Careful attention to technique, such as avoiding the superior portion of the intercostal space, never puncturing medial to the midclavicular line, and not penetrating too deeply into the thorax during needle insertion should be practiced. Hemothorax may be diagnosed by the rapid accumulation of

reaccumulation of fluid as noted on a postthoracentesis upright chest film. If this occurs, evacuation through a thoracostomy tube is usually indicated according to the criteria indicated in Chapter 9. Hemoperitoneum may result from puncture of the spleen or liver through the diaphragm. This may occur when thoracentesis is performed with a low posterior approach during expiration. If laceration of intraabdominal contents is suspected, close observation is essential. A surgical consultation is usually in order, and an exploratory laparotomy may be indicated. Computed tomography may be helpful as an alternative diagnostic approach for suspected intra-abdominal solid organ injury.

As with all surgical procedures, there is the potential for infection. The risk of infection is estimated at 2 per cent.[8] The risk is kept low with proper attention to patient preparation and sterile technique. In the case of rapid relief of a tension pneumothorax, preparation is minimal; however, any risk of infection is greatly outweighed by the risk of cardiopulmonary collapse from a tension pneumothorax.

Inadvertent shearing of the plastic catheter may occur when a through-the-needle catheter technique is used. This complication is prevented by securing the needle with a needle guard after it has been withdrawn from the chest. In addition, the catheter should not be withdrawn back through the needle at any time. Should a catheter tip be left in the chest, a method of percutaneous retrieval using a bent needle tip under fluroscopy has been described.[113] Some other technical problems of thoracentesis may be encountered. The most common are "traumatic" taps contaminated by blood (11 per cent) and "dry" taps in which no fluid or inadequate fluid is obtained (9 per cent).[85] Grogan and associates found fewer pneumothoraces and dry taps when thoracentesis for pleural effusion was guided by ultrasonography.[114] Air embolus could occur if the thoracentesis device is left open to air and if the needle or catheter is inadvertently inserted into a pulmonary or intrathoracic blood vessel. Hypoproteinemia may occur after removal of a large pleural effusion. A thick pleural "peel" may accumulate secondary to inadequate drainage of a hemothorax or an empyema. This complication is avoided by using tube thoracostomy to drain blood or empyema more completely rather than using thoracentesis. Pleural "peels" may occasionally require thoracotomy and chest decortication.

References

1. Garrison FH: An Introduction to the History of Medicine. 4th ed. Philadelphia, WB Saunders Co, 1929.
2. Wagner RB: History of non-penetrating chest trauma and its treatment. Md Med J 37:297, 1988.
3. Glinz W: Chest Trauma. New York, Springer-Verlag, 1981.
4. Bowditch HI: Paracentesis thoracis. Am J Med Sci 23:103, 1852.
5. Hewett FC: Thoracentesis: The plan of continuous aspiration. Br Med J 1:317, 1876.
6. Valle AR: An analysis of 2811 chest casualties of the Korean conflict. Dis Chest 26:623, 1964.
7. McNamara JJ, Messersmith JK, Dunn RA, et al: Thoracic injuries in combat casualties in Vietnam. Ann Thorac Surg 10:389, 1970.
8. Light RW: Pleural Diseases. Philadelphia, Lea & Febiger, 1983.
9. Vukich DJ: Pneumothorax. Emerg Med Clin North Am 1:431, 1983.
10. Bense L, Eklund G, Wiman L: Smoking and the increased risk of contracting spontaneous pneumothorax. Chest 92:1009, 1987.
11. Anderson HJ, Hansen LG, Block AV: Catamenial pneumothorax. J Thorac Cardiovasc Surg 35:238, 1987.
12. Donovan PJ: Bilateral spontaneous pneumothorax: A rare entity. Ann Emerg Med 16:1277, 1987.
13. Zimmerman JE, Dunbar BS, Klingenmaier CH: Management of subcutaneous emphysema, pneumomediastinum, and pneumothorax during respiration therapy. Crit Care Med 3:69, 1975.
14. Steier M, Ching N, Roberts EB, et al: Pneumothorax complicating continous ventilatory support. J Thorac Cardiovasc Surg 67:17, 1974.
15. McLoud TC, Barash PG, Ravin CE: PEEP: Radiographic features and associated complications. AJR 129:209, 1977.
16. Reinstein L, Twardzik FG, Mech KF: Pneumothorax: A complication of

needle electromyography of the supraspinatous muscle. Arch Phys Med Rehabil 68:561, 1987.

17. Arisio R, Carbone G, Maina A, et al: Pneumothorax as a complication of fine needle aspiration of the breast. Panminerva Med 30:58, 1988.

18. Wisdom K, Nowak RM, Richardson, HH, et al: Alternate therapy for traumatic pneumothorax in "pocket shooters". Ann Emerg Med 15:428, 1986.

19. Savader SJ, Omori M, Martinez CR: Pneumothorax, pneumomediastinum, and pneumopericardium: Complications of cocaine smoking. J Fla Med Assoc 75:151, 1988.

20. Orriols R: A new physical sign in pneumothorax. (Letter.) Ann Intern Med 107:255, 1987.

21. Cooke DAP, Cooke JC: The supine pneumothorax. Ann R Coll Surg Engl 69:130, 1987.

22. Tocino IM, Miller MH, Fairfax WR: Distribution of pneumothorax in the supine and semirecumbant critically ill adult. AJR 144:901, 1985.

23. Wall SD, Federle MP, Jeffrey RB, et al: CT diagnosis of unsuspected pneumothorax after blunt abdominal trauma. AJR 141:919, 1983.

24. Tocino IM, Miller MH, Frederick DR, et al: CT detection of occult pneumothorax in head trauma. AJR 143:987, 1984.

25. Rhea JT, DeLuca SA, Greene RE: Determining the size of pneumothorax in the upright patient. Radiology 144:733, 1982.

26. Ross DS: Chest trauma. In Levy RC, Hawkins HH, Barsan WG (eds): Radiology in Emergency Medicine. St. Louis, CV Mosby Co, 1986.

27. Stradling P, Poole G: Conservative management of spontaneous pneumothorax. Thorax 21:145, 1966.

28. Kircher LT, Jr, Swartzel, RL: Spontaneous pneumothorax and its treatment. JAMA 155:24, 1954.

29. Raja OG, Labor AJ: Simple aspiration of spontaneous pneumothorax. Br J Dis Chest 75:207, 1981.

30. Talbot-Stern J, Richardson H, Tomlanovich MC, et al: Catheter aspiration for simple pneumothorax. J Emerg Med 4:437, 1986.

31. Vallee P, Sullivan M, Richardson H, et al: Sequential treatment for a simple pneumothorax. Ann Emerg Med 17:936, 1988.

32. Crouch JD, Keagy BA, Delany DJ: "Pigtail" catheter drainage in thoracic surgery. Am Rev Respir Dis 136:174, 1987.

33. Fuhrman BP, Landrum BG, Ferrara TB, et al: Pleural drainage using modified pigtail catheters. Crit Care Med 14:575, 1986.

34. Lawless S, Orr R, Killian A, et al: New pigtail catheter for pleural drainage for pleural drainage in pediatric patients. Crit Care Med 17:173, 1989.

35. Rutherford RB, Holcombe HH, Brickman RD, et al: The pathophysiology of progressive tension pneumothorax. J Trauma 8:212, 1968.

36. Hurewitz AN, Sidhu U, Bergofsky EH, et al: Cardiovascular and respiratory consequences of tension pneumothorax. Bull Eur Physiopathol Respir 22:545, 1986.

37. Gough D, Rust D: Nasogastric intubation: Morbidity in an asymptomatic patient. Am J Emerg Med 4:511, 1986.

38. Zwillich CW, Pierson DJ, Creogh CE, et al: Complications of assisted ventilation. Am J Med 57:161, 1974.

39. McLoud TC, Barsash PG, Ravin CE, et al: Elevation of pulmonary artery pressure as a sign of pulmonary barotrauma (pneumothorax). Crit Care Med 6:81, 1978.

40. Lernau O, Bar-Moor JA, Nessan S: Traumatic diaphragmatic hernia simulating acute tension pneumothorax. J Trauma 14:880, 1974.

41. Blair E, Topazlu C, Davis JH: Missed diagnosis in blunt chest trauma. J Trauma 11:129, 1971.

42. Gobien RP, Reines HD, Schabel SJ: Localized tension pneumothorax: Unrecognized form of barotrauma in adult respiratory distress syndrome. Radiology 142:15, 1982.

43. Glinz W: Priorities in diagnosis and treatment of blunt chest injuries. Injury 17:318, 1986.

44. Heimlich JH: Valve drainage of the pleural cavity. Dis Chest 53:282, 1968.

45. McSwain NE: A thoracostomy tube for field and emergency department use. JACEP 6:324, 1977.

46. Bayne CG: Pulmonary complications of the McSwain Dart. Ann Emerg Med 11:136, 1982.

47. Peitzman AB, Paris P: Thoracic trauma. In Campbell JE (ed): Basic Trauma Life Support—Advanced Prehospital Care. 2nd ed. Englewood Cliffs, NJ, Prentice-Hall, Inc, 1988.

48. Wiener-Kronish JP, Matthay MA: Pleural effusions associated with hydrostatic and increased permeability pulmonary edema. Chest 93:852, 1988.

49. Hills BS, Bryan-Brown CW: Role of surfactant in the lung and other organs. Crit Care Med 11:951, 1983.

50. Verreault J, Lepoge, S, Bisson G, et al: Ascites and right pleural effusion: Demonstration of a peritoneo-pleural communication. J Nucl Med 27:1706, 1986.

51. Robinov K, Stein M, Frank H: Tension hydrothorax: An unrecognized danger. Thorax 21:465, 1966.

52. Bennett MR, Chaudhry RM, Owens GR: Elevated pleural fluid glucose: A risk for tension hydrothorax. South Med J 79:1287, 1986.

53. Shin MS, Rahn NH, Ho KJ: Tension hydrothorax: Roentenographic characteristics and pathogenetic consideration. South Med J 74:498, 1981.

54. Collins JD, Burwell D, Furmanski S, et al: Minimum detectable pleural effusions: A roentgen pathology model. Radiology 105:51, 1972.

55. Fishman NH: Thoracic Drainage: A Manual of Procedures. Chicago, Year Book Medical Publishers, Inc, 1983, pp 21–25.

56. Moskowitz H, Platt RT, Schachar R, et al: Roentgen visualization of minute pleural effusion. Radiology 109:33, 1973.

57. Hollerman JJ, Simms SM: The contralateral decubitus chest film. Ann Emerg Med 15:198, 1986.

58. Woodring JH: Recognition of pleural effusion on supine radiographs: How much fluid is required. AJR 142:59, 1984.

59. Kohan JM, Poe RH, Israel RH, et al: Value of chest ultrasonography versus decubitus roentgenography for thoracentesis. Am Rev Respir Dis 133:1124, 1986.

60. Maffessati M, Tommasi M, Pelligrini P: Computed tomography of free pleural effusion. Eur J Radiol 7:87, 1987.

61. Griffin DJ, Gross BH, McCracken S, et al: Observations on CT differentiation of pleural and peritoneal fluid. J Comput Assist Tomogr 8:24, 1984.

62. Federle MP, Mark AS, Guillaumin ES: CT of subpulmonic pleural effusions and atelectasis: Criteria for differentiation from subphrenic fluid. AJR 146:685, 1986.

63. Health and Public Policy Committee, American College of Physicians: Diagnostic thoracentesis and pleural biopsy in pleural effusions. Ann Intern Med 103:799, 1985.

64. Houston MC: Pleural fluid pH: Diagnostic, therapeutic and prognostic value. Am J Surg 154:333, 1987.

65. Brooke MP, Dupree DW: Bilateral traumatic chylothorax. Ann Emerg Med 17:69, 1988.

66. Gilmartin JJ, Wright AJ, Gibson GJ: Effects of pneumothorax or pleural effusion on pulmonary function. Thorax 40:60, 1985.

67. DeSouza R, Lipsett N, Spagnolo SV: Mediastinal compression due to tension hydrothorax. Chest 72:782, 1977.

68. Perpina M, Benllock E, Marco V, et al: Effect of thoracentesis on pulmonary gas exchange. Thorax 38:747, 1983.

69. Light RW, Stansbury DW, Brown SE: The relationship between pleural pressure and changes in pulmonary function after therapeutic thoracentesis. Am Rev Respir Dis 133:658, 1986.

70. Little AG, Ferguson MK, Golomb HM, et al: Pleuroperitoneal shunting for malignant pleural effusions. Cancer 48:2740, 1986.

71. Weil PH, Margolis IB: Systematic approach to traumatic hemothorax. Am J Surg 142:692, 1981.

72. Cordice JWV, Cabezon J: Chest trauma with pneumothorax and hemothorax. J Thorac Cardiovasc Surg 50:316, 1965.

73. Drummond DS, Craig RH: Traumatic hemothorax: Complications and management. Am Surg 33:403, 1967.

74. Shashy SS, Jones BC, Kitchens CS: Spontaneous hemothorax in a patient with Osler-Weber-Rendu disease. South Med J 78:1393, 1985.

75. Opperman HC, Wille L: Hemothorax in the newborn. Pediatr Radiol 9:129, 1980.

76. Wood RP, Tazkis A, Shaw BW, et al: A simplified technique for the treatment of simple pleural effusions. Surg Gynecol Obstet 164:283, 1987.

77. Sahn SA: Evaluation of pleural effusions and pleural biopsy. In Petty TL (ed): Pulmonary Diagnostic Techniques. Philadelphia, Lea & Febiger, 1975.

78. Stackhouse C: How to perform safe thoracentesis. Hospital Physician, October 1982, p 45.

79. O'Moore PV, Mueller PR, Simeone JF, et al: Sonographic guidance in diagnostic and therapeutic interventions in the pleural space. AJR 149:1. 1987.

80. Westcott JL: Percutaneous catheter drainage of pleural effusion and empyema. AJR 144:1189, 1985.

81. Velardocchio JM, Boutin C, Irisson M: Pleural pressure during thoracocentesis in patients with cancerous pleural effusion. Bull Eur Physiopathol Respir 20:61, 1984.

82. Clarke JM: A new instrument for thoracentesis. Surg Gynecol Obstet 159:587, 1984.

83. Cooper CMS: Pleural aspiration with a central venous catheter. Anaesthesia 42:217, 1987.

84. Sahn SA: The differential diagnosis of pleural effusions. West J Med 137:99, 1982.

85. Collins TR, Sahn SA: Thoracocentesis: Clinical value, complications, technical problems and patient experience. Chest 91:817, 1987.

86. Peterman TA, Speicher CE: Evaluating pleural effusions: A two-stage laboratory approach. JAMA 252:1051, 1984.

87. Light RW, MacGregor I, Ruchsinger PC, et al: The diagnostic separation of transudates and exudates. Ann Intern Med 77:507, 1972.

88. Light RW, Erozan YS, Ball WC: Cells in pleural fluid: Their value in differential diagnosis. Arch Intern Med 132:854, 1973.

89. Dines DE, Pierre RV, Franzen SJ: The value of cells in the pleural fluid in the differential diagnosis. Mayo Clin Proc 50:571, 1975.

90. Light RW, Ball WC: Glucose and amylase in pleural effusions. JAMA 225:257, 1973.

91. Salcedo JR: Urinothorax: Report of 4 cases and review of the literature. J Urol 135:805, 1986.

92. Stark DD, Shanes JG, Baron RL, et al: Biochemical features or urinothorax. Arch Intern Med 142:1509, 1982.

93. Gastrin B, Lovestad A: Diagnostic significance of pleural fluid lactate concentration in pleural and pulmonary diseases. Scand J Infect Dis 20:85, 1988.

94. Hamm H, Braham U, Bohmer R, et al: Cholesterol in pleural effusions: A diagnostic aid. Chest 92:296, 1987.
95. Yu VY, Lieu SW, Robertson NR: Pneumothorax in the newborn: Changing patterns. Arch Dis Child 50:449, 1975.
96. Kuban KCK, Leviton A, Brown ER, et al: Respiratory complications in low-birth-weight infants who received phenobarbital. Am J Dis Child 141:996, 1987.
97. Ryan CA, Barrington KJ, Phillips HJ, et al: Contralateral pneumothoraces in the newborn. Incidence and predisposing factors. Pediatrics 79:417, 1987.
98. Stern RC, Behrman RE: Diseases of the pleura. In Vaughan VC, Nelson WE (eds): Nelson Textbook of Pediatrics. 13th ed. Philadelphia, WB Saunders Co.
99. Scanlin TF: Cystic fibrosis. In Fleisher GR, Ludwig S (eds): Textbook of Pediatric Emergency Medicine. 2nd ed. Baltimore, Williams & Wilkins, 1988.
100. Athreya BH, Yancey CL, Eichenfield AH: Rheumatologic emergencies. In Fleisher GR, Ludwig S (eds): Textbook of Pediatric Emergency Medicine. 2nd ed. Baltimore, Williams & Wilkins, 1988.
101. Templeton JM: Thoracic emergencies. In Fleischer GR, Ludwig S (eds): Textbook of Pediatric Emergency Medicine. 2nd ed. Baltimore, Williams & Wilkins, 1988.
102. Hoffer FA, Albow RC: The cross-table lateral view in neonatal pneumothorax. AJR 142:1283, 1984.
103. Barkin RM, Rosen P (eds): Emergency Pediatrics: A Guide to Ambulatory Care. 3rd ed. St. Louis, CV Mosby Co, 1990.
104. Broennle AM, Gewitz MH, Flandler SD, et al: Illustrated techniques of pediatric emergency procedures. In Fleischer GR, Ludwig S (eds): Textbook of Pediatric Emergency Medicine. 2nd ed. Baltimore, Williams & Wilkins, 1988.
105. Ziskind MM, Weil H, George RA: Acute pulmonary edema following the treatment of spontaneous pneumothorax with excessive negative intrapleural pressure. Am Rev Respir Dis 92:632, 1965.
106. Murphy K, Tomlanovich MC: Unilateral pulmonary edema after drainage of a spontaneous pneumothorax: Case report and review of the world literature. J Emerg Med 1:29, 1983.
107. Trapnell DH, Thurston JGB: Unilateral pulmonary edema after pleural aspiration. Lancet 1:1367, 1970.
108. Bainton R, Mostafa SM: Re-expansion pulmonary edema: Slow decompression. Br J Anaesth 60:116, 1988.
109. Pavlin DJ, Raghu G, Rogers TR, et al: Reexpansion hypotension: A complication of rapid evacuation of prolonged pneumothorax. Chest 89:70, 1986.
110. Pavlin DJ, Nessly ML, Cheney FW: Hemodynamic effects of rapidly evacuating prolonged pneumothorax in rabbits. J Appl Physiol 62:477, 1987.
111. Branstetter RD, Cohen RP: Hypoxemia after thoracentesis: A predictable and treatable condition. JAMA 242:1060, 1979.
112. Brahams D: Perforation of the heart during attempt to drain pleural cavity. Lancet 2:586, 1986.
113. Sibbitt RR, Palmaz JC, Garcia F: A method for retrieval of retained subcutaneous catheter fragments. AJR 147:1017, 1986.
114. Grogan DR, Irwin RS, Channick R, et al: Complications associated with thoracentesis: A prospective, randomized study comparing three different methods. Arch Intern Med 150:873, 1990.

Chapter 9

Tube Thoracostomy

*Kenneth Frumkin
and Seth W. Wright*

INTRODUCTION

Tube thoracostomy is a commonly performed procedure that is used to evacuate an abnormal collection of air or fluid from the pleural space. Normally, the visceral and parietal pleurae are closely approximated. This potential space between the two layers is occupied by only a thin layer of fluid that acts as a lubricant. The addition of air, blood, or other fluids to this space disrupts the normal ventilatory mechanism, producing subjective dyspnea and interference with normal gas exchange. The amount of pulmonary and cardiovascular dysfunction is generally proportional to the amount of the abnormal collection and the rate at which it accumulates. Respiratory and cardiovascular embarrassment result from multiple mechanisms, including intrapulmonary shunting; mechanical compression of the mediastinum, the heart, and the great vessels; increased intrathoracic pressure; and altered diaphragmatic motion.[1]

Continuous intercostal drainage with a water seal for the treatment of empyema was described in the English literature by Playfair in 1872.[2] However, the technique was not widely performed until 1917 when it was used in treating postinfluenzal empyema.[3] It is believed that the increased use of such tubes as both initial and definitive treatment of wartime thoracic trauma led to much of the decrease in mortality from such injuries in battles following World War II.[4, 5] Today the procedure is used in individuals who have sustained penetrating chest trauma during violent crimes or blunt trauma in highway accidents. Tube thoracostomy is also used frequently in cases of spontaneous pneumothorax. Other indications are listed in Table 9–1.

INDICATIONS

Traumatic Pneumothorax, Hemothorax, or Hemopneumothorax

PATHOPHYSIOLOGY

Pneumothorax and hemopneumothorax are common after blunt or penetrating thoracic trauma. Pneumothorax alone occurs in 15 to 50 per cent of significant injuries resulting from blunt chest trauma and is usually attributed to lung puncture from a rib fracture. Following trauma, a definite rib fracture may not always be evident on radiographs. In the absence of fractures, pneumothorax is believed to result from rupture of an alveolus secondary to abrupt increases in intrathoracic and intra-alveolar pressures against a closed glottis. The air leak may be self-limited, or a ball-valve mechanism may lead to a tension pneumothorax (see later discussion).

Table 9–1. Indications for Tube Thoracostomy

Traumatic conditions
  Pneumothorax
  Hemothorax
  Hemopneumothorax
  Open pneumothorax
  Conditions requiring "prophylactic" surgical management
Iatrogenic complications (hemo- or pneumothorax) from
  Central venous line placement
  Thoracentesis
  Pleural biopsy
  Intercostal block
  Bronchoscopy
  Bronchoalveolar lavage
  Feeding tube placement
Spontaneous pneumothorax
Tension pneumothorax
Drainage of recurrent pleural effusion
Empyema
Chylothorax

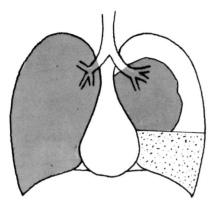

Figure 9–1. Hemopneumothorax. Note that the fluid level produces a straight line as opposed to a meniscus when a pneumothorax is present with the pleural fluid.

Air in the pleural space is not always secondary to primary lung pathology. Esophageal rupture and injuries to the tracheobronchial tree may also be responsible for pneumothorax and are often manifested by persistent air leaks or food particles in the thoracostomy tube drainage.[6] Penetrating injuries result in simple pneumothorax by allowing air to enter the chest, either through a persistent chest wall defect or by direct injury to underlying lung.

Hemothorax may result from bleeding from the heart, lungs, great vessels or their branches, intercostal arteries or veins, mediastinal veins, diaphragm, chest wall vessels, fractured ribs, or torn pulmonary adhesions. Bleeding from the lung parenchyma is usually self-limited because of the relatively low-pressure vascular supply of the lung and the high concentration of tissue thromboplastins. In addition, reexpansion of the collapsed lung generally tamponades the low-pressure bleeding sites. Partially severed intercostal arteries bleed particularly briskly, because all but the first two come directly from the aorta. In addition, the partially lacerated internal mammary artery will rarely cease bleeding without surgical intervention.

Diagnosis

Physical Examination. Alert patients with a pneumo-, hemo-, or hemopneumothorax may complain of chest pain, usually pleuritic in character, and shortness of breath. Pneumothorax alone may be manifested by increased resonance to percussion, decreased tactile fremitus, decreased or absent breath sounds, or subcutaneous emphysema. As a general rule, air in the subcutaneous tissues (subcutaneous emphysema) originates from an internal structure, such as lung, bronchi, or esophagus, and does not represent air introduced from the ambient environment because of a penetrating thoracic wound. With an isolated hemothorax, breath sounds will be decreased as well, but the percussion note is dull. A succussion splash has been described when air *and* fluid are both present. It is important to note that physical examination is often misleading, and many pneumothoraces may go undetected by physical examination alone.

Hemothorax alone may also be difficult to detect. Patients can rapidly lose 30 to 40 per cent of their blood volume into the pleural space with little resistance from the compliant lung. They may then present primarily with signs of shock.[7] The presence of shock in a patient with a chest injury should also raise the question of pericardial tamponade, which may not be manifested by distended neck veins in the hypovolemic patient (see Chapter 16). Evidence of

mediastinal shift or compression (distended neck veins, shifted trachea) may represent massive blood or fluid accumulation or, more likely, tension pneumothorax. In contrast, a small hemothorax (less than 400 ml) may produce few clinical findings. Physical findings of a hemothorax include dullness to percussion or loss of breath sounds at the lung base.

Radiographic Diagnosis. A standard, 6-foot posteroanterior (PA) upright chest radiograph is the diagnostic procedure of choice for hemo- or pneumothorax. A pneumothorax is diagnosed more readily on the *expiratory* x-ray because the lung collapses further. A pneumothorax may also be accentuated with a lateral decubitus film (unaffected side down, injured side up). One can often obtain a sitting (portable) 6-foot PA film in patients (who may require some assistance) by having them sit up and "hug" the x-ray plate to their chest. The machine is placed at the standard distance behind the patient. This view more closely approximates standard technique and allows a better evaluation of mediastinal size. Otherwise, anteroposterior (AP) films should be taken with the patient sitting in as erect a position as possible.

When one is interpreting a supine chest film, it is important to compare the relative densities of both lung fields. On a supine chest radiograph, even as much as 1000 ml of blood may be manifested only as a slight homogeneous increase in the density of one hemithorax. Up to 500 ml of blood may be required to produce blunting of the costophrenic angle on an upright film. Subpulmonic collections can resemble an elevated hemidiaphragm. Lateral decubitus films may be required to demonstrate either of these findings. If an air-fluid level (straight line to the top of the fluid collection), as opposed to a fluid meniscus, is seen, a pneumothorax must also be present (Fig. 9–1).

The size of the pneumothorax can be estimated by the method outlined in Figure 9–2.[8] The area of the collapsed lung is subtracted from the area of the involved hemithorax. One calculates the area of the collapsed lung in the figure, using the area of a rectangle drawn to include the extreme superior (*a*), lateral (*b*), and inferior (*c*) margins of the collapsed lung and the center of the mediastinum (*d*). One then subtracts this number from the area of a rectangle encompassing the entire affected hemithorax, measured

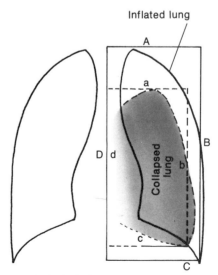

Figure 9–2. Method of calculating the area of a pneumothorax. [Area of hemithorax (A × B) − Area of collapsed lung (a × b)] ÷ Area of hemithorax (A × B).[44] The shaded area is the collapsed lung.

from the inferior border of the first rib *(A)*, the inner border of the midlateral chest wall *(B)*, the tip of the costophrenic angle *(C)*, and the center of the mediastinum *(D)*. One divides the difference between the area of the hemithorax and the area of the collapsed lung by the area of the hemithorax to yield the percentage of the pneumothorax.

Alternatively, the size of a pneumothorax can also be estimated by calculating the average interpleural distance as described in Figure 9–3.[9] The average interpleural distance is the mean of the maximal apical interpleural distance and the interpleural distances of the upper and lower lung fields. The average interpleural distance is then correlated with the percentage of the pneumothorax size by means of the nomogram in Figure 9–4.

A simpler way of monitoring the size of the pneumothorax involves measuring from the lateral lung margin to the lateral chest wall on full inspiration. It is important to have some easily reproducible means of repeatedly recording the size of a pneumothorax, particularly if the patient is to be examined by different physicians and management is to be based on serial measurements of pneumothorax size.

TREATMENT

In a patient in extremis with evidence of major thoracic trauma (subcutaneous emphysema, palpable rib fractures, flail chest), no further diagnostic studies need be undertaken. Needle aspiration may confirm the diagnosis but can be misleading or even cause a pneumothorax. If a tension pneumothorax is suspected, needle aspiration may be a temporary solution, but subsequent tube thoracostomy is indicated on the suspected side of injury. In the case of gunshot wounds or severe closed chest trauma, bilateral chest tubes may be required.

Tube thoracostomy allows egress of the fluid or air and provides a means of continuous drainage and monitoring of the pleural space. Further drainage can be quantified, and the need for other intervention can thus be assessed. Observation of the drainage and collection devices allows for the diagnosis of persistent air leak or other problems that may require additional treatment.

Small pneumothoraces and hemothoraces (less than 400

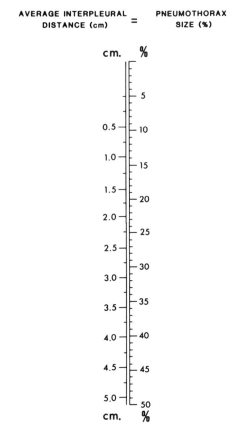

AVERAGE INTERPLEURAL DISTANCE (cm) = PNEUMOTHORAX SIZE (%)

Figure 9–4. Nomogram for the prediction of pneumothorax size from an average interpleural distance. (From Rhea JT, DeLuca SA, Greene RE: Determining the size of pneumothorax in the upright patient. Radiology 144:733, 1982.)

ml) have been treated with observation alone if the patient is relatively asymptomatic, otherwise healthy, and not likely to require positive-pressure ventilation. Resolution occurs in 10 to 14 days.[6] Patients with larger or more symptomatic traumatic hemo-, pneumo-, or hemopneumothoraces should have a thoracostomy tube placed.

A tube should be placed "prophylactically" in a patient with evidence of a penetrating injury to the chest even without demonstrable intrathoracic injury if anesthesia and positive-pressure ventilation are required or if the patient will be transported a long distance for definitive care of other injuries. Such patients are at high risk for developing a tension pneumothorax when subjected to positive airway pressures. They may also develop a simple or tension pneumothorax during transport when diagnostic adjuncts are suboptimal or definitive treatment may be difficult or impossible.

Early institution of blood replacement is recommended in patients with massive hemothorax (more than 2000 ml) before evacuation is begun. The blood in the chest may be functioning to tamponade a briskly bleeding vessel, and marked hypotension can result from precipitous evacuation without prior fluid resuscitation.[9, 10] A number of commercial devices are available for the collection, filtration, anticoagulation, and autotransfusion of blood obtained by tube thoracostomy (see Chapter 34). Autotransfusion is indicated in instances of massive hemothorax when such facilities are available.

Seventy-two to 82 per cent of patients with traumatic hemothorax can have their injuries managed successfully by tube thoracostomy and volume replacement alone.[5, 11, 12] In the remaining patients, immediate or delayed elective tho-

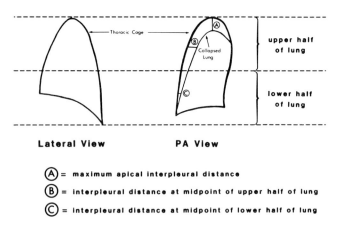

ⓐ = maximum apical interpleural distance

ⓑ = interpleural distance at midpoint of upper half of lung

ⓒ = interpleural distance at midpoint of lower half of lung

$$\text{Average Interpleural Distance} = \frac{A \cdot B \cdot C}{3}$$

Figure 9–3. Calculation of per cent pneumothorax using the average interpleural distance method. The base of the lung is not seen in the posteroanterior (PA) view. The total height of the PA view is assumed to be the same as that shown on the lateral view. (From Rhea JT, DeLuca SA, Greene RE: Determining the size of pneumothorax in the upright patient. Radiology 144:733, 1982.)

Table 9–2. Indications for Surgery After Tube Thoracostomy*

Massive hemothorax (more than 1000 ml)
Bleeding
    Rapid (more than 300 to 500 ml in first hour)
    Continued (more than 200 ml per hour for first 3 or more
      hours)
    Increasing size of hemothorax on chest film
Persistent hemothorax
    After two functioning tubes placed
    Clotted hemothorax
Large air leak preventing effective ventilation
Persistent air leak after placement of second tube or inability to
    expand lung fully
Documented bronchial injury
Ruptured esophagus
Ruptured diaphragm
Upper mediastinal entrance wound
Pericardial tamponade
Cardiac arrest; secondary to penetrating trauma
Great vessel injury
Cardiac injury
Open pneumothorax
Gross intrapleural contamination from a foreign body

*Data from references 5, 6, 7, 12, 40, 64.

racotomy may be required. There is disagreement among different researchers concerning the indications for surgery. Table 9–2 provides a summary of surgical indications.

Open Pneumothorax

Open pneumothorax ("sucking chest wound"; Fig. 9–5) most commonly results from shotgun or combat injuries with a loss of chest wall integrity. Such wounds can produce markedly deficient gas exchange and cardiovascular function when the negative intrapleural pressure is replaced with atmospheric pressure. If the chest wall defect is larger in cross-sectional area than the trachea, air will move preferentially through the chest wall with diaphragmatic excursions, and no ventilation will occur. With smaller defects, a tension pneumothorax (see subsequent discussion) may develop. Clinically, a chest wall defect and subcutaneous emphysema are seen in a patient with marked respiratory distress. Emergency (prehospital) treatment involves the application of a (preferably sterile) dressing to act as a one-way (flap) valve, allowing air to exit the pleural space while blocking reentry. In the field, anything (palm, plastic wrap, gauze) can be used. The patient is instructed to perform a Valsalva maneuver after deep inspiration or to cough just as the dressing is placed. Ideally, a sterile dressing of petrolatum-impregnated gauze extending 3 to 5 inches beyond the wound in all directions is used. This underlying dressing should be covered by gauze dressings and secured on *three* sides only. An airtight dressing could predispose to tension pneumothorax in the presence of a continued intrapleural air leak. This dressing may be sealed after tube thoracostomy through a separate site is performed to allow continued evacuation of air or fluid. The presence of the open wound is an indication for operative debridement and closure of the chest wall defect with continued tube drainage of the pleural space.[6, 9, 13]

Spontaneous Pneumothorax

PATHOPHYSIOLOGY

Spontaneous pneumothorax (Fig. 9–6) is the cause of one in every 1000 general hospital admissions and usually occurs in males less than 40 years of age.[14] Although as many as 40 per cent of affected patients do not have *known* underlying lung disease, the most common predisposing factor is emphysema.[15, 16] A Swedish study found that smoking is a major risk factor for spontaneous pneumothorax.[17] They determined that the life span risk of developing a spontaneous pneumothorax for heavy smokers is approximately 12 per cent, with a risk of only 1 in 1000 in people who have never smoked. Other associated potential etiologic factors are chronic bronchitis, asthma, tuberculosis, pneumonia, bronchiectasis, atelectasis, pulmonary fibrosis, lymphoma, trauma (exertion, cough, injuries), and various connective tissue diseases such as scleroderma or eosinophilic granuloma. Tuberous sclerosis, rupture of a hydatid cyst, pulmonary infarct, foreign body, and alpha$_1$-antitrypsin deficiency have all been implicated. Neoplasm is a consideration in older patients. Recurrent pneumothoraces attributed to pleural diagphragmatic endometriosis occur in some women at the time of menstruation.[14, 15, 18] Patients with acquired immune deficiency syndrome and *Pneumocystis carinii* pneumonia have also been found to be at increased risk for spontaneous pneumothorax.[19]

The rupture of an emphysematous bleb, an alveolar septum, or the bronchial wall causes air to flow freely into the pleural space. Seventy to 80 per cent of cases occur when

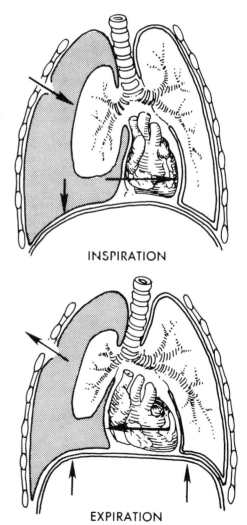

INSPIRATION

EXPIRATION

Figure 9–5. Simple open pneumothorax without tension. (Reproduced by permission from Vukich DJ, Markovchick VJ: Pulmonary and chest wall injuries. In Rosen P, et al (eds): Emergency Medicine: Concepts and Clinical Practice. St Louis, CV Mosby Co, 1988.)

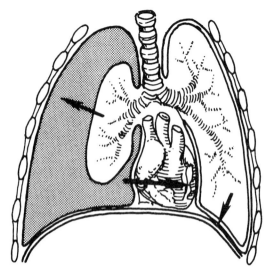

Figure 9–6. Simple closed spontaneous pneumothorax. (Reproduced by permission from Vukich DJ, Markovchick VJ: Pulmonary and chest wall injuries. In Rosen P, et al (eds): Emergency Medicine: Concepts and Clinical Practice. St Louis, CV Mosby Co, 1988.)

the patients are at rest; and 70 per cent of affected individuals seek medical attention within 24 hours of onset. Five to 7 per cent of cases are bilateral. The symptoms correlate with the amount of collapse, the mobility of the mediastinum, the amount of respiratory reserve, the presence of underlying disease, and the degree of compression of the rest of the lung.

DIAGNOSIS

Almost all patients with a spontaneous pneumothorax (95 per cent) complain of chest or shoulder (or, rarely, back or abdominal) pain that is usually sudden in onset, sharp, pleuritic, and cutting. Tightness may be described. Sixty per cent have dyspnea in addition to these symptoms, and 12 per cent have a mild cough.[18] Breathlessness and anxiety are more common in older patients, and the morbidity and mortality are increased in patients with underlying disease.[20] Half may attribute the onset of pain to a sudden mild exertion (cough, sneeze) or trauma. Varying degrees of respiratory distress may be manifested. Subcutaneous emphysema rarely occurs. Decreased breath sounds, decreased tactile fremitus, and hyperresonance to percussion may be noted in an uncomplicated spontaneous pneumothorax, although the physical examination may reveal no abnormalities if the pneumothorax is small.

The diagnosis is made on a standard upright PA chest film. Small pneumothoraces are best seen by radiography with the patient in full expiration. During expiration, the volume of air in the pleural space remains the same, but the expiratory decrease in the volume of the collapsed lung on the affected side increases the apparent relative size of the pneumothorax. A lateral film helps rule out complications (see later discussion) and may help define the etiology when the pneumothorax is secondary to some other intrathoracic pathology. In pediatric patients or in those who are uncooperative for other reasons, radiographs in both decubitus positions may successfully demonstrate a small pneumothorax. If the patient is placed in the lateral decubitus position with the affected side up, air will collect in the uppermost portion of the pleural space, and the pneumothorax may be more perceptible.

In the patient with chest pain, pneumothorax must be differentiated from myocardial infarction, dissecting aneurysm, pericarditis, pneumonia, pulmonary embolus, spontaneous esophageal rupture, perforated peptic ulcer, and biliary or renal colic. Radiographically, giant bullae or lung cysts may mimic a pneumothorax and these must be carefully differentiated, occasionally with tomography.

TREATMENT

The treatment varies with the age of the patient, the symptoms, the degree of respiratory compromise, the bilaterality, the need for general anesthesia, the size of the pneumothorax, and whether the current episode represents a recurrence. From a purely physiologic viewpoint, all patients with a pneumothorax do not automatically require pleural space aspiration. However, exactly when to treat becomes a clinical judgment issue, and compliance, the need for close follow-up, or other mitigating circumstances may be such that placing a chest tube is the safest and most expedient course. Otherwise healthy and asymptomatic patients with small (less than 10 per cent or less than 1 cm collapse laterally) pneumothoraces may be treated by observation alone. A period of hospital observation (with the length depending on the amount of time the pneumothorax has been present) is recommended to ensure that the pneumothorax is not expanding. Reexpansion is estimated to occur at 1.25 per cent of lung volume daily.[8] Affected patients must be instructed to return immediately if symptoms increase, to minimize their activities, and to have follow-up chest films to document resolution. Needle or catheter aspiration of a pneumothorax has been advocated by some and has had a variable degree of success.[21–32] Needle aspiration does carry a slight chance of increasing the size of the pneumothorax if the lung is punctured. Traditional therapy of a spontaneous pneumothorax is tube thoracostomy and water seal drainage with or without the addition of suction. The tube evacuates the intrapleural air, prevents further accumulation, and allows monitoring for persistent air leaks. The local irritation of the tube is believed to aid in scar formation and in preventing recurrence. The tube is left for 24 hours after all evidence of continued air leak has disappeared.

A number of investigators have reported successful outpatient management of chest tubes in 74 to 88 per cent of their patients with spontaneous pneumothorax.[33–36] Stable patients are selected; these individuals should be free of significant underlying disease or persistent air leaks and should have satisfactory lung reexpansion after 1 to 12 hours of observation in the emergency department. They are sent home with a flutter (Heimlich) valve attached and are seen 3 to 4 days later for tube removal if complete reexpansion is maintained.

Surgical treatment (usually thoracotomy with abrasion of pleural surfaces) is advocated at the time of the first or second recurrence.[14] Patients who have had one pneumothorax have a 30 to 50 per cent chance of ipsilateral recurrence within 1 to 2 years. After a second spontaneous pneumothorax, the probability of a third rises to 50 to 80 per cent.[15, 18, 37] Surgery may be recommended on the occasion of a patient's first pneumothorax in a number of situations: life-threatening tension pneumothorax, massive air leaks with incomplete reexpansion, an air leak persisting 4 to 5 days after a second intercostal tube has been placed, associated hemothorax with complications (see later discussion), cases of identifiable bullous disease, and failure of easy reexpansion in patients with cystic fibrosis.[15, 38]

Tension Pneumothorax

ETIOLOGY

Tension pneumothorax (Fig. 9–7) may be a complication of both spontaneous pneumothorax and traumatic hemopneumothorax. Rarely, a pneumothorax that has been stable for a number of days will rapidly develop tension. Fractures of the trachea or the bronchi, the presence of an occlusive dressing over an open pneumothorax, or a ruptured esophagus may also result in tension pneumothorax. The risk is markedly increased in patients with chest trauma undergoing positive-pressure ventilation. Because of this, a patient with penetrating thoracic injury (even without immediate evidence of intrathoracic bleeding or air) may be a candidate for "prophylactic" chest tube placed before surgery. A "tension *hemo*thorax" does not occur in the absence of massive fluid replacement, because the volume of blood required to produce a shift of mediastinal structures requires nearly total exsanguination into the chest.

PATHOPHYSIOLOGY

Classically, a pulmonary parenchymal or bronchial tear creates a ball-valve mechanism. The increased endobronchial

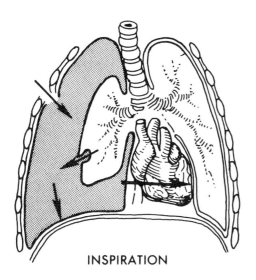

INSPIRATION

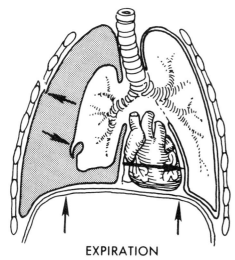

EXPIRATION

Figure 9–7. Tension pneumothorax. (Reproduced by permission from Vukich DJ, Markovchick VJ: Pulmonary and chest wall injuries. In Rosen P, et al (eds): Emergency Medicine: Concepts and Clinical Practice. St Louis, CV Mosby Co, 1988.)

diameter and intrathoracic negative pressure during inspiration allow air to pass into the pleural space. The decrease in bronchial diameter and the relatively elevated intrathoracic pressure during expiration cause the leak to close. This mechanism traps increasing amounts of air in the pleural space with each respiratory cycle. As intrapleural pressure rises, venous return to the right heart declines and cardiac output drops. The mediastinum shifts toward the uninvolved side, mechanically interfering with right atrial filling. Ventilation of both the involved lung and the opposite lung is compromised, and hypoxemia or acidosis, or both, result from ventilation-perfusion inequalities. Tension pneumothorax may develop at any time after injury, during resuscitation, or with cardiopulmonary resuscitation (CPR). It should be considered as a possible cause for deterioration in any susceptible patient, particularly if positive-pressure ventilation is being used.

DIAGNOSIS

Clinically, patients with tension pneumothorax may present with or rapidly develop restlessness, dyspnea, agitation, or cyanosis. Hypotension, tachypnea, tachycardia, nasal flaring, and retractions may occur. Pulsus paradoxus may be evident. There is hyperresonance to percussion and decreased breath sounds on the affected side. Obvious chest trauma, rib fractures, or subcutaneous emphysema should alert one to the possibility of tension pneumothorax. The trachea and the cardiac apex are displaced toward the uninvolved side. Neck veins may be distended but can be flat in the hypovolemic patient. The prominent, fixed, and overinflated hemithorax may be obvious when the semisitting patient is inspected from the head or the foot of the bed.[35] Increased airway resistance in an intubated patient (one of the first signs of a tension pneumothorax) may be manifested by increased difficulty in manual ventilation or increased ventilatory pressures when a volume-cycled respirator is used. If there is time, a chest radiograph that shows a depressed hemidiaphragm and lung collapse on the affected side with a shift of the mediastinum to the opposite side is confirmatory.

Pericardial tamponade figures strongly in the differential diagnosis and should be considered in the trauma patient when mediastinal shift, hyperresonance, and decreased breath sounds are not prominent clinical features or when needle aspiration of the hemithorax fails to bring prompt relief.

TREATMENT

If the patient is in extremis and the diagnosis is suspected clinically, needle aspiration of the involved side should be undertaken without further delay (see Chapter 8). Even if no facilities are available for chest tube placement, a large needle inserted into the chest to convert a tension pneumothorax to an open pneumothorax can be life saving. A 14-gauge needle is commonly placed in the second anterior intercostal space but is effective anywhere in the pleural space. A temporary flutter valve may be fashioned from the fingers of a rubber surgical glove until definitive treatment is available. The definitive treatment of a tension pneumothorax is tube thoracostomy.

Other Indications

DRAINAGE OF RECURRENT PLEURAL EFFUSIONS

Initially, most pleural effusions can be managed by thoracentesis (see Chapter 8), but recurrent effusions may require tube thoracostomy.

EMPYEMA

Empyema was one of the first recorded indications for continuous intercostal drainage in adults[39] and children[2] and remains a prominent one today.

CHYLOTHORAX

Chylothorax can be a rare complication of thoracic trauma. It may result directly from penetrating injury or from a fall from a height. Chyle will collect extrapleurally, and 2 to 10 days may elapse before it enters the pleural cavity. Initially, the few clinical manifestations may be masked by other injuries. As fluid accumulates in large amounts, dyspnea and the physical findings of a pleural effusion become prominent. Thoracentesis reveals a milky white liquid with a high lymphocyte count, 4 to 5 gm/dl of protein, and a high fat content. Repeated thoracentesis or tube thoracostomy is combined with bed rest and parenteral alimentation until the volume of chyle declines.[6]

POSTOPERATIVE THORACOTOMY

Chest tubes are nearly always placed under direct vision when open thoracotomy is performed.

CONTRAINDICATIONS

A list of contraindications may be found in Table 9–3. There are probably no absolute contraindications in the compromised patient who requires the procedure, although some relative contraindications exist. Multiple pleural adhesions, emphysematous blebs, and scarring should mandate caution in a stable patient. *It is important to note that a giant emphysematous bleb or bulla in adults and congenital lobar emphysema in infants may be extremely difficult to differentiate from a pneumothorax on chest films.* A second or third spontaneous pneumothorax in a stable patient may be an indication to proceed directly to surgery instead of attempting another tube thoracostomy. A patient requiring immediate open thoracotomy (i.e., in the case of cardiac arrest after penetrating trauma) may not benefit from chest tube placement. The presence of a massive hemothorax usually requires rapid blood or crystalloid replacement with or without immediate surgery. Tube thoracostomy before fluid replacement is believed by some to promote further bleeding.[9, 40] Treatment of respiratory distress because of a massive hemothorax, however, must take precedence over the theoretic risk of aggravating bleeding by immediate institution of chest tube drainage. The setting of bleeding dyscrasias before clotting factor replacement may be a relative contraindication.

EQUIPMENT

Instruments

The instruments required for performing tube thoracostomy by the method detailed below are listed in Table 9–

Table 9–3. Relative Contraindications to Tube Thoracostomy

Multiple adhesions, blebs
Recurrent pneumothorax mandating surgical treatment
Need for immediate open thoracotomy
Massive hemothorax without adequate volume replacement
Bleeding dyscrasia

Table 9–4. Instrument Tray for Tube Thoracostomy

Preparation razor
Sterile towels—4
Basin for preparation solution
Gauze pads
Towel clips (optional)—4
10- to 20-ml syringe and assorted needles for infiltration of local anesthetic
Medicine cup for local anesthetic
Large, straight (suture) scissors
Large, curved (Mayo) scissors
Large clamps (Kelly)—2
Medium clamps (Kelly)—2 to 4
Needle holder
Number 0 or 1–0 silk on large cutting needles—several
Knife handle #4—1
Number 10 scalpel blades
Forceps

4. Prepared "trays" are available in hospitals and often contain many more instruments than are required or described here. In addition to the instruments, a number of other materials are needed; these are listed in Table 9–5. All the necessary items should be assembled and tested before the start of the procedure. If the tape is torn as desired, the solutions are poured, the packages are opened, and a check list (mental or written) is reviewed before beginning, the procedure will go much more smoothly.

Chest Tubes

The size, shape, and characteristics of tubes used for thoracostomy vary considerably. The most commonly used devices are clear plastic straight tubes (Argyle) with a series of holes at one end. They have a radiopaque strip that is commonly interrupted by the last fenestration. Angled (90 degrees) tubes are also available. A wide variety of soft rubber tubes (including Malecot, de Pezzer, and Foley catheters) have been used, most commonly for simple pneumothoraces. They are particularly useful for second anterior intercostal space placement, in which the fenestrated segment of the standard tubes may be too long and may project outside the skin. Sizes used for adults have varied from 12 to 42 French. Most authorities believe that 20 to 32 French is adequate for a pneumothorax alone, although small catheters (8 French) have been suggested, especially if the patient is to be treated and released. Larger tubes (a minimum of

Table 9–5. Other Materials Required for Tube Thoracostomy

Local anesthetic
Antiseptic solution
Arm restraints (padded)
Vaseline-impregnated gauze
Tincture of benzoin
Adhesive tape—cloth-backed
Chest tubes
   28 to 36 French for adults
   16, 20, 24 French for children
   Right-angled tubes (36 French)
Plastic tubing—clear, sterile in 6-foot lengths; ½-inch diameter
Hard plastic serrated connectors
Drainage apparatus with sterile water for water seal
High-flow, high-volume regulated suction pump (Emerson)
Y connectors

36 French) are best when blood or pus is to be drained. It is a mistake to attempt to drain a hemothorax with a small chest tube. For pediatric patients, 16, 20, and 24 French tubes are adequate.[41] The right-angled tubes are used in various ways—most often to fit in the posterior costophrenic sulcus when a single straight tube fails to drain a dependent fluid accumulation adequately.

PROCEDURE

The ideal procedure performed under ideal circumstances is described. The degree of urgency as determined by the patient's condition and the available resources will dictate how closely to the ideal any one chest tube insertion will come. Under the best circumstances, the diagnosis should be established before the procedure and the appropriate radiographs should be taken. The preferred films are upright PA and lateral chest radiographs. The nature and necessity of the procedure should be explained to the patient as completely as possible, and (preferably) informed consent should be obtained and documented.

Tube Location

The classic approach has always been to place tubes anteriorly in the second intercostal space, midclavicular line (usually 2 inches from the lateral border of the sternum) for pneumothorax alone, and dependently in the mid- or posterior axillary line and directed posteriorly for fluid removal (Fig. 9–8). *In an emergency, a tube placed anywhere in the pleural space should be adequate.* The second intercostal space is nearly always mentioned as a location for tube placement but in practice is less often used. Disadvantages include the need to dissect through several inches of muscle mass and the resulting unsightly and highly visible scar, which is particularly undesirable in women. Some sources have advocated using the lateral insertion for women but retaining the anterior site for men.[34]

Some investigators have suggested avoiding the second intercostal space entirely and recommend a midaxillary line placement for all indications. It is cosmetically preferable and better tolerated and is believed to result in increased pleural involvement and scarring.[15, 38] If the tube is placed slightly anteriorly, the patients may lie on their backs more comfortably. Gill and Long have stated, however, that the "practice of attempting to drain both air and fluid through a single tube inserted in the mid-axillary line has been unsatisfactory and often leads to multiple tube insertions and reinsertions."[42] Hegarty randomly placed tubes in either the second intercostal space, midclavicular line or the fifth intercostal space, midaxillary line in 131 cases of pneumo- or combined hemopneumothorax. He found that the time of removal of the tube was not influenced by location, regardless of whether air, blood, or both were being drained.[43] Duponselle studied 156 randomly placed chest tubes and found no unsatisfactory results with pneumothorax regardless of tube position.[44] Logically, as the collapsed lung expands and the parietal and visceral pleurae become more tightly opposed, either air or fluid will follow the path of least resistance and will enter a functioning drainage tube, regardless of its location. Although some clots may remain in the pleural space because of brisk bleeding and rapid clotting, Broadie and coworkers[45] demonstrated that blood that is drained from the chest cavity has no demonstrable fibrinogen and is thus *incoagulable.* Therefore, a tube anywhere in the pleural space should adequately drain a hemothorax of unclotted blood, as long as there are no adhesions.

Specific recommendations for lateral placement have varied from anterior to posterior axillary lines and from the fourth to the eighth intercostal space. If time permits and the physician who will subsequently be caring for the patient can be consulted, his or her preference should be followed. For all indications for "routine" placement in the emergency department, the fourth or fifth intercostal space slightly anterior to the midaxillary line is suggested for chest tube placement. This is roughly at the level of the nipple or the inferior scapular border in most patients. The tube is directed posteriorly and toward the apex of the lung. This has proved satisfactory for drainage of either fluid or air. If fluid continues to accumulate, a second tube may be placed in the posterior axillary line at the same interspace or one interspace lower. Obviously, the location of the diaphragm varies with the position of the patient and can rise quite high when the patient is supine. The phase of respiration and other associated injuries (diaphragmatic hernia, abdominal distention) can also alter its position. The most reliable means of preventing inadvertent damage to lung or abdominal viscera is a thorough digital exploration of the pleura before tube insertion. If the patient breathes during this procedure, the location of the diaphragm can often be verified and intrapleural placement can be ensured.

Tube Insertion

PATIENT PREPARATION

For axillary insertions, the patient is ideally placed with the head of the bed elevated 30 to 60 degrees (Fig. 9–9). Inserting a chest tube while the patient is lying flat increases the chances of injury to the diaphragm, the spleen, or the liver and presents a more difficult operating position for the practitioner. When the patient is lying down, the diaphragm may rise as high as the third intercostal space. The arm on the affected side is placed over the patient's head and restrained in that position with wide strips of adhesive tape or by other means. The other arm can be restrained comfortably at the patient's side. (Even in the conscious and seemingly cooperative patient, judicious use of comfortable restraints before painful or frightening procedures often allows more rapid and efficient completion.) For anterior midclavicular line placements, the patient's arms may be placed at the sides.

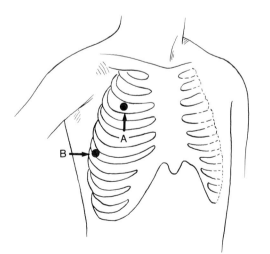

Figure 9–8. Standard sites for tube thoracostomy. *A,* Second intercostal space, midclavicular line. *B,* Fifth intercostal space, midaxillary line.

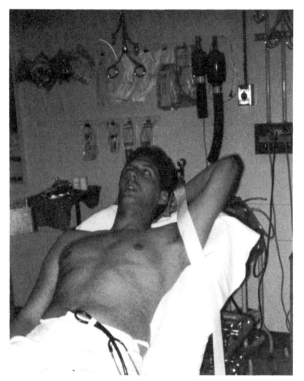

Figure 9–9. Position of the patient for axillary chest tube insertions. Whenever possible, the patient should be semi-erect at a 30- to 60-degree angle.

After identifying the area of tube placement, the surrounding skin should be shaved if necessary. The area is sterilized with a povidone-iodine solution or another suitable antiseptic and draped with sterile towels. Nasal oxygen may be helpful for the patient with subjective dyspnea.

ANESTHESIA

A local anesthetic should be used generously; *careful anesthesia can render the procedure nearly painless* (Fig. 9–10). One half to 1 per cent lidocaine (Xylocaine) with epinephrine (1:100,000) is most commonly used. The maximum dose of 5 mg/kg should not be exceeded.[46] A skin wheal should be raised with a 25- to 26-gauge short (½- to ⅝-inch) needle

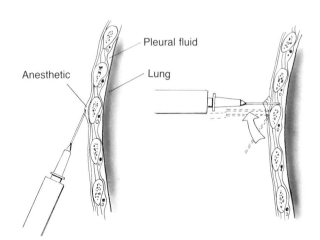

Figure 9–10. Infiltration of the skin and pleura with local anesthetic. (Redrawn from Hughes WT, Buescher ES: Pediatric Procedures. 2nd ed. Philadelphia, WB Saunders Co, 1980, p 234.)

in the area of the skin incision. Many physicians advocate locating the skin wound one intercostal space below the one through which the tube will pass. The "tunneling" up and over the next rib that is required if this is to be done is believed to provide a better seal against air leaks both while the tube is in place and during and after its removal (Fig. 9–11). A larger (23-gauge, 1½-inch) needle is used to infiltrate the subcutaneous tissues, the muscle, the periosteum, and the parietal pleura in the areas through which the tube will pass. The sterile syringe should be kept readily available because further anesthesia is often required. *A common error is inadequate local anesthesia.* Intercostal nerve (rib) blocks above and below the incision and insertion rib spaces are also helpful. The anesthetic needle and syringe should be used to aspirate the pleural cavity in the area of insertion (Fig. 9–12). If air or fluid is not obtained and the patient's condition is stable, the diagnostic evaluation may need to be repeated or the insertion site changed. This simple and extremely useful technique to verify the location and the character of the intrapleural accumulation is often forgotten.

Intravenous analgesia and sedation should be considered for the hemodynamically stable patient. Many practi-

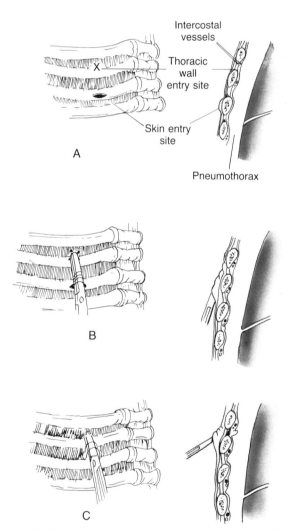

Figure 9–11. The skin wound is made one intercostal space below the space through which the tube will pass (A). Blunt dissection is carried subcutaneously (B) and into the pleural space (C). A common error in technique is to attempt to insert a large chest tube through a skin incision that is too small. (Redrawn from Hughes WT, Buescher ES: Pediatric Procedures. 2nd ed. Philadelphia, WB Saunders Co, 1980, p 237.)

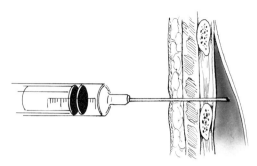

Figure 9–12. Use of the anesthetic needle to puncture the pleura and establish the presence of blood or air in the pleural space. This procedure not only is diagnostic but also may be a *temporary* therapeutic maneuver in a tension pneumothorax. (Redrawn from Richards V: Tube thoracostomy. J Fam Pract 6:631, 1978.)

tioners advocate the careful use of a narcotic combined with a benzodiazepine for pain control, sedation, and amnesia. Careful dosing and slow titration to the desired clinical effect are mandatory when these potent agents are used. In elective situations, 2 to 3 μg/kg of the short-acting narcotic fentanyl, either alone or supplemented with 1 to 3 mg of the amnestic short-acting benzodiazepine midazolam is helpful. Once the tube is in place, intramuscular meperidine can be used for long-term pain relief.

INSERTION

One measures the length of the tube to be inserted by holding it near the chest wall. The distance from the incision site to the apex of the lung is estimated, and a clamp is placed on the tube at the point at which it should enter the chest wall. This position must be proximal enough from the last drainage hole to ensure that all holes are within the pleural space. The beveled end of the tube is often cut squarely at this time so that it better fits the commonly available connectors.

A *generous* 2- to 4-cm transverse skin incision is made through the skin and the subcutaneous tissues directly over the rib one interspace beneath the rib the tube will pass over. *It is a common error to attempt to place a chest tube through an incision of inadequate size.* This incision is extended by *blunt* dissection to the fascia overlying the intercostal muscles. A scalpel is needed *only* to make the skin incision. Care must be taken to avoid the intercostal vessels and the nerve located on the inferior margin of each rib (Fig. 9–13). One uses a large Kelly clamp to tunnel superiorly through the subcutaneous tissues over the rib above, pushing forward with the closed points and then spreading and pulling back with the points spread (see Fig. 9–11). Some physicians used a curved Mayo scissors in the same manner as a Kelly clamp as a blunt dissecting instrument. The closed points of the heavy clamp are then pushed with some force through the muscles, and the parietal pleura immediately overlying the rib and the pleural cavity is entered. A twisting or drilling motion will enhance pleural penetration. A rush of air or fluid should occur at this point. If pleural fluid is under enough pressure it may be expelled with considerable force and cover the unwary (and subsequently embarrassed) practitioner with blood or pus. Appropriate gown, glove, and goggle precautions should be observed by the practitioner as well. The tips of the clamp, still within the pleural cavity are spread widely and withdrawn (Fig. 9–14). One must be certain to make an adequate opening in the pleura.

Next is one of the most important parts of the procedure: *the insertion of a gloved finger into the chest to verify that*

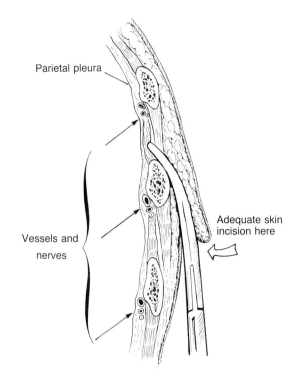

Figure 9–13. Location of the intercostal neurovascular bundle. (From Millikan JS, et al: Complications of tube thoracostomy for acute trauma. Am J Surg 140:739, 1980.)

the pleura has been entered and that pleural adhesions are absent. The finger should sweep completely around the hole in the chest wall. Dense adhesions may mandate an alternative site for tube placement. The finger is left in the pleural space. The tube is then grasped with the curved clamp, with the tube tip protruding from the jaws (Fig. 9–15). (Another technique is to pass one jaw of the clamp inside the tube through a distal fenestration.) *With the finger in the chest cavity as a guide,* the tip is placed into the pleural space (Fig. 9–

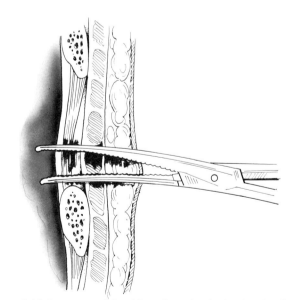

Figure 9–14. One accomplishes blunt dissection by forcing the closed points of the clamp forward and then spreading the tips and pulling back with the points spread. One must be certain to make an adequate opening in the parietal pleura. (From Bricker DL: Safe, effective tube thoracostomy. E.R. Reports 2:49, 1981.)

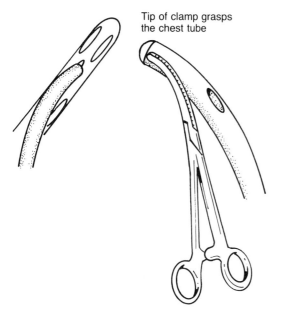

Tip of clamp grasps
the chest tube

Figure 9–15. The tube is grasped with the curved clamp, with the tube tip protruding from the jaws.

16). The finger is used to verify intrapleural placement of the chest tube. The curve in the clamp is used to guide the tip superiorly and posteriorly. The clamp is released, and the tube is pushed superiorly, medially, and posteriorly until marker clamp that was previously attached to measure the insertion distance touches the chest wall. All the holes in the chest tube *must* be within the pleural space. A common error, especially in obese patients, is to fail to advance the chest tube far enough into the pleural space, leaving the drainage holes either in the subcutaneous tissues or outside the skin.

Alternatively, the tube may be advanced until pain is

felt or until resistance is met and then pulled back 2 to 3 cm. It is surprisingly easy to misdirect the chest tube even though the pleural space has been opened. Subcutaneous placement is a frequent complication, and dissection of tissue planes in the chest wall by an advancing chest tube can simulate entry into the chest cavity (Fig. 9–17). Therefore, following placement a finger is again inserted if possible to verify that the tube has entered the pleural space. Entry into the thoracic cavity is suggested by the appearance of condensation on the inside of the tube coincident with respiratory movements, the audible movement of air through the tube during respiration, the free flow of blood or fluid, and the ability of the operator to rotate the tube freely after insertion. The tube is attached to the previously assembled water seal or suction set-up by means of a sterile serrated connector before the clamp is released. Asking the patient to cough and observing bubbles in the water seal device is a good way to check system patency.

SECURING THE TUBE

Before elaborate steps are taken to secure the tube, be certain that the chest tube position is verified on a chest film. There are as many ways of fastening a chest tube in place as there are physicians who place the device. More important than the individual technique chosen is the need to communicate the method used effectively to the person who will be caring for the patient, particularly the one who will be removing the tube. A reasonable approach is as follows: A number 0 or 1-0 silk suture on a cutting needle is used. Flimsy suture material, such as size 3-0 or finer, should be avoided. The first suture is placed next to the tube to close the lateral margin of the skin incision and is tied firmly (Fig. 9–18). The ends of this suture are left long, and these are then tied repeatedly around the chest tube and knotted securely to hold it in place. The sutures must be tied tightly enough to indent the chest tube slightly to avoid slippage (Fig. 9–19). A horizontal mattress suture is then placed around the tube approximately 1 cm across the incision on either side of the tube (Fig. 9–20). This will be used to close the incision after the tube is removed. No knots are tied

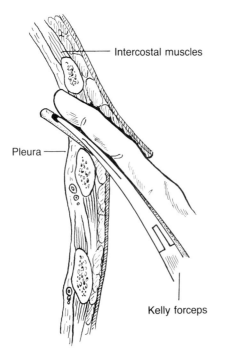

Intercostal muscles

Pleura

Kelly forceps

Figure 9–16. Using the finger as a guide, one places the tip into the pleural cavity. (From Millikan JS, et al: Complications of tube thoracostomy for acute trauma. Am J Surg 140:739, 1980.)

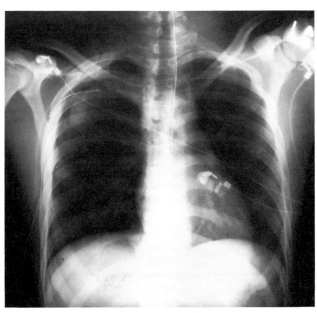

Figure 9–17. Subcutaneous placement of a chest tube. The incorrect placement was not appreciated until the radiograph was taken.

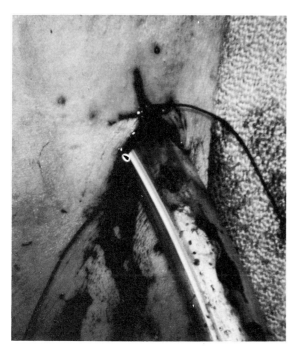

Figure 9–18. A suture is placed next to the tube to close the skin incision. The ends are left long.

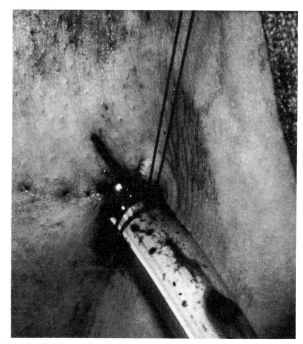

Figure 9–19. The ends of the suture are wound twice about the tube tightly enough to indent the tube slightly and are tied securely.

initially, but the skin should be pulled snugly together and held with a surgeon's knot (double throw). The loose ends are repeatedly wound tightly around the chest tube as it enters the skin with occasional repeated surgeon's knots tied tightly enough to indent the tube gently. The final knot is a bow, which should clearly identify the suture as one not to be cut.

An occlusive dressing of Vaseline-impregnated gauze

should be placed where the tube enters the skin. Overlying this should be two or more gauze pads with a Y-shaped cut from the middle of one side to the center. These are oriented at 90 degrees to each other (Fig. 9–21). The shaved skin and the tube may be coated with tincture of benzoin and wide (3-inch) cloth adhesive tape used to hold the tube more securely in place. Two strips of tape applied with an "elephant-ear" technique at 90 degrees to each other provide

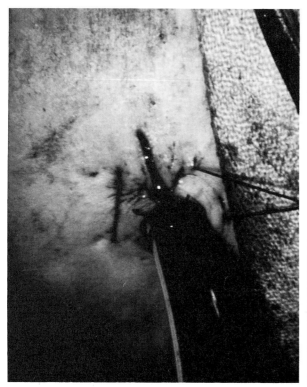

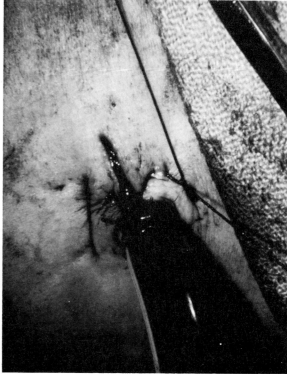

Figure 9–20. A horizontal mattress suture is placed around the tube and is held only with a surgeon's knot.

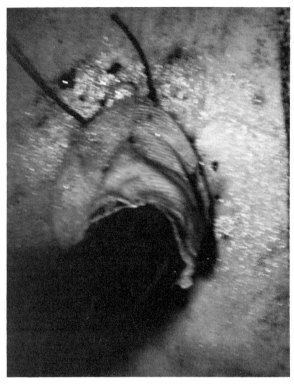

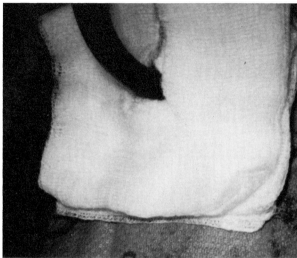

Figure 9–21. A dressing consisting of Vaseline-impregnated gauze and gauze sponges is applied to the entry site.

an excellent method of securing the tube in place (Fig. 9–22). The tape is torn so that one end is split into three pieces extending halfway to the center. The two outside pieces are placed on the skin on either side of the tube site, and the center piece is wrapped tightly around the tube. This is repeated with a second piece of tape, which is torn similarly and placed at 90 degrees to the first. A third simple piece of tape may be used elsewhere on the chest to prevent the tube from being pulled loose accidentally. The connections are then securely taped.

Confirmation of Tube Placement

Repeat PA (and occasionally a lateral) radiographs must be taken to confirm tube placement and to document the degree of resolution. In a stable patient, it is often better to obtain the postprocedure films with a less elaborate temporary dressing in place, in case tube repositioning is required. It is important to note that a simple pneumothorax should be completely reexpanded within a few minutes of continual suction. If the film taken following chest tube insertion shows that the lung is still collapsed, one should consider

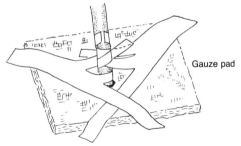

Gauze pad

Figure 9–22. The tube is secured with two strips of wide adhesive tape. (Redrawn from Suratt PM, Gibson RS: Manual of Medical Procedures. St. Louis, CV Mosby Co, 1982.)

three possibilities: (1) The tube may be in the wrong place or the proximal hole is outside the chest cavity. (This is the most easily corrected problem.) (2) A persistent air leak, usually from a large bronchus or the trachea, may be delaying expansion. (3) Plugging of a main bronchus with blood, mucus, or aspirated material may be delaying resolution of the pneumothorax.

Drainage System

Physicians who place chest tubes infrequently or who do not participate in the ongoing care of patients who have undergone this procedure may have little familiarity with the physiology and mechanics of chest tube drainage systems. Life-threatening complications may arise from improper use of these devices, however, and the physician must be knowledgeable about the salient features of the system.

With the availability of modern closed drainage systems, the classic glass bottle collection system is rather cumbersome and largely antiquated. Nevertheless, the principles of the various drainage systems are discussed here. The simplest drainage device is a flutter (Heimlich) valve (commonly used only for pneumothorax) attached to the end of the chest tube itself (Fig. 9–23). Such valves allow one-way flow of air from the chest but collapse to prevent air from passing back into the chest. Normal respiration (assisted by coughing) gradually removes the excess air from the pleural space, and the lung reexpands to fill the thoracic cage. The one-way Heimlich valve does not require a suction source when its purpose is the drainage of a pneumothorax. Therefore, it can be used in the treatment of outpatients. This valve is not generally used in conjunction with a closed suction-driven collection system to drain a hemothorax because backflow is not a problem during continuous suction.

The simplest device to remove small amounts of either fluid or air is the underwater seal (single-bottle) device (Fig. 9–24). The chest tube is connected to a second plastic tube, which runs into a closed glass or plastic container. The tube

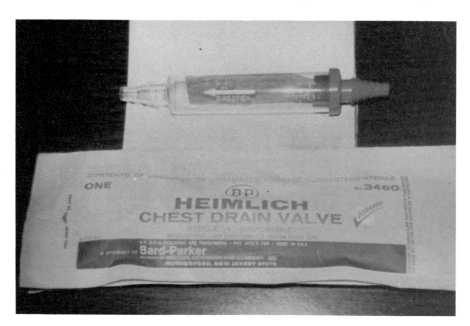

Figure 9–23. Heimlich valve.

extends 2 to 4 cm below the surface of the (sterile) water placed in the drainage bottle. The water provides a "seal" against the entering of further air into the chest. The water also acts as a one-way valve. The intrathoracic pressure need only be greater than the depth of immersion of the tip of the drainage tube in the collection bottle to cause the intrathoracic air or fluid to exit into the bottle. This is easily accomplished with simple coughing.

For air to enter back into the pleural space through the chest tube, the patient must generate enough negative intrathoracic pressure to pull the water in the collection bottle up to the height of the chest. Normal inspiration is not forceful enough to do this *if the bottle is kept on the floor*. The normal fluctuation in the height of the fluid level in the long tube during respiration provides proof that free communication exists with the pleural space and that the tube is functioning normally. An absence of respiratory fluctuation or a decrease in the drainage implies blockage or, if the tube has been in for a long enough period, full expansion of the lung and obliteration of the pleural space. The two situations (blockage and full expansion) should be distinguishable by clinical and radiographic means.

On the other hand, an *increase* in respiratory fluctuation may imply an increased inspiratory effort due to airway obstruction or atelectasis. If blocked, the tube and collecting tubing may be changed or "milked" or "stripped" to dislodge clots.[35] *Milking* refers to forcing air or fluid back into the chest by pinching or clamping the tube distally and, with the other hand, compressing the tube and forcing the contents proximally. This can dislodge a blocking intrathoracic clot and can obviate the need for tube replacement when radiographic or clinical examination suggests incomplete expansion or drainage. *Stripping* involves proximal pinching or clamping and progressive distal compression followed by release of the proximal aspect. This allows the tube to spring open. The sudden increase in negative pressure may extract clots and fluid from a more proximal location. These procedures are more effective with soft latex tubing than with clear plastic tubes. Persistent bubbling in the tube in both expiration and inspiration implies an air leak, *the most common source of which is the drainage system connections*. These should be taped thoroughly and rechecked frequently.

Another source of leakage may be failure to get the last opening of the chest tube inside the chest wall so that ambient air is sucked into the exposed hole. One may best manage leaking at the skin incision site by initially tunneling up one interspace and by using effective suture technique and a Vaseline-impregnated gauze dressing. Of course, the bottle must always remain dependent, because gravity contributes a great deal to the proper drainage of the pleural space. Elevating the bottle above the chest can cause fluid to reenter the chest and can increase the probability of infection. If a bronchopleural fistula exists, drowning can also occur with bottle elevation.[20] The length of the tubing must be carefully controlled so that dependent loops of fluid do not form. Such loops of accumulated liquid must be displaced before more air or fluid can pass. The amount of positive intrapleural pressure required for air to pass through a dependent loop of fluid is greater than the vertical elevation of the fluid in the loop (Fig. 9–25). If the fluid loop becomes high enough (15 to 25 cm of water), egress of air may be blocked to a degree sufficient to cause a tension pneumothorax.[47] Similarly, as fluid accumulates in the water seal, the immersed tip of the tube must be raised so that it

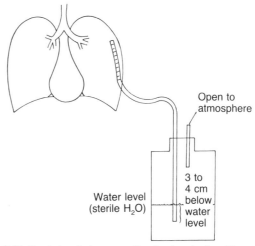

Figure 9–24. Single-bottle (water seal) collection device. (From Bricker DL: Safe, effective tube thoracostomy. E.R. Reports 2:49, 1981.)

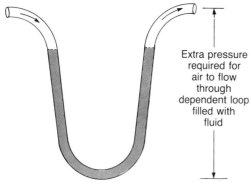

Figure 9–25. Dependent loops of fluid-filled tubing require positive intrapleural pressure greater than the vertical height of the fluid-filled loop for drainage to occur. (From Batchelder TL, Morris KA: Critical factors in determining adequate pleural drainage in both the operated and non-operated chest. Am Surg 28:298, 1962.)

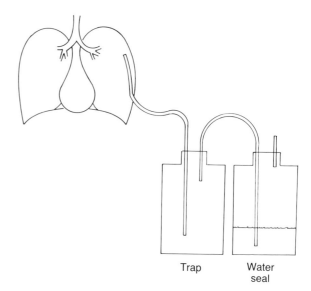

Figure 9–26. A "trap" proximal to the water seal is sometimes used. (From Bricker DL: Safe, effective tube thoracostomy. E. R. Reports 2:49, 1981.)

stays 2 to 4 cm below the water surface. Otherwise, a similarly progressive increase in intrathoracic pressure will be required to continue emptying the pleural space.

Sometimes a second "trap," or collecting bottle, is placed proximally to the water seal (Fig. 9–26). This has the advantage of keeping the level of fluid in the water seal bottle constant and allows for better measurement of collected drainage. A disadvantage is that air can enter the chest tube from the first bottle with accidental disconnection of any of the tubes or with a significant increase in negative intrapleural pressure. The dead space provided by the dry trap can produce an air-lock effect and can lead to to-and-fro pressure changes with ventilation without effective drainage.[35] More commonly, when a two-bottle system is used, it is connected to suction. The amount of suction in tube 1 is regulated not by the pressure reading on the wall suction valve but by the depth of water in the second bottle above tube 3 and by the depth of tube 1 (Fig. 9–27). When suction exceeds the depth of the water in bottle 2, air enters from the top of the third tube to prevent further increases. The internal diameter of the various tubes (especially 3) also contributes to the amount of suction that can be created.

The more complex the system, the more problems that can occur. Evaporation occurs quickly, and fluid levels must be maintained to keep pressures from steadily decreasing. Vigorous bubbling in the first bottle may cause foam to rise

and to be suctioned into the second, either breaking the water seal or changing the pressure regulation. A few drops of a chemical agent (caprylic alcohol) can be used in bottle 1 to prevent this. As the first bottle fills with fluid, the effective suction decreases because of an increase in hydrostatic pressure at the bottom of tube 1. Although a two-bottle system (water seal plus suction regulator) is adequate for nearly all emergency department applications,[41] a number of self-contained set-ups that avoid the bulky bottle system are commercially available.

Some add a third bottle for fluid collection (Fig. 9–28). Commercially available chest drainage systems that mimic the three-bottle system are now used by most hospitals. These units are plastic, lightweight, compact, easily transported, and easily assembled. Currently available models (Fig. 9–29) collect up to 2500 ml of fluid, allow easy regulation of suction, and can be used for autotransfusion. Because glass bottles are cumbersome and time consuming to assemble, the editors *strongly* urge emergency departments to use the convenient, disposable chest drainage collection systems.

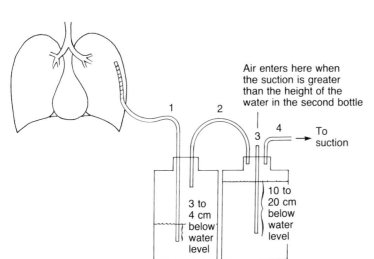

Air enters here when the suction is greater than the height of the water in the second bottle

To suction

3 to 4 cm below water level

10 to 20 cm below water level

Bottle 1

Bottle 2

Figure 9–27. A two-bottle system for applying regulated suction to the pleural space. The height of the column of water in bottle 2 regulates the amount of suction applied, independent of the pressure on the suction valve. (From Bricker DL: Safe, effective tube thoracostomy. E. R. Reports 2:49, 1981.)

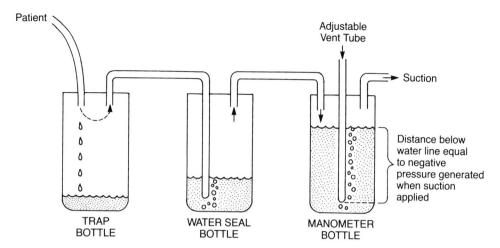

Figure 9–28. A three-bottle system with fluid trap bottle, water seal, and adjustable vent tube. (From Miller KS, Sahn SA: Chest tubes: Indications, technique, management and complications. Chest 91:258, 1987.)

Occlusive clamping of chest tubes should be performed only with great trepidation and physician supervision, particularly in the first 24 hours after the tubes are placed. Clamping with a persistent intrathoracic air leak or fluid accumulation may lead rapidly to a tension pneumo- or hemothorax. Clamping is appropriate only to change the underwater seal bottle rapidly. Patients with chest tubes in place are best transported without clamping—on water seal only, with the bottle placed well below chest level.

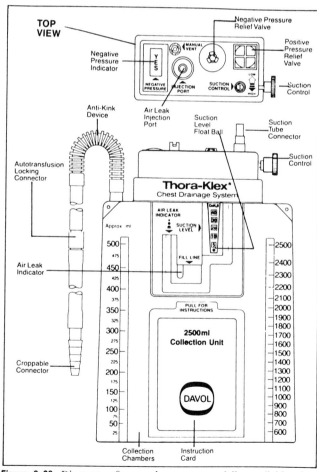

Figure 9–29. Diagram of a modern commercially available chest drainage system. Included is a 2500-ml fluid collection chamber, a suction control device, an air leak indicator, and a fluid sampling port. A separate attachment is available for autotransfusion. (Courtesy of Davol, Inc., Division of C. R. Bard, Cranston, R.I.)

Role of Suction

Most sources recommend suction at least initially in all patients with chest tubes placed for either pneumo- or hemothorax.[6, 14, 15, 48] Ideally, a suction machine must have high flow (up to 20 liters per minute) and a regulated constant suction (0 to 60 cm of water). Gill and Long recommend suction only if the air leak is massive, if the lung fails to reexpand, or if bleeding continues.[42] The continuous bubbling and the lack of respiratory variation with suction can mask the presence of air leak. With extensive bleeding, excessive suction may actually increase the rate of blood loss, particularly when the bleeding is from a relatively low-pressure pulmonary vessel. Intermittent clamping or water seal use may be preferred. With a massive air leak, excess suction may cause respiratory distress by removing inspired air before alveolar gas exchange can occur.[1] Suction may be useful for rapid initial expansion and drainage. Because of the added complexity and complications, suction should be replaced by simple underwater seal drainage as long as expansion and drainage are satisfactory and no persistent air leak exists. *When suction is applied, 20 cm of water is normally used.*

Prophylactic Antibiotics

The routine use of prophylactic antibiotics in patients requiring tube thoracostomy is controversial. Patients with associated injuries who are at high risk for infection (e.g., open fractures, perforated viscus, esophageal injury) are always given antibiotics. Whether patients with isolated chest trauma or spontaneous pneumothorax require antibiotic prophylaxis has yet to be definitively determined. Grover and coworkers[49] conducted a prospective randomized double-blind study of 75 patients with penetrating chest injuries and found that 2.6 per cent treated with clindamycin developed empyema. In contrast, 16.2 per cent of patients given placebo developed empyema. LoCurto and coworkers[50] used cefoxitin in patients with blunt and penetrating chest trauma and found one infectious complication among 30 (3.0 per cent) patients. The chest infection rate in patients not receiving antibiotics was 29 per cent. However, in another series of 80 patients with penetrating chest injuries, none of 40 patients treated with doxycycline and only one of 40 who were not given antibiotics demonstrated infections.[51] Neubauer and colleagues[52] actually demonstrated a higher rate of infection in patients with spontaneous pneumothoraces who were given antibiotics (0 versus 3.1 per cent). Their report is limited in that the type, dosage, schedule, route, and duration of antibiotic were not stated.

Probably more important than the use of antibiotic prophylaxis is ensuring that when time permits strict aseptic technique is performed when the tube is initially placed. If antibiotics are used, the first dose is given as soon as possible, preferably before the tube is inserted, and continued until the tube is removed. The chosen antibiotic should cover *Staphylococcus aureus* because this is the most common organism causing empyema, but gram-negative bacteria coverage is also desirable. A first- or second-generation cephalosporin is probably a good choice because they have a wide spectrum of activity and easily pass into the pleural space. A reasonable approach would be to administer prophylactic antibiotics when the tube is placed in an emergency situation and the possibility of infection is greater because of possible contamination. Stable patients who receive a chest tube in controlled and elective situations probably do not require antibiotic prophylaxis.

Tube Removal

Recommendations vary, but chest tubes should generally be removed when there has been no drainage of fluid or air for a minimum of 24 hours, when respiratory variations in the water seal have ceased, and when high-quality radiographs reveal satisfactory resolution. Because of pleural irritation, small amounts of serous fluid (less than 200 ml per day) may continue to drain without contraindicating removal.

To remove a chest tube, the patient should be placed in a semierect position, and the dressings should be removed. Sedation or restraints may be helpful. The area should be sterilized and draped, and sterile technique should be followed. The only instruments required are sterile basins, heavy scissors to cut the suture, dressing materials, and instruments to tie the previously placed purse-string suture or to place a new one. Facilities and equipment should be available to reinsert a new chest tube promptly if it should become necessary. The suture holding the tube to the skin should be removed from the tube, and the purse-string suture that was placed previously should be loosened and readied for tying. A second (gloved) assistant is helpful. The tube should be clamped, and the connecting tubing should be removed. A Vaseline-or antibiotic- impregnated gauze dressing should be prepared. The patient should inhale fully and should perform a mild Valsalva maneuver. The tube is removed in one swift motion while the patient holds the breath. Two fingers hold the skin edges shut, and the purse-string suture is tied. The occlusive dressing is placed and taped securely. A period of observation (minimum 2 to 6 hours) is recommended if the patient is to be sent home, with a chest film at the end of that time. Any increase in symptoms should call for prompt reevaluation. After 48 hours, the dressing may be removed and the wound managed as any sutured skin wound would be.

Pneumothorax in Pediatric Patients

INCIDENCE

Pneumothorax occurs more commonly during the neonatal period than at any other time of life. When chest radiographs are taken of all newborns in large series, the incidence of pneumothorax is high (1 to 2 per cent). The incidence does not seem to change when normal (term) vaginal deliveries are compared with premature births or with delivery by cesarean section. The incidence of *symptomatic* pneumothorax in newborn infants, however, is consis-

tently only 0.05 to 0.07 per cent. Of newborns with pneumothorax, several studies report twice as many males as females. Some studies report more instances of right-sided collapse. Ten to 20 per cent of cases are bilateral.[53–56]

It should be noted that lobar emphysema in a newborn may cause severe respiratory symptoms shortly after birth (Fig. 9–30). The physical examination may detect decreased breath sounds in a hemithorax and even evidence of mediastinal shift. Lobar emphysema often looks like a tension pneumothorax radiographically, and the unwary physician may rush to insert a chest tube. The treatment in this case is surgical removal of the diseased lobe, and a chest tube may worsen the clinical condition.

PATHOPHYSIOLOGY

There seem to be two groups of newborns who develop pneumothorax. The first are term or postterm neonates with a history of fetal distress; difficult delivery; need for resuscitation; or aspiration of meconium, amniotic fluid, or blood. These infants tend to become symptomatic within the first 2 hours of life and generally fare quite well. The mechanism in this group is believed to be an excess intra-alveolar pressure generated at birth. With the first breath, the transpulmonary pressure rises from 40 to as much as 100 cm of water. Compression of the chest during vaginal delivery places the diaphragm and the muscles of respiration at a marked mechanical advantage. With mechanical obstruction of some alveoli or bronchioles, as can occur with aspiration, the intense transpulmonary pressure is transmitted to the normally aerated alveoli, which can overdistend and rupture. Mechanical ventilation, end-expiratory pressure, and resuscitative efforts can also precipitate alveolar rupture.

The second group of newborns with pneumothorax are those who have underlying pulmonary disease (most notably hyaline membrane disease [respiratory distress syndrome]) or congenital abnormalities. These infants commonly develop their pneumothoraces in the second day of life, often while being treated with positive airway pressures. The prognosis in these cases is much worse.[54, 56]

CLINICAL FINDINGS

The physical examination of the newborn with pneumothorax can yield findings ranging from no abnormalities whatsoever to complete cardiovascular collapse. Grunting respirations and tachypnea (to a respiratory rate as high as

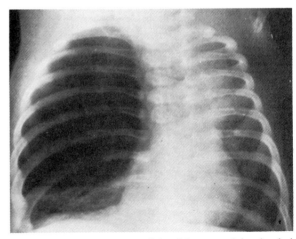

Figure 9–30. Lobar emphysema of the right upper lobe simulating a tension pneumothorax. (From Harris JH, Harris WH: The Radiology of Emergency Medicine, 2nd ed. Baltimore, Williams & Wilkins, 1981. © Williams & Wilkins, 1981.)

120) are often seen. Retractions or nasal flaring can be seen. Crepitus in the neck may be present. Cyanosis may be present or may occur only with crying or feeding. Irritability, restlessness, apneic periods, bradycardia, or tachycardia may be the only manifestation. Distention and tympany of the affected side may be found. A decrease in breath sounds is difficult to appreciate in the newborn. With tension pneumothorax, the cardiac impulse and the trachea may be shifted away from the affected side.

DIAGNOSIS

The definitive diagnosis is made with high-quality radiographs taken in both the AP and the horizontal beam (crosstable) lateral projections. Small pneumothoraces may be seen only on the lateral view, as the air collects at the top of the thoracic cavity. Bilateral tension pneumothorax can appear as microcardia, without any mediastinal shift. Further radiologic studies may be needed to differentiate this condition from lung cysts, lobar emphysema, and skin folds.

Transillumination of the chest with a high-intensity fiberoptic light source has been used with great success to detect and follow pneumothorax and pneumomediastinum in newborns.[57]

Monin and Vert have noted that abrupt changes in transthoracic impedance in infants on respiratory monitors have been related to the appearance of pneumothorax.[54] Such changes should initiate prompt reevaluation of the patient's respiratory status.

TREATMENT

In general, tube thoracostomy is the treatment of choice. When signs of tension pneumothorax are present, aspiration with a plastic catheter over-the-needle device is recommended (see Chapter 8). Small pneumothoraces (less than 20 per cent of the hemithorax) in relatively asymptomatic infants (who are without other problems and who do not require positive airway pressures) can be merely monitored by close observation.

Repeated films or transillumination and frequent monitoring of vital signs and arterial blood gases are indicated. Breathing 100 per cent oxygen is believed to hasten reabsorption by as much as sixfold.[53, 58] The risks of retrolental fibroplasia and pulmonary oxygen toxicity must be carefully assessed, however.

When evacuation of the pleural space is elected, needle aspiration using a 50-ml syringe, an 18-gauge catheter over-the-needle device, and a three-way stopcock may be attempted once (see Chapter 8).[59] This may suffice in patients without a continued air leak, although the risk of lung puncture is considerable.

TECHNIQUE

The technique of tube thoracostomy in pediatric patients varies little from that already described. Small, commercially available thoracostomy tubes (Argyle) or standard "red rubber" catheters with extra holes cut in the tip can be used. Numbers 8 to 10 French catheters are used in premature infants, and 10 to 12 French catheters are used in larger newborns. Blunt dissection minimizes the complications of lung puncture, hemorrhage, and traumatic fistula formation, which are seen more often with trocar insertion.[60, 61]

Various tube locations have been proposed. In their controlled trial, Allen and associates compared the effectiveness of lateral (fourth to fifth intercostal space, anterior axillary line) and superior (first to third intercostal space, midclavicular line) placements of 149 chest tubes for their effectiveness in evacuating pneumothorax.[63] The most important factor was the eventual location of the tube rather than the site of insertion. Anterior tubes were effective 96 per cent of the time, whereas only 42 per cent of the tubes directed posteriorly functioned satisfactorily.

Placement in the third intercostal space, midaxillary line with the tip directed under the sterum appears to be a good compromise.[54] Care must be taken to avoid the nipple, which can be difficult to identify in the premature infant. Water seal with 10 to 20 cm of water for suction is usually recommended until reexpansion occurs and the absence of continued air leakage is verified.

Smaller collecting bottles are recommended to measure drainage more accurately. Hughes and Beuscher have described a miniature water seal apparatus using a 50-ml multiple-use saline bottle, standard intravenous tubing, and one long and one short needle (Fig. 9–31).[63]

Other Techniques

TROCAR INSERTION

The blunt dissection technique described previously is the one that is commonly advocated by authorities on chest tube placement. Many practitioners have become proficient in using a trocar for the percutaneous introduction of chest tubes. The trocar device that is currently commercially available consists of a siliconized plastic catheter that is generally smaller than 34 French and has fewer fenestrations than do the other (Argyle) tubes. It fits over a central pointed steel or aluminum rod with a plastic ball handle at one end and a small portion of the sharpened tip protruding through the fenestrated end. The positioning, preparation, and local

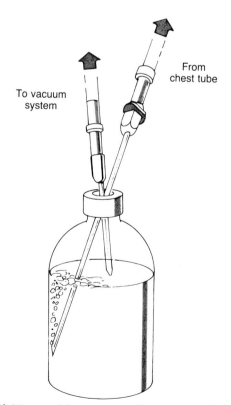

Figure 9–31. Water seal for newborns. (Redrawn from Hughes WT, Beuscher ES: Pediatric Procedures. 2nd ed. Philadelphia. WB Saunders Co, 1980, p 239.)

anesthesia that were described previously are used. A skin incision as before is made with a number 11 blade. With the tip of the catheter held firmly in one hand for control and the ball held in the other hand, one forces the trocar point through the intercostal muscles and the parietal pleural. As the pleural space is entered, the catheter is pushed from the stylet into the pleural space and is secured in the usual fashion.[64] Other trocars contain a sharp obturator and a hollow metal tube through which a rubber catheter may be passed and secured.[6] Millikan and coworkers reviewed 1249 patients undergoing tube thoracostomy for acute trauma from 1967 to 1978. The researchers abandoned the trocar in 1974 in favor of a blunt technique because of "major technical complications," such as damage to lung and solid organs, and concluded that "the trocar should never be used."[48] Bricker in his recent review also noted that "most authorities condemn" such devices.[1] We do *not* recommend the use of the trocar technique to puncture the pleura, although the trocar may be used instead of a Kelly clamp to introduce or guide the chest tube *after the pleura has been opened* (Fig. 9–32). While the use of trocars for insertion of large bore tubes is fraught with danger, new mini-catheter systems that combine the trocar approach with a guide wire dilator system appear promising for management of pneumothoraces. These catheter systems are used in the fashion described below.

CATHETER ASPIRATION

Indications and Contraindications. Numerous studies[21–32] have demonstrated that a simple uncomplicated pneumothorax can be treated safely and effectively with small-caliber catheter aspiration. This procedure is done in lieu of a formal chest tube drainage. After successful reexpansion of the lung, selected patients may have the catheter removed and be treated as outpatients. Patients with iatrogenic pneumothorax (e.g., after pulmonary artery catheter, thoracentesis, bronchoscopy), those who have intravenous drug abuse-induced pneumothoraces, victims of minor chest trauma, and patients with spontaneous pneumothoraces are potential candidates for catheter aspiration. Those with tension pneumothorax, hemothorax, hemodynamic instability, and patients with serious associated injuries requiring surgery should receive conventional tube thoracostomy. Patients with underlying lung pathology such as pneumonia, congestive heart failure, asthma, or emphysema are generally not candidates for this procedure.

Equipment. Equipment suggested for the technique includes a number 14 through-the-needle Intracath, a 14-gauge intravenous catheter, or an 8.5 French Arrow trauma catheter inserted with the Seldinger (guide wire) technique. An 8 Fr guide-wire commercial system (CCASP-FORD-110485, Cook Catheter, Bloomington, Ind.) also is popular. A 14 Fr introducer (Introstat, Hart Medical, Clearwater, Fla.) and 12 Fr polyvinylchloride chest tube system (Argyle, Sherwood Medical, St. Louis, Mo.) has been used as a compromise between the smaller catheters and a full-sized chest tube.[64a]

Procedure. Placement of a catheter into the pleural space is relatively simple. The patient is prepared with sterile procedures at either the fourth or fifth intercostal space at the anterior axillary line or the second or third intercostal space at the midclavicular line (either site is acceptable.) After the generous local infiltration of lidocaine, a thin-walled 16-gauge needle is advanced cephalad over the top of the rib at a 60-degree angle. When the pleural space is entered (identified by the aspiration of air into the syringe), a guide wire is inserted and the needle removed. A nick is

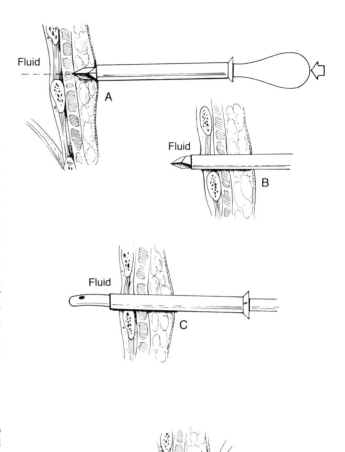

Figure 9–32. Sequence of steps in the use of a hollow metal trocar to insert a catheter into the pleural space. Before starting, one must determine that the entire length of the catheter can pass through the trocar. Newer trocar sets use a chest tube over the trocar system without a hollow tube. After entry of the trocar into the pleural space, the chest tube is slid over the trocar into the pleural space. *Note:* Although the trocar apparatus may be used to introduce the chest tube *after the pleura has been opened,* we do not recommend the use of the trocar method to puncture the pleura. (Redrawn from Cosgriff JH: An Atlas of Diagnostic and Therapeutic Procedures for Emergency Personnel. Philadelphia, JB Lippincott Co, 1978, pp 257–258.)

made in the skin with a number 11 blade, and a small-caliber radiopaque catheter is threaded over the guide wire into the pleural space. (*Note:* Slight variations in catheter insertion technique [e.g., use of a dilator in entering the pleural space] have been described for some commercial aspiration systems.) The wire is removed and a three-way stopcock is attached along with a 60-ml syringe. Air is then aspirated until resistance is felt. A surprising amount of air can be removed. Occasionally air cannot be aspirated, because the catheter is kinked or blocked with soft tissue. If no air is obtained, place the patient in the full upright position, have the patient cough or take a deep breath or walk around (if the condition warrants this stress), or withdraw the catheter slightly. This often results in successful aspiration, when no additional air can be aspirated, a chest radiograph is obtained to document full expansion of the lung. If residual pneumothorax is present, an attempt at further aspiration is made.

Vallee and colleagues[32] have proposed a protocol utilizing this technique as the first step in treating simple pneumothoraces (Fig. 9–33). Patients with successful aspiration are observed in the emergency department for 4 hours, and if a repeat radiograph shows no reaccumulation of air, the catheter is removed. After 2 more hours of observation another chest radiograph is obtained and the patient is discharged home if there is no recurrent pneumothorax. A Heimlich valve is attached to the catheter if a patient has more than a 10 per cent residual apical pneumothorax. The valve is placed on suction only if this does not result in full expansion. Patients with continued residual pneumothorax then receive a conventional tube thoracostomy.

Using this protocol, Vallee and colleagues[32] report a 59 per cent success rate with simple aspiration in 35 patients with a total of 37 pneumothoraces. An additional 27 per cent responded to the use of a Heimlich valve with or without suction. Only five patients (14 per cent) required a tube thoracostomy; two of these were patients initially responsive to catheter aspiration who returned with a recurrent pneumothorax on follow-up visits. This technique appears to be useful in patients with selected simple pneumothoraces, but further study is warranted.

COMPLICATIONS

As with any surgical procedure, complications can and will occur (Table 9–6).[48, 65] Local infection at the site of insertion is common and may reflect the often hurried performance of this procedure in the emergency setting. Osteomyelitis has been reported in settings in which tubes have been kept in place for a long time. Empyema is uncommon, because tube thoracostomy remains a useful treatment for this problem. Documented cases of empyema

Table 9–6. Complications of Tube Thoracostomy

Infection
  Pneumonia
  Empyema
  Local incision infection
  Osteomyelitis
Bleeding
  Local incision hematoma
  Intercostal artery or vein laceration
  Internal mammary artery laceration (with midclavicular line placement)
  Pulmonary vein or artery injury
  Great vessel injury (rarely)
Laceration or puncture of nerves or solid organs
  Lung
  Liver
  Spleen
  Diaphragm
  Stomach
  Colon
  Long thoracic nerve
  Intercostal nerve (may result in intercostal neuritis/neuralgia)
  Intercostal muscles (intercostal myalgia)
Mechanical problems
  Chest tube dislodgement from chest wall
  Incorrect tube position
    Subcutaneous placement
    Intra-abdominal placement
Air leaks
  Leaks from tubing or drainage bottles
  Last tube fenestration not entirely within pleural space
  Leaks from skin site
Flow of drainage bottle contents into chest from inadvertently elevating drainage bottles
Blocked drainage
  Kinked chest tube or drainage tubes
  Clots
Miscellaneous
  Allergic reactions to surgical preparation or anesthesia
  Pulmonary atelectasis
  Persistent pneumothorax
  Retained hemothorax
  Clotted hemothorax or fibrothorax
  Subcutaneous or mediastinal emphysema
  Reexpansion pulmonary edema
  Reexpansion hypotension
  Recurrence of pneumothorax after chest tube removal

developed in only 1.3 to 2.7 per cent of patients in recent studies.[48, 66] Empyema tends to occur in patients with a loculated effusion and in those who are inadequately drained. Pneumonia and atelectasis are attributed to a decrease in coughing and failure to clear secretions because of pain. As for any postoperative patient, early ambulation and vigorous pulmonary toilet are indicated.

A local hematoma may occasionally develop at the incision site but may be prevented by careful dissection. Intercostal arteries or veins may be lacerated at the time of tube insertion. These lacerations can be minimized if sharp dissection is carried only to the fascia and the tube is carefully placed just above the rib. The tube may adequately tamponade such bleeding, but if tamponade is insufficient, the incision may need to be extended to expose or ligate the bleeding vessel. If a lacerated intercostal artery does not stop bleeding, one may attempt to insert a Foley catheter into the incision, inflate the balloon, and withdraw the catheter to tamponade the vessel. Anterior chest wall tube placement carried to the midline may result in internal mammary artery laceration. This is notoriously difficult to control and may require thoracotomy. Great vessel injury is uncommon.

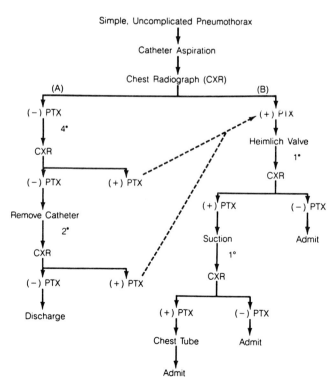

Figure 9–33. Suggested protocol for catheter aspiration of pneumothorax. *PTX*, pneumothorax present on chest radiograph (*CXR*). (From Vallee P, Sullivan M, Richardson H, et al: Sequential treatment of a simple pneumothorax. Ann Emerg Med 17:936, 1988.)

Millikan and colleagues[48] noted a 1 per cent incidence of technical complications (visceral perforation) in their series of 447 patients undergoing tube thoracostomy for trauma. Daly and coworkers[66] reported a 1.8 per cent rate of errors related to the placement of the chest tube in 164 patients in their series. Damage to the lung parenchyma or the intrapulmonary vessels can occur readily. This was more common with the trocar insertion technique, which has now been largely abandoned in favor of blunt dissection. The use of digital exploration of the pleura to exclude or free adhesions is mandatory before tube placement. Careful attention to the anatomy, with recognition of exactly how high the diaphragm may rise (especially if the abdomen is filled with blood), can minimize injuries to the diaphragm or the intra-abdominal organs.

Reexpansion pulmonary edema is a rare and potentially fatal complication of thoracentesis or tube thoracostomy.[67–69] Pulmonary edema, usually ipsilateral, can appear as soon as 1 to 2 hours after lung reexpansion. Edema commonly occurs when collapse has been present for longer than 72 hours and when 1000 ml or more of pleural fluid is removed. Suction seems to worsen the edema. The exact pathogenesis of reexpansion pulmonary edema has yet to be adequately determined but is likely multifactorial.[69] Increased pulmonary vascular permeability appears to be a major factor and is probably related to hypoxic injury to the capillary beds and alveolar membranes. Increased pulmonary capillary pressure and blood flow, decreased surfactant levels, and mechanical damage to the lung also play a role. The rapid removal of air or fluid may result in an abrupt return of circulation and transudation of protein and fluid into the alveolar space. Occasionally an associated shock-like state will occur with hypotension and evidence of decreased organ perfusion.[70] Treatment includes supportive care, oxygenation, and positive-pressure ventilation when indicated. Patients with hypotension are given volume replacement and inotropic agents as needed. Invasive monitoring is frequently required. The best course is to prevent this complication by slow, staged removal of large effusions or collections of air (especially if they have been present for several days) and by avoidance of suction, if possible.

Mechanical problems commonly result in air leaks with failed reexpansion or inadequate drainage. Tension pneumothorax can occur if a blockage in the drainage system at any point is associated with an air leak. Failure of reexpansion or incomplete reexpansion of a pneumothorax may be due to a mechanical air leak, but it may also indicate a bronchopleural fistula, a continued parenchymal lung leak, or a bronchial injury. Retained hemothorax may result from clotting or poor tube function. The largest possible tube should be used for drainage of a hemothorax. Reinsertion or placement of a second tube may be indicated if the first tube is not functioning properly. Often, an angled tube in the posterior diaphragmatic sulcus will promote drainage of a dependent fluid collection. Clotted hemothorax or fibrothorax is an indication for elective decortication and pleurodesis. Subcutaneous emphysema can occur if the chest tube is partially extruded or plugged.

If a chest tube is not functioning properly or has not reversed the pathologic condition as expected, one must carefully reevaluate the position of the chest tube. In an emergency situation, the tube may have been placed subcutaneously, and the incorrect placement may not be obvious to the physician. If the tube dissects in a fascial plane posteriorly along a rib, even the postinsertion film may appear to confirm proper placement. Such a condition may be lethal. As a general rule, if a chest tube is not functioning properly and the patient is deteriorating, the tube should be removed and inserted again, or another tube should be inserted.

REFERENCES

1. Bricker DL: Safe effective tube thoracostomy. Part I: Pathophysiology, diagnosis, indications. Part II: Insertion, collection, transport, complications. E. R. Reports 2:45, 1981.
2. Playfair WS: On the treatment of empyema in children. Obstet Trans 14:4, 1872.
3. Graham EA, Bell RD: Open pneumothorax: Its relation to the treatment of empyema. Am J Med Sci 156:839, 1918.
4. Brewer LA: Wounds of the chest in war and peace, 1943–1968. Ann Thorac Surg 7:387, 1969.
5. McNamara JJ, Messersmith JK, Dunn RA, et al: Thoracic injuries in combat casualties in Vietnam. Ann Thorac Surg 10:389, 1970.
6. Kirsh MM, Sloan H: Blunt Chest Trauma. Boston, Little, Brown & Co, 1977, pp 4979.
7. Jones KW: Thoracic trauma. Surg Clin North Am 60:957, 1980.
8. Kircher LT Jr, Swartzel RL: Spontaneous pneumothorax and its treatment. JAMA 155:24, 1954.
9. Rhea JT, DeLuca SA, Greene RE: Determining the size of the pneumothorax in the upright patient. Radiology 144:733, 1982.
10. Bayne CG: Pulmonary complications of the McSwain Dart. Ann Emerg Med 11:136, 1982.
11. Beall AC, Crawford HW, DeBakey ME: Considerations in the management of acute traumatic hemothorax. J Thorac Cardiovasc Surg 52:351, 1966.
12. Siemons R, Polk HC, Gray LA, Jr., et al: Indications for thoracotomy following penetrating thoracic injury. J Trauma 17:493, 1977.
13. Shefts LM: The Initial Management of Thoracic and Thoraco-abdominal Trauma. Springfield, IL, Charles C Thomas, 1956.
14. DeVries WC, Wolfe WG: The management of spontaneous pneumothorax and bullous emphysema. Surg Clin North Am 60:851, 1980.
15. Brooks JW: Thoracotomy in the management of spontaneous pneumothorax. Ann Surg 177:798, 1973.
16. Ruckley CV, McCormack RJ: The management of spontaneous pneumothorax. Thorax 21:139, 1966.
17. Bense L, Eklund G, Wiman L: Smoking and the increased risk of contracting spontaneous pneumothorax. Chest 92:1009, 1987.
18. Clark TA, Hutchison DE, Deaner RM, et al: Spontaneous pneumothorax. Am J Surg 124:728, 1972.
19. Fleisher AG, McElvaney G, Lawson L, et al: Surgical management of spontaneous pneumothorax in patients with acquired immunodeficiency syndrome. Ann Thorac Surg 45:21, 1988.
20. Borrie J: Management of Thoracic Emergencies. 3rd ed. New York, Appleton-Century-Crofts, 1980.
21. Bjork L: The use of the Seldinger technic for percutaneous introduction of drainage tubes into thoracic cavities. Scand J Thor Cardiovasc Surg 3:67, 1969.
22. Raja OG, Lalor AJ: Simple aspiration of spontaneous pneumothorax. Br J Dis Chest 75:207, 1981.
23. Bevelaqua FA, Aranda C: Management of spontaneous pneumothorax with small lumen catheter manual aspiration. Chest 81:693, 1982.
24. Hamilton AAD, Archer GJ: Treatment of pneumothorax by simple aspiration. Thorax 38:934, 1983.
25. Mukherjee D, Lyon JL: A simple treatment for pneumothorax. Surg Gynecol Obstet 156:499, 1983.
26. Obeid FN, Shapiro MJ, Richardson HH, et al: Catheter aspiration for simple pneumothorax in the outpatient management of simple traumatic pneumothorax. J Trauma 25:882, 1985.
27. Jones JS: A place for aspiration in the treatment of spontaneous pneumothorax. Thorax 40:66, 1985.
28. Talbot-Stern J, Richardson H, Tomlanovich MC, et al: Catheter aspiration for simple pneumothorax. J Emerg Med 4:437, 1986.
29. Wisdom K, Nowak RM, Richardson H, et al: Alternate therapy for traumatic pneumothorax in "pocket shooters." Ann Emerg Med 15:428, 1986.
30. Conces DJ, Tarver RD, Gray WC, et al: Treatment of pneumothoraces utilizing small caliber chest tubes. Chest 94:55, 1988.
31. Casola G, vanSonnenberg E, Keightley A, et al: Pneumothorax: Radiologic treatment with small catheters. Radiology 166:89, 1988.
32. Vallee P, Sullivan M, Richardson H, et al: Sequential treatment of a simple pneumothorax. Ann Emerg Med 19:936, 1988.
33. Cannon WB, Mark JBD, and Jamplis RW: Pneumothorax: A therapeutic update. Am J Surg 142:26, 1981.
34. Mercier C, Page A, Verdant A, et al: Outpatient management of intercostal tube drainage in spontaneous pneumothorax. Ann Thorac Surg 22:163, 1976.
35. Von Hippel A: A Manual of Thoracic Surgery. Springfield, IL, Charles C Thomas, 1978.
36. Guyton SW, Pauli DL, Anderson RP: Introducer insertion of minithoracostomy tubes. Am J Surg 155:693, 1988.

37. Seremetis MG: The management of spontaneous pneumothorax. Chest 57:65, 1970.
38. Gazzaniga AB: Surgical considerations in pulmonary disease. In Burton GG, Gee GN, Hodgkin JE (eds): Respiratory Care. Philadelphia, JB Lippincott Co, 1977.
39. Hewett FC: Thoracentesis: The plan of continuous aspiration. Br Med J 1:317, 1876.
40. American College of Surgeons Committee on Trauma: Advanced Trauma Life Support Course, 1981.
41. Munnell ER, Thomas EK: Current concepts in thoracic drainage systems. Ann Thorac Surg 19:261, 1975.
42. Gill W, Long WB (eds): Shock Trauma Manual. Baltimore, Williams & Wilkins, 1979.
43. Hegarty MM: A conservative approach to penetrating injuries of the chest. Injury 8:53, 1976.
44. Duponselle EFC: The level of the intercostal drain and other determinant factors in the conservative approach to penetrating chest injuries. Cent Afr J Med 26:52, 1980.
45. Broadie TA, Glover JL, Bang N: Clotting competence of intracavitary blood in trauma victims. Ann Emerg Med 10:127, 1981.
46. Gilman AG, Goodman LS, Gilman A (eds): Goodman and Gilman's The Pharamacological Basis of Therapeutics. 6th ed. New York, Macmillan Publishing Co, Inc., 1980.
47. Batchelder TL, Morris KA: Critical factors in determining adequate pleural drainage in both the operated and non-operated chest. Am Surg 28:296, 1962.
48. Millikan JS, Moore EE, Steiner E, et al: Complications of tube thoracostomy for acute trauma. Am J Surg 140:738, 1980.
49. Grover FL, Richardson J, Fewel JG, et al: Prophylactic antibiotics in the treatment of penetrating chest wounds: A prospective double-blinded study. J Thorac Cardiovasc Surg 74:528, 1977.
50. LoCurto JJ, Tischler CD, Swan KG, et al: Tube thoracostomy and trauma: Antibiotics or not? J Trauma 26:1067, 1986.
51. Mandal AK, Montano J, Thadepalli H: Prophylactic antibiotics and no antibiotics compared in penetrating chest trauma. J Trauma 25:639, 1985.
52. Neubauer MK, Fishburg GR, Trummer JM: Routine antibiotic therapy following pleural space intubation: a reappraisal. J Thorac Cardiovasc Surg 61:882, 1971.
53. Chernick V, Reed MH: Pneumothorax and chylothorax in the neonatal period. J Pediatr 76:624, 1970.
54. Monin P, Vert P: Pneumothorax. Clin Perinatol 5:335, 1978.
55. Steele RW, Metz JR, Bass JW, et al: Pneumothorax and pneumomediastinum in the newborn. Radiology 98:629, 1971.
56. Yu VYH, Liew SW, Robertson NRC: Pneumothorax in the newborn. Changing pattern. Arch Dis Child 50:449, 1975.
57. Kuhns LR, Bednarek FJ, Wyman ML, et al: Diagnosis of pneumothorax or pneumomediastinum in the neonate by transillumination. Pediatrics 56:355, 1975.
58. Chernick V, Avery ME: Spontaneous alveolar rupture at birth. Pediatrics 32:816, 1963.
59. Moore GC, Mills LJ, Mast CP: Thoracentesis and chest tube insertion. In Levin DL, Moriss FC, Moore GC (eds): A Practical Guide to Pediatric Intensive Care. St. Louis CV Mosby Co, 1979, pp. 415–422.
60. Banagale RC, Outerbridge EW, Aranda JV: Lung perforation: A complication of chest tube insertion in neonatal pneumothorax. J Pediatr 94:973, 1979.
61. Moessinger AC, Driscoll JM Jr, Wigger HJ: High incidence of lung perforation by chest tube in neonatal pneumothorax. J Pediatr 92:635, 1978.
62. Allen RW Jr, Jung AL, Lester PD: Effectiveness of chest tube evacuation of pneumothorax in neonates. J Pediatr 99:629, 1981.
63. Hughes WT, Buescher ES: Pediatric Procedures. 2nd ed. Philadelphia, WB Saunders Co., 1980.
64. Richardson JD: Management of noncardiac thoracic trauma. Heart Lung 7:286, 1978.
64a. Guyton SW, Paull DL, Anderson RP: Introducer insertion of minithoracostomy tubes. Am J Surg 155:693, 1988.
65. Artz CP, Hardy JD: Management of Surgical Complications. 3rd ed. Philadelphia, WB Saunders Co., 1975.
66. Daly RC, Mucha P, Pairolero PC, et al: The risk of percutaneous chest tube thoracostomy for blunt thoracic trauma. Ann Emerg Med 14:865, 1985.
67. Johnstone W: Reexpansion pulmonary edema. Va Med 107:790, 1980.
68. Sewell RW, Fewel JC, Grover FT, et al: Experimental evaluation of reexpansion pulmonary edema. Ann Thorac Surg 26:126, 1978.
69. Mahfood S, Hix WR, Aaron BL, et al: Reexpansion pulmonary edema. Ann Thorac Surg 45:340, 1988.
70. Pavlin DJ, Raghu G, Rogers TR, et al: Reexpansion hypotension: A complication of rapid evacuation of prolonged pneumothorax. Chest 89:70, 1986.

Cardiac Procedures

Chapter 10

Carotid Sinus Massage

Stephen Gazak

INTRODUCTION

In 1961, Bernard Lown stated that "in recent years, insufficient attention has been given to the carotid sinus test."[1] This statement continues to apply to practice today. Generally speaking, carotid sinus massage (CSM) is either glossed over hastily or neglected entirely during the training of medical students and house officers alike. In the clinical setting, this safe, simple, and relatively effective maneuver is often neglected in favor of the immediate use of expensive and occasionally dangerous drug therapy.

The human cardiovascular system is richly supplied with specialized sensory nerve endings, known as baroreceptors, which autoregulate heart rate and blood pressure. The carotid sinus is part of this autoregulatory system, along with additional baroreceptors located at the level of the aortic arch, the atria, the ventricles, and the pulmonary veins. The carotid sinus, however, maintains a privileged position by virtue of its unique accessibility to external manipulation.

The word *carotid* is derived from the Greek *karos*, meaning deep sleep.[2] The soporific properties of carotid sinus stimulation have been exploited by warriors and physicians alike since antiquity. Carotid sinus massage remains an important diagnostic and therapeutic maneuver in modern-day medicine because of its profound effects on the cardiovascular system. With practice and continual refinement of technique, it is a safe and potentially useful tool for any physician summoned regularly to evaluate patients with cardiac dysrhythmias.

ANATOMY AND PHYSIOLOGY

The bifurcation of the common carotid artery possesses an abundant supply of sensory nerve endings located within the adventitia of the vessel wall (Fig. 10–1). These nerves have a characteristic spiral configuration, continually intertwining along their course and eventually uniting to form the sinus nerve of Hering. This small nerve travels but a short distance before joining the glossopharyngeal nerve, which then terminates in the cardiac and vasomotor centers of the medulla.[3] This pathway constitutes the afferent loop in the carotid sinus circuit. The efferent loop, in turn, has two parts. The vagus nerve exits the dorsal motor nucleus of cranial nerves IX and X in the medulla to supply the sinus node and the atrioventricular (AV) node. In addition, there are sympathetic inhibitory fibers that leave the med-

ullary vasoconstrictor center and travel, by way of the sympathetic chain, to supply the heart and the peripheral vasculature. Hering initially delineated these anatomic pathways in the 1920s.[1]

The afferent nerve endings located within the carotid sinus are sensitive to mean arterial pressure as well as the rate of change of pressure.[4] Generally speaking, pulsatile stimuli are more effective than sustained pressure in evoking a response.[1] Increasing stretch on the baroreceptors, which occurs in the presence of relative hypertension, leads to increased firing of the afferent nerve endings. The reverse occurs when pressures are low.[5] The sensitivity is greater in response to hypotensive states, a phenomenon that seems teleologically sound.[6]

Both the parasympathetic and the sympathetic nervous systems play a role in the carotid sinus reflex. Increased firing of the carotid sinus results in reflex stimulation of vagal activity, while simultaneously there is a reflex reduction in sympathetic output. From a clinical standpoint, the vagal effect has the most significance. The parasympathetic effect is almost immediate, occurring within the first second. The sympathetic effect, however, becomes manifest only after several seconds and may not take effect until 1 minute has elapsed.[7]

Carotid sinus stimulation has a variety of effects. The two of greatest clinical importance are the cardioinhibitory and vasodepressor effects. These are independent phenomena. The fall in heart rate is blocked by the administration of atropine, whereas epinephrine blocks the reduction in blood pressure. A third effect of carotid sinus stimulation is a cerebral response, manifested by varying degrees of alteration of consciousness; the cerebral response is independent of the reduction in heart rate and blood pressure.[8] The cerebral effect is not blocked by the administration of atropine or epinephrine.[9] The etiology of this response remains controversial, although many feel that it is a reflection of carotid occlusive disease that is exacerbated by the application of carotid sinus pressure that is too vigorous.[2, 10] The respiratory effects of carotid sinus stimulation include bronchoconstriction (CSM may induce wheezing), a decrease in respiratory rate, and pulmonary hypotension.

The parasympathetic branch of the carotid sinus reflex supplies the sinus node and the AV node. The sinoatrial pacemaker is more likely to be affected than is the AV node, except when digitalis has been administered. In order of decreasing frequency, the changes seen clinically with CSM include (1) sinoatrial slowing, occurring in approximately 75 per cent of cases and leading to sinus arrest approximately 3 per cent of the time; (2) atrial conduction defects, manifested by an increase in width of the P wave on the electrocardiogram; (3) prolongation of the PR interval and higher degrees of AV block, seen in approximately 10 per cent of cases; (4) nodal escape rhythms; (5) complete asystole, defined as sinus arrest without ventricular escape lasting greater than 3 seconds, occurring in 4 per cent of cases; and (6) premature ventricular contractions.[1, 11] Although evi-

AFFERENT   EFFERENT

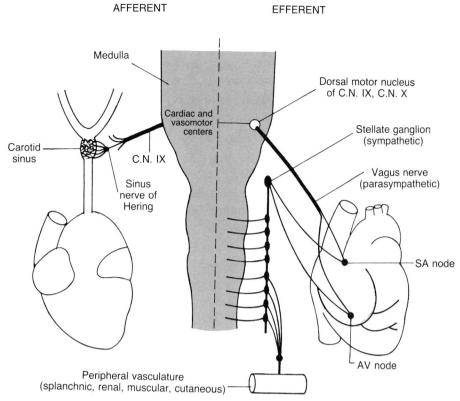

Figure 10–1. Anatomy of the carotid sinus reflex. Carotid receptors send impulses to the medulla by way of the sinus nerve of Hering and cranial nerve IX. Efferent nerves are shown on the right. (Adapted from Scher AM. Control of arterial blood pressure. In Ruch TC, Patton HD: Physiology and Biophysics. 20th ed. Vol 2. Philadelphia, WB Saunders Co, 1974.)

dence suggests some degree of vagal innervation to the ventricle, CSM has not been observed to alter the configuration of the QRS complex.[12]

The sympathetic branch of the reflex during stimulation is less important from a clinical standpoint. It exerts its effect through the stellate ganglion by sending inhibitory fibers to the sinus node and the AV node and thus further decreases heart rate. Efferents to heart muscle fibers cause a generalized decrease in cardiac contractility. Nerve endings supplying the peripheral vasculature cause a generalized vasodilation of the splanchnic, renal, muscular, and cutaneous arterial circulation.[4]

Although the carotid sinus mechanism has been described as "one of the oldest and best known of the cardiovascular reflexes,"[1] much controversy and uncertainty still exists regarding its total function. Early literature, for example, implicated the carotid sinus reflex in the development of essential hypertension, speculating that chronic elevation of blood pressure might simply reflect a basic defect in the autoregulatory capacity of the cardiovascular system. This theory was never substantiated, and it is now apparent that the carotid sinus pressor reflex acts as a "shock absorber" within the cardiovascular tree, reducing the minute-to-minute fluctuations in blood pressure to approximately 50 per cent of what they would be if the system were not operative.[4] It plays a minimal role in the long-term control of hypertension. Current topics of interest include the role of the carotid sinus in the regulation of body fluids[13] and its effect on renin secretion.[14]

CLINICAL USE OF CAROTID SINUS MASSAGE

The most valuable application of CSM is in the diagnosis and treatment of tachydysrhythmias, particularly when the QRS complex is wide and the differentiation between supraventricular and ventricular tachycardia must be made quickly.[15] It should be emphasized, however, that CSM is potentially useful when one is confronted with a dysrhythmia at any rate, including bradycardias.[1]

Lown and Levine summarize the indications for CSM with the statement that "when a patient shows a rhythm disorder that is not readily deciphered, complete investigation requires determination of the response of the heart to vagal stimulation. Carotid sinus massage is usually the simplest and safest way of achieving this."[1] Although CSM is primarily used in the management of dysrhythmias, at one time the indications for it were broader, and the technique was used in the management of angina pectoris and pulmonary edema.[1, 16] It may also be helpful in the evaluation of the patient with palpitations and a normal electrocardiogram (ECG), during auscultation of the heart in the patient with tachycardia, and in the investigation of syncope.

Bradycardia

At rates between 30 and 60 beats per minute when the rhythm is regular, CSM may differentiate between sinus bradycardia and various degrees of partial or complete heart block. If smooth, gradual slowing of the ventricular rate is achieved, then the mechanism is sinus. Under these circumstances, cessation of CSM is accompanied by a gradual return to the original heart rate. A jerky or irregular decrease in heart rate suggests the presence of second-degree heart block. The irregular slowing is a consequence of increasing AV block, and nonconducted P waves may be demonstrated. An additional clue to the presence of second-degree heart block is the precipitation of paradoxical acceleration of the

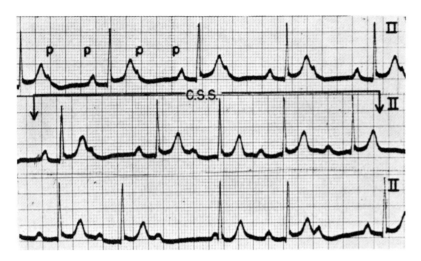

Figure 10–2. Acceleration of ventricular rate by carotid sinus stimulation (CSS). Continuous tracing. Upper strip shows 2:1 atrioventricular block: atrial rate = 102; ventricular rate = 51. The second and third strips were recorded during and after CSS, when the atrial rate was reduced to 68; a 1:1 response occurs. (From Lown B, Levine SA: Carotid sinus—clinical value of its stimulation. Circulation 23:766, 1961. Reproduced by permission.)

ventricular rate during CSM. As was discussed earlier, the carotid sinus reflex is more likely to affect the sinoatrial pacemaker rather than the AV node. In the presence of AV block, the initial response to CSM is likely to be slowing of the atrial rate by slowing of the sinoatrial node. The previously blocked impulse now reaches the AV node when it is no longer refractory to conduction. Theoretically, this could convert 2:1 conduction to 1:1 conduction and could actually increase the heart rate (Fig. 10–2).

The ventricular rate in complete heart block is unaffected by CSM, and complete heart block is ruled out if some effect on ventricular rate is achieved with the procedure. If the procedure has no effect, an independent ventricular source for the dysrhythmia is suggested. The lack of a response to carotid sinus massage is essentially nondiagnostic, however, because the failure of response may be a result of other factors as well, including an insensitive carotid sinus reflex or faulty technique on the part of the examiner. CSM may be helpful in the diagnosis of complete heart block if the procedure affects the atrial but not the ventricular rate. If the atrial rate is slowed but the ventricular rate is unaffected, previously hidden P waves may now be demonstrated. A decreased atrial rate is easily measured on a rhythm strip. CSM is useful both in slow ventricular rates and in the investigation of ventricular tachycardia (Fig. 10–3).

Normal Heart Rate

At normal rates, carotid sinus massage is also helpful diagnostically. Smooth, gradual alterations in the heart rate suggest a sinus mechanism. An abrupt slowing or an exact halving of the heart rate may occur in the presence of either paroxysmal atrial tachycardia (PAT) with block or atrial flutter. Atrial flutter with 2:1 conduction may be indistinguishable on the ECG from a sinus tachycardia. If the rate is 150 to 160 beats per minute with a sinus mechanism, the P wave will be hidden in the QRS complex but will be demonstrated if CSM slows the ventricular rate. PAT with block is often an elusive and misleading rhythm that is commonly a result of digitalis toxicity. PAT caused by digitalis toxicity is suggested by the emergence of nonconducted P waves when CSM increases AV block (Fig. 10–4). The *atrial* rate in PAT with block is characteristically less than 200 beats per minute, whereas the *atrial* rate in atrial flutter is characteristically 300 beats per minute and in a sawtooth pattern. It is important to note that the underlying cause of atrial tachycardia is almost always digitalis toxicity if CSM changes AV block to a higher degree without affecting the atrial mechanism.[17]

Tachycardia

At rapid heart rates, CSM has its greatest clinical application, because it is useful from both a diagnostic and a therapeutic standpoint (Table 10–1). If ventricular slowing is achieved with CSM, then ventricular tachycardia is most probably ruled out. The procedure may be helpful in diagnosis of ventricular tachycardia if the atrial rate is slowed while the ventricular rate remains constant or if P waves can be demonstrated to indicate AV dissociation (see Fig. 10–3). Ventricular tachycardia is not terminated by CSM in the vast majority of cases. It is generally believed that autonomic tone has little effect on ventricular dysrhythmias, but Hess and associates[18] reported two cases of ventricular tachycardia that were terminated by CSM. Other sporadic cases[19] have been reported, and the consensus that CSM will not terminate ventricular tachycardia is not an absolute rule. In the

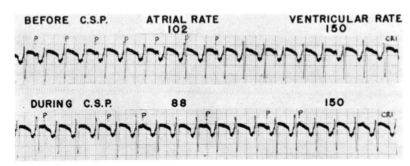

Figure 10–3. Carotid sinus pressure (CSP) slows atria but not ventricles, thus establishing the presence of atrioventricular dissociation, supporting the diagnosis of ventricular tachycardia. The QRS measures 0.16 second. Note the atrial rate slowing from 102 to 88 while the ventricular rate is unaffected. (From Lown B, Levine SA: Carotid sinus—clinical value of its stimulation. Circulation 23:766, 1961. Reproduced by permission.)

Table 10–1. *Effects of Carotid Sinus Massage on Various Cardiac Rhythms*

Cardiac Rhythm	Usual Response to Carotid Sinus Massage (CSM)
Sinus rhythm	1. Smooth and gradual slowing of ventricular rate with return to original rate with termination of CSM. (The procedure may bring out diagnostic P waves.) 2. Occasionally produces varying degrees of heart block. 3. *Caution:* Possible prolonged asystole with hypersensitive carotid sinus syndrome.
Atrial flutter or atrial fibrillation	1. Irregular slowing of ventricular rate by increasing atrioventricular (AV) block. 2. An effect is rarely absent. 3. CSM does not terminate the rhythm but may bring out diagnostic flutter or fibrillation waves. 4. *Caution:* Ventricular standstill may occur if CSM is prolonged.
Paroxysmal atrial tachycardia (PAT)	1. No effect or abrupt termination of dysrhythmia.
Paroxysmal atrial tachycardia (Wolff-Parkinson-White syndrome)	1. Varying results (slowing, no effect, termination). 2. CSM may unmask Wolff-Parkinson-White syndrome by increasing anomalous AV conduction.
Paroxysmal AV junctional tachycardia	1. No effect or termination of dysrhythmia.
Nonparoxysmal junctional tachycardia	1. No response 2. *Caution:* CSM may be dangerous if rhythm results from digitalis toxicity.
Ventricular tachycardia	1. No response in ventricular rate. 2. CSM may uncover AV dissociation by demonstrating P waves or a decrease in atrial rate. 3. If rhythm is ventricular parasystole, response may be variable.
Digitalis-toxic rhythms	1. CSM should not be attempted.

Hess cases the termination of ventricular tachycardia was thought to be secondary to CSM-induced AV nodal echo beats in one patient and direct vagal effects on the ventricular muscle or the ventricular conduction system in the other. The vast majority of cases of ventricular tachycardia, however, will not be terminated by CSM.

Smooth slowing of a rapid ventricular rate with gradual resumption of the original rate following termination of CSM indicates a sinus mechanism. Slowing may unmask P waves that were hidden in the QRS complex of a rapid sinus tachycardia (Fig. 10–5). Occasionally, varying degrees of heart block may be precipitated during CSM with an underlying sinus rhythm (Fig. 10–6). If the tachycardia stops abruptly and sinus rhythm is maintained, either paroxysmal atrial or nodal tachycardia was present (Fig. 10–7). If PAT or paroxysmal nodal tachycardia is known to be present and the response to CSM is a decrease in AV conduction without conversion, the dysrhythmia is usually secondary to digitalis excess.[15] CSM has no effect on nonparoxysmal junctional tachycardia and should not be attempted if this rhythm is known to exist, because more serious dysrhythmias may be precipitated. Nonparoxysmal junctional tachycardia is often seen with digitalis toxicity. If slowing of the heart rate is abrupt but temporary with a jerky, irregular return, then atrial flutter, atrial fibrillation, or PAT with block is present. The ventricular rate of PAT with block is rarely more than 100 beats per minute, and hence PAT with block is unlikely to be confused with the more common tachydysrhythmias.

In the presence of fast but *irregular* rhythms, the major conditions to be ruled out are atrial fibrillation, atrial flutter with varying block, sinus tachycardia with premature atrial contractions (PACs), and PAT with variable block. Atrial fibrillation, atrial flutter, and PAT with block respond to CSM in a similar fashion, with an increase in AV block. The diagnosis of atrial flutter is confirmed if CSM slows the ventricular rate and demonstrates typical flutter waves. The atrial rate in atrial flutter is characteristic—300 beats per minute (Fig. 10–8). A regular rhythm of 150 to 160 beats per minute with a narrow QRS complex should always raise the suspicion of atrial flutter with 2:1 conduction. Atrial

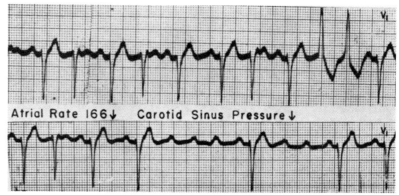

Figure 10–4. Carotid sinus pressure uncovers P waves hidden in the ventricular complex. The upper strip resembles atrial flutter or atrial fibrillation with ventricular ectopic beats. The lower strip shows paroxysmal atrial tachycardia with variable block at an atrial rate of 166. (From Lown B, Levine SA: Carotid sinus—clinical value of its stimulation. Circulation 23:766, 1961. Reproduced by permission.)

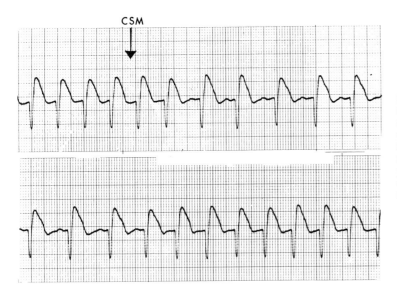

Figure 10–5. Sinus tachycardia. The sinus P wave is obscured within the descending limb of the T wave. Carotid sinus massage (CSM) transiently slows the sinus rate and exposes the P wave. The rate then increases. The strips are continuous. (From Silverman ME: Recognition and treatment of arrhythmias. In Schwartz GR, et al: Principles and Practice of Emergency Medicine. Vol. 2. Philadelphia, WB Saunders Co, 1978. Reproduced by permission.)

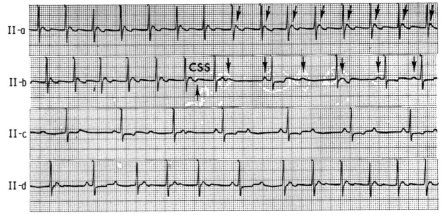

Figure 10–6. Arrows indicate sinus P waves. Strips II-a to II-d are continuous. The basic rhythm is sinus, but marked first-degree atrioventricular block is present. High-degree (advanced) atrioventricular block associated with transient slowing of sinus rate is produced by carotid sinus stimulation (CSS). (From Chung EK: Electrocardiography. 2nd ed. New York, Harper & Row, Publishers, 1980. Reproduced by permission.)

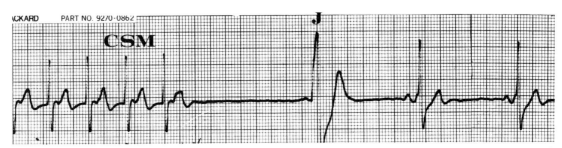

Figure 10–7. Paroxysmal atrial tachycardia. Carotid sinus massage (CSM) abolishes the dysrhythmia and results in a period of sinus suppression with a junctional (J) escape beat. Prolonged periods of asystole may produce anxiety in the physician who is waiting for the resumption of a sinus pacemaker. (From Silverman ME: Recognition and treatment of arrhythmias. In Schwartz GR, et al: Principles and Practice of Emergency Medicine. Vol 2. Philadelphia, WB Saunders Co, 1978. Reproduced by permission.)

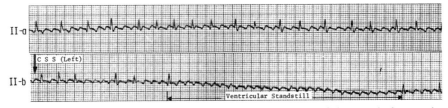

Figure 10–8. Carotid sinus stimulation (CSS, *downward arrow*) produces marked slowing of the ventricular rate in atrial flutter. Note the obvious flutter waves with an atrial rate of 300 and a long period of ventricular standstill. Strips are continuous. (From Chung EK: Electrocardiography. 2nd ed. New York, Harper & Row, Publishers, 1980. Reproduced by permission.)

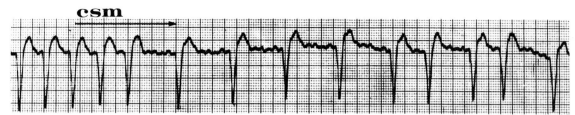

csm

Figure 10–9. Atrial fibrillation. Carotid sinus massage (CSM) slows the ventricular response transiently, revealing the fibrillating baseline. The ventricular rate will subsequently accelerate. (From Silverman ME: Recognition and treatment of arrhythmias. In Schwartz GR, et al: Principles and Practice of Emergency Medicine. Vol. 2. Philadelphia, WB Saunders Co, 1978. Reproduced by permission.)

flutter may closely resemble sinus tachycardia on the ECG and may be differentiated only with CSM. In atrial fibrillation, CSM transiently slows the ventricular rate and reveals a fibrillating baseline (Fig. 10–9). Long periods of ventricular standstill may occur following CSM in both atrial flutter and atrial fibrillation. As a rule, neither atrial flutter nor atrial fibrillation converts to a sinus rhythm with CSM. Sinus tachycardia with PACs responds in the usual fashion, with gradual slowing of the ventricular rate.

The following six "rules of massage" essentially summarize the clinical features of carotid sinus massage at any heart rate:

1. A positive effect on the ventricular rate generally rules out a ventricular dysrhythmia,[18] except in the rare instances, such as ventricular tachycardia secondary to a parasystolic mechanism. (CSM may slow the heart rate in this circumstance).[15] CSM may slow the atrial rate in ventricular tachycardia or complete heart block and may demonstrate P waves or obvious AV dissociation.

2. Abrupt changes in the heart rate without conversion are a result of increasing AV block.

3. Gradual slowing of the ventricular rate suggests the presence of a sinus rhythm. Only rarely will CSM decrease AV conduction in the presence of a sinus mechanism.

4. The dysrhythmias most likely to convert to sinus rhythm are PAT and paroxysmal nodal tachycardia.

5. Dysrhythmias that are associated with AV conduction defects (PAT with block, atrial flutter, atrial fibrillation) infrequently convert to a sinus rhythm,[15] but the ventricular rate invariably slows.

6. A negative response to CSM is nondiagnostic.

Other Clinical Considerations

The success rates for conversion of PAT and paroxysmal nodal tachycardia to sinus rhythm vary considerably in the literature. White reported only a 10 per cent rate of conversion,[20] whereas others noted success in 80 per cent of cases. Success rates are even higher when parasympathomimetic agents, such as edrophonium (Tensilon), are used in con-

junction with CSM.[4] Young patients with recurrent attacks of PAT can be taught CSM to abolish attacks without fear of producing serious side effects.[21]

CSM may also be helpful in those patients who present with palpitations, or "fluttering in the chest," and a normal ECG.[1] The differentiation between an organic and a functional etiology is difficult at times, and the temptation often is to diagnose the disorder as functional in origin. CSM may supply useful information in these cases. Because the sinus rate is slowed, an ectopic focus may emerge, or AV conduction defects may be unmasked (Fig. 10–10). In patients with Wolff-Parkinson-White syndrome, reflex vagal stimulation impairs conduction down the normal AV bundle, thus favoring conduction through the accessory pathway. Actual (antegrade) tachycardia associated with this syndrome can frequently be terminated by CSM, according to Chung,[22] but the effects of CSM in Wolff-Parkinson-White syndrome are variable. Because CSM impairs conduction in the normal AV pathways in Wolff-Parkinson-White syndrome, the favoring of conduction through the anomalous bundles may facilitate the diagnosis of this syndrome.

CSM can be a diagnostic aid during auscultation of the heart in the presence of tachycardia. If the rate is fast, it may be impossible to distinguish between the first and second heart sounds. By slowing the heart rate and lengthening diastole, CSM facilitates the differentiation. Likewise, CSM has been useful in eliciting the diastolic rumble of mitral stenosis, a murmur that is often difficult to appreciate.

In their extensive review of CSM, Lown and Levine pointed out an interesting but little appreciated phenomenon, namely, that this maneuver is helpful diagnostically and therapeutically in the evaluation of the patient with suspected angina pectoris.[1] CSM has been supplanted by newer pharmacologic agents and more sophisticated studies, such as cardiac catheterization and myocardial scanning. Nevertheless, from a physiologic and historical standpoint, the relationship between CSM and "chest pain of uncertain etiology" deserves brief discussion.

According to Wasserman, "carotid sinus massage may provide relief unobtainable by other means" in the presence of angina pectoris and may be followed by complete disap-

Figure 10–10. Carotid sinus stimulation (CSS) reveals ventricular extrasystoles, thereby explaining the cause of palpitation in this case. (From Lown B, Levine SA: Carotid sinus—clinical value of its stimulation. Circulation 23:766, 1961. Reproduced by permission.)

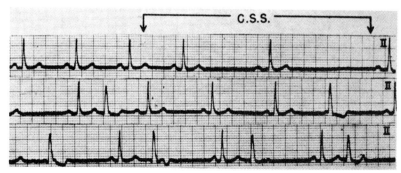

C.S.S.

pearance of the pain after only a few seconds.[23] According to Lown and Levine, relief of pain is a function of cardiac slowing.[1] More recent work has shown that relief is not accompanied by slowing of the heart rate in all cases. Bronk further suggested that relief may be secondary to inhibition of sympathetic discharge from the stellate ganglion.[24] Certainly, the speed with which relief is obtained favors a reflex neurogenic mechanism. Lown and Levine state that if chest pain is relieved by CSM, then it is anginal in origin. Pain from gastrointestinal disorder is not affected by CSM, and functional chest pain may be worsened by this procedure.[1] If there is no relief with CSM, then the test is inconclusive. These considerations suggest that CSM could have a role in the emergency department's evaluation of the patient with chest pain of uncertain etiology. One should be aware that patients with coronary artery disease, especially during an acute anginal attack, may be exquisitely sensitive to CSM and are at risk for the development of dangerous cardiac dysrhythmias.[3, 25]

According to Alzamora-Castro and colleagues, relief can be obtained in 80 per cent of patients with pulmonary edema through the use of CSM.[16] The proposed mechanism is peripheral vasodilation secondary to reflex sympathetic inhibition as well as relative bradycardia leading to more efficient diastolic filling. The following quotation from Lown and Levine reflects the enthusiasm that earlier clinicians had for this procedure in the presence of acute pulmonary edema:

> The patient is promptly able to lie flat. Pain, dyspnea, and chest oppression disappear, perspiration lessens, and pallor vanishes. Pulmonary rales decrease or clear entirely, respirations become less labored, heart sounds diminish in intensity, and the apex impulse becomes less forceful. The episode is frequently completely reversed.[1]

Despite this, CSM is not generally advocated as a first-line treatment of pulmonary edema. CSM must be maintained for extended periods in this setting, thus increasing the risk of side effects. Furthermore, the disorder can usually be handled adequately by more conventional means.

An uncommon cause of dizziness and actual syncope may be the hypersensitive carotid sinus syndrome (Fig. 10–11). Most affected patients are older and have associated diabetes or vascular disease. Some clinicians advocate the controlled use of CSM in the work-up of syncope to investigate this syndrome as a cause for clinical symptoms. Specific cautions for the diagnostic use of CSM under these circumstances are listed later.

CONTRAINDICATIONS

CSM is essentially contraindicated in two groups of patients: (1) those at significant risk for the development of a cerebrovascular accident during the procedure because of atherosclerosis of the carotid arteries, and (2) those at risk for the development of life-threatening dysrhythmias as a

manifestation of a hypersensitive carotid sinus reflex.[26, 27] Patients in this latter category may develop a syncopal episode simply by coughing, sneezing, or quickly turning the head.[9] A hypersensitive carotid sinus reflex is defined as (1) asystole lasting longer than 3 seconds and unaccompanied by the emergence of a ventricular escape rhythm, (2) a fall in the systolic blood pressure by 50 mm Hg, and (3) reproducible results following CSM. Slowing of the heart rate by 30 to 50 per cent of the original value or a decrease in the systolic blood pressure by 30 mm Hg is considered a borderline response.[26] Patients lacking a history of carotid sinus hypersensitivity should nevertheless be carefully evaluated before the procedure is attempted if the history and physical examination uncover any of the factors known to enhance the sensitivity of the carotid sinus reflex, particularly the presence of coronary artery disease or a history of digitalis use. A standby transcutaneous pacemaker (see Chapter 15) should be available when CSM is used in the setting of a suspected hypersensitive carotid sinus reflex.

A basic list of contraindications to CSM include (1) the presence of carotid bruits on physical examination; (2) age above 75; (3) a history or suspicion of sick sinus syndrome (a hypersensitive carotid sinus may be the presenting feature of previously undiagnosed sick sinus syndrome); (4) possible digitalis toxicity; and (5) the presence of nonparoxysmal junctional tachycardia (this rhythm is unresponsive to carotid sinus massage, and, more importantly, it is frequently a manifestation of digitalis toxicity).[15] CSM should be used cautiously in patients with a history or suspicion of a hypersensitive carotid sinus. The presence of coronary artery disease or ingestion of drugs known to heighten the sensitivity of the carotid sinus may render the carotid sinus hypersensitive. The use of CSM under controlled circumstances may be the only definitive test to diagnose a hypersensitive carotid sinus and may be required when a patient with debilitating symptoms is evaluated. Cardiac pacing may be indicated in such patients.

TECHNIQUE OF CAROTID SINUS MASSAGE

Given an examiner who knows how and when to massage the carotid sinus, the procedure is effective and carries minimal risk to the patient. It works best in patients with long, narrow necks.[21] In any situation, however, it is essential to have a relaxed patient. A tense platysma muscle makes palpation of the carotid sinus difficult. Furthermore, an anxious patient will be less sensitive to carotid sinus massage as a result of heightened sympathetic tone. Mild sedation of selected patients has been recommended by some physicians.[21]

Before attempting CSM, the clinician should start an intravenous line; normal saline is preferred as a precaution against hypotension. Atropine and lidocaine should be readily available at the bedside as well as resuscitative equipment, including a transvenous or transcutaneous pacemaker, in the event that a life-threatening dysrhythmia occurs.

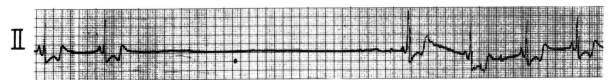

Figure 10–11. Hyperreactive carotid sinus reflex. Gentle pressure was applied to the carotid sinus for 3 seconds (indicated by the black bar over the electrocardiographic tracing), resulting in a pause in sinus rhythm of approximately 7 seconds. This syndrome may be the cause of syncope. (From Bigger JT Jr: Mechanisms and diagnosis of arrhythmias. In Braunwald E: Heart Disease. Vol. 1. Philadelphia, WB Saunders Co, 1980. Reproduced by permission.)

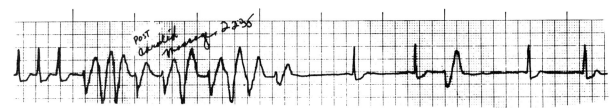

Figure 10–12. A run of ventricular tachycardia is seen immediately after a supraventricular dysrhythmia is terminated by carotid sinus massage. The patient remained asymptomatic, and a normal sinus rhythm was established spontaneously within a few seconds.

One should always auscultate for carotid bruits on both sides of the neck before attempting CSM, *because the detection of bruits is a contraindication to massage.* The patient requires continuous electrocardiographic monitoring. One should monitor a lead that is most likely to demonstrate a P wave. This is usually lead II or lead V_1 or V_2. One may use the Lewis lead modification, in which the right and left arm leads are placed at the second and fourth intercostal spaces, respectively, just to the right of the sternum. With the Lewis leads in place, the ECG machine should record on the lead I setting. It is preferable to have an assistant available at the bedside; this person can document on the monitor strip the times of initiation and termination of massage.

The patient should be in the *supine or Trendelenburg position if it can be tolerated.* Occasionally PAT will convert merely by lowering the back of the bed, presumably because the supine position results in a stretching of the carotid bulb, giving maximum baroreceptor sensitivity. The supine position may also prevent syncope. Hauswald and Tandberg have demonstrated that the mean carotid sinus diameter is increased by the Trendelenburg position and is maximum during a headstand.[28] They suggest that these positions may enhance the sensitivity of the carotid bulb through activation of stretch receptors. The pneumatic anti-shock garment (PASG) has also been used to similarly increase vagal tone (see Chapter 35).

The examiner should begin on the right side[29] and should stand slightly behind the patient, with the cardiac monitor always in full view. It is conventional to begin massage on the right side for two reasons. First, the success rate is higher with right-sided massage,[9] and second, there is a greater incidence of escape rhythms associated with right-sided carotid sinus massage.[30] Escape rhythms are generally a desirable safety mechanism should CSM produce asystole, although the precipitation of ventricular tachycardia has been observed (Fig. 10–12). The explanation for these clinical observations remains a mystery but may reflect a subtle asymmetry of neural input from side to side.[4] Simultaneous bilateral CSM is absolutely contraindicated, because no data indicate that it is more effective than unilateral CSM, and cerebral circulation may be severely compromised.

The examiner should observe the monitor, not the patient, during CSM. An assistant may watch the patient, or the examiner may have the patient count aloud to ten during the procedure.[21] This serves several purposes: First, it places an upper limit on the duration of massage; second, it continually monitors the patient's level of consciousness during CSM (as long as the patient is counting, the examiner knows that he is awake); and third, it may distract the patient from the occasional discomfort associated with the procedure.

The patient should assume the recumbent position as a precaution against syncope.[1] The head is tilted backward and slightly to the opposite side,[31] until the expansile body is readily palpated in the neck. This is usually accomplished just below the angle of the mandible at the upper level of the thyroid cartilage and anterior to the sternocleidomastoid

muscle.[1] Once the expansile body is identified, one should use the thumb[9] or the tips of the fingers to administer CSM in a posteromedial direction, aiming toward the vertebral column.[29] At this point, it must be reemphasized that the procedure is truly *massage.*[8] Simple compression of the vessel is contraindicated, because it is more dangerous and less effective. Prolonged compression has been implicated in clot formation that is due to stasis.

CSM should be firm, yet not so vigorous as to occlude the pulse of the carotid artery. One can check this tendency by simultaneously palpating the superficial temporal artery with the opposite hand.[2, 8] As long as this vessel can be felt, patency of the carotid artery is ensured. CSM should be administered up and down the length of the vessel—a distance of approximately 3 cm.[21] The massage should be continued until the desired effect is achieved, asystole develops, or 5 to 10 seconds elapse. If unsuccessful, CSM may be repeated after 30 seconds. If the procedure is still unsuccessful, the opposite carotid sinus may be massaged in a similar fashion.

If the initial CSM is ineffective, a simultaneous Valsalva maneuver may enhance carotid sinus sensitivity. In an interesting programmed electrical stimulation study by Mehta and colleagues, the Valsalva maneuver performed in the supine position was significantly more effective in terminating junctional tachycardia than a Valsalva maneuver in the standing position, CSM, or facial immersion in ice water.[31] The PASG has also been suggested as a method to enhance vagal tone during CSM. In fact, inflating the PASG in itself has been reported to terminate PAT.[33–35] If the CSM, coupled with a Valsalva maneuver in the supine or Trendelenburg position, is unsuccessful, the CSM can be repeated after the administration of digitalis, edrophonium (Tensilon), propranolol, or verapamil. CSM may be more effective following the administration of these medications and may result in termination of the dysrhythmia on a second attempt after the medication renders the carotid sinus more sensitive. However it is suggested that a Valsalva maneuver in the supine or Trendelenburg position be done in conjunction with CSM before drug therapy is instituted.

The literature reflects a lack of full standardization of the technique of CSM. Massage is advocated for anywhere from 5 to 30 seconds, and occasionally even longer.[29] In this discussion, the lower limits of time are recommended, simply because CSM should be effective within the first few seconds if done properly. In any event, the greatest obstacle to successful CSM is faulty technique, not duration of massage. Many observers believe that high failure rates reflect carotid *artery* massage, rather than massage of the sinus.[4] As Greenwood stated, "the drama of effective carotid sinus pressure by the fingers of a skilled physician is impressive."[36] This skill is certainly within the reach of any physician willing to practice and refine the technique.

COMPLICATIONS

There are two major deleterious side effects of CSM: further deterioration in the cardiac rhythm with decreased level of consciousness and a transient ischemic attack or a cerebrovascular accident as a result of interference with cerebral circulation. Lown and Levine stated that "permanent cessation of the heartbeat or serious ventricular arrhythmias are almost unheard of."[1] Since that statement was made, however, it has become apparent that in rare cases prolonged asystole or ventricular fibrillation may result from CSM. It is common, for instance, to have 3 to 5 seconds of asystole, a few escape PVCs, or a short run of ventricular beats following conversion of PAT with carotid sinus massage; the straight line or ventricular tachycardia on the ECG will invariably disappear but can produce a few anxious moments.

Dysrhythmias are largely preventable by proper patient selection. Avoidance of CSM in patients with a history or suspicion of a hypersensitive carotid sinus reflex or use of a standby transcutaneous cardiac pacemaker should eliminate cases of prolonged asystole. Furthermore, *all* cases of ventricular fibrillation following CSM have occurred in patients taking digitalis glycosides. Ventricular fibrillation should not occur if massage is withheld in patients who have digitalis toxicity. No clear danger of CSM has been demonstrated in patients with *therapeutic* levels of digitalis, but the procedure is definitely contraindicated in the presence of digitalis *toxicity.*

From time to time, authors have commented on the risk of precipitating permanent neurologic sequelae by performing CSM.[37] In 1945, Askey conducted an extensive review of this issue, presenting case reports of seven patients who became hemiplegic following CSM.[38] All patients in his series were elderly and had a history of advanced atherosclerosis. Bastulli and Orlowski reported a stroke (hemispheric infarct) temporally related to CSM in a 77-year-old patient without angiographic evidence of carotid artery disease.[39] Beal and colleagues demonstrated a probable CSM-related cerebral atheromatous embolism on autopsy in an elderly diabetic with peripheral vascular disease.[40] Interestingly, neither patient had a clinically detectable carotid bruit. Vascular stasis during prolonged CSM or an atheromatous embolism or both were postulated as the cause of these neurologic deficits. Some authors have recommended that CSM be totally avoided in the elderly, even if auscultation fails to detect a bruit. Although age itself is not a contraindication to CSM, it would seem prudent to use the technique with caution in elderly patients with known atherosclerotic vascular disease.

FACTORS AFFECTING SENSITIVITY OF THE CAROTID SINUS

The presence of diffuse, advanced atherosclerosis is associated with increased sensitivity of the carotid sinus reflex, particularly when the coronary or cerebral arteries are involved. The association between coronary artery disease and carotid sinus hypersensitivity is profound.[3,41] The exaggerated response of affected patients reflects the increased vagal tone that is invariably present. The hypersensitivity is further augmented during an anginal attack or an acute myocardial infarction. An article by Brown and co-workers showed that the degree of carotid sinus hypersensitivity was directly proportional to the severity of coronary artery disease documented by cardiac catheterization in a study of 66 patients.[42] Increased sensitivity of the carotid sinus reflex is likewise associated with hypertension and the sick sinus syndrome.

The response of the cardiovascular system to CSM is markedly age-related. A positive effect is seen in approximately 80 per cent of patients older than 40 years of age, as opposed to approximately 20 per cent of patients under 40 years old.[1] Whether this is strictly a function of age or whether it is caused by some other factor (such as atherosclerosis, which is associated with the process of aging) remains open to discussion. Males are somewhat more sensitive than females at any given age. Organic diseases that enhance vagal tone, such as cholecystitis, are associated with increased carotid sinus sensitivity.[43] Other miscellaneous conditions cited in the literature that enhance the sensitivity of the carotid sinus include fatigue, inflamed cervical lymph nodes, and the presence of acidosis.

Because carotid sinus baroreceptors are stimulated by mechanical distention of the carotid bulb, the diameter of the carotid sinus may have a great influence on vagal tone. When measured by ultrasound, the carotid sinus diameter is significantly affected by patient positioning and pneumatic anti-shock garment (PASG) inflation (Table 10–2). Hauswald and Tandberg predict a more successful response to CSM when the carotid sinus is massaged while at its greatest diameter, making a case for the clinical use of both the PASG and the Trendelenburg position during CSM.[28]

A wide variety of pharmacologic agents may render the carotid sinus hypersensitive. Digitalis must be mentioned first, because in addition to sensitizing the carotid sinus to the effects of CSM, it is a precipitating factor in the development of dysrhythmias and is frequently "on board" in those patients under consideration for therapeutic carotid sinus massage. Carotid sinus massage should not be used in patients with possible digitalis toxicity, although it may be used cautiously in patients with therapeutic digitalis levels. Other agents that may render the carotid sinus hypersensitive to massage include cholinergic agents, such as edrophonium (Tensilon), methyldopa (Aldomet),[44] propranolol,[22] morphine sulfate, nitrites, calcium, salicylates, and insulin.[45]

Conditions predisposing to sinus tachycardia or creating a state of heightened sympathetic tone are associated with a decreased sensitivity of the carotid sinus reflex. Such conditions include fever, anemia, thyrotoxicosis, pneumonia, chronic obstructive pulmonary disease, anxiety states, and hyperventilation.[9] Several drugs, including the sympathomimetics, alcohol, quinidine, and vagolytic agents, have been implicated in the production of an insensitive carotid sinus reflex. Other miscellaneous factors include hypocalcemia, hypoxia, and high spinal anesthesia.

ALTERNATIVES TO CAROTID SINUS MASSAGE

In addition to PASG and Valsalva maneuvers, other techniques have been used successfully to terminate supraventricular tachycardias. Like CSM they are based on an enhancement of vagal tone. Digital rectal massage has been reported to terminate SVT.[46] Immersing the face in an ice

Table 10–2. **Effect of Position and Mast Inflation on Carotid Sinus Diameter**[28]

Position	Mean Carotid Sinus Diameter (mm)*
Supine	5.7
Trendelenburg position	6.1
PASG inflated in supine position	6.5
PASG inflated in Trendelenburg position	7.0
Headstand	7.3

*Each mean value is significantly different (p <0.01).

water bath for 20 to 30 seconds may enhance vagal tone via the diving reflex, but this maneuver has met with varying degrees of success and requires significant patient cooperation.[47] An alternative is to place an iced washcloth on the face. Other methods, such as gagging, passing a nasogastric tube, and ocular compression have been suggested but are not routinely recommended.

CONCLUSION

CSM, the "oldest and best known cardiovascular reflex," can be useful diagnostically and therapeutically when the physician is confronted with a cardiac dysrhythmia. The major limitation to its usefulness seems to be improper technique. If the procedure is to be helpful and simultaneously is to do no harm, it must be performed properly and in the correct clinical setting. CSM is often included early in the protocol for management of cardiac dysrhythmias. CSM is to be avoided in patients with carotid bruits or suspicion of digitalis toxicity. The procedure must be used cautiously in the elderly and in those with a history of coronary artery disease.

REFERENCES

1. Lown B, Levine SA: Carotid sinus—clinical value of its stimulation. Circulation 23:766, 1961.
2. Silverstein A, et al: Manual compression of the carotid vessels, carotid sinus hypersensitivity and carotid artery occlusions. Ann Intern Med 52:172, 1960.
3. Sigler LH: Hyperactive cardioinhibitory carotid sinus reflex as an aid in the diagnosis of coronary disease—its value compared with that of the electrocardiogram. N Engl J Med 226:46, 1942.
4. Scher A: Carotid and aortic regulation of arterial blood pressure. Circulation 56:521, 1977.
5. Bjursted H, Rosenhamer G, Tyden G: Cardiovascular responses to changes in carotid sinus transmural pressure in man. Acta Physiol Scand 94:497, 1975.
6. Mancia G, Ferrari A, Gregorini L, et al: Controls of blood pressure by carotid sinus baroreceptors in human beings. Am J Cardiol 44:895, 1979.
7. Wang SC, Borison HL: An analysis of the carotid sinus mechanism. Am J Physiol 150:712, 1947.
8. Toole JF: Stimulation of the carotid sinus in man. 1. The cerebral response. 2. The significance of head positioning. Am J Med 17:952, 1959.
9. Evans E: The carotid sinus: Its clinical importance. JAMA 149:46, 1952.
10. Gurdjian EJ, Webster JE, Linder DW: On the nonexistence of the cerebral form of "irritable carotid sinus." Trans Am Neurol Assoc 49, 1958.
11. Purks WK: Electrocardiographic findings following carotid sinus stimulation. Ann Intern Med 13:270, 1939.
12. Waxman MB, Cupps CL, Cameron DA: Modulation of an idioventricular rhythm by vagal tone. J Am Coll Cardiol 11:1052, 1988.
13. Lindblad L: Circulatory effects of carotid sinus stimulation and changes in blood volume distribution in hypertensive man. Acta Physiol Scand 111:299, 1981.
14. Cunningham SC, et al: Carotid sinus reflex influence on plasma renin activity. Am J Physiol 234:H670, 1978.
15. Read EA, Scott JC: Factors influencing the carotid sinus cardioinhibitory reflex. Am J Physiol 181:21, 1955.
16. Alzamora-Castro V, Battiliana G, et al: Acute left ventricular failure and carotid sinus stimulation. JAMA 157:266, 1955.
17. Chung EK (ed): Electrocardiography: Practical Applications with Vectorial Principles. 2nd ed. New York, Harper & Row, 1980.
18. Hess DS, Hanlon T, Scheinman M, et al: Termination of ventricular tachycardia by carotid sinus massage. Circulation 65:627, 1982.
19. Waxman MB, Wald RW: Termination of ventricular tachycardia by an increase in cardiac vagal drive. Circulation 56:385, 1977.
20. White PD: Alternation of the pulse—still a common and important clinical condition. Concepts of Cardiovasc Dis 22:174, 1953.
21. Prinzmetal M: The Auricular Arrhythmias. Springfield, Ill, Charles C Thomas, 1952.
22. Chung E: Cardiac Emergency Care. 2nd ed. Philadelphia, Lea & Febiger, 1980.
23. Wasserman S: Acute Cardiac Pulmonary Edema. Springfield, Ill, Charles C Thomas, 1959.
24. Bronk DW, et al: Inhibition of cardiac accelerator impulses by the carotid sinus. Proc Soc Exp Biol Med 31:579, 1933–34.
25. Sigler LH: The hyperactive cardioinhibitory carotid sinus reflex: A possible aid in the diagnosis of coronary artery disease. Arch Inter Intern Med 67:177, 1941.
26. Trout HH III, Brown LL, Thompson JE: Carotid sinus syndrome—treatment by carotid sinus denervation. Ann Surg 189:575, 1979.
27. Chughtai A, Yans J, Kwatra M: Carotid sinus syncope. Report of two cases. JAMA 237:2320, 1977.
28. Hauswald MD, Tandberg D: The effect of patient position and MAST inflation on carotid sinus diameter. Ann Emerg Med 14:1065, 1985.
29. Gould L, et al: Usefulness of carotid sinus pressure in detecting the sick sinus syndrome. J Electrocardiography 11:261, 1978.
30. Rizzon P, DiBase M: Effect of carotid sinus reflex on cardiac impulse formation and conduction: Electrophysiologic study. In Schwartz PJ, Brown AM, Milliani A, Zanchetti A (eds): Neural Mechanisms in Cardiac Arrhythmias. New York, Raven Press, 1978.
31. Sigler LH: The cardioinhibitory carotid sinus reflex—its importance as a vagocardiosensitivity test. Am J Cardiol 12:175, 1963.
32. Mehta D, Wafa S, Ward DE, et al: Relative efficacy of various physical maneuvers in the termination of junctional tachycardia. Lancet 1:1188, 1988.
33. Walker LA, MacMath TL, Chipman H, et al: MAST application in the treatment of paroxysmal supraventricular tachycardia in a child. Ann Emerg Med 17:529, 1988.
34. Tandberg D, Rusnak R, Sklar D, et al: Successful treatment of paroxysmal supraventricular tachycardia with MAST. Ann Emerg Med 13:1068, 1984.
35. Tandberg D, Hauswald M, Rusnak R: MAST conversion of paroxysmal supraventricular tachycardia in Wolff-Parkinson-White syndrome. Ann Emerg Med 16:712, 1987.
36. Greenwood RJ, Dupler DA: Death following carotid sinus pressure. JAMA 181:605, 1962.
37. Brannon ES: Hemiplegia following carotid sinus stimulation. Am Heart J 36:299, 1948.
38. Askey JM: Hemiplegia following carotid sinus stimulation. Am Heart J 31:131, 1946.
39. Bastulli JA, Orlowski JP: Stroke as a complication of carotid sinus massage. Crit Care Med 13:869, 1985.
40. Beal MF, Parks TS, Fisher CM: Cerebral atheromatous embolism following carotid sinus pressure. Arch Neurol 38:310, 1981.
41. Reed EA, Scott JC: Factors influencing the carotid sinus cardioinhibitory reflex. Am J Physiol 181:21, 1955.
42. Brown KA, Maloney JD, Smith CH, et al: Carotid sinus reflex in patients undergoing coronary angiography: Relationship of degree and location of coronary artery disease to response to carotid sinus massage. Circulation 62:697, 1980.
43. Engel GL, Engel FL: Significance of the carotid sinus reflex and biliary tract disease. N Engl J Med 227:470, 1942.
44. Bauernfeind R, et al: Carotid sinus hypersensitivity with alpha methyldopa. Ann Intern Med 88:214, 1978.
45. Rudnikoff I: Insulin and the carotid sinus. Arch Intern Med 34:1382, 1951.
46. Roberge R, Anderson E, MacMath T, et al: Termination of paroxysmal supraventricular tachycardia by digital rectal massage. Ann Emerg Med 16:1291, 1987.
47. Peters RW, Scheinman MM: Emergency treatment of supraventricular tachycardia. Med Clin North Am 63:73, 1979.

Chapter 11

Direct Current Electrical Cardioversion

Stephen Gazak

INTRODUCTION

Cardioversion is the use of direct current electricity to convert a cardiac dysrhythmia to a sinus mechanism. The use of electrical current to terminate ventricular fibrillation is termed *defibrillation*. Cardioversion is performed with the aid of a synchronizer, which ensures a timed discharge of electrical current during a specific phase of the cardiac cycle. In defibrillation, electrical current is immediately discharged asynchronously, that is, regardless of the underlying cardiac activity.

In many cases, direct current cardioversion has specific advantages over drug therapy. The speed and simplicity of electrical cardioversion enhance its usefulness in the emergency department setting. Cardioversion is effective almost immediately, has few side effects, and is often more successful than drug therapy in terminating dysrhythmias. In addition, the effective dose of many antidysrhythmic medications has not been standardized, and there is often a small margin between therapeutic and toxic dosages. Although they suppress an undesired rhythm, drugs may also suppress a normal sinus mechanism or may create toxic manifestations that are more severe than the dysrhythmia being treated. In the clinical setting of hypotension or acute cardiopulmonary collapse, cardioversion may be life saving.

The earliest recorded experimentation in "therapeutic" electroshock was performed by Abildgaard in 1775, when he demonstrated that dead fowl could be revived by means of an electrical shock of a certain amplitude.[1] In 1899, Provost and Batelli observed that a relatively small current of electricity induced ventricular fibrillation, whereas a stronger current discharged over a short interval terminated ventricular fibrillation.[2]

In 1947, Beck was the first to defibrillate the human heart successfully, and in the early 1960s, electrical energy was used to treat dysrhythmias other than ventricular fibrillation for the first time. Alternating current remained in vogue until 1962, when Lown and colleagues advocated direct current countershock as the method of choice for terminating atrial fibrillation.[3] This advance culminated years of investigation that had suggested that direct current was safer and more effective than alternating current in the treatment of dysrhythmias. Ventricular fibrillation follows alternating current countershock in an alarming number of cases. The switch to direct current immediately led to a tenfold decrease in the incidence of ventricular fibrillation following countershock.

BACKGROUND

In 1934, King noted that discharge of a low-intensity current would precipitate ventricular fibrillation only when current was applied during a specific phase of the cardiac cycle. This 30-msec interval immediately preceding the apex of the T wave on the electrocardiogram was termed the "vulnerable period." The vulnerable period represents the phase of early repolarization in the cardiac cycle. During this phase, a variably excitable field results from asynchronous recovery of individual myocardial cells. An electrical impulse interspersed during this period may precipitate a reentrant dysrhythmia, which can degenerate into ventricular fibrillation. The synchronizer on the cardioverter is programmed to discharge a direct current shock, which is timed to avoid the vulnerable period of the T wave. At delivered currents exceeding

1 ampere (greater than 100 joules), the entire ventricle is depolarized, and the risk of ventricular fibrillation by stimulation in the vulnerable period is thus eliminated.

The relative safety of direct current countershock is easily explained. The duration of direct current discharge is exceedingly brief (1.5 to 4 msec) and thus can be programmed to avoid the vulnerable period. In contrast, the standard 60-Hz sinusoidal waveform of alternating current has a duration of 0.2 second. Because of the relatively lengthy duration of this waveform, it is difficult to guarantee discharge of alternating current shock outside the vulnerable period during cardioversion (Fig. 11–1).

The basic concept of cardioversion is that electrical shock momentarily causes depolarization of the majority of cardiac cells and allows the sinus node to resume normal pacemaker function. In reentrant dysrhythmias, such as paroxysmal supraventricular tachycardia and ventricular tachycardia, cardioversion restores sinus rhythm by interrupting a self-perpetuating reentrant circuit. Reentry is similar to an advancing wavefront that "chases its tail" in a cyclic journey around the conducting tissue of the heart. This advancing wavefront is separated from its tail by a stretch of nonrefractory tissue, the so-called excitable gap (Fig.11–2). Cardioversion succeeds by depolarizing a segment of the excitable gap, which is then refractory when the wave of depolarization arrives.[2] The self-perpetrating cardiac dysrhythmia is thus abolished, and the sinus node resumes its function as a pacemaker. Cardioversion is much less effective in terminating tachycardias resulting from augmented normal automaticity, such as digitalis-induced dysrhythmias.

INDICATIONS AND CONTRAINDICATIONS

Cardioversion is indicated on an emergency basis when cardiac dysrhythmias are complicated by the presence of significant hypotension, congestive heart failure, chest pain suggesting myocardial ischemia, or evidence of cerebral

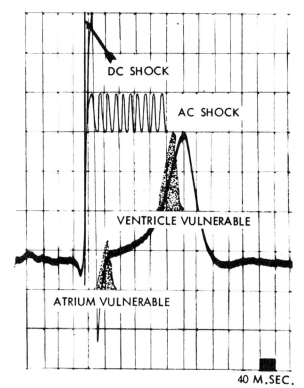

Figure 11–1. Phases of vulnerability for atrium and ventricle. Note that an alternating current shock of 0.20 second may end at the T wave even when synchronized with the R wave of the electrocardiogram. (From Resnekov L: Theory and practice of electroversion in cardiac dysrhythmias. Med Clin North Am 60:325, 1976. Reproduced by permission.)

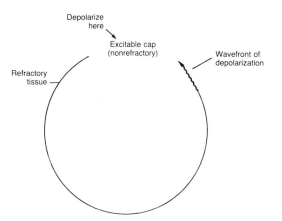

Figure 11–2. Schematic representation of the mechanism of termination of a cardiac dysrhythmia by cardioversion. See text.

ischemia. Rapid cardioversion is also advocated when the ventricular rate exceeds 180, especially in the elderly patient, because of the risk of imminent hemodynamic compromise.[5] Cardioversion is useful on a less urgent basis in the patient with a cardiac dysrhythmia refractory to conventional drug therapy. It is a common tendency and a common error to delay cardioversion in a compromised patient in the hope that drug therapy will prove successful. Such a timid approach should be avoided, because the outcome of procrastination may be cardiac arrest.

A history or suspicion of digitalis toxicity is a relative contraindication to the use of emergency cardioversion; alternatives to cardioversion are preferable in this case. A therapeutic digitalis level, however, is not a contraindication to cardioversion. Slow atrial fibrillation, usually secondary to ischemic heart disease if not digitalis related, is also a relative contraindication. Restoration of sinus rhythm in this setting may result in an even slower ventricular rate, which may worsen the patient's condition. Likewise, patients known to be in the tachycardiac phase of sick sinus syndrome may develop asystole following cardioversion, and thus the procedure is also contraindicated in this instance. Intravenous overdrive pacing is preferable in these settings. The presence of myocardial infarction is *not* a contraindication to cardioversion.

EQUIPMENT AND PREPARATION FOR CARDIOVERSION

The cardioverter device consists of five components (Fig. 11–3): (1) a direct current depolarizer, which provides varying amounts of electrical current; (2) an oscilloscope screen for monitoring heart rate and rhythm; (3) access to a continuous electrocardiogram (ECG) readout to document the patient's course and response to treatment; (4) two removable electrode paddles, which can be applied easily to the patient's chest wall; and (5) a synchronizer, permitting discharge of energy outside the vulnerable period of the cardiac cycle. The synchronizer permits triggering of the electrical discharge by the R or S wave of the ECG.

The actual size of the electrode paddle is of no great significance, but paddles must be large enough to depolarize the majority of heart fibers simultaneously. In addition, because current is discharged over a greater surface area, larger paddles limit the risk of myocardial injury by decreasing the current density passing through each unit of myocardium. Most conventional paddles have an electrode diameter of at least 4 inches.

The ideal placement of the paddle on the chest wall has

been debated ever since the inception of cardioversion. Two systems have been used traditionally in clinical practice: (1) the anterolateral position, with one paddle placed in the left fourth to fifth intercostal space, midaxillary line, and the other just to the right of the sternal margin in the second to third intercostal space (Fig. 11–4); and (2) the anteroposterior position, with one paddle placed anteriorly over the sternum and the other on the back between the scapulae (Fig. 11–5). Many of the newer cardioverter-defibrillators are specifically designed for anterolateral paddle placement. Anteroposterior paddle placement may be more convenient in elective cases, the operator manipulates only one paddle during the procedure of cardioversion, but this position of paddle placement may be inconvenient in an emergency. Either method of paddle placement is acceptable in clinical practice. Kerber and associates demonstrated that transthoracic resistance, paddle size, or paddle position has no relationship to the energy required or the incidence of successful elective cardioversion in patients with atrial flutter or atrial fibrillation.[6]

Generous use of ECG paste or defibrillator gel pads on the underside and, especially, along the edges of the electrode paddles is essential, both to reduce transthoracic impedance and to prevent skin burns. Paste should be applied liberally but must never run between paddles if the anterolateral approach is used, because the paste may cause current (which always seeks the path of least resistance) to be diverted over the skin surface and away from the heart. This is a crucial consideration, because (even under ideal circumstances) only 10 to 30 per cent of the total current passes through the heart. Saline-soaked pads are generally not practical or safe for the aforementioned reasons.

Before cardioversion, the patient should assume the supine position and should be as relaxed as possible, with an intravenous line and supplemental oxygen in place. The use of analgesia (e.g., 50 to 150 μg fentanyl) and sedative agents (e.g., 50 to 120 mg methohexital) just before initiating the procedure (when time permits) is *strongly* recommended. The cardiac rhythm is under constant surveillance by the oscilloscope on the cardioverter. To ensure discharge of the current at the appropriate time, one should choose the lead that displays the highest R wave amplitude. When it is activated in the synchronized mode, the cardioverter will automatically discharge when it "reads" a regular recurrent R wave. It is preferable to have the monitor sense the electrical activity through standard electrode leads rather than through the paddles.

The provision of adequate analgesia and amnesia is an absolute prerequisite in the stable conscious patient. Stressing the need for premedication, Kowey has emphasized the significant adverse psychologic impact of the procedure in the awake patient, citing insomnia, fear of physicians, depression, nightmares, panic attacks, and multiple somatic complaints after undergoing cardioversion.[7] Intravenous midazolam (Versed) is an excellent short-acting amnestic, and it is preferred by many physicians. The dosage is 2 to 5 mg initially, given intravenously over 1 to 2 minutes, followed by increments of 1 mg every 1 minute until adequate sedation is achieved. Slurred speech, nystagmus, or obtundation should be present to enhance amnesia. The average dose required for effective amnesia and sedation is 5 to 15 mg, but variability among patients is considerable, and clinical evaluation is the best judge of adequate premedication. Suitable alternatives are diazepam or lorazepam in doses sufficient to produce adequate sedation.[8, 9] Because of their depressant effect on respiration, however, benzodiazepines must be used cautiously in the elderly and in patients with congestive heart failure or pulmonary disease. Some clinicians prefer a short-acting barbiturate, such as metho-

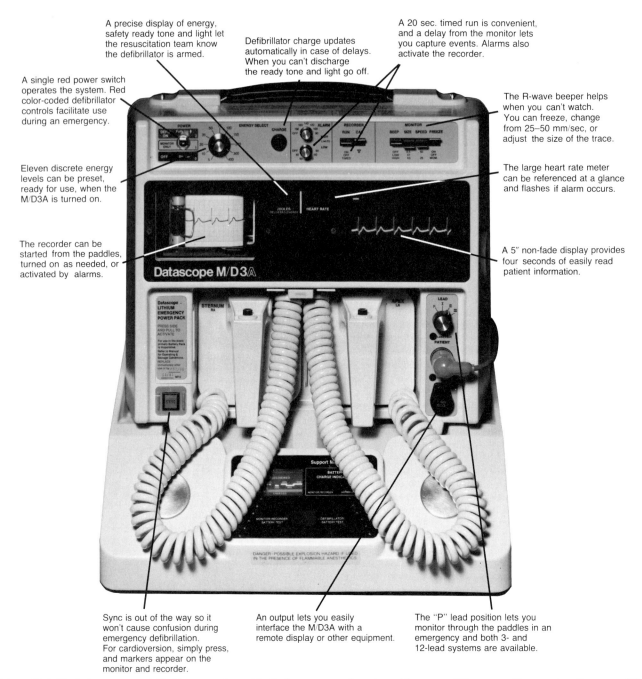

A precise display of energy, safety ready tone and light let the resuscitation team know the defibrillator is armed.

Defibrillator charge updates automatically in case of delays. When you can't discharge the ready tone and light go off.

A 20 sec. timed run is convenient, and a delay from the monitor lets you capture events. Alarms also activate the recorder.

A single red power switch operates the system. Red color-coded defibrillator controls facilitate use during an emergency.

The R-wave beeper helps when you can't watch. You can freeze, change from 25–50 mm/sec, or adjust the size of the trace.

Eleven discrete energy levels can be preset, ready for use, when the M/D3A is turned on.

The large heart rate meter can be referenced at a glance and flashes if alarm occurs.

The recorder can be started from the paddles, turned on as needed, or activated by alarms.

A 5″ non-fade display provides four seconds of easily read patient information.

Datascope M/D3A

Sync is out of the way so it won't cause confusion during emergency defibrillation. For cardioversion, simply press, and markers appear on the monitor and recorder.

An output lets you easily interface the M/D3A with a remote display or other equipment.

The "P" lead position lets you monitor through the paddles in an emergency and both 3- and 12-lead systems are available.

Figure 11–3. Typical converter–defibrillator monitor with display screen and readout. (Courtesy of Datascope Corporation, Paramus, NJ).

hexital sodium (Brevital), for anesthesia because this agent is more effective than diazepam as an amnestic and has a shorter duration of action. The dosage of methohexital is 5 to 12 ml of a 1 per cent solution (50 to 120 mg), given by slow intravenous push.

Ancillary Equipment

Resuscitation equipment (including bag-valve-mask apparatus) and ampules of lidocaine, atropine, and other antidysrhythmics must be immediately available should respiratory depression or life-threatening ventricular ectopy or bradycardia ensue during or following attempts at cardioversion.

TECHNIQUE OF CARDIOVERSION

The technique of cardioversion is essentially the same regardless of the dysrhythmia.[10] One proceeds to the cardioverter, turning the power on and setting the unit on the synchronized mode. A common error in an emergency is to neglect to set the machine in the synchronized mode, because most equipment is routinely stored in the nonsynchronized mode in anticipation of ventricular fibrillation. Two to 10 seconds are required for the capacitor to warm up and the charge button to light up. One selects the desired energy by choosing the corresponding number on the dial labeled "energy select." One should begin at the lowest practical energy for the specific dysrhythmia and should increase the power gradually if cardioversion is unsuccessful and the clinical situation permits. A useful rule of thumb in elective

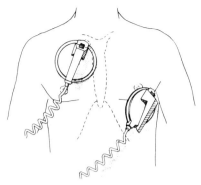

Figure 11–4. Anterolateral paddle electrode position. (From Suratt, PM, Gibson RS: Manual of Medical Procedures. St. Louis, CV Mosby Co, 1982. Reproduced by permission).

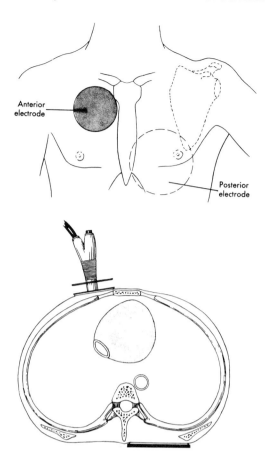

Figure 11–5. Anteroposterior paddle electrode position. (From Suratt PM Gibson RS: Manual of Medical Procedures. St. Louis, CV Mosby Co, 1982. Reproduced by permission.)

cases is to begin at 25 joules in adults, increasing to 50, 100, 150, 200, 250, 300, 350, and 400 joules in succession as needed. If the patient is taking digitalis, one should begin at 5 to 10 joules and should proceed in increments of 5 to 10 joules.[4] In the clinical setting of acute coronary or cerebral ischemia, myocardial infarction, pulmonary edema, or cardiovascular collapse, that has been aggravated or caused by the patient's dysrhythmia, one should select an energy that is most likely to produce immediate cardioversion. In the adult, a 150- to 200-joule initial shock is acceptable. In a child, the initial energy setting of 2 joules per kg is satisfactory. *Note: One should always be prepared for the development of ventricular fibrillation or asystole following cardioversion.*

Irregular rhythms, such as atrial fibrillation or atrial flutter with variable block, may not be converted with the synchronized mode and may require unsynchronized shock. The chance occurrence of ventricular fibrillation following unsynchronized cardioversion is approximately 2 per cent,[4] although some physicians routinely use no synchronizer during the procedure.[11] If no synchronizer is used, it is important to use a higher energy level to ensure depolarization of all myocardial fibers and to lessen the chance for ventricular fibrillation.

Before attempting cardioversion, with the monitor sensing the rhythm through standard leads, the operator should check the accuracy of discharge within the cardiac cycle by placing the paddles against each other and discharging the current.[3] One should observe where the blip discharge artifact occurs on the monitor. The blip must coincide with the peak of the R wave. One must be absolutely certain that the monitor screen is free of artifact before proceeding to the patient. The capacitor may inadvertently interpret artifact as R waves, with potentially disastrous results. Likewise, improper synchronization may occur in the patient with tall T waves or in the presence of right bundle branch block. The lead that best shows the R wave should always be chosen for monitoring, because the cardioverter only "senses" the QRS complex that appears on the screen.

The patient's skin must never be in contact with metal on the stretcher, and all bystanders must remove themselves from the stretcher before cardioversion. The operator should place the well-lubricated paddles firmly against the chest wall in the appropriate positions. Firm paddle contact is essential to minimize transthoracic impedance and to ensure proper contact. Approximately 20 pounds of contact pressure is desirable. *The operator should not be in contact with the stretcher or the patient at the time of cardioversion to avoid the potential of self-injury.* One should warn ancillary staff that countershock is imminent by shouting "all clear." The operator should press the buttons on the paddles to discharge current during exhalation when the thoracic impedance is

minimized. There will be a delay of a few moments before the current is discharged, so one must maintain constant contact with the chest wall. The patient's response is heralded by a twitch of the thoracic muscles, a jerk of the arms, and an audible sigh. If cardioversion is successful, the monitor will usually reveal sinus bradycardia initially. This will be followed by a gradually accelerating rate as the sinus node warms up.[5] If normal sinus rhythm is obtained, the operator should stop. If the dysrhythmia persists, patient clinical status permitting, one should wait at least 3 minutes before proceeding to the next energy level. If ventricular fibrillation occurs, one should *switch off the synchronizer* and defibrillate *immediately.* Following successful cardioversion, the patient should be monitored in a critical care setting for at least 24 hours; proper antidysrhythmic medication should be given to prevent recurrence.

DRUG THERAPY AND CARDIOVERSION

All efforts should be made to ensure that there is a proper electrolyte and acid-base balance and adequate oxygenation before cardioversion is attempted.

There is no convincing evidence that quinidine or any other antidysrhythmic drug given *routinely* immediately before cardioversion reduces the energy requirements, increases the chance for success, or helps maintain sinus rhythm afterward. Medication may, however, prevent premature beats following cardioversion. In elective cases, some physicians prefer to have patients receive maintenance quinidine therapy before cardioversion of atrial fibrillation and to withhold digitalis for 48 hours before cardioversion. Such protocols are impossible in the unstable patient who requires emergency cardioversion.

As a routine approach to patients requiring emergency cardioversion of *non–digitalis-toxic* rhythms, no prophylactic medications are given. If premature ventricular beats occur following unsuccessful cardioversion, they should be suppressed with intravenous lidocaine in 50- to 75-mg bolus injections (or equivalent doses of procainamide) before one proceeds to the next higher energy level. Such drugs may depress pacemaker function as well as suppress ectopic beats. If persistent after successful cardioversion, premature ventricular contractions (PVCs) may indicate digitalis toxicity or electrolyte disturbance and should be treated accordingly. Lidocaine, procainamide, or phenytoin may be helpful. A few transient PVCs frequently occur following cardioversion and need not be treated. Persistent bradycardia or asystole following cardioversion should be treated with intravenous atropine (1.0 to 2.0 mg).

Patients with *digitalis-toxic* rhythms present a particularly difficult problem. Fortunately, most digitalis-toxic rhythms need not be treated with cardioversion. Digitalis significantly lowers the direct current threshold for ventricular tachycardia and ventricular fibrillation in dogs, but direct current cardioversion appears safe in converting supraventricular dysrhythmias in patients receiving maintenance digitalis therapy who have no evidence of digitalis toxicity, acute myocardial ischemia, or electrolyte disturbance.[12] The potential for dangerous ventricular rhythms or ventricular fibrillation following cardioversion in the presence of digitalis toxicity has long been recognized (Fig. 11–6). When emergency cardioversion is required in patients with digitalis toxicity, it appears prudent to pretreat with prophylactic intravenous lidocaine (75 to 100 mg), phenytoin (100 to 200 mg), or procainamide (75 to 100 mg) *before* cardioversion and to check serum potassium levels on a stat basis. Magnesium sulfate (1 to 2 gm over 2 minutes intravenously) also may be helpful. Propranolol has been advocated, but it should be administered with the concomitant use of atropine to prevent asystole or bradycardia following cardioversion. The availability of rapidly acting digitalis-specific antibodies (Digibind) has reduced significantly the morbidity and mortality from digitalis poisoning. This agent should be used in the setting of digitalis-toxic rhythms and may obviate the need for electrical cardioversion. In addition to administering prophylactic medication, one should reduce the energy used in this situation by 10 to 15 joules.[13–15]

ENERGY REQUIREMENTS FOR SPECIFIC DYSRHYTHMIAS

Cardioversion is effective in terminating a variety of cardiac dysrhythmias. In an emergency situation, any dysrhythmia associated with a rapid ventricular rate may be treated with cardioversion. General energy requirements for specific dysrhythmias are discussed in the following paragraphs.

Ventricular Tachycardia

Cardioversion is successful in converting ventricular tachycardia in more than 95 per cent of cases.[4] In the stable patient, drug therapy is advocated as the first-line treatment. The energy required for effective termination of ventricular tachycardia is almost always less than 100 joules, and 10 joules will convert approximately 80 per cent of cases. An initial setting of 25 to 50 joules is suggested.

If ventricular tachycardia occurs at rapid rates with bizarre and widened QRS intervals, a broad, prominent T wave may not be distinguished from the QRS complex. This has been termed "ventricular tachycardia of the vulnerable period," or ventricular flutter.[2] In such a setting, the cardioverter apparatus may not be able to separate the T wave from the QRS complex. Synchronized cardioversion under these circumstances may be dangerous, because there is a 50 per cent chance that current will be discharged during the peak of the T wave or the vulnerable period of the cardiac cycle. Nonsynchronized cardioversion of at least 100 joules is preferable in these instances. The chance occurrence of ventricular fibrillation in association with asynchronized cardioversion is 2 per cent, and one may minimize this small risk further by delivering a shock of sufficient energy to depolarize all myocardial fibers instantaneously. This requires an electrical current of at least 1 ampere. In clinical practice, a shock of 100 joules or greater will accomplish this. Immediately following conversion of ventricular tachycardia, antidysrhythmic medication should be given to prevent recurrence.

Atrial Flutter

Atrial flutter is ideally suited to cardioversion. Atrial flutter is difficult to convert with drug therapy, which must often be given to the point of toxicity, but sinus rhythm is easily achieved through cardioversion. Success has been reported in 72 to 100 per cent of cases,[2, 4, 6, 7] with most investigators reporting success in more than 90 per cent of patients. Cardioversion is now considered the treatment of choice for atrial flutter, even in stable patients. Low energies generally will suffice, and a shock of 25 to 50 joules is usually successful on the first attempt.[2] Some cases of atrial flutter that do not immediately change to sinus rhythm may instead convert to atrial fibrillation,[18] especially after an initial countershock of low intensity (10 to 20 joules). These cases will usually convert to sinus rhythm with the use of higher energies.

Atrial Fibrillation

Cardioversion is effective in the majority of cases of atrial fibrillation, the most common disorder of the heart beat, although there is a smaller immediate and long-term success rate than that in cases of atrial flutter.[2–4, 19–22] If atrial

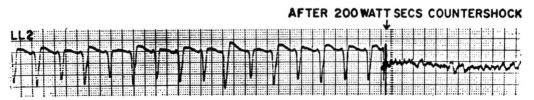

Figure 11–6. Ventricular fibrillation following countershock in the presence of digitalis toxicity (lead 2). Control shows junctional paroxysmal tachycardia (rate, 150 beats per minute), probably the result of digitalis toxicity. Note the occurrence of ventricular fibrillation following countershock (*arrow*) (From Bellet S: Clinical Disorders of the Heart Beat. 3rd ed. Philadelphia, Lea & Febiger, 1971. Reproduced by permission.)

fibrillation in the absence of demonstrable heart disease (idiopathic, or "lone," atrial fibrillation) is excluded, success rates approach 90 per cent. Atrial fibrillation seldom requires cardioversion on an emergency basis, and chronic or recurrent cases are best managed with drug therapy.

Duration of the rhythm is the single most important factor affecting successful cardioversion of atrial fibrillation. An average of 100 joules is required when atrial fibrillation has been present for less than 3 months, in contrast to an average of 150 joules when the rhythm has persisted for more than 6 months.[2] The chance of successful conversion or the maintenance of sinus rhythm is decreased in the presence of an enlarged left atrium, atrial fibrillation of longer than 1 year's duration, chronic mitral valve disease, and atrial fibrillation in the setting of left ventricular failure. If slow atrial fibrillation is encountered in the absence of cardiac medication, the use of cardioversion is dangerous, and the procedure should not be attempted because serious bradycardia may result.

The size of the fibrillatory, or F, wave in the V_1 lead is a reliable predictor of the energy requirements for conversion of atrial fibrillation to sinus rhythm.[2] The energy is inversely proportional to the size of the F wave. On the average, a shock of 140 joules is needed when the F wave is 1 mm in height, whereas one of approximately 90 joules is required when the F wave measures 2 mm.

Supraventricular Tachycardia

Most cases of supraventricular tachycardia can be treated with carotid sinus massage (see Chapter 10) or drug therapy, but in a series studied by Vassaux and Lown, cardioversion was successful in terminating 70 per cent of cases of supraventricular tachycardia (paroxysmal atrial tachycardia [PAT] with block, paroxysmal atrial tachycardia, and junctional tachycardias).[23] Most failures occurred in the presence of PAT with block, a rhythm that is often a manifestation of digitalis toxicity. When PAT with block is successfully converted to sinus rhythm, it often occurs at low energies. Patients who fail to convert generally respond as though they are overdigitalized, with further deterioration of the rhythm.

The most important factor complicating the approach in the case of the patient with supraventricular tachycardia is the presence of digitalis. Cardioversion is dangerous in the patient who is taking digitalis, and low energies must always be used in this setting.[13–15]

Cardioversion may actually be helpful diagnostically in determining whether a dysrhythmia is digitalis related.[24] If attempts at cardioversion are met with increasing degrees of atrioventricular block or PVCs, then digitalis toxicity should be suspected. If the atrial rate increases following unsuccessful cardioversion, then digitalis toxicity is invariably present.

Paroxysmal atrial tachycardia is a common dysrhythmia during pregnancy, especially in the third trimester. Schroeder and Harrison used cardioversion successfully during all three trimesters of pregnancy without serious side effects to mother or fetus.[25] Fetal rhythm should be monitored when cardioversion is attempted during the third trimester of pregnancy, although the risk of inducing fetal dysrhythmias is small, because the effective energy reaching the fetus is exceedingly low.[2]

COMPLICATIONS

In 1970, Resnekov reported a 14.5 per cent overall incidence of complications following cardioversion, excluding minor complications, such as superficial skin burns, slight

muscle discomfort, and transient bradycardia immediately after shock. The complication rate is profoundly dose related (Fig. 11–7). At 150 joules, the incidence of complications is only 6 per cent, whereas at 400 joules, the incidence rises to greater than 30 per cent.[4]

Dysrhythmias are a frequent complication following cardioversion.[26] Usually they are benign and transient. The establishment of a temporary nodal rhythm before the sinus node takes over is quite common, as are PVCs and bigeminy. These transient dysrhythmias need not be treated if they follow conversion of a supraventricular rhythm. Frequent or multifocal PVCs are a warning of impending ventricular dysrhythmias and should be abolished with intravenous medication. Antidysrhythmic medication should always be given following cardioversion of ventricular tachycardia.

The incidence of serious ventricular dysrhythmias following cardioversion is proportional to the energy requirement.[26] Lown and colleagues observed that the risk of ventricular tachycardia in dogs was 3 per cent at 100 joules, rose to 25 per cent at 200 joules, and was 65 per cent at 400 joules. They likewise reemphasized the danger of cardioversion in the presence of digitalis by demonstrating an 8000-fold increase in sensitivity to electrical shock in dog models following administration of toxic doses of ouabain.[2] Patients with enlarged hearts are also at increased risk of developing ventricular dysrhythmias following cardioversion.

The incidence of ventricular fibrillation has been reported to be 0.8 per cent following synchronized cardioversion and is essentially of two types. The first (more benign) variety occurs immediately after countershock and is easily reversed by a second, nonsynchronized shock. This type of ventricular fibrillation results from improper synchronization, with discharge of current occurring during the vulnerable period. The second variety, which is more ominous, occurs approximately 30 seconds to a few minutes following attempted cardioversion. This dysrhythmia is characteristically preceded by the development of PAT with block or a junctional rhythm. In affected patients, it may be very difficult to convert the dysrhythmia to a sinus rhythm. This phenomenon occurs in patients who have been taking digitalis glycosides and is presumably a manifestation of digitalis toxicity.[27, 28]

An increase in serum enzyme levels (CK, LDH, SGOT) may also occur following cardioversion, and the incidence has been reported to be between 10 and 70 per cent.[2, 4, 27]

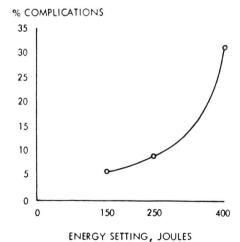

Figure 11–7. Percentage of complications in 220 patients treated by countershock related to the maximum energy setting used ≤ 150 joules, 108 patients; ≤ 250 joules, 55 patients; ≤ 400 joules 37 patients. (From Resnekov L: Theory and practice of electroversion in cardiac dysrhythmias. Med Clin North Am 60:325, 1976. Reproduced by permission.)

The enzyme rise is usually a consequence of skeletal muscle injury rather than myocardial damage. Transient ST segment elevation occurs in 3 per cent of cases but does not necessarily indicate myocardial injury, as subsequent cardiac scanning of these patients has shown.[29] Cardioversion does not alter the enzyme profile of patients with myocardial infarction.[30]

Myocardial damage may occur as a consequence of countershock and is usually subepicardial in location.[2] The risk is a function of many variables, including the strength and number of shocks; impedance of the heart, the ribs, and the skin; the size of the electrodes; the use of ECG paste versus saline pads and creams; and the interval between successive shocks.[31] In general, smaller and fewer shocks, lower impedance, large electrodes, use of ECG paste or gel pads, and intervals of at least 3 minutes between shocks will minimize the risk of myocardial injury.

Pulmonary and systemic embolization occurs in approximately 1.5 per cent of patients following cardioversion.[2, 4, 22] This risk, however, is negligible in patients who have previously undergone anticoagulation therapy. Lown and colleagues reported that the incidence of embolism following cardioversion of atrial fibrillation was 1.2 per cent in a series of 450 patients, with a zero incidence in the 100 patients who received anticoagulation therapy before countershock.[3] Such observations raise the issue of the value of prophylactic anticoagulation before cardioversion. Although this measure may be impractical in the emergency situation the use of intravenous heparin has been advocated when there is an increased risk of embolism, such as in patients with myocardial infarction, coronary artery disease, mitral valve disease, cardiomyopathy, prosthetic heart valves, or history of a previous embolic event.[2]

A puzzling complication of cardioversion that has been reported periodically is the development of pulmonary edema approximately 1 to 3 hours following successful cardioversion.[32–35] With the exception of one case, it has occurred exclusively following conversion to normal sinus rhythm, thus developing paradoxically in cases in which improved cardiac output would be expected. Myocardial damage secondary to countershock was originally implicated in these cases of pulmonary edema, but it has since been shown that this complication occurs regardless of the strength or the number of shocks, factors that are known to increase the risk of myocardial injury. One of the more popular current theories is that the development of pulmonary edema represents a defect in contractile capacity of the left atrium relative to the right atrium.

Other miscellaneous complications that have been reported in the literature include pericarditis,[36] pneumonitis, hypotension, ocular damage,[37] transient left recurrent laryngeal nerve paralysis, and compression fractures of the thoracic vertebrae.[38]

CONCLUSION

The overall success rate of direct current cardioversion in the presence of cardiac dysrhythmias approaches 90 per cent. Countershock is a relatively recent therapeutic method that combines safety, ease of operation, and efficacy when used properly. It is an invaluable tool in the emergency department setting when cardiac dysrhythmias are complicated by the presence or threat of hemodynamic compromise. Extreme caution must be exercised in patients who are taking digitalis as well as those with sick sinus syndrome, and electrical cardioversion is relatively contraindicated in these groups. Cardioversion is most effective in the presence of ventricular tachycardia and atrial flutter, although it is also frequently successful in cases of atrial fibrillation and various supraventricular tachycar-

dias. The lowest practical energy setting should be used initially, because complications are directly proportional to shock strength.

REFERENCES

1. Driscol T, Ratnoff O, Nygaard OF: The remarkable Dr. Abildgaard and countershock. Ann Intern Med 83:878, 1972.
2. DeSilva RA, et al: Cardioversion and defibrillation. Am Heart J. 100:881, 1980.
3. Lown B, et al: "Cardioversion" of atrial fibrillation. N Engl J Med 269:325, 1963.
4. Resnekov L: Theory and practice of electroversion in cardiac dysrhythmias. Med Clin North Am 60:325, 1976.
5. Isselbacher KJ, et al (eds): Harrison's Principles and Practice of Internal Medicine. 9th ed. New York, McGraw-Hill Book Co, 1980, pp 1072–1073.
6. Kerber RE, et al: Elective cardioversion: Influence of paddle-electrode location and size on success rates and energy requirements. N Engl J Med 305:658, 1981.
7. Kowey PR: The calamity of cardioversion of conscious patients Am J Cardiol 13:1106, 1988.
8. Orko R: Anesthesia for cardioversion: A comparison of diazepam, thiopentone, and propanidid. Br J Anaesth 48:257, 1976.
9. Kahler RI, Burrow FJ, Felig P: Diazepam-induced amnesia for cardioversion. JAMA 200:997, 1967.
10. Lown B, Klieger R, Wolff G: The technique of cardioversion. Am Heart J 67:282, 1964.
11. Kreus KE, Salokannel SJ, Waris EK: Nonsynchronized and synchronized direct-current countershock in cardiac arrhythmias. Lancet 2:405, 1966.
12. Ditchey RV, Karlinger JS: Safety of electrical cardioversion without digitalis toxicity. Ann Intern Med 95:676, 1981.
13. Hagemeijer F, Van Houwe E: Titrated energy cardioversion of patients on digitalis. Br Heart J 37:1303, 1975.
14. Szekely P, Wynne NA, Pearson DT, et al: Direct current shock and digitalis. Br Heart J 31:91, 1969.
15. Klieger R, Lown B: Cardioversion and digitalis II: Clinical studies. Circulation 33:878, 1966.
16. Morris JJ, Kong Y, North WC, et al: Experience with cardioversion of atrial fibrillation and flutter. Am J Cardiol 14:94, 1964.
17. Frithz G, Aberg H: Direct current cardioversion of atrial flutter. Acta Med Scand 187:271, 1970.
18. Guiney TE, Lown B: Electrical conversion of atrial flutter to atrial fibrillation-flutter mechanism in man. Br Heart J 34:1215, 1972.
19. Morris JJ, Peter RH, MacIntosh HD: Electrical conversion of atrial fibrillation—immediate and long term results and selection of patients. Ann Intern Med 65:216, 1966.
20. Szekely P, Batson G, Stark DC: Direct current shock treatment of cardiac arrhythmias. Br Heart J 28:366, 1966.
21. Bjerkelund C, Ornig OM: Evaluation of direct current shock therapy of atrial arrhythmias. Acta Med Scand 184:481, 1968.
22. Razavi M, Duarte E, Tahmooressi P: Cardioversion: Ten year Cleveland Clinic experience. Cleve Clin Q 43:175, 1976.
23. Vassaux C, Lown B: Cardioversion of supraventricular tachycardia. Circulation 39:791, 1969.
24. Gilbert R, Cuddy RP: Digitalis intoxication following cardioversion to sinus rhythm. Circulation 32:58, 1965.
25. Schroeder JS, Harrison DC: Repeated cardioversion during pregnancy. Am J Cardiol 27:445, 1971.
26. Donoso E, Cohn LJ, Friedberg CK: Ventricular arrhythmias after precordial shock. Am Heart J 73:595, 1967.
27. Aberg H, Cullhed I: Direct current countershock complications. Acta Med Scand 183:415, 1968.
28. Ross EM: Cardioversion causing ventricular fibrillation. Arch Intern Med 114:811, 1964.
29. Chun P, Davia J, Donohue D: ST-segment elevation with elective DC cardioversion. Circulation 63:220, 1981.
30. Reiffel J, McCarthy DM, Leahey EB: Does DC cardioversion affect isoenzyme recognition of myocardial infarction? Am Heart J 97:6, 1979.
31. Dahl CF, Ewy GA, Warner ED, Thomas ED: Myocardial necrosis from direct current discharge. Effect of paddle electrode size and time interval between discharges. Circulation 50:956, 1974.
32. Sutton RB, Tsagaris TO: Pulmonary edema following direct current cardioversion. Chest 57:191, 1970.
33. Resnekov L, McDonald L: Pulmonary edema following treatment of arrhythmias by direct current shock. Lancet 1:506, 1965.
34. Budow J, Natarajan P, Kroop IG: Pulmonary edema following direct current cardioversion for atrial arrhythmias. JAMA 218:1803, 1971.
35. Lindsey J Jr: Pulmonary edema following cardioversion. Am Heart J 74:434, 1967.
36. Strom S: Pericarditis following cardioversion. A case report. Acta Med Scand 195:431, 1974.
37. Berger RO: Ocular complications of cardioversion. Ann Ophthalmol 10:161, 1978.
38. Okel BB: Vertebral fracture from cardioversion shock (letter). JAMA 203:369, 1968.

Jerris R. Hedges and Michael I. Greenberg

Chapter 12

Defibrillation

INTRODUCTION

Defibrillation is the conversion of ventricular fibrillation to an alternative (preferably supraventricular) rhythm. Ventricular fibrillation (VF) is incompatible with life. It is often associated with myocardial ischemia or infarction, marked electrolyte disturbances, electrical injuries, pronounced hypothermia, or drug toxicity (e.g., that caused by tricyclic antidepressants, quinidine, and digitalis). Although brief periods of VF with spontaneous reversion to a sinus rhythm have been recorded, VF is usually irreversible without electrical countershock.[1]

Ventricular fibrillation is the primary cause of sudden cardiac death.[2] The majority of victims of sudden death have *not* suffered a myocardial infarction, although most have advanced coronary disease and often have poor ventricular function.[2-4] Furthermore, survivors of sudden death attributable to VF are at increased risk of suffering a recurrence, although this chance may be lessened with the use of long-term β-blocker therapy.[2,4,5]

With the advent of portable defibrillation units and prehospital cardiac resuscitation teams, the challenge of early defibrillation of the potential victim of sudden death in VF is being aggressively addressed. Up to 40 per cent of prehospital VF cardiac arrest victims can be saved if cardiac massage and ventilation are provided promptly (in less than 4 minutes) and followed by advanced cardiac resuscitation (within 8 minutes).[6-8] It has been demonstrated consistently that the *timeliness of defibrillation* is the single most important factor determining the prognosis in out-of-hospital cardiac arrest. Prompt, effective defibrillation is equally important for inhospital VF cardiac arrests; physicians and nurses alike must be thoroughly familiar with this procedure.

BACKGROUND

The concept of electrical shock therapy in resuscitation can be traced to the experiments of Abildgaard in the eighteenth century. Abildgaard described chickens as "lifeless" following electrical shocks and noted successful resuscitation after the use of additional shocks. Subsequent animal studies were reported by Preust and Batell.[9] In 1947 the first successful human defibrillation using the direct application of electrical current to the heart was reported by Beck and coworkers.[10] Nine years later, Zoll and associates reported the first successful cardiac defibrillation using an alternating current (AC) electrical shock applied externally to the thorax.[11]

Portable direct current (DC) defibrillators were introduced by Lown and colleagues[12] and Edmark and coworkers[13] during the 1960s. DC defibrillators opened the way for prehospital defibrillation.[2,4,6,14] Although the basic design of modern defibrillators has changed little since the 1960s, modifications in paddle size, energy delivered, energy waveform, conducting materials, and pharmacologic enhancement of defibrillation have been recent areas of research. These topics are discussed later in this chapter.

INDICATIONS AND CONTRAINDICATIONS

Electrical defibrillation of the heart in VF is indicated whenever immediate spontaneous conversion to a perfusing rhythm does not occur. "Quick-look" paddles, which permit immediate monitoring of the cardiac arrest patient's rhythm before electrical defibrillation are helpful; unresponsive patients with regular tachydysrhythmias are best treated with synchronized cardioversion (see Chapter 11), although if monitoring capabilities are not immediately available, an initial unsynchronized countershock may be life saving.

Although the timing of defibrillation has been debated, an initial electrical shock applied to the victim of sudden death before drug administration is currently recommended.[15] In most resuscitations, cardiac massage and ventilations are initiated while the defibrillator is being readied. If the patient is unconscious, apneic, and pulseless, it is reasonable to assume that an episode of VF is taking place if cardiac monitoring is not available. In such instances, an immediate attempt at defibrillation is warranted. Although asystole and, more rarely, ventricular tachycardia may appear clinically similar, an immediate countershock is unlikely to affect either clinical situation adversely. Defibrillation countershock is otherwise contraindicated in the patient with a rhythm other than VF, or perhaps ventricular flutter.

Because "fine" VF can occasionally masquerade as ventricular standstill or asystole, monitoring paddle electrodes should be rotated 90 degrees from their original position or the monitor lead changed before the decision *not* to defibrillate the victim of sudden death is made (Fig. 12–1).[16] Low-voltage VF likewise is *not* a contraindication to defibrillation, because it may reflect low monitor gain or a problem with monitor lead or paddle placement. More than three *repeated* countershocks are contraindicated before efforts to optimize oxygenation and body temperature are initiated, because these derangements may make the heart refractory to countershock. In addition, repeated countershocks may produce tissue damage.

CHARACTERISTICS OF VENTRICULAR FIBRILLATION

Electrocardiographically, VF is characterized by the presence of low-amplitude baseline undulations that are variable in both amplitude and periodicity. Although often considered to represent an electrically random process, electrical directionality to depolarization (i.e., wavefronts) may exist.[16] Mechanically, VF represents an uncoordinated, disorderly contractile process. The absence of effective contractile function abolishes tissue perfusion and leads to death.

At the tissue level, VF represents a disorganization of the orderly depolarization sequence that usually occurs in the ventricles. Normally, the refractory period of depolarized muscle prevents the development of reentrant ventricular rhythms. When ischemia, electrolyte disorders, cardiac drug toxicities, rapid ventricular rates, hypothermia, and certain other disorders exist, refractory periods may shorten or conduction velocities may increase in certain areas of the ventricle. Wandering depolarization wavefronts that become self-perpetuating can develop. A combination of disorders of impulse formation (automaticity) and impulse conduction (reentry) generally contribute to the development of VF.[17,18] The tendency for VF is enhanced by, but is not dependent on, premature ventricular impulses that occur during the "vulnerable" period of the cardiac cycle represented by early ventricular repolarization (T wave).[19]

Asynchronous ventricular depolarization may be confined to a small area of the ventricle if the remaining ventricle is refractory to further stimulation. Several studies have shown that a critical muscle mass is required for VF to be self-sustaining.[20,21] A large mass of muscle involved in asynchronous depolarization having a brief refractory period

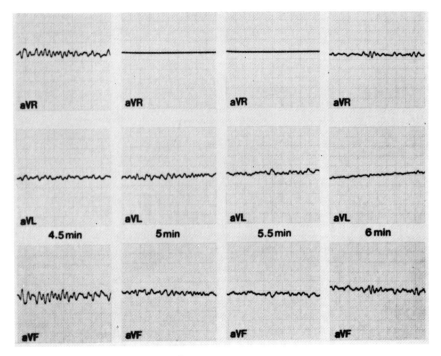

Figure 12–1. Leads aVR, aVL, and aVF from an animal with electrically induced ventricular fibrillation (VF). From onset to 4½ minutes, VF waves were obvious in all six frontal plane leads. At 5 minutes and 5½ minutes, lead aVR was a straight line. Note that aVR is the electrical sum of leads aVL and aVF. By 6 minutes, the null vector had changed and VF was again evident in all six frontal plane leads. (From Ewy GA, Dahl CF, Zimmerman M, et al: Ventricular fibrillation masquerading as ventricular standstill. Crit Care Med 9:841, 1981. © by Williams & Wilkins, 1981. Reproduced by permission.)

and a slow conduction velocity increases the tendency for the ventricles to fibrillate.

Cummins and coworkers[22, 23] have classified ventricular fibrillation on the basis of average peak-to-trough wave amplitude (Table 12–1). They note that the amplitude of the VF waveform is associated positively with the probability of resuming a perfusing rhythm. Signals that have an amplitude of less than 1 mm (when the monitor is calibrated at 10 mm/mV) should be considered asystole[23] because countershock of such low amplitude rhythms is only rarely associated with conversion to a perfusing rhythm.[24, 25]

Basis for Defibrillation

Electrical defibrillation represents the simultaneous depolarization of sufficient ventricular tissue to render the

Table 12–1. Classification of Ventricular Fibrillation (VF) Based on Mean Waveform (Peak to Trough Averaged over a 3-to 6-second Interval) Amplitude

Terminology	Average Amplitude (mm)
Asystole	0 to <1
Fine VF	1 to <3
Medium VF	3 to <7
Coarse VF	7 to <12
Extra Coarse VF (V Flutter)	≥12

Historically, it has been taught that coarse VF is easier to defibrillate than fine VF, and one of the functions of epinephrine in the setting of cardiac arrest is to coarsen fine VF to facilitate defibrillation. However, when subjected to study, this contention has been difficult to prove. Weaver and colleagues (Ann Intern Med 102:53, 1985) studied 394 patients with prehospital cardiac arrest and found that epinephrine did not augment the amplitude of VF. Although patients with coarse VF were not successfully defibrillated more often than those with fine VF, the postdefibrillation rhythm was frequently asystole (survival rate 6%) in patients with fine VF and a supraventricular rhythm (survival rate 36%) in those with coarse VF. In a canine study Jones and coworkers (J Electrocard 17:393, 1984) found more electrical similarities than differences in coarse and fine VF and concluded that the wave amplitude in early VF is due to electrocardiogram lead orientation rather than differences in the synchronization of electrical activity. The clinical importance of fine versus coarse VF is still unsettled.

(Modified from Cummins RO, Stults KR, Haggar B, et al: A new rhythm library for testing automatic external defibrillators: Performance of three devices. J Am Coll Cardiol 11:597, 1988. Reprinted with permission from the American College of Cardiology.)

tissue ahead of the VF wavefronts refractory to further electrical conduction. Following generalized depolarization, the sinus node or other pacemaker region of the heart with the highest degree of automaticity can then acquire dominance of a well-ordered depolarization-repolarization sequence.

DEFIBRILLATOR CHARACTERISTICS

General standards[26] and product evaluations[27] for cardiac defibrillation devices are beyond the scope of this chapter. This section discusses the major components and design configurations of a defibrillator and how they relate to effective defibrillation.

Waveforms

Although the first successful human defibrillation was performed using alternating current,[10] Lown and coworkers were able to demonstrate that direct current is more effective than alternating current in defibrillation and produces a much lower incidence of postcardioversion dysrhythmias.[12] Only DC defibrillators are in clinical use today. Most of the modern defibrillators use a damped half-sinusoidal waveform or a trapezoidal (truncated exponential decay) waveform. The trapezoidal waveform can be modified to resemble a square waveform. The more square the waveform, the more effective it is for experimental defibrillation.[28, 29] Furthermore, in a comparison of square waveforms and damped half-sinusoidal waveforms for animal defibrillation, it was found that less peak current per kilogram was needed with the square waveforms, although the average current levels were equivalent.[30] Furthermore, the delivered waveform is dependent on thoracic resistance.[29] In clinical practice, however, there is little difference in the effectiveness of the currently available waveforms.

Stored Energy

Because the ability to defibrillate is dependent on current delivered to the myocardium,[31] the stored energy is one factor that, coupled with transthoracic impedance and internal defibrillator energy loss, contributes to successful defibrillation. Each defibrillator is calibrated by measuring the current delivered as a function of time across a 50-ohm impedance. Defibrillators do not always deliver the energy indicated on the device. With a "stored" energy of 400 joules (1 joule = 1 watt-sec), from 155 to 410 joules may be delivered.[32–34] The current (for a square waveform) delivered to the myocardium is related to the energy delivered by the defibrillator, the electrical impedance in the device and chest, and the duration of current flow:

$$\begin{array}{cccc} \text{Energy} = & \text{current}^2 & \times \text{ impedance} & \times \text{ duration} \\ \text{(joules)} & \text{(amperes)}^2 & \text{(ohms)} & \text{(seconds)} \end{array}$$

Obviously, any increase in transthoracic impedance will further reduce delivered current.

Device Switches

Many portable (capable of battery operation) defibrillators have separate power switches for the accompanying monitor and recorder and for the defibrillator. Before attempting defibrillation, the physician must be familiar with the location and operation of the controls to avoid attempting to defibrillate a patient when the defibrillator portion is not yet turned on. One defibrillator in common usage is shown in Figure 11–3.

Defibrillators also have a control permitting synchronous cardioversion. The physician must be sure that the control is set to the *asynchronous* mode to permit defibrillation; otherwise, the device in the synchronous mode would wait indefinitely for a nonexistent repetitive series of R waves before discharging.

Energy settings may be determined by a switch or a dial setting or may be read off a meter permitting a continuous range of settings. In each case the physician must be aware of the need for charging the device initially and recharging after each discharge. The mechanism of charging the device may be intrinsic to the setting of the dial or meter but more commonly requires the use of a separate charge button on the device control panel or paddle handle. Full charge accumulation usually takes 2 to 5 seconds following activation of the charging mechanism.

Discharge controls are generally present on the paddle handles, allowing the operator to place the paddles and to deliver the charge as desired. Alternatively, there may be a separate control on the panel. Usually the simultaneous activation of the control on both paddles is required for energy discharge.

Monitor controls permit alteration of lead-monitored image size and often allow the selection of chest lead electrode versus paddle electrode monitoring. The latter is desirable when an initial "quick-look" rhythm evaluation is desired before placement of the chest lead electrodes. A hard copy paper recorder for documenting rhythms may operate in a real-time, delay, or standby mode.

Paddles or Electrode Pads

Most commercial defibrillator devices have adult paddle electrodes with diameters between 8 and 9 cm. Canine studies have shown that slightly larger (12.8 cm diameter) paddles are more effective for defibrillation[35] and produce less myocardial injury.[36] Paddles that are slightly smaller (4.5 cm diameter) produce greater damage at the same energies. The larger paddles may permit a greater amount of muscle to be depolarized while minimizing the potentially damaging

current density. If the paddles are too large with respect to the heart (e.g., if adult paddles are used during infant resuscitation), the current density may be less and the defibrillator may be less effective.[37] The recommended minimum diameter for infant transthoracic paddles is 2.2 cm.[26] Atkins and colleagues suggest that because of their reduction in transthoracic impedance, the larger adult electrodes should be used whenever a child's thorax is large enough to permit electrode-to-chest contact over the entire paddle surface.[38] This transition occurs at an approximate weight of 10 kg. The time delay required to change from adult to pediatric paddles may be excessive. The routine use of adult paddles on any child who weighs more than 10 kg is recommended.

Some defibrillators have a flat posterior ground shield rather than a second paddle for lateral chest wall placement. With the two-paddle system, charge and discharge controls are generally present on the paddles.

The metal composition of the paddle electrode will affect transthoracic impedance to the defibrillation discharge. Most modern defibrillators use stainless steel because of its durability, although copper alloys and several other metals provide a lower transthoracic impedance.[39]

Defibrillation can also be performed with self-adhesive electrode pads applied to the skin. The self-adhesive monitor or defibrillator pads appear to perform as well or better than hand-held paddles.[40–42] Stults and colleagues in a controlled prehospital study found that the use of self-adhesive pads shortened the time to successful defibrillation, reduced the number of countershocks, reduced the amount of rhythm artifact, and improved survival to hospital admission over the use of standard hand-held paddles.[42] The expense of self-adhesive defibrillator pads has limited their general acceptance. If future studies support their superiority in other clinical settings, it is likely that the pads will gain acceptance.

Conductive Materials

Transthoracic impedance varies with the type of conductive material applied between the paddles and the chest wall.[43, 44] For paddles that are 8.0 cm in diameter, the transthoracic impedance is 91 ± 20 ohms for bare contact, 71 ± 11 ohms for saline-soaked gauze, and 64 ± 15 ohms for Redux Paste.[45] Ewy and Taren recommend that Corgel, Redux Paste, American Writer, GE Gel, Electrode Jelly, or Trucon Electrode Paste be used to minimize impedance.[44] Saline-soaked gauze pads may be used, although one must be careful not to allow the saline to bridge the skin between the electrodes. Some form of coupling medium (e.g., paste, cream, gel, pad) should be used to reduce impedence, but data are conflicting regarding which product is ideal. Although Redux paste (Hewlett-Packard) has been associated with significantly lower transthoracic impedence, a statistically significant increase in the success of defibrillation, has not been demonstrated with any specific product.

Hummell and coworkers investigated conductive materials for their potential to overheat and to spark. They found that the products that offer lower impedance (e.g., Redux Paste, Signagel) remained stable and did not spark after four or five defibrillation discharges as seen with the higher impedance products (e.g., Redux Cream, Aquasonic 100, EKG Sol, Spectra 360, and Derma-Jel).[46]

PROCEDURE

Sudden death victims suspected to be in VF should be defibrillated as soon as possible (Fig. 12–2). When adequate

Initiate CPR if additional rescuers are present

↓

Verify VF[a]

↓

Defibrillate (200 J adult; 2 J/kg child)

↓

Defibrillate (200 to 300 J adult; 2 to 3 J/kg child)

↓

Defibrillate (360 J adult—maximum; 4 J/kg child)

↓

Initiate or resume CPR

↓

Intubate if not yet done

↓

Epinephrine (1 mg IV adult; 0.01 mg/kg IV child)
(Repeat every 3 to 5 minutes)

↓

Defibrillate (360 J adult or maximum; 4 J/kg child)

↓

Lidocaine (1 mg/kg IV)

↓

Defibrillate (360 J adult or maximum; 4 J/kg child)

↓

Bretylium (5 mg/kg IV)

↓

Defibrillate (360 J adult or maximum; 4 J/kg child)

↓

Consider the following in conjunction with repeated attempts at defibrillation depending on the clinical situation[b]:

1. Lidocaine (1 mg/kg IV)
2. Bretylium (10 mg/kg IV)
3. Epinephrine (0.1 to 0.2 mg/kg IV)
4. Magnesium sulfate (1 to 2 gm IV push)
5. Potassium chloride (10 mEq IV over 15 to 30 minutes)
6. Sodium bicarbonate (1 to 2 mEq/kg IV)
7. Calcium chloride (20 mg/kg IV push)
8. Digitalis antibody (Digobind)

[a]Consider electrical countershock of systole (see text).
[b](1 and 2): Consider further anyidysrhythmics when the patient develops ectopy (following defibrillation) leading to reccurent VF. (3): Consider high-dose epinephrine (up to 15 mg) when the patient cannot sustain perfusion (following defibrillation) leading to recurrent VF. Avoid further epinephrine in the setting of postdefibrillation tachydysrhythmias. (4): Consider magnesium replacement in the setting of recurrent VF, prior diuretic therapy, malnutrition (including chronic alcoholism), or digitalis toxicity. (5): Consider potassium chloride in a setting of hypokalemia (e.g., prior diuretic therapy). (6 and 7): Consider sodium bicarbonate and calcium chloride therapy in the setting of hyperkalemia (e.g., prior renal failure, dialysis, iatrogenic overdose, broad complexes between VF episodes). (8): If digitalis toxic, administer 5 to 10 vials of digitalis-binding antibody (Digibind).

Figure 12–2. Algorithm for management of unwitnessed ventricular fibrillation (VF) or witnessed VF not responsive to precordial thump. After each therapy, the rhythm is reassessed, and the rescuer must evaluate the need for continued treatment for VF. If VF persists, the rescuer continues through the protocol. *CPR,* cardiopulmonary resuscitation; *IV,* intravenously.

personnel are available, cardiopulmonary resuscitation (CPR) should be initiated while the defibrillator device is being readied.

After applying conductive material to the entirety of the paddle conductive surface, the paddles should be firmly applied to the chest. One paddle should be positioned to the right of the upper sternum below the clavicle; the second paddle is placed just to the left of the nipple in the midaxillary line and is centered in the fifth intercostal space (see Fig. 11–4). Ideally the current should pass through the heart. One should *avoid* placing both paddles close together on the anterior chest wall. In some paddle sets, each paddle is labeled "sternum" or "apex" so that any rhythm detected on the monitor can be properly aligned. This is irrelevant for defibrillation but is important for cardioversion. Antero-

posterior paddle positioning is also acceptable and may deliver more current to the heart.[47, 48] The anterior paddle is placed to the left of the sternum over the precordium and the posterior electrode is placed just to the left of the spine directly posterior to the heart (see Fig. 11–5).

With the monitor turned on and set to display the "paddle" electrodes, the rhythm is evaluated. If a flatline rhythm is detected, the monitor gain is increased fully to rule out a "fine VF" tracing. Should the tracing remain flat during a pause in closed-chest cardiac massage, the paddles are rotated 90 degrees from the original position and the rhythm is reassessed. The incidence of VF masquerading as asystole was approximately 2.5 per cent in one prehospital study of patients with an initial flatline monitor rhythm.[49] Cummins[23] recommends that the rescuer check all monitor cable connections to the patient and defibrillator, check the electrocardiogram (ECG) size control, check the power supply, and rotate the monitor leads as discussed. If VF is observed during any of these maneuvers, defibrillation should follow. Should a bradycardiac or asystolic rhythm be detected, standard resuscitation measures, including basic CPR, correction of hypoxia, administration of catecholamines, correction of volume or cardiac filling deficiencies, and emergency cardiac pacing (see Chapters 13 to 15), should be initiated. Although defibrillation should have no theoretic benefit for asystole, the use of countershock will result in the development of a QRS rhythm in a small percentage of patients who are given shocks when thought to be asystolic. Presumably such cases represent fine VF simulating a flatline on the EGG.

In cases of "fine" VF when a patient is wearing an implanted (subcutaneous) pacemaker, the pacer spikes may initially appear to be a paced but nonconducted rhythm; attention to the baseline and lack of ST changes characteristic of capture should reveal the true nature of the dysrhythmia. Because injury to the pacemaker pulse generator[50] and to the myocardium can occur by transmission of current down the pacing electrode,[51] the physician must be careful to situate the defibrillator paddle at least 12 cm away from the pulse generator.

In the presence of VF, the paddles should be immediately charged to a stored energy of 2 joules/kg for children and 200 joules for adults. Separate power switches may be needed to turn on the defibrillator and to store the charge. The amount of charge is usually set by a button or a dial on the control panel. In most devices, the preset level of charge (energy) can be stored if a button on the "apex" paddle is pressed. The physician must check to be certain that the defibrillator is *not* in the synchronous mode.

Once the paddles are charged, the physician should instruct all personnel to stand back from the patient and the stretcher to avoid stray discharge. The operator in particular must be sure that the only contact being made is with dry paddle handles. The patient is allowed to exhale passively to minimize transthoracic impedance[52] while firm (25 pound) pressure is applied through the paddles to the thorax.[53, 54] The energy in the paddles is discharged through the chest as soon as possible following charging to minimize energy decay inside the device. Simultaneous depression of both paddle discharge buttons is essential for discharge. Anticipation of patient extremity motion subsequent to discharge of the paddles will minimize operator injury.

Should no skeletal muscle contraction occur following simultaneous depression of the discharge buttons, the physician should ensure that firm chest wall contact is made (some devices will not discharge without adequate contact), that the device is in the asynchronous mode, that a charge has been stored and the defibrillator (not just the monitor) is turned on, and that the battery is not low (when operating off the storage battery). If there is no muscle contraction even when these factors have been ruled out, a back-up defibrillator should be brought into use.

After the first countershock, the paddles should remain in place for 5 to 10 seconds to enable the physician to check for an organized rhythm while ventilation is continued. While waiting to analyze the rhythm, the rescuer should recharge the paddles for an immediate second defibrillation (200 to 300 joules for adults, 2 to 3 joules/kg for children) should VF persist. Should VF continue after the second shock, an immediate third defibrillation (360 to 400 joules for adults; 4 joules/kg for children) should be given. If the third defibrillation is unsuccessful, closed-chest cardiac massage should be continued, hypoxia corrected, and α-agonist catecholamines administered to elevate the diastolic pressure and to improve coronary perfusion.[55–58] Following circulation of the catecholamine agent, an attempt at defibrillation should be repeated. A porcine CPR study[55–59] and anecdotal case reports[60] suggest that high doses of catecholamines (e.g., 0.2 mg/kg of epinephrine) may be required in certain cases.

Infants who develop VF are often taking digitalis preparations. Because excessive defibrillation energy may produce irreversible VF in the digitalis-toxic patient, the lowest available energy level should be used for the initial defibrillation. If the initial energy dose is unsuccessful, the energy level can be increased cautiously for successive countershocks.

Additional therapy can be undertaken to enhance defibrillation; this is discussed in the following section. Adequate ventilation, cardiac massage, and correction of electrolyte disorders are intrinsic to every resuscitation and are not discussed further. In addition, evaluation of the patient for hypothermia and rapid core rewarming when indicated (see Chapter 91) should not be overlooked.

When practical, electronic monitoring devices and transvenous pacemakers should be turned off or, preferably, disconnected from the patient to avoid equipment damage. Recently manufactured patient monitoring devices, however, have built-in protective filter circuitry, which makes equipment damage an unlikely occurrence.

ENHANCING DEFIBRILLATION SUCCESS

Early Defibrillation

Energy requirements for conversion of VF may increase dramatically shortly after the onset of VF.[61, 62] The rationale for early defibrillation is that in the absence of adequate coronary perfusion, cellular metabolism continues with the depletion of energy substrates and the accumulation of toxic metabolites. Electrophysiologic changes secondary to cellular ischemia develop and contribute to continued asynchronous transmission of VF wavefronts.

Clinical investigation of immediate defibrillation rather than drug therapy preceding defibrillation is limited. Martin and coworkers in a retrospective analysis of prehospital VF resuscitations found that survival to hospital discharge was greater when CPR followed by immediate defibrillation was used rather than CPR and drug therapy before countershock.[63] The group receiving drug therapy first had a longer mean time until defibrillation (12 minutes additional), which was explained in part by the time required for intravenous line placement, drug administration, and drug circulation. Nonetheless, until further clinical studies are available, immediate defibrillation for VF appears to be appropriate.

Transthoracic Impedance

Delivery of current to the heart is dependent on the energy supplied to the paddles and the impedance to transmission of that energy. Reported values for human transthoracic impedance using electrodes 8.0 cm in diameter range from 50 to 100 ohms with a mean of 75 ohms.[67] We have previously discussed the importance of paddle electrode composition[39] and size,[35] conductive materials,[43–45] applied paddle-to-chest-wall pressure,[53, 54] state of ventilation,[52] and location of the paddle on the chest wall.[47, 48]

The transthoracic impedance of direct current discharge also decreases with higher energy shocks,[65] increasing number of previous countershocks delivered,[54, 66, 67] and decreasing interval between the discharges.[67] Unfortunately, each of the aforementioned maneuvers is also associated with an increased *potential* for myocardial injury.

Nonetheless, one may be faced with the need to defibrillate a very obese patient who is unresponsive to standard paddle placement and maximum device energies. Should such a situation exist, the patient can be rolled on the side and anteroposterior defibrillation attempted. Should this prove unsuccessful, a second defibrillating device can be simultaneously charged and used to administer countershock *immediately* following discharge of the first defibrillator. Interestingly, a canine study of *internal* defibrillation indicates that two sequential shocks over different pathways reduce both total energy and peak voltage required to terminate VF.[68] Hence, sequential defibrillation using slightly different paddle placements may be beneficial independent of the concurrent reduction in transthoracic impedance.

Energy Choice

Clinicians often refer to a *defibrillation energy threshold* for converting VF. Davy and coworkers suggest that no unique defibrillation energy threshold exists for the in vivo heart.[69] Experimentally they found that successful defibrillation was related to delivered energy by a "dose-response" curve. However, there is evidence for a defibrillation *current* threshold.[31]

Successful defibrillation is dependent on the simultaneous depolarization of a sizable mass of the myocardium by the passage of current through the heart. For a given thorax, defibrillation device, and defibrillation technique, more current is passed through the heart and, hence, more tissue is depolarized with larger energies. Once sufficient tissue has been depolarized, however, additional current is not desirable and may in fact produce additional tissue injury. Kerber and coworkers have suggested that the use of defibrillators that adjust defibrillation energy for the patient's transthoracic impedance (measured by the device just before charging) may be one means to deliver an adequate current to the myocardium while minimizing potential harm.[70] Such devices are not in routine use at present but may be helpful in the future for both the identification of high impedance situations and adjustment of delivered energy.[71]

Several studies have supported the concept that when current needs cannot be predicted nor current delivery measured, a weight-adjusted dosage of energy is preferred for converting VF.[72, 73] Indeed, a dose based on the patient's weight has been found clinically useful for treating children in VF.[74] Other prospective human adult studies have questioned the importance of dose strength to conversion of VF.[75–78] Weaver and coworkers alternated treatment protocols to determine prospectively the merits of 175 watt-sec (200 joules stored energy) versus 320 watt-sec (400 joules stored) countershocks for defibrillation.[79] On test days, VF patients were shocked initially with one or two 175 watt-sec discharges, and all subsequent shocks needed were 320 watt-sec. On alternate days, only 320 watt-sec shocks were given. The investigators found that 73 per cent (n = 76) of the patients were defibrillated following the first two shocks in the low-energy group, whereas 81 per cent (n = 77) of the patients were initially defibrillated in the high-energy group (difference not statistically significant). Asystole occurred in 19 per cent of patients receiving high energy and in 12 per cent receiving low energy. Transient or persistent heart block occurred in 25 per cent of patients shocked with high energy versus 11 per cent of patients shocked with low energy. Survival to hospital discharge was inversely related to the number of shocks required; no patients requiring more than eight shocks survived.

Weaver and associates concluded that low-energy (175 watt-sec delivered) countershocks were safe, effective, and less cardiotoxic. Obviously, many factors besides discharged energy play a role in successful defibrillation. Kerber and colleagues have found that defibrillation success rate is a unimodal function of transthoracic current.[80] The maximum defibrillation rate for their patients with a brief duration of VF (less than 1 minute) occurred at a peak transthoracic current of 38 to 41 amp. Whether a similar optimum transthoracic current is found in patients with prolonged VF remains to be determined. Until energy levels based on measured transthoracic impedance are shown to be predictive of defibrillation success in a variety of settings, most authorities recommend using an initial 200-joule energy setting in adults and a 2-joule/kg energy setting in children. When two sequential defibrillations at this setting are unsuccessful, countershock at 360 joules (or maximum output if needed) is recommended.

Drug Therapy

The role of correcting hypoxia and electrolyte disorders in the treatment of VF has been discussed previously. The benefit of α-agonist catecholamines to enhance aortic diastolic pressure and to improve coronary perfusion has also been mentioned. Further discussion of the role of sodium bicarbonate, adrenergic agents, and antidysrhythmic agents follows:

Sodium Bicarbonate. The administration of sodium bicarbonate during CPR is controversial and previous recommendations are currently undergoing reappraisal.[82] Although acidosis can reduce the responsiveness of the myocardium and vascular system to catecholamines, *no clinical studies have supported the use of sodium bicarbonate for treatment of VF.* Yakaitis and colleagues found that although acidosis did not affect defibrillation success in a canine model of brief VF (75 seconds), prearrest acidosis or hypoxia (in the absence of exogenous epinephrine) was rarely associated with resumption of perfusion.[83] Guerci and coworkers used a prolonged VF (20 minutes of CPR) canine model with epinephrine administration before defibrillation to assess the potential benefit of sodium bicarbonate administration. They failed to show an advantage from the use of sodium bicarbonate in either defibrillation success or maintenance of perfusion after defibrillation.[84] The influence of acidosis on catecholamines appears to be most prominent at low doses and may not apply to the large amounts of epinephrine used during CPR.[85] Although sodium bicarbonate therapy should be considered for the patient with suspected or proven extreme acidosis, hyperkalemia, or both, *it cannot be recommended routinely for VF therapy.*

There are a number of reasons to avoid sodium bicar-

bonate therapy during cardiac arrest. Aside from the fact that it does not facilitate defibrillation and may not be associated with a better final outcome, alkalosis will shift the oxyhemoglobin dissociation curve to inhibit oxygen release, induce hyperosmolar and hypernatremic states, produce paradoxical acidosis through an acceleration of carbon dioxide production, and exacerbate central venous acidosis.

Adrenergic Agents. Drugs that stimulate α-adrenergic receptors have been advocated during cardiac arrest to increase myocardial and central nervous system blood flow during CPR. These agents may not enhance the ability to defibrillate VF, but they do enhance the development of a perfusing rhythm following defibrillation.[81] It is important to note that α agonists are potent vasopressors and that these drugs increase systemic vascular resistance and elevate aortic diastolic pressure, resulting in increased coronary and carotid blood flow. This enhanced perfusion, and not direct β-adrenergic stimulation, is credited with increased survival rates.[86, 87] In fact, the β-adrenergic properties of epinephrine and isoproterenol have been postulated to be harmful because these pharmacologic effects increase myocardial oxygen consumption and reduce subendocardial perfusion. When used alone, isoproterenol, a potent β agonist without alpha effects, does not favorably influence resuscitation rates. Epinephrine has been the vasopressor of choice during CPR, administered in Advanced Cardiac Life Support (ACLS) recommended doses of 0.5 to 1.0 mg every 5 minutes. Large doses of epinephrine (0.2 mg/kg), 10 to 15 times higher than currently recommended, may provide better initial resuscitation rates.[88, 89] However, other investigators have suggested an adverse outcome associated with high-dose epinephrine in patients with ventricular fibrillation.[90] Long-term survival may *not* be improved with high-dose epinephrine.

A number of pure α agonists have been advocated to overcome the theoretic disadvantages of epinephrine. For example, Silvast noted similar resuscitation rates from out of hospital cardiac arrest (e.g., from VF, asystole, and Electrical Mechanical Dissociation [EMD]) when phenylephrine (one or two 1.0-mg boluses) was used in place of standard doses of epinephrine.[91] Methoxamine (10 to 20 mg) has also been used with success rates similar to those of epinephrine.[92] There is concern, however, that although pure α agonists favorably augment peripheral vascular resistance, they do so at the expense of cerebral perfusion and myocardial blood flow.[93] One inadequacy of the available literature is that all forms of cardiac arrest (VF, EMD, asystole) have been treated, and a specific effect of the alpha agents on defibrillation is unclear. The exact role of either high-dose epinephrine or pure α agonists in facilitating defibrillation is currently unsettled, and adherence to standard ACLS guidelines is advocated until the benefits of alternative therapies are clarified.

Bretylium Tosylate. Bretylium tosylate has been used to facilitate ventricular defibrillation.[94–96] Bretylium (Bretylol) has been shown in one animal model to decrease the threshold shock strength required for defibrillation.[97] Other investigators have found no significant effect on the defibrillation threshold.[98–101] The drug increases the effective refractory period in normal ventricular muscle and Purkinje fibers[102] and enhances electrical uniformity throughout the myocardium, thus tending to terminate conditions supportive of reentrant rhythms.[103] Bretylium raised the threshold for electrically induced VF in a canine CPR model within 10 minutes after administration.[104] Bretylium appears to elevate the VF threshold by adrenergic neuronal blockade.[105] One canine study has shown an increased potential for electromechanical dissociation with bretylium following defibrillation.[106]

Spontaneous chemical defibrillation has been reported

in myocardial infarction patients who were given bretylium by intravenous drip rather than by bolus perfusion during cardiopulmonary resuscitation.[107] A retrospective study suggests that the early use of bretylium tosylate during VF sudden death may enhance survival.[108]

For VF, 5 to 10 mg/kg of bretylium is given by rapid intravenous push, and cardiac massage is performed for 1 to 2 minutes to permit circulation of the drug before defibrillation attempts. If after 2 minutes the initial therapy is unsuccessful, a repeat dose of 10 mg/kg is given, and defibrillatory efforts are continued. Successful defibrillation may be followed by hypotension; the physician must be prepared to administer volume or pressor agents to support the blood pressure.

Lidocaine. Lidocaine has long been used to facilitate defibrillation.[109] The rationale for use of lidocaine in VF is primarily based on anecdotal experience. Two nonischemic canine studies have demonstrated that lidocaine *increases* the energy required for electrical defibrillation.[110, 111] Kerber and coworkers suggest that the elevation of the defibrillation threshold noted by others may be a function of the anesthetic used in the animal model and not a factor clinically.[112]

Lidocaine has complex effects on membrane responsiveness—little change in conduction velocity occurs in normal myocardium, whereas conduction in ischemic tissue is decreased.[113] Lidocaine increases uniformity of the action-potential duration and refractory period throughout the ventricles[114] and can terminate ventricular reentrant rhythms.[115] Lidocaine also raises the threshold for electrically induced VF in a canine CPR model within 5 minutes after administration, although the antifibrillatory effect is not sustained with a single bolus dose.[98]

One retrospective study of prehospital VF arrests documented a small but statistically *insignificant* improvement in both defibrillation rate and survival when patients refractory to conventional therapy for VF were given lidocaine during the course of their resuscitation.[116] Unfortunately, strict drug and therapy protocols were not followed, and variations in treatment may have masked a beneficial effect of lidocaine administration. Comparison studies of prehospital lidocaine and bretylium use for refractory VF showed similar conversion and survival rates in the two drug treatment groups.[117, 118] Although the role of lidocaine and bretylium in the facilitation of defibrillation remains to be defined more clearly, clinical experience suggests that both drugs have value in aiding defibrillation. Although one drug may be more beneficial than the other in a given patient, broader generalizations cannot be made. Certainly both drugs are useful for preventing degeneration of a supraventricular rhythm once effective defibrillation occurs. Lidocaine is initially given as a bolus of 1 mg/kg to the VF sudden death victim who is refractory to conventional defibrillatory efforts. A second 1 mg/kg bolus can be given in 10 to 15 minutes.

COMPLICATIONS

The major complications of direct current defibrillation are (1) injury to skin and other soft tissue, (2) myocardial injury, and (3) cardiac dysrhythmias.

Soft Tissue Injury

When skin contact is firm and a conductive material is applied between the paddles and the chest wall, contact burns are minimal. Nonetheless, repeated countershocks can produce erythema resembling superficial skin burns. The presence of liquids (e.g., blood, intravenous solutions, vomitus, urine, excessive sweat) may permit the passage of current across the trunk. This electrical arcing will produce thermal burns (third-degree at times) and ineffective defibrillation. Hummel and coworkers have shown that repeated defibrillations using certain high-impedance conducting gels is associated with sparking and represents a fire hazard in an oxygen-enriched environment[46] and an explosion hazard in the presence of nitroglycerin ointment or patches.[119–121] Intrathoracic injuries (extrinsic to the heart) are likely to occur but are difficult to document during the postresuscitative period and to separate from cardiac injury (e.g., pulmonary edema).[122–124]

Myocardial Injury

The direct application of electrical countershock to the heart has long been known to produce epicardial and myocardial injury.[125] Lown and coworkers demonstrated that closed-chest defibrillation could produce cardiac injury. This suggested that electrical current rather than direct thermal injury produced injury.[12] Multiple countershocks have been shown in animals to produce ST segment elevation and gradual cell necrosis (over days) with subsequent fibrosis.[126, 127] The lesions are primarily subepicardial at the points of current entrance and exit wounds. Animals receiving less than twice the defibrillation threshold value do not develop significant necrosis.[128] The degree of cardiac injury correlates with increasing energy exposure.

Jones and coworkers using an in vitro model have created transient sarcolemmal microlesions (45–60 Å) during high-intensity electric field stimulation identical to that of defibrillation.[129] These lesions result in a "short-circuit" depolarization of the cells by loss of the normal sodium-potassium gradient across the sarcolemma. When the lesions are limited, the cell can recover after about 1 minute. However, with extensive lesions, shock-induced cytosolic calcium overload can occur and can result in postshock contracture.

The ability to document anatomic injury to the human heart is limited by the natural reparative process, concurrent ischemic processes producing similar microscopic changes, and the fact that several days are needed for the injuries to manifest themselves. Cardiac isoenzyme (CK MB) levels were shown to rise in patients undergoing elective cardioversion only if the cumulative *delivered* energy was greater than 475 joules.[130] Therefore, *standard* defibrillation does not invalidate enzymatic diagnosis of myocardial infarction, given that defibrillations were not excessive and that isoenzymes are measured. Although myocardial scintigraphy with technetium 99m pyrophosphate is a sensitive means of demonstrating canine myocardial injury due to transthoracic countershocks,[131] Werner and associates were unable to detect injury in defibrillated sudden death victims who received standard delivered energies.[132] Nonetheless, it is likely that cardiac injury from defibrillation is possible, and data from animal injury studies are expected to be valid for patients.

Animal studies have shown that ST segment elevation and pathologic changes are increased with more rapidly delivered discharges (1 or 3 seconds versus 15 seconds between discharges).[126] Furthermore, the cumulative energy correlates with myocardial injury for a given dosing schedule.[126–128, 133]

Cardiac Dysrhythmias

The rhythm that one obtains following defibrillation may be ventricular, supraventricular, or flatline (asystole).

Laboratory studies have suggested a correlation between the severity of postdefibrillation dysrhythmias and the degree of myocardial damage produced.[134, 135] Reducing the peak current delivered to the heart by changing the waveform of the discharge was associated with fewer dysrhythmias.[136] Weaver and coworkers noted that asystole occurred in 19 per cent of prehospital VF patients receiving high energy and in 12 per cent of patients receiving low energy. Furthermore, transient heart block occurred significantly more frequently (25 per cent versus 11 per cent) in the patients shocked with high energy. Gueze and Koster also found that postdefibrillation dysrhythmias were more common following prolonged VF and higher energy level countershocks.[137]

Injuries to Health Care Providers

All electrical devices, including defibrillators when improperly grounded or insulated, can cause injury to the device operator.[138, 139] Other participants in a resuscitation who touch the patient or the stretcher can also serve as a ground for the defibrillator charge and can sustain electrical injury. Gibbs and coworkers[140] estimate that the rate of paramedic injury during patient defibrillation is one per 1700 defibrillatory shocks. They found only one paramedic who required hospital admission for therapy and monitoring of countershock ectopy. Improper use of the device for cranial countershock can also produce short-term memory loss.[141] Explosions and fires resulting from defibrillator sparks[46] in the presence of nitroglycerin patches or ointment,[119–121] flammable gases, or an oxygen-enriched environment can also injure health care personnel.

SPECIAL TOPICS IN DEFIBRILLATION

Thump Defibrillation

The precordial thump is a firm, rapid blow applied to the midsternum with a closed fist from a height of 30 to 38 cm above the pulseless patient. Such a blow delivers approximately 5 joules of energy.

The precordial thump is of value in VF. Miller and associates noted no VF conversion in 15 prehospital patients who had suffered cardiac arrest.[142] They did note that rhythm was improved in two of the ten ventricular tachycardia patients after a precordial thump, although the rhythm deteriorated in six of the ten and did not change in the other two. Caldwell and colleagues reported the results of a precordial thump in 68 cases of ventricular tachycardia and 248 cases of ventricular fibrillation.[143] They reported 26 favorable cardioversions, including five patients in VF. Because successful internal defibrillation can occur with as little as 1 joule following cardiopulmonary bypass,[144] a vigorous precordial thump may create sufficent current flow to defibrillate the heart when the duration of arrest has been brief (i.e., witnessed cardiac arrest).

Automatic Implantable Cardioverter Defibrillators

Automatic implanted defibrillators are in limited clinical use, although they hold great promise for patients with recurrent VF who are unresponsive to drug therapy. The current models (manufactured by Medrad, Inc., Pittsburgh, Pa.) physically resemble early pacemakers. The defibrillator is surgically placed with one electrode passed transvenously in the superior vena cava and the other a concave ventricular patch, is placed over the cardiac apex extrapericardially.[145] A third lead placed into the apex of the right ventricle is used with some devices to record and synchronize the device with the R wave. These units are capable of cardioverting tachydysrhythmias.[146] Recently, units with two epicardial patches (generally placed anterior and posteriorly) have been implanted.

Although the device discharges internally at a potential of 700 volts, the surface voltage at the time of discharge is on the order of tens of volts.[147] A discharge during cardiopulmonary resuscitation is likely to startle the rescuer, although injury is unlikely. Standard rhythm monitoring devices should also be well protected electrically in the event that the device discharges.[147]

The device is programmed to provide a set number of discharges. Following this series of discharges, it will not discharge again until it senses an organized rhythm. In the event that the implanted cardioverter-defibrillator continues to discharge during resuscitation and interferes with rhythm stabilization, the device can be inactivated with a (ring-shaped, toroidal) pacemaker-type magnet.[146] The magnet is advanced perpendicularly over the upper right corner of the device generator, assuming the header (lead attachment end) is cephlad. The generator is usually located in the left abdominal wall. Proper positioning of the magnet results in an audible tone. When in the active mode, the device will emit a series of intermittent tones. After approximately 30 seconds the tones become continuous, indicating that the device is no longer activated. Removal of the magnet while the tone is continuous renders the device inactive; reversal of the procedure results in device activation. When the device is reactivated, the magnet should be left in place until confirmed QRS-sensed tones are clearly heard.[148]

Theoretically, the presence of epicardial patch electrodes (with insulation on the back of the patch) could shield the heart from external defibrillation. Defibrillation should therefore be performed perpendicular to a line between the patch electrodes if known. A right sternal-apex external defibrillation approach is recommended with anteroposterior patch electrodes. An anteroposterior approach may be best when the sole patch electrode is cupped over the ventricular apex.

Automatic External Defibrillators

Automatic external defibrillators have been developed with sophisticated digital software to take advantage of algorithms that can reliably recognize VF.[22] These small portable battery-operated devices permit nonparamedic prehospital providers to defibrillate cardiac arrest patients without human rhythm interpretation.[149]

Because the devices monitor and defibrillate through the same skin electrodes, the user must simply place the adhesive electrode pads at the standard locations (right upper sternal and left anterior axillary line below the nipple), turn on the device, and heed warnings to avoid contact with the patient or surface in contact with the patient. Detailed discussion of the operation of these devices is beyond the scope of this chapter. The reader is referred to the instruction manual for the respective devices.

REFRACTORY VENTRICULAR FIBRILLATION

The major determinants of successful defibrillation are the early use of countershock, adequate oxygenation, lack of serious metabolic derangements, and general health of the patient.

Hargarten and colleagues note that few prehospital patients who remain in VF after the fifth shock are subsequently converted to a perfusing rhythm.[150] Kerber and colleagues note that patients who never defibrillated despite multiple shocks had a prolonged duration of CPR preceding the first shock (21 ± 14 minutes) and systemic hypoxia and acidosis.[151] These conditions tended to occur in their patients whose initial cardiac arrest rhythm was asystole, severe bradycardia, or electromechanical dissociation.

A number of clinical conditions may result in the inability to convert VF initially or the recurrence of VF following the first successful defibrillation. Patients with severe hypothermia are often refractory to initial defibrillation and require rapid core rewarming to be treated effectively. Severe bradycardia will predispose to lethal escape rhythms, and emergency cardiac pacing may be required. Severe electrolyte disturbances, such as hypokalemia, hypomagnesemia, and hypocalcemia may precipitate refractory VF and be amenable only to the rapid infusion of the deficient electrolyte. Such cases may be seen in fad dieters or abusers of diuretics. Uncorrected acidosis or hypoxia, such as seen with drowning, may be the cause of persistent VF. In addition, excessive adrenergic stimulation, such as seen with cocaine or amphetamine overdose, may require the use of propranolol infusion before successful defibrillation. As a final note, following defibrillation all patients should be treated with prophylactic lidocaine (or other appropriate antidysrhythmic therapy) to minimize the chance of recurrent VF.

CONCLUSION

Electrical defibrillation is the preferred treatment for VF sudden death. Treatment should be initiated early with attention to proper energy selection and minimization of transthoracic impedance. Although repetitive high-energy shocks may be associated with myocardial injury, this feature has not been clinically found to be common at the currently recommended energy levels.

REFERENCES

1. Bigger JT: Mechanism and diagnosis of arrhythmias. In Braunwald E (ed): Heart Disease: A Textbook of Cardiovascular Medicine. Philadelphia, WB Saunders Co, 1980, pp 609–670.
2. Cobb LA, Baum TLS, Alvarez H III et al: Resuscitation from out-of-hospital ventricular fibrillation: 4 years follow-up. Circulation 52(Suppl III):223, 1975.
3. Liberthson RR, Nagle EL, Hirschman JC, et al: Prehospital ventricular defibrillation; prognosis and follow-up course. N Engl J Med 291:317, 1974.
4. Schaffer WA, Cobb LA: Recurrent ventricular fibrillation and modes of death in survivors of out-of-hospital ventricular fibrillation. N Engl J Med 293:259, 1975.
5. Myerburg RJ, Kessler KM, Zaman L, et al: Survivors of prehospital cardiac arrest. JAMA 247:1485, 1982.
6. Eisenberg MS, Bergner L, Hallstrom A: Cardiac resuscitation in the community. Importance of rapid provision and implications for program planning. JAMA 241:1905, 1979.
7. Thompson RG, Hallstrom AP, Cobb LA: Bystander initiated cardiopulmonary resuscitation in the management of ventricular fibrillation. Ann Intern Med 90:737, 1979.
8. Lund I, Skulberg A: Cardiopulmonary resuscitation by lay people. Lancet 2:702, 1976.
9. Preust JL, Batelli F: Sur quelques effets des décharges électriques sur le coeur des mammiferers. CR Acad Sci (Paris) 129:1267, 1899.
10. Beck CS, Pritchard WH, Feil H: Ventricular fibrillation of long duration abolished by electrical shock. JAMA 135:985, 1947.
11. Zoll PM, Linenthal AJ, Gibson W, et al: Termination of ventricular fibrillation in man by an externally applied electric countershock. N Engl J Med 254:727, 1956.
12. Lown B, Neuman J, Amarasingham R, et al: Comparison of alternating current with direct current countershock across the closed chest. Am J Cardiol 10:223, 1962.
13. Edmark KW, Thomas GI, Jones TW: DC pulse defibrillation. J Thorac Cardiovasc Surg 51:326, 1966.
14. Eisenberg MS, Copass MK, Hallstrom AP, et al: Treatment of out-of-hospital cardiac arrests with rapid defibrillation by emergency medical technicians. N Engl J Med 302:1379, 1980.
15. Parmley WH, Hatcher CR, Ewy GA, et al: Thirteenth Bethesda Conference: Emergency cardiac care, task force V.: Physical interventions and adjunctive therapy. Am J Cardiol 50:409, 1982.
16. Ewy GA, Dahl DF, Zimmerman M, et al: Ventricular fibrillation masquerading as ventricular standstill. Crit Care Med 9:841, 1981.
17. Zipes DP: Electrophysiological mechanisms involved in ventricular fibrillation. Circulation 52(Suppl. III):120, 1975.
18. Cranefield PF: Ventricular fibrillation. N Engl J Med 289:732, 1973.
19. Wiggers CJ, and Wegria R: Ventricular fibrillation due to a single, localized induction and condenser shocks applied during the vulnerable phase of ventricular systole Am J Physiol. 128:500, 1940.
20. Garrey WE: The nature of fibrillatory contraction of the heart—its relation to tissue mass and form. Am J Physiol 33:397, 1914.
21. Zipes DP, Fisher J, King RM, et al: Termination of ventricular fibrillation in dogs by depolarizing a critical amount of myocardium. Am J Cardiol 36:37, 1975.
22. Cummins RO, Stults KR, Haggar B, et al: A new rhythm library for testing automatic external defibrillators: Performance of three devices. J Am Coll Cardiol 11:597, 1988.
23. Cummins RO: Defibrillation. Emerg Med Clin North Am 6:217, 1988.
24. Stults KR, Brown DD, Kerber RE: Ventricular fibrillation amplitude predicts ability to defibrillate (abstract). Am J Emerg Med 4:423, 1986.
25. Weaver WD, Cobb LA, Dennis D, et al: Amplitude of ventricular fibrillation waveform and outcome after cardiac arrest. Ann Intern Med 102:53, 1985.
26. American National Standard for Cardiac Defibrillator Devices. Arlington, V, Association for the Advancement of Medical Instrumentation, 1981.
27. Battery-powered defibrillator monitors. Health Devices, April 1980, pp 135–163.
28. Schuder JC, Rahmoeller GA, Stueckle H: Transthoracic ventricular defibrillation in the triangular and trapezoidal waveforms. Circ Res 19:689, 1966.
29. Tacker WA, Geddes LA, Bourland JD, et al: The effect of tilt on the strength duration curve for trans-chest ventricular defibrillation. In Proceedings of the 12th Annual Meeting, Association for the Advancement of Medical Instrumentation, 1977, p 403.
30. Geddes LA, Tacker WA, Bourland MD, et al: Comparative efficacy of square and damped sine wave current for ventricular defibrillation. In Proceedings of the 12th Annual Meeting, Association for the Advancement of Medical Instruments, 1977, p 404.
31. Lerman BB, Halperin HR, Tsitlik JE, et al: Relationship between canine transthoracic impedance and defibrillation threshold: Evidence for current-based defibrillation. J Clin Invest 80:797, 1987.
32. Ewy GA, Fletcher RD, Ewy MD: Comparative analysis of direct current defibrillators. J Electrocardiol 5:349, 1972.
33. Ewy GA: Defibrillation output. In Proceedings of the Cardiac Defibrillation Conference. West Lafayette, Ind, Purdue University, 1975, p 33.
34. Sloman G, Storckey J, Kowadlow E, et al: Direct current defibrillator testing. Med J Aust 1:597, 1983.
35. Thomas ED, Ewy GA, Dahl CF, et al: Effectiveness of direct current defibrillation: Role of paddle electrode size. Am Heart J 93:436, 1977.
36. Dahl CF, Ewy GA, Warner ED, et al: Myocardial necrosis from direct current countershock. Circulation 50:956, 1974.
37. Ewy GA, Horan WJ: Effectiveness of direct current defibrillation: Role of paddle electrode size II. Am Heart J 93:674, 1977.
38. Atkins DL, Sirna S, Kieso R, et al: Pediatric defibrillation: Importance of paddle size in determining transthoracic impedance. Pediatrics 82:914, 1988.
39. Ewy GA, Eerman SG, Alferness C, et al: Effect of electrode metal on the transthoracic impedance to defibrillator discharge. In Proceedings of the 15th Annual Meeting, Association for the Advancement of Medical Instrumentation. San Francisco, April 13–17, 1980, p 43.
40. Kerber RE, Martins JB, Kelly KJ, et al: Self-adhesive preapplied electrode pads for defibrillation and cardioversion. J Am Coll Cardiol 3:815, 1984.
41. Aylward PE, Kieso R, Hite P, et al: Defibrillator electrode-chest wall coupling agents: Influence on transthoracic impedance and shock success. J Am Coll Cardiol 6:682, 1985.
42. Stults KR, Brown DD, Cooley F, et al: Self-adhesive monitor/defibrillation pads improve prehospital defibrillation success. Ann Emerg Med 16:872, 1987.
43. Ewy GA, Taren D: Impedance to transthoracic direct current discharge: A model for testing interface material. Med Instrum 12:47, 1978.
44. Ewy GA, Taren D: Relative impedance of gels to defibrillation discharge. Med Instrum 13:295, 1979.
45. Connell PN, Ewy GA, Dahl CF et al: Transthoracic impedance to defibrillation discharge; effect of electrode size and electrode-chest wall interface. J Electocardiol 6:313, 1973.
46. Hummel RS, Ornato JP, Weinberg SM, et al: Spark-generating properties of electrode gels used during defibrillation: A potential fire hazard. JAMA 260:3021, 1988.

47. Nachlas MM, Bix HH, Mower MM, et al: Observations on defibrillation and synchronized countershock. Progr Cardiovasc Dis 9:64, 1966.
48. Dolan AM, Horucek BM, Rantaharju PM: Evaluation of cardiac defibrillation using a computer model of the thorax (abstract). Med Instrum 12:54, 1978.
49. Cummins RO, Austin D, Jr: The frequency of "occult" ventricular fibrillation masquerading as a flat line in prehospital cardiac arrest: Ann Emerg Med 17:813, 1988.
50. Lan FYK, Bilitch M, Wintrab AJ: Protection of implanted pacemakers from excessive electrical energy of DC shock. Am J Cardiol 23:244, 1969.
51. Aylward P, Blood R, Tonkin A: Complications of defibrillation with permanent pacemaker in situ. Pace 2:462, 1979.
52. Ewy GA, Hellman DA, McClung S, et al: Influence of ventilation place on transthoracic impedance and defibrillation effectiveness. Crit Care Med 8:164, 1980.
53. Kerber RE, Grayzel J, Hoyt R, et al: Transthoracic resistance in human defibrillation: Effects of body weight, chest size, serial same energy shocks, paddle size, and paddle contact pressure (abstract). Med Instrum 14:156, 1980.
54. Kerber P, Hoyt R, Grayzel J, et al: Transthoracic resistance in defibrillation: Effects of repeated same energy shocks and paddle contact pressure. Circulation 59 and 60(Suppl. II):127, 1979.
55. Yakaitis RW, Ewy GA, Otto W, et al: Influence of time and therapy on ventricular defibrillation in dogs. Crit Care Med 8:147, 1980.
56. Chandra N, Tsitlik J, Weisfeldt ML: Coronary flow during cardiopulmonary resuscitation in the dog (abstract). Crit Care Med 9:165, 1981.
57. Yakaitis RW, Otto EW, Blitt CB: Relative importance of α and β adrenergic receptors during resuscitation. Crit Care Med 7:293, 1979.
58. Redding JG, Pearson JW. Evaluation of drugs for cardiac resuscitation. Anesthesiology 24:203, 1963.
59. Brown CG, Werman HA, Davis EA, et al: The effects of graded doses of epinephrine on regional myocardial blood flow during cardiopulmonary resuscitation in swine. Circulation 75:491, 1987.
60. Koscove EM, Paradis NA: Successful resuscitation from cardiac arrest using high-dose epinephrine therapy. JAMA 259:3031, 1988.
61. Wolff GA, Veith F, Lown B: Vulnerable period for ventricular tachycardia following myocardial infarction. Cardiovasc Res 2:111, 1968.
62. Kerber RE, Sarnat W: Factors influencing the success of ventricular defibrillation in man. Circulation 60:226, 1979.
63. Martin TG, Hawkins NS, Weigel JA, et al: Initial treatment of ventricular fibrillation: Defibrillation or drug therapy. Am J Emerg Med 6:113, 1986.
64. Ewy GA, Ewy MD, Nuttall AJ, et al: Canine transthoracic resistance. J Appl Physiol 32:91, 1972.
65. Ewy GA: Defibrillation. In Harwood AL (ed): Cardiopulmonary Resuscitation. Baltimore, Williams & Wilkins, 1982, pp 89–126.
66. Geddes LA, Tacker WA, Cabler P, et al: The decrease in transthoracic impedance during successive ventricular defibrillation trials. Med Instrum 9:139, 1975.
67. Dahl CF, Ewy GA, Ewy MD, et al: Transthoracic impedance to direct current discharge: Effect of repeated countershocks. Med Instrum 10:151, 1976.
68. Chang M-S, Inoue H, Kallok MJ, et al: Double and triple sequential shocks reduce ventricular defibrillation threshold in dogs with and without myocardial infarction. J Am Coll Cardiol 8:1393, 1986.
69. Davy J-M, Fain ES, Dorian P, et al: The relationship between successful defibrillation and delivered energy in open-chest dogs: Reappraisal of the "defibrillation threshold" concept. Am Heart J 113:77, 1987.
70. Kerber RE, McPherson D, Charbonnier F, et al: Automatic impedance-based energy adjustment for defibrillation: Experimental studies. Circulation 71:136, 1985.
71. Kerber RE, Martins JB, Kienzle MG, et al: Energy, current, and success in defibrillation and cardioversion: Clinical studies using an automated impedance-based method of energy adjustment. Circulation 77:1038, 1988.
72. Geddes LA, Tacker WA, Rosborough JP, et al: Electrical dose for ventricular defibrillation of large and small animals using precordial electrodes. J Clin Invest 53:310, 1974.
73. Tacker WA, Galiato FM, Giuliani E, et al: Energy dosage for human trans-chest electrical ventricular defibrillation. N Engl J Med 290:214, 1974.
74. Gutzesell HP, Tacker WA, Geddes LA, et al: Energy dose for defibrillation in children. Pediatrics 58:898, 1976.
75. Partridge JR, Adgey AAJ, Webb SW, et al: Electric requirements for ventricular defibrillation. Br Med J 2:313, 1975.
76. Adgey AA: Electrical energy requirements for ventricular defibrillation. Br Heart J 40:1197, 1978.
77. Gasche JA, Crampton RS, Cherwek ML, et al: Determinants of ventricular defibrillation in adults. Circulation 60:231, 1979.
78. Crampton JA, Crampton RS, Sipes JN, et al: Energy levels and patient weight in ventricular defibrillation. JAMA 242:1380, 1979.
79. Weaver WD, Cobb LA, Copass MK, et al: Ventricular defibrillation— a comparative trial using 175 J and 320 J shocks. N Engl J Med 307:1101, 1982.
80. Kerber RE: Energy requirements for defibrillation. Circulation 74:IV-117, 1986.
81. Otto CW, Yakaitis RW, Ewy GA: Effect of epinephrine on defibrillation in ischemic ventricular fibrillation. Am J Emerg Med 3:285, 1985.
82. Jaffe AS: Cardiovascular pharmacology I. Circulation 74:IV-70, 1986.
83. Yakaitis RW, Thomas JD, Mahaffey JE: Influence of pH and hypoxia on the success of defibrillation. Crit Care Med 3:139, 1975.
84. Guerci AD, Chandra N, Johnson E, et al: Failure of sodium bicarbonate to improve resuscitation from ventricular fibrillation in dogs. Circulation 74:IV-75, 1986.
85. Andersen MN, Borden JR, Mouritzen CV: Acidosis, catecholamines, and cardiovascular dynamics: When does acidosis require correction. Ann Surg 166:344, 1967.
86. Yakaitis RW, Otto CW, Blitt CD: Relative importance of alpha and beta adrenergic receptors during resuscitation. Crit Care Med 7:293, 1979.
87. Ralston SH: Alpha agonist drug usage during CPR. Ann Emerg Med 13:786, 1984.
88. Koscove EM, Paradis NA: Successful resuscitation from cardiac arrest using high-dose epinephrine therapy: Report of two cases. JAMA 259:303, 1988.
89. Gonzalez ER, Ornato JP, Garnett AR, et al: Dose dependent vasopressor response to epinephrine. Ann Emerg Med 18:920, 1989.
90. Marwick TH: Adverse effect of early high-dose adrenaline on outcome of ventricular fibrillation. Lancet 2:66, 1988.
91. Silvast T: Comparison of adrenaline and phenylephrine in out of hospital cardiopulmonary resuscitation: Double blind study. Acta Anaethesiol Scand 29:610, 1985.
92. Brown CG, Davis EA, Werman HA, et al: Methoxamine versus epinephrine on regional cerebral blood flow during cardiopulmonary resuscitation. Crit Care Med 15:682, 1987.
93. Brown CG, Werman HA, Davis EA, et al: The effect of high-dose phenylephrine versus epinephrine on regional cerebral blood flow during CPR. Ann Emerg Med 16:743, 1987.
94. Heissenbuttel TLH, Bigger JR: Bretylium tosylate: A newly available antiarrhythmic drug for ventricular arrhythmias. Ann Intern Med 91:229, 1979.
95. Bernstein JG, Koch-Weser J: Effectiveness of bretylium tosylate against refractory ventricular arrhythmias. Circulation 45:1024, 1972.
96. Holder DA, Sniderman AD, Fraser G, et al: Experience with bretylium tosylate by a hospital cardiac arrest team. Circulation 55:541, 1977.
97. Tacker WA, Niebauer MJ, Babbs CF, et al: The effect of newer antiarrhythmic drugs on defibrillation threshold. Crit Care Med 8:177, 1980.
98. Chow MSS, Kluger J, DiPersio DM, et al: Antifibrillatory effects of lidocaine and bretylium immediately post-cardiopulmonary resuscitation. Am Heart J 110:938, 1985.
99. Dorian P, Fain ES, Davy J-M, et al: Effect of quinidine and bretylium on defibrillation energy requirements. Am Heart J 112:19, 1986.
100. Chow MSS, Kluger J, Lawrence R, et al: The effect of lidocaine and bretylium on the defibrillation threshold during cardiac arrest and cardiopulmonary resuscitation. Proc Soc Exp Biol Med 182:63, 1986.
101. Kerber RE, Pandian NG, Jensen SR, et al: Effect of lidocaine and bretylium on energy requirements for transthoracic defibrillation: Experimental studies. J Am Coll Cardiol 7:397, 1986.
102. Bigger JT Jr, Jaffee CC: The effects of bretylium tosylate on the electrophysiologic properties of ventricular muscle and Purkinje fibers. Am J Cardiol 27:82, 1971.
103. Cardinal R, Sasyniuk BJ: Electrophysiological effects of bretylium tosylate on subendocardial Purkinje fibers from infarcted canine hearts. J Pharmacol Exp Ther 204:159, 1978.
104. Hanyok JJ, Chow MSS, Kluger J, et al: Anti-fibrillatory effects of high dose bretylium and a lidocaine-bretylium combination during cardiopulmonary resuscitation. Crit Care Med 16:691, 1988.
105. Euler DE, Scanlon PG: Mechanism of the effect of bretylium on the ventricular fibrillation threshold in dogs. Am J Cardiol 55:1396, 1985.
106. Euler DE, Zeman TW, Wallock ME, et al: Deleterious effects of bretylium on hemodynamic recovery from ventricular fibrillation. Am Heart J 112:25, 1986.
107. Sanna G, Arcidiacono R: Chemical ventricular defibrillation of the human heart with bretylium tosylate. Am J Cardiol 32:982, 1973.
108. Harrison EE, Amey BD. The use of bretylium in prehospital ventricular fibrillation. Am J Emerg Med 1:1, 1983.
109. Goldberg AH. Cardiopulmonary arrest. N Engl J Med 290:1974.
110. Babbs CF, Yim GKW, Whistler ST, et al: Elevation of ventricular defibrillation threshold in dogs by antiarrhythmic drugs. Am Heart J 98:345, 1979.
111. Dorian P, Fain ES, Davy JM, et al: Lidocaine causes a reversible, concentration-dependent increase in defibrillation energy requirements. J Am Coll Cardiol 8:327, 1986.
112. Kerber RE, Pandian NG, Jensen SR, et al: Effect of lidocaine and bretylium on energy requirements for transthoracic defibrillation: Experimental studies. J Am Coll Cardiol 7:397, 1986.
113. Kupersmith J, Antman EM, Hoffman BF: In vivo electrophysiological effects of lidocaine in canine acute myocardial infarction. Circ Res 36:84, 1975.
114. Wittig J, Harrison LA Wallace AG: Electrophysiological effects of lidocaine on distal Purkinje fibers of canine heart. Am Heart J 86:69, 1978.
115. El-Sherif N, Scherlag BJ, Lazzara R, et al: Reentrant ventricular arrhyth-

mias in the late myocardial infarction period. IV. Mechanism of action of lidocaine. Circulation 56:395, 1977.

116. Harrison EE: Lidocaine in prehospital countershock refractory ventricular fibrillation. Ann Emerg Med 10:420, 1981.

117. Hayes RE, Chinn TL, Copass MR, et al: Comparison of bretylium tosylate and lidocaine in the management of out-of-hospital ventricular fibrillation: A randomized clinical trial. Am J Cardiol 48:353, 1981.

118. Olson DW, Thompson BM, Darin JC, et al: A randomized comparison study of bretylium tosylate and lidocaine in resuscitation of patients out-of-hospital ventricular fibrillation in a paramedic system. Ann Emerg Med 13, 807, 1984.

119. Parke JD, Higgins SE: Hazards associated with chest application of nitroglycerin ointments. JAMA 248:427, 1982.

120. Babka JC: Does nitroglycerin explode? N Engl J Med 309:379, 1983.

121. Kuhnen R, Nitsch J, Luderitz B: Explosion of transdermal nitroglycerin during defibrillation. Dtsch Med Wochenschr 110:37, 1985.

122. Resnekov L, McDonald L: Pulmonary oedema following treatment of arhythmias by direct current therapy. Lancet 1:506, 1965.

123. Honey M, Nicholls TT, Towers MK : Pulmonary oedema following direct current defibrillation. Lancet 1:765, 1965.

124. Palcheimo JA: Pulmonary oedema after defibrillation. Lancet 2:439, 1965.

125. Tedeschi CG, White CW Jr: Morphologic study of canine hearts subjected to fibrillation, electrical defibrillation and manual compression. Circulation 9:916, 1954.

126. Dahl CF, Ewy GA, Warner ED, et al. Myocardial necrosis from direct current countershock. Circulation 50:956, 1974.

127. Warner ED, Dahl C, Ewy GA: Myocardial injury from transthoracic defibrillation countershock. Arch Pathol 99:55, 1975.

128. Davis JS, Lie JT, et al: Cardiac damage due to electric current and energy. In Proceedings of the Cardiac Defibrillation Conference. West Lafayette, Ind, Purdue University, 1975, p 27.

129. Jones JL, Jones RE, Balsky G: Microlesion formation in myocardial cells by high-intensity electric field stimulation. Am J Physiol 87:H480, 1987.

130. Ehsani A, Ewy GA, Sobel BE: Effects of electrical countershock on serum creatinine phosphokinase (CPK) isoenzyme activity. Am J Cardiol 87:12, 1976.

131. DiCala UC, Freedman GS, Downing SE, et al: Myocardial uptake of technetium-99m stannous pyrophosphate following direct current transthoracic countershock. Circulation 54:980, 1976.

132. Werner JA, Potkin RT, Botvinick EH, et al: Scintigraphic and enzymatic findings in survivors of sudden cardiac death. Clin Res 1:73A, 1977.

133. Ewy GA, et al: Comparison of myocardial damage from defibrillator discharge at various dosages. Med Instrum 14:10, 1980.

134. Peleska B: Cardiac arrhythmias following condenser discharges and their dependence upon strength of current and phase of cardiac cycle. Circ Res 13:21, 1963.

135. Jones JL, Jones RE: Postshock arrhythmias: A possible cause of unsuccessful defibrillation. Crit Care Med 8:167, 1980.

136. Peleska B: Cardiac arrhythmias following condenser discharge led through an inductance; comparison with effects of pure condenser discharges. Circ Res 16:11, 1965.

137. Gueze RH, Koster RW: Ventricular fibrillation and transient arrhythmias after defibrillation in patients with acute myocardial infarction. J Electrocard 17:353, 1984.

138. Hopps JA: The electric shock hazard in hospitals. Can Med Assoc J 21:1002, 1968.

139. Edmark KW, Proctor RL, Thomas GI, et al: DC defibrillator failure. J Thorac Cardiovasc Surg 5:741, 1968.

140. Gibbs W, Eisenberg M, Damon SK: Dangers of defibrillation: Injuries to emergency personnel during patient resuscitation. Am J Emerg Med 8:101, 1990.

141. Iserson EV, Barsan WG: Accidental "cranial" defibrillation. JACEP 7:24, 1979.

142. Miller J, Tresch D, Horwitz L, et al: The precordial thump—useful or detrimental? (abstract). Ann Emerg Med 12:246, 1983.

143. Caldwell G, Millar G, Quinn E, et al: Simple mechanical methods for cardioversion: Defence of the precordial thump and cough version. Br Med J 291:627, 1985.

144. Lake CL, Sellers TD, Nolan SP, et al: Low-energy defibrillation: Safe and effective. Am J Emerg Med 3:104, 1985.

145. Mirowski M, Mower MM, Bhagavan BS, et al: The implantable automatic defibrillator. Cardiovasc Med 4:851, 1979.

146. Mirowski M: The automatic implantable cardioverter-defibrillator: An overview. J Am Coll Cardiol 6:641, 1985.

147. Tacker WA: Problems of clinical significance—current clinical trends in cardiac defibrillation: Monitors and defibrillators. In Cardiac Monitoring in a Complex Patient Care Environment. AAMI Technology Assessment Report. Arlington, V, Association for the Advancement of Medical Instrumentation, 1982, pp 13–14.

148. Chapman PD, Veseth-Rogers JL, Duquette SE: The implantable defibrillator and the emergency physician. Ann Emerg Med 18:579, 1989.

149. Cummins RO, Eisenberg MS, Litwin PE, et al: Automatic external defibrillators used by emergency medical technicians. JAMA 257:1605, 1987.

150. Hargarten KM, Stueven HA, Olson DW, et al: Prehospital experience with defibrillation of coarse ventricular fibrillation (abstract). Ann Emerg Med 19:157, 1990.

151. Kerber RE, Jensen SR, Gascho JA, et al: Determinants of defibrillation: Prospective analysis of 183 patients. Am J Cardiol 52:739, 1983.

Chapter 13

Emergency Transvenous Cardiac Pacing

Georges C. Benjamin

INTRODUCTION

The purpose of transvenous cardiac pacing is to restore or ensure effective cardiac depolarization. Several approaches to pacing exist, including transcutaneous, transthoracic, epicardial, endocardial, and, most recently, esophageal (see also Chapters 14 and 15). The transvenous method of endocardial pacing is used most frequently and is both safe and effective. In skilled hands, the semifloating transvenous catheter is successfully placed under electrocardiographic guidance in 80 per cent of patients.[1] The technique can be performed in less than 20 minutes in 72 per cent of patients and in less than 5 minutes in 30 per cent of patients. As with other medical procedures, it should not be performed without a thorough understanding of both its indications and contraindications.

BACKGROUND

The ability of muscle to be artificially depolarized was recognized as early as the eighteenth century. Over the succeeding years, several scattered experiments were reported, and in 1951, Callaghan and Bigelow first used the transvenous approach to stimulate the asystolic heart in hypothermic dogs.[2] Zoll demonstrated the first clinical use of cardiac pacing in humans in 1952.[3] He reported the successful use of an external transcutaneous electrical stimulator in two patients with ventricular standstill.

Furman and Schwedel demonstrated the transvenous endocardial approach in humans in 1959.[4] They treated two patients with complete heart block and Stokes-Adams seizures, reconfirming that low-voltage pacing could completely control myocardial depolarization. The catheter remained in their second patient for 96 days without complication. Other clinical studies by Muller and Bellet,[5] Siddons and Davies,[6] and DeSanctis[7] have proved that transvenous pacing is a valuable procedure in medicine. Fluoroscopic guidance was used for placement of the pacing catheter in all these studies.

In 1964, Vogel and colleagues demonstrated the use of a flexible catheter passed without fluoroscopic guidance for intracardiac electrocardiography.[8] One year later, this technique was used by Kimball and Killip to insert an endocardial pacemaker at the bedside.[9] They noted technical difficulties, including intermittent capture, difficulty passing the catheter, and catheter knotting, in 20 per cent of their patients. During the same year, Harris and associates confirmed the ease and speed with which this procedure could be accomplished.[10]

Before 1965, all intracardiac pacing was done asynchronously, which meant that the pacing catheter could cause electrical stimulation during any phase of the cardiac cycle. Asynchronous pacing frequently resulted in the pacemaker firing during the vulnerable period of an intrinsic depolarization; this occasionally caused ventricular tachycardia or fibrillation. In 1966, Goetz and coworkers demonstrated a pacing generator that sensed intrinsic depolarizations and inhibited the pacemaker for a predetermined period of time.[11] In 1967, this form of *demand* pacemaker was used successfully by Zuckerman and associates in six patients.[12]

A further improvement in the pacing catheter was made by Rosenberg and colleagues when they introduced the Elecath semi-floating pacing wire.[1] The Elecath was stiffer than the Flexon steel wire electrode. Rosenberg and coworkers achieved pacing in 72 per cent of patients, with an average procedure time of 18 minutes. They also noted that 30 per cent of their patients were paced in 5 minutes or less. Bedside insertion resulted in successful pacing for an average of 4 days. Six of 111 patients developed minor complications, including pneumothorax, local infection, and arterial bleeding, resulting in a complication rate of 7 per cent. Inconsistent pacing occurred in 14 per cent of patients and required simple bedside repositioning.[1]

The technique of heart catheterization using a flow-directed balloon-tipped catheter was introduced by Swan and associates in 1970.[13] This concept was used successfully by Schnitzler and coworkers for the placement of a right ventricular pacemaker in 15 of 17 patients.[14]

In 1981, Lang and colleagues compared the bedside use of the flow-directed balloon-tipped catheter with insertion of a semirigid electrode catheter in 111 patients.[15] These researchers found a significantly shorter insertion time (6 minutes 45 seconds compared with 13 minutes 30 seconds), a lower incidence of serious arrhythmias (1.5 per cent compared with 20.4 per cent), and a lower incidence of catheter displacement (13.4 per cent compared with 32 per cent) with the balloon-tipped catheter. They concluded that the balloon-tipped catheter was the method of choice for temporary transvenous pacing (Table 13–1).

Kruger and associates reviewed retrospectively the experience of general internists with transvenous pacemaker placement under electrocardiogram (ECG) guidance.[16] A 4 per cent risk of complications and a 14 per cent incidence of electrode malfunction was reported, and these percentages were noted to be similar to those reported by university cardiologists. They concluded that pacemaker placement by primary care physicians was safe and effective when done under ECG guidance without fluoroscopy.

INDICATIONS

The purpose of cardiac pacing is to resume effective cardiac depolarization. In most cases, the specific indications

Table 13–1. History of Transvenous Pacing

Date	Investigator	Event
1700	Early investigators	First restimulation studies
1951	Callaghan and Bigelow	First transvenous approach in dogs
1952	Zoll	Transcutaneous cardiac stimulator
1958	Falkmann and Walkins	Implanted pacing wires after surgery
1959	Furman and Robinson	First transvenous pacer in humans
1964	Vogel and associates	Flexible electrocardiographic catheter without fluoroscopy
1965	Kimball and Killip	First bedside transvenous pacing
1966	Goetz and associates	Demand pacemaker developed
1967	Zuckerman and associates	Use of demand pacemaker clinically
1969	Rosenberg and associates	Semifloating pacing catheter
1973	Schnitzler and associates	Balloon-tipped pacers

Table 13–2. Indications for Cardiac Pacing

Bradycardias
Without myocardial infarction
  Symptomatic sinus node dysfunction (sinus arrest, tachybrady [sick sinus] syndrome, sinus bradycardia)
  Second-degree and third-degree heart block
  Atrial fibrillation with slow ventricular response
With myocardial infarction
  Symptomatic sinus node dysfunction
  Mobitz II second-degree and third-degree heart block
  Left bundle branch block (LBBB), right bundle branch block (RBBB), bifascicular block, and alternating bundle branch block
Trauma patient with hypotension and unresponsive bradycardia
Prophylaxis—cardiac catheterization, after open heart surgery, threatened bradycardia during drug trials for tachydysrhythmias
Malfunction of implanted pacemaker
Asystolic arrest patient—not clear

Tachycardias
Supraventricular dysrhythmias
Ventricular dysrhythmias
Prophylaxis—cardiac catheterization, after open heart surgery

for cardiac pacing are clear; however, some controversial areas remain. The decision to pace on an emergent basis requires knowledge of the presence or absence of hemodynamic compromise, the etiology of the rhythm disturbance, the status of the atrioventricular (AV) conduction system, and the type of dysrhythmia. In general, the indications can be grouped into those that cause either tachycardias or bradycardias (Table 13–2).

Bradycardias

Sinus Node Dysfunction. In a review of 200 initial pacemaker implants at Montefiore Hospital during 1975, 36.5 per cent were used for sinus node dysfunction, 11.3 per cent were used for sinus arrest, 20.2 per cent were used for tachybrady (sick sinus) syndrome, and 5 per cent were used for sinus bradycardia.[17] Patients without myocardial infarction who present with symptomatic sinus node dysfunction should be promptly paced if medical therapy fails. Escher and Furman note that pacing is indicated until the etiology of the dysrhythmia is clarified and stability is ensured.[18]

In the asymptomatic patient, a more intensive cardiac evaluation is required to decide whether pacing will be beneficial. This evaluation frequently includes 24-hour Holter monitoring, noting sinus node recovery times, and coronary care unit monitoring.

Sinus bradycardia occurs in an average of 17 per cent of patients with acute myocardial infarction.[19-22] Sinus bradycardia occurs more frequently in inferior than in anterior infarction and has a relatively good prognosis when accompanied by a hemodynamically tolerable escape rhythm. Sinus bradycardia is not a benign rhythm in this situation; it has a mortality rate of 2 per cent with inferior infarction and 9 per cent with anterior infarction.[23] Several mechanisms have been suggested to explain sinus node dysfunction with infarction. Among these, ischemia of the node[21] or its neurologic controls[22-25] and reflex slowing secondary to pain play dominant roles.[26] Sinus node dysfunction frequently responds to medical therapy but requires prompt pacing if this fails.

Asystolic Arrest. The role of transvenous pacing in the asystolic or bradyasystolic patient remains unclear. In one study of 13 patients who had suffered cardiac arrest, capture of the myocardium was noted in four patients, but there were no survivors.[27] Transvenous pacing alone may also not be effective in postcountershock pulseless bradyarrhythmias.[28, 29] This failure of pacing has also been demonstrated with transcutaneous pacemakers, suggesting that failure of effective pacing is primarily related to the state of the myocardial tissue.[28] Other causes of failure to pace include catheter malposition and dislodgment of the pacing wire during closed chest massage.[27] Frequently, cardiac pacing is used as a "last ditch" effort in bradyasystolic or asystolic patients. Some studies suggest that early pacing is essential to improving on these low rates of effective pacing.[30] A more complete discussion of pacing in bradyasystolic cardiac arrest appears in Chapter 15.

Atrioventricular Block. Atrioventricular block is the classic indication for pacemaker therapy. In symptomatic patients without myocardial infarction and in the asymptomatic patient with a ventricular rate below 40, pacemaker therapy is indicated.[31]

In patients with acute myocardial infarction, 15 to 19 per cent progress to heartblock: approximately 8 per cent develop first-degree block, 5 per cent develop second-degree block, and 6 per cent develop third-degree block.[32, 33] First-degree block progresses to second- or third-degree block 33 per cent of the time, and second-degree block progresses to third-degree block about one third of the time.[34]

Atrioventricular block occurring during anterior infarction is believed to occur because of diffuse ischemia to the septum and conduction tissue infranodally. Patients with atrioventricular block tend to progress to high degree block without warning and should be prophylactically paced temporarily if conduction abnormalities develop, even without hemodynamic compromise.

During inferior infarction, early septal ischemia is the exception, and block develops serially from first degree to Mobitz type I second degree, then to third degree. These conduction abnormalities frequently result in hemodynamically tolerable escape rhythms because of sparing of the bundle branches. The hemodynamically unstable patient who is unresponsive to medical therapy should be paced promptly. When the stable patient should be paced has not been determined.

One study in which the indications for temporary and permanent pacemaker insertion were reviewed in 432 patients with myocardial infarction concluded that patients with second- or third-degree atrioventricular block should be paced, because a higher incidence of sudden death or recurrent high degree block over the following year was found in patients who were not continuously paced.[35]

Bundle Branch Block. Bundle branch block, occurring in acute myocardial infarction, is associated with a higher mortality rate and a greater incidence of third-degree heart block than uncomplicated infarction. Atkins and associates noted that 18 per cent of patients had bundle branch block with myocardial infarction.[36] Of these patients, complete heart block developed in 43 per cent who had right bundle branch block and left axis deviation, 17 per cent who had left bundle branch block, 19 per cent who had left anterior hemiblock, and 6 per cent who had no conduction block. The investigators concluded that right bundle branch block with left axis deviation should be prophylactically paced.

A later study by Hindman and colleagues confirmed the natural history of bundle branch block during myocardial infarction.[37] In their study, the presence or absence of first-degree atrioventricular block, the type of bundle branch block, and the age (new versus old) of the block were used to determine the relative risk of progression to type II second-degree or third-degree block (Table 13–3).

Table 13–3. The Influence of Different Variables on Risk of High-Degree Atrioventricular Block in Patients with Bundle Branch Block During Myocardial Infarction

	Patients	High-Degree AVB (%)
Infarct location		
Anterior	272	25
Indeterminate	77	12
Inferior or posterior	83	20
PR Interval		
>0.20 sec	169	25
≤0.20 sec	263	19
Type BBB		
LBBB	163	13
RBBB	48	14
RBBB + LAFB	149	27
RBBB + LPFB	45	29
ABBB	27	44
Onset BBB		
Definitely old	91	13
Possibly new	95	25
Probably new	65	26
Definitely new	181	23

Hi° AVB, high-degree atrioventricular block; BBB, bundle branch block; LBBB, left bundle branch block; RBBB, right bundle branch block; LAFB, left anterior fascicular hemiblock; LPFB, left posterior fascicular hemiblock; ABBB, alternating bundle branch block. (Reprinted by permission of the American Heart Association from Hindman MC, Wagner GS, JaRo M, et al: The clinical significance of bundle branch block complicating acute myocardial infarction. 2. Indications of temporary and permanent pacemaker insertion. Circulation 58:690, 1978.)

Because of the increased risk, most physicians would pace new onset left bundle branch block, right bundle branch block with left axis deviation or other bifascicular block, and alternating bundle branch block.[35–38] One authority recommends prophylactic pacing for all new bundle branch blocks when myocardial infarction is evident.[39]

Whether to place a transvenous pacemaker prophylactically in patients with left bundle branch block before insertion of a flow-directed pulmonary artery catheter remains controversial. Some researchers strongly advocate this procedure because of the risk of transient right bundle branch block and life-threatening complete heart block.[40, 41] One study notes that this risk is low in patients with prior left bundle branch block but continues to recommend temporary catheter placement for all cases of new left bundle branch block.[42] One solution to this problem is to place an external pacemaker before catheterization as an emergency measure should heart block develop. In these cases a temporary transvenous pacemaker can be placed in a semielective manner when needed.[43]

Trauma. In the patient with nonpenetrating chest trauma, several rhythm and conduction disturbances have been documented.[44–46] In these patients, traumatic injury to the specialized conduction system may predispose the patient to life-threatening dysrhythmias and blocks that can be treated by cardiac pacing.[47]

Hypovolemia and hypotension can cause ischemia of conduction tissue and cardiac dysfunction.[48, 49] Continued marked bradydysrhythmias after vigorous volume replacement may respond to cardiac pacing in patients with such trauma.[50]

Tachycardias

Hemodynamically compromising tachycardias are usually treated by medical means or cardioversion (see Chapters

10 and 11). Over the last 15 years, there has been an increasing interest in pacing therapy for symptomatic tachycardias. In 1960, two groups reported that asynchronous pacing prevented ventricular tachycardia and fibrillation in patients with bradycardia and heart block.[51, 52] Over the next 4 to 5 years, several investigators noted that supraventricular dysrhythmias could be suppressed, even in the absence of heart block.[53–55] It was also learned that pharmacologic and pacing therapies could augment each other when used concurrently.

Supraventricular dysrhythmias, with the exception of atrial fibrillation, respond well to atrial pacing. By pacing the atria at rates 10 to 20 beats per minute faster than the underlying rhythm, the atria become intrained, and when the rate is slowed, the rhythm frequently returns to normal sinus. A similar procedure is done for ventricular dysrhythmias.[53, 56–58]

Overdrive pacing is especially useful for recurrent prolonged Q-T interval arrythmias such as those seen with quinidine toxicity or torsade de pointes.[59] Transvenous pacing also is useful in patients with digitalis-induced dysrhythmias in whom direct current (DC) cardioversion may be dangerous or in patients in whom there is further concern about myocardial depression with drugs.[57]

EQUIPMENT

Several items are required to insert a transvenous pacemaker adequately. Like most special procedures, a prearranged tray is convenient. The usual components required to insert a transvenous cardiac pacemaker are listed in Table 13–4.

Many different pacing generators are available, but in general, they all have the same basic features. The on/off switch frequently will have a locking feature to prevent the generator from inadvertently being switched off. An amperage knob allows the operator to control the amount of electrical current delivered to the myocardium and usually ranges from 0.1 to 20 milliamperes (mA). The pacing control mode is the gain control for the sensing function of the generator. By moving this knob, one can convert the unit from a fixed rate (asynchronous mode) to a demand (synchronous mode) pacemaker. In the fixed rate mode, the unit fires despite the underlying intrinsic rhythm; the unit

does not sense any intrinsic electrical activity. In the full demand mode, however, the pacemaker senses the underlying ventricular depolarizations, and the unit does not fire as long as the patient's ventricular rate is equal to or faster than the set rate of the pacing generator. A sensing indicator meter and rate control knob are also present. An example of a pacing generator is shown in Figure 14–2.

Several sizes and brands of pacing catheters are available. In general, most range from 3 French to 5 French in size and are approximately 100 cm in length. Along the catheter surface, there are lines that are marked at approximately 10 cm intervals, which can be used to estimate catheter position during insertion. Two basic types of pacing catheters are currently in use: the flexible semifloating or floating catheter and the rigid fixed-position catheter.[60]

The flexible catheters are more advantageous than the rigid catheter in their ability to be inserted in low flow states as well as in their decreased tendency to perforate the ventricle. For emergency pacing, the 4 French semifloating bipolar electrode with or without the balloon tip is used most frequently (Fig. 13–1). The balloon holds approximately 1.5 ml of air or carbon dioxide, and some of them have a locking lever to secure balloon expansion. Before insertion, the balloon is checked for air leakage by inflating it and immersing it in sterile water (Fig. 13–2). The presence of an air leak is noted by a stream of bubbles arising at the surface of the water. An inflated balloon helps the catheter "float" into the heart in low flow states but is obviously not advantageous in the cardiac arrest situation.

For all practical purposes, temporary transvenous pacing is accomplished with a bipolar pacing catheter. The terms *unipolar* and *bipolar* refer to the number of electrodes in contact with that portion of the heart that is to be stimulated. All pacemaker systems must have both a positive (anode) and a negative (cathode) electrode, and all stimulation is *bipolar*. The typical bipolar catheter that is used for temporary transvenous pacing has the cathode (stimulating electrode) at the tip of the pacing catheter. The anode is located 1 to 2 cm proximal to the tip, and the two electrodes may be separated by a balloon or an insulated wire. The electrodes are usually platinum rings that encircle the pacing catheter. When properly positioned, both electrodes will be within the right ventricle so that a field of electrical excitation is set up between the electrodes. With the bipolar catheter, the cathode does not need to be in direct contact with the endocardium for pacing to occur, although it is preferable to have direct contact.

Table 13–4. Equipment
Pacemaker Tray
10-ml syringe
1% lidocaine
Alcohol wipes
Betadine
Several gauze pads
4 sterile drapes
No. 11 scalpel blade
0.9 normal saline—2 ampules
Sterile gloves
Needle holder
2 22-gauge needles
Scissors (suture)
2 4–0 silk sutures on needles
Sterile basin
Electrical Hardware
Spare 9-volt battery
Medtronic pacing unit No. 5375
3F Balectrode Pacing Kit (catalog No. 11—KBE1)
12 lead electrocardiographic machine (well grounded)

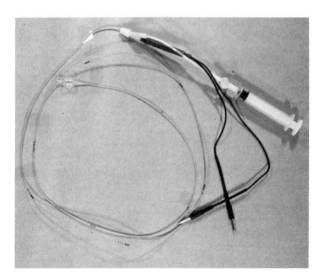

Figure 13–1. Balloon-tipped pacing catheter.

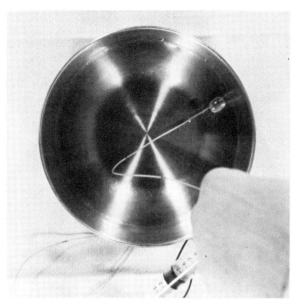

Figure 13–2. Testing the balloon for leakage.

A unipolar system is also effective but is infrequently used for temporary transvenous pacing. In a unipolar system, the cathode is at the tip of the pacing catheter, and the anode is located either in the pacing generator itself, more proximal on the catheter (outside the ventricle), or underneath the skin on the patient's chest. The bipolar system may be converted to a unipolar system by simply disconnecting the positive proximal connection of the bipolar catheter from the pacing generator and running a new wire from the positive terminal to the patient's chest wall. Such a conversion may be required in the unlikely event of failure of one lead of the bipolar system.

Theoretically, the field of electrical stimulation of a pacing catheter is equal to the distance between the electrodes. If the field of excitation is not close enough to the myocardium, depolarization will not occur. When a catheter is passed blindly in an emergency, it seems advantageous to ensure the best chance of capture by separating the electrodes more than the standard 1 to 2 cm. A pacing catheter that uses this configuration (Davison pacing lead, Electro-Catheter Corp.) is a hybrid of the standard bipolar and unipolar catheters. This catheter has the cathode at the tip, but the anode is situated 19 cm proximal to the tip. This configuration allows pacing with a very wide field of excitation. Pacing has been reported to occur with this catheter when the catheter is placed anywhere within the thoracic venous system.[61] The catheter is a hybrid because both electrodes are present on the same catheter (bipolar), but both electrodes will not be positioned in the same cardiac chamber (unipolar).

An electrocardiograph can be used to record the heart's inherent electrical activity during pacer insertion and to aid in localization of the catheter tip without fluoroscopy. The electrocardiograph machine must be well grounded to prevent leakage of alternating current, which can cause ventricular fibrillation. Such leakage should be suspected if 50 to 60 cycles per second (Hz) interference is noted on the electrocardiograph.

The electrocardiograph machine should be placed in such a manner to allow easy visibility of the rhythm during insertion. One method is to place the machine on the same side of the patient as the operator at the level of the midthorax (Fig. 13–3). Note that the operator stands at the head of the patient during internal jugular or subclavian

vein passage of the catheter and at the midabdomen for femoral or brachiocephalic vein insertion.

An introducer set or sheath is required for venous access (see Chapter 23). Some pacing catheters are prepackaged with the appropriate equipment, whereas others require a separate set. The introducer set is used to enhance passage of the pacing catheter through the skin, subcutaneous tissue, and vessel wall. To allow passage of the pacing catheter, the sheath must be one size larger than the pacing catheter. A makeshift sheath can be made with an appropriate sized intravenous catheter. For the 3 French balloon-tipped catheter, a 14-gauge, 1.5- to 2-inch intravenous catheter is suitable.

A balloon-directed pulmonary artery catheter (Paceport pacing system; American Edwards Laboratories; American Hospital Supply Corp.) has been developed that has a separate lumen that allows the passage of a transvenous pacing catheter.[62] This catheter is 7.5 French and has an opening 19 cm from the catheter tip that allows passage of the 2.4 French pacing wire. This stainless steel wire is Teflon coated for easy passage and has a flexible tip. Combination pulmonary artery or pacemaker catheters are also available but are not widely used in the emergency setting.

Overall, the key to success with this procedure is preparation. It is imperative that one examines all the components of the tray before starting the procedure and ensures that all wires, sheaths, dilators, and syringes fit as expected.

PROCEDURE

Patient Preparation

Patient instruction is an extremely important aspect of any procedure. Frequently, there is not enough time to give patients a detailed explanation. Nonetheless, sufficient information should be provided so that the patient feels at ease. Patients should be assured that they will feel no discomfort after the venipuncture site has been anesthetized and that they will feel better when the catheter is in place and is functional. Continued reassurance is required during the procedure, because patients are usually facing away from the operator; because their faces are often covered, they may be unsure of what is occurring.

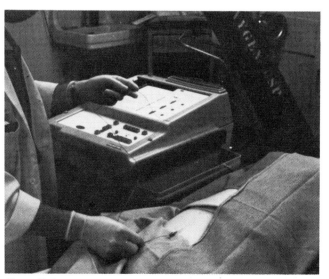

Figure 13–3. Position of an electrocardiogram device during femoral vein insertion of a pacemaker catheter.

Whenever possible, all operators should wear surgical masks, caps, gloves, and gowns to decrease the risk of infection before catheter placement. This aseptic precaution should also be explained to the patient.

Site Selection

The four venous channels that provide an easy access to the right ventricle are the brachial, subclavian, femoral, and internal jugular veins (Table 13–5). The route selected is often one of personal or institutional preference. The right internal jugular and the left subclavian veins have the straightest anatomic pathway to the right ventricle and are generally preferred for temporary transvenous pacing. In some centers, a particular site is preferred for *permanent* transvenous pacemaker placement, and, if possible, this site should be avoided for temporary placement.

The subclavian vein can be accessed by both an infraclavicular and a supraclavicular approach; the infraclavicular approach is most commonly reported for all temporary transvenous pacemaker insertions. This route is preferred because of its easy accessibility, close proximity to the heart, and ease in catheter maintenance and stability. The supraclavicular approach, although described in the literature for several years, has only recently gained popularity among some physicians.[63] The left subclavian vein is preferred because of the less acute angle traversed when compared with the right-sided approach.

Some physicians believe the internal jugular approach is as easy as and safer than subclavian catheterization.[64] The right internal jugular vein is preferred because of the direct line to the superior vena cava. Problems with this approach include dislodgment of the pacemaker with movement of the head, carotid artery puncture, and thrombophlebitis (see Chapter 26).

During cardiopulmonary resuscitation, the use of the right internal jugular vein and the left subclavian veins for pacemaker insertion have been demonstrated to result in the highest rates of proper placement in the right ventricle.[65, 66] The right internal jugular vein is the more direct route of the two and may be the most appropriate site.[65] Because of the extremely low flow state during cardiopulmonary resuscitation, a larger (5 French), semirigid catheter may be a more appropriate choice than the 3 to 4 French catheters commonly used.[65]

Femoral veins, like neck veins, are reusable and easily catheterized. Problems include easy dislodgment, infection, and increased risk of thrombophlebitis.[67–69a]

Brachial vein catheterization is easy to perform but results in a high incidence of infection and vessel thrombosis.[70] In addition, the catheter is easily dislodged with arm motion. This approach is seldom used in the emergency setting.

Skin Preparation

The skin over the venipuncture site is cleaned twice with an antiseptic solution such as povidone-iodine and isopropyl alcohol. A wide area is prepared because of the tendency for guide wires and catheters to spring from the hands of the unsuspecting operator. For the infraclavicular approach to the subclavian, the skin between the opposite sternal border, the nipple line, the anterior axillary line, and the posterior aspect of the clavicle must be cleaned (Fig. 13–4). For the supraclavicular and internal jugular approach, an area enclosing the sternal notch, clavicle, midshoulder, and lateral neck from the midline to the ramus of the mandible (Fig. 13–5) should be prepared. For the femoral approach, skin preparation includes an area 2 inches above and 6 inches below the inguinal ligament, from the mid inner thigh to its lateral border (Fig. 13–6).

Similarly, wide draping is carried out in the standard manner to maintain a sterile field and to allow clear visibility of the venipuncture site.

Obtaining Venous Access

The infraclavicular approach is used in this chapter to illustrate venous access, although the mechanics are generally the same for other vascular approaches. The reader is referred to Chapters 25 and 26 for the specific techniques of venous access.

Occasionally, a patient who already has a central venous line in place requires the emergent placement of a pacing catheter. An existing central venous pressure (CVP) line can be used to place the pacing catheter if the catheter lumen is large enough to accept a guide wire. The CVP line should be withdrawn 1 to 2 inches to expose an area of sterile tubing. The tubing is transected through a sterile area while being held firmly at the skin level (Fig. 13–7). A guide wire can then be passed through the tubing, and the tubing can be withdrawn, leaving only the wire in the vein (Fig. 13–8). The guide wire and the tubing should never be released, because embolization may result. An introducer unit can then be passed over the guide wire, as is done in the Seldinger technique (see Chapter 23), and the pacing catheter can be placed (Fig. 13–9).

Table 13–5. Advantages and Disadvantages of Pacemaker Placement Sites

Venous Channels	Advantages	Disadvantages
Brachial	Very safe route Vessel easily accessible—either by cutdown or percutaneous approach	Often requires cutdown Easily displaced and poor patient mobility Not reusable if cutdown technique is performed Catheter is more difficult to advance than with central or larger vessels
Subclavian	Direct access to right heart (especially via left subclavian) Rapid insertion time Reusable Good patient mobility	Pneumothorax and other intrathoracic trauma is possible
Femoral	Direct access to right heart Rapid insertion time Reusable	Increased incidence of thrombophlebitis Can be dislodged by leg movement and poor patient mobility Infection
Internal jugular	Direct access to right heart (especially via right internal jugular) Rapid insertion time Reusable	Possible carotid artery puncture Dislodgment with movement of the head Thrombophlebitis

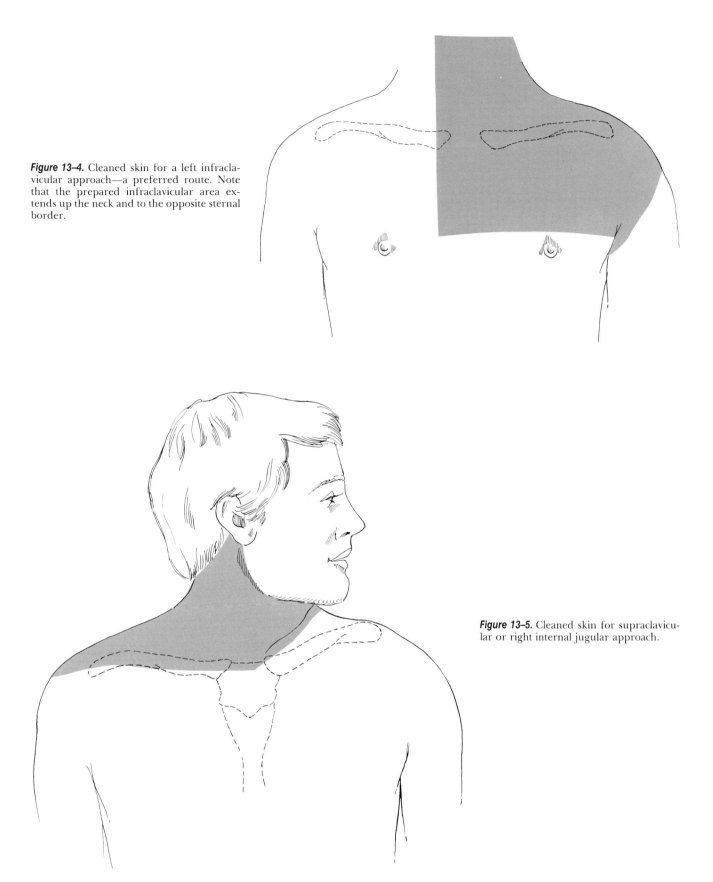

Figure 13–4. Cleaned skin for a left infraclavicular approach—a preferred route. Note that the prepared infraclavicular area extends up the neck and to the opposite sternal border.

Figure 13–5. Cleaned skin for supraclavicular or right internal jugular approach.

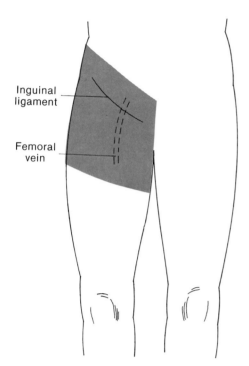

Figure 13–6. Area of skin preparation for femoral approach.

Pacemaker Placement (Electrocardiographic Guidance)

The patient should be connected to the limb leads of an ECG machine, and the indicator should be turned to record the chest (V) lead. The pacing wire should be inserted about 10 to 12 cm into the selected vein. The *distal* terminal of the pacing catheter must be connected to the V lead of the ECG machine by a male-to-male connector (Fig. 13–10) or by an insulated wire with an alligator clip on each end (Fig. 13–11). The pacing catheter is thus an exploring electrode that creates a unipolar electrode for intracardiac electrocardiographic recording. The ECG recorded from the electrode tip localizes the position of the tip of the pacing electrode. If a balloon-tipped catheter is used, the balloon is inflated with air or carbon dioxide *after* the catheter enters the superior vena cava. Carbon dioxide is preferred because of its rapid absorption if balloon rupture occurs, although carbon dioxide is not usually available.

The pacing catheter should be advanced both quickly and smoothly. The V lead should be monitored, and the P wave and QRS complex should be observed to ascertain the location of the pacing catheter tip. The use of an ECG to guide the placement of a pacing catheter is based on two concepts. First, the complex will vary in size depending on which chamber is entered. For example, when the tip of the pacing catheter is in the atrium, one will see large P waves, often larger than the corresponding QRS complex. Second, the sum of the electrical forces will be negative if the depolarization is moving away from the catheter tip and will be positive if the depolarization is moving toward the catheter tip. Therefore, if the catheter tip is *above* the atrium, both the P wave and the QRS complex will be negative. As the tip progresses inferiorly in the atrium, the P wave will become isoelectric (biphasic) and will eventually become positive as the wave of atrial depolarization advances toward the catheter tip. The electrocardiogram resembles an aVR lead initially when in the left subclavian vein (Fig. 13–12A) or midsuperior vena cava (Fig. 13–12B). At the high right

atrium, both the P wave and QRS complex are negative; the P wave is larger than the QRS complex and is deeply inverted (Fig. 13–12C and D). As the center of the atrium is approached, the P wave becomes large and biphasic (Fig. 13–12E). As the catheter approaches the lower atrium (Fig. 13–12F), the P wave becomes smaller and upright. The QRS complex is fairly normal. When striking the right atrial wall, an injury pattern with a P–Ta segment is seen (Fig. 13–12G). As the electrode passes through the triscupid valve, the P wave becomes smaller and the QRS complex becomes larger (Fig. 13–12H). Placement in the inferior vena cava may be recognized by a change in the morphology of the P wave and a decrease in the amplitude of both the P wave and the QRS complex (Fig. 13–12I).

Once the pacing catheter is in the desired position, the balloon is deflated by unlocking it and allowing the air to passively fill the syringe. One should avoid drawing back on the syringe, because this may cause balloon rupture. If the plunger does not move back spontaneously, assume that the balloon ruptured and do not subsequently place more air into the port. The pacing catheter should be withdrawn, and the balloon should be checked for leaks. If a leak is found, the pacing catheter should be replaced.

After successful placement of the catheter within the right ventricle, the tip should be advanced until contact is made with the endocardial wall. When this occurs, the QRS segment will show ST segment elevation (Fig. 13–12J). Ideally, the tip of the catheter should be lodged in the trabeculae at the apex of the right ventricle; however, pacing may be successful if the catheter is in various other positions within the ventricle or outflow tract.

If the pacer enters the pulmonary artery outflow tract, the P wave again becomes negative and the QRS amplitude diminishes (Fig. 13–12K). If the catheter is in the pulmonary artery, the pacing catheter should be withdrawn into the right ventricle and readvanced. Sometimes a clockwise or counterclockwise twist of the catheter will redirect its path in a more favorable direction. If catheter-induced ectopy develops, the catheter should be slightly withdrawn until the ectopy stops; then it should be readvanced. Occasionally, an

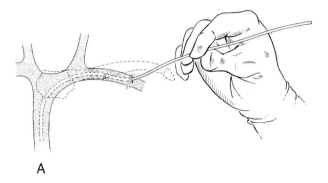

A

Figure 13–7. Preparing the central line for guide wire insertion. The existing central venous pressure (CVP) line is grasped *(A)*, withdrawn a few inches *(B)*, and transected *(C)*. Note that the remaining CVP line must be considerably shorter than the guide wire to permit continuous control of the guide wire. Once the central line is transected, the lumen must be kept occluded until guide-wire passage (see Fig. 13–8).

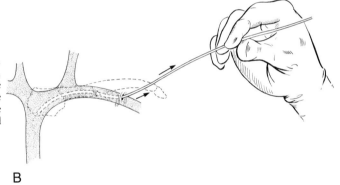

B

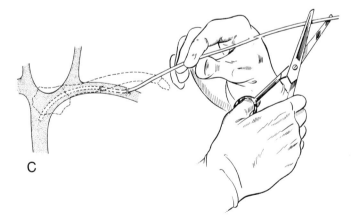

C

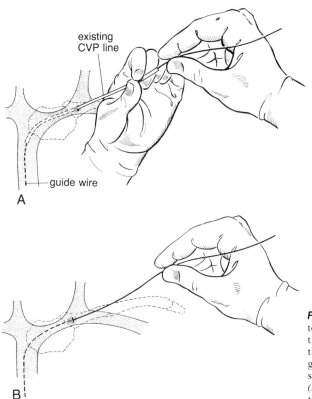

A

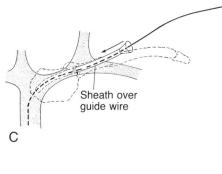

C

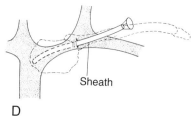

D

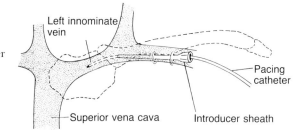

B

Figure 13–8. Using the central venous pressure (CVP) line to insert the guide wire. The guide wire is passed through the transected CVP line into the central circulation *(A)*, and the existing CVP line is then withdrawn, leaving only the guide wire in the vein *(B)*. *C,* The passage of an introducer sheath over the guide wire. The guide wire is then removed *(D),* and the pacemaker is subsequently inserted through the sheath (see Fig. 13–9). The lumen of the sheath should be occluded by its intrinsic seal during this process.

Figure 13–9. Insertion of the pacing catheter through the introducer sheath.

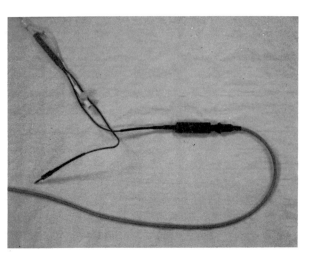

Figure 13–10. Connecting the temporary pacemaker to the V lead of an electrocardiographic machine with a male-to-male connector.

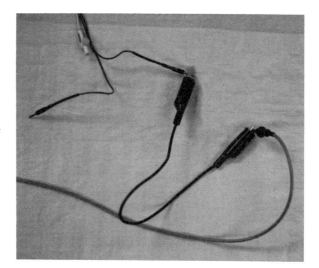

Figure 13–11. Using alligator clips to connect the pacemaker to the V lead of an electrocardiographic machine.

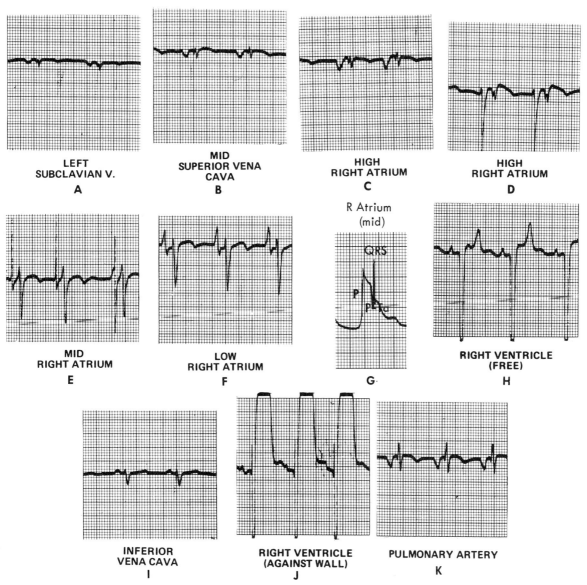

Figure 13–12. *A–K,* Intracardiac electrocardiography. (*A–F* and *H–K* from Bing OH, McDowell JW, Hantman J, et al: Pacemaker placement by electrocardiographic monitoring. N Engl J Med 287:651, 1972. *G* from Goldberger E: Treatment of Cardiac Emergencies. 3rd ed. St. Louis, CV Mosby Co, 1982, p 252.)

antidysrhythmic drug such as lidocaine may need to be given to desensitize the myocardium. Once ventricular endocardial contact is made, the catheter is disconnected from the ECG machine. The proximal positive and negative leads are connected to their respective terminals on the pacing generator. The pacing generator is then set to a rate of 80 beats per minute or 10 beats per minute faster than the underlying ventricular rhythm, whichever is higher. The full demand mode is selected with an output of about 5 mA. The pacing generator is then turned on. If complete capture does not occur or if it is intermittent, the pacer will need to be repositioned. When proper capture occurs, the pacer is tested for optimal positioning. This is done by testing the thresholds for sensing and pacing, by chest radiographs, by physical examination, and by electrocardiograph.

Catheter Placement (Without an Electrocardiograph)

Occasionally, it is necessary to use a transvenous pacemaker in an emergency setting when a well-grounded electrocardiograph machine is not available.

EMERGENCY BLIND PLACEMENT

Blind insertion of the transvenous pacing catheter is a safe and effective alternative to electrocardiographic guidance. In this technique, the pacing catheter is placed 10 to 12 cm into the venous port and is connected to the pacing generator as noted previously. The pacing rate is selected at *twice* the intrinsic heart rate, and the output is set at an amperage that is too low to capture the ventricle, usually less than 0.2 mA. The unit is then turned on, and the pacing is begun in order to *sense* but *not* to pace. On entering the ventricle, the pacer will sense on every other beat. The balloon can then be deflated, the amperage can be increased to 4 to 5 mA, and the pacemaker can be advanced to capture the ventricle. If this does not occur within an additional 10 cm, the pacing catheter should be withdrawn to its original position and then advanced again. As with electrocardiographic placement, proper positioning must be ensured.

Fluoroscopy is a valuable tool in the placement of transvenous pacemakers. Its use depends on the operator's preference, the patient's condition, and its availability. Pacemakers should not be inserted under fluoroscopy without electrocardiographic monitoring because of the high incidence of ventricular dysrhythmias.[60]

If the cardiac output is too low to "float" a pacing catheter or if the patient is in extremis, there often is not enough time to advance a pacing catheter under ECG guidance. Such a situation would be asystole or complete heart block with malignant ventricular escape rhythms (although one can make a case for transthoracic or transcutaneous pacing in such conditions). In the emergency blind placement technique, the pacing catheter is connected to the energy source, the output is turned to the maximum amperage, and the asynchronous mode is selected. The catheter is then blindly advanced, in hopes that it will enter the right ventricle and that pacing will be accomplished. The pacing catheter is rotated, advanced, withdrawn, or otherwise manipulated according to the clinical response. The right internal jugular approach is the most practical access route in this situation. In such instances, there is the theoretic advantage of using the previously described Davison catheter, because one is only interested in rapid capture until the patient is stabilized.

Testing Threshold

The threshold is the minimum current necessary to obtain capture. Ideally, this is less than 1.0 mA, and usually it is between 0.3 and 0.7 mA. If the threshold is in this ideal range, good contact with the endocardium can be presumed.

To determine the threshold, the pacing generator should be placed in the full demand mode at 5 mA with a rate of approximately 80 beats per minute. The amperage (output) should then be reduced slowly until capture is lost. This current is the threshold. This maneuver should be carried out two or three times to ensure that this value is consistent; the amperage should then be increased to two and one half times the threshold to ensure consistency of capture (usually between 2 and 3 mA).

If one reduces the output to below the threshold and then slowly increases it, there may be a difference in the point at which capture returns. This difference is called hysteresis and represents the time interval between sensing and pacemaker firing. If the difference in capture current is greater than 20 per cent, the pacing catheter should be repositioned, because serious dysrhythmias may result if the pacemaker fires during the vulnerable period of repolarization.[60, 71]

Testing Sensing

The sensing function should be tested in patients who have underlying rhythms. The pacemaker system is again set in full demand mode with complete capture, and the rate is decreased until it is suppressed by the patient's intrinsic rhythm. This is done several times to ensure accuracy of the sensing function.

In bipolar systems, another method of evaluating the sensing mode is to take a unipolar electrocardiogram from each end of the bipolar lead on a chest lead at one-fourth standardization to permit observation of the entire complex.[60] The voltage of the QRS complex is multiplied by four and, if adequate, should be greater than the sensing threshold by more than 1 mV (Fig. 13–13). Another method is to set the electrocardiograph machine on lead I and to connect the wires from the proximal electrode to the right arm lead and the left arm lead to the distal electrode (Fig.

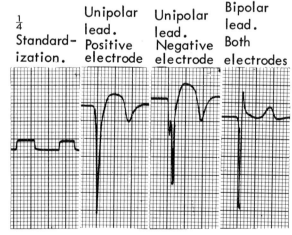

Figure 13–13. Testing unipolar sensing with a bipolar system. (From Goldberger E: Treatment of Cardiac Emergencies. 3rd ed. St. Louis, CV Mosby Co, 1982.)

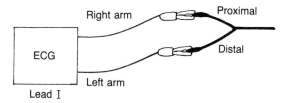

Figure 13–14. Pacemaker lead attachment to electrocardiographic machine for lead I monitoring of sensing function.

13–14). A lead I is created, which, when the QRS voltage is multiplied by four, should also be at least 1 mV greater than the sensing threshold.

Securing and Final Assessment

After the pacemaker's position has been tested for electrical accuracy, the introducer sheath should be withdrawn (Fig. 13–15) and the catheter should be secured to the skin with 4–0 silk suture. A fastening suture should be sewn to the skin, and the catheter should be tied securely in place. The excess pacing catheter should be coiled and secured in a sterile manner along with the introducer (Fig. 13–16). A large sterile dressing should be applied. Pacemaker function should again be assessed, and a chest film should be taken to ensure proper positioning. Ideal positioning of the pacing catheter is at the apex of the right ventricle (Fig. 13–17).

A 12 lead electrocardiogram should be obtained after placement. If the catheter is within the right ventricle, a left bundle branch pattern with left axis deviation should be evident in paced beats (Fig. 13–18). If a right bundle branch block pattern is noted, coronary sinus placement or left ventricular pacing due to septal penetration should be suspected.

With a properly functioning ventricular pacemaker, large cannon waves will be noted on inspection of the venous pulsations at the neck. This is caused by the atria contracting against a closed tricuspid valve. On auscultation of the heart, a slight murmur secondary to tricuspid insufficiency from the catheter interfering with the tricuspid valve apparatus may be evident.[72] A clicking sound heard best during expiration following each pacemaker impulse may also be noted here and is believed to represent either intercostal or diaphragmatic muscular contractions caused by the pacemaker.[73–75] Note that this can also be a sign of cardiac perforation.[76] On auscultation of the second heart sound, paradoxical splitting may be noted. This represents a delay in closure of the aortic valve because of delayed left ventricular depolarization.

As in any procedure, the patient should then be assessed for improvement in his clinical status. An evaluation of vital signs, mentation, improvement in congestive symptoms, and urinary output must be noted. In addition, complications secondary to the procedure should be sought and treated as needed.

COMPLICATIONS

The complications of emergency transvenous cardiac pacing are numerous and represent a compendium of those related to central venous catheterization, those related to right heart catheterization, and those unique to the pacing catheter itself (Table 13–6).

Problems Related to Central Venous Catheterization

Inadvertent arterial puncture is a well-known complication of the percutaneous approach to the venous system.[77]

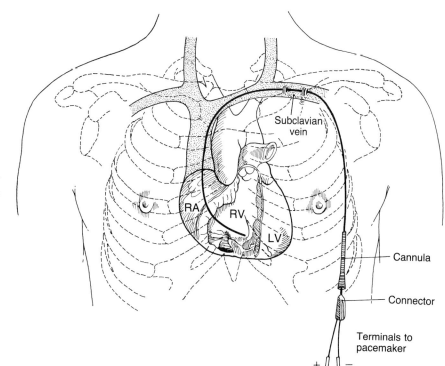

Figure 13–15. Pulling back the introducer sheath (cannula). *RA,* right atrium; *RV,* right ventricle; *LV,* left ventricle.

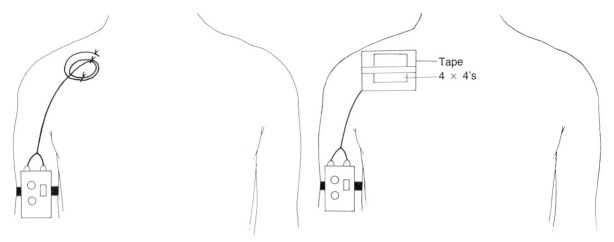

Figure 13–16. Securing the pacemaker.

This problem is usually recognized quickly because of the rapid return of arterial blood. Firm compression over the puncture site will almost always result in hemostasis in 5 minutes or less.

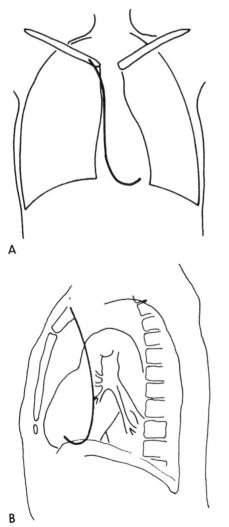

Figure 13–17. Normal pacemaker position on posteroanterior (A) and lateral (B) chest films. (From Goldberger E: Treatment of Cardiac Emergencies. 3rd ed. St. Louis, CV Mosby Co, 1982.)

Venous thrombosis and thrombophlebitis are also potential problems with central venous catheterization. Thrombophlebitis, which occurs early after insertion, is said to be a rare complication. Some experts believe that it can be managed without removal of the catheter or anticoagulation.[70] When thrombophlebitis occurs in long-term implanted pacemakers, removal and anticoagulation may be required. In one series, only 0.1 per cent of permanent pacemakers were in this category, and, in a small percentage of these, occult malignancies were found.[70] Complete thrombosis of the innominate vein is also a rare problem, with pulmonary embolism an even more uncommon event.[78] Femoral vein thrombosis, however, appears to be a much more common event associated with femoral vein catheterization.[67–69] Studies using noninvasive techniques have shown a 37 per cent incidence of femoral vein thrombosis, with 55 per cent of these having ventilation-perfusion scan evidence of pulmonary embolism.[68] Thrombosis in the right atrium may also occur and has been treated successfully with thrombolytic agents.[79]

Pneumothorax is consistently a problem with the various approaches to the veins at the base of the neck. Various techniques have been introduced to lessen the chance of pneumothorax, but in general, this complication probably relates to the lack of skill and patience of the operator and to the presence of anatomic variation, such as the apex of the lung being located higher than expected. The decision to place a chest tube in patients with this complication depends on the extent of the air leak and the clinical status of the patient (see Chapter 9). In addition, laceration of the subclavian vein with hemothorax, thoracic duct laceration with chylothorax, air embolism, wound infections, pneumomediastinum and hemomediastinum, phrenic nerve injury, fracture of the guide wire with embolization, and catheter or guide wire knotting are all potential complications.[60, 80–88]

Complications of Right Heart Catheterization

A very common complication of the pacing catheter is dysrhythmia, with premature ventricular contractions being a common occurrence in my experience. One study noted a 1.5 per cent incidence of serious dysrhythmias with a balloon-tipped catheter using electrocardiographic guidance compared with a 32 per cent incidence rate with the semirigid catheter and fluoroscopic guidance, suggesting that the balloon catheter was the preferred type of catheter.[15] An-

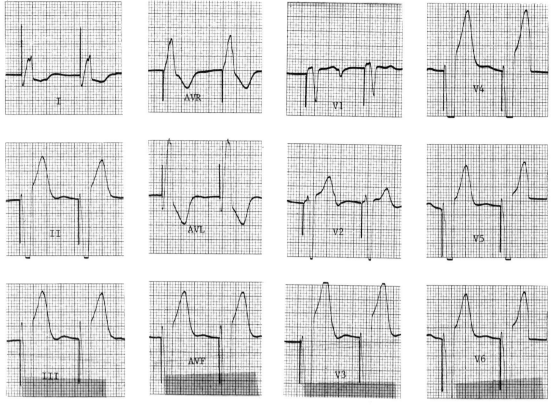

Figure 13–18. Electrocardiogram pattern of right ventricular pacemaker.

Table 13–6. Complications of Transvenous Cardiac Pacing

Year	Author	Patients	Catheter	Route	Result
1969	Rosenberg AS, et al[1]	111	Flexon steelwire vs. unipolar semifloating (ECG)	96 subclavian 5 basilic 1 external jugular	12 inconsistent pacing, 3 local infection, 2 pneumothorax, 1 subclavian artery puncture; 16% complication rate
1973	Schnitzler RN, et al[14]	17	3F bipolar semifloating balloon (ECG)	Antecubital vein	2 PVCs, stable pacing, no thrombophlebitis
1973	Weinstein J, et al[69a]	100	6F bipolar (fluoroscopy)	Femoral	2 ventricular tachycardia, 2 perforations, 2 required repositionings, 1 questionable thrombophlebitis and pulmonary embolism, 1 local infection
1973	Lumia FJ, Rios JC[125]	142 insertions in 113 patients	Bipolar (fluoroscopy)	61 brachial 81 femoral	12 ventricular tachycardia and fibrillation in 9 patients, 3 perforations in 2 patients; local hematoma, abscess, and bleeding in 30%; 16.9% complication rate
1980	Pandian NG, et al[69]	20	5F bipolar (fluoroscopy)	Femoral	25% deep venous thrombosis
1980	Nolewajka AT, et al[68]	29	6F cordis (fluoroscopy)	Femoral	34% venous thrombosis by venogram with 60% of these with pulmonary embolism by VQ scan
1981	Lang R, et al[15]	111	Balloon, semifloating vs. semirigid	Subclavian	Serious dysrhythmia: 1.5% balloon-tipped, 20.4% semirigid Catheter displacement: 13.6% ± 4.4 days balloon-tipped; 32% ± 1.9 day semirigid
1982	Austin JL, et al[67]	113 insertions in 100 patients	4–7F bipolar (fluoroscopy)	Brachial Femoral	Failure to sense or pace in 37%; repositioning in 37% of brachial insertions; repositioning in 9% of femoral insertions; fever, sepsis, local infection only in femoral insertions; 20% complication rate

ECG, electrocardiogram; PVC, premature ventricular contraction; VQ, ventilation perfusion.

other study noted a 6 per cent incidence of ventricular tachycardia during insertion.[67] It is well known that the ischemic heart is more prone to dysrhythmias than the nonischemic heart.[89, 90] The therapy for catheter-induced ectopy involves withdrawing the catheter from the ventricle. This usually stops the ectopy; however, if after repeated attempts it is found that the catheter cannot be passed without ectopy, myocardial suppressant therapy may be used to desensitize the myocardium.

Misplacement of the pacing catheter has been well studied. Passage of the catheter into the pulmonary artery can be diagnosed cardiographically by observing the return of an inverted P wave and the decrease in the voltage of the QRS complex. Misplacement in the coronary sinus may occur and should be suspected in the patient in whom a paced right bundle branch pattern on the electrocardiogram is seen with right ventricular pacing (Fig. 13–19). Rarely, a right bundle branch pattern can be seen with a normal right ventricular position; therefore, all right bundle branch patterns do not represent coronary sinus pacing.[91] Further evidence for coronary sinus location can be obtained by viewing the lateral chest film. Normally, the catheter tip should point anteriorly toward the apex of the heart; however, with coronary sinus placement, the catheter tip is displaced posteriorly and several centimeters away from the sternum (Fig. 13–20). Other potential forms of misplacement include left ventricular pacing through an atrial septal defect or ventricular septal defect, septal puncture, extraluminal insertion, and arterial insertions.[92]

Perforation of the ventricle is also a well-described complication that can result in loss of capture, hemopericardium, and tamponade.[93–95] Reported symptoms and signs of this problem include chest pain, pericardial friction rub, and diaphragmatic or chest wall muscular pacing.[96] At least one case of a postpericardiotomy-like syndrome and two cases of endocardial friction rub have been reported without perforation.[97, 98]

Pericardial perforation is suggested radiographically when the pacing catheter is outside or abuts the cardiac silhouette and is not in proper position within the right ventricular cavity (Fig. 13–21).[99] Electrocardiographic clues include a change in the QRS and T wave axis or a failure to properly sense. In suspected cases, a two-dimensional echocardiogram usually demonstrates the catheter's extracardiac position. Uncomplicated perforation can usually be treated by simply pulling back the catheter and repositioning it in the right ventricle.

During the insertion of a permanent pacing catheter when a temporary catheter is in place, there is a small risk of entanglement or knotting. This potential also exists with other central lines and Swan-Ganz catheters. Frequently, these lines can be untangled under fluoroscopy using specialized catheters.

Although local infection does not always require removal of a permanent pacing catheter, systemic infection always does. The most common organism responsible for this infection is *Staphylococcus aureus* followed by *Staphylococcus epidermidis*.[70] One should be certain of the diagnosis of bacteremia before removing the pacing catheter. Therapy for bacteremia usually requires removal of the catheter, placement of a temporary transvenous pacemaker, and 6 weeks of intravenous antibiotics.[100, 101] Sometimes it is difficult to remove a permanent catheter because of entrapment from endothelialization and scar formation. A technique for removing these pacing catheters using a constant traction device has been described.[102] This method may be useful before considering open thoracotomy.

Balloon rupture, pulmonary infarction, phrenic nerve pacing, and rupture of the chorda tendineae are also potential complications.[103–105]

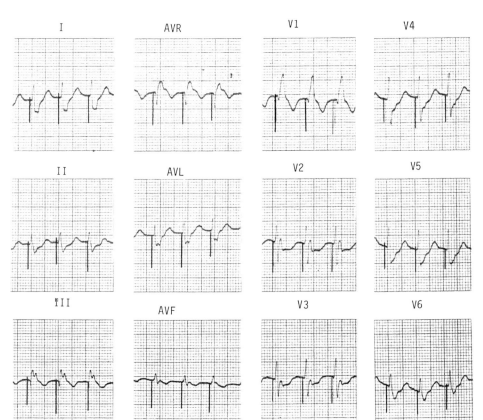

Figure 13–19. Coronary sinus pacing. Note the paced right bundle branch block pattern.

Complications of the Pacing Electrode

The complications related to the pacing electrode can be separated into three groups: mechanical, organic, and electrical.

Mechanical failures include displacement, fracture of the catheter, and loose leads. Displacement can result in intermittent or complete loss of capture or improper sensing, malignant dysrhythmias, diaphragmatic pacing, or perforation. Displacement should be suspected with changes in amplitude, with vector changes greater than 90 degrees, or with a change in threshold.[106] Fracture of the catheter or loose leads have been reported after chest trauma or even after physical exertion.[107, 108] Frequently, catheter fractures may be detected by a careful review of the chest film or may be suspected because of a change in the sensing threshold. As with displacement, intermittent or complete loss of capture may result. This problem usually does not occur until 30 or more days after placement of permanent pacemakers; however, it may occur sooner with temporary units.

Organic causes of pacemaker failure result in changes in the threshold or sensing function. Progressive inflammation, fibrosis, and thrombosis may result in more than doubling of the original threshold. This may occur in 3 to 4 weeks and should be expected in prolonged temporary or permanent pacemakers. Physiologic and pharmacologic factors that affect the threshold have been studied. Sleeping, eating a heavy meal, lowered aldosterone concentration,

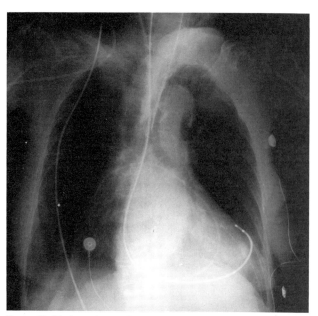

Figure 13–21. A pacing catheter that is outside or abuts the cardiac silhouette and is not properly positioned within the right ventricular cavity suggests myocardial perforation. (From Tarber RD, Gillespie KR: The misplaced tube. Emerg Med, February 29, 1988, p 97.)

potassium infusions, and myxedema all increase the threshold by raising the resting membrane potential. The threshold to cardiac pacing tends to decrease with exercise, sympathetic amines, glucocorticoids, and toxic levels of procainamide.[109–113]

In some patients, the atrial contribution to ventricular filling is extremely important. Transvenous ventricular pacing results in the loss of the atrial kick and ultimately a decrease in left ventricular stroke volume. This phenomenon is called *postpacer syndrome* and occasionally is severe enough to preclude the use of a pacemaker.[114] A sequential pacemaker that stimulates the atria and ventricles in sequential fashion is a viable alternative for patients unable to tolerate the loss of the atrial kick. Atrioventricular sequential pacers are now available for temporary transvenous pacing. Their use requires a dual-chamber pulse generator and significant experience with catheter placement. Placement of this type of pacemaker should be done only by experienced operators.[115]

Electrical problems with pacing include battery failure, dysrhythmias, and outside interference. Battery failure is usually detected by a slowing of the heart rate.[109] With the old mercury battery system, sensing capability was usually lost first, followed by a relatively rapid loss in capture. With the new lithium and nuclear units, a slow, progressive rate decrease occurs naturally. These units found in permanent pacemaker systems are usually replaced electively after the rate decreases approximately 10 per cent. When they do fail, however, the underlying intrinsic rhythm may require emergency pacing. Occasionally, runaway pacing with rates greater than 200 may be a manifestation of battery failure. In an emergency situation, the skin pocket that contains the pacemaker generator can be opened under sterile technique. The wires may be cut close to the generator and connected to a temporary unit. The pacemaker generator can then be replaced electively.

In the first type of units available, outside interference, caused by television transmitters, electric tooth brushes, electric razors, magnetic fields, microwave ovens, and airport surveillance equipment, frequently resulted in pacemaker inhibition because of inappropriate sensing.[116–121] Although current models are designed to prevent this type of compli-

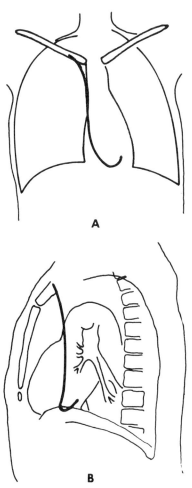

Figure 13–20. Coronary sinus position. *A,* Posteroanterior view. *B,* Lateral view. (From Goldberger E: Treatment of Cardiac Emergencies. 3rd ed. St. Louis, CV Mosby Co, 1982.)

cation, problems still occur.[122] Usually converting the unit to a fixed mode will permit continued pacing.

Although ventricular tachycardia and ventricular fibrillation have been reported to result from pacemakers, these dysrhythmias are rare. Because of this, patients who present with such dysrhythmias should be evaluated for a nonpacemaker etiology.[123]

Direct current cardioversion and electroshock therapy are safe procedures to carry out in patients who have pacemakers as long as the current does not go directly over the generator pack.[109, 124]

CONCLUSION

Temporary transvenous pacing is a rapid, safe, and reliable method for achieving effective electrical stimulation of the heart. It can and should be mastered by any physician who is responsible for the care of the critically ill or injured patients. Symptomatic bradycardias unresponsive to pharmacologic means and some tachycardias are indications for its use. In acute myocardial infarction, it serves both a therapeutic and prophylactic function. Transvenous pacing in the trauma patient may be advocated more frequently in the future.

REFERENCES

1. Rosenberg AS, Grossman JI, Escher DJW, et al: Bedside transvenous cardiac pacing. Am Heart J 77:697, 1969.
2. Callaghan JC, Bigelow WG: Electrical artificial pacemaker for standstill of heart. Ann Surg 134:8, 1951.
3. Zoll PM: Resuscitation of the heart in ventricular standstill by external electrical stimulation. N Engl J Med 247:768, 1952.
4. Furman S, Schwedel JB: Intracardiac pacemaker for Stokes-Adams seizures. N Engl J Med 261:943, 1959.
5. Muller OF, Bellet S: Treatment of intractable heart failure in the presence of complete atrioventricular heart block by the use of internal cardiac pacemaker. Report of two cases. N Engl J Med 265:768, 1961.
6. Siddons H, Davies JG: A new technique for internal cardiac pacing. Lancet 2:1204, 1963.
7. DeSanctis RW: Short-term use of intravenous electrode in heart block. JAMA 184:130, 1963.
8. Vogel JHK, Tabari K, Averill KH, et al: A simple technique for identifying P waves in complex arrhythmias. Am Heart J 67:158, 1964.
9. Kimball JT, Killip T: A simple bedside method for transvenous intracardiac pacing. Am Heart J 70:35, 1965.
10. Harris CW, Hurlburt JC, Floyd WL, et al: Percutaneous technique for cardiac pacing with a platinum-tipped electrode catheter. Am J Cardiol 15:48, 1965.
11. Goetz RH, Dormandy MD, Berkovits BV: Pacing on demand in the treatment of atrioventricular conduction disturbances of the heart. Lancet 1:599, 1966.
12. Zuckerman W, Zaroff L, Berkovits BV, et al: Clinical experience with a new implantable demand pacemaker. Am J Cardiol 20:232, 1967.
13. Swan HJ, Gantz W: Catheterization of the heart in man with use of a flow-directed balloon-tipped catheter. N Engl J Med 283:447, 1970.
14. Schnitzler RN, Caracta AR, Damato AN: "Floating" catheter for temporary transvenous ventricular pacing. Am J Cardiol 31:351, 1973.
15. Lang R, David D, Herman HO, et al: The use of the balloon-tipped floating catheter in temporary transvenous cardiac pacing. PACE 4:491, 1981.
16. Kruger BK, Rakes S, Wilkerson J, et al: Temporary pacemaking by general internists. Arch Intern Med 143:1531, 1983.
17. Furman S: Cardiac pacing and pacemaker. I. Indications for pacing bradyarrhythmias. Am Heart J 93:523, 1977.
18. Escher DJ, Furman S: Emergency treatment of cardiac arrhythmias. Emphasis on use of electrical pacing. JAMA 214:2028, 1970.
19. Julian DG, Valentine DA, Miller GG: Disturbances of rate, rhythm, and conduction in acute myocardial infarction: A prospective study of 100 consecutive unselected patients with the aid of electrocardiographic monitoring. Am J Med 37:915, 1965.
20. Adgey AAJ, Geodes JS, Mulholland HC, et al: Incidence, significance, and management of early bradyarrhthmias complicating acute myocardial infarction. Lancet 2:1097, 1968.
21. Haden RF, Langsjoen H, Rapoport M, et al: The significance of sinus bradycardia in acute myocardial infarction. Dis Chest 44:168, 1963.
22. Rotman M: Bradyarrhythmias in acute myocardial infarction. Circulation 45:703, 1972.
23. Baba N: Experimental cardiac ischemia, observation of the sinoatrial and atrioventricular node. Lab Invest 23:168, 1970.
24. James TN: Cardiac innervation: Anatomic and pharmacologic relations. Bull NY Acad Med 43:1041, 1967.
25. Constantin L: Extracardiac factors contributing to hypotension during coronary occlusion. Am J Cardiol 11:205, 1963.
26. Wolf S: Bradycardia of the dive reflex: A possible mechanism of sudden death. Trans Am Clin Climatol Assoc 76:142, 1964.
27. Hazard PB: Transvenous cardiac pacing in cardiopulmonary resuscitation. Crit Care Med 9:666, 1981.
28. Niemann JT, Adomian GE, Garner D, et al: Endocardial and transcutaneous cardiac pacing, calcium chloride, and epinephrine in postcountershock asystole and bradycardias. Crit Care Med 13:699, 1985.
29. Niemann JT, Haynes KS, Garner D, et al: Postcountershock pulseless rhythms: Response to CPR, artificial cardiac pacing, and adrenergic agonists. Ann Emerg Med 15:112, 1986.
30. Syverund SA, Dalsey WC, Hedges JR: Transcutaneous and transvenous cardiac pacing for early bradyasystolic cardiac arrest. Ann Emerg Med 15:121, 1986.
31. Conklin EF, Giannelli S, Nealon TF: Four hundred consecutive patients with permanent transvenous pacemakers. J Thorac Cardiovasc Surg 69:1, 1975.
32. Escher DJ: The use of artificial pacemakers in acute myocardial infarction. In Chung EK (ed): Controversy in Cardiology: A Practical Clinical Approach. New York, Springer-Verlag, 1976, p 51.
33. Simon AB, Steinke WE, Curry JJ: Atrioventricular block in acute myocardial infarction. Chest 62:156, 1972.
34. Resuekov L, Lipp H: Pacemaking in acute myocardial infarction. Prog Cardiovasc Dis 14:475, 1972.
35. Hindman MC, Wagner GS, JaRo M, et al: The clinical significance of bundle branch block complicating acute myocardial infarction. 2. Indications of temporary and permanent pacemaker insertion. Circulation 58:689, 1978.
36. Atkins JM, Leshin SJ, Blumquist G, et al: Ventricular conduction blocks and sudden death in acute myocardial infarction. N Engl J Med 288:281, 1978.
37. Hindman MC, Wagner GS, JaRo M: The clinical significance of bundle branch block complicating acute myocardial infarction. 1. Clinical characteristics, hospital mortality, and one year follow-up. Circulation 58:679, 1978.
38. Jocobson CB, Lester RM, Scheinman MM: Management of acute bundle branch block and bradyarrhythmias. Med Clin North Am 63:93, 1979.
39. Escher DJ: The use of cardiac pacemakers. In Braunwald E (ed): Heart Disease: A Textbook of Cardiovascular Medicine. Philadelphia, WB Saunders Co, 1980, p 749.
40. Abernathy WS: Complete heart block caused by the Swan Gantz catheter. Chest 65:349, 1974.
41. Thompson JR, Dolton BC, Lapis DG, et al: Right bundle branch block in complete heart block caused by Swan Gantz catheter. Anesthesiology 51:359, 1979.
42. Morris D, Mulvihill D, Lew WYW: Risk of developing complete heart block during bedside pulmonary artery catheterization in patients with left bundle-branch block. Arch Intern Med 147:2005, 1987.
43. Buran MJ: Transcutaneous pacing as an alternative to prophylactic transvenous pacemaker insertion. Crit Care Med 15:623, 1987.
44. Bharati S, Chervony A, Gruhn J, et al: Atrial arrhythmias related to trauma to sinoatrial node. Chest 61:331, 1972.
45. Dreifus LS: Dysrhythmias related to cardiac trauma. Chest 61:310, 1972.
46. Miller MS, Scott SF: Cardiac contusion and right bundle branch block. JACEP 6:504, 1974.
47. Bognolo DA, Rabow RI, Vijayanagar RR, et al: Traumatic sinus node dysfunction. Ann Emerg Med 11:319, 1982.
48. Mazor A, Roger S: Cardiac aspects of shock. Ann Surg 178:128, 1973.
49. White BC, Hoehner PJ, Petinga TJ, et al: HIS electrocardiographic characterization of terminal arrhythmias of hemorrhagic shock in dogs. JACEP 8:298, 1979.
50. Millikan JS, Moore EE, Dunn EL, et al: Temporary cardiac pacing in traumatic arrest victims. Ann Emerg Med 9:591, 1980.
51. Schwedel JB, Furman S, Escher D: Use of intracardiac pacemaker in treatment of Stokes-Adams seizures. Prog Cardiovasc Dis 3:170, 1960.
52. Zoll PM, Limenthal AJ, Zarsky LRN: Ventricular fibrillation: Treatment and prevention by external electric currents. N Engl J Med 262:105, 1960.
53. Haft JL: Treatment of arrhythmias by intracardiac electrical stimulation. Prog Cardiovasc Dis 16:539, 1974.
54. Cheng TO: Transvenous ventricular pacing in the treatment of paroxysmal atrial tachyarrhythmias alternating with sinus bradycardia and standstill. Am J Cardiol 22:874, 1968.
55. Kastor JA: Transvenous atrial pacing in the treatment of refractory ventricular irritability. Ann Intern Med 66:439, 1967.
56. Barold SS, Linhart JW: Recent advances in the treatment of ectopic tachycardias by electrical pacing. Am J Cardiol 25:698, 1970.
57. Weiner I: Pacing techniques in the treatment of tachycardias. Ann Intern Med 93:326, 1980.
58. DeSanctis RW, Kastor JA: Rapid intracardiac pacing for treatment of recurrent ventricular arrhythmias in the absence of heart block. Am Heart J 76:168, 1968.

59. Disegni E, Klein HO, David D, et al: Overdrive pacing in quinidine syncope and other long QT-interval syndromes. Arch Intern Med 140:1036, 1980.
60. Goldberger E: Temporary cardiac pacing. *In* Goldberger E, Wheet MW Jr (eds): Treatment of Cardiac Emergencies. 3rd ed. St. Louis, CV Mosby Co, 1982, p 233.
61. Personal communication with Electro-Catheter Corp.
62. Simoons ML, Demey HE, Bossaert LL, et al: The paceport catheter: A new pacemaker system introduced through a Swan Gantz catheter. Cath Cardiol Diag 15:66, 1988.
63. Dronen S, Thompson B, Nowak R, et al: Subclavian vein catheterization during cardiopulmonary resuscitation. JAMA 247:3227, 1982.
64. Mostert MD, Kenny GM, Murphy GP: Safe placement of central venous catheter into the internal jugular veins. Arch Surg 101:431, 1970.
65. Syverund SA, Dalsey WC, Hedges JR: Radiographic assessment of transvenous pacemaker placement during CPR. Ann Emerg Med 15:131, 1986.
66. Bartecchi LE: Emergency transvenous (subclavian) cardiac pacing in elderly patients. J Am Geriatrics Soc 27:208, 1979.
67. Austin JL, Preis LK, Crampton RS, et al: Analysis of pacemaker malfunction and complications of temporary pacing in the coronary care unit. Am J Cardiol 44:301, 1982.
68. Nolewajka AT, Goddard MD, Brown TG: Temporary transvenous pacing and femoral vein thrombosis. Am J Cardiol 45:459, 1980.
69. Pandian NG, Kosowsky BD, Gurewich V: Transfemoral temporary pacing and deep vein thrombosis. Am Heart J 100:847, 1980.
69a. Weinstein J. Gnoj J, Mazzara JT, et al: Temporary transvenous pacing via the percutaneous femoral approach: A prospective study of 100 cases. Am Heart J 85:695, 1973.
70. Furman S: Pacemaker emergencies. Med Clin North Am 63:113, 1979.
71. Thompson ME, Shaver JA: Undesirable cardiac arrhythmias associated with rate hysteresis pacemakers. Am J Cardiol 38:685, 1976.
72. Nachnani GH, Gooch AS, Hsu I: Systolic murmurs induced by pacemaker catheters. Arch Intern Med 24:202, 1969.
73. Kluge WF: Pacemaker sound and its origin. Am J Cardiol 25:362, 1970.
74. Korn M, Schoenfeld CD, Ghahramani A, et al: The pacemaker sound. Am J Med 49:451, 1970.
75. Pupillo GA, Talley RC, Linhart JW: "Pacemaker heart sound" caused by diaphragmatic contractions. Am Heart J 82:711, 1971.
76. Kramer DH, Moss AJ, Shah PM: Mechanisms and significance of pacemaker-induced extracardiac sound. Am J Cardiol 25:367, 1970.
77. Herbst CA: Indications, management, and complications of percutaneous subclavian catheters. Arch Surg 113:1421, 1978.
78. Sethi GK, Bhayana JN, Scott SM, et al: Innominate venous thrombosis: A rare complication of transvenous pacemaker electrodes. Am Heart J 87:770, 1974.
79. May KJ, Cardone JT, Stroebel PP, et al: Streptokinase dissolution of a right atrial thrombus associated with a temporary pacemaker. Arch Intern Med 148:903, 1988.
80. Johnson CL, Jazarchick J, Lynn HB: Subclavian venipuncture, preventable complications. Mayo Clin Proc 45:719, 1970.
81. Woods RR: Technique of subclavian vein cannulization to eliminate danger of pneumothorax. South Med J 70:1111, 1977.
82. Arbitman M, Kart BH: Hydromediastinum after aberrant central venous catheter placement. Crit Care Med 7:27, 1979.
83. Drachler DH, Koepte GH, Wey JG: Phrenic nerve injury from subclavian vein catheterization. JAMA 236:2880, 1976.
84. Cope C: Intravascular breakage of seldinger spring guide wires. JAMA 180:1061, 1962.
85. Schwartz AJ, Harrow JC, Jobes DR, et al: Guide wires—a caution. Crit Care Med 9:347, 1981.
86. Johansson L, Malmstrom G, Uggla LG: Intracardiac knotting of the catheter in heart catheterization. J Thorac Surg 27:605, 1954.
87. Boal BH, Keller BD, Ascheim RS, et al: Complication of intracardiac electrical pacing—knotting together of temporary and permanent electrodes. N Engl J Med 280:650, 1969.
88. Lipp H, O'Donoghue K, Resnekov L: Knotting of a flow-directed balloon catheter. N Engl J Med 284:220, 1971.
89. Mehra R, Furman S, Crump J: Vulnerability of the mildly ischemic ventricle to cathodal, anodal, and bipolar stimulation. Circ Res 41:159, 1977.
90. Chatterjee K, Harris A, Leatham A: The risk of pacing after infarction and current recommendations. Lancet 2:1061, 1969.
91. Abernathy WS, Crevey BJ: Right bundle branch block during transvenous ventricular pacing. Am Heart J 90:774, 1975.
92. Campo I, Garfield GJ, Escher DJW, et al: Complications of pacing by pervenous subclavian semifloating electrodes including extraluminal insertions. Am J Cardiol 26:627, 1970.
93. Goswani M, Gould L, Gompiecht RF, et al: Perforation of the heart by flexible transvenous pacemaker. JAMA 216:2013, 1971.
94. Danielson GK, Shabetai R, Bryant LR: Failure of endocardial pacemaker due to myocardial perforation. J Thorac Cardiovasc Surg 54:42, 1967.
95. Kalloor GJ: Cardiac tamponade. Report of a case after insertion of transvenous endocardial electrode. Am Heart J 88:88, 1974.
96. Jorgensen EO, Lyngborg K, Wennevold A: Unusual sign of perforation of a pacemaker catheter. Am Heart J 74:732, 1967.
97. Kaye D, Frankl W, Arditi LI: Probable postcardiotomy syndrome following implantation of a transvenous pacemaker: Report of the first case. Am Heart J 90:627, 1975.
98. Glassman RD, Noble RJ, Tavel ME, et al: Pacemaker-induced endocardial friction rub. Am J Cardiol 40:811, 1977.
99. Tarver RB, Gillespie KR: The misplaced tube. Emerg Med 20:97, 1988.
100. Furman RW, Hiller AJ, Playforth RH, et al: Infected permanent cardiac pacemaker. Management with removal. Ann Thorac Surg 14:54, 1972.
101. Kennelly BM, Diller LW: Management of infected transvenous permanent pacemakers. Br Heart J 36:1133, 1974.
102. Bilgulay AM, Jensen NK, Schmidt WR, et al: Incarceration of transvenous pacemaker electrode. Removal by traction. Am Heart J 77:377, 1969.
103. Foote GA, Schabel SI, Hodges M: Pulmonary complications of the flow-directed balloon-tipped catheter. N Engl J Med 290:927, 1974.
104. Sprinkle JD, Takaro T, Scott SM: Phrenic nerve stimulation as a complication of implantable cardiac pacemaker. Circulation 28:114, 1963.
105. Escher DJ, Furman S, Solomon N, et al: Transvenous pacing of the phrenic nerve. Am Heart J 72:283, 1977.
106. Preston TA: Electrocardiographic diagnosis of pacemaker catheter displacement. Am Heart J 854:445, 1973.
107. Kronzon I, Mehta SS: Broken wire in multiple trauma: A case report. J Trauma 14:82, 1974.
108. Ohm O: Displacement and fracture of pacemaker electrode during physical exertion: Report of three cases. Acta Med Scand 192:33, 1972.
109. Smith ND: Pacemaker dysfunction. *In* Greenberg MI, Roberts JR (eds): Emergency Medicine: A Clinical Approach to Challenging Problems. Philadelphia, FA Davis Co, 1982, p 355.
110. Preston TA, Fletcher RD, Lucchesi BR, et al: Changes in myocardial threshold, physiologic, and pharmacologic factors in patients with implanted pacemakers. Am Heart J 74:235, 1967.
111. Gay RJ, Brown DF: Pacemaker failure due to procainamide toxicity. Am J Cardiol 34:728, 1974.
112. Walker WJ, Elkins JT, Wood LWW: Effect of potassium in restoring myocardial response to a subthreshold cardiac pacemaker. N Engl J Med 271:12, 1964.
113. Basu D, Chatterjee K: Unusually high pacemaker threshold in severe myxedema. Decrease with thyroid hormone therapy. Chest 70:677, 1976.
114. Haas JM, Strait GB: Pacemaker-induced cardiovascular failure. Am J Cardiol 33:295, 1974.
115. Guzy PM: Emergency Cardiac Pacing. Emerg Clin North Am 4:745, 1986.
116. D'Cunha GF, Nicoud T, Pemberton AH, et al: Syncopal attacks arising from erratic demand pacemaker function in the vicinity of a television transmitter. Am J Cardiol 31:789, 1973.
117. Escher DJ, Parker B, Furman S: Pacemaker triggering (inhibition) by electric toothbrush. Am J Cardiol 38:126, 1976.
118. Furman S: Electric razor interference with cardiac pacemakers. JAMA 222:1658, 1972.
119. Escher DJ, Parker B, Furman S: Influence of alternating magnetic fields on triggered pacemakers: Circulation 44:162, 1971.
120. Microwaves and pacemakers: Just how well do they go together? (editorial) JAMA 221:957, 1972.
121. Mitchell JC, Hurt WD, Walters WH, et al: Empirical studies of cardiac pacemaker interference. Aerospace Med 45:189, 1974.
122. Sumchai A, Sternbach G, Eliastam M, et al: Pacing hazards in helicopter aeromedical transport. Am J Emerg Med 6:236, 1988.
123. Leung FW, Oill PA: Ticket of admission unexplained syncopal attacks in patients with cardiac pacemaker. Ann Emerg Med 9:527, 1980.
124. Youmans RC, Bourianoff G, Allensworth DC, et al: Electroshock therapy and cardiac pacemakers. Am J Surg 118:931, 1969.
125. Lumia FJ, Rios JC: Temporary transvenous pacemaker therapy: An analysis of complications. Chest 64:604, 1973.

Chapter 14

Emergency Transthoracic Cardiac Pacing*

James R. Roberts

INTRODUCTION

The history of electrical stimulation of the heart began in the mid-eighteenth century when crude attempts were made to revive dead animals and humans with electrical current from a Leyden jar.[1] The first successful clinical application of external cardiac pacing was accomplished by Zoll (1952) using a method of externally applied closed-chest pacing for Stokes-Adams disease.[2] In the 1960s, a popular technique involved the use of percutaneous wires implanted directly into the myocardium through the chest wall.[3] The apparatus most commonly used today for *transthoracic* pacing is the transmyocardial pacemaker, a bipolar pacing wire that is placed into the ventricular cavity using an intracardiac stick with a needle introducer.

With the development of sophisticated transvenous pacemaker electrodes, the technique of transthoracic wire implantation for emergency pacing became less prevalent. Advancements in technology and the development of the specialty of emergency medicine sparked a temporary interest in the concept of emergency transthoracic pacing in the 1970s, but the procedure has been largely replaced with transcutaneous techniques (Chapter 15).

In most textbooks the use of the transthoracic route is mentioned only briefly or not at all[4–7] and it is unlikely that this procedure will be used frequently. A complete presentation is presented, however, for physicians who find the technique useful or must rely on it for lack of suitable alternatives. In general, transthoracic pacing should be used only if transcutaneous pacing is unavailable.

This chapter reviews the development, concepts, and technique of transthoracic pacemaker insertion and offers a rational approach to current application of the procedure in the emergency department. All references to transthoracic pacing that follow apply to percutaneous pacing wires introduced through a transthoracic needle and do not apply to electrodes inserted into the myocardium by a thoracotomy or under direct vision.

BACKGROUND

Clinical experience with any form of emergency cardiac pacing for the treatment of cardiac arrest has been disappointing (see Chapter 15 for a complete discussion), and it is unlikely that many patients will be resuscitated from asystole even with the early use of transthoracic pacing.[2, 7–17] Before the development of reliable transvenous electrodes, initial attempts at transthoracic pacing consisted of two external needle electrodes placed subcutaneously on the chest wall with the wires attached to an external energy source.[2, 15, 16] Pacing of the heart through the chest wall by this minimally invasive method was generally successful, although extremely high voltages were sometimes required and capture was intermittent. With this technique, the entire thorax and the diaphragm were also stimulated, resulting in painful muscle contractions. Skin burns occasionally occurred, and the unsedated patient had difficulty tolerating the discomfort. Although clinically successful, this impractical technique was short lived.

Thevenet and associates[3] published the first description of a *transthoracic* technique that incorporated the percutaneous implantation of a unipolar wire electrode (cathode) into the myocardial wall of the right ventricle. The uninsulated wire was inserted through a spinal needle using a left parasternal approach. The indifferent electrode (anode) was a wire placed subcutaneously in the chest wall near the cardiac apex. The experimental animals in this study had surgical interruption of the atrioventricular node and bundle of His and were in complete heart block. Transthoracic pacing was successful in controlling the heart rate in all the experimental animals, and no harmful effects to the myocardium or pericardium were noted at autopsy. One dog was paced for 10 days. In addition, a percutaneous wire was successfully placed in the ventricles of seven human cadavers, thus demonstrating the clinical feasibility of the technique. Thevenet and coworkers concluded that the procedure was safe, easy, and effective and that it had no significant associated morbidity. Other investigators reported success with percutaneous pacing in experimental animals and in humans when a wire was implanted into the ventricular wall, although the procedure and equipment varied slightly with each report.[8–12]

Tintinalli and White[17] reported a retrospective series of 21 unsuccessful resuscitations in which the transthoracic pacer was used in bradyasystolic arrest. The study used an older model of the transthoracic pacer, and the device was used for some conditions for which a pacer could not have been expected to be of benefit. In addition, the device was used as a last resort, approximately 30 to 45 minutes into the resuscitation and only after extensive drug therapy had failed. Despite the late use of the pacer in the study, capture occurred in eight of 21 patients, and a transient blood pressure was recorded in two patients. A cardiac tamponade occurred in one patient, and this complication may have contributed to an unsuccessful outcome. The investigators concluded that the transthoracic pacer did not alter outcome in bradyasystolic arrest when standard advanced cardiac life support (ACLS) therapy was unsuccessful.

Roberts and Greenberg[18] reported the successful use of the transthoracic pacemaker in six patients with bradyasystolic cardiac arrest. Pathologic rhythms included asystole, atrioventricular dissociation, and supraventricular bradycardia. The severity of the underlying disease did not allow for long-term survival in three patients, but the initial resuscitation of all patients was attributed to the technique of transthoracic pacing.

Ornato and coworkers reported on patients in bradyasystolic cardiac arrest who had failed standard pharmacologic therapy and were treated with transthoracic cardiac pacing.[19] Electrical capture was noted in 30 of 48 patients (63 per cent); two of the patients developed a pulse; and one of the patients survived to admission but died in the hospital. Although electrical capture was more likely if the patient was paced shortly after cardiac arrest, the researchers were unable to show statistical significance to this trend. White and Brown reported a prospective trial of transthoracic pacing that was used as an initial method of emergency department therapy for 48 asystolic arrest patients.[20] Their patients had failed pharmacologic resuscitation in the prehospital phase, and they did not report the duration of cardiac arrest before transthoracic pacing. White and Brown demonstrated electrical capture in 23 per cent of the patients and a palpable pulse in 17 per cent. With subsequent intracardiac sodium bicarbonate and epinephrine therapy, the capture rate rose to 46 per cent with a transient pulse or blood pressure in 33 per cent. One of their patients survived to be admitted but there were no long-term survivors. They concluded that *immediate* transthoracic pacing is *temporarily effective in restoring electrical activity* in a substantial number of asystolic patients but that the procedure does not change mortality rates. In a series of patients reported by Eisner and associates, emergency transthoracic pacing was given highest priority in the treatment of cardiac arrest.[21] Despite the ability to obtain a pulse in three of seven witnessed asystolic arrest patients paced within 12 minutes of collapse, no patient survived to leave the hospital.

INDICATIONS FOR EMERGENCY TRANSTHORACIC PACING

Although the absolute indications for emergency transthoracic pacing are not described, most physicians express a

---

*Modified with permission from Roberts JR, Greenberg MI: Emergency transthoracic pacemaker. Ann Emerg Med 10:600, 1981.

consensus about contraindications. General guidelines suggest that when the time and clinical situation permit, cardiac pacing should be done using the transcutaneous method (see Chapter 15) or the transvenous route with fluoroscopy or flow-directed pacemaker catheters (see Chapter 13). The transthoracic route is contraindicated in the stable or awake patient or in situations in which the cardiac emergency can be managed quickly and easily by drug therapy.[4] Obviously, these are imprecise criteria that are subject to various interpretations. For the sake of discussion concerning the use of emergency transthoracic pacing, patients can be divided into two general categories: those who are "unstable" but perfusing, including critically ill patients in heart block, recurrent ventricular tachycardia, or profound bradycardia; and all patients in cardiac arrest.

Unstable Patients

The specific use of transthoracic pacing in unstable patients is poorly addressed in the modern literature. Early studies demonstrated the efficacy of the procedure in animals and in a few patients with complete heart block. With the current knowledge of drug therapy and with the development of transcutaneous pacing or sophisticated transvenous pacing methods, it is questionable whether the transthoracic route is currently indicated for unstable patients with third-degree atrioventricular block or with other forms of symptomatic bradycardia. Because the procedure has been shown to be relatively safe, rapid, and effective in complete heart block, I believe that it is reasonable to consider emergency transthoracic pacing in patients with severe *drug-resistant* ventricular bradycardias that produce pulmonary edema, seizures, recurrent ventricular fibrillation, or ventricular tachycardia. *These are patients in whom a transvenous pacemaker cannot be inserted rapidly or for whom transcutaneous pacing may be unsuccessful or unavailable.*

Transthoracic pacing is a simple procedure when compared with transvenous pacemaker placement. Transthoracic pacing can be accomplished rapidly when one considers the time required for a cutdown or for securing a large-bore central cannula. Therefore, the transthoracic route may be advantageous in selected situations that produce an unstable clinical picture. A special advantage is that no blood flow is required to float the transthoracic pacemaker into proper position.

A *rapidly deteriorating patient* with complete atrioventricular dissociation or other type of ventricular bradycardia should be considered a candidate for emergency transthoracic pacing if transcutaneous or transvenous pacing cannot be instituted immediately. The ability to institute such therapy is dependent on the availability of consultation and the expertise of the emergency physician.

Cardiac Arrest

The use of transthoracic pacing during cardiac arrest is a controversial subject. Cardiology texts usually dismiss the procedure with brevity. One text on pacing states that the procedure is "dangerous and should be used only in an emergency."[22] Because cardiac arrest is an emergency, one would assume that the technique would be supported in such cases.[23]

Many physicians report poor results with transthoracic pacing in cardiac arrest, whereas others have reasonable (although largely anecdotal) success. Preston[24] estimates a 40 per cent success rate in achieving pacing by the transthoracic route and attributes this low rate to the moribund condition of most patients in whom the procedure is used. Iseri and associates[25] suggest that because bradyasystolic cardiac arrest is associated with an almost certain fatal outcome, transthoracic pacing may be one of the techniques that can be explored to alter this rather dismal prognosis. Accurate statistics are not available concerning the efficacy of emergency transthoracic pacing. Because resuscitation from cardiac arrest is successful in only approximately 15 per cent of the cases[26] (range 8.5 to 28.6 per cent[27–29]), any technique or drug therapy will be associated with a poor result. The issue of transthoracic pacing during cardiac arrest becomes even more controversial when one considers two additional questions: When during the resuscitation is pacing attempted? What constitutes the underlying cause of the cardiac arrest?

Rationale for Use in Cardiac Arrest

The routine use of any form of emergency cardiac pacing will not significantly alter the survival rate of bradyasystolic cardiac arrest, and emergency pacing of any sort should not be considered a panacea for cardiac arrest. Emergency pacing, however, may be life saving in selected clinical situations. The effectiveness of pacing in cardiac arrest is dependent upon the time during the arrest at which pacing is instituted. Bellet and colleagues[9] demonstrated that a pacemaker was ineffective in patients with prolonged cardiac arrest. Patients with cardiac arrest for more than 5 to 10 minutes could not be resuscitated with the use of pacing, but patients who had a pacemaker placed within 2 to 7 minutes after cardiac standstill were successfully resuscitated.

Pacing should be instituted as soon as possible, rather than after exhaustive medical therapy has failed. The standard argument against the use of transthoracic pacing is that anecdotal clinical experience indicates a lack of appreciable success with the procedure after all other methods and drug therapies have failed.[17] This "last ditch" or "final effort" approach may have led to much of the negativism associated with the procedure.

Not all rhythms encountered during cardiac arrest are amenable to pacing. One would not expect pacing by any route to be effective in the treatment of electromechanical dissociation. Electromechanical dissociation, which can result from primary cardiac disease or from hypovolemia or cardiac tamponade from trauma, can be defined as electrical activity at an appropriate rate (occasionally a relatively normal-looking QRS complex on electrocardiogram [ECG] is seen) with the absence of a pulse, blood pressure, or audible heart sounds. Because electrical stimulation is believed to be intact in this primarily mechanical derangement, the addition of another electrical stimulation would not be beneficial[4, 28] unless the electrical activity occurred at an unacceptably slow rate.[4, 30] Pacing is without value in the treatment of ventricular fibrillation. With the onset of ventricular fibrillation, the heart becomes insensitive to pacemaker activity, and a pacemaker spike may be observed to "march" through an ECG.

Although trauma frequently results in death from electromechanical dissociation secondary to anoxia, acidosis, or hypovolemia, cardiac collapse from trauma occasionally is manifested as severe drug-resistant bradycardia.[31, 32] Millikan and colleagues[33] reported life-saving benefit from emergency pacing (epicardial pacemaker used during surgery) in two patients with penetrating thoracic injuries with bradycardia unresponsive to cardioactive medication and volume replacement. Although it is unlikely that most trauma-related cardiac arrests will be responsive to pacing, when bradycardia persists despite correction of the underlying pathology, the

Table 14–1. Recommendations for Emergency Transthoracic Pacing When Transvenous or Transcutaneous Pacing Is Not Immediately Available

Indications*	Contraindications
Asystole from permanent pacemaker failure†	Stable patient
Any severe bradycardia	Pathology quickly and easily corrected by medication
Pulseless idioventricular rhythm	Presence of functioning transvenous pacemaker
Atrioventricular dissociation with inadequate ventricular response or recurrent V-fibrillation or V-tachycardia	**Cannot Be Expected to Benefit**
Unstable sinus bradycardia/ junctional bradycardia/ atrial fibrillation with high-degree atrioventricular block	Electromechanical dissociation Ventricular fibrillation

*Consider the use of pacing in trauma arrest if the patient is unresponsive to other forms of therapy. (From Roberts JR, Greenberg MI: Emergency transthoracic pacemaker. Ann Emerg Med 10:603, 1981.)

†Changes in survival rate not proven.

use of temporary emergency pacing to correct conduction abnormalities secondary to prolonged ischemia during hypovolemic shock may be life saving.

Certain rhythms that arise during cardiac arrest may benefit from emergency transthoracic cardiac pacing. These are any form of heart block and slow idioventricular rhythm. Both heart block and the wide, slow, bizarre QRS complex rhythm without pulses (termed *pulseless idioventricular rhythm*) are associated with high mortality rates. Both rhythms may benefit from emergency pacing,[23, 34, 35] and both lend themselves to the rapid transthoracic approach. The severely hypoxic or acidotic heart has little chance for resuscitation by any method; thus it is reasonable to institute pacing efforts in the early stages of therapy, when the heart is most likely to respond to pacemaker stimulation. Simultaneous measures to correct anoxia should be started. A summary of clinical recommendations for transthoracic pacing is shown in Table 14–1.

EQUIPMENT

The most widely used instrumentation for transthoracic pacing is a sterile, one-time use, prepackaged kit. A representative device is the Elecath Pacejector (Fig. 14–1). The Pacejector consists of a 13-cm 17-gauge needle, a 10-ml syringe, and a 30-cm bipolar pacing wire that is preloaded via a side port in the needle hub. The syringe is used to withdraw blood to suggest, *but not prove*, intracavitary placement of the needle tip and to inject intracardiac medications, if so desired. Because the pacing wire is already threaded to the tip of the needle, one simply advances the wire a few centimeters once the cardiac chamber has been entered. The entire introducing assembly is then removed, leaving the pacing wire in the right ventricle. A variety of external pacemaker energy sources are available (Fig. 14–2). In the standard bipolar pacing wire, the negative electrode (cathode), situated at the tip of the pacing wire, and the positive electrode (anode), situated 10 cm proximal to the tip, are separated by an insulating sleeve. The separation of the electrodes in this configuration theoretically develops a wider field of electrical excitation than did the older models that placed the electrodes adjacent at the tip of the pacing stylet.

One model has the trademark "transmyocardial" as opposed to "transthoracic" pacer (Electro-Catheter Corp.). When the transmyocardial pacing wire is positioned properly, the cathode lies within the ventricle, and the anode lies within the myocardium or on the outer surface of the heart. Although the tip of the pacing wire is situated within the ventricular cavity, direct contact with the endocardium is not necessary for successful pacemaker function, and the tip often floats freely within the ventricle.

PROCEDURE

The transmyocardial pacing wire can be positioned properly by an experienced physician in approximately 30 to 45 seconds. Cardiopulmonary resuscitation (CPR) can be continued during most of the procedure but should be stopped while the intracardiac needle is being placed to minimize possible myocardial or lung damage.

The most accurate method for the proper placement of percutaneous transthoracic pacing wires is not known (Figs. 14–3 and 14–4). Clinical reports do not document or address the location of the pacing wire, and the only data available to date are from a cadaver study by Brown and associates.[36] In their study transthoracic pacing stylets were placed via three parasternal and three subxiphoid routes, and the position was verified at autopsy. The fifth intercostal space was entered immediately to the left of the sternum and at a site 4 or 6 cm to the left of the midsternal line. Parasternal needles were directed medially, dorsally, and cephalad toward the second right costochondral junction at an angle of 30 degrees to the skin. The subxiphoid needles were all

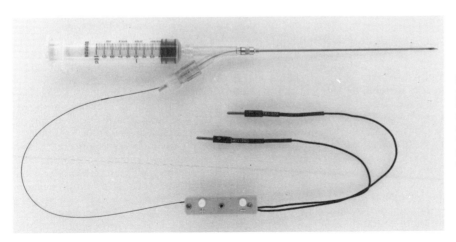

Figure 14–1. Elecath Pacejector transthoracic pacemaker. A bipolar pacing wire is preloaded through a side port and threaded to the tip of the needle. The pacing wire, as shown, is attached to the connector, which will be hooked up to the pacing energy source. (Courtesy of Electro-Catheter Corporation, Rahway, NJ.)

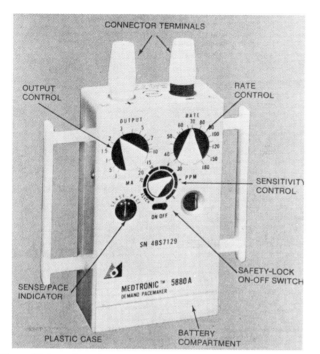

Figure 14–2. Medtronic pacemaker energy source. Unit has (+) and (–) connector terminals, rate control, output control, and sensitivity control.

placed through the left xiphocostal notch at a 30-degree angle to the skin and directed toward the right shoulder, sternal notch, or left shoulder.

The accuracy of all of the techniques was disappointing—ventricular placement was successful in 65 to 90 per cent of cases—and many of the pacing wires were placed in the pulmonary artery, vena cava, or right atrium. All three parasternal approaches had a higher success rate than that of the subxiphoid–right shoulder or sternal notch techniques. The success of the subxiphoid–left shoulder approach was statistically equal to that of the parasternal approaches. In this study blood was not aspirated before wire passage, and although the aspiration of blood may signify intraventricular placement during cardiac arrest, it does not ensure proper blind placement. From this study, the parasternal approach or the subxiphoid–left shoulder approaches appear to be superior to other subxiphoid routes, but the data are insufficient to recommend categorically any specific technique.

The ideal position for the wire is within the right ventricular cavity. Atrial pacing or left ventricular pacing also may be successful. Atrial pacing is of no value in heart block. The left ventricle is not easily accessible through the transthoracic route, and its thick wall may be an obstacle to positioning of the electrode. Certain conditions, such as dextrocardia, severe emphysema, or scoliosis, make successful placement more difficult. It is imperative that the angle between the skin and the needle not exceed 45 degrees if one is using the subxiphoid approach. A greater angle may direct the needle too far posteriorly and miss the heart or risk injury to the left lobe of the liver or the stomach, both of which are dangerously close to the xyphoid.

The needle is advanced approximately three fourths of its length. Aspiration of blood with the syringe suggests, but does not confirm, proper positioning. (As an aside, an intracardiac injection of cardioactive drugs may be given through the intracardiac needle at this time if a central intravenous line has not already been obtained.) If no blood is aspirated, the needle is withdrawn and reinserted. When

the intracavitary placement of the needle tip is suggested by the aspiration of blood, the pacing wire is advanced a few centimeters via the side port. The introducing needle is now withdrawn and CPR is again instituted.

Some physicians prefer to insert an introducing needle with an inner trocar as a unit directly into the ventricle. Removal of the trocar reveals free-flowing or easily aspirated blood when the transthoracic needle is correctly located in the ventricle. A pacing wire is then passed, and the introducing needle is withdrawn as before. If one stabilizes the pacing wire, the pacing wire will not be pulled accidentally out as the needle is withdrawn. Now only the pacing wire exits from the chest.

The proximal end of the pacing wire is inserted into the plastic connector and secured by the screws in the body of the connector. The pacing wire must be inserted all the way into the connector to ensure proper contact. The positive and negative wire from the plastic connector is then secured to the respective terminals on the external energy source, and electrical stimulation is initiated (Fig. 14–5).

The external energy source should be used initially as

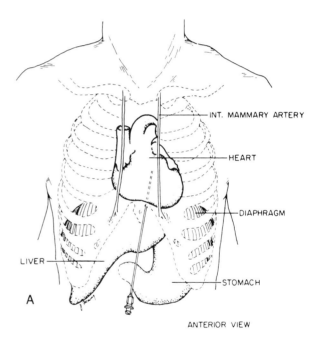

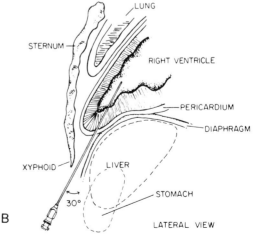

Figure 14–3. Subxiphoid approach to the right ventricle. It is suggested that the needle be aimed toward the left shoulder. *A,* Frontal view. *B,* Lateral view. Note the proximity of the stomach and the liver to the entrance point.

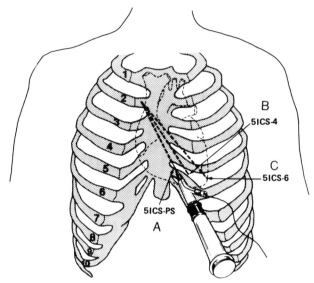

Figure 14–4. Placement of percutaneous transthoracic pacemakers via parasternal approaches. All entry sites are in the fifth intercostal space—parasternally *(A)*, and 4 cm *(B)* and 6 cm *(C)* lateral to the midsternal line. In autopsy studies, all of the parasternal approaches result in more accurate placement than the subxiphoid routes (unless the needle is aimed toward the left shoulder).[36]

a fixed-rate (asynchronous) pacemaker, with pacing initiated without regard for the intrinsic rate of the patient. The rate is set at 70 to 90 beats per minute. The current output control is turned to the maximum milliamperes possible to facilitate capture. The sensitivity control (which senses the patient's R wave) is turned to the "off" or "asynchronous" position.

There is no real danger of injuring the heart from too strong a stimulating current with commercial pacemaker generators. If spontaneous cardiac activity becomes apparent, the fixed-rate pacemaker can easily become a demand pacemaker by activating the sensitivity control, which senses the patient's electrical complex and inhibits the pacemaker's own output. The pacemaker should be disconnected during defibrillation whenever possible. A summary of the operation of the pacemaker energy source is given in Table 14–2.

If pacing is not successful, the pacing wire should be manipulated to change its position, and the connections should be checked. Regardless of the clinical situation, a pacing spike should be noted on the ECG, although the spike may fail to capture. One must be careful not to interpret an artifact on the ECG as a paced beat (Fig. 14–6). Failure to observe a pacing spike on the ECG generally results either from poor contact between the pacing wire and the electrical connector or from rundown batteries in the pacemaker energy source.

The position of the pacing wire should be verified with both anteroposterior and lateral chest films (Fig. 14–7). It is imperative to examine the chest film for evidence of a pneumothorax. A 12-lead ECG should be obtained to document capture. The position of the pacing wire can be confirmed by the QRS configuration in the ECG. If the stylet is pacing from the right ventricle, there should be a positive QRS complex in leads I and V_6 and a negative QRS in lead V_1 (Fig. 14–8). This occurs because depolarization is from the right to the left ventricle and simulates a left bundle branch block pattern. If the stylet is pacing from the left ventricle, a right bundle branch block pattern is observed, and because depolarization is from left to right, the QRS complex is positive in V_1 and negative in I and V_6.

When the pacemaker is functioning properly, the entire apparatus should be taped securely to the patient (Fig. 14–9). Should the pacing box fall from the patient, the pliable pacing wire will be pulled out accidentally. The entire apparatus should remain in place until a transvenous pacing lead is in place and functioning.

Occasionally during cardiac arrest from trauma, an emergency thoracotomy is performed in the emergency department or in the operating room. If pacing is required in such a situation on a truly emergent basis, a sew-in epicardial pacing wire as pictured in Figure 14–10 may be used, as opposed to placing a transthoracic pacer under direct vision. The material is a steel wire with a curved needle on one end and a straight needle on the other end. The needles are separated by an insulating material along the length of the suture material. One sews two wires into the epicardium approximately 2 cm apart, using the curved needles. The straight needles are then inserted into the terminals on the pacing power source. These electrodes are often used prophylactically after cardiac surgery.

COMPLICATIONS

The type and incidence of complications from emergency transthoracic pacing cannot be assessed accurately. Although potentially dangerous injuries have been inferred from autopsy studies that demonstrate errant pacing wire placement, the clinical relevance of these cadaver studies is unknown.[36, 37] Even though animal studies have not demonstrated serious complications from the procedure and clinical trials have found limited morbidity or mortality directly related to transthoracic pacing, the procedure must not be used indiscriminately. One might expect complications similar to those associated with other conditions requiring intracardiac injections of drugs, such as pericardial tamponade, pneumothorax, myocardial laceration, or coronary artery or other major vessel laceration. Although intracardiac injections are much maligned and the technique is usually not recommended,[38–40] data in the literature do not support this hard-line approach.

Amey and colleagues[41] demonstrated that intracardiac

Table 14–2. Operation of an External Pacemaker (Medtronic Model 5880-A)

To operate the external pacemaker in the *asynchronous* or fixed-rate mode:

1. Set the *rate* between 70 and 90 or at a rate to exceed the intrinsic rate of the patient.
2. Turn the *current* output control clockwise to maximum.
3. Turn the *sensitivity* control to "off" or to the "async" mode.
4. Turn the pacemaker to the "on" position.
5. Check for activation of the pacing indicator needle, which should deflect to the "PACE" indication.

To convert to a *demand* mode:

1. Turn the *sensitivity* control to the maximum clockwise position. This will then sense the R wave if there is intrinsic electrical activity.
2. Turn the *rate* control to 10 beats lower than the patient's intrinsic rate. This should stop the pacemaker, and the needle indicator should deflect to the "SENSE" indication or "PACE" if the patient's rate drops below the reading set on the rate control.

Note: The pacemaker should be disconnected during defibrillation whenever possible.

(From Roberts JR, Greenberg MI: Emergency transthoracic pacemaker. Ann Emerg Med 10:607, 1981.)

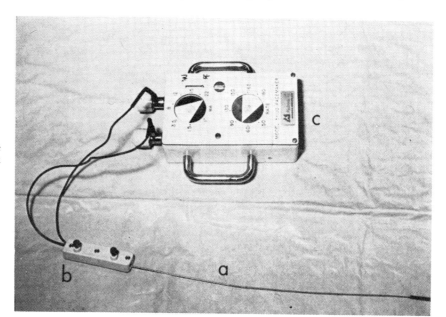

Figure 14–5. Proper connection of pacing wire *(A)*, plastic connector *(B)*, and pacemaker box *(C)*.

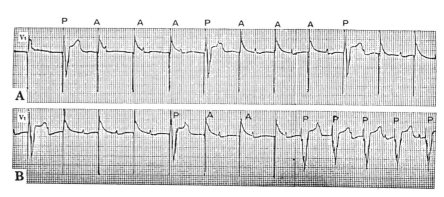

Figure 14–6. Pacemaker spike with failure to pace. Only beats marked "P" are paced beats. During decay of a pacer spike of high voltage, an artifact may be produced that can simulate a QRS complex *(A)*.

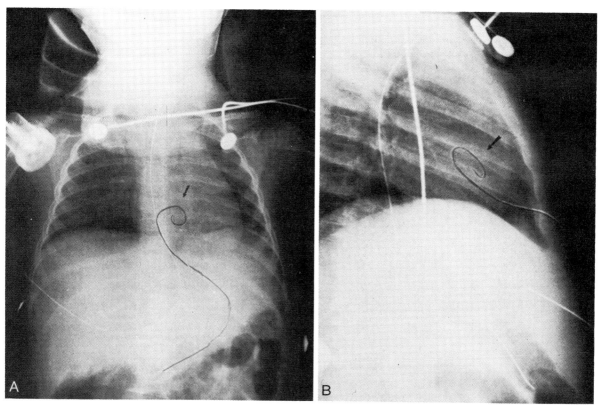

Figure 14–7. Chest films demonstrating transthoracic pacing wire *(arrow)* in right ventricle. *A*, Anteroposterior view. *B*, Lateral view.

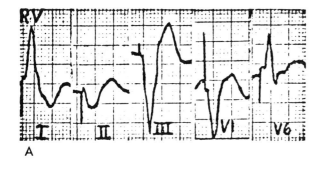

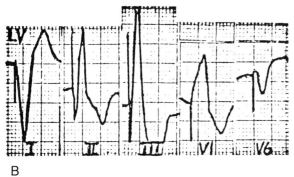

Figure 14–8. QRS configuration seen with pacing wire in right *(A)* and left *(B)* ventricles.

injections by paramedics in the prehospital care of cardiac arrest patients are accomplished with ease and with only a slight increase in complications over control groups. In this small series of 47 intracardiac injections, there were no cases of endocarditis, air embolism, or pericardial effusion. There were four cases of pneumothorax, but these were associated with vigorous CPR and rib fractures.

In a series of 147 intracardiac injections during CPR for the purpose of transthoracic pacemaker insertion or drug therapy, Davidson and coworkers[42] demonstrated that percutaneous puncture of the heart using the subxiphoid

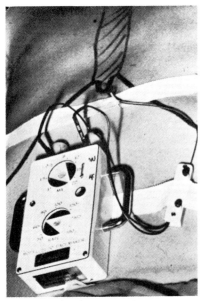

Figure 14–9. Secured pacemaker and wire.

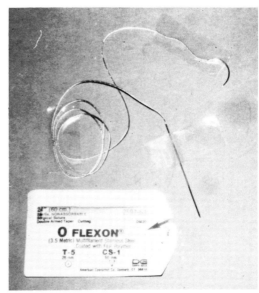

Figure 14–10. Sew-in epicardial pacing wires. This material is Flexon from Davis and Geck Company. The curved needle is used to sew in the wire. The straight wire was designed to guide the wire through the chest wall for easy pull out of the wire. Once the curved needle is used to penetrate the myocardium, the needle is cut off so that only the wire remains attached. During an emergency thoracotomy, the straight needle can be inserted into the pacemaker box to give contact.

approach seldom results in complications of any serious consequence. In this study, small pericardial effusions secondary to bleeding were relatively common (about 30 per cent of the cases), but there were no cases of pericardial tamponade or myocardial or coronary artery laceration. In addition, only one of the 40 patients in whom circulation had been restored had a pneumothorax, even though most patients (62 per cent) continued to receive positive-pressure ventilation after CPR.

Tintinalli and White[17] and Roberts and Greenberg[18] have each reported a case of pericardial tamponade that probably was a direct result of a transthoracic pacer and may have contributed to the death of the patient. Ma[43] reported one case where the needle lumen was obstructed by tissue preventing recognition of ventricular placement. The use of an obturator or the expulsion of lumenal contents using a saline-filled syringe may help avoid this problem.

Considering the dismal outcome of cardiac arrest, an intracardiac needle puncture for the purpose of pacemaker insertion is justified if the procedure itself is assumed to be of potential value. If the pacer were inserted during CPR, the complication rate would be expected to be greater. Especially worrisome would be the development of a tension pneumothorax if the lung were punctured during positive-pressure ventilation or a pericardial tamponade if the patient were anticoagulated or had another bleeding diathesis. Although a small amount of pericardial bleeding may be common in patients receiving transthoracic pacing and CPR, pericardial tamponade appears uncommon.

CONCLUSION

The technique of transthoracic cardiac pacing has been clinically feasible for the past 20 years, yet the procedure remains somewhat controversial. Although the transthoracic pacemaker is associated with potentially serious complications and the procedure should not be used indiscriminately, transthoracic placement of pacing wires is accomplished rapidly and easily and may be effective in selected clinical situations.

There is no debate that cardiac pacing itself is a valuable clinical procedure, although most nonarrest situations can be best handled with transcutaneous or transvenous pacing.

REFERENCES

1. Registers of the Royal Humane Society of London. Nichols & Sons, 1774–1784.
2. Zoll PM: Resuscitation of the heart in ventricular standstill by external electric stimulation. N Engl J Med 247:768, 1952.
3. Thevenet A, Hodges PC, Lillehei CW: The use of myocardial electrode inserted percutaneously for control of complete atrioventricular block by an artificial pacemaker. Dis Chest 34:621, 1958.
4. Braunwald E (ed): Heart Disease. Philadelphia, WB Saunders Co, 1980.
5. Schwartz G, Safar P, Stone D, et al (eds): Principles and Practice of Emergency Medicine. Philadelphia, WB Saunders Co, 1978.
6. Gottlieb R, Chung EK: Techniques of temporary pacing. In Chung EK (ed): Artificial Cardiac Pacing—A Practical Approach. Baltimore, Williams & Wilkins, 1978, pp 150–160.
7. Daicoff GR, Miscia VE: Shock, pacemakers, and surgical therapy. In Eliot RS (ed): The Acute Cardiac Emergency. Mount Kisco, NY, Futura Publishing Co, Inc, 1972, p 253.
8. Ross SM, Hoffman BE: A bipolar pacemaker for immediate treatment of cardiac arrest. J Appl Physiol 154:974, 1960.
9. Bellet S, Muller OF, DeLeon AC, et al: The use of an internal pacemaker in the treatment of cardiac arrest and slow heart rates. Arch Intern Med 105:361, 1960.
10. Lillehei CW, Levy MJ, Bonnabeau RC, et al: Direct wire electrical stimulation for acute postsurgical and postinfarction complete heart block. Ann NY Acad Sci 111:938, 1964.
11. Roe BB: Intractable Stokes-Adams disease: A method of emergency management. Am Heart J 69:470, 1965.
12. Roe BB, Katz HJ: Complete heart block with intractable asystole and recurrent ventricular fibrillation with survival. Am J Cardiol 15:401, 1965.
13. Kodjababian GH, Gray RE, Keenan RL, et al: Percutaneous implantation of cardiac pacemaker electrodes. Am J Cardiol 19:372, 1967.
14. Morris JH, Gillette PC, Barrett FF: Atrioventricular block complicating meningitis: Treatment with emergency cardiac pacing. Pediatrics 58:866, 1976.
15. Zoll PM, Linenthal AJ, Norman LR: Treatment of Stokes-Adams disease by external electric stimulation of the heart. Circulation 9:482, 1954.
16. Zoll PM, Linenthal AJ, Norman LR, et al: Use of the external electric pacemaker in cardiac arrest. JAMA 159:1428, 1955.
17. Tintinalli JE, White BC: Transthoracic pacing during CPR. Ann Emerg Med 10:113, 1981.
18. Roberts JR, Greenberg MI: Emergency transthoracic pacemaker. Ann Emerg Med 10:600, 1981.
19. Ornato JP, Carveth WL, Windle JR, et al: Pacemaker insertion for prehospital bradyasystolic cardiac arrest. Ann Emerg Med 13:101, 1984.
20. White JD, Brown CG: Immediate transthoracic pacing for cardiac asystole in an emergency department setting. Am J Emerg Med 3:125, 1985.
21. Eisner RF, Barreca RS, Cooke D: Value of transthoracic pacing in the face of ventricular asystole (abstract). Ann Emerg Med 15:627, 1986.
22. Dreifus LS, Chaudry KR, Otawa S: Temporary and emergency cardiac pacing. In Varriate P, Naclerio E (eds): Cardiac Pacing. Philadelphia, Lea & Febiger, 1979, pp 133–143.
23. Johnson RA, Haber E, Austen WG (eds): The Practice of Cardiology. Boston, Little, Brown, & Co, 1981, p 28.
24. Preston TA: The use of pacemaking for the treatment of acute arrhythmias. Heart Lung 6:249, 1977.
25. Iseri LT, Humphrey SB, Siner EJ: Prehospital brady-asystolic cardiac arrest. Ann Intern Med 88:741, 1978.
26. Schriver JA: Results of cardiopulmonary resuscitation: A review. Top Emerg Med 1:103, 1979.
27. Lund I, Skulberg A: Resuscitation of cardiac arrest outside hospitals: Experience with a mobile intensive care unit in Oslo. Acta Anaesthesiol Scand 53:13, 1973.
28. Hollingsworth JH: The result of cardiopulmonary resuscitation: A three-year university hospital experience. Ann Intern Med 71:459, 1969.
29. Lemire JG, Johnson AL: Is cardiac resuscitation worthwhile? A decade of experience. N Engl J Med 286:970, 1972.
30. Raizes G, Wagner G, Hackel D: Instantaneous non-arrhythmic cardiac death in acute myocardial infarction. Am J Cardiol 39:1, 1977.
31. Mazor A, Rogel S: Cardiac aspects of shock. Ann Surg 178:128, 1973.
32. White B, Hoehner PJ, Petinga TJ, et al: His electrocardiographic characterization of terminal arrhythmias of hemorrhagic shock in dogs. JACEP 8:298, 1979.
33. Millikan JS, Moore EE, Dunn EL, et al: Temporary cardiac pacing in trauma arrest victims. Ann Emerg Med 9:591, 1980.
34. Meltzer LE, Cohen HE: The incidence of arrhythmias associated with acute myocardial infarction. In Meltzer LE, Dunning AJ (eds): Textbook of Coronary Care. Philadelphia, Charles Press, 1972.
35. Escher DJ, Furman S: Emergency treatment of cardiac arrhythmias. Emphasis on use of electrical pacing. JAMA 214:228, 1970.
36. Brown CG, Hutchins GM, Gurley HT, et al: Placement accuracy of percutaneous transthoracic pacemaker. Am J Emerg Med 3:193, 1985.
37. Brown CG, Gurley HT, Hutchins GM, et al: Injuries associated with percutaneous placement of transthoracic pacemakers. Ann Emerg Med 14:223, 1985.
38. Schechter DC: Transthoracic epinephrine injection in heart resuscitation is dangerous. JAMA 234:1184, 1975.
39. Goldberg AH: Cardiopulmonary arrest. N Engl J Med 290:381, 1974.
40. Vijay NK, Schoonaker FW: Cardiopulmonary arrest and resuscitation. Am Fam Phys 26:85, 1975.
41. Amey BD, Harrison EE, Staub EJ, et al: Paramedic use of intracardiac medications in pre-hospital sudden cardiac death. JACEP 7:130, 1978.
42. Davison R, Barresi V, Parker M, et al: Intracardiac injections during cardiopulmonary resuscitation—a low risk procedure. JAMA 244:111, 1980.
43. Ma FH: Transthoracic pacemaker insertion failure caused by needle lumen obstruction. Am J Emerg Med 7:124, 1989.

Chapter 15

Emergency Transcutaneous and Transesophageal Cardiac Pacing

Scott A. Syverud

TRANSCUTANEOUS CARDIAC PACING

Introduction

Transcutaneous cardiac pacing is a rapid, minimally invasive method of treating severe bradycardias and asystole. Electrodes are applied to the skin of the anterior and posterior chest walls, and pacing is initiated with a portable pulse generator. In an emergency setting, this pacing technique is faster and easier to initiate than transvenous or transthoracic pacing. Pulse generators are sufficiently portable to be used in emergency departments, hospital wards, intensive care units, and mobile paramedic vehicles.

In 1872, Duchenne reported a successful resuscitation of a child by attaching one electrode to a limb while a second electrode was rhythmically touched to the precordium of the thorax.[1] Successful overdrive pacing of the human heart, using a precordial electrode, was reported by VonZiemssen in 1882.[2]

In 1952, Zoll introduced the first practical means of transcutaneous cardiac pacing. Using a ground electrode attached to the skin and a subcutaneous needle electrode over the precordium, he reported the successful resuscitation of two patients in ventricular standstill.[3] One patient was paced for 5 days and subsequently was discharged from the hospital. Zoll later introduced a machine that delivered impulses lasting 2 msec through 3-cm–diameter paddles pressed firmly against the anterior chest wall. This device was the first commercial transcutaneous cardiac pacemaker. During the 1950s, Zoll and Leatham demonstrated the effectiveness of transcutaneous pacing in patients with bradycardia and asystole.[4–7] Leatham used larger electrodes (4 × 6 cm) and a longer pulse duration (20 msec) to successfully pace two patients with bradydysrhythmias.[7]

Until the late 1950s, transcutaneous pacing was the only clinically accepted method of cardiac pacing. The technique had adverse effects, including local tissue burns, muscle contraction, and severe pain.[3, 7] With the development of the first implantable pacemakers, from 1958 through 1960, and the improvement of transvenous electrodes during the early 1960s, transcutaneous pacing was rapidly discarded.[8]

Transvenous pacing requires access to the central venous circulation and is difficult and time consuming when trying to resuscitate patients with severe bradycardia or asystole. Flow-directed catheters are difficult to advance in patients with hypotensive states, and the catheter tip frequently does not seat in the right ventricle. Successful capture and ultimate survival using transvenous or transthoracic pacing for cardiac arrest remain poor with current techniques.[9, 10] Conventional pharmacologic therapy for asystolic or bradycardic arrests is rarely successful. In one series of patients who suffered cardiac arrest while paramedics were on the scene and in whom conventional Advanced Cardiac Life Support guidelines were followed, there was not a single survivor whose initial rhythm was asystole or pulseless bradycardia.[11] The limitations of invasive emergency pacing techniques, the poor efficacy of pharmacologic therapy, and an interest in prehospital pacing led contemporary investigators to reexamine transcutaneous pacing as an emergency procedure.[12, 13]

Early transcutaneous pacemakers used short impulse durations (2 msec), high current outputs ($>$ 100 mA), and small surface electrodes (3-cm diameter).[4, 12] The resulting electrical stimulus, although successful in producing cardiac capture, was extremely painful and produced marked muscle contraction and cutaneous burns (especially with prolonged use).[4, 12] Because no other pacing techniques were available in the early 1950s, the clinician who used the transcutaneous pacing technique for resuscitation was frequently left with a pacemaker-dependent patient who was in severe pain from the technique and for whom no permanent pacing modality was available.[13]

Refinements in electrode size and pulse characteristics have led to the reintroduction of transcutaneous pacing into clinical practice.[12, 14] Increasing the pulse duration from 2 to 20 msec or longer was found to decrease the current output required for cardiac capture.[15, 16] Longer impulse durations also make the induction of ventricular fibrillation less likely.[15] Larger surface area electrodes (8-cm diameter) decrease the current density at the underlying skin and therefore decrease pain and the possibility of tissue burns.[12]

Trials of transcutaneous pacemakers using the newer impulse and electrode characteristics have demonstrated the success of these modifications in overcoming the limitations of earlier transcutaneous pacemakers. Falk and colleagues studied 16 normal male volunteers who were paced without sedation and reported the volunteers' threshold for cardiac capture and subjective "discomfort level."[17] The mean current required for electrical capture was 54 mA (range 42 to 60). Most subjects could tolerate pacing at their capture threshold; only one subject required discontinuation of pacing at 60 mA because of intolerable pain. Heller compared subjective pain perception and capture thresholds in ten volunteers paced with five different transcutaneous pacers.[18] Capture rates (40 to 80 per cent), thresholds (66.5 to 104 mA), and subjective discomfort varied from pacemaker to pacemaker.

A variety of transcutaneous pacing units are now commercially available.[19] These units range from small, inexpensive units with asynchronous pacing only and no monitoring capability to large, expensive demand/asynchronous pacemakers with monitoring and defibrillation capability.[20–22] At least two major manufacturers have incorporated transcutaneous pacing into their newer defibrillator models. Dillon has reviewed the features, product clinical trials, and cost of the various commercial units.[19]

Studies in animals have shown transcutaneous pacing of up to 1 hour duration to be safe.[13, 23] Cardiac and tissue damage caused by pacing during this interval is clinically insignificant.[23, 24] Longer use of transcutaneous pacing has not been investigated fully. The potential for cardiac and cutaneous damage does exist with prolonged pacing at these higher output levels. For this reason, transcutaneous pacing should be used for temporary stabilization only and should always be followed as soon as feasible by an internal pacing technique (usually transvenous). Theoretically, one may induce ventricular fibrillation by stimulating the myocardium during an electrically vulnerable period, but this complication has not yet been encountered clinically.[15] In animal studies of chronic complete heart block, transcutaneous pacing produces a hemodynamic re-

sponse that compares favorably with that produced by transvenous pacing.[25, 26]

Clinical studies have demonstrated improved survival in bradyasystolic arrest patients who recieve pacing within 5 minutes of arrest onset.[27, 28] Syverud and coworkers compared emergency department patients who were paced transcutaneously within 5 minutes of the onset of bradyasystolic arrest (group 1) with those paced more than 5 minutes after arrest onset (group 2).[27] In the first group, two of five patients recovered full neurologic and cardiac function. None of the 14 patients in group 2 survived to hospital discharge. Zoll and colleagues reported a larger study of inhospital bradyasystolic cardiac arrest patients with similar results.[28] Transcutaneous pacing produced survivors in eight of 16 patients paced within 5 minutes of the onset of arrest as compared with four of 44 patients paced 5 to 30 minutes after the onset of arrest. Dalsey and associates have demonstrated that the use of transcutaneous pacing late in the course of bradyasystolic arrest (greater than 20 minutes after arrest onset) may produce electrical capture but does not result in long-term survivors.[29] Clearly, if transcutaneous pacing is to be of benefit in the setting of bradyasystolic arrest, it must be used early.

This observation has led to trials of transcutaneous pacing in prehospital settings. Large numbers of patients received prehospital transcutaneous pacing in two studies. Paris and coworkers reported the use of transcutaneous pacing for 112 prehospital patients found either in asystole, pulseless idioventricular rhythm, or complete heart block.[30] Although the pacemaker was used as soon as possible, the mean delay to application of the pacemaker was 29 minutes. Furthermore, these researchers did not use the pacemaker for complete heart block until all pharmacologic means of therapy had been exhausted. Electrical capture was obtained in 52 per cent of patients found in bradyasystolic arrest; mechanical capture was obtained in 18 per cent. Interestingly, none of the patients in complete heart block showed mechanical capture. Eitel and colleagues reported a series of 91 patients with cardiac arrest who received prehospital transcutaneous pacing.[31] The delay from the onset of arrest to pacing was 24 minutes in this series. Electrical capture was obtained in 11 per cent. Neither of these studies reported any long-term survivors.

Hedges and associates reported a controlled randomized prehospital trial of transcutaneous pacing for 202 patients in bradyasystolic cardiac arrest.[21] Patients in the control group (even days) were treated with standard pharmacologic therapy; patients in the treatment group received pacing along with drug therapy. Although a short time to the initiation of pacing showed a trend toward hospital admission in this study, there was no improvement in outcome in the paced group over the control group. The mean delay from arrest onset to pacing was 21 minutes in the paced group. A similar study design was used by Barthell and coworkers in a prehospital study of 239 patients in bradyasystolic arrest or hemodynamically significant bradycardia.[32] Although no improvement in outcome was observed in patients in asystolic arrest, patients with bradycardia were more likely to survive with pacing (six of six survivors in the paced group versus two of seven controls). The mean delay to pacing was 23 minutes in this study.

Delay from the onset of arrest to the initiation of pacing is a major problem limiting the usefulness of transcutaneous pacing in prehospital care. Some investigators have suggested that delays could be reduced by incorporating the transcutaneous pacer into a prehospital defibrillator.[21] The results of a small study by Jaggarao and coworkers using an automatic prehospital defibrillator-pacer supports this concept.[22] It also appears likely that as transcutaneous pacemakers become standard resuscitation equipment, providers will begin to use them earlier in resuscitation. In a follow-up study, Hedges and colleagues reported that everyday availability of pacing increased the number of patients who received pacing within 10 minutes of hemodynamic decompensation and increased long-term patient survival as well.[33] Prehospital pacing may be most useful in treatment of the patient with a hemodynamically significant bradycardia who has not yet progressed to cardiac arrest (e.g., heart block in the setting of acute myocardial infarction) or in the patient who arrests after the arrival of prehospital providers.[11, 21, 32, 34]

Equipment

Few medical product lines have changed as rapidly as commercial transcutaneous pacemakers. Patent controversy, corporate acquisitions, and rapid product evolution have all contributed to this rapid change.[35] Of eight commercial transcutaneous pacemakers reviewed in a 1988 product review,[19] four are no longer available. Several manufacturers no longer produce transcutaneous pacemakers or have gone out of business.

In spite of this instability in the marketplace, transcutaneous pacemaker sales continue to increase. The devices are now standard equipment in most emergency departments and are rapidly spreading to inhospital and prehospital care settings. The pacemakers introduced in the early 1980s tended to be asynchronous devices with a limited selection of rate and output parameters. Units introduced more recently have demand mode pacing, more output options, and are more likely to be combined with a defibrillator in a single unit. Combined defibrillator-pacers offer advantages in both cost and ease and rapidity of use when compared with stand-alone devices. An example of a recently introduced combined unit is shown in Figure 15–1. A full-featured stand-alone pacemaker is illustrated in Figure 15–2.

All transcutaneous pacemakers have similar basic features. Most allow operation in either a fixed rate (asynchronous) or a demand mode. Most allow rate selection in a range from 30 to 200 beats per minute. Current output is usually adjustable from zero to 150 mA. If an electrocardiograph (ECG) monitor is not an integral part of the unit, *an output adapter to a separate monitor is required* to "blank" the large electrical spike from the pacemaker impulse to allow interpretation of the much smaller ECG complex. Without blanking protection, the standard ECG machine is swamped by the pacemaker spike and is uninterpretable. This could be disasterous because the large pacing artifacts *can mask treatable ventricular fibrillation* (Fig. 15–3). Pulse durations on available units vary from 20 to 40 msec and are not adjustable by the operator.

Two sets of patient electrodes are usually required for operation of the device. One set of standard ECG electrodes is used for monitoring. The much larger pacing electrodes

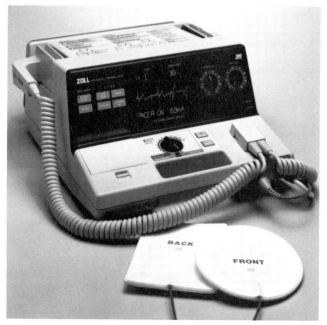

Figure 15–1. Combined defibrillator-transcutaneous pacemaker unit (Zoll-PD). The unit defibrillates through standard hand-held paddles and has additional cable connections for electrocardiograph monitoring electrodes and for pacing electrodes. (Courtesy of ZMI Corp., Cambridge, Mass.)

deliver electrical impulses through an 8-cm–diameter conducting surface. One pacing electrode is placed over the middorsal spine, and the other is placed over the left anterior chest. The posterior electrode serves as the ground.

One currently marketed combined defibrillator-pacemaker (Medac ALS System 4) uses a single set of electrodes for ECG monitoring, pacing, and defibrillation. Although this approach makes use of the device simpler, its clinical utility remains to be proved. Because the impedance characteristics of the ideal pacing electrode differ from those of the ideal ECG and defibrillation electrode, this approach may not prove to be ideal.[15, 16]

Indications for Transcutaneous Cardiac Pacing

Transcutaneous pacing is technically the fastest and easiest method of emergency pacing. This technique is useful for initial stabilization of the patient in the emergency department who requires emergency pacing while arrangements for transvenous pacemaker insertion are being made. The use of the equipment is readily mastered, and the procedure is fast and minimally invasive.[14, 20] Refinements in the equipment have made transcutaneous pacing the emergency pacing procedure of choice. Transcutaneous pacing also is gaining widespread prehospital use in helicopter ambulance programs and inhospital use in the cardiac catheterization laboratory, operating room, intensive care unit, and on general medical floors.[36–38] The technique may be preferable to transvenous pacing in patients who have received thrombolytic agents. No central venous puncture, with the attendant risk of hemorrhage, is required. Limited experience suggests that transcutaneous pacing also may be useful in the treatment of refractory tachydysrhythmias by overdrive pacing.[39–40a] Although small pediatric electrodes for transcutaneous pacing have been developed, experience with pediatric transcutaneous pacing has been limited.[41]

Transcutaneous pacing is indicated for the treatment of hemodynamically significant bradydysrhythmias that have not responded to atropine therapy. *Hemodynamically significant* implies hypotension, anginal chest pain, pulmonary edema, or evidence of decreased cerebral perfusion. This technique is a *temporary* technique that is indicated for short intervals as a bridge until transvenous pacing can be initiated or until the underlying cause of the bradyarrhythmia (e g, hyperkalemia, drug overdose) can be reversed. Although often unsuccessful, transcutaneous pacing may be attempted in the treatment of asystolic cardiac arrest. The technique will only be efficacious if used early after arrest onset (within 10 minutes) in this setting. It is not indicated for treatment of prolonged arrest victims with a final morbid rhythm of asystole.

In conscious patients with hemodynamically stable bradycardias, transcutaneous pacing may not be necessary. It is reasonable to attach electrodes to such patients and to leave the pacemaker in standby mode against the possibility of hemodynamic deterioration while further efforts at treatment of the patient's underlying disorder are being made. This approach has been used successfully in patients with new heart block in the setting of cardiac ischemia.[28]

Technique

The pacing electrodes are applied as shown in Figure 15–4 and are attached to the instrument cable. The anterior electrode (cathode or negative electrode) is placed as close as possible to the point of maximal impulse on the left anterior chest wall. This 8-cm–diameter electrode adheres

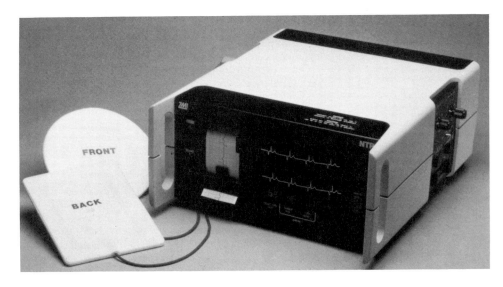

Figure 15–2. "Stand alone" transcutaneous pacemaker (Zoll NTP). This unit has a built-in monitor and strip chart recorder. (Courtesy of ZMI Corp., Cambridge, Mass.)

to the skin and has a large surface area for electrical contact. The second electrode is placed directly posterior to the anterior electrode. Failure to capture may be due to misplacement of the electrodes, and failure to pace may be rectified with a small change in anterior electrode position. Electrocardiogram electrodes are placed on the chest wall and connected to the instrument cable. Some physicians prophylactically apply electrodes to all critically ill patients

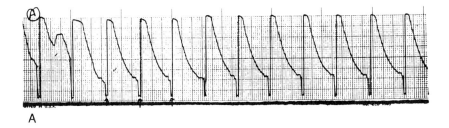

A

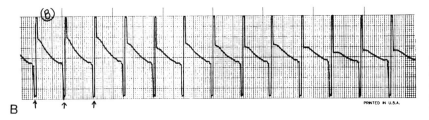

B

Figure 15–3. The top three rhythm strips (A, B, C) are taken from a standard wall-mounted electrocardiograph monitor. They all demonstrate large pacer spikes without capture. The underlying rhythm cannot be determined and could be treatable ventricular fibrillation. The bottom rhythm strip (D) demonstrates a tracing on the same patient with the external pacer monitor (special dampening). Note that the pacing spikes are much smaller, and it is easily seen that the underlying rhythm is asystole, without pacer capture.

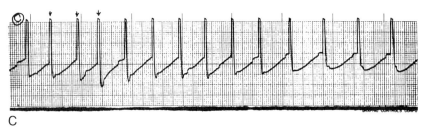

C

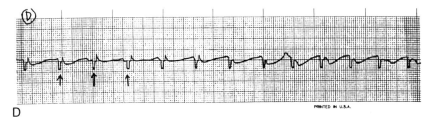

D

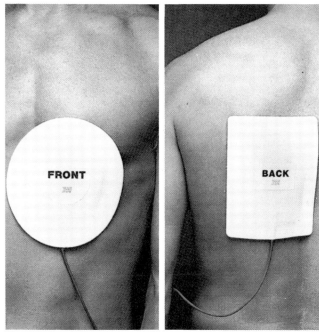

Figure 15–4. Correct placement of transcutaneous pacemaker electrodes (see text). (Courtesy of ZMI Corp., Cambridge, Mass.)

to facilitate immediate transcutaneous pacing should decompensation occur.

There is little risk of electrical injury to health care providers during transcutaneous pacing. Power delivered during each impulse is less than 1/1000 of that delivered during defibrillation.[42] Chest compressions (cardiopulmonary resuscitation) can be administered directly over the insulated electrodes while pacing.[29] Inadvertent contact with the active pacing surface results only in a mild shock.

To initiate transcutaneous pacing, the electrodes are applied, and the device is activated. In the setting of brady-asystolic arrest, it is reasonable to turn the stimulating current to maximal output, then decrease the output if capture is achieved. In the setting of a patient with a hemodynamically compromising bradycardia (but not in cardiac arrest), the operator should slowly increase the output from the minimal setting until capture is achieved. Rate and output selections are adjustable as shown (Fig. 15–5). Assessment of capture can be made by monitoring the electrocardiogram on the filtered monitor of the pacing unit (Fig. 15–6). The hemodynamic response to pacing also must be assessed, either by blood pressure cuff or arterial catheter. Ideally, pacing should be continued at an output level just above the threshold of initial electrical capture.

Failure to capture with transcutaneous pacing may be related to electrode placement or patient size. Patients with barrel-shaped chests and large amounts of intrathoracic air conduct electricity poorly and may prove refractory to capture. A large pericardial effusion or tamponade also will increase the output required for capture.[23] Failure to electrically capture with a transcutaneous device in these settings is an indication to consider immediate transvenous or transthoracic pacer placement.

Patients who are conscious or who regain consciousness during transcutaneous pacing will experience discomfort because of muscle contraction.[17, 18, 28] Analgesia with incremental doses of a narcotic, sedation with a benzodiazepine, or both will make this discomfort tolerable until transvenous pacing can be instituted.

Complications

The major potential complication of transcutaneous pacing is *failure to recognize the presence of underlying treatable ventricular fibrillation.* This complication is primarily due to the size of the pacing artifact in the ECG screen, a technical problem inherent in systems without appropriate dampening circuitry.

Other *potential* complications of transcutaneous pacing include induction of dysrhythmias, pain from stimulation, and tissue damage. With epicardial electrodes, the threshold current required to induce ventricular fibrillation decreases as impulse duration increases. At a 10-msec impulse duration, ventricular fibrillation can be induced with currents as low as 25 mA delivered through epicardial electrodes.[15] Because transcutaneous pacing impulses are of even longer duration (20 msec) and of higher current (50 to 200 mA), there has been concern about possible induction of ventricular fibrillation during transcutaneous pacing. Studies of fibrillation thresholds using large *precordial* electrodes have shown the relationship of threshold to impulse duration to be the opposite of that seen with *epicardial* electrodes. With *cutaneous* precordial electrodes, the current required to induce fibrillation *increases* as pulse duration *increases.*[16] The apparent paradox may be explained by the differing nature of the electrodes. Epicardial electrodes are localized on one small area of the myocardium, whereas transcutaneous electrodes deliver a broad electrical charge to the myocardium as a whole. The implication is that longer impulse durations, although more dangerous with internal pacing, seem to decrease the chance of inducing ventricular fibrillation with transcutaneous pacing.

Pain from electrical skin and muscle stimulation was a significant complication of earlier transcutaneous pacemakers. In recent studies of the Zoll transcutaneous pacemaker, only two of 30 subjects (patients and volunteers) who were paced while conscious required discontinuation of pacing owing to discomfort.[17] Most reported the discomfort as "mild or moderate and easily tolerable." Sedation would presumably improve a conscious patient's ability to tolerate transcutaneous pacing. Pride and McKinley have reported one 7-week-old child who was paced for 45 hours without a pad change and developed third-degree burns.[42a]

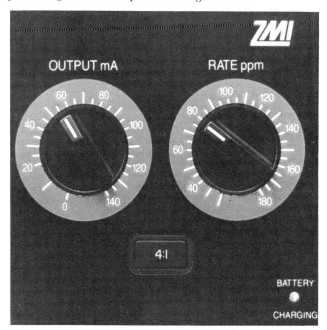

Figure 15–5. Rate and output selections.

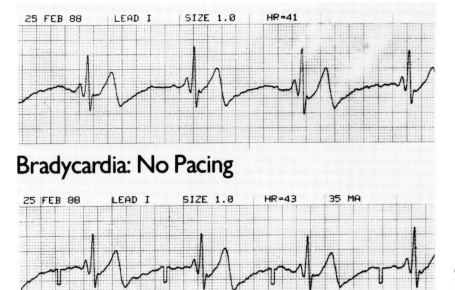

Bradycardia: No Pacing

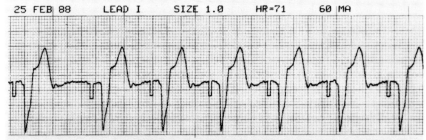

Pacing below Threshold (35 mA): No Capture

Pacing above Threshold (60 mA): with Capture (Pacing-Pulse Marker ⊔)

Figure 15–6. Assessing electrocardiogram capture with transcutaneous pacing. Note that the monitor has been adapted to accommodate the large pacing artifact so as not to obscure the underlying ventricular activity.

Previous experience with transcutaneous pacing in humans has not been extensive. Zoll and colleagues reported 25 humans paced for up to 108 hours with impulses of a 20-msec duration.[6] Pacer-induced dysrhythmias did not occur. Leatham and associates paced one patient for 68 hours with impulses of a 20-msec duration.[7] The patient died 2 days after pacing was discontinued. Pathologic examination revealed no evidence of pacer-induced myocardial damage. Madsen and colleagues paced ten healthy volunteers at threshold for 30 minutes and found no enzyme or echocardiographic abnormalities.[43]

Studies of repetitive direct current countershocks in dogs have induced tissue damage with energy levels that are 1000 times greater than those required to pace the heart transcutaneously. In a canine study, ten animals with chronic heart block that were paced for 60 minutes (20-msec duration at 80 beats per minute with 8-cm–diameter cutaneous electrodes) did not develop pacer-related dysrhythmias. Serial cardiograms and cardiac enzymes revealed no evidence of ischemia or infarction.[13] Examination of the canine hearts after the dogs were sacrificed 72 hours after pacing did not reveal clinically significant myocardial damage.[24] A single primate paced for 1 hour with 20-msec impulses of 400 mA had no evidence of tissue damage at autopsy and at microscopic examination after sacrifice 24 hours later.[44] Based on these studies, transcutaneous pacing appears to be safe for short-term use in humans.

Conclusions

Devices that pace the heart have been available for clinical use since 1952. Technologic improvements have minimized the complications associated with earlier use of the transcutaneous route and have enabled the reapplication of this relatively old pacing technique to a selected subset of cardiac emergencies. The introduction of combined defibrillator-pacemakers promises to make pacing more available in prehospital and health care settings. Although the technique is still not universally available, it is rapidly becoming "standard of care" for resuscitation protocols and equipment. Instituting pacing earlier in the course of bradycardic rhythms, including the prehospital phase of care, may improve the poor survival rate now associated with these rhythms.

TRANSESOPHAGEAL CARDIAC PACING

Introduction

Another method of rapid, minimally invasive cardiac pacing involves passing a pacing electrode down the esophagus to the area just behind the right atrium. Transesophageal resistance is high (approximately 600 ohms) requiring high voltages (up to 30 volts) for cardiac capture. The close proximity of the esophagus to the heart keeps current requirements for capture relatively low (5 to 20 mA). An emergency transesophageal pacing system is commercially available in Europe, but at present, none has been approved for use in humans in the United States. Several case reports of successful resuscitation using transesophageal pacing have appeared in the medical literature.[45–48]

Procedure

Transesophageal pacing requires passage of an electrode-bearing nasogastric tube and correct positioning of the tube so that the electrode lies directly behind the right atrium. This technique may be more difficult to use during a cardiac arrest than transcutaneous pacing. Even when properly placed in the esophagus behind the heart, the electrode could be displaced by chest compressions or patient movement during transport. This technique offers advantages over transvenous and transthoracic pacing in terms of the ease and rapidity with which pacing can be established. The nasogastric pacing catheter can be passed by paramedics at the scene of cardiac arrests. Lower current is required for transesophageal pacing than for transcutaneous pacing. Prophylactic insertion of the nasogastric pacing catheter during surgical procedures in which bradycardia might be encountered seems to be the most immediate practical application of transesophageal emergency pacing.[49] Investigations of its use during cardiac arrest have not as yet been carried out. Further development and investigation of transesophageal pacing await commercial availability of pulse generators and catheters as well as approval of the technique by the United States Food and Drug Administration.

REFERENCES

1. Duchenne de Boulogne: De l'électrisation localise et son application a la pathologique et a la therapeutique. Paris, Bailliere, 1872.
2. VonZiemssen H: Studien über die Bewegungsvorgänge am menschlichen Herzen, sowie über die mechanische und elektrische Erregbarkeit des Herzens und des Nervus, 1882.
3. Zoll PM: Resuscitation of the heart in ventricular standstill by external electric stimulation. N Engl J Med 247:768, 1952.
4. Zoll PM, Linenthal AJ, Norman LR, et al: Treatment of unexpected cardiac arrest by external electric stimulation of the heart. N Engl J Med 254:541, 1956.
5. Zoll PM, Linenthal AJ, Norman LR: Treatment of Stokes-Adams disease by external stimulation of the heart. Circulation 9:482, 1954.
6. Zoll PM, Linenthal AJ, Norman LR, et al: External electric stimulation of the heart in cardiac arrest. Arch Intern Med 96:639, 1955.
7. Leatham A, Cook P, Davis JG: External electric stimulator for treatment of ventricular standstill. Lancet Dec 8, 1956, p 1185.
8. Chardack WM, Gage AA, Greatbatch W: A transistorized self-contained, implantable pacemaker for the long-term correction of complete heart-block. Surgery 48:643, 1960.
9. Hazard PB, Benton C, Milnor P: Transvenous cardiac pacing in cardiopulmonary resuscitation. Crit Care Med 9:666, 1981.
10. Tintinalli JE, White BC: Transthoracic pacing during CPR. Ann Emerg Med 10:113, 1981.
11. Iseri LT, Siner EF, Humphrey SB, et al: Prehospital cardiac arrest after arrival of the paramedic unit. JACEP 6:530, 1977.
12. Zoll PM: External noninvasive electric stimulation of the heart. Crit Care Med 9:393, 1981.
13. Syverud SA, Dalsey WC, Hedges JR, et al: Transcutaneous cardiac pacing: Determination of myocardial injury in a canine model. Ann Emerg Med 12:261, 1983.
14. Dalsey WC, Syverud SA, Trott A: Transcutaneous cardiac pacing. J Emerg Med 1:201, 1984.
15. Jones M, Geddes LA: Strength duration curves for cardiac pacemaking and ventricular fibrillation. Cardiovasc Res Bull 15:101, 1977.
16. Varghese PJ, Bren G, Ross A: Electrophysiology of external cardiac pacing: A comparative study with endocardial pacing. Circulation 66:349, 1982.
17. Falk RH, Zoll PM, Zoll RH: Safety and efficacy of noninvasive cardiac pacing: A preliminary report. N Engl J Med 309:1166, 1983.
18. Heller MB, Kaplan RM, Peterson J, et al: Comparison of performance of five transcutaneous pacing devices (abstract). Ann Emerg Med 16:493, 1987.
19. Dillon DJ: Transcutaneous pacemakers. Health Devices 17:39, 1988.
20. Clinton JE, Zoll PM, Zoll R, et al: External noninvasive cardiac pacing. J Emerg Med 2:155, 1985.
21. Hedges JR, Syverud SA, Dalsey WC, et al: Prehospital trial of emergent transcutaneous pacing. Circulation 76:1337, 1987.
22. Jaggarao NSV, Grainger R, Heber M, et al: Use of an automated external defibrillator-pacemaker by ambulance staff. Lancet 2:73, 1982.
23. Hedges JR, Syverud SA, Dalsey WC, et al: Threshold enzymatic and pathologic changes associated with prolonged transcutaneous pacing in a chronic heart block model. J Emerg Med 7:1, 1989.
24. Kicklighter EJ, Syverud SA, Dalsey WC, et al: Pathologic aspects of transcutaneous cardiac pacing. Am J Emerg Med 3:108, 1985.
25. Niemann JT, Rosborough JP, Garner D, et al: External noninvasive cardiac pacing: A comparative study of two techniques with conventional endocardial pacing. PACE 7:230, 1984.
26. Syverud SA, Hedges JR, Dalsey WC, et al: Hemodynamics of transcutaneous cardiac pacing. Am J Emerg Med 4:17, 1986.
27. Syverud SA, Dalsey WC, Hedges JR: Transcutaneous and transvenous cardiac pacing for early bradyasystolic cardiac arrest. Ann Emerg Med 14:121, 1986.
28. Zoll PM, Zoll RH, Falk RH, et al: External non-invasive temporary cardiac pacing: Clinical trials. Circulation 71:937, 1985.
29. Dalsey WC, Syverud SA, Hedges JR: Emergency department use of transcutaneous cardiac pacing for cardiac arrests. Crit Care Med 13:399, 1985.
30. Paris PM, Stewart RD, Kaplan RM, et al: Transcutaneous pacing for bradyasystolic cardiac arrests in prehospital care. Ann Emerg Med 14:320, 1985.
31. Eitel DR, Guzzardi LJ, Stein SE, et al: Noninvasive transcutaneous cardiac pacing in prehospital cardiac arrest. Ann Emerg Med 16:531, 1987.
32. Barthell E, Troiano P, Olson D, et al: Prehospital external cardiac pacing: A prospective, randomized, controlled clinical trial. Ann Emerg Med 17:1221, 1988.
33. Hedges JR, Shultz B, Easter R, et al: Prehospital transcutaneous cardiac pacing. Phase II: Daily pacing availability (abstract). Ann Emerg Med 18:469, 1989.
34. Dalsey WC, Syverud SA, Ross DS, et al: Transcutaneous cardiac pacing (letter). Ann Emerg Med 13:410, 1984.
35. Heller MB: Of pacing, patents, and patients (editorial). Am J Emerg Med 6:78, 1988.
36. Berliner D, Okun M, Peters RW, et al: Transcutaneous pacing in the operating room. JAMA 254:84, 1985.
37. Johnson DQ, Vukov LF, Farnell MB: External transcutaneous pacemakers in air medical transport services (abstract). Aeromedical J 2:23, 1987.
38. Noe R, Cockrell W, Moses HW, et al: Transcutaneous pacemaker use in a large hospital. PACE 9:101, 1986.
39. Rosenthal ME, Stamato NJ: Noninvasive cardiac pacing for termination of sustained, uniform ventricular tachycardia. Am Heart J 561, 1986.
40. Sharkey SW, Chaffee V, Kapser S: Prophylactic external pacing during conversion of atrial tachyarrhythmias. Am J Cardiol 55:1632, 1985.
40a. Altamura G, Bianconi L, Boccadamo R, et al: Treatment of ventricular and supraventricular tachyarrhythmias by transcutaneous cardiac pacing. PACE 12:331, 1989.
41. Beland MJ, Hesslein PS, Finlay CD, et al: Noninvasive transcutaneous cardiac pacing in children. PACE 10:1262, 1987.
42. Syverud SA, Dalsey WC, Hedges JR: Transcutaneous cardiac pacing (letter). Ann Emerg Med 13:982, 1984.
42a. Pride HB, McKinley DF: Third-degree burns from the use of an external cardiac pacing device. Crit Care Med 18:572, 1990.
43. Madsen JK, Pedersen F, Grande P, et al: Normal myocardial enzymes and normal echocardiographic findings during noninvasive transcutaneous pacing. PACE 11:1188, 1988.
44. Varghese J, Bren G, Ross A: Absence of Tissue Injury After Prolonged Transcutaneous Pacing. The Scientific and Technical Basis of External Cardiac Pacing. Wilsonville, Oreg, Cardiac Resuscitator Corporation, 1982.
45. Burack B, Furman S: Transesophageal cardiac pacing. Am J Cardiol 23:149, 1969.
46. Rowe CG, Ward T, Neblett I: Cardiac pacing with an esophageal electrode. Am J Cardiol 24:549, 1969.
47. Shaw RJ, Berman LH, Hinton JM: Successful emergency transesophageal cardiac pacing with subsequent endoscopy. Br Med J 284:309, 1982.
48. Colquhoun M: Emergency transesophageal cardiac pacing. Br Med J 284:1263, 1982.
49. Hartley JM: Transesophageal cardiac pacing. Anaesthesia 37:192, 1982.

Chapter 16

Pericardiocentesis

Michael L. Callaham

INTRODUCTION

The experimental induction of cardiac tamponade from infusion of intrapericardial fluid was first reported in 1889.[1] However, pericardiotomy under direct vision was first done in 1815, and in 1840, the first blind approach using a trocar was carried out successfully on a patient with tamponade from malignancy.[2] By the end of the nineteenth century, the trocar and cannula method of pericardiocentesis was commonly used. The subxiphoid approach was described in 1911. In the past three decades, there has been little change in the technique of pericardiocentesis until the recent advent of two-dimensional ultrasound.

Pericardiocentesis is a procedure that is occasionally life saving and should be thoroughly understood by all physicians, although few will actually perform it. The medical literature concerning pericardiocentesis tends to fall into two distinct categories: studies of traumatic hemopericardium and studies of pericardial effusion from other causes. This separation is not entirely artificial, because these two clinical entities are quite different in their time course, etiology, and treatment. In the following section, these two categories, traumatic and nontraumatic, respectively, are discussed, with the understanding that patients with the former usually present with an acute hemopericardium, and those with the latter present with a pericardial effusion that may be bloody but is not composed of whole blood.

CAUSES OF PERICARDIAL EFFUSION AND TAMPONADE

Many disease processes can cause pericardial effusion, ranging from the common to the rare (Table 16–1). The etiology, natural history, and clinical course of pericardial effusions vary widely and must be considered when choosing a mode of therapy.

Traumatic

In trauma, a discrete event (such as a knife wound to the heart or a misdirected cardiac catheter) causes bleeding into the pericardial sac. Blood from a penetrating wound or blood from a bleeding myocardium usually accumulates in the pericardial space much faster than exudate or transudate. Tamponade from hemorrhage occurs frequently because often such bleeding does not stop spontaneously and the pericardial sac cannot change size immediately to accommodate the extra volume.

If tamponade develops following penetrating trauma, the patient or the physician is usually aware immediately of an abnormal state, and looks for a cardiac injury. However, there are deceptive exceptions to the "self-declaring" nature of traumatic tamponade. These include tamponade as a complication of closed-chest cardiopulmonary resuscitation (CPR), cardiac catheterizations, bleeding diathesis, and dissecting aortic aneurysm.

Traumatic tamponade is the most acutely life-threatening form of tamponade, because it may occur very rapidly.

Table 16–1. Causes of Pericardial Effusion	
Neoplasm	Mesothelioma
	Lung
	Breast
	Melanoma
	Lymphoma
Pericarditis	Radiation (especially after Hodgkin disease)
	Viral
	Bacterial
	Fungal
	Tuberculosis
	Amebiasis
	Toxoplasmosis
	Idiopathic
	Staphylococcus
	Pneumococcus
	Haemophilus
Connective Tissue Disease	Systemic lupus erythematosus
	Scleroderma
	Rheumatoid arthritis
	Acute rheumatic fever
Metabolic Disorders	Myxedema
	Uremia
	Cholesterol pericarditis
	Bleeding diatheses
Cardiac Disease	Acute myocardial infarction
	Dissecting aortic aneurysm
	Congestive heart failure
	Coronary aneurysm
Drugs	Hydralazine
	Phenytoin
	Anticoagulants
	Procainamide
	Minoxidil
Trauma	Blunt
	Major trauma
	Closed-chest CPR
	Penetrating
	Major penetrating trauma
	Intracardiac injections
	Transthoracic and transvenous pacing wires
	Pericardiocentesis
	Cardiac catheterization
	CVP catheter
Miscellaneous	Serum sickness
	Chylous effusion
	Löffler's syndrome
	Reiter's syndrome
	Behçet's syndrome
	Pancreatitis
	Postpericardiotomy
	Amyloidosis
	Ascites

(Data from Guberman BA, Fowler NO, Engel PJ, et al: Cardiac tamponade in medical patients. Circulation 64:633, 1981; and Pories WJ, Gaudiani VA: Cardiac tamponade. Surg Clin North Am 55:573, 1975.)

Most commonly, tamponade is the result of a stab wound to the heart,[3] presumably because the pericardium seals itself after a stab wound but cannot do so after gunshot wounds.[3, 4] Approximately 80 to 90 per cent of stab wounds to the heart demonstrate tamponade,[3, 5] compared with 20 per cent of gunshot wounds. Larger pericardial wounds from gunshots generally drain into the pleural space and produce a hemothorax.[6] Cardiac tamponade is often suspected with anterior chest wounds, but it is imperative that one remember that any penetrating wound of the lateral chest, back, or upper abdomen may involve the heart.

Theoretically, CPR can cause effusions secondary to the

blunt trauma of overenthusiastic CPR, broken ribs, or intracardiac injections. Early studies of CPR survivors reported pericardial effusion in 1 to 3 per cent.[7] Echocardiographic studies showed small cardiac effusions (but not tamponade) in 12 per cent of survivors, only 4 per cent of whom had received intracardiac injections.[8] A study of 53 patients who received 147 intracardiac injections during CPR showed no lacerations of coronary arteries or ventricles, but half of the 17 patients who had echocardiograms demonstrated insignificant effusions.[9] Thus it would appear that CPR and intracardiac drug injections are unlikely to cause significant effusion, much less tamponade.

A bleeding diathesis may cause spontaneous bleeding into the pericardial sac. The incidence of spontaneous pericardial tamponade in anticoagulated patients has been reported to range from 2.5 to 11 per cent.[10, 11] If patients are anticoagulated, pericardial blood will not clot and can be easily aspirated, unlike the situation in traumatic tamponade in which clots are frequent, making diagnosis more difficult and pericardiocentesis less beneficial.

An aneurysm of the ascending aorta may dissect around the base of the aorta into the pericardial sac, causing dramatic, rapid, and often fatal tamponade. Such aneurysms may be caused by syphilis, Marfan syndrome, atherosclerosis, or deceleration injuries in motor vehicle accidents. Infection may create pseudoaneurysms of the aorta, which can also present as tamponade.[12] Diagnosis of this mechanism of tamponade depends on maintaining a high index of suspicion. The possibility of aneurysm should always be entertained in the hypotensive patient in general and when hemorrhagic pericardial effusion is found in particular.

Iatrogenic causes of cardiac tamponade are relatively uncommon but are well-known complications of invasive or diagnostic procedures. Pacemaker insertion (either transthoracic or transvenous) and cardiac catheterization are two of the main causes, resulting in tamponade when cardiac chambers or coronary vessels are inadvertently penetrated.[6, 13] Such penetration of vascular structures is very common during transthoracic pacemaker placement.[14] Tamponade is also seen as a complication after cardiac surgery, although it is usually anticipated, and mediastinal or pericardial drainage helps to control and prevent it.[13, 15] Pericardiocentesis itself can cause tamponade by lacerating myocardium or coronary vessels.[16, 17]

Cardiac tamponade may result from perforation of the right atrium or, less commonly, of the right ventricle or superior vena cava, by a central venous pressure (CVP) catheter or subclavian hemodialysis catheter.[18] This event is usually not diagnosed early and is therefore usually fatal.[19] Perforation may occur during placement or, more commonly, 1 to 2 days later when the catheter erodes through tissue, particularly if a catheter of stiff material is used or when the left internal jugular vein approach is used.[20] Fatal mediastinal tamponade also can occur if fluid infused through a misplaced catheter enters the mediastinum.[19] Tamponade from CVP line placement is seldom seen in the emergency department but must always be considered when there is sudden decompensation in a patient with a CVP line in place. In this situation, immediate pericardiocentesis (or placing the intravenous fluid bag below the patient to aspirate solution from the pericardium) may be the only effective treatment, but it is usually not thought of until it is too late. Tamponade should always be considered when a patient deteriorates hemodynamically after an invasive diagnostic or therapeutic procedure involving the heart.

Blunt trauma may cause hemopericardium; significant trauma (e.g., from a motor vehicle crash) is usually required. The presence of a major chest injury with associated bruises or rib and sternal fractures is often obvious. Cases have been

reported, however, in which tamponade occurred in major blunt trauma with no immediate obvious signs of injury to the thorax.[21] Such incidents may be more common than is clinically recognized, judging by the reports of constrictive pericarditis and pericardial defects found months to years later in trauma patients who were not originally noted to have effusion.

Severe deceleration injury may cause aortic dissection and tamponade. However, less than 14 per cent of people with severe aortic injury reach the hospital alive.[22] In one series, only one of 28 patients with aortic injury developed tamponade. Interestingly, in the same series, five of 72 victims of blunt trauma without aortic injuries developed tamponade. In another series, only one of 43 patients with aortic injury had hemopericardium; thus tamponade is a relatively uncommon development of aortic deceleration injury.[23]

An interesting but rare cause of cardiac tamponade is pneumopericardium. Pneumopericardium is most commonly seen with pneumothorax and pneumomediastinum as a complication of respiratory therapy in infants, but it may also occur from similar barotrauma in adults.[24] Pneumopericardium also occurs spontaneously in asthma,[25] following blunt chest injury,[26] and even after high-speed motorcycle rides.[27] Pneumopericardium is usually benign, but tension pneumopericardium has been reported as a cause of life-threatening tamponade after blunt chest trauma[28] and after pericardiectomy.[29] The appearance of life-threatening pneumopericardium and tamponade have also been described immediately[30] and 6 days after penetrating chest trauma.[31]

Nontraumatic

The difference between nontraumatic and traumatic tamponade is usually obvious but is a distinction that must be made, because the etiology determines the aggressiveness, type, and speed of treatment. Patients with nontraumatic etiologies usually accumulate effusions slowly, which allows the pericardium to stretch to accommodate up to 2000 ml of fluid.[32] This slower accumulation (compared with the rapid accumulation of blood in traumatic tamponade) means that even in a moderately hypotensive patient more time may be available for workup. Infrequently, the patient with nontraumatic tamponade may be severely ill when first seen and may require immediate therapy. More often the patient is stable enough that pericardiocentesis (or another therapeutic procedure) can be performed under controlled conditions. In many cases of nontraumatic effusion, tamponade does not occur and the effusion may resolve with treatment of the underlying disease or may be managed successfully by pericardiocentesis.

The cause of nontraumatic tamponade may not be obvious on examination in the emergency department, and tamponade is frequently misdiagnosed as congestive heart failure or respiratory disease. There are many causes of nontraumatic pericardial effusion (see Tables 16–1 and 16–2). Nontraumatic effusions can be of tremendous size, because their gradual development over weeks or months usually allows time for the pericardium to stretch to accommodate the fluid.[33, 34] The pericardium is not able to stretch immediately, although there is a minor relaxation effect within minutes after the first increase in intrapericardial pressure, which slightly decreases pressure.[35]

Cancer is a prominent cause of nontraumatic effusions; the pericardium is involved in 20 per cent of patients with disseminated tumors[1] and 8 per cent of all patients with cancer.[36] There is primary pericardial involvement in 69 per

Table 16-2. Etiology of Pericardial Effusion in Two Studies

	Krikorian[11] (120 patients) (%)	Guberman[10] (56 patients) (%)
Neoplastic disease	—	32
Pericardial invasion	16	—
Radiation pericarditis	7.5	4
Etiology uncertain	18	—
Traumatic hemopericardium	9	—
Hemopericardium, nontraumatic	2.5	—
Rheumatic disease	12	2
Uremia/dialysis	5	9
Bacterial infection	2.5	12.5
Congestive heart failure (CHF)	1.5	—
Uncertain etiology	12.5	—
Idiopathic pericarditis	13.5	14
Cardiac infarction	—	—
Iatrogenic diagnostic procedures	—	7.5
Myxedema	—	4
Aneurysm	—	4
Anticoagulation and cardiac disease	—	11
Postpericardiotomy	—	2

cent of acute leukemias, in 64 per cent of malignant melanomas, and in 24 per cent of lymphomas; however, the incidence of actual tamponade in these malignancies is not known. Of metastases to the pericardium, 35 per cent originate in the lung, 35 per cent in the breast, 15 per cent in lymphomas, and less than 3 per cent in each of the other cancers.[36] Thus any patient who is known to have one of these malignancies should be considered at risk for tamponade. Metastasis to the heart is usually a late finding in cancer, and other foci located elsewhere are usually evident.[37] Classic findings of tamponade, such as pulsus paradoxus, are frequently absent in cancer patients with tamponade, and their symptoms are usually attributed to their malignancy.[36]

Radiation pericarditis, particularly after treatment for Hodgkin's disease, is a common cause of effusion.[32] Effusion occurs in approximately 5 per cent of those patients who receive 4000 rads to the heart.

Cardiac tamponade was the presenting manifestation of pericarditis in 81 per cent of Guberman and coworkers' patients; however, most of those patients also had chest pain. Thirty per cent of myxedema patients may have pericardial effusions, but few have tamponade.[10]

Approximately 15 to 20 per cent of patients on dialysis for renal failure develop pericarditis, and 35 per cent of those with pericarditis develop tamponade.[38, 39] Up to 7 per cent of patients on chronic dialysis may have effusions, sometimes of a liter or more.[39] Some series have reported tamponade in 34 per cent of uremic patients who have effusions.[39] Pericardial effusion in renal failure may be managed with dialysis alone in many cases (discussed later).

Most of the other etiologies listed in Table 16-1 are isolated case reports, and their exact incidences have not been determined.

PATHOPHYSIOLOGY OF TAMPONADE

The pericardium is a tough, leathery sac that encloses the heart. The pericardium is not elastic, although it does demonstrate stress relaxation within minutes of increased intrapericardial pressure, providing a slight ability to accommodate sudden increases in fluid.[35] With chronic effusions over weeks, the pericardium lengthens circumferentially to a huge size and can accommodate liters of fluid. Pericardial compliance varies considerably in different individuals and disease states. This compliance helps to determine the pressure-volume response curves shown in Figures 16–1 and 16–2.[40]

The pericardial sac normally contains about 25 to 35 ml of serous fluid.[40] As more fluid accumulates, the first 80 to 120 ml are easily accommodated without significantly affecting pericardial pressure (see Fig. 16–1).[41] An additional 20 to 40 ml, however, almost doubles the intrapericardial pressure, often leading to sudden decompensation. This pressure-volume relationship demonstrates hysteresis; the withdrawal of a quantity of fluid drops the pressure more than its addition raised it (see Fig. 16–2).[33] For example, adding 160 ml of fluid raises pressure about 9 mm Hg, but only 80 ml has to be removed to return the pressure to the original value.[1]

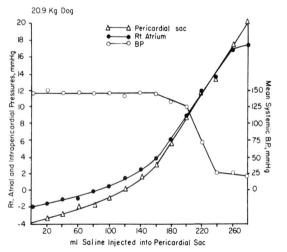

Figure 16–1. Production of cardiac tamponade by injections of saline into the pericardial sac. Note steep increases in pressure and drop in blood pressure at about 200 ml of saline. (From Fowler NO: Physiology of cardiac tamponade and pulsus paradoxus. II: physiological, circulatory, and pharmacological responses in cardiac tamponade. Mod Concepts Cardiovasc Dis 47:116, 1978. Reproduced by permission of the American Heart Association, Inc.)

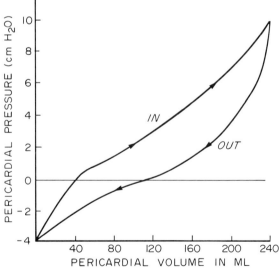

Figure 16–2. Relationship of intrapericardial pressure to volume of pericardial fluid. Note that pressure drops more rapidly when fluid is removed than when it accumulates. (From Pories W, Gaudiani V: Cardiac tamponade. Surg Clin North Am 55:573, 1975. Reproduced by permission.)

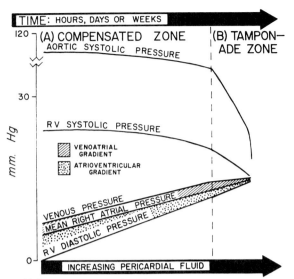

Figure 16–3. Summary of physiologic changes in tamponade. *RV*, right ventricle. (From Shoemaker WC, Carey SJ, Yao ST, et al: Hemodynamic monitoring for physiological evaluation, diagnosis, and therapy of acute hemopericardial tamponade from penetrating wounds; and Spodick D: Acute cardiac tamponade: Pathologic physiology, diagnosis, and management. Prog Cardiovasc Dis 10:65, 1967. Reproduced by permission.)

As fluid accumulates, the increased intrapericardial pressure is transmitted across the myocardial wall and causes compression of the atria and perhaps the vena cava and pulmonary veins. This reduces right ventricular filling in diastole, with a resultant decreased stroke volume and cardiac output.[42–44] A change in intrapericardial pressure of 10 mm Hg produces significant tamponade and can cause a 60 per cent decrease in cardiac output.[45] Severe tamponade is produced with intrapericardial pressures of only 15 to 20 mm Hg.[46] The increased atrial pressure is reflected in increased CVP. Pulse pressure narrows as reflex sympathetic stimulation increases. In chronic effusion and in early tamponade, cardiac contractility is not affected.[42, 47]

Because stroke volume is decreased, heart rate increases to maintain cardiac output. Sympathetic discharge causes both arterial and venous vasoconstriction.[44, 48] Vasoconstriction increases venous pressure, which helps to restore the normal venous-atrial and atrioventricular filling gradients. These mechanisms are often very effective and may permit establishment of a new homeostasis with normal cardiac output.

Increased pericardial pressure also decreases coronary perfusion pressure, so in its later stages, tamponade is an ischemic event for the heart. Ischemia is not significant in early tamponade when systemic blood pressure is still well maintained.[49] However, by the time hypotension is measurable, left ventricular blood flow has already decreased 37 per cent.[50] There is a proportionally greater drop in subendocardial blood flow compared with subepicardial blood flow. For comparable degrees of hypotension, experimental animals in hemorrhagic shock have five times greater coronary blood flow than animals in cardiac tamponade.[50] This ischemia of the myocardium decreases contractility and diastolic relaxation, which further impedes diastolic coronary perfusion. Acute severe experimental tamponade is followed by large increases in creative kinase-MB and microscopic evidence of cardiac injury due to ischemia.[51] Furthermore, the increased sympathetic discharge increases cardiac work and oxygen consumption, hastening the time to electromechanical dissociation and cardiovascular collapse; this effect can be reversed by propranolol.[52]

As intrapericardial pressure continues to rise, the heart's compensatory mechanisms fail. Myocardial ischemia and perhaps lactic acidosis from poor tissue perfusion may be the triggering event that disrupts the uneasy equilibrium.[53] Atrial pressure rises rapidly (Fig. 16–3; also see Fig. 16–1). The atria and pulmonary circulation, being at much lower pressure than the systemic arterial pressure, are more vulnerable to the rising intrapericardial pressure. A "pressure plateau" occurs in which right atrial pressure, right ventricular diastolic pressure, pulmonary artery diastolic pressure, and pulmonary capillary wedge pressure are virtually identical. In fact, the diagnosis of tamponade should not be made if the filling pressure of the two sides of the heart differs by much more than 2 to 3 mm Hg.[46] The exception to this is the patient with reduced left ventricular diastolic compliance and increased left ventricular diastolic pressure, such as the dialysis patient, who can have tamponade with unequal pressures in the two sides of the heart.

This equalization of pressures leads to the echocardiographic hallmark of tamponade, right ventricular collapse. At this point hypotension is severe, bradycardia is common, and so-called electromechanical dissociation (EMD) may occur (although arterial pressure monitoring will show a pulse). Unless intrapericardial pressure is immediately decreased, pulmonary blood flow ceases and cardiac arrest follows.[53]

Total blood volume intimately affects cardiac compensation, and it is possible to encounter a "low pressure" cardiac tamponade. The hypovolemic patient with tamponade will have a decreased venous pressure. This not only decreases cardiac output but also may obscure the diagnosis, because distended neck veins or an elevated CVP will not be present (Fig. 16–4). Conversely, increasing blood volume in hypovolemia will increase CVP enough to provide a higher filling pressure, thus, at least temporarily, offsetting increased intrapericardial and ventricular pressure. In a patient with a chronic pericardial effusion, the onset of hypovolemia can lower filling pressure enough to precipitate tamponade. The result is tamponade in the presence of low right atrial pressure and low CVP, despite the fact that tamponade is usually associated with an elevated CVP.[54]

Effects of CO₂ Levels in Tamponade

Ventilation, and blood carbon dioxide levels, have significant effects in cardiac tamponade. This is of particular

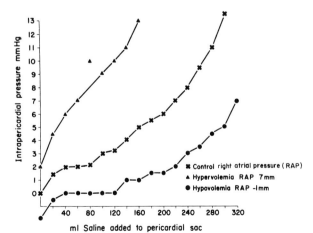

Figure 16–4. Experimental pericardial pressure-volume curve in three states: control, hypovolemia, and hypervolemia. (From Fowler NO: Physiology of cardiac tamponade and pulsus paradoxus. II: physiological, circulatory, and pharmacological responses in cardiac tamponade. Mod Concepts Cardiovasc Dis 47:117, 1978. Reproduced by permission of the American Heart Association, Inc.)

Table 16–3. Shoemaker System of Grading Cardiac Tamponade

Grade	Pericardial Volume (ml)	Cardiac Index	Stroke Index	Mean Arterial Pressure	CVP	Heart Rate	Beck's Triad
I	< 200	normal or ↑	normal or ↓	normal	↑	↑	Venous distention, hypotension, muffled heart sounds usually not present
II	≥ 200	↓	↓	normal or ↓	↑ (≥ 12 cm H_2O)	↑	May or may not be present
III	> 200	↓ ↓	↓ ↓	↓ ↓	↑ ↑ (up to 30–40 cm H_2O)	↓	Usually present

(From Shoemaker WC, Carey SJ, Yao ST, et al: Hemodynamic monitoring for physiologic evaluation, diagnosis, and therapy of acute hemopericardial tamponade from penetrating wounds. J Trauma 13:36, 1973.)

significance because trauma and other patients with tamponade may also have respiratory impairment. In addition, such patients often need intubation, mandatory ventilation, and general anesthesia, all of which can have profound effects on cardiac output.[55] Pericardial pressure decreases 3 to 6 mm Hg with hypocarbia of 24 mm Hg, and increases 2 to 4 mm Hg when P_{CO_2} reaches 57 mm Hg.[45] This degree of hypercarbia-induced pericardial pressure rise can decrease cardiac output 25 per cent. Similarly, fluctuations in intrapleural pressure induced by intermittent positive-pressure ventilation are transmitted to the pericardial space and can reduce cardiac output another 25 per cent.[56]

The clinical implications of these findings are that patients suspected of having tamponade should normally be allowed to breathe spontaneously and should not be ventilated with positive pressure unless it is absolutely necessary, as their hemodynamic status may deteriorate precipitously. (This is particularly true of the hypovolemic trauma patient, whose venous return will be additionally impaired by positive-pressure ventilation.) However, blood gases should be monitored meticulously for these patients, and they should not be allowed to become hypercarbic. It is also well known that general anesthesia induction often worsens hypotension, so the suspected tamponade patient who is intubated and induced for anesthesia is at particular risk of hemodynamic collapse. This risk makes the use of preanesthetic "therapeutic" pericardiocentesis an important therapeutic option.

DIAGNOSIS OF CARDIAC TAMPONADE

Patient Profile and Symptoms

The diagnosis of pericardial effusion can be difficult. Pericardial tamponade may be diagnosed on clinical grounds alone, but clinical signs of any kind are often inaccurate. As an example, 37 to 46 per cent of patients with cardiac injury and blood in the pericardial sac had no clinical signs of tamponade.[57, 58] In the setting of potential traumatic tamponade the clinician needs access to cardiac ultrasound to make the diagnosis rapidly.

A number of classical clinical findings are described for tamponade. However, these findings represent the legacy of preultrasound medicine, when effusion and tamponade were routinely diagnosed late and often only when the patient was in extremis. Currently the clinician strives to diagnose tamponade early when the patient suffers no more than dyspnea, weakness, or sometimes right heart failure. A common pitfall is when respiratory symptoms, such as dyspnea on exertion, suggest heart failure or pulmonary pathology, and pericardial effusion is not suspected until the classic late signs appear, including hypotension.[59]

Acute pericardial tamponade may resemble tension pneumothorax, acute hemothorax, hypovolemia, pulmonary edema, or pulmonary embolism. The patient is often agitated or panic stricken, confused, uncooperative, restless, cyanotic, diaphoretic, and acutely short of breath. In the late stages, the patient is moribund. Hypotension in the presence of severe cyanosis and distended neck veins is a helpful finding, but diagnosis of tamponade on purely clinical grounds may be difficult to ascertain. When the patient is rapidly deteriorating in a clinical setting that does not immediately bring tamponade to mind (e.g., aortic dissection or CVP catheter eroded into the pericardial sac), the diagnosis is easily overlooked until it is too late.

Physical Signs

The classic physical findings of tamponade were first characterized by Beck in 1935. He described two triads, one for acute and one for chronic compression.[60] The chronic compression triad consists of high CVP, ascites, and a small, quiet heart. The triad in acute compression consists of high CVP, decreased arterial pressure, and muffled heart sounds. Unfortunately, in most major trauma series, only about one third of the patients demonstrate the complete acute triad,[53, 61] although almost 90 per cent have one or more signs.[3] The simultaneous occurrence of all three physical signs is a very late manifestation of tamponade and is usually seen only shortly before cardiac arrest (see Fig. 16–3).

Careful hemodynamic monitoring reveals much earlier changes that indicate the progression of tamponade (Table 16–3).[62] In grade I tamponade, cardiac output and arterial pressure are normal, but CVP and heart rate are increased. In grade II tamponade, blood pressure is normal or slightly decreased, CVP is increased, and tachycardia persists. In grade III tamponade, the classic findings of Beck's acute triad occur. Although this sequence represents the natural history of acute tamponade, the time course varies. Some patients are stable at a given stage for hours; others proceed to cardiac arrest within minutes.[53, 62]

The clinical diagnosis of tamponade requires a high index of suspicion and careful evaluation using the physical signs and imaging techniques described below. Two-dimensional echocardiography represents the ultimate standard for diagnosis.

PULSUS PARADOXUS

Pulsus paradoxus is defined as an exaggeration of the normal inspiratory fall in blood pressure.[48, 61] A paradoxical pulse (pressure) is one of the classic physical signs of tamponade, but it is not pathognomonic. It is also caused by

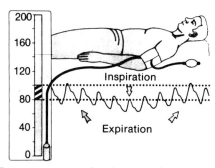

Figure 16–5. Measurement of pulsus paradoxus. (From Stein L, Shubin H, Weil M: Recognition and management of pericardial tamponade. JAMA 225:504, 1973. Copyright 1973, American Medical Association. Reproduced by permission.)

pulmonary emphysema, asthma, labored respirations, obesity, cardiac failure, constrictive pericarditis, pulmonary embolism, and cardiogenic shock.[3, 33, 53] To measure a paradoxical pulse, the patient should be lying comfortably, at a 30- to 45-degree angle, breathing normally and in an unlabored fashion—unusual conditions in a patient suspected of cardiac tamponade.[48] The blood pressure cuff is inflated well above systolic pressure and slowly deflated until one first hears the systolic sounds that are synchronous with expiration (Fig. 16–5). Initially, one will hear the arterial pulse only during expiration, and it will disappear during inspiration. The cuff is then further deflated until arterial sounds are heard throughout the respiratory cycle. If the difference between these two pressures is greater than 10 mm Hg, the paradoxical pulse is considered significant (abnormal). Most patients with proven tamponade will have a difference of 20 to 30 mm Hg or more during the respiratory cycle,[3, 33, 53] but this absolute figure is not reliable. Patients with very narrow pulse pressures (typical of grade III tamponade) will have a deceptively "small" paradoxical pulse of 5 to 15 mm Hg. This occurs because the paradoxical pulse is a function of actual pulse pressure, and the inspiratory systolic pressure may be below the level at which diastolic sounds disappear.[48] For this reason, the ratio of paradoxical pulse to the pulse pressure is a more reliable measure. A paradoxical pulse greater than 50 per cent of the pulse pressure is abnormal.[48]

The mechanism of pulsus paradoxus is unknown, but two physiologic principles have traditionally been thought to be contributory factors. During inspiration, blood is preferentially drawn into the right ventricle. This increase in right ventricular volume shifts the intraventricular septum to the left, and, by this shift in the septum, the compression of the left ventricle may decrease left ventricular filling enough to diminish left ventricular outflow. Second, with inspiration, blood pools in the pulmonary veins, thereby reducing left ventricular filling enough to have an effect on left ventricular output. Pressure in the pericardial space secondary to pericardial fluid may accentuate these normal physiologic events enough to be clinically evident.

Measuring the paradoxical pulse is difficult and time consuming, and any frightened, hypotensive patient with labored breathing can have it. Although the mean paradoxical pulse was 49 mm Hg in one series of nontraumatic tamponade,[10] 23 per cent of the patients had a paradoxical pulse of less than 20 mm Hg and one had no measurable paradoxical pulse. One half of the uremic patients with tamponade had no abnormal pulsus paradoxus, because these patients typically have poor left ventricular compliance and often do not demonstrate the equalization of heart pressures normally seen in tamponade.[39, 46]

An abnormal pulsus paradoxus has been reported to be absent in tamponade when there is an atrial septal defect,

aortic insufficiency, localized collections of pericardial blood, extreme tamponade with hypotension, or when left ventricular diastolic pressure is intrinsically elevated (owing to poor left ventricular compliance).[54] In traumatic tamponade, it is deemed unreliable.[3, 46, 63, 64] In one study, only 35 per cent of trauma patients had an abnormal paradoxical pulse when elevated CVP and decreased heart sounds were present.[64] In another study of 197 traumatic cases, only 8.6 per cent of the diagnoses of tamponade were made by finding an abnormal pulsus paradoxus.[65]

Absolute pulsus paradoxus has been correlated with cardiac output and the severity of tamponade.[66] The correlation with cardiac output is 0.87, about the same as the correlation with intrapericardial pressure and stroke volume.[67] Based on this data, the upper 95 per cent confidence interval limit for normal pulsus paradoxus is 12 mm Hg systolic.[66] This limit had an accuracy of about 90 per cent in separating patients with tamponade from those without. Even more useful was the correlation between the degree of pulsus paradoxus and the amount of impairment of cardiac output by tamponade (Fig. 16–6). This study of patients without trauma demonstrated that the absence of a measurable pulsus paradoxus is fairly strong evidence against tamponade, and certainly strong evidence against severe impairment of cardiac output due to tamponade. A similar study of right ventricular diastolic collapse by echocardiography found that an abnormal pulsus paradoxus had a sensitivity of 79 per cent, specificity of 40 per cent, positive predictive value of 81 per cent, and negative predictive value of 40 per cent.[67] All these values were markedly inferior to the accuracy of echocardiography, but nonetheless the degree of pulsus paradoxus correlates with the degree of hemodynamic compromise.

A paradoxical pulse can be palpated if it is very large; during palpation, the pulse may completely disappear during inspiration. When present, this technique is a quick bedside confirmation of the possibility of severe tamponade. Palpation for this purpose is best done at peripheral arteries such as the radial or femoral. If arterial pressure monitors are already in place, paradoxical pulse can be measured rapidly and accurately. The absence of a paradoxical pulse rules against severe tamponade, but does not completely rule it out. Whether time is taken to determine pulsus paradoxus depends on the patient's status. If the patient is moribund or rapidly deteriorating, taking time to check is obviously a poor choice of priorities.

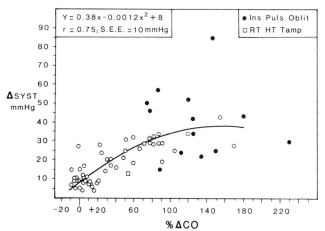

Figure 16–6. Relationship between pulsus paradoxus and per cent change in cardiac output. *Closed circle,* inspiratory pulse obliteration; *open square,* right heart tamponade only. (From Curtiss E, Reddy P, Uretsky B, Cecchetti A: Pulsus paradoxus: Definition and relation to the severity of cardiac tamponade. Am Heart J 115:391, 1988. Reproduced by permission.)

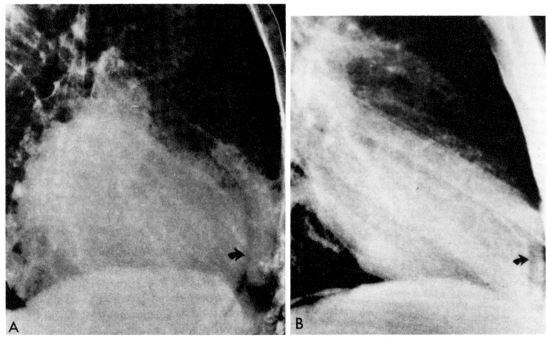

Figure 16–7. Epicardial fat pad sign. The water-density space between the radiolucent epicardial fat and the mediastinal fat represents the pericardium and its contents and should be 2 mm or less. An increase suggests pericardial fluid or thickening. *A,* Left anterior-oblique chest film. *B,* Lateral chest film.

VENOUS DISTENTION

Venous distention, reflecting increased CVP, is also a late sign in cardiac tamponade (see Fig. 16–3). It may be masked by venoconstriction due to vasopressors (such as dopamine), intrinsic sympathetic discharge, or hypovolemia.[33, 53, 62, 63] Neck vein distention may be obvious clinically, but the measured CVP is more reliable than the presence of venous distention. A CVP line may be placed immediately in all patients who have penetrating chest trauma, and the position should be verified by radiologic examination. The CVP reading should take into account positive-pressure ventilation and the effects of a Valsalva maneuver. Most patients with significant tamponade will have a CVP of 12 to 14 cm H_2O or greater.[63] *Hypovolemia changes the intrapericardial pressure-volume curve in tamponade and will lower the CVP reading at any given stage in the tamponade process.*

Animal studies have documented that right atrial pressure can be normal in tamponade when hypovolemia is present. One case of low-pressure cardiac tamponade was reported in a patient with no jugular venous distention, no paradoxical pulse, and a right atrial pressure of 8 mm Hg.[54] Thus although the initial CVP reading is useful and diagnostic if grossly elevated—for example, 20 to 30 cm H_2O[29, 63] —it is actually the trend of CVP readings that is the most sensitive diagnostic tool.[63] A rising CVP, especially when there is persistent hypotension, is extremely suggestive of tamponade in the trauma patient. In the rare case of the hypovolemic patient who is suspected of tamponade but who demonstrates a low CVP, a fluid challenge will help clarify the situation and will also improve the cardiac output at least temporarily.[54]

Chest Radiographs

Chest radiographs are not useful in the diagnosis of acute traumatic tamponade, because the cardiac size and shape does not change acutely. They may, however, reveal hemothorax, bullet location, or even pneumopericardium.

In the unstable trauma patient with clinical tamponade, time should not be wasted obtaining films. In the nontrauma patient with chronic effusion, a chest film will often reveal an enlarged sac-like "water bottle" cardiac shadow. Unfortunately, radiographic findings cannot accurately differentiate pericardial from myocardial enlargement, nor can they distinguish between simple pericardial effusion and tamponade. The value of a chest film is that it may suggest the diagnosis (to those with a low level of suspicion) and indicate further investigation.

Another useful finding on the plain chest film is the epicardial fat pad sign, seen in 41 per cent of lateral and 23 per cent of frontal chest films in proven pericardial effusion.[68] The water-density space between the radiolucent epicardial fat and the mediastinal fat represents the pericardial tissues and is normally less than 2 mm. An increase in this width suggests pericardial fluid or thickening (Fig. 16–7).

Electrocardiogram

The electrocardiogram is seldom of diagnostic value, because most changes of tamponade, such as altered ST segments, low-voltage QRS complexes, and T inversions, are nonspecific.[33] If low voltage is defined as the sum of the limb lead QRS amplitudes being 30 mm or less, this test has a sensitivity of 55 per cent and a specificity of 67 per cent for effusions of 300 to 700 ml, and 68 per cent and 75 per cent, respectively, for effusions greater than 700 ml.[69] If low voltage is defined as 5 mm or less in each limb lead, the sensitivity is 32 per cent and specificity 83 per cent for smaller effusions, and 44 per cent and 92 per cent, respectively, for the larger ones.[69] However, none of these findings differentiate tamponade from effusion.

Electrical alternans is caused by pendular motion of the heart within the pericardial sac.[70] Alternans of the QRS complex was seen in about 22 per cent of medical tamponade cases[59] but only 5 per cent of cancer patients with tamponade.[36] Electrical alternans of both the P wave and the QRS complex (total electrical alternans) is a rare finding but, when seen, is thought to be pathognomonic of tamponade (Fig. 16–8).[33, 71] Alternans does not always appear in the standard electrocardiograph (ECG) leads; a bipolar chest lead (Lewis lead) may be needed to detect it. Electromechanical dissociation and profound bradycardia are terminal events, and one hopes that the physician observing such findings would already have pericardiocentesis needle or scalpel in hand.[72]

Echocardiography

Echocardiography is the gold standard for diagnosing pericardial effusion, and has the further advantage of being noninvasive. The availability of echocardiography and skilled interpretation vary from institution to institution; however, when it is available, echocardiography is a benign, noninvasive procedure that can rapidly determine the presence of an effusion and tamponade with great accuracy.[73] In one series, 42 per cent of patients with an echocardiographically proven diagnosis of tamponade had not had the diagnosis made clinically before echocardiography.[59] Pericardiocentesis guided by echocardiography has a much lower complication rate than traditional pericardiocentesis.[74]

The disadvantages of echocardiography are that it takes the availability of ultrasound equipment and at least a moderately skilled operator. In most hospitals, it is difficult to obtain cardiac ultrasound on short notice, particularly during evening and weekend hours. Even when immediately available, echocardiography takes at least 5 to 10 minutes, which may be too much time for patients who are deteriorating rapidly.

One article has described the use of ultrasound in emergency situations by emergency physicians.[75] It does not take much training to recognize a large pericardial effusion, but many of the signs of tamponade are much more subtle. The accuracy of diagnosis by nonechocardiographers is completely unstudied and should be viewed with caution. The physician wishing to learn echocardiography for emergency purposes would be wise to obtain formal training before entrusting the patient's outcome to his or her interpretations.

Although M-mode ultrasound was originally used, it has been largely supplanted by two-dimensional echo for diagnosis of pericardial effusion and tamponade.[74–77] The diagnosis of effusion is easily made by visualizing a large area of fluid, often best seen behind the heart. This view will also demonstrate the ventricular wall, and quickly distinguishes the patient with a large effusion and tamponade from the patient with congestive heart failure and a dilated ventricle. However, effusion is not synonymous with tamponade, and the volume of fluid needed to produce tamponade in an individual depends on the thickness of the ventricular myocardium, the rate of fluid accumulation, and the thickness of the pericardium. The diagnosis of actual tamponade is best made on the observation of right ventricular diastolic collapse, which only occurs during tamponade and is accompanied by significant hemodynamic compromise.[78, 79] Right ventricular collapse has a sensitivity of 93 per cent, specificity of 100 per cent, positive predictive value of 100 per cent, and negative predictive value of 83 per cent for the presence of cardiac tamponade.[67] The duration of collapse is proportional to the hemodynamic compromise; for example, it has a negative correlation of 0.992 with stroke volume and 0.899 with cardiac output.[67] However, it should be noted that right ventricular diastolic collapse will not occur in the presence of severe right ventricular hypertrophy.[78] This once again emphasizes the fact that echocardiographic diagnosis of tamponade requires considerable expertise and the ability to identify more than simple pericardial effusion.

Other useful echocardiographic suggestions of tamponade are observing the heart swinging rhythmically in the pericardial effusion, excessive respiratory variation in the size of the ventricles, greatly decreased right ventricular size, and pseudoprolapse of the mitral valve.[46]

Echocardiography has become equally useful in directing pericardiocentesis itself. With ultrasound, the area of the heart with the greatest fluid accumulation can be accurately identified, and its relationship to the body wall clarified.[77, 80] An entry site and angle of penetration can then be chosen that has the greatest likelihood of obtaining fluid while simultaneously avoiding vital structures. Without ultrasound, pericardiocentesis is blind, and vital structures are vulnerable to injury (see "Complications"). Echo-directed pericardiocentesis series suggest that the intercostal space near the heart apex is usually the best site for puncture, rather than the traditional subxiphoid approach.[80] Echocardiography also allows identification of loculated fluid and localized accumulations, which are quite common; solid material (such as tumor) within the pericardial sac can be identified and avoided. Ultrasound is used to decide on the angle of approach and can also be used to identify when the needle tip enters the pericardial space, but visualizing the needle with ultrasound is difficult and cannot be relied on to avoid complications.[76]

The risk of performing pericardiocentesis without echocardiographic determination of pericardial fluid is shown in the Krikorian series.[11] Of patients with a clinical picture of tamponade, 17 per cent actually had constrictive pericarditis, 16 per cent had congestive heart failure and fluid overload, and 5 per cent had obstruction of the superior vena cava. None of these patients could be expected to benefit from pericardiocentesis and all were at risk for complications.

Rarely, echocardiography may reveal a pericardial effusion but not clearly diagnose tamponade (e.g., in dialysis patients). In this case it may be helpful to directly measure pericardial, right atrial and systemic arterial pressure, and cardiac output before and after removal of pericardial fluid by pericardiocentesis.[46]

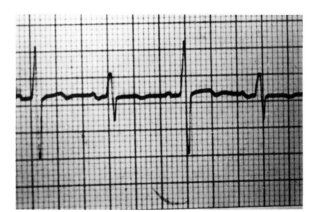

Figure 16–8. Lewis lead electrocardiogram showing total electrical alternans of both amplitude and configuration of P and QRS complexes. This is pathognomonic of tamponade. (From Sotolongo RP, Horton JD: Total electrical alternans in pericardial tamponade. Am Heart J 101:854, 1981. Reproduced by permission.)

Other Imaging Techniques

Fluoroscopy, radiograph contrast techniques, and radioisotope techniques have been used but are too slow and difficult to arrange for emergency purposes. These techniques have all been supplanted by echocardiography.

INDICATIONS FOR PERICARDIOCENTESIS

There are two indications for pericardiocentesis: (1) to diagnose the cause or presence of a pericardial effusion and (2) to relieve tamponade.

Diagnostic Pericardiocentesis

The use of pericardiocentesis for diagnosis of the etiology of nontraumatic effusions is widespread and frequently recommended.[32, 81] Neoplastic cells, blood, bacteria, and chyle can be sought. pH can be helpful because inflammatory fluid is significantly more acidotic than noninflammatory.[82]

The results of a large series of pericardiocenteses for nontraumatic effusions cast some doubt on diagnostic accuracy, however. Although fluid was obtained in 90 per cent of the taps, specific etiologic diagnoses were obtained from only 24 per cent of the fluid specimens.[11] In patients with normal venous pressure, only 14 per cent of the taps provided a diagnosis.[11] Fluid was falsely negative for cytology in several cases of lymphoma and mesothelioma. Overall it was concluded that although 68 per cent of the patients with elevated venous pressure benefited in some hemodynamic manner from the procedure, only 11 per cent of those with normal venous pressure received any benefit. There were several complications, including death, delays of surgery, purulent pericarditis, hemopericardium secondary to the procedure, and ventricular tachycardia. The risks were thought to exceed those of other methods of diagnosis.

By comparison, subxiphoid pericardiotomy seems to be a much safer technique than pericardiocentesis and involves few major complications in experienced hands. Pericardial biopsy provides a definite diagnosis in virtually all cases and can be obtained safely without general anesthesia by this method.[83, 84] Some investigators believe that diagnostic pericardiocentesis is inappropriate and that pericardiocentesis is indicated only for the emergency relief of tamponade.[85]

The use of pericardiocentesis to make a definitive diagnosis of traumatic tamponade is inappropriate. As a diagnostic measure to determine the presence of pericardial bleeding in trauma, the procedure has a false-negative rate of between 20 and 40 per cent.[5, 63, 64, 86–88] An "inconclusive" tap is one in which no fluid is obtained (although many researchers have equated a dry tap with a negative tap). A true negative tap recovers a few milliliters of clear serous fluid, but such fluid is almost never obtained because of the very small amount of fluid that is normally present in the pericardial sac. The reason for the high false-negative rate (defined as no blood aspirated) is well demonstrated by typical stab wounds of the heart.[5, 89] Ninety-six per cent of the patients had blood in the pericardium, but it was clotted in 41 per cent of the patients and partially clotted in another 24 per cent. In only 19 per cent was the blood completely fluid and thus capable of giving a true-positive result on pericardiocentesis. Obviously, pericardiocentesis will be negative in the presence of clotted blood, and it will fail to fully relieve tamponade when the tamponade is secondary to clotted blood.

Therapeutic Pericardiocentesis

TAMPONADE CAUSED BY NONTRAUMATIC EFFUSIONS

Pericardiocentesis is often at least temporarily therapeutic in cardiac tamponade, and can be life saving. Most nontraumatic effusions are liquids that can be drained easily through a small needle. Removal of even a small amount of fluid can immediately and dramatically improve blood pressure and cardiac output (Fig. 16–9). Pericardiocentesis relieves tamponade due to nontraumatic effusions in 60 to 90 per cent of the cases.[10, 11, 36] Patients in whom it failed often had purulent pericarditis or malignant invasion of the pericardium; the latter can be detected by echocardiography in advance. In these patients subxiphoid pericardiotomy may be preferable.

Pericardiocentesis is much less useful for long-term management of these patients; 26 per cent of the patients in Guberman's series eventually required pericardial resection.[10] In Krikorian's series, 24 per cent of the patients were managed successfully with one pericardiocentesis, 37 per cent needed multiple taps or an indwelling catheter, and 39 per cent required surgical drainage. Fifty-five per cent of the last-mentioned group had traumatic hemopericardium.

Patients with renal failure may be better managed by methods other than pericardiocentesis. Approximately 7 per cent of all dialysis patients will develop a large pericardial effusion. In one series, 63 per cent of these patients were successfully managed with dialysis alone, and only 6 per cent needed surgical treatment over the long term.[11] Tamponade is less frequent with pericarditis when it occurs within the first months of dialysis, and such patients are much more likely to be successfully managed without invasive interven-

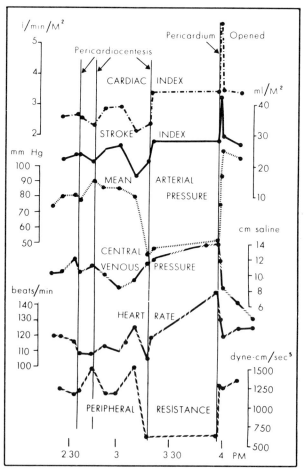

Figure 16–9. Effect of pericardiocentesis in a patient with tamponade. On two of the three occasions, pericardiocentesis was productive of 30 ml of nonclotting blood, with favorable effects on hemodynamic parameters. (From Shoemaker WC: Algorithm for early recognition and management of cardiac tamponade. Crit Care Med 3:62, 1975. © 1975, Williams & Wilkins.)

tion.[38] Dialysis should be tried first; invasive treatment is usually needed if echocardiography shows either progression of the effusion over several weeks or persistence of anterior or posterior effusion.[38] Patients with a temperature higher than 102° F, rales, blood pressure less than 100 mm Hg systolic, jugular venous distention, and leukocytosis are less likely to respond to dialysis, but the echocardiographic findings of large effusion and anterior plus posterior effusion are more accurate predictors of dialysis failure than all these factors.[90] When invasive treatment is needed, pericardiocentesis is probably a poor choice; nine of ten patients who received it had complications in one series, and it was the only invasive treatment that resulted in death.[38]

In summary, pericardiocentesis is therapeutic in many patients with nontraumatic tamponade, because their effusions are more frequently liquid and are more easily tapped. Ultrasound when available should be obtained first in these patients to ensure accurate diagnosis and optimal anatomic approach. Pericardiocentesis generally should be performed under controlled situations, such as in a catheterization lab or intensive care unit, under ultrasound guidance. Uremic patients may be more safely managed by dialysis. An algorithm for the emergency management of nontraumatic cardiac tamponade is shown in Figure 16–10.

USE IN TRAUMATIC TAMPONADE

In distinct contrast to its significant role in the therapy of nontraumatic tamponade, pericardiocentesis may be misleading or perhaps even dangerous in traumatic effusion. The high incidence of pericardial clots has already been discussed. Failure to obtain fluid does not rule out pericardial bleeding, and the false-negative rate in trauma is high.

Even if the pericardiocentesis confirms the suspicion of pericardial bleeding, it is never definitive treatment in traumatic tamponade.[91, 92] Although aspiration of a small quantity of fluid may cause dramatic improvement, blood usually reaccumulates.[33, 71] Repeated taps will be necessary, increasing the risk of complications. A plastic catheter may be left in place, but it cannot prevent or remove intrapericardial clots. Such a catheter may give a false sense of security. A positive tap does not provide information regarding the size or nature of the cardiac injury. Thus, ultimately, patients with pericardial hemorrhage require thoracotomy to explore and repair the cardiac wound.

One of the greatest potential drawbacks of pericardiocentesis in traumatic tamponade is that significant time may be spent with nondefinitive therapy, either delaying thoracotomy or creating a false sense of security. In one study of 25 trauma patients with cardiac injury,[91] all those who were operated on within 2 hours of injury survived, regardless of age or type of wound. With greater delay, none survived. Sugg and colleagues, in a study of 459 similar patients, found a mortality rate of 43 per cent when pericardiocentesis was the sole treatment but a mortality rate of only 16 per cent when surgery was performed.[87] Most investigators agree that with early thoracotomy and little or no reliance on pericardiocentesis the number of deaths due to stab wounds has decreased.[5, 13, 63, 86, 88, 92, 93] Mortality rates dropped from 26 to 5 per cent in one series.[87]

With a similar change in approach, Symbas and coworkers reported a drop in the mortality rate, from 17.6 per cent when relying heavily on pericardiocentesis to 5 per cent with surgery, using pericardiocentesis only to gain time.[3] By comparison, Sugg and associates report that 10 of 18 patients with traumatic tamponade who were managed by repeated

Figure 16–10. Management of *nontraumatic* cardiac tamponade. *IV,* intravenous line; *CVP,* central venous pressure; *ECG,* electrocardiogram.

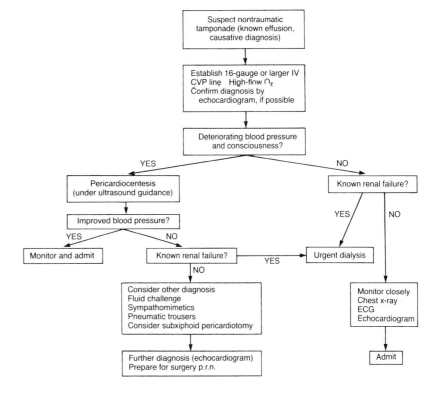

pericardiocentesis alone died within 1 to 2 hours.[87] At autopsy, all patients had completely repairable wounds.

Thoracotomy has a low complication rate and low mortality (see Chapter 18).[72, 94] Emergency department thoracotomy can resuscitate 73 per cent of patients with penetrating cardiac injuries and no detectable vital signs or cardiac activity on arrival.[89] Emergency thoracotomy is reported to result in an infection rate of 6.8 per cent or less,[93] with most studies reporting no infection.[3, 70, 87, 89, 92] Thus pericardiocentesis is not an acceptable alternative to rapid surgical treatment.

Pericardiocentesis is, however, the mandated treatment of last resort when the physician is faced with a deteriorating patient, when other treatments have been unsuccessful (Fig. 16–11), when surgical consultation has already been initiated, and when other surgical approaches are not possible for one reason or another. If a patient with clinical signs of tamponade is deteriorating to the stage of unconsciousness as a result of hypotension, cardiac arrest is not far off. At this point, doing nothing is not an option. The emergency physician who is not experienced in emergency thoracotomy must attempt therapeutic pericardiocentesis, because it is the only option available and it may be life saving.

Ideally, pericardiocentesis should be carried out in such a situation before the patient's condition has deteriorated to unconsciousness. Experimental studies have shown that tamponade is an ischemic event for the heart that causes myocardial decompensation, which contributes to the tamponade process.[50, 95] Intrapericardial pressure rapidly exceeds diastolic and even right ventricular systolic pressure. Combined with decreased aortic pressure and tachycardia, this results in reduced coronary flow and ventricular work.[48, 50]

Some clinical evidence supports the usefulness of pericardiocentesis as a temporizing measure while preparing for definitive surgical treatment. In a study of 174 patients with tamponade from penetrating trauma, 96 had operating room (OR) thoracotomy, 44 had emergency department (ED) thoracotomy, and 34 received only pericardiocentesis and were observed.[65] Of those with OR thoracotomy, 68 per cent were hemodynamically unstable and preoperative pericardiocentesis decreased the mortality rate from 25 to 11 per cent. Ninety-one per cent of those with ED thoracotomy were unstable, and prethoracotomy pericardiocentesis decreased the mortality rate from 94 to 63 per cent. Of those observed after pericardiocentesis, 50 per cent were unstable and the mortality rate was 15 per cent. Thirty-five per cent of the latter group had recurrent tamponade, which was treated with repeat pericardiocentesis. (This latter group probably had small cardiac wounds that sealed themselves off without surgery.)

Pericardiocentesis has no role as the definitive treatment of traumatic tamponade. Nonetheless, while other temporizing treatments (such as fluid challenge, vasopressors, and perhaps pneumatic antishock garment inflation) are instituted and while arrangements for definitive surgical treatment are being made, pericardiocentesis may help reduce myocardial ischemia and improve the outcome. Pericardiocentesis should be used only to temporize. For the unconscious and hypotensive or agonal patient, emergency thoracotomy is the preferred treatment (see Chapter 18). Subxiphoid pericardiotomy is an alternative only for the relatively stable patient and only in the hands of an experienced physician. *No penetrating trauma victim should die of presumed hypovolemic shock unresponsive to volume therapy without cardiac tamponade first being ruled out.*

CONTRAINDICATIONS

The contraindications to pericardiocentesis are relative, not absolute. They include lack of familiarity with the procedure and its complications, absence of proper equipment (especially monitors, defibrillators, and resuscitation equipment), and the immediate availability of a better treatment modality (e.g., dialysis for uremic patients and immediate surgery for trauma patients). For diagnostic or nonemergency pericardiocentesis, absence of echocardiographic diagnosis is a relative contraindication, because the complication rate increases dramatically under such circumstances.

EQUIPMENT FOR PERICARDIOCENTESIS

Although the procedure can be performed with only a syringe and a spinal needle, electrocardiographic monitoring is desirable. An alligator clamp is used to connect the needle to the V lead of a properly grounded ECG device (Fig. 16–12). Whenever possible, two-dimensional echocardiographic equipment should be used in advance to identify the safest path for the needle.

The traditional needle choice has been a 3- to 5-inch 18-gauge needle, ideally of the spinal type, with an obturator. Recently, the shorter Teflon-sheathed "intracath"-type needle has been used. Alternatively, one can use the Seldinger technique, inserting a plastic catheter over a flexible guide or J wire. With this technique only a small, 18-gauge, thin-walled needle is used for placement of the wire. The catheter (after removal of the accompanying introducer) may be left in place for prolonged drainage if needed.[96, 97]

For drainage of blood, pus, or other viscous effusions, a large catheter such as a 7 to 9 French Cordis sheath should be inserted.[74] Alternatively, the Seldinger technique can be used to insert a radiopaque, 16-gauge, flexible, fenestrated, central venous catheter, which can then be connected to closed suction drainage and left in place for long periods of time.[98] Pigtail catheters with side and end holes, or nephrostomy drainage catheters, can also be used.[97] Multilumen catheter patency can be maintained by very slow continuous flush with heparinized saline solution.[97]

A three-way stopcock may be attached to the needle or catheter to allow removal of more than one syringeful without much movement of the needle. The continuous motion of the heart may require minor changes in needle or catheter position during the procedure. Lengthy or repeat drainage is much safer if the steel needle is withdrawn and a plastic catheter is left in place.

PROCEDURE

All necessary equipment must be checked and laid out in advance. Full resuscitation equipment must be on hand, including a defibrillator. The patient must have an intravenous line in place and be attached to a cardiac monitor. The nonemergency patient may require sedation, but on an emergency basis, pericardiocentesis is usually performed on patients who are already obtunded or unresponsive as a result of low cardiac output. Use of sedation in these patients not only is unnecessary but carries a high risk of hemodynamic or respiratory deterioration. Premedication of the patient with atropine may help to prevent vasovagal reactions. If possible, the presence of pericardial effusion and the optimal anatomic approach should be determined in advance by echocardiography. If surgery may be needed, preparations should already be under way to ensure prompt availability of both an operating room and a surgeon.

If the patient's clinical condition permits, the patient's chest should be elevated at a 45-degree angle to bring the heart closer to the anterior chest wall. If the abdomen is distended because of gastric contents or previous CPR, a

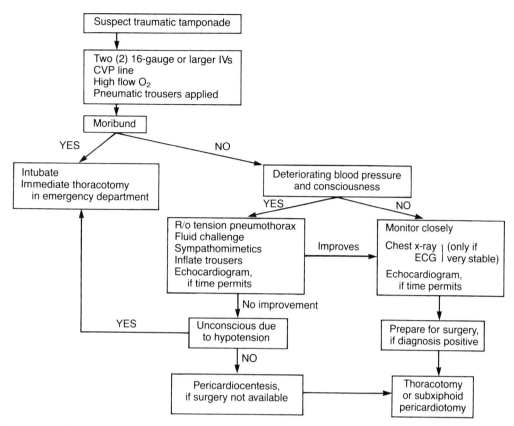

Figure 16–11. Management of *traumatic* cardiac tamponade. *IV*, intravenous lines; *CVP*, central venous pressure; *ECG*, electrocardiogram; *R/O*, rule out.

nasogastric tube should be used to decompress the stomach. The entire lower xiphoid and epigastric area should be carefully prepared with povidone-iodine (10 per cent solution) and sterilely draped, if time permits.

If the patient is awake, the skin and the proposed route of the pericardial needle should be anesthesized by infiltration with 1 per cent plain lidocaine or 0.5 per cent bupivicaine. The pericardium is very sensitive and should be anesthesized in patients who are awake.[96]

The choice of anatomic approach in the past has been governed largely by conjecture and theory, not by actual study of patients with pericardial effusion. The xiphosternal approach was preferred under these considerations and is widely touted in most texts and articles as by far the optimal choice. Two-dimensional echocardiography allows direct visualization in the individual patient of both the areas of maximal effusion and location of vital structures. Studies of echo-directed pericardiocentesis found that the intercostal space near the heart apex is usually the best site for puncture, not the traditional subxiphoid approach.[74, 80] Careful cadaver studies have corroborated this finding, demonstrating greater safety with a parasternal approach in the fifth intercostal space and showing that the greatest number of injuries (usually to the right atrium) occurred with any variant of the subxiphoid approach.[14] Clinicians should consider the intercostal approach the preferred one, but optimal results in an individual patient can only be obtained by performing two-dimensional echocardiography, which should be the standard whenever time and the patient's condition permit.

In the *intercostal approach,* the needle is inserted perpendicular to the skin in the left fifth intercostal space medial to the border of cardiac dullness (Fig. 16–13). It has always been taught that the puncture site should be at least 3 to 4

cm lateral to the sternal border to avoid the internal thoracic artery, but when actual anatomic study was done, it was found that penetration immediately lateral to the sternum was in fact least likely to cause this complication.[14] Previously, it was thought that pneumothorax was more common by this route, or that the left coronary artery or its branches could be lacerated,[33] but more recent echocardiographic and anatomic studies show that this route is the safest in the greatest number of patients.[14, 74, 80] Best results are always obtained when ultrasound is used before pericardiocentesis to identify the maximal areas of effusion and the location of vital structures and their relationship to the body wall in the individual patient.

Another method is the *apical approach;* the needle is

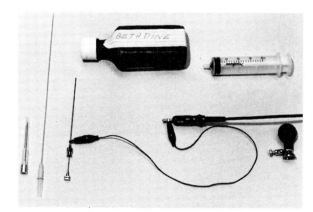

Figure 16–12. Equipment for pericardiocentesis: bactericidal solution (povidone-iodine); long, 18-gauge spinal needle; wire with alligator clips for connection to the electrocardiograph machine; and syringe (three-way stopcock optional). A local anesthetic is also required.

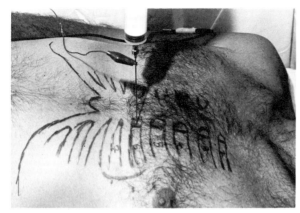

Figure 16–13. Parasternal approach for pericardiocentesis. The patient is depicted in a supine position, although a preferable position would be that of sitting at a 45-degree angle, if the patient's clinical condition permits.

inserted 1 cm outside the apex beat in the intercostal space below it, within the area of cardiac dullness, and aimed toward the right shoulder.[96] If the apex cannot be palpated, the needle is inserted just inside the area of cardiac dullness. This area is very close to the lingula and left pleural space, and pneumothorax is more frequent; a concomitant pleural effusion may be inadvertently tapped. In theory, this technique is used because the coronary vessels are small at the apex, and if the ventricle is entered, it is the thick-walled left ventricle and more likely to seal off any ventricular injury. There are insufficient data to state whether these theoretical advantages are important.

In the traditional *xiphosternal approach* recommended in the preechocardiographic literature, the needle is inserted between the xiphoid process and the left costal margin at a 30- to 45-degree angle to the skin (Fig. 16–14). Because the heart is an anterior structure, an angle greater than 45 degrees may intercept the liver or stomach. In this approach, the needle enters the pericardium at the angle at which it becomes the diaphragmatic pericardium. Recommendations as to where to aim the needle vary from the right shoulder to the left shoulder and all points in between, including the sternal notch.[85, 96] The only anatomic study done demonstrated that in fact the xiphosternal approach is very likely to injure the thin-walled right atrium and that aiming for the right shoulder is much more likely to do this than aiming for the left.[14]

After the skin has been punctured but before the pericardial needle is advanced, ECG monitoring is begun by attaching a sterile cord with alligator clips (see Fig. 16–12) from the pericardial needle to the precordial lead (V lead) of the ECG machine. The V lead is then recorded, as the needle becomes an "exploring electrode." The machine must be properly tested and internally grounded; small current leaks can induce dysrhythmias.[33] The purpose of the ECG monitoring is to prevent ventricular puncture. When the needle touches the epicardium, a current of injury pattern is noted on the ECG (Fig. 16–15). This current of injury may be local and could be missed if a lead other than the V lead is monitored. Usually one notes ST segment elevation on contact with the heart or pericardium in the absence of an effusion, but a premature contraction or other ventricular dysrhythmia may also be induced by the direct mechanical stimulation of the ventricular epicardium by the needle. Contact with the atrium can cause atrial dysrhythmias, marked elevation of the PR segment, or atrioventricular dissociation.[16] If there is abnormal myocardial scarring secondary to infarction or other diseases or if there is malignant

infiltration of myocardium, no current of injury may be generated.[17] Thus ECG monitoring is not infallible in preventing myocardial penetration. In addition, the incessant motion of the heart makes it almost impossible to merely *touch* the epicardium.

In the unlikely event that ECG monitoring is not available and pericardiocentesis must be carried out immediately, one author has suggested placing a large 14-gauge needle over a 20-gauge spinal needle.[99] The pericardium is entered with the small needle; once fluid is aspirated, the large needle is advanced. There seems little justification for this unstudied technique in the era of the Seldinger guide wire method.

With constant ECG monitoring, the operator slowly advances the needle and syringe, aspirating constantly. The needle will penetrate the pericardium (a barrier whose penetration usually cannot be palpated) at about 6 to 8 cm below the skin in adults and 5 cm or less below the skin in children.[40] The patient who is awake may complain of sharp chest pain as the sensitive pericardium is entered. When a current of injury is noted (see Fig. 16–15), the needle is touching epicardium and can easily lacerate myocardium or coronary vessels. The needle should be withdrawn a few millimeters until the current of injury disappears. At this point, the needle should be safely positioned in the pericardial space, although heart motion may quickly bring it back into contact with the myocardium. This is particularly a risk if the presence of a large effusion has not been demonstrated by ultrasound.

An attempt is then made to drain pericardial fluid or blood. If blood is obtained, a hematocrit can be done on both the presumed pericardial sample and venous blood. Hemorrhagic pericardial fluid should have a lower hemato-

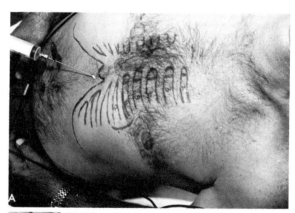

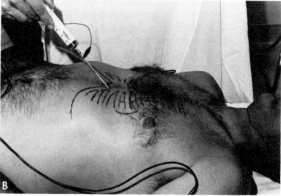

Figure 16–14. Xiphosternal approach for pericardiocentesis. The needle is aimed for the sternal notch or the left shoulder. Note the electrocardiograph monitoring. Although the patient is shown in the supine position, a preferable position would be that of sitting at a 45-degree angle, if the patient's clinical condition permits.

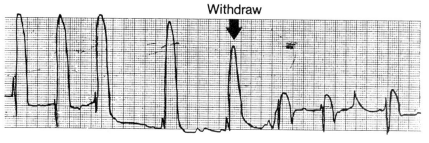

Withdraw

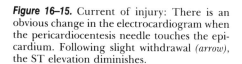

Figure 16–15. Current of injury: There is an obvious change in the electrocardiogram when the pericardiocentesis needle touches the epicardium. Following slight withdrawal *(arrow)*, the ST elevation diminishes.

crit measurement than venous blood, and substantially different values rule out the possibility that the needle was in a cardiac chamber. Hemorrhagic pericardial fluid also usually is about 0.10 pH units more acid than simultaneously obtained arterial blood.[82] Bloody pericardial fluid may clot, particularly in traumatic situations when bleeding is brisk, so clotting of the aspirated blood does not eliminate the possibility of a pericardial source. Nonclotting blood is indicative of defibrinated pericardial blood. Most ventricular punctures during the procedure occur in the lower aspect of the right ventricle. Because the pressure is lower here than in the left ventricle,[40] there should be less bleeding; however, the ventricular wall is also thinner and more vulnerable to laceration.

As much fluid as possible should be aspirated from the pericardium. The removal of even 30 to 50 ml may result in a marked clinical improvement in patients with tamponade. If diagnosis of the effusion is a consideration, fluid should be taken for cell counts, Gram stain, cytology, culture, pH, and other routine tests. Air can be injected into the pericardium to allow delineation of the pericardial space on a chest film. Repeat films will allow monitoring of the reaccumulation of fluid.[39] This should be done only if the fluid obtained contained no blood; injection of air into the heart can cause fatal air embolism. An indwelling plastic catheter with attached stopcock may be left in place if continued drainage is desired. A chest film should be obtained after the procedure to rule out iatrogenic pneumothorax. Patients should be monitored closely for 24 hours for signs of reaccumulating fluid or iatrogenic complications from the procedure. Repeat ultrasound examination is wise.

COMPLICATIONS

One of the most common complications of pericardiocentesis is the high false-negative rate, which was discussed previously. Another major complication is the consumption of time by this procedure in a deteriorating patient who needs definitive immediate surgical treatment.

The pericardial needle can injure any organ within its reach, causing pneumothorax or myocardial or coronary vessel laceration and thus hemopericardium.[93] Venous air embolism may be caused by air entering the heart.[100] The pericardial needle can also induce dysrhythmias from direct irritation of the epicardium or from small currents leaking from the connected ECG machine.[2]

Although many complications of pericardiocentesis have been reported anecdotally in the literature since 1896,[2] only during the last 50 years has the incidence of complications been reported in large series of patients. The first series was that of Kotte and McGuire,[101] who reported that 18 of 21 physicians polled had seen at least one fatality due to pericardiocentesis. Bishop and associates[102] reported six ventricular punctures in 40 procedures. Kilpatrick and Chapman[2] reported seven ventricular punctures in 20 procedures, with three patients developing hypotension and one

death. Frederiksen and colleagues[103] reported three cardiac chamber punctures in 21 procedures. Pradham and Ikins[104] reported one iatrogenic tamponade in five procedures, and Silverberg and coworkers[105] reported one cardiac arrest in 21 procedures. Many of these smaller studies were not detailed.

It is important to separate the problems inherent in a potentially fatal process such as tamponade from those caused by the procedure itself. Six studies summarized in Table 16–4 demonstrate that the risks of pericardiocentesis are quite significant. However, pericardiocentesis guided by echocardiography is much safer than that carried out before the echocardiographic era.[74, 106] The major complications will be discussed individually.

Cardiac Arrest and Death

Cardiac arrest and death occurred in approximately 2 per cent of patients in the larger series listed in Table 16–4, but in none of a series of patients whose pericardiocentesis was directed solely by ultrasound. An exact causal relationship between pericardiocentesis and sudden death, however, is difficult to substantiate. In Wong's series of 52 patients, the one death occurred in a patient in cardiogenic shock who had a nonproductive pericardiocentesis and who, on postmortem examination, had severe arteriosclerotic heart disease, not tamponade.[106a] There was an additional case of cardiac arrest in Wong's series that was successfully resuscitated, also in a patient with a nonproductive pericardiocentesis; the cause of the arrest was not discussed.

In Guberman's series of 56 patients, there was also one death during pericardiocentesis; details were not given.[10] Another patient with tamponade had right ventricular laceration by the pericardial needle, causing cardiac arrest; she was resuscitated and had emergency pericardiotomy but suffered hypoxic brain damage and died 2 weeks later.

In Krikorian's series of 123 patients, there were two deaths reported, both in seriously ill patients who had other medical problems.[11] One suffered right ventricular laceration and iatrogenic tamponade. Another patient with large effusion but no tamponade died shortly after pericardiocentesis was performed; the exact cause of death was not known. A third patient, in whom an indwelling catheter was left for 5 days to drain pericardial effusion, developed purulent pericarditis and died shortly after pericardiocentesis was performed; the exact cause of death was not known. Two additional patients in Krikorian's series died after pericardiocentesis; the time spent performing the procedure delayed definitive surgery and was believed to contribute substantially to death. If these patients are included, the mortality rate in this series rises to 3.2 per cent.

Most deaths associated with pericardiocentesis occur in patients who were already seriously ill. It should be noted that Wong found the most complications in patients who in retrospect had no effusion at all. With use of echocardiography to direct pericardiocentesis, the rate of complications

Table 16–4. Incidence of Complications of Pericardiocentesis

	Permanyer-Miralda[106] (1985)	Wong[106a] (1979)	Guberman[10] (1981)	Krikorian[11] (1978)	Kwasnik[39] (1978)	Callahan[74] (1985)
Number of cases	80	52	56	123	34	117
Environment	Cardiology service in Spain, all echoed	Cath lab with echo, fluoroscopy no trauma	Cardiology service with echo, fluoroscopy, etc., no trauma	University hospital, most in cath lab, 9% trauma	All uremic patients	Mostly medical, all echo-directed
Success in obtaining fluid (%)	88	69	87	86	—	98
Diagnosis from taps (%)	19	50	60 (malignancy only)	18	—	—
Cardiac arrest (% resuscitated)	0	2	2	—	—	0
Death (%)	0	2	2	1.6(3.2)*	—	0
Ventricular puncture or laceration (%)	1.2	9	6.5	—	—	1.5 (minor)
False-negative taps (%)	5.3	7.6	—	—	—	0.8
Surgery needed for tamponade (%)	1.2	—	26	39	—	—
New hemopericardium (%)	1.2	—	—	10.5	—	0
Major dysrhythmias (%)	0	—	—	0.08	—	0
Hypotensive episode (% vasovagal)	—	—	—	2	—	0.8
Pneumothorax (%)	0	—	—	—	3	0.8
Pneumoperitoneum (%)	0	—	—	—	3	0.8

*1.6% indicates directly attributable deaths; 3.2% also includes contributory deaths.

decreased significantly. A summary of studies of pericardiocentesis in cancer patients shows a mortality rate of less than 1 per cent with echocardiographic guidance. In the two most recent studies comprising 197 patients under echocardiographic guidance, there have been no cardiac arrests or deaths.[74, 106]

Cardiac Chamber, Vessel, or Lung Laceration

Cardiac chamber, vessel, or lung laceration occurs in 6 to 9 per cent of patients, even in the hands of experienced physicians under controlled situations. Nonfatal cardiac puncture, pneumothorax, and pneumoperitoneum have been reported,[39] as well as suppurative costochondritis. In the Krikorian series, 13 of 123 patients developed hemopericardium as a result of pericardiocentesis, one as a result of a lacerated coronary artery. One patient died from a punctured ventricle. Surgical control was necessary for four patients who developed tamponade, whereas eight patients did not develop tamponade and were managed conservatively. Several cases of induced tamponade occurred in patients with platelet counts greater than 50,000/ml.

Guberman reported three right ventricular lacerations in 46 patients; one was fatal. Wong found five right ventricular punctures, four in patients with nonproductive pericardiocentesis, but none causing "any adverse sequelae." In a series of dialysis patients, nine of ten receiving pericardiocentesis had serious complications, including three deaths and two myocardial lacerations.[38]

A review of the earlier literature reveals 22 ventricular punctures and six iatrogenic tamponades caused by 230 pericardiocenteses, for an overall ventricular puncture rate of 10 per cent. Researchers differ in their opinions as to the adverse effects of ventricular puncture. Atrial puncture has also been reported.[16]

In a series of patients whose pericardiocentesis was exclusively directed by ultrasound, ventricular puncture still occurred in 1.5 per cent, but was without consequence due to small needle size.[74] No vessels were injured, and a major reason for the low complication rate was that echocardiography revealed nontraditional, parasternal approaches to be

the safest for the majority of patients. However, in another study, right ventricular laceration occurred in one patient despite the use of echocardiography, producing tamponade and necessitating emergency surgery.[106]

A small number of pneumothoraces and pneumopericardium have been reported in various series (see Table 16–4) but have been without clinical consequence. A single case of tension pneumothorax has been reported after pericardiocentesis, but the cause and effect relationship was unclear.[107]

Dysrhythmias

Serious dysrhythmias induced by pericardiocentesis are rare. Premature ventricular contractions (PVCs) occur commonly during the procedure and are benign in most cases. Wong, Guberman, Callahan, and Kwasnik reported no dysrhythmias. Krikorian reported only one episode of ventricular tachycardia and "several" hypotensive vasovagal reactions, which were associated with bradycardia and responded to atropine and fluid loading.

Adverse Physiologic Consequences

There have been a few case reports of adverse consequences even when pericardiocentesis inflicts no injury. Most of these have to do with the fact that during pericardiocentesis the previously collapsed right ventricle's stroke volume increases 77 per cent with the first 200 ml of fluid removed.[42] Generally, this increase in stroke volume is greater initially than that demonstrated by the left ventricle. This can have significant consequences for both right and left ventricular function. In three of six patients in whom large effusions were removed by pericardiocentesis, there was right ventricular dilation and overload, with abnormal septal motion and either no increase in right ventricular ejection fraction, or a decrease.[108] In effect, these patients acted as if the normal restraining action of the pericardium itself had been removed, and returned to normal hemodynamic status slowly. Sudden pulmonary edema has also been reported after

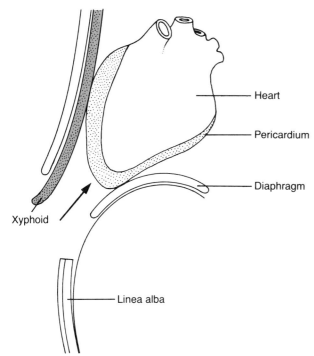

Figure 16–16. Anatomic approach of subxiphoid pericardiotomy. (From Alcan K, Zabetakis P, Marino N: Management of acute cardiac tamponade by subxiphoid pericardiotomy. JAMA 247:1143, 1982. Copyright 1982, American Medical Association.)

pericardiocentesis, presumably due to a sudden increase in venous return to the left ventricle at a time when peripheral vascular resistance is still high from compensatory catecholamine secretion.[109] Supporting evidence for this explanation is that right ventricular stroke volume increased 76 per cent after relief of tamponade, greater than the stroke volume increase of the left ventricle.[47] Only a single such case has been reported, however, so the admonitions to remove fluid slowly may not be necessary.

A case of brief profound bradycardia and rebound hypertension has also been reported after surgical relief of tamponade.[110] Such responses have not been noted in large series of patients receiving pericardiocentesis.

SUBXIPHOID PERICARDIOTOMY

Although most pericardial effusion is removed either by pericardiocentesis or by thoracotomy, there is a third alternative. The subxiphoid surgical approach to the pericardium is a relatively minor operation that takes about 30 minutes in experienced hands.[83, 111, 112] The procedure can be done under local anesthesia, although usually this is successful only in the stable, nontrauma patient.[58]

Indications

A crucial question is what role subxiphoid pericardiotomy should play in the patient with immediately life-threatening tamponade. Textbooks are contradictory; one recommends the procedure only if the patient is cardiovascularly stable.[113] Another recommends the procedure "when death is imminent and the presence of tamponade uncertain," suggesting putting a finger into the pericardial cavity but pointing out that "massive bleeding, however, may quickly ensue."[94] Large studies by trauma surgeons recommend this procedure for the stable patient (who has re-

sponded to fluid resuscitation) who is suspected of cardiac injury but does not otherwise warrant thoracotomy.[57, 58] It is not clear that the diagnostic benefit of the procedure cannot be duplicated by echocardiography.[57] Reports of pericardiostomy performed in the operating room by experienced surgeons indicate that only 18 to 28 per cent of all patients and only 22 per cent of patients with signs of tamponade actually had blood in the pericardial sac (indicating cardiac trauma).[57, 58] However, 37 to 46 per cent of patients with positive pericardiotomy and cardiac injury had no signs of tamponade. Not surprisingly, pericardiotomy has occasionally been positive in patients with negative pericardiocentesis. The use of pericardiotomy in trauma is well documented, and its role is mainly as an operating room alternative to exploratory thoracotomy to rule out occult cardiac injury in high-risk patients.[114, 115] It is not generally advocated in the treatment of tamponade or in the acutely deteriorating patient.

There is only one case report in which subxiphoid pericardiotomy is recommended for relief of tamponade in the emergency department.[112] The place for this procedure in the patient with traumatic tamponade has been argued to be the patient "in the middle of the spectrum" who is not unstable enough to need immediate thoracotomy, nor stable enough to wait for formal thoracotomy in the operating room.[112] In these patients, the investigator recommends subxiphoid pericardiotomy "if pericardiocentesis shows no abnormality, if it does not adequately decompress the tamponade, or if the physician wishes to avoid its uncertainty." Although the investigators admit that the procedure requires more time and surgical expertise than pericardiocentesis, they state that it should not be difficult for the emergency physician to learn and use in the emergency department. There is no literature on this procedure in the hands of emergency physicians, and two of the more experienced centers state that subxiphoid pericardial window procedures should not be performed with patients under local anesthesia or in the emergency department.[57, 115]

What are the advantages of subxiphoid pericardiotomy over pericardiocentesis? Chiefly, when the procedure is performed by experienced surgeons it has a lower complication rate, less serious complications, and a much lower false-positive and false-negative rate. Its disadvantages are that it takes much more time, it still does not allow repair of cardiac injury (which necessitates thoracotomy), it takes much more training and experience, and, despite claims that it can be done under local anesthesia, its use in trauma patients necessitates general anesthesia.

Although this procedure may have a limited place in the emergency department, it will not often be used, and is best done by an experienced surgeon. Having performed it myself, I doubt that the emergency physician who does it once every few years will ever do it speedily or well. Emergency physicians who wish to include this procedure in their armamentarium should arrange for formal training by a local surgeon and prospectively establish criteria with the local surgical staff as to when, where, and by whom the procedure will be done.

Procedure (Overview)

The procedure takes advantage of the fact that the pericardial sac lies relatively close to the abdominal wall in the subxiphoid region (Figs. 16–16 and 16–17). The abdominal skin and the linea alba are incised and then the entire xiphoid process is removed, which exposes the pericardial sac underneath. The pericardium can then be entered for removal of effusion, biopsy, or placement of large drainage

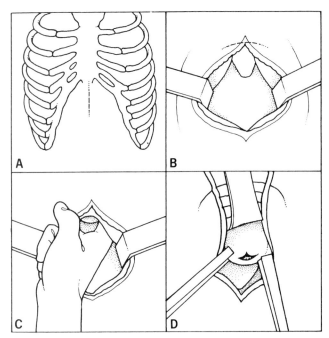

Figure 16–17. Technique of forming a subxiphoid pericardial window. (From Brewster S, Thirlby R, Snyder W: Subxiphoid pericardial window and penetrating cardiac trauma. Arch Surg 123:937, 1988. Copyright 1988, American Medical Association.)

catheters (such as 28 French chest tubes). This procedure is excellent for terminal patients with malignant effusions, diagnostic tap of purulent pericarditis, and sometimes for pericardial biopsy.[117] In trauma cases, the subxiphoid incision can be extended for a median sternotomy or a laparotomy.[57]

Complications

This procedure has a low infection rate and the most common complication is postpericardiotomy syndrome. Its disadvantages are that it provides very poor visualization of the heart itself, it can occasionally produce false-positive results, and it is often poorly tolerated under local anesthesia by trauma patients.[57] The last-mentioned problem has led experienced surgeons to perform it under light general anesthesia with intubation, diazepam, and fentanyl,[57] or under general anesthesia.[58] In addition, the procedure takes about 30 minutes even in experienced hands and therefore could better be considered an "urgent" procedure than an "emergency" one. In inexperienced hands, this procedure not only would probably delay definitive treatment, but it could lead to the major complications of inadvertent opening of the peritoneal cavity and pulmonary injury.

CONCLUSION

In *nontraumatic patients*, tamponade should always be considered in the differential diagnosis of shock, especially in patients who are on anticoagulants, who have had recent myocardial infarction, or who have had pericardial disease; when malignancy is present; when aortic dissection is suspected; or when a CVP catheter is in place. Tamponade should also be considered in the differential diagnosis when hypotension persists following closed-chest CPR or attempts at cardiac pacing.

In any patient with blunt or penetrating chest or upper abdominal trauma, the possibility of *traumatic tamponade* must also be considered. If clinical deterioration occurs in the emergency de-

partment pending operative care, temporizing pericardiocentesis should be considered if other therapy fails. When such a patient arrives with no obtainable blood pressure or in profound shock and unconscious, immediate thoracotomy and pericardiotomy is indicated after intubation.[92, 118, 119] Pericardiocentesis may cause a dangerous delay in this situation and has a low success rate. There seems to be little role for the use of subxiphoid pericardiotomy in such patients.

Management of either traumatic or nontraumatic tamponade requires a sound understanding of pathophysiology, an ever-vigilant attitude, and the willingness, if it is necessary, to perform relatively high-risk procedures such as pericardiocentesis on critically ill or injured patients.

REFERENCES

1. Stein L, Shubin H, Weil M: Recognition and management of pericardial tamponade. JAMA 225:503, 1973.
2. Kilpatrick Z, Chapman C: On pericardiocentesis. Am J Cardiol 16:622, 1965.
3. Symbas P, Harlafhs N, Waldo W: Penetrating cardiac wounds: A comparison of different therapeutic methods. Ann Surg 183:377, 1976.
4. Clarke D: The heart and great vessels. In Dudley H (ed): Hamilton Bailey's Emergency Surgery. 11th ed. Bristol, England, Wright Publishers, 1986, pp. 235–247.
5. Borja A, Lansing A, Randell H: Immediate operative treatment for stab wounds of the heart. Ann Thorac Cardiovasc Surg 59:662, 1970.
6. Blair E, Tapuzla C, Dean R: Chest trauma. In Hardy J (ed): Critical Surgical Illness. Philadelphia, WB Saunders, 1971, pp 175–185.
7. Atcheson S, Fred H: Complications of cardiac resuscitation. Am Heart J 89:263, 1975.
8. Glasser S, Harrison E, Amey B: Echocardiographic incidence of pericardial effusion in patients resuscitated by emergency medical technicians. JACEP 8:6, 1979.
9. Davison R, Barresi V, Parker M, et al: Intracardiac injections during cardiopulmonary resuscitation. JAMA 244:1110, 1980.
10. Guberman B, Fowler N, Engel P: Cardiac tamponade in medical patients. Circulation 64:633, 1981.
11. Krikorian J, Hancock E: Pericardiocentesis. Am J Med 65:808, 1978.
12. Olson L, Edwards W, Olney B, et al: Hemorrhagic cardiac tamponade: A clinicopathologic correlation. Mayo Clin Proc 59:785, 1984.
13. Thomas T: Emergency evacuation of acute pericardial tamponade. Ann Thorac Surg 10:566, 1970.
14. Brown C, Gurley H, Hutchins G, et al: Injuries associated with percutaneous placement of transthoracic pacemakers. Ann Emerg Med 14:223, 1985.
15. Frater R: Intrapericardial pressure and pericardial tamponade in cardiac surgery. Ann Thorac Surg 10:563, 1970.
16. Kerber R, Ridges J, Harrison D: Electrocardiographic indications of atrial puncture during pericardiocentesis. N Engl J Med 282:1142, 1979.
17. Sobol S, Thomas H, Evans R: Myocardial laceration not demonstrated by continuous electrocardiographic monitoring occurring during pericardiocentesis. N Engl J Med 292:1222, 1979.
18. Barton B, Hermann G, Weil R: Cardiothoracic emergencies associated with subclavian hemodialysis catheters. JAMA 250:2660, 1983.
19. Sheep RE, Guiney WB: Fatal cardiac tamponade: Occurrence with other complications after left internal jugular vein catheterization. JAMA 248:1632, 1982.
20. Edwards H, King T: Cardiac tamponade from central venous catheters. Arch Surg 117:965, 1982.
21. Ramp J, Harkins J, Mason G: Cardiac tamponade secondary to blunt trauma. J Trauma 14:767, 1974.
22. Roe B: Cardiac trauma including injury of great vessels. Surg Clin North Am 52:573, 1972.
23. Kirsh M, Behrendt D, Orringer M: The treatment of acute traumatic rupture of the aorta. Ann Surg 184:308, 1976.
24. Hurd T, Novak R, Gallagher T: Tension pneumopericardium: A complication of mechanical ventilation. Crit Care Med 12:200, 1984.
25. Toledo T, Moore W, Nash D: Spontaneous pneumopericardium in acute asthma: Case report and review of the literature. Chest 16:118, 1972.
26. Hacker P, Dorsey D: Pneumopericardium and pneumomediastinum following closed chest injury. JACEP 8:409, 1979.
27. Frascone R, Cicero J, Sturm J: Pneumopericardium occurring during a high-speed motorcycle ride. J Trauma 23:163, 1983.
28. McDougal C, Mulder G, Hoffman J: Tension pneumopericardium following blunt chest trauma. Ann Emerg Med 14:167, 1985.
29. Khan R: Air tamponade and tension pneumopericardium. J Thorac Cardiovasc Surg 68:328, 1974.
30. Robinson M, Markovchick V: Traumatic tension pneumopericardium: A case report and literature review. J Emerg Med 2:409, 1985.
31. Lynn R: Delayed post-traumatic pneumopericardium producing acute cardiac tamponade. Can J Surg 26:62, 1983.

32. Hancock E: Management of pericardial disease. Mod Concepts Cardiovasc Dis 48:1, 1979.
33. Pories W, Gaudiani A: Cardiac tamponade. Surg Clin North Am 55:573, 1975.
34. LeWinter M, Pavelec R: Influence of the pericardium on left ventricular end-diastolic pressure-segment length relations during early and later phases of experimental chronic volume overload in dogs. Circ Res 50:401, 1982.
35. Lee M, Fung Y, Shabetai R: Biaxial mechanical properties of human pericardium and canine comparisons. Am J Physiol 253:H75, 1987.
36. Press O, Livingston R: Management of malignant pericardial effusion and tamponade. JAMA 257:1088, 1987.
37. Hanfling S: Metastatic cancer in the heart. Circulation 22:474, 1960.
38. Rutsky E, Rostand S: Treatment of uremic pericarditis and pericardial effusion. Am J Kidney Dis 10:2, 1987.
39. Kwasnick E, Kostes J, Lazarus J: Conservative management of uremic pericardial effusions. J Thorac Cardiovasc Surg 76:629, 1978.
40. Baue A, Blakemore W: The pericardium. Ann Thorac Surg 14:81, 1972.
41. Shabetai R, Fowler N, Guntheroth W: The hemodynamics of cardiac tamponade and constrictive pericarditis. Am J Cardiol 26:480, 1970.
42. Grose R, Greenberg M, Steingart R, Cohen M: Left ventricular volume and function during relief of cardiac tamponade in man. Circulation 66:149, 1982.
43. Fowler N, Gabel M: The hemodynamic effects of cardiac tamponade: Mainly the result of atrial, not ventricular, compression. Circulation 71:154, 1985.
44. Spodick D: The normal and diseased pericardium: Current concepts of pericardial physiology, diagnosis, and treatment. J Am Coll Cardiol 1:240, 1983.
45. Koller J, Smith R, Sjostrand U, Breivik H: Effects of hypo-, normo-, and hypercarbia in dogs with acute cardiac tamponade. Anesth Analg 62:181, 1983.
46. Shabetai R: Changing concepts of cardiac tamponade. Mod Concepts Cardiovasc Dis 52:19, 1983.
47. Manyari D, Kostuk W, Purves P: Effect of pericardiocentesis on right and left ventricular function and volumes in pericardial effusion. Am J Cardiol 52:159, 1983.
48. Spodick D: Acute cardiac tamponade. Pathologic physiology, diagnosis, and management. Prog Cardiovasc Dis 10:64, 1967.
49. Crystal G, Bashour F, Downey H, Parker P: Myocardial blood flow and oxygen consumption during moderate cardiac tamponade: Role of reflex vasoconstriction. Proc Soc Exper Biol Med 160:65, 1979.
50. Wechsler A, Auerbach B, Graham T: Distribution of intramyocardial blood flow during pericardial tamponade correlated with microscopic anatomy and intrinsic myocardial contractility. J Thorac Cardiovasc Surg 68:847, 1974.
51. Wertheimer W, Bloom S, Hughes R: Myocardial effects of pericardial tamponade. Ann Thorac Surg 14:494, 1972.
52. Kostreva D, Castaner A, Kampine J: Role of autonomics in the initiation of electromechanical dissociation. Am J Physiol 241:R213, 1981.
53. Shoemaker W, Carey S, Yao S: Hemodynamic monitoring for physiologic evaluation, diagnosis, and therapy of acute hemopericardial tamponade from penetrating wounds. J Trauma 13:36, 1973.
54. Antman E, Cargill V, Grossman W: Low-pressure cardiac tamponade. Ann Intern Med 91:403, 1979.
55. Symbas P: Blunt and penetrating trauma to the heart. In Glenn W (ed): Thoracic and Cardiovascular Surgery Norwalk, CT, Appleton-Century-Crofts, 1983, pp 1480–1489.
56. Moller C, Schoonbee C, Rosendorff C: Haemodynamics of cardiac tamponade during various modes of ventilation. Br J Anaesth 51:409, 1979.
57. Miller F, Bond S, Shumate C, et al: Diagnostic pericardial window. A safe alternative to exploratory thoracotomy for suspected heart injuries. Arch Surg 122:605, 1987.
58. Brewster S, Thirlby R, Snyder W: Subxiphoid pericardial window and penetrating cardiac trauma. Arch Surg 123:937, 1988.
59. Markiewicz W, Borovik R, Ecker S: Cardiac tamponade in medical patients: Treatment and prognosis in the echocardiographic era. Am Heart J 111:1138, 1986.
60. Beck C: Two cardiac compression triads. JAMA 104:715, 1935.
61. DiPasquale J, Pluth J: Penetrating wounds of the heart and cardiac tamponade. Postgrad Med 49:114, 1971.
62. Shoemaker W, Carey J, Jao S: Hemodynamic alterations in acute cardiac tamponade after penetrating injuries of the heart. Surgery 67:754, 1970.
63. Shoemaker W: Algorithm for early recognition and management of cardiac tamponade. Crit Care Med 3:59, 1975.
64. Trinkle J, Marcas J, Grover F: Management of the wounded heart. Ann Thorac Surg 17:230, 1974.
65. Breaux E, Dupont J, Albert H: Cardiac tamponade following penetrating mediastinal injuries: Improved survival with early pericardiocentesis. J Trauma 19:461, 1979.
66. Curtiss E, Reddy P, Uretsky B, Cecchetti A: Pulsus paradoxus: Definition and relation to the severity of cardiac tamponade. Am Heart J 115:391, 1988.
67. Singh S, Wann L, Klopfenstein H, et al: Usefulness of right ventricular diastolic collapse in diagnosing cardiac tamponade and comparison to pulsus paradoxus. Am J Cardiol 57:652, 1986.
68. Carsky E, Azimi F, Maucer R: Epicardial fat sign in the diagnosis of pericardial effusion. JAMA 244:2762, 1980.
69. Parameswaran R, Maniet A, Goldberg S, Goldberg H: Low electrocardiographic voltage in pericardial effusion. Chest 85:631, 1984.
70. Sotolongo R, Horton J: Total electrical alternans in pericardial tamponade. Am Heart J 101:853, 1981.
71. Spodick D: Electrical alternans of the heart. Its relation to the kinetics and physiology of the heart during cardiac tamponade. Am J Cardiol 10:155, 1962.
72. Friedman H, Gomer J, Tardio A: The electrocardiographic features of acute cardiac tamponade. Circulation 50:260, 1974.
73. Ansinger R, Rourke T, Hodges M: Role of echocardiography in emergencies. Minn Med 63:855, 1980.
74. Callahan J, Seward J, Nishimura R, et al: Two-dimensional echocardiographically guided pericardiocentesis: Experience in 117 consecutive patients. Am J Cardiol 55:476, 1985.
75. Mayron R, Gaudio F, Plummer D, et al: Echocardiography performed by emergency physicians: Impact on diagnosis and therapy. Ann Emerg Med 17:150, 1988.
76. Preis L, Taylor G, Martin R: Traumatic pericardiocentesis: Two-dimensional echocardiographic visualization of an unfortunate event. Arch Intern Med 142:2327, 1982.
77. Callahan J, Seward J, Tajik A: Cardiac tamponade: Pericardiocentesis directed by two-dimensional echocardiography. Mayo Clin Proc 60:344, 1985.
78. Singh S, Wann L, Schuchard G, et al: Right ventricular and right atrial collapse in patients with cardiac tamponade: A combined echocardiographic and hemodynamic study. Circulation 70:966, 1984.
79. Klopfenstein H, Schuchard G, Wann L, et al: The relative merits of pulsus paradoxus and right ventricular diastolic collapse in the early detection of cardiac tamponade: An experimental echocardiographic study. Circulation 71:829, 1985.
80. Clarke D, Cosgrove D: Real-time ultrasound scanning in the planning and guidance of pericardiocentesis. Clin Radiol 38:119, 1987.
81. Memon A, Zawadski Z: Malignant effusions: Diagnostic evaluation and therapeutic strategy. Curr Probl Cancer 5:1, 1981.
82. Kindig J, Goodman M: Clinical utility of pericardial fluid pH determination. Am J Med 75:1077, 1983.
83. Prager R, Wilson C, Bender H: The subxiphoid approach to pericardial disease. Ann Thorac Surg 34:6, 1981.
84. Alcan K, Zabetakis P, Marino N: Management of acute cardiac tamponade by subxiphoid pericardiotomy. JAMA 247:1143, 1982.
85. Fowler N: Recognition and management of pericardial disease and its complications. In Hurst J (ed): The Heart. 4th ed. New York, McGraw-Hill Book Co, 1978.
86. Bolanowksi P, Swaminathan A, Neville W: Aggressive surgical management of penetrating cardiac injuries. J Thorac Cardiovasc Surg 66:52, 1973.
87. Sugg W, Rea W, Ecker R: Penetrating wounds of the heart: An analysis of 459 cases. J Thorac Cardiovasc Surg 56:531, 1968.
88. Arom K, Richardson J, Webb G: Subxiphoid pericardial window in patients with suspected traumatic pericardial tamponade. Ann Thorac Surg 23:545, 1977.
89. Ivatury R, Shah P, Ito K, Ramirez-Schon G, Suarez F, Rohman M: Emergency room thoracotomy for the resuscitation of patients with "fatal" penetrating injuries of the heart. Ann Thorac Surg 32:377, 1981.
90. DePace N, Nestico P, Schwartz A, et al: Predicting success of intensive dialysis in the treatment of uremic pericarditis. Am J Med 76:38, 1984.
91. Boyd T, Strieder J: Immediate surgery for traumatic heart disease. J Thorac Cardiovasc Surg 50:305, 1965.
92. Siemens R, Polk H, Gray L: Indications for thoracotomy following penetrating thoracic injury. J Trauma 17:493, 1977.
93. Beall A, Gasior R, Bricker D: Gunshot wounds of the heart: Changing patterns of surgical management. Ann Thorac Surg 11:523, 1972.
94. Spencer F, Culliford A: Acquired heart disease: Cardiac trauma. In Schwartz S, Shires G, Spencer F, Storer E (eds): Principles of Surgery. 4th ed. New York, McGraw-Hill Book Co, 1984, pp 807–873.
95. Friedman H, Sakura H, Choe S: Pulsus paradoxus: A manifestation of a marked reduction of left ventricular end-diastolic volume in cardiac tamponade. J Thorac Cardiovasc Surg 79:74, 1980.
96. Treasure T, Cottler L: Practical procedures: How to aspirate the pericardium. Br J Hosp Med 24:488, 1980.
97. Patel A, Kosolcharoen P, Nallasivan M, et al: Catheter drainage of the pericardium. Practical method to maintain long-term patency. Chest 92:1018, 1987.
98. Stewart J, Gott V: The use of a Seldinger wire technique for pericardiocentesis following cardiac surgery. Ann Thorac Surg 35:467, 1983.
99. Kaye W: Invasive therapeutic techniques: Emergency cardiac pacing, pericardiocentesis, intracardiac injections, and emergency treatment of tension pneumothorax. Heart Lung 12:300, 1983.
100. Kizer K, Goodman P: Radiologic manifestations of venous air embolism. Diag Radiol 144:35, 1982.
101. Kotte J, McGuire J: Pericardial paracentesis. Mod Concepts Cardiovasc Dis 20:102, 1951.
102. Bishop L, Estes E, McIntosh H: The electrocardiogram as a safeguard in pericardiocentesis. JAMA 62:264, 1956.

103. Fredericksen R, Cohen L, Mullins C: Pericardial windows or pericardio-centesis for pericardial effusion. Am Heart J 82:158, 1971.
104. Pradham D, Ikins P: The role of pericardiectomy in the treatment of pericarditis with effusion. Am Surg 42:257, 1976.
105. Silverberg S, Oreopoulos D, Wise D: Pericarditis in patients undergoing long-term hemodialysis and peritoneal dialysis. Am J Med 63:874, 1977.
106. Permanyer-Miralda G, Sagrista-Sauleda J, Soler-Soler J: Primary acute pericardial disease: A prospective series of 231 consecutive patients. Am J Cardiol 56:623, 1985.
106a. Wong B, Murphy J, Chang CJ: The risk of pericardiocentesis. Am J Cardiol 44:1110, 1979.
107. Ewer M, Ali M, Frazier O: Open chest resuscitation for cardiopulmonary arrest related to mechanical impairment of the circulation. Crit Care Med 10:198, 1982.
108. Armstrong W, Feigenbaum H, Dillon J: Acute right ventricular dilatation and echocardiographic volume overload following pericardiocentesis for relief of cardiac tamponade. Am Heart J 107:1266, 1984.
109. Vandyke WJ, Cure J, Chakko C, Gheorgeiade M: Pulmonary edema after pericardiocentesis for cardiac tamponade. N Engl J Med 309:595, 1983.
110. Prida X, Cody R: Profound bradycardia following release of cardiac tamponade. Chest 83:148, 1983.
111. Osuch J, Khandekar J, Fry W: Emergency subxiphoid pericardial decompression for malignant pericardial effusion. Am Surg 51:298, 1985.
112. Courcy P, Stair T, Brotman S: Subxiphoid pericardial window in traumatic pericardial tamponade. Am J Emerg Med 2:153, 1984.
113. Kirsh M: Trauma protocols for resuscitation and evaluation. In Siegel J (ed): Trauma: Emergency Surgery and Critical Care. New York, Churchill Livingstone, 1987, pp 805–823.
114. Karrel R, Shaffer M, Franaszek J: Emergency diagnosis, resuscitation, and treatment of acute penetrating cardiac trauma. Ann Emerg Med 11:504, 1982.
115. Duncan AO, Scalea TM, Sclafani SJA, et al: Evaluation of occult cardiac injuries using subxiphoid pericardial window. J Trauma 29:955, 1989.
116. Brewster SA, Thirlby RC, Snyder WH: Subxiphoid pericardial window in penetrating cardiac trauma. Arch Surg 123:937, 1988.
117. Sinzobahamvya N: Results of subxiphoid pericardiostomy in pericardial effusion. Acta Chir Belg 88:175, 1988.
118. Mattox K, Beall A, Jordan G: Cardiography in the emergency center. J Thorac Cardiovasc Surg 68:886, 1974.
119. Fulton R: Penetrating wounds of the heart. Heart Lung 7:262, 1978.

Chapter 17

Artificial Perfusion During Cardiac Arrest

Carol S. Federiuk and Arthur B. Sanders

INTRODUCTION

The modern era of cardiopulmonary resuscitation (CPR) was introduced by Kouwenhoven and colleagues[1] in 1960 in a classic paper that brought together the concepts of mouth-to-mouth ventilation, closed-chest compression, and external defibrillation. An increased understanding of the mechanism of blood flow during CPR has led to periodic revision of the recommended standards for CPR and to development of alternate methods of CPR. This chapter discusses the current understanding of the mechanism of blood flow during CPR, standard and alternate techniques of CPR, and methods for evaluation of these techniques by assessment of perfusion during CPR.

MECHANISM OF BLOOD FLOW

Kouwenhoven, in his 1960 paper, proposed the traditional "cardiac" pump mechanism of blood flow.[1] Pressure on the chest compresses the heart between the sternum and the vertebrae, forcing out blood (Fig. 17–1).[2] The relaxation phase of CPR allows the heart to fill. This model assumes that compression of the ventricles raises intraventricular pressure above that of the aorta and pulmonary artery, creating a pressure gradient that generates forward blood

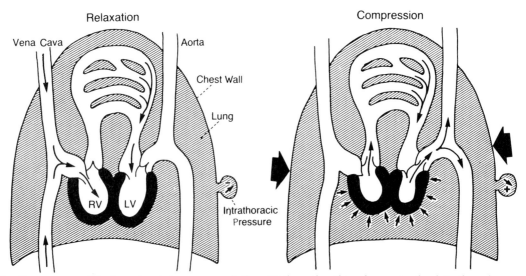

Figure 17–1. Cardiac pump model of cardiopulmonary resuscitation. During relaxation phase, negative intrathoracic pressure enhances blood return to heart. During closed-chest compression, the heart is squeezed between sternum and spine, a pressure gradient is developed between ventricles and great vessels, and antegrade flow occurs because of the one-way arrangement of heart valves. RV indicates right ventricle; LV, left ventricle. (From Luce JM, Cary JM, Ross BK, et al: New developments in cardiopulmonary resuscitation. JAMA 244:1366, 1980. Copyright 1980, American Medical Association.)

flow. Closure of the atrioventricular valves during chest compression was thought to prevent retrograde blood flow.

This intuitively obvious model of blood flow has been the subject of much debate since its introduction. Weale and Rothwell-Jackson, in 1962, showed that chest compression induces almost equivalent increases in arterial and venous pressures in animals.[3] They hypothesized that closed-chest compression creates a generalized increase in intrathoracic pressure that is transmitted equally to the heart and intra- and extrathoracic vessels, because the atrioventricular valves remain open. In a human study, MacKenzie and coworkers demonstrated that right atrial and aortic root pressures were elevated equally in three patients undergoing external chest compression for cardiac arrest.[4] Wilder, in 1963, showed that simultaneous ventilation and compression produced higher blood pressures than alternating ventilation and compression, supporting the idea that increased intrathoracic pressure produces forward flow of blood.[5] These early studies questioning the "cardiac" mechanism of blood flow had been forgotten until a few years ago, when researchers hypothesized that by elucidating the mechanism of blood flow they may be able to improve the technique of CPR.

Recent studies have focused on the "thoracic" pump mechanism of blood flow (Fig. 17–2).[2] Rudikoff and associates raised intrathoracic pressures in dogs by clamping the endotracheal tube at end-inspiration, thus keeping the lungs inflated during chest compression.[6] This technique was found to increase significantly aortic systolic pressure and carotid blood flow. These results were confirmed in humans by Chandra and colleagues, who used a technique of simultaneous compression ventilation CPR (SCV-CPR) in a study involving 11 patients in cardiac arrest.[7] SCV-CPR significantly increased mean systolic radial artery pressure and carotid blood flow compared with standard CPR. Other methods of increasing intrathoracic pressure, such as abdominal binding, have also been shown to increase these parameters.[6, 8]

Rudikoff also studied blood pressure in the right atrium, pulmonary artery, left ventricle, and aorta during external massage in dogs and demonstrated generation of identical pressures.[6] These observations are consistent with the idea that a generalized increase in intrathoracic pressure rather than direct cardiac compression induces forward blood flow during CPR.

Several investigators have noted that the increase in intrathoracic pressure generated by coughing may by itself generate blood flow during cardiac arrest. Criley and co-workers demonstrated that coughing early in cardiac arrest enabled patients to maintain enough forward blood flow to remain conscious until definitive treatment could be initiated.[9] Niemann and associates confirmed these observations and showed that coughing during cardiac arrest produces systemic blood flow.[10]

The idea that increased intrathoracic pressure is responsible for blood flow while the heart remains a passive conduit raises the question of why forward rather than reverse blood flow should occur during CPR. Niemann and colleagues demonstrated that little retrograde flow is observed in the jugular venous system during chest compression.[11] These investigators postulated that intrathoracic pressure was transmitted unequally to the arterial and venous vessels by the functioning of venous valves at the thoracic inlet. Forward rather than backward flow may be enhanced for several other reasons. Arterial resistance to vessel collapse is greater than that of veins, thus venous collapse under increased intrathoracic pressure may prevent back flow. Additionally, venous capacitance is greater than arterial capacitance, so that greater pressures are generated in the arteries for an equal volume of blood.[12]

Other studies, however, dispute the idea that compression of the thorax is the primary determinant of forward blood flow during CPR. In echocardiographic studies, Deshmukh and colleagues demonstrated cardiac valve motion and a change in left ventricular dimensions during the early phases of CPR in mini pigs.[13] Sanders and coworkers compared the success rate of conventional CPR with a technique of simultaneous compression ventilation and abdominal binding for resuscitation of dogs in cardiac arrest.[14] This study showed that five of six dogs could be resuscitated with conventional CPR, but none of six dogs were resuscitated with simultaneous ventilation and compression.

Although the debate over the exact mechanism of blood flow during CPR persists, Maier and associates shed light on the subject in their study of the effect of varying the rate, force, and duration of compressions in CPR on large dogs.[15] These investigators demonstrated that the relative contribution of the thoracic pump and direct cardiac compression models to blood flow varied with the CPR technique utilized.

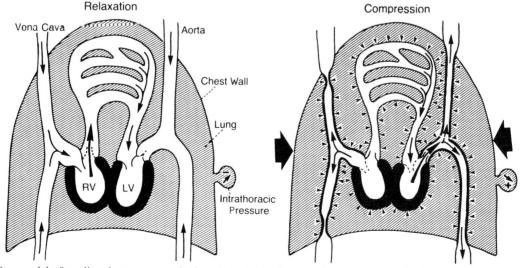

Figure 17–2. New model of cardiopulmonary resuscitation. Closed-chest compression causes generalized increase in intrathoracic pressure that squeezes all structures, including pulmonary reservoir, which is filled during relaxation phase. A pressure gradient is developed, and blood flows into the head because the thick-walled carotid artery remains patent while the thin-walled jugular vein is squeezed shut, or because of a venous valve. RV indicates right ventricle; LV, left ventricle. (From Luce JM, Cary JM, Ross BK, et al: New developments in cardiopulmonary resuscitation. JAMA 244:1366, 1980. Copyright 1980, American Medical Association.)

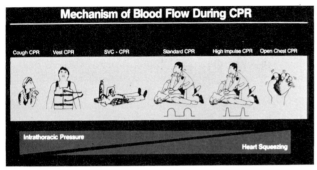

Figure 17–3. Contribution of direct cardiac compression and intrathoracic pressure mechanisms to blood flow during cardiopulmonary resuscitation. (Courtesy of Physio-Control Corp., Redmond, Wash.)

Direct cardiac compression was shown to play a greater role when chest compressions are delivered at higher rates (high-frequency CPR), and the thoracic pump mechanism predominated in low-momentum compression techniques, such as simultaneous compression and ventilation CPR. In addition, Babbs and coworkers noted that the optimal technique of CPR varied with the size of the experimental animal and the size of the pad performing chest compressions.[16] Large animals were more likely to benefit from SCV-CPR, whereas smaller animals did not. Direct cardiac compression was proposed to play a greater role in smaller animals.

In summary, the mechanism of forward blood flow during closed chest compression has not been clearly elucidated. Figure 17–3 shows a spectrum of mechanisms based on several factors:

1. Body size of patient
2. Chest configuration, particularly anterior-posterior diameter
3. Previous thoracic surgery
4. Molding of the chest with continued CPR
5. Size of hand or paddle performing chest compressions
6. Rate and force of chest compressions

Knowledge of the mechanism(s) of blood flow during CPR may allow the clinician to use alternative techniques that provide better perfusion pressures during cardiac arrest. The optimal technique for CPR may not be the same in every patient. For example, obese patients with large anterior-posterior diameters may benefit more from simultaneous ventilation and compression; thin patients may benefit from faster compression rates. The key to clinically implementing these changes is being able to assess perfusion during ongoing CPR. Advances in this area are discussed later in this chapter.

TECHNIQUE OF CPR

Guidelines for the performance of CPR have been recommended by the American Heart Association and are revised periodically to reflect ongoing research.[17] Current guidelines are summarized in Table 17–1.

External chest compression is performed two finger widths above the xiphoid process, compressing the sternum 3.8 to 5.0 cm in the normal-sized adult. The pressure is released completely after each compression and an equivalent amount of time is allotted for relaxation as for compression. The chest compression rate is 80 to 100 per minute. Two ventilations are given after each 15 chest compressions in one-rescuer CPR, and 1 to 1.5 seconds are allowed for each breath in order to provide good chest expansion. In two-rescuer CPR, one ventilation is performed after every five compressions during a 1 to 1.5-second pause. Once the patient is endotracheally intubated, the rescuer need not stop compressions for the ventilatory pause.[17]

In children, compressions are performed with the heel of one hand two finger widths above the xiphoid process. The chest is compressed to a depth of 2.5 to 3.8 cm at a rate of 80 to 100 per minute. At the end of every fifth compression, a 1 to 1.5-second pause is allowed for ventilation in both one- and two-rescuer CPR.[17]

Chest compressions in infants currently are performed two finger widths below the intramammary line. Recent studies, however, suggest that the heart lies under the lower third of the sternum in all age groups, and hand position may not need to vary between infants and adults.[18, 19] The chest is compressed with two to three fingers to a depth of 1.3 to 2.5 cm. The recommended compression rate in infants is at least 100 per minute. A 5:1 compression to ventilation ratio is maintained for both one- and two-rescuer CPR.[17] An alternative technique for the resuscitation of neonates involves encircling the chest of the neonate with the rescuer's hands and compressing the sternum with the two apposed thumbs.[20, 21] The sternum of a neonate is compressed 1.3 to 2.0 cm at the rate of 120 per minute.[20]

MECHANICAL DEVICES FOR STANDARD CPR

Mechanical resuscitators have been developed that can provide standard chest compressions and ventilations during CPR. Clinical studies have demonstrated that mechanical CPR devices are comparable to standard manual CPR. Taylor and colleagues compared manual and mechanical CPR in 50 patients in cardiac arrest.[22] Resuscitation, survival, and complication rates were similar in both groups of patients. McDonald compared the hemodynamics of mechanical and manual CPR techniques in 15 patients.[23] He found that manual CPR produced higher systolic arterial pressures, but mechanical CPR resulted in higher mean arterial pressures.

The advantages of mechanical devices include controlled, constant chest compressions, the elimination of operator fatigue, and the freeing up of personnel to perform other functions.

Manually operated devices were initially developed to give the resuscitator a mechanical advantage for performing chest compressions. These have been largely replaced by gas-powered resuscitators that automatically deliver chest

Table 17–1. Standard CPR Guidelines				
	Adult	**Child**	**Infant**	**Neonate**
Rate of compression	80–100	100	≥ 100	120
Compression depth	1.5–2 in	1–1.5 in	0.5–1 in	0.5–0.75 in
Compression duration	50% of cycle	50% of cycle	50% of cycle	50% of cycle
Compression mode	Both hands	Heel of one hand	2–3 fingers	Apposed thumbs
Compression to ventilation ratio	15:2 (one rescuer)	5:1 (one rescuer)	5:1 (one rescuer)	5:1 (one rescuer)
	5:1 (two rescuers)	5:1 (two rescuers)	5:1 (two rescuers)	5:1 (two rescuers)

compression and ventilations. The two devices currently in common use are (1) the Thumper Cardiopulmonary Resuscitator manufactured by Michigan Instruments, Inc., and (2) the HLR Quick Fit manufactured by Brunswick Manufacturing Company.

Thumper

The Thumper is a gas-powered mechanical device that is in relatively broad use. This device consists of a compressed-gas–powered plunger mounted on a backboard and a time-pressure cycled ventilator (Fig. 17–4).

The Thumper delivers 60 chest compressions per minute with a compression duration that is 50 per cent of the cycle length. Every fifth compression is followed by a ventilation at adjustable airway pressure. The Thumper can be driven off wall oxygen at 50 psi or by standard portable oxygen tanks.

Procedure for Setup of Thumper[24]

The Thumper can be positioned from either side of the patient. Care should be taken to ensure that the base plate is positioned horizontally under the patient's posterior thorax with the patient lying near the center of the base plate. After the cylindric column and piston are fitted on the base plate, the piston pad position should be adjusted so that the pad lies over the lower one third of the sternum. The compressor piston is positioned after the oxygen hose has been connected; therefore, CPR is not interrupted during assembly of the Thumper. The piston column is calibrated with rings; each ring indicates 1.25 cm of piston excursion. Before starting the device, the piston height should be adjusted so that one ring is just visible on the piston column. With the Thumper operational, chest compressions should be adjusted to 5 to 6.25 cm ("four rings," of sternal displacement) or 20 to 25 per cent of the patient's anterior-posterior diameter, once the machine is in operation. The device should not be set to function at a predetermined chest compression force.

The ventilation hose can be connected to an endotracheal tube, to an esophageal obturator, or a face mask. Airway pressure should be adjusted to 40 to 50 cm H_2O

during ventilation as displayed on the airway pressure gauge when the patient is intubated. Otherwise the airway pressure limit should be set at 30 cm H_2O to avoid gastric distention. Airway pressure is maintained for 1.5 to 1.8 seconds.

While using the Thumper one must operate three key switches: (1) the main on/off switch; (2) the ventilation on/off switch; and (3) the piston activator switch. When a pause in compressions is required for other procedures, the operator can easily stop compressions by turning off the third switch. Subclavian or jugular central lines can be placed with the Thumper in position, although it is recommended that the device be turned off during needle advancement to avoid arterial or lung injury. Defibrillation should be performed during the compression phase, when thoracic impedance is minimized.

HLR Quick Fit

The HLR Quick Fit device also delivers standard American Heart Association CPR. The compression plate is strapped onto the sternum (Fig. 17–5). Thus the device must be removed for attempts at electrical defibrillation. The force of chest compression is adjustable. Ventilations after every fifth compression are provided through a volume cycled ventilator. The ventilation hose can be attached to a mask or, with an adapter, to an endotracheal tube. There is concern about the amount of dead space when low inspiratory volumes are used because the nonrebreathing valve is located at the base plate.[24]

Procedure for Setup of HLR Device[24]

When the HLR device is used, care should be taken to position the patient near the center of the base plate. As is the case when the Thumper is used, the piston assembly should not be positioned until the oxygen hose and the ventilation hose are connected to avoid unnecessary interruption of chest compression. After the piston assembly has been appropriately placed so that the piston head lies on the lower end of the sternum, the positioning straps should be tightened and secured. It is important not to tighten these straps excessively, since this may restrict chest expansion during ventilation.

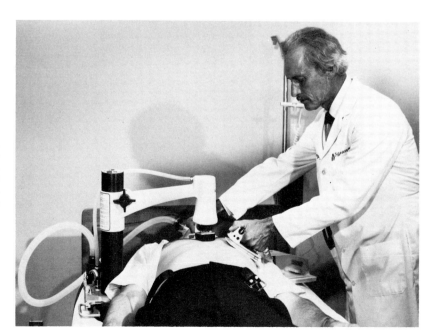

Figure 17–4. The Thumper is a gas-powered chest compressor. The device consists of a back plate with a cylindric column. On the column fits the sliding arm, with the compressor piston to be positioned over the lower sternum. The force of chest compression is adjustable, and defibrillation can be easily performed with the device in place. (With permission of Dixie USA.)

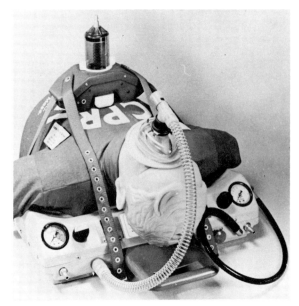

Figure 17–5. The HLR device is a gas-powered chest compressor. The device consists of a wedge-shaped base plate and a piston assembly to be positioned over the sternum. The piston is held in place by four straps that engage with the base plate.

Once the piston assembly is secured, the device is turned on. The chest compression force is adjusted to produce 5 cm of piston displacement (as gauged from the piston indentations) or until four indentation lines are visible. The ventilation volume should then be adjusted so that adequate chest excursion is ensured.

Central line placement can be performed with the HLR device in place, although only the internal and external jugular routes lend themselves to easy and safe access. The device should be momentarily turned off when the needle is being advanced to avoid arterial or lung injury. In excessively large patients, the maximum chest compression force may produce inadequate sternal displacement. In such cases the device should be removed and manual CPR reinstituted.

ALTERNATIVE CPR TECHNIQUES

Modifications of the standard CPR technique have been proposed over the last decade. Although each technique has initially been promising when investigated in one or two laboratories, none has demonstrated improved survival in clinical trials when compared to standard CPR.

Simultaneous Compression Ventilation CPR

The SCV-CPR method of CPR was designed to take advantage of the thoracic pump mechanism of forward blood flow. It maximizes intrathoracic pressure by generating a high airway pressure during the compression phase of chest massage. During the relaxation phase, the airway pressure is released. As discussed previously in this chapter, simultaneous compression and ventilation has been shown to improve arterial pressure and carotid blood flow in some animal studies.[6] Because SCV-CPR has not been demonstrated to have a beneficial effect on clinical outcome, the technique should be regarded as experimental.[24a]

Interposed Abdominal Compression CPR

The technique of IAC-CPR interposes abdominal compressions between the chest compressions of CPR (Fig.

17–6).[25–27] CPR is performed using American Heart Association guidelines; however, during the relaxation phase, the abdomen is compressed by pressure on a partially inflated, folded blood pressure cuff connected to a transducer to monitor applied pressure.

Several animal studies have demonstrated that IAC-CPR increases arterial systolic and diastolic pressures, cardiac output, and the arteriovenous diastolic pressure difference compared with standard CPR.[25–27] Despite these results, IAC-CPR has not been shown to improve *survival* in animal studies.[28]

In humans, IAC-CPR has been demonstrated to increase the mean arterial pressure, but not the diastolic arteriovenous pressure difference.[29] Mateer and coworkers compared IAC-CPR with standard CPR on patients treated in the field by paramedics following endotracheal intubation.[30] They found no difference in successful resuscitation with the use of IAC-CPR. In addition, questions regarding the safety of this technique have been raised. The risk of hypoventilation, aspiration in patients with unprotected airways, and abdominal injuries such as liver lacerations have not been fully studied.[31] IAC-CPR thus remains an experimental technique whose clinical efficacy has yet to be demonstrated.

High Frequency (Rapid Manual) CPR

Rapid manual CPR uses standard CPR techniques, but chest compressions are performed at a rate of 120 per minute. Maier and colleagues demonstrated that increasing the compression rate to 120 compressions per minute in an animal model resulted in increased cardiac output, aortic pressure, and coronary blood flow.[15] These studies provided the impetus for revision of the American Heart Association CPR standards to increase the chest compression rate to 80 to 100 per minute.

Studies by Feneley and associates demonstrated that a compression rate of 120 per minute resulted in improved resuscitation and more successful 24-hour survival in dogs compared with a compression rate of 60.[32] Additional studies are needed to determine whether rapid rates of chest compression will improve the efficacy of CPR for humans in cardiac arrest.

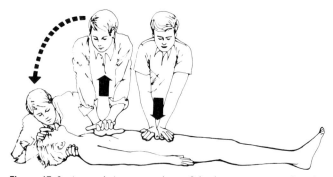

Figure 17–6. An artist's conception of basic rescuers performing interposed abdominal compression–cardiopulmonary resuscitation. For clarity, both rescuers are shown on the same side of the victim. With two rescuers, the first compresses the chest and ventilates while the second compresses the abdomen. With three rescuers, ventilation, chest compression, and abdominal compression are performed by separate individuals. (From Voorhees WD, Nicbauer MJ, Bubbs CF: Improved oxygen delivery during cardiopulmonary resuscitation with interposed abdominal compressions. Ann Emerg Med 12:128, 1983. Reproduced by permission.)

Pneumatic Antishock Garment

The pneumatic antishock garment (PASG), commonly referred to as military antishock trousers or the MAST suit, consists of a double-layered fabric with inflatable bladders that surround the legs and abdomen. The PASG has been used extensively as a therapeutic modality in hypovolemic shock and generally produces an increase in mean arterial pressure when inflated (see Chapter 35). The mechanism for this effect on blood pressure has been shown to be an increase in peripheral vascular resistance.[33]

Use of the PASG in animal models of cardiac arrest has produced mixed results. Redding and Rudikoff demonstrated that pneumatic abdominal binding increased aortic diastolic and systolic pressure and carotid blood flow during CPR.[6, 34] Harris and colleagues, however, found a high incidence of liver lacerations when abdominal binding was used in conjunction with CPR in dogs.[35] Mahoney and Mirick studied the efficacy of PASG during CPR in patients undergoing out-of-hospital resuscitation.[36] No difference in overall resuscitation or survival rate was demonstrated by the use of PASG. PASG, therefore, cannot be recommended for routine use in patients undergoing CPR.

Vest Cardiopulmonary Resuscitation

Mechanical devices have been developed to simulate "cough CPR" in the animal model. The vest or binder device produces pulsatile simultaneous increases in intrathoracic, intraabdominal, and airway pressure through simultaneous inflation of a pneumatic vest, abdominal binder, and endotracheal tube. Niemann and coworkers demonstrated improved hemodynamics and 24-hour survival for those animals receiving vest/binder CPR compared with standard CPR.[37] In contrast, Kern and colleagues could find no improvement in resuscitation or 24-hour survival when vest CPR was compared with standard mechanical CPR.[38] Further studies using these devices must be done to clarify their role in the treatment of patients in cardiac arrest.

ASSESSMENT OF ONGOING CARDIOPULMONARY RESUSCITATION

The prognosis for resuscitation of patients in cardiac arrest depends upon down time before CPR is initiated, time to advanced life support (defibrillation), and the initial cardiac rhythm. Once the resuscitation efforts are initiated, there is no ideal criterion to judge the efficacy of CPR. In most animal and clinical studies, outcome (i.e., resuscitation or death) is the only criterion used. Recent studies in the literature have focused attention on the problem of assessing effectiveness of ongoing resuscitation efforts.

Hemodynamics

Studies in experimental arrest models have demonstrated the importance of the aortic diastolic and myocardial perfusion pressures for successful resuscitation. Crile and Dolley first noted, in 1906, that resuscitation in a canine arrest model depended on producing a coronary perfusion pressure of 30 to 40 mm Hg.[39] Redding, in a series of classic experiments, showed that the aortic diastolic pressure must be raised over 40 mm Hg to successfully resuscitate animals in cardiac arrest (Fig. 17–7).[34] He suggested that α-catecholamine agents were crucial for resuscitation because they help

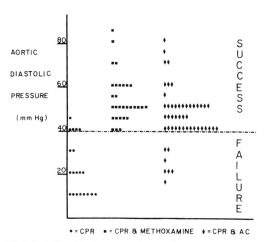

Figure 17–7. Relationship between the maximal aortic diastolic pressure during resuscitation and success in restoring spontaneous circulation. CPR, cardiopulmonary resuscitation. AC, abdominal compression. (From Redding JS: Abdominal compression in cardiopulmonary resuscitation. Anesth Analg 50:668, 1971.)

raise the aortic diastolic pressure.[34, 40–42] More recently, Sanders and associates demonstrated that animals could be resuscitated even after 30 minutes of ventricular fibrillation, providing the aortic diastolic and myocardial perfusion pressures were maintained at adequate levels.[43] Coronary blood flow has been shown to correlate well with the diastolic pressure difference between the aorta and right atrium.[44–46]

Although data confirming these observations are limited for humans undergoing CPR, one can extrapolate that CPR will be most effective when it provides adequate myocardial perfusion. In the setting of cardiac arrest, coronary blood flow and myocardial perfusion are directly related to the aortic to right atrial diastolic pressure gradient. The critical level of perfusion pressure needed for humans in cardiac arrest is unknown.[46a] It may be impossible to generate adequate blood flow to some areas of the myocardium in patients with severe coronary artery obstruction. These patients probably have a poor prognosis for resuscitation unless they are placed on emergency cardiopulmonary bypass and their coronary lesions promptly corrected.

In summary, the aortic diastolic pressure and myocardial perfusion pressure appear to be the best available criteria for assessing perfusion during cardiopulmonary resuscitation and correlate with survival in animal models. Thus the clinician should attempt to optimize these hemodynamic parameters during CPR. In most practice settings, however, the clinician will not have the opportunity to measure aortic and right atrial pressures during cardiopulmonary resuscitation. Therefore simpler, less invasive parameters are needed to guide resuscitation efforts in most patients suffering cardiac arrest.

Arterial Blood Gases

Clinicians often use arterial blood gas results to confirm the adequacy of their CPR efforts. Studies in experimental models have not shown a correlation of arterial blood gas results to successful resuscitation.[47] Physiologically, one would not expect the arterial pH, P_{O_2}, and P_{CO_2} to reflect tissue perfusion pressures. In fact, patients who suffer sudden ventricular fibrillation with no systemic perfusion will have normal aortic pH, P_{O_2}, and P_{CO_2} for several minutes following the arrest.

More recently, attention in the literature has focused on mixed venous gases. In the setting of cardiac arrest, venous gases will frequently show severe hypercarbia and acidosis, while arterial blood gases are relatively normal.[48] The extent of this venous-arterial P_{CO_2} gap may be reflective of poor perfusion pressures. Evaluation of the venous-arterial P_{CO_2} gap, however, must be considered an experimental technique. Pending further clinical evaluation, this invasive approach is not recommended for routine practice.

Pulses

Another commonly used technique for assessing the adequacy of CPR efforts is the presence or absence of femoral or carotid pulses. There are no studies indicating the clinical utility of pulses during CPR. The pulse represents a pulse pressure or the systolic to diastolic pressure gradient. As discussed previously, the key hemodynamic parameter associated with successful resuscitation is the aortic diastolic pressure. Thus the presence or absence of a pulse does not necessarily provide information regarding the aortic diastolic or myocardial perfusion pressures. In addition, reliance on femoral pulses can be misleading. Since there are no valves in the inferior vena cava, blood frequently flows in a retrograde fashion to the lower half of the body during chest compression. Thus the *palpable femoral pulse may represent venous rather than arterial blood flow.* The presence of carotid pulses may indicate some forward blood flow with chest compression. However, the extent of blood flow and, more important, tissue perfusion cannot be gauged by the presence or absence of a pulse.

Oximetry

Monitoring of the oxygen tension in the skin or conjunctiva is a potentially useful tool for assessing the adequacy of CPR. The literature has focused predominantly on the use of transconjunctival oximetry for patients in cardiac arrest. Abraham and Fink have shown that conjunctival oxygen tension as well as the ratio of conjunctival to arterial oxygen index promptly falls when a patient goes into cardiac arrest and returns to baseline when the patient is resuscitated.[49] They have also demonstrated that when a new rescuer with more vigorous chest compressions begins CPR the oxygen tension increases. Transconjunctival oximetry shows promise as an assessment criterion for monitoring patients in cardiac arrest. More research needs to be done, however, to determine whether conjunctival oxygen tension will reflect changes in perfusion pressures during the low output states accompanying CPR. Its clinical utility as a prognostic indicator for successful resuscitation remains to be determined.

Capnometry

INTRODUCTION

An area that has received considerable recent investigation is the use of capnometry to monitor ongoing CPR efforts. Capnometers use infrared spectroscopy to measure carbon dioxide in exhaled air. The sensor or sampling port is attached to the endotracheal tube. Carbon dioxide concentration in exhaled air is dependent on (1) its production by systemic metabolism, (2) its circulation, specifically pulmonary blood flow or cardiac output, and (3) the ventilatory system for excretion. In the setting of cardiac arrest and CPR where systemic metabolism and ventilation are held relatively constant, exhaled carbon dioxide reflects primarily lung perfusion and cardiac output.

Investigators have demonstrated in the experimental model that end-tidal carbon dioxide concentration during CPR correlates well with cardiac output and myocardial perfusion pressure.[50, 51] Studies in animal models have shown that CO_2 monitoring during CPR can distinguish those animals who will be successfully resuscitated from those that die.[52, 53] Swine in ventricular fibrillation for 12 minutes that were resuscitated had higher end-tidal CO_2 concentrations than if they did not have spontaneous perfusion restored (1.7 ± 0.2 per cent versus 0.5 ± 0.1 per cent).[53] In a similar study, swine in ventricular fibrillation were more often successfully defibrillated if their $P_{ET_{CO_2}}$ exceeded 16 mm Hg.[54]

There have been few studies evaluating the clinical use of capnometry for monitoring patients in cardiac arrest. Kalenda reported three patients who suffered cardiac arrest while being monitored by capnometry.[55] He found that when a rescuer fatigued while performing CPR, the CO_2 concentration fell; however, the CO_2 promptly increased again when a fresh rescuer took over. These observations led to the concept of using capnometry as a prognostic guide to ongoing resuscitation.

INDICATIONS

While capnometry remains an experimental technique, it shows promise as a means of noninvasively monitoring perfusion during CPR. Animal[53] and clinical studies[56, 57] suggest that capnometry may be the first indicator of restoration of spontaneous circulation. The technique may also prove helpful for quantifying the probability of developing a perfusing rhythm as a result of resuscitative efforts. The technique is noninvasive and is relatively contraindicated only when pharmacologic therapy may affect proper interpretation of the resuscitative efforts.

EQUIPMENT AND PROCEDURE

A variety of manufacturers supply capnometry equipment. Most capnometers use infrared absorption spectroscopy to measure carbon dioxide. Operation of each monitor and recorder should follow its manufacturer's instructions. Calibration of the monitor should be performed periodically with a known CO_2 source.

A sampling port slips between the endotracheal tube and a resuscitation bag. Some devices provide in-line continuous CO_2 readings, whereas others suction off samples of air from the endotracheal tube to a sensor in the body of the machine. The clinician is interested in the end-tidal CO_2 (or peak) level, since this most closely approximates the alveolar CO_2 concentration.

INTERPRETATION

End-tidal CO_2 measurements are given either as a concentration in percentage CO_2 (ETCO$_2$) or as the partial pressure of CO_2 in mm Hg ($P_{ET_{CO_2}}$). Measurement of the $P_{ET_{CO_2}}$ varies slightly with the altitude at which the reading is taken. Animal studies have indicated that end-tidal CO_2 measurements correlate with cardiac output,[51] myocardial perfusion pressure,[50, 52] and resuscitation from cardiac arrest.[52, 53]

Clinical studies assessing end-tidal CO_2 during CPR have been limited. In one series of 18 adults in late cardiac arrest, an ETCO$_2$ concentration of 1.7 to 1.8 per cent was associated with a mean arterial diastolic pressure of 22 to 25 mm Hg.[58] None of the patients were resuscitated. Another study of 23 arrest victims by the same group including ten patients attaining spontaneous circulation did not find a difference in ETCO$_2$ concentration between those resuscitated and those without return of spontaneous circulation.[56]

Falk and associates used capnometry to monitor 13 cardiac arrests in 10 critically ill patients.[57] The investigators noted a prompt fall in ETCO$_2$ from 1.4 ± 0.9 per cent to 0.4 ± 0.4 per cent at the onset of cardiac arrest, an increase in $ETCO_2$ to 1.0 ± 0.5 per cent once precordial compressions were begun, and a rapid increase of $ETCO_2$ to 3.7 ± 2.1 per cent in the seven patients in whom spontaneous circulation was restored.[57] No significant differences were noted in the $ETCO_2$ concentration for resuscitated and nonresuscitated patients during CPR. Lepilin noted a similar pattern of $ETCO_2$ for arrest and resuscitation in four postoperative patients.[59]

Recent clinical studies have addressed differences in carbon dioxide excretion during ongoing CPR as a predictor of effectiveness of resuscitation. Callaham and Barton correlated initial end-tidal CO_2 with the return of a palpable pulse in 55 emergency department patients. The 14 patients who had a return of palpable pulse had a mean PET_{CO_2} of 19 mm Hg compared with 5 mm Hg for the 41 patients who did not develop pulses.[60] Another clinical study of 35 adult cardiac arrests demonstrated a difference in PET_{CO_2} during ongoing CPR in those patients who were successfully resuscitated and survived to discharge compared with those who died.[61] The nine patients who were successfully resuscitated also had a higher average PET_{CO_2} during CPR than those who could not be resuscitated (15 ± 4 versus 7 ± 5 mm Hg). All nine resuscitated patients had an average PET_{CO_2} of 10 mm Hg or greater and the three who survived to hospital discharge had an average PET_{CO_2} of 17 mm Hg.

Caution must be used in interpreting end-tidal CO_2 values. Experimentally, the administration of sodium bicarbonate has been shown to increase the excretion of CO_2 and hence adversely affect the correlation of end-tidal CO_2 with perfusion during CPR. Therefore, end-tidal CO_2 readings are not reflective of perfusion pressures during CPR for 5 minutes following the administration of bicarbonate. Additionally, alterations in ventilations during CPR may affect end-tidal CO_2 readings. The effect of pressor agents during ongoing CPR on end-tidal CO_2 is variable.[62, 63] Experimentally, high doses of epinephrine will lower the end-tidal CO_2 and cardiac output during cardiac arrest while myocardial perfusion pressures and coronary blood flow increase.[64, 65]

CONCLUSIONS

While explicit values for end-tidal CO_2 that reflect effective artificial cardiac perfusion cannot be given at this time, capnometry appears to have potential as a noninvasive barometer of artificial perfusion. The use and limitations of capnometry in the management of patients in cardiac arrest will be determined by further clinical studies.

SUMMARY

Assessment of ongoing cardiopulmonary resuscitation efforts will allow clinicians to rationally manage patients in cardiac arrest. It would also allow researchers to evaluate alterations in the technique of CPR and changes in resuscitation protocols.

Hemodynamic monitoring, especially the aortic diastolic pressure and aortic to right atrial perfusion gradient, is currently the best indicator of adequate cardiac perfusion during ongoing CPR. It is often impractical to measure these hemodynamic parameters in the setting of a cardiac arrest. Therefore, indirect indices of perfusion such as capnometry may be useful in the overall evaluation of patients in cardiac arrest.

REFERENCES

1. Kouwenhoven WB, Jude JR, Knickerbocker GG: Closed-chest cardiac massage. JAMA 173:1064, 1960.
2. Luce JM, Cary JM, Ross BK, et al: New developments in cardiopulmonary resuscitation. JAMA 244:1366, 1980.
3. Weale FE, Rothwell-Jackson RL: The efficiency of cardiac massage. Lancet 1:990, 1962.
4. MacKenzie GJ, Taylor SH, McDonald AH, Donald KW: Haemodynamic effects of external cardiac compression. Lancet 1:1342, 1964.
5. Wilder RJ, Weir D, Rush BF, Ravitch MM: Methods of coordinating ventilation and closed-chest cardiac massage in the dog. Surgery 53:186, 1963.
6. Rudikoff MT, Maughan WL, Effron M, et al: Mechanisms of blood flow during cardiopulmonary resuscitation. Circulation 61:345, 1980.
7. Chandra N, Rudikoff M, Weisfeldt ML: Simultaneous chest compression and ventilation at high airway pressure during cardiopulmonary resuscitation. Lancet 1:351, 1980.
8. Chandra N, Snyder LD, Weisfeldt ML: Abdominal binding during cardiopulmonary resuscitation in man. JAMA 246:351, 1981.
9. Criley JM, Blaufuss AH, Kissel GL: Cough induced cardiac compression. JAMA 236:1246, 1976.
10. Niemann JT, Rosborough JP, Niskonen RA, et al: Mechanical cough cardiopulmonary resuscitation during cardiac arrest in dogs. Am J Cardiol 55:199, 1985.
11. Niemann JT, Rosborough JP, Hausknecht M, et al: Pressure-synchronized cineangiography during experimental cardiopulmonary resuscitation. Circulation 64:985, 1981.
12. Weisfeldt MI, Chandra N, Tsitlik JE, Rudikoff M: New attempts to improve blood flow during CPR. In Schluger J, Lyon AF (eds): CPR and Emergency Cardiac Care: Looking to the Future. New York, EM Books, 1980.
13. Deshmukh HG, Weil MH, Rackow EC, et al: Echocardiographic observations during cardiopulmonary resuscitation: A preliminary report. Crit Care Med 13:904, 1985.
14. Sanders AB, Ewy GA, Alferness CA, et al: Failure of one method of simultaneous chest compression, ventilation, and abdominal binding during CPR. Crit Care Med 10:509, 1982.
15. Maier GW, Tyson GS, Olsen CO, et al: The physiology of external cardiac massage: High impulse cardiopulmonary resuscitation. Circulation 70:86, 1984.
16. Babbs CF, Tacker WA, Paris RL, Murphy RJ: CPR with simultaneous compression and ventilation at high airway pressure in 4 animal models. Crit Care Med 10:501, 1982.
17. American Heart Association Standards and Guidelines for Cardiopulmonary Resuscitation and Emergency Cardiac Care. JAMA 255:2841, 1986.
18. Orlowski JP: Optimum position for external cardiac compression in infants and young children. Ann Emerg Med 15:667, 1986.
19. Finholt DA, Ketterick RG, Wagner HR, Swedlow PB: The heart is under the lower third of the sternum. AJDC 140:646, 1986.
20. Chameides L, ed: Textbook of Advanced Life Support. Dallas, American Heart Association, 1988.
21. David R: Closed-chest cardiac massage in the newborn infant. Pediatrics 18:552, 1988.
22. Taylor GJ, Rubin R, Tucker M, Greene HL, Rudikoff MT, Weisfeldt ML: External cardiac compression. JAMA 240:644, 1978.
23. McDonald JL: Systolic and mean arterial pressures during manual CPR in humans. Ann Emerg Med 11:292, 1982.
24. Chandra N: Mechanical adjuncts for CPR. In Roberts JR, Hedges JR (eds): Clinical Procedures in Emergency Medicine. 1st ed. Philadelphia, WB Saunders Co, 1985, pp 231–240.
24a. Krisher JP, Fine EG, Weisfeldt ML, et al: Comparison of prehospital conventional and simultaneous compression-ventilation cardiopulmonary resuscitation. Crit Care Med 17:1263, 1989.
25. Babbs CF, Ralston SH, Voorhees WD III: Improved cardiac output during CPR with interposed abdominal compressions. Ann Emerg Med 12:527, 1983.
26. Voorhees WD, Niebauer MJ, Babbs CF: Improved oxygen delivery during cardiopulmonary resuscitation with interposed abdominal compressions. Ann Emerg Med 12:128, 1983.
27. Ralston SH, Babbs CF, Niebauer MJ: Cardiopulmonary resuscitation with interposed abdominal compressions in dogs. Anesth Analg 61:645, 1982.
28. Kern KB, Carter AB, Showen RL, et al: Twenty-four hour survival in a canine model of cardiac arrest comparing three methods of manual cardiopulmonary resuscitation. J Am Coll Cardiol 7:859, 1986.
29. Howard M, Carrubba C, Foss F, et al: Interposed abdominal compression CPR: Its effects on parameters of coronary perfusion in human subjects. Ann Emerg Med 16:253, 1987.
30. Mateer JR, Stueven HA, Thompson BM, et al: Prehospital IAC-CPR versus standard CPR. Am J Emerg Med 8:143, 1985.
31. Bircher NG, Abramson NS: Interposed abdominal compression CPR (IAC-CPR). Am J Emerg Med 2:177, 1984.
32. Feneley MP, Maier GW, Kern KB, et al: Influence of compression rate on initial success of resuscitation and 24 hour survival after prolonged manual cardiopulmonary resuscitation in dogs. Circulation 77:240, 1988.
33. Kaback KR, Sanders AB, Meislin HW: MAST suit update. JAMA 252:2598, 1984.
34. Redding JS: Abdominal compression during cardiopulmonary resuscitation. Anesth Analg 50:668, 1971.
35. Harris LC, Kirimli B, Safar P: Augmentation of artificial circulation during cardiopulmonary resuscitation. Anesthesiology 28:730, 1967.
36. Mahoney BD, Mirick MJ: Efficacy of pneumatic trousers in refractory prehospital cardiopulmonary arrest. Ann Emerg Med 12:8, 1983.
37. Niemann JT, Rosborough JP, Niskanen RA, et al: Mechanical "cough"

cardiopulmonary resuscitation during cardiac arrest in dogs. Am J Cardiol 55:199, 1985.

38. Kern KB, Carter AB, Showen RL, et al: Comparison of mechanical techniques of cardiopulmonary resuscitation. Am J Emerg Med 5:190, 1987.
39. Crile G, Dolley DH: Experimental resuscitation of dogs killed by anesthetics and asphyxia. J Exp Med 6:713, 1906.
40. Redding JS, Pearson JW: Resuscitation from ventricular fibrillation drug therapy. JAMA 203:93, 1968.
41. Redding JS, Pearson JW: Evaluation of drugs for cardiac resuscitation. Anesthesiology 24:203, 1963.
42. Pearson JW, Redding JS: Influence of peripheral vascular tone on cardiac resuscitation. Anesth Analg 44:746, 1965.
43. Sanders AB, Ewy GA, Taft TV: Prognostic and therapeutic importance of the aortic diastolic pressure in resuscitation from cardiac arrest. Crit Care Med 12:871, 1984.
44. Ditchey RV, Winkler JV, Rhodes CA: Relative lack of coronary blood flow during closed-chest resuscitation in dogs. Circulation 66:297, 1982.
45. Michael JR, Guerci AD, Koehler RC, et al. Mechanisms by which epinephrine augments cerebral and myocardial perfusion during cardiopulmonary resuscitation in dogs. Circulation 69:822, 1984.
46. Ralston SH, Voorhees WD, Babbs CF. Intra-pulmonary epinephrine during prolonged cardiopulmonary resuscitation: Improved regional flow and resuscitation in dogs. Ann Emerg Med 13:79, 1984.
46a. Paradis NA, Martin GB, Rivers EP, et al: Coronary perfusion pressure and the return of spontaneous circulation in human cardiopulmonary resuscitation. JAMA 263:1106, 1990.
47. Sanders AB, Ewy GA, Taft TV: Resuscitation and arterial blood gas abnormalities during prolonged cardiopulmonary resuscitation. Ann Emerg Med 13:676, 1984.
48. Weil MH, Rackow EC, Trevino R, et al: Difference in acid base state between venous and arterial blood during cardiopulmonary resuscitation. N Engl J Med 315:153, 1986.
49. Abraham E, Fink S: Conjunctival oxygen tension monitoring in emergency department patients. Am J Emerg Med 6:549, 1988.
50. Sanders AB, Atlas M, Ewy GA, et al: Expired CO_2 as an index of coronary perfusion pressure. Am J Emerg Med 3:147, 1985.
51. Weil MH, Bisera J, Trevino RR, Rackow EC: Cardiac output and end-tidal carbon dioxide. Crit Care Med 13:907, 1985.
52. Sanders AB, Ewy GA, Bragg S, et al: Expired P_{CO_2} as a prognostic

indicator of successful resuscitation from cardiac arrest. Ann Emerg Med 14:948, 1985.
53. Gudipati CV, Weil MH, Bisera J, et al: Expired carbon dioxide: A noninvasive monitor of cardiopulmonary resuscitation. Circulation 77:234, 1988.
54. Von Planta M, von Planta I, Weil MH, et al: End-tidal carbon dioxide for monitoring blood flow during CPR (Abstract). Crit Care Med 16:388, 1988.
55. Kalenda Z: The capnogram as a guide to the efficacy of cardiac massage. Resuscitation 6:259, 1978.
56. Garnett AR, Ornato JP, Gonzales ER, Johnson EB: End-tidal carbon dioxide monitoring during cardiopulmonary resuscitation. JAMA 257:512, 1987.
57. Falk JL, Rackow EC, Weil MH: End-tidal carbon dioxide concentration during cardiopulmonary resuscitation. N Engl J Med 318:607, 1988.
58. Ornato JP, Gonzalez ER, Garnett R, et al: Effect of cardiopulmonary resuscitation compression rate on end-tidal carbon dioxide concentration and arterial pressure in man. Crit Care Med 16:241, 1988.
59. Lepilin MG, Vasilyev AV, Bildinor OA, Rostovtsen NA: End tidal carbon dioxide as a non-invasive monitor of circulatory status during cardiopulmonary resuscitation: A preliminary study. Crit Care Med 15:958, 1987.
60. Callaham M, Barton C: Prediction of outcome of cardiopulmonary resuscitation from end-tidal carbon dioxide concentration. Crit Care Med 18:358, 1990.
61. Sanders AB, Kern KB, Otto CW, et al: End-tidal carbon dioxide monitoring during cardiopulmonary resuscitation: A prognostic indicator for survival. JAMA 262:1347, 1989.
62. Paradis NA, Goetting MG, Rivers EP, et al: Increases in coronary perfusion pressure after high-dose epinephrine result in decreases in end-tidal CO_2 during CPR in human beings (Abstract). Ann Emerg Med 19:491, 1990.
63. Callaham M, Barton C: Effect of epinephrine administration on ability of end-tidal carbon dioxide readings to predict outcome of cardiac arrest (Abstract). Ann Emerg Med 19:490, 1990.
64. Chase PB, Kern KB, Saunders AB, et al: The effect of high and low dose epinephrine on myocardial perfusion, cardiac output and end-tidal carbon dioxide during prolonged CPR (Abstract). Ann Emerg Med 19:466, 1990.
65. Martin GB, Gentile NT, Paradis NA, et al: Effect of epinephrine on end-tidal carbon dioxide monitoring during CPR. Ann Emerg Med 19:396, 1990.

Chapter *18*

Resuscitative Thoracotomy

Robert L. Bartlett

INTRODUCTION

As a multidisciplinary specialist, the emergency physician at times finds it necessary to use procedures previously considered to be the province of one of the surgical specialities. The emergency thoracotomy is the most invasive and controversial of these procedures.[1–7] "The days when an individual specialty could restrict the use of a technical skill are long gone. Pertinent to technical skills are appropriate training, skills maintainance, and judgment as to when to apply them or when to withhold them."[8]

In the past two decades, the development of sophisticated emergency medical systems using well-trained paramedics, advanced life support, and rapid transport has increased the number of patients arriving at the emergency department in various stages of shock.[9–11] With increasing frequency, emergency physicians are being given the opportunity to resuscitate patients who previously

would have expired at the scene. For some, survival is possible if an aggressive approach using emergency thoracotomy is taken. Therefore, knowing who may respond to thoracotomy becomes an important issue.[12–18]

This chapter discusses the factors that influence the outcome of an emergency thoracotomy and the pathophysiology, diagnosis, and treatment of those injuries that require such an invasive procedure. The heart, the lungs, and the great vessels are the three vital structures in which injuries may require the use of a resuscitative thoracotomy. The mechanism of injury, prehospital vital signs, and systolic blood pressure following thoracotomy form the basic structure of a resuscitative algorithm.

Although this chapter provides considerable detail of the rationale for and the technique of resuscitative thoracotomy, the emergency physician should be aware of the *specific goals to be attained after opening the chest*. In the trauma patient receiving a resuscitative thoracotomy, the physician seeks to relieve any cardiac tamponade; to support cardiac function (with direct cardiac compressions, cross-clamping of the aorta to improve coronary perfusion, and internal defibrillation when indicated); and to control hemorrhage from the heart, pulmonary vessels, thoracic wall, and great vessels. While certain circumstances may require this sequence of resuscitation to be altered, the emergency physician should be cognizant of these goals upon opening the chest.

Additionally, each institution should establish guidelines for the initiation of resuscitative thoracotomy and subsequent patient care in the emergency department. Ideally a preestablished plan of chest wound management and postthoracotomy care should be established with the service providing the emergency physician's surgical backup for those times when members of the surgical team cannot be onsite at the time of the resuscitation. With such a plan, a team approach to resuscitation and optimal patient care is possible.

INDICATIONS AND CONTRAINDICATIONS

The current trend toward more aggressive management of trauma was pioneered in the mid-1960s and early 1970s by Sugg and colleagues,[19] Mattox and associates,[20, 21] and others. Most simply, the indication for thoracotomy in the emergency care unit has been the absence of vital signs on admission or the loss of pulse and blood pressure during the resuscitation of a trauma victim. In the past, thoracotomy with cross-clamping of the aorta was performed on all moribund patients, regardless of the mechanism of injury. The high success rates for the initial resuscitation (75 per cent) and the long-term survival rates (8 to 31 per cent) were cited as support for such indiscriminate use of emergency thoracotomies. A closer review of these early reports reveals the mechanism of injury and prehospital vital signs as the major determinants of a successful outcome.[21–23] Blunt and penetrating trauma are the two categories of injury that will be considered. The importance of making this distinction becomes apparent when published survival rates are reviewed.

Resuscitative Thoracotomy in Blunt Trauma

When other methods of resuscitation failed, it was thought that victims of *blunt* trauma would be helped by a thoracotomy. Unfortunately, the *survival* rate for these patients is negligible. In the past 10 years there have been seven published reports evaluating the role of emergency thoracotomy in blunt trauma.[7, 20, 22–27] The overall survival rate was only 2.9 per cent. Patients rarely survived when their vital signs were lost before admission, and there were no survivors when the electrocardiogram (ECG) demonstrated asystole.[20, 24]

To date, Bodai and coworkers have published the most detailed study of blunt trauma resuscitation with emergency thoracotomy.[25] Only those patients who exhibited a pulse or respiratory efforts at the scene were studied. Half of the patients arrived in the emergency department within 30 minutes of injury, yet more than 85 per cent of patients had no obtainable vital signs or were *agonal* upon arrival. *Agonal* was defined as having irregular respiration or thready pulse without measurable blood pressure. From this group of 38 patients, 56 per cent were resuscitated following thoracotomy and transferred to the operating room. This initial resuscitation rate is impressive; however, only 10 per cent (4 of 38) survived the surgical procedures, and each of these individuals expired shortly thereafter. Two died from brain injuries, one from multiple organ failure, and one from disseminated intravascular coagulation. Thus there were no long-term survivors in this series.

In summary, emergency thoracotomy for *blunt* trauma is limited in its ability to resuscitate patients who develop cardiac arrest or who arrive with agonal signs. Until more encouraging results are advanced, this resuscitative procedure generally should be reserved for those patients sustaining *blunt* trauma who arrive in the emergency care unit with pulse, respiratory efforts, and reactive pupils.[22, 25, 28]

Emergency Thoracotomy for Penetrating Trauma

Following the unsuccessful attempts of Capplelen[29] and Farina[30] to repair a wound of the heart in 1896, Page stated that "the surgery of the heart has probably reached the limits set by nature to all surgery. No new method or discovery can overcome the natural difficulties that attend a wound of the heart."[31] Yet that same year Rehn[32] successfully relieved a pericardial tamponade and repaired an actively bleeding wound of the right ventricle. Over the next 50 years, the effectiveness of cardiorrhaphy for penetrating wounds of the heart and the great vessels was firmly established, with survival figures ranging from 50 per cent to 65 per cent.[33–44] These reports, however, involved patients who were transported directly to the operating theater and tolerated their wounds in the absence of prehospital emergency care.

The prehospital mortality for penetrating chest wounds depends on the structures involved. For heart wounds in particular, the prehospital mortality is approximately 80 per cent. Nonetheless, if any signs of life are present during the prehospital phase, these patients may be salvaged. Recently, the vital importance of speed and the use of the emergency department as the site of thoracotomy has been emphasized. Mattox and colleagues, in describing 37 emergency thoracotomies in emergency center patients in cardiac arrest shortly before or after arrival, stated that there was "no question that these patients could not have survived the short trip to the operating room. This group represents patients who, in former years, probably would have died at the scene or en route to the hospital."[21] MacDonald, commenting on his series of 28 emergency thoracotomies in a community hospital, observed that "resuscitation can be hampered by significant delays in assembling the necessary operating room staff. These delays sometimes mean that a trauma patient will be detained for a significant amount of time in the emergency department before a definitive procedure can be performed in the operating room."[7]

When the patient's vital signs suggest that cardiac arrest is imminent despite airway control and the initiation of volume replacement, a thoracotomy should be performed immediately. A tragic death may result if the physician allows a cardiac arrest to occur while waiting for a possible response to ancillary therapy or while transporting the patient to the operating table. Beall and coworkers[45] compared the mortality figures for emergency thoracotomies performed for penetrating cardiac injuries in patients with inhospital cardiac arrest. For the group receiving thoracotomies before cardiopulmonary arrest the mortality was 15 per cent. If the thoracotomy was performed after cardiopulmonary arrest, the mortality increased to 60 per cent. Reul and colleagues[46] compared the mortality figures for emergency thoracotomies performed on patients with mixed trauma (blunt and penetrating) to the thoracic great vessels. Again, only those patients whose arrest had occurred in the hospital were studied. When the thoracotomy preceded the arrest, the mortality was 18 per cent. If arrest occurred before the thoracotomy, the mortality was 73 per cent.

Unfortunately, the observations by Reul and associates do not permit a more detailed analysis, and it must be acknowledged that patients who suffer cardiac arrest may have more severe injuries. Nonetheless, it should be clear that every effort, including thoracotomy, should be made to avert a cardiac arrest. As stated by Siemens and coworkers, "delay and observation in the shocked, bleeding, or tamponading injury can only lead to prolongation of hypotension, acidosis, excessive requirement of blood and crystalloids, and on occasion sudden ventricular fibrillation or standstill."[47] If the etiology of the patient's deterioration is hemorrhage, "surgery should not await resuscitation but is an integral part of resuscitation, as only when bleeding is controlled can the circulating blood volume be restored adequately."[48]

With penetrating thoracic trauma, the frequency of organ injury corresponds to the relative exposure of each organ. The lung is the most commonly injured organ, followed by the heart, the great vessels, the tracheobronchial tree, and the esophagus. Approximately 80 per cent of penetrating chest injuries can be managed conservatively with tube thoracostomy if the only significant injury is a pneumothorax[47, 49–51] (see Chapter 9).

When heart wounds in particular are considered, the distribution of injuries reflects the relative exposure of each chamber and the intracardiac vessels. A review of the distribution of 1802 cardiac wounds showed an incidence of 43 per cent for right ventricular injuries, 33 per cent for left ventricular injuries, 14 per cent for right atrial injuries, and 5 per cent for injuries to the intrapericardial vessels.[52, 53] The percentage of anterior chest wall exposure of these structures is 55 per cent for the right ventricle, 20 per cent for the left ventricle, 10 per cent for the right atrium, 10 per cent for the great vessels, and 5 per cent for the vena cava.[53, 54]

The combined survival rate in nine reports of penetrating chest injuries requiring emergency department thoracotomy was 34 per cent for gunshot wounds and 45 per cent for stab wounds.[52, 53] Gunshot wounds are the most common form of penetrating injury. When they involve the heart, the associated blast effect usually results in exsanguination rather than tamponade.[55] In contrast, 80 to 90 per cent of stab wounds to the heart will result in tamponade. The development of tamponade may be temporizing during the prehospital phase. If tamponade does not occur, most patients with myocardial stab wounds will exsanguinate.[56, 57]

Two additional factors that influence the development of tamponade are wound size and chamber involvement. Wounds of the myocardium less than 1 cm may spontaneously seal, depending on the location. Wounds larger than 1 cm will usually continue to bleed regardless of the chamber involved.[57, 58] The low-pressured atria will usually clot off before tamponade develops.[54] However, a wound of the right ventricle is often associated with tamponade. This is the result of a thin wall (3 mm) with little occlusive potential and a higher systolic pressure than that of the atria. In contrast, the thicker-walled left ventricle (120 mm Hg average) may spontaneously seal stab wounds up to 1 cm in length. Thus tamponade may be absent even though the left ventricle has been lacerated.[57]

HEMODYNAMIC RESPONSE TO EMERGENCY THORACOTOMY

A report of emergency department thoracotomies for blunt and penetrating trauma from Denver General Hospital related the hemodynamic response to thoracotomy to patient outcome.[22] Of the 146 cases reviewed, 45 patients (31 per cent) were transferred to the operating room following initial resuscitation and aortic cross-clamping when necessary. For those patients surviving with full neurologic recovery, the average systolic blood pressure after the first 30 minutes of resuscitation was 110 mm Hg. In those who were long-term survivors but had developed significant brain damage, the average systolic blood pressure was 85 mm Hg. There were no survivors when the mean systolic blood pressure was less than 70 mm Hg. Thus the blood pressure response to emergency thoracotomy becomes predictive of survival. For those patients who remain lifeless with systolic blood pressures below 70 mm Hg despite control of hemorrhage, volume replacement, and cross-clamping for 30 minutes, we recommended that "heroic measures should be discontinued." Transfer of these patients to the operating suite for definitive repair would be nonproductive.

SUMMARY

Improved survival figures support the selective use of emergency department thoracotomy. *This procedure is most effective when it is used to prevent a cardiac arrest rather than to treat it.* Four factors are closely associated with patient outcome following resuscitative thoracotomy: (1) mechanism of injury; (2) presence or absence of pulse, pupil reactivity, and respiratory effort at the scene and on admission; (3) ECG activity; and (4) systolic blood pressure after cross-clamping. The following guidelines should be considered:

1. Blunt trauma victims who lose their vital signs while en route to the emergency department rarely survive, despite thoracotomy.

2. Penetrating trauma victims who lose their vital signs while en route to the emergency department may still survive and should receive an immediate thoracotomy.

3. Thoracotomy should be considered when the systolic blood pressure cannot be maintained above 70 mm Hg with aggressive management and use of the pneumatic anti-shock garment.

4. Further efforts generally should be discontinued following thoracotomy when patients do not exhibit cardiac activity or tamponade.

5. Further efforts should be discontinued following thoracotomy if the systolic pressure cannot be raised above 70 mm Hg.

Cardiac Tamponade

DIAGNOSIS AND PATHOPHYSIOLOGY

Cardiac tamponade is defined as the *decompensated* phase of cardiac function resulting from increased intrapericardial pressure (see also Chapter 16).[59] The clinical diagnosis of pericardial tamponade in the unstable trauma patient is difficult because of the combined effect of hemorrhagic and cardiogenic shock. The classic signs of Beck triad (distended neck veins, hypotension, and decreased heart sounds) have limited diagnostic value for acute penetrating cardiac trauma. In most series, the complete triad was found in only 35 per cent of patients.[60–63] Additional signs of tamponade include tachycardia; pulsus paradoxus; elevated central venous pressure; agitation and confusion (reflecting decreased cerebral perfusion); air hunger; and cold, clammy skin.[64–66]

Three mechanisms may partially compensate for the cardiac tamponade state. The first is a reactive tachycardia. Reactive tachycardia during the hypotensive phase of tamponade is the usual finding, but for some patients a bradycardia may be present. Several studies involving rapid induction of cardiac tamponade failed to find significant changes in heart rate.[67] These findings may reflect vagally mediated cardiac depressor reflexes. Receptors for these reflexes have been identified in the left and right atria, the left coronary artery, the myocardium, and the epicardium.[67–70]

A second compensatory mechanism is the elevation of central venous pressure (CVP). Although this is partially a reflection of poor atrioventricular filling, it is primarily the result of increased venomotor tone, which improves the effective filling pressure of the ventricles. In the acute situation with persistent hypotension one cannot rely on the CVP. Many affected patients have marked volume depletion and are incapable of elevating their CVP despite advanced tamponade. If hypotension persists and the CVP rises, the patient should be presumed to have cardiac tamponade. One should be aware that in some cases there may be a poor correlation between the CVP and the extent of tamponade even when the blood volume has been corrected.[71, 72]

The third compensatory mechanism is an increased peripheral vascular resistance that preserves arterial pressure in the face of falling cardiac output. When hypotension does appear, it is an ominous sign, and the emergency physician must respond quickly.

TREATMENT OF CARDIAC TAMPONADE

The definitive therapy for acute tamponade is surgical decompression and repair. The adjunctive therapies include rapid volume expansion, atropine, pericardiocentesis or a subxiphoid window (see Chapter 16), and the use of a vasopressor with alpha activity *during* the induction of anesthesia.

Because of the steep slope of the curve relating blood pressure to intrapericardial pressure, cardiac tamponade may behave in a very labile manner, depending on the treatment used.[60, 73] Rapid volume expansion with blood or colloids should be the first form of therapy. In spite of severe tamponade, volume expansion alone, which further increases the venous pressure, may temporarily normalize cardiac output and arterial pressure.[74] A high CVP is not necessarily a sign of fluid overload but rather is a sign of poor ventricular filling and increased venous tone. Improved circulatory dynamics may occur with only minimal increases (5 to 6 cm H_2O) in CVP.[73]

Pulmonary Injuries and Emergency Thoracotomy

Pulmonary injuries can be divided into three types: parenchymal, tracheobronchial, and large vessel. Parenchymal and tracheobronchial injuries rarely create a situation requiring thoracotomy in the emergency department. The vast majority of these injuries can be treated adequately by tube thoracostomy during initial resuscitation (see Chapter 9).

Tracheobronchial injuries may be incurred from penetrating trauma; however, blunt trauma is the more usual cause. Most patients with this injury expire at the scene. A comprehensive study of 1178 motor vehicle fatalities revealed the presence of this injury in 33 cases.[76] Unfortunately, because this injury is not always associated with severe thoracic trauma, it may be overlooked. In 12 of 80 bronchial tears reported by Hood and Sloan,[77] the tracheobronchial injury was the only major intrathoracic wound.

With this injury, the airway is usually maintained, even in the face of a complete transection. The stiff tracheobronchial cartilage tends to hold the lumen open while the peritracheal and peribronchial fasciae preserve the relationship of proximal to distal bronchi.[78] Ninety per cent of tracheobronchial tears occur within 1 inch of the carina.

These tears most commonly involve the main stem bronchi. Less frequently, vertical tears may occur along the membranous cartilage line of the trachea. Complete division of the trachea is extremely rare. Depending on the size and the location of the injury, patients may present with one or more of the following: massive hemoptysis when bronchial vessels are involved, airway obstruction, and pneumomediastinum or pneumothorax with or without tension.

Fatalities are the result of associated injuries or a tension pneumothorax. The buildup of pleural air under pressure impairs venous return directly by partially or fully collapsing the vena cava and indirectly by mediastinal shifts that distort the caval-atrial junction.[79] A large chest tube is usually sufficient treatment. If the leak is large, a point is reached at which the rate of removal of pleural air prevents adequate intake of air into the lungs. In this event, the emergency physician must settle for a pneumothorax without tension and must discontinue further attempts to expand the lung fully. Affected patients require urgent thoracotomy in the

operating suite. Relief of the tension pneumothorax should allow sufficient time for safe transfer. If hemorrhaging is profuse or if the site of injury can be determined, the use of a bifid endotracheal tube or the unilateral intubation of a main stem bronchus will secure the airway.

Lacerations of the parenchyma unaccompanied by major vessel injuries also respond well to a tube thoracostomy. Although the associated hemothorax may be significant, the pulmonary vascular system is of sufficiently low pressure that reexpansion of the lung will often halt or reduce bleeding. Reduction of parenchymal bleeding by negative pressure coaptation of the pleural surfaces is successful in 72 to 98 per cent of cases.[47, 80] If the initial chest tube drainage is more than 800 ml with continued drainage at a rate of 50 ml every 10 minutes or if there is persistent hypotension, immediate thoracotomy should be considered.[47, 81] Such patients rarely have simple parenchymal injuries; major vascular structures are usually involved. A complication of parenchymal injuries that will require immediate thoracotomy is the development of air embolism.

Air Embolism

Suspicion of air embolism following trauma is considered to be an indication for emergency thoracotomy. Until recently, the occurrence of air embolism following penetrating injuries of the lung had not been widely recognized, although it may be a significant cause of morbidity and mortality.[82, 83]

The preoperative and postmortem diagnosis of air embolism is difficult. Air embolism is confirmed at thoracotomy by needle aspiration of a foamy air-blood admixture from the left or right heart or by visualization of air within the coronary arteries. Preoperative demonstration of air by aspiration from a central venous catheter or the femoral artery is rare but has been reported.[83, 84]

Air embolism may appear in either the right or the left side of the circulatory system. Involvement of the right side of the circulation is referred to as *venous* or *pulmonary* air embolism. Generally, venous air is well tolerated, but death may occur when the volume of air reaches 5 to 8 ml/kg. The rate at which air moves into the circulation and the body position are important determinants of the volume that can be tolerated. Death usually results from obstruction of the right ventricle or the pulmonary circulation. If the mean pulmonary arterial pressure exceeds 22 mm Hg, air may pass into the systemic circulation. Paradoxical air embolism may also occur in the 15 to 25 per cent of patients who have a potentially patent foramen ovale.

The most common cause of venous air embolism is management error with intravenous therapy.[83, 85, 86] Air embolism fatalities have been reported with subclavian venipuncture.[85] A pressure difference of 5 cm H_2O across a 14-gauge needle will allow the introduction of 100 ml of air per second. Injuries of the vena cava or the right heart would also create obvious portals of entry into the right circulatory system.

Air embolism involving the left side of the circulatory system is referred to as *arterial* or *systemic* air embolism. The lethal volume depends on the organs to which it is distributed. As little as 0.5 ml of air in the left anterior descending coronary artery has led to ventricular fibrillation. Arterial air will traverse systemic capillaries more readily than those in the pulmonary system. The pressure threshold for the passage of air through these capillaries is usually less than that of the normal systemic arterial pressure.[87] Air can pass from the femoral artery to the femoral vein with pressures as low as 20 mm Hg. The required pressure for visceral capillaries is higher and has a much larger range. Experimental pressures as high as 180 mm Hg have occasionally been required. Unfortunately, not all of the air will traverse the capillaries, and some will remain and obstruct blood flow. Air that passes through to the right side of the circulation is referred to as *secondary venous embolism*. Clinical manifestations of arterial air embolism are related to the involvement of the coronary or cerebral circulation. The distribution of arterial air is partly a function of body position.

Systemic air embolism following injury of the lung has only recently been described.[87-89] The formation of traumatic bronchovenous fistulas creates the potential entry points for air to move into the left side of the circulatory system. The only requirement is the formation of an air-blood gradient conducive to the inward movement of air. Although a lowered intravascular pressure from hemorrhage is a risk factor, the most important element in all reports of air embolism has been the use of positive-pressure ventilation.[84]

Air embolization has even been shown to occur in the absence of penetrating lung injuries. In the canine model, the threshold airway pressure for systemic air embolism is 65 mm Hg with or without a penetrating injury. For intratracheal pressures less than 65 mm Hg, air embolism does not occur. In the canine model, the presence of a penetrating lung injury does not appear to alter the threshold for embolization. It does, however, increase significantly the volume of air embolized for any given pressure beyond the threshold pressure.[90, 91]

In a review of 447 cases of major thoracic trauma, Yee and colleagues found adequate chart data to diagnose air embolism in 61 patients.[82] This incidence of 14 per cent is remarkable in light of the small number of reported cases before 1973.[87] A mechanism of blunt injury should not preclude a consideration of this diagnosis, because 25 per cent of patients with air embolism reported by Yee had blunt trauma with associated lung injury secondary to multiple rib fractures or hilar disruption.[82] The overall mortality was 56 per cent (34 of 61 patients). Refractory cardiac arrest accounted for 63 per cent of the operative deaths, with exsanguination or severe brain trauma as the cause in the remaining 37 per cent.

The diagnosis of air embolism is easily overlooked because of the similarity of the signs and symptoms to those of hypovolemic shock. Two valuable signs that were present in 36 per cent of patients were hemoptysis and the occurrence of cardiac arrest after intubation and ventilation. The diagnosis of air embolism should also be considered when unconsciousness develops suddenly and is followed by convulsions in a lung injury patient on positive-pressure ventilation.[92]

TREATMENT OF AIR EMBOLISM

A high index of suspicion with rapid control of the source of air embolism is vital. The patient should immediately be placed in the Trendelenburg (head-down) position to minimize cerebral involvement by directing the air emboli to less critical organs. This step should be followed by a left anterolateral thoracotomy. The exposed thorax should be flooded with sterile saline. Peripheral bronchovenous fistulas can be identified by the bloody froth created during positive-pressure ventilation. A quick search for hilar injuries should be carried out in the patient with blunt trauma. If the source of air embolism is not readily apparent, a contralateral thoracotomy should be performed. Once the bronchovenous communication is controlled, needle aspiration of the residual air that commonly remains in the left heart and the aorta should be performed. If the patient is hypotensive,

the aorta may now be cross-clamped or compressed with the hand. "Reflex" cross-clamping of the aorta before control of bronchovenous fistulas and removal of residual air will result in further dissemination of air to the heart and the brain.

Adjunctive Therapy. As mentioned earlier, air emboli will traverse capillary beds if the blood pressure is high enough.[87] A brief period of proximal aortic hypertension can be produced by cross-clamping of the decending aorta. Systemic arterial pressure should be maintained with adequate fluid resuscitation. If vasopressors are required, metaraminol (Aramine) appears to be the drug of choice.[89]

Left atrial pressure should be maintained at a high level. The ventilator inspiratory pressures should be kept as low as possible, and 100 per cent oxygen should be used to facilitate diffusion of nitrogen from emboli. Pharmacotherapy may include steroids, mannitol, aspirin, and barbiturates in conjunction with hypothermia.[92-97] The most important adjunct therapy will be the use of a hyperbaric chamber.[92-95]

Hyperbaric oxygen therapy is beneficial because it (1) compresses air bubbles, (2) establishes a high diffusion gradient that greatly speeds the dissolution of the bubbles, and (3) improves the oxygenation of ischemic tissues and lowers intracranial pressure. Hyperbaric oxygen therapy should be sought even though it may be many hours before it can be initiated. The effectiveness of hyperbaric oxygen therapy is illustrated by cases of success and improvement even when as many as 36 hours elapsed before pressurization.

Major Vascular Injuries

Major vascular injury resulting in rapid deterioration following blunt or penetrating trauma will require the use of an emergency thoracotomy for diagnosis, resuscitation, and control of hemorrhage. Mavroudis and associates reviewed 76 patients with thoracic vascular injury from mixed trauma who received an emergency department thoracotomy because they were moribund or an immediate thoracotomy in the operating suite for hemodynamic instability.[98] The three most common sites of vascular injuries are the pulmonary artery (28 per cent of cases), intercostal artery (23 per cent of cases), and pulmonary vein (20 per cent of cases). Aortic injuries account for only 12 per cent of the injuries requiring immediate surgical intervention. However, even with immediate intervention, survival rates are low (14 to 29 per cent). Air embolism was the cause of death in 18 per cent of cases.

The clinical approach to patients with suspected vascular injury depends on their hemodynamic status, the mechanism of injury, and the presence of associated injuries. If the patient is sufficiently stable, angiography is a valuable diagnostic measure, although the risk of sudden deterioration necessitates constant monitoring. If the patient is deteriorating rapidly and vascular injury is suspected, emergency thoracotomy will play a dual role as a diagnostic and a resuscitative procedure. It must be emphasized that patients with seemingly trivial penetrating wounds can appear stable and yet may precipitously exsanguinate and suffer an arrest from 5 minutes to 2 hours after admission.[50, 98]

In the setting of penetrating abdominal injury, thoracotomy with cross-clamping of the thoracic aorta to control hemorrhage from the injury has been advocated, but survival rates have been poor for those undergoing this procedure. The collective survival rate in 194 cases described in the literature is only 5 per cent.[7, 21-24, 26] Three factors contribute to this low figure. First, aortic occlusion will not substantially affect the rate and volume of bleeding from major venous injuries. Second, most patients had lost all vital signs by the time of thoracotomy. Third, multiple collateral pathways around the cross-clamped aorta diminish the effectiveness of this procedure.[99]

Aortic cross-clamping for massive hemoperitoneum was originally conceived as a preoperative "prophylactic" procedure to prevent sudden hypotension following abdominal decompression.[100, 101] In this role, it has clearly been beneficial when systolic pressure cannot be raised above 80 mm Hg prior to laparotomy.[101]

Open-Chest Resuscitation for Nontraumatic Arrest

Failure to resuscitate patients from cardiac arrest is a result of (1) a delay in the onset of cardiopulmonary resuscitation (CPR), (2) the use of less than optimal resuscitative techniques, or (3) the intractability of the underlying disease process.[102] The development of closed-chest resuscitation, which is quickly and easily applied, coupled with the development of more advanced prehospital care has dramatically reduced the number of failures caused by a delay in the onset of CPR.[103] The new frontier is now in the area of improving resuscitative techniques. Evidence suggests that in adults, after the first 5 minutes, closed-chest compression provides inadequate cerebral blood flow and almost no myocardial perfusion.[104–109] Consequently, some investigators are calling for a critical reevaluation of current CPR techniques—a first step, they hope, toward something better.

Current studies have focused attention on the changes in intrathoracic pressure during closed-chest resuscitation.[110–116] It is now generally accepted that blood flow during adult CPR is commonly the result of intrathoracic pressure changes rather than direct cardiac compression, as was previously thought (see Chapter 17). During CPR the heart is essentially a conduit. Such a concept has important implications for coronary blood flow because it suggests that closed-chest resuscitation does not provide an effective perfusion gradient for coronary circulation. The work of Ditchey and colleagues and Niemann and coworkers supports this hypothesis.[104, 105] In canine models using standard CPR, the coronary blood flow is less than 1 per cent of prearrest values. For practical purposes there is no coronary blood flow when standard closed-chest resuscitation is used.

Disappointing results were also found when investigators evaluated common carotid blood flows using standard CPR methods. In animal models, carotid blood flows vary from 7 to 17 per cent of the prearrest value.[106–109] Irreversible brain damage occurs quickly when carotid blood flow cannot be maintained at more than 10 per cent of normal.[108, 117] It is important to recall that the common carotid artery contributes to both the external and the internal carotid. Thus changes in common carotid blood flows do not necessarily correlate with changes in cerebral blood flow. Measurements of regional cerebral cortical blood flow during CPR by Jackson and associates suggest that adequate cortical perfusion is *not* achieved.[118] Jackson and coworkers found cortical blood flows to be less than 10 per cent of normal. This value is in agreement with previous microsphere studies that found cerebral blood flows to be only 5 per cent of normal when conventional CPR was used.[106]

There is no question that closed-chest resuscitation has saved countless lives. The length of time that closed-chest resuscitation can maintain life, however, appears to be more limited than was previously suspected. Observations by Eliastam and associates, Jeresaty and colleagues, and others suggest that there are rarely any long-term survivors after 30 minutes of *continuous* advanced cardiac life support.[119–125]

The two exceptions to this rule are those patients suffering from hypothermia or drug overdose.

In view of the results of these studies, open-chest methods of resuscitation are being reconsidered.[126–128] Direct compression of the heart produces higher arterial pressures and greater blood flows than do current closed-chest techniques.[107–109, 129–139] Del Guercio and coworkers measured the comparative hemodynamics of open and closed methods during cardiac resuscitation of patients.[135, 137, 138] The cardiac index was more than doubled by open-chest massage. The cardiac index produced by the closed-chest method was 0.6 liters per minute per m². With an open-chest method, the cardiac index increased to 1.3 liters per minute per m². Equally important is the return of coronary blood flow with open-chest resuscitation.[104, 109]

In a comparative study of closed- and open-chest resuscitation using a canine model, Bartlett and coworkers demonstrated improved survival and neurologic outcome with the open-chest cardiac compression method. Only 10 per cent of the control animals could be resuscitated after 50 minutes of closed-chest resuscitation, and all had fixed and dilated pupils. An experimental group received 10 minutes of closed-chest resuscitation followed by 40 minutes of open-chest resuscitation for a total arrest time of 50 minutes. *All* of these dogs were resuscitated; equally important was the preservation of the pupillary light reflex in 90 per cent of these animals.[140]

At present the precise role of open-chest resuscitation for nontraumatic arrests is poorly defined. Although several indications have been suggested, only two can be readily accepted. The first indication is for resuscitation of patients with hypothermic arrest (see Chapter 91). When cardiopulmonary bypass is not readily available, asystole unresponsive to pacing or ventricular fibrillation unresponsive to cardioversion may be treated with internal massage and direct rewarming of the heart.[141–144] The second indication is for use in medical arrests unresponsive to external resuscitation. Unfortunately, there is no clear method for determining the point at which unresponsiveness occurs, nor is it easy to determine when signs of tissue perfusion exist.[127, 145–148] A palpable pulse does not ensure flow.[145]

There have been several reports of successful open-chest resuscitation occurring after closed-chest resuscitation had failed.[129, 137, 138, 145, 146] Cohn and Del Guercio reported long-term survival in 11 patients who were resuscitated after closed chest resuscitation was abandoned in favor of the direct internal approach.[137, 138] Sykes and Ahmed reported four survivors out of 36 patients resuscitated with internal massage after external massage had failed.[146] The renewal of coronary perfusion with internal massage may supply sufficient oxygen and substrate to restore effective electrical or mechanical activity.[145] Based on the previously mentioned observations, the following guidelines may be helpful.

Duration of Closed-Chest Resuscitation. There are rarely any long-term survivors when the duration of closed-chest resuscitation is *continuous* for more than 30 minutes without cardiac response. The probability of long-term survival for witnessed medical arrests is approximately 86 per cent during the first 10 minutes of resuscitation.[119] This is reduced to 30 per cent by 16 minutes[121] and becomes less than 1 per cent after 30 minutes.[122–125] (This analysis assumes that basic life support begins within 4 minutes and that advanced life support is initiated within 8 minutes.)

A publication by Kern attempted to address the optimum timing of open-chest cardiac massage following closed-chest compression using a canine model.[132] It appears that if initiation of open-chest cardiac massage is delayed for more than 20 minutes from the onset of cardiac arrest, few or no successful outcomes can be expected despite the prompt institution of closed-chest compression. On the other hand, beginning direct cardiac massage after 15 minutes of closed-chest massage could still produce a 75 per cent success rate, which is very significant when compared with the 12 per cent success rate in the control group in which 15 minutes of closed-chest compression was not followed by direct cardiac massage. A clinical study from San Francisco also suggests that open-chest resuscitation has little value in humans after more than 20 minutes of arrest. Geehr compared the use of internal versus external cardiac massage and did not find any difference in survival in 49 cardiac arrest victims brought to the emergency department.[134] It should be noted that the time of arrest to the onset of direct cardiac massage was more than 20 minutes in all cases.

Onset of Asystole. When asystole occurs, regardless of the resuscitation duration, there will rarely be any survivors if standard methods are used. In most large series, the fatality rate for asystole is 100 per cent.[149, 150] Shocket and Rosenblum observed that some affected patients actually are in fine ventricular fibrillation.[145] The return of coronary blood flow with internal massage may restore coordinated electrical and mechanical activity[145] or may convert the fine ventricular fibrillation into the more responsive coarse fibrillation.

Onset of Electromechanical Dissociation (EMD) or Pulseless Idioventricular Rhythm. Possible causes of EMD, such as tension pneumothorax, volume depletion, and pericardial tamponade, should be rapidly excluded. If the patient does not respond immediately to conventional therapy, the outcome is generally fatal.[150] Therefore, open-chest methods should be considered.

Onset of Nonreactive Pupils. The pupillary light reflex should be noted as soon as possible and should be observed continually. Loss of this reflex during resuscitation indicates inadequate cerebral and brain stem perfusion. During resuscitation, this is the only clinical sign of perfusion that can be assessed. Although complete neurologic recovery is possible, the loss of this reflex is an ominous sign[151] and should not be tolerated for more than a few minutes. Unfortunately, the administration of pharmacologic agents during resuscitation may alter the value of this parameter.

Presence of Hypoxia. Arterial blood gases should be determined before attempting open-chest resuscitation. If significant hypoxia has developed, internal massage will be of little benefit. The relationship of hypoxia to arteriovenous shunting and its reversibility with increased blood flow is unknown.

Although closed-chest resuscitation continues to be the first-line method of handling medical cardiac arrests, there is sufficient experimental and clinical evidence to support the use of open-chest resuscitation if standard closed-chest methods fail. At present, the criteria for and the timing of open-chest resuscitation must rest with the individual physician.[128, 136]

EQUIPMENT FOR RESUSCITATIVE THORACOTOMY

The physician must carefully consider the instruments to be included in a resuscitation thoracotomy tray. The inclusion of too many instruments makes the tray cumbersome and delays the procedure. Nonessential instruments are best kept available in the resuscitation room in case they are needed for specific repair (e.g., Foley catheter for stellate wound tamponade).

The following items are essential for a thoracotomy tray:

Scalpel with attached number 20 blade,
Mayo scissors,
Rib spreaders,
Tissue forceps (10 inch),
Vascular clamps (two needed, Satinsky),
Needle holder (10 inch, Hegar),
2–0 or larger silk on large-curve needle,
Suture scissors, and
Aortic tamponade instrument.

The following items are optional for the tray and can be supplied as needed by an assistant:

Towel clips (six),
Hemostats (four to six, curved and straight),
Metzenbaum scissors,
Right-angled clamp,
Liebsche knife (or sternal osteotome with hammer),
Foley catheter (20 French, 30-ml balloon),
Chest tube (number 30, Argyle),
Lap sponges (12) or gauze pads,
Towels (six),
Cloth tape, and
Teflon patches.

In addition, functioning suction and sterile suction tips, antiseptic solution, sterile gloves, a defibrillator with internal paddles, and overhead surgical lights are needed in the resuscitation room. In the unlikely event that the patient awakens during the procedure, diazepam and narcotics can be administered for sedation, amnesia, and pain control.

PROCEDURE

If a potential survivor is to benefit from a resuscitative thoracotomy, the emergency physician must act swiftly and skillfully. A thoracotomy per se does not save lives; it is the repairs and adjunctive therapies used that determine the outcome.

Preliminary Considerations

In the urban setting in which a trauma center is less than 15 minutes away, patients with penetrating thoracic injuries should receive immediate transportation with the least possible field time. Two studies suggest that this "scoop and run" approach provides a better survival rate.[152, 153]

For all trauma victims presenting to the emergency department with hypotension, the initial working diagnosis must be one of volume depletion. Other possibilities should be rapidly excluded, such as tension pneumothorax, cardiac tamponade, air embolism, and neurogenic or cardiogenic shock. An algorithmic overview of the approach to chest trauma is shown in Figure 18–1.[154–156]

Because a large amount of blood may be lost into the chest, an autotransfusion system should be available (see Chapter 34). The use of autotransfusion has several benefits.[157, 158] The most important advantages are (1) immediate availability of "compatible," warm blood, (2) significantly higher levels of 2,3-DPG than in stored blood, and (3) less risk of exhausting the banked supply of the patient's blood type. This third point can be crucial when there are blood bank shortages or when there are cross-match problems.

Another factor to be considered is ensuring adequate ventilation and oxygenation of the hypotensive patient. Intubation with controlled ventilation is desirable for all agonal patients and crucial in the management of the thoracotomy patient. Antiseptic preparation of the chest wall by necessity is abbreviated during resuscitative thoracotomy and is best

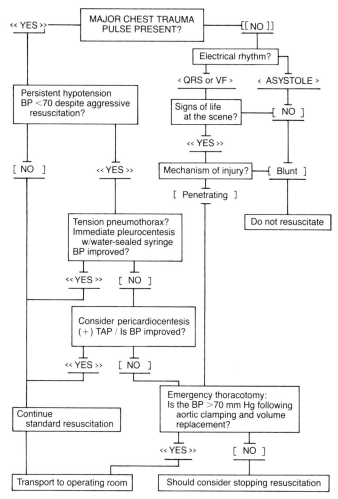

Figure 18–1. An approach to chest trauma. BP, blood pressure; VF, ventricular fibrillation; (+) TAP, pericardial tap yielding blood.

performed by an assistant while the physician is putting on surgical gloves.

Subxiphoid Pericardial Window. Most patients with suspected cardiac injury should receive a subxiphoid pericardial window for diagnosis and decompression (see also Chapter 16).[65, 159–162] This procedure is best performed in the operating suite.

Anterolateral Thoracotomy Incision

When the site of injury is unknown and the patient's status requires immediate intervention for possible intrathoracic injuries, a left anterolateral incision over the fifth rib with dissection into the fourth intercostal space provides the best access to the heart and the great vessels. In the setting of cardiac arrest, time should not be taken to count the rib spaces. An incision just beneath the nipple in the male or along the inframammary fold in the female will approximate the fourth intercostal space. Closed-chest compressions are continued during the initial incision. The first sweep of the scalpel (number 20 blade) should separate skin, subcutaneous fat, and the superficial portions of the pectoralis and serratus muscles. When dividing the intercostal muscles with a scalpel or Mayo scissors, one should be careful not to lacerate the lung. With the first opening of the pleura, ventilations should be stopped momentarily. This will allow the lung to collapse away from the chest wall. The intercostal incision just over the top of the fifth rib can then be carried

quickly and safely to completion. Some surgeons prefer to begin the thoracotomy incision over the sternum, whereas others begin 2 cm lateral to the edge of the sternum, hoping to avoid the internal mammary artery. Should the internal mammary artery be transected during the procedure, hemorrhage is generally minimal until after perfusion is reestablished. At that time the patient can exsanguinate from a lacerated internal mammary artery. Therefore, all internal mammary artery lacerations should be ligated once perfusion is established.

The intercostal space is spread and a chest wall retractor (rib spreader) is placed with the handle and ratchet bar down (Fig. 18–2). If the retractor is placed with the handle up, the ratchet bar will prevent extension of the incision into the right chest. When the site of injury is to the right of the heart and cannot be reached, a transsternal extension into the right chest is performed with a Liebsche knife or a sternal osteotome.

It is important to establish wide exposure from the outset by extending the skin incision past the posterior axillary line. One can facilitate this by quickly wedging towels or sheets under the left posterior chest and by placing the patient's left arm above the head. Inadequate exposure, rib fractures, and additional delays occur when the skin incision is too limited. In patients with suspected left subclavian vessel injuries or aortic arch injuries, better exposure and control will be obtained when the third intercostal space is used. If access is still difficult, the superior ribs may be separated at the costochondral junction.

Pericardiotomy

If cardiac arrest has occurred, the question of whether to open the pericardial sac arises. If the myocardium cannot be visualized, the pericardium should be opened, but in the majority of cases the myocardium can be evaluated through the intact pericardium. If a tamponade is not present, it is usually best to leave the pericardial sac closed. From a physiologic standpoint, compression of the heart is more efficient when it is performed with the pericardium open, because pressure is transmitted only to the ventricles. Opening the pericardium, however, will only increase the risk of added complications. The delay in beginning cardiac compressions will add to the risk of cerebral damage. The myocardium or a coronary vessel may be injured. The left phrenic nerve may be cut by mistake and if there has been previous pericardial disease, adhesions may be present. If attempts are made to separate these adhesions rapidly, tears of the atrial or right ventricular wall can occur. The incidence of traumatic rupture of the atria or the right ventricle during massage is greater when the pericardium is open. With an intact pericardium, pressure is distributed over a larger area and the pericardial fluid seldom allows the compression fingers to remain in one spot for a prolonged period.

Patients with tamponade will require pericardiotomy. This is performed in a location anterior and parallel to the left phrenic nerve. The incision should start near the diaphragm to avoid possible injury of the coronary arteries. When the pericardium is under tension, it may be very difficult to grasp the pericardium with forceps. In that case, sharp, straight Mayo scissors are used to divide the pericardium by layers. If the heart is in arrest, speed is important, and sharp scissors should be used to "catch" the pericardium and to start the pericardiotomy. To do this, the point of the scissors is held almost parallel to the surface of the heart with enough pressure to create a wrinkle in the pericardium that can be punctured as the scissors are moved forward.

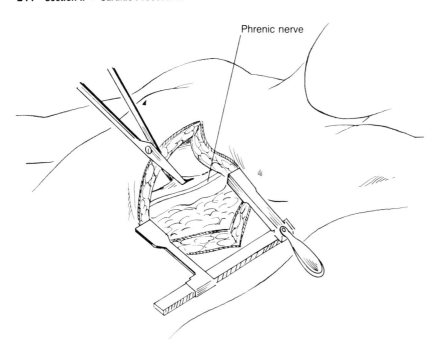

Phrenic nerve

Figure 18–2. Left anterolateral thoracotomy. An incision is made between the fourth and fifth interspaces. It is important to stay as close to the top of the fifth rib as possible to avoid the intercostal artery. The rib spreader should be placed with the handle lateral. Pericardiotomy is started near the diaphragm and anterior to the phrenic nerve.

Moderate pressure must be used to puncture the fibrous pericardium. The sudden give that occurs when the pericardium opens may result in a laceration of the myocardium if the point of the scissors is unnecessarily angled toward the heart. Clots of blood are removed from the pericardial sac by the sweeping motion of a gloved hand or with sterile lap sponges or gauze pads.

Direct Cardiac Compressions

Three techniques for cardiac compression have been advocated: one-handed compression, one-handed with sternal compression, and two-handed (bimanual) compression (Fig. 18–3). One-handed compression is performed with the thumb placed over the left ventricle, the opposing fingers over the right ventricle, and the apex of the heart resting in the palm of the hand. The one-handed technique with sternal compression is also performed with the fingers flat. The fingers of the hand are held tightly together to form a flat surface over the left ventricle while compressing the heart up against the sternum. To perform the two-handed technique, the left hand is cupped and placed over the right ventricle. The fingers of the right hand are held tightly together to form a flat surface over the left ventricle that compresses the heart against the cupped surface of the left hand. Of these three, the bimanual technique is consistently superior, and whenever possible, it is the preferred method.[163, 164]

A difference of opinion exists regarding the optimal rate at which the heart should be compressed. Most of the literature has recommended a rate of 50 to 60 compressions per minute; however, there is nothing to support such a recommendation. Johnson and Kirby studied the relationship of compression rate to cardiac output and blood pressure and found these parameters to be directly related.[163] Although their work has been disputed,[165] a more recent study has confirmed these findings.[166] Using an animal model, compression rates of 60 and 90 were compared. The cardiac index and mean arterial pressure were increased by almost 20 per cent and 25 per cent, respectively, when the compression rate was increased to 90 per minute.[166]

It is important to remember the following points while performing cardiac compression:

1. Fingertip pressure should be avoided at all times. Compression is performed using the entire palmar surface of the fingers.

2. Whichever technique is used, the force of compression should be perpendicular to the plane of the septum. The anterior descending coronary artery is located over the interventricular septum and is a helpful landmark to orient proper hand placement. It is clearly seen, with or without the pericardium open.

3. The fingers should be positioned so that the coronary arteries will not be occluded.

4. Venous filling of the heart is especially sensitive to changes in position. It is important to maintain a relatively normal anatomic position of the heart to prevent kinking of the great vessels. The heart should not be angled more than 30 degrees into the left chest.

5. It is also essential to completely relax the heart between compressions. If present, intraarterial pressure monitoring is of tremendous value for assessing the consistency and effectiveness of compressions.

Control of Hemorrhagic Cardiac Wounds

One may partially control active bleeding from ventricular wounds by placing the finger of one hand over the wound while using the other hand to stabilize the beating heart. The wound is repaired by placement of several horizontal mattress sutures under the tamponading finger (Fig. 18–4). Nonabsorbable 2–0 silk sutures are customarily used. Smaller sutures should *not* be used, and nylon sutures should be avoided. Some physicians prefer to use even larger silk sutures, such as number 1 or 2 (note that this is *not* 0 [1–0] or 0–0 [2–0]). When multiple sutures are needed, they should all be in place before they are tied. This allows for a rapid and equal distribution of wound tension, which prevents tearing of the myocardium.[57, 167] Passing the suture through Teflon pledgets also prevents the suture from cutting through the myocardium. It is especially important to use Teflon pledgets for reinforcement when the myocar-

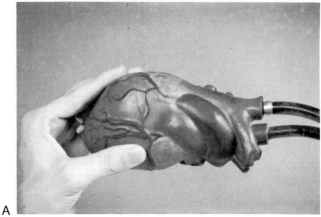

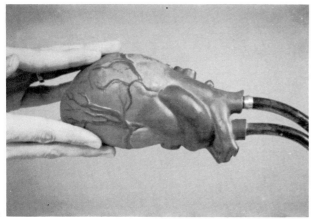

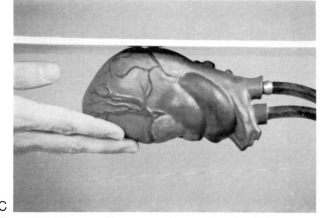

Figure 18–3. Direct cardiac compressions. *A,* One-handed compression. *B,* Two-handed compression. *C,* One-handed, with sternal compression.

dium has been weakened by the blast effect of a bullet.[64, 65] With large wounds that cannot be palpably controlled, an incomplete horizontal mattress suture should be placed on either side of the wound (Fig. 18–5). The free ends are then crossed to stop the bleeding. The actual reparative sutures can then be accurately placed. It must be stressed that suturing the myocardium requires good technique. Excessive tension may tear the myocardium and aggravate the situation. Keys to success include the use of an appropriate-sized suture, a generous "bite" with the needle, and the application of only enough tension as needed to control bleeding.

If exsanguinating hemorrhage is not controlled by the aforementioned methods, temporary inflow occlusion can be used. Inflow occlusion may be applied intermittently for 60 to 90 seconds. During occlusion the heart shrinks, hem-

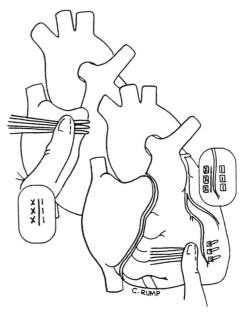

Figure 18–4. Technique of repair. Multiple horizontal mattress sutures are placed 6 mm from the wound edge before tying. The wound is closed just enough to stop the bleeding. Teflon pledgets are used for reinforcement. For repairs near a coronary artery, care is taken to pass the suture under the artery.

orrhage is controlled, and sutures can be placed in a decompressed injury. Three techniques have been described: (1) vascular clamping of the superior and inferior vena cava for partial inflow occlusion,[168] (2) use of the Sauerbruch grip (Fig. 18–6) for occlusion of the vena cava between the ring and the middle finger of the left hand for partial inflow occlusion,[44] and (3) use of a venous mesocardial snare for total inflow occlusion.[169] The mesocardial snare for total inflow occlusion is formed with heavy cloth tape (Fig. 18–7). The tape is passed through the transverse sinus and encircles the inferior surface of the heart. The oblique sinus is then packed with gauze pads. Constriction of the umbilical tape will now compress the horseshoe-shaped venous mesocardium against the gauze tampon. This particular method has several advantages: (1) preliminary placement of a venous mesocardial snare before opening the pericardium allows the physician to "shut off" the entire circulation instantly in the event of uncontrollable hemorrhage; (2) one can perform the procedure intermittently by simply tightening and relaxing the snare; (3) with total inflow occlusion, venous return from the lungs will not be lost through left

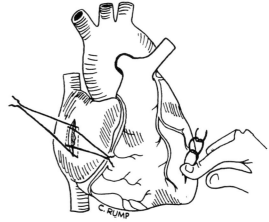

Figure 18–5. Control of bleeding by using digital pressure and by crossing two widely placed incomplete mattress sutures.

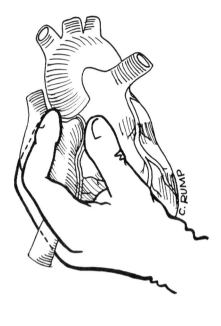

Figure 18–6. Sauerbruch maneuver: Venous inflow occlusion is achieved by using the first and second or second and third fingers as a clamp.

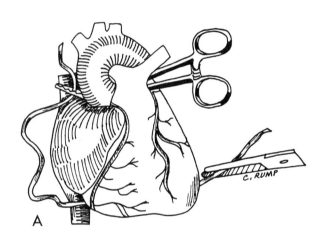

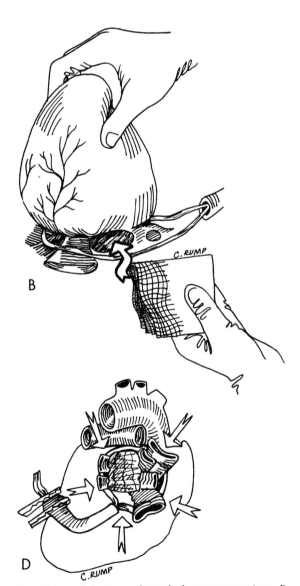

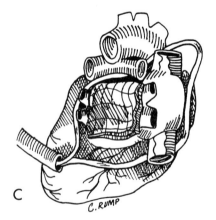

Figure 18–7. Venous mesocardial snare for total inflow occlusion. *A,* A hemostat is used to pull the snare through the transverse sinus. *B,* Inferior view. Arrow indicates the shallow oblique sinus, which is packed with gauze. The heart has been elevated for illustration. Clinically, excessive lifting of the heart can produce cardiac arrest. *C,* Posterior view, with snare and tampon in place. *D,* Posterior view during venous occlusion.

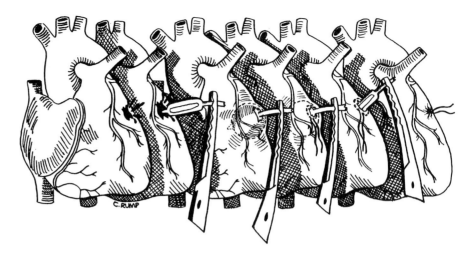

Figure 18–8. Serial illustration. Gentle traction on an inflated Foley catheter will control hemorrhage and allow easy repair. The balloon is inflated with saline, and care is taken to avoid rupturing the balloon with the suture needle. This technique is particularly useful with injuries of the inferior caval-atrial junction, with posterior wounds, and during cardiac massage. Volume loading can be obtained by infusion of blood or crystalloid solutions through the lumen of the catheter. Care should be taken to avoid an air embolus through the lumen of the catheter during placement.

heart wounds; and (4) it does not interfere with the operative field.

Insertion of a Foley catheter (20 French with a 30-ml balloon) through a wound is another technique for controlling hemorrhage.[55, 57, 170–173] Following insertion of the catheter, the balloon is inflated, the catheter is clamped, and gentle traction is applied (Fig. 18–8). Enough traction is applied to slow the bleeding to an acceptable level for visualization and repair. Attempts to achieve complete hemostasis with excessive traction may pull the catheter out and potentially enlarge the wound. The balloon will effectively occlude the wound internally. When repairing the wound, the operator must be careful with the suture needle to prevent rupturing the balloon. Temporarily pushing the balloon into the ventricular lumen during needle passage is helpful. It is important to use normal saline when inflating the balloon. Use of air will result in air embolism if the balloon is ruptured by the suture needle.

Foley catheters have several advantages over other methods of controlling cardiac wounds. With the digital method, the fingertip will often slip if there is a strong heartbeat, the wound cannot be visualized during repair, and digital pressure significantly interferes with cardiac massage. Total venous inflow occlusion is an effective method of controlling bleeding and decompressing the heart, but such control will be at the expense of a poor cardiac output. Comparatively, the Foley catheter causes very little cardiovascular interference, although inflation

near the base of the ventricle may obstruct blood flow. Attempts to elevate the heart for control and repair of posterior cardiac wounds will often result in cardiac arrest by reduction of both venous and arterial flows. With posterior injuries, one cannot continuously view the wound for digital control of bleeding. Use of a catheter does not require continued viewing after the initial placement. If bleeding can be controlled, repairs in this location should await full volume expansion or cardiopulmonary bypass.[23, 65, 174] Regardless of location, the most valuable feature of using a Foley catheter is its ability to control hemorrhage without interfering with cardiac compression.

Shamoun and colleagues have reported the use of surgical staples for ventricular wound closure.[174a] They prefer the Ethicon Proximate Quantum Skin Stapler (Model PQW-35, Ethicon, Inc., Sommerville, NJ). The staples may be left in place or replaced upon further wound exploration in the operating room.

Deliberate fibrillation should be considered as a last resort for repair of difficult wounds of the ventricle or the proximal aorta. Elective cardiac arrest is best tolerated if there is adequate blood volume and oxygenation before fibrillation.[21] For fibrillation, the internal cardiac paddles are placed perpendicular ("on-edge") to the surface of the heart and discharged at 20 watt-sec (Fig. 18–9).[168] This produces a local area of depolarization. The resulting disparity in relative refractory periods sets up a circus movement producing ventricular fibrillation. The heart should be massaged intermittently during repair, and the duration of fibrillation should not exceed 3 to 4 minutes.

Defibrillation is accomplished while the internal paddles are firmly pressed *tangentially* over the right and left ventricles. Following repair, the epicardium is often dry and should be moistened with saline to improve electrical conduction. An energy level of 20 watt-sec is used. If the initial attempt is unsuccessful, repeated shocks at the same setting should be used. Higher energy levels can cause myocardial necrosis.[175] Defibrillation through an intact pericardium also should begin with 20 watt-sec. If unsuccessful, the shock should be repeated once and then increased to between 40 to 60 watt-sec.

Management of the wounded heart that has spontaneously arrested is controversial. Some physicians have recommended a rapid repair of ventricular wounds while the heart is arrested. Others consider immediate cardiac massage and reversal of cardiac arrest to be more important. Immediate cardiac massage to maintain blood flow is probably the best approach. When cardiac arrest occurs, physiologic reserves have been depleted, and a delay for repair during

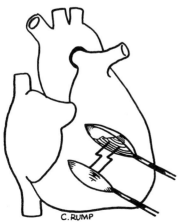

Figure 18–9. Technique for elective fibrillation. Twenty joules (watt-sec) are delivered through internal defibrillating paddles placed perpendicular to the epicardium. Coronary vessels should be avoided during paddle placement.

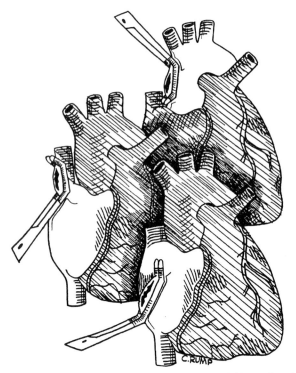

Figure 18–10. Use of a partial occluding clamp in different locations for control of bleeding and repair.

arrest would only diminish the chance of a successful resuscitation.

Wounds of the atria are managed with partial occlusion clamps (Fig. 18–10). Because of the thin structure and instability of the atrial wall, digital pressure will not effectively stop bleeding. Injuries near the caval-atrial junction are not amenable to clamping. In this location a Foley catheter should be used to tamponade the wound (Fig. 18–11).[171–174] Care must be exercised to avoid obstruction of atrial filling with the inflated balloon. During wound closure, the catheter should be pushed away from the ventricular wall to avoid rupture of the balloon.

Wounds of the septa, valves, and coronary arteries require definitive repair in the operating suite. Hemorrhage

from a coronary artery can generally be controlled with digital pressure. Ligation of a coronary artery should be avoided when possible.

Control of Hemorrhagic Great Vessel Wounds

Wounds of the great vessels can be controlled with digital pressure or partial occlusion clamps.[174] Exsanguinating hemorrhage from the left subclavian artery can be prevented by cross-clamping of the intrathoracic portion of the artery. Cross-clamping of the right subclavian artery is very difficult. For injuries of this vessel, compression with laparotomy pads in the apex of the pleura from below and the supraclavicular fossa from above (Fig. 18–12) will prevent further bleeding as the patient is stabilized and moved to the operating suite.[176]

Large or difficult vena caval injuries should be controlled with a temporary intravascular shunt to maintain venous return while providing vascular isolation of the injured segment.[171, 176] Ideally, heparin-bonded tubing should be used.[23] If this is not available, a number 30 Argyle plastic chest tube will be a satisfactory alternative.[171] The tube is placed through a pursestring suture in the right atrium, and the tip is advanced beyond the site of the injury (Fig. 18–13). Flow is established by creation of several large ports in the proximal portion of the tube, which is then advanced into the atrium. Next, a clamp is placed across the tube just outside the atrium. Finally, vascular isolation of the injury is completed by placement of tourniquets above and below the site of injury (Fig. 18–14).

The usual technique for placing atrial catheters using a pursestring suture in the right atrium has several disadvantages. First, it is relatively time consuming for a patient in cardiac arrest, and cardiac massage is often interrupted to allow suture placement. In addition, the suture may tear the atrial appendage, the suture holes are frequently associated with fluid leaks through the thin atrial wall, and the catheter can slide out of place.

Samuelson and coworkers described an innovative technique utilizing an umbilical cord clamp with a center hole (Fig. 18–15A).[177] A standard umbilical cord clamp (Laugh-

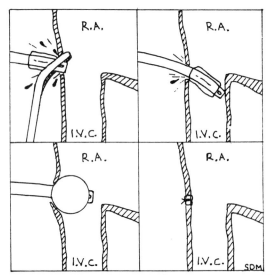

Figure 18–11. Wounds of the inferior caval-atrial junction are difficult to manage with simple vascular clamping. Use of a Foley catheter will provide satisfactory control.

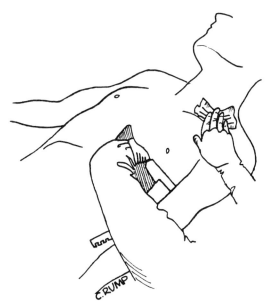

Figure 18–12. Cross-clamping for control of subclavian bleeding is difficult and time consuming. Compression with laparotomy pads in the apical pleura from below and the supraclavicular fossa from above will control hemorrhage while the patient is stabilized.

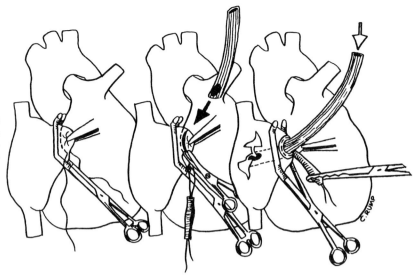

Figure 18–13. Technique for placing an atrial line or vascular shunt. A pursestring suture is placed, the atrial appendage is clamped, and an incision is made. A catheter or intravascular shunt is inserted, and the pursestring is tightened.

erty Corp.) is modified by drilling a hole through the center to match the size of standard intravenous tubing or whatever catheter is to be used. The diameter of the hole should hold the catheter firmly enough to prevent slippage. These clamps, by necessity, must be prepared in advance and gas sterilized.

To place a catheter utilizing this technique, the right atrial appendage is gently grasped between the left thumb and index finger. Scissors are used to create a small opening in the atrial appendage and a previously flushed catheter is inserted into the right atrium. The umbilical cord clamp is placed over the catheter at the edge of the appendage and snapped shut (Fig. 18–15B). The cord clamp holds the catheter securely, provides good hemostasis, and does not interfere with the operative field.

When the systolic pressure cannot be raised above 70 mm Hg, temporary occlusion of the descending thoracic aorta will maintain myocardial and cerebral perfusion (Fig. 18–16). Selective clamping will be necessary when the aorta has been injured with blunt trauma (Fig. 18–17). Aortic occlusion has a limited role in controlling hemorrhage below the diaphragm.[28, 99] When there is a tense abdomen with massive hemoperitoneum, aortic cross-clamping is clearly beneficial when applied just before laparotomy. This has been referred to as *prophylactic cross-clamping* to prevent a sudden drop in blood pressure when the abdomen is decom-

pressed.[100, 101] As a preoperative procedure, cross-clamping should be applied when the systolic pressure is less than 80 mm Hg in the setting of a tense abdomen.[101]

To expose the descending aorta, the left lung is retracted in a superior-medial direction by an assistant. To achieve adequate exposure, it is sometimes necessary to divide the inferior pulmonary ligament (Fig. 18–18). The aorta can be quickly identified by advancement of the fingers of the left hand along the thoracic cage toward the vertebral column. On some occasions, the operator may choose to have an assistant simply occlude the aorta with digital pressure. To locate the aorta, one uses a DeBakey aortic clamp or a curved Kelly clamp for blunt dissection and spreads open the pleura above and below the aorta (Fig. 18–19). The esophagus, which lies medially and slightly anteriorly, is separated from the vessel. When the aorta is completely isolated, the index finger of the left hand is flexed around the vessel and a vascular clamp is applied with the right hand. The brachial blood pressure should be checked immediately after the occlusion. If the systolic pressure is more than 120 mm Hg, the clamp should be slowly released and adjusted to maintain a systolic pressure of 120 mm Hg.[101]

Perhaps a simpler approach to aortic occlusion is to use the aortic tamponade instrument (Fig. 18–20).[178] The application of vascular clamps is fraught with complications, which include inadvertent dislodgment or inadequate occlu-

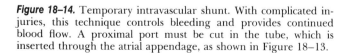

Figure 18–14. Temporary intravascular shunt. With complicated injuries, this technique controls bleeding and provides continued blood flow. A proximal port must be cut in the tube, which is inserted through the atrial appendage, as shown in Figure 18–13.

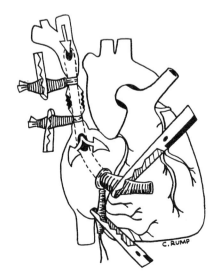

A

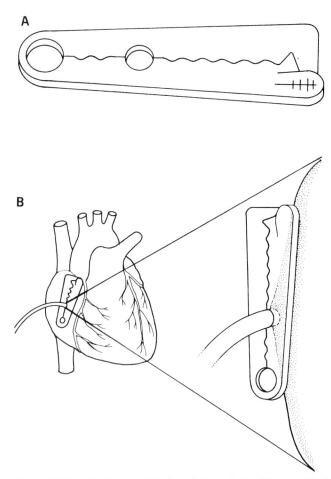

B

Figure 18–15. *A,* Modified umbilical cord clamp. *B,* Modified umbilical cord clamp securing a catheter in the right atrial appendage.

sion as a result of improper application. The aortic tamponade instrument, on the other hand, may be applied blindly to the vertebral column, permitting safe, quick, and complete aortic occlusion. The instrument's unique shape allows it to remain in place and provide atraumatic occlusion. The degree of occlusion can be varied by the amount of pressure exerted by the operator.

The issue of whether aortic cross-clamping is beneficial in hypovolemia because it increases coronary perfusion or whether it is detrimental because it increases afterload to an ischemic heart has been addressed. Dunn and colleagues,[179] using a canine shock model, measured ventricular contractility before and after aortic occlusion. Contractility was impaired during the period of hypotension before cross-clamping. Following aortic occlusion, contractility returned to normal.

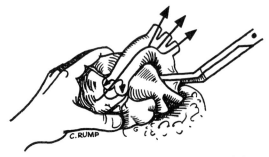

Figure 18–16. Manual massage and cross-clamping of the aorta to increase coronary and cerebral perfusion selectively.

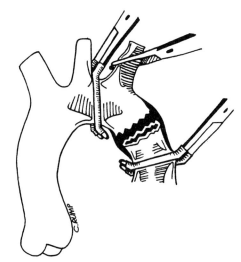

Figure 18–17. Traumatic rupture of the aorta. Three clamps are required for control. Back-bleeding will occur if fewer than three clamps are used.

Potential complications of aortic cross-clamping are multiple: ischemia of the spinal cord, liver, bowel, and kidneys as well as iatrogenic injury of the aorta and the esophagus may occur.[101] Failure to monitor blood pressure every 60 seconds during aortic occlusion may result in cerebral hemorrhage or left ventricular failure if there is excessive elevation of pressure. Fortunately, these complications are infrequent. In a report of 12 patients surviving emergency department thoracotomy with cross-clamping for as long as 60 minutes, there were no lasting impairments of renal, myocardial, or neurologic function.[180] Whenever possible, the aorta was unclamped for 30 to 60 seconds every 10 minutes to increase renal perfusion. Final release of the aorta is always performed gradually.

Treatment of Hypothermia

Prolonged resuscitation and the administration of cold crystalloid solutions or blood can lead to hypothermia in the traumatic and nontraumatic arrest situation. Under such conditions, core rewarming may be required before reestab-

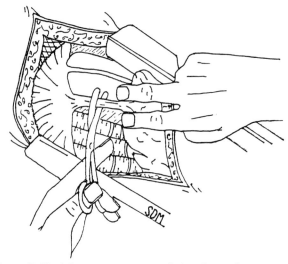

Figure 18–18. Adequate exposure of the descending aorta may require division of the inferior pulmonary ligament.

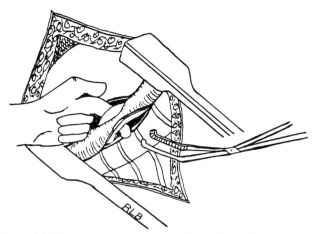

Figure 18–19. Aortic cross-clamping: Using blunt dissection, one spreads the pleura above and below the aorta. The vessel should be fully mobilized and clearly separated from the esophagus before clamping.

lishment of cardiac function.[143–145] Tap water at a temperature of 40° C can be infused directly about the heart and thorax during open-chest cardiac compression to enhance rewarming. Sterile saline heated in a microwave oven to the same temperature is equally effective and somewhat more hygienic. Other therapeutic maneuvers for management of the hypothermic patient are discussed in Chapter 91.

COMPLICATIONS

There are a variety of postoperative complications that may occur in patients surviving emergency thoracotomy.[19, 23, 181, 182] Most of these complications stem from the particular injuries of each patient and must be considered on an individual basis. The complications of open-chest resuscitation are relatively insignificant when compared with a fatal outcome. There are two postthoracotomy complications that are frequently discussed. One is thoracic sepsis. This is a rare complication, and excessive concern with preparation may unnecessarily delay a thoracotomy.[183] In a combined series of 142 emergency department thoracotomies there were no reports of wound infections.[47, 158, 167] It should be noted that most patients received antibiotics just before or during the procedure. Thus the concern for infection as a complication of a thoracotomy performed with less than

sterile technique is unwarranted, although a short course of antibiotics should be administered as soon as possible.

A second complication that is frequently feared and may actually deter a life-saving thoracotomy is the imagined threat that the patient will survive but will be in a vegetative neurologic state. This complication is also rare and such apprehension appears unjustified. Likewise, the concern of "tying up intensive care unit beds" with patients who have "fatal" injuries has been overemphasized. The first 24 hours following injury will rapidly separate those patients who will become long-term survivors; most patients with fatal injuries expire within 24 hours. The San Francisco experience with 168 emergency thoracotomies for mixed trauma illustrates this point.[184] Of those patients surviving the first 24 hours, 80 per cent (33 of 41) recovered and left the hospital. Full neurologic recovery occurred for 90 per cent of these survivors. Overall, only 2.4 per cent (4 of 168) remained severely disabled or in a persistent vegetative state. Of these four patients, only one (0.6 per cent) lived beyond 2 months; he eventually expired at 14 months from sepsis.

The report by Moore and colleagues[22] in Denver describing 146 emergency thoracotomies for mixed trauma was comparable with the report from San Francisco. Moore reported 15 patients who survived the surgical repairs in the operating suite. Eighty per cent (12 of 15) of these patients went on to become long-term survivors; 75 per cent had full neurologic recovery. In the Denver study, two valuable observations were made regarding the presence or absence of various signs. First, all survivors with full neurologic recovery had respiratory efforts at the scene; in 75 per cent of these patients respiratory efforts were still present on arrival in the emergency care unit. Second, the presence or absence of a palpable pulse is not a reliable prognostic indicator. Sixty-six per cent of long-term survivors (11 patients with penetrating trauma and 1 with blunt trauma) had no detectable pulse on arrival in the emergency care unit.

AIRWAY CONTROL DURING EMERGENCY DEPARTMENT THORACOTOMY

Patients undergoing resuscitative thoracotomy in the emergency department obviously require assisted ventilation. Airway control is best obtained with standard oral tracheal intubation, but exposure of the thoracic organs and surgical repairs or procedures may be hampered by frequent inflations of the left lung. Selective one-lung ventilation using a specialized double-lumen endotracheal tube is an established technique in thoracic surgery, but the availability of these devices is limited. Most emergency physicians have no experience with this technique. Lui and Johnson[184] have demonstrated that the right lung can be selectively intubated by merely blindly advancing a standard single-lumen endotracheal tube to a depth of 30 cm (measured at the corner of the mouth) in adult patients. Although the left lung and the right upper lobe are not ventilated with the tracheal tube in this position, animal studies and preliminary data from humans suggest that selective right lung ventilation provides adequate oxygenation and ventilation for at least 60 minutes, thereby expediting the thoracotomy by minimizing the technical problems encountered by continual left lung inflation.

ANESTHESIA AND AMNESIA

Comatose patients undergoing resuscitation may regain consciousness during a successful emergency thoracotomy, but the use of paralyzing agents may mask the return of

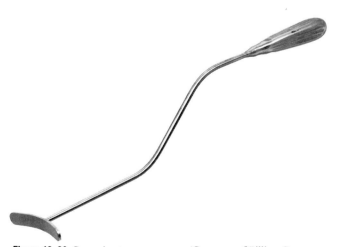

Figure 18–20. Conn Aorta compressor. (Courtesy of Pilling Company, Ft. Washington, Pa.)

awareness. The physician must be cognizant of this phenomenon and administer adequate analgesia and amnestic agents to the paralyzed patient. We recommend the judicious use of narcotics and generally the frequent use of benzodiazepines, especially midazolam, until paralyzing agents have worn off and the level of awareness can be assessed adequately.

CONCLUSION

Advances in prehospital care have increased the number of patients requiring advanced resuscitation. For selected patients, an emergency thoracotomy will substantially reduce morbidity and mortality. The effectiveness of using this procedure for resuscitation has been well documented. The mechanism of injury and the status of vital signs "at the scene" and on arrival to the hospital should be considered before an emergency thoracotomy is performed. Victims of penetrating trauma who had any vital signs present at the scene are candidates for resuscitative thoracotomy and have a chance of survival. In contrast, the survival rates for victims of blunt trauma are negligible. With blunt trauma, resuscitative thoracotomy generally should be considered only when vital signs are still present on arrival to the emergency care unit. Following emergency thoracotomy, the systolic blood pressure after the first 30 minutes of resuscitation may be used as a decision point for further treatment. This response of blood pressure to thoracotomy applies to both blunt and penetrating trauma. With injuries of the heart, the lungs, and the great vessels, successful resuscitation will depend on rapid restoration of an effective blood volume and surgical intervention through a thoracotomy. The pathophysiology and treatment of those injuries that require resuscitative thoracotomy have been discussed. Pericardial tamponade, hemorrhagic shock, air embolism, and cardiac arrest may all require this procedure.

Debate over who should perform an emergency thoracotomy is not necessary. It stands to reason that whoever uses this resuscitative procedure must be prepared to manage the patient. Emergency physicians must possess the knowledge and skills necessary to enable the optimal survival of as many patients as possible. Whenever possible, a preestablished plan of chest wound management and postthoracotomy care should be established with the emergency physician's surgical backup. With such a plan, a team approach to resuscitation and, hence, optimal patient care will be possible.

REFERENCES

1. Mattox KL: Emergency department thoracotomy (editorial). JACEP 7:455, 1978.
2. Denny MK: Emergency department thoracotomy question raises larger issues. JACEP 8:385, 1979.
3. MacDonald JR: Emergency department thoracotomy (correspondence). JACEP 8:441, 1979.
4. Page JR: Emergency department thoracotomy (correspondence). JACEP 8:441, 1979.
5. Johnson LS: Emergency department thoracotomy (correspondence). JACEP 8:441, 1979.
6. Mattox KL: Emergency department thoracotomy (correspondence). JACEP 8:441, 1979.
7. MacDonald FR, McDowell RM: Emergency department thoracotomies in a community hospital. JACEP 7:423, 1978.
8. Rosen P, Baker FJ, Braen RG, et al: Emergency Medicine: Concepts and Clinical Practic. St. Louis, CV Mosby Co, 1983, p 3.
9. Hirshman JC, Nussenfeld SR, Nagel EL: Mobile physician command: A new dimension in civilian telemetry-rescue systems. JAMA 230:255, 1974.
10. Cobb LA, Conn RD, Samson WE: Prehospital coronary care: The role of a rapid mobile intensive care system. Circulation 43 and 44 (Suppl 2):45, 1971.
11. American Medical Association: Recommendations of the Conferences on the Guidelines for the Categorization of Hospital Emergency Capabilities. Chicago, American Medical Association, 1971.
12. Champion HR: Emergency thoracotomy. Arch Emerg Med 3:95, 1986.
13. Donovan PJ: Emergency thoracotomy. J Emerg Med 6:75, 1988.
14. Feliciano DV: Liberal use of emergency center thoracotomy. Am J Surg 152:654, 1986.
15. Hoffman JR: Emergency department thoracotomy. Am J Emerg Med 4:574, 1986.
16. Mattox KL: Symposium paper: Penetrating wounds of the thorax. Injury 17:313, 1986.
17. Ordog GJ: Emergency thoracotomy. Am J Emerg Med 5:312, 1987.
18. Powell RW: Resuscitative thoracotomy in children and adolescents. Am Surg 54:188, 1988.
19. Sugg WL, Rea WJ, Ecker RR, et al: Penetrating wounds of the heart: An analysis of 459 cases. J Thorac Cardiovasc Surg 56:531, 1968.
20. Mattox KL, Espanda R, Beall AC, et al: Performing thoracotomy in the emergency center. JACEP 3:13, 1974.
21. Mattox KL, Beall AC, Jordan GL, et al: Cardiorrhaphy in the emergency center. J Thorac Cardiovasc Surg 68:886, 1974.
22. Moore EE, Moore JB, Gallaway AC, et al: Post injury thoracotomy in the emergency department: A critical evaluation. Surgery 86:590, 1979.
23. Baker CC, Thomas AN, Trunkey DD: The role of emergency room thoracotomy in trauma. J Trauma 20:848, 1980.
24. Harnar TJ, Oreskovich, MR, Copass MK, et al: Role of emergency thoracotomy in the resuscitation of moribund trauma victims. Am J Surg 142:96, 1981.
25. Bodai BI, Mith JP, Blaisdell RW: The role of emergency thoracotomy in blunt trauma. J Trauma 22:487, 1982.
26. Flynn TC, Ward RE, Miller PW: Emergency department thoracotomy. Ann Emerg Med 11:413, 1982.
27. Ivatury RR: Emergency department thoracotomy for trauma: A collective review. Resuscitation 15:23, 1987.
28. Bodai BI, Smith PJ, Ward RE, et al: Emergency thoracotomy in the management of trauma. JAMA 249:1981, 1983.
29. Capplelen A: Vulnus cordis sutur of hjertet. Nord Mag f Laegenvid 11:285, 1896.
30. Farina G: Discussion (cited by Durante). Zentralbl Chir 23:1224, 1896.
31. Page CH: Operative treatment of heart wounds. Ann Surg 50:101, 1909.
32. Rehn L: Veber Penetriren den Herzwunden and Hertnacht. Arch Chn Chir 55:315, 1897.
33. Bigger IA: Heart wounds. J Thorac Surg 8:239, 1939.
34. Bigger IA: Diagnosis and treatment of heart wounds with summary of 34 cases. Med Ann Distr Columbia 9:390, 1940.
35. Demetriades D: Emergency room thoracotomy for stab wounds to the chest and neck. J Trauma 27:483, 1987.
36. Elkin DC: Diagnosis and treatment of cardiac trauma. Ann Surg 114:169, 1941.
37. Demetriades D: Indications for thoracotomy in stab injuries of the chest: A prospective study of 543 patients. Br J Surg 73:888, 1986.
38. Elkin DC: Wounds of the heart. Ann Surg 120:817, 1944.
39. Baillot R: Penetrating chest trauma: A 20-year experience. J Trauma 27:994, 1987.
40. Griswald RA, Maguire CH: Penetrating wounds of the heart and pericardium. Surg Gynecol Obstet 74:517, 1943.
41. Nelson H: Penetrating wounds of the heart. Arch Surg 47:517, 1943.
42. Linder H, Hodo H: Stab wounds of the heart and pericardium. South Med J 37:261, 1944.
43. Blau MH: Wounds of the heart. Am J Med Sci 210:252, 1945.
44. Maynard ADI, Cordice JW, Naclerio EA: Penetrating wounds of the heart. A report of 81 cases. Surg Gynecol Obstet 94:605, 1952.
45. Beall AC, Diethrich EB, Crawford HW, et al: Surgical management of penetrating cardiac injuries. Am J Surg 112:686, 1966.
46. Reul BJ, Beall AC, Jordan BL, Mattox KL: The early operative management of injuries to the great vessels. Surgery 74:862, 1973.
47. Siemens R, Polk MC Jr, et al: Indications for thoracotomy following penetrating thoracic injury. J Trauma 17:493, 1977.
48. Beall AC, Diethrich EB, Cooley DS, DeBakey ME: Surgical management of penetrating cardiovascular trauma. South Med J 60:698, 1967.
49. Beall AC, Bricker DL, Crawford HW, et al: Considerations in the management of penetrating thoracic trauma. J Trauma 8:408, 1968.
50. Oparah SS, Mandal AK: Operative management of penetrating wounds of the chest in civilian practice. Review of indications in 125 cases. J Thorac Cardiovasc Surg 77:162, 1979.
51. Oparah SS, Mandal AK: Penetrating stab wounds of the chest: Experience with 200 consecutive cases. J Trauma 16:868, 1976.
52. Karrel R, Shaffer MA, Franasek JB: Emergency diagnosis, resuscitation and treatment of acute penetrating cardiac trauma. Ann Emerg Med 11:504, 1982.
53. Ivatury RR: Penetrating cardiac injuries: Twenty-year experience. Am Surg 53:310, 1987.
54. Symbas PN: Trauma to the Heart and the Great Vessels. New York, Grune & Stratton, 1976, p 17.
55. Tassi A, Davies AL: Pericardial tamponade due to penetrating fragment wounds of the heart. Am J Surg 118:535, 1969.
56. Carrasguilla C, Wilson RF, Wait AF, et al: Gunshot wounds of the heart. Ann Thorac Surg 13:208, 1972.
57. Asfaw I, Austin A: Penetrating wounds of the pericardium and heart. Surg Clin North Am 57:37, 1977.
58. Beach PM, Bognolo E, Hutchison JE: Penetrating cardiac trauma: Experience with 34 patients in hospital without cardiopulmonary bypass capability. Am J Surg 131:411, 1976.
59. Spodick D: Acute cardiac tamponade: Pathophysiology, diagnosis, and management. Prog Cardiovasc Dis 10:64, 1967.
60. Shoemaker WC, Carey JS, Yao ST, et al: Hemodynamic alterations in

acute cardiac tamponade after penetrating injuries of the heart. Surgery 67:754, 1970.

61. Beall AC, Ochsner JL, Morris GC, et al: Penetrating wounds of the heart. J Trauma 1:195, 1961.

62. Naclerio EA: Penetrating wounds of the heart: Experience with 249 patients. Dis Chest 46:1, 1964.

63. Wilson RF, Basset JS: Penetrating wounds of the pericardium and its contents. JAMA 195:513, 1966.

64. Evans J, Gray LA, Rayner A, et al: Principles for the management of penetrating cardiac wounds. Ann Surg 189:777, 1979.

65. Symbas PN, Harlaffis N, Waldo WJ: Penetrating cardiac wounds. A comparison of different therapeutic methods. Ann Surg 183:377, 1976.

66. Broja AR, Ransdell HT: Treatment of penetrating gunshot wounds of the chest: Experience with 145 cases. Am J Surg 122:81, 1971.

67. Jarisch A, Zotterman Y: Depressor reflexes from the heart. Acta Physiol Scand 16:31, 1948.

68. Coleridge HM, Coleridge JCG, Kidd C: Cardiac receptors of the dog with particular reference to two types of afferent endings in the ventricular wall. J Physiol 174:323, 1964.

69. Brown AM: The depressor reflex arising from the left coronary artery of the cat. J Physiol 184:825, 1966.

70. Sleight P, Widdicomb JG: Action potentials in fibers from receptors in the epicardium and myocardium of the dog's left ventricle. J Physiol 181:235, 1965.

71. Roe BB: Cardiac trauma including injury of the great vessels. Surg Clin North Am 52:573, 1972.

72. Beall AC, Wilson RF: Penetrating wounds of the heart: Changing patterns of surgical management (correspondence). J Trauma 12:6, 1972.

73. Shoemaker WC: Algorithm for early recognition and management of cardiac tamponade. Crit Care Med 3:59, 1975.

74. Carey JS, Yao ST, Kho LK, et al: Cardiovascular responses to hemopericardium, compression by balloon tamponade and acute coronary occlusion. J Thorac Cardiovasc Surg 54:65, 1967.

75. Arom KV, Richardson JD, Webb G, et al: Subxiphoid pericardial window in patients with suspected traumatic pericardial tamponade. Ann Thorac Surg 23:545, 1977.

76. Bertelsen S, Howitz P: Injuries of the trachea and bronchi. Thorax 27:188, 1972.

77. Hood RM, Sloan HE: Injuries of the trachea and major bronchi. J Thorac Cardiovasc Surg 38:458, 1959.

78. Guest JL, Anderson JN: Major airway injury in closed chest trauma. Chest 72:63, 1977.

79. Rutherford RB, Hurt HH, Brickman Rd, Tubb JM: The pathophysiology and treatment of progressive tension pneumothorax. J Trauma 8:212, 1968.

80. Schwartz GR, Wagner DJ: Emergency therapy: Penetrating trauma to the chest, heart, and great vessels. JACEP 2:196, 1973.

81. Borja AR, Ransdell H: Treatment of thoracoabdominal gunshot wounds in civilian practice: Experience with 44 cases. Am J Surg 121:580, 1971.

82. Yee ES, Verrie Ed, Thomas AN: Management of air embolism in blunt, and penetrating thoracic trauma. J Thorac Cardiovasc Surg 85:661, 1983.

83. Thomas NA, Stephens GB: Air embolism: A cause of morbidity and death after penetrating chest trauma. J Trauma 14:633, 1974.

84. Graham JJ, Beall CA, Mattox KL, et al: Systemic air embolism following penetrating trauma to the lung. Chest 72:449, 1977.

85. Flanagan JP, Frandisaria IA, Gross RJ, et al: Air embolism: A lethal complication of subclavian venipuncture. N Engl J Med 281:488, 1969.

86. Doblar DD, Hinkel JC, Fay ML, et al: Air embolism associated with pulmonary artery catheter introducer kit. Anesthesiology 53:307, 1982.

87. Thomas AN, Roe BB: Air embolism following penetrating lung injuries. J Thorac Cardiovasc Surg 66:553, 1973.

88. King MW: Fatal air embolism following penetrating lung trauma: An autopsy study. J Trauma 24:753, 1984.

89. Goldstone J, Towan HJ, Ellis RJ: Rationale for use of vasopressors in treatment of coronary air embolism. Surg Forum 29:237, 1978.

90. Meier GH, Symbas PN: Systemic air embolization: Factors involved in its production following penetrating lung injury. Am J Surg 12:765, 1978.

91. Meier GH, Wood WJ, Symbas PN: Systemic air embolization from penetrating lung injury. Ann Thorac Surg 27:161, 1978.

92. Halpern P, Greenstein A, Malamed Y, et al: Arterial air embolism after penetrating lung injury. Crit Care Med 11:392, 1983.

93. Peirce EC: Specific therapy for arterial air embolism. Ann Thorac Surg 29:300, 1980.

94. Tomatis L, Nemiroff M, Riahi M, et al: Massive arterial air embolism due to rupture of pulsatile assist device: Successful treatment in the hyperbaric chamber. Ann Thorac Surg 32:604, 1981.

95. Warren PA, Phillips RB, Inwood MJ: The ultrastructural morphology of air embolism platelet adhesion to the interface and endothelial damage. Br J Exp Pathol 54:163, 1973.

96. Diethrich EB, Koopot R, Maze A, Dyess N: Successful reversal of brain damage from iatrogenic air embolism. Surg Gynecol Obstet 154:572, 1982.

97. Mills NL, Ochsner JL: Massive air embolism during cardiopulmonary bypass. J Thorac Cardiovasc Surg 80:708, 1980.

98. Mavroudis C, Roon AJ, Baker C, et al: Management of acute cervicothoracic vascular injuries. J Thorac Cardiovasc Surg 80:342, 1980.

99. Brotmans S, Oster-Granite M, Cox EF: Failure of cross clamping the thoracic aorta to control intraabdominal bleeding. Ann Emerg Med 11:147, 1982.

100. Sankaran S, Lucas C, Walt AJ: Thoracic aortic clamping for prophylaxis against sudden cardiac arrest during laparotomy for acute massive hemoperitoneum. J Trauma 15:290, 1975.

101. Ledgerwood AM, Krazmers M, Lucas EC: The role of thoracic aortic occlusion for massive hemoperitoneum. J Trauma 16:610, 1976.

102. Babbs CF: A renaissance of CPR research. Crit Care Med 8:119, 1980.

103. Kouwenhoven WB, Jude JR, Knickerbocker GG: Closed-chest cardiac massage. JAMA 173:94, 1960.

104. Ditchey RV, Winkler JV, Rhodes CA: Relative lack of coronary blood flow during closed-chest resuscitation in dogs. Circulation 66:297, 1982.

105. Niemann JT, Rosborough JP, Ung S, et al: Coronary perfusion pressure during experimental cardiopulmonary resuscitation. Ann Emerg Med 11:127, 1982.

106. Luce JM, Ross BK, O'Quinn RJ, et al: Regional blood flow during cardiopulmonary resuscitation in dogs using simultaneous and nonsimultaneous compression and ventilation. Circulation 67:258, 1983.

107. Bircher N, Safer P, Stewart R: A comparison of standard, "MAST"-augmented, and open-chest CPR in dogs. Crit Care Med 8:147, 1980.

108. Bircher N, Safar P: Comparison of standard and "new" closed-chest CPR and open-chest CPR in dogs. Crit Care Med 9:384, 1981.

109. Byrne D, Pass HI, Neely WA, et al: External versus internal cardiac massage in normal and chronically ischemic dogs. Am Surg 46:657, 1980.

110. Babbs CF: Knowledge gaps in CPR. Crit Care Med 8:181, 1980.

111. Criley JM, Niemann JT, Rosborough JP, et al: The heart is a conduit in CPR. Crit Care Med 9:373, 1981.

112. Weisfeldt ML, Chandra N, Tsitlik J: Increased intrathoracic pressure—not direct heart compression—causes the rise in intrathoracic vascular pressures during CPR in dogs and pigs. Crit Care Med 9:377, 1981.

113. Babbs CF: New versus old theories of blood flow during CPR. Crit Care Med 8:191, 1980.

114. Chandra N, Guerci A, Weisfeldt ML, et al: Contrasts between intrathoracic pressures during external chest compression and cardiac massage. Crit Care Med 9:789, 1981.

115. Rudikoff MT, Maughan WL, Effron M, et al: Mechanisms of blood flow during cardiopulmonary resuscitation. Circulation 61:345, 1980.

116. Niemann JT, Rosborough JP, Hausknecht M, et al: Pressure-synchronized cineangiography during experimental cardiopulmonary resuscitation. Circulation 64:985, 1981.

117. Kovach AGB, Sandor P: Cerebral blood flow and brain function during hypotension and shock. Annu Rev Physiol 38:571, 1976.

118. Jackson RE, Joyce K, White B, et al: Blood flow in the cerebral cortex during cardiac resuscitation in dogs. Ann Emerg Med 12:257, 1983.

119. Szczygiel M, Wright R, Wagner E, et al: Prognostic indicators of ultimate long-term survival following advanced life support. Ann Emerg Med 10:566, 1981.

120. DeBard M: Cardiopulmonary resuscitation: Analysis of six years' experience and review of the literature. Ann Emerg Med 10:408, 1981.

121. Eisenberg M, Bergner L, Hallstrom A: Cardiac resuscitation in the community. JAMA 241:1905, 1979.

122. Eliastam M, Duralde T, Martinez F, et al: Cardiac arrest in the emergency medical service system: Guidelines for resuscitation. JACEP 6:525, 1977.

123. Eliastam M: When to stop cardiopulmonary resuscitation. In Budassi SA, Bander JJ, et al (eds): Cardiac Arrest and CPR. Rockville, Md, Aspen Systems Corp, 1980, p 161.

124. Jeresaty RM, Godar TJ, Liss JP: External cardiac resuscitation in a community hospital. Arch Intern Med 124:588, 1969.

125. Bedell SE: Survival after cardiopulmonary resuscitation in the hospital. N Engl J Med 309:569, 1983.

126. Bartlett RL, Raymond JI, Anstadt GL, et al: Clinical research: Use of direct mechanical ventricular assistance in cardiopulmonary resuscitation. Richland Memorial Hospital Investigational Review Board, Columbia, SC, 1982.

127. Stephenson HE: An increasing role for surgeons in cardiac resuscitation. Surg Gynecol Obstet 152:822, 1981.

128. Alifimoff JK, Babbs C, Del Guercio L, et al: Resuscitative thoracotomy symposium—panel discussion. Resuscitation 15:59, 1987.

129. Del Guercio LRM: Open chest cardiac massage: An overview. Resuscitation 15:9, 1987.

130. Eldor J: Open chest cardiac massage: A review. Resuscitation 16:155, 1988.

131. Barsan WG, Levy RC: Experimental design for study of cardiopulmonary resuscitation in dogs. Ann Emerg Med 10:135, 1981.

132. Kern KB: Open-chest cardiac massage after closed-chest compression in a canine model: When to intervene. Resuscitation 15:51, 1987.

133. Weiser FM, Adler LN, Kuhn LA: Hemodynamic effects of closed and open chest cardiac resuscitation in normal dogs and those with acute myocardial infarction. Am J Cardiol 10:555, 1962.

134. Geehr EC, Lewis FR, Auerbach PS: Failure of open-heart massage to improve survival after prehospital nontraumatic cardiac arrest. N Engl J Med 314:1189, 1986.

135. Del Guercio LRM, Coomarswamy RP, State D: Cardiac output and other hemodynamic variables during external cardiac massage in man. N Engl J Med 269:1398, 1963.

136. Osborn HH: Introduction [Editorial introduction to issue on resuscitative thoracotomy]. Resuscitation 15:1, 1987.
137. Del Guercio LRM, Feins NR, Cohn JD, et al: Comparison of blood flow during external and internal cardiac massage in man. Circulation 31 (Suppl 1):171, 1965.
138. Cohn JD, Del Guercio LRM: Cardiorespiratory analysis of cardiac arrest and resuscitation. Surg Gynecol Obstet 23:1066, 1966.
139. Redding JS, Cozine RA: A comparison of open-chest and closed-chest cardiac massage in dogs. Anesthesiology 22:280, 1961.
140. Bartlett RL, Stewart NJ, Raymond JI, Martin SD: A comparative study of closed and open resuscitation: Effects on survival and neurologic damage. Ann Emerg Med 13 (Part 2):773, 1983.
141. Miller JW, Danzl DF, Thomas DM: Urban accidental hypothermia: 135 cases. Ann Emerg Med 9:456, 1980.
142. Wickstrom P, Ruix R, Lija GP, et al: Accidental hypothermia. Am J Surg 131:622, 1976.
143. Truscott DG, Firor WB, Clein LJ: Accidental profound hypothermia. Arch Surg 106:216, 1973.
144. Althaus U, Aeberhard P, Schupbach P, et al: Management of profound accidental hypothermia with cardiorespiratory arrest. Ann Surg 195:492, 1982.
145. Shocket E, Rosenblum R: Successful open cardiac massage after 75 minutes of closed massage. JAMA 200:157, 1967.
146. Sykes MK, Ahmed N: Emergency treatment of cardiac arrest. Lancet 2:347, 1963.
147. Bayer MJ: Emergency thoracotomy and internal cardiac massage. Topics Emerg Med 1:95, 1979.
148. Alifimoff JK: Open versus closed chest cardiac massage in non-traumatic cardiac arrest. Resuscitation 15:13, 1987.
149. Castagna J, Weil MH, Shubin J: Factors determining survival in patients with cardiac arrest. Chest 65:527, 1974.
150. Iseri LT, Siner EJ, Humphrey SB, Mann S: Prehospital cardiac arrest after arrival of the paramedic unit. JACEP 6:530, 1977.
151. Longstreth WT, Diehr P, Inui TS: Prediction of awakening after out-of-hospital cardiac arrest. N Engl J Med 308:1378, 1983.
152. Clevenger FW, Yarbrough DR, Reines HD: Resuscitative thoracotomy: The effect of field time on outcome. J Trauma 28:441, 1988.
153. Ivatury RR, Nallathambi MN, Roberge RJ, et al: Penetrating thoracic injuries: In-field stabilization vs prompt transport. J Trauma 27:1066, 1987.
154. Brautigan MW, Tietz G: Emergency thoracotomy in an urban community hospital: Initial cardiac rhythm as a new predictor of survival. Am J Emerg Med 3:311, 1985.
155. Jones TK, Barnhart GR, Greenfield LJ: Cardiopulmonary arrest following penetrating trauma: Guidelines for emergency hospital management of presumed exsanguination. J Trauma 27:24, 1987.
156. Hollingsworth AB: Emergency thoracotomy in the emergency department or the operating room? Emerg Decisions 4:30, 1988.
157. Young GP: Emergency autotransfusion. Ann Emerg Med 12:180, 1983.
158. Reul GJ, Mattox KL, Beall AC, et al: Recent advances in the operative management of massive chest trauma. Ann Thorac Surg 16:52, 1973.
159. Snow N, Lucas AE: Subxiphoid pericardiotomy. Am Surg 49:249, 1983.
160. Santos GH, Frater RWM: The subxiphoid in the treatment of pericardial effusion. Ann Thorac Surg 23:467, 1977.
161. Miller FB: Diagnostic pericardial window: A safe alternative to exploratory thoracotomy for suspected heart injuries. Arch Surg 122:605, 1987.
162. Alcan KE, Zabetakis PM, Marino ND, et al: Management of acute cardiac tamponade by subxiphoid pericardiotomy. JAMA 247:1143, 1982.
163. Johnson J, Kirby CK: An experimental study of cardiac massage. Surgery 26:472, 1949.
164. Barnett WM: Comparison of open-chest cardiac massage techniques in dogs. Ann Emerg Med 15:408, 1986.
165. Stephenson HE: Cardiac Arrest and Resuscitation. 5th ed. St. Louis, CV Mosby Co, 1974.
166. Bartlett RL, Stewart NJ, Raymond JI, Martin SD: Open chest resuscitation: The relationship of compression rate to cardiac output and blood pressure (submitted for publication).
167. Mattox KL, Von Kock L, Beall AC Jr, et al: Logistic and technical considerations in the treatment of the wounded heart. Circulation 51, 52:210, 1975.
168. Trinkle JK, Toon RS, Franz JL, et al: Affairs of the wounded heart: Penetrating cardiac wounds. J Trauma 19:467, 1979.
169. Cooper P: The Craft of Surgery. 2nd ed, vol 1. Boston, Little, Brown & Co, 1971, pp 29–31.
170. McQuillan RF, McCormack T, Heligan MC: Penetrating left ventricular stab wound: A method of control during resuscitation and prior to repair. Injury 12:63, 1980.
171. Levitsky S: New insights in cardiac trauma. Surg Clin North Am 55:43, 1975.
172. Pearce CW, McCool E, Schmidt FE: Control of bleeding from cardiovascular wounds. Ann Surg 163:257, 1966.
173. Wilson SM: In extremis use of a foley catheter in a cardiac stab wound. J Trauma 26:400, 1986.
174. Reul GJ, Beall AC, Jordan GL, Mattox KL: The early operative management of injuries to the great vessels. Surgery 74:862, 1973.
174a. Shamoun JM, Barraza KR, Jurkovich GJ, et al: In extremis use of staples for cardiorrhaphy in penetrating cardiac trauma: Case report. J Trauma 29:1589, 1989.
175. Kerber RE, Carter J, Klein S, et al: Open chest defibrillation during cardiac surgery. Am J Cardiol 46:393, 1980.
176. Bricker DL, Morton JR, Okies JE, et al: Surgical management of injuries to vena cava: Changing patterns of injury and newer techniques of repair. J Trauma 11:725, 1971.
177. Samuelson SL: A new method of rapid fluid resuscitation during thoracotomy performed in the emergency room. Surg Gynecol Obstet 165:175, 1987.
178. Schwab CW: Emergency department thoracotomy (EDT): A 26-month experience using an "agonal" protocol. Am Surg 52:20, 1986.
179. Dunn EL, Moore EE, Moore JB: Hemodynamic effects of aortic occlusion during hemorrhagic shock. Ann Emerg Med 11:238, 1982.
180. Garcia-Rinaldi R, Defore WW, Mattox KL, Beall AC: Unimpaired renal, myocardial and neurologic function after cross clamping of the thoracic aorta. Surg Gynecol Obstet 143:249, 1976.
181. Symbas PN, Diorio DA, Tyras DH, et al: Penetrating cardiac wounds: Significant residual and delayed sequelae. J Thorac Cardiovasc Surg 66:526, 1973.
182. Heller RF, Rahimtolla SH, Ehsani A, et al: Cardiac complications: Results of penetrating chest wounds including the heart. Arch Intern Med 134:491, 1974.
183. Mandal AK: Prophylactic antibiotics and no antibiotics compared in penetrating chest trauma. J Trauma 25:639, 1985.
184. Lui RC, Johnson FE: Selective right-lung ventilation during emergency department thoracotomy. Crit Care Med 17:1057, 1989.

Vascular Techniques and Volume Support

Chapter 19

Arterial Puncture and Cannulation

William J. Barker

INTRODUCTION

Arterial blood gas evaluation provides useful information that is essentially unavailable by other means. The respiratory status and acid-base equilibrium of individuals with pulmonary disorders, drug overdoses, and metabolic diseases may be evaluated through this procedure. The current sophistication of critical care medicine would be impossible without arterial access, permitting continuous arterial pressure monitoring and frequent blood sampling for metabolic and hematologic indices.

Access to the arterial system may now be obtained easily in most patients. Many improvements in arterial access methodology and equipment have occurred since Hales, in 1733, first used a technique similar to today's cutdown technique to attach a fluid column for measurement of the blood pressure of a horse.[1] J. L. M. Poiseuille first introduced the use of a mercury manometer for the measurement of blood pressure in 1828. In 1847, Karl Ludwig graphically recorded blood pressure fluctuations by placing a float with a pointer on the mercury column, permitting the pointer to scratch a smoked drum rotating adjacent to the column. Today's manometers, transducers, and recorders use electronics rather than simple mechanics, thus permitting mathematical waveform analysis in addition to visual analysis.

INDICATIONS AND CONTRAINDICATIONS

Many patients who are seen in the emergency department benefit from arterial puncture or cannulation (see Table 19–1). Most commonly, arterial blood gases are used to evaluate individuals who have significant respiratory pathology. Although most patients with respiratory illness may be managed without arterial puncture, arterial blood gas determination is imperative when they are severely ill. Critically ill patients with nonrespiratory disease may need frequent metabolic and electrolyte monitoring. For instance, the patient with severe diabetic ketoacidosis cannot be managed properly without frequent pH, electrolyte, and glucose measurements. Although arterial blood gas analysis is the most frequent indication for arterial puncture, all blood chemistries can be performed from an arterial sample. Blood cultures may also be obtained through an indwelling arterial line with sensitivity and specificity equal to cultures from a venipuncture site.[2, 3] When frequent blood sampling is required, it is easier and certainly more humane to insert an indwelling arterial cannula. The nurse who is caring for the patient may then sample the blood as needed.

The most common indication for long-term arterial cannulation is continuous monitoring of arterial blood pressure. An electromechanical pressure transducer attached to an oscilloscope screen allows continuous observation of arterial systolic and diastolic pressures. This capability is most useful in a critical care unit but is also helpful when available in an emergency department. Many situations, such as during the use of vasoactive drugs (e.g., nitroprusside and dopamine), require continuous arterial pressure monitoring. The response of trauma and cardiac patients to resuscitative efforts also may be more easily followed in this manner.

Another common use of arterial puncture is radiologic diagnostic imaging of the arterial system. Obviously, this is an uncommon indication in the emergency department but may be considered for suspected cases of peripheral arterial trauma or embolism. Although this procedure is fairly simple to perform, arterial access for diagnostic imaging is most often performed by a radiologist. Arterial puncture is also used by cardiologists and radiologists for coronary, cerebral, renal, and other central arterial angiography. Aortography can be very important for chest trauma and suspected cases of dissecting or leaking aneurysms.

Few contraindications to arterial puncture exist; none are absolute. Arterial puncture performed in patients who are anticoagulated or who have other coagulopathies should be undertaken with extreme care. Luce and associates reported seven patients with compression neuropathies secondary to hematoma after arterial puncture, all of whom were anticoagulated at the time of puncture.[4] Repeated arterial sampling in these patients may necessitate insertion of an indwelling cannula to minimize the number of puncture sites in the arterial wall. Arterial cannulation or puncture should be used in a patient receiving thrombolytic therapy *only* if it will provide essential data that cannot be obtained in any other fashion.

The presence of severe atherosclerosis, with or without diminution of flow, is a relative contraindication to arterial

Table 19–1. Arterial Puncture and Cannulation

Indications	Relative Contraindications
Blood gas sampling	Previous surgery in the area,
Continuous pressure monitoring	especially cutdown
Frequent blood sampling for	Anticoagulation
any purpose	Coagulopathy
Diagnostic angiography	Skin infection at site
Therapeutic embolization	Atherosclerosis
	Decreased collateral flow

puncture, especially when followed by cannulation. The existence of a bruit or a palpable decrease in the pulse should warn the physician of the presence of intravascular disease. If either is noted and if the arterial puncture is imperative, an alternative site should be considered.

Evidence of decreased or absent collateral flow in areas in which flow normally exists should also lead one to consider an alternative site. A positive Allen test (discussed in the technique section) may possibly eliminate the radial and ulnar arteries as sites of cannulation. One should also avoid puncture of an artery when infection, burn, or other damage to cutaneous defenses exists in the overlying skin.

EQUIPMENT

The equipment used for arterial cannulation has a great influence on the accuracy of pressure measurements. Frequency responses of tubing, transducers, and other components of the monitoring system influence the measurement accuracy of systolic and diastolic pressures.

The dynamic response characteristics of the monitoring system are of minimal importance if the clinician is interested primarily in the mean arterial pressure (MAP).[5] In the emergency department, trends in the MAP are more useful than absolute values for systolic and diastolic pressures.

The various catheter types have demonstrated similar frequency response characteristics, but studies have shown more variable effects on complication rates. Teflon catheters have been implicated as a factor associated with increased thrombosis in one study,[6] whereas the results of other studies deny any such effect.[7–9] The diameter of the indwelling cannula seems to have a more consistent effect; the incidence of thrombosis is inversely related to the ratio of vessel lumen to catheter diameter.[10] Thus for a given vessel size, the incidence of thrombosis will increase as the catheter diameter decreases. Catheter choice should be influenced by availability and convenience of use of a particular brand. A short catheter is ideal for peripheral artery cannulation, whereas a longer over-the-needle catheter is preferable for the femoral artery (Fig. 19–1). Downs and associates suggest that thrombosis is less likely with a nontapered catheter.[11] An 18- to 20-gauge catheter should be used in adults. Small children and infants require a 22- to 24-gauge catheter, which may need to be inserted through a cutdown technique.

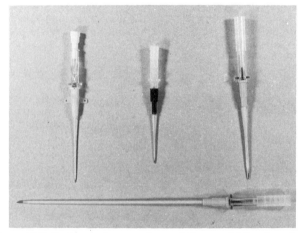

Figure 19–1. Catheters that may be used for arterial line insertion. Short, small-gauge over-the-needle catheters are ideal for peripheral artery cannulation (*top*). The long over-the-needle catheter is used for femoral arterial lines (*bottom*).

The tubing that connects the catheter to the pressure transducer has a significant effect on monitoring systems. The higher the frequency response of the whole system, the more accurate is the determination of systolic and diastolic pressure.[5, 12] A stiff, low-capacitance plastic tubing should be used, and the manometer should be placed as close as possible to the patient, because the frequency response of a tube is inversely related to its length.[12–14]

After the pressure wave is transmitted from the artery through the catheter and connecting tubing, a measuring device is required to obtain a numerical value for the arterial pressure. Most commonly used today is an electromechanical pressure transducer that changes a mechanical pressure pulse, the fluid wave, into an electrical signal, which is then displayed on an oscilloscope. Additional circuitry can be added to display the systolic and diastolic pressure as numerical values. Various minicomputer systems that allow computation of mean arterial pressure, trend monitoring, and other capabilities in addition to displaying the systolic and diastolic pressures are available. So many transducer and oscilloscope combinations exist that a discussion of their relative merits is beyond the scope of this chapter.

Intravascular transducers are also available but have many potential disadvantages and are used infrequently. They are fragile, temperature sensitive, of variable quality, and much more difficult to place into a vessel than is a catheter. Fibrin deposition on the device is also a common finding. The greatest, and possibly only, advantage of these intravascular transducers is the elimination of potential error induced by catheters, stopcocks, and connecting tubing.

Less expensive means of deriving a number representative of the arterial pressure are available, especially if one is interested in determining only the MAP. Zorab describes the use of an anaeroid manometer connected to the arterial system by a catheter filled with heparinized saline.[15] The catheter is arranged to have a fluid meniscus at the same level as the heart when there is no pressure input. The meniscus is below an air column in a vertical tube that is long enough to avoid saline contamination of the manometer at maximal pressures (Fig. 19–2). A mercury manometer, especially a J tube, may also be used in place of an anaeroid manometer in the previously described system for measurement of MAP.

For continuous arterial pressure monitoring, some method of flushing the system is necessary to maintain patency of the catheter lumen. This may be as simple as a three-way stopcock through which the tubing is intermittently flushed with heparinized saline. There are continuous flush devices that are designed to push a set amount of fluid (usually 2 to 3 ml per hour) through the line. A typical monitoring system that includes this device is shown in Figure 19–3. The pressure transducer is usually mounted at the level of the patient's heart on a bedside pole.

The equipment needed to percutaneously obtain a single sample for arterial blood gas analysis is simple and readily available in any hospital, often in the form of a prepackaged kit (Fig. 19–4). The necessary items for arterial line placement are listed in Table 19–2 and referred to in the section that describes the procedures. Obtaining a sample from an indwelling arterial line requires only two syringes, one of which has been heparinized.

SITE SELECTION

Selection of an arterial site is the first step in placing an indwelling cannula or in obtaining a sample of arterial blood

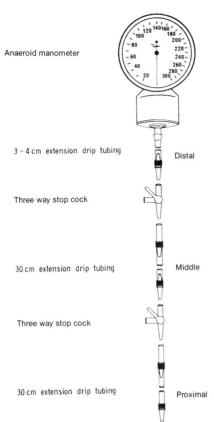

Figure 19–2. Assembly technique for anaeroid manometer system. The middle and proximal extension tubings contain heparinized saline. The middle extension tubing is arranged to form a fluid meniscus at the same level as the heart when the proximal stopcock is closed to the middle tubing (i.e., no pressure input). The distal extension tubing is filled with air and held vertically so that there is no saline contamination of the manometer at maximal pressures. Approximately 10 to 12 cm of air in the distal and middle tubings is optimal. The same system can be used with a mercury manometer in place of the anaeroid manometer. Sterility of the extension tubing and stopcocks is essential. (From Zorab JSM: Continuous display of the arterial pressure: A simple manometric technique. Anaesthesia 24:433, 1969. Copyright © 1969 by the Association of Anaesthetists of Great Britain and Ireland. Reproduced by permission.)

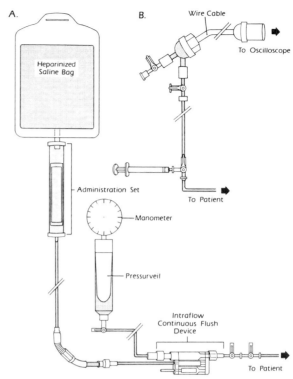

Figure 19–3. Arterial pressure monitoring systems. *A,* System for continuous flush. Heparin (2 ml of 1:1000 unit solution) is added to a 1-liter bag of normal saline, and the bag is pressurized to 300 mm Hg using a metered blood pump (not shown). The continuous flush device is set to deliver 3 ml of the heparinized saline per hour. A mechanical pressure transducer (Pressurveil, Concept Co.) is depicted. The transducer device is a sterile, inexpensive, fully assembled monitor that can be used during patient transfer. Alternatively, the electronic transducer depicted in *B* may be used. *B,* System for manual flush. A heparinized saline flush solution can be injected manually through a syringe at the proximal or distal port. The transducer dome should be maintained at the level of the patient's heart. (From Beal JM (ed): Critical Care for Surgical Patients. New York, Macmillan Publishing Co, Inc., 1982. Reproduced by permission.)

for a blood gas analysis. Successful cannulation of the radial, ulnar, brachial, axillary, dorsalis pedis, and femoral arteries in children and adults is possible. The temporal and umbilical arteries are often cannulated in infants and neonates. However, radial artery cannulation is also very safe for these patients.[16] (See also Chapter 20.) The radial, brachial, and femoral arteries are usually punctured for blood gas sampling in adults.

The potential consequence of total loss of blood flow through a vessel due to intraluminal thrombosis is one of several variables that must be considered when choosing a site for arterial puncture. Arteries known to have good collateral blood flow, such as the radial and dorsalis pedis, are thus favored. Determining the effect of the site chosen on the ease of patient care will be appreciated by those who will subsequently be providing direct care. An arterial line in the lower extremities may be preferred during a procedure on the upper body, whereas a femoral or axillary line may be poorly tolerated by patients who are capable of positioning themselves. Characteristics of the common arterial sites are discussed following general descriptions of the techniques of arterial puncture and cannulation.

Table 19–2. Equipment for Insertion and Maintenance of an Indwelling Arterial Cannula

Percutaneous insertion
    Alcohol or iodophor solution
    1% lidocaine or other local anesthetic solution
    4–0 nylon or silk suture on skin needle
    10-cm by 10-cm dressing sponges
    Adhesive tape
    Iodophor ointment
    Arm board for brachial, radial, or ulnar cannulations
    Syringes
    Pressure tubing
    Two three-way stopcocks
    Pressure transducer
    Connecting wire
    Oscilloscope, thermal graph, or other output display
    Heparinized saline
    Pressure blood infusor, set up with continuous flush device
Additional equipment required for cutdown insertion technique
    Scalpel blade (No. 10)
    0-silk sutures (2 or more)
    Small hemostat
    Forceps

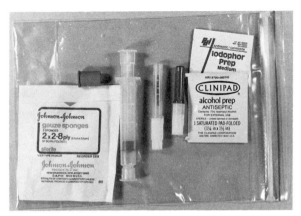

Figure 19–4. Arterial blood gas kit. Contents include skin preparation pads, prefilled heparinized syringe, stopper for syringe, needles, gauze sponges, and plastic bag for crushed ice.

TECHNIQUES

Percutaneous Technique for Single Arterial Puncture

To obtain a single sample of arterial blood by the percutaneous method, a small (5 ml) syringe is attached to a 20- to 22-gauge needle. A smaller needle may be required for young children or individuals who have had many previous punctures. To prevent clotting of the sample, 1 or 2 ml of a heparinized saline solution (1000 IU per ml) are drawn into the syringe to coat the barrel and needle and are then ejected through the needle shortly before puncture. All the visible heparin is ejected, so that all that remains is enough anticoagulant to coat the barrel and fill the dead space of the syringe and needle, minimizing heparin-related errors.[17]

Because of the air-fluid boundary in the heparin storage bottle, heparin solution has a higher P_{O_2} and a lower P_{CO_2} than blood, and changes in these parameters reflect a dilutional effect. The addition of 0.4 ml of heparin solution to a 2-ml sample of blood (dilution of 20 per cent) will lower the P_{CO_2} by 16 per cent. A falsely low P_{CO_2} is the most clinically significant change caused by excess heparin.[18, 19] P_{O_2} levels are not significantly altered by the addition of heparin in most instances, although a slight increase in P_{O_2} has been reported. The pH is affected (lowered) only if high concentrations of heparin are used (25,000 IU per ml), but generally the tremendous buffering capacity of blood maintains a normal pH. The dead space of a 5-ml Luer-Lok glass syringe and a 22-gauge, 3.8-cm needle is 0.2 ml. Therefore, to minimize heparin-related error, *at least 3 ml of blood should be collected,* even though blood gas analysis equipment requires only a 0.5-ml sample. Some packaged blood gas syringes contain a powdered heparin that mixes with the arterial blood. Although thrombosis of the needle may be more common with this system, smaller volumes (1 ml) of blood can be used.

The arterial pulse is palpated to ascertain the location of the vessel, and the overlying skin is prepared sterilely with an iodophor or other antiseptic solution. The patient's skin should then be anesthetized with a wheal of local anesthetic without epinephrine placed through a small-gauge (25 or 27) needle. If the patient is unresponsive to pain in the area, this step may be omitted. Care must be taken to use a small amount of local anesthetic, because a large wheal may obscure the pulse.

The arterial pulsation is then isolated between the index and middle fingers of the *gloved* nondominant hand (Fig. 19–5). The skin should be punctured through the anesthetic wheal, and the needle should be advanced toward the pulsating vessel. The needle should form an angle of about 15 to 20 degrees with the skin. A larger angle is required for femoral artery puncture. Once the needle has entered the arterial lumen, the syringe plunger should be allowed to rise with the arterial pressure to minimize the chance of venous sampling. If no blood flow is obtained, the needle should be withdrawn slowly, because both walls of the vessel may have been punctured. A sample may be obtained during withdrawal. Redirection of the needle should occur only when the needle has been retracted to a location just deep to the dermis.

Maher and Dougherty describe the use of a hand-held Doppler ultrasound probe to aid arterial puncture.[19a] The probe is held over the artery proximal to the puncture site. Loss of audible pulsations suggests vessel compression with imminent arterial puncture.

After a sample of at least 3 ml of blood has been obtained, the needle is removed from the artery and firm pressure is applied at the puncture site for a minimum of 5 minutes. Ten to 15 minutes of pressure is required if the patient is on anticoagulant therapy or has another coagulopathy.

Proper handling of the sample is very important. When the needle is withdrawn, it is imperative to expel any air bubbles that are present in the syringe to avoid false elevation of the P_{O_2}.[20] Air in the sample will significantly increase the P_{O_2} (mean increase of 11 mm Hg) after 20 minutes of storage, even if kept at 4° C. The pH and P_{CO_2} are not significantly altered by air bubbles if the blood is stored at 4° C for 20 minutes.

Removal of air is neatly and easily accomplished by placing an alcohol wipe or gauze sponge on the needle and tapping the inverted syringe to force any air to the top. Air is then pushed out of the needle, and any blood that is spilled will be caught by the sponge (Fig. 19–6). The needle is then plugged or removed, and the syringe is capped to ensure anaerobic conditions. Blood gas analysis is ideally performed immediately, but if this is not feasible, the sample may be stored in ice water for 1 hour with limited deterioration.[20, 21] If the sample is stored anaerobically, regardless

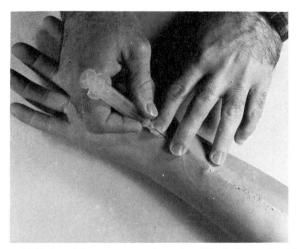

Figure 19–5. Arterial puncture at the wrist. The index and middle fingers are used to isolate the pulsating artery before insertion of the needle. Contrary to the illustration, latex gloves should be worn during the procedure.

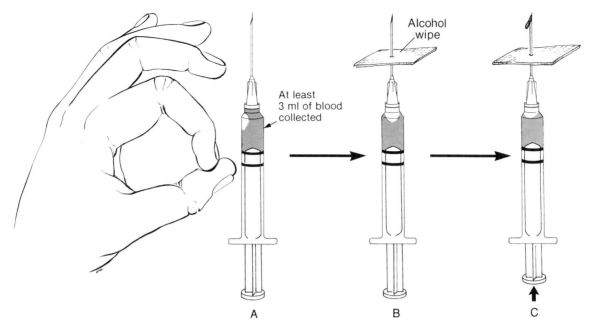

Figure 19–6. Removal of air bubbles from the syringe. *A,* Air bubbles are finger-tapped to the top of the syringe. *B,* An alcohol swab is placed over the top of the needle. *C,* The plunger is advanced to expel air while drops of blood are collected on the alcohol swab. After removal of the bubbles, the syringe is capped and sent to the laboratory.

of the temperature, the P_{O_2}, P_{CO_2}, and pH are relatively stable for up to 20 minutes. If blood is stored at room temperature for longer than 20 minutes, the P_{CO_2} will increase and the pH will decrease, probably as a result of leukocyte metabolism. In a stored sample, the P_{O_2} varies to such an extent that the change is unpredictable for chemical interpretation at 30 minutes, regardless of storage method. High leukocyte or thrombocyte counts, such as those seen in leukemic patients, may shorten acceptable storage intervals.[22, 23] Local anesthesia will make the procedures of arterial puncture easier for both the patient and the physician; however, one study found no significant alteration of P_{CO_2} or pH from the pain or anxiety of an unanesthetized arterial puncture (Table 19–3).[24]

Percutaneous Technique for Arterial Cannulation

Percutaneous puncture is the preferred method for arterial cannulation. It is also the method of choice for obtaining an isolated blood gas sample (see the preceding section) when an indwelling cannula has not been placed.

Once the site has been selected, the skin should be prepared with iodophor or other antiseptic solution, and sterile drapes should be placed around the area. Sterile technique should be meticulously maintained throughout the procedure. Levy and colleagues describe an alternative skin preparation method for central venous catheters that uses a 1 minute isopropyl alcohol scrub followed by catheter placement through an iodophor-impregnated adherent film (Ioban Z antimicrobial film, 3M Co., St. Paul, Minn.).[25] Catheter tip and glove tip contamination were virtually eliminated. This technique may be considered for arterial cannulation as well.

The artery is entered as described in the preceding section, using a catheter-over-the needle apparatus. Once the artery has been entered, bright red blood should be visible in the flash chamber of the cannula. Advance the

needle approximately 1 mm into the vessel lumen (Fig. 19–7), then fix the needle while threading the catheter further into the lumen. When the needle is withdrawn, blood will pulsate from the catheter hub. Inadvertent puncture of the back wall of the artery can occur, and indeed, a variation of the percutaneous technique is to puncture both walls of the vessel with a single pass. If the back wall is punctured, the needle is withdrawn from the catheter and the catheter is slowly pulled back until a steady stream of blood flows from its hub. The catheter is then advanced carefully further into the lumen. The double puncture method is especially useful for cannulating small vessels. Jones and colleagues report no increase in complications when both walls, rather than one, are punctured.[26]

Once the vessel has been entered, occasionally one will encounter difficulty advancing the catheter into the lumen.

Table 19–3. *Parameters That Affect Interpretation of Arterial Blood Gases*

Parameter	Heparin*	Air Bubble in Sample	Delayed Analysis‖
P_{O_2}	No significant change†	Elevated	Variable¶
P_{CO_2}	Lowered‡	No significant change§	Elevated**
pH	Unchanged‡	No significant change§	Lowered**

*Use only 1000 IU per ml concentration; fill dead space of needle and syringe only, and collect 3 ml of blood.

†There are reports of slight increases in P_{O_2} with excessive heparin.

‡The falsely lowered P_{CO_2} that occurs with added heparin is the most clinically significant change noted. pH may be decreased if a large volume of concentrated heparin (25,000 IU/ml) is used.

§If stored at 4° C for 20 minutes.

‖Anaerobic storage at room temperature for 20 minutes results in no significant change.

¶Changes unpredictable at 30 minutes, regardless of storage method.

**Minimal changes up to 2 hours, if stored at 4° C.

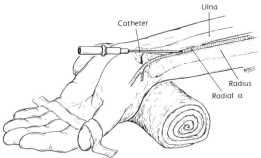

Figure 19–7. Percutaneous arterial cannulation at the wrist. The catheter unit is advanced 1 to 2 mm into the vessel lumen after blood first appears in the flash chamber. While the needle is fixed, the catheter is threaded over the needle. (From Beal JM (ed): Critical Care for Surgical Patients. New York, Macmillan Publishing Co, Inc, 1982. Reproduced by permission.)

The "liquid stylet" method may aid further passage of the catheter.[27] A 10-ml syringe should be filled with about 5 ml of sterile normal saline. The syringe is then attached to the catheter hub, and 1 to 2 ml of blood should be easily aspirated to confirm intraluminal position. The fluid from the syringe is then slowly injected, and the catheter is advanced behind the fluid wave. Catheter sets are available with a wire stylet that permits a modified Seldinger technique for catheter placement; the over-the-needle catheter follows the self-contained guide wire during cannulation (Fig. 19–8). One readily available device of this type is the Arrow Arterial Catheterization System (Arrow International, Inc., Reading, Pa.). This device is available alone, in catheter exchange sets, and in complete single-use kits that are packaged in a container that can serve as a disposable wrist support.

Once the catheter has been placed successfully, it should be advanced until the hub is in contact with the skin. The catheter is then secured by fastening it to the skin with suture material. Silk (4–0) or nylon (5–0) sutures provide the best anchoring. To accomplish this, a moderate bite of skin is taken with the needle and a knot is tied in the suture. Care should be taken to avoid pinching the skin too tightly. The loose ends of the suture are then tied around the catheter or its hub without occluding the lumen by constriction (Fig. 19–9).

After tying the catheter in place, a drop of antibiotic ointment is applied to the puncture site, and a self-adhesive dressing is applied over the area. The catheter and its connecting tubing are further secured with sterile sponges

General instructions for use of Radial Artery set.

1. Prepare puncture site in preferred manner.
2. Peel open package and remove entire unit.
3. Remove protective shield. Trial advance and retract spring-wire guide through needle via actuating lever to ensure proper feeding. *Note:* Catheter hub wing clip can be "snapped" out of groove and removed if desired. This allows suture ring on hub to be optionally used for attachment to skin after placement.
   CAUTION: Before insertion, actuating lever must be retracted proximally as far as possible so as not to inhibit blood flashback.
4. Puncture vessel using a continuous, controlled, slow forward motion, being careful to avoid transfixing both vessel walls. Blood flashback in clear hub of introducer needle indicates successful entry into vessel *(A).*
   CAUTION: If both vessel walls are punctured, advancement of spring-wire guide could result in inadvertent subarterial placement.

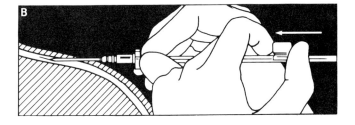

6. Advance the entire placement unit a maximum of 1 to 2 mm farther into the vessel.
7. Firmly hold clear introducer needle hub in position and advance catheter forward to track spring-wire guide into vessel. If difficulty is encountered during catheter advancement, a slight rotating motion of catheter hub may be helpful *(C).*

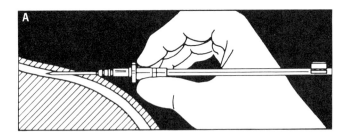

5. Stabilize position of introducer needle and carefully advance spring-wire guide (via actuating lever) distally as far as possible into vessel *(B).* Reference mark on clear feed tube indicates approximate actuating lever advancement position at which soft tip of spring-wire guide coincides with tip of needle.
   CAUTION: If resistance is encountered while advancing spring-wire guide, *do not force feed and do not retract spring-wire guide while in vessel* (to avoid damaging wire). Withdraw entire unit and attempt new puncture.

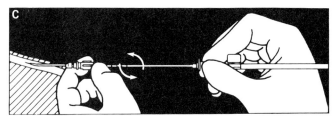

8. Hold catheter in place and remove introducer needle, spring-wire guide, and feed tube assembly. Free blood flow indicates successful placement in vessel.
   CAUTION: Do not reinsert needle into catheter.
9. Attach desired stopcock, injection cap, or connecting tubing to catheter hub.
10. Secure catheter to patient in preferred manner, using wing clip or suture ring as described in Step 3.
11. Cover puncture site with suitable dressing.

Figure 19–8. Step-by-step arterial cannulation, using the guide wire technique (Arrow Arterial Catheterization Kit). (Courtesy of Arrow International, Inc., Reading, Pa.)

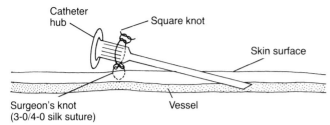

Figure 19–9. Illustration of a technique for securing a vascular catheter to adjacent skin.

and adhesive tape. All tubing connections must be tight and secure. If the tubing becomes disconnected inadvertently, the patient may exsanguinate rapidly.

When successful arterial cannulation has been performed, the catheter should be attached to a pressurized fluid-filled system. If the catheter has been placed for monitoring arterial blood pressure, it should be connected to a mechanical or electrical transducer by a short length of rigid plastic tubing filled with saline. A three-way stopcock is interposed between the patient and the transducer for blood gas sampling and to allow flushing of the system with heparinized saline (2 ml 1:1000 heparin per liter of saline). Flushing can be periodic or continuous at a rate of 3 to 4 ml per hour through a continuous flow device (see Fig. 19–3).

Procurement of a blood sample from this system is easily performed. A syringe is attached to the three-way stopcock, and blood is aspirated and discarded to clear the line. Studies examining the necessary discard volume of flush-blood solution have found considerable variation dependent on the volume of the system.[28, 29] Short lengths of tubing between the catheter and aspiration port minimize the discard volume. For a tubing length of 91 cm (36 inches), 4 to 5 ml should be aspirated;[29] for a tubing length of 213 cm (84 inches), 8 ml should be aspirated.[28] A second syringe, which has been heparinized, is then attached, and 3 ml of blood are aspirated and sent for blood gas analysis. If the blood is to be used for other tests, the second syringe does not need to be heparinized. The stopcock and line should be flushed after sampling to avoid clotting.

Seldinger Technique for Arterial Cannulation

An alternative method of placing an indwelling cannula is by the Seldinger technique,[30] which is described in detail for venipuncture in Chapter 23. A needle is percutaneously placed into the arterial lumen, as described previously. A guide wire is then placed through the needle into the vessel lumen, and the needle is removed. A catheter is then threaded over the wire, and the wire is pulled out. As mentioned before, one commercial catheter permits the Seldinger technique to be performed without separate guide wire manipulation.

Cutdown Technique for Arterial Cannulation

The cutdown technique is another common method of obtaining arterial access. Cannulation is performed after direct visualization of the vessel. A cutdown can be performed on any artery but is most commonly reserved for the brachial and other distal limb arteries. After a site has been selected, the overlying skin should be surgically pre-

pared with an iodophor solution. The physician then puts on sterile gloves and drapes the extremity. Local anesthetic solution is injected subcutaneously in a horizontal line 2 to 3 cm long and perpendicular to the artery. Local anesthesia is not necessary if the patient is unconscious or is otherwise anesthetic at the cutdown site.

Using a scalpel with a No. 10 or 15 blade, the skin is incised along the anesthetic wheal. Underlying tissues are spread parallel to the artery with a mosquito hemostat. The pulse is palpated repeatedly throughout the procedure to ensure proper positioning. Once the surrounding soft tissue has been removed, exposing the artery for a distance of approximately 1 cm, the artery should be isolated by passing two silk sutures underneath it, using the hemostat. Strip away only enough perivascular tissue to expose the artery. Perivascular tissue will help to limit bleeding at the time of catheter removal. A catheter-over-the-needle device, such as that used in the percutaneous method, is now introduced through the skin just distal to the incision and advanced into the surgical site (Fig. 19–10).[31] The arterial wall is punctured with the needle tip, and the catheter is threaded into the vessel lumen. When this has been accomplished, the two silk sutures, which have been used only to control the vessel, are removed and the skin incision is closed. The artery is not tied off as the vessel would be during a venous cutdown. Firm pressure, as used following arterial puncture, should be applied over the cutdown site. The separation of the soft tissue during the procedure may allow considerable hemorrhage into the tissue if pressure is not applied. The catheter is secured to the skin in the same manner as with the percutaneous method (see Fig. 19–9).

ARTERIES

Radial and Ulnar

The radial artery is the artery that has most frequently been used for prolonged cannulation. A widespread collateral flow exists in the wrist. There are two major palmar anastomoses, known as *arches* (Fig. 19–11). The superficial palmar arch lies between the aponeurosis palmaris and the tendons of the flexor digitorum sublimis. The arch is formed mainly by the terminal ulnar artery and the superficial palmar branch of the radial artery. The other major communication of these two vessels, the deep palmar arch, is formed by connections of the terminal radial artery with the deep palmar branches of the ulnar artery.[32] Some collateral flow is almost always present at the wrist, with the deep arch alone being complete in 97 per cent of 650 hand dissections.[33] In spite of Coleman and Anson's findings at autopsy, Friedman noted the absence of palpable ulnar pulses in 10

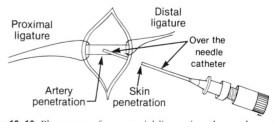

Figure 19–10. Placement of an arterial line using the cutdown technique. Note that the catheter enters the surgical wound percutaneously to minimize bacterial entry into the healing wound and to permit better stabilization of the catheter. Catheter entry of the vessel is more parallel to the vessel than is illustrated.

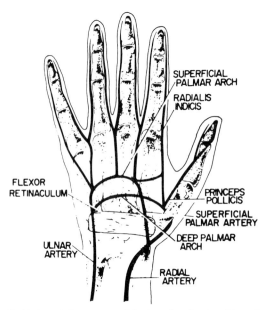

Figure 19–11. Arterial anatomy of the hand and wrist. (From Raman-athan S, Chalon J, Turndorf H: Determining patency of palmar arches by retrograde radial pulsation. Anesthesiology 42:758, 1975. Reproduced by permission.)

of 290 (3.4 per cent) healthy children and young adults.[34] Interestingly, this was always a bilateral finding. The radial pulses were present in 100 per cent of the subjects.

A simple test has been recommended to determine the presence of collateral flow in the hand. This procedure has seen many modifications[35, 36] since being described by Allen in 1929.[37] In a cooperative patient, the basic Allen test is performed as follows: The examiner occludes the radial and ulnar arteries with digital pressure, and the patient is asked to tightly clench the fist repetitively to exsanguinate the hand. The hand is then opened, and the examiner releases the occlusion of the ulnar artery (Fig. 19–12). After several minutes, the test is repeated with release of the radial artery. Rubor should rapidly return to the hand with release of either vessel.

An abnormal (positive) Allen test, indicative of inadequate collateralization, is defined as the continued presence of pallor 5 to 15 seconds after release of the artery.[10, 32, 38, 39] If the return of color takes longer than 5 to 10 seconds, radial artery puncture should not be performed. One must be careful to avoid overextension of the hand with wide separation of the digits, because this may compress the palmar arches between fascial planes and give a false-positive result.[38] Barber and associates[35] report a modified Allen test that is useful in unconscious or anesthetized patients who cannot clench their fists. An Esmarch bandage is used to exsanguinate the hand, and the test is performed as previously described. Time permitting, performance of some variation of the Allen test is desirable before ulnar or radial puncture for cannulation or blood gas sampling.

A study by McGregor has shown that abnormal Allen tests may be false positives when further evaluated by intra-arterial fluorescein angiography.[40] Slogoff and colleagues in a study of 1700 radial artery cannulations for monitoring purposes report 16 cases of radial artery cannulation in patients with abnormal Allen tests, none of whom developed ischemia or abnormality of radial flow after cannulation.[41] Of note, the Allen test was only performed on 411 of their 1700 patients, giving an abnormal result 4 per cent of the time. Cardiovascular surgical patients of the Texas Heart

Institute have been monitored with radial artery cannulation for 20 years without routine performance of the Allen test. Nonetheless, at this time the results of an Allen test should be documented on the chart for medicolegal reasons, and an abnormal result suggests that an alternative site be used, if available. A normal Allen test is desirable, but it is not a guarantee against digital ischemia following radial artery cannulation.[42]

Once adequate collateral flow has been ascertained, arterial puncture may be performed. At the wrist, the radial artery rests on the flexor digitorum superficialis, flexor pollicus longus, the pronator quadratus, and against the radius.[33] Just distal to the styloid process of the radius, the artery winds around the lateral aspect of the wrist to the dorsum of the hand. The pulsation of the artery should be isolated on the palmar surface of the wrist where it is superficial. Dorsiflexing the wrist at about a 60-degree angle over a towel or sandbag, with or without fixing the wrist to

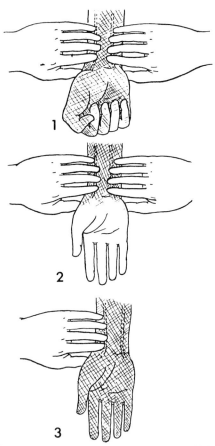

Figure 19–12. Allen test. Before puncturing the radial artery it is important to be sure that a competent ulnar artery is present. This can be done as follows:

1. The examiner compresses both arteries, and the patient repeatedly makes a tight fist to squeeze all the blood out of the hand.

2. The patient then extends the fingers, and the examiner observes the blanched hand.

3. Compression of the ulnar artery is released, and the examiner observes the hand fill with blood. If filling does not occur within 5 to 10 seconds, radial artery puncture should not be done. If brisk filling occurs, the test is then repeated with release of the radial artery to assess radial artery patency. If both radial and ulnar arteries demonstrate patency, the wrist may be used for arterial puncture. (From Schwartz GR (ed): Principles and Practice of Emergency Medicine. Philadelphia, WB Saunders Co, 1978, p. 354. Reproduced by permission.)

an armboard, will help isolate and fix the artery (see Fig. 19–7).[10, 43, 44]

The ulnar artery may occasionally be used but is technically more difficult to puncture than the radial artery because of its smaller size. At the wrist, the ulnar artery runs along the palmar margin of the flexor carpi ulnaris in the space between it and the flexor digitorum sublimis.[33] In this area, it is in intimate contact with the ulnar nerve. The ulnar nerve and artery pass into the hand just radial to the pisiform bone. The ulnar artery can often be made more accessible with dorsiflexion of the wrist.

Brachial

Barnes and colleagues[8] monitored 54 patients with an 18- or 20-gauge Teflon catheter percutaneously placed in the left brachial artery at the antecubital fossa. None of these patients developed Doppler evidence of brachial artery obstruction; however, partial to complete obstruction of the radial artery was noted in two patients and of the ulnar artery in one patient. None of these three patients exhibited ischemic symptoms. These researchers also noted no clinical evidence of ischemia in 1000 brachial catheterizations over a period of 3 years. Thus the brachial artery appears to be a safe site for arterial puncture, although collateral circulation in this area is not as great as in the hand.

The brachial artery begins as the continuation of the axillary artery and ends at the head of the radius, where it splits into the ulnar and radial arteries. The preferred site of puncture of the brachial artery is in or just proximal to the antecubital fossa. In this region, the vessel lies on top of the brachialis muscle and enters the fossa underneath the bicipital aponeurosis (Fig. 19–13). The median nerve runs along the medial side of the artery. Owing to reduced collateral circulation and the necessity of maintaining the arm in extension for puncture or prolonged cannulation, more distal vessels are preferred when the upper extremity is chosen for cannulation.

Axillary

Axillary artery cannulation as described by Adler and coworkers[45] is also a safe means of monitoring arterial blood pressure for a long period of time. The left axillary artery is preferred in order to decrease the possibility of cerebral embolization of flush solution or thrombus. The path from the left subclavian to the left carotid artery is less direct than on the right side, whereas the vertebral arteries are equally vulnerable.

To cannulate the axillary artery, the arm is held in 90-degree abduction. The axillary pulse is then palpated high in the axilla between the insertion of the pectoralis major and the deltoid muscles. The artery may then be cannulated percutaneously with or without a Seldinger guide wire. This site is technically more difficult and time consuming and probably should be avoided in the emergency department. No studies have been reported regarding large numbers of axillary punctures; therefore, the relative safety of this location cannot be determined.

Dorsalis Pedis

The dorsalis pedis artery is a continuation of the anterior tibial artery. Anterior to the ankle joint, the dorsalis pedis runs from approximately midway between the malleoli

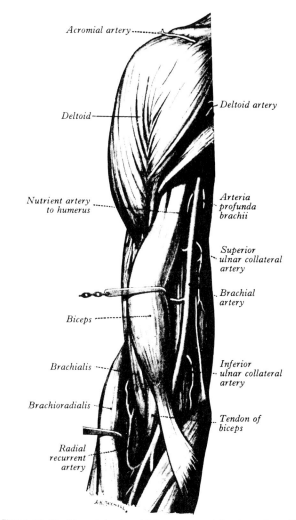

Figure 19–13. The right brachial artery and its branches. (From Warwick R, Williams PL (eds): Gray's Anatomy. 35th ed. Edinburgh, Churchill Livingstone, 1973, p 650. Reproduced by permission.)

to the posterior end of the first metatarsal space, where it forms the dorsal metatarsal and deep plantar arteries. The lateral plantar artery, which is a branch of the posterior tibial, passes obliquely across the foot to the base of the fifth metatarsal. The plantar arch is completed where the lateral plantar artery joins the deep plantar artery between the first and second metatarsals. On the dorsum of the foot, the dorsalis pedis artery lies in the subcutaneous tissue parallel to the extensor hallucis longus tendon, between it and the extensor digitorum longus (Fig. 19–14).[5] The artery should be cannulated in the midfoot region. Although this vessel is amenable to cutdown, the vascular anatomy of the foot is quite variable. This is of no consequence if a pulse can be palpated, but, Huber, in his dissection of 200 feet, noted the dorsalis pedis artery to be absent in 12 per cent.[46] In 16 per cent of patients, the dorsalis pedis artery provides the main blood supply to the toes.[47] Collateral flow can be determined with a modified Allen test using the posterior tibial and dorsalis pedis arteries, but this is not as easily performed in the foot as in the hand. The pressure wave obtained with an electronic transducer attached to the dorsalis pedis artery will be 5 to 20 mm Hg higher than that of the radial artery, and in addition, it will be delayed by about one tenth of a second.[48]

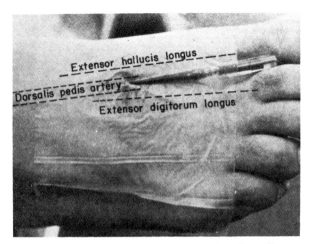

Figure 19–14. A 20-gauge catheter in the dorsalis pedis artery, illustrating the relationship to surrounding tendons. The catheter is secured with Steri-drape. Splinting is not needed. (From Johnstone RE, Greenhow DE: Catheterization of the dorsalis pedis artery. Anesthesiology 39:655, 1973. Reproduced by permission.)

Femoral

Currently, the femoral artery is the second most commonly used vessel for prolonged arterial cannulation. Several studies have demonstrated the efficacy and safety of using this vessel, and, indeed, several investigators suggest that it should be the vessel of choice.[49-52] The femoral artery is the direct continuation of the iliac artery. The femoral artery enters the thigh after passing behind the inguinal ligament, where, in most patients, it may be easily palpated at a point midway between the pubic symphysis and the anterior superior iliac spine. When puncturing this vessel, care must be taken to avoid the femoral nerve and vein, which are in close proximity to the artery on the lateral and medial sides, respectively (Fig. 19–15).

A longer cannula is required for the femoral artery owing to the relatively greater depth at which it lies. The Seldinger technique is especially useful for this site, enabling the placement of a 15- to 20-cm plastic catheter for prolonged monitoring. Catheter-over-the-needle devices may also be used but should be at least 10 cm long. Use of catheter-through-the-needle devices has been reported[51] but should be avoided because of the possibility of leakage around the catheter, which may occur with high arterial pressures owing to the loose fit of the cannula in the hole in the vessel wall. Regardless of the device used, the needle should enter the skin at an angle of about 45 degrees instead of the usual 15- to 20-degree angle.

The extremely large ratio of arterial diameter to that of the catheter is felt to beneficially reduce the incidence of thrombosis, particularly total occlusion. However, occlusions have been reported with femoral cannulation for monitoring purposes.[33]

A commonly postulated disadvantage of this site is the possibility of increased bacterial contamination because of its proximity to the warm, moist groin and perineum; however, no studies confirm this hypothesis.[54] The femoral area is inconvenient for the patient who is awake and mobile, especially if the patient is capable of sitting in a chair. In spite of these theoretic difficulties, some large hospitals use femoral arterial lines almost exclusively, and the intensive care nursing staff is often more comfortable caring for these lines than those at other sites.

Umbilical and Temporal

In the neonate, arterial access can be accomplished through the umbilical artery for a short period of time. After this artery closes, the temporal artery provides a safe alternative. Prian describes the use of the temporal artery, noting its accessibility and the lack of clinical sequelae if it undergoes thrombosis.[55] The cutdown method should be used with a 22-gauge catheter after the artery's course has been traced with an ultrasonic flow detector. Because of the increasing accuracy of ear oximeters and the use of capillary blood gases for pH determination, prolonged arterial cannulation will become less frequent during infant care. Further discussion of infant arterial cannulation is provided in Chapter 20.

COMPLICATIONS

Long-term arterial cannulation is safe if care is taken to avoid complications. Almost all the difficulties one may encounter can be avoided or their incidence markedly decreased if one adheres to a few simple principles. Reported clinical sequelae of arterial puncture and cannulation range from simple hematomas to life-threatening infections and exsanguination. The incidence of complications varies with the site and method of cannulation and with the skill and concern of the patient's physicians and nurses. It is difficult to compare complication rates at various sites, because most published studies have primarily used the radial artery. Many studies also report complications of puncture for arteriography and other procedures unrelated to long-term cannulation.

A commonly encountered problem is hematoma formation at the puncture site. Zorab[15] reported this complication in 50 per cent of catheterizations. The bruising was of minimal clinical significance in Zorab's study, but leakage, when it occurs, around the catheter or from the puncture site after its removal can be of danger to the patient. Compression neuropathy secondary to bleeding has been reported after brachial artery puncture in anticoagulated patients; in some cases, surgical decompression was necessary.[4] The large amount of soft tissue surrounding the femoral artery makes bleeding in this area difficult to control.[56] Large hematomas are not uncommon after femoral artery catheterization; indeed, Soderstrom and associates[49] report two cases of bleeding that required transfusion after femoral puncture. Another patient suffered a large hematoma that became infected and required incision and drainage.

Prevention of bleeding complications may be accomplished with frequent careful inspection of the puncture site and with the use of prolonged compression after removal of the catheter or needle. Firm pressure should be maintained for at least 10 minutes after removal of a peripheral artery catheter and for a longer period of time after femoral cannulation or if the patient is anticoagulated. Five minutes of pressure is sufficient after puncture for a blood gas sample in an individual with normal coagulation. Exsanguination, a related complication, may occur if the arterial line apparatus becomes disconnected. This is more common in the obtunded or combative patient, and restraints are often required for patients with indwelling arterial cannulas. Exsanguination should not occur if tight connections are maintained throughout the system and if frequent, careful inspections of both the circuit and the patient are made.

Serious infections rarely complicate arterial cannulation. However, the incidence of catheter-related infections in-

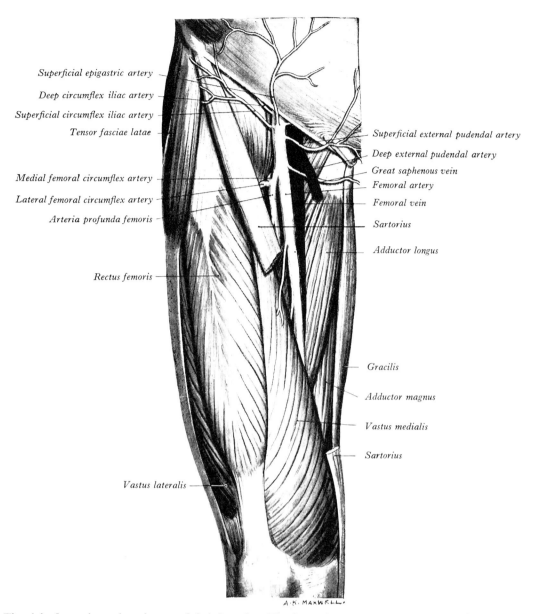

Superficial epigastric artery

Deep circumflex iliac artery

Superficial circumflex iliac artery

Tensor fasciae latae

Medial femoral circumflex artery

Lateral femoral circumflex artery

Arteria profunda femoris

Rectus femoris

Vastus lateralis

Superficial external pudendal artery

Deep external pudendal artery

Great saphenous vein

Femoral artery

Femoral vein

Sartorius

Adductor longus

Gracilis

Adductor magnus

Vastus medialis

Sartorius

A·K·MAXWELL·

Figure 19–15. The right femoral vessels and some of their branches. The femoral nerve (not shown) lies lateral to the artery and may be deep to the artery. (From Warwick R, Williams PL (eds): Gray's Anatomy. 35th ed. Edinburgh, Churchill Livingstone, 1973, p 676. Reproduced by permission.)

creases with prolonged cannulation.[54, 57] Catheters placed with sterile technique have an extremely low rate of infection up to 96 hours. Catheters changed over a guide wire every 96 hours have an infection rate of about 10 per cent at the radial and femoral sites.[54]

Most begin as local infections at the puncture site and remain localized, although systemic sepsis has been reported.[36] Radial and femoral sites have a similar incidence of complications, but axillary cannulations seem to have a much higher incidence of infection, although no large studies of this site exist.[54, 57] Arterial cannulas are more prone to infectious complications than other vascular catheters. Many mechanisms have been proposed for this.[58–60] The arterial pressure monitoring system usually consists of a long column of fairly stagnant fluid and is subject to frequent manipulation. Stamm and colleagues[59] found that patients were at greater risk for systemic infection if they had an arterial line and required frequent blood gas determinations than if they

had the cannula alone. The sampling stopcock is a site of frequent bacterial contamination.

The risk of infection also increases as the duration of cannulation is prolonged. Catheters should be changed after 4 days if continued monitoring is necessary.[57, 61] In addition, Makai and associates[60] recommend changing the entire fluid-filled system, including transducer chamber-domes and continuous flow devices, every 48 hours. Shinozaki and coworkers[62] demonstrated a marked reduction in equipment contamination when the continuous flush device was located just distal to the transducer, as opposed to the device being positioned closer to the three-way stopcock used for sampling. This set-up reduces the length of the static column of fluid between the sampling stopcock and the transducer. As mentioned previously, a drop of iodophor or antibiotic ointment applied to the puncture site decreases the incidence of local wound infection.[61]

Thrombosis of the vessel in which the cannula is placed

is another frequently encountered problem. The incidence with which this occurs varies with the method used to determine the presence of the clot. Bedford and Wollman[7] found a greater than 40 per cent occlusion rate when radial artery catheters were left in place for more than 20 hours. All these occluded vessels eventually recanalized. Angiographic studies show deposition of fibrin on 100 per cent of the catheters left in place for more than 1 day, although clinical evidence of ischemia secondary to occlusion with thrombus is present in less than 1 per cent in most studies.[6] Most reports of nonangiographic catheterizations that mention thrombosis study the radial artery. Therefore, it is difficult to compare the incidence of thrombosis at other sites, although during the 176 femoral catheterizations of Soderstrom and Ersoz,[49, 51] dorsalis pedis pulses were decreased in only two patients and no clinical signs of ischemia were noted. Larger catheter sizes, trauma during cannulation, and the presence of atherosclerosis have all been postulated to increase the incidence of thrombosis; however, conflicting studies abound. Downs and colleagues associated tapered catheters with an increased incidence of thrombosis.[11]

Arterial spasm after puncture can predispose to thrombus formation and can even lead to ischemic changes without fibrin deposition. Successful reversal of spasm after intra-arterial lidocaine, reserpine, and phentolamine has been reported, but no reliable studies of efficacy in this situation have been published.[63] Thrombosis can be minimized by decreasing the duration of catheterization, by proper flushing, and by using larger arteries. Surgical embolectomy or thrombectomy is rarely required, because the smaller vessels that are most likely to occlude usually have good collateral circulation. A normal (negative) Allen test or a similar test suggests but does not ensure adequate collateral flow.[42] The larger femoral artery, which has poor collateralization, rarely occludes with catheterization for monitoring purposes.

Another complication of thrombosis is occlusion of the catheter. Times until occlusion of radial and femoral artery catheters have been compared, and it was noted that radial cannulas became occluded at an average of 3.8 days, whereas femoral cannulas occluded after 7.3 days.[49] The importance of this comparison is minimal if the clinician follows infection prophylaxis guidelines and changes arterial catheters after 4 days.

A few less common complications are easily prevented. One such complication, which occurs only with the percutaneous catheter-through-the-needle method, is catheter embolization. Once the catheter has been placed through the needle, it should never be pulled back, because the end of the catheter may be sheared off by the sharp needle bevel. If this occurs, surgical removal of the catheter tip is necessary.

Skin necrosis is a complication of radial artery cannulation, involving an area of the volar forearm proximal to the cannula.[64, 65] Wyatt and colleagues[64] believe this is secondary to the poor blood supply of this area and state that taking the precautionary steps described previously prevents or decreases the incidence of necrosis. One feared complication of indwelling radial and brachial arterial catheters is the occurrence of a cerebrovascular accident secondary to embolization from flushing of the catheters.[11, 66] As little as 3 to 12 ml of flush solution has been shown to reflux to the junction of subclavian and vertebral arteries.[66] A fatality due to air embolism from a radial artery catheter has been reported and was recreated in a macaque model.[67] Although these animals are much smaller (7 kg) than an adult human, as little as 2.5 ml of air at a relatively low flush rate was found to embolize in a retrograde fashion to the brain. Cerebral embolization can be prevented with the use of

continuous flush systems (3 ml per hour) and by ensuring the integrity of the tubing and transducer systems to prevent air entry. Additionally small volumes (<2 ml) of intermittent flush solution should be used.

Complication rates also vary according to the method of arterial cannulation. Mortensen[68] studied the three main techniques, discussed in the section entitled "Techniques," but unfortunately, most of his arterial cannulations were for angiographic purposes. The complications associated with prolonged cannulation time are therefore underrepresented. For Mortensen's series, cutdown arteriotomy exhibited the lowest incidence of complications (7.7 per cent), whereas the Seldinger technique had a complications incidence of 17.7 per cent. Complications of percutaneous cannulation were 11.3 per cent. Apparently, false passage of the guide wire, the catheter, or both were associated with increased intimal damage and complications. *It is imperative to advance the wire or catheter only if no resistance is met!*

In actuality, arterial puncture and cannulation are safe procedures when care is taken and when basic principles are kept in mind. The operator should be skilled and should seek an atraumatic insertion. Once the monitoring system has been set up, it should be manipulated as little as possible. Any handling should be performed with a flawless aseptic technique. The tubing and other fluid-filled devices should be changed every 48 hours, and catheters should be inserted into a vessel that provides a vessel-to-catheter ratio that is as great as possible without compromising other needs. If these principles are followed and if the patient and system are carefully inspected at frequent intervals, complications of arterial puncture and cannulation can be minimized.

INTERPRETATION

An indwelling arterial cannula can provide valuable information about the hemodynamic status of a patient (continuous pressure monitoring) and about the patient's respiratory and metabolic status (through intermittent sampling for blood gas analysis and other blood tests). The partial pressure of carbon dioxide and pH of the blood can be used to define four major groups of metabolic derangement: respiratory acidosis or alkalosis, and metabolic acidosis or alkalosis. Rarely will a disorder be strictly classified into one of these groups; however, a simple chart such as that shown in Figure 19–16 will assist one in determining the relative effects of metabolic and respiratory influence on the blood pH. A rough estimate of the contribution of respiratory factors may be made by assuming that for every 10 mm Hg that the P_{CO_2} varies from 40, the pH will inversely vary 0.08 pH unit from 7.4. Adequacy of oxygenation of the blood can be determined from the measured P_{O_2} of the arterial blood and from the known concentration of oxygen that the patient is inspiring. To avoid iatrogenic complications of intensive care, one must be absolutely certain that the data are from an arterial sample that has been properly analyzed before basing one's treatment decisions on the numbers obtained. Not uncommonly, one may accidentally puncture a vein when attempting to obtain an arterial blood sample. Furthermore, false readings may result if the sample is not free of air bubbles, not promptly chilled, and not analyzed within 20 to 30 minutes. Although still controversial, blood gas values that are *uncorrected* for body temperature appear more appropriate for guiding therapy in hypothermic patients.[69, 70]

An indwelling arterial catheter also provides continuous blood pressure monitoring. The trend of a patient's pressure helps one assess the effect of various therapeutic interventions. The absolute systolic and diastolic pressures measured

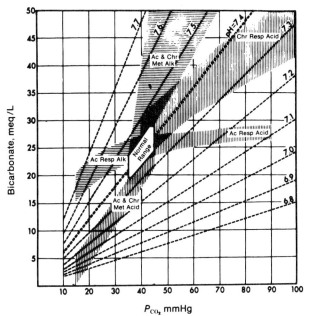

Figure 19–16. In vivo nomogram showing bands for uncomplicated respiratory or metabolic acid-base disturbances. Each "confidence" band represents the mean ± 2 SD for the compensatory response of normal subjects or patients to a given primary disorder. Ac, acute. Chr, chronic. Resp, respiratory. Met, metabolic. Alk, alkalosis. Acid, acidosis. (From Thorn GW, Adams RD, Braunwald E, et al (eds): Harrison's Principles of Internal Medicine. 8th ed. New York, McGraw-Hill Book Co, Inc, 1977, p 377. Reproduced by permission.)

will vary at different catheter sites, with higher peak systolic pressures measured at the periphery; the pressures will also be higher when measured in the distal lower limb.[12, 48] A wide variance between direct arterial pressure and that measured with a standard pneumatic cuff will always exist in some patients. Data averaged over a population group, however, compare fairly well.[12] For this reason, the cuff pressure and that displayed on the monitor should be compared regularly. A change in their relationship may be the first indication of difficulties with the direct measuring system. Auscultatory methods usually give a slightly lower value than direct measuring systems.

Waveform analysis may also provide an early indication of thrombosis in the arterial catheter. Many variables affect the waveform, including cardiac valvular disease, arteriosclerosis, and other peculiarities of an individual's cardiovascular system that may contribute to pulse wave reflections.[71] Waveforms may vary tremendously among patients, but after an adequate monitoring system has been established, a change in an individual's pressure wave is usually indicative of thrombosis or other malfunction in the monitoring system. A change in waveform may also indicate a change in the patient's cardiovascular status, such as a papillary muscle rupture. Once again, before making a therapeutic decision based on an electronically generated number, the patient should be rechecked with a pneumatic cuff; this device is less fallible than the electromechanical system.

CONCLUSION

As intensive care knowledge and technology grow and develop, cannulation of the arterial system may become a more routine procedure. Nonetheless, devices have been developed, which, in some cases, may decrease the frequency with which this procedure

is performed. Oximeters can determine the quality of oxygenation of the blood percutaneously and are becoming more accurate and sophisticated (see Chapter 5). Electronic sphygmomanometers are being refined for continuous indirect blood pressure monitoring. However, these devices will not soon replace the indwelling arterial cannula, because of the need for frequent blood sampling for chemical and hematologic analysis.

Arterial puncture and cannulation are invaluable aids to the emergency and critical care physician. Long-term catheterization is a safe procedure when the catheter is placed, maintained, and removed with care. The radial artery is the most favored location for puncture, but as more experience is gained and reported with femoral artery catheterization, the latter may become a more frequently used site. Selection of either site is associated with a low complication rate and should be determined by the skill of the physician and the nursing team and the relative convenience and comfort of the patient.

REFERENCES

1. Geddes LA: The Direct and Indirect Measurement of Blood Pressure. Chicago, Year Book Medical Publishers, Inc, 1970.
2. Thomas F, Orme JF, Clemmer TP, et al: A prospective comparison of arterial catheter blood and catheter-tip cultures in critically ill patients. Crit Care Med 12:860, 1984.
3. Zaret PH, Crump JM, Van Raalte BA, et al: Accuracy of blood cultures drawn through indwelling arterial lines. Crit Care Med 14:353, 1986.
4. Luce EA, Futrell JW, Wilgis EF, et al: Compression neuropathy following brachial arterial puncture in anticoagulated patients. J Trauma 16:717, 1976.
5. Gardner RM: Direct blood pressure measurement. Dynamic response requirements. Anesthesiology 54:227, 1981.
6. Formanek G, Frech RS, Amplatz K: Arterial thrombus formation during clinical percutaneous catheterization. Circulation 41:833, 1970.
7. Bedford RF, Wollman H: Complications of percutaneous radial-artery cannulation: An objective prospective study in man. Anesthesiology 38:228, 1973.
8. Barnes RW, Foster EJ, Janssen GA, et al: Safety of brachial arterial catheters as monitors in the intensive care unit: Prospective evaluation with the Doppler ultrasonic velocity detector. Anesthesiology 44:260, 1976.
9. Brown AE, Sweeney DB, Lumley J: Percutaneous radial artery cannulation. Anaesthesia 24:532, 1969.
10. Bedford RF: Radial arterial function following percutaneous cannulation with 18 and 20 gauge catheters. Anesthesiology 47:37, 1977.
11. Downs JB, Rackstein AD, Klein EF, et al: Hazards of radial-artery catheterization. Anesthesiology 38:283, 1973.
12. Bruner JM, Krenis LJ, Kunsman JM, et al: Comparison of direct and indirect methods of measuring arterial blood pressure (Parts I, II, III). Med Instrum 15:11–21, 97–101, 182–188, 1981.
13. McCutcheon EP, Evans JM, Stanifer RR: Direct blood pressure measurement: Gadgets vs progress. Anesth Analg 51:746, 1972.
14. Rothe CF, Kim KC: Measuring systolic arterial blood pressure. Possible errors from extension tubes or disposable transducer domes. Crit Care Med 18:683, 1980.
15. Zorab JSM: Continuous display of the arterial pressure: A simple manometric technique. Anaesthesia 24:431, 1969.
16. Selldén H, Nilsson K, Larson LE, et al: Radial artery catheters in children and neonates: A prospective study. Crit Care Med 15:1106, 1987.
17. Ordog GJ, Wasserberger J, Balasubramaniam S: Effect of heparin on arterial blood gases. Ann Emerg Med 14:233, 1985.
18. Goodwin NM, Schreiber MT: Effects of anticoagulants on acid-base and blood gas estimations. Crit Care Med 7:473, 1979.
19. Dake MD, Peters J, Teague R: The effect of heparin dilution on arterial blood gas analysis. West J Med 140:792, 1984.
19a. Maher JJ, Dougherty JM: Radial artery cannulation guided by Doppler ultrasound. Am J Emerg Med 7:260, 1989.
20. Madiedo G, Sciacca R, Hause L: Air bubbles and temperatures effect on blood gas analysis. J Clin Pathol 33:864, 1980.
21. Beetham R: A review of blood pH and blood gas analysis. Ann Clin Biochem 19:198, 1982.
22. Hess CE, Nichols AB, Hunt WB, et al: Pseudohypoxemia secondary to leukemia and thrombocytosis. N Engl J Med 301:361, 1979.
23. Shohat M, Schonfield T, Zaizov R, et al: Determination of blood gases in children with extreme leukocytosis. Crit Care Med 16:787, 1988.
24. Morgan EJ: The effects of unanesthetized arterial puncture on P_{CO_2} and pH. Am Rev Respir Dis 120:795, 1979.
25. Levy JH, Nagle DM, Curling PE, et al: Contamination reduction during central venous catheterization. Crit Care Med 16:165, 1988.
26. Jones RM, et al: The effect of method of radial artery cannulation on postcannulation blood flow and thrombus formation. Anesthesiology 55:76, 1981.
27. Stirt JA: "Liquid Stylet" for percutaneous radial artery cannulation. Can Anaesth Soc J 29:492, 1982.

28. Dennis RC, Ng R, Yeston NS, et al: Effect of sample dilutions on arterial blood gas determinations. Crit Care Med 13:1067, 1985.
29. Al-Ameri MW, Kruse JA, Carlson RW: Blood sampling from arterial catheters: Minimum discard volume to achieve accurate laboratory results. Crit Care Med 14:399, 1986.
30. Seldinger SI: Catheter replacement of the needle in percutaneous angiography: A new technique. Acta Radiol 39:368, 1953.
31. Bradley MN: A technique for prolonged intra-arterial catheterization. Surg Gynecol Obstet 119:117, 1964.
32. Ramanathan S, Chalon J, Trundorf H: Determining patency of palmar arches by retrograde radial pulsation. Anesthesiology 42:756, 1975.
33. Coleman SS, Anson JJ: Arterial patterns in the hand based upon a study of 650 specimens. Surg Gynecol Obstet 113:409, 1961.
34. Friedman SA: Prevalence of palpable wrist pulses. Br Heart J 32:316, 1970.
35. Barber JD, Wright DJ, Ellis RH: Radial artery puncture: A simple screening test of the ulnar anastomotic circulation. Anaesthesia 2:291, 1973.
36. Ryan JF, Raines J, Dalton BC, et al: Arterial dynamics of radial artery cannulation. Anesth Analg 52:1017, 1973.
37. Allen EV: Thromboangitis obliterans; Methods of diagnosis of chronic occlusive arterial lesions distal to the wrist with illustrative cases. Am J Med Sci 178:237, 1929.
38. Palm T: Evaluation of peripheral arterial pressure on the thumb following radial artery cannulation. Br J Anaesth 49:819, 1977.
39. Greenhow DE: Incorrect performance of Allen's test: Ulnar artery flow erroneously presumed inadequate. Anesthesiology 37:356, 1972.
40. McGregor AD: The Allen test: An investigation of its accuracy by fluorescein angiography. Hand Surg 12-B:82, 1987.
41. Slogoff S, Keats AS, Arlund C: On the safety of radial artery cannulation. Anesthesiology 59:42, 1983.
42. Baker RJ, Chunprapaph B, Nyhus LM: Severe ischemia of the hand following radial artery catheterization. Surgery 80:449, 1976.
43. Llamas R, Gupta SK, Baum GL: A simple technique for prolonged arterial cannulation. Anesthesiology 31:289, 1969.
44. Brown AE, Sweeney DB, Lumley J: Percutaneous radial artery cannulation. Anaesthesia 24:532, 1969.
45. Adler DC, Bryan-Brown CW: Use of the axillary artery for intravascular monitoring. Crit Care Med 1:148, 1973.
46. Huber JF: The arterial network supplying the dorsum of the foot. Anat Rec 80:373, 1941.
47. Spoerel WE, Deimling P, Aitkin R: Direct arterial pressure monitoring from the dorsalis pedis artery. Can Anaesth Soc J 22:91, 1975.
48. Johnstone RE, Greenhow DE: Catheterization of the dorsalis pedis artery. Anesthesiology 39:654, 1973.
49. Soderstrom CA, Wasserman DH, Dunham CM, et al: Superiority of the femoral artery for monitoring: A prospective study. Am J Surg 144:309, 1982.
50. Gurman G, Schachar J: Femoral artery cannulation in critically ill patients (abstr). Crit Care Med 9:202, 1981.
51. Ersoz CJ, Hedden M, Lain L: Prolonged femoral arterial catheterization for intensive care. Anesth Analg 49:160, 1970.
52. Russell JA, Joel M, Hudson RJ, et al: Prospective evaluation of radial and femoral artery catheterization sites in critically ill adults. Crit Care Med 11:936, 1983.
53. Sessler CN, Alford P: Arterial occlusion after femoral artery cannulation. Crit Care Med 14:520, 1986.
54. Norwood SH, Cornier B, McMahon NG, et al: Prospective study of catheter-related infection during prolonged arterial catheterization. Crit Care Med 16:836, 1988.
55. Prian GW: Temporal artery catheterization for arterial access in the high risk newborn. Surgery 82:734, 1977.
56. Berneus B, Carlsten A, Holmgren A, et al: Percutaneous catheterization of peripheral arteries as a method for blood sampling. Scand J Clin Lab Invest 6:217, 1954.
57. Damen J, Verhoef J, Bolton DT, et al: Microbiologic risk of invasive hemodynamic monitoring in patients undergoing open-heart operations. Crit Care Med 13:548, 1985.
58. Makai DG: Nosocomial bacteremia: An epidemiologic overview. Am J Med 70:719, 1981.
59. Stamm WE, Colella JJ, Anderson RL, et al: Indwelling arterial catheters as a source of nosocomial bacteremia: An outbreak caused by flavobacterium species. N Engl J Med 292:1099, 1975.
60. Makai DG, Hassemer CA: Endemic rate of fluid contamination and related septicemia in arterial pressure monitoring. Am J Med 70:733, 1981.
61. Makai DG, Bank JD: A comparative study of polyantibiotic and iodophor ointments in prevention of vascular catheter-related infection. Am J Med 70:739, 1981.
62. Shinozaki T, Deane RS, Mazuzan JE, et al: Bacterial contamination of arterial lines. A prospective study. JAMA 249:223, 1983.
63. Dalton B, Laver M: Vasospasm with an indwelling radial artery cannula. Anesthesiology 34:194, 1971.
64. Wyatt R, Glaves I, Cooper DJ: Proximal skin necrosis after radial-artery cannulation. Lancet 1:1135, 1974.
65. Johnson RW: A complication of radial-artery cannulation. Anesthesiology 40:598, 1974.
66. Lowenstein E, Little JW, Lo HH: Prevention of cerebral embolization from flushing radial-artery cannulas. N Engl J Med 285:414, 1971.
67. Chang C, Dughi J, Shitabata P, et al: Air embolism and the radial arterial line. Crit Care Med 16:141, 1988.
68. Mortensen JD: Clinical sequelae from arterial needle puncture, cannulation, and incision. Circulation 35:1118, 1967.
69. Swain JA: Hypothermia and blood pH: A review. Arch Intern Med 148:1643, 1988.
70. Danzl DF, Pozos RS, Hamlet MP: Accidental hypothermia. In Auerbach PS and Geehr EC (eds): Management of Wilderness and Environmental Emergencies. 2nd ed. St Louis, CV Mosby Co, 1989, pp 44–46.
71. O'Rourke MF, Yaginuma T: Wave reflections and the arterial pulse. Arch Intern Med 144:366, 1984.

Chapter 20

Vascular Access and Blood Sampling Techniques in Infants and Children

William A. Engle and Frederick J. Rescorla

INTRODUCTION

The need for repeated blood sampling and vascular access remains one of the most challenging aspects of patient care in infancy and childhood. Invasive monitoring with arterial catheters and central venous catheters is commonplace in contemporary pediatric care. This chapter reviews the basic principles and techniques of blood sampling as well as selection and placement of intravenous and intra-arterial catheters in infants and children. The use of umbilical catheters in neonates is also reviewed. Although rarely required, emergency cutdown is occasionally life saving, and a section of the chapter is devoted to this technique. Many patients require long-term parenteral nutrition delivered through a centrally placed venous catheter; the techniques for placement of these catheters from peripheral and central venous insertion sites are also described.

BLOOD SAMPLING TECHNIQUES

Although blood samples for biochemical and hematologic analyses and blood gases may be obtained from indwelling vascular lines, capillary, arterial, and venous blood sampling are the principal methods for obtaining blood samples (especially blood cultures) from patients presenting with acute clinical crises. In the sick neonate and young infant, procuring blood samples may be difficult because many clinicians are not experienced in the techniques of blood sampling in this age group.[1] This section reviews these techniques as they pertain to the neonate and young infant.

Capillary Blood Sampling

INDICATIONS AND CONTRAINDICATIONS

Capillary blood sampling, or heel stick puncture, is a frequently used technique to obtain blood samples in young infants. In older children and adults, this technique may be employed to obtain blood samples from the finger, toes, and ear lobe. It is most appropriate for patients who require repeated sampling because the number of times small arteries and veins can be entered successfully is limited, as is the total number of vessels available in small infants. Capillary blood sampling is most often indicated whenever an adequate sample of blood can be obtained by the heel stick puncture technique and when an alternative technique (i.e., indwelling catheter) is not more readily available. It is especially useful for obtaining "arterialized" blood for blood gas analysis when arterial access is unavailable, as in many chronically ill neonates and young infants. Noninvasive monitoring techniques such as pulse oximetry and transcutaneous oxygen monitoring (see Chapter 5) have reduced the frequency with which these samples must be taken.

Sampling from an area of inflammation should be avoided. Repetitive sampling from the same site may induce inflammation and subsequent scarring and hence should be avoided. In general, heel stick sampling is *not* ideal for blood gas analysis in the following situations: (1) when the infant is hypotensive, (2) when the heel is markedly bruised, or (3) when there is evidence of peripheral vasoconstriction. Capillary blood does not always produce an accurate analysis of arterial P_{O_2}. When the capillary P_{O_2} is greater than 60 mm Hg, the arterial P_{O_2} may be considerably higher, with possibly dangerous consequences to infants receiving supplemental oxygen. In this situation, the use of either a transcutaneous oxygen saturation or a transcutaneous P_{O_2} monitor may allow adjustment of the inspired oxygen concentration until either an arterial P_{O_2} or a repeat capillary P_{O_2} can be obtained.[2, 3]

PROCEDURE

A 3-mm lancet should be used to perform this procedure; a scalpel blade should never be used. After the heel is cleansed with alcohol and allowed to dry, the skin is punctured with the lancet on the lateral or medial portion[4] of the plantar surface of the heel (anterior to the posterior margin of the heel) (Fig. 20–1). The use of a 3-mm lancet will prevent the puncture from penetrating more than the maximum safe distance. The *full 3 mm of the lancet should be used;* a more superficial incision will not bleed adequately. Prewarming the foot in a hot towel will produce hyperemia and will enhance blood flow. *Squeezing of the foot should be avoided,* since this may inhibit capillary filling and may actually decrease blood flow. Furthermore, squeezing may dilute the sample with serum or tissue fluid and may make analysis less accurate. If blood does not flow freely, another puncture may be required.

The first small drop of blood is wiped away with gauze, and another drop is allowed to form. A heparinized capillary tube is placed in the drop of blood, and the proximal end of the inverted tube is allowed to fill by capillary action. The tube (or tubes, if several tests will be needed) is sealed at one end by sticking the end into wax before being sent to the laboratory. A dry dressing is applied to the puncture site.

When a heel stick is performed for arterialized blood samples, the technique used is similar to that discussed previously for routine blood sampling, with the following differences: The infant's foot *must* be wrapped with a warm cloth for a few minutes. The first drop of blood *must* be discarded and the remaining blood allowed to flow freely

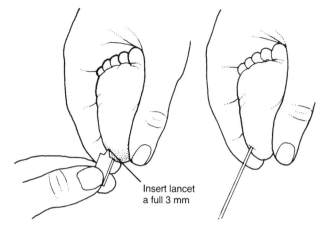

Figure 20–1. The heel stick is performed on the lateral or medial aspect of the heel. Blood is allowed to flow into the capillary tube, thereby avoiding air bubbles. Avoid squeezing the foot, and keep the proximal end of the capillary tube below the puncture site. Contrary to the illustration, latex gloves should be worn during the procedure.

into a heparinized capillary tube. The tip of the tube should be placed as near the puncture site as possible to minimize exposure of the blood to environmental oxygen. Collection of air in the tube as well as excessive squeezing of the foot should be avoided, because this may artificially lower the P_{O_2}. Approximately 0.2 to 0.3 ml of blood should be collected in the heparinized capillary tube.

COMPLICATIONS

When properly performed, heel sticks are associated with a low incidence of complications. Lacerations should not occur when the procedure is performed with a lancet rather than a scalpel blade. Heel sticks may cause infection (local infection, bacteremia,[5] or osteomyelitis[6]), scarring, and calcified nodules.[7] When the heel stick technique is used for the procurement of "arterialized" blood for pH, P_{CO_2}, and P_{O_2} analysis, the most important potential error is that false information (inaccurate P_{O_2}) may result in the exposure of the infant to improper amounts of supplemental oxygen.

INTERPRETATION

Numerous studies have compared the reliability of the capillary blood with that of arterial blood for determination of pH, P_{CO_2}, and P_{O_2}. Although the results have been quite variable,[8–13] most investigations have documented a close correlation between the arterial and capillary samples for pH and P_{CO_2} determinations (except when the patient is in shock or has an extremely high P_{CO_2}). Unfortunately, the P_{O_2} determination has not been found to be as reliable when performed on blood obtained by capillary or "arterialized" sampling. Most studies indicate that the capillary (heel stick) P_{O_2} correlates poorly with the arterial P_{O_2}, especially if the arterial P_{O_2} is greater than 60 mm Hg. For example, a capillary P_{O_2} of 70 mm Hg may reflect an arterial P_{O_2} of 70 to 200 mm Hg. In nearly all situations, the capillary P_{O_2} is equal to or less than the arterial P_{O_2}, but in any individual case, one does not know how closely the capillary value approximates the arterial level. Therefore, *reliance on a capillary sample of blood for P_{O_2} measurement in an acutely sick infant may be fraught with potential risks.* "Arterialized" blood samples obtained from finger and toe sticks might be more reliable for P_{O_2} determination than those obtained from heel sticks, but the data are controversial.[14–17]

Venous Sampling

VENIPUNCTURE

Although many laboratory tests for the small infant may be performed on blood obtained by heel sticks, a larger volume of blood than is obtainable by heel stick may be necessary. Venipuncture is the usual method used for obtaining large quantities of blood as well as samples for blood culture. In an emergency or if venous access sites are limited, blood for laboratory analysis may be obtained from an arterial puncture.

Procedure. Sites that are reasonably accessible for obtaining venous blood include the antecubital veins (Fig. 20–2) or any easily visible peripheral vein (e.g., on the scalp, the hands, or the feet); the external jugular veins and femoral veins are rarely used. When venous access is unavailable, arterial blood may be used for most laboratory tests, including blood cultures. If an extremity vein is to be used, a tourniquet should be applied proximal to the selected vein; in small infants, a rubber band will serve as an adequate tourniquet, but one must be certain to remove the rubber band following venipuncture. The tourniquet should not be so tight that arterial filling is obstructed. The area surrounding the planned site of penetration of the skin is cleansed with alcohol. An appropriate-sized syringe (approximately 3 ml) should be available to attach to a butterfly scalp vein needle or straight needle (usually 21 to 25 gauge). A small-gauge butterfly needle is usually preferred over a needle and syringe for obtaining blood in infants. It is difficult to

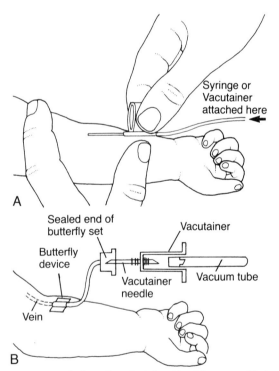

Figure 20–2. *A,* Technique for obtaining blood by antecubital venipuncture with a butterfly needle and a syringe. Once blood is obtained, the butterfly needle may serve as an infusion site. Note that this procedure often requires two persons to carry it out—one to hold the arm and insert the needle and the other to aspirate the blood. *B,* As an alternative to a syringe, a Vacutainer system may be used to apply suction. The Vacutainer needle punctures the sealed end of the butterfly set. Using this method helps to prevent the premature clotting of blood that may occur if there is a delay in filling the collection tubes.

manipulate standard needles and syringes in tiny veins, and better control is obtained with the butterfly needle. Suction is also more controlled with the butterfly needle and syringe. The butterfly needle may also serve as an infusion line once adequate amounts of blood are obtained. If a straight needle and syringe are used, the technique is similar to that described later for percutaneous arterial puncture, except that a peripheral vein is punctured.

Once the needle penetrates through the skin and into the vein, one must apply suction by *gently and slowly withdrawing the plunger of the syringe.* Alternatively, suction may be applied with a Vacutainer system where the Vacutainer needle punctures the sealed end of the butterfly device (see Fig. 20–2*B*). If the suction is excessive, the vein will collapse and blood flow will stop. If a butterfly or scalp vein needle technique is used, the procedure is similar to that described later for placement of a peripheral intravenous line. Drawing blood from a small infant is usually a two-person procedure. An assistant should attach the syringe to the catheter of the butterfly needle apparatus and withdraw the blood while the physician concentrates on keeping the needle within the vein and immobilizing the arm. After the required amount of blood is withdrawn, the needle is removed, and a sterile dressing is applied to the skin.

It should be emphasized that immobilization of the extremity is mandatory. Prior stabilization of the extremity on a board is especially important if the butterfly scalp vein needle is to be used for subsequent infusion.

The external jugular and femoral veins also may be used in infants for the performance of a venipuncture, although peripheral venous (antecubital, scalp, hand) and arterial sampling are preferable. The external jugular vein lies in a line from the angle of the jaw to the middle of the clavicle and is usually visible on the surface of the skin. The vein is more prominent when the baby is crying. An assistant is needed to restrain the infant in a supine position with the head and neck extended over the edge of the bed. The head is turned approximately 40 to 70 degrees from the midline (Fig. 20–3), and the skin surrounding the area to be punctured is cleansed with alcohol. Lidocaine (0.1 ml of 1 per cent solution) may then be infiltrated into the skin. A finger may be placed just above the clavicle to distend the jugular vein. Using a 21- to 25-gauge straight needle with a syringe, a 21- to 25-gauge butterfly scalp vein needle attached to a syringe, or a 19- to 24-gauge plastic catheter (Angiocath, Medicut, or another similar catheter), the clinician punctures the skin and advances the needle slowly until the jugular vein is entered. The syringe is connected to the needle or the catheter at all times to maintain a constant negative pressure to avoid an air embolism. After the appropriate amount of blood is obtained, the needle is withdrawn and slight pressure is applied to the vessel. The infant should be placed in an upright position after the needle is removed, and slight pressure should be continued for 3 to 5 minutes. Close observation of the puncture site should follow.

The femoral vein lies medial to the femoral artery and inferolateral to the inguinal ligament (Fig. 20–4). The use of this vein for blood sampling is reserved for situations in which patients present in extremis and no other sampling sites are present. An assistant positions the hips in mild abduction and extension while the artery is palpated and its location is identified by placing a mark on the abdomen just superior to the femoral triangle (see Fig. 20–4). The femoral triangle is then prepared with alcohol; a betadine scrub is also recommended when obtaining blood cultures. The skin puncture site may then be infiltrated with 0.1 ml of 1 per cent lidocaine. The technique of needle or catheter insertion is similar to that for external jugular venipuncture (see Fig. 20–3). The clinician punctures the skin and then directs the

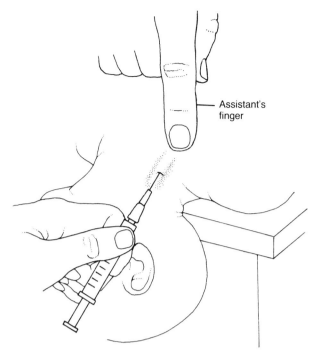

Figure 20–3. External jugular venipuncture. Either a syringe or a butterfly needle may be used. This vein becomes distended when the infant cries and the neck is extended over the side of the bed. This procedure requires two persons to perform it. Contrary to the illustration, both the clinician and assistant should wear latex gloves.

Assistant's finger

needle or catheter toward the umbilicus at a 30- to 45-degree angle to the skin, remaining medial to the femoral artery pulsation. A slight constant negative pressure is applied throughout insertion. After the needle or catheter enters the femoral vein, the desired blood samples are withdrawn, and the needle or catheter is removed (unless venous access with an intravenous catheter is desired). Pressure is applied to the femoral triangle for a minimum of 5 minutes, and the site is observed closely for recurrent bleeding.

Complications. Complications of venipuncture include hematoma formation, local infection, injury to structures adjacent to vessels, and phlebitis. All of these complications

are uncommon. Special care should be used when puncture of the external jugular vein or femoral vein is attempted. Inadvertent deep puncture in the neck can produce injury to the carotid artery, the vagus or phrenic nerve, or the apex of the lung. In the femoral triangle injury to the femoral artery, femoral nerve, and hip capsule may occur. Such structures are unlikely to be injured if proper technique is practiced, however.

Blood Cultures

Although the heel stick capillary tube procedure has been used in some centers for the procurement of blood from infants for cultures,[18, 19] there is a significant incidence of false-positive results with the technique, and therefore it is not recommended if venous blood is available. Venipunctures continue to be the main source of blood for culture in small infants. In the newborn infant, blood may be obtained for culture from an umbilical arterial or venous catheter, if it is obtained immediately after sterile insertion; even then, there is considerable controversy concerning the incidence of false-positive cultures. Arterial blood may also be used to obtain blood cultures.

Procedure. The technique of venipuncture for a blood culture is similar to that described previously for general blood sampling, with the following differences: The puncture site should be doubly prepared, first with a povidone-iodine solution and then with alcohol (see also Chapter 90). (Following completion of the procedure, all of the iodine solution should be removed from the infant's skin to prevent irritation.) The volume of blood required for a blood culture depends on the size of the infant. In the neonate with bacteremia there is a greater number of organisms per milliliter of blood;[20] a sample size of 0.5 to 1 ml is probably sufficient. In older infants, 2 to 3 ml of blood is ideal. After the appropriate volume of blood is withdrawn, the needle that was used to penetrate the skin is removed, and a sterile needle is attached to the syringe. Half of the specimen should be placed in an anaerobic culture bottle and half in an aerobic bottle.

Arterial Blood Sampling

The arterial blood gas is an important laboratory test for evaluation of an infant or child with respiratory distress (see also Chapter 19). Arterial blood may also be used for routine laboratory analysis if venous blood cannot be obtained. In fact, if venous access is unavailable, an artery may be used to obtain all laboratory specimens. Possible sites of arterial blood sampling include (1) radial, brachial, temporal, dorsalis pedis, and posterior tibial arteries; (2) umbilical arteries in the newborn infant; and (3) capillaries ("arterialized"). Femoral arteries should not be used for obtaining routine blood samples from the infant or child.[21] Transcutaneous electrodes for P_{O_2}, P_{CO_2}, and oxygen saturation analyses may provide a useful adjunct to arterial sampling in many patients. Nonetheless, they do not replace intermittent arterial sampling, which remains necessary for the stabilization of infants and for verification of the accuracy of these noninvasive methods.

Peripheral Artery Puncture

Peripheral artery punctures may be performed in the radial, brachial, temporal, dorsalis pedis, and posterior tibial arteries. No vein or nerve is immediately adjacent to the radial artery, which minimizes the risk of obtaining venous blood or damaging a nerve. This is not the case with the

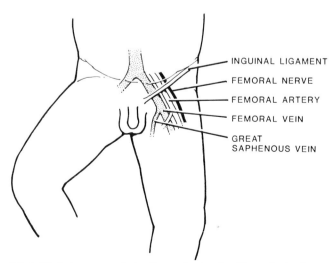

Figure 20–4. Anatomy of the femoral triangle. The vein is always medial to the artery.

INGUINAL LIGAMENT
FEMORAL NERVE
FEMORAL ARTERY
FEMORAL VEIN
GREAT SAPHENOUS VEIN

brachial artery, and the risk of both complications appears to be greater when this artery is used.[22] The temporal artery is also adjacent to a vein, and if the patient's head is in an oxygen hood it is nearly impossible to obtain a sample in a steady state.

The radial artery (Fig. 20–5) is most frequently used to obtain intermittent arterial samples from infants and children. We prefer not to use the ulnar artery for arterial puncture to preserve the collateral circulation to the hand, although some clinicians advocate performing punctures and catheterization of the ulnar artery. The median nerve is in the midline and the ulnar nerve is near the ulnar artery; these areas should therefore be avoided.

Procedure. In preparation for a radial artery puncture, one should first heparinize a tuberculin syringe. All heparin should be ejected from the syringe; a 25- or 26-gauge needle should then be attached to the syringe. The amount of heparin coating the barrel of the syringe is adequate to anticoagulate the sample; excess heparin may result in inaccurate P_{CO_2} determinations because of dilution of the blood sample.[23-26]

The clinician should hold the infant's wrist and hand in the left hand (if the clinician is right-handed) and should palpate the pulsations of the radial artery just proximal to the transverse wrist creases. Some clinicians prefer to immobilize the wrist by taping it to a sandbag or another restraint.[27] The area is cleansed with alcohol. Some practitioners advocate the use of subcutaneous lidocaine. The skin is penetrated at a 30- to 45-degree angle (Fig. 20–6), and while the plunger of the syringe is withdrawn, the needle is advanced slowly until the radial artery is punctured or until resistance is met (Fig. 20–7). In contrast to the procedure with adults, it is necessary with infants to provide continuous suction on the plunger of the syringe. One can be sure that the radial artery is punctured when blood appears in the hub of the needle. Some clinicians prefer to use a 25-gauge scalp vein butterfly needle connected to a syringe. This allows better control of the needle while an assistant aspirates the syringe and may also permit a larger volume of blood to be withdrawn. Other clinicians prefer to attach the syringe to the butterfly needle only after blood return is noted; suction is thereafter applied. One may place a transillumi-

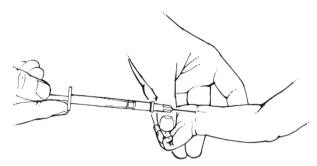

Figure 20–6. For arterial blood gas analysis, the needle should be inserted under the skin at a 30- to 45-degree angle. A butterfly needle and syringe are used if larger volumes of blood are required. Contrary to the illustration, latex gloves should be worn during the procedure.

nator on the underside (dorsum) of the wrist to visualize the radial artery.

If one meets resistance while pushing the needle deeper, one slowly withdraws the needle to the point at which only the distal needle tip remains beneath the skin and then repeats the procedure. After 0.3 ml of blood is obtained, the needle is removed, and light pressure is applied for 5 minutes or longer to prevent any bleeding.[28]

A simulator (Medical Plastics Laboratory, Gatesville, Tex.) may be used to teach and practice the technique of radial artery puncture in infants.[28]

Complications. The complications of radial artery puncture include infection, hematoma formation, scar formation, tendon injury, arteriovenous fistula formation, and nerve damage.[29, 30] With the use of proper technique, however, the complication rate is extremely low. The most common concern with puncture of a radial artery (or any peripheral artery) in infants is that the baby may start to cry before blood is obtained, thus changing the P_{O_2} and P_{CO_2} from the values of the quiet state.[31, 32]

Another potential problem is the dilutional effect of heparin on the P_{CO_2}. The heparin in the dead space of the tuberculin syringe may decrease the P_{CO_2} by 15 to 25 per cent when 0.2 ml of blood is obtained and by approximately 10 per cent with 0.4 ml of blood. This emphasizes the need for all heparin to be ejected from the dead space of the syringe *before the needle is applied*. The use of a syringe (e.g., Becton-Dickinson 1-ml U-100 insulin syringe) with minimal dead space or the use of lyophilized heparin eliminates this problem[33] (see also Chapter 19).

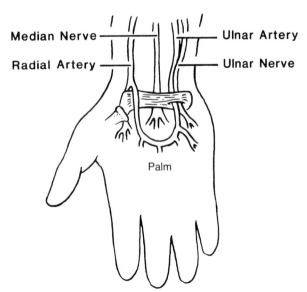

Figure 20–5. Anatomy of the volar surface of the wrist and the palm.

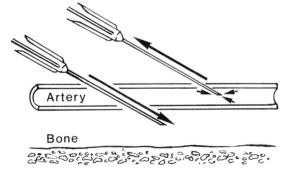

Figure 20–7. If resistance is met during passage of the blood gas needle, it usually indicates contact with the bone. The needle should be withdrawn slowly. If the needle has traversed both walls of the artery, blood will be obtained as the needle is slowly withdrawn into the arterial lumen.

VASCULAR LINE PLACEMENT: VENOUS AND ARTERIAL

Intravascular lines are indicated when access to the venous or arterial circulations is necessary. Intravenous (IV) lines may be positioned in peripheral veins (scalp, hand, forearm, foot, ankle, axilla, thigh) or central veins (superior vena cava via the internal jugular, axillary, superficial temporal, posterior auricular, or subclavian venous approach,[34, 35] and inferior vena cava via the umbilical or femoral venous approach) (Fig. 20–8). Likewise, intra-arterial lines may be positioned peripherally (radial, posterior tibial, dorsalis pedis, superficial temporal arteries) or centrally (abdominal or thoracic aorta via an umbilical or femoral artery approach). Techniques to secure access to these intravascular spaces are discussed in the following sections. Note that 50 per cent nitrous oxide in oxygen administration to the patient (see Chapter 42) may facilitate these vascular procedures by reducing pain and anxiety.[35a]

Peripheral Intravenous Placement: Percutaneous

INDICATIONS

Peripheral IV lines are used for maintenance of fluid balance, administration of medication, nutrition, and prevention of hypoglycemia. In general, peripheral IV lines are indicated when the patient is unable to attain medical and nutritional goals with enteral therapy. (See also Chapter 21.)

EQUIPMENT

Materials needed for placement of a peripheral IV line in an infant include: (1) a 21- to 27-gauge butterfly scalp vein infusion set or a 21- to 24-gauge plastic catheter, such as Angiocath, Medicut, or Quikcath; (2) a roll of ½-inch tape; (3) a plastic medicine cup; (4) a bottle of intravenous fluid; (5) an intravenous fluid chamber with microdrip; and (6) a continuous infusion pump. One must carefully monitor fluid administration in an infant. *Macrodrip tubing and liter bottles should not be used;* inadvertent infusion of large amounts of fluids to an infant may be disastrous. An infusion pump is an ideal way of limiting fluid infusion while keeping the vein open.

PROCEDURE

A number of IV sites are available for the placement of a peripheral intravenous needle or catheter in the infant.[34, 35] The scalp veins are probably the easiest to cannulate, but many clinicians prefer the veins on the dorsa of the hands and feet. The antecubital veins are often easily cannulated in the older infant. If one is using a peripheral vein on the hands, the feet, or the antecubital fossa, one should first immobilize the extremity by taping it to an armboard, a padded splint, a full plastic intravenous fluid bag, or a sandbag. The particular site is a matter of preference, and the physician should choose the vein that appears to be the easiest to cannulate. If percutaneous central venous catheter placement is contemplated, the clinician may choose to avoid the antecubital veins for peripheral IV line placement.

If the scalp veins are used, the area surrounding the planned site of insertion should be shaved and cleansed with an iodine solution. Arteries and veins can usually be differentiated on the scalp by the fact that arteries are more tortuous than veins. In addition, the flow of blood is away

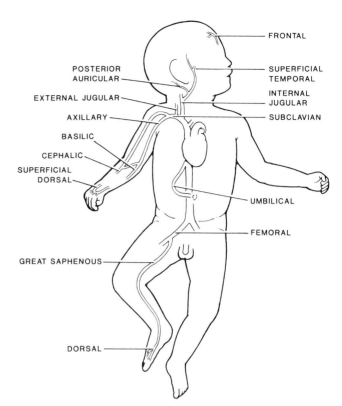

Figure 20–8. Venous access sites in the neonate and young infant. If venous access is unavailable, arterial blood may be used for most laboratory tests, including blood cultures.

from the heart in arteries and toward the heart in veins. If an artery is entered during placement of the needle and fluid is infused, blanching will occur in the area. If this happens, the catheter or needle should be removed, light pressure should be maintained for several minutes, and the procedure should be repeated in another site. A rubber band may be used as a tourniquet around the head to produce venous dilation. One should always check that the rubber band is removed after venous cannulation.

When removing this rubber band, it should be carefully slipped over the catheter or butterfly needle or cut with a pair of scissors. Although cutting the rubber band with scissors is often the easiest technique, the clinician must take care to hold both ends of the cut rubber band to avoid having the infant "snapped" by one or both ends of the rubber band. If a peripheral extremity is used, a tourniquet may be placed proximal to the planned site of entry. Although not in widespread use, nitroglycerin ointment (0.4–0.8 mg) is advocated by some physicians to induce local vasodilation, thereby aiding venous cannulation.[36]

The tubing of the scalp vein butterfly infusion set or the catheter should be flushed before venipuncture with a sterile intravenous solution, such as D_5W or normal saline, to prevent air embolism. If a plastic catheter is used,[37] the catheter with stylet in place is directed through the skin at a 10- to 20-degree angle. The catheter with stylet is slowly advanced until blood return is noted. One then advances the catheter over the stylet into the vein.

If a scalp vein butterfly infusion set is used, the wings of the butterfly are grasped between the thumb and forefinger and the needle is introduced beneath the skin approximately 0.5 cm distal to the anticipated site of vein entrance (Fig. 20–9). The needle is advanced slowly toward the vessel

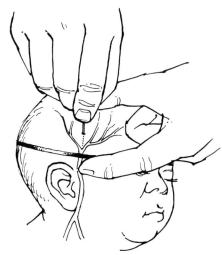

Figure 20–9. The needle is introduced approximately 0.5 cm distal to the anticipated site of the vessel puncture in a scalp vein. Contrary to the illustration, latex gloves should be worn.

until blood appears in the tubing, indicating that the vessel has been entered. The tourniquet should then be removed. The needle should be flushed with 0.5 to 2 ml of intravenous fluid such as D_5W or normal saline to ensure that the needle is properly in place within the vein. If infiltration occurs, as noted by a subcutaneous bump, the IV line should be removed, and the process should be repeated at another site.

The needle assembly may be taped, as shown in Figure 20–10. After the wings are secured with tape, the tubing of the butterfly set should be taped in a loop on the scalp so that it is not accidentally pulled. A wisp of cotton may be placed under the wings of the butterfly if the infusion is positional. A small plastic medicine cup or half of a paper cup may be taped over the wings and the needle to protect the IV line (Fig. 20–11). The catheter of the butterfly set should then be connected to the tubing from the intravenous system, and the IV pump should be started.

If a catheter is used for placement of the IV line, the stylet is removed and the IV line is connected to the hub of the catheter by means of a T piece connector. The catheter is fixed to the skin with a piece of ½-inch tape placed adhesive side uppermost under the catheter hub and crossed

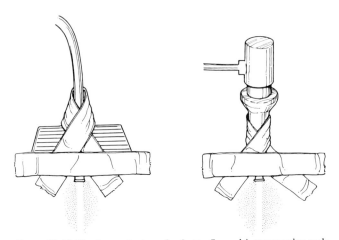

Figure 20–10. Taping technique for butterfly and intravascular catheters.

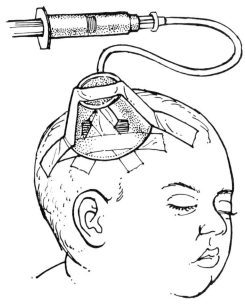

Figure 20–11. Protecting the intravenous line with a plastic medicine cup.

over the catheter in a V shape. A second piece of tape is passed around and over the catheter hub and is fixed to the skin (see Fig. 20–10).

COMPLICATIONS

Complications of intravenous fluid therapy include infection,[38] injection of sclerosing agents into the subcutaneous space with resultant necrosis and sloughing of the skin[39] (especially in small infants), air embolism,[40] and administration of inappropriate volumes of fluid. The incidence of infection secondary to peripheral intravenous therapy may be decreased by routine periodic replacement of the needles. Because the life span of an IV needle or catheter is usually fairly short (less than 72 hours) in the small infant, the decision concerning elective removal and replacement of the intravenous system is not usually a problem. Of course, it is important to pay meticulous attention to sterility during insertion and maintenance of the intravenous system to decrease the risk of infection.

A simulator (Medical Plastics Laboratory, Gatesville, Tex.) is available to demonstrate and practice the proper technique of placement of peripheral IV needles in infants.[41]

Central Intravenous Line Placement: Percutaneous

Percutaneous placement of central venous lines (CVLs) has become the technique of choice of many clinicians in securing central venous access in neonates and young infants (see also Chapters 25 and 26).[42–50] This technique has largely supplanted the conventional technique of venous cutdown catheterization. Both percutaneous and venous cutdown techniques require central venous catheters, which can be purchased separately or within self-contained kits (Arrow International, Inc., Reading, Pa.; Gesco International, San Antonio, Tex.). However, CVL placement requires little additional equipment, whereas venous cutdown catheterization requires a set of sterile instruments. Percutaneous CVL placement also preserves the access veins for repeated use, whereas the venous cutdown technique has traditionally included ligation of the access vein. Finally, the percutaneous approach avoids the tissue injury associated with surgical incision and dissection.[50] This percutaneous technique may be used for rapid venous access in emergency situations as well as to secure central venous access when peripheral venous access is limited (e.g., in low-birth-weight infants).[43, 47]

INDICATIONS AND CONTRAINDICATIONS

Percutaneous intravenous line placement is indicated to secure vascular access (1) when peripheral venous access is limited, (2) during cardiac arrest, hypotensive crises, and shock, (3) when hyperalimentation and intravenous infusions are required for days to weeks, and (4) when low-birth-weight neonates and young infants require central venous access. After placing intravenous lines, some investigators use them to draw blood samples; this procedure must be performed with caution because the risk of contamination increases each time the system is opened. Contraindications to percutaneous placement of central venous catheters include local infections or burns at insertion sites; malformations or deformations that may distort vascular anatomy; vascular insufficiency of an extremity; obstruction or compression of the access veins by tumor, abnormal vessels, hematoma, thrombus, abscess, or malformation; absence of access veins; or a planned future transfemoral cardiac catheterization.[49] Bacterial septicemia is a relative contraindication; we generally recommend delaying placement of central venous access until cultures have been sterile for 48 hours.

EQUIPMENT

Percutaneous venous catheterization in a small infant or neonate requires a selection of sterile catheters ranging in size from 24 gauge to 16 gauge; the catheters are typically made of a silicone elastomer, polyvinyl chloride, or polyethylene (Gesco International, Inc., San Antonio, Tex.; Arrow International, Inc., Reading, Pa.; Cook, Inc., Bloomington, Ind.). The length of catheter is variable, and from 1- to 3-lumen catheters are available. Other necessary equipment includes sterile forceps and scissors, povidone-iodine solution, gauze pads, sterile drapes, gowns, gloves, caps and masks, syringes (3 ml, 5 ml, and 10 ml), Tegoderm (Medical Products, Inc., St. Paul, Minn.), Opsite (Smith and Nephew Medical, Massilon, Ohio), or other sterile transparent skin coverings, Luer-Lok three-way stopcocks, 0.25 to 1.0 per cent lidocaine, and flush solution (1 to 2 units sodium heparin per milliliter normal saline or D_5W). Depending on the access vein to be used, restraint of the extremity, pelvis, or head may require a padded support, an assistant, or both.

TECHNIQUES

Percutaneous placement of central venous catheters can be accomplished using two methods that differ only in the use of a guide wire. We prefer to use the guide wire technique (see also Chapter 23) when catheters are inserted into the femoral vein or subclavian vein. When using the basilic or cephalic vein of the forearm and antecubital space, axillary vein, or superficial temporal or posterior auricular scalp vein, we prefer to insert the catheter through an introducer needle. Some investigators may use the saphenous vein as an access vein. See Chapters 25 and 26 for procedural details for these approaches. Details for the pediatric femoral and antecubital approaches follow.

Femoral Access. Central venous catheters are often required for monitoring central venous pressure and venous blood gases in critically ill infants and children, administration of parenteral nutrition, and for venous access when peripheral venous access becomes unavailable. Some infants require the administration of vasoactive agents in addition to numerous other medications and fluids; insertion of a multi-lumen catheter for these infusions may be advantageous in these instances. Previously, central venous catheters were most commonly inserted by cutdown on the external or internal jugular vein or high saphenous vein or by percutaneous cannulation of the subclavian or internal jugular vein.[51]

The safety and efficacy of percutaneous femoral venous access have been demonstrated.[43, 46, 52, 53] Advantages of this technique include bedside performance and avoidance of specific risks associated with subclavian and internal jugular vein catheterization (pneumothorax and carotid or subclavian artery puncture). Inadvertent entry into the femoral artery can be controlled by direct pressure. Risks of the procedure include thrombosis and infection, as occur with all venous catheters.

Procedure. The child must be adequately restrained to permit exposure of the inguinal region. Sedation may be useful. We have found it helpful to use an ultrasonic Doppler flow detector to locate the femoral artery and then place a heavy ink mark on the abdomen in the line of the femoral artery. This may be useful if edema makes palpation of the artery difficult or if the artery is difficult to locate when wearing gloves. Both groins are generally prepared with betadine in the event that the initial attempt is unsuccessful.

The introducer needle supplied with the kit can be used with or without a syringe to enter the femoral vein. The femoral artery is palpated with one finger, and the needle is placed in the skin just medial to the artery. One enters the skin at a 30- to 45-degree angle approximately 1 cm below the inguinal ligament. The general course of the needle is in a line directed toward the umbilicus. When blood return is noted, the wire is gently passed through the needle into the proximal vein. An alternative method that we have found useful when placing the 4 French double-lumen Arrow catheter is to remove the tubing from a 21-gauge butterfly needle (Abbott Hospitals, Inc., North Chicago, Ill.) and use the needle to enter the vein (Fig. 20–12A). The butterfly needle is very easy to hold in a stable position and is also shorter than the needles supplied with the assembled kits. When blood return is obtained, the wire is passed through the butterfly needle into the proximal vein.

A small incision (1 to 2 mm) is then made along the wire to allow passage of the vein dilator (Fig. 20–12B). The dilator is removed; the catheter, which has been flushed with saline, is advanced over the wire into the vein; and the wire is then removed (Fig. 20–12C).[54] We occasionally find it useful to rotate and advance the catheter simultaneously as it enters the vein. Blood return is noted from the catheter ports, which are then flushed with a heparinized saline solution (10 units/ml). The catheter is subsequently secured with silk or nylon sutures (Fig. 20–12D). A sterile transparent skin covering placed over the exit site may be used as an impermeable dressing.

We found this technique useful in children as small as 1000 gm. When one is placing femoral venous catheters in children less than 1500 gm, a smaller single-lumen catheter (3 French or 24 gauge) should be used, because a larger catheter may occlude blood flow in the femoral vein.

Antecubital Access. Percutaneous insertion of central catheters by way of peripheral antecubital veins is used most frequently to obtain central venous access in patients with

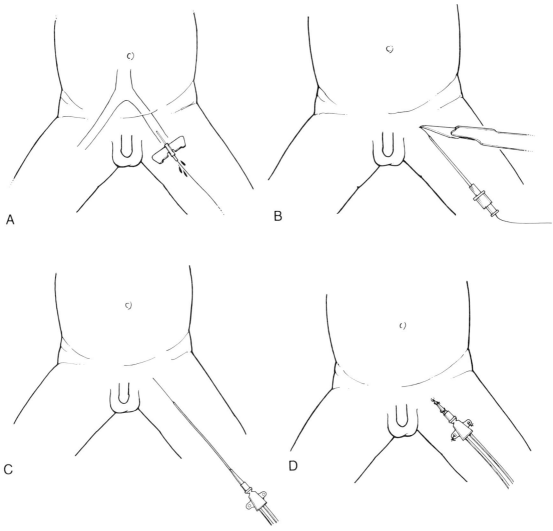

Figure 20–12. Technique for inserting a femoral venous catheter. *A,* A 21-gauge butterfly catheter is used to enter the femoral vein, and the guide wire is passed into the proximal vein. Note that the tubing has been removed from a standard butterfly set. *B,* A small incision is made alongside the wire, and the dilator is advanced over the wire into the vein. *C,* The catheter is advanced over the wire into the vein. *D,* The wire is removed and the catheter secured. Note that many commercial kits have a self-contained 21-gauge needle, making modification of a butterfly needle catheter unnecessary.

very small-caliber vessels, for example, low-birth-weight neonates and very young infants.

 Procedure. The vessel to be cannulated is initially stabilized using a support board or the help of an assistant. The remainder of the procedure requires sterile technique. Betadine is used to cleanse the skin overlying the vessel to be cannulated, and 0.25 to 1 per cent lidocaine is infiltrated at the skin site to be punctured. This skin site is punctured with an 18-gauge needle to ease introduction of the introducer through the skin. The catheter to be inserted is chosen based on the size of the access vessel.

 Typically we use a 23-gauge silicone elastomer catheter found with other needed accessories in a kit prepared by Gesco International, Inc. (San Antonio, Tex.). Advantages of this catheter include (1) a double-wing silicone adapter, which precludes the need to make homemade blunt-end adapters to fit small cannulas and simplifies the taping procedure, and (2) an introducer needle that is breakaway so it can be peeled off the catheter, thereby precluding the need for sliding the introducer off the catheter and placing an adapter. Because the length of this catheter (33.5 cm) is

longer than needed in low-birth-weight neonates and young infants, the distance from the insertion site to the superior vena cava–right atrial junction is estimated (measure the distance between insertion site and the right nipple, Fig. 20–13A) and the catheter cut 1 to 3 cm longer than the estimated distance to compensate for variability between the estimated and actual needed length of the catheter. The end of this catheter is then connected to a Luer-Lok stopcock and syringe and filled with flush solution; the catheter is then ready for use.

 The 20-gauge breakaway introducer needle (Gesco International, Inc., San Antonio, Tex.) is also filled with flush solution and then directed slowly through the insertion site and into the access vein. When blood return occurs, the catheter is picked up approximately 1 cm from its tip and guided into the introducer needle (Fig. 20–13B). The catheter is advanced in 1-cm increments until reaching the previously estimated distance such that the catheter tip is at the superior vena cava–right atrial junction. The breakaway introducer needle is then withdrawn several centimeters from the insertion site before peeling the introducer off the catheter to avoid accidental catheter laceration. If accidental laceration occurs, blunt-end adapters should be readily available. Immediately after catheter placement and withdrawal of the introducer needle, the clinician will be able to manipulate the position of the catheter. Once clotting occurs around the catheter at the insertion site, however, the catheter becomes difficult to manipulate. In addition, after the sterile field is discontinued, the catheter should never be advanced. The function of the catheter is checked by withdrawal of blood, residual air bubbles within the catheter, or both. After the clinician is assured that no air bubbles remain in the line, the catheter is flushed; this catheter should be "easy" to flush. If it is not easy to flush, the clinician should reposition the catheter and recheck its function. If the catheter remains difficult to flush, it should be considered clotted and removed. Alternatively, position may be confirmed by chest radiograph, and if considered appropriate, the use of fibrinolytic therapy employed.

A transparent skin covering is placed and is removed only when the catheter is removed; it is not routinely removed as are coverings of some surgically placed central venous catheters. Stabilization sutures are not routinely placed during this procedure. Occasionally a small amount of bleeding occurs at the insertion site, which generally stops spontaneously or with gentle pressure. With the three-way stopcock in place, central venous pressure measurement and infusion of medications, intravenous fluids, and hyperalimentation solutions can be performed.

COMPLICATIONS

The incidence of complications from indwelling central venous catheters ranges from 0 to 11 per cent.[46] Infection and thromboses are the major risks associated with these catheters.[46, 50, 55, 56] Other complications include accidental displacement, phlebitis, hemorrhage, hematoma, dysrhythmia, air embolus, vascular obstruction or perforation, right atrial perforation, and localized edema. Morbidity from complications can be minimized by removal of catheters as soon as they are no longer needed. Occasionally infections associated with central venous lines can be successfully treated with antibiotics alone. In the majority of catheter-associated infections, however, the catheters must be removed to resolve the infection. Colonization of the catheter tip is related to in situ time, younger age, and inotropic support.[57] Central venous catheters are generally free of colonization if used for no more than 3 days in infants under 1 year and no more than 6 days in older children. Right atrial and major vessel thrombus formation can be monitored using echocardiography; treatment with fibrinolytic agents is occasionally successful in restoring catheter patency.[58] These types of catheters have been used for up to 80 days with mean duration as long as 34 days in very-low-birth-weight neonates.[49, 50] Most clinicians find that the majority of these catheters are discontinued because they are no longer needed.[43]

Emergency Vascular Access

Pediatric resuscitation requires prompt access to the intravascular space. The difficulty of obtaining venous access during cardiac arrest is appreciated by all emergency physicians and pediatricians. At least three studies have demonstrated that the average time required to obtain such access during pediatric cardiac arrest is a frustrating 7 to 8 minutes.[59–61] In the review by Rossetti and colleagues,[61] 6 per cent of cases never had an intravenous line established before attempts at resuscitation were halted.

If no venous line is available, appropriate drugs should be given via the endotracheal tube while attempts at venous access are initiated. *The initial attempts at venous access should be peripheral placement by percutaneous venipuncture;* however, if unsuccessful within the first 1 to 2 minutes, we advocate insertion of a percutaneous femoral venous catheter.[59] *A common mistake is to persist with futile attempts at a peripheral site instead of quickly progressing to central alternatives.* If experienced personnel are available, a simultaneous cutdown of the greater saphenous vein at the ankle or the groin is advisable. One advantage of a cutdown at the groin level is that the saphenous vein can be cannulated and a double-lumen catheter advanced into the femoral vein for rapid fluid infusions through one port and medication administration through the other port. Depending on the experience of the physicians involved in the resuscitation effort, a subclavian or internal jugular catheter insertion may be attempted; however, this is not an easy procedure if chest compressions are in progress or if other physicians are

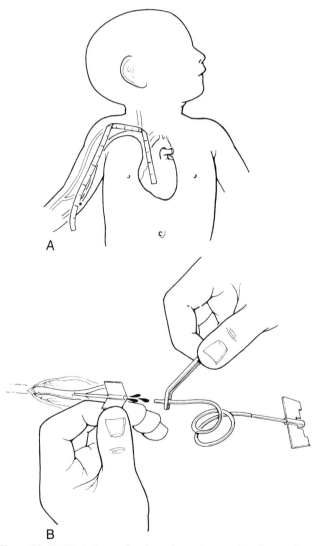

Figure 20–13. Techniques for insertion of central catheters from peripheral veins. *A,* A tape measure is used to determine the catheter length. *B,* The placement of the catheter through the introducer needle.

simultaneously attempting to secure the airway. Venkataraman and associates have reported a 92 per cent success rate with percutaneous subclavian vein catheterization in critically ill infants using a Seldinger technique.[60] If access by these routes is unavailable, intraosseous administration of fluids should be attempted (see Chapter 29). Vascular access should generally be obtained within 5 minutes following this protocol.[61–63]

Venous Cutdown Catheterization

With the development of small intravenous catheters and scalp vein needles, peripheral venous cutdown is rarely used in infants. Nonetheless, when rapid venous access is needed in an infant (particularly for the infant in shock, in whom few veins are visible), venous cutdown can be life saving. For the purpose of illustration, the exposure and cannulation of the saphenous vein are discussed (Fig. 20–14). The same principles apply when a cutdown is performed on an arm vein (see also Chapter 24).

EQUIPMENT

Successful venous catheterization in the small infant requires sterile instruments, an assistant, good lighting, and a selection of catheters. Previous clinical experience is helpful. The use of self-retaining retractors is a personal preference. Because of temperature instability, a warming light or an overhead radiant warmer is frequently useful. Silastic catheters, which can be obtained in 2, 3, and 4 French sizes

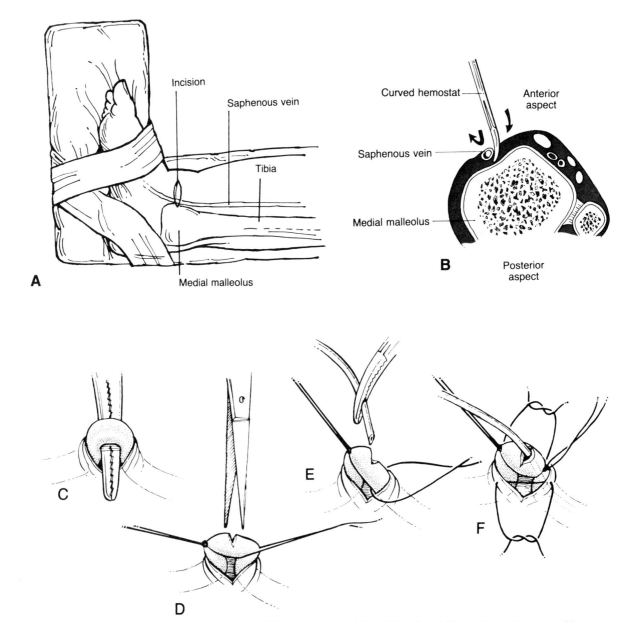

Figure 20–14. Venous cutdown (saphenous vein). *A*, Immobilization of the ankle and the site of skin incision. *B*, A curved hemostat scoops up the vein. The point of the hemostat should be kept against the bone. *C*, The vein is dissected free. (From Suratt PM, Gibson RS: Manual of Medical Procedures. St. Louis, CV Mosby Co, 1982. Reproduced by permission.) *D*, With a proximal and distal tie to stabilize the vein and to control bleeding, an incision is made in the upper one third of the vein. *E* and *F*, The infusion catheter is threaded into the vein lumen and advanced.

(Dow-Corning Co.), seem to remain patent longer and can be sterilized with the instruments to make a "cutdown tray." Standard 18- to 22-gauge intravenous catheters (Angiocath, Deseret Medical, Inc., Sandy, Utah) are also useful.

PROCEDURE

The clinician should begin with complete immobilization of the thigh, the leg, the ankle, and the foot by taping them to a padded armboard, which in turn is attached to the table or bed where the procedure is being performed (see Fig. 20–14A) (see also Chapter 24). The area around the medial malleolus is prepared with a povidone-iodine solution and draped with sterile towels. Local anesthesia is accomplished by a superficial infiltration with 0.25 to 1 per cent lidocaine in an area proximal and anterior to the superior portion of the medial malleolus. Fortunately, there are no major nerves or tendons that accompany the vein in this location.

A tourniquet is placed in the midleg, and a transverse skin incision is made; a small mosquito hemostat is inserted into the wound, with the concavity of the clamp upward. The tip of the hemostat is advanced to the bone in one corner of the wound, and all tissues lying against the bone and in the subcutaneous region are "scooped up" with the hemostat (see Fig. 20–14B). This will invariably lift the vein out of the wound with surrounding tissues. Fine forceps or a mosquito hemostat is used to separate and remove all nonvenous structures, leaving only the saphenous vein tented over the hemostat (see Fig. 20–14C). To avoid injury to the vein during dissection, one spreads the ends of the hemostat parallel to the direction of the vein—never transversely.

Two 4–0 silk sutures are passed under the vein; one silk suture is pulled distal to stabilize the vein, and the other suture is pulled proximal to the site of venipuncture. The distal suture is commonly tied. Some clinicians will not tie the distal suture, however, using it only for stabilization. Removal of the untied distal suture following vein cannulation may allow for subsequent vein recannulation following eventual catheter removal. If the distal suture is left untied, longitudinal traction on it permits hemostasis and continued exposure of the vein above the wound. Fine scissors or a scalpel blade may be used to make an oblique or V-shaped incision in the anterior (superficial) vein wall between the

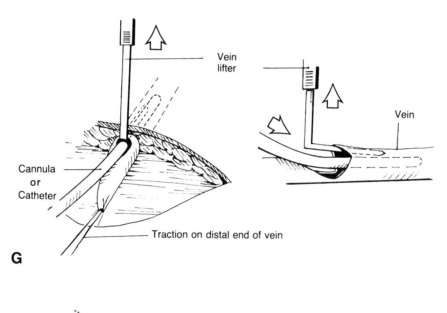

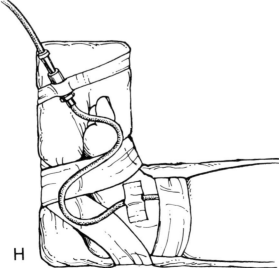

Figure 20–14 *Continued G,* A vein lifter/dilator facilitates the placement of the catheter into the vein lumen. *H,* The incision is sutured, and the catheter is secured.

sutures (see Fig. 20–14*D*). The catheter (beveled at its tip) is then filled with saline.

The catheter is grasped with forceps and is advanced into the vein for a distance of 2 to 3 cm (see Fig. 20–14*E* and *F*). This is usually the most difficult and time-consuming portion of the procedure. A vein dilator or forceps may be used to hold open the incision in the vein (see Fig. 20–14*G*). Downward pull on the distal tie will give countertraction and will stabilize the vein during catheter advancement. The tourniquet is then removed. One ties the proximal suture around the vein with the catheter inside, taking care not to occlude the catheter by tying the suture too tight. If the distal suture was tied, the free ends of the suture can be tied around the catheter, providing additional stability to the catheter. If it was not tied, the distal suture is now removed. When the distal suture is left untied, the proximal suture is still tied to secure the catheter, but the ends are left long so that the suture can be pulled out of the incision and removed to allow recannulation once the infusion catheter is removed.

Continued infusion of saline through the catheter from an attached syringe will ensure patency. The catheter is oriented into either corner of the incision, and the incision is closed with interrupted 4–0 nylon sutures. The skin suture nearest the catheter is wrapped around the catheter and tied to hold the catheter in place. Bleeding can be controlled with direct pressure. Antibiotic ointment is placed over the wound, and a sterile, occlusive dressing is applied. The intravenous tubing is connected and taped securely to the footboard to prevent inadvertent removal of the catheter (see Fig. 20–14*H*).

One should change the dressing carefully every day, using sterile technique with reapplication of antibiotic ointment. When cared for properly, the catheters can remain in place for as long as 7 to 10 days. Generally, though, a line is replaced using another site after 3 to 4 days. Obviously, at the first sign of infiltration or infection the catheter must be removed. Unfortunately, once the vein has been used for a cutdown, it is usually rendered useless for future venous cannulation.

Mini-cutdown. The cannulation of a small vein with a catheter or tube may be difficult and very time consuming if one is not experienced in the technique. As an alternative, the mini-cutdown procedure may be used. Once the vein is exposed through a skin incision and subcutaneous dissection, it is cannulated directly with a standard intravenous catheter (Medicut, Angiocath) rather than nicked with a scalpel (Fig. 20–15). A silk suture or hemostat may be placed under the vein to immobilize it during puncture, but with the mini-cutdown technique the vein is not tied off after being cannulated. The catheter will not be as secure with this modification, but the technique is useful when time is critical. The vein is not destroyed with this technique. In essence, the mini-cutdown uses the percutaneous technique of cannulation, except that venipuncture is performed through a skin incision under direct visualization (see also Chapter 24).

SUGGESTIONS

In an emergency situation, if a percutaneous peripheral or central venous access is not available within several minutes, a saphenous cutdown should be performed (see previous discussion). The technique requires practice and may consume 5 to 15 minutes of resuscitation time. One common error is making an improper skin incision. The incision must be made through all layers of the skin without severing the vein. Subcutaneous fat should be visible through the incision. The subcutaneous incision should be carried to the end of the skin incision so that the clinician can take full advantage

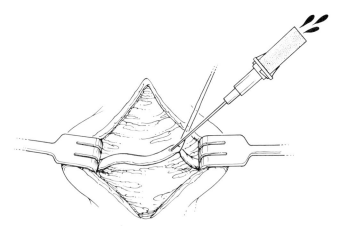

Figure 20–15. The mini-cutdown procedure using a standard intravenous catheter over the needle system is technically easier than the full cutdown and may be preferred in an emergency.

of the skin incision. A 2-cm incision is usually required, and one should not try to work through a skin incision that is too small.

One should perform dissection only with a blunt technique, spreading the hemostat parallel to the course of the vein. Inadvertent severance of the vein may occur during dissection, and one can best control bleeding by pulling the silk ties taut. The incision in the vessel may be a source of frustration. One must incise completely into the lumen of the vessel; a superficial nick, although it will bleed, will not allow for catheter passage. If the vein is severed completely, it will retract from view and will be difficult to find. Generally, an incision should include one third of the vessel diameter. Placing the catheter into the vessel lumen is usually the most difficult part of the procedure, and it is easy to create a false lumen. Small plastic vein dilators are available to facilitate entering into the lumen. If a valve is encountered during passage, one should increase the rate of fluid administration while gently advancing the catheter.

COMPLICATIONS

In addition to the problems discussed previously, venous cutdowns can result in wound infections and phlebitis. Adjacent structures may be injured during the incision and subsequent blunt dissection. When the mini-cutdown technique without ligatures is used, extravasation of infusate may result. Light pressure on the closed wound will generally prevent continued extravasation.

Umbilical Vein Catheterization

The major indication for umbilical vein catheterization is access to the vascular system for emergency resuscitation and stabilization of the newborn. The umbilical vein may also be used for exchange transfusions and short-term central venous access in newborns. The umbilical vein may be cannulated up to the age of 5 to 7 days, but after 1 week of life the technique is not generally used. The procedure is technically easier than umbilical artery cannulation. *Umbilical vein catheterization is not an acceptable alternative after the baby leaves the hospital* (for example, the procedure would not be used should a 2- to 4-week-old infant present to the emergency department).

PROCEDURE

The supplies and equipment for catheterization are listed in Table 20–1. The infant is placed beneath a radiant warmer, and the extremities are restrained. The skin temperature is maintained at 35.8° C (96.5° F). Oxygen is administered as needed, and the audible beep on the cardiac monitor is turned on. The operator should wear a surgical cap and mask and a sterile gown and gloves.

The umbilicus is scrubbed with a bactericidal solution. Pooling of liquid at the infant's side should be avoided, because this may be associated with blistering of the skin under a radiant warmer. The umbilical area is draped in a sterile fashion with the infant's head left exposed for observation.

To provide hemostasis and to anchor the line after placement, a pursestring suture is placed at the junction of the skin and the cord (Fig. 20–16). Alternatively, a constricting loop of umbilical tape in the same position may be used. The cord is cut 3 to 5 mm from the skin, and the vessels are identified. The vein is usually located at 12 o'clock and has a thin wall and large lumen, whereas the two arteries have thicker walls and smaller lumina. Occasionally, a persistent urachus may be mistaken for the umbilical vein, but the return of urine should identify the mistake.

The catheter (3.5 to 8.0 French), which has been flushed with heparinized saline, is placed in the lumen of the umbilical vein and is advanced gently. The catheter is inserted only 4 to 5 cm in a term-sized infant, and the suitable length should be marked before the catheter is advanced. If the catheter is pushed farther than 4 to 5 cm, it will do one of two things: (1) It may enter the ductus venosus and then move into the inferior vena cava. The catheter must be inserted approximately 10 to 12 cm in a term-sized infant to reach the inferior vena cava; this may be a desirable location in some newborn infants whose peripheral vascular access is limited and for whom central venous access is desired for central venous pressure monitoring or infusion of medications, high concentrations of glucose (>10 per cent), intravenous fluids, and hyperalimentation solutions. (2) It may enter a branch of the portal vein within the liver (evidenced by obstruction at 5 to 10 cm). Ideally, radiographs should be obtained to document the placement of the catheter; an umbilical venous catheter will proceed directly cephalad (without making a downward loop) until it passes through the ductus venosus (Fig. 20–17). Of course, in a resuscitation, radiographic documentation may not be possible. Therefore, it is generally recommended that the catheter be inserted approximately 4 to 5 cm to minimize the risk of injecting sclerosing solutions into the liver.

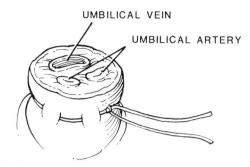

Figure 20–16. A pursestring suture or umbilical tape is passed around the base of the cord to provide hemostasis.

Air embolism may occur at the time of catheter removal if the infant generates sufficient negative intrathoracic pressure (as during crying) to cause air to be drawn into the patent umbilical vein. Therefore, caution must be used during catheter removal to ensure that the vein is promptly occluded (by tightening a pursestring suture or applying pressure on or just cephalad to the umbilicus).

COMPLICATIONS

Complications of umbilical venous catheters include hemorrhage, infection, injection of sclerosing substances into the liver (resulting in hepatic necrosis), air embolism, and vessel perforation. It is most important that one follow careful technique in insertion and maintenance of catheters to minimize such complications.

Umbilical Artery Catheterization

Umbilical artery catheterization is a useful procedure in the care of newborn infants who require frequent arterial blood gas and blood pressure assessment, although it is imperative for the clinician to remain aware of potential complications.[64-66] One of the two umbilical arteries may be cannulated for resuscitation purposes, but an umbilical vein is generally technically easier to cannulate and may be preferred in an emergency.

Table 20–1. Umbilical Vein and Artery Catheterization Equipment

Line fluid usually consists of $D_{5-10}W$ with electrolytes. Some physicians also add 1 unit of heparin per ml fluid (to "prevent" clotting in the catheter).
Fluid chamber, intravenous tubing, infusion pump, filter (0.22 μ), short length of intravenous tubing, three-way stopcock.
Umbilical artery catheter (3.5 to 5 French).
3–0 silk suture on a curved needle.
Curved iris forceps without teeth.
Small clamps, forceps, scissors, needle holder.
Sterile drapes.
Light source.
10 ml of heparinized solution for flush (1 to 2 units Na^+ heparin per ml fluid).
Surgical cap, mask, gown, and gloves.

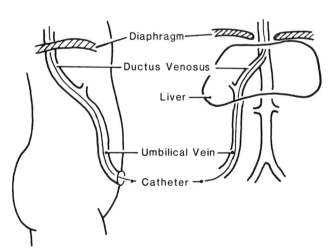

Figure 20–17. An umbilical vein catheter is directed toward the head and remains anterior until it passes through the ductus venosus into the inferior vena cava.

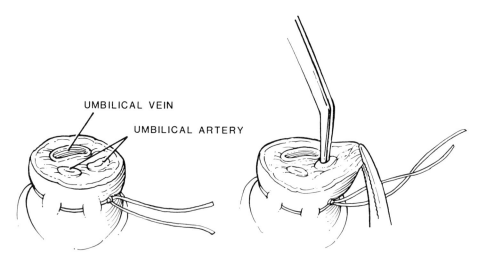

UMBILICAL VEIN

UMBILICAL ARTERY

Figure 20–18. The umbilical cord is grasped with a curved hemostat near the selected artery. The umbilical artery is then dilated with curved iris forceps.

PROCEDURE

The technique of umbilical artery catheterization is similar to that described for the umbilical vein catheterization in the preceding section. After the umbilical arteries have been located, the cord is grasped with a curved hemostat near the selected artery (Fig. 20–18). This maneuver is important because it provides clear visualization and stabilization of the vessel. Using the curved iris forceps without teeth, one gently dilates the artery. Umbilical artery spasm may make the procedure difficult. A 3.5 to 5 French catheter is attached to a three-way stopcock and is flushed with the sterile heparinized solution. The catheter may then be introduced into the dilated artery. A 3.5 to 4 French catheter is recommended for infants weighing less than 2 kg and a 5 French catheter for those weighing more than 2 kg.

When the catheter is being inserted, tension should be placed cephalad on the cord, and the catheter should be advanced with slow, constant pressure toward the feet (Fig. 20–19). Resistance is occasionally felt at 1 to 2 cm. Resistance should be overcome by gentle, sustained pressure. If the catheter passes 4 to 5 cm and meets resistance, this generally indicates that a "false passage" through the vessel wall has occurred. Occasionally, one may bypass the perforation by attempting catheterization with the larger 5 French catheter.

If a low (L-3 to L-4) position is desired, the catheter may be advanced 7 to 8 cm in a 1-kg premature infant or 12 to 13 cm in a full-term infant. Graphs are available to estimate the proper length of insertion for a high or low

catheter location.[67, 68] Once sterile technique is broken, the line may not be advanced. It is therefore preferable to position the catheter too high and to withdraw as necessary according to the location on a radiograph. After it has been positioned appropriately, the catheter should be tied with the previously placed suture (see Fig. 20–19) and taped to the abdominal wall (Fig. 20–20). A radiograph should be obtained, and the catheter should be repositioned, if necessary, with the tip at the lower border of the L-3 vertebra. Some clinicians prefer to place the catheter high (T-6 to T-9 vertebrae). There are no unequivocal data to support either preference.[69, 70]

Radiographs of an arterial catheter (Fig. 20–21) will show the catheter proceeding from the umbilicus down toward the pelvis, making an acute turn into the internal iliac artery, continuing toward the head into the bifurcation of the aorta, and then moving up the aorta slightly to the left of the vertebral column.[71]

Most unsuccessful umbilical artery catheterization attempts fail because the catheter perforates the arterial wall approximately 1 cm below the umbilical stump where the umbilical artery begins curving toward the feet.[72] In this instance, the catheter is advanced in the extraluminal space, and resistance is met at 4 to 6 cm. The following maneuvers make it possible to avoid perforating the umbilical arterial wall in most cases:

1. The catheter should be advanced slowly. When slight resistance is met at approximately 1 cm, the catheter should

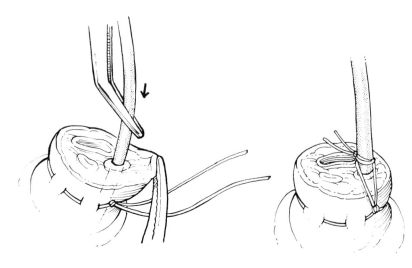

Figure 20–19. The catheter is introduced into the dilated artery and advanced toward the feet. The suture placed around the base of the cord is tied to the catheter.

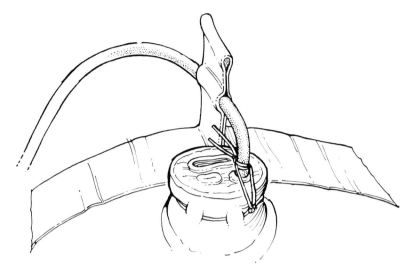

Figure 20–20. The tape is pleated above and below the catheter.

be advanced very gently with steady pressure. The catheter should never be forced, because it will likely perforate the wall. A catheter or feeding tube with a molded tip should be used. A catheter tip that has been cut with scissors is more difficult to insert and advance.

2. Because the artery curves toward the feet, the umbilical stump should be held with a curved clamp and should be pulled toward the head so that the catheter is inserted toward the feet in as straight a direction as possible.

The use of a placenta[73] or a commercially available simulator[74] (Medical Plastics Laboratory, Gatesville, Tex.) makes it relatively easy to demonstrate and practice the proper technique of umbilical artery catheterization.

COMPLICATIONS

If the catheter becomes plugged or fails to function properly or if there is blanching or discoloration of the buttocks, the heels, or the toes, the catheter should be removed at once. Umbilical arteries are most easily cannulated in the first few hours of life but may be a viable vascular route as late as 5 to 7 days of age.

Complications include hemorrhage,[75, 76] infection,[77–80] thromboembolic phenomena (especially to the kidneys, the gastrointestinal tract, and the lower extremities),[81-86] vasospasm, air embolism, vessel perforation, peritoneal perforation, hypertension,[87–89] and possible effects of plasticizers.[90]

Percutaneous Arterial Catheterization

A percutaneous peripheral arterial catheter may be indicated when there is a need for frequent blood gas sampling or continuous arterial pressure monitoring, or both (see also Chapter 19). Arteries used for peripheral catheters in infants include the radial,[91–94] ulnar,[93] temporal,[95, 96] and posterior tibial arteries.

Only the procedure for radial artery cannulation is described here, but cannulation of other vessels is similar. The procedure should be performed with good lighting and an adequate work area while the infant's heart and respiratory rates are monitored closely.

CONTRAINDICATIONS

The following are contraindications to peripheral arterial catheterization: (1) situations in which adequate peripheral arterial samples can be obtained by percutaneous punctures, (2) situations in which circulation of the extremity to be catheterized is compromised, (3) situations in which occlusion of the vessel to be catheterized results in compromised perfusion of that extremity, (4) the presence of an ongoing bleeding diathesis, (5) the presence of localized infection or inflammation overlying the artery to be cannulated, and (6) situations in which intensive monitoring of line function is not available.

Figure 20–21. The umbilical artery catheter makes a loop downward before heading cephalad (schematic drawing of an x-ray interpretation).

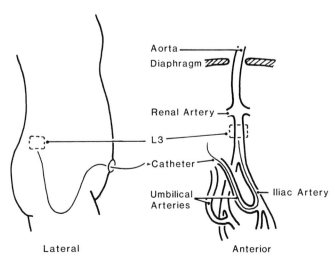

PROCEDURE

The radial artery may be palpated proximally to the transverse wrist crease on the palmar surface of the wrist, medial to the styloid process of the radius. The artery is then compressed, and the hand and fingers are observed for color change. If blanching or cyanosis is noted (indicating poor collateral circulation), catheterization is not performed.

A fiber optic transilluminator may be used to localize the artery. With the overhead lights off, the transilluminator head (with a rubber shield or filter to prevent overheating the skin[97, 98]) is positioned beneath the wrist, and the artery is visualized as a dark, pulsatile shadow.

The equipment includes a 22- or 24-gauge catheter with hollow metal stylet, T-piece connector, and stopcock. One should connect the T piece and the stopcock, and then fill them with an isotonic solution.

The area over the radial artery is prepared with a povidone-iodine solution and washed with alcohol. With the infant's hand and forearm held firmly between the thumb and forefingers of one of the clinician's hands, the catheter with stylet is inserted through the skin just proximal to the transverse wrist crease at a 10- to 20-degree angle (Fig. 20–22). It should be noted that this is less of an angle than is used for simple arterial puncture. The catheter with stylet is advanced slowly until blood return is noted from the hollow metal stylet. One then pushes the catheter over the stylet. The stylet is removed, and the stopcock and T piece connector are attached to the catheter hub. The stopcock is opened to the syringe to confirm pulsatile blood return. It is then flushed with 0.5 ml heparinized flush solution very gently to clear the catheter while the fingers and the hand are observed for evidence of blanching or cyanosis.

The catheter is fixed to the skin by a thin piece of tape placed adhesive side uppermost under the catheter hub and crossed over the catheter in a V shape. A second piece of tape is passed around and over the catheter hub and is fixed to the wrist. If not previously restrained, the hand and wrist are stabilized on a tongue depressor splint with the hand slightly dorsiflexed and the palmar surface uppermost and with a gauze pad or a cotton ball underneath the wrist (Fig. 20–23). A small piece of tape is used to attach the T piece connector to the wrist area or to the splint. The fingers should be easily visible.

An isotonic solution of either glucose or electrolytes is used for infusion. Some clinicians prefer to add 1 to 2 units of heparin per milliliter of infusion solution infused at 1 to 2 ml per hour. *Medications, blood or blood products, amino acid*

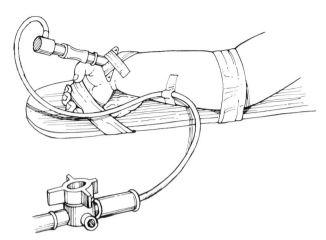

Figure 20–23. One technique of taping the arterial catheter. The armboard should be well padded and secured.

solutions, intravenous fat solutions, or hypertonic solutions are not infused through the catheter.

The catheter must be removed when there is evidence of blanching or cyanosis or when it is impossible to withdraw blood from the catheter or difficult to flush the catheter.

COMPLICATIONS

Complications, which have been reported with every type of arterial catheter,[99–104] include hemorrhage, thrombosis, spasm, infection, scars, air embolism, retrograde blood flow, transient elevation in blood pressure with rapid (less than 1 second) infusion, and nerve damage. Thrombosis or spasm may result in blanching or cyanosis of the extremity or skin. There is potential for loss of digits, an entire extremity, or large areas of skin, as well as cerebral infarction with temporal artery catheters. Malposition of the catheter such that infusion of a glucose solution flows into the celiac artery may also precipitate hypoglycemia on discontinuation of the glucose infusion. Saladino and colleagues note that complications from emergency department–placed arterial lines are uncommon and generally minor.[104a]

Arterial Cutdown Catheterization

INDICATIONS AND CONTRAINDICATIONS

Arterial catheterization by cutdown on the posterior tibial artery,[105] radial artery, and temporal artery[106–108] may be indicated when the need exists for frequent monitoring of arterial blood gases or blood pressure and when percutaneous access is not possible. Arterial cutdowns are contraindicated when (1) adequate peripheral blood gas samples can be obtained by percutaneous punctures or catheterization, (2) circulation of the extremity to be catheterized is compromised, and (3) occlusion of the vessel to be catheterized results in compromised perfusion of that extremity.

PROCEDURE

The anatomy and technique for posterior tibial arterial cutdown are described in detail (Fig. 20–24). The same technique is applicable for the radial artery. The clinician stabilizes the foot in a neutral position by taping the externally rotated lower leg to a splint. The posterior tibial artery is then localized by Doppler ultrasound just *posterior* to the medial malleolus. The operator prepares for the procedure

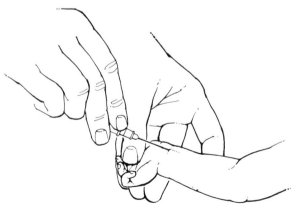

Figure 20–22. The catheter assembly is introduced into the radial artery through skin at a 10- to 20-degree angle. This is less of an angle than is used for simple arterial *puncture*. Contrary to the illustration, latex gloves should be worn.

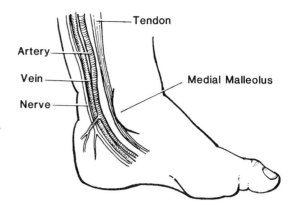

Figure 20–24. Anatomy of the posterior tibial artery and surrounding structures.

by scrubbing and donning a gown and gloves; the foot is prepared with a povidone-iodine solution. The following materials may be used: T connector, stopcock, and syringe filled with flush solution (D$_5$W with 1 to 2 units of heparin per ml); silk suture ties; and a 22- or 24-gauge Angiocath (Deseret Medical, Inc., Sandy, Utah).

Following subcutaneous injection of 1 per cent lidocaine, a 5- to 7-mm transverse incision is made in the skin over the artery posterior to and at the midlevel of the medial malleolus (Fig. 20–25). With blunt dissection in a vertical direction (parallel to the vessels) the tissue is separated with a small, curved forceps, and the artery is identified. The artery courses with the vein just anterior and superficial to the nerve and is usually pulsatile. One isolates the artery by sliding a small, curved forceps beneath it and gently elevating the vessel (see Fig. 20–25). Excessive manipulation of the artery can cause spasm; if this occurs, a few drops of 1 per cent lidocaine applied locally may result in dilation. A silk tie (without a needle) is then placed beneath the artery to stabilize it during cannulation.

At a 10-degree angle, a 22-gauge Angiocath with the catheter bevel down is inserted into the artery over the surface of the forceps. When blood return is seen, the catheter is advanced over the stylet to its full length (Fig. 20–26). The needle stylet is then removed, the catheter is connected to the T connector, and the three-way stopcock is prefilled with heparinized flush solution. Patency is checked by observation of blood return with pulsations; the catheter is then flushed slowly and gently. The silk suture is removed, and the skin incision is sutured. The catheter is sutured to the skin over the heel. The catheter and connector are then secured to the heel with tape (Fig. 20–27). The stopcock is then connected to the infusion line.

COMPLICATIONS

The complications of arterial cutdown are similar to those of percutaneous arterial catheterization. They include hemorrhage, thrombosis, or spasm resulting in loss of tissue; infections; permanent scars; and nerve damage. Complications have been reported with all types of arterial cutdown. Follow-up data and computed tomography data suggest an association between temporal artery catheterization by the cutdown technique and cerebral infarct that may result in hemiparesis.[105] Therefore, we advocate that temporal artery catheterization be the last choice for arterial catheterization.

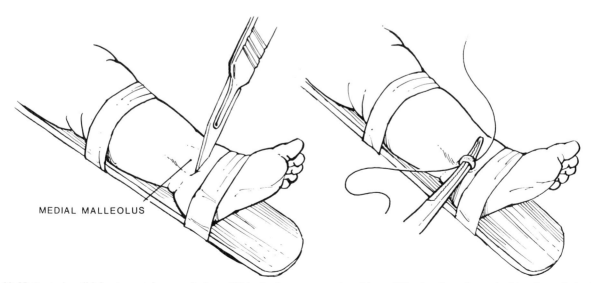

Figure 20–25. Posterior tibial *artery* cutdown technique. With the foot prepared and immobilized, a 5- to 7-mm incision is made in the skin posterior to and at the midline of the medial malleolus. Curved forceps and a silk suture are inserted beneath the posterior tibial artery, which courses just posterior to the medial malleolus.

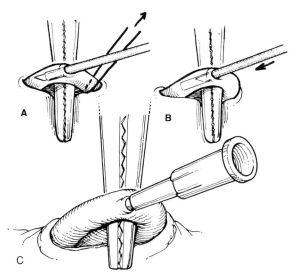

Figure 20–26. Technique of inserting the arterial catheter. A silk tie is used to stabilize the artery during cannulation. One inserts the catheter under direct vision without making an incision in the vessel.

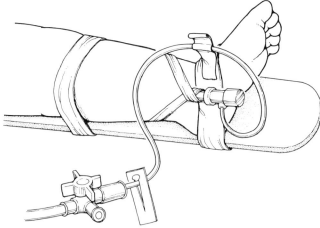

Figure 20–27. The skin incision is closed and the catheter and connector secured to the heel with tape.

REFERENCES

1. Schreiner RL, Lemons JA, Weber TR: Vascular access and blood sampling techniques in infants and children. In Roberts JR, Hedges JR (eds): Clinical Procedures in Emergency Medicine. Philadelphia, WB Saunders Co, 1985, pp 268–286.
2. Krauss AN, Waldman S, Frayer WW, Auld PAM: Noninvasive estimation of arterial oxygenation in newborn infants. J Pediatr 93:275, 1978.
3. Duran AM, Ramanathan R: Pulse oximetry for continuous oxygen monitoring in sick newborn infants. J Pediatr 109:1052, 1986.
4. Blumenfeld TA, Turi GK, Blanc WA: Recommended site and depth of newborn heel skin punctures based on anatomical measurements and histopathology. Lancet 1:230, 1979.
5. Lauer BA, Altenburger KM: Outbreak of staphylococcal infections following heel puncture for blood sampling. Am J Dis Child 135:277, 1981.
6. Lilien LD, Harris VJ, Ramamurthy RS, Pildes RS: Neonatal osteomyelitis of the calcaneus: Complication of heel puncture. J Pediatr 88:478, 1976.
7. Sell EJ, Hansen RC, Struck-Pierce S: Calcified nodules on the heel: A complication of neonatal intensive care. J Pediatr 96:473, 1980.
8. Folger GM, Kouri P, Sabbah HN: Arterialized capillary blood sampling in the neonate: A reappraisal. Heart Lung 9:521, 1980.
9. Hunt CE: Capillary blood sampling in the infant: Usefulness and limitations of two methods of sampling, compared with arterial blood. Pediatrics 51:501, 1973.
10. Desai SD, Holloway R, Thambiran AK, Wesley AG: A comparison between arterial and arterialized capillary blood in infants. S Afr Med J 41:13, 1967.
11. Glasgow JFT, Flynn DM, Swyer PR: A comparison of descending aortic and "arterialized" capillary blood in the sick newborn. Can Med Assoc J 106:660, 1972.
12. Banister A: Comparison of arterial and arterialized capillary blood in infants with respiratory distress. Arch Dis Child 44:726, 1969.
13. Koch G, Wendel H: Comparison of pH, carbon dioxide tension, standard bicarbonate and oxygen tension in capillary blood and in arterial blood during the neonatal period. Acta Paediatr Scand 56:10, 1967.
14. Corbet AJS, Burnard ED: Oxygen tension measurements on digital blood in the newborn. Pediatrics 46:780, 1970.
15. Duc GV, Cumarasamy N: Digital arteriolar oxygen tension as a guide to oxygen therapy of the newborn. Biol Neonate 24:134, 1974.
16. Karna P, Poland RI: Monitoring critically ill newborn infants with digital capillary blood samples: An alternative. J Pediatr 92:270, 1978.
17. Power WF: Digital capillary sampling. J Pediatr 93:729, 1978.
18. Knudson RP, Alden ER: Neonatal heelstick blood culture. Pediatrics 65:505, 1980.
19. Holt RJ, Frankcombe CH, Newman RL: Capillary blood cultures. Arch Dis Child 49:318, 1974.
20. Fischer GW, Crumrine MH, Jennings PB: Experimental *Escherichia coli* sepsis in rabbits. J Pediatr 85:117, 1974.
21. Feldman S, Goodgold J, Levy H, Zaleznak BD: Acute thrombosis of the femoral artery in an infant. J Pediatr 38:498, 1951.
22. Pape KE, Armstrong DL, Fitzhardinge PM: Peripheral median nerve damage secondary to brachial arterial blood gas sampling. J Pediatr 93:852, 1978.
23. Gast LR, Scacci R, Miller WF: The effect of heparin dilution on hemoglobin measurement from arterial blood samples. Resp Care 23:149, 1978.
24. Fan LL, Dellinger KT, Mills AL, Howard RE: Potential errors in neonatal blood gas measurements. J Pediatr 97:650, 1980.
25. Bageant RA: Variations in arterial blood gas measurements due to sampling techniques. Resp Care 20:565, 1975.
26. Accurso FJ, Bailey DL, Cotton EK: Effect of syringe heparinization technique on arterial blood gas determination. Pediatr Res 14:588, 1980.
27. Curran JS, Ruge W: A restraint and transillumination device for neonatal arterial/venipuncture: Efficacy and thermal safety. Pediatrics 66:128, 1980.
28. Schreiner RL, Gresham EL, Gosling CG, Escobedo MB: Neonatal radial artery puncture: A teaching simulator. Pediatrics (Suppl 6) 59:1054, 1977.
29. Koenigsberger MR, Moessinger AC: Iatrogenic carpal tunnel syndrome in the newborn infant. J Pediatr 91:443, 1977.
30. Skoglund RR, Giles EE: The false cortical thumb. Am J Dis Child 140:375, 1986.
31. Speidel BD: Adverse effects of routine procedures on preterm infants. Lancet 1:864, 1978.
32. Long JG, Philip AGS, Lucey JF: Excessive handling as a cause of hypoxemia. Pediatrics 65:203, 1980.
33. Crockett AJ, McIntyre E, Ruffin R, Alpers JH: Evaluation of lyophilized heparin syringes for the collection of arterial blood for acid base analysis. Anaesth Intens Care 9:40, 1981.
34. Clarke TA, Reddy PG: Intravenous infusion technique in the newborn. Clin Pediatr 18:550, 1979.
35. Hanid TK: Intravenous injections and infusions in infants. Pediatrics 56:1080, 1975.
35a. Henderson JM, Spence DG, Komocar LM, et al: Administration of nitrous oxide to pediatric patients provides analgesia for venous cannulation. Anesthesiology 72:269, 1990.
36. Vaksmann G, Rey C, Breviere GM, et al: Nitroglycerine ointment as aid to venous cannulation in children. J Pediatr 111:89, 1987.
37. Filston HC, Johnson DG: Percutaneous venous cannulation in neonates and infants: A method for catheter insertion without "cut-down." Pediatrics 48:896, 1971.
38. Stamm WE, Kolff CA, Dones EM, et al: A nursery outbreak caused by *Serratia marcescens*—scalp-vein needles as a portal of entry. J Pediatr 89:96, 1976.
39. Gaze NR: Tissue necrosis caused by commonly used intravenous infusions. Lancet 2:417, 1978.
40. Willis J, Duncan C, Gottschalk S: Paraplegia due to peripheral venous air embolus in a neonate: A case report. Pediatrics 67:472, 1981.
41. Hildebrand WL, Schreiner RL, Yacko MS, et al: Placing a needle in an infant's scalp vein. Am Fam Physician 21:139, 1980.
42. Oriot D, Defawe G: Percutaneous catheterization of the axillary vein in neonates. Crit Care Med 16:285, 1988.
43. Newman D, Jewett TC Jr, Karp MP, Looney DR: Percutaneous central venous catheterization in children: First line choice for venous access. J Pediatr Surg 21:685, 1986.
44. Dolcourt JL, Bose CL: Percutaneous insertion of Silastic central venous catheters in newborn infants. Pediatrics 70:484, 1982.
45. Vdassin R, Vinograd I, Alpan G, Arad I: Percutaneous subclavian venous catheters in premature infants less than 1500 grams. Am J Perinatol 2:118, 1985.
46. Kanter RK, Zimmerman JJ, Strauss RH, et al: Central venous catheter insertion by femoral vein: Safety and effectiveness for the pediatric patient. Pediatrics 77:845, 1986.

47. Kanter RK, Zimmerman JJ, Strauss RH, et al: Pediatric emergency intravenous access. Am J Dis Child 140:132, 1986.
48. Irwin G Jr, Fifield G, Clinton J: Emergency catheterization of the superior vena cava in pediatric patients. Am J Emerg Med 2:494, 1984.
49. Durand M, Ramanathan R, Martinelli B, Tolentino M: Prospective evaluation of percutaneous central venous Silastic catheters in newborn infants with birthweights of 510 to 3920 grams. Pediatrics 78:245, 1986.
50. Puntis JWL: Percutaneous insertion of central venous feeding catheters. Arch Dis Child 11:1138, 1986.
51. Fonkelsrud EW, Gerguist W, Burke M, Ament ME: Long-term hyperalimentation in children through saphenous central venous catheterization. Am J Surg 21:685, 1986.
52. Swanson RS, Uhlig PN, Gross PL, McCabe CJ: Emergency intravenous access through the femoral vein. Ann Emerg Med 13:244, 1984.
53. Shulman RJ, Pokorny WJ, Martin CG, et al: Comparison of percutaneous and surgical placement of central venous catheters in neonates. J Pediatr Surg 21:348, 1986.
54. Seldinger SI: Catheter replacement of the needle in percutaneous arteriography. Acta Radiol 39:368, 1953.
55. Thomas F, Burke JP, Parker J, et al: The risk of infection related to radial vs femoral sites for arterial catheterization. Crit Care Med 11:807, 1983.
56. Morgan BC: Complications from intravascular catheters. Am J Dis Child 138:425, 1984.
57. Damen J, Van Der Tweel I: Positive tip cultures and related risk factors associated with intravascular catheterization in pediatric cardiac patients. Crit Care Med 16:221, 1988.
58. Kellam B, Fraze D, Kanarck KS: Clot lysis for thrombosed central venous catheters in pediatric patients. J Perinatol 8:242, 1986.
59. Brunette DD, Fischer R: Intravascular access in pediatric cardiac arrest. Am J Emerg Med 6:577, 1988.
60. Venkataraman ST, Orr RA, Thompson AE: Percutaneous infraclavicular subclavian vein catheterization in critically ill infants and children. J Pediatr 113:480, 1988.
61. Rossetti V, Thompson BM, Aprahamian C, et al: Difficulty and delay in intravascular access in pediatric arrests. Ann Emerg Med 13:406, 1984.
62. Kanter RK, Zimmertman JJ, Strauss RH, Stoekel KA: Pediatric emergency intravenous access. Evaluation of a protocol. Am J Dis Child 140:132, 1986.
63. Randolph J: Technique for insertion of plastic catheter into saphenous vein. Pediatrics 24:631, 1959.
64. Lemons JA, Honeyfield PR: Umbilical artery catheterization. Perinatal Care 2:17, 1978.
65. Dorand RD, Cook LN, Andrews BF: Umbilical vessel catheterization—the low incidence of complications in a series of 200 newborn infants. Clin Pediatr 16:569, 1977.
66. Tooley WH, Myerberg DZ: Should we put catheters in the umbilical artery? Pediatrics 62:853, 1978.
67. Weaver RL, Ahlgren EW: Umbilical artery catheterization in neonates. Am J Dis Child 122:499, 1971.
68. Rosenfeld W, Biagtan J, Schaeffer H, et al: A new graph for insertion of umbilical artery catheters. J Pediatr 96:735, 1980.
69. Mokrohisky ST, Levine RL, Blumhagen JD, et al: Low positioning of umbilical-artery catheters increases associated complications in newborn infants. N Engl J Med 299:561, 1978.
70. Harris MS, Little GA: Umbilical artery catheters: High, low, or no. Perinatal Med 6:15, 1978.
71. Paster SB, Middleton P: Roentgenographic evaluation of umbilical artery and vein catheters. JAMA 231:742, 1975.
72. Clark JM, Jung AL: Umbilical artery catheterization by a cutdown procedure. Pediatrics (Suppl 6) 59:1036, 1977.
73. Clarke TA, Levy L, Mannino F: Use of the placenta as a teaching model. Pediatrics 62:234, 1978.
74. Schreiner RL, Gresham EL, Escobedo MB, Gosling CG: Umbilical vessel catheterization—a teaching simulator. Clin Pediatr 17:506, 1978.
75. Hilliard J, Schreiner RL, Priest J: Hemoperitoneum associated with exchange transfusion through an umbilical arterial catheter. Am J Dis Child 133:216, 1979.
76. Miller D, Kirkpatrick BV, Kodroff M, et al: Pelvic exsanguination following umbilical artery catheterization in neonates. J Pediatr Surg 14:264, 1979.
77. Krauss AN, Albert RF, Kannan MM: Contamination of umbilical catheters in the newborn infant. J Pediatr 77:965, 1970.
78. Bard H, Albert G, Teasdale F, et al: Prophylactic antibiotics in chronic umbilical artery catheterization in respiratory distress syndrome. Arch Dis Child 48:630, 1973.
79. Cowett RM, Peter G, Hakanson DO, et al: Prophylactic antibiotics in neonates with umbilical artery catheter placement—a prospective study of 137 patients. Yale J Biol Med 50:457, 1977.
80. Lim MO, Gresham EL, Franken EA Jr, Leake RD: Osteomyelitis as a complication of umbilical artery catheterization. Am J Dis Child 131:142, 1977.
81. Goetzman BW, Stadalnik RC, Bogren HG, et al: Thrombotic complications of umbilical artery catheters: A clinical and radiographic study. Pediatrics 56:374, 1975.
82. Neal WA, Reynolds JW, Jarvis CW, Williams HJ: Umbilical artery catheterization: Demonstration of arterial thrombosis by aortography. Pediatrics 50:6, 1972.
83. Purohit DM, Levkoff AH, deVito PC: Gluteal necrosis with foot-drop—complications associated with umbilical artery catheterization. Am J Dis Child 132:897, 1978.
84. Rudolph N, Wang H, Dragutsky D: Gangrene of the buttock: A complication of umbilical artery catheterization. Pediatrics 53:106, 1974.
85. Aziz EM, Robertson AF: Paraplegia: A complication of umbilical artery catheterization. J Pediatr 82:1051, 1973.
86. Krishnamoorthy KS, Fernandez RJ, Todres ID, DeLong GR: Paraplegia associated with umbilical artery catheterization in the newborn. Pediatrics 58:443, 1976.
87. Bauer SB, Feldman SM, Gellis SS, Retik AB: Neonatal hypertension—a complication of umbilical-artery catheterization. N Engl J Med 293:1032, 1975.
88. Merten DF, Vogel JM, Adelman RD, et al: Renovascular hypertension as a complication of umbilical arterial catheterization. Radiology 126:751, 1978.
89. Plumer LB, Kaplan GW, Mendoza SA: Hypertension in infants—a complication of umbilical arterial catheterization. J Pediatr 89:802, 1976.
90. Hillman LS, Goodwin SL, Sherman WR: Identification and measurement of plasticizer in neonatal tissues after umbilical catheters and blood products. N Engl J Med 292:381, 1975.
91. Adams JM, Rudolph AJ: The use of indwelling radial artery catheters in neonates. Pediatrics 55:261, 1975.
92. Amato JJ, Solod E, Cleveland RJ: A "second" radial artery for monitoring the perioperative pediatric cardiac patient. J Pediatr Surg 12:715, 1977.
93. Barr PA, Sumners J, Wirtschafter D, Porter RC, Cassady G: Percutaneous peripheral arterial cannulation in the neonate. Pediatrics (Suppl 6) 59:1058, 1977.
94. Todres ID, Rogers MC, Shannon DC, Moylan FMB, Ryan JF: Percutaneous catheterization of the radial artery in the critically ill neonate. J Pediatr 87:273, 1975.
95. Schlueter MA, Johnson BB, Sudman DA, et al: Blood sampling from scalp arteries in infants. Pediatrics 51:120, 1973.
96. Au-Yeung YB, Sugg VM, Kantor NM, et al: Percutaneous catheterization of scalp arteries in sick infants. J Pediatr 91:106, 1977.
97. McArtor RD, Saunders BS: Iatrogenic second-degree burn caused by a transilluminator. Pediatrics 63:422, 1979.
98. Pearse RG: Percutaneous catheterization of the radial artery in newborn babies using transillumination. Arch Dis Child 53:549, 1978.
99. Randel SN, Tsang BHL, Wung JT, et al: Experience with percutaneous indwelling peripheral artery catheterization in neonates. Am J Dis Child 141:848, 1987.
100. Rao HKM, Elhassani SB: Iatrogenic complications of procedures performed on the newborn. Perinatology-Neonatology (Sept-Oct) 25, 1980.
101. Adams JM, Speer ME, Rudolph AJ: Bacterial colonization of radial artery catheters. Pediatrics 65:94, 1980.
102. Cartwright GW, Schreiner RL: Major complication secondary to percutaneous radial artery catheterization in the neonate. Pediatrics 65:139, 1980.
103. Mayer T, Matlak ME, Thompson JA: Necrosis of the forearm following radial artery catheterization in a patient with Reye's syndrome. Pediatrics 65:141, 1980.
104. Ducharme FM, Gauthier M, Lacroix J, et al: Incidence of infection related to arterial catheterization in children: A prospective study. Crit Care Med 16:272, 1988.
104a. Saladino R, Bachman D, Fleisher G: Arterial access in the pediatric emergency department. Ann Emerg Med 19:382, 1990.
105. Spahr RC, MacDonald HM, Holzman IR: Catheterization of the posterior tibial artery in the neonate. Am J Dis Child 133:945, 1979.
106. Prian GW: Temporal artery catheterization for arterial access to the high risk newborn. Surgery 82:734, 1977.
107. Prian GW: Complications and sequelae of temporal artery catheterization in the high-risk newborn. J Pediatr Surg 12:829, 1977.
108. McGovern G, Baker AR: Temporal artery catheterization for the monitoring of blood gases in infants. Surg Gynecol Obstet 127:601, 1968.
109. Bull MJ, Schreiner RL, Garg BP, et al: Neurologic complications following temporal artery catheterization. J Pediatr 96:1071, 1980.

Chapter 21

Peripheral Intravenous Access

Edith L. Hambrick and Georges C. Benjamin

INTRODUCTION

Peripheral intravenous catheterization is one of the mainstays of modern medicine. It is a common procedure done by all levels of health care professionals, including physicians, nurses, physicians' assistants, nurse practitioners, and emergency medical technicians. The procedure allows access to the peripheral circulation for blood sampling, fluid and nutrition administration, and administration of medications. Generally peripheral intravenous catheterization can be accomplished in adults and children in less than 5 minutes if the patient has adequate peripheral circulation and normal veins.[1, 2, 3]

Although bloodletting has been described since the time of Hippocrates around 460 B.C.,[4, 5] one of the first documented descriptions of intravenous therapy, in the form of a blood transfusion, was made by an Italian physician, Giovanni Francisco Colle, in 1628.[6-8] In 1654, Dr. Francesco Folli was said to have used a combination of a silver tube, bone cannula, and animal blood vessel to accomplish a blood transfusion.[4] In the late 1650s (dates vary from 1656 to 1659), Christopher Wren and Robert Boyle injected opium and crocus metallorum using a quill and bladder into the vein of a dog.[6] In 1662, Johann Daniel Major, a German physician, is credited with being the first to inject a medicinal substance into the vein of a human successfully.[7] Richard Lower, an English physician, is credited with being the first to transfuse blood from animal to animal in February 1665.[9] Animal (lamb)-to-human transfusions were accomplished by Dr. Jean Dennis on June 25, 1667; as a result of the transfusion, a transfusion reaction was noted.[4]

In 1829, Dr. J. Blundell performed pioneering work on human-to-human blood transfusion. During the Franco-Prussian War (1870–1871), Dr. J. Roussell is credited with performing the first battlefield transfusions.[4] Dr. Moses Swick first described intravenous urography in 1929, and the first blood transfusion using the slow-drip method was described in 1935 by Drs. Hugh Marriot and Alan Kekuck.[4] Initially steel needles were used for catheterization; however, in the early 1950s, plastic catheters were introduced for continuous intravenous infusions and over time have largely replaced those made of steel.[10, 11]

INDICATIONS AND CONTRAINDICATIONS

Peripheral intravenous cannulation is performed to provide access to the patient's circulatory system. This access can be used for phlebotomy, delivery of medication and fluids, and short-term nutrition (primarily intralipid and dextrose). Peripheral lines are also placed in patients who have potentially life-threatening conditions as a means of ensuring adequate venous access should a problem develop.[12]

Establishment of intravenous access is essential during cardiac arrest and major trauma. The setting for intravenous line placement and the role of high-volume resuscitation before hemorrhage is controlled and definitive care is avail-

able remain controversial.[13] Intravenous fluids, blood, and crystalloid administered through large-bore catheters (16 gauge or less) are important for fluid resuscitation (see Chapter 22) and vital for the delivery of medications. In patients with normal perfusion, delivery times to the central circulation with peripheral venous access is similar to that with central venous access.[14] During closed-chest cardiopulmonary resuscitation (CPR), medication is delivered to the left ventricle more than a minute faster with central venous lines than with peripheral venous access. The former is the preferred route when available.[15–17] Short-term nutrition and hyperalimentation, primarily intralipids, can be administered peripherally. However, all other hyperalimentation must be given through a central intravenous line because of the high tonicity of the solution.

The use of a heparin lock is preferable when access to the circulation is needed for medication delivery and limited intravenous fluid administration is anticipated. This is especially useful in cardiac, renal, or hepatic failure. It has been recommended by one group for use in the prehospital setting when prophylactic access or access only for administration of bolus medications is desired.[18]

Peripheral intravenous lines should not be started in an extremity in which massive edema, burns, traumatic injury, sclerosis, phlebitis, or thrombosis is present because of the potential for fluid extravasation or inadequate volume flow. In addition, the ipsilateral arm of a patient with a mastectomy, neck trauma, or indwelling fistula should also be avoided if possible. In patients with chest, abdominal, and proximal extremity trauma, the vein selected for an intravenous line should not empty into the affected area because the integrity of the proximal veins cannot be ensured. For example, it is preferable for patients with gunshot wounds to the abdomen to have intravenous lines started in their upper extremities, neck, or chest.

The potential risk of inoculating the central circulation with bacteria is increased when an intravenous line is started in an area in which cellulitis is present, and therefore local cutaneous infection is a contraindication. Patients who have renal shunts or fistulas should have intravenous lines placed in the opposite extremity because of the risk of infection or thrombosis of the shunt or fistula. The extremity with a shunt or fistula can be used by an experienced practitioner in an emergency situation if extreme aseptic precautions are used and arterial delivery of the solution is not contraindicated.

EQUIPMENT

The necessary items for achieving intravenous access are shown in Table 21–1. Povidone-iodine, 70 per cent alcohol, or both should be used to clean the skin. A tourniquet is necessary to occlude the venous blood flow; a flexible

Table 21–1. Materials Required for Peripheral Insertion
Povidone-iodine swabs
70% alcohol pads
Tourniquet or blood pressure cuff
Gauze sponges
Arm board
Tape
Antibiotic ointment or film barrier
Intravenous catheter
1-inch tape
¼-inch tape
Latex gloves

The authors wish to give special thanks to the Photography Department of the Howard University College of Medicine for their assistance. Mr. Jeffrey Fearing was particularly helpful.

rubber tube, a commercial rubber tourniquet with Velcro, or a sphygmomanometer inflated to 10 to 15 mm Hg below the systolic blood pressure serves this purpose. Sterile gauze pads are used to wipe away excess povidone-iodine or alcohol and to stop any bleeding from the phlebotomy site after withdrawal of a catheter. An arm board may be necessary if the line is placed over a joint or if the line requires stabilization. Additional items such as tape, topical antibiotics, and appropriate dressings are also required.

Several catheter types are commonly used to gain peripheral venous access: a hollow steel needle, a plastic catheter over a hollow steel needle, a plastic catheter inserted through a hollow steel needle, or a plastic catheter over a flexible metal guide wire[12] (Fig. 21–1). The catheter over the needle is the most common type used today for peripheral access (Fig. 21–2). Multilumen catheters (for example, Twin-Cath, Arrow International, Reading, Pa.) are useful when multiple medicines must be administered simultaneously.

PREPARATION

To allay patient fears, reduce apprehension, and correct misinformation, the purpose, methods, and outcome of the procedure should be explained clearly at the onset by the practitioner when the patient is conscious and time permits. Before initiating intravenous lines, all of the items necessary for performing the procedure should be assembled and placed in convenient proximity to the practitioner. This is especially important if the practitioner is performing the procedure alone. As with all invasive procedures, universal blood precautions should be taken, which includes wearing latex gloves, at a minimum.[19]

Site Selection

Straight, large, bifurcated, easily accessible peripheral veins with healthy subcutaneous tissue are ideal for cannulation (Fig. 21–3). The veins of the upper extremity are generally chosen to initiate intravenous lines because many potential sites are available and because the patient will be more comfortable. The most distal vein should be selected first if several sites are available. This strategy allows the practitioner to use a more proximal site in the event that

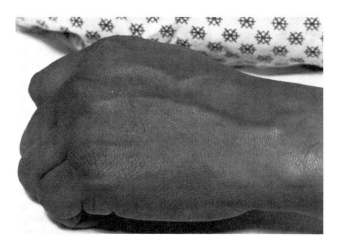

Figure 21–2. Plastic catheter over a hollow needle.

the initial attempt is unsuccessful and avoids proximal fluid leakage from a previous puncture wound during fluid infusion. The veins of the hand and volar aspect of the forearm are the preferred sites. The veins of the antecubital space or other upper extremity joints, although popular, are best avoided as a primary site because of vein tortuosity and the

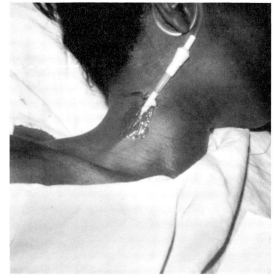

Figure 21–3. *A,* Prominent veins on the dorsum of the hand. *B,* The external jugular vein may be cannulated in the same manner as any other peripheral vein, which often negates the need for central venous catheterization. This site is especially useful in obese adults, infants, and intravenous drug addicts. The major disadvantages are that flow is very dependent on the position of the neck (a significant problem in children and obtunded or restless adults), and valves may abut against the tip of the catheter. Air embolism is another potential hazard with this access route.

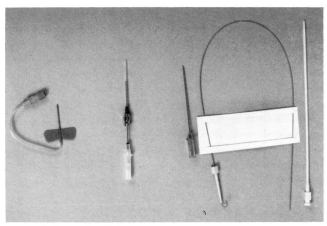

Figure 21–1. Catheters used for intravenous access. *Left to right:* hollow steel needle, plastic catheter over hollow needle, plastic catheter inserted through a hollow needle with a guide wire.

need to immobilize the patient's arm to prevent kinking of the catheter. The foot and lower leg are acceptable secondary sites. The external jugular vein may also serve as a site for venous access, particularly in infants and adults without suitable arm veins. This site may negate the need for central venous catheterization in intravenous drug addicts (Fig. 21–3B). A percutaneous approach to the brachial vein has been described and is useful in patients who lack other peripheral sites.[20] Evidence in dogs suggests that 90 per cent of peripheral intravenous fluid reaches the central circulation even when it is injected under an inflated pneumatic anti-shock garment (PASG).[21] The injected fluid must be infused under a pressure greater than that in the PASG.

ANATOMY (See also Chapters 24 to 26)

In the upper extremity, on the dorsal surface of the hand, the veins collect blood from dorsal and oblique communicating veins of the fingers, which form the dorsal plexus. These in turn drain into the superficial radial and ulnar veins on the lateral and medial sides of the forearm, respectively (see Fig. 26–8). The cephalic vein is located on the radial border of the forearm and receives branches from the small veins in the forearm (see Fig. 24–2). The cephalic vein ascends the arm, gives off the median cephalic vein, and empties into the axillary vein (see Fig. 26–9).

The basilic vein collects blood from the ulnar portion of the veins of the ulnar portion of the posterior forearm. It then joins the median cubital vein and ascends on the medial portion of the arm. The axillary vein begins at the lower border of the teres major muscle as a continuation of the basilic vein. It ends at the outer border of the first rib, where it becomes the subclavian vein. The subclavian vein unites with the internal jugular to form the brachiocephalic (innominate) vein. The right and left brachiocephalic veins join to form the superior vena cava, which empties into the right atrium of the heart (see Fig. 26–8).

In the lower extremity, on the dorsal surface of the foot, the dorsal digital veins receive blood from the plantar veins and then join with the dorsal metatarsal veins to form the dorsal venous arch. On the sole of the foot, superficial veins form a plantar cutaneous arch, which drains into the medial and lateral marginal veins. The medial marginal vein drains into the great (long) saphenous vein at the ankle, which as it ascends collects tributaries from superficial and deep veins and ends at the femoral vein in the proximal thigh (see Fig. 24–1). The palmar digital veins drain into the plantar metatarsal veins, forming the deep plantar venous arch.

The arch then drains into the medial and lateral plantar veins, which receive tributaries from the great and small saphenous veins to form the posterior tibial vein. The posterior and anterior tibial veins unite and form the popliteal vein (Fig. 21–4). The femoral vein is a continuation of the popliteal vein. After passing behind the inguinal ligament, the femoral vein becomes the external iliac vein. The internal iliac, which arises from a confluence of veins draining the pelvis, joins with the external iliac to form the common iliac. The inferior vena cava is formed by the union of the common iliac veins and in turn empties into the right atrium of the heart.

Intravenous Line Assembly

Intravenous fluid, an intravenous tubing set, and a primary administration set are selected appropriately for the clinical situation. A standard nonshock resuscitation set is shown in Figure 21–5. If medication is being administered

intravenously, a shorter secondary administration set is also needed (Fig. 21–6). The cap and protective tabs should be removed from the container and drip chamber end of the intravenous tubing. After closing the regulating clamp, the spiked end of the tubing is then inserted fully into the receptacle on the solution container (Fig. 21–7). The container is then turned over so that the tubing is dangling from below. The drip chamber should be pinched so that it fills halfway (Fig. 21–8). The regulating clamp is then opened, and fluid is allowed to fill the tubing completely, expelling all air bubbles. The bottle is then hung from an intravenous pole higher than the level of the insertion site.

Placement of the Tourniquet

The tourniquet is placed 3 to 4 cm proximal to the site of the phlebotomy, taking care not to pinch the patient's skin (Fig. 21–9A). It is applied so that arterial blood continues to flow into the extremity but venous flow is occluded.

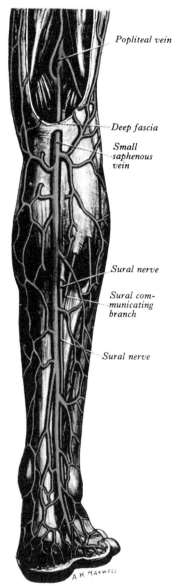

Popliteal vein

Deep fascia

Small saphenous vein

Sural nerve

Sural communicating branch

Sural nerve

Figure 21–4. The small saphenous vein and its tributaries. (From Warwick R, Williams PL [eds]: Gray's Anatomy. 35th ed. Edinburgh, Churchill Livingstone, 1973, p 705. Reproduced by permission.)

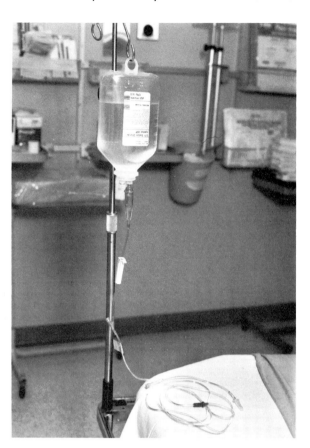

Figure 21–5. Standard nonshock resuscitation set.

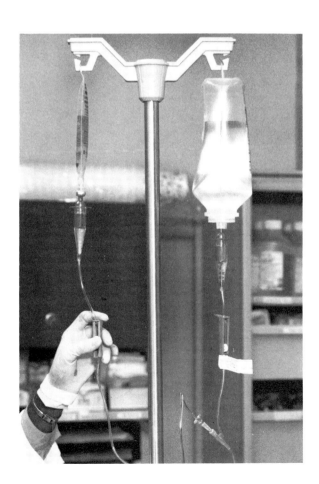

Figure 21–6. Secondary administration set.

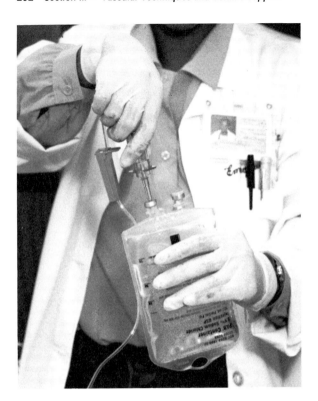

Figure 21–7. Insertion of the spiked end of tubing into an intravenous fluid bottle.

Figure 21–8. Pinching of the drip chamber.

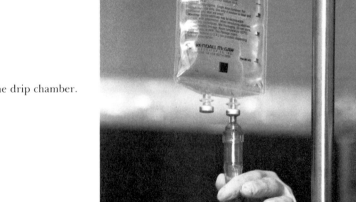

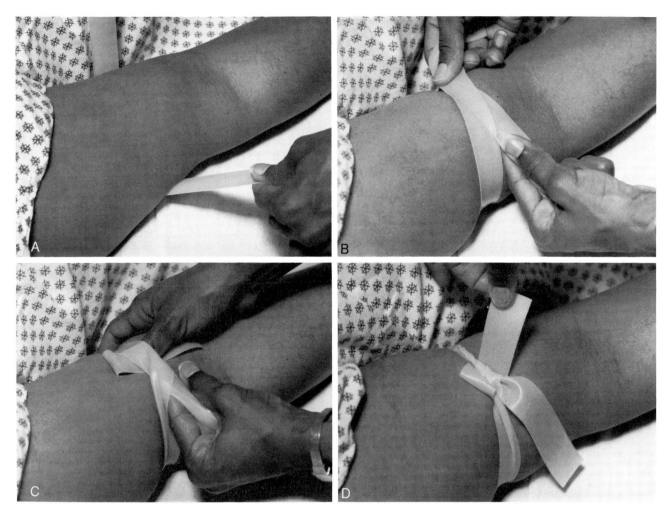

Figure 21–9. Application of a tourniquet. *A,* Placement of a tourniquet 3 to 4 cm proximal to the planned insertion site. *B,* Crossing of the ends of the tourniquet under tension. *C,* Tucking the longer end under the "X" to make a loop. *D,* One-handed technique for releasing the tourniquet.

Often, the practitioner must start the intravenous line without assistance. Therefore, the flexible rubber tube should be tied so that it can be released with one hand as the practitioner steadies the catheter with the other (Fig. 21–9D). The rubber tube is stretched and, while maintaining tension (Fig. 21–9A), crossed in front of the extremity, making an "X," and leaving one portion longer than the other (Fig. 21–9B).[22] The middle of the longer end is tucked under the stretched tube, creating a loop and leaving the tip dangling free (Fig. 21–9C and 21–9D).

After application of the tourniquet, the veins may not become prominent or the practitioner may not adequately feel the distended veins subcutaneously. Several explanations are possible. The tourniquet may be too tight, occluding both the venous and arterial blood flow; the patient may have inadequate blood volume; or the veins may be sclerosed. To determine whether the tourniquet is too tight, the practitioner should feel the pulses distal to the tourniquet. If absent, the tourniquet should be released and reapplied so that only the venous flow is occluded. If a sphygmomanometer is used, the cuff is inflated to 10 to 15 mm Hg less than the systolic pressure. A blood pressure cuff tourniquet has been shown to produce greater venous distention than an elastic tube tourniquet.[23]

The patient's veins should be checked again for sclerosis or thrombosis. If venous pathology is the cause of inade-

quate venous prominence, another site should be selected. If inadequate volume or shock is suspected as the cause of peripheral venous collapse, central venous lines, peripheral venous cutdown, or interosseous infusion can be used until peripheral veins become more prominent.

Adjuncts for Venous Dilation

The practitioner may still have difficulty locating a vein even though the patient has a normal blood pressure, no previous exposure to irritating medications and the tourniquet is applied properly. Other techniques for vein location can be used. A warm moist towel can be applied to the site for several minutes, or an infrared light can be allowed to radiate over the site (not in contact with the skin) to cause vasodilation of the veins.[22] If this method is chosen, patients should have normal skin and sensation to avoid burns. Tapping sharply over the vein can result in mechanical reflex dilation of the vascular walls.[22] The tapping must be light enough to avoid reflex vasoconstriction from pain. Active or passive pumping of the extremity can also distend the veins by enhancing flow. Although rarely used, reactive hyperemia can be created by completely occluding the circulation with a sphygmomanometer for a few minutes and then releasing the sphygmomanometer to 10 to 15 mm below the diastolic pressure.[22] This technique should not be used in patients at risk for peripheral vascular disease or coagulopathies.

Four-tenths per cent nitroglycerin ointment applied to the venipuncture site has been shown to facilitate venous dilation in children younger than 1 year of age.[24] In adults, a 2 per cent nitroglycerin ointment increases the success rate of cannulation of small-caliber veins without significant side effects.[25] This is accomplished by placing one-quarter inch of the ointment over the planned puncture site to an area 2.5 cm² for 2 minutes and then removing the ointment before skin preparation.

A venous distention device has been used to augment venous filling in the nonemergency patient.[23] By using this device, peripheral venous cannulation can be achieved in 90 per cent of patients who have difficult veins.[26] Complications with its use are minimal and include mild discomfort and petechiae. This device is still experimental and is not available for common use. Its role in the care of critical patients remains undefined.

Site Preparation

The skin should be cleaned with a povidone-iodine solution in a circular motion, starting over the planned site of insertion and spiraling outward for 4 to 5 cm. After allowing this area to dry, 70 per cent (isopropanol) alcohol is applied by using the same motion. Patients with iodine sensitivity can be cleaned with 70 per cent alcohol alone if necessary, but this method may be less effective than that using povidone-iodine.[27]

Most catheters can be placed without anesthesia. When many punctures are anticipated, large-bore catheters are placed, or patient anxiety is a factor, 0.5 or 1 per cent lidocaine (Xylocaine), 0.1 ml intradermally (using a 27-gauge needle and 1-ml syringe), can be used at the puncture site to provide local anesthesia for approximately 20 minutes.[28] A more temporary anesthetic effect (3 minutes) can also be obtained by intradermal injection of 0.1 ml of sterile normal saline.[28] A solution of 0.9 per cent benzyl alcohol and normal saline has been shown in one study to be superior to normal saline alone for this purpose.[29] In general, topical anesthetics are of little value because of poor penetration through the skin. A mixture called eutectic mixture of local anesthetics (EMLA) is a topical mixture of lidocaine and prilocaine base and may be an exception to this generalization; in children, the mixture seems to be well tolerated and effective.[30] Disadvantages to its use include the long application time (1 hour), the need for an occlusive dressing, and the occasional local irritation, probably from the adhesive tape.

CATHETER INSERTION

The skin should be grasped and *pulled taut to stabilize the vein* with the nondominant hand (Fig. 21–10A). The intravenous catheter is held in the dominant hand and the skin rapidly punctured by a sterile catheter, bevel up, at a 30-degree angle and parallel to the vein. After entering the subcutaneous space, the needle should be aligned in a parallel fashion with the surface of the extremity and along the long axis of the vein (Fig. 21–10B). This will lessen the chances of perforating the back wall of the vein. A technique favored by many practitioners is to enter at the junction of two veins as a means of ensuring cannulation. Once into the skin, the catheter is advanced until a pop is felt and blood is seen in the flash chamber of the catheter or in the syringe (Fig. 21–10C). The catheter is then advanced over the needle to the hub, and the needle is removed (Fig. 21–10D) with

pressure being placed on the proximal vein over the catheter tip. A syringe can then be connected to the catheter hub for phlebotomy before infusion (Fig. 21–10E). The intravenous tubing is then attached to the hub of the needle or catheter (Fig. 21–10F), the tourniquet is released, and after opening the regulating clamp, fluids are infused at the preselected rate.

Occasionally the catheter system will not advance because of the size or a spasm of the vessel wall. The practitioner can remove the needle and connect the intravenous tubing. The infusion is started, and the catheter is advanced slowly. This technique may be especially valuable in infants or in adults with limited available veins. This procedure is used only when partial cannulation is ensured and the solution is a nonirritant. If a heparin lock is desired, the hub of the catheter is sealed with a heparin lock, and 1 ml (100 units/ml) of heparin sodium or saline is injected to fill the lock (Fig. 21–11). Interestingly, 0.9 per cent sodium chloride has been found to be as effective as heparin and does not carry the minor risks of heparin.[31, 32]

After the indwelling catheter has been placed, an antibiotic ointment should be applied at the site of skin penetration (povidone-iodine or multiple antibiotic ointment such as Neosporin or Bacitracin). An adhesive bandage or other sterile dressing (gauze pads or transparent polyurethane) is commonly placed over the puncture site, and the hub of the catheter and intravenous tubing are then taped securely. Alternatively, a piece of one-fourth-inch tape with the sticky side facing upward may be placed under the hub (Fig. 21–12A) and crossed in front of it making an "X" (Fig. 21–12B). Clear polyurethane dressings allow direct examination of the site for signs of complications, such as thrombophlebitis and extravasation of intravenous fluid, and are used in many centers instead of tape (Fig. 21–13A). However, there is evidence that the plastic dressing has a higher incidence of phlebitis than gauze dressing and despite its convenience may be inferior to gauze.[33] After making a loop, the tubing should be taped down (Fig. 21–13B). This loop helps prevent the tubing or catheter from being dislodged accidentally if it is pulled. In many centers the dressing is dated, and the type and size of the catheter are recorded along with the practitioner's initials. As an additional measure, a short piece of stockinette or elastic netting can be applied over the insertion site and distal tubing to help prevent dislodgment (Fig. 21–14).

Percutaneous Brachial Vein Cannulation

An alternative technique is percutaneous brachial vein cannulation. This technique is recommended for patients who do not have easily accessible peripheral intravenous veins and is successful in 70 per cent of cases.[20, 34] In one study, complications included transitory paresthesias in 18 per cent, brachial artery puncture in 8 per cent, and hematomas in 1.6 per cent.[34] All of these complications were without long-term effects.

The practitioner first locates the brachial artery in the antecubital fossa by palpation. A tourniquet is then applied to the upper arm, and the skin is prepared as noted earlier. The brachial artery is again located, and a puncture site lateral or medial to the pulse is selected. The optimal side of the artery to use varies with the individual. An intravenous catheter attached to a syringe is advanced at a 30- to 45-degree angle to the patient's arm (Fig. 21–15) while the practitioner maintains suction on the syringe. After penetration of the vessel, the assembly is advanced 2 to 3 mm to ensure cannulation. The catheter is then advanced into the vein and secured.[20]

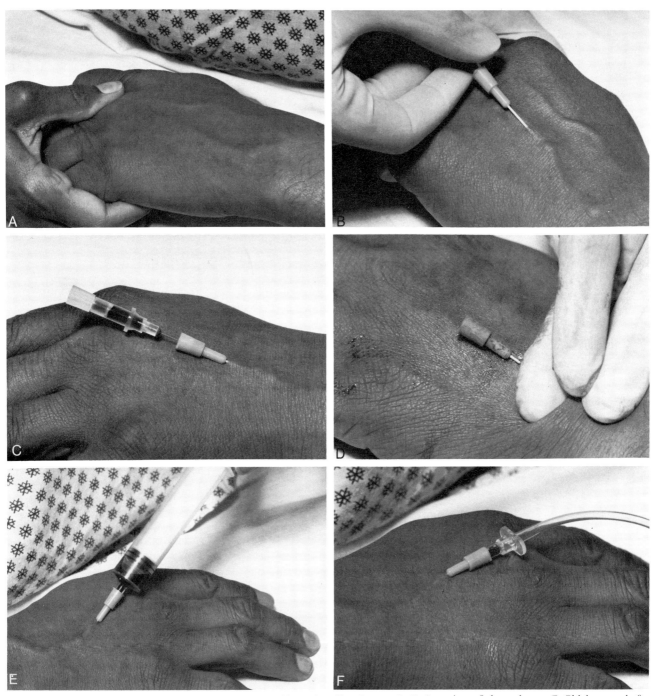

Figure 21–10. Insertion of the catheter. *A,* Grasping the skin and pulling it taut. *B–D,* Insertion of the catheter. *E,* Phlebotomy before attaching the intravenous tubing. *F,* Attaching the intravenous tubing to the catheter.

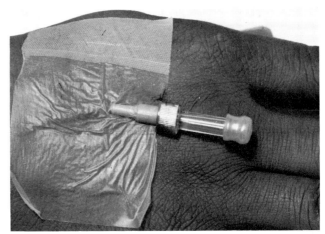

Figure 21–11. Application of a heparin lock.

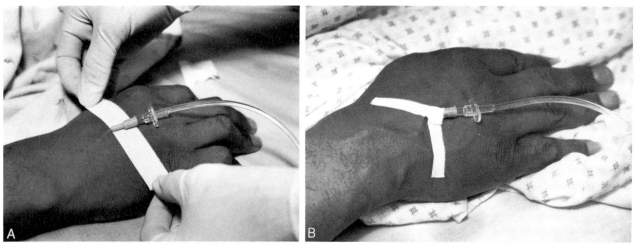

Figure 21–12. Securing the intravenous tubing. *A*, Placing the tape under the hub of the catheter sticky side up. *B*, Crossing the ends of the tape over the hub, forming an "X."

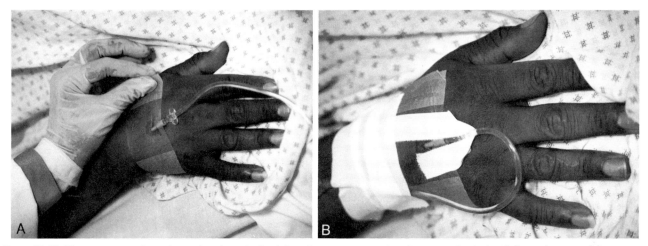

Figure 21–13. Transparent polyurethane dressing. *A*, Applying the transparent dressing over the hub of the catheter and intravenous tubing. *B*, Taping the intravenous tubing securely, making a loop.

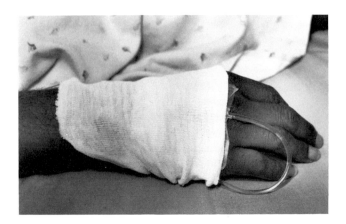

Figure 21–14. Application of a stockinette to prevent dislodgment.

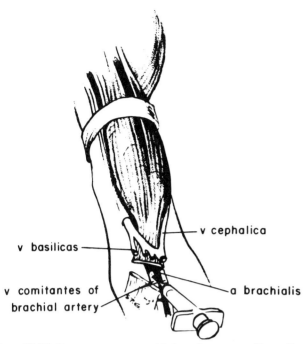

Figure 21–15. Percutaneous antecubital venipuncture. (From Roseman JM: Deep percutaneous antecubital venipuncture: An alternative to surgical cutdown. Am J Surg 146:285, 1983. Reproduced by permission.)

Seldinger Technique

Occasionally a smaller gauge intravenous catheter (e.g., 20 gauge) must be exchanged for one that is larger. This exchange is made using the Seldinger technique (see Chapter 23). This procedure may be necessary when other venous access sites are unavailable or more rapid access is required using a larger bore catheter. Such a catheter exchange set is made by Arrow, Inc. (Product No. RC-09850). The site is prepared by swabbing povidone-iodine solution over the puncture site, indwelling catheter, and intravenous connector assembly. The administration tubing is disconnected from the indwelling catheter, and the flexible end of the guide wire is inserted through the lumen of the catheter. The catheter is then removed over the guide wire. The cutaneous puncture site is enlarged with a number 11 scalpel blade, and a larger catheter is placed over the guide wire. The dilator is removed if a sheath-dilator assembly is used, and the catheter is checked for free-flowing blood. After successful cannulation, the catheter is attached to the intravenous tubing and secured.

DIAGNOSTIC PHLEBOTOMY

Often the health care provider is unable to perform a diagnostic phlebotomy from a site away from the patient's intravenous line. This occurs when the patient has limited veins, multiple intravenous lines, amputated extremities, or relative contraindications such as mastectomy and renal shunts. In these situations, the practitioner must draw blood from the same extremity in which the intravenous line is placed. Phlebotomy can be done while the intravenous line is infusing if it is done *well below the infusion site*.[35, 36] This will not result in dilution of most serum chemistries; however, the serum glucose will be elevated if a glucose-containing solution is infusing.[35] A tourniquet can be placed in between the intravenous and phlebotomy sites for venous distention.[37]

Blood can also be drawn directly from the intravenous catheter after stopping the infusion and waiting for 2 minutes.[35, 37a] Another technique for diagnostic phlebotomy directly from the intravenous line has been described by Isaacson and colleagues.[36] The intravenous line is clamped above the injection port for 1 minute, and a tourniquet is applied above the intravenous site. A 10-ml Vacutainer tube and needle is inserted into the injection port, and 5 ml of blood is collected and discarded (Fig. 21–16). Uncontaminated blood should now be available for collection using the Vacutainer system. Tapping the vein at the catheter tip has been described as a method of restoring the blood flow by breaking away the seal between the vein and the catheter if the flow decreases. After collection of blood, the tourniquet and clamp are removed, and the tubing is flushed with a few milliliters of saline. Glucose and potassium levels may be elevated significantly by this technique if glucose- or potassium-containing solutions are infusing. This potential error should be taken into account when using this technique.

COMPLICATIONS

Complications of intravenous therapy may be local or systemic (Table 21–2). Local complications include extravasation of fluids with local swelling, hematomas, phlebitis, cellulitis, and thrombosis. Hematomas are usually caused when the posterior wall of the vein is punctured during cannulation or after the cannula is removed. Bruising can be minimized in the antecubital fossa after venipuncture by leaving the elbow extended and applying direct pressure over the venipuncture site instead of flexing the elbow.[38] If the vein is not properly cannulated with resultant unrecognized subcutaneous tissue placement and intravenous fluids are begun, the fluids will infuse into the tissues, causing swelling and pain. To avoid this, the practitioner should be careful to observe for blood in the flash chamber on insertion; check the intravenous drip chamber for flow; and check the intravenous site periodically for swelling, pain, and tenderness.

Extravasation of irritants or medications can result in tissue destruction with resultant sloughing, thrombophlebitis, cellulitis, or venous thrombosis. If extravasation occurs, the cannula must be removed and replaced at another site as appropriate.[39] Significant skin sloughing that occasionally

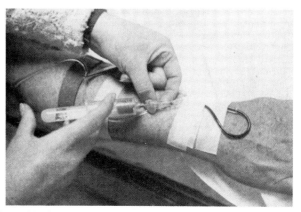

Figure 21–16. Drawing venous blood from an intravenous line. Contrary to the illustration, latex gloves should be worn. (From Isaacson G, Mansfield PF, Kirkland ML: An atraumatic technique for diagnostic phlebotomy. N Engl J Med 313:1478, 1985. Reprinted by permission of the New England Journal of Medicine.)

Table 21–2. Complications from Peripheral Intravenous Lines

Air embolism
Catheter embolism
Cellulitis
Hematoma
Hemorrhage
Infiltration, possibly tissue necrosis
Phlebitis
Sepsis
Thrombophlebitis
Thrombosis
Volume overload

Table 21–4. Examples of Intravenous Solutions with High Osmolalities That May Cause Tissue Necrosis When Extravasation Occurs

Intravenous Injection	mOsm/L
Potassium chloride 2 mEq/ml	4000
Dextrose 50% in water	2525
Calcium chloride 10%	2096
Sodium bicarbonate 8.4%	2000
Crystalline amino acids 4.25%/dextrose 25%	1675
Crystalline amino acids 4.25%/dextrose 10%	925
Dextrose 10% in water	505
Dextrose 5% in sodium chloride 0.45% with potassium chloride 40 mEq/L	486

(Adapted from MacCara ME: Extravasation: A hazard of intravenous therapy. Drug Intell Clin Pharm 17:713, 1983.)

requires skin grafting may occur with the extravasation of certain medications, such as hypertonic solutions, vasopressors, and chemotherapy agents. Occasionally an "antidote" is available, such as in the instance of the extravasation of vasopressors, in which the resulting injury may be ameliorated by the local subcutaneous injection of phentolamine (Regitine) (Tables 21–3, 21–4, and 21–5).

Phlebitis may occur in up to 75 per cent of hospitalized patients.[31] The risk of phlebitis is increased by the infusion of irritant solutions, mechanical irritation from the catheter, infection, prolonged placement, catheter type (steel carries more risk than plastic), and large catheter size.[39, 40, 41] It is generally agreed that catheters should not be left in place for longer than 3 days because of the risk of a mechanical phlebitis.[39, 40] To identify infection or phlebitis, the insertion site should be checked daily for erythema, tenderness, and swelling. If inflammation is found, the intravenous catheter should be discontinued and a new catheter placed in another site. To avoid phlebitis or thrombosis from irritant medications, the medications should be dissolved in a large volume of fluid or administered through a central intravenous line.

Table 21–3. Suggested Antidotes for Drugs Causing Extravasation Injury*

Extravasated Drug	Suggested Antidote†	Dose	Mechanism of Antidote
Aminophylline	Hyaluronidase 15 U/ml‡	5 × 0.2 ml	Increased absorption
Calcium solutions	Hyaluronidase 15 U/ml‡	5 × 0.2 ml	Increased absorption
Carmustine	Sodium bicarbonate 8.4%	5 ml	Chemical deactivation
Dactinomycin	Sodium thiosulfate 10%	4 ml	Decreased DNA binding
	+ sterile water	6 ml	
	Ascorbic acid injection	50 mg	Decreased DNA binding
Daunorubicin	Sodium bicarbonate 8.4%	5 ml	Decreased DNA binding
	+ dexamethasone	4 mg	Decreased inflammation
Dextrose 10%	Hyaluronidase 15 U/ml‡	5 × 0.2 ml	Increased absorption
Dobutamine	Phentolamine	5–10 mg	α-adrenergic blockade
Dopamine	Phentolamine	5–10 mg	α-adrenergic blockade
Doxorubicin	Hydrocortisone sodium succinate	50–200 mg	Decreased inflammation
	+ hydrocortisone cream 1%	Apply twice a day	
	Sodium bicarbonate 8.4%	5 ml	Decreased DNA binding
	+ dexamethasone	4 mg	Decreased inflammation
Epinephrine	Phentolamine	5–10 ml	α-adrenergic blockade
Mechlorethamine	Sodium thiosulfate 10%	4 ml	Rapid alkylation
	+ sterile water	6 ml	
Metaraminol	Phentolamine	5–10 mg	α-adrenergic blockade
Mithramycin	Sodium edetate	150 mg	Decreased DNA binding
Mitomycin	Sodium thiosulfate 10%	4 ml	Direct inactivation
	+ sterile water	6 ml	
Nafcillin	Hyaluronidase 15 U/ml‡	5 × 0.2 ml	Increased absorption
Norepinephrine	Phentolamine	10–15 mg	α-adrenergic blockade
Parenteral nutrition solutions	Hyaluronidase 15 U/ml‡	5 × 0.2 ml	Increased absorption
Potassium solutions	Hyaluronidase 15 U/ml‡	5 × 0.2 ml	Increased absorption
Radiocontrast media	Hyaluronidase 15 U/ml‡	5 × 0.2 ml	Increased absorption
Vasopressin	Guanethidine 10 mg in sodium chloride 0.9% 10 ml + heparin 1000 U		Vasodilation
Vinblastine	Sodium bicarbonate 8.4%	5 ml	Chemical precipitation
	Hyaluronidase + heat	150 U	Increased absorption
Vincristine	Hyaluronidase sodium succinate	25–50 mg/ml extravasate	Decreased inflammation
	Sodium bicarbonate 8.4%	5 ml	Chemical precipitation
	Hyaluronidase + heat	150 U	Increased absorption
Vindesine	Hyaluronidase + heat	Not stated	Increased absorption

*Antidote administered either via the offending intravenous cannula or via multiple subcutaneous injections with the catheter removed.
†Apply ice to extravasated antitumor agents but heat to others.
‡Hyaluronidase: use a 1:10 dilution of a 150-unit vial in saline, giving multiple subcutaneous injections of 0.2 ml each.
(Adapted from MacCara ME: Extravasation: A hazard of intravenous therapy. Drug Intell Clin Pharm 17:713, 1983.)

Table 21–5. Other Drugs Known to Cause Tissue Damage When Extravasated

Hyperalimentation solutions
Renografin-60
Sodium thiopental
Phenytoin
Nafcillin
Tetracycline
Propylene glycol
Ethyl alcohol
Nitroglycerine
Chlordiazepoxide
Diazepam
Colchicine

Heparin and steroids may reduce the incidence of thrombophlebitis and may be useful in appropriate settings.[31, 42–45] Buffering of acidic infusions with sodium bicarbonate may also reduce the incidence of phlebitis.[45–47] Peripheral intravenous lines placed in the prehospital care setting should be replaced when possible because of the high incidence of phlebitis when compared with the incidence associated with intravenous lines placed in the emergency department.[1] Therapy for noninfectious phlebitis includes moist heat, elevation of the extremity, and anti-inflammatory agents.

Thrombosis can occur if intravenous fluids are allowed to run out or if the heparin lock is not flushed periodically. Infiltrated intravenous lines should not be irrigated because of the risk of central embolism.[48] If infiltration occurs, a 3-ml syringe is connected to the cannula using aseptic technique and gentle aspiration. If a bloody return is achieved, discard the return and flush the catheter gently with 3 ml of sterile saline. The infusion is then resumed. If a bloody return is not achieved, flush the catheter gently, as noted earlier. If resistance is felt, the procedure is discontinued, and the catheter should be placed at another site.[49]

Nerve, tendon, or arterial damage may occur if these structures are directly punctured by the needle.[50–52] Additionally, large hematomas may cause nerve damage and arterial insufficiency indirectly by compressing those structures and interrupting the blood supply.

Suppurative phlebitis is a rare complication and can result in sepsis and death.[53] This complication is suspected when phlebitis is associated with fever or purulent drainage.[53] Catheter-related infections of this type can be caused by the absence of aseptic skin preparation before cannula insertion, contaminated intravenous equipment, bacterial colonization, phlebitis, or contaminated infusate.[41] When these infections occur, any purulent drainage should be Gram stained and cultured, and the catheter tip should be sent to the laboratory to be cultured. Treatment includes removal of the catheter, intravenous antibiotics, moist heat, elevation, and venectomy.

Systemic complications include sepsis or embolism due to catheter, air, or clot. Bacteremia and sepsis can occur in 7 per cent of patients with plastic catheters.[54] These infections are generally caused by common organisms such as *Staphylococcus aureus* and *Staphylococcus epidermidis*.[55, 56] As with noninfectious phlebitis, the incidence of catheter colonization and bacteremia increases significantly after 3 days. Hand washing and aseptic technique on insertion (or system manipulation) and changing the intravenous sites every 3 days generally prevents this complication. Topical antibiotics such as povidone-iodine should be applied to the insertion site and may decrease the incidence of infection.[56–59] Despite earlier claims, frequent dressing changes are not necessary to prevent infection. In all cases, the site should be checked at least every 48 hours, and if infection or phlebitis is present, the catheter should be removed and placed at a new site.[39, 40, 54, 58–60]

Air embolism is a rare complication that occurs when air is introduced into the patient's blood stream through the catheter, either through a syringe when improperly used to draw blood or more commonly through intravenous tubing when the container with intravenous fluids has been allowed to empty. Air embolism through an intravenous line is most common when fluids are delivered under pressure. Prevention is the key and is best done by ensuring the absence of air in the intravenous lines, keeping the intravenous container vertical during patient transfers, not allowing the intravenous containers to run dry, filling the drip chamber halfway before moving the patient, and paying careful attention to technique when changing tubing or containers.

If air becomes trapped in the intravenous line, the least invasive method should be used to remove it. Boykoff and colleagues have described six ways to remove air from an intravenous line.[61] If the air is near the top of the intravenous line, it can be removed by holding the air-filled tubing taut and tapping on it with the finger. The air bubbles should rise into the drip chamber. Another technique is to curl a section of the tubing below the bubbles around a pen or syringe. The pen is then rolled upward toward the drip chamber, removing the bubbles.

If the bubbles are in the upper section of tubing, the bag can be lowered and the roller clamp opened to allow backflow of blood into the tubing. This may push the air back into the drip chamber. The "Y" connector can be used as a port from which to aspirate and is especially useful to remove air found directly above the connector. To accomplish this, clamp the tubing below both the "Y" connector and the air. Clean the "Y"-connector port with 70 per cent alcohol and insert a 10-ml syringe with a small-gauge needle into the port and release the roller clamp. Aspirate the fluid and air into the syringe. The syringe is then removed, followed by the clamp. Using a similar technique, one can inject a sterile solution into the "Y" connector, pushing the bubbles into the drip chamber. This technique is especially useful if the drip chamber has collapsed. Finally, the tubing can be disconnected and flushed by opening up the rolling clamp. The intravenous tubing can be reattached directly to the catheter, or a heparin lock can be attached to the catheter and the intravenous tubing reattached using a sterile needle.

The use of inline filters to prevent phlebitis is controversial.[62, 63] Filters are quite effective in removing particulate matter and reducing postinfusion phlebitis but are subject to filter clogging, air locking, and drug binding.[64] Drug binding is especially a problem when the amount of drug injected is small. In most cases, the modern processing of parenteral materials, the frequent changing of intravenous tubing and catheters, and the use of dilute solutions are effective in preventing phlebitis.

CONCLUSIONS

The use of peripheral intravenous access when performed correctly and appropriately is easy, safe, and life-saving with few disadvantages. It can be performed by any health care provider with minimal training within minutes.

REFERENCES

1. Lawrence DW, Lauro AJ: Complications From IV therapy: Results from field-started and emergency department-started IVs compared. Ann Emerg Med 17:314, 1988.
2. Jones SE, Nespert P, Alcoaloumre E: Prehospital intravenous line placement: A prospective study. Ann Emerg Med 18:244, 1989.

3. Cwinn AA, Pons PT, Moore EE: Prehospital advanced life support for critical blunt-trauma victims. Ann Emerg Med 16:399, 1968.
4. McGrew RE: Encyclopedia of Medical History. New York, McGraw-Hill Book Co, 1985, p 33.
5. Dreyfus C: Some Milestones in the History of Hematology. New York, Grune & Stratton, Inc, 1957, p 117.
6. Farr AD: The first human blood transfusion. Med History 24:143, 1980.
7. Schmidt JE: Medical Discoveries Who and When. Springfield, Ill, Charles C Thomas, 1959, p 61.
8. Mettler CC, Mettler FA: History of Medicine. York, Pa, The Blackiston Co, 1947, p 207.
9. Garrison FH: History of Medicine. Philadelphia, WB Saunders Co, 1913, p 268.
10. Ladd M, Schreiner GE: Plastic tubing for intravenous alimentation. JAMA 145:642, 1951.
11. Anderson LH: Venous catheterization for fluid therapy: A technique and results. J Lab Clin Med 36:645, 1950.
12. Standards and Guidelines for Cardiopulmonary Resuscitation (CPR) and Emergency Cardiac Care (ECC). JAMA 255:2905, 1986.
13. Lloyd S: Mast and IV infusion: Do they help in prehospital management? Ann Emerg Med 15:565, 1987.
14. Barson WG, Hedges JR, Nishiyama H, et al: Differences in drug delivery with peripheral and central venous injections: Normal perfusion. Am J Emerg Med 4:1, 1986.
15. Hedges JR, Barsan WB, Doan LA, et al: Central versus peripheral intravenous routes in cardiopulmonary resuscitation. Am J Emerg Med 2:385, 1984.
16. Kuhn GJ, White BC, Swetnam RE, et al: Peripheral vs central circulation times during CPR: A pilot study. Ann Emerg Med 10:417, 1981.
17. Barsan WG, Levy RC, Weir H: Lidocaine levels during CPR: Differences after peripheral venous, central venous, and intracardiac injections. Ann Emerg Med 10:73, 1981.
18. Schwarzman P, Rottman SJ: Prehospital use of heparin locks: A cost-effective method for intravenous access. Am J Emerg Med 5:475, 1987.
19. Center for Disease Control: Recommendations for prevention of HIV transmission in health care settings. MMWR 36:2s, 1987.
20. Roseman JM: Deep, percutaneous antecubital venipuncture: An alternative to surgical cutdown. Am J Surg 146:285, 1983.
21. Mullin MJ, Krohmer JR, McCabe JB: Intravenous fluid flow beneath inflated antishock trousers in a canine hemorrhagic shock model. Ann Emerg Med 16:153, 1987.
22. Newman EV: The technic of venipuncture and intravenous injection. Am J Nurs 52:418, 1952.
23. Hedges JR, Weinshenker E, Dirksing R: Evaluation of venous distension device: Potential aid for intravenous cannulation. Ann Emerg Med 15:540, 1986.
24. Vaksmann G, Rey C, Breviere GM, et al: Nitroglycerine ointment as aid to venous cannulation in children. J Pediatr 111:89, 1987.
25. Roberge RJ, Kelly M, Evans TC, et al: Facilitated intravenous access through local application of nitroglycerin ointment. Ann Emerg Med 16:546, 1987.
26. Amsterdam JT, Hedges JR, Weinshenker E, et al: Evaluation of venous distension device: Phase II: Cannulation of nonemergency patients. Am J Emerg Med 6:224, 1988.
27. Jakobsen C-JB, Grabe N, Damm MD: A trial of povidone-iodine for prevention of contamination of intravenous cannulae. Acta Anaesthesiol Scand 30:447, 1986.
28. Millam DA: How to insert an IV. Am J Nurs 79:1268, 1979.
29. Wrightman MA, Vaughan RW: Comparison of compounds for intradermal anesthesia. Anesthesiology 45:687, 1976.
30. Hallen B, Uppfeldt A: Does lidocaine-prilocaine cream permit painfree insertion of IV catheters in children? Anesthesiology 57:340, 1982.
31. Bass J, Freeman JB, Makarewicz P, et al: Preventing superficial phlebitis during infusion of crystalloid solutions in surgical patients. Can J Surg 28:124, 1985.
32. Hamilton RA, Plis JM, Clay C, et al: Heparin sodium versus 0.9% sodium chloride injection for maintaining patency of indwelling intermittent infusion devices. Clin Pharm. 7:439, 1988.
33. Littenberg B, Thompson L: Gauze versus plastic for peripheral intravenous dressings: Testing a new technology. J Gen Intern Med 2:411, 1987.
34. Kramer DA, Staten-McCormick MD, Freeman SB: Percutaneous brachial

vein catheterization: An alternative site for IV access. Ann Emerg Med 12:247, 1983.
35. Watson KR, O'Kell RT, Joyce JT: Data regarding blood drawing sites in patients receiving intravenous fluids. J Clin Pathol 79:119, 1983.
36. Isaacson G, Mansfield PE, Kirland ML: An atraumatic technique for diagnostic phlebotomy. N Engl J Med 313:1478, 1985.
37. Ong YY, Boykin SF, Barnett RN: You can draw blood from the "IV arm" below the intravenous needle if you put a tourniquet in between. Am J Clin Pathol 72:101, 1979.
37a. Herr RD, Bossart PJ, Blaylock RC, et al: Intravenous catheter aspiration for obtaining basic analytes during intravenous infusion. Ann Emerg Med 19:789, 1990.
38. Dyson D, Bogod D: Minimising bruising in the anticubital fossa after venipuncture. Br Med J 294:1659, 1987.
39. Hershey CO, Tomford JW, McLaren CE, et al: The natural history of intravenous catheter-associated phlebitis. Arch Int Med 144:1373, 1984.
40. Maki DE, Botticelli JT, LeRoy ML, et al: Prospective study of replacing administration sets for intravenous therapy at 48 vs 72 hour intervals. JAMA 258:1777, 1987.
41. Lodge JP, Chisholm EM, Brennan TG, et al: Insertion technique, the key to avoiding infusion phlebitis: A prospective clinical trial. Br J Clin Pract 41:816, 1987.
42. Daniell HW: Heparin in the prevention of phlebitis. JAMA 226:1317, 1973.
43. Schafermeyer RW: Prevention of phlebitis. JAMA 228:695, 1974.
44. Fonkalsrud EW, Pederson BM, Murphy T, et al: Reduction of infusion thrombophlebitis with buffered glucose solutions. Surgery 63:280, 1968.
45. Turco SJ: Hazards associated with parenteral therapy. Am J IV Ther & Clin Nutri 8:9, 1981.
46. Clemetson CAB, Moshfeghi MM: Strange effects of dextrose 5% in water. N Engl J Med 280:332, 1969.
47. Elfving G, Saikku K: Effect of pH on the incidence of infusion thrombophlebitis. Lancet 1:953, 1966.
48. McFarland M: Irrigating clotted IV lines: A potential hazard. Focus on Crit Care 10:45, 1983.
49. Barrus DH, Danek G: Should you irrigate an occluded IV line? Nursing 17:63, 1987.
50. Preston DP, Logigian E: Iatrogenic needle-induced peroneal neuropathy of the foot. Ann Int Med 109:921, 1988.
51. Selander D, Dhuner KG, Lunborg G: Peripheral nerve injury due to injection needles used for regional anesthesia: An experimental study of the acute effects of needle point trauma. Acta Anesthesiol Scand 21:182, 1977.
52. Yuan RT, Cohen MJ: Lateral antebrachial cutaneous nerve injury as a complication of phebotomy. Plast Reconstr Surg 76:299, 1985.
53. Stein JM, Pruitt BA: Suppurative thrombophlebitis. A lethal iatrogenic disease. N Engl J Med 282:1452, 1970.
54. Maki DG, Goldman DA: Infection control in intravenous therapy. Ann Intern Med 79:867, 1973.
55. Stamm WE: Infections related to medical devices. Ann Intern Med 89:764, 1978.
56. Tully JL, Friedland GH, Baldini IM, et al: Complications of intravenous therapy with steel needles and teflon catheters. Am J Med 70:702, 1981.
57. Maki DG, Band JD: A comparative study of polyantibiotic and iodophor ointments in prevention of vascular catheter-related infection. Am J Med 70:739, 1981.
58. Maki DG, Marilyn R: Evaluation of dressing regimens for prevention of infection with peripheral intravenous catheters. JAMA 258:2396, 1987.
59. Richard P, Martin R, Marcoux JA: Protection of indwelling vascular catheters: Incidence of bacterial contamination and catheter-related sepsis. Crit Care Med 13:541, 1985.
60. Center for Disease Control Working Group: Guidelines for prevention of intravenous related infections. Infect Control 3:62, 1981.
61. Boykoff SL, Boxwell AO, Boxwell JJ: Six ways to clear the air from an IV line. Nursing 18:46, 1988.
62. Gurevich I: Are IV inline filters worth the price? Nursing 16(7):42, 1986.
63. Friedland G: Infusion related phlebitis: Is the in-line filter the solution? N Engl J Med 312:113, 1985.
64. Rapp RP, Bivins BA, DeLuca P: Filtration and intravenous therapy. Am J IV Ther & Clin Nutri 7:36, 1980.

Chapter **22**

High-Flow Infusion Techniques

Kenneth V. Iserson

INTRODUCTION

Physicians since earliest history have tried to access the vascular system; early efforts were made to drain blood rather than to infuse blood or fluids. One of the first experiments relating to the infusion of fluids and medications was carried out at Oxford University in 1656. Christopher Wren and Robert Boyle, both later to gain fame in other fields, demonstrated in a series of experiments the efficacy of intravenous injection of various compounds in dogs. They used an animal bladder as an intravenous bag.[1] In 1666, Dr. Richard Lower of Oxford performed the first documented transfusion between dogs.[2] Subsequently, blood transfusions from animals to humans were carried out but quickly lost favor.

In more recent times, Dr. J. Blundell of the United Hospitals of St. Thomas and Guy, is generally given credit for having been the pioneer of human-to-human blood transfusion. His first "success" was in 1829; a mere 240 ml of blood was infused into a woman with postpartum hemorrhage. Blood transfusion was thereafter used only as a last resort for patients dying of postpartum hemorrhage and trauma. The technique was used both during the Crimean War and the American Civil War, but very little blood was normally infused. Furthermore, because two of any three transfusions will randomly be of a suitable blood group, hemolytic reactions were rarely seen. During this period, infusions of not only human blood but also milk and animal blood were attempted regularly.[3] The infusion of blood and fluids did not become an accepted mode of medical practice until World War I, when anticoagulation gave rise to the transfusion of donor blood. Over the past half century, the Russians have had success transfusing blood from deceased victims of myocardial infarction, electrocution, and hypertensive heart disease (but not trauma victims with significant tissue injury).[4]

High-flow infusion techniques date back to the Viet Nam era. Intravenous tubing was surgically placed in veins to facilitate rapid high-volume infusions. A difficulty in describing high-flow techniques is that there has been a progressive increase in what is meant by "high flow." Whereas 1 liter per hour of isotonic fluid was at one time considered a rapid infusion, isotonic fluids can now be placed through peripheral intravenous lines into normovolemic adults with commercially available equipment at rates exceeding 800 milliliters per minute.[5]

"High-volume" infusion of crystalloids may be set arbitrarily at 500 milliliters per minute. Massive transfusion of blood has been defined traditionally as transfusion of an amount at least equal to the recipient's blood volume within a 24-hour period.[6] However, with commercially available equipment the in vitro flow rate of admixed erythrocytes can exceed 800 milliliters per minute through one line.[7] There is one reported case of a patient surviving after having received more than 12 units of blood product per hour for 30 hours.[8]

Importance of Technique. There often is little time in which to restore effective circulating intravascular volume in a patient who has lost the volume acutely, through traumatic or nontraumatic hemorrhage, septic or anaphylactic shock, or other reasons for third-spacing fluid. The principle of fluid resuscitation is to replace the fluid at the same rate and over the same period of time in which it was lost. In patients who have lost this fluid in the space of minutes, as is seen with acute injury and illness, the methods used must, by necessity, be those of high-flow infusion.

Hypovolemic shock also results in an increase in intravascular capacity, requiring much more intravenous fluid to be replaced than the volume of blood lost.[9] It is essential to restore sufficient intravascular volume (preferably with adequate oxygen-carrying capacity) to supply nutrients for cellular metabolism.

The techniques of rapid high-volume infusion that can be used successfully with only one large-bore intravenous line in place gain added significance in situations in which multiple lines can be established only with difficulty, such as in patients in severe shock, patients with a history of intravenous drug abuse, patients with massive swelling, or patients who are obese.[10]

ROLE OF HIGH-FLOW INFUSION

High-flow infusion has the potential to be used by all clinicians who treat critically ill patients. Trauma patients, patients with gastrointestinal bleeding, and those in septic or anaphylactic shock are prime candidates. Physicians, paramedical personnel, and nurses can use these techniques. The techniques involved are relatively easy to learn, and the equipment is both inexpensive and similar enough to that already being used for standard intravenous fluid therapy that there should be no major barriers to using high-flow techniques when they are indicated.

Some of the techniques, especially those using the automated external pressurization devices, reduce the time needed by the personnel to infuse fluid by conventional intravenous techniques (Table 22–1).[11] Paramedical personnel have demonstrated that the larger peripheral intravenous catheters are not much more difficult to place than the 14- or 16-gauge catheters that are routinely recommended. Furthermore, placement of large intravenous catheters en route to the hospital, even if large amounts of fluid cannot be infused, facilitates the institution of rapid fluid replacement on the patient's arrival at the emergency department. In addition, when transit times are long, large amounts of intravenous fluids can be infused en route.[12] It has been suggested, at least for the pediatric population, that performing venous cutdowns, whether to place intravenous tubing or catheters, takes a significant amount of time and skill.[13] Although venous cutdown lines (see Chapters 20 and 24) can be used in conjunction with high-flow infusion systems, cutdown lines are not addressed further in this chapter.

INDICATIONS AND CONTRAINDICATIONS

The primary indication for high-volume infusion is the presence of hypovolemic shock. Although they may be needed only for a short period of time until vital signs stabilize, the techniques involved can be easily maintained on standby in case the patient deteriorates progressively.

Occasionally it is unclear whether the patient is actually in need of high-volume resuscitation. Patients may arrive overloaded with fluid after prolonged transport and high-volume infusions if vital signs are not obtained or not interpreted accurately. In field or hospital situations, if any doubt exists regarding the need for high-volume infusion, short, rapid boluses (10 to 20 ml/kg) of fluid can be given and the patient reassessed.

The goal of shock resuscitation is to maintain organ perfusion until the pathophysiologic state can be reversed. In hemorrhagic shock, control of ongoing blood loss is essential. When the blood loss is internal, excessive volume resuscitation accompanied by elevation of blood pressure may exacerbate the blood loss preoperatively. The classic clinical example of this phenomenon is the patient with a leaking aortic aneurysm. Hence volume resuscitation must be closely monitored.

Rapid high-volume infusion is relatively contraindicated in cases of spinal shock following trauma. Because the

Table 22–1. Flow Rates Through Common Intravenous Catheters

Catheter (g = gauge)	Tubing*	Flow Rate Saline—Gravity (ml/min)	Flow Rate Saline—300 mm Hg Pressure (ml/min)	Flow Rate Dilute Red Blood Cells —Gravity (ml/min)
Deseret angiocatheter				
14-g; 2-inch	3 mm	93	301	300
16-g; 2-inch	3 mm	75	248	200
16-g; 5¼-inch	3 mm	64	199	
18-g; 1¼-inch	3 mm	55	164	
Desilets-Hoffman sheath				
16-g; 3½-inch	3 mm	77	228	
Intramedicut				
16-g; 8-inch	3 mm	31	97	
18-g; 8-inch	3 mm	13	51	
Argyle Medicut				
14-g; 2-inch	3 mm	92	319	
16-g; 2-inch	3 mm	81	280	200
18-g; 2-inch	3 mm	62	214	
Travenol				
14-g; 2-inch	3 mm	134	429	
14-g; 2-inch	Fenwal	211	500	
16-g; 2-inch	3 mm	88	270	
16-g; 2-inch	Fenwal	110	333	
UMI				
8 French; 4¼-inch	3 mm	171	545	
8 French; 4¼-inch	Fenwal	387	1263	
Vygon				
12-g; 3¼-inch	3 mm	169	522	
12-g; 3¼-inch	Fenwal	333	889	
16-g; 2-inch	3 mm	102	324	
16-g; 2-inch	Fenwal	136	369	

*The internal diameter of both the Fenwal Y-type Blood-Solution Set and Delmed Y-Blood Solution Set is 3 mm (9 French); the Fenwal large-bore blood tubing has an internal diameter of 3.66 mm (11 French). Catheter lengths are for that portion of the catheter designed to be inside the patient.
(Adapted from references 5, 19, and 20.)

hypotension of spinal shock is not due to hypovolemia, hemodynamics will not improve as a result of large amounts of fluid. Rather, the fluid will often collect in the patients' lungs and lead to pulmonary edema. Patients who can be recognized as having hypotension that is due to a pericardial tamponade may do well with short, rapid boluses of fluid until a pericardiocentesis or definitive repair is performed, but large volumes of fluid do not appear to be beneficial. Patients whose hypotension is not due to hypovolemia (e.g., those who experience myocardial contusion, tension pneumothorax) can be harmed severely by the fluid overload that would accompany a rapid, high-volume infusion.

EQUIPMENT

The key to performing effective rapid infusion therapy and obtaining the proper equipment is to consider the entire infusion system, rather than just the individual parts. Each part of the infusion system must be able to meet the desired flow and time requirements (see Table 22–1).

Unfortunately, *manufacturers' claims often cannot be relied on*, especially in this unregulated portion of the medical equipment field.[14, 15] Likewise, intravenous catheters with exactly the same "measurements" deliver fluid at surprisingly different rates. (Note from Table 22–1 that three different manufacturers make 14-gauge 2-inch catheters, and the flow rates by gravity range from 93 to 134 milliliters per minute.) Therefore, once a system is set up, it should be tested to ensure that the system and all components perform as advertised.

Catheter. Fluid flow through a tube, as in the case of an intravenous catheter, generally behaves in a fashion described by Poiseuille's law:

$$\text{Rate of Flow} = \frac{\pi \times (\text{catheter radius})^4 \times \text{pressure gradient}}{8 \times \text{dynamic fluid viscosity}}$$

With all elements of a high-flow infusion system, it is the *internal diameter* (ID) that is overwhelmingly important in determining flow rates. Internal diameter affects flow rates to the *fourth* power, whereas all other elements affect flow only to a small extent. Therefore, to obtain a maximal flow rate, the constant consideration must be the ID of each piece of the system.

Although a difference in IDs of intravenous catheters could be inferred from the differing flow rates in previous studies dating back to 1973, it was not until 1987 that actual measurements were made of intravenous catheters sold for medical use.[14, 16–18] Sizable discrepancies were discovered between the labeled size (outside diameter, OD) of the catheters and their true OD. More important, sizable discrepancies also were found between the ID of catheters supposedly of the same size and flow rates.[14] This finding suggests that interpreting the results of some of the studies that measure comparative flow rates in intravenous catheters may be difficult.[19]

Although some very large experimental catheters, exceeding 4.5 mm (14 French) ID, have been developed and used successfully for human infusions,[20–22] large, commercially available percutaneous intravenous catheters have a maximum ID of 2.16 mm (12 gauge, Vygon Mosquito 123) or 3 mm (9 French).[14] The French-sized Swan-Ganz introducers are not tapered and have a very thin-walled construction. Because they are designed to accommodate the size catheter for which they are labeled, the labeled size is usually their ID.

Since the pressure gradient in a tube is inversely proportional to its length, Poiseuille's law indicates that catheter length affects the rate of fluid flow only minimally. This is true even with longer catheters; the inside diameter is much more important than the length. Catheter length is significant primarily because the catheter must be long enough to mechanically remain in place within the vascular space.

Theoretically, an intravenous catheter for rapid fluid replacement should have a maximum ID maintained throughout its length. This means not only that the main portion of the catheter should have a maximum ID consistent with structural stability, but also that the reduction in internal diameter from narrowing at the catheter tip should be minimal. Some catheters lose more than 36 per cent of their ID in this taper. Although a minimal taper is desirable, the overall shape of the catheter must also be consistent with rapid entry into the vascular system.[14]

A major exception to using the catheter ID to extrapolate the resultant flow rate is when an intraosseous approach is chosen. Even though large ID catheters are placed, studies have not shown a flow rate adequate for hypovolemic resuscitation in adults and larger children. The resistance to flow out of the intraosseous space appears to limit rapid, high-volume infusion at this site.

Intravenous Tubing and Extension Tubing. Poiseuille's law applies to intravenous tubing as well as to indwelling catheters. Most standard intravenous tubing for blood transfusions has an ID of 3 mm.[5, 23] Larger tubing is now available, some with an ID of 3.66 mm (11 French) to 4.0 mm. It has been amply demonstrated that the inclusion of even a short segment of the 3-mm tubing in an infusion system markedly diminishes flow rates.[23] A more recent development is the Medex Hi-Flow Trauma Quad system tubing, with an ID of 5.7 mm. Although this large-bore tubing can sustain flows of more than 1 liter per minute of admixed blood, it essentially ceases to function because of obstruction of its own filter after three units of packed cells have been infused. This defect can be overcome successfully by using an in-line Pall filter.[6]

What is immediately apparent is that even the standard-sized blood tubing is as large or larger than the ID of most commonly used catheters. Why, therefore, use larger sized tubing? Using even the 3.66 mm tubing can increase flow rates of saline from 70 per cent (12-gauge catheter, pressurized) to 126 per cent (8 French catheter, no pressure) over rates with the 3-mm tubing.[5] A comparable difference would be expected with blood products.

Even if a large-diameter intravenous tubing is used, adding a smaller sized extension tubing can reduce the ID of the system enough to make this element the rate-limiting step, negating the benefit of the other components of the system. If a large ID intravenous tubing is used, it is essential that similarly sized extension tubing also be available.

Even when crystalloid is infused, all intravenous tubing must be of the "Y" type. That is, there must be at least two attachments for intravenous bags. This allows one bag to be changed while the other is infusing. At the flow rates achieved by rapid high-flow systems, not having a Y-type tubing will normally *cut the overall system infusion rate by at least half*. Y-type tubing is also necessary to admix blood with warmed saline as described later.

Solution Container. All fluids used in the resuscitation of hypovolemic patients are now available in compressible, soft plastic containers. The more rigid plastic and glass containers should be avoided, because they are much more difficult to externally pressurize in the former case and present the danger of breaking in the latter case. To conserve the number of bag changes that personnel have to perform, a time-consuming element of infusion, liter bags are preferable to smaller sizes for the adult patient. Blood, generally in the form of "packed" red blood cells, is packaged in standard plastic containers that can accommodate up to 600 ml of fluid (see "Blood Warmers").

External Pressure Device. *Pressurizing* the fluid that is being infused intravenously increases the fluid flow rate dramatically.[5, 10] There are two main methods by which pressure can be applied to intravenous fluids. The first, and least practical in an emergency situation, is pumping the fluid through a form of bypass machine. This technique has significant drawbacks, including difficult vascular access, the necessity for a skilled technician to run the machine, and the significant possibility of air embolism.

The most practical means of adding pressure to a high-flow intravenous system is through the use of external pressure devices (Fig. 22–1). The standard maximal external pressure exerted by these units is 300 mm Hg. Until recently, most centers were still using pneumatic pressurization devices, with the inflow and outflow of air controlled by a screw-down mechanism—the blood pump.[24] This device is not only cumbersome, but also unreliable in either maintaining pressure or releasing pressure so that a new bag of fluid or blood can be placed.[11] More recently, somewhat less expensive pressure bags with three-way stopcocks have become available. These appear to be easier to use but still have the problem of not maintaining a constant pressure on the fluid while the bag empties. Some pressure bags (Infusable, Biomedical Dynamics Corp., Minneapolis, Minn.) are considered to be disposable, even though many uses can be obtained from each unit.

Other more elaborate external pressure devices have also been advocated. Initially they were the blood pumps attached to a constant air pressure source.[25] More recently they not only have been powered by wall air, but also have been contained in a rigid metal or plastic container for safety, more rapid access, and extremely rapid pressurization and depressurization (Infuser-1; and Alton Dean Infuser, North Salt Lake City, Utah). They have the advantage of maintaining a constant pressure on the fluid container during emptying. It has been shown that using the air pressure devices dramatically decreases the time needed for changing bags during infusions (Table 22–2), thus enhancing the effective flow rate during high-volume infusion situations.[11, 26]

Some initial work has been done with devices exerting a higher external pressure on the fluid containers. Pressures of 600 mm Hg have been obtained. As expected from Poiseuille's law, the larger the ID of the tubing and catheters in the system, the greater the increase in flow rate achieved with increased pressure. Although there was no significant damage noted to the equipment, it is unclear whether blood cells may have been damaged.[10]

Blood Warmers. In nearly all high-volume infusions, blood products are administered. This poses the problem of infusing blood products at or around 4° C, the temperature at which blood is stored, or using a blood warmer in the system. Rapid infusion of cold blood is associated with an increase in ventricular fibrillation and cardiac arrest,[27, 28] and hypothermia is a major, yet often unappreciated, problem during the resuscitation of seriously ill patients, particularly those who require multiple blood transfusions. Several blood warmers that are commonly available significantly slow the flow rates of high-flow systems.[28, 29] Some blood warmers

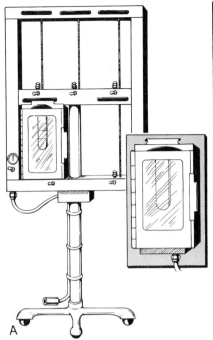

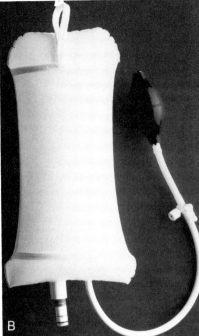

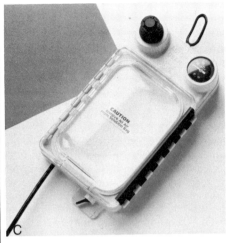

Figure 22–1. Three types of external pressure devices. *A,* Infuser-1. (As modified in Iserson KV, Reeter A, Woods W, Criss E: Pressurization of IV bags: A new configuration and evaluation for use. J Emerg Med 3:89, 1985.) *B,* Infusable (Biomedical Dynamics Corp., Minneapolis, Minn.). *C,* Alton Dean Infuser (North Salt Lake City, Utah).

have been developed that have more rapid flow rates, but hese are not readily available.[30] One proposed method for keeping flow rates high while warming blood to approximately body temperature is to dilute the blood with an equivalent volume of 70° C saline.[31–33] This technique, because of the rapid equilibration of temperatures between the two mixing fluids, does no damage to the erythrocytes. Of course, because of the resulting warm temperature of the blood (approximately 37° C), it must be infused rapidly. In addition, *the 70° C saline must never be used for direct infusion* (Fig. 22–2).

One commercial system combines warmed saline at 45° C with cold blood in a single pressurized mixing bag and delivers the admixed solution through a high-flow infusion set (Sangui-Stat System, Ackard Laboratories, Cranford, NJ). This system is designed specifically for the rapid warming and transfusion of packed erythrocytes in the emergency department (Fig. 22–3).

Fluids. Although a great deal of experimental work has been done to compare lactated Ringer solution and normal saline in hypovolemic resuscitation, the solutions seem to be equivalent in clinical settings. Since World War II, there has been a resurgence of interest in resuscitation through the use of small amounts of *hypertonic* saline rather than larger amounts of isotonic saline or blood products. The success of hypertonic saline in the resuscitation of hypovolemic shock is promising but remains to be determined and continues to be experimental.[34, 35]

When transfusing cellular blood products rapidly, it is essential not only to warm the fluid but also to dilute it adequately to reduce the incidence of erythrocyte hemolysis. Cellular destruction in blood flow systems is directly proportional to the magnitude of shear stress and cellular-solid surface interactions. These are affected directly by hematocrit and plasma protein concentration. The more the dilution of the blood product, the less hemolysis.[36]

New Equipment. Although a number of newer pieces of equipment have been developed to assist in high-volume infusion, they all are limited by the same essential principle—that the minimum ID of the system must be as large as possible.[20–22] Equipment that only offers increased pressure, decreased set-up and takedown time, or decreased system length of flow will do little to improve rapid fluid delivery if the system's ID is not sufficiently large.

Inadequate equipment that restricts fluid flow at some part of the system or has excessive set-up delays will fail to

Table 22–2. *Mean Time (Minutes:Seconds) for Two Fluid Systems*

Systems	Pump-up/Drain (first liter)	Take Down/ Set Up	Pump-up/Drain (second liter)	Total Time
System 1: 3.66-mm ID tubing Pneumatic pressure device 12 gauge (0.0839-inch maximum ID) intravenous catheter	1:16	0:22	1:10	2:48
System 2: 3.0-mm ID tubing Hand-pumped pressure device 14-gauge (0.0563-inch maximum ID) intravenous catheter	4:19	1:37	3:37	9:33
p values: <0.0005		<0.0005	<0.0005	<0.0005

ID, internal diameter.
(Adapted from Iserson KV, Criss E: Combined effect of catheter and tubing size on fluid flow. Am J Emerg Med 4:238, 1986; and Iserson KV, Newberg CE, Clemans SB: Non-standardization of the manufacture of intravenous catheters. J Clin Engineering 12:367, 1987.)

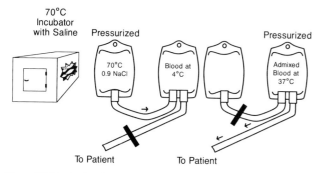

Figure 22–2. *(1)* During all handling of blood, standard universal precaution procedures should be followed.

(2) Remove a 250-ml bag of normal saline from the 70° C incubator. Check the bag for clarity, discoloration, particulates, obvious decreased volume, and cracking of the outer wrapper. Do not use if problems are found.

(3) Check the thermometer of the incubator to ensure that the incubator temperature is between 65° and 75° C. Do not use if above 75° C.

(4) "Spike" the PRBC unit from the blood bank with one end of a Fenwal plasma transfer set (#4C2243). Spike the other end of the transfer set into the 70°C 250-ml normal saline bag. Open the clamp, raise the saline bag above the level of the PRBC bag, and manually squeeze (or use external pressure bag or other external pressure device) the saline into the PRBC bag. (PRBC, packed red blood cells.)

(5) A towel or pot-holder-type kitchen glove may be used to squeeze the 70° C saline bag, if desired.

(6) After all of the 70° C saline is transferred into the PRBC bag, tightly close the clamp on the transfer set tubing.

(7) Do not remove the transfer set tubing spike from the PRBC bag (to prevent contamination). The now-empty saline bag may be removed from the other end of the transfer set and discarded, or simply left in place.

(8) On the patient's side, spike the unused part of the PRBC bag (now admixed with 70° C saline) with one limb of the Y-type blood set already attached to the patient. The admixture temperature will be approximately 37° C.

(9) Close the clamp on the other limb of the Y set, which has been infusing standard warm or room-temperature normal saline in to the patient.

(10) If the blood is to be rapidly infused, pressurize the external pressure bag or device.

(11) Open the clamp on the PRBC admixture bag to begin infusion of 37° C PRBC into the patient.

(12) Additional units of warm-admixed PRBC may be prepared using the same technique. Remove the empty admixed PRBC bag from the Y set, after closing its clamp and replace with the second unit. Open the clamp and begin infusing the second unit.

(13) Infuse the blood into the patient as rapidly as necessary.

(14) For each unit of warm-admixed PRBC infused, document in the patient's record that the patient received "1 U of PRBC admixed with 250 ml of normal saline at an infusion temperature of approximately 37° C," and include start and stop times of infusion and the name of the person preparing and administering the infusion. (Illustration and text from Iserson KV, Knaut MA, Anhalt D: Rapid admixture blood warming: Technical advances. Crit Care Med 18:1138, 1990. © 1990, Williams & Wilkins, Baltimore.)

Following admixture, the infused blood will be between 35 and 40° C. Many studies have been performed that demonstrate the safety of this procedure. It is designed to avoid the problems of hypothermia with multiple transfusions. *Note:* Keep the blood bag hanging when adding saline.

If the blood is admixed, it must be infused or wasted to avoid contamination.

There is no need to mix the blood manually or shake the bag.

Do not directly infuse 70° C saline into patients!

deliver large amounts of fluid rapidly. Alternative equipment, such as a pump for internal pressurization of the fluid system rather than an external pressure device, introduces an unnecessary major risk—that of air embolus.

PROCEDURE

Usually the most difficult parts of initiating a rapid, high-volume fluid system are overcoming the inadequate inservice training of physician and nursing personnel, keeping the components on hand, and having these components set up conveniently for use. Although the set-up and ease of availability of the components vary from hospital to hospital, a basic principle is to have all equipment located conveniently around the patient and in reach of the practitioners. When this obstacle has been overcome, the next difficulty is establishing intravenous access with a large-bore catheter. Even if initially only a smaller catheter can be placed, a larger catheter can be inserted through this access using the Seldinger technique (see Chapter 23).[37] Ideally a 10- or 12-gauge, 9 French, or larger catheter is placed in either a peripheral or femoral vein. Central veins about the neck should be avoided if possible, because all of the complications inherent in errant central lines are magnified many times with the larger catheters and the more rapid flow rates.

Once the catheters are in place, large-bore Y-type tubing, no less than 3.66-mm ID should be attached. If an extension tube is needed, it must have at least as large an ID as the rest of the tubing. Prewarmed 1-liter bags of crystalloid solutions (ideally at 37° C) should be initially hung in an external pressure device. Either an easily used manually operated pressure bag (Infusable, Biomedical Dynamics Corp, Minneapolis, Minn.) or a wall-operated pneumatic device (Infuser-1; and Alton Dean Infuser, North Salt Lake City, Utah) is acceptable.

When erythrocyte units are available, they should be diluted 1:1 with 70° C preheated 0.9 saline (*Note:* do not use lactated Ringer solution). Dilution should use a special system (e.g., Fenwal Plasma Transfer Set, #4C2243, Fenwal Laboratories, Deerfield, Ill.) to guarantee that the hot saline will *not* be directly infused into the patient.[38] Many types of laboratory incubators can be used for preheating the saline. A constant temperature monitor should be available to ensure adequate heating. According to tests by the manufacturer, bacterial growth within the unopened heated saline units should not occur for at least 2 weeks if the units are left in their overwrap packaging.[33] When the 1:1 dilution is used, the admixed blood is then at approximately 37° C and ready for rapid infusion. Mistakes may be minimized by preheating only one particular-sized bag (250 ml is appropriate and usually the right amount for diluting the erythrocyte unit) and premarking the bags for dilution with bright orange or yellow tape. Heated saline bags should be discarded if not used after 2 weeks to avoid chemical leaching from prolonged heating.[38]

If a rapid infusion system is used in one part of an institution, it is essential not only that other interactive units, such as the operating room and intensive care unit, be made aware of it, but also that any equipment these other units use in managing critical care patients be compatible with that used for rapid infusion.

Vascular Access Sites Affecting Flow in Vivo. The limitation to placing large venous catheters in an adult or a larger child is generally the skill of the operator. Any large peripheral or central vein is large enough to accommodate, with the natural distention that occurs, very large catheters. *There is virtually no obstruction to flow from any venous site.*[21]

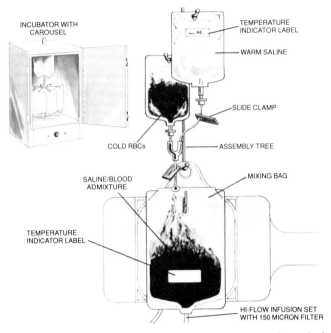

Figure 22–3. The concept of adding warmed saline to cold packed red blood cells to facilitate the rapid infusion of blood is illustrated by the FDA-approved Sangui-Stat system (Ackrad Laboratories, Cranford, New Jersey). With this system, saline at 45° C is mixed with banked blood in a separate collection bag, and the warmed solution is delivered under pressure via a high-flow infusion set (infusion rate of 400 to 500 ml/minute). The final temperature of the mixture is about 33° C. (Courtesy of Ackrad Laboratories.)

However, placing catheters in veins distal to an area of vascular injury, such as in a lower extremity in a patient with abdominal bleeding, may limit the usefulness of the fluid resuscitation.

Intravascular Volume Affecting Flow in Vivo. It does not appear that intravascular volume limits the flow rate of rapid replacement of intravenous fluid significantly. Although the estimated back pressure is 15 to 18 mm Hg in supine, normovolemic males, this seems only to decrease the flow rate from that measured in vitro by a negligible 5 to 6 per cent.[5]

COMPLICATIONS

The complications of high-volume infusion usually are related to one of three problems. The catheter may be in the wrong location so that large amounts of fluid enter into a closed space, such as the chest or pericardium, with untoward effect. Rather than being resuscitated by the rapid fluid infusion, the patient will deteriorate as a result of and in proportion to the fluid infused. This complication is one excellent reason not to use the central veins around the neck or shoulders for high-volume infusions.[21] The second problem occurs when too much fluid is inadvertently and unknowingly infused.

Unfortunately, there is no totally satisfactory way of monitoring intravascular volume in the acute setting and excessive fluid resuscitation is surprisingly easy. Close attention to vital signs, pulmonary status, and urine output is important. Although occasionally it has been suggested otherwise, in most centers techniques such as central venous pressure monitoring and Swan-Ganz catheter monitoring have either proved inadequate or too unwieldy to be used effectively in the acute setting.[39] Additionally, there are the

problems related to massive blood transfusions. The major and most immediate problems relate to hypothermia (with resultant dysrhythmias) and coagulopathies. These may be mostly ameliorated with the use of warmed blood and the timely use of fresh frozen plasma (see Chapter 33).

The complication rate of high-volume fluid therapy in patients with severe hypovolemia is unknown. The patient's condition—hypovolemic shock—usually implies a poor outcome from the start. Limited information on massive, rapid fluid boluses in otherwise healthy animals suggests that there are few problems that do not resolve once the infusion is stopped.[40] In the injured patient, however, cellular changes accompanying injury (e.g., pulmonary, neurologic) may not allow reversal of fluid-induced changes as easily.

If a patient is found to have been overloaded with fluid, normal techniques to reduce the amount of fluid such as stopping the infusion, using diuretics, and—if necessary—initiating cardiovascular or respiratory support should be instituted.

INTERPRETATION

Success with rapid intravenous infusion techniques is often fleeting. Often the goal is only to buy enough time to institute definitive operative intervention. Interpretation of one's fluid resuscitation, at least at the present time, is largely clinical. Evaluation of the entire clinical picture, including vital signs, urine output, peripheral perfusion, and mentation, is necessary to determine the success of infusion therapy. Occasionally, of course, when a thoracotomy has been done, direct observation of the central circulation allows an accurate determination of the state of vascular filling.

With rapid infusion consisting primarily of crystalloid solutions, patients sometimes have enough blood loss to leak "water" from bleeding sites. This is essentially a visual hematocrit and indicates a nearly hopeless prognosis. Otherwise, hematocrit measurements are virtually useless in assessing the intravascular status of unstable patients. Some patients, especially younger ones, continue to have enough vascular tone to appear to stabilize after an initial large bolus of fluid. These patients must be very carefully observed and evaluated, because they can deteriorate again without warning.

CONCLUSION

Success with rapid, high-flow intravenous infusion does not guarantee a successful outcome for the patient. Often, the severity of injury precludes a successful outcome despite adequate volume replacement. In the emergency department or prehospital care setting, it is often impossible to assess immediately the severity of major injuries. Therefore, rapid, high-flow infusion therapy should be begun, in conjunction with other therapies, to maximize each shock patient's chance at survival.

High-volume infusion techniques allow more seriously injured trauma patients to get to the operating theater. These patients challenge the current technical capabilities of trauma surgeons. But as more of these patients arrive in the operating arena with some chance of survival, technical advances are expected to save ever more seriously injured patients. Finally, a readily usable, on-line method for measuring intravascular volume during infusion needs to be developed to complement rapid, high-volume infusion techniques; such a development represents an area of active ongoing investigation.

REFERENCES

1. Sprat T: The History of the Royal Society of London, for the Improving of Natural Knowledge. Cited in Mollison PL, Engelfriet CP, Contreras

M: Blood Transfusion in Clinical Medicine. 8th ed. Oxford, Blackwell Scientific, 1987.

2. Keynes G: The history of blood transfusion. In Keynes G: Blood Transfusion. Bristol, John Wright and Sons, 1949.

3. Rutman RC, Miller WV: Transfusion Therapy: Principles and Procedures. 2nd ed. Rockville, Md., Aspen Systems, 1985, pp 5–6.

4. Tarasov MM: Cadaveric blood transfusion. Ann NY Acad Science 87:512, 1960.

5. Iserson KV, Reeter AK, Criss E: Comparison of flow rates for standard and large-bore blood tubing. West J Med 143:183, 1985.

6. Reiner A, Kickler TS, Bell WR: How to administer massive transfusions effectively. J Crit Illness 2:15, 1987.

7. Krivchenia A, Knauf MA, Iserson KV: Flow characteristics of admixed erythrocytes through medex tubing with a Pall filter. J Emerg Med 6:269, 1988.

8. Brotman S, Lamonica C, Cowley RA: Massive transfusion without major complications after trauma. Am J Emerg Med 4:514, 1986.

9. Hardaway RM: Expansion of the intravascular space in severe shock. Am J Surg 142:258, 1981.

10. Mateer JR, Thompson BM, Tucker J, et al: Effect of high infusion pressure and large bore tubing on intravenous flow rates. Am J Emerg Med 3:187, 1985.

11. Iserson KV, Criss E: Combined effect of catheter and tubing size on fluid flow. Am J Emerg Med 4:238, 1986.

12. Gervin AS: Peripheral large-bore IV lines by prehospital providers (abstract). Ann Emerg Med 17:880, 1988.

13. Iserson KV, Criss EA: Pediatric venous cutdowns: Utility in emergency situations. Pediatr Emerg Care 2:231, 1986.

14. Iserson KV, Newberg CE, Clemans SB: Non-standardization of the manufacture of intravenous catheters. J Clin Engineering 12:367, 1987.

15. Iserson KV: Intravenous equipment—Caveat emptor. J Emerg Med 7:201, 1989.

16. Dailey RH: Flow rate variance of commonly used IV units. JACEP 2:341, 1973.

17. Graber D, Dailey RH: Catheter flow rates updated. JACEP 6:518, 1977.

18. Dula DJ, Muller HA, Donovan JW: Flow rate variance of commonly used IV infusion techniques. J Trauma 21:480, 1981.

19. Hodge D, Fleisher G: Pediatric catheter flow rates. Am J Emerg Med 3:403, 1985.

20. Iserson KV, Reeter AK: Rapid fluid replacement: A new methodology. Ann Emerg Med 13:97, 1984.

21. Iserson KV, Reeter AK: Rapid fluid replacement for severe hypovolemia—human subject trials. West J Med 146:313, 1987.

22. Reeter AK, Iserson KV: A new device for rapid fluid replacement. J Clin Engineering 9:37, 1984.

23. Cross GD: Evaluation of 3-mm diameter intravenous tubing for the rapid infusion of fluids. Arch Emerg Med 4:173, 1987.

24. Ready LB: An aid to rapid intravenous infusion. Anesth Analg 58:155, 1979.

25. Houghton IT: A constant pressure infusor. Anaesthesia 31:73, 1976.

26. Iserson KV, Reeter A, Woods W, Criss E: Pressurization of IV bags: A new configuration and evaluation for use. J Emerg Med 3:89, 1985.

27. Boyan CP: Cold or warmed blood for massive transfusion. Am Surg 160:282, 1964.

28. Russell WJ: A review of blood warmers for massive transfusion. Anaesth Intens Care 2:109, 1974.

29. Millikan JS, Cain TL, Hansbrough J: Rapid volume replacement for hypovolemic shock: A comparison of techniques and equipment. J Trauma 24:428, 1984.

30. Fried SJ, Bhagwan CT, Zeeb P: Normothermic rapid volume replacement for hypovolemic shock: An in vivo and in vitro study utilizing a new technique. J Trauma 26:183, 1986.

31. Wilson EB, Knauf MA, Donohoe K, Iserson KV: Red blood cell survival following admixture with heated saline: Evaluation of a new blood warming method for rapid transfusion. J Trauma 28:1274, 1988.

32. Wilson EB, Iserson KV: Admixture bloodwarming: A technique for rapid warming of erythrocytes. Ann Emerg Med 16:413, 1987.

33. Wilson EB, Iserson KV, Knauf MA: Red cell tolerance of admixture with heated saline. Transfusion 28:170, 1988.

34. Maningas PA, DeGuzman LR, Tilman FJ, et al: Small-volume infusion of 7.5% NaCl in 6% dextran 70 for the treatment of severe hemorrhagic shock in swine. Ann Emerg Med 15:1131, 1986.

35. Holcroft JW, Vassar MJ, Turner JE, et al: 3% NaCl and 7.5% NaCl/Dextran 70 in the resuscitation of severely injured patients. Ann Surg 206:279, 1987.

36. Calkins JM, Vaughan RW, Cork RC, et al: Effect of dilution, pressure, and apparatus on hemolysis and flow rate in transfusions of packed erythrocytes. Anesth Analg 61:776, 1982.

37. Seldinger SL: Catheter replacement of the needle in percutaneous arteriography. Acta Radiol 39:368, 1953.

38. Iserson KV, Knauf MA, Anhalt D: Rapid admixture blood warming: Technical advances. Crit Care Med 18:1138, 1990.

39. Dailey RH: "Code red" protocol for resuscitation of the exsanguinated patient. J Emerg Med 2:373, 1985.

40. Cornelius LM, Finco DR, Culver DH: Physiologic effects of rapid infusion of Ringer's lactate solution into dogs. Am J Vet Res 39:1185, 1978.

Chapter 23

Seldinger (Guide Wire) Technique for Venous Access

Alfred D. Sacchetti

INTRODUCTION

The expedient placement of large-bore or central venous catheters can be a difficult task, especially in the unstable, critically ill patient. Frequently the physician is faced with the problem of being unable to locate a suitable vein or, more frustrating, being unable to cannulate a vein that is found. The Seldinger or guide wire technique of catheter introduction may be the optimal solution to difficult vascular access problems in the emergency department.

There are four basic intravenous access systems: the metal needle system, the catheter-over-the-needle system, the catheter-through-the-needle system, and the Seldinger wire guide technique. Each of these approaches has its own advantages and disadvantages (Fig. 23–1).

Metal (butterfly) needles are of value in *transient* vascular access in pediatric patients or immunosuppressed patients. Their major use is in obtaining blood samples rather than in serving as long-term indwelling lines, because even in the best of circumstances these needles are unstable and prone to dislodgment or infiltration.

Catheter-over-the-needle devices (e.g., Angiocath, Jelco) are usually the first choice for vascular access because of their ease of placement, stability, and size options. Catheters as small as 24 gauge to as large as 12 gauge are readily available and represent the quickest, most stable intravenous routes in the emergency department patient. These systems can be used for central lines or for peripheral venous access but have two disadvantages. The first relates to the design of the system. Successful vein entry is signaled by a flash of blood in the proximal chamber of the needle. However, it is possible for the needle to enter the vessel and a blood return to be observed while the catheter is still outside the vessel (Fig. 23–2). If the needle is removed at this point, the catheter will remain outside the vein, resulting in an unsuccessful cannulation. The proper technique is to advance the catheter off the needle when a blood return is observed. Even with this approach, however, the catheter may push the vein ahead of it and still not enter the lumen. The second drawback to this system is that the size of the needle relates directly to the size of the catheter. A 14-gauge catheter requires approximately a 14-gauge needle. This is of little concern in peripheral veins but is a major consideration when multiple insertions are made in a search for hidden vessels in the chest or neck; structural injury is more common when a larger bore needle is used to locate the central veins.

The catheter-through-the-needle set-ups (e.g., Intracath) are designed primarily for central venous cannulations. The probability of advancing the catheter into the lumen successfully is much greater with this system because the catheter is threaded through the needle. However, the risk of catheter embolism is also present because the catheter may be sheared off if it is withdrawn through the needle. In a tense, rushed environment this can happen quite easily and is of genuine concern. In addition, because the catheter must fit

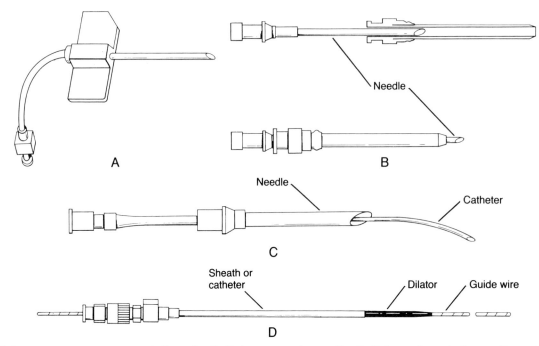

Figure 23–1. Intravenous access systems. *A*, Butterfly. *B*, Catheter over the needle. *C*, Catheter through the needle. *D*, Seldinger-type catheter and guide wire (sheath-type with vein dilator).

through the introducing needle, its size is directly proportional to the size of the catheter. A large-bore catheter requires a larger needle. As a result, the puncture site in the vessel wall is larger than the final indwelling device. Because of these disadvantages, these devices have little place in current vascular access systems.

The Seldinger technique offers the advantage of rapid intravenous access without the aforementioned hazards. The technique is also excellent for placement of introducers for transvenous pacemakers or Swan-Ganz catheters.

The guide wire-through-the-needle technique was originally described in 1953 by Seldinger as a method for catheter placement in percutaneous arteriography.[1] The basic approach is extremely simple and has been adapted for placement of a catheter in any hollow-lumened structure or body cavity. A needle much smaller than the infusion catheter is used to enter a vessel. Once the introducing needle is positioned within the vessel's lumen, a wire is threaded, and the needle is removed. The wire, which is now within the vessel, serves as a guide over which the selected catheter is advanced.

INDICATIONS

The primary advantage to the Seldinger technique of vascular access is that a relatively small needle can be used to place any size or shape of catheter into a vessel. Table 23–1 lists the various sizes of vascular catheters along with the sizes of their introducer needles. A very large 8.5 French high-flow infusion catheter or introducer sheath can be placed through a 22-gauge puncture. This flexibility is extremely valuable when attempting to place catheters in deep vessels such as central veins. Subclavian, internal jugular, external jugular, brachial, and femoral veins can all be cannulated utilizing this technique.[2–5] The use of the smaller introducer needle increases the probability of finding a hidden or collapsed vessel while at the same time theoretically reducing resultant injury should the wrong vessel, such as an artery or an adjacent structure, be entered.

Guide wire approaches also allow for the rapid percutaneous placement of many catheters that might otherwise require a cutdown. A number of large-bore infusion catheters can be placed within the central circulation without the need for surgical exposure of the femoral, saphenous, or

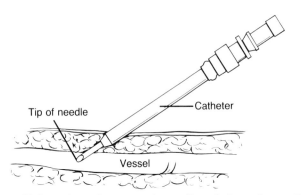

Figure 23–2. In the catheter-over-the-needle technique, the needle will enter the vessel lumen, and a blood return may be observed while the catheter is still outside the vessel wall.

Table 23–1. Needle Sizes for Venous and Arterial Catheters*	
Standard Full-Length Coil Guide Wire **Catheter Size**	**Needle Gauge†**
3 French	21
4.0–4.5 French	20
5.0–6.0 French	20–19
6.0–8.5 French	19–18

*Any sized catheter from 3.0 to 8.5 French may be introduced using a 22-gauge needle if a solid wire (Cor-Flex, Cook Critical Care) is used.
†All needle gauges are for thin-walled needles only.

brachial veins.[4, 5] In addition, this technique can be used to quickly convert small peripheral intravenous catheters to larger flow systems without the need for recannulation.[6, 7]

Modifications of the Seldinger approach have expanded the indications for this technique beyond those of vascular access. Guide wire systems exist now for almost every catheter system used in medicine. Table 23–2 presents a list of available guide wire systems relevant to emergency medicine along with some of their manufacturers.

EQUIPMENT

The equipment needed for the Seldinger guide wire technique of vascular access is listed in Table 23–3. All of these items, with the exception of the needle, the wire, and the catheter, are part of the standard emergency department stock. *The syringe in these systems should be a non–Luer-Lok or slip tip type.* The added twisting needed to remove a Luer-Lok syringe from the introducer needle may actually dislodge a needle tenuously located in a vein. One system permits passage of the guide wire through a hollow syringe plunger, obviating the need for removal of the syringe from the needle (Safety Syringe, Arrow International, Reading, Pa.).

Needle

Virtually any needle or catheter can be used to introduce a guide wire into a vessel, provided a few precautions are remembered. Obviously, the needle must be large enough to accommodate the desired wire. The needles contained in prepared sets are usually *thin walled*, and therefore a smaller gauge can accommodate a larger wire. If a needle that is not thin walled is chosen, a size that is one gauge smaller (larger bore) than that listed in Table 23–1 should be used. In standard peripheral intravenous systems that use a catheter-over-the-needle design, an 18-gauge or larger bore catheter will generally accept the standard guide wire that fits an 18-gauge thin-walled needle. Another factor in the selection of the introducing needle is the taper of the lumen at the proximal end. Seldinger needles have a funnel-shaped taper that guides the wire directly into the needle (Fig. 23–3). Ordinary needles may have a straight-bore lumen that leads squarely into the needle. These needles can present a problem if the wire abuts against the flat end plate surface.

Table 23–2. Emergency Department Catheters and Devices Placed with Guide Wire Technique*
Single-lumen central venous catheters (1,2,3,6)
Multilumen central venous catheters (1,2,3,6)
Arterial line catheters (1,2,3,5,6)
Sheath introducers (e.g., for pacemaker insertion) (1,2,4,5)
Large-bore infusion catheters (1,2,4,5)
Tracheostomy sets (1)
Peritoneal lavage catheters (1,2)
Tube thoracostomy (chest tubes) (1)
Pneumothorax aspiration catheters (1)
Cricothyrotomy sets (1)
Cystostomy sets (1)

*Included is only a partial list of manufacturers; other companies may produce similar items. Manufacturers: (1) Cook Critical Care; (2) Arrow International; (3) Burron Medical, Inc.; (4) Bard, Inc.; (5) Cordis Corp.; and (6) Deseret.

Table 23–3. Necessary Equipment for Seldinger Technique	
Introducing needle	Number 11 scalpel
Guide wire	Lidocaine
Catheter or sheath introducer	3-ml syringe (for anesthetizing)
Prep solution (iodine)	3- to 5-ml syringe
Sterile gloves	(*not* Luer-Lok)
Small anesthetizing needle	Suture (0–00)
(1.5 inch, 25 gauge)	Sterile drapes
Gauze pads	Antibiotic ointment
Prep razor	Completed radiograph request

Guide Wire

Two basic types of guide wires are used: straight or J-shaped. The straight wires are for use in vessels with a linear configuration, whereas the J wires are for use in tortuous vessels. Both wires have essentially the same internal design (Fig. 23–4A). The flexibility of the wire is a result of a stainless steel coil or helix that forms the bulk of the guide wire. Within the central lumen of the helix is a straight central core wire, called a *mandrel*. The mandrel is fixed at one end of the helix and terminates between 0.5 and 3.0 cm from the other end. It adds rigidity to the portion of the wire surrounding it, whereas the remainder of the wire without the mandrel is the flexible or floppy end. Many guide wires also contain a straight safety wire that runs parallel to the mandrel to keep the wire from kinking or shearing.

Wires with two flexible ends contain the mandrel only in the central portion of the wire. In these systems one end is usually straight and the other end J shaped.

The most common size for these wires is from 0.025 to 0.035 inch (0.064 to 0.089 cm) in diameter. Wire in this size range is generally introduced through an 18-gauge thin-walled needle. A modification of this standard wire utilizes a bare mandrel with the flexible coil soldered to its end. This construction provides a wire with a diameter of only 0.018 inches (0.047 cm) but with the same rigidity as the larger wires. Such a wire can be introduced through a 22-gauge thin-walled needle, yet still guide an 8.5 French catheter.[8]

The flexible end of the guide wire allows the wire to flex on contact with the wall of a vessel. If the contact is tangential, as in an infraclavicular approach to the subclavian vein, the straight wire is generally preferred. If the angle is

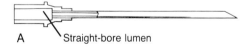

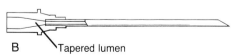

Figure 23–3. Introducing needles. *A*, Ordinary needle with a straight-bore lumen. *B*, Seldinger needle with a tapered lumen.

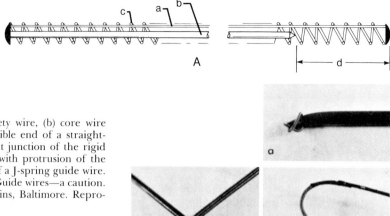

Figure 23–4. *A,* Guide wire internal structure: (a) safety wire, (b) core wire (mandrel), (c) coiled wire, (d) flexible tip. *B,* (a) Flexible end of a straight-spring guide wire knotted on a vessel dilator, (b) bent junction of the rigid and flexible portions of a straight-spring guide wire with protrusion of the central core *(arrow),* (c) partially fractured tip *(arrow)* of a J-spring guide wire. (From Schwartz AJ, Horrow JL, Jobes DR, Ellison N: Guide wires—a caution. Crit Care Med 9:348, 1981. © 1981 Williams & Wilkins, Baltimore. Reproduced by permission.)

more acute, as in an external jugular approach to the subclavian vein or if the vessel is particularly tortuous or the valves must be transversed, the J wire is used. The more rounded leading edge of the J wire provides a broader surface to manipulate within the vessel and a decreased risk of perforation. This is an especially advantageous characteristic when attempting to thread a wire through a vessel with valves.

One easily introduces the straight wire by threading the flexible end of the wire into the proximal hub of the indwelling needle. To introduce the J wire, a plastic sleeve contained in the kit is advanced to the floppy end of the wire to straighten out the J shape. This straightened end is now introduced into the proximal hub of the indwelling needle. Once the J wire has been advanced, the sleeve is removed and discarded (Fig. 23–5). *Caution:* In an emergency this sleeve may be misplaced, making insertion of the J wire very difficult.

It is important to emphasize that guide wires are delicate and may bend, kink, or unwind. A force of 4 to 6 pounds may result in rupture of a wire. Embolization of portions of the guide wire is possible, and sharp defects in the wire may perforate vessel walls (see Fig. 23–4). One should carefully inspect wires before use for defects such as kinks, sharp ends or spurs, and weak points.[9] *Wires should thread easily and smoothly and never be forced.*

Catheters

Once the guide wire is in place and the needle is removed, any number of catheter devices may be introduced, including triple-lumen catheters and sheath introducers. Multilumen catheters are discussed elsewhere, and only the sheath introducers are discussed in detail here. The Desilets-Hoffman–type sheath introducer was designed by D. T. Desilets and R. Hoffman in 1965 to aid in arteriography

procedures that required many catheter changes.[10] The sheath introducer unit consists basically of two catheters, one inside the other (Fig. 23–6). The first catheter, termed the *dilator,* is hard, with an inner lumen that fits over the guide wire. This catheter is longer and thinner than its sheath and has a tapered end that serves as a dilator when the unit is passed through subcutaneous tissue and into the vessel. The dilator serves no other function than to facilitate placement of the sheath. The second catheter, termed the *sheath* or *introducer,* has a blunt end and is simply a catheter with a large diameter. This sheath is usually used as a large-bore infusion catheter, but it may serve as a guide (introducer) for the passage of a pacemaker or a Swan-Ganz catheter.

Many modifications of the sheath exist, with side arms and diaphragms to aid in placement of nonlumen devices. Care must be taken in the use of side-arm sets for rapid fluid administration, because some catheters may be 8.5 French but may have only a 5 French side arm. If faced with this problem, one can either remove the diaphragm or introduce an 8 French feeding tube through the diaphragm at the catheter hub for rapid fluid administration.

Another modification is the so-called soft catheter. These catheters, designed for long-term placement, are too flexible to be threaded directly through the subcutaneous tissue into a vein. To introduce these catheters, a separate dilator is passed over the guide wire first. Leaving the wire in place, the dilator is removed, creating a tract through which the soft permanent catheter can be introduced.

PROCEDURE FOR THE SELDINGER TECHNIQUE

The actual procedure for placement of Seldinger-type guide wire catheters is quite simple. The vessel is first cannulated with a needle or an indwelling intravenous cath-

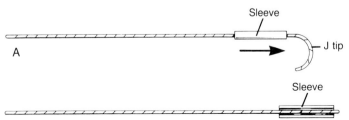

Figure 23–5. J wire. *A,* Plastic sleeve in retracted position, demonstrating the J tip. *B,* Plastic sleeve is advanced to straighten the curve to allow easy introduction into the needle hub.

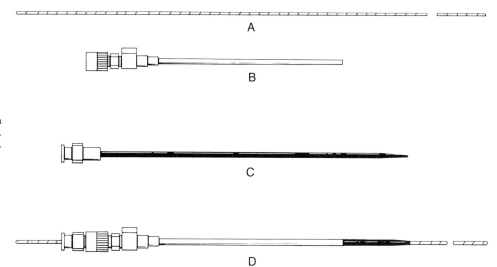

Figure 23–6. Desilets-Hoffman sheath introducer. *A,* Guide wire. *B,* Sheath or introducer. *C,* Dilator. *D,* Assembled device.

eter. A guide wire is threaded through the needle or catheter and the needle or catheter is removed, leaving only the wire within the vessel. A catheter or introducer-sheath unit (often with a dilator) is passed over the guide wire through the skin and into the vessel. Once the infusion device is in place, the guide wire and introducer are removed. These steps are detailed in the following discussion.

Guide Wire Placement

Sterile technique is maintained, and the area of vascular access should be prepared and cleaned as described in the chapters on central venous access.

An introducing needle or a standard over-the-needle catheter that is large enough to accommodate the guide wire is selected. The needle is attached to a small syringe (Fig. 23–7). The needle and syringe are introduced together, and the selected vessel is cannulated. Once a free return of blood is obtained, the syringe is removed, and the needle is stabilized by its hub to prevent displacement from the vessel lumen. When cannulating a central vein, the needle hub is capped with one's thumb before passing the guide wire; this minimizes the potential for air embolism. Next, the flexible end of the guide wire is threaded through the needle. If an intravenous catheter is already in place, the wire is simply passed through it before the catheter is removed from the vein.

The wire should thread smoothly into the vein. If resistance is met, the wire should not be forced but should be removed from the needle and the syringe reattached to confirm intravascular placement. It is extremely important for the wire to slip easily from the needle during removal. If any resistance to removal of the wire is felt, *the wire and the needle should be removed as a single unit* to prevent shearing off the wire. Despite its necessity, this last maneuver is often disregarded. It is not that removal of both the wire and needle as a unit is technically difficult; rather there is often a reluctance on the physician's part to abandon a needle already in a vein.

Manipulation of the wire within an introducer needle should be done only with the standard coil wire guides; manipulation should be avoided when using the solid wire sets in which the coil is soldered onto the mandrel. In the solid wire sets the taper of the mandrel to the wire creates a very small lip that can become caught on the edge of the needle tip and shear off the coil portion of the wire. These

wires must thread freely on the first attempt or the entire wire and needle assembly must be removed.

Some physicians recommend applying these restrictions to all guide wires and believe that no wire should ever be withdrawn through the introducing needle.[11] One method of avoiding this problem is to cannulate the vessel with a catheter-over-the-needle system and then use the soft catheter, rather than a sharp needle, as the entry source for the guide wire. The limitation of this approach is that the catheter itself cannot be advanced to relocate a vessel if the initial attempt at wire passage fails.

Occasionally a wire must be teased into the vessel; rotating the wire or needle often helps in difficult placements. If the wire does not thread easily, another helpful maneuver is to pull back slightly on the needle itself just before advancing the wire. This helps if the opening of the needle is abutted against the vessel's inner wall, blocking the wire's entry, or the vein is compressed by introduction of the needle. Changing wire tips from a straight to a J wire or vice versa may also solve an advancement problem. If the inner lumen of a vessel is smaller than the diameter of the J, it will prevent the wire from reforming its natural shape, causing the spring in the coil to generate resistance. Any advantages of a J wire will be negated if the wire fails to regain its intended shape. In this instance, a straight tip should be introducible without problems. Alternately, if the angle of entry of the needle and the vessel is more acute than was suspected, the straight wire may not be able to bend appropriately as it encounters the vessel's far wall. A J-tipped wire may be used and threaded in such a manner that the wire resumes its J shape away from the far wall. There is no way the operator can know for certain that this is the problem but may attempt a solution by repeatedly withdrawing the wire, rotating it, and readvancing it. All of these maneuvers are performed with gentle free motions of the wire within the needle. If at any time the wire cannot be advanced freely, improper placement must be suspected and the attempt reevaluated.

If it is threading easily, the guide wire should be advanced until at least one quarter of the wire is within the vessel. The further into the vessel the wire extends the more stable its location when the catheter is introduced. Occasionally a wire threads easily past the tip of the needle and then suddenly does not advance any farther. If the introducer needle demonstrated free blood return at the time of wire entry and the initial advancement of the wire met no resistance, the wire is most likely located properly in the

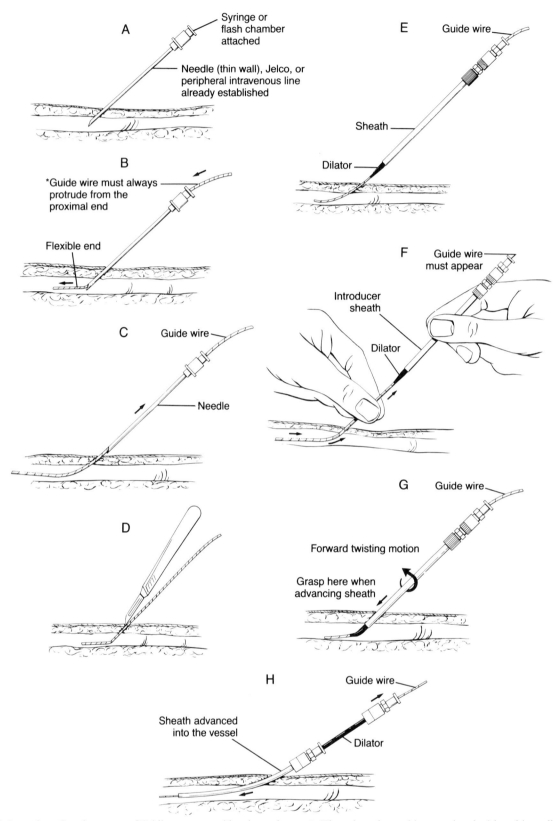

Figure 23–7. Procedure for placement of Seldinger-type guide wire catheter. *A,* The selected vessel is cannulated with a thin-walled needle, or an existing intravenous catheter is chosen to be changed with the wire technique. *B,* The guide wire is threaded through the vessel, with the flexible end first into the lumen of the vessel. If a J wire is used, a sleeve will facilitate entry into the needle (see Fig. 23–5). *C,* The needle is removed so that only the wire now exits from the vessel. *D,* The skin entry site is enlarged with a number 11 scalpel. *E,* The catheter sheath and the dilator are threaded over the wire and advanced to the skin. The wire must be visible through the back of the device. *F,* If the proximal wire is *not* visible, it is pulled from the skin through the catheter until it appears at the back of the catheter. *G,* The sheath and the dilator are advanced as a unit into the skin with a twisting motion. It is best to grasp the unit at the junction of the sheath and the dilator to prevent bunching up of the sheath. *H,* Once the sheath and the dilator are well within the vessel, the guide wire and the dilator are removed. Contrary to the illustration, latex gloves should be worn.

vessel and can serve as a guide for the catheter. If further confirmation is needed, the needle may be removed, and a radiograph showing wire placement can be made before passing the catheter. This confirmation may be advisable if the location of a wire is suspect and the introduction of a large-sized sheath is planned. A freely advancing wire may suddenly stop once it is well within a vessel if the vessel makes an unsuspected bend or is being compressed or deviated by another structure such as a rib or muscle.

Catheter and Introducer Unit Placement

Once the wire is placed into the vessel, the needle is removed and the physician is now ready to pass the desired catheter (see Fig. 23–7). A small skin incision is made at the site of the wire. The incision should be approximately the size of the catheter to be introduced and should extend completely through the dermis. Precisely placing this skin incision directly over the wire entry site may be difficult if a very small aspirating needle was used. A wire-guided scalpel that may help alleviate this problem is currently under development. Alternately, some physicians prefer to make the skin nick first and to introduce the needle through this incision. The disadvantage of this approach is that if the vessel is displaced, the physician is forced to attempt a difficult entry through the existing incision or make a second incision.

Once the incision is made, the catheter or sheath with the dilator is threaded over the wire to a point 1 cm from the surface of the skin. The guide wire should be stabilized at the point of skin entry by the clinician during advancement of the introducer unit over the guide wire. *The wire should protrude from the back end of the introducer before advancement into the vessel.* This is a critically important procedural point. If the wire is not protruding from the proximal end of the introducer, it may be lost in the vessel and migrate to the central circulation. If the wire is not visible at the proximal end of the introducer, the guide wire is carefully withdrawn at the site of skin entry until it exits from the proximal end of the introducer unit. The wire must always be visible and graspable from the back end of the introducer throughout the remainder of the procedure. Guide wires are always longer than their catheters, and with experience it becomes easy to judge the optimal distance to thread the wire to ensure good introducer placement as well as to leave enough wire protruding from the proximal end of the introducer unit.

Once the wire is visible, it is grasped and held. The introducer unit is threaded into the skin with a twisting motion until it is well within the vessel. When one uses the sheath and dilator, it is best to grasp the unit at the junction of the sheath and dilator. This prevents the thinner sheath from kinking or bending at the tip or from bunching up at the coupler end. The dilator need only be advanced a few centimeters into the vessel, because it only serves to dilate the vessel so that it will accept the sheath. Once the vessel has been dilated, the sheath is advanced over the dilator to its full length within the vessel. The wire and the dilator are then removed, leaving the sheath in the selected vessel. Precautions are again taken to cover the sheath hub to avoid air embolism after removal of the wire and dilator before attachment of the infusion tubing. Once in place the device is usually affixed with one or two sutures, and infusion or monitoring is begun.

If a single small catheter is used instead of a sheath with an inner dilator, the wire is removed simply from the catheter after passing the catheter. The wire must be easily removed from the catheter. If any resistance is met, both the wire and catheter must be removed as a single unit and the procedure reattempted. The most common cause of this problem is a small piece of adipose tissue wedged between the wire and the lumen of the catheter. This can be avoided by creating a deep enough skin nick before insertion of the catheter.

When this technique is used for subclavian line placement, the dilator may be curved slightly in its center (i.e., it has a banana shape) to facilitate guidance into the superior vena cava.

Replacement of Existing Catheters

In addition to placing new catheters, the Seldinger technique can be used to change existing devices. The utility of this technique in converting a peripheral small-gauge catheter to a larger infusion catheter is obvious. Within a few seconds, an existing peripheral or central 18-gauge intravenous catheter can be changed to an 8.5 French infuser, saving valuable time that would be lost trying to find another vein. A guide wire technique can also be used to change single-lumen central venous catheters to triple-lumen or sheath introducer sets. In these instances the guide wire for the new device is inserted into the existing central venous catheter until approximately a few centimeters are protruding and graspable from the proximal end. With one hand holding the wire securely, the catheter and wire are removed as a single unit until the tip of the catheter just clears the patient's skin. The wire is grasped at the point at which it exits the skin, and only then is the other end of the wire released. The catheter is then slid off the wire, and the new device is inserted in the normal fashion. Caution must be exercised with this technique because catheter embolization has occurred during placement of the guide wire into an existing catheter that had been cut to facilitate guide wire placement.[11]

Self-Contained Guide Wire Catheter Systems

One modification of the Seldinger technique is a self-contained system in which the wire is maintained within a side sleeve of the needle and need not be introduced into the aspiration needle separately (Fig. 23–8). Such a system permits a more rapid placement of the wire once the vessel is cannulated. Although quicker, such systems sacrifice operator sensitivity in teasing difficult wires into place. The location of the introducer directly over the aspiration needle is also designed to permit more rapid catheter placement because it eliminates the step of threading the catheter or introducer unit onto the wire. In this regard these designs resemble catheter-over-the-needle systems with the potential problem of carrying the larger introducer along with the needle when searching for the intended vessel. If the correct vessel is entered, this is an advantage; however, if the wrong structure is punctured, the larger hole produced by the introducer may result in more injury.

The Seldinger technique is readily adapted to placement of catheters in any body cavity. The technique in these situations is identical except that blood is not aspirated through the introducing needle. Other situations in which this technique is used include intra-abdominal abscess drainage, peritoneal lavage, percutaneous nephrostomy and cystostomy, cricothyrotomy, pericardiocentesis, tube thoracostomy, and many others.[12, 13] These procedures are discussed more fully elsewhere in this text.

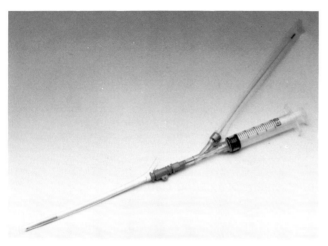

Figure 23–8. Arrow EID catheter with self-contained wire and catheter-introducer unit. (Courtesy of Arrow International, Inc., Reading, Pa.)

COMPLICATIONS

Vascular access using the Seldinger technique has gained wide acceptance in emergency and critical care units. Any complication inherent in the performance of central or peripheral vascular access with other systems may also occur with this technique. Although intuitively this approach with small needles should be safer than that with the larger needles used in the catheter-through-the-needle systems, the only comparison study between these two techniques failed to demonstrate any significant decrease in complications with the guide wire technique.[14] However, in another study in which only the Seldinger technique was used, fewer complications were noted in central venous catheter placements than found in previous reports without guide wire use.[15]

Some complications unique to guide wire use may also occur. Wires have been reported to form knots or to perforate vessels if forcibly introduced. Lost wires have embolized when the technique was not performed correctly and the wire was not grasped at all times or easily removed from the introducer needle. Experience has shown that the wire will indeed kink or separate when ego exceeds wisdom and removal of the wire from a catheter is forcibly attempted rather than removal of the two as a unit.

The use of the Seldinger technique has also allowed the introduction of a number of new catheter styles, each with its own complications. Multilumen central venous catheters tend to be larger and stiffer than their single-lumen counterparts, making them more susceptible to vessel perforations. In addition to size, the configuration of the catheter affects its tendency to perforate. A model comparing the relative perforating potential of various catheters revealed that pigtailed or flexible-tipped catheters were less likely to perforate a simulated vessel wall than straight catheters.[16]

Sheath introducers have also demonstrated some unique complications. Thin-walled sheaths may collapse or crimp from external tissue pressure or from being forced into a severe bend. This is not a problem if the sheath is being used to introduce a pacemaker, but if it is being placed for fluid resuscitation, its efficacy decreases markedly. Newer devices with internal supports or flexible sections do not create this problem and allow much greater freedom in the bending of these sheaths.

Another complication of such devices concerns the adaptors used to seal the proximal ends. Because of the large size of these catheters the chance for air entry into the system is greater if the caps or diaphragms are not fitted properly. Air leakage and actual air emboli have been reported to result from improperly sealed devices.[17]

CONCLUSION

The development of the Seldinger guide wire technique for catheter placement has made possible a simple, rapid, percutaneous system for entry of almost any desired vessel or cavity. Because it can be learned quickly and it presents minimal complications, this approach is well suited to emergency and critical care vascular access.

REFERENCES

1. Seldinger SI: Catheter replacement of needle in percutaneous arteriography. Acta Radiol 39:369, 1953.
2. Dailey RH: External jugular vein cannulation and its use for CVP monitoring. J Emerg Med 6:133, 1988.
3. Dailey RH: Use of wire guided (Seldinger-type) catheters in the emergency department. Ann Emerg Med 12:489, 1983.
4. Jones TK, Barnhart GR, Gervin AS: Tandem 8.5 French subclavian catheters: A technique for rapid volume replacement. Ann Emerg Med 16:1369, 1987.
5. Dailey RH: "Code red" protocol for resuscitation of the exsanguinated patient. J Emerg Med 2:373, 1985.
6. Falcone RE, Zeeb P, Satiani B: Resuscitation without risk (letter). Ann Emerg Med 17:1130, 1988.
7. Aedem MI, Crung JP, Rhodes JM: Technical limitations in the rapid infusion of intravenous fluids. Ann Emerg Med 14:307, 1985.
8. Micropuncture Introducer Sets and Trays with Cor-Flex Wire Guides. Bloomington, Ind, Cook Critical Care, 1984.
9. Schwartz A, Horrow J, Jobes D, Ellison N: Guidewires—a caution. Crit Care Med 9:4, 1981.
10. Desilets DT, Hoffman R: A new method of percutaneous catheterization. Radiology 85:145, 1965.
11. Propp DA, Cline D, Hennenfent BR: Catheter embolism. J Emerg Med 6:17, 1988.
12. Campbell CT, Harris RC, Cook MH, et al: A new device for emergency percutaneous transtracheal ventilation in partial and complete airway obstruction. Ann Emerg Med 17:927, 1988.
13. Semrad N: A new technique for closed thoracostomy insertion of chest tube. Surg Gynecol Obstet 166:171, 1988.
14. Schug CB, Culhane DE, Knopp RK: Subclavian vein catheterization in the emergency department: A comparison of guidewire and nonguidewire techniques. Ann Emerg Med 15:769, 1986.
15. Ramoska EA, Sacchetti AD, Warden TD: Credentialing of emergency physicians: Support for delineation of privileges in invasive procedures. Am J Emerg Med 6:278, 1988.
16. Gravenstein N, Blackshear R: Relative perforating potential of 7-Fr. triple-lumen catheters. Crit Care Med 16:435, 1988.
17. Kondo K, O'Reily L, Chiota J: Air embolism associated with an introducer for pulmonary arterial catheters. Anesth Analg 63:871, 1984.

Chapter **24**

Venous Cutdown

Steven C. Dronen

INTRODUCTION

"The standard cutdown is well known to all surgeons and needs no description."[1] Were this a true statement, the remainder of this chapter would be superfluous; however, physician training in the technique of venous cutdown has been largely informal. For four decades, the mechanics of venous cutdown have been handed down from house officer to house officer as one of the rites of internship. There are, in fact, few detailed descriptions of the procedure in the medical literature, and the scientific data documenting its usefulness or complication rate are sparse.

The frequency with which the venous cutdown is performed is impossible to estimate. The growing popularity of central venous cannulation by the internal jugular and subclavian routes has most probably decreased the frequency of venisection. Nevertheless, the cutdown remains an excellent method of obtaining venous access in several emergent clinical situations. Although a cutdown is mechanically simple to perform, ease of performance does not guarantee that the procedure will be performed efficiently and without complications. This can be achieved only by a thorough knowledge of the procedure and by attention to its many details.

An early description of the technique of venous cutdown was provided by Keeley in 1940. He offered the procedure as an alternative to venipuncture in patients in shock or in individuals with small, thin veins.[2] In 1945, Kirkham gave the first detailed description of the saphenous vein cutdown at the ankle.[3] Although the article is now somewhat dated, most of the steps remain unchanged today.

The most significant changes over the past four decades have involved not the technique itself but the cannulas that are used. Keeley and Kirkham used metal needles. With the advent of plastic cannulas in the mid-1940s, the cutdown became more popular as a means of providing long-term intravenous (IV) infusion. Physicians have used IV tubing, feeding tubes, and even nasogastric tubes as cannulas in the management of hypovolemic patients. Currently, large-bore catheters (10 gauge, 8 French) are often inserted by cutdown in the management of hypovolemic shock.[4]

INDICATIONS

There are no absolute indications for venous cutdown, simply because several options for venous access usually exist. The indications for use of the procedure are relative, depending to a great extent on physician experience and preference. There are several clinical situations in which the venous cutdown may be used.

Venous Access in Infants. Small children present a unique challenge to the clinician who does not perform pediatric venipuncture regularly (see also Chapter 20). The challenge is greater still if the procedure must be performed rapidly in a critically ill child. The distal saphenous vein is large enough to cannulate in most children and has a predictable anatomic location. Consequently, venous cutdown at the ankle is commonly used for both emergent and long-term venous access.[5, 6]

A venous cutdown may be performed when all accessible peripheral sites have been exhausted. Alternatively, many physicians would use intraosseous infusion under these circumstances, and some would cannulate the femoral, subclavian, or internal jugular veins. In selected circumstances, such as in the treatment of status epilepticus with diazepam, the rectal route with mucosal absorption is an effective alternative to a cutdown.

Hypovolemic Shock. The rapid percutaneous insertion of large-bore (14 gauge) catheters is appropriate in most cases of hypovolemic shock. Unfortunately, peripheral vessels frequently collapse in hypovolemia or have been rendered useless by intravenous drug abuse or previous venous catheterization. The venous cutdown is an acceptable alternative in these instances, although the insertion of a large-bore introducer device into a central vein can usually be performed more rapidly. When the cutdown can be performed quickly, it offers the advantage of direct visualization of the vessel during cannulation. The use of the cutdown as a vehicle for the insertion of intravenous extension tubing and rapid transfusion was popularized during the Vietnam war.[7] The technique also has been found useful in civilian practice for the resuscitation of patients with profound hypovolemia.[8]

The superiority of large-bore lines is determined by physical laws, which state that flow is proportional to the fourth power of the cannula radius and inversely proportional to the cannula length and fluid viscosity. The flow rate for saline through a standard IV extension set (3 mm inside diameter) cut to a length of 28 cm (12 inches) and inserted directly into the vein is 15 to 30 per cent greater than that through a 5 cm, 14-gauge catheter. The difference is greater if pressure is applied to the system. The improvement in flow rate through large-bore lines is greater for blood than for crystalloid solutions because the viscous characteristics of blood greatly impede its passage through small-bore tubing.[8, 9] One can transfuse a unit of blood in 3 minutes using IV extension tubing inserted intravenously. Consequently, large-bore lines placed by venous cutdown are an excellent mechanism for the treatment of severe hypovolemia. These factors are discussed further in Chapter 22.

CONTRAINDICATIONS

Venous cutdown is contraindicated when less invasive alternatives exist or when excessive delay would be required for the procedure to be performed.[10] Although highly skilled operators may perform a cutdown in less than 60 seconds,[11] studies by Rhee and colleagues[12] and Iserson and Criss[13] have shown that, on the average, the procedure requires 5 to 6 minutes to complete. Percutaneous insertion of large-bore catheters is the preferred method of fluid resuscitation unless very high flow rates are required or peripheral vessels are collapsed. Another method of rapid fluid infusion that is technically easier than venisection is the percutaneous insertion of large-bore introducer devices into the subclavian, internal jugular, or large peripheral veins (see Chapters 21, 25, and 26). The use of these vessels is also preferable to the cutdown for long-term applications.

Other contraindications are relative. In the presence of coagulation disorders, impaired healing, or compromised host-defense mechanisms, the need to perform a cutdown should be weighed carefully against the potential complications.

ANATOMY

Detailed knowledge of anatomy is critically important to the success of this procedure. Veins in both the upper and the lower extremities may be used. The choice of a particular vein should be governed by its accessibility and size and by the physician's experience and training. The anatomy of individual vessels and their relative merits as cutdown sites are described in the following paragraphs.

The Greater Saphenous Vein. The greater saphenous vein is the longest vein and runs subcutaneously throughout much of its course (Fig. 24–1). It is most easily accessible at the ankle but may also be cannulated above the knee and below the femoral triangle. The greater saphenous vein begins at the ankle, where it is the continuation of the medial marginal vein of the foot. The vein crosses 1 cm anterior to the medial malleolus and continues up the anteromedial aspect of the leg.[14] At the level of the malleolus, the vein lies adjacent to the periosteum and is accompanied by the relatively insignificant saphenous nerve, which if transected causes sensory loss in a small area along the medial aspect of the foot. At the ankle, the vessel can be exposed with minimal blunt dissection. The vein's superficial, predictable, and isolated location has made the distal saphenous vein the classic pediatric cutdown site.[15]

The saphenous vein lies superficially on the medial aspect of the knee. A cutdown performed 1 to 4 cm below the knee and immediately posterior to the tibia is described in the pediatric literature.[5] This site is distal enough to avoid interference with the performance of other resuscitative procedures, yet proximal enough to allow the passage of a long line into the central circulation.[16] This site of venous cutdown is seldom used, however. Disadvantages of this technique include kinking of the line as the knee is flexed and the risk of injury to associated structures. Improper

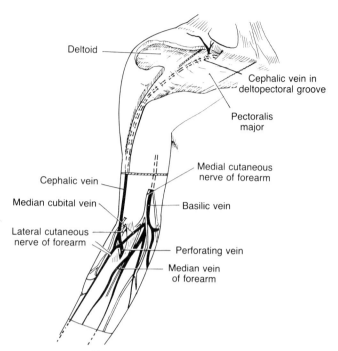

Figure 24–2. Veins of the upper limb.

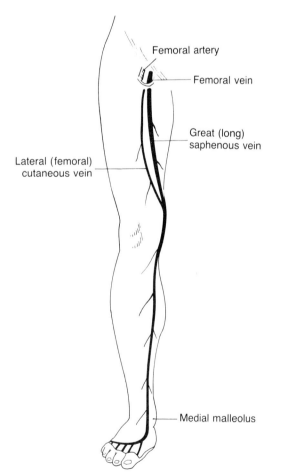

Figure 24–1. Superficial veins of the lower limb.

placement of the incision may injure the saphenous branch of the genicular artery and the saphenous nerve.[17]

In the thigh, the saphenous vein begins on the medial aspect of the knee and crosses anterolaterally as it ascends toward the femoral triangle. Proximally, it enters the fossa ovalis and joins the femoral vein. Three to 4 cm distal to the inguinal ligament the saphenous vein is of large caliber (4 to 5 mm outside diameter) and is easily isolated from the surrounding fat. Also lying anteromedially in the thigh is the lateral femoral cutaneous vein, which has a smaller diameter (2 to 3 mm) and lies lateral to the greater saphenous vein.[18, 19] The accessibility and large diameter of the greater saphenous vein in the thigh make it an excellent choice in the treatment of profound hypovolemia.[8]

The Basilic Vein. The basilic vein is a preferred site for venous cutdown in the upper extremity. Veins of the dorsal venous network of the hand unite to form the cephalic and basilic veins, traveling along the radial and ulnar sides of the forearm, respectively (Fig. 24–2). At the level of the mid forearm, the basilic vein crosses anterolaterally and is consistently found 1 to 2 cm lateral to the medial epicondyle on the anterior surface of the upper arm. The medial cubital vein crosses over from the radial side of the arm to join the basilic vein just above the medial epicondyle. The basilic vein then continues proximally, occupying a superficial position between the biceps and pronator teres muscles. In this segment it lies in close association with the medial cutaneous nerve, which supplies sensation to the ulnar side of the forearm. The vein penetrates the brachial fascia in the distal third of the upper arm and then occupies a deeper position.[20]

The basilic vein is generally cannulated at the antecubital fossa 2 cm above and 2 to 3 cm lateral to the medial epicondyle. It is exposed through a transverse incision on the medial aspect of the proximal antecubital fossa. This vein is of sufficient size to be located easily even in the hypotensive or hypovolemic patient. Large catheters, such as intravenous extension tubing and pediatric feeding tubes, can generally be passed without difficulty. The median cubital vein is accessible through the same incision. Superficially at this level there are no important associated structures, but the brachial artery and the median nerve are found deep to the basilic vein.

A more proximal insertion site has been recommended by Simon and colleagues[21] to avoid the network of interconnecting veins at the level of the antecubital fossa. However, in the distal third of the upper arm, there is a closer association between the basilic vein and the medial cutaneous nerve. Transection of this nerve produces a sensory loss on the ulnar side of the forearm.

The Cephalic Vein. This vessel begins on the radial aspect of the wrist and crosses anteromedially, ascending toward the antecubital fossa (see Fig. 24–2). In the forearm it lies in close association with the lateral cutaneous nerve, which supplies sensory innervation to the radial aspect of the forearm. In the antecubital fossa it lies subcutaneously, just lateral to the midline, and then ascends in the upper arm, overlying the lateral aspect of the biceps muscle. At the shoulder the cephalic vein lies in the deltopectoral groove. Just below the clavicle, it passes deep to end in the axillary vein.[20]

Venisection is easily performed on the cephalic vein because of its large diameter and superficial location. In the forearm it is important to avoid the lateral cutaneous nerve. A good location is in the antecubital fossa at the distal flexor crease. Cutdown on the cephalic vein at the wrist has also been reported,[23] but the thin skin overlying the vein at this level usually permits simple percutaneous cannulation when the vein is available for cannulation. The cephalic vein may also be entered in the deltopectoral groove. The slightly deeper position and physical interference with the performance of other procedures make this approach more difficult.

The Brachial Veins. The brachial veins are small, paired vessels lying on either side of the brachial artery. In contrast to the vessels described earlier, these are not superficial and will not accommodate large cannulas. Their most superficial location is 1 to 2 cm above the antecubital fossa just medial to the biceps muscle. Palpation of the brachial pulse serves as a useful landmark, but the artery may be inadvertently cannulated in the pulseless patient. Additionally, there is the risk of injury to the closely associated median nerve. Time-consuming blunt dissection is generally required. Consequently, the brachial vein cutdown is not recommended as an emergency venous access route[10] and should be used only in the absence of a suitable alternative. This site may be acceptable when time and vessel size are not critical factors, but it is difficult to justify the deep dissection that is required.

The External Jugular Vein. The external jugular vein begins below the angle of the mandible formed by confluence of the posterior auricular and retromandibular veins. It descends posterolaterally across the surface of the sternocleidomastoid muscle and then pierces the fascia to join the subclavian vein deep to the clavicular head of this muscle. The greater auricular nerve, which supplies sensation to the external ear, travels parallel to the external jugular vein.[14]

A venous cutdown may be performed on the external jugular vein at its superficial location on the sternocleidomastoid muscle. This is not recommended as a first-line means of venous access for the following reasons: (1) there is risk of injury to the greater auricular nerve; (2) performance of a cutdown may cause physical interference with airway management and central venous cannulation; (3) it is difficult to immobilize the area adequately; and (4) it is a hazardous procedure in the uncooperative patient.[10] As a general rule, cutdown on the external jugular vein should be performed only when other means of venous access are exhausted. The external jugular vein is an acceptable site for emergency *percutaneous* venous cannulation, especially in children.

EQUIPMENT

The materials required to perform a venous cutdown are listed in Table 24–1. All necessary instruments should be available on a sterile tray before the procedure is begun. The standard cutdown tray is shown in Figure 24–3. A time-consuming search for the proper instrument can be avoided if only necessary instruments are included. The appropriate catheter should also be placed on this tray. Catheter choice depends on the function of the venous line. When a central position is required, the catheter chosen must be long enough to reach the superior vena cava. The average distance from the antecubital fossa to the superior vena cava is 54 cm in the adult male. One can approximate this distance by aligning the catheter over the chest with the tip at the level of the manubrial-sternal junction. Lumen size is relatively unimportant when the line is intended to measure central venous pressure (CVP) or to infuse drugs, but it is a critical factor in the treatment of hypovolemia. Short, large-bore catheters are preferred when fluids must be delivered rapidly. Silastic catheters are preferred by some over plastic tubing. A pediatric 5 or 8 French feeding tube may also be used as an infusion catheter. Tables 24–2, 24–3, and 24–4 list the flow rate of fluids through some of the commonly used devices. Knowledge of relative flow rates is essential if maximal benefit is to be obtained from the time spent performing the cutdown. One can achieve excellent flow rates by threading intravenous tubing (sterile tubing may be cut to the appropriate length) directly into the vein or by using a 5 cm, 10-gauge intravenous catheter.[4, 11]

TECHNIQUE

The technique of venous cutdown is essentially the same regardless of the vessel cannulated (Figs. 24–4 through 24–13). Detailed knowledge of the local anatomy is important if the procedure is to be performed rapidly without injury to associated structures. Even in emergency situations, reasonable precautions should be taken to avoid infection. The area of the skin incision should be widely prepared with an antiseptic solution and then draped. A tourniquet placed proximal to the cutdown site helps in the visualization of the vein.

In the conscious patient, the site is infiltrated with 1 per cent lidocaine (Xylocaine). A skin incision is made transverse to the course of the vessel (see Fig. 24–4). A longitudinal incision may decrease the risk of transecting neurovascular

Table 24–1. Materials Required for Venous Cutdown*

Curved Kelly hemostat
Scalpel with number 11 blade
Small mosquito hemostat
Tissue spreader
Iris scissors
Plastic venous dilator or lifter
4–0 silk suture ties
4–0 nylon suture on cutting needle
Antibiotic ointment
Gauze sponges
1-inch tape
Armboard
Intravenous catheter
Rolled gauze bandage

*See Figure 24–3.

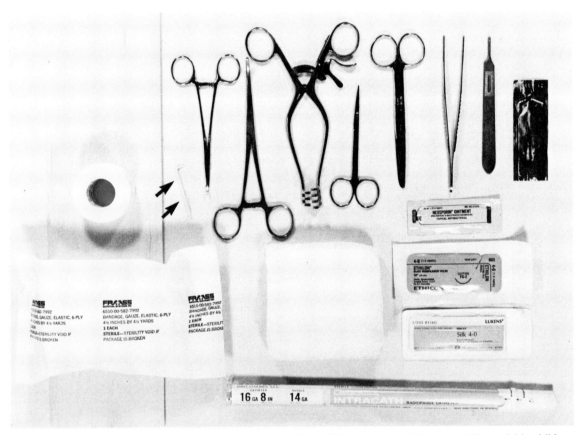

Figure 24–3. Venous cutdown tray. Note the small plastic vein dilator-lifter *(arrows)*, which is especially useful in children.

Table 24–2. Comparative Average Flow Rates (ml/min) for Tap Water*

Catheter	Pressure 200 mm Hg (95% CI)†	Gravity (95% CI)
Central Venous Catheters		
USCI 9 French Introducer Internal diameter 0.117 in., length 5½ in.	566 (± 16)	247 (± 2)
USCI 8 French Introducer Internal diameter 0.104 in., length 5½ in.	540‡	243 (± 5)
Deseret Angiocath Gauge 14, length 5¼ in.	341 (± 6)	157 (± 6)
Deseret Angiocath Gauge 16, length 5¼ in.	195 (± 4)	91 (± 2)
Deseret Subclavian Jugular Catheter Gauge 16, length 12 in.	142 (± 4)	54 (± 3)
Peripheral Venous Catheters		
Intravenous tubing Internal diameter 0.12 in., length 12 in.	500 (± 21)	222 (± 4)
Argyle Medicut Gauge 14, length 2 in.	484 (± 8)	194 (± 5)
Deseret Angiocath Gauge 14, length 2 in.	405 (± 2)	173 (± 4)
Vicra Quick-Cath Gauge 14, length 2¼ in.	—	167 (± 1)
Argyle Medicut Gauge 16, length 2 in.	353 (± 4)	151 (± 3)
Deseret Angiocath Gauge 16, length 2 in.	231 (⊥ 1)	108 (± 1)
Vicra Quick-Cath Gauge 16, length 2 in.	—	108 (± 1)

*Mean of three trials with hydrostatic pressure head of 1 m.
†CI, confidence interval.
‡95% confidence interval not calculated because all three trials resulted in 11.1 sec for 100-ml flow.
(From Mateer JR, Thompson BM, Aprahamian C, Darin JC: Rapid fluid resuscitation with central venous catheters. Ann Emerg Med 12:150, 1983. Reproduced by permission.)

Table 24–3. Comparative Average Flow Rates (ml/min, 200 mm Hg Pressure) for Red Blood Cells

Catheter	Diluted PRBCs Hct 45% (95% CI)	Diluted PRBCs Hct 45% Through Blood Warmer (95% CI)	PRBCs Hct 65% (95% CI)
Central Venous Catheters			
USCI 9 French Introducer Internal diameter 0.117 in., length 5½ in.	343 (±21)	218 (±26)	124 (±2)
USCI 8 French Introducer Internal diameter 0.104 in., length 5½ in.	324 (±23)	—	—
Deseret Angiocath Gauge 14, length 5¼ in.	210 (±7)	171 (±9)	63 (±6)
Deseret Angiocath Gauge 16, length 5¼ in.	125 (±4)	—	—
Peripheral Venous Catheters			
Intravenous extension tubing Internal diameter 0.12 in., length 12 in.	312 (±1)	—	—
Argyle Medicut Gauge 14, length 2 in.	287 (±21)	192 (±15)	96 (±6)
Deseret Angiocath Gauge 14, length 2 in.	257 (±11)	—	—
Argyle Medicut Gauge 16, length 2 in.	220 (±5)	—	—
Deseret Angiocath Gauge 16, length 2 in.	158 (±14)	—	—

(From Mateer JR, Thompson BM, Aprahamian C, Darin JC: Rapid fluid resuscitation with central venous catheters. Ann Emerg Med 12:151, 1983. Reproduced by permission.)

Table 24–4. Comparative Average Flow Rates in Milliliters per Minute

Catheter	Tap Water at 200 mm Hg	Diluted PRBCs at 200 mm Hg	Tap Water Gravity	Diluted PRBCs Blood Warmer at 200 mm Hg	PRBCs at 200 mm Hg
Central Venous Catheters					
USCI 9 French Introducer Internal diameter 0.117 in., length 5½ in.	566 (±16)	343 (±21)	247 (±2)	218 (±26)	124 (±2)
USCI 8 French Introducer Internal diameter 0.104 in., length 5½ in.	540*	324 (±23)	243 (±5)	—	—
Deseret Angiocath Gauge 14, length 5¼ in.	341 (±6)	210 (±7)	157 (±6)	171 (±9)	63 (±6)
Peripheral Venous Catheters					
Intravenous extension tubing Internal diameter 0.12 in., length 12 in.	500 (±21)	312 (±1)	222 (±4)	—	—
Argyle Medicut Gauge 14, length 2 in.	484 (±8)	287 (±21)	194 (±5)	192 (±15)	96 (±6)
Argyle Medicut Gauge 16, length 2 in.	353 (±4)	220 (±5)	151 (±3)	—	—

*95% confidence interval not calculated because all three trials resulted in 11.1 sec for 100-ml flow.
(From Mateer JR, Thompson BM, Aprahamian C, Darin JC: Rapid fluid resuscitation with central venous catheters. Ann Emerg Med 12:151, 1983. Reproduced by permission.)

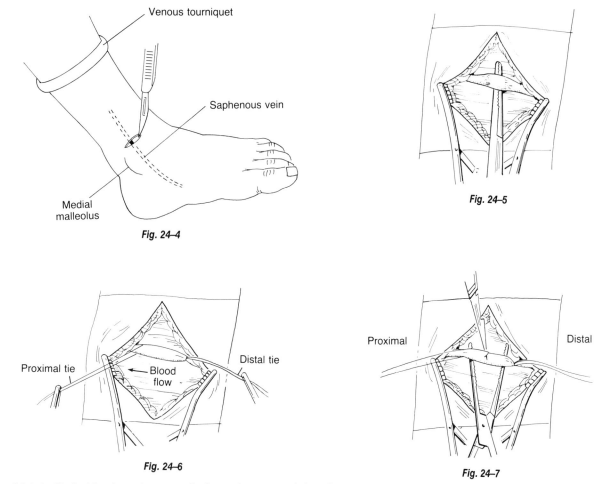

Fig. 24–4

Fig. 24–5

Fig. 24–6

Fig. 24–7

Figure 24–4. A skin incision is made perpendicular to the course of the vein.

Figure 24–5. Skin retracted and vein exposed. (From Vander Salm TJ, et al: Atlas of Bedside Procedures. Boston, Little, Brown & Co, 1979. Reproduced by permission.)

Figure 24–6. Proximal and distal ties are passed under the vein. If the vein is to be sacrificed, the distal suture is tied to prevent bleeding, and the ends are left long to help stabilize the vein during cannulation. The proximal tie is not tied at this point, but traction on it will control back bleeding. (From Vander Salm TJ, et al: Atlas of Bedside Procedures. Boston, Little, Brown & Co, 1979. Reproduced by permission.)

Figure 24–7. The vein is stretched flat and incised at a 45 degree angle. Approximately one third of the lumen must be exposed. Traction on the proximal tie will control back bleeding.

structures but does not provide sufficient exposure. A transverse incision involving all layers of the skin is the best approach. Subcutaneous fat should bulge from the incision. One bluntly dissects subcutaneous tissue by spreading the tissue gently with a curved hemostat. The tissue is spread in a direction parallel to the course of the vein. Bleeding is usually minimal, unless the vein is nicked. A tissue spreader or a self-retaining retractor may be used to provide a wider field. The vein is then isolated from the adjacent tissue and mobilized for 1 to 3 cm (see Fig. 24–5).

After the vein is mobilized, proximal and distal silk ties are passed under it. The distal ligature may or may not be tied at this point, but if it is tied it should not be cut, because it is useful in controlling the vein (see Fig. 24–6). Using a hemostat, one then elevates the vessel and stretches it flat. This provides good visualization and control of the vessel and limits bleeding when the vessel is incised. Alternatively, placing gentle traction on the proximal tie will control oozing around the puncture site. The vessel is incised at a 45-degree angle, through one third to one half of its diameter (see Fig. 24–7). A number 11 blade (as illustrated) or a pair of iris

scissors may be used to incise the vessel. Too small an incision may cause threading of the catheter into a false channel in the adventitia; conversely, the vessel may be torn completely and may retract from the field if the incision is too large.[23] A longitudinal incision is sometimes made to avoid transecting the vessel, but the lumen is more difficult to identify with this technique. The vessel incision must enter the actual lumen of the vein, although some bleeding will occur after the vein has merely been nicked. Incision of the vessel is unnecessary when an IV catheter with an introducing needle is used. The vessel is simply punctured, as in percutaneous venous cannulation. (See the section on the mini-cutdown procedure.)

Before being introduced into the vessel, the cannula is beveled at a 45-degree angle, unless a cannula with a tapered tip is used. A short bevel is preferred, and a sharply pointed tip is to be avoided, because it may pierce the posterior wall or otherwise damage the vein. The rounded tip of a feeding tube may be more difficult to introduce, but it may be advanced less traumatically. The cannula may be introduced directly through the skin incision or through a separate stab

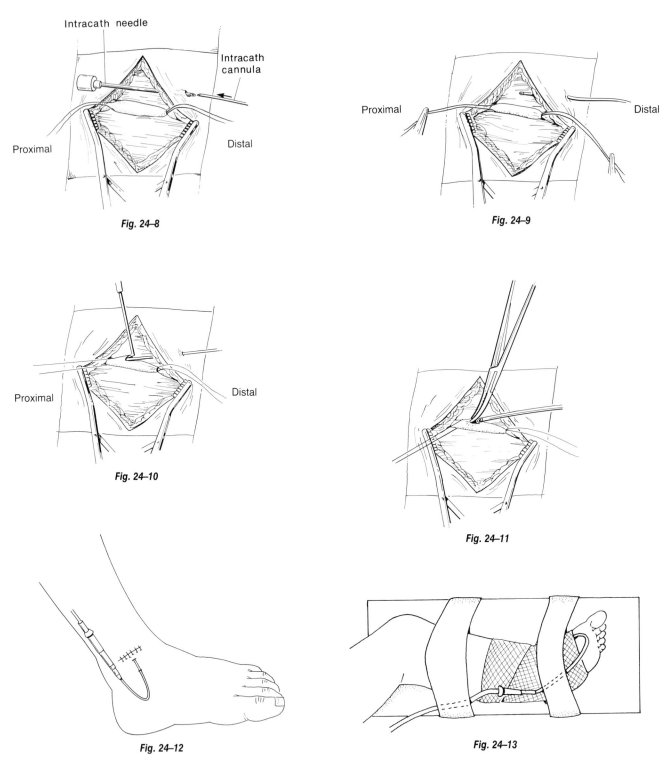

Fig. 24–8

Fig. 24–9

Fig. 24–10

Fig. 24–11

Fig. 24–12

Fig. 24–13

Figure 24–8. Use of the Intracath needle to produce a separate stab incision. The cannula is introduced into the wound by retrograde passage through the introducing needle. (From Vander Salm TJ, et al: Atlas of Bedside Procedures. Boston, Little, Brown & Co, 1979. Reproduced by permission.)

Figure 24–9. A cannula threaded through the stab incision. The intracath needle has been withdrawn following introduction of the cannula into the wound. (From Vander Salm TJ, et al: Atlas of Bedside Procedures. Boston, Little, Brown & Co, 1979. Reproduced by permission.)

Figure 24–10. Threading the catheter with the aid of a venous dilator (lifter). This is technically the most difficult part of the procedure. The lifter is especially helpful in small veins.

Figure 24–11. In larger veins, a mosquito hemostat can facilitate the placement of the cannula by opening the lumen and providing countertraction.

Figure 24–12. The incision is closed, and the catheter is sutured in place.

Figure 24–13. The cutdown site is securely dressed and splinted.

wound. The latter method is illustrated in Figures 24–8 and 24–9. Theoretically, the percutaneous approach reduces the risk of infection.[24] The beveled catheter is then threaded into the vessel lumen. Threading the catheter into the vein is usually the most difficult portion of the procedure and is often time-consuming.

Difficulty in threading may be encountered for several reasons. The lumen may have been incorrectly identified, or a false passage may have been created. This frequently occurs and may be difficult to recognize, because the catheter can easily advance between layers of the vessel wall. Other causes of difficult threading are penetration of the posterior vessel wall or use of a catheter that is too large for the vessel being cannulated. Identification of the vessel lumen may be facilitated through use of a plastic venous dilator or lifter (Becton-Dickinson X10152). The small, pointed tip of the device is threaded into the vessel to expose the lumen in advance of the catheter (see Fig. 24–10). This device is useful in pediatric cutdowns but is generally unnecessary in adults. One can facilitate the threading of very large catheters in adults by grasping the proximal surgical edge of the vessel with small forceps or a mosquito hemostat. Countertraction is applied as the catheter is advanced (see Fig. 24–11). At no time should one force a catheter that will not advance.

Once the catheter is advanced into the lumen, air is back-bled from the cannula, and the cannula is connected to IV tubing. The proximal ligature is tied around the vessel wall and the intraluminal cannula. The distal tie may be removed instead of tied, but oozing at the puncture site often occurs. The tourniquet is now removed, the catheter is affixed to the skin, and the incision is closed (see Fig. 24–12). An antibiotic ointment is applied at the point at which the catheter passes through the skin, and the wound is dressed. Adequate immobilization must be provided to prevent displacement of the line. This is especially important in children (see Fig. 24–13).

Mini-Cutdown

An alternative method that is designed to preserve the vein[25] and to bypass the time-consuming step of placing a catheter into the vessel has been described. A skin incision and blunt dissection are used to locate the vessel. Once identified, the vein is punctured under direct vision with a standard percutaneous venous catheter. Alternatively, a large-bore introducer device could be threaded over a guide wire using this technique. The needle may be introduced through a separate stab incision or through the skin incision. If a separate incision is used, the cannula is threaded through the needle into the vein, and the needle is withdrawn to the skin surface (Fig. 24–14). A guard is placed on the needle tip, the catheter device is fixed to the skin, and the incision is closed. An over-the-needle device (Angiocath, Medicut) may also be used, in which case the needle would be withdrawn and discarded. This method eliminates the need for tying or cutting the vein, thereby permitting repeated catheterization. Venipuncture is easier, and the technique uses the same equipment as for percutaneous venous cannulation. The mini-cutdown is therefore used in the treatment of chronically ill patients who require long-term intravenous therapy or in children who have limited accessible veins. A simple skin incision may also permit direct visualization of veins in the obese patient and may facilitate standard percutaneous venipuncture.

Hansbrough and coworkers[4] described the mini-cutdown procedure with a 10-gauge intravenous catheter (Deseret 10-gauge Angiocath). The flow rates of blood and saline with this catheter are equal to the rates obtained when intravenous extension tubing is placed in a vein using the more time-consuming standard venous cutdown technique. This catheter allows one to infuse a unit of whole blood in 2 to 3 minutes if pressure and oversized intravenous tubing (urology irrigating tubing) are used.

Shockley and Butzier describe a further modification whereby the guide wire technique is modified by passage of the guide wire, dilator, and sheath system following standard cutdown and venotomy.[25a] They found this technique to save more than 2 minutes' time over the standard technique when performed by novices.

Removal of catheters inserted by cutdown requires only cutting of skin stitches holding the catheter in place, followed by withdrawal of the catheter. Back-bleeding from the proximal venous end is controlled by a simple pressure dressing and is generally not a significant problem.

COMPLICATIONS

The complications of venous cutdown include local hematoma and infection, sepsis, phlebitis, embolization, wound dehiscence, and injury to associated structures. An indirect, but significant, complication is deterioration of an unstable patient during a time-consuming cutdown attempt. Documentation of complications and their frequency has been sparse. Bogen reported a 15 per cent complication rate in 234 cases.[26] Infection and phlebitis each occurred at a rate of 4 per cent. Infectious complications may result from the introduction of pathogens during line placement, transcutaneous invasion along the course of the cannula, or deposition of blood-borne organisms on the catheter tip.[27] A clear correlation exists between the incidence of infectious complications and the length of time that a catheter is left in place. Moran and associates found that the infection rate rose from 50 per cent to 78 per cent when a catheter was left in place for more than 48 hours.[28] Druskin and Siegel, studying a mixed population of patients who had undergone cutdowns and those who had had catheters percutaneously inserted, found that the incidence of culture-positive catheter tips rose from 0 to 52 per cent after 48 hours.[27] In Moran, Atwood, and Rowe's study, *Staphylococcus albus* was the predominant organism that was isolated, but organisms more commonly thought of as pathogenic (*S. aureus*, enterococcus, and *Proteus*) were isolated with greater frequency from cutdowns that had been in place for long periods.[28] Rhee and colleagues reported a 1.4 per cent infection rate (one episode of cellulitis) following 73 cutdown attempts.[12] All catheters were removed within 24 hours.

There is some evidence that the rate of infectious complications decreases when a broad-spectrum antibiotic ointment is applied to the cutdown site. Moran and coworkers found a rate of infectious complications of 18 per cent when topical Neosporin was used, compared with a 78 per cent rate in a placebo-treated group.[28] In this study, it was also shown that topical antibiotic use results in only a moderate decrease in the incidence of phlebitis (from 53 to 37 per cent) but a significant decrease in the incidence of phlebitis associated with positive cultures (from 86 to 14 per cent). This suggests that phlebitis is primarily a chemical or an irritative process rather than an infective process.[28] Whatever the cause, the incidence of phlebitis is clearly related to the duration of catheterization.[7, 26, 29] Early removal is a key factor in the prevention of both phlebitis and the infectious complications of venous cutdown. This is especially true of lines inserted during emergency resuscitative treatment. Such lines should be removed as soon as the patient's condition stabilizes and alternative routes exist.[8, 10]

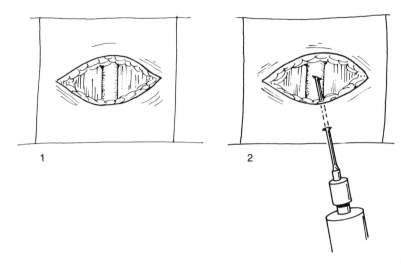

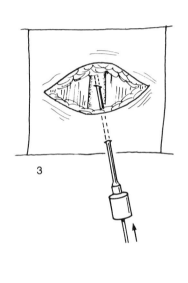

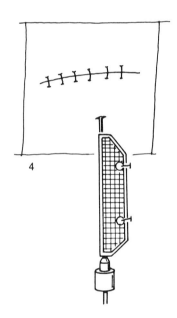

Figure 24–14. The mini-cutdown technique is an alternative to the venous cutdown method. The vein is cannulated under direct vision using standard percutaneous catheters. A separate entry site (shown) may be used, or the vein can be cannulated through the skin incision. Note that the vein is not tied off with this technique.

Proper attention to the details of surgical technique will limit the occurrence of minor complications, such as local hematoma, abscess, and wound dehiscence. One can avoid injury to associated structures by selecting a site in which the vein is isolated and, specifically, avoiding brachial vein cutdown.

CONCLUSION

The venous cutdown is a time-honored, simple surgical technique that is useful in the management of seriously ill patients. It is an excellent means of venous access in children and in markedly hypovolemic patients. Complications are potentially serious but can be controlled by good surgical technique and prompt removal of the line following clinical improvement.

REFERENCES

1. Craig RG, Jones RA, Sproul GL: The alternate methods of central venous system catheterization. Am Surg 3:131, 1968.
2. Keeley JL: Intravenous injections and infusions. Am J Surg 50:485, 1940.
3. Kirkham JH: Infusion into the internal saphenous vein at the ankle. Lancet 2:815, 1945.
4. Hansbrough JF, Cain TL, Millikan JS: Placement of 10 gauge catheter by cutdown for rapid fluid replacement. J Trauma 23:231, 1983.
5. Aldeman S: An emergency intravenous route for the pediatric population. JACEP 5:596, 1976.
6. Alexander E, Small W, Campbell JB: A dependable method for constant intravenous therapy in infants using polyethylene tubing. Ann Surg 127:1212, 1948.
7. Dudley HAF (ed): Hamilton Bailey's Emergency Surgery. 10th ed. Bristol, John Wright & Sons, 1977, p 28.
8. Dronen SC, Yee AS, Tomlanovich MC: Proximal saphenous vein cutdown. Ann Emerg Med 10:328, 1981.
9. Westaby S: Ryle's tube for rapid intravenous transfusion. Lancet 1:360, 1979.
10. Knopp R: Venous cutdowns in the emergency department. JACEP 7:429, 1978.
11. Posner M, Moore EE: Distal saphenous vein cutdown—technique of choice for rapid volume resuscitation. J Emerg Med 3:395, 1985.
12. Rhee KJ, Derlet RW, Beal SL: Rapid venous access using saphenous vein cutdown at the ankle. Am J Emerg Med 7:263, 1989.
13. Iserson KV, Criss EA: Pediatric venous cutdowns: Utility in emergency situations. Pediatr Emerg Care 2:231, 1986.
14. Hollinshead WH (ed): Textbook of Anatomy. 2nd ed. New York, Harper & Row, 1967, p 442.
15. Randolph J: Technique for insertion of plastic catheters into the saphenous vein. Pediatrics 24:631, 1959.
16. Preston G: Emergency venous access and cannulation. JACEP 11:642, 1982.
17. Anderson JE (ed): Grant's Atlas of Anatomy. 7th ed. Baltimore, Williams & Wilkins, 1978, pp 4.6, 4.11.
18. Ficcara BJ: Saphenous vein alimentation. Angiology 21:563, 1970.
19. Gray H: The veins. *In* Goss CM (ed): Anatomy of the Human Body. 29th ed. Philadelphia, Lea & Febiger, 1973, p 717.

20. Warwick R, Williams P: Gray's Anatomy. 35th ed. Philadelphia, WB Saunders Co, 1973, p 669.
21. Simon RR, Hoffman JR, Smith M: Modified new approaches for rapid intravenous access. Ann Emerg Med 16:44, 1987.
22. Talan DA, Simon RR, Hoffman JR: Cephalic vein cutdown at the wrist: Comparison to the standard saphenous vein ankle cutdown. Ann Emerg Med 17:38, 1988.
23. Stanley-Brown EG: The venous cutdown. Arch Pediatr 75:480, 1958.
24. Priouleau WH: Technique of venesection in infants. Surg Gynecol Obstet 122:838, 1966.
25. Shiu MH: A method for conservation of veins in the surgical cutdown. Surg Gynecol Obstet 134:315, 1972.

25a. Shockley LW, Butzier DJ: A modified wire-guided technique for venous cutdown access. Ann Emerg Med 19:393, 1990.
26. Bogen JE: Local complications in 167 patients with indwelling venous catheters. Surg Gynecol Obstet 110:112, 1960.
27. Druskin MS, Siegel PD: Bacterial contamination of indwelling intravenous polyethylene catheters. JAMA 185:966, 1963.
28. Moran JM, Atwood RP, Rowe M: A clinical and bacteriologic study of infections associated with venous cutdown. N Engl J Med 272:554, 1963.
29. Collins RN, Braun PA, Zinner SH, et al: Risk of local and systemic infection with polyethylene intravenous catheters. N Engl J Med 279:340, 1968.

Chapter **25**

Central Venous Catheterization: Subclavian Vein Approach

Steven C. Dronen

INTRODUCTION

The popularity of subclavian venipuncture has paralleled the medical advances of recent years. The development of sophisticated monitoring techniques, transvenous pacemaker devices, total parenteral nutrition, and emergency resuscitative protocols has created a need for rapid and reliable methods of central venous access. Peripheral venous sites can be used for some of these procedures, but the choice of these sites necessitates the use of long catheters that must be threaded accurately into the superior vena cava. Peripheral veins may be collapsed, thrombosed, buried in subcutaneous fat, or otherwise difficult to locate. The subclavian vein has a predictable relationship to easily identified anatomic landmarks and can be cannulated within minutes. Consequently, subclavian venipuncture has become a common practice in a variety of clinical settings. Supraclavicular (SC) and infraclavicular (IC) approaches have been described.

BACKGROUND

The technique of subclavian venipuncture was first described in the French literature in 1952, and numerous articles soon appeared to support the use of the technique.[1–8] Wilson and colleagues, who described the role of central venous pressure (CVP) monitoring in the maintenance of optimal blood volume, are credited with popularizing the procedure in the United States. They used the subclavian vein for the introduction of CVP catheters, arguing that this approach is easier, safer, and more accurate than that of other methods.[9]

Numerous reports of clinical experience with the IC technique followed Wilson's article. These stressed the clinical usefulness of the procedure, the ease with which it is performed, and the low complication rate. Subclavian venipuncture was described as useful in the management of hypovolemia, burns, cardiac arrest, chronic intravenous (IV) therapy, and septic shock.[10–14]

Early enthusiasm for IC subclavian venipuncture was countered by a growing awareness of serious and occasionally fatal complications. Yarom was the first to warn of the potential dangers in 1964.[15] A year later, Matz called for the abandonment of the technique, labeling it a "disease of medical progress." He encountered six complications, including two fatalities, in 1 week.[16] Smith and co-

workers reported eight complications over a 2-year period and concluded that the subclavian vein should be cannulated only when other means have been exhausted.[17]

The reported complications of the IC subclavian approach suggested the need for a safer method. In 1965, Yoffa described the SC approach. Anatomic dissections had shown that the route to the subclavian vein is more direct when approached from above the clavicle. In a series of 130 patients, he reported no fatalities or serious complications when the SC approach was used.[18] Other studies have substantiated the utility of this approach.[19–25] Dronen and associates compared the two approaches during the performance of cardiopulmonary resuscitation (CPR) and found a significant decrease in catheter tip malposition and CPR interruption when the SC approach was used.[26]

Irrespective of the approach that is used, subclavian vein cannulation has increased dramatically over the past 25 years. It would be difficult to estimate the frequency with which this procedure is performed today, but it is a commonplace practice in hospitals throughout the world. Other methods of central venous cannulation have been developed simultaneously. These include the passage of long lines through the basilic vein and cannulation of the internal jugular vein (see Chapter 26). Each has its relative merits (Table 25–1). Any physician involved in the care of critically ill patients should master several of these techniques.

INDICATIONS

Infraclavicular Approach

There are no absolute indications for IC subclavian venipuncture. Because this technique is one of several venous access routes, its use depends to a great extent on physician experience. There are several clinical situations in which its use is applicable. Although generally reserved for adults, the IC approach is a reasonable option for emergency or long-term venous access in infants and children when alternative techniques are unsuitable.

CVP Monitoring. Wilson and colleagues described the placement of a catheter into the superior vena cava as a means of assessing blood volume.[9] Although supplanted to some extent by more sophisticated methods, this remains a useful tool in the treatment of hypovolemic patients (see Chapter 27).

Volume Loading. Subclavian venipuncture has been widely used as a vehicle for rapid volume resuscitation. Unfortunately, it is often misused in this regard. The flow rate of saline through a peripheral 5-cm, 14-gauge catheter is roughly twice the rate of that through a 20-cm, 16-gauge central venous catheter, with equivalent pressure heads.[27, 28] The difference in flow is even greater for blood products because of viscosity factors, which slow the passage of red cells through small-gauge catheters.[28, 29] Consequently, *the placement of peripheral large-bore catheters is the preferred method of rapid volume loading, unless time would be lost searching for venipuncture sites, or unusually large volumes need to be infused.*

Table 25–1. Advantages and Disadvantages of Techniques

Technique	Advantages	Disadvantages
Basilic (peripheral) puncture	Low incidence of major complications Performed under direct visualization of vein Allows large quantities of fluid to be given rapidly	Greater incidence of minor complications of infection, phlebitis, and thrombosis Hinders free movement of arms More difficult to place catheter in correct position for central venous pressure monitoring
Internal jugular puncture	Good external landmarks Lesser risk of pneumothorax than with subclavian puncture Bleeding can be recognized and controlled Malposition of catheter is rare Almost a straight course to the superior vena cava on the right side Carotid artery easily identified Useful alternative approach to cutdown in children under the age of 2 years	"Blind" procedure Has a slightly higher incidence of failures than subclavian More difficult and inconvenient to secure
Infraclavicular subclavian puncture	Good external landmarks	Higher incidence of complications, especially in hypovolemic shock "Blind" procedure Should not be attempted in children under 2 years of age
Supraclavicular subclavian puncture	Good landmarks Less risk of pneumothorax than with infraclavicular puncture Most practical method of inserting a central line in cardiorespiratory arrest Malposition of catheter is uncommon	"Blind" procedure

(Modified from Knopp R, Dailey RH: Central venous cannulation and pressure monitoring. JACEP 6:358, 1977.)

than routine subclavian venipuncture but uses a catheter that exceeds even the flow capabilities of commonly used IV tubing.[30] In trained hands this is a useful method of rapid fluid resuscitation, although it is associated with significant risk if the catheter is misplaced (see Chapter 22). Dutky and colleagues note that kinking of the large-bore introducer catheter may halve the flow rate.[30a] They found that catheter kinking was common when long introducer catheters are placed via the IC route at the junction of the medial and middle thirds of the clavicle.

Emergency Venous Access. The predictable anatomic location of the subclavian vein and the speed with which it can be cannulated (15 to 30 seconds) have prompted its use in cardiac arrest and other emergency situations. Although subclavian venipuncture by the infraclavicular route is an ideal means of rapid venous access, it may not be the best technique to use during CPR. Chest wall motion and physical interference with the performance of effective CPR make IC venipuncture more difficult and perhaps more dangerous in this setting.[26] The need for a central line during CPR is controversial, although many clinicians advocate use of a central line routinely. It has been suggested that therapeutic drug levels are reached more rapidly if given centrally. This claim has been verified in animal studies,[31–33] although differences are small when cardiac output is high[31] or small animals are used.[33] A cadaver study demonstrated significant delay in the arrival of peripherally injected dye in the arterial circulation.[34] When easily obtained, central venous cannulation is preferred over peripheral venous access because it provides a rapid and reliable route for the administration of drugs to the central circulation of the patient in cardiac arrest.

Routine Venous Cannulation. Drug abusers, burn victims, and obese or long-term hospitalized patients may have inadequate peripheral IV sites. Subclavian vein cannulation may be indicated under these circumstances.

Routine Blood Drawing. Despite the claim of Kalcev that subclavian venipuncture is a "safe and easy method" of obtaining blood specimens,[8] the potential complications of this procedure do not justify its use in routine blood sampling. Lines already in place may be used for this purpose if they are properly cleared of IV fluid. A 20-cm, 16-gauge catheter contains 0.3 ml of fluid, so at least this much must be withdrawn to avoid dilution of blood samples. Because of the increased risk of infectious complications, air embolus, and venous back-bleeding, the IV tubing should not be repeatedly disconnected from the catheter hub. Interposition of a three-way stopcock in the IV tubing simplifies access and is an acceptable method of blood sampling in the intensive care unit setting.

Hyperalimentation. In 1969, Dudrick and colleagues described beneficial results of long-term parenteral nutrition in patients with various gastrointestinal disorders. Intravenous hyperalimentation by way of the subclavian vein was found to be safe and reliable.[35] Use of the IC technique frees the patient's extremities and neck; this procedure is therefore well suited to long-term applications.[36] Strict aseptic technique is necessary to minimize infectious complications.[37]

Infusion of Concentrated Solutions. Hyperosmolar or irritating solutions that have the potential to cause thrombophlebitis if given through small peripheral vessels are frequently infused by way of the subclavian vein. Examples are potassium chloride (greater than 40 mEq/L), hyperosmolar saline, and acidifying solutions, such as ammonium chloride.

Other indications for central venous access include the placement of a Swan-Ganz catheter or a temporary transvenous pacemaker, the performance of cardiac catheterization and pulmonary angiography, and hemodialysis. Catheters such as the Uldall can be inserted within minutes, permitting use of the subclavian vein for emergency or short-term hemodialysis[38] (see also Chapter 28).

Supraclavicular Approach

The indications for SC venipuncture are essentially the same as those for the IC procedure. During CPR the SC route is often preferred, however, because it minimizes physical interference with the functions of chest compression and airway management. The IC technique requires deep penetration of a moving chest wall and frequently demands an interruption of chest compression. Supraclavicular subclavian venipuncture can be performed without cessation of CPR and involves superficial penetration of the relatively motionless neck.[26] This technique also avoids interference with airway management, which commonly occurs when the internal jugular vein is cannulated.[39] When a true central location is required, the SC approach is superior to the IC and long peripheral line insertion techniques because of the low incidence of catheter tip malposition with the SC approach.[22, 26] Additionally, the SC technique has been performed in the sitting position in patients with severe orthopnea. Placement of a central line with a patient in the sitting position is virtually impossible with other central venous access routes.[19, 40] Finally, the low complication rate reported for SC subclavian venipuncture makes it a more attractive alternative, especially in the seriously ill patient.[18–23]

CONTRAINDICATIONS

The contraindications to subclavian venipuncture have been described in several reviews.[39, 41, 42] They are listed in Table 25–2. Subclavian venipuncture is generally contraindicated in patients with distortion of the local anatomy or landmarks. These include patients who have undergone previous surgery or trauma involving the clavicle, the first rib, or the subclavian vessels; patients who have undergone previous radiation therapy to the clavicular area; patients with significant chest wall deformities; and those with marked cachexia or obesity. Physicians in many burn centers routinely place a central catheter through a burned area, however. Patients with unilateral deformities not associated with pneumothorax (e.g., fractured clavicle) should be catheterized on the opposite side.

Table 25–2. Contraindications to Subclavian Venipuncture

Distorted local anatomy*
Chest wall deformities
Extremes of weight
Vasculitis
Prior long-term subclavian cannulation
Prior injection of sclerosing agents
Suspected superior vena cava injury
Suspected subclavian vessel injury*
Previous radiation surgery*
Pneumothorax†
Bleeding disorders
Anticoagulant therapy
Combative patients
Inexperienced, unsupervised physician

---

*May cannulate contralateral side.
†May cannulate ipsilateral side.

Subclavian venipuncture is not contraindicated in patients who have penetrating thoracic wounds unless the injuries involve the superior vena cava. Generally, the vein on the *same side* as the chest wound should be cannulated to avoid the possibility of bilateral pneumothoraces, unless one suspects that subclavian vessels have been injured. In such instances, the opposite side is cannulated.[43] In penetrating wounds that may involve the superior vena cava, neither subclavian vessel should be cannulated, and venous access below the diaphragm should be sought. Use of the subclavian approach in patients with coagulation disorders or in those receiving heparin therapy is contraindicated. A more visible and accessible site should be chosen (preferably percutaneous cannulation of a peripheral vein), because it is impossible to apply direct pressure to an oozing subclavian vein. The procedure should not be performed in combative patients because of the greater possibility of pneumothorax, vessel laceration, air embolism, and septic complications. Subclavian venipuncture is not generally recommended for use in small children because of the higher risk of complications. Kron and colleagues[44] report a 72 per cent success rate with no complications in 32 children less than 2 years of age. Similar results should not be expected unless the physician has a detailed knowledge of pediatric anatomy and performs the procedure frequently. Bonventre and coworkers[45] noted that vascular placement was less successful and the complication rate higher in the younger child. Internal jugular cannulation is an acceptable alternative in young children. Other relative contraindications include those conditions predisposing to sclerosis or thrombosis of the central veins, such as vasculitis, long-term subclavian cannulation, or intravenous drug abuse via the jugular system. Finally, the procedure should not be performed by unsupervised physicians who are inexperienced in the technique.

ANATOMY

The subclavian vein begins as a continuation of the axillary vein at the outer edge of the first rib (Figs. 25–1 and 25–2). It joins the internal jugular vein to become the innominate vein 3 to 4 cm proximally. It has a diameter of 10 to 20 mm and is valveless. After crossing the first rib, the vein lies posteriorly to the medial third of the clavicle. It is only in this area that there is an intimate association between the clavicle and the subclavian vein. The costoclavicular ligament lies anterior and inferior to the subclavian vein, and the fascia contiguous to this ligament invests the vessel. Posterior to the vein, separating it from the subclavian artery, lies the anterior scalene muscle, which has a thickness of 10 to 15 mm. The phrenic nerve passes over the anterior surface of the scalene muscle and runs immediately behind the junction of the subclavian and internal jugular veins. The thoracic duct (on the left) and the lymphatic duct (on the right) pass over the anterior scalene muscle and enter the subclavian vein near its junction with the internal jugular vein. Superior and posterior to the subclavian artery lies the brachial plexus. The dome of the *left* lung may extend above the first rib, but the right lung rarely extends this high.

EQUIPMENT

The materials required for subclavian venipuncture are listed in Table 25–3. The catheter may be of the "over-the-needle" or "through-the-needle" variety, or it may be a component in a guide wire system that combines both technologies (Fig. 25–3). Over-the-needle devices (such as

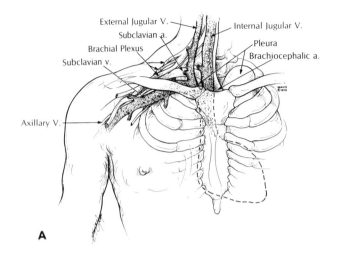

A

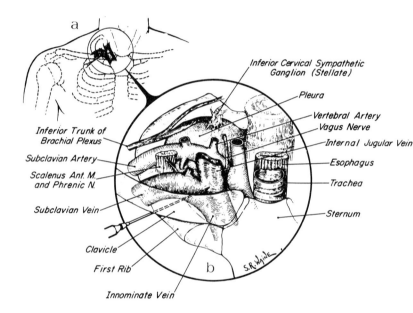

Figure 25–1. *A* and *B*, Subclavian vein and local anatomy. (Part *A* from Linos D, Mucha P, von Heerden J: The subclavian vein: A golden route. Mayo Clin Proc 55:316, 1980. Part *B* from Davidson JJ, Ben-Hur N, Nathan H: Subclavian venepuncture. Lancet 2:1140, 1963. Reproduced by permission.)

B *a,* **Point of insertion and direction of needle.**
b, **Oblique anterosuperior view of root of neck.**

the Angiocath) use a tapered plastic catheter that passes through the vessel wall into the lumen using the needle tip as a guide. There are several advantages of this system. The catheter does not pass through a sharp needle, and the risk

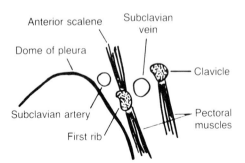

Figure 25–2. Subclavian area, sagittal section. (From Brahos G: Central venous catheterization, SC approach. J Trauma 17:873, 1977. Copyright 1977, The Williams & Wilkins Company, Baltimore. Reproduced by permission.)

of shearing with resultant catheter embolization is thus decreased. The needle is removed following cannulation, making a guard unnecessary. The hole made by the needle in the vessel wall is smaller than the catheter, producing a tighter seal. The main disadvantage is the length of the catheter, which is generally limited to 5 to 8 cm. Also, catheter threading is made more difficult by the longer length of the needle relative to the catheter. With over-the-needle catheters, the needle extends a few millimeters past the tip of the catheter. A blood return will be obtained when the tip of the needle is in the vein, but the catheter may actually be outside the lumen. If the needle is withdrawn before the catheter is advanced, the catheter tip will remain outside the vein. One must be certain to keep the needle steady and to advance the catheter forward over the needle to ensure intravascular placement.

Through-the-needle devices (such as the Intracath) use a catheter of smaller gauge than the puncturing needle. Generally, the needle is 14-gauge and the catheter is 16-gauge. This catheter is threaded through the lumen of the needle after the vessel is entered by the needle tip. After the threading, the needle is withdrawn and is left on the

Table 25–3. Materials for Subclavian Venipuncture
1 per cent lidocaine (Xylocaine)
26-gauge needle
2-ml Luer-Lok syringe
10-ml non–Luer-Lok syringe
Swabs
Preparation solution
Gloves
Drapes
Catheter device
Intravenous tubing
Intravenous solution
Needle holder
4–0 silk sutures
Suture scissors
Antibiotic ointment
Gauze pads
Tincture of benzoin
Cloth tape

skin surface with a plastic guard protecting the patient and the catheter. A modification of this system uses a detachable hub on the catheter so that the needle can be removed. The main advantage of through-the-needle systems is that catheters of any length may be used. Also, the rate of successful entry of the catheter into the vessel lumen is generally higher. The main disadvantage of this system is the potential for catheter shearing during or after insertion. Systems using a detachable catheter hub (Deseret 755) allow the needle to be removed completely following insertion but require assembly of small plastic parts. This is undesirable in an emergency situation. Another disadvantage of through-the-needle devices is that the caliber of the catheter must be smaller than that of the needle. Standard catheters are 16-gauge, a size not optimal for rapid infusion of blood.

Recently introduced catheters tend to combine through-the-needle and over-the-needle technology. The Argyle Intramedicut catheter has a short over-the-needle catheter that serves as an introducer for a longer (30 cm) infusion catheter. Following successful cannulation of the vein with the introducing catheter, the needle is withdrawn and the infusion catheter is advanced through the introducing catheter.

Further refinement of this system was made possible by the development of thin-walled 18-gauge needles that permit passage of a flexible guide wire. The Arrow Central Vein Catheterization Set (CS-04300) uses a 6.4-cm, 16-gauge catheter inserted over an 18-gauge thin-walled needle. Either the catheter or the needle may be used as a conduit for the introduction of a 45-cm guide wire over which is passed a 20-cm infusion catheter (see also Chapter 23).

Physicians inexperienced in the use of these systems frequently encounter difficulty passing the guide wire. This may be caused by motion of the thin-walled needle as it is detached from the syringe with resultant loss of its intravascular position. The need to detach the syringe can be eliminated by use of the Arrow Safety Syringe. This is a recently introduced product that incorporates a hollow syringe through which the guide wires can be passed directly into the thin-walled needle without detachment. In addition, this reduces the risk of air embolism that may occur when the needle is open to the air.

The combination of over-the-needle and through-the-needle technology offers the theoretic advantage of greater safety because these systems use needles of smaller diameter (18 gauge) than those typically found in through-the-needle devices. There is no evidence, however, that the complications of subclavian cannulation are related to the size of the

puncturing needle. Moreover, the initial small vessel puncture is usually enlarged with a venous dilator before catheter insertion. Schug and colleagues[46] compared subclavian venipuncture performed with a standard through-the-needle device (Deseret Intracath 3162) to a system using a thin-walled needle and guide wire (Arrow AK 04300). They found no difference in the success or complication rates, but there was a significantly higher incidence of catheter misplacement or nonfunction when the guide wire technique was used.

The real advantage of the combined system is increased flexibility. Although more steps are required with the guide wire technique, it has several uses once it is mastered. Minor modification of the process and the equipment used permits the insertion not only of standard infusion catheters but also of multilumen catheters, large-bore rapid infusion catheters, and introducer devices. If this degree of flexibility is desired, use of the new combined systems may be advantageous despite their significantly greater cost.

Catheter length and size are also important considerations. The superior vena cava begins at the level of the manubrial-sternal junction and terminates in the right atrium, approximately 5 cm lower. *The proper position of the catheter is in the superior vena cava, not the right atrium or ventricle.* Therefore, the catheter should be threaded approximately 2 cm below the manubrial-sternal junction. One can estimate this distance by placing the catheter parallel to the chest wall before insertion. The standard catheters marketed for subclavian venipuncture are 20 to 30 cm long. Thirty-centimeter catheters should not be inserted directly into the subclavian vein because the catheter tip is likely to terminate in the right atrium or ventricle. Twenty centimeters is an appropriate length for the average adult male, but it may be appropriate to advance the catheter less than its full length in smaller adults. Proper placement is best assessed by a chest film, not by predetermined measurements.

Subclavian veins are often cannulated in seriously ill patients who will require subsequent Swan-Ganz monitoring or transvenous pacemakers. Any CVP catheter that is initially inserted should have a lumen that is large enough to accept the guide wire for an introducer sheath (Seldinger technique) that can be used to insert the aforementioned devices. Not all of the commercially available CVP catheters will accept a guide wire through the lumen. As long as one is cannulating the vein, it is reasonable to use a catheter that can later be converted via the Seldinger technique for other purposes.

A number of different subclavian catheters are currently manufactured. It is *not* advisable to stock several different catheter types. This practice adds unnecessary confusion to the duties of supply clerks and nurses, not to mention the physician who might be handed an unfamiliar brand during patient resuscitation. It is better to use one brand routinely and to see that all medical personnel are thoroughly schooled in its use.

TECHNIQUE

The technique of subclavian venipuncture has been described in several reports.[14, 39, 47–54] Undue attention has been given to descriptions of angles and landmarks and to myths concerning the effects of patient positioning. The important factors governing success or failure are knowledge of the anatomy and meticulous attention to the details of the procedure.[55]

Strict adherence to the principles of sterile technique is important if septic complications are to be avoided. Violation of these principles for the sake of speed is seldom justified.

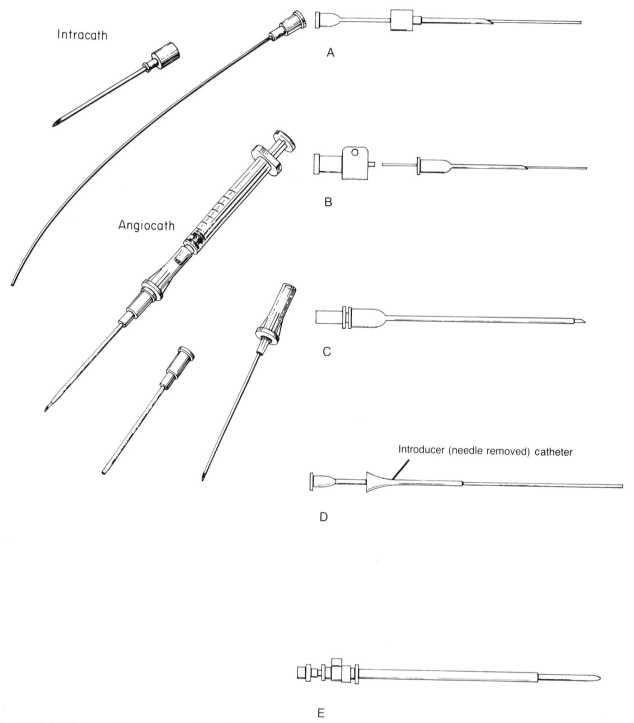

Figure 25–3. Subclavian catheter types. *A*, Through the needle; a 16-gauge catheter is threaded through a 14-gauge needle. Any length catheter may be used, but the gauge is generally limited. This is a poor choice for rapid fluid infusion and has the potential for catheter embolization. Example: Intracath *(upper left)*. *B*, Deseret 3162. Through the needle, detachable hub. Modification of *A* in which the needle is withdrawn over the catheter before the hub is attached. This eliminates the need for a needle guard, but assembly of small parts is required. *C*, Deseret 755. Over-the-needle 14-gauge catheter is advanced over a 16-gauge needle. This permits the use of a larger bore catheter than those illustrated in *A*, *B*, or *D*, but the catheter length is limited. Threading is more difficult than with the through-the-needle devices. Example: Angiocath *(lower left)*. *D*, Intramedicut. A long 16-gauge catheter is threaded through a short 14-gauge catheter previously advanced over a 16-gauge needle. This eliminates the risk of catheter shearing and the need for a needle guard. It has the same low flow rate as do the through-the-needle devices. Example: Argyle Intramedicut. *E*, Introducer set. A large-bore catheter advanced over a venous dilator. This permits very rapid fluid infusion, but insertion is more complicated than with other devices.

The few extra seconds required to put on gloves and to swab and drape the chest will rarely make a critical difference in patient survival. It is recognized that the optimum practice of aseptic technique often cannot take place during a resuscitation. For this reason, all central lines placed in this setting should be replaced at the earliest possible opportunity.

The area of the needle puncture should be widely prepared with an iodophor solution. In iodine-allergic patients, pHisoHex is an acceptable alternative. The area that is prepared should include puncture sites for the IC and SC subclavian and internal jugular approaches. This permits the physician to change the site following an unsuccessful attempt without repeating the preparation. A standard preparation should include the ipsilateral anterior neck, the supraclavicular fossa, and the anterior chest 3 to 5 cm past the midline and the same distance above the nipple line.

The need to perform an operating suite–style preparation (gowns, surgical scrub, and so forth) in patients receiving hyperalimentation is unproven. In a study of 63 patients with long-term subclavian catheterization for hyperalimentation, Merk reported only one infection using a simple iodophor spray preparation. He emphasized the role of experienced personnel as having prime importance in the prevention of infection.[35]

Infraclavicular Approach

The patient is placed in the supine position with the head in a neutral position and the arm adducted. Placing the patient in the Trendelenburg position (10 to 15 degrees) decreases the risk of air embolism. The claim that this position distends the vein[52] is controversial at best. Land has demonstrated by venographic studies that there is no change in the diameter of the subclavian vein associated with the Trendelenburg position.[56] Because his patients were normovolemic, this finding cannot necessarily be extrapolated to hypovolemic patients. Nonetheless, the vessel is hemmed by the semirigid costoclavicular ligament on its anterior-inferior aspect and therefore will not distend in a direction that facilitates IC venipuncture.[18] Further support for this concept can be found in a cadaver and volunteer study by Jesseph and colleagues.[57] Magnetic resonance imaging clearly demonstrated that the caliper of the subclavian vein is determined by its attachment to adjacent structures, and is not affected by the central venous pressure. These findings are in conflict with those of Fortune and colleagues,[58] who noted mild dilation of the subclavian vein on B-mode ultrasound of normal subjects during Trendelenberg positioning.

Abduction of the arm has been recommended to flatten the deltoid bulge.[59] This is sometimes a helpful maneuver in muscular individuals but is not generally necessary. Land has demonstrated that abduction moves medially the point at which the subclavian vein passes beneath the clavicle.[56]

Turning the head to the opposite side, as advocated by Borja and Hinshaw,[47] has no effect on the vessel size or on the relative positions of the vessel and the clavicle.[56] This maneuver does change the relative positions of the subclavian and internal jugular veins and has been postulated to cause an increased incidence of catheter malposition in the jugular vein.[57] Placing a pillow under the back is commonly recommended to make the clavicle more prominent, but as the shoulder falls backward the space between the clavicle and first rib narrows, making the subclavian vein less accessible.[59] Jesseph and colleagues demonstrated significant compression of the subclavian vessel between these bony structures as the shoulders retract.[57]

The right subclavian vein is usually cannulated because of the lower pleural dome on the right and because of the

need to avoid the left-sided thoracic duct. The anatomically more direct route between the left subclavian vein and the superior vena cava is a theoretic advantage of left-sided subclavian venipuncture over the right-sided approach. It is as yet unproved if there is a higher incidence of catheter malposition when the right IC approach is used.

In the conscious patient, the point of needle entry is anesthetized with 1 per cent lidocaine. Subcutaneous infiltration to the periosteum of the clavicle will make the procedure painless but is not always necessary. When using a through-the-needle device, one attaches the 14-gauge needle to a 10-ml non–Luer-Lok syringe. It is advised that the needle not be left attached to the catheter as it is packaged (Deseret 3162), because this gives less control over the needle tip. It also makes catheter threading more difficult, because the catheter slides back and forth in the plastic envelope (Fig. 25–4).

Opinions vary as to the best point of needle entry. The junction of the middle and medial thirds of the clavicle is the standard site. There the vein lies just posteriorly to the clavicle and just above the first rib, which acts as a barrier to penetration of the pleura. This protective effect is lost when a more lateral location is chosen. Westreich advocates entry just laterally and inferiorly to the junction of the clavicle and the first rib, with the needle aiming at this junction.[42] Simon advocates entry at the site of a small tubercle in the medial aspect of the deltopectoral groove.[54] In my opinion, the point of entry is less important than the direction taken by the needle after entry. Points lateral to the midclavicle should be avoided, because this location requires a deeper puncture and potentially increases the risk of pneumothorax. Orientation of the needle bevel is important. It should be oriented inferomedially to direct the catheter toward the innominate vein rather than toward the opposite vessel wall or up the internal jugular vein (Fig. 25–5). Alignment of the needle bevel with markings on the barrel of the syringe permits awareness of bevel orientation

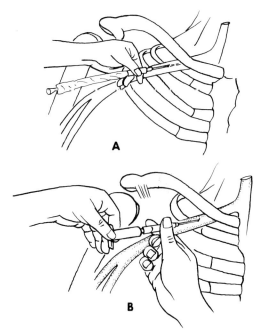

Figure 25–4. *A,* Insertion of a through-the-needle device, as packaged. *B,* It is advisable to remove the packaged catheter and to puncture the vein with a syringe attached to the needle. Contrary to the illustration, latex gloves should be worn. (Redrawn from Gallitano AL, Kondi ES, Deckers PJ: A safe approach to the subclavian vein. Surg Gynecol Obstet 135:97, 1972. Reproduced by permission of Surgery, Gynecology & Obstetrics.)

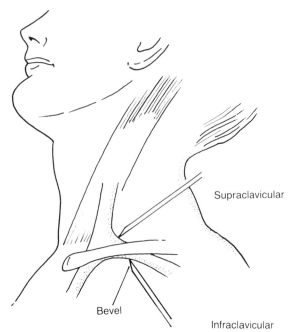

Figure 25–5. Needle bevel orientation using supraclavicular and infraclavicular venipuncture. The orientation of the needle bevel may help in positioning the catheter properly by guiding the direction of the catheter during advancement.

immediately above and posteriorly to the index finger. Vessel entry, signaled by a flashback of dark venous blood, usually occurs at a depth of 3 to 4 cm. If the needle tip is truly intraluminal, there will be a free flow of blood. The return of a pulsatile flow signifies arterial puncture. A single arterial puncture without laceration rarely causes serious harm. Use of this technique eliminates the need to measure angles, to "walk" the clavicle, or to concentrate excessively on maintaining the needle parallel to the chest wall. All of these techniques are based on fear of complications rather than knowledge of anatomy.[60] Mogil and colleagues have advocated changing the direction of the needle after it passes posteriorly to the lower edge of the clavicle.[14] In my opinion, this adds a step that is not only unnecessary but also dangerous. One should avoid any sweeping motions of the needle tip to prevent unseen injuries. In patients who are being ventilated with positive pressure, it is advisable to halt ventilations for a moment as the needle penetrates the chest wall. Interruptions should be kept to a minimum and should not exceed the 30-second standard.[61]

After a venous flashback is obtained, the syringe is detached from the needle. Removing the syringe is a step that causes frustration for many physicians. Removal of the syringe may displace the needle tip from the vein lumen, necessitating repuncture. If the syringe is tightly attached to the needle, a hemostat can be used to grasp and secure the needle during detachment of the syringe. Needle tip dis-

after skin puncture. Some investigators advise puncturing the skin with a number 11 scalpel blade to avoid skin plugs in the needle. Others suggest filling the syringe with a few milliliters of local anesthetic both to anesthetize the subcutaneous tissue and to flush the needle.

The mechanics of IC subclavian venipuncture using a through-the-needle device are illustrated in Figures 25–6 through 25–9. Before insertion, the left index finger is placed in the suprasternal notch and the thumb is positioned at the costoclavicular junction.[42] These serve as reference points for the direction of needle travel. The needle is aimed

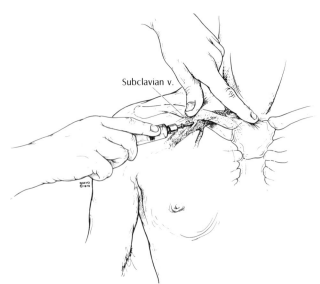

Figure 25–6. Hand position during subclavian venipuncture. Note that surgical gloves should be worn during this procedure, in contrast to the illustration. (From Linos D, Mucha P, von Heerden J: Subclavian vein: A golden route. Mayo Clin Proc 55:318, 1980. Reproduced by permission.)

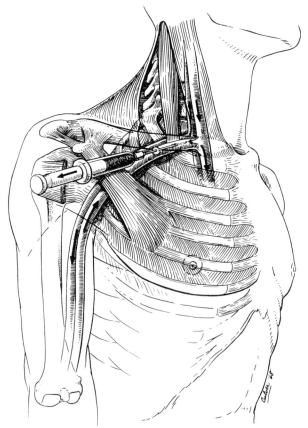

Figure 25–7. Subclavian venipuncture, venous backflow. After venipuncture, the syringe is removed carefully to avoid inadvertent motion of the needle tip, which may dislodge the needle from the vein lumen. A hemostat may help hold the needle hub to prevent motion during withdrawal of the syringe. (From Phillips SJ: Technique of percutaneous subclavian vein catheterization. Surg Gynecol Obstet 127:1080, 1968. Reproduced by permission of Surgery, Gynecology & Obstetrics.)

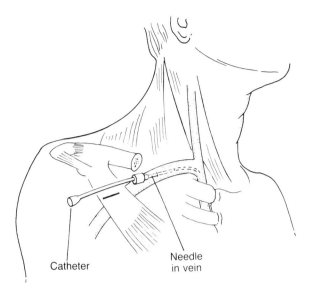

After removal of syringe,
thread catheter fully into needle

Figure 25–8. Catheter threading.

placement may also occur if blood specimens are drawn at this stage in the procedure. Blood drawing should be delayed until the catheter is threaded well into the vessel lumen. *The needle hub should be covered with the thumb at this time to prevent air embolus.* Additionally, the patient may be asked to exhale, hum, or perform a Valsalva maneuver to raise intrathoracic pressure. The catheter is then threaded through the needle.

At no time should the catheter be withdrawn through the needle or forced when it will not thread. Should it thread smoothly into the vessel, it is advanced fully into the needle hub, and the needle is withdrawn from the skin. The guard should be placed immediately. The wire stylet is then re-

moved, and the IV tubing is connected. When a detachable hub (through-the-needle system) is used, the catheter is threaded through the needle to 5 cm from its proximal end. The needle is then withdrawn over the catheter, and the catheter hub is attached (Fig. 25–10).

The guard is sutured to the chest wall parallel to and just below the clavicle (Fig. 25–11). A silk suture (4–0) is used to fix the guard at two points. This prevents excessive motion, which would kink the catheter at the point at which it exits the guard. Fixation also limits to-and-fro catheter motion, which is postulated to traumatize the vessel and to increase the risk of thrombophlebitis, infection, and vascular perforation.[62, 63] It is important to be certain that the catheter fits into the groove in the needle guard. Occasionally, the catheter is misplaced, and when the guard is clamped it occludes the catheter lumen.

When an over-the-needle system is used, the needle is advanced into the vein until there is free venous backflow. At this point the needle tip, but not necessarily the catheter, is in the vessel lumen. The needle is not withdrawn; rather, the catheter is advanced over the needle into the vessel lumen. Once threaded, the needle and the syringe are removed, with the thumb kept over the open catheter hub, until the IV tubing is attached.

Systems combining over-the-needle and through-the-needle technology use an initial approach identical to the

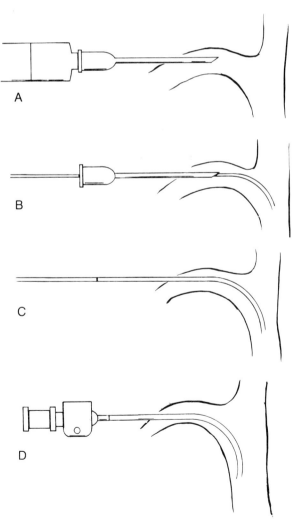

Figure 25–10. Detachable hub catheter system. *A,* Puncture vein, aspirate blood. *B,* Detach syringe, thread catheter. *C,* Withdraw needle over catheter end. *D,* Attach Luer-Lok adapter to catheter.

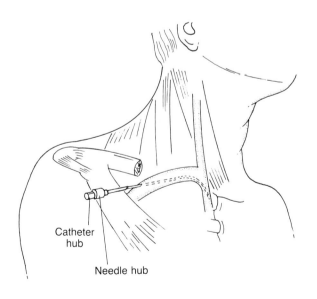

Withdraw needle tip from skin,
leaving catheter in vein

Figure 25–9. Withdrawal of the needle to the catheter hub leaves only the infusion catheter exiting from the skin. (From James P, Myers R: Central venous pressure monitoring. Ann Surg 175:695, 1972. Reproduced by permission.)

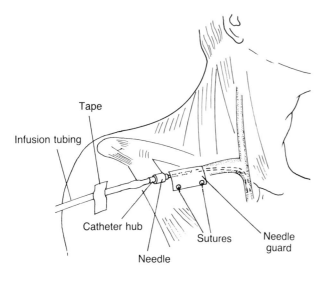

Tape

Infusion tubing

Catheter hub

Needle

Sutures

Needle guard

Place guard and suture beneath clavicle

A

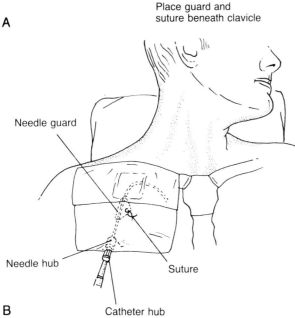

Needle guard

Needle hub

Suture

Catheter hub

B

Figure 25–11. *A,* Suture the guard to the skin. *Note:* Be sure that the catheter fits into the specially designed groove in the plastic needle guard to avoid crushing the catheter when the guard is closed. *B,* Alternative method of securing the subclavian catheter to allow free use of the arm. Note the slight bend in the catheter as it exits from the skin. Also note that the needle guard is sutured to the skin with a single suture. A second suture for fixation should be placed near the needle hub. (From Vander Salm TJ, et al: Atlas of Bedside Procedures. Boston, Little, Brown & Co, 1979. Reproduced by permission.)

over-the-needle method. Typically a 16-gauge, 6.4-cm length catheter is advanced intraluminally over an 18-gauge, thin-walled needle. The needle is then withdrawn, and a flexible 45-cm catheter is advanced through the catheter 15 to 20 cm into the vein. The catheter is then withdrawn and a vessel dilator is passed over the guide wire and into the vessel. It is usually necessary to first enlarge the skin puncture with a number 11 scalpel. Some systems use a catheter-over-the-dilator technique (introducer catheter), whereas others require withdrawal of the dilator and passage of a 20-cm, 16-gauge catheter over the guide wire into the vessel. Continuous control of the guide wire is essential (see also Chapter 23).

A properly placed catheter should thread easily. Difficulty in catheter threading may be caused by passage out of the vessel lumen, trapping against the opposite vessel wall, kinking, or angulation up the internal jugular vein. Rotating the needle bevel may alleviate catheter trapping.

Before the infusion of fluids, the intravenous bottle is lowered below the patient, and the line is checked for backflow of blood. *The free backflow of blood is suggestive, but not diagnostic, of intravascular placement.* Backflow may occur with a hematoma or a hemothorax if the catheter is free in the pleural space. One may attach a syringe directly to the catheter hub to check for the free aspiration of blood, which also *suggests* intraluminal catheter tip placement.

An antibacterial ointment can be applied to the skin puncture site. Antibiotic ointment has been shown to reduce the rate of infectious complications following venous cutdown[64] and may have a beneficial effect in percutaneous venous cannulation.[62, 65] Alternatively, a silver-impregnated cuff (VitaCuff, Vitaphore Corporation, San Carlos, Calif.) may be used to create a subcutaneous barrier to bacteria.[66] This cuff is recommended when long-term use of the catheter (i.e., more than 3 to 4 days) is expected. The device must be placed onto the catheter before the catheter is placed over the guide wire. The catheter hub must be firmly secured to prevent dislodgment, disconnection of the catheter–intravenous tubing junction, or skin maceration. A small gauze pad placed between the plastic guard or catheter hub and the skin protects against skin maceration. Tincture of benzoin is applied 3 cm in all directions around the insertion site and then the area is taped securely. Transparent dressings such as Op-Site also work well. The catheter hub is included within the tape; this prevents accidental disconnection and allows future use of this site for routine blood drawing.

Following the procedure, the lungs should be auscultated to detect inequality of lung sounds that suggest a pneumo- or hemothorax. One should obtain a chest film as soon as possible, checking for hemothorax, pneumothorax, and catheter tip position. Because small amounts of fluid or air may layer out parallel to the x-ray plate with the patient in the supine position, the film should be taken in the upright or semiupright position whenever possible. Proper catheter tip position is shown in Figure 25–12. *Misplaced catheters should be repositioned.*

Supraclavicular Approach

The goal of the supraclavicular technique is to puncture the subclavian vein in its superior aspect just as it joins the internal jugular vein. The needle is inserted above and behind the clavicle, lateral to the sternocleidomastoid muscle. It advances in an avascular plane, away from the subclavian artery and the dome of the pleura. The right side is preferred because of the lower pleural dome, because it is the direct route to the superior vena cava, and because the thoracic duct is on the left side. The Trendelenburg position may be helpful in distending the vein, because the vein is not bound by fasciae on its superior aspect.[22] The patient's head may be turned to the opposite side to help identify the landmarks.

The technique has been well described by Brahos.[22] After the area of the supraclavicular fossa has been prepared and draped, a point is identified 1 cm lateral to the clavicular head of the sternocleidomastoid and 1 cm posterior to the clavicle (Fig. 25–13). The area is anesthetized with 1 per cent lidocaine. If a 3-cm needle is used for anesthesia, it may also be used to locate the vessel in a relatively atraumatic manner. The subclavian vein can almost always be located

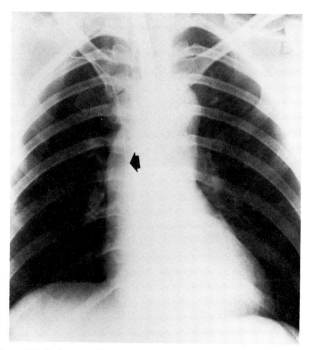

Figure 25–12. A chest film showing the proper catheter tip placement in the superior vena cava *(arrow)*. The tip should *not* lie within the right atrium or the right ventricle.

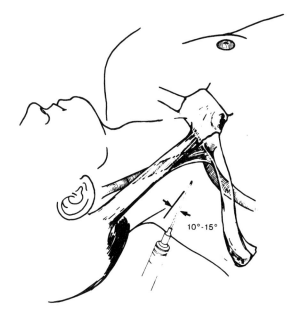

1. Insert needle at a point 1 cm lateral to the sternocleidomastoid muscle and 1 cm cephalad to the clavicle.
2. Direct needle at a 45° angle from the transverse and sagittal planes, angling slightly upward (10°-15°) from the horizontal plane toward the contralateral nipple (in the male).
3. If vein is not entered, withdraw the needle and redirect it in a slightly more cephalad direction.
4. Ensure blood flow and thread catheter.

A

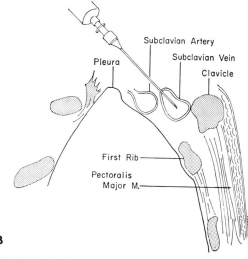

B

Figure 25–13. *A,* Technique for the supraclavicular subclavian approach. (From Dronen S, Thompson B, Nowak RM, Tomlanovich M: Subclavian vein catheterization during cardiopulmonary resuscitation. JAMA 247:3228, 1982. Copyright 1982, American Medical Association. Reproduced by permission.) *B,* Sagittal section.

with this needle because of its superficial location and the absence of bony structures in the path of the needle. A 14-gauge needle (or 18-gauge thin-walled needle) is then advanced with gentle negative pressure applied to an attached syringe. The needle is aimed so as to bisect the clavicosternomastoid angle, with the tip pointing just caudad to the contralateral nipple. The bevel is oriented medially to prevent catheter trapping against the inferior vessel wall. The axis of the syringe is pointed 10 degrees above the horizontal. Successful vessel puncture generally occurs at a depth of 2 to 3 cm. The mechanics of catheter insertion are the same as for the IC technique. Generally, a shorter length of catheter is needed for superior vena caval placement with the SC approach. The guard or catheter hub is best secured to the skin in the supraclavicular fossa parallel to the clavicle. As in the IC technique, a chest film must always be obtained following this procedure. *Misplaced catheters should be repositioned.*

MULTIPLE OR UNSUCCESSFUL ATTEMPTS

Cannulation of the subclavian vein may not be successful on the first attempt. It is reasonable to try again, but after three or four unsuccessful attempts it is best to try another approach or to allow a colleague to attempt the procedure. One must use a new set-up each time blood is obtained, because clots and tissue will clog the needle and will mislead the physician even if subsequent procedures are performed correctly. If several attempts are made, the admitting physician or anesthesiologist must be informed so that proper precautions are taken to identify subsequent complications. It is advisable to obtain radiographs of the chest even after unsuccessful attempts if multiple needle punctures were made. For aesthetic reasons, one should use the same needle hole for subsequent attempts to avoid an embarrassing pincushion appearance of the upper chest. If the subclavian route is unsuccessful on one side, it is best to attempt an internal jugular catheterization on the *same side* rather than

attempt a subclavian catheterization on the opposite side. In this manner, bilateral complications are avoided.

REDIRECTION OF MISPLACED CATHETERS

One common complication of central venous line placement is misdirection of the catheter into an inappropriate vein. Although infusions can still be made, CVP readings are inaccurate, and irritating solutions may produce phlebitis. Most commonly, the catheter is misdirected into the internal jugular vein. A number of options are available to remedy this problem. Schaefer[67] has described a novel technique in which a 2 French Fogarty catheter is inserted through the lumen of the central line and advanced 3 cm beyond the tip. The entire assembly is withdrawn until only the Fogarty catheter is in the subclavian vein. One milliliter of air is injected into the balloon, and the Fogarty catheter is advanced. It is hoped that the blood flow will direct the assembly into the superior vena cava. The balloon is deflated and the central line is advanced over the Fogarty catheter, which is then withdrawn. Other manipulations with guide wires have been suggested, but often reinsertion with another puncture is required for the misplaced catheter to be positioned correctly.

COMPLICATIONS

The medical literature is replete with reports of the complications of subclavian venipuncture. Initial descriptions of the procedure stressed its clinical usefulness rather than its potential complications.[1–3, 9–13, 51] Shortly after subclavian venipuncture became popular as a route for CVP monitoring, reports of serious and occasionally fatal complications began to appear.[15–17] Reports have continued to appear, prompting the United States Food and Drug Administration to issue recommendations intended to limit complications.[68] Some have called for strictly limiting the use of subclavian venipuncture in the emergency department,[69, 70] ignoring the well-documented principle that complication rates fall as the level of experience increases.[71, 72] Others have cited the need for improved house officer training and supervision if a low complication rate is to be maintained.[73, 74]

Infraclavicular Approach

Although more commonly used, the IC approach has been shown to have a consistently higher complication rate than the SC approach. Large series have reported complication rates ranging from 0.4 to 11.1 per cent.[75] The average complication rate is about 5 per cent. To date, at least 30 different complications of the IC technique have been described.[59, 75, 76] These are listed in Table 25–4. One can anticipate potential problems by reviewing the anatomic structures associated with the subclavian vein (Table 25–5). These can be categorized according to the major organ system involved.

Pulmonary. Pulmonary complications of subclavian venipuncture include pneumothorax, hemothorax, hydrothorax, hemomediastinum, hydromediastinum, tracheal perforation, and endotracheal tube cuff perforation. Pneumothorax is the most frequently reported complication, occurring in up to 6 per cent of subclavian venipunctures.[76] Initially the importance of this complication was minimized, but reports of fatalities caused by tension pneumothorax, bilateral pneumothorax, and combined hemopneumothorax followed.[16, 77, 78] One would expect a higher incidence of pneumothorax if the procedure were performed during CPR or positive-pressure ventilation. A small pneumothorax can quickly become a life-threatening tension pneumothorax under positive-pressure ventilation. Hemothorax may occur following subclavian vein or artery laceration,[17, 79] pulmonary artery puncture,[80] or intrathoracic infusion of blood.[15, 17, 81] Hydrothorax occurs as a result of infusion of IV fluid into the pleural space.[16, 75] Hydromediastinum is an uncommonly reported complication that is potentially fatal.[82] I have observed this complication on two occasions in patients receiving IV fluids through introducer devices in the subclavian vein. Both patients recovered without significant sequelae.

Vascular. Air embolism is a potentially fatal complica-

Table 25–4. Complications of Subclavian Venipuncture

Pulmonary
Pneumothorax
Hemothorax
Hydrothorax
Hemomediastinum
Hydromediastinum
Tracheal perforation
Endotracheal cuff perforation
Intrathoracic catheter fragmentation

Vascular
Air embolus
Subclavian artery puncture
Pericardial tamponade
Thrombophlebitis
Catheter embolus
Volume depletion
Arteriovenous fistula
Superior vena cava obstruction
Thoracic duct laceration
Local hematoma
Mural thrombus formation

Infectious
Generalized sepsis
Local cellulitis
Osteomyelitis
Septic arthritis

Neurologic
Phrenic nerve injury
Brachial plexus injury
Cerebral infarct

Miscellaneous
Dysrythmias
Ascites
Catheter knotting
Catheter malposition
Chest pain

tion of subclavian venipuncture.[75, 83–86] There were 5 fatalities in 13 reported cases.[76] The first case was reported by Flanagan and colleagues, who determined that a 14-gauge needle can transmit 100 milliliters of air per second with a 5-cm H_2O pressure difference across the needle.[83] This is a potential complication of several invasive procedures about the head and the neck and is not specifically a result of subclavian venipuncture. Air embolism may occur if the line is left open to air during catheterization or if it subsequently becomes disconnected. The recommended treatment is to place the patient in the left lateral decubitus position to relieve the air bubble occlusion of the right ventricular outflow tract.[87] If this is unsuccessful, aspiration with a catheter advanced into the right ventricle has been advocated.[88, 89]

Catheter embolization resulting from shearing of the catheter by the needle tip is a serious and avoidable complication. This occurs when the catheter is withdrawn through the needle or if the guard is not properly secured. It is more likely to occur when using catheters that are not permanently fixed to the catheter hub. Complications occur frequently following embolization, including arrhythmias, venous thrombosis, endocarditis, myocardial perforation, and pulmonary embolus.[90] Mortality in patients who did not have catheters removed has been reported as high as 60 per cent.[91] As might be expected, retrieval of the catheter is associated with a dramatic reduction in mortality. Transvenous retrieval techniques are usually attempted and are followed by surgery if they are unsuccessful.[92]

Table 25–5. *Anatomic Structures That Can Be Injured by Subclavian Cannulation*

Structure	Anatomic Relation to Subclavian Vein (SV)	Error in Procedure	Injury
Subclavian artery	Posterior and slightly superior, separated by scalenus anterior—10 to 15 mm in adults, 5 to 8 mm in children	Insertion too deep or lateral	Hemorrhage, hematoma, and possible hemothorax
Brachial plexus	Posterior to and separated from SV by the scalenus anterior and the subclavian artery (20 mm)	Same as with subclavian artery	Possible motor or sensory deficits of hand, arm, or shoulder
Parietal pleura	Contact with posterior inferior side of the SV, medial to the attachment of the anterior scalenus muscle to the first rib	Needle penetrates beneath or through both walls of the SV	Pneumothorax
Phrenic nerve	Same as with parietal pleura	Placement of needle above or behind the vein or by penetration of both its walls	Paralysis of the ipsilateral hemidiaphragm
Thoracic duct	Cross the scalenus anterior and enter the superior margin of the SV near the internal jugular junction	Same as with phrenic nerve	Soft tissue lymphedema or chylothorax on left

(From Knopp R, Dailey RH: Central venous cannulation and pressure monitoring. JACEP 6:358, 1977. Reproduced by permission.)

Perforation or laceration of vascular structures may cause hemothorax, hemomediastinum, and volume depletion. These are rarely serious complications, but fatalities have been reported.[79] Surgical repair is occasionally required.[93] Arteriovenous fistula formation has also been reported.[94]

Perforation of the myocardium is a very rare but generally fatal complication of central venous cannulation by any route.[95–101] The presumed mechanism is prolonged contact of the rigid catheter tip with the beating myocardium.[100–102] The catheter perforates the myocardial wall and causes a tamponade by either bleeding from the involved chamber or infusion of IV fluid into the pericardium. The right atrium is involved more commonly than the right ventricle.[102] This complication can be prevented by determining the catheter tip position on a postinsertion chest film and repositioning improperly placed catheters. Cardiac tamponade can also occur with misplacement of the central venous line in the pericardiophrenic vein.[103] Premature atrial or ventricular beats may be observed if the catheter tip is in contact with the endocardium. Serious dysrhythmias do not occur, and the ectopic beats may be abolished if the catheter is repositioned.

Catheter knotting or kinking may occur if the catheter is forced or repositioned or if an excessively long catheter is used.[104] The most common result of kinking is poor flow of intravenous fluids. Johnson and associates reported a case of superior vena caval obstruction caused by a kinked catheter.[105]

Thrombosis and thrombophlebitis occur rarely because of the large caliber and high flow rates of the vessels involved.[60] It is important to determine that the catheter tip rests in the superior vena cava, especially during the infusion of irritating or hypertonic fluids.[105] Thrombi may also form secondary to prolonged catheter contact against the vascular endothelium. Ducatman and colleagues[106] reported a 29 per cent incidence of mural thrombi in the innominate vein, superior vena cava, and right ventricle of patients who had central lines in place an average of 8 days before death. No complications were directly attributable to these small, firmly adherent thrombi.

Thoracic duct laceration is a frequently discussed complication of left-sided subclavian venipuncture; however, it is extremely uncommon. McGoon and coworkers cite this as a complication of internal jugular cannulation but not subclavian cannulation.[76]

Infectious. Infectious complications include local cellulitis, thrombophlebitis, generalized septicemia, osteomyelitis, and septic arthritis.[76] The incidence of septic complications varies from 0 to 25 per cent.[107, 108] In a retrospective audit, Herbst documented only one culture-proven infectious complication in a series of 117 patients.[71] The frequency with which infectious complications are seen is directly related to the attention given to aseptic technique in insertion and aftercare of the catheter.

Neurologic. Neurologic complications are extremely rare and are presumably caused by direct trauma from the needle during venipuncture. Brachial plexus palsy[17] and phrenic nerve injury with paralysis of the hemidiaphragm[109, 110] have been reported.

Miscellaneous. Improper catheter tip position occurs commonly. Conces and Holden[111] reported that only 71 per cent of subclavian catheters were located in the superior vena cava on the initial chest film. Complications of improper placement include myocardial perforation,[99] hydrothorax,[75] hemothorax,[17] ascites,[112] chest wall abscesses,[113] embolization to the pleural space,[114] and chest pain.[115] More commonly, improper location yields inaccurate measurements of the central venous pressure[116] or is associated with poor flow caused by kinking. An unusual complication caused by improper tip position is cerebral infarction. Hurwitz and Posner reported two patients who developed fatal cerebral infarcts following inadvertent cannulation of the subclavian artery.[117]

Supraclavicular Approach

The claim by Moosman[59] that the SC approach is more likely to be accompanied by complications is not substantiated by the medical literature. In all reported series the complication rate has been low, ranging from 0 to 6 per cent.[18–23, 25] A compilation of the data from these series yields an overall complication rate of 1.3 per cent. In a randomized prospective comparison of supraclavicular and infraclavicular venipuncture in 500 emergency department patients, Sterner and colleagues reported complication rates of 2.0 and 5.1 per cent, respectively.[118] The most significant complications have been pneumothorax and subclavian artery puncture; the highest incidence of pneumothorax is 2.4 per cent.[19] Adherence to Yoffa's technique[18] decreases the risk of these complications, because the needle is directed away from the pleural dome and the subclavian artery. The relatively superficial location of the vein when approached from above (1.5 to 3.5 cm) lessens the risk of puncture or laceration of deep structures.

Catheter tip malposition is also quite low because of the more direct path to the superior vena cava. For those series in which malposition has been reported, the overall rate is 1.1 per cent.[19, 22, 26] Fischer and coworkers noted a malposition rate of 27.6 per cent using the IC technique,[119] and Herbst has reported a range of 1.7 to 24 per cent.[71] Similarly, Sterner[118] reported malposition rates of 0.4 per cent for the SC approach and 8.2 per cent for the IC approach. The highest incidence of malposition using the SC technique is 7 per cent and occurred during the performance of CPR.[26] In the same series, a 26 per cent malposition rate was reported for the IC technique.

The incidence of failure to establish a functioning SC intravenous line ranges from 0 to 5 per cent,[18–26] with an overall rate of 4 per cent. The failure rate reported for the IC technique ranges from 2.5 to 8 per cent.[60] One death has been reported as a result of air embolism, a complication not specifically related to the SC technique.[20]

PREVENTION OF COMPLICATIONS

The reference to subclavian venipuncture as "a favorite clinical whipping boy" made two decades ago[120] remains appropriate today. It is unfortunate that a procedure that is clinically useful, easy to perform, and relatively safe has been criticized to such a great extent. It is clear that many of the reported complications are avoidable when proper technique is used. Attention to specific details of patient selection, anatomy, surgical technique, and equipment must be stressed, since this *will* prevent complications. Adherence to the following guidelines is particularly important:

1. Patients should be selected properly. Obese, cachectic, emphysematous, and combative patients are poor candidates.

2. The physician should know the anatomy in detail. A poor understanding of the relationship of the subclavian vessels to the clavicle and the first rib is a major cause of complications, especially pneumothorax.[42]

3. Inexperienced personnel should not be allowed to perform the procedure unsupervised. The complication rate is inversely proportional to the level of physician experience.[72–75] The many small steps designed to prevent complications are often forgotten or ignored by the novice. A study by Sznajder and colleagues recommends that inexperienced physicians learn the technique in mechanically ventilated, unconscious patients because of a lower complication rate in this less mobile patient group.[74]

4. The procedure should be performed frequently or not at all. In Herbst's retrospective audit, 46 per cent of the procedures during which complications occurred were performed by physicians who attempted an average of only one subclavian venipuncture in a year.[71] Complications were also higher among gynecologists, who started an average of only 8 subclavian lines during the year.

5. Aseptic technique should be practiced throughout, and lines placed during resuscitations should be removed as soon as possible. Antibiotic ointments placed at the skin puncture site may have a role in limiting septic complications.[62, 64, 65]

6. All measures designed to prevent air embolus should be practiced. These include use of the Trendelenburg position, active exhalation, occlusion of the open needle hub, and adequate measures to prevent air entry into IV tubing.

7. One should never pull the catheter through the needle or use through-the-needle devices without the needle guard.

8. One should always lower the IV bag and check for venous backflow or withdraw blood directly from the catheter before infusing fluids. It should be noted that a blood return is only suggestive of intravascular placement.

9. The procedure should always be followed by a chest film. The physician should personally check the film for the presence of hemo- or pneumothorax and for catheter position.

10. Kinked or malpositioned lines should always be replaced or repositioned.

11. During CPR, the supraclavicular technique should be used when a subclavian line is indicated.[26]

12. Excessive punctures should not be made if initial attempts are unsuccessful. An alternative route should be used. If multiple punctures are required, the admitting physician should be alerted for possible complications.

13. Individuals placing and maintaining central lines should be thoroughly familiar with the catheter and the manufacturer's recommendations regarding its use.

CONCLUSION

Subclavian venipuncture is a widely used clinical tool despite reports of potentially fatal complications. Its usefulness has been demonstrated in a variety of clinical settings. It is a relatively safe and simple procedure that should be associated with few significant problems. The keys to successful application of this technique are in-depth knowledge of the anatomy and meticulous attention to the details of the procedure.

REFERENCES

1. Aubaniac R: L'injection intraveineuse sous-claviculaire. Avantages et techniques. Press Med 60:1456, 1952.
2. Aubaniac R: Une nouvelle voie d'injection ou de ponction veineuse: La voie sous-claviculaire. Sem Hop Paris 28:3445, 1952.
3. Aubaniac R: L'intraveineuse sous-claviculaire: Avantages et technique. Afr Fr Chir 3–4:131, 1952.
4. Lepp H: Uber eine neue intravenose Injektions und Punktions-methode; die infraklavikulare Punktion der vena subclavia. Dtsch Kahnaerztl Z 8:511, 1953.
5. Lepp H: Die infraklavikulare Punktion der vena subclavia nach Aubaniac. Munch Med Wochenschr 96:1392, 1954.
6. Villafane PE: Technica de la transfusion por via subclavicular. Prensa Med Argent 40:2379, 1953.
7. Keeri-Szanto M: The subclavian vein, a constant and convenient intravenous injection site. Arch Surg 72:179, 1956.
8. Kalcev B: Subclavian venepuncture (letter to the editor). Lancet 1:45, 1964.
9. Wilson JW, Grow JB, Demong CV: Central venous pressure in optimal blood volume maintenance. Arch Surg 85:563, 1962.
10. Ashbaugh D, Thompson JWW: Subclavian-vein infusion. Lancet 2:1138, 1963.
11. Davidson JT, Ben-Hur N, Nathen H: Subclavian venepuncture. Lancet 2:1139, 1963.
12. Malinak LR, Gulde RE, Faris AM: Percutaneous subclavian catheterization for central venous pressure monitoring. Applications in obstetrical and gynecological problems. Am J Obstet Gynecol 92:477, 1965.
13. Giles HV: The subclavian vein: Its usefulness in burn cases. Plast Reconstr Surg 38:519, 1966.

14. Mogil RA, DeLaurentis DA, Rosemond GP: The infraclavicular venepuncture: Value in various clinical situations including central venous pressure monitoring. Arch Surg 95:320, 1967.
15. Yarom R: Subclavian venepuncture (letter to the editor). Lancet 1:45, 1964.
16. Matz R: Complications of determining the central venous pressure. N Engl J Med 273:703, 1965.
17. Smith BE, Modell JH, Gaub ML: Complications of subclavian vein catheterization. Arch Surg 90:228, 1965.
18. Yoffa D: Supraclavicular subclavian venepuncture and catheterisation. Lancet 2:614, 1965.
19. Garcia JM, Mispireta LA, Pinho RV: Percutaneous supraclavicular superior vena caval cannulation. Surg Gynecol Obstet 134:839, 1972.
20. James PM, Myers RT: Central venous pressure monitoring: Misinterpretation, abuses, indications and a new technique. Ann Surg 175:693, 1972.
21. Nugent RP: Supraclavicular catheterization of the subclavian vein. Aust N Z J Surg 43:41, 1973.
22. Brahos GJ: Central venous catheterization via the supraclavicular approach. J Trauma 17:872, 1977.
23. Craig RG, Jones RA, Sproul GL: The alternate method of central venous system catheterization. Am Surg 34:131, 1968.
24. Defalque RJ: Subclavian venepuncture: A review. Anesth Analg 47:677, 1968.
25. Brahos GJ, Cohen MJ: Supraclavicular central venous catheterization: Technique and experience in 250 cases. Wis Med J 80:36, 1981.
26. Dronen SC, Thompson B, Nowak R: Subclavian vein catheterization during cardiopulmonary resuscitation. JAMA 247:3227, 1982.
27. Graber D, Dailey RH: Catheter flow rates updated (letter to the editor). JACEP 6:518, 1977.
28. Dronen SC, Yee AS, Tomlanovich MC: Proximal saphenous vein cutdown. Ann Emerg Med 10:328, 1981.
29. Westaby S: Ryles tube for rapid intravenous transfusion. Lancet 1:360, 1979.
30. Haynes BE: Catheter introducers for hypovolemic patients (letter to the editor). Ann Emerg Med 11:642, 1982.
30a. Dutky PA, Stevens SL, Maull KI: Factors affecting rapid fluid resuscitation with large-bore introducer catheters. J Trauma 29:856, 1989.
31. Barsan WG, Levy RC, Weir H: Lidocaine levels during CPR: Differences after peripheral venous, central venous, and intracardiac injections. Ann Emerg Med 10:73, 1981.
32. Hedges JR, Barsan WG, Doan LA, et al: Central versus peripheral intravenous routes in cardiopulmonary resuscitation. Am J Emerg Med 2:385, 1984.
33. Fleisher G, Caputo G, Baskin M: Comparison of external jugular and peripheral venous administration of sodium bicarbonate in puppies. Crit Care Med 17:251, 1989.
34. Kuhn GJ, White BC, Swetnam RE, et al: Peripheral vs. central circulation times during CPR: A pilot study. Ann Emerg Med 10:417, 1981.
35. Dudrick SJ, Wilmore DW, Vars HM: Can intravenous feeding as the sole means of nutrition support growth in the child and restore weight loss in an adult? Ann Surg 169:974, 1969.
36. Dudrick SJ, Wilmore DW: Long term parenteral feeding. Hosp Pract 3:65, 1968.
37. Merk EA, Rush BF: Emergency subclavian vein catheterization and intravenous hyperalimentation. Am J Surg 129:266, 1975.
38. Fares LG, Tzu-Chi H, Leva R: A subclavian cannulation: Valuable dialysis access alternative. Am Surg 50:283, 1984.
39. Knopp R, Dailey RH: Central venous cannulation and pressure monitoring. JACEP 6:358, 1977.
40. Nowak RM: Personal communication, Detroit, Michigan. April, 1981.
41. Mitty WF, Nealon TF: Complications of subclavian sticks. JACEP 4:24, 1975.
42. Westreich M: Preventing complications of subclavian vein catheterization. JACEP 7:368, 1978.
43. Simpson ET, Aitchison JM: Percutaneous infraclavicular subclavian vein catheterization in shocked patients: A prospective study in 172 patients. J Trauma 22:781, 1982.
44. Kron IL, Rheuban K, Miller ED, et al: Subclavian vein catheterization for central line placement in children under two years of age. Am Surg 51:272, 1985.
45. Bonventre EV, Lally KP, Chwals WJ, et al: Percutaneous insertion of subclavian venous catheters in infants and children. Surg Gynecol Obstet 169:203, 1989.
46. Schug CB, Culhane DE, Knopp RK: Subclavian vein catheterization in the emergency department. A comparison of guide wire and nonguide wire techniques. Ann Emerg Med 15:769, 1986.
47. Borja AR, Hinshaw JR: A safe way to perform infraclavicular subclavian vein catheterization. Surg Gynecol Obstet 130:673, 1970.
48. Tofield JJ: A safer technique of percutaneous catheterization of the subclavian vein. Surg Gynecol Obstet 128:1069, 1969.
49. Sullivan R, Pomerantz M: Central venous pressure monitoring: The subclavian approach. Surg Clin North Am 49:1489, 1969.
50. Gallitano AL, Kondi ES, Deckers PJ: A safe approach to the subclavian vein. Surg Gynecol Obstet 135:96, 1972.
51. Longerbeam JK, Vannix R, Wagner W, et al: Central venous pressure monitoring. Am J Surg 110:220, 1965.
52. Phillips SJ: Technique of percutaneous subclavian vein catheterization. Surg Gynecol Obstet 127:1079, 1968.
53. Buchman RJ: Subclavian venipuncture. Milit Med 134:451, 1969.
54. Simon RR: A new technique for subclavian puncture. JACEP 7:409, 1978.
55. Feiler EM, de Alva WE: Infraclavicular percutaneous subclavian vein puncture. Am J Surg 118:906, 1969.
56. Land RE: Anatomic relationships of the right subclavian vein. Arch Surg 102:178, 1971.
57. Jesseph JM, Conces DJ, Augustyn GT: Patient positioning for subclavian vein catheterization. Arch Surg 122:1207, 1987.
58. Fortune JB, Kupinski AM, Wallace JR, et al: The effect of patient position on size and location of the subclavian vein for percutaneous puncture (abstract). J Trauma 29:1725, 1990.
59. Moosman DA: The anatomy of infraclavicular subclavian vein catheterization and its complications. Surg Gynecol Obstet 136:71, 1973.
60. Borja AR: Current status of infraclavicular subclavian vein catheterization. Ann Thorac Surg 13:615, 1972.
61. American Heart Association: Standards and guidelines for cardiopulmonary resuscitation and emergency cardiac care. JAMA 244:453, 1980.
62. Collins RN, Braun PA, Zinner SH, et al: Risk of local and systemic infection with polyethylene intravenous catheters. N Engl J Med 279:340, 1968.
63. Feliciano D: Complications of percutaneous subclavian vein catheters. Curr Concepts Trauma Care 9:Fall 1980.
64. Moran JM, Atwood RP, Rowe MI: A clinical and bacteriologic study of infections associated with venous cutdowns. N Engl J Med 272:554, 1963.
65. Henzel JH, DeWeese MS: Morbid and mortal complications associated with prolonged central venous cannulation. Am J Surg 121:600, 1971.
66. Maki DG, Cobb L, Garman JK, et al: An attachable silver-impregnated cuff for prevention of infection with central venous catheters: A prospective randomized multicenter trial. Am J Med 85:307, 1988.
67. Schaefer CJ: Redirection of misplaced central venous catheters. Arch Surg 115:789, 1980.
68. Willis JL (ed): Precautions necessary with central venous catheters. FDA Drug Bulletin, July 1989, pp 15–16.
69. Abraham E, Shapiro M, Podolsky S: Central venous catheterization in the emergency setting. Crit Care Med 11:515, 1983.
70. Ferguson M, Max MH, Marshall W: Emergency department infraclavicular subclavian vein catheterization in patients with multiple injuries and burns. South Med J 81:433, 1988.
71. Herbst C: Indications, management and complications of percutaneous subclavian catheters. Arch Surg 113:1421, 1978.
72. Sloan E, Hart R, Zalut T, et al: The clinical practice of central venous catheterization (CVC) in the emergency department (abstract). J Emerg Med 6:371, 1988.
73. Fares LG, Block PH, Feldman SD: Improved house staff results with subclavian cannulation. Am Surg 52:108, 1986.
74. Sznajder JI, Zuiebil FR, Bitterman H, et al: Central vein catheterization: Failure and complication rate by three percutaneous approaches. Arch Intern Med 146:259, 1986.
75. Feliciano D, Mattox K, Graham J, et al: Major complications of percutaneous subclavian vein catheters. Am J Surg 138:869, 1979.
76. McCoon M, Benedetto P, Greene B: Complications of percutaneous central venous catheterization: A report of 2 cases and a review of the literature. Johns Hopkins Med J 145:1, 1979.
77. Schapira M, Stern W: Hazards of subclavian vein cannulation for CVP monitoring. JAMA 201:111, 1967.
78. Maggs PR, Schwaber JR: Fatal bilateral pneumothoraces complicating subclavian vein catheterization. Chest 71:552, 1977.
79. Goldman LI: Another complication of subclavian puncture: Arterial laceration. JAMA 217:78, 1971.
80. Holt S, Kirkham N, Myerscough E: Hemothorax after subclavian vein cannulation. Thorax 32:101, 1977.
81. Fontanelle LJ, Dooley BN, Cuello L: Subclavian venipuncture and its complications. Ann Thorac Surg 11:331, 1971.
82. Adar R, Mozes M: Hydromediastinum. JAMA 214:372, 1970.
83. Flanagan J, Gradisar I, Gross R: Air embolus—a lethal complication of subclavian venipuncture. N Engl J Med 281:488, 1969.
84. Lucas C, Irani F: Air embolus via subclavian catheter. N Engl J Med 281:966, 1969.
85. Levinsky W: Fatal air embolism during insertion of CVP monitoring apparatus. JAMA 209:1721, 1969.
86. Peters JL, Armstrong R: Air embolism as a complication of central venous catheterization. Ann Surg 187:375, 1978.
87. Durant TM, Long JW, Oppenheimer MJ: Pulmonary (venous) air embolism. Am Heart J 33:269, 1947.
88. Michenfelder JD, Terry HR, Daw EF: Air embolism during neurosurgery. A new method of treatment. Anesth Analg 45:390, 1966.
89. Sink JD, Comer PB, James PM, et al: Evaluation of catheter placement in the treatment of venous air embolism. Ann Surg 183:58, 1976.
90. Propp DA, Cline D, Hennenfent BR: Catheter embolism. J Emerg Med 6:17, 1988.

91. Blair E, Hanziker R, Flanagan ME: Catheter embolism. Surgery 67:457, 1970.
92. Meng RL, Delaria CA, Goldin MD: Transjugular forceps removal of catheter embolus. Ann Thorac Surg 29:575, 1980.
93. Lefrak E, Noon G: Management of arterial injury secondary to attempted subclavian vein catheterization. Ann Thorac Surg 14:294, 1972.
94. Farhat K, Nakhjavan K, Cope C, et al: Iatrogenic arteriovenous fistula. A complication of percutaneous subclavian vein puncture. Chest 67:480, 1975.
95. Thomas CS, Carter JW, Lowden SC: Pericardial tamponade from central venous catheters. Arch Surg 98:217, 1969.
96. Fitts CT, Barnett LT, Webb CM, et al: Perforating wounds of the heart caused by central venous catheters. J Trauma 10:764, 1970.
97. Bone DK, Maddrey WC, Eagen J, et al: Cardiac tamponade: A fatal complication of central venous catheterization. Arch Surg 106:868, 1973.
98. Brandt RL, Foley WJ, Fink GH, et al: Mechanism of perforation of the heart with production of a hydropericardium by a venous catheter and its prevention. Am J Surg 119:311, 1970.
99. Friedman BA, Jurgeleit HC: Perforation of the atrium by polyethylene central venous catheters. JAMA 203:1141, 1968.
100. Collier PE, Ryan JJ, Diamond DL: Cardiac tamponade from central venous catheters: A report of a case and review of the English literature. Angiology 35:595, 1984.
101. Tapson JS, Udall PR: Fatal hemothorax caused by a subclavian hemodialysis catheter. Thoughts on prevention. Arch Intern Med 144:1685, 1984.
102. Sheep RE, Guiney WB: Fatal cardiac tamponade. JAMA 248:1632, 1982.
103. VanHaeften TW, vanPampus ECM, Boot H, et al: Cardiac tamponade from misplaced central venous line in pericardiophrenic vein. Arch Intern Med 148:1649, 1988.
104. Nicolas F: Knotting of subclavian central venous catheters. JAMA 214:373, 1970.
105. Johnson CL, Lazarchick J: Subclavian venipuncture: Preventable complications, report of two cases. Mayo Clin Proc 45:712, 1970.
106. Ducataman BS, McMichan JC, Edwards WD: Catheter-induced lesions of the right side of the heart. A one-year prospective study of 141 autopsies. JAMA 253:791, 1985.
107. Wilmore DW, Dudrick SJ: Safe long term venous catheterization. Arch Surg 98:256, 1967.
108. Wilmore DW, Dudrick SJ: Guarding against complications in subclavian vein catheterization. Hosp Phys 6:82, 1970.
109. Drachler D, Koepke G, Weg J: Phrenic nerve injury from subclavian vein catheterization: Diagnosis by electromyography. JAMA 236:2880, 1976.
110. Obel IW: Transient phrenic nerve paralysis following subclavian venipuncture. Anesthesiology 33:369, 1970.
111. Conces DJ, Holden RW: Aberrant locations and complications in the initial placement of subclavian vein catheters. Arch Surg 119:293, 1984.
112. Allsop JR, Askew AR: Subclavian vein cannulation: A new complication. Br Med J 4:262, 1975.
113. Oakes DD, Wilson RE: Malposition of subclavian lines. JAMA 233:532, 1975.
114. Hegarty MM: The hazards of subclavian vein catheterization: Practical considerations and an unusual case report. S Afr Med J 52:240, 1977.
115. Webb JG, Simmonds SD, Chan-Yan C: Central venous catheter malposition presenting as chest pain. Chest 89:309, 1986.
116. Thomas T: Location of catheter tip and its importance on central venous pressure. Chest 61:668, 1972.
117. Hurwitz BJ, Posner JB: Cerebral infarction complicating subclavian vein catheterization. Ann Neurol 1:253, 1977.
118. Sterner S, Plummer DW, Clinton J, et al: A comparison of the supraclavicular approach and the infraclavicular approach for subclavian vein catheterization. Ann Emerg Med 15:421, 1986.
119. Fischer J, Lundstrom J, Ohand, HG: Central venous cannulation: A radiological determination of catheter positions and immediate intrathoracic complications. Acta Anaesthesiol Scand 21:45, 1977.
120. Russo J: The subclavian catheter (letter to the editor). N Engl J Med 281:1425, 1969.

Chapter 26

Central Venous Catheterization: Internal Jugular Approach and Alternatives

William J. Barker

INTRODUCTION

There are several alternatives to subclavian vein cannulation when access to the central venous circulation is needed. The venae cavae may be reached readily from the internal and external jugular, femoral, basilic, and cephalic veins. The internal jugular (IJ) route is the most commonly used by the emergency physician, although all of these alternative methods have their merit.

The IJ approach was first mentioned in the United States in a pediatric handbook by Silver and coworkers in 1963.[1] Although puncture of the superior jugular bulb at the base of the skull had been used by neurologists for quite some time, the approach was too dangerous for use in routine catheterization.[2] Internal jugular vein catheterization in the adult was first described by Hemosura in 1966.[3] He discussed a variation of what is now commonly termed the central approach. Over the next several years, other methods were proposed.[4-10] Defalque reviewed 17 methods in 1974 and grouped them into three major approaches: central, anterior, and posterior.[2] These methods are discussed in detail later in the chapter.

The femoral, basilic, and cephalic approaches developed primarily as routes for passage of transvenous pacemakers and Swan-Ganz pressure catheters. The development of commercial flexible wire introducer sets (Seldinger technique) has also permitted central venous cannulation by way of the external jugular vein.[11, 12]

All of these techniques have a place in the practice of emergency medicine, and often the choice of a certain method is determined solely by the confidence of the individual physician in his or her ability to perform them. Kanter and colleagues,[13] Arrighi and coworkers,[14] Senagore and associates,[15] and others have demonstrated that success rates are higher and complications occur less frequently for technically more experienced clinicians.[16, 17] The IJ, femoral, and subclavian (supraclavicular and infraclavicular) approaches are favorites of the emergency physician because of the rapid manner in which access can be obtained.

INDICATIONS AND CONTRAINDICATIONS

General indications for central venous cannulation are discussed for subclavian vein catheterization in Chapter 25. Specific sites are preferred for certain applications, and relative indications and contraindications for specific sites are discussed later in this chapter.

In the past the use of central venous cannulation for volume resuscitation was thought to be poor practice. As more experience with alternative central venous techniques has been gained, and larger, safer catheters have been developed, central venous cannulation for volume resuscitation has become more accepted.[14, 18-21] High-flow volume resuscitation, however, should not use intrathoracic lines unless proper line placement and vascular integrity have been verified.

Before the following techniques are attempted, a thorough understanding of the principles of central venous catheterization is required. The reader is referred to Chapter 25 for a comprehensive discussion of these principles.

Internal Jugular Approach

As is true of the supraclavicular subclavian approach, the IJ technique is useful for securing routine central venous access and for emergency venous access during cardiopulmonary resuscitation (CPR). The approach is desirable during CPR because the site is removed from the area of chest compressions.[15, 22–24] Comparisons of IJ and subclavian cannulation by Kaiser and associates[22] found a significantly greater incidence of proper venipuncture and catheter passage with the infraclavicular subclavian approach as compared with the posterior IJ method (98 per cent versus 84 per cent). A 20 per cent rate of catheter malposition was noted with each method. In a retrospective study, Eisenhauer and colleagues[23] found that only 0.4 per cent of 248 IJ cannulations resulted in clinically significant morbidity compared with 4.2 per cent of 298 subclavian insertions, even though the overall complication rate was similar. Senagore and colleagues[15] and Patel and associates[24] found a similar incidence of significant complications with either route. However, both of the pneumothoraces that occurred in the latter study were in the subclavian group. Although there may be a slight difference in complications between the two routes, in the absence of specific contraindications the physician should use the technique of central venous cannulation with which he or she is most familiar. The IJ route is slightly more difficult technically than the subclavian route, but it is faster and easier than a venous cutdown.

Cervical trauma with swelling or anatomic distortion at the intended site of IJ venipuncture is a specific contraindication to the IJ approach. Neck motion is limited when the IJ central line is in place and represents a relative contraindication in the conscious patient. Furthermore, a short, thick neck may preclude the necessary needle manipulation for IJ catheterization. Although bleeding disorders are relative contraindications to central venous cannulation, the IJ approach is preferred in patients with a coagulopathy, because the area may be compressed directly if bleeding occurs; compression of the subclavian vein is not possible. Carotid artery disease (plaque or obstruction) is a relative contraindication to IJ cannulation. Inadvertent puncture of the artery may dislodge a plaque. Additionally, prolonged compression of the artery to control bleeding may impair cerebral circulation if collateral blood flow is compromised. If a preceding subclavian catheterization has been unsuccessful, the ipsilateral IJ route is generally preferred for a subsequent attempt. In this manner, bilateral iatrogenic complications are avoided.

External Jugular Approach

In instances in which alternative methods of central venous catheterization are not possible, one may obtain access to the central venous system by way of the external jugular vein.[11, 12, 25, 26] Although the external jugular vein is a ready emergency intravenous access route when standard peripheral intravenous catheters are used, the valves and tortuosity of the external jugular system often preclude or delay placement of standard central venous catheters. Successful central vein cannulation is generally possible only with the use of guide wires. The external jugular vein must be readily visible for percutaneous cannulation to be successful. When time is available for a careful, deliberate attempt, this technique is valuable because it avoids the complications of pneumothorax, carotid artery puncture, and hidden hemorrhage that occur not infrequently with other methods of central venous cannulation.

The procedure can be used in both children and adults, but success is more common in adults.[26–28] Central venous catheterization by the external jugular route is technically more difficult than internal jugular cannulation, but it is successful 76 to 100 per cent of the time in adults.[11, 12, 25, 28, 29] Both the straight guide wires and the J-tipped wires have been used. Use of the J-tipped wires is more reliable and is the preferred technique.[12, 25, 28] The J wires are more easily advanced because the rounded tip bounces off vessel walls and navigates sharp angulations in the vessel course more easily.

Despite the increased success of central cannulation via the external jugular route with J wires, the technique is extremely time consuming.[12] Hence, this approach is contraindicated when immediate central access is desired (e.g., cardiac arrest, shock). Nonetheless, simple external jugular cannulation without attempts to pass a central venous catheter serves as a useful alternative for the rapid administration of fluid and drugs.

Femoral Approach

The cannulation of the femoral vein for central venous access has become increasingly popular in the last several years, especially for the passage of transvenous pacemakers and pressure measurement catheters in critically ill patients.[30, 31] With the increasing collective experience with this technique, complication rates have been found to be well within acceptable limits, and more indications for its use are being developed. Mangiante and associates[19] have had such success with femoral catheters for trauma patients that all hypotensive patients have a femoral line established with an 8.5 French Teflon catheter connected to genitourinary irrigation tubing immediately after two peripheral antecubital catheters are established. They report no significant iliofemoral thrombosis, major hematoma, or infectious complications due to the catheters. Getzen and Pollak[18] reported 759 successful femoral catheterizations in 796 attempts during military casualty resuscitations with an acceptable complication rate. More recent indications for urgent femoral cannulation include emergency cardiopulmonary bypass for resuscitation purposes, charcoal hemoperfusion for severe drug overdoses, and dialysis access.[32, 33] Advantages of the femoral site over other central venous access sites are that the femoral area is less congested with monitoring and airway equipment than the head and neck area and that the conscious patient, who is still bedridden, may turn the head and use the arms without danger to the central line. Obviously, the femoral site is strongly contraindicated in the ambulatory patient who requires central access.

Infection of catheters in the femoral area has been feared, perhaps because of the proximity to the genitalia and rectum. Thomas and associates[34] found no significant difference in infection rates when comparing radial and femoral sites for arterial cannulation. Other studies have consistently found acceptably low infection rates for femoral venous catheterizations.[13, 18, 19, 31, 35]

A contraindication for femoral catheterization is significant trauma to the groin area or suspected trauma to the inferior vena cava or iliac veins. Percutaneous femoral line placement is not recommended in a patient who is in cardiac arrest or a patient with an absent femoral pulse for any reason unless other alternatives have been exhausted.[19, 36–38] The origin of the palpable femoral pulse in a canine model of cardiopulmonary arrest was found to be the femoral artery and vein each approximately 50 per cent of the time.[39] Whereas Kaye and Bircher[40] suggest successful use of the femoral vein during CPR, most investigators have reported low success rates.[36–38] In addition, unless a long catheter is used, drug delivery may not be as efficient, owing to delayed flow from below the diaphragm during CPR.[41–43]

As with any venous cannulation, skin abnormalities such as burns, deep abrasions, or severe dermatitis at or in close proximity to the puncture site are a strong relative contraindication.[44]

Basilic-Cephalic Approach

When rapidity of access to the central venous circulation is not important, the basilic-cephalic approach should be considered, because it has the lowest incidence of major complications. The location of the basilic and cephalic veins away from vital organs and major arteries accounts for this low incidence of major problems. When the patient is upright, the basilic vein is preferred over the cephalic vein because of a higher incidence of successful central catheter passage, although the overall success rate of superior vena cava cannulation is similar for both techniques in the supine patient.[45–47] Nonetheless, both veins have valves, which may impede catheter advancement.[48–51]

In a cardiac arrest situation in which access for drug or fluid delivery is of primary concern, cannulation of these veins with a standard intravenous (short) large-bore catheter (14 to 18 gauge, 3 cm) is preferred over cannulation with longer central catheters. Drug delivery to the heart is almost as expeditious with the shorter catheters, and fluid volume delivery is more rapid.[52, 53] The presence of previous phlebitis and shoulder or proximal extremity trauma is a contraindication to placement of a basilic or a cephalic central line. Furthermore, the prolonged use of the catheter may induce phlebitis and hence render the vessel useless for future cannulation. Therefore, the intended future use of the basilic and cephalic vessels for other purposes (e.g., transvenous pacemaker placement or venipuncture) is a relative contraindication to basilic and cephalic catheterization. The arm should also be immobilized following catheter placement to minimize catheter motion or kinking caused by extremity motion. The technique is therefore undesirable in the combative patient.

PROCEDURE

Equipment

The equipment for IJ, femoral, and basilic-cephalic cannulation is the same as that used for the subclavian route (see Table 25–3), with the addition of a 22-gauge locator needle and a 90-cm (36-inch) catheter for the femoral and basilic-cephalic approaches. As stated earlier, central venous cannulation via the external jugular approach should be undertaken with the guide wire (Seldinger) technique, using a curved wire (J wire). In fact, many clinicians believe that all approaches are generally performed more easily using the guide wire technique (see Chapter 23).

Internal Jugular Vein Cannulation Technique

Anatomy of the Internal Jugular Vein. The anatomy of the IJ vein is relatively constant, regardless of body habitus. The vein drains the cranium, beginning as the superior jugular bulb, which is separated from the floor of the middle ear by a delicate bony plate. The IJ vein emerges deep to the posterior belly of the digastric muscle. At its origin the IJ vein courses adjacent to the spinal accessory, vagus, and hypoglossal nerves as well as the internal carotid artery. Several tributary veins enter the IJ vein at the level of the hyoid bone. The IJ vein, the internal (and, later, the common) carotid artery, and the vagus nerve course together in the carotid sheath. The IJ vein occupies the anterior lateral position in the carotid sheath.[54] The only structure that maintains a fixed anatomic relationship with the IJ vein is the carotid artery. The vein invariably lies lateral and slightly anterior to the carotid artery, and the course of the artery serves as a guide to venous cannulation. At the level of the thyroid cartilage, the IJ vein can be found just deep to the sternocleidomastoid muscle (Fig. 26–1).

The IJ vein emerges from under the apex of the triangle of the two heads of the sternocleidomastoid muscle and joins the subclavian vein behind the clavicle. As the vein approaches its supraclavicular junction with the subclavian vein, it assumes a more medial position in the triangle formed by the two heads of the sternocleidomastoid muscles following the anterior border of the lateral head. In this lower cervical region, the common carotid artery assumes a deep paratracheal location. The brachial plexus is separated from the IJ vein by the scalenus anterior muscle. The phrenic nerve is anterior to the scalenus anterior muscle. Although quite deep, the stellate ganglion lies anterior to the lower brachial plexus.

Unlike the subclavian vein, the IJ vein is quite distensible. The vessel diameter is increased with the performance of a Valsalva maneuver and the assumption of the head-down (Trendelenburg) tilt position. The diameter of the vein should theoretically increase with the application of the pneumatic anti-shock garment (PASG), although this has not been studied. The PASG minimally increases venous return but can significantly increase intrathoracic pressure and hence decrease emptying of the IJ vein. Prolonged palpation of the carotid pulse will decrease the diameter of the IJ vein.[54] Rotating the head 90 degrees toward the opposite side or extending the neck will not change the size of the IJ vessel significantly. Severe rotation of the head, however, will bring the sternocleidomastoid muscle anterior or medial to the IJ vein. Severe rotation may make it impossible to cannulate the IJ vein without first traversing the carotid artery when the anterior approach is used. The diameter of the IJ vessel is largest below the cricoid ring,[54] where it may reach 2 to 2.5 cm.

Preparation. Defalque[2] reviewed methods of IJ cannulation and organized the approaches into three groups defined by the anatomy of the sternocleidomastoid muscle. In preparation for all three methods, the patient is tilted 15 to 30 degrees in the Trendelenburg position and the head is turned slightly away from the side of venipuncture. The internal jugular vein is distensible, and tilting the patient increases the diameter of the vessel. If the patient is awake, he or she should be instructed to perform a Valsalva maneuver during vessel cannulation. In the unconscious patient, abdominal compression by an assistant can be used to help distend the vein.

Familiarity with the anatomy of the neck is important both to increase the probability of successful cannulation and to avoid complications. Most authors favor cannulation of the right side of the neck, which provides a more direct route to the superior vena cava and avoids the thoracic duct. Although it is probably clinically insignificant, the cupola of the pleura is also slightly lower on the right side. The left internal jugular approach is more circuitous and, when used with a stiff Teflon catheter, may result in a major venous puncture leading to hydrothorax, hydromediastinum, or even pericardial tamponade.[55–58] When time permits, the skin is prepared with a povidone-iodine solution and is

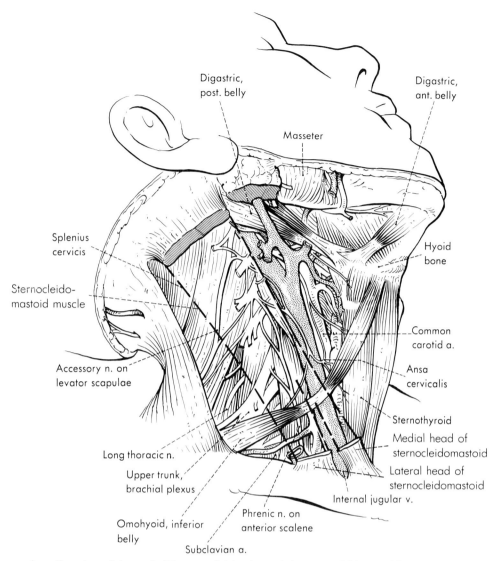

Figure 26–1. Structures in a dissection of the neck. The superficial veins and the sternocleidomastoid muscle have been removed, as have the submandibular gland and a segment of the facial vein. The cutaneous nerves have been cut down to short stumps arising from the second, third, and fourth cervical nerves. The internal jugular vein is drawn somewhat more medial in this illustration than is commonly found. (From Hollinshead WH: Textbook of Anatomy. 3rd ed. New York, Harper & Row, 1974, p 765. Reproduced by permission)

draped with sterile towels. Levy and associates[59] described the virtual elimination of catheter contamination by inserting the catheter through a previously placed iodophor-impregnated sterile film after the usual sterile preparation and draping. Preparation should include the subclavian area in case of failure of the IJ approach. Interestingly, Clayton and colleagues[60] found no statistical difference in catheter contamination rates during 137 insertions using an aseptic technique versus a "standard nonsterile" technique of insertion. The patients and their skin were prepared similarly in both groups except for the presence or absence of sterile towels for draping. Physicians in the aseptic group prepared as if for surgery with a 5-minute scrub and full gown, hat, mask, and gloves, whereas the "nonsterile" physicians did not necessarily even wash their hands or use sterile gloves. The contaminating organism in 87.1 per cent of the overall cases was *Staphylococcus epidermis.*

The procedure should be described briefly to the conscious patient, and each step should be restated as it is about to be performed. The area to be punctured should be anesthetized with a local anesthetic and a 25-gauge needle. As noted previously, it is advisable to attempt a subclavian approach on the same side if the IJ approach is unsuccessful (rather than to attempt an IJ route on the opposite side) to avert bilateral iatrogenic injuries.

Central Route. This approach is favored by Daily and associates[5] and Kaplan and Miller,[61] who believe that the incidence of cannulation of the carotid artery is decreased and the cupola of the lung is avoided with this method. The triangle formed by the clavicle and the sternal and clavicular heads of the sternocleidomastoid muscle is first palpated and identified. The lateral border of the carotid pulse can be marked by a local anesthetic skin wheal or a marking pen, and all subsequent needle puncture can be performed laterally to that point.

Some practitioners prefer to attempt cannulation with the catheter apparatus initially. Other clinicians use a small-gauge "locator" needle to locate the vein. The smaller needle allows one to ascertain the location of the vein and minimizes injury to the deep structures by an incorrectly placed larger needle. Use of a locator needle can be time consuming in a cardiac arrest situation. With the exploring technique, a 22-gauge, 3-cm needle attached to a 5- to 10-ml syringe is introduced near the rostral apex of the triangle and is

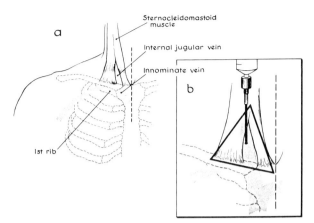

Figure 26–2. Central approach to the internal jugular vein. *a,* Relationship of the sternocleidomastoid muscle to the chest. *b,* Course of the internal jugular vein; note its sagittal course. (From Daily PO, Griepp RB, Shumway NE: Percutaneous internal jugular vein cannulation. Arch Surg 101:534, 1970. Copyright 1970, American Medical Association. Reproduced by permission.)

directed caudally at an angle 30 to 40 degrees to the skin. The needle should initially be directed parallel and slightly laterally to the course of the carotid artery (Fig. 26–2). If three fingers are lightly placed over the course of the carotid artery, the parallel course of the IJ vein can be estimated. The vein consistently lies just lateral to the carotid artery. Prolonged deep palpation of the carotid artery may decrease the size of the vein, and the three-finger technique should be used only long enough to identify the course of the artery.

Negative pressure should be maintained on the syringe at all times as the needle is advanced or retracted. The vein is more superficial than might be expected, and deep probing with the needle should be avoided; the vein is usually encountered at a depth of 1 to 1.5 cm. If the internal jugular vein is not entered at a depth of 3 to 5 cm, the needle should be withdrawn to just below the skin surface and directed toward the ipsilateral nipple underneath the medial border of the lateral (clavicular) head of the sternocleidomastoid muscle. During any type of central venous cannulation a needle must always be withdrawn to the surface before being redirected to avoid lacerating or otherwise damaging important nerves, vessels, or other structures. The vein should be entered at 1 to 3 cm, and dark blood should be easily aspirated. (Bright red blood indicates carotid artery penetration and the need for needle repositioning.) The locator needle is withdrawn and is replaced with a 14-gauge, 5-cm needle attached to a syringe.[4] A drop of the aspirated blood from the locator needle can be placed at the edge of the sterile field in line with the point of vessel entry, thus serving as a guide to recannulation.

The larger needle is advanced through the skin along the path determined by the smaller needle until blood is aspirated. Care must be taken to cover the needle hub with a gloved thumb whenever the needle lumen is exposed to air. This practice will prevent an air embolus when the patient inspires.[62] A catheter and stylet are then passed through the needle into the superior vena cava. Alternatively, an over-the-needle catheter may be used. The over-the-needle catheter is less desirable, because it may not reach the intrathoracic central venous circulation. Once the catheter is felt to be in the central circulation, the intravenous fluid set-up should be attached and the bag or bottle of fluid lowered to below the position of the patient's right atrium. With proper positioning of the catheter, blood return into

the IV tubing should be noted. This test is usually reliable even several days after the line is initially placed.[63] A pulsatile blood column may be noted if the catheter has been inadvertently placed into the carotid artery. Less pronounced pulsations may also occur if the catheter is advanced too far and reaches the right atrium or ventricle. Pulsations may also occasionally be noted with changes in intrathoracic pressure due to respirations, although one hopes this will be at a much slower rate than the arterial pulse!

One secures the catheter in place by placing a suture through the skin, tying three square knots, and then tying the suture around the catheter. The catheter will be both secure and functional if the knot is tied tightly enough to slightly indent the catheter; the stylet may be left in place while the knot is tied to prevent catheter occlusion. Two other skin sutures should be placed on either side (or through standard openings) of the needle guard. To avoid crimping of the catheter, one usually loops the catheter around the ipsilateral ear (Fig. 26–3). Antibiotic ointment is then applied to the puncture site, and a sterile dressing is placed. The intravenous tubing should be securely fastened to the catheter with tape to prevent air embolism or blood loss.

Posterior and Anterior Routes. The techniques of manipulating needles, syringes, and catheters for these approaches are identical to those for the central route; only the landmarks and needle directions vary. For the posterior approach, the skin is entered at the lateral edge of the sternocleidomastoid muscle one third of the way from the clavicle to the mastoid process (Fig. 26–4). The locator needle is directed caudally and medially under the lateral border of the sternocleidomastoid muscle toward the sternal notch until blood is aspirated.

To perform the anterior approach described by Mostert and coworkers,[7] the course of the carotid artery is identified (Fig. 26–5). The small needle should then enter the skin at the midpoint of the medial aspect of the sternocleidomastoid muscle. The needle is directed at an angle of 30 to 45 degrees to the coronal plane caudad toward the ipsilateral nipple. Kaplan and Miller[61] alter this approach by starting at the level of the thyroid notch. The proximity of the carotid artery in the anterior approach may prohibit venous

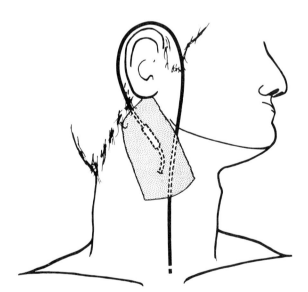

Figure 26–3. Internal jugular line secured by looping around the ear. (From Boulanger M, et al: Une nouvelle voie d'abord de la veine jugulaire interne. Can Anaesth Soc J 23:609, 1976. Reproduced by permission.)

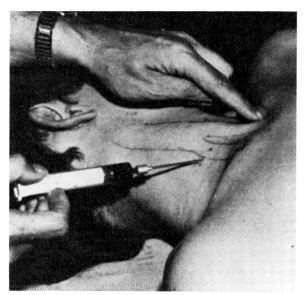

Figure 26–4. Posterior approach to the internal jugular vein. Contrary to the illustration, surgical gloves should be worn during the procedure. (From Delfaque RJ: Percutaneous catheterization of the internal jugular vein. Anesth Analg 53:116, 1974. Reproduced by permission.)

cannulation without carotid puncture.[54] Legler and Nugent[64] report the use of Doppler ultrasound to facilitate difficult IJ cannulation. This technique is obviously restricted to non-emergency cannulations.

Internal Jugular Vein Catheterization in Infants and Children. Prince and coworkers[65] reported a high success rate (40 of 54 cases) in patients from the ages of 6 weeks to 14 years. Nicolson and associates[26] reported an 86 per cent success rate for IJ cannulations in pediatric surgical patients with 99 per cent of those catheters found to be in proper position in the thorax. Success was dependent on infant size

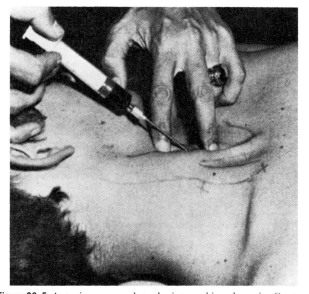

Figure 26–5. Anterior approach to the internal jugular vein. Contrary to the illustration, surgical gloves should be worn during the procedure. (From Delfaque RJ: Percutaneous catheterization of the internal jugular vein. Anesth Analg 53:116, 1974. Reproduced by permission.)

(better above 10 kg) and central venous pressure (better over 10 cm H_2O). Using the central approach of Daily and coworkers[5] with needle puncture at the apex of the triangle bordered by the two heads of the sternocleidomastoid muscle and the clavicle, one passes a 22-gauge needle attached to a 2- to 5-ml non–Luer-Lok syringe into the skin at a 45-degree angle and directs it caudally and laterally toward the ipsilateral nipple. The vessel is usually entered at a depth of 1 to 2 cm. The locator needle is then withdrawn, and a 17- to 19-gauge needle is inserted into the skin and passed along the track of the 22-gauge needle until the IJ vein is penetrated. A catheter is inserted through the needle and is secured in place.

External Jugular Vein Technique

With the patient prepared and in the Trendelenburg position, the external jugular vein is entered with a 16- to 18-gauge needle or a standard over-the-needle peripheral intravenous catheter. Local anesthesia should be used in the conscious patient. The needle or catheter must be able to accept a guide wire through its lumen. The vein is first distended by instructing the patient to perform a Valsalva maneuver and then tamponading the vein just cephalad to the clavicle with a finger. The vein is approached from the side while slight traction is placed on the vein to stabilize it. The needle is advanced following an acute angle with the vessel until it is felt to pop into the lumen of the vein. The needle or catheter should be advanced slightly after feeling the pop to ensure intraluminal placement. When the vein has been cannulated with a needle or a catheter, a J wire is passed through the lumen and into the central venous circulation.[25] If an introducing needle is used, it is now withdrawn to avoid shearing off the guide wire during manipulation. A Teflon over-the-needle catheter is preferred over a needle because it may stay in the vein during guide wire passage or may serve as a temporary peripheral venous line if the central circulation cannot be cannulated.

One advances the guide wire into the thorax by rotating, teasing, or otherwise manipulating the tip until the wire is within the central venous circulation (Fig. 26–6). Guide wire advancement is the most difficult and time-consuming portion of the procedure, and this time constraint limits the usefulness of the technique in an emergency. A small-radius J-tipped wire, a distended vessel lumen, and exaggeration of patient head tilt coupled with skin traction may facilitate successful guide wire passage. Partially withdrawing the wire and twisting it 180 degrees before re-advancing the tip may also be helpful. Once the wire is in the correct position, a standard central venous catheter may be threaded over the wire, or a sheath introducer may be passed (with the aid of a vein dilator, as described in Chapter 23) to facilitate the introduction of a transvenous pacemaker or a pulmonary artery catheter. Even with central placement of the guide wire, the catheter may not pass centrally. After catheter placement, the guide wire is removed and the intravenous line is attached.

Central venous cannulation via the external jugular vein is time consuming and often difficult. It also sometimes results in significant complications, especially with the use of the left external jugular vein.[26, 56] For these reasons, it is not recommended in an emergency. Nonetheless, the external jugular approach does provide central venous access in selected stable patients. Furthermore, simple cannulation with a short catheter is useful for fluid and drug administration during an emergency when peripheral veins cannot be cannulated.

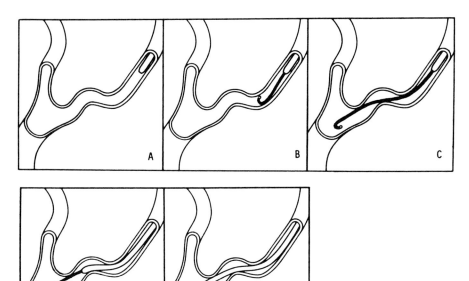

Figure 26–6. Insertion of a catheter over a wire via the external jugular vein. (From Blitt CD, Wright WA, Petty WC: Central venous catheterization via the external jugular vein, a technique employing the J-wire. JAMA 229:817, 1974. Reproduced by permission.)

Femoral Vein Catheterization Technique

The femoral vein is most easily cannulated percutaneously in patients with a palpable femoral pulse. The femoral vein lies just medially to the artery in the femoral canal below the inguinal ligament. Beneath the femoral vessels lie the psoas muscle and the hip (Fig. 26–7).

After skin preparation, the pulse should be palpated briefly, and the femoral vein should be approached medial to the pulse. The femoral vein is a large vessel, and in adults the puncture should be made 5 to 15 mm medial to the pulse.[18, 38] Ultrasound studies of the inguinal anatomy in infants suggests puncture will be most successful when made 5 to 6 mm medial to the pulse, 1 cm below the inguinal crease.[66] During CPR, palpable pulsations may represent venous pressure waves.[39] Hence, if the femoral vein must be used and initial attempts are unsuccessful in a cardiac arrest, a more lateral approach over the pulsation is recommended. When the femoral artery pulsation is not palpable, the femoral artery bisects a line that can be drawn from the anterior superior iliac crest to the pubic symphysis.

After local anesthesia is used in the conscious patient, a 14-gauge, 5-cm needle attached to a saline-filled syringe may be inserted 1 cm medial to the artery. Negative pressure is maintained with the syringe at all times while the needle is under the skin. The needle is directed posteriorly and is advanced until the vein is entered, as identified by a flash of dark, nonpulsating blood. If the vessel is penetrated when the syringe is not being aspirated, the blood flash may be seen only as the needle is being withdrawn.

Once in the vein, the needle is stabilized; often a hemostat is helpful for holding the needle during removal of the syringe. A premeasured section of a 90-cm catheter may then be inserted through the needle. One determines the appropriate length by holding the catheter over the patient's body and estimating the distance from the skin puncture site to the right atrium. Contamination of the catheter must be avoided while this maneuver is performed. Once the catheter is placed, it is secured with sutures and is dressed in the same manner as other central lines. A locator needle with or without a guide wire may minimize vessel injury during location and cannulation of the femoral vein.

The guide wire technique (see Chapter 23) is generally preferred to direct use of a 14-gauge needle.

In situations requiring rapid volume infusion, in the absence of intra-abdominal trauma, the femoral vein may be cannulated with the Seldinger technique. The sheath introducer will allow the rapid transfusion of large volumes of blood or crystalloid solution for fluid resuscitation.[19] Various catheters are available with single large-bore lumens or as many as three lumens for infusion of separate intravenous solutions and medications. One study[67] suggested a higher incidence of contamination with triple-lumen catheters; however, Kelly and associates[35] reported an acceptably low incidence of bacteremia and sepsis (3.1 per cent) using this device. The femoral vessels may also be cannulated under direct visualization using a cutdown technique (see Chapter 24).

Basilic and Cephalic Cannulation

Anatomy of the Basilic and Cephalic Veins. Considerable variation is present in the venous vasculature of the upper extremities. Nonetheless, the cephalic and basilic veins can usually be located in the volar antecubital region (Fig. 26–8). The interconnecting median antecubital vein is often the most prominent, thus making it a popular site for venipuncture during blood sampling. The basilic vein merges proximally with the brachial vein to form the axillary vein, which subsequently meets the cephalic vein to form the subclavian vein near the distal clavicle. The internal and external jugular veins join the subclavian vein to form the innominate vein bilaterally. Many venous valves exist in the peripheral vessels. Vascular anastomoses may permit aberrant advancement of a long line from the upper extremity. In particular, lines threaded up the cephalic vein may dead-end in a venous plexus or may enter the external jugular vein (Fig. 26–9). Furthermore, lines passed through the basilic vein may easily enter the internal jugular vein.

Technique. Basilic and cephalic venous systems are entered through the large veins in the antecubital fossa (see Fig. 26–8). Tourniquet placement aids venous distention and initial venous puncture. Cannulation can often be per-

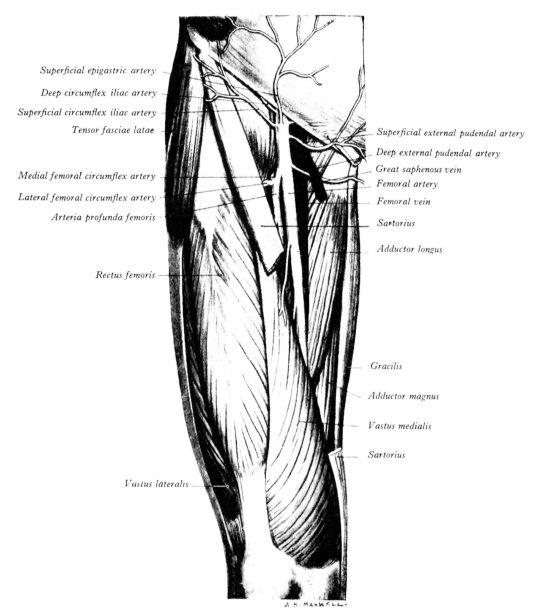

Figure 26–7. The right femoral vessels and some of their branches. The femoral nerve (not shown) lies lateral to the artery and may be deep to the artery. (From Warwick R, Williams PL (eds): Gray's Anatomy. 35th ed. Edinburgh, Churchill Livingstone, 1973, p 676. Reproduced by permission.)

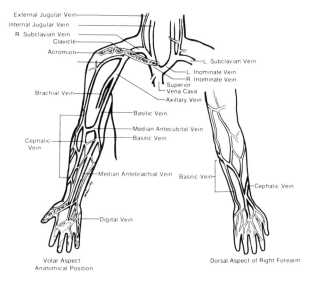

Figure 26–8. Major veins of the upper half of the body. (From Hedges JR: Vascular access. Curr Top Emerg Med 2:1, 1981. Reproduced by permission.)

formed percutaneously with a 14-gauge needle under direct visualization or by using the guide wire technique. When veins are not visible, they may be reached with a cutdown procedure, as described in Chapter 24. The basilic vein, located on the medial aspect of the antecubital fossa, is generally larger than the radially located cephalic vein. Furthermore, the basilic vein generally provides a more direct route for passage into the axillary subclavian vein and superior vena cava. Once a vein has been entered, a pre-measured length of a 90-cm catheter is threaded aseptically into the superior vena cava. Catheter length is estimated using the combined distance from the puncture site to the axilla and from the axilla to the middle of the manubrium.

Inability to pass the catheter is common. The cephalic vein may terminate inches above the antecubital fossa or may bifurcate before entering the axillary vein, sending a branch to the external jugular vein. The cephalic vein may also enter the axillary vein at right angles, defeating any

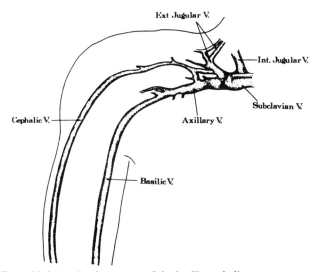

Figure 26–9. Proximal anatomy of the basilic-cephalic venous system. (From Webre DR, Arens JF: Use of the cephalic and basilic veins for introduction of central venous catheters. Anesthesiology 33:389, 1973. Reproduced by permission.)

attempt to pass the catheter centrally. Furthermore, both the basilic system and the cephalic system contain valves that may impede catheterization. Abduction of the shoulder may help to advance the catheter if resistance near the axillary vein occurs. The incidence of failure to place the catheter in the superior vena cava ranges from a high of 40 per cent to a low of 2 per cent.[47, 48, 50] Holt[48] believes that there is a higher incidence of success if crystalloid solution is continuously infused during the passage of the catheter. This contention is not supported by Bridges and coworkers,[47] who found an 80 to 84 per cent success rate with slow catheter advancement without infusion versus a 44 per cent success rate with crystalloid infusion in the supine patient.

The greatest success rate (98 per cent) reported was obtained with slow catheter advancement with the patient in a 45- to 90-degree upright position.[47] Flexible Bard (C.R. Bard, Inc., Murray Hill, NJ) (16 gauge) catheters were introduced into the basilic vein until the tip was judged to be proximal to the junction of the cephalic and basilic veins and distal to the junction of the internal jugular vein with the innominate vein (see Fig. 26–9). The wire stylet was withdrawn 18 cm, and the catheters were advanced slowly 1 cm at a time, with 2 seconds allowed between each 1 cm insertion. The natural flexibility of the Bard catheters contributed to negotiation into the superior vena cava when the patient was upright. Obviously, this time-consuming technique is contraindicated when the patient cannot tolerate an upright position.

Further Comments

All of the percutaneous methods of central venous cannulation can be performed with the Seldinger (guide wire) technique described in Chapter 23. Furthermore, when puncturing the skin with a large-bore needle, one should start with 1 to 2 ml of normal saline in the attached syringe. After the skin has been entered, a small amount of this fluid should be expelled to remove any plug of skin that might be present and that could interfere with subsequent aspiration of blood. The needle bevel should routinely be aligned with the numeric markings on the syringe to aid in bevel location once the skin is entered.

Immediately after any central line has been placed, blood should be aspirated from the catheter. Alternatively, one should place the intravenous bag at a level below the patient to check for blood return in the intravenous tubing. It should be noted that blood return is presumptive evidence of intravascular placement and does not substitute for radiographic confirmation. When this gravity flow method is used, it is important to check the intravenous tubing for the presence of a one-way flow valve. A one-way valve will prevent a flashback of blood. The flashback of blood should also be observed for pulsations that may indicate line placement in an artery, tricuspid regurgitation, atrial fibrillation, or ventricular tachycardia. A chest film should also be obtained after central line placement to confirm catheter placement and to rule out hemothorax or pneumothorax. An interesting technique using a Fogarty catheter to convert a central venous line into a flow-directed balloon catheter has been described by Laufer.[68] If the central line is found to be malpositioned, such as a subclavian catheter that has ascended into the IJ vein, an appropriately sized Fogarty catheter is introduced through the central line. Both catheters are then withdrawn past the junction where the incorrect turn occurred. The Fogarty balloon is then inflated and the catheter advanced with the assistance of blood flow to draw it into proper position. The Fogarty catheter is then deflated and removed.

COMPLICATIONS

The methods of preventing complications of subclavian venipuncture that were discussed in Chapter 25 should be heeded when the approaches to central venous access mentioned in this chapter are used. Several cautions in particular need to be reemphasized. When performing any of these procedures, an individual should have a thorough knowledge of the anatomy or should be supervised by someone who does. One must also remember to replace as soon as possible all lines that were placed during a cardiac arrest or in other less than optimally sterile situations. Furthermore, all central lines should be discontinued at the earliest clinical opportunity. Finally, it is incumbent on the physician who placed the line to check the chest film personally for proper catheter position and possible complications. The following discussion is supplemental to the complication section of Chapter 25.

Internal Jugular Vein Approach Complications

Many of the complications of IJ cannulation are similar to those that have been discussed in the preceding chapter for the supraclavicular approach to the subclavian vein. Infection, catheter malposition, thrombosis, and damage to surrounding structures are complications common to all puncture sites for central venous cannulation. The reported rates of thrombosis for internal jugular vein catheterizations range from a report of no significant thrombosis in one study to a high of 66 per cent of patients exhibiting some thrombosis in a study of 33 medical intensive care unit patients.[69, 70] No reports of significant pulmonary embolus directly attributable to an IJ catheter were found. Such wide variation in the reported incidence of complications is common, in part because of the different methods of detecting and reporting complications and the widely varying experience with a specific technique of individual institutions and physicians. The number of complications increases, especially those due to thrombosis and infection, with longer durations of catheterization and increasing severity of the patient's illness.[14, 70] Complications also seem to be higher with the use of the left IJ vein as opposed to the right.[54–56] Reported complications felt to be due at least in part to the use of the left-sided approach include mediastinal migration of the catheters and at least one instance of fatal pericardial tamponade.

Although at least one study has found no significant difference in the incidence of major complications between the IJ and subclavian routes, one fairly common complication unique to the IJ approach is a hematoma in the neck.[15] With the IJ approach, pressure can be maintained easily on the area of swelling, and most hematomas will resolve spontaneously. If carotid arterial puncture is recognized and treated with compression, it rarely causes significant morbidity in the absence of marked atherosclerotic disease, although arteriovenous fistulas have been reported after IJ puncture.[71–75] Several neurologic complications unique to the IJ site of venipuncture have also been reported as a result of hematomas or of direct injury.[76, 77] These complications include damage to the phrenic nerves, an iatrogenic Horner syndrome, trauma to the brachial plexus, and even an instance of the passage of a catheter into the thecal space of the spinal canal.[78–81] If the carotid artery is punctured, one may again attempt IJ or subclavian cannulation on the same side after appropriate, prolonged (15 to 20 minutes) compression.

Arterial puncture is a contraindication to attempting the IJ route on the opposite side, because bilateral hemorrhage may occur with resultant airway compromise. The physician should be prepared to rapidly intubate should this occur. Even in the face of a coagulopathy, however, the IJ approach has been found to be successful (99.3 per cent of cases) and safe (less than 1 per cent complication rate).[82]

Femoral Vein Approach Complications

Femoral lines are generally associated with less severe complications than are IJ or subclavian approaches because of the avoidance of thoracic trauma. The peritoneum can, however, be violated with possible resulting perforation of the bowel. Bowel penetration is especially likely if the patient has a femoral hernia.[83] Injury to the bowel is likely to be minimal and is unlikely to require specific treatment. Nonetheless, the potential bacterial contamination of the femoral puncture site may pose a significant problem. The aspiration of air on placement of a femoral line necessitates removal of the catheter and reinsertion at another site. Bonadio and associates[84] reported a case in which a patient developed clinical signs of peritonitis, which were found to be due to the infiltration of intravenous fluids into the anterior abdominal wall from a femoral catheter. A psoas abscess may result from penetration posteriorly of the underlying psoas fascia.[83] The bladder, when distended, can also be punctured during femoral cannulation, although bladder puncture is unlikely to require therapy beyond removal of the aberrantly placed catheter. Strict aseptic technique should be maintained to prevent septic arthritis in the unlikely event that the hip capsule is punctured. This complication has been reported in infants.[85]

The most common complications of femoral venipuncture are accidental arterial and venous perforation. As mentioned in the "Indications" section, arterial puncture is more common in the patient who is in a low- or no-flow circulatory status. Emerman and colleagues reported that during cardiac arrest, the success rate for femoral catheterization was only 77 per cent compared with 94 per cent for subclavian vein catheterization.[36] Prolonged (greater than 15 minutes) pressure should stop any arterial hemorrhage in a patient with normal clotting mechanisms. The femoral nerve can also be injured by an errant needle puncture.[82, 84] Complications will be minimized if the patient has a pulse and the femoral vein is approached medial to the femoral pulsations. A helpful mnemonic is NAVEL, which describes the anatomy of the region from lateral to medial: nerve, artery, vein, empty space, and inguinal ligament. One report[86] of 5306 femoral vein cannulations using the Seldinger technique reported five severe complications (three episodes of severe retroperitoneal bleeding after external iliac artery puncture, one case of fatal femoral artery hemorrhage, and one reversible femoral nerve injury).

Getzen and Pollak,[18] in a large study of military casualties, reported a 1.6 per cent incidence of major hematomas, a 3.3 per cent incidence of infection, and a 5.6 per cent incidence of thrombophlebitis. Thrombophlebitis does occur more frequently with femoral lines than with IJ and supraclavicular methods.[83] Thrombophlebitis is usually seen only with prolonged cannulation. There have even been reports (two of 24 patients) of pulmonary emboli thought to result from the thrombosis caused by prolonged (3 to 14 days) femoral cannulation.[87] Kanter and coworkers[13] reported an 11 per cent incidence of leg swelling or documented thrombosis in a series of pediatric patients. Another complication that occurs at femoral and other sites with the use of catheter through-the-needle devices is catheter tip embolism.[88, 89] This complication can be prevented by avoiding withdrawal of the catheter through a needle, even slightly, while the needle is still in the skin.

Basilic-Cephalic Approach Complications

Cannulation of the central venous system through the arm veins has the lowest major complication rate of all. Superficial local infections are common (10 to 20 per cent incidence) and rarely may lead to more serious problems including sepsis. Catheter malposition is common, and studies have shown this to happen in 10 to 40 per cent of placements.[48–50] One nuisance with this type of catheter is the need to immobilize an entire extremity and the shoulder to prevent catheter movement and kinking.

CONCLUSION

There is no "ideal" location for cannulation of the central venous circulation. Factors such as urgency, availability of access sites, duration of catheterization, and skill of the physician are the most important determinants of cannulation route.

The major advantage of IJ cannulation compared with subclavian cannulation is the decreased incidence of pleural puncture. If a hematoma occurs as a result of inadvertent puncture of the carotid artery, compression is easily maintained with the IJ approach. In addition, the right IJ route provides a straight anatomic course to the right atrium, thus helping to ensure successful placement of the catheter tip. This is an obvious advantage if a pacemaker or a Swan-Ganz catheter will be passed.

Cannulation of the IJ vein is more difficult than cannulation of the subclavian vein, because the IJ vein is more variable in size, more easily displaced, and more difficult to locate than the subclavian vein. In patients with short, thick necks, the IJ route can be virtually impossible, because the needle and the syringe cannot be manipulated in the small area between the head and the clavicle.

Peripheral insertion of a catheter through the basilic-cephalic vein systems is generally free from major complications but is time consuming. In addition, the final catheter tip location is variable. External jugular insertion using a guide wire avoids the hazards of carotid puncture, brachial plexus injury, and pneumothorax. Frequent cannulation of the superior vena cava from the external jugular vein indicates that this technique can minimize risk and maximize central location of the catheter tip.[11, 12, 27] Unfortunately, the external jugular approach using guide wires can be prohibitively time consuming, especially if one is unfamiliar with the method. Schwartz and coworkers found that central cannulation through the external jugular vein with the guide wire technique took 5 to 25 minutes.[12] The same group had a significantly better success rate with curved J wires rather than straight guide wires (86 per cent versus 61 per cent).

Insertion of a central line during cardiac arrest and resuscitation should be secondary in importance to peripheral venous cannulation. Central venous cannulation is indicated when venous collapse or vasoconstriction makes peripheral cannulation impossible, when the need for a rapid central access for drug administration is imperative, or when central venous cannulation can be accomplished more quickly than peripheral venous cannulation in an emergency. In a cardiac arrest situation, a cutdown on a peripheral vein may be too time consuming. Furthermore, both external and internal jugular cannulation may be difficult, because access to the head is limited by the need to maintain an airway and to ventilate the patient. Cardiac massage may interfere with the placement of a subclavian catheter and increases the risk of a pneumothorax or subclavian vein or artery laceration. Femoral cannulation may be a safe alternative, but cannulation can be difficult in the absence of an easily palpable pulse.[36] Each technique of central cannulation has its drawbacks during a cardiac arrest. Thus every physician who may be faced with venous cannulation of the cardiac arrest patient should be familiar with at least one of these techniques for placement of an appropriate line within a short period. Ideally, emergency physicians and others who deal with these extremely urgent situations should familiarize themselves fully with as many alternatives as possible.

REFERENCES

1. Silver JH, Kemp CH, Bruyn HB: Handbook of Pediatrics. 5th ed. Los Altos, Calif, Lange Medical Publications, 1963, pp 37–38.
2. Defalque RH: Percutaneous catheterization of the internal jugular vein. Anesth Analg 53:116, 1974.
3. Hemosura B: Measurement of pressure during intravenous therapy. JAMA 195:181, 1966.
4. Civetta JM, Gabel JC, Gemer M: Internal jugular vein puncture with a margin of safety. Anesthesiology 36:622, 1972.
5. Daily PA, Griepp RB, Shumway NE: Percutaneous internal jugular vein cannulation. Arch Surg 101:534, 1970.
6. Jernigan WR, Gardener WC, Mahr MM, Milburn IL: Use of the internal jugular vein for placement of central venous catheter. Surg Gynecol Obstet 130:520, 1970.
7. Mostert JW, Kenny GM, Murphy GP: Safe placement of cardiovascular catheters into the jugular vein. Arch Surg 101:431, 1970.
8. English ICW, Frew RM, Pigott JEG, Zaki M: Percutaneous cannulation of the internal jugular vein. Thorax 24:496, 1969.
9. English ICW, Frew RM, Pigott JF, Zaki M: Percutaneous catheterization of the internal jugular vein. Anaesthesia 24:521, 1969.
10. Craig RG, Jones RA, Sproul GJ, Kinyon GE: The alternate methods of central venous system catheterization. Am Surg 34:131, 1968.
11. Blitt CD, Wright WA, Petty WC: Central venous catheterization via the external jugular vein: A technique employing the J-wire. JAMA 229:817, 1974.
12. Schwartz AJ, Jobes DR, Levy WJ, et al: Intrathoracic vascular catheterization via the external jugular vein. Anesthesiology 56:400, 1982.
13. Kanter RK, Zimmerman JJ, Strauss RH, et al: Central venous catheter insertion by femoral vein: Safety and effectiveness for the pediatric patient. Pediatrics 77:842, 1986.
14. Arrighi DA, Farnell MB, Mucha P, et al: Prospective randomized trial of rapid venous access for patients in hypovolemic shock. Ann Emerg Med 18:927, 1989.
15. Senagore A, Waller J, Bonnell BW, et al: Pulmonary artery catheterization: A prospective study of internal jugular and subclavian approaches. Crit Care Med 15:35, 1987.
16. Sznajder JI, Zveibil FR, Bitterman H, et al: Central vein catheterization: Failure and complication rates by three percutaneous approaches. Arch Intern Med 146:259, 1986.
17. Bo-Linn GW, Anderson DJ, Anderson KC, et al: Percutaneous central venous catheterization performed by medical house officers: A prospective study. Cathet Cardiovasc Diagn 8:23, 1982.
18. Getzen LC, Pollak EW: Short term femoral vein catheterization. Am J Surg 138:875, 1979.
19. Mangiante EC, Hoots AV, Fabian TC: The percutaneous common femoral vein catheter for volume replacement in critically injured patients. J Trauma 28:1644, 1988.
20. Demetriades D: Internal jugular vein catheterization in shocked patients. S Afr Med J 63:969, 1983.
21. Hodge D, Delgado-Paredes C, Fleisher G: Central and peripheral catheter flow rates in "pediatric" dogs. Ann Emerg Med 15:1151, 1986.
22. Kaiser CW, Koornick AR, Smith N, Soroff HS: Choice of route for central venous cannulation: Subclavian or internal jugular vein? A prospective randomized study. J Surg Oncol 17:345, 1981.
23. Eisenhauer ED, Derveloy RJ, Hastings PR: Prospective evaluation of central venous (CVP) catheters in a large city-county hospital. Ann Surg 196:560, 1982.
24. Patel C, Laboy V, Venus B, et al: Acute complications of pulmonary artery catheter insertion in critically ill patients. Crit Care Med 14:195, 1986.
25. Dailey RH: External jugular vein cannulation and its use for CVP monitoring. J Emerg Med 6:133, 1988.
26. Nicolson SC, Sweeney MF, Moore RA, et al: Comparison of internal and external jugular cannulation of the central circulation in the pediatric patient. Crit Care Med 13:747, 1985.
27. Humphrey MJ, Blitt CD: Central venous access in children via the external jugular vein. Anesthesiology 57:50, 1982.
28. Blitt CD, Carlson GL, Wright WA, et al: J-wire versus straight wire for central venous system cannulation via the external jugular vein. Anesth Analg 61:536, 1982.
29. Belani KG, Buckley JJ, Gordon JR, et al: Percutaneous cervical central venous line placement: A comparison of the internal and external jugular vein routes. Anesth Analg 59:40, 1980.
30. Bozetti F: Percutaneous femoral vein catheterization. Anesthesia 33:761, 1978.
31. Dailey RH: Femoral vein cannulation: A review. J Emerg Med 2:367, 1985.
32. Safar P, Abramson NS, Angelos M, et al: Exposure and cannulation of femoral artery and vein via cutdown within 5 minutes with external CPR. Am J Emerg Med 8:55, 1990.
33. Koffler A, Bernstein M, LaSette A, et al: Fixed bed charcoal hemoperfusion: Treatment of drug overdose. Arch Intern Med 138:1691, 1978.

34. Thomas F, Burke JP, Parker J, et al: The risk of infection related to radial vs femoral sites for arterial catheterization. Crit Care Med 11:807, 1983.
35. Kelly CS, Ligas JR, Smith CA, et al: Sepsis due to triple lumen central venous catheters. Surg Gynecol Obstet 163:14, 1986.
36. Emerman CL, Bellon EM, Lukens TW, et al: A prospective study of femoral versus subclavian vein catheterization during cardiac arrest. Ann Emerg Med 19:26, 1990.
37. Jastremski MS, Matthias HD, Randall PA: Femoral venous catheterization during cardiopulmonary resuscitation: A critical appraisal. J Emerg Med 3:387, 1984.
38. Swanson RS, Uhlig PN, Gross PL, et al: Emergency intravenous access through the femoral vein. Ann Emerg Med 13:244, 1984.
39. Coletti RH, Hartjen B, Gozdziewskis S, et al: Origin of canine femoral pulses during standard CPR (abstract). Crit Care Med 11:218, 1983.
40. Kaye W, Bircher NG: Access for drug administration during cardiopulmonary resuscitation. Crit Care Med 16:179, 1988.
41. Dalsey WC, Barsan WG, Joyce SM, et al: Comparison of superior vena cava vs inferior vena cava access using a radioisotope technique during normal perfusion and cardiopulmonary resuscitation. Ann Emerg Med 13:881, 1984.
42. Emmerman CL, Pinchak EE, Hagan J, et al: The effect of injection site on circulation times during cardiac arrest. Crit Care Med 16:1138, 1988.
43. Niemann JT, Rosborough J, Hausknelti M, et al: Blood flow without cardiac compression during closed chest CPR. Crit Care Med 9:380, 1981.
44. Franceschi D, Gerding RL, Phillips G, et al: Risk factors associated with intravascular catheter infections in burned patients: A prospective, randomized study. J Trauma 29:811, 1989.
45. Woods DG, Lumley J, Russell WJ, et al: The position of central venous catheters inserted through the arm veins: A primary report. Anaesth Intensive Care 2:43, 1947.
46. Lumley J, Russell WJ: Insertion of central venous catheters through arm veins. Anaesth Intensive Care 3:101, 1975.
47. Bridges BB, Carden E, Takacs FA: Introduction of central venous pressure catheters through arm veins with a high success rate. Can Anaesth Soc J 26:128, 1979.
48. Holt MH: Central venous pressures via peripheral veins. Anesthesiology 25:1093, 1967.
49. Johnston AO, Clark RG: Malpositioning of central venous catheters. Lancet 2:1395, 1972.
50. Longston LS: The aberrant central venous catheter and its complications. Radiology 100:55, 1971.
51. Webre DR, Arens JF: Use of the cephalic and basilic veins for introduction of central venous catheters. Anesthesiology 38:389, 1973.
52. Barsan WG, Levy RC, Weir H: Lidocaine levels during CPR: Differences after peripheral venous, central venous, and intracardiac injections. Ann Emerg Med 10:73, 1981.
53. Graber D, Daily RH: Catheter flow rates updated (letter to the editor). JACEP 6:518, 1977.
54. Bazaral M, Harlan S: Ultrasonographic anatomy of the internal jugular vein relevant to percutaneous cannulation. Crit Care Med 9:307, 1981.
55. Sheep RE, Guiney WB: Fatal cardiac tamponade: Occurrence after left internal jugular vein catheterization. JAMA 248:1632, 1982.
56. Moortay SS, McCammon RL, Deschner WP, et al: Diagnosis and management of mediastinal migration of central venous pressure catheters. Heart Lung 14:80, 1985.
57. Albertson TE, Fisher CJ, Vera Z: Accidental mediastinal entry via (L) internal jugular vein cannulation. Intensive Care Med 11:154, 1985.
58. Chute E, Cerra FB: Late development of hydrothorax and hydromediastinum in patients with central venous catheters. Crit Care Med 10:868, 1982.
59. Levy JH, Nagle DM, Curung PE: Contamination reduction during central venous catheterization. Crit Care Med 16:165, 1988.
60. Clayton DG, Shanahan EC, Ordman AJ, et al: Contamination of internal jugular cannulae. Anaesthesia 40:523, 1985.
61. Kaplan JA, Miller ED: Internal jugular vein catheterization. Anesth Rev 21, 1976.

62. O'Quin RJ, Lakshminaraan S: Venous air embolism. Arch Intern Med 142:2173, 1982.
63. Malenka J, Ross JM: Perforation by central venous catheters: A new testament to an old test. J Parenter Enter Nutr 13:309, 1989.
64. Legler D, Nugent M: Doppler localization of the internal jugular vein facilitates central venous cannulation. Anesthesiology 60:481, 1984.
65. Prince SR, Sullivan RL, Hackel A: Percutaneous catheterization of the internal jugular vein in infants and children. Anesthesiology 44:170, 1976.
66. Kanter RK, Gorton JM, Palmier IK: Anatomy of femoral vessels in infants and guidelines for venous catheterization. Pediatrics 83:1020, 1989.
67. Miller JJ, Venus B, Mathru M: Comparison of the sterility of long term central venous catheterization using single lumen, triple lumen and pulmonary artery catheters. Crit Care Med 12:634, 1984.
68. Laufer E: Simple way to reposition a wandering central venous catheter. J Trauma 25:438, 1985.
69. Perkins NAK, Cail WS, Bedford RF, et al: Internal jugular vein function after Swan-Ganz catheterization. Anesthesiology 61:456, 1984.
70. Chastre J, Cornud F, Bouchama A, et al: Thrombosis as a complication of pulmonary artery catheterization through the internal jugular vein. N Engl J Med 306:278, 1982.
71. Ortiz J, Dean WF: Arteriovenous fistula as a complication of percutaneous internal jugular vein catheterization: Case report. Milit Med 141:171, 1976.
72. Hayward R, Swanton H, Treasure T: Acquired arteriovenous communication: Complication of cannulation of internal jugular vein. Br Med J 21:1195, 1984.
73. Hansbrough JF, Narrod JA, Rutherford R: Arteriovenous fistulas following central venous catheterization. Intensive Care Med 9:287, 1984.
74. Sato O, Tada Y, Sudo K, et al: Arteriovenous fistula following central venous catheterization. Arch Surg 121:729, 1986.
75. Robinson PN, Jewkes DA, Kendall B: Vertebrovertebral arteriovenous fistula: A complication of internal jugular catheterization. Anaesthesia 39:46, 1984.
76. Frasquet FJ, Belda FJ: Permanent paralysis of C-5 after cannulation of the internal jugular vein. Anesthesiology 54:528, 1981.
77. Briscoe CE, Bushman JA, McDonald WI: Extensive neurological damage after cannulation of internal jugular vein. Br Med J 1:314, 1974.
78. Topaz O, Sharon M, Rechavia E, et al: Traumatic internal jugular vein cannulation. Ann Emerg Med 16:1394, 1987.
79. Parikh RK: Horner's syndrome. A complication of percutaneous catheterizations of internal jugular vein. Anaesthesia 27:327, 1972.
80. Paschall RM, Mandel S: Brachial plexus injury from percutaneous cannulation of the internal jugular vein (letter to editor). Ann Emerg Med 12:58, 1983.
81. Nagai K, Kemmotzu O: An inadvertent insertion of a Swan-Ganz (R) catheter into the intrathecal space. Anesthesiology 62:848, 1985.
82. Goldfarb G, Lebrec D: Percutaneous cannulation of the internal jugular vein in patients with coagulopathies: An experience based on 1000 attempts. Anesthesiology 56:321, 1982.
83. Bosch DT, Kengeter JP, Beling CA: Femoral venipuncture. Am J Surg 79:722, 1950.
84. Bonadio WA, Losek JD, Meltzer-Lange M: An unusual complication from a femoral venous catheter. Pediatr Emerg Care 4:27, 1988.
85. Agnes RS, Arendar GM: Septic arthritis of the hip: A complication of femoral venipuncture. Pediatrics 38:837, 1966.
86. Fuchs JH, et al: Percutaneous puncture of the femoral vein for hemodialysis: Report of 5000 punctures. Dtsch Med Wochenschr 102:1280, 1977.
87. Walters MB, Stanger HAD, Rotem CE: Complications with percutaneous central venous catheters. JAMA 220:1455, 1972.
88. Propp DA, Cline D, Hennenfent RR: Catheter embolism. J Emerg Med 6:17, 1988.
89. Fischer HBJ, Ward G: Catheter tip embolism: A continuing complication of central venous catheterization. Intensive Care Med 9:127, 1983.

Chapter 27

Central Venous Pressure Measurement

Alice M. Donahue and Jerris R. Hedges

INTRODUCTION

For the past two decades, central venous pressure (CVP) monitoring has been used to assess cardiac performance and to guide fluid therapy for critically ill patients. Although the concept was first demonstrated by Forssman in 1931, it was not until the early 1960s that cannulation of the central veins and measurement of the CVP became commonplace.[1, 2]

Simply stated, the CVP is the pressure exerted by the blood against the walls of the intrathoracic venae cavae. Because the pressure in the great veins of the thorax is generally within 1 mm Hg of the right atrial pressure, the CVP reflects the pressure under which blood is returned to the right atrium.[3, 4] The pressure in the central veins has two significant hemodynamic effects. First, the pressure promotes filling of the heart during diastole, a factor that helps determine cardiac output. Second, the CVP is also the back pressure of the systemic circulation, opposing the return of blood from the peripheral blood vessels into the heart.[4] The CVP therefore affects both the ability of the heart to pump blood and the tendency for blood to flow from the peripheral veins.[3, 5] The CVP reading is determined by a complex interaction of intravascular volume, right atrial and ventricular function, venomotor tone, and intrathoracic pressure.[2]

One can measure CVP accurately by placing the tip of a pressure-monitoring catheter into any of the great systemic veins of the thorax or into the right atrium.[4] Because the risks of catheter placement in the atrium include atrial perforation and cardiac dysrhythmias, any large vein within the thorax is preferred.[6] The catheter is commonly connected to a water manometer, and pressure is expressed in relation to the height, in centimeters, of a column of water above the level of the tricuspid valve. Electronic manometers can also be used and appear more accurate, especially when the patient is being mechanically ventilated.[7] The level of the tricuspid valve is chosen as the standard reference point for measurement, because at this point the hydrostatic pressure does not affect the measurement significantly.[3]

Clinically, CVP measurements are most frequently used as a guide for determination of a patient's volume status and fluid requirements and for investigation of the possibility of cardiac tamponade.[8–11] Critical commentaries have been written by some researchers who regard CVP monitoring as ineffective, outmoded, and unreliable.[12–15] The astute clinician, however, can maximize the usefulness of this diagnostic tool by careful consideration of its indications and limitations. The CVP is one of many variables that must be correlated in the development of an overall management plan for the care of critically ill patients.

INDICATIONS AND CONTRAINDICATIONS FOR CENTRAL VENOUS PRESSURE MONITORING

The major indications for CVP monitoring include the following clinical situations:

1. Acute circulatory failure
2. Anticipated massive blood or fluid replacement therapy
3. Cautious fluid replacement in patients with compromised cardiovascular status
4. Suspected cardiac tamponade

The procedure is contraindicated when other resuscitation therapeutic and diagnostic interventions take priority over central venous access and CVP manometer or transducer set-up and calibration.

LIMITATIONS OF CVP MONITORING

The greatest misconception is the incorrect assumption that CVP consistently reflects pressures found in the left side of the heart.[14] The measurement that best reflects left ventricular pressure changes and reserve is the left atrial pressure, or the nearly equivalent pulmonary capillary wedge pressure (PCWP). The development of the flow-directed pulmonary artery catheter has allowed repeated measurements of PCWP, thus permitting accurate assessment of left atrial pressure.

The CVP is most helpful in patients without significant preexisting cardiopulmonary disease. No consistent correlation between isolated CVP and left atrial pressure measurements has been demonstrated in patients with significant cardiopulmonary disease. Forrester and coworkers, in a study of 50 patients with myocardial infarction, demonstrated that CVP measurements had no consistent relationship to PCWP.[15] DiLaurentis and associates, in their study of 32 surgical patients without myocardial infarction, found that CVP and pulmonary arterial pressure correlated in only 50 per cent of their patients.[14] James and Myers[16] studied three parameters—CVP, pulmonary arterial pressure, and PCWP—in 116 patients who either were in shock or had undergone major surgery. In 76 of 116 instances, the PCWP differed significantly from the CVP. An early rise in the PCWP was noted before the rise in the CVP. Samii and coworkers[13] studied 13 relatively elderly patients (mean age of 62) without obvious cardiac or respiratory disease and found a disparity between the right and left ventricular filling pressures. They concluded that CVP may be a misleading index for predicting PCWP in elderly patients.

Toussaint and associates[17] reported a significant *correlation* between CVP and PCWP in 14 patients with no prior history of cardiopulmonary disease. Yet in the same study, a poor correlation between CVP and PCWP was shown in 13 patients with a history of cardiopulmonary disease. Interestingly, Rajacich and colleagues found that CVP accurately predicted left atrial pressure in 17 cardiac bypass graft patients even in the setting of high positive end-expiratory pressure.[18] Their patients had well-preserved cardiac function and normal valvular function. These findings suggest that *CVP provides a reliable assessment of cardiac function only in the absence of cardiopulmonary disease.*

PROCEDURE

The CVP is usually expressed as centimeters of water, indicating the height of a column of water above the zero point on the manometer. Although CVP measurements can be obtained electronically from the level of the right atrium, manometric measurements are more frequently used in the emergency situation and are the focus of this discussion.[7, 19] The reading on a properly placed CVP catheter will fluctuate 1 to 3 cm of H_2O during normal respiration. The reading decreases with inspiration and increases with expiration, straining, or coughing.

Readings should be taken at the end of *inspiration* of a normal breath. If the patient is on a respirator, the CVP changes during the respiratory cycle are reversed, rising with positive-pressure inspiration and decreasing with expi-

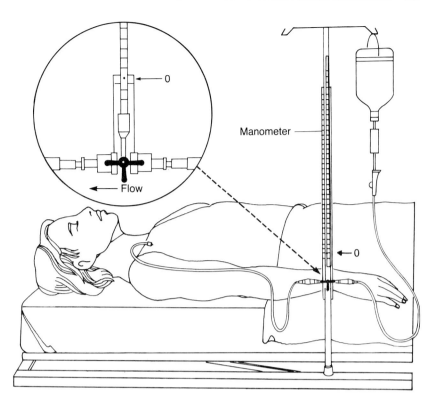

Figure 27–1. The stopcock is turned to direct the flow to the patient, bypassing the manometer. This is the position that is maintained to keep the catheter patent. The tubing is always flushed before connecting it to the patient's central venous pressure catheter.

ration. Readings should be taken near the end of *expiration*, when the patient is being mechanically ventilated.[7] That is, during both normal and mechanical ventilation, the lowest reading is a useful estimate of mean CVP, although some clinicians prefer to visually average the high and low readings. Visual averaging generally leads to overestimation of the mean CVP, especially in mechanically ventilated patients.[7] Regardless of the technique used, a consistent reading method is essential for patient monitoring. When possible the same observer should make or oversee all of the readings.

A prepackaged disposable plastic or glass manometer with a three-way stopcock and standard infusion tubing is most commonly used for measuring CVP (Fig. 27–1). The equipment is connected to a standard intravenous solution bottle. One fills the tubing by turning the stopcock to the position that directs flow of the intravenous solution through the distal end of the catheter, bypassing the manometer. One then primes the manometer with fluid by turning the stopcock to direct the fluid flow from the intravenous solution bottle to the manometer (Fig. 27–2). The distal end of the primed set is now connected to the central catheter, and the stopcock (closed to the manometer) directs fluid from the intravenous bottle to the patient (Fig. 27–3). To obtain a reading, the stopcock (closed to the bottle) is directed to open the system from the patient to the manometer. The patient's CVP is reflected by the height of the water in the manometer. The fluid level is allowed to fall spontaneously until it stabilizes before a reading is taken. Between readings, the fluid is turned off to the manometer, and the CVP catheter serves as a standard intravenous infusion site (see Fig. 27–1). The rate of infusion should be capable of maintaining catheter patency and meeting fluid needs of the patient. A small amount of heparin (1000 units per liter) may be added to the intravenous solution bottle to minimize catheter tip clotting without altering systemic coagulation.[2]

When preparing the CVP manometer system, one must be certain to remove all air bubbles from the manometer. Bubbles in the manometer fluid column will decrease the accuracy of the reading. The manometer column is initially raised to approximately 20 to 25 cm. Care must be taken so the water column does not reach the top. Water at the manometer top dampens the cotton and impedes air movement into and out of the chamber. The wet cotton is also a potential source of contamination. If the water column reaches the manometer top, a new set-up should be prepared. The addition of multiple vitamins (such as Berocca-C) has been suggested to color the fluid and to enhance the visibility of the fluid column in the manometer. The manometer is preferably secured to an intravenous pole that is attached to the patient's bed. A floor model intravenous pole is less desirable because of its instability.[20]

A reading may be taken after proper assembly of the equipment and after accurate placement of the tip of the

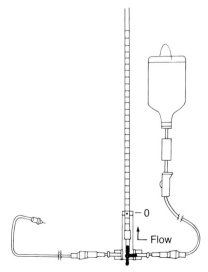

Figure 27–2. The stopcock is turned to fill the manometer to 25 cm H_2O.

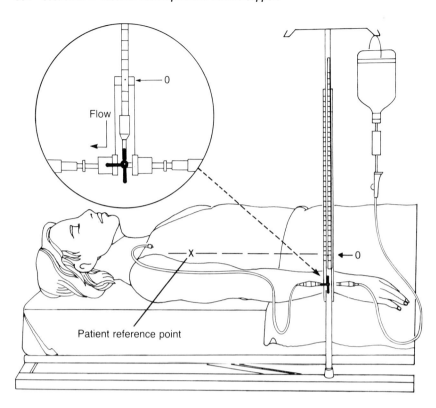

Figure 27–3. The stopcock is opened to the patient, and the column of water in the manometer is allowed to fall and stabilize before a reading is taken. Note that the zero mark is horizontally aligned with the tricuspid valve (midaxillary line in a supine patient).

catheter has been established. Proper catheter placement is best checked by chest film. The presence of respiratory fluctuations does not ensure superior vena caval placement. Fluctuations with movement of the head suggest improper placement of the catheter in the internal jugular system.

To ensure optimal measurement, the patient should be in a supine position. Two points have been identified in CVP measurements:[21, 22]

1. The patient reference point: This is the point on the patient's lateral chest wall that indicates the position of the tip of the CVP catheter.
2. The zero mark on the manometer: This is the zero line on the manometer, which is aligned with the reference point of the patient's chest.

One determines the patient reference point by locating an external landmark on the thorax at the approximate level of the right atrium.[23] Although a number of anatomic sites have been described[4, 5, 21, 22] and recommended, the most frequently used site is the midaxillary line in the fourth intercostal space. One should clearly mark the reference point with a marking pen, placing a line or an X on the patient's thorax.

Because the absolute zero level is less important than maintaining consistency in serial measurements, all readings should be taken at the same location and in the same manner. Readings are taken with the zero point on the manometer matched with the horizontal level of the patient reference point (see Fig. 27–3). All readings are ideally taken while the patient is supine.[24] If the patient cannot tolerate this position, however, the two reference points are matched in the midaxillary line at the estimated base of the heart. The position of the patient is noted, and measurements are recorded. Serial measurements must reflect the identical position of the patient for meaningful interpretation of CVP variation with therapy.

FACTORS AFFECTING ACCURACY OF READING

A number of extrinsic factors may alter the accuracy of the CVP reading (Table 27–1).[2, 5, 25, 26] In addition to the position of the patient, changes in intrathoracic pressure affect the CVP reading.[24] A patient on a respirator has an elevated intrathoracic pressure, which elevates the CVP reading. Usually, positive-pressure ventilation raises the CVP reading by only a few centimeters of water. If disconnection can be tolerated, the patient should be temporarily disconnected from the respirator to provide a more reliable measurement. Activities that increase intrathoracic pressure, such as coughing and straining, may cause spuriously high measurements. The patient should be relaxed at the time of measurement and should be breathing normally. The position of the manometer must also be consistent. The zero point on the manometer must be opposite the patient reference point at the level of the right atrium. Use of varied reference points may result in inaccurate measurements that may be interpreted as a change in the patient's status when none has actually occurred.[2, 21, 22, 25]

Another reason for faulty readings is malposition of the catheter tip. If the catheter tip is not passed far enough into the central venous system, peripheral venous spasm and

Table 27–1. Faulty Central Venous Pressure Readings

Increased intrathoracic pressure (ventilator, straining, coughing)
Reference points in error
Malposition of catheter tip
Blocking or ball valve obstruction of catheter
Air bubbles in the manometer
Readings during wrong phase of ventilation
Reading by different observers
Vasopressors (presumed)

venous valves may yield pressure readings that are inconsistent with the true CVP.[5, 25]

If the catheter tip is passed into the right ventricle, a falsely high CVP is obtained. This situation should be suspected when excessive fluctuations (6 to 10 cm H_2O) of the manometer fluid column are observed. Such fluctuations may also be seen in correctly placed CVP lines when tricuspid regurgitation or atrioventricular dissociation is present.

Inaccurate low venous pressure readings are seen when a valve-like obstruction at the catheter tip occurs either by clot formation or by contact against the vein wall. Negative intrathoracic pressures seen during inspiration drop the manometer water level, but when the catheter is occluded during expiration, the manometer is unable to sense the true CVP.[19, 25] Air bubbles in the manometer or tubing also lead to faulty readings.

Some investigators mention a falsely elevated CVP in patients who are receiving vasopressors, but controlled data on this aberration are lacking. One animal study suggests that fluid can be infused into one lumen of a multilumen catheter without affecting the CVP reading at another lumen.[27]

INTERPRETATION OF THE CENTRAL VENOUS PRESSURE MEASUREMENT

Because determination of the CVP aids the clinician in assessment of the critically ill patient, it is paramount that the clinician know the normal values and the variables that may alter these values and recognize the pathologic conditions that correlate with abnormal values.

Although early articles reported varying normal ranges for CVP measurements, recent cardiac catheterization studies have demonstrated that the normal range extends from -2 to $+7$ cm H_2O.

Gowen reports from his clinical experience that a reading of 7 cm H_2O is the upper limit of normal, and a reading of 8 to 10 cm H_2O is a borderline elevation, whereas levels greater than 12 cm H_2O are consistent with impending heart failure.[28] Weil and coworkers, however, describe the normal CVP as ranging from 2 to 10 cm H_2O and consider a high CVP to be greater than 15 cm H_2O.[10] Knobel and associates note that a CVP of less than 6 cm H_2O is rarely associated with a PCWP of more than 12 cm H_2O in septic patients.[29] A rough guideline that reflects a consensus in the literature[5, 10, 11, 28, 29] and informal opinions of colleagues follows:

Low	Less than 6 cm H_2O
Normal	6 to 12 cm H_2O
High	Greater than 12 cm H_2O

In the late stages of pregnancy (30 to 42 weeks), the CVP is physiologically elevated, and normal readings are 5 to 8 cm H_2O higher in pregnant than in nonpregnant women.

A CVP reading of less than 6 cm H_2O is consistent with low right atrial pressure and reflects a decrease in the return of blood volume to the right heart. This may indicate that the patient requires additional fluid or blood. A low CVP reading is also obtained when vasomotor tone is decreased, as in sepsis, an anaphylactic reaction, or another form of sympathetic interruption.[10, 11, 28, 29]

A CVP reading falling within a normal range is viewed in relationship to the clinical situation. A reading of greater than 12 cm H_2O indicates that the heart is not effectively circulating the volume presented to it. This situation may occur in the case of either a normovolemic patient with cardiac decompensation or a patient with a normal heart

who is overhydrated or overtransfused. A high CVP is also related to variables other than pump failure, which include pericardial tamponade, restrictive pericarditis, pulmonary stenosis, and pulmonary embolus.[28]

Changes in blood volume, vessel tone, and cardiac function may occur alone or in combination with one another; therefore, it is possible to have a normal or a high CVP in the presence of normovolemia, hypovolemia, and hypervolemia. One must interpret the specific CVP values with respect to the entire clinical picture; *the response of the CVP to an infusion is more important than the initial reading.*

Fluid Challenge

Monitoring of the CVP is helpful as a practical guide for fluid therapy.[9, 10] Serial CVP measurement provides a fairly reliable indication of the capability of the right heart to accept an additional volume load. Although the PCWP is a more sensitive index of left heart fluid needs (and in some clinical situations PCWP measurement is absolutely essential), the serial measurement of CVP can provide significant information.

A fluid challenge can help assess both volume deficits and pump failure. Although a fluid challenge can be used with either PCWP monitoring or CVP monitoring, only the fluid challenge for CVP monitoring is discussed here. Slight variations in the methodology of fluid challenge are reported in the literature. Generally, aliquots of 50 to 200 ml of crystalloid fluid (isotonic saline or lactated Ringer solution) or smaller aliquots of colloid (5 per cent albumin solution) are sequentially administered, and measurements of CVP levels are obtained after a 10-minute observation period.[10, 11, 16, 28]

The fluid challenge as described by Weil[10] is generally carried out in the following manner: Fluid is administered by a route other than that used for monitoring. An initial CVP reading is taken, and fluid is infused at a rate of 20 milliliters per minute over a 10-minute period. The infused volume is allowed to equilibrate for 10 minutes, and a reading is again taken. If the CVP is greater than 5 cm of H_2O over the initial measurement, the fluid challenge is discontinued, and one assumes that the right ventricle is unable to handle an additional fluid load. Increases of between 3 and 5 cm H_2O over the initial CVP reading arc equivocal, and additional measurements are taken over the next 30 minutes if this reading is obtained. Increases of less than 2 cm H_2O over the original reading or a return of higher readings to this level within 30 minutes is indicative of volume depletion. The fluid challenge is repeated until measurements indicate that adequate volume expansion has been obtained. The fluid challenge is discontinued as soon as hemodynamic signs of shock are reversed or signs of cardiac incompetence are evident.

Cardiac Tamponade

In cardiac tamponade, *pericardial* pressure rises to equal right ventricular end-diastolic pressure. The *pericardial* pressure encountered in pericardial tamponade characteristically produces an elevated CVP. The degree of CVP elevation is variable, and one must interpret measurements cautiously; CVP readings in the range of 16 to 18 cm H_2O are typically seen in acute tamponade,[10, 30] but elevations of up to 30 cm H_2O may be encountered. The exact CVP reading is often lower than one might intuitively expect, and it is not uncommon to encounter tamponade with a CVP of 10 to 12 cm H_2O. A normal, or even a low, CVP reading may be seen if the tamponade is associated with significant hypovolemia.

An excessive rise in CVP following a fluid challenge may be more important than a single reading in the diagnosis of pericardial tamponade. It is interesting to note that Shoemaker and associates[30] reported a decrease in CVP just before cardiovascular collapse in patients with pericardial tamponade.

Excessive straining, agitation, pneumatic anti-shock garment inflation, positive-pressure ventilation, or tension pneumothorax may raise intrathoracic pressure, producing a high CVP reading, and may erroneously suggest the diagnosis of pericardial tamponade. Increases in vascular tone as seen with the use of dopamine or other vasopressors may also elevate the CVP, mimicking tamponade and complicating volume estimation.

CONCLUSION

With the introduction of the pulmonary artery catheter and the ability to measure pulmonary capillary wedge pressure, some clinicians have discouraged the use of CVP monitoring. Nonetheless, CVP monitoring continues to be an important adjunct in the care of the critically ill patient in the acute phase of volume resuscitation.

Measurements of CVP performed in the appropriate clinical situation can be useful. Initial readings, serial measurements, and trends following fluid infusion provide a guide to therapy in acutely ill or injured patients. Proper interpretation of specific readings requires knowledge of the cardiovascular dynamics as well as an appreciation for extrinsic factors that may alter CVP readings. The clinician is reminded to evaluate the data in relation to the entire clinical situation.

REFERENCES

1. Huberty J, Schwartz R, Emich J: Central venous pressure monitoring. Obstet Gynecol 30:842, 1967.
2. Wilson JN, et al: Central venous pressure in optimal blood volume maintenance. Arch Surg 85:563, 1962.
3. Guyton AC: Textbook of Medical Physiology. 4th ed. Philadelphia, WB Saunders Co, 1971, p 227.
4. Guyton A, Jones C: Central venous pressure: Physiological significance and clinical implications. Am Heart J 86:431, 1973.
5. Knopp R, Dailey RH: Central venous cannulation and pressure monitoring. JACEP 6:358, 1977.
6. Dunbar RD, Mitchell R, Lavine M: Aberrant locations of central venous catheters. Lancet 1:711, 1981.
7. Clayton DG: Inaccuracies in manometric central venous pressure measurement. Resuscitation 16:221, 1988.
8. Cohn JN: Central venous pressure as a guide to volume expansion. Ann Intern Med 66:1283, 1967.
9. MacLean LD, Duff JH: The use of central venous pressure as a guide to volume replacement in shock. Dis Chest 48:199, 1965.
10. Weil MH, Shubin H, Rosoff L: Fluid repletion in circulatory shock. Central venous pressure and other practical guides. JAMA 192:668, 1965.
11. Greenall MJ, Blewitt RW, McMahon MJ: Cardiac tamponade and central venous catheters. Br Med J 2:595, 1975.
12. Swan HJC: Central venous pressure monitoring is an outmoded procedure of limited practical value. In Ingelfinger FJ, et al (eds): Controversy in Internal Medicine II. Philadelphia, WB Saunders Co, 1974, pp 185–193.
13. Samii K, Conseiller C, Viars P: Central venous pressure and pulmonary wedge pressure. A comparative study in anesthetized patients. Arch Surg 111:1122, 1976.
14. DeLaurentis D, Hayes M, Matsumoto T: Does central venous pressure accurately reflect hemodynamic and fluid volume patterns in the critical surgical patient? Am J Surg 126:415, 1973.
15. Forrester JS, Diamond G, McHugh TJ, et al: Filling pressures in the right and left sides of the heart in acute myocardial infarction. N Engl J Med 285:190, 1971.
16. James P, Myers R: Central venous pressure monitoring. Ann Surg 175:693, 1972.
17. Toussaint GPM, Burgess JH, Hampson LG: Central venous pressure and pulmonary wedge pressure in critical illness. A comparison. Arch Surg 109:265, 1974.
18. Rajacich N, Burchard KW, Hasan FM, et al: Central venous pressure and pulmonary capillary wedge pressure as estimates of left atrial pressure: Effects of positive end-expiratory pressure and catheter tip malposition. Crit Care Med 17:7, 1989.
19. Mann RL, Carlon GC, Turnbull AD: Comparison of electronic and manometric central venous pressures. Influence of access route. Crit Care Med 9:98, 1981.
20. Fisher RE: Measuring central venous pressure: How to do it accurately and safely. Nursing 79:74, 1979.
21. Pennington LA, Smith C: Leveling when monitoring central blood pressures: An alternative method. Heart Lung 9:1053, 1980.
22. Debrunner F, Bühler F: "Normal central venous pressure," significance of reference point and normal range. Br Med J 3:148, 1969.
23. Winsor T, Bruch GE: Phlebostatic axis and phlebostatic level, reference levels for venous pressure measurements in man. Proc Soc Exp Biol Med 58:165, 1945.
24. Woods SL, Mansfield LW: Effect of body position upon pulmonary artery and pulmonary capillary wedge pressures in noncritically ill patients. Heart Lung 5:87, 1976.
25. Wilson J, Owens J: Pitfalls in monitoring central venous pressure. Hosp Med 5:86, 1970.
26. Haughey B: CVP lines: Monitoring and maintaining. Am J Nurs 78:635, 1978.
27. Ikeda S, Schweiss JF: Maximum infusion rates and CVP accuracy during high-flow delivery through multilumen catheters. Crit Care Med 13:586, 1985.
28. Gowen F: Interpretation of central venous pressure. Surg Clin North Am 86:432, 1973.
29. Knobel E, Akamine N, Fernandes CJ Jr, et al: Reliability of right atrial pressure monitoring to assess left ventricular preload in critically septic patients. Crit Care Med 17:1344, 1989.
30. Shoemaker WC, Carey JS, Yao ST: Hemodynamic monitoring for physiologic evaluation, diagnosis, and therapy of acute hemopericardial tamponade from penetrating wounds. J Trauma 13:36, 1973.

Chapter 28

Accessing Indwelling Lines

John M. Howell

INTRODUCTION

Many therapies require the use of intravenous catheters that afford indwelling access to the central circulation. Indwelling central venous access is essential to those who require lengthy chemotherapy,[1, 2] hyperalimentation,[3, 4] extended antimicrobial therapy,[5] and hemodialysis.[6-8] An ever-increasing number of individuals care for these devices as outpatients. Consequently, indwelling lines are now available to emergency department staff to draw blood and administer medications, blood products, and intravenous fluids with minimal patient discomfort. Further, an awareness of attendant complications should help minimize the risk of line sepsis and central vein thrombosis.

One of the earliest recorded vascular procedures occurred during the 1660s when Lower[9] connected the carotid artery of one dog to the jugular vein of another. This early attempt at vascular surgery predated the development of hemodialysis by three centuries. During the 1950s Kolff[10] described the first successful attempt at hemodialysis. Soon thereafter Scribner[11] designed the first arteriovenous shunt, and parenteral hyperalimentation was introduced during the early 1960s.[12] Later attempts at extended parenteral feedings spurred improvements in catheter technology.

In 1973, after unsuccessful efforts with arteriovenous shunts, Broviac designed an intravenous catheter that afforded prolonged access for hyperalimentation patients.[3] This Silastic catheter was 90 cm long and passed through the subclavian vein to the mid-right atrium. Broviac's initial description fashioned a template for several products in use today.

Hickman altered Broviac's prototype in 1979[1] for the treatment of leukemia patients receiving chemotherapy (Fig. 28–1). His modified catheter was larger in diameter and lacked a surrounding sheath. This bigger lumen facilitated the drawing of blood as well as the infusion of chemotherapeutic agents, blood, and intravenous solutions. More recent approaches to the dilemma of prolonged access include multilumen external catheters[13] and surgically implanted subcutaneous infusion devices (e.g., Port-A-Cath, Infuse-A-Port, and Mediport).[14] These products are beneficial in that they obviate the need for multiple peripheral intravenous lines; however, their use may lead to complications. Wound sepsis and central

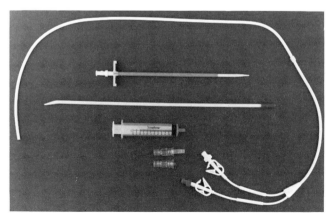

Figure 28–1. Hickman double-lumen catheter (12 French), injection caps (2), attached clamps (2), sheath introducer with vessel dilator, syringe, and 33-cm tunneler.

venous thrombosis are among the more common difficulties encountered by patients tending their catheters at home.[5, 15] Timely recognition of these complications may avert morbidity in a population composed largely of immunocompromised individuals.

INDICATIONS

Patient Populations with Indwelling Lines

Central venous and right atrial catheters are commonly placed in patients with cancer to deliver chemotherapy[1, 2] and to prevent tissue infiltration of these destructive chemicals.[14, 16] They are useful in treating both hematologic and solid malignancies and have been placed to facilitate daily radiation therapy of brain tumors in children.[17] Many patients opt to perform local care at home and return only periodically to a clinic or hospital for intravenous chemotherapy.

Otherwise healthy individuals with soft tissue or bony infections receive intravenous antimicrobials in the same manner.[5, 18] Alternate indications include ambulatory heparin therapy[19] and parenteral hyperalimentation,[3] especially in those with short bowel syndrome and malnutrition.[4] McDowell and colleagues[7] and Schanzer and associates[8] report good results using double-lumen, cuffed central venous catheters as an alternative to arteriovenous shunts in patients who need long-term hemodialysis.

Although the predominant indication for arteriovenous fistulas and shunts is hemodialysis,[19] they have also been used for parenteral hyperalimentation[20] and chemotherapy.[21] However, right atrial catheters are more widely accepted for parenteral hyperalimentation and chemotherapy owing to their ease of insertion and the ability of patients to self-administer medications at home. Double-lumen, subclavian Uldall catheters[22, 23] are frequently positioned to deliver hemodialysis for up to 8 weeks while a peripheral fistula matures.

Emergency Department Access

Indications for accessing right atrial and multilumen catheters in the emergency department include phlebotomy and administration of intravenous fluids and medications. Arteriovenous fistulas, shunts, and Uldall catheters are used only in emergency situations because infection and shunt malfunction may result and necessitate additional surgical procedures to obtain access for hemodialysis.

INDWELLING CATHETER, SHUNT, AND FISTULA DEVICES

The majority of techniques designed to allow prolonged intravenous access form the following categories: long-term venous access catheters; implantable venous access devices; percutaneous multilumen catheters; and methods to deliver hemodialysis that include arteriovenous shunts, fistulas, and Uldall catheters.

Long-Term Venous Access Catheters

Long-term venous access catheters are made by several manufacturers and include Broviac, Hickman, Leonard, Raaf, and Hermed catheters (see Fig. 28–1). They are positioned in the right atrium either during an operation or at the bedside.[7, 14, 19] Access to the central circulation is

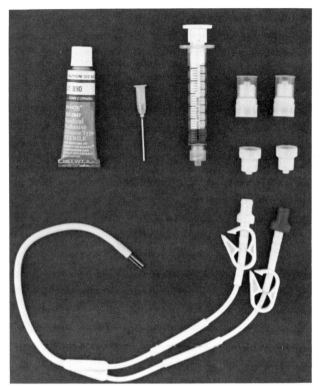

Figure 28–2. Hickman catheter repair kit, with tube of adhesive, 18-gauge needle, plastic syringe, injection caps (2), Luer-Lok caps (2), and external catheter segment with attached clamps.

achieved by various methods, including cephalic,[24] external jugular,[17, 19] saphenous,[19] internal jugular,[17] brachiocephalic,[25] subclavian,[19, 26] and translumbar[4] approaches. They are generally tunneled subcutaneously from the venous access point to a position on the anterior chest wall. Many kits include a 33-cm tunneler to pull catheters through subcutaneous tissues. A Dacron cuff is positioned midcatheter to anchor and prevent the spread of infection.[19]

Manufacturers produce right atrial catheters in various lengths and diameters.[19] Single-lumen Broviac catheters are popular for children and vary in size from 2 to 6 French. Many Hickman catheters provide a double-lumen alternative up to 19 French. Weese[27] produced a triple-lumen variation by placing Hickman and double-lumen Raaf catheters through the same venotomy. Individual lumen widths in double-lumen devices vary between 0.7 and 1.6 mm. Repair kits are available (Evermed, Inc.) that include silicone adhesive and a 12 French catheter segment (Fig. 28–2).

Home care of long-term venous access catheters is generally performed on a daily basis.[19] The skin site is cleansed with alcohol and povidone-iodine before applying a sterile dressing (e.g., Tegaderm). Two to 3 ml of 100 U/ml heparin are then flushed to prevent catheter thrombosis.[19, 28, 29] The injection cap is changed weekly after first clamping the catheter.[19] Breaks in sterile procedure or overlooking the heparin flush may result in thrombosis or line sepsis.

Implantable Venous Access Devices

Implantable venous access devices (Port-A-Cath, Infus-A-Port, and Mediport) are surgically implanted circular, subcutaneous chambers in continuity with a central Silastic catheter (Fig. 28–3).[14, 19, 30, 31] The major difference between these two systems is that access to implantable venous access

devices is obtained by inserting a tapered needle through the skin into a diaphragm approximately 7 to 11 mm in diameter (Fig. 28–4).[19] The chamber is palpable as well as visible on the anterior chest wall. Catheter widths are between 2.2 and 2.8 mm.[19]

In contrast to long-term venous access catheters, implantable venous access devices are accessed through a 20- or 22-gauge tapered (Huber) needle to limit cylinder damage.[19] Although this technique allows approximately 2000 punctures,[19] it also hinders the rapid delivery of blood and blood products. Implantable venous access devices are initially more expensive than long-term venous access catheters: however, they also require less frequent home care. Weekly or monthly[19, 28] flushing with 4 to 5 ml of heparin (1000 U/ml) is adequate to prevent thrombosis.

Percutaneous Multilumen Catheters

Triple-lumen catheters (Arrow) are inserted percutaneously into the central circulation to allow for phlebotomy and the simultaneous delivery of medication and blood products. They are approximately 7 French in caliber and deliver these substances through 16-gauge and 18-gauge lumens. Drawbacks include daily wound care, heparinization, and relative brevity of use. Multilumen catheters are usually left in place less than 3 weeks,[13, 19] although extended use may approach several months.[19] In contrast, Hickman catheters have been left in place for 474 days,[32] Port-A-Cath catheters up to 351 days.[30]

Arteriovenous Shunts, Fistulas, and Uldall Catheters

Arteriovenous shunts are external Silastic bridges between the arterial and venous circulations. When placed in extremities they facilitate hemodialysis during acute renal insufficiency and failure.[19] However, subclavian and femoral vein access have recently subverted their use in the intensive

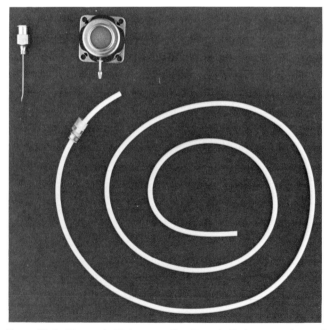

Figure 28–3. Tapered Huber needle, Port-A-Cath reservoir, and catheter segment.

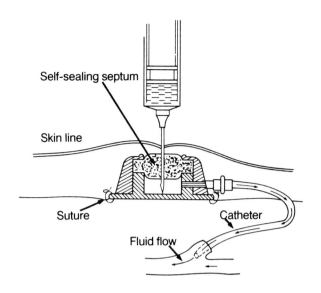

Figure 28–4. Port-A-Cath system. The Port-A-Cath system is accessed by inserting a Huber-point needle through the skin and portal septum. (Courtesy of Pharmacia Nutech, Pharmacia Laboratories, Piscataway, NJ.)

care unit settings of hemorrhagic shock and sepsis. Additionally, central venous catheters are now used frequently as a temporizing measure until permanent arteriovenous access sites mature. Consequently, emergency physicians are less likely to encounter arteriovenous shunts in their daily routine.

Peripheral arteriovenous fistulas, on the other hand, represent the procedure of choice for permanent vascular access in end-stage renal disease.[19] They are produced by anastomosing the peripheral venous and arterial circulations. In this way a superficial, dilated vein serves as a permanent access site for large-bore hemodialysis needles. Vessels commonly used for fistulas are the radial artery and cephalic vein or the ulnar artery and basilic vein.[19] Patent fistulas, generally located near the wrist, are easily discerned by their characteristic bruit and thrill. Arteriovenous fistulas have been inadvertently produced by penetrating vascular injury[33] and superficial phlebotomy.[34]

Large-bore Uldall catheters[22, 23] are generally placed in the subclavian vein and provide hemodialysis access for up to 8 weeks while a peripheral site matures. These double-lumen catheters are tunneled subcutaneously and lack the Dacron cuff present on most central venous access catheters. They are capped after dialysis with approximately 2500 units of heparin in each luminal "arm."

EQUIPMENT

Long-Term Venous Access Catheters[29]

1. Sterile gloves, mask, and eyewear
2. Povidone-iodine solution (10 per cent)
3. Sterile drapes
4. One 10-ml syringe filled with normal saline
5. One 10-ml syringe containing 5 ml of heparin solution (100 U/ml)
6. One catheter clamp or hemostat without teeth

7. Fluids and medications to be administered

Implantable Venous Access Devices[29]

1. Sterile gloves, mask, and eyewear
2. Povidone-iodine solution (10 per cent)
3. Sterile drapes
4. One 10-ml syringe filled with normal saline
5. One 10-ml syringe containing 5 ml of heparin solution (1000 U/ml)
6. Two Huber needles with a 90-degree bend (19-gauge, 20-gauge, or 22-gauge) or in an emergency, a standard 19-gauge needle
7. Extension tubing with a slide clamp
8. 4-inch by 4-inch gauze and 1-inch silk tape adequate to reinforce and stabilize the Huber needle
9. Fluids and medications to be administered

Percutaneous Multilumen Catheters[29] (including Uldall catheters)

1. Sterile gloves, mask, and eyewear
2. Povidone-iodine solution (10 per cent)
3. Sterile drapes
4. One 10-ml syringe filled with normal saline
5. One 10-ml syringe containing 5 ml of heparin solution (100 U/ml)
6. Three standard needles (18-gauge, 19-gauge, or 20-gauge)
7. Fluids and medications to be administered

Arteriovenous Fistulas and Shunts (*access only in emergencies*)

1. Sterile gloves, mask, and eyewear
2. Povidone-iodine solution (10 per cent)
3. Sterile drapes
4. Standard large-bore needles and intravenous catheters
5. Two 10-ml syringes
6. Fluids and medications to be administered

PROCEDURES

Accessing Long-Term Venous Access Catheters

Sterile technique is mandatory at all times when accessing indwelling lines.[28] The catheter is first clamped to prevent air embolism. Patients usually carry their own clamps; however, a hemostat without teeth will suffice. In an emergency, sterile tape or tubing wrapped around the teeth of a hemostat also protects the catheter. The cap is removed, and a 10-ml syringe of sterile water or normal saline is attached. Three to 5 ml of solution are injected and then withdrawn to ensure patency. This procedure is done slowly with a syringe at least 10 ml in volume to avoid damage to the cap area.[29]

Phlebotomy is accomplished by withdrawing dead space solution, reclamping, and using a separate syringe to remove the desired amount of blood.[29] Bolus medications are then injected and intravenous solutions infused through the catheter, which is clamped whenever unattached. A 5-ml normal saline flush should be delivered between medications. On completion, 3 to 5 ml of heparin (100 U/ml) are injected, the line is clamped, and the cap is repositioned.[19, 29]

Difficulty in drawing blood from a long-term venous access catheter may be due to catheter position, catheter malfunction, or a fibrinous clot on the catheter tip.[29] Maneuvers to facilitate blood flow include Valsalva, reverse Trendelenburg, slight tension on the catheter, and having the patient raise his or her arms above head level.[28, 29] *Overzealous withdrawal on the syringe will collapse the catheter and make the demonstration of patency difficult.*[19] If these measures are unsuccessful, a clot may be present on the catheter tip. A gentle 3- to 5-ml heparin flush is often successful in dislodging a clot. Haimov[19] reports no clinical pulmonary emboli after 70 such attempts at declotting. Streptokinase[19, 35] and urokinase[19, 29] are reasonable next steps. One half to 1 ml of urokinase (5000 U/ml) may be injected and aspiration attempted after a 10-minute interval.[19, 29] A urokinase flush may successfully declot the line in up to 95 per cent of cases.[19]

Accessing Implantable Venous Access Devices

The procedure for accessing implantable venous access devices is unique because these devices are not externalized. Instead, a circular reservoir lies subcutaneously on the anterior chest wall. The cylinder is first palpated, and the overlying skin is prepared with povidone-iodine solution. A 10-ml syringe filled with sterile water or normal saline is attached to connecting tubing, which in turn is applied to a 20-gauge or 22-gauge, 90-degree tapered (Huber) needle. A clamp should be applied to the connecting tubing whenever the system is open. Air is expelled, and the Huber needle is inserted through the reservoir septum. The needle is inserted slowly and steadily through the diaphragm to the back of the reservoir. Although incomplete perforation of the septum will block flow, substantial pressure may also damage the back of the device. The clamp is removed slowly, and 5 ml of solution is injected to ensure patency. If patency is not easily demonstrated, the same measures described under "Accessing Long-Term Venous Access Catheters" may be used, to include positioning, Valsalva maneuver, heparin flush, and low-dose thrombolytic therapy.[19, 29]

Once the solution has been injected, gentle negative pressure is applied to demonstrate the backflow of blood. The Huber needle is then stabilized by building 4-inch by 4-inch gauze about the needle and further reinforcing with 1-inch silk tape. Phlebotomy is performed through the extension tubing after first removing 8 to 9 ml of blood with a separate syringe. Intravenous solutions may also be delivered through extension tubing, although the rate of flow will be limited by the Huber needle's radius. A standard 19-gauge needle may be used in emergency circumstances; however, one risks shortening the device's lifetime. A 5-ml normal saline flush should be delivered between medications. The procedure is completed with a 3- to 5-ml heparin (1000 U/ml) flush[29] and removal of the Huber needle.

Accessing Percutaneous Multilumen Catheters

Percutaneous multilumen central catheters are used infrequently by outpatients. They are usually placed in the subclavian vein to facilitate patient comfort. One port is available for each lumen, and, after povidone-iodine preparation is completed, access is gained by either inserting a needle or syringe into the protective cap or removing the cap entirely. A 5-ml normal saline or sterile water flush and verification of backflow precede all subsequent procedures. Phlebotomy is performed through the proximal 18-gauge lumen to prevent mixture with medications being delivered through the other two ports. The proximal lumen port of the Arrow multilumen catheter is white in color and the longest of the three tails. Tails attached to the more distal lumens are blue and brown in color. Intravenous infusions are delivered in similar fashion, and a normal saline flush is injected between medications. The procedure is terminated with a 3- to 5-ml heparin (100 U/ml) flush.

Accessing Arteriovenous Fistulas, Shunts, and Uldall Catheters

Arteriovenous fistulas, shunts, and Uldall catheters are placed in patients who require long-term hemodialysis and represent the sole access for that purpose. Consequently, routine use of these sites for phlebotomy and fluid administration is condemned. In fact, venipuncture of any type in the same extremity as a patent arteriovenous fistula is not recommended. When standard intravenous access cannot be obtained under emergency circumstances, however, fistulas, shunts, and Uldall catheters may all be used to administer intravenous solutions and medications. If possible, fistula patency should first be ascertained by noting a bruit and palpable thrill, although these signs may not be appreciable if the patient is in extremis.

Prepare the area with povidone-iodine solution and access the fistula with the smallest gauge needle appropriate to the task. When complete, monitor the area for hemorrhage, and apply local pressure to avoid significant bleeding. Arteriovenous shunts are accessed similarly by placing the smallest needle possible into the catheter, bridging arterial and venous circulations. Local pressure should be applied for 5 minutes after completing the procedure. Uldall catheters are used in much the same way that multilumen central catheters are accessed. The retaining cap on each arm may be either removed or injected. Up to 5000 units of heparin are present within the two lumens, and so it is imperative that aspiration be performed before administering fluid or medications.

AFTERCARE INSTRUCTIONS

Before discharge, each patient should be reminded of those aspects of catheter care that prevent complications and prolong the device's lifetime.[29] Patients with implantable venous access devices should avoid direct pressure on the reservoir and report local bruising or bleeding immediately. Although they may bathe and swim normally, heparin flushes are essential to prevent thrombosis in patients with these indwelling devices.

Long-term venous access catheters and multilumen catheters must be sterilely dressed and flushed on a routine basis,[29] and patients should never force the delivery of heparin. An inability to flush any indwelling catheter should be reported immediately to a physician. All indwelling catheters must be observed daily for bleeding and signs of infection, to include fever, pain, redness, swelling, and purulent drainage.

CONTRAINDICATIONS

Right atrial and multilumen catheters should not be accessed in the emergency department if patency cannot be demonstrated using the maneuvers described under "Procedures."[28, 29] Medications that are known to be incompatible (e.g., calcium and bicarbonate) should not be administered concurrently through multilumen catheters because turbulence at the catheter tip permits mixture (personal communication, Arrow). Medications should not be delivered through indwelling lines without intercurrent normal saline flushes. Arteriovenous fistulas, shunts, and Uldall catheters are used only in emergency situations in which more standard methods of intravenous access are unobtainable.

Taylor[29] states that diazepam and diphenylhydantoin crystallize on contact with the silicone catheter walls of long-term venous access catheters and implantable venous access devices, thereby necessitating catheter replacement. In contradistinction, the manufacturers (Evermed, Pharmacia) hold that crystallization does not occur and that the silicone catheter wall absorbs these drugs without damage or the need for removal. Acetone and tincture of iodine products, however, are injurious to catheter walls (personal communication, Evermed) and should not be used topically in the area of right atrial or triple-lumen catheters. Povidone-iodine and alcohol are perfectly acceptable.

COMPLICATIONS

Complications of Emergency Department Access

Line sepsis, discussed in more depth later, occurs when sterile technique is not strictly maintained (Table 28–1).[28, 29, 36] Gloves, mask, and goggles should be donned before accessing indwelling lines and arteriovenous fistulas. Also, maintaining a closed system by clamping the catheter appropriately prevents the delivery of air into the venous circulation. Air embolism[37] is heralded by tachypnea, hypotension, and coma. When air embolism is suspected clinically, the patient should be positioned on the left side in the Trendelenburg position, and supportive measures should be undertaken, to include high-flow oxygen and secure intravenous access.

The externalized portion of a right atrial catheter may be cut with scissors[5] or perforated during clamping, especially if an improper clamp is used.[37] The catheter should be reclamped immediately between the patient's skin and the location of the injury.[29] At this point an alternate method of intravenous access may be sought. Repair kits (Evermed) are available that contain silicone adhesive, plastic clamps, injection caps, and a 12 French catheter replacement segment (see Fig. 28–2). Familiarity with this technique is necessary to avoid further injury. Information may be obtained from Evermed at 1-800-626-8266.

Embolization of catheter thrombi during flushing and injection of solutions is a concern. Anderson and colleagues[15] prospectively evaluated the size and frequency of catheter thrombi in 43 patients by aspirating after a urokinase flush. Clots were noted in 40 of 43 subjects and 153 of 508 total specimens. Thrombus fragments varied in size from fragments to 5 cm. No clinical sequelae were noted; however, the investigators discuss the potential for pulmonary embolism. Haimov[19] reported no clinical pulmonary emboli after heparin flushes in 70 patients; however, Zureikat and associates reported one case of pulmonary embolus associated with Broviac catheterization in a 2-month-old.[38] Emergency

---

Table 28–1. Complications of Accessing Indwelling Lines in the Emergency Department

Line sepsis
Pulmonary embolism
Air embolism
Perforation of externalized catheter
Displacement of catheter
Cardiac dysrhythmias

---

department personnel should be vigilant for symptoms of pulmonary embolus and should inject fluids with care.

Catheter displacement may occur when patients do not remain still during the procedure. Harvey and colleagues[32] reported two cases of Hickman catheters being withdrawn accidentally by patients. Chardavoyne and coworkers[39] described a similar case in which an implantable venous access device (Infuse-A-Port) spontaneously withdrew from the central circulation after documented placement. Care must be taken when handling both long-term venous access catheters and implantable venous access devices, especially in active patients.

General Complications of Indwelling Lines and Arteriovenous Fistulas and Shunts

INFECTIOUS COMPLICATIONS

Emergency department personnel must remain vigilant for catheter sepsis in this largely immunocompromised population. Long-term venous access catheter infection rates in adults are between 1.5 and 19 per cent.[5, 14, 32] whereas implantable venous access device sepsis may be less frequent at 3 per cent.[14] Among children, 2.8 Hickman catheter infections occur every 1000 catheter days,[40] and children between 1 and 4 years of age have a greater risk of multiple septic complications.[40] Catheter infections occur at the skin exit site, subcutaneous tunnel, and skin overlying the catheter (venous) insertion site.[32] The subcutaneous tunnel and exit site seem to be involved more frequently.[32] Clinical manifestations include local erythema, tenderness, fever, and purulent drainage;[5] however, generalized immune suppression may mask these signs.[32] Harvey and coworkers[32] found catheter infections common among leukemia patients who were neutropenic at the time of infection; however, Couch and associates[5] noted a lower infection rate and no such correlation when considering the total white blood cell count at the time of insertion into osteomyelitis patients.

Staphylococci, streptococci, and diptheroid organisms are cultured most frequently from infected indwelling catheters (Table 28–2).[17, 26, 35, 40] *Staphylococcus aureus* and *S. epidermidis*[5, 17, 42, 43] are common, as are *S. faecalis, S. bovis,* and viridans group strep.[43] Group C streptococci have also been implicated.[44] Gram-negative bacteria occur less frequently and may be associated with a neutropenic state.[42] These organisms include *Pseudomonas aeruginosa, Klebsiella* sp., *Acinetobacter* sp., and *Serratia* sp.; *Corynebacterium* sp.,[42, 46] *Bacillus* sp.,[45] and atypical mycobacteria[47, 48] have also been implicated.

Fungal infections occur less frequently; however, they are nonetheless virulent. Premature infants requiring prolonged hyperalimentation seem to be at greatest risk,[49, 50] and organisms cultured include *Candida* sp., *Malassezia pachydermatis,* and *M. furfur,* the causative agent of tinea versicolor.[46, 49–52] These children present with low-grade fever, bradycardia, thrombocytopenia, apnea, and a predominance of immature polymorphonucleocytes.[51] Adults may develop primary cutaneous aspergillosis near a long-term venous access catheter exit site with erythema, induration, and black cutaneous necrosis.[53] One adult with acute nonlymphocytic leukemia presented with a mycotic aortic aneurysm while receiving outpatient chemotherapy through a Hickman catheter.[51] Appropriate antifungal therapy includes ketoconazole, itraconazole, flucytosine, and amphotericin B on an inpatient basis.[51, 53] Management of indwelling catheter infections must be coordinated through the patient's primary physician (e.g., hematologist, oncologist). After supportive measures have

Table 28–2. Microorganisms Causing Indwelling Catheter Infection

Bacterial	
Gram-positive cocci	*Staphylococcus aureus, S. epidermidis, Streptococcus faecalis, S. bovis,* group C streptococci, and viridans streptococcus
Gram-negative bacilli	*Pseudomonas aeruginosa, Klebsiella* sp., *Acinetobacter* sp., *Serratia* sp.
Gram-positive bacilli	*Bacillus cereus, B. laterosporus, Corynebacterium* sp.
Atypical	*Mycobacterium neoaurum, M. fortuitum, M. chelonae*
Mycotic	*Malassezia furfur, M. pachydermatis, Aspergillus fumigatus, A. flavus, Candida albicans*

been undertaken, the primary considerations are (1) the choice of antimicrobial, (2) the decision to remove the indwelling line, and (3) the decision to hospitalize. Selected patients may not require catheter removal.[5, 46, 47, 54] Couch and associates[5] removed only five of 105 Hickman catheters from infected sites before completion of antimicrobial therapy. Further, a portion of those treated without catheter removal may be followed as outpatients.[5] Criteria for outpatient management of indwelling catheter infections include (1) a competent immune system, (2) an intelligent patient with adequate outpatient support, (3) an infection localized to the skin exit site, and (4) an absence of fever, leukocytosis, granulocytopenia, tachycardia, and hypotension.

Cultures are obtained of local purulent discharge, blood drawn through the catheter, and blood drawn from a distant site. An oral antimicrobial should then be chosen that covers both staphylococcus and streptococcus organisms; semisynthetic penicillins and first-generation cephalosporins are adequate to the task. Finally, the patient may be discharged only after consultation with the primary physician and assurance that 24- to 48-hour follow-up will occur to ensure clinical reassessment and review of culture results.

All patients with indwelling catheter infections falling outside of this narrow spectrum are hospitalized. Those who are hemodynamically stable may have cultures taken and be treated with intravenous antimicrobials that are effective against gram-positive and gram-negative organisms. Vancomycin is effective[26, 32, 55] because of its gram-positive spectrum and efficacy against diptheroids, which may be resistant to other antimicrobials. Aminoglycosides provide adequate gram-negative coverage;[55] however, broad-spectrum triple antimicrobial therapy may be necessary in neutropenic patients. Strong consideration should be given to catheter removal when hypotension supervenes. Before an indwelling line is removed, cultures should be obtained of blood drawn through the device as well as the catheter tip itself. The decision to remove a catheter should be made in concert with the consultant, as these devices are both surgically implanted and expensive.

Arteriovenous shunts are seen less frequently in the emergency department owing to the increased use of femoral and subclavian Uldall catheters for temporary hemodialysis. Localized shunt infections are generally due to staphylococci and streptococci.[56] Gram-negative organisms are implicated less frequently, and antimicrobial coverage may be extended to include them.[57] Arteriovenous fistula infections are rare but when present may lead to thrombosis and massive bleeding.[19] Overlying cellulitis without involvement of the fistula itself may be treated on an outpatient basis

with a single intravenous dose of vancomycin. Involvement of the fistula itself mandates hospital admission and observation for hemorrhagic complications.

NONINFECTIOUS COMPLICATIONS

Catheter thrombosis seems to occur more frequently in long-term venous access catheters (22 per cent) than in implantable venous access devices (1 per cent),[14] and pulmonary embolism associated with indwelling lines has been reported.[38, 58, 59] Flushing these catheters with heparin, urokinase, and streptokinase should be done with great care and vigilance. A potentially fatal pulmonary embolus may be heralded by the sudden onset of chest pain, shortness of breath, tachycardia, and tachypnea. Continuous urokinase therapy has been effective in resolving pulmonary emboli in the setting of a large right atrial thrombus.[38] Inability to clear an indwelling line using the measures described under "Procedures" necessitates peripheral venous access and referral for possible catheter replacement.

Additional complications of indwelling lines include mediastinitis, cardiac dysrhythmias, superior vena cava syndrome, subcutaneous tunnel hematoma, central vein stenosis, and septic atrial thrombosis associated with Budd-Chiari malformation.[5, 59, 61] Erosion of the subcutaneous tissue by the Dacron cuff, causing a superficial ulcer, has also been reported.[62] In addition, pneumothorax, cardiac tamponade, lymphatic duct puncture, air embolism, and brachial plexus injury may worsen among outpatients if the result of catheter insertion is not recognized immediately.[61]

The most life-threatening complication of arteriovenous fistulas is bleeding, due either to trauma or infection. Massive blood loss is possible because the arterial system is violated; treatment includes local pressure, intravenous access, oxygen, supportive therapy, and immediate vascular surgery referral to obtain definitive control of the bleeding site. In addition to hemorrhaging, arteriovenous fistulas may also thrombose, a complication usually related to dehydration (e.g., after hemodialysis), hypotension, recent surgery, local trauma, or a superficial ulcer.[19] Thrombectomy may salvage the fistula once these precipitating factors have been addressed. The steal syndrome occurs when blood passes preferentially through a low-resistance arteriovenous fistula at the expense of distal arteries.[63] It generally occurs within 24 hours of fistula surgery in 1 to 3 per cent of patients.[64, 65] Symptoms include pain, paresthesia, and weakness of the fingers and hand.[19] Again, surgical evaluation of the fistula is indicated. Venous hypertension distal to a forearm fistula may lead to painful hand swelling, stasis changes, and hyperpigmentation. The fistula may need to be closed if symptoms persist. Finally, venous aneurysms develop commonly; however, they are not life threatening if the overlying skin remains intact.[19]

CONCLUSION

Numerous methods of vascular access are currently available to include indwelling catheters and arteriovenous anastomoses. Facility with these devices enables emergency department staff to access the venous circulation in a safe and painless manner. However, vigilance during these procedures is necessary to avert potentially life-threatening complications. Knowledge and recognition of these complications among outpatients may prevent sepsis and life-threatening hemorrhage.

REFERENCES

1. Hickman RO, Buckner CD, Clift RA, et al: A modified right atrial catheter for access to the venous system in marrow transplant recipients. Surg Gynecol Obstet 148:871, 1979.

2. Thompson WR, Alexander HR, Martin AJ, et al: Percutaneous subclavian catheterization or prolonged systemic chemotherapy. J Surg Oncol 29:184, 1985.

3. Broviac JW, Cole JJ, Scribner BH: A silicone rubber atrial catheter for prolonged parenteral alimentation. Surg Gynecol Obstet 136:602, 1973.

4. Denny DF, Dorfman GS, Greenwood LH, et al: Translumbar inferior vena cava Hickman catheter placement for total parenteral nutrition. AJR 148:621, 1987.

5. Couch L, Cierny G, Mader JT: Inpatient and outpatient use of the Hickman catheter for patients with osteomyelitis. Clin Orthop 219:226, 1987.

6. Hunter DW, So SK: Dialysis access: Radiographic evaluation and measurement. Radiol Clin North Am 25:249, 1987.

7. McDowell DE, Lakshmikumar P, Goldstein RM: A simplified technique for percutaneous insertion of permanent vascular access catheters in patients requiring chronic hemodialysis. J Vasc Surg 7:574, 1988.

8. Schanzer H, Kaplan S, Bosch J, et al: Double-lumen, silicone rubber, indwelling venous catheters. Arch Surg 121:229, 1986.

9. Lower R: Tractus de corde (1669). Early Science in Oxford. 9, 1932.

10. Kolff WJ: The first clinical experience with the artificial kidney. Ann Intern Med 62:508, 1965.

11. Quinton W, Dillard D, Scribner B: Cannulation of blood vessels for prolonged hemodialysis. Trans Am Soc Artif Intern Organs 6:104, 1960.

12. Dudrick JJ, Wilmore DW, Vars HM, et al: Long-term total parenteral nutrition with growth development and positive nitrogen balance. Surgery 64:134, 1968.

13. Schuman E, Brady A, Gross G, et al: Vascular access options for outpatient cancer therapy. Am J Surg 153:487, 1987.

14. Greene FL, Moore W, Strickland G, et al: Comparison of a totally implantable access device for chemotherapy (Port-A-Cath) and long-term percutaneous catheterization (Broviac). South Med J 81:580, 1988.

15. Anderson AJ, Krasnow SH, Boyer MW, et al: Hickman catheter clots: A common occurrence despite daily heparin flushing. Cancer Treat Rep 71:651, 1987.

16. Raaf JH: Results from use of 826 vascular access devices in cancer patients. Cancer 55:1312, 1985.

17. Harrison CA, Filshie J: The use of Hickman-Broviac catheters for paediatric radiotherapy. Ann R Coll Surg Engl 68:312, 1986.

18. Williams PJ, Lee AS, McCaffrey F, et al: Use of the Hickman catheter for the treatment of lower extremity infections. J Foot Surg 24:355, 1985.

19. Haimov M: Vascular Access: A Practical Guide. New York, Futura Publishing Co, 1987.

20. Engels LG, Slotnick SH, Buskins FG, et al: Home parenteral nutrition via arteriovenous fistula. JPEN 7:412, 1983.

21. Raaf JH: Vascular access grafts for chemotherapy. Ann Surg 190:614, 1979.

22. Uldall PR, Woods F, Merchant N, et al: Two years' experience with the subclavian cannula for temporary vascular access for haemodialysis and plasmapharesis. Proc Dial Transplant Forum 9:32, 1979.

23. Uldall PR, Dyck RF, Woods F, et al: A subclavian cannula for temporary vascular access for haemodialysis or plasmapharesis. Dial Transplant 8:963, 1979.

24. Chutter T, Starker PM: Placement of Hickman-Broviac catheters in the cephalic vein. Surg Gynecol Obstet 166:163, 1988.

25. LaBerge MT, Deppe G, Malviya VK: A simplified technique of Hickman catheter insertion at the bedside in gynecology oncology patients. Gynecol Oncol 26:298, 1987.

26. Jacobs MB, Yeager M: Thrombotic and infectious complications of Hickman-Broviac catheters. Arch Intern Med 144:1597, 1984.

27. Weese JL, Trigg ME: Triple lumen venous access for pediatric bone marrow transplantation candidates. J Surg Oncol 36:55, 1987.

28. Karrei I: Hickman catheters: Your guide to trouble free use. Can Nurs 78(11):25, 1982.

29. Taylor JP, Taylor JE: Vascular access devices: Uses and aftercare. J Emerg Nurs 13:160, 1987.

30. Bothe A, Piccione W, Ambrosino JJ, et al: Implantable central venous access system. Am J Surg 147:565, 1984.

31. Wurzel CL, Halom K, Feldman JG, et al: Infection rates of Broviac-Hickman catheters and implantable venous devices. AJDC 142:536, 1988.

32. Harvey MP, Ramsey-Stewart G, Trent RJ, et al: Complications associated with indwelling venous Hickman catheters in patients with hematological disorders. Aust NZ J Med 16:211, 1986.

33. Rich NM, Spencer FC: Arteriovenous fistulas. In Vascular Trauma. Philadelphia, WB Saunders Co, 1978.

34. Norcross WA, Shackford SR: Arteriovenous fistula: A potential complication of venipuncture. Arch Intern Med 148:1815, 1988.

35. Zajko AB, Reilly JJ, Bron KM, et al: Low-dose streptokinase for occluded Hickman catheters. AJR 141:1311, 1983.

36. Howser DM, Meade CD: Hickman catheter care: Developing organized teaching strategies. Cancer Nurs 10:70, 1987.

37. Flanagan JP, Frandisaria IA, Gross RJ, et al: Air embolism: A lethal complication of subclavian venipuncture. N Engl J Med 281:488, 1969.

38. Zureikat GY, Martin GR, Silverman NH, et al: Urokinase therapy for a catheter-related right atrial thrombus and pulmonary embolism in a 2-month-old infant. Pediatr Pulmonol 2:203, 1986.

39. Chardavoyne R, Auguste LJ, Wise L: Spontaneous withdrawal of an implantable venous catheter (letter). N Engl J Med 13:996, 1985.

40. Johnson PR, Edwards KM, Wright PF: Frequency of Broviac catheter infections in pediatric oncology patients. J Infect Dis 154:170, 1986.

41. King DR, Komer M, Hoffman J, et al: Broviac catheter sepsis: The natural history of an iatrogenic infection. J Pediatr Surg 20:728, 1985.

42. Kumar A, Brar SS, Murray DL, et al: Central venous catheter infections in pediatric patients in a community hospital. Infection 16(2):86, 1988.

43. Kaye BR, Kearns PJ: Streptococcus bovis catheter infection and the short bowel syndrome. Am J Med 80:735, 1988.

44. Kuskie MR: Group C streptococcal infections. Pediatr Infect Dis J 6:856, 1987.

45. Saleh RA, Marchall AS: Bacillus sp. sepsis associated with Hickman catheters in patients with neoplastic disease. Pediatr Infect Dis J 6:851, 1987.

46. Schuman ES, Winters V, Gross GF, et al: Management of Hickman catheter sepsis. Am J Surg 149:627, 1985.

47. Davison BD, McCormack JG, Blacklock ZM, et al: Bacteremia caused by *Mycobacterium neoaurum*. J Clin Microbiol 26:762, 1988.

48. Flynn PM, Van Hooser B, Gigliotti F: Atypical mycobacterial infections of Hickman catheter exit sites. Pediatr Infect Dis J 7:510, 1988.

49. Mickelson PA, Viano-Paulson MC, Stevens DA, et al: Clinical and microbiological features of infections with *Malassezia pachydermatis* in high risk infants. J Infect Dis 157:1163, 1988.

50. Powell DA, Aungst D, Snedden S, et al: Broviac catheter related *Malassezia furfur* sepsis in five infants receiving intravenous fat emulsions. J Pediatr 105:987, 1984.

51. Tchekmedyian S, Newman K, Moody MR, et al: Case report: Special studies of the Hickman catheter of a patient with recurrent bacteremia and candidemia. Am J Med Sci 291:419, 1986.

52. Redline RW, Redline SS, Boxerbaum B, et al: Systemic *Malassezia furfur* infections in patients receiving intralipid therapy. Hum Pathol 16:815, 1985.

53. Allo MD, Miller J, Townsend T, et al: Primary cutaneous aspergillosis associated with intravenous catheters. N Engl J Med 317:1105, 1987.

54. Tenney JH, Moody MR, Newman KA, et al: Adherent microorganisms on lumenal surfaces of long-term intravenous catheters. Arch Intern Med 146:1949, 1986.

55. Olson TA, Fischer GW, Lupo MC, et al: Antimicrobial therapy of Broviac catheter infections in pediatric hematology oncology patients. J Pediatr Surg 22:839, 1987.

56. Eykyn S, Plillips I, Evans J: Vancomycin for staphylococcal shunt site infections in patients on regular hemodialysis. Br Med J 1:80, 1970.

57. Simmons RL, Foker JE, Lower RR, et al: Transplantation. In Schwartz SI, Shires GT, Spencer FC (eds): Principles of Surgery. 4th ed. New York, McGraw-Hill Book Co, 1984

58. Rockoff MA, Gang DL, Vacanti JP: Fatal pulmonary embolism following removal of a central venous catheter. J Pediatr Surg 19:307, 1984.

59. Firor HV: Pulmonary embolism complicating total intravenous hyperalimentation. J Pediatr Surg 7:81, 1972.

60. Haddad W, Idowu J, Georgeson K, et al: Septic atrial thrombosis. Am J Dis Child 140:778, 1986.

61. Ferrara BE: Thrombotic complications of the Hickman catheter. J Fla Med Assoc 74:255, 1987.

62. Fisher WB: Complication of a Hickman catheter. JAMA 254:2934, 1985.

63. Khalil IM, Livingston DH: The management of steal syndrome occurring after access for dialysis. J Vasc Surg 7:572, 1988.

64. Guillou PJ, Leveson SH, Kesler RC: The complications of vascular access. Br J Surg 67:517, 1980.

65. Kinneart P, Struyven J, Mathiew J, et al: Intermittent claudication of the hand after creation of arterio-venous fistulas in the forearm. Am J Surg 139:838, 1980.

Chapter **29**

Intraosseous Infusion

William H. Spivey

INTRODUCTION

Obtaining vascular access in a critically ill pediatric patient can be one of the most difficult and frustrating procedures a physician may have to perform. For example, in a review of intravascular access in pediatric cardiac arrest, Brunette and Fischer noted that the average time needed to establish venous access was a disappointing 7.9 ± 4.2 minutes.[1] Although peripheral percutaneous venous access was the fastest method (mean time 3.0 minutes), it was successful in only 17 per cent of cases. Success rate was highest for an intraosseous infusion (83 per cent), followed by surgical cutdown (81 per cent), and central venous catheterization (77 per cent). The mean time required to obtain a functioning intraosseous line was 4.7 minutes, followed by 8.36 minutes for a central line, and 12.7 minutes for a cutdown.

Small peripheral vessels in children often collapse during shock, and the child's increased body fat makes peripheral cannulation time consuming and at times impossible. Central vein cannulation can be equally difficult and has a risk of pneumothorax or arterial injury. Alternative routes for drug administration, such as the endotracheal and rectal routes, do not provide rapid, reliable drug absorption during cardiac arrest. For example, epinephrine administered by the endotracheal route, although effective in a normally functioning cardiovascular system, is poorly absorbed and produces minimal physiologic response when administered during cardiac arrest.[2, 3]

In light of the need for rapid vascular access in pediatric patients, the previously abandoned technique of intraosseous infusion has been reintroduced. It provides a safe, reliable method of accessing the cardiovascular system for administration of fluids and drugs during cardiac arrest and other resuscitations.

BACKGROUND

One of the earliest references describing the intraosseous route was by Drinker and colleagues, who in 1922 examined the circulation of the sternum and suggested it as a site for transfusion.[4] The sternum was a common site for bone marrow aspiration at that time, and it seemed logical that blood could be administered via the same route. The route was not used clinically until 1934 when Josefson, a Swedish physician, administered liver concentrate into the sternum of 12 patients with pernicious anemia and reported that all 12 improved.[5] Subsequently, the technique became widespread in the Scandinavian countries.

In 1940 the technique was introduced to American physicians by Tocantins, who described a series of animal and clinical studies that demonstrated fluid was rapidly transported from the medullary cavity of long bones to the heart.[6-8] Over the next two decades, thousands of cases of intraosseous infusion of blood, crystalloid substances, and drugs were reported.[9-11] Relatively few complications were reported, considering the needles were often left in place for 24 to 48 hours. Heinald and coworkers in 1947 reviewed 982 cases of intraosseous infusion and reported only 18 failures and five cases of osteomyelitis.[11] None of the cases of osteomyelitis occurred in patients who received isotonic solutions.

With the introduction of plastic catheters and improved cannulation skills, the need for intraosseous infusion as an alternative route of access diminished, and the technique was all but abandoned. Although Turkel continued to advocate the technique for resuscitation in children and adults,[12-14] it was not until the mid-1980s that the technique was reintroduced in response to the need for immediate vascular access during cardiopulmonary resuscitation.[15, 16] Use of the technique during cardiac arrest was supported by experiments that demonstrated sodium bicarbonate was effectively transported to the heart during cardiac arrest.[17] Since then, the technique has become widespread throughout the United States.

ANATOMY AND PHYSIOLOGY

Long bones are richly vascular structures with a dynamic circulation that is capable of accepting large volumes of fluid and rapidly transporting fluids or drugs to the central circulation. The bone, like most organs, is supplied by a major artery (nutrient artery). The artery pierces the cortex and divides into ascending and descending branches, which further subdivide into arterioles that pierce the endosteal surface of stratum compactum to become capillaries. The capillaries drain into medullary venous sinusoids throughout the medullary space that in turn drain into a central venous channel (Fig. 29–1). The medullary sinusoids accept fluid and drugs during intraosseous infusion and serve as a route for transport to the central venous channel, which exits the bone as nutrient and emissary veins.[18] Radiographic studies have demonstrated that radiopaque dye spreads only a few centimeters in the medullary space before being transported to the venous system.[19]

Almost every drug and fluid commonly used in resuscitation has been reported in clinical and preclinical intraosseous studies. Crystalloid, blood, 50 per cent dextrose, epinephrine, dopamine, atropine, sodium bicarbonate, succinylcholine, diazepam, and antibiotics are just a few of the substances that have been administered by this route.[20-25] Crystalloid infusion studies in animals have demonstrated that infusion rates of 10 to 17 milliliters per minute may be achieved with gravity infusion and rates as high as 42 milliliters per minute with a pressure infusion.[26-28] Intraosseous crystalloid infusion has been shown to produce a significant increase in blood pressure in a hemorrhagic shock model in rabbits.[29] In small animals (7 to 8 kg) the size of the marrow cavity is the rate-limiting factor, whereas in larger animals (12 to 15 kg), the size of the needle determines the flow.[28] Blood under pressure can be infused approximately two thirds as fast as crystalloid fluids.[28]

Comparisons of intraosseous and venous infusion of drugs have demonstrated that the drugs reach the central circulation by both routes in similar concentrations and at

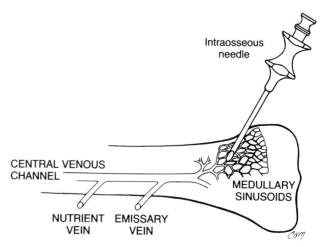

Figure 29–1. Schematic diagram illustrating the venous drainage from the marrow of a long bone with an intraosseous needle in place.

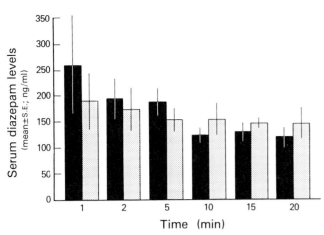

Figure 29–2. Serum diazepam levels (mean ± standard error; ng/ml) graphed for the intraosseous *(shaded area)* and intravenous *(blackened area)* groups as a function of time when injected during normal perfusion. Initially the intravenous drug level is slightly higher, but overall the difference between the two routes of administration is not significant.

the same time[6, 20] (Fig. 29–2). This holds true even during cardiopulmonary resuscitation, in which sodium bicarbonate has been shown to provide a greater buffering capacity when administered by the intraosseous route than by the peripheral venous route.[17]

INDICATIONS AND CONTRAINDICATIONS

Intraosseous infusion is a means of achieving rapid temporary vascular access until a patient can be stabilized and traditional vascular access obtained. It is indicated when fluid or drugs must be introduced into the circulation rapidly and venous access is not readily available. The primary indication is cardiac arrest in an infant or child. The route has been used in adults, but vascular access is usually easily obtainable and alternatives are not often needed in adults. In pediatric patients, it may be used as a first line of vascular access if peripheral vascular access does not appear to be readily obtainable. Other indications include shock, trauma, extensive burns, severe dehydration, and status epilepticus or any situation in which the emergency administration of fluids or drugs is necessary but not feasible by other routes.[25] Intraosseous infusion also has been used as a site for lower extremity venography.[30]

In addition to serving as a route for fluid administration, the intraosseous needle may be used for obtaining blood for type and cross match and blood chemistries from the marrow cavity. Serum electrolyte, blood urea nitrogen (BUN), creatinine, glucose, and calcium levels are very similar to samples obtained from an intraosseous aspirate.[31, 32] A complete blood count may not be reliable, because it reflects the marrow cell count rather than the cell count in the peripheral circulation. Furthermore, the aspirated blood usually clots within seconds even if it is placed in a tube that contains heparin.

The only absolute contraindications to intraosseous infusion are an infection at the intended puncture site and a fracture of the bone. Osteogenesis imperfecta is associated with a high fracture potential; the procedure should be avoided when this diagnosis is known. A fractured bone is avoided because as fluid is infused, it increases the intramedullary pressure and forces fluid to extravasate at the fracture site. This may slow the healing process or cause a

nonunion of the bone. A similar extravasation of fluid can occur through recent intraosseous puncture sites placed in the same bone. Hence, recent prior use of the same bone for intraosseous infusion represents a relative contraindication. Another relative contraindication is generalized sepsis. There are, however, many case reports of septic infants who have received intraosseous fluid and antibiotics without complications.[21, 33] The potential for osteomyelitis with intraosseous infusion must be weighed against the potential delay in obtaining traditional vascular access for administering antibiotics in a life-threatening situation.

EQUIPMENT

The only equipment necessary for establishing intraosseous access is a sturdy needle with a stylet and a syringe for aspiration. Needles range in size from 20 to 13 gauge and are made by several companies. Standard needles for drawing blood or administering medications are generally *not adequate* for interosseous infusions; they are simply not sturdy enough to penetrate bone. In the past, an 18-gauge spinal needle was commonly used for children under 12 to 18 months of age. This needle, although readily available in most emergency departments, often bends and is too long for rapid fluid infusion. Several needles are currently employed in emergency departments for intraosseous infusion (Fig. 29–3). Bone marrow aspiration needles such as the Rosenthal or Osgood needles are the best choice. They are large enough (16 gauge) to be used on older children or adults and are good for fluid administration. The Illinois sternal/iliac aspiration needle (Monoject, Division of Sherwood Medical, St. Louis, Mo.) is a 16-gauge needle that has an adjustable plastic sleeve to prevent the needle from penetrating too deeply or through the opposite cortex. Its disadvantage is that it has a long shaft and cumbersome handle that make it vulnerable to dislodgment from the bone during transport or other procedures. The Cook intraosseous needle (Cook Critical Care, Bloomington, Ind.) comes in 18- and 16-gauge sizes and has a detachable handle that decreases the likelihood of its being dislodged. A useful feature of this needle is a line located 1 cm from the tip of the needle to serve as a depth marker. The Sur-Fast needle (Cook Critical Care, Inc., Bloomington, Ind.) has a threaded shaft to permit a more secure needle placement. A 13-gauge needle is manufactured by MedSurg Industries (Rockville, Md.) and is good for fluid resuscitation. However, like the

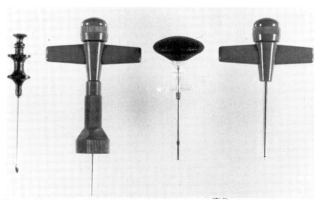

Figure 29–3. Needles used for intraosseous infusion. *Left to right:* Rosenthal bone marrow aspiration needle, Illinois sternal/iliac aspiration needle, Cook intraosseous needle, MedSurg Industries bone marrow aspiration needle. See text for needle manufacturers.

Illinois sternal/iliac aspiration needle, this latter product has a large handle that makes it cumbersome.

SITE

Originally the sternum was used as a site for intraosseous infusion. After several cases of osteomyelitis and mediastinitis in children, the site was abandoned.[34] Other sites, such as the clavicle and humerus, have been used, but neither has gained popularity. Today, the site of choice is the proximal tibia, followed by the distal tibia and distal femur.

The tibia is popular because it is a large bone with a thin layer of subcutaneous tissue that allows landmarks to be readily palpated. On the proximal tibia, the broad, flat anteromedial surface is used with the tibial tuberosity serving as a landmark. The index finger is placed over the tibial tuberosity, the medial surface of the tibia is grasped with the thumb, and an imaginary line is drawn between them (Fig. 29–4). Halfway between these two points and 1 or 2 cm distally is the optimal site for needle placement. This is far enough from the growth plate to prevent damage but in an area in which the bone is still soft enough to allow easy penetration of a needle. This site is good for newborns, infants, and children up to school age. It may be used in adults but is more difficult and requires a 16- to 13-gauge needle to penetrate.

Another site that is popular and recommended by some as even better than the proximal tibia is the distal tibia.[35] The site of needle insertion is the medial surface at the junction of the medial malleolus and the shaft of the tibia (Fig. 29–5). This is the preferred site for adults but is also

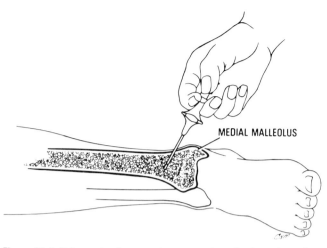

Figure 29–5. Schematic diagram demonstrating the insertion of an intraosseous needle into the distal tibia. Landmarks are the junction of the medial malleolus and the shaft of the tibia.

good for infants and children.[36] No study to date has compared flow from the proximal tibia with flow from the distal tibia, but the difference is probably not significant. Interestingly, one hypovolemic swine study found that flow rates were slightly better at the distal tibia, although access at the femur was better than at either tibial site.[37]

The distal femur is occasionally used, but because of thick overlying muscle and soft tissue, it is difficult to palpate bony landmarks. If it is chosen, the dorsal surface in the region in which the condyles taper into the shaft of the bone is the site of penetration.

PROCEDURE

Once a site has been identified, the area is prepared with a povidone-iodine solution or alcohol. Local anesthesia is not usually required because the patient is in a state of cardiac arrest or shock; however, if the patient is conscious, the skin and periosteum should be anesthetized. The intraosseous needle is then inserted with the needle pointing away from the joint space. The needle should be grasped in the palm of the hand and with the index finger that was used to stabilize it during the procedure (Fig. 29–6). This also helps keep the needle from penetrating too deeply or through the bone. A twisting or rotary motion is used to cut the bone and facilitate puncture of the cortex. Once the cortex has been pierced, there is decreased resistance and a crunching feeling as the needle moves through the bony trabeculae in the marrow cavity. The stylet is then removed, and a 5- to 10-ml syringe is used to aspirate blood and marrow contents for confirmation of position. Many times, particularly during cardiac arrest, blood aspiration does not occur. If the needle is felt to be in the proper place, the physician may cautiously infuse 2 to 3 ml of sterile saline while palpating the area of the limb for extravasation. If there is none, the needle may be used for fluid and drug administration. When fluid is infused, there will be slight resistance, much like injecting water into a balloon. If there is excessive resistance, the needle should be pulled back a few millimeters, and another attempt should be made to infuse fluid. If continued resistance is met, the needle may be advanced further (with stylet in place) or a new site may be chosen.

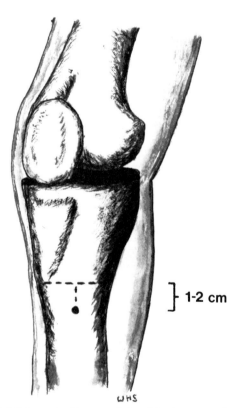

1-2 cm

Figure 29–4. Schematic diagram of the tibia, demonstrating an imaginary line between the tibial tuberosity and medial aspect of the tibia. This area is bisected, and the intraosseous needle is inserted 1 to 2 cm distally. The bevel of the needle is directed away from the joint space.

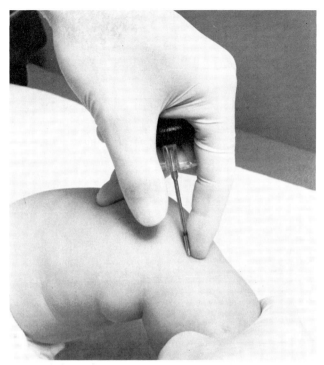

Figure 29–6. Insertion of an intraosseous needle. The handle is grasped in the palm, and a rotary motion is applied with moderate pressure. The index finger is used to stabilize the shaft and prevent it from being forced too deeply into the bone or through the bone.

COMPLICATIONS

As with any procedure, complications may arise when attempting to use the bone for vascular access. Complications may be divided into two categories: technical and latent soft tissue or bone problems. Technical difficulties are the most common, but these decrease as familiarity with the technique increases (Fig. 29–7). The most common mistake is to place excessive pressure on the needle during insertion and force it through the bone. This may be avoided by placing the index finger against the skin to prevent the needle from going in too deeply. Also, attention to depth of the needle or use of a sheath on the needle to prevent excess penetration will decrease occurrences of this problem. Incomplete penetration of the bone may also occur, in which case, blood will not be aspirated and fluid will extravasate if infused. Serum levels of medication are decreased when intraosseous infusion is performed through bones with multiple cortical defects.[38] If several attempts are made to place a needle in the same bone, fluid may extravasate from previous puncture wounds. If extravasation occurs, the needle should be removed and pressure applied.

The needle may be blocked periodically by clots forming around the bevel or by bony spicules obstructing the flow of fluid. This complication may require that the line be flushed with 3 to 5 ml of sterile saline every 10 to 15 minutes to keep it open. Pressure infusions usually do not require taking this step.

A major concern of any person using intraosseous infusion is infection. This concern often leads physicians to shy away from using the bone and to continue searching for other methods of vascular access. Although the potential for infection is real, its actual incidence is low. A literature review of more than 4000 cases from 1942 to 1977 found a 0.6 per cent incidence of infection.[15] Although most of the affected access sites were not placed under emergency con-

ditions, the needles were often left in 1 to 2 days, thus increasing the likelihood of infection. A survey of more than 1000 U.S. and foreign medical schools found the incidence of infection for intraosseous needles placed in emergency conditions less than 3 per cent (Spivey, Hodge, unpublished data).

The most common infection is cellulitis at the puncture site, which usually responds well to antibiotics. Osteomyelitis is less common, but it also usually responds to antibiotics. Heinild and colleagues[11] reported three cases of osteomyelitis in 25 patients who received infusions of undiluted $D_{50}W$. Undiluted $D_{50}W$ injected into rabbit femurs produces edema and pyknotic marrow nuclei that improve within 1 month.[39] In addition to infection, inflammatory reactions of the bone may be seen. These are most common when hypertonic or sclerosing agents are used and may produce an elevation of the periosteum with a positive bone scan (Fig. 29–8). Unlike the clinical appearance of a patient with osteomyelitis due to bacteria, a child with a sterile inflammatory reaction does not look toxic. One hypertonic sclerosing drug that is routinely used during cardiac arrest is sodium bicarbonate. Heinild and coworkers reported 78 cases of bicarbonate infusion with no complications.[11] Animal studies have reported a decrease in cellularity with edema and destruction of some cells, but these changes are temporary and completely resolve in a few weeks.[39, 40] Phenytoin has not been found to damage the marrow of piglets.[41, 42]

Another complication that has been reported is necrosis and sloughing of the skin at the site of infusion.[43] This occurs if fluid or drugs extravasate from the puncture site into the surrounding tissues. Care should be taken when infusing drugs such as calcium chloride, epinephrine, and sodium bicarbonate to prevent dislodgment of the needle and extravasation into the tissue. It is best to infuse drugs gently and not under pressure, because pressure frequently causes extravasation.

Injury of the growth plate and developmental abnormalities of the bone are ongoing concerns. These fears have not been supported in the literature, however. There have been no reports of growth plate damage or permanent abnormalities of the bone. One animal study specifically examined damage to the epiphysis by injecting sodium bicarbonate directly into the epiphysis and found no radiologic evidence of epiphyseal injury.[44] By pointing the needle

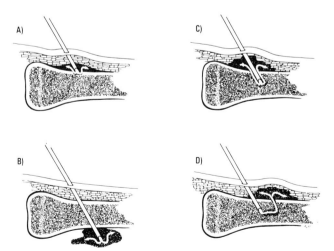

Figure 29–7. Schematic diagram of possible problems encountered with intraosseous infusion. *A,* Incomplete penetration of the bony cortex. *B,* Penetration of the posterior cortex. *C,* Fluid escaping around the needle through the puncture site. *D,* Fluid leaking through a nearby previous cortical puncture site.

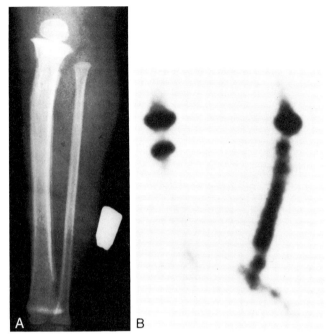

Figure 29–8. Radiograph *(A)* and bone scan *(B)* of the tibia, demonstrating an inflammatory reaction 4 days after the patient received intraosseous phenytoin and phenobarbital. The periosteum is elevated the length of the bone, mimicking osteomyelitis on the plain films and the bone scan. A diagnosis of osteomyelitis requires either clinical evidence of infectious toxicity or positive cultures (blood or periosteal aspirate).

away from the joint space and using the previously mentioned landmarks for insertion, the danger of epiphyseal injury is remote.

Fat embolism is frequently mentioned as a potential complication.[15, 35] However, this condition is rare and only reported for adult patients.[45] Two animal studies addressing this issue found no changes in blood gases during intraosseous infusion and limited evidence of fat globule collection in the lungs.[46, 47] Because the marrow in infants and children is primarily hematopoietic, this potential complication is unlikely to occur.

A case of compartment syndrome following intraosseous line use during cardiac resuscitation has been reported.[48] Tibial fractures have also been reported.[49] Follow-up radiographs of patients with intraosseous needle placement or attempts are indicated.

INTERPRETATION

The determination of whether an intraosseous infusion is functioning may be made by assessing the ease with which fluid infuses and the clinical response of the patient. If the needle is properly placed, fluid should flow smoothly with only occasional flushes necessary to keep it open. A clinical response to fluid or drugs should be seen at approximately the same time and in the same magnitude as with intravenous administration.

CONCLUSION

Intraosseous infusion provides a means of rapidly accessing the cardiovascular system in emergencies. The technique is not intended to replace traditional venous access; instead it should serve as a temporizing measure for resuscitation until venous access can be obtained. It is now used widely throughout the United States and Canada and has been reviewed extensively in the emergency medicine and pediatric literature. The technique also is used by prehospital care personnel, who have demonstrated a high success rate in the field.[50]

Complications are most commonly related to technical mistakes. By carefully locating landmarks, staying away from the growth plate, and paying attention to the depth of the needle, complications can be minimized. Finally, as with any technique, practice on cadaver or animal leg bones (e.g., chicken, pig) greatly improves one's skill.

REFERENCES

1. Brunette DD, Fischer R: Intravascular access in pediatric cardiac arrest. Ann Emerg Med 6:577, 1988.
2. Ralston SH, Tacker WA, Showen L, et al: Endotracheal versus intravenous epinephrine during electromechanical dissociation with CPR in dogs. Ann Emerg Med 14:1044, 1985.
3. Crespo SG, Spivey WH, Schoffstall JM: Absorption of epinephrine by endotracheal tube during cardiac arrest (abstract). Ann Emerg Med 17:878, 1988.
4. Drinker CK, Drinker KR, Lund CC: The circulation in the mammalian bone marrow. Am J Physiol 62:1, 1922.
5. Josefson A: A new method of treatment—intraosseous injections. Acta Med Scand 81:550, 1934.
6. Tocantins LM: Rapid absorption of substances injected into the bone marrow. Pro Soc Exp Biol Med 45:292, 1940.
7. Tocantins LM, O'Neil JF: Infusions of blood and other fluids into the general circulation via the bone marrow. Surg Gynecol Obstet 73:281, 1941.
8. Tocantins LM, O'Neil JF, Jones HW: Infusions of blood and other fluids via the bone marrow. JAMA 117:1229, 1941.
9. Elston JT, Jayne RV, Kaump DH, et al: Intraosseous infusions in infants. Am J Clin Pathol 17:143, 1947.
10. Arbeiter HI, Greengard J: Tibial bone marrow infusion in infancy. J Pediatr 25:1, 1944.
11. Heinild S, Sondergaard T, Tudvad F: Bone-marrow infusion in childhood: Experiences from a thousand infusions. J Pediatr 30:400, 1947.
12. Turkel H: Intraosseous infusion. Am J Dis Child 137:706, 1983.
13. Tarrow AB, Turkel H, Thompson MS: Infusion via the bone marrow and biopsy of the bone and bone marrow. Anesthesiology 13:501, 1952.
14. Turkel H: Intraosseous infusions. JAMA 151:1108, 1953.
15. Rossetti VA, Thompson BM, Miller J, et al: Intraosseous infusion: An alternative route of pediatric intravascular access. Ann Emerg Med 14:885, 1985.
16. Parrish GA, Turkewitz D, Skiendzielewski JJ: Intraosseous infusions in the emergency department. Am J Emerg Med 4:59, 1986.
17. Spivey WH, Lathers CM, Malone DR, et al: Comparison of intraosseous, central, and peripheral routes of sodium bicarbonate administration during CPR in pigs. Ann Emerg Med 14:1135, 1985.
18. Kelly PJ: Pathways of transport in bone. In Handbook of Physiology—The Cardiovascular System III. London, Oxford University Press, 1985.
19. Begg AC: Intraosseous venography of the lower limb and pelvis. Br J Radiol 27:318, 1954.
20. Spivey WH, Unger HD, Lathers CM, et al: Intraosseous diazepam suppression of pentylenetetrazol-induced epileptogenic activity in pigs. Ann Emerg Med 16:156, 1987.
21. McNamara RM, Spivey WH, Unger HD, et al: Emergency applications of intraosseous infusion. J Emerg Med 5:97, 1987.
22. Valdes MM: Intraosseous fluid administration in emergencies. Lancet 1:1235, 1977.
23. Berg RA: Emergency infusion of catecholamines into bone-marrow. Am J Dis Child 138:810, 1985.
24. Macht DI: Absorption of drugs through the bone marrow. Pro Soc Exp Biol Med 47:299, 1941.
25. Papper EM: The bone marrow route for injecting fluids and drugs into the general circulation. Anesthesiology 3:307, 1942.
26. Shoor PM, Berryhill RE, Benumof JL: Intraosseous infusions. Pressure flow relationship in pharmacokinetics. J Trauma 19:772, 1979.
27. Hodge D, Delgado-Paredes C, Gleisher G: Intraosseous infusion flow rates in hypovolemic "pediatric" dogs. Ann Emerg Med 16:305, 1987.
28. Schoffstall JM, Spivey WH, Davidheiser S, et al: Intraosseous crystalloid and blood infusion in a swine model. J Trauma 29:384, 1989.
29. Morris RE, Schonfeld N, Haftel AJ: Treatment of hemorrhagic shock with intraosseous administration of crystalloid fluid in the rabbit model. Ann Emerg Med 16:27, 1987.
30. Wegner GP, Flaherty TT, Crummy AB: Intraosseous lower extremity venography. Am Surg 98:105, 1969.
31. Spivey WH, McNamara RM, Lathers CM: Comparison of intraosseous and intravenous CBC and ASTRA 8 in swine (abstract). Ann Emerg Med 15:647, 1986.
32. Orlowski JP, Porembka DT, Gallagher JM, et al: The bone marrow as a source of laboratory studies. Ann Emerg Med 18:1348, 1989.

33. Glaeser PW, Losek JD: Emergency intraosseous infusions in children. Am J Emerg Med 4:34, 1986.
34. Tocantins LM, O'Neil JF: Complications of intraosseous therapy. Ann Surg 122:266, 1945.
35. Iserson KV, Criss E: Intraosseous infusions: A usable technique. Am J Emerg Med 4:540, 1986.
36. Iserson KV: Intraosseous infusions in adults. J Emerg Med 7:587, 1989.
37. Warren DW, Kissoon N, Sommerauer JF, et al: Multiple intraosseous sites vs peripheral intravenous: Comparison of infusion rates in normovolemic and hypovolemic pigs (abstract). J Emerg Med 8:381, 1990.
38. Brickman K, Rega P, Choo M, et al: Comparison of serum phenobarbital levels after single versus multiple attempts at intraosseous infusion. Ann Emerg Med 19:31, 1990.
39. Wallden TM, Lennart W: On injuries of bone marrow after intraosseous injections: An experimental investigation. Acta Chir Scand 96:152, 1947.
40. Spivey WH, Unger HD, McNamara RM, et al: The effect of intraosseous sodium bicarbonate on bone in swine. Ann Emerg Med 16:773, 1987.
41. Vinsel PJ, Moore GP, O'Hair KC, Comparison of intraosseous versus intravenous loading of phenytoin in pigs and effect on bone marrow. Am J Emerg Med 8:181, 1990.
42. Jaimovich DG, Shabino CL, Ringer TV, et al: Comparison of intraosseous

and intravenous routes of anticonvulsant administration in a porcine model. Ann Emerg Med 18:842, 1989.
43. Rimar S, Westry JA, Rodriguez RL: Compartment syndrome in an infant following an emergency intraosseous infusion. Clin Pediatr 27:259, 1988.
44. Brickman KR, Rega P, Koltz M, et al: Analysis of growth plate abnormalities following intraosseous infusion through the proximal tibial epiphysis in pigs. Ann Emerg Med 17:121, 1988.
45. Thomas ML, Tighe JR: Death from fat embolism as a complication of intraosseous phlebography. Lancet ii:1415, 1973.
46. Plewa MC, Kaplan RM, LaCowey D, et al: Fat embolism following intraosseous infusion. Ann Emerg Med 17:407, 1988.
47. Orlowski JP, Julius CJ, Petras RE, et al: The safety of intraosseous infusions: Risks of fat and bone marrow emboli to the lungs. Ann Emerg Med 18:1062, 1989.
48. Moscati R, Moore GP: Compartment syndrome with resultant amputation following intraosseous infusion (letter). Am J Emerg Med 8:470, 1990.
49. LaFleche F, Slepin M, Vargas J, et al: Iatrogenic bilateral tibial fractures after intraosseous infusion attempts in a 3-month old infant. Ann Emerg Med 10:1099, 1989.
50. Smith RJ, Keseg DP, Manley LK, et al: Intraosseous infusions by prehospital personnel in critically ill pediatric patients. Ann Emerg Med 17:97, 1988.

Chapter **30**

Endotracheal Drug Administration

J. Thomas Ward, Jr.

INTRODUCTION

The endotracheal administration of certain medications is a simple, rapid, and effective alternative means of drug delivery to the central circulation in certain settings. This technique of drug administration should be reserved for use in those situations in which a patient's condition warrants immediate pharmacologic intervention and a more conventional means of drug delivery, such as intravenous access, is not readily available. Such settings occur infrequently; however, when they do occur, knowledge of the appropriate drugs and dosages that can be delivered effectively by this route may prove to be life saving. It is therefore mandatory that physicians be familiar with the concept and method of endotracheal drug therapy.

The history of endotracheal drug administration dates back to the mid-1800s, when the ability of the lung to absorb solutions rapidly was first demonstrated. In 1857 Bernard performed an experiment in which he instilled a solution of curare into the upper respiratory tract of dogs by way of a tracheostomy.[1] After the dogs were tilted to an upright position, they died within 7 to 8 minutes, and Bernard concluded that the alveoli must be permeable to curare. Over the next several decades, other investigators expanded this work and demonstrated that solutions containing salicylates, atropine, potassium iodide, strychnine, and chloral hydrate were also absorbed rapidly from the lung and excreted in the urine after injection of their aqueous solutions into the tracheas of experimental animals.[2]

In 1915, Kline and Winternitz and Smith provided experimental data that suggested the "direct medication" of the lung in pulmonary disease might prove to be an effective therapeutic route.[3, 4] This philosophy of treating pulmonary disease then gained further acceptance in 1935 when Graeser and Rowe demonstrated that the inhalation of epinephrine mist dramatically relieved the symptoms of asthma.[5]

During the late 1930s and early 1940s, certain chronic suppurative disorders of the lung failed to respond to the parenteral use of the antibiotics penicillin and sulfa, and once again the philosophy of "direct medication" of the lung was instituted. Initially, antibiotics were delivered by inhaled mist[6-18] and later by solutions injected intratracheally.[16-22] During this period of time, two important observations were made concerning endotracheal drug therapy: (1) penicillin delivered by the endotracheal route demonstrated a "depot effect," resulting in therapeutic blood levels that lasted twice as long as those noted with intramuscular injection[16]; and (2) various diluents mixed with penicillin could affect both the rate and the degree of absorption of penicillin from the lungs.[17]

In the 1950s, other important research concerning the endotracheal administration of drugs was carried out by investigators who were attempting to elucidate the mechanism responsible for "anesthetic reactions."[23-26] Results from this research demonstrated several important points. First, the rate of absorption of drugs from the mucous membranes varied with the location of their application: drugs that were delivered endotracheally were absorbed much more rapidly than those applied to the posterior pharynx.[26, 27] Second, the rapid absorption of drugs applied locally to the larynx and trachea resulted in blood levels significant enough to be considered a cause of some of the "anesthetic reactions."[26, 27]

In 1967, Redding, Asuncion, and Pearson considered the possibility of using the endotracheal route of drug delivery as a primary means of rapid systemic drug administration.[28] They administered epinephrine by the intravenous, intracardiac, and intratracheal routes, and then evaluated its effectiveness in the resuscitation of dogs that had undergone both respiratory and circulatory arrests secondary to hypoxia. Redding and coworkers found that the intravenous, intracardiac, and intratracheal (diluted) routes of drug administration were equally effective in restoring the circulation of dogs in cardiac arrest. They concluded that "whichever of these routes is most immediately available should be used."[28] Thus it was demonstrated that the endotracheal route of drug delivery provided an effective window to the systemic circulation.

A decade then passed before further research was published concerning the use of endotracheal drug therapy as an alternative means of systemic drug administration. Roberts and associates revived the study of endotracheal drug delivery with a series of papers concerning both the experimental and clinical administration of endotracheal epinephrine.[29-33] Since that time, a number of important animal studies,[34-55] human studies,[56-59] and case reports[60-67] have appeared in the literature, providing new and valuable information regarding the endotracheal method of drug delivery.

These investigations, combined with work from previous studies, have helped to identify several important issues regarding various aspects of endotracheal drug therapy. These issues, some of which still require further elucidation, include (1) the most appropriate single dose volume of drug solution; (2) the most

Table 30–1. Endotracheally Administered Emergency Drugs Found to Be Effective Experimentally and Clinically

Epinephrine	Naloxone
Atropine	Diazepam*
Lidocaine	

*One animal study found pulmonary inflammation secondary to the diluent of this agent.[46]

Table 30–2. Endotracheally Administered Emergency Drugs That Appear to Be Effective Experimentally But That Are Not Clinically Proven

Midazolam
Propranolol
Metaraminol

appropriate diluent solution to be mixed with a drug for delivery; (3) the effects of "pharmacologically active" diluent solutions; (4) the most effective technique for endotracheal drug delivery; and (5) the effects certain conditions, such as hypoxemia, hypotension, pulmonary edema, shock, acidosis, and cardiopulmonary arrest, have on the absorption and distribution of endotracheally administered drugs. Many of these issues are likely to be the subject of future investigations.

INDICATIONS

The basic indication for endotracheal drug therapy is the need for rapid pharmacologic intervention in a setting in which a more reliable access to the circulation, such as the intravenous route, is not readily available. Indications for the delivery of a specific drug endotracheally are generally the same indications as those for intravenous administration. However, not all drugs that can be given safely by the intravenous route can also be given safely and effectively by the endotracheal route. The classic example of this is sodium bicarbonate, which appears to inactivate pulmonary surfactant when given endotracheally.[68]

At present only a limited number of drugs have been shown to be effective when delivered by the endotracheal route (Tables 30–1 and 30–2). A large portion of the data on these drugs, however, comes from experimental animal models[29, 30, 36, 40–48, 68] or human studies[59, 69, 70] performed in nonshock or non–cardiopulmonary resuscitation (CPR) settings (Table 30–3). It appears that the pharmacokinetics of endotracheally administered drugs in a setting of shock, hypoxemia, or cardiopulmonary arrest may differ significantly from those of the nonshock or non–CPR state (Table 30–4).[39, 49–51, 54, 57, 58] A number of case reports do exist, however, that demonstrate endotracheal drug therapy to be beneficial, if not life saving, when given in the near-arrest or CPR setting (Table 30–5).[32, 33, 60–67]

Emergency drugs that have been administered endotracheally and found to be effective in both experimental animal models and human studies or case reports include epinephrine,[28–33, 39–41, 49, 52, 63, 65, 66] atropine,[45, 47, 59, 60, 62, 65, 66, 68] lidocaine,[42–44, 50, 51, 56, 69, 70] naloxone,[34, 61] and diazepam.[35, 46, 64] Several other endotracheally delivered drugs that appear to be effective in animal models but remain clinically unproven

at this time include midazolam,[48] propranolol,[47] and metaraminol.[71]

Specific recommendations concerning the most appropriate dosage for drugs administered by the endotracheal route in an arrest or near-arrest state are difficult to make at present. It is reasonable to state that the endotracheal dosage of a medication should at least be equal to the intravenous dosage of that same drug given for the same indication. It appears, however, that at least two drugs may require higher dosages endotracheally than intravenously to be effective. Lidocaine has been shown to yield therapeutic serum levels when administered endotracheally in doses of approximately 3 mg/kg,[56, 69, 70] a dose which has been recommended for use by some investigators.[57] Also, both animal[49] and human studies[58] suggest that the presently recommended endotracheal dose of 1 mg of epinephrine for an adult may not be sufficient, leading some sources to recommend a 2-mg dose when endotracheal delivery is necessary for adults in cardiopulmonary arrest.[71, 72] One should be concerned, however, about the postresuscitative hypertension that this larger dose of epinephrine may produce in conjunction with the observed "depot effect" of the drug.[32, 39, 49] Once an appropriate dose has been selected, it should then be delivered in a volume of 5 to 10 ml for adults and 1 ml for infants, using normal saline for a diluent when needed.

CONTRAINDICATIONS

At present, the only true contraindication to the endotracheal delivery of an *appropriate* drug is the presence of another access to the systemic circulation through which the needed drug can be delivered rapidly and effectively. As noted earlier, the pharmacokinetics and effectiveness of endotracheally delivered drugs given in various states of cardiovascular or pulmonary compromise are to a large extent unknown, and for that reason, more conventional routes of rapid and effective drug administration should be used when available.

A complete list of drugs that are "contraindicated" relative to their delivery by the endotracheal method is not available. Thus far, those drugs shown to be detrimental or ineffective when delivered by the endotracheal route include sodium bicarbonate,[68] calcium chloride,[32] bretylium tosy-

Table 30–3. Human Studies in Nonshock or Non–Cardiopulmonary Resuscitation Settings

Drug	Dose	Volume	Technique	Findings	Comments
Atropine[59]	0.6 mg	1 ml	Through catheter in endotracheal tube	Maximum increase in heart rate at 45 seconds; amplitude of response same as intravenous dose; duration of effect was 4.3 minutes	Study compared effects of intravenous versus endotracheal atropine
Lidocaine[56, 69, 70]	2.4–7.7 mg/kg	<5 ml	Sprayed directly into trachea or translaryngeally	Therapeutic levels reached in 5 minutes and maintained for 30–60 minutes	Drugs delivered before intubation

Table 30–4. *Human Studies in a Cardiopulmonary Resuscitation (CPR) Setting*

Drug	Dose	Volume	Technique	Findings	Comments
Epinephrine[58]	1 mg	10 ml	Instilled through endotracheal tube	No change in serum epinephrine levels found over 3-minute sampling period	Epinephrine delivered by this method not found to be effective in animal CPR setting either[39]
Lidocaine[57]	1.1–3.1 mg/kg	3.75–10 ml	Squirted or poured down endotracheal tube	Therapeutic levels not consistently reached; 8–10 minutes required to reach therapeutic levels; study recommended 3 mg/kg dose	Too few drug samplings; too many variables present to interpret data clearly

late,[36] and isoproterenol.[47] No drug should be delivered by the endotracheal route without experimental or clinical evidence to support its effectiveness and safety.

It should be noted that the endotracheal delivery of at least one drug in solution (diazepam) has resulted in a transient decrease in the arterial partial pressure of oxygen (P_{O_2}).[35] However, a number of human case reports have not documented any significant deterioration in the respiratory status of patients receiving endotracheal drug therapy that could be directly attributable to the method of drug delivery.[32, 60–67]

EQUIPMENT

Patients in need of endotracheal drug therapy first require management of their airways, usually in the form of tracheal intubation. Once this procedure has been performed (see Chapter 1), little other equipment is needed for the endotracheal delivery of a drug.

Under the section on procedure, several different techniques for endotracheal drug administration are described. The equipment listed in what follows is all that is required to perform any of the four different techniques described in the next section.

1. Manual bag ventilation device capable of delivering a fraction of inspired oxygen (FI_{O_2}) of at least 50 per cent. In most circumstances in which endotracheal drug delivery is indicated, the nature of the patient's condition also warrants supplemental oxygen.[32, 60–67] Although a number of experimental studies[49, 44, 46, 10] and case reports[64, 67] have shown no significant deterioration in the respiratory status of patients after endotracheal drug therapy and no decrease in arterial oxygen content when measured, it is still advisable to administer additional oxygen after drug delivery if oxygen is not already being supplied. It should also be noted that experimental work suggests that several rapid insufflations immediately after drug delivery will help to deliver the drug distally, where it may be absorbed more rapidly and effectively.[37]

2. A fine-bore catheter, preferably at least 8 French in size and at least 35 cm (14 inches) in length. Several studies have suggested that the use of such a catheter placed through the endotracheal tube for the purpose of drug injection improves drug absorption and effectiveness.[30, 39, 42] The most effective length or diameter of the catheter has not yet been determined, but it appears that to be most beneficial, the catheter should be long enough to protrude past the distal end of the endotracheal tube. Some investigators have even used catheters long enough to deliver the drug solution endobronchially.[39, 52] As for the diameter of the catheter, it must be large enough to allow for the rapid delivery of a 10-ml volume of solution.

Several different types of catheters commonly available to emergency department personnel might be considered for this purpose: (1) a 16-gauge central venous pressure or cutdown catheter; most of these are only 30 cm in length, however, and the proximal end of the endotracheal tube requires shortening to allow the catheter to protrude past the distal end; (2) an 8 French 35-cm catheter (e.g., Cook, Inc., P.O. Box 489, Bloomington, Ind. 47402), commonly used as a vessel dilator by radiologists; it also comes in a number of different sizes and lengths; and (3) an 8 French (or larger) pediatric pulmonary suction catheter without the control port (e.g., Pharmaseal Tri-Flo Suction Catheter: PT64). This third type of catheter is made to extend past the tip of the endotracheal tube, and it has several holes in the distal end that conveniently produce a spray when solutions are injected through it. The tip of a Luer-Lok syringe also will fit nicely on the catheter's proximal end. The only drawback to this type of catheter is that it is not quite as stiff as one might need for rapid insertion through an endotracheal tube.

3. An intravenous adapter lock (e.g., Argyle Intermittent Infusion Plug or Travenol PRN Adaptor). These can be placed on the end of any of the three catheters listed previously (including the suction catheter) to convert them for use with the prefilled syringes in which most emergency medications now come. Of course, the intravenous adapter lock is unnecessary if a standard syringe is used.

4. A 10- to 20-ml syringe, preferably a Luer-Lok–type of syringe big enough to deliver the desired volume of drug solution plus an additional 5 ml of air. Unfortunately (for endotracheal drug therapy), most of the medications now prescribed for emergency situations come in prefilled syringes with long built-in needles. This type of apparatus usually does not allow one to draw up an additional volume of air to empty the catheter of solution. Also, the needle on the prefilled syringe may reduce the effectiveness of endotracheal drug delivery. One study showed decreased absorption of lidocaine when the drug was administered into the endotracheal tube with a syringe and attached needle versus a syringe alone.[42]

5. Desired drug solution. The optimal volume of solution for endotracheal drug therapy has yet to be determined, but it appears that a volume of 5 to 10 ml for adults and 1 ml for infants is appropriate. When a drug must be diluted to reach an adequate volume, most investigators have chosen to use normal saline because it does not appear to have any adverse effects on the lung when delivered in small volumes (10 ml or less). However, similarly small volumes of distilled water (10 ml or less) have not yet been adequately studied and should not be completely ruled out as a diluent because water appears to be absorbed more rapidly into the circulation than normal saline.[73]

6. A number 18- or 19-gauge needle for use in drawing

Table 30–5. Human Case Reports

Drug	Dose	Volume	Technique	Setting	Results and Comments
Epinephrine[32]	1 mg	10 ml	ET Needle	Pulseless bradycardia 57-year-old female asthmatic	Sinus tachycardia at 150 and pulse within 1 minute. Hypertensive period postresuscitation. Discharged alive in good condition.
Epinephrine[32, 33]	0.01 mg	1 ml	ET Syringe	CPR—asystole 13-day-old infant	Strong apical pulse and respirations within 45 seconds. Developed sinus tachycardia at 160. Died of intraventricular bleeding 3 days later.
Epinephrine[63]	0.025–0.1 mg	0.25–1 ml	ET Needle	Bradycardic infants not responsive to 100% O_2; some with CPR	All infants developed sinus tachycardia at 140–180 within 5 to 10 seconds. Three infants later died of intraventricular bleeding.
Epinephrine[65] Atropine[65]	0.10 mg ? mg	1 ml 0.5 ml	ET ET	3-month-old CPR Asystole	Initial doses repeated at 5 minutes. Heart rate of 48 noted 10 minutes later but no pulses. Infant died next day. Unclear effect of ET drugs.
Epinephrine[66] Atropine[66]	0.02 mg/kg 0.015 mg/kg	0.2 ml/kg ?	ET ET	7-month-old CPR—burn and smoke inhalation ? initial rhythm	Ventricular bradycardia 30 seconds after ET epinephrine. Sinus arrhythmia and blood pressure of 69/56 after ET atropine. ET epinephrine dose repeated. Time frame for drugs and responses uncertain.
Atropine[60]	1 mg	?	ET Syringe	74-year-old female CPR; initial rhythm bradycardia	30 seconds after ET atropine, heart rate of 100. At 90 seconds, supraventricular rhythm with rate of 100 and blood pressure of 170/90. Blood levels of atropine obtained. Patient discharged without pulmonary complications after hospitalization.
Atropine[62]	0.6 mg	?	ET	Patient of unknown age in unit; ventricular tachycardia, asystole, ventricular fibrillation, sinus bradycardia	"Rapid improvement in rate" in about 10 seconds. Many other drugs given before ET atropine, including IV atropine. Possible effect of ET atropine.
Diazepam[64]	5 mg	1 ml	Tracheostomy	76-year-old female with generalized seizures for 90 minutes	Seizure activity stopped within 2 minutes. Intramuscular phenobarbital had been given previously—unreported time frame. No complications noted on chest x-ray or by arterial blood gases.
Diazepam[46]	1 mg	0.2 ml	ET	7-month-old infant in status epilepticus	Seizure activity stopped within 2 minutes; no pulmonary complications noted in follow-up.
Naloxone[61]	0.8 mg × 2	2 ml × 2	ET Syringe	24-year-old male, comatose, apneic, heroin overdose, with sinus bradycardia of 40	Some of solution expelled with cough. Patient awake and alert within 60 seconds of first dose. Naloxone blood levels obtained.
Albuterol[67]	2.5 mg 5.0 mg	3 ml 4 ml	ET ET	67-year-old female asthmatic in respiratory distress	Extubation possible 25 minutes after second dose; improvement in arterial blood gases; no transient drop in Pa_{O_2}.

ET, endotracheal; CPR, cardiopulmonary resuscitation.
Where data was not supplied, a question mark is shown.

up the drug solution (and possibly for injecting the solution through the endotracheal tube wall into the lumen of the tube). Also, a number 21- or 22-gauge needle is required if the translaryngeal technique of drug administration is used.

7. An alcohol wipe.

PROCEDURE

Several factors have been identified that may modify the manner and degree of drug absorption after endotracheal drug therapy: use of a diluent solution, type of diluent solution used, pharmacologic activity of diluent solution, total volume of solution, technique or method of drug delivery, and use of rapid, forceful ventilations after drug delivery.[74, 74a] It also appears that simple variations in the technique of drug delivery may have significant effects on drug absorption.[42] Hypovolemic shock has been shown to correlate with higher lidocaine levels following endotracheal delivery of the drug.[74a]

Use of a Catheter

Several different techniques of endotracheal drug administration have been reported in the literature.[29, 35, 36, 39, 42, 49, 56, 57, 70, 75-78] At present, the most effective technique for drug delivery and absorption appears to be the injection of the drug solution through a catheter placed within the endotracheal tube, its tip protruding beyond the distal end of the endotracheal tube. Apparently, this method of drug delivery minimizes the loss of drug solution within the endotracheal tube and promotes more distal delivery of the drug into the lung, thereby improving absorption.[29, 39]

Once the patient has been intubated (see Chapter 1), the endotracheal tube should be secured by tape or string so that the tube is not likely to be expelled during a forceful cough. In addition, the cuff of the tube, when present, should be inflated. The patient should then be ventilated with a ventilation device using supplemental oxygen while the required drug dose is drawn up in either a 10- or a 20-ml syringe, preferably of the Luer-Lok type. If necessary, the drug should be diluted with normal saline to a total volume of 5 to 10 ml (for adults). The plunger of the syringe should then be drawn back further so that an equal volume of air is present in the barrel of the syringe with the solution. The syringe can be attached to a catheter at this time or once the catheter has been placed within the endotracheal tube (Fig. 30–1).

The connection between the proximal end of the endotracheal tube and the ventilation device should then be interrupted and the catheter placed within the lumen of the endotracheal tube so that the proximal end of the catheter is just outside of, but near, the proximal end of the endotracheal tube. The proximal ends of the catheter and the endotracheal tube should be held in one hand while the syringe is attached to the catheter (if not already) with the other hand. The drug solution should then be injected rapidly and forcefully through the catheter into the trachea followed by the 5 to 10 ml of air needed to flush the catheter of any remaining drug solution. The syringe and catheter should then be promptly removed from the endotracheal tube. If the patient makes an effort to cough, one should place the thumb (preferably gloved) over the opening of the endotracheal tube to prevent expulsion of the solution. If the endotracheal tube has not been properly secured by this time, the tube itself can be expelled during reflex coughing.

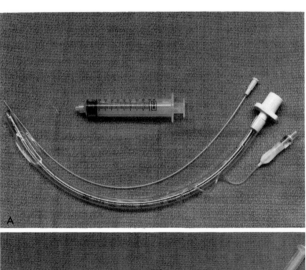

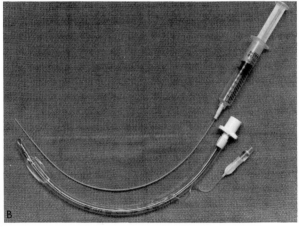

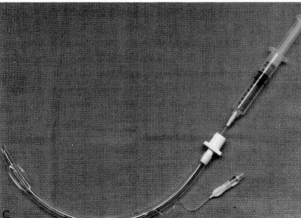

Figure 30–1. Use of a central venous catheter for endotracheal drug delivery.

If external cardiac massage is being performed, it should be interrupted for a few seconds during drug delivery so that chest compressions do not expel the drug.

As soon as possible after drug delivery the bag ventilation device with supplemental oxygen should be reattached to the endotracheal tube, and five rapid insufflations should be performed to promote more distal delivery of the drug.

Use of Prefilled Syringes

As noted previously, emergency drugs frequently come in prefilled syringes of the Abboject type (Fig. 30–2) that are designed to save the time needed to draw up drug dosages. Most of these drugs already come in convenient volumes of 5 to 10 ml. Although they do have the disadvantages discussed previously, the prefilled syringes can still be used by either attaching the intravenous adapter lock to the catheter or by breaking off the needle near the hub so that the syringe tip will fit into the proximal end of the catheter. When these prefilled syringes are used, one should note that the flow rate of solution exiting the distal tip of the catheter is not as great as the rate when a syringe without the needle is used.

Probably the most frequently used method of endotracheal drug administration is simply squirting the drug solution into the proximal end of the endotracheal tube and then following it with several rapid insufflations of the bag ventilation device connected to the supplemental oxygen. Although a number of experimental animal studies[29, 30, 34, 40, 42, 44] and human studies[69, 70] have shown this method of drug delivery to be effective, these investigations were all performed in nonshock or non-CPR settings. Studies done on human subjects undergoing CPR have demonstrated that drugs delivered endotracheally by this method are not absorbed consistently.[57, 58] Also, animal data obtained from a CPR model have shown this method of drug delivery to be ineffective, whereas lesser doses of the same drug produced physiologic effects in the same model after being delivered deeper into the bronchial tree by means of a catheter placed through the endotracheal tube.[39] The aggregate of this data suggests that in low-flow states, absorption of drugs delivered into the larger airways is not as great as that of drugs delivered deeper into the pulmonary tree.

Injection Through the Endotracheal Tube Wall

A third method of drug delivery that has not yet been evaluated scientifically but has been suggested by several authors[76, 77] provides for the use of a number 18- or 19-

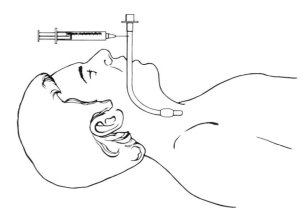

Figure 30–3. Method for drug injection through the endotracheal tube wall.

gauge needle inserted into the side of the endotracheal tube proximally (Fig. 30–3). The drug solution is then injected into the endotracheal tube during the inspiratory phase of ventilation. This method of drug delivery does not require interruption of the connection between the ventilation device and the endotracheal tube and has the theoretic advantage of having the solution "blown down the tube into the lungs." To what degree these theoretic considerations affect the delivery and absorption of the administered drug is unknown.

Translaryngeal Administration

One final method of endotracheal drug therapy is more properly termed *translaryngeal drug administration*. Drug administration by this technique has been reported to produce therapeutic blood levels of at least one drug (lidocaine) in the same amount of time as that for the methods described earlier.[56] The primary purpose of this form of drug delivery has been to provide local anesthesia to the larynx and trachea before intubation.[79, 80] Because experience with this form of drug delivery is limited to local anesthetics such as lidocaine, it cannot be recommended for use with other emergency drugs at present (see Chapters 3 and 7).

The volume of solution required for translaryngeal drug delivery seems to be less than that required for endotracheal drug delivery. Frequently, 1.5 to 3.5 ml of a 4 per cent solution of lidocaine is used for the purpose of translaryngeal anesthesia; however, as much as 9 ml of anesthetic has been delivered by this method.[56, 79, 80]

COMPLICATIONS

It is difficult to obtain accurate information concerning the complications of endotracheal drug therapy, in part because of the infrequent use of this method of drug administration. In addition, most patients who receive this form of drug therapy are either critically ill or have sustained cardiopulmonary arrest. In such a setting, it becomes difficult to determine whether the endotracheal delivery of a drug has any adverse effect on the patient's status because of the large number of variables involved.

With regard to the techniques of endotracheal drug administration, no serious complications have been reported. A theoretic complication is the loss of a needle or catheter during forceful administration of the drug. If translaryngeal anesthesia is included as a method of endotracheal drug

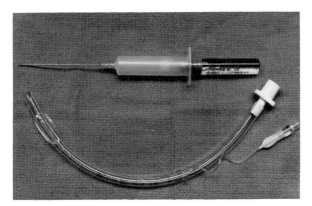

Figure 30–2. Example of a prefilled syringe frequently used in endotracheal therapy.

delivery, other complications can arise, although their frequency is low. Gold and Buechel reviewed 17,500 cricothyroid punctures for translaryngeal anesthesia and noted eight complications with no fatalities.[79] There were two cases of severe laryngospasm, four soft tissue infections of the neck, and two broken needles that were retrieved. Thus the techniques of endotracheal drug administration seem to provide a safe method of drug delivery.

As for the adverse effects of endotracheal drug administration, one potentially serious side effect has been reported in the literature. Epinephrine administered by the endotracheal route during CPR in animal models[39, 49] and in a human case report[32] has been noted to produce a period of prolonged hypertension of varying degrees during the postresuscitative state, after the return of a perfusing rhythm. It appears that this side effect is related to the "depot effect" observed with certain endotracheally administered medications. In at least one of these animal models,[49] the period of hypertension appeared to be dose related. No serious sequelae were reported, however, in regard to this period of hypertension.

The potential for drug toxicity with any medication delivered by the endotracheal route during CPR should be a concern during the postresuscitative state, when the improved hemodynamic status of the patient might enhance the absorption of drugs previously delivered to the lungs. The pharmacokinetics of endotracheally administered drugs during CPR is an area that requires further investigation.

A second area of potential concern with endotracheal drug therapy is a transient decrease in arterial oxygen content during or after drug delivery. A number of animal studies[35, 36, 42–44, 46, 48] have addressed this issue by reviewing arterial blood gas measurements before and after the endotracheal delivery of drug solutions. In most of these studies no significant change in values was noted.[42–44, 46, 48] In a few animal studies, however, some evidence of mild respiratory dysfunction was noted, primarily when large volumes (2 ml/kg) of solution were administered endotracheally[38] or in association with the endotracheal delivery of diazepam.[35, 46]

Greenberg and associates reported a study in which 2 ml/kg of normal saline was instilled endotracheally in dogs.[38] The arterial P_{O_2} was noted to decrease to a level of approximately 80 per cent of baseline values for about 20 minutes. Also, it was reported that 2 ml/kg of distilled water instilled endotracheally in dogs produced a drop in arterial P_{O_2} to a level of approximately 60 per cent of baseline values, which persisted for at least 20 minutes. Although the volume of fluid used in this experiment represents a dose of fluid much greater than that usually delivered endotracheally as a single dose to humans, the findings do show that if large enough volumes of fluid are delivered endotracheally, a resultant decrease in arterial P_{O_2} develops.

In an animal study by Barsan and colleagues that assessed the endotracheal administration of diazepam, a 12.2 mm Hg decrease in the mean arterial P_{O_2} from the mean control value was noted after drug delivery.[35] This change occurred at 60 minutes after drug delivery and returned toward control values at 90 minutes. It should be noted that the diluent utilized in this study was 95 per cent ethanol, because diazepam is not readily soluble in normal saline. Another study, by Rusli and associates, reported an increased incidence of pneumonitis at postmortem in a group of dogs that were administered diazepam endotracheally compared with those administered the same volume of normal saline.[46] No significant changes in arterial blood gas values were noted in this study.

In human subjects, information regarding the possible decrease in arterial oxygen content secondary to endotra-

cheal drug therapy is minimal and comes primarily from case reports. In these reports, endotracheal drug delivery was not found to be associated with any adverse respiratory effects clinically, radiographically, or by arterial blood gas determinations.[64, 67]

It thus appears that in most instances of endotracheal drug therapy, transient hypoxemia does not develop; the only transient decreases in arterial oxygen content were noted in association with large volumes of endotracheally administered fluid (2 ml/kg) or with the endotracheal administration of diazepam. It should be remembered, however, that any decrease of arterial P_{O_2} in a critically ill patient, regardless of how small or how transient, may have deleterious effects. The potential for this adverse effect should always be considered when administering drugs by the endotracheal route, and supplemental oxygen should always be administered in an effort to improve oxygenation and offset any transient drop in arterial oxygen content that might develop.

CONCLUSION

Endotracheal drug therapy has been shown to be a safe and effective means of drug administration to the central circulation in nonshock or non-CPR settings. However, the setting in which endotracheal drug therapy is most often used is one of shock or cardiopulmonary arrest. Information has been obtained that suggests the pharmacokinetics of certain endotracheally administered drugs in a setting of shock or cardiopulmonary arrest may differ significantly from the pharmokinetics of the drugs in a nonshock or non-CPR state. At present, further investigation is necessary to determine the most appropriate drug dosages as well as more accurate pharmacokinetic profiles of drugs administered by the endotracheal route in patients in arrest or near-arrest states. Despite this lack of knowledge, endotracheal drug therapy in dosages similar to those administered intravenously has been shown to be effective, and even life saving, in humans. For that reason it is of utmost importance that physicians be familiar with this method of drug therapy.

REFERENCES

1. Bernard C: Leçons sur les effets des substances toxiques et méditcamenteuses. Paris, 286, 1857.
2. Mutch N: Inhalation of chemotherapeutic substances. Lancet 2.775, 1944.
3. Kline BS, Winternitz MD: Studies upon experimental pneumonia in rabbits. VIII. Intra vitam staining in experimental pneumonia, and the circulation in the pneumonic lung. J Exp Med 21:311, 1915.
4. Winternitz MC, Smith GH: Preliminary Studies in Intratracheal Therapy: Collected Studies on the Pathology of War Gas Poisoning. New Haven, Conn, Yale University Press, 1920.
5. Graeser JB, Rowe AH: Inhalation of epinephrine for the relief of asthmatic symptoms. J Allergy 6:415, 1935.
6. Barach AL, Molomut N, Soroka M: Inhalation of nebulized Promin in experimental tuberculosis. Am Rev Tuberc 46:268, 1942.
7. Stacey JW: The inhalation of nebulized solution of sulfonamides in the treatment of bronchiectasis. Dis Chest 9:302, 1943.
8. Harris TN, Sommer HE, Chapple CC: The administration of sulfonamide micro-crystals by inhalation. Am J Med Sci 205:1, 1943.
9. Chapple CC, Lynch HM: A study of sulfonamide aerosol inhalation: A supplemental note. Am J Med Sci 205:488, 1943.
10. Applebaum IL: The treatment of bronchial lesions by the inhalation of nebulized solution of sodium sulfathiazole. Dis Chest 10:415, 1944.
11. Edlin JS, Bobrowitz ID, Safford FK, et al: Promin inhalation therapy in pulmonary tuberculosis. Am Rev Tuberc 50:543, 1944.
12. Bryson V, Sansome E, Laskin S: Aerosolization of penicillin solutions. Science 100:33, 1944.
13. Barach AL, Silberstein FH, et al: Inhalation of penicillin aerosol in patients with bronchial asthma, chronic bronchitis, bronchiectasis, and lung abscess. A preliminary report. Ann Intern Med 22:485, 1944.
14. Segal MS, Ryder CM: Penicillin aerosolization in the treatment of serious respiratory infections. N Engl J Med 233:747, 1945.
15. Segal MS, Levinson L, Miller D: Penicillin inhalation therapy in respiratory infections. JAMA 134:762, 1947.

16. Gaensler EA, Beakey JF, Segal MS: Pharmacodynamics of pulmonary absorption in man. I. Aerosol and intratracheal penicillin. Ann Int Med 31:582, 1949.
17. Beakey JF, Gaensler EA, Segal MS: Pharmacodynamics of pulmonary absorption in man. II. The influence of various diluents on aerosol and intratracheal penicillin. Ann Int Med 31:805, 1949.
18. Gaensler EA, Beakey JF, Segal MS: Relative effectiveness of parenteral, intratracheal, and aerosol penicillin in chronic suppurative diseases of the lung. J Thorac Surg 18:546, 1949.
19. May HB, Floyer MA: Infected bronchiectasis treated with intratracheal penicillin. Br Med J 1:907, 1945.
20. Norris CM: Sulfonamides in bronchial secretion. JAMA 123:667, 1943.
21. Vinson PP: Treatment of chronic non-tuberculous pulmonary infection by bronchoscopy and insufflation of sulfonamide compounds. Ann Otol Rhinol Laryngol 53:787, 1944.
22. Kay EB, Meade RH: Penicillin in the treatment of chronic infections of the lungs and bronchi. JAMA 129:200, 1945.
23. Derbes VJ, Englehardt HT: Deaths following the use of local anesthetics in transcricoid therapy: A critical review. J Lab Clin Med 29:478, 1944.
24. Rubin HJ, Kully BM: Speed of administration as related to the toxicity of certain topical anesthetics. Ann Otol Rhinol Laryngol 69:627, 1951.
25. Steinhaus JE: A comparative study of the experimental toxicity of local anesthetic agents. Anesthesiology 13:577, 1952.
26. Adriani J, Campbell D: Deaths following topical application of local anesthetics to mucous membranes. JAMA 162:1527, 1956.
27. Campbell D, Adriani J: Absorption of local anesthetics. JAMA 168:873, 1958.
28. Redding JS, Asuncion FS, Pearson JW: Effective routes of drug administration during cardiac arrest. Anesth Analg 46:253, 1967.
29. Roberts JR, Greenberg MI, Knaub M, et al: Comparison of the pharmacological effects of epinephrine administered by the intravenous and endotracheal routes. JACEP 7:260, 1978.
30. Roberts JR, Greenberg MI, Baskin SI: Blood levels following intravenous and endotracheal epinephrine administration. JACEP 8:53, 1979.
31. Greenberg MI, Roberts JR, Krusz JC, et al: Endotracheal epinephrine in a canine anaphylactic shock model. JACEP 8:500, 1979.
32. Roberts JR, Greenberg MI, Baskin SI: Endotracheal epinephrine in cardiorespiratory collapse. JACEP 8:515, 1979.
33. Greenberg MI, Roberts FR, Baskin SI: Use of endotracheally administered epinephrine in a pediatric patient. Am J Dis Child 135:767, 1981.
34. Greenberg MI, Roberts JR, Baskin SI: Endotracheal naloxone reversal of morphine-induced respiratory depression in rabbits. Ann Emerg Med 9:289, 1980.
35. Barsan WG, Ward JT, Otten ET: Blood levels of diazepam after endotracheal administration in dogs. Ann Emerg Med 11:242, 1982.
36. Murphy KM, Caplen SM, Nowak RM, et al: Endotracheal bretylium tosylate in a canine model. Ann Emerg Med 13:87, 1984.
37. Greenberg MI, Spivey W: Comparison of deep vs. shallow endotracheal medication administration in dogs. Ann Emerg Med 14:209, 1985.
38. Greenberg MI, Baskin SI, Kaplan AM, et al: Effects of endotracheally administered distilled water and normal saline on the arterial blood gases of dogs. Ann Emerg Med 11:600, 1982.
39. Ralston SH, Voorhees WD, Babbs CF: Intrapulmonary epinephrine during prolonged cardiopulmonary resuscitation: Improved regional blood flow and resuscitation in dogs. Ann Emerg Med 13:79, 1984.
40. Chernow B, Holbrook P, D'Angona DS, et al: Epinephrine absorption after intratracheal administration. Anesth Analg 63:829, 1984.
41. Schuttler J, Hornchen U, Stoeckel H: Pharmacokinetics and dynamics of epinephrine administered endobronchially. Anesthesiology 63:A117, 1985.
42. Mace SE: Effect of technique of administration on plasma lidocaine levels. Ann Emerg Med 15:552, 1986.
43. Mace SE: Effect of total fluid volume administered on plasma lidocaine levels with endotracheal drug therapy (abstract). Am J Emerg Med 4:420, 1986.
44. Mace SE: The effect of dilution on plasma lidocaine levels with endotracheal administration. Ann Emerg Med 16:522, 1987.
45. Prete MR, Hannan CJ, Burkle FM: Plasma atropine concentrations via intravenous, endotracheal, and intraosseous administration. Am J Emerg Med 5:101, 1987.
46. Rusli M, Spivey WH, Bonner H, et al: Endotracheal diazepam: Absorption and pulmonary pathologic effects. Ann Emerg Med 16:314, 1987.
47. Scott B, Martin FG, Matchett J, et al: Canine cardiovascular responses to endotracheally and intravenously administered atropine, isoproterenol, and propranolol. Ann Emerg Med 16:1, 1987.
48. Gaddis GM, Sheets CA, Gaddis ML, et al: Endotracheal midazolam pharmacokinetics in dogs (abstract). Ann Emerg Med 17:879, 1988.
49. Ralston SH, Tacker WA, Showen L, et al: Endotracheal versus intravenous epinephrine during electromechanical dissociation with CPR in dogs. Ann Emerg Med 14:1044, 1985.
50. Mace SE: Endotracheal drug therapy during hypovolemic shock (abstract). Ann Emerg Med 15:633, 1986.
51. Mace SE: Effect of hypoxemia on endotracheal lidocaine in a canine model (abstract). Ann Emerg Med 16:1103, 1987.
52. Hornchen U, Schuttler J, Stoeckel H, et al: Endobronchial instillation of epinephrine during cardiopulmonary resuscitation. Crit Care Med 15:1037, 1987.
53. Crespo SG, Spivey WH, Schoffstall JM: Absorption of epinephrine by endotracheal tube during cardiac arrest (abstract). Ann Emerg Med 17:878, 1988.
54. Orlowski JP, Gallagher JM, Porembka DT: Intratracheal epinephrine is unreliable (abstract). Crit Care Med 16:389, 1988.
55. Brickman K, Rega P, Guinness M: Comparison of intraosseous, intratracheal, and central venous administration of lidocaine in pigs (abstract). Ann Emerg Med 17:435, 1988.
56. Boster SR, Danzl DF, Madden RJ, et al: Translaryngeal absorption of lidocaine. Ann Emerg Med 11:461, 1982.
57. McDonald JL: Serum lidocaine levels during cardiopulmonary resuscitation after intravenous and endotracheal administration. Crit Care Med 13:914, 1985.
58. Quinton DN, O'Byrne G, Aitkenhead AR: Comparison of endotracheal and peripheral intravenous adrenaline in cardiac arrest. Lancet 1:828, 1987.
59. Bray BM, Jones HM, Grundy EM: Tracheal versus intravenous atropine. Anaesthesia 42:1188, 1987.
60. Greenberg MI, Mayeda DV, Chrzanowski R, et al: Endotracheal administration of atropine sulfate. Ann Emerg Med 11:546, 1982.
61. Tandberg D, Abercrombie D: Treatment of heroin overdose with endotracheal naloxone. Ann Emerg Med 11:443, 1982.
62. Welik K, LaGana GM: Successful ET administration of atropine (letter). Ann Emerg Med 12:516, 1983.
63. Lindemann R: Resuscitation of the newborn: Endotracheal administration of epinephrine. Acta Paediatr Scand 73:210, 1984.
64. Pasternak SJ, Heller MB: Endotracheal diazepam in status epilepticus (letter). Ann Emerg Med 14:485, 1985.
65. McNamara RM, Spivey WH, Sussman C: Pediatric resuscitation without an intravenous line. Am J Emerg Med 4:31, 1986.
66. Polin K, Brown DH, Leikin JB: Endotracheal administration of epinephrine and atropine. Pediatr Emerg Care 2:168, 1986.
67. Verbeek PR, Gareau AB, Rubes CJ: Treatment of asthma-related respiratory arrest with endotracheal albuterol (salbutamol). Ann Emerg Med 17:358, 1988.
68. Elam JO: The intrapulmonary route for CPR drugs. In Safar P (ed): Advances in Cardiopulmonary Resuscitation. New York, Springer-Verlag, 1977, p 132.
69. Telivuo L: An experimental study on the absorption of some local anaesthetics through the lower respiratory tract. Acta Anaesth Scand 16(Suppl):121, 1965.
70. Chu SS, Rah KH, Brannan MD, et al: Plasma concentration of lidocaine after endotracheal spray. Anesth Analg 54:438, 1975.
71. Raehl CL: Endotracheal drug therapy in cardiopulmonary resuscitation. Clin Pharm 5:572, 1986.
72. Marchant B: Endotracheal adrenaline in cardiac arrest. Lancet 1:1098, 1987.
73. Courtice FC, Phipps PJ: The absorption of fluids from the lungs. J Physiol 105:186, 1946.
74. Ward JT: Endotracheal drug therapy. Am J Emerg Med 1:71, 1983.
74a. Mace SE: Plasma lidocaine levels occurring with endotracheal administration during hemorrhagic shock. Resuscitation 19:291, 1990.
75. Simon JS: Device for endotracheal route medication (letter). Ann Emerg Med 10:341, 1981.
76. Feferman I, Leblanc L: A simple method for administering endotracheal medication (letter). Ann Emerg Med 12:196, 1983.
77. Stewart RD, Lacovey DC: Administering endotracheal medication (letter). Ann Emerg Med 14:711, 1985.
78. Jones HM, Bray B: Intratracheal drug administration (letter). Anaesthesia 40:921, 1985.
79. Gold MI, Buechel DR: Translaryngeal anesthesia: A review. Anesthesiology 20:181, 1959.
80. Danzl DF, Thomas DM: Nasotracheal intubations in the emergency department. Crit Care Med 8:677, 1980.

Chapter **31**

Chapter **31**

Intracardiac Injections

Thomas G. Frohlich and Richard Davison

INTRODUCTION

Successful resuscitation from cardiac arrest has been shown to depend on the speed with which spontaneous, effective circulation is restored.[1] The prompt administration of certain drugs is an important part of advanced cardiac life support (ACLS) and seems to play a crucial role in the termination of circulatory arrest.[2, 3] It is estimated that each year, in the United States more than 300,000 deaths from cardiac arrest occur outside the hospital, and surely many others involve hospitalized patients without an intravenous line at the time of the arrest.[4] In these patients, rapid intravascular access is critical to a successful resuscitation.

Throughout the 1960s, intracardiac injection (ICI) was recommended as the most expeditious route of drug administration during cardiac arrest.[3, 5] In the years that followed, the technique fell into disfavor for several reasons. (1) Several investigators emphasized the potential for serious complications resulting from ICI.[6–8] (2) Safe and simple percutaneous techniques were developed that allowed entry into the central venous circulation (subclavian, internal jugular, or femoral vein puncture and intraosseous infusion). (3) Concern was expressed about the cessation of cardiopulmonary resuscitation (CPR) maneuvers during the performance of ICI.[6] (4) Experimental evidence suggested that the administration of drugs through ICI offered no advantage over injection into peripheral veins.[9] (5) The endotracheal route of drug administration was validated.[10, 11]

We believe that although ICI is not the preferred route for drug administration during CPR, intracardiac injection can still be useful in those cases in which prompt intravenous (IV) access is unattainable or when drug administration by other routes has proved ineffective. The technique of ICI is easily taught and requires little equipment. Studies suggest that when properly performed, ICI carries a low risk of clinically significant complications.[12, 13]

Most likely, the frequency with which intracardiac injection is performed will depend on the skill of the operator in the initiation of IV lines. Intracardiac injection may be necessary only in exceptional circumstances; nonetheless, it behooves those individuals involved in the delivery of ACLS to be familiar with this technique.

BACKGROUND

The technique of ICI appears to have originated in the latter part of the nineteenth century. Fantus attributed its first use to a German physiologist, Schiff, around 1880.[14] Over the next 40 years, scattered case reports appeared of successful resuscitation from cardiac arrest with the use of various intracardiac medications.[15, 16] In a 1923 case report, Bodon[17] reviewed the literature and found 90 cases of intracardiac administration of medication, with 24 successful resuscitations. The technique of the injection varied widely, and so did the substances injected, including camphor, caffeine, strophanthin, Pituitrin, strychnine, and epinephrine, the last of which Bodon recommended as the most effective.

By 1930, more than 250 case reports had appeared in the literature; taken together, these reports note an approximate 25 per cent success rate with ICI in terms of prolonged survival. Many of these cases were instances of cardiac arrest secondary to chloroform anesthesia. Yet use of ICIs remained controversial. A JAMA editorial in 1930 proclaimed that "reports of resuscitation by intra-cardiac injection belong with the miracles."[18] In that same year, the Special Committee on Intracardiac Therapy of the Witkin Foundation published its report.[19] Hyman, the author of this detailed paper, concluded that the beneficial effect of intracardiac injection was not from the medication itself but from the irritant effect of the needle on the myocardium. He recommended that right atrial puncture (without injection of medication) be used in the treatment of all cases of cardiac arrest. Hyman's point of view was still popular 17 years later, when Beecher and Linton reported a case of intraoperative cardiac arrest that failed to respond to repeated right atrial punctures until two injections of epinephrine into the right atrium restored a normal sinus rhythm.[20] They concluded that the epinephrine, and not the puncture itself, was responsible for the successful resuscitation.

In 1951, Kay published the results of one of the first modern experimental studies of the treatment of cardiac arrest.[21] Following the induction of asystole and ventricular fibrillation in dogs, he performed open chest cardiac massage and injected different substances into the cardiac chambers. He concluded that ventricular standstill was effectively treated by cardiac massage plus ICI of epinephrine, but he did not recommend epinephrine for the treatment of ventricular fibrillation. By the mid-1950s, intracardiac epinephrine had become part of the standard treatment for cardiac arrest,[5, 22] and with the advent of closed-chest cardiac massage in the 1960s, the intracardiac route of drug administration remained popular.[8, 23, 24] By the mid-1970s, the popularity of ICI had declined. Goldberg warned of the numerous potential complications and advised against the use of ICI, except when it was "absolutely necessary" or during open chest cardiac massage.[6] Schechter, in a letter to JAMA in 1975, harshly condemned the intracardiac injection of epinephrine and stated that "the technique has been obsolete for about 20 years."[25]

INDICATIONS AND CONTRAINDICATIONS

The circulation time during CPR has been measured in a few instances and has been shown to be quite prolonged,[26] suggesting that the beneficial effect of a drug could be considerably delayed when the agent is administered into a peripheral site. Kuhn and associates[27] have demonstrated that, during CPR in humans, medications injected into a central vein reach the systemic arteries more rapidly than medications injected peripherally. This possible time advantage was confirmed by two experimental studies of circulation time in dogs during closed- and open-chest CPR.[28, 29] The clinical significance of these differences in delivery times is unknown.

To date, no experimental or clinical data suggest an advantage of the intracardiac route for drug delivery during cardiac resuscitation. Thus the primary indication for the intracardiac injection of medications during cardiopulmonary resuscitation is restricted to the circumstance in which the administration of an essential drug by other routes would result in an intolerable delay.

Based exclusively on anecdotal information, several researchers have suggested that the intracardiac administration of epinephrine may be more effective than the intravenous route in treatment of asystole or electromechanical dissociation.[30–34] As a secondary indication, then, if intravenous epinephrine fails to reverse asystole or electromechanical dissociation, it would seem appropriate to readminister it by intracardiac puncture.

In either of the aforementioned two circumstances, there are no true contraindications to this technique. Certain associated conditions, such as the presence of a preexistent pneumothorax or the hyperinflated chest of chronic lung disease, make the procedure more difficult. Anticoagulation has been shown to be associated with a greater incidence of hemopericardium, but this rarely results in hemodynamic embarrassment.[24]

EQUIPMENT AND DRUGS

An 8.75-cm-long 18-gauge needle is most often used for the performance of ICI. Syringes prefilled with a standard dose of epinephrine (1 mg in 10 ml) and calcium chloride (1 gm in 10 ml = 14 mEq of calcium) are provided by the manufacturer with an "intracardiac needle" (Abboject or Bristoject). If these are not available, an 18-gauge spinal needle can be fitted to the end of a regular medication syringe (Fig. 31–1). Spinal needles of narrower gauge may be used, but they are more prone to bending and occlusion by tissue plugs; we discourage their use.

Sodium bicarbonate given by the intracardiac route is well described in the pediatric literature.[34–36] In the adult,[13] the relatively large volume of solution that is required imposes a lengthy injection time and a dangerous prolongation of the period during which CPR maneuvers are withheld. Furthermore, the usual commercial syringes containing bicarbonate are prefitted with short needles. If one believes that the intracardiac administration of bicarbonate in an adult is desirable, one can break off the short needle by grasping it with the needle guard and bending the needle close to the hub from side to side. Once the short needle is broken off, an 18-gauge spinal needle can be fitted onto the hub of the syringe.

PROCEDURE

For many years, the "correct" technique for ICI was in dispute. In fact, there was even disagreement concerning the appropriate cardiac chamber to enter. Hyman's contention[19] that a right atrial injection would be as effective as a ventricular injection and would be less likely to cause ventricular fibrillation has never been confirmed and retains only historical interest. In the 1950s and 1960s, many investigators recommended that the injections be made into the left ventricle.[2, 8, 21, 37] Theoretically, this approach has the advantage of a more direct delivery of the drugs into the coronary arteries. In addition, the thick left ventricular wall is more likely to seal off a puncture hole and is less susceptible to being torn than the thinner right ventricular wall. In spite of these considerations, no clear difference in effectiveness between right and left ventricular injections has been demonstrated.[38] In fact, based on observations accumulated during the performance of transthoracic cardiac ventriculography, it is at times difficult to predict which chamber will be entered during the insertion of the transthoracic needle into the heart.[39]

The Subxiphoid Approach

A needle entering the heart through its diaphragmatic surface is unlikely to encounter a large epicardial coronary artery or interposed lung tissue. Two studies that relied mainly on the subxiphoid technique showed it to be associated with a low incidence of complications.[12, 13] It is therefore the preferred approach for the performance of ICI. This route of injection usually involves the right ventricle.

Technique. Without interrupting CPR, the left costoxiphoid area is prepared with an antiseptic solution. The syringe with the drug to be injected is freed of all air bubbles. At this point, the lungs are allowed to deflate, and CPR maneuvers are stopped. With the bevel up, the tip of the needle is inserted in the xiphocostal notch (approximately 1 cm to the left of the tip of the xiphoid process). The needle is directed cephalad toward the middle of the left clavicle at a 30- to 45-degree angle with the skin of the abdominal wall (Fig. 31–2). As soon as the skin is punctured, constant negative pressure is applied to the syringe, and the needle is advanced rapidly. When blood spurts into the syringe, the needle advancement is stopped, and the medication is injected as quickly as possible. The needle is withdrawn immediately, and CPR is resumed. *An intracardiac injection should not interrupt CPR for more than 5 to 10 seconds.* If after full insertion of the needle there is no blood return, the needle must be withdrawn immediately, and CPR must be resumed before another attempt is made. One may then attempt penetration again, this time with the needle directed straight up toward the suprasternal notch. If this fails, a third attempt with the needle directed toward the mid-right clavicle is recommended. If this is also unsuccessful, the left parasternal approach should be tried.

The Left Parasternal Approach

Although with this technique the chance of entering the cardiac chambers may be greater, the potential for complications has historically been considered greater. Specific risks include laceration of the internal mammary artery, damage to the left anterior descending coronary, and pneumothorax secondary to puncture of the lingula.

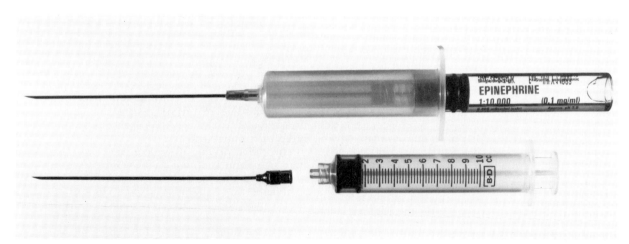

Figure 31–1. Equipment for intracardiac injections. "Intracardiac" needles are available in prefilled syringes *(top)*. An 8.75-cm, 18-gauge spinal needle can be fitted onto a regular syringe *(bottom)*.

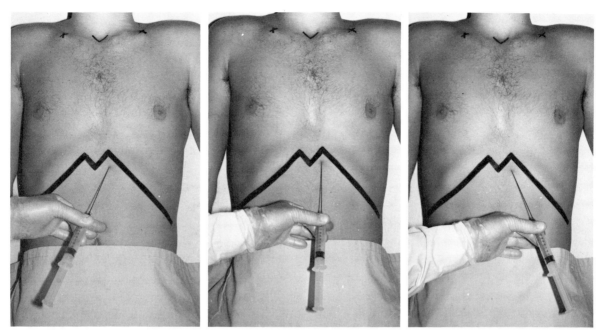

Figure 31–2. The subxiphoid approach. *A*, The initial attempt is performed with the needle directed toward the middle of the left clavicle. If this attempt is unsuccessful, the needle should be redirected straight up *(B)*. *C*, One can make a third attempt by aiming toward the mid-right clavicle.

Technique. For this approach, an area surrounding the left fourth intercostal space along the sternal border is prepared with antiseptic solution. After the lungs are allowed to deflate passively, the needle is inserted just over the fifth rib, two fingerbreadths from the left sternal border. The needle is perpendicular to the frontal plane or angled slightly medially (Fig. 31–3). While exerting suction on the syringe, one rapidly advances the needle until an abrupt blood return is observed. At this time, the medication is injected as rapidly as possible, the needle is withdrawn, and CPR is resumed immediately.

A study by Brown and coworkers examined injuries caused by transthoracic pacemaker leads that were inserted experimentally into cadavers just before autopsy.[40] They found fewer potential complications if a more medial parasternal approach was used. For this technique, the insertion site is in the fifth intercostal space just to the left of the sternal border. The needle is directed medially, dorsally, and cephalad, toward the right second costochondral junction at an angle of 30 degrees to the skin. Aside from the trajectory of the needle, the technique is identical to the parasternal approach described earlier. Although the possible advantages of this parasternal border approach have not been validated by clinical studies during resuscitation, the technique may be of value, especially if subxiphoid and traditional parasternal approaches have failed.[41]

Intracardiac Injections in Infants and Children

The injection technique for infants and children is essentially the same as that for adults. Both the left parasternal and the subxiphoid routes may be used. The chest wall in children is thinner and more pliable than in adults, and injection with a 20- or 22-gauge spinal needle has been recommended.[35, 36] Prepackaged pediatric doses of cardiac drugs are also available with an "intracardiac needle." For the subxiphoid approach, the point of insertion and the angulation of the needle are identical to those used in adult patients.[36] If the left parasternal approach is used, the needle is inserted in the fourth or fifth intercostal space, 2 to 5 cm from the left sternal border; the younger the child, the closer to the sternum.[35] The needle may be angled slightly medially and cephalad. Because of the relative difficulty in obtaining intravenous access in infants and children, ICI is used more frequently in these age groups.

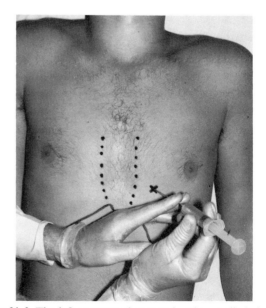

Figure 31–3. The left parasternal approach. The needle is inserted at a point perpendicular to the frontal plane, just over the sixth rib, two fingerbreadths from the left sternal border.

COMPLICATIONS

A reviewer of the literature on ICI will probably be baffled by the disparity between the anticipated high frequency of complications and the paucity of instances in which they have actually been documented (Table 31–1).

Coronary artery laceration is one of the most feared and frequently mentioned potential complications of ICI. Bodon, in his 1923 review of 90 cases,[17] found no instance of coronary artery laceration and quoted Brunning's calculation that the area occupied by the coronaries is less than 1/1000 of the area of the free walls of the heart. In 1954 Smith and coworkers, reporting on percutaneous ventriculography experiments in dogs, found one instance of left anterior descending artery laceration following 15 left parasternal injections.[42] Subsequently, 60 subxiphoid injections were accomplished without laceration. In more than 300 human ventriculographies involving subxiphoid injection, Lehman found no evidence of coronary artery laceration.[43] At a symposium on resuscitation in 1968, Holmdahl mentioned two instances of coronary artery laceration in his group's experience with human CPR, but the technique of injection was not specified. At that same symposium, Jude and associates reported never having seen this complication.[44] Amey and colleagues studied 29 survivors of cardiac arrests who had received a total of 47 ICIs. They compared this group with 67 patients who had survived cardiac arrest without the use of intracardiac medication. There were no significant differences between these two groups in the incidence of acute myocardial infarctions.[13] Davison and coworkers studied 53 patients who had received a total of 147 ICIs during cardiac arrest.[12] In the 24 nonsurvivors in whom an autopsy was performed, no evidence of coronary artery laceration was found. In the 29 survivors there was no clinical evidence to suggest coronary artery puncture or laceration. Saphir found no coronary artery lacerations at autopsy in 62 patients who had received a total of 155 ICIs during unsuccessful resuscitation attempts.[24] Similarly, Sabin and associates found no autopsy evidence of coronary lacerations in his group of 18 nonsurvivors who had received a total of 46 attempts at ICI.[45]

Coronary lacerations have been described, however, in two studies that used cadavers for experimental cardiac puncture. Sabin and colleagues found no coronary injuries in 17 cadavers following subxiphoid puncture, whereas four of 17 parasternal punctures resulted in laceration of the left anterior descending artery.[45] Brown and coworkers compared injuries produced by transthoracic pacemaker insertion, using six different techniques in each of 20 cadavers.[40] Six of 60 subxiphoid attempts lacerated the right coronary artery and three of 60 parasternal attempts produced lacerations of the left anterior descending artery. There are several possible explanations for the increased incidence of coronary injury seen in these studies. The experimental protocols may have allowed for a more careful search for needle injuries than would be possible in postmortems after clinical ICI during unsuccessful CPR. An immobile, contracted, postmortem heart may be more vulnerable to coronary laceration than the fibrillating, more dilated organ found during cardiac arrest. Moreover, postmortem anatomic relationships (with deflated lungs and a contracted heart) may differ significantly from those in life, making it difficult to apply results from cadaver studies to patients undergoing CPR.

Thus although coronary artery laceration is frequently mentioned as a hazard of ICI,[6–9, 42, 46] and has been reported during experimental postmortem injections,[40, 45] there is very little evidence to suggest that coronary laceration is a significant hazard of the clinical use of ICI during resuscitation.

Hemopericardium, however, appears to be relatively common following intracardiac injection. In a series of left ventriculographies using the intercostal approach, Bjork and colleagues found four instances of hemopericardium among 27 patients who underwent surgery following cardiac puncture.[47] In the same series were six instances of cardiac tamponade among 138 patients. Lehman found three instances of tamponade in more than 300 patients receiving transthoracic ventriculography by the subxiphoid approach.[43] Saphir reported nine cases of hemopericardium at autopsy in 62 patients following unsuccessful CPR and noted that this complication is associated with ICI.[24] Another study found evidence of hemopericardium in 12 of 39 patients by echocardiography or postmortem but no clinical evidence of tamponade in 29 survivors.[12]

Intuitively, one would expect *pneumothorax* to be a common occurrence following ICI. Bjork and coworkers reported pneumothorax in 8 of 138 patients in whom contrast was injected into the heart by the left parasternal approach.[47] McCaughan and Pate found two instances of this complication in 134 patients studied by the subxiphoid approach.[48] Chen identified a pneumothorax in five of 16 patients receiving left parasternal injections during CPR.[41] In the study by Amey and colleagues, three of 29 patients receiving ICI developed a pneumothorax, compared with only one of

Table 31–1. Complications of Intracardiac Injections

Study	Technique	Coronary Laceration*	Hemopericardium	Tamponade	Pneumothorax	Intramyocardial Injection
Pondsmenech, 1951[49]	subxiphoid	0(30)	0(30)	0(30)	0(30)	0(30)
Lehman et al, 1957[39]	subxiphoid	0(60)	11(35)	0(60)	0(60)	0(60)
McCaughan, Pate, 1957[48]	subxiphoid	0(29)	—	0(29)	2(29)	2(29)
Lehman, 1959[43]	subxiphoid	0(300)	—	3(300)	—	2(300)
Bjork et al, 1961[47]	parasternal	1(137)	4(27)	6(137)	8(137)	—
Amey et al, 1978[13]	parasternal and subxiphoid	0(33)	1(8)	0(8)	3(33)	—
Davison et al, 1980[12]	subxiphoid	0(53)	12(39)	0(29)	1(29)	—
Chen, 1981[41]	parasternal	—	—	—	5(16)	—
Sabin, 1983[45]	parasternal and subxiphoid	0(18)	—	—	2(18)	—
Total		1(660)	28(139)	9(593)	21(352)	4(419)

*Numbers in parentheses indicate number of patients examined for evidence of each complication.

64 who did not receive ICIs during CPR.[13] Davison and coworkers found only one instance of pneumothorax in 40 patients receiving ICI.[12]

The cadaver study by Brown and colleagues found no lung injuries following 60 subxiphoid and 20 parasternal border pacemaker insertions.[40] Lung puncture was found in 15 per cent of the cadavers subjected to a more lateral parasternal approach. The clinical significance of such puncture and its expected frequency in living subjects are unknown. In any case, the incidence of pneumothorax complicating ICI appears to be relatively low, especially if the subxiphoid approach is used.

The *intramyocardial injection* of contrast material has been associated with intractable ventricular fibrillation and death.[43] The combined results of two ventriculography series involving the subxiphoid approach showed that four of 434 patients underwent intramyocardial injections with subsequent ventricular fibrillation.[43, 48] This situation is probably not comparable with ICIs during CPR when the heart is not beating and injection must be made without the benefit of fluoroscopic guidance. It is unlikely that the true incidence of this dire complication, which may result in the same rhythm as was originally being treated, will ever be known.

Laceration of other organs is a potential complication that has rarely been reported as a consequence of ICI during human resuscitation. The subxiphoid approach brings the injecting needle close to the stomach and the left lobe of the liver, and Smith and colleagues reported hepatic laceration during subxiphoid injection in dog experiments.[42] Although Brown and coworkers reported 14 liver punctures in cadavers following 60 subxiphoid pacemaker insertions, no reports of liver or stomach laceration resulting from the clinical use of ICI are found in the literature. Brown and associates also found a high incidence of inadvertent right atrial puncture that complicated the subxiphoid approach. Based on evidence from clinical studies, it appears that this complication is either rare or of little clinical significance during human resuscitation.[12, 13, 45]

Punctures of the pulmonary artery and aorta have been reported by Sabin and coworkers following atypical parasternal approaches utilizing the second or third intercostal space.[45] Other potential complications include infection and air embolism. Although Bodon in 1923 described a case of fulminant pericarditis following intracardiac injection,[17] no subsequent incidence of pericarditis or endocarditis has been documented. Similarly, air embolism has not been reported.

Careful attention to technique minimizes the risk of some of these complications. During subxiphoid injection, the needle should form an angle of 30 to 45 degrees with the skin of the abdominal wall. A more vertical position may cause the needle to pass posterior to the heart and cause damage to the liver or the stomach. Applying constant suction on the syringe during insertion of the needle is necessary to ensure proper intracavitary positioning and thus to prevent intramyocardial injection. One may lessen the risk of pneumothorax by using the subxiphoid approach and by allowing passive deflation of the lungs before injection. Following a successful resuscitation, a chest film should be examined for evidence of pneumothorax.

By far the most common error in technique that we have observed is the repeated attempt at ICI after an initial failure *without the reinstitution of CPR*.

CONCLUSION

For more than 100 years, the intracardiac route has been used to deliver medication during cardiac arrest. Although the technique has been shown to be effective, its popularity declined because of the availability of other effective routes for drug administration and

the fear of potential complications. A review of the literature suggests that these fears are overstated. Although intracardiac puncture is not recommended as the initial route of injection, it should be retained as a valid technique for the administration of emergency drugs during CPR when other routes are not readily available.

REFERENCES

1. Eisenberg MS, Bergner L, Hallstrom A: Cardiac resuscitation in the community. JAMA 241:1905, 1979.
2. Redding JS, Pearson JW: Evaluation of drugs for cardiac resuscitation. Anesthesiology 24:203, 1963.
3. Pearson JW, Redding JS: Epinephrine in cardiac resuscitation. Am Heart J 66:210, 1963.
4. McIntyre KM, Lewis AJ (eds): Textbook of Advanced Cardiac Life Supports. Dallas, American Heart Association, 1981.
5. Massey FC (ed): Clinical cardiology. Baltimore, Williams & Wilkins, 1953, p 872.
6. Goldberg AH: Cardiopulmonary arrest. N Engl J Med 290:381, 1974.
7. Enarson DA, Gracey DR: Complications of cardiopulmonary resuscitation. Heart Lung 5:805, 1976.
8. Philips JH, Burch GE: Management of cardiac arrest. Am Heart J 67:265, 1964.
9. Redding JS, Asuncion FS, Pearson JW: Effective routes of drug administration during cardiac arrest. Anesth Analg 46:253, 1967.
10. Roberts JR, Greenberg MI, Baskin SI: Endotracheal epinephrine in cardiorespiratory collapse. JACEP 8:515, 1979.
11. Roberts JR, Greenberg MI, Baskin SI: Blood levels following intravenous and endotracheal epinephrine administration. JACEP 8:53, 1979.
12. Davison R, Barresi V, Parker M, et al: Intracardiac injections during cardiopulmonary resuscitation. JAMA 244:1110, 1980.
13. Amey BD, Harrison EE, Staub EJ, et al: Paramedic use of intracardiac medication in prehospital sudden cardiac death. JACEP 7:130, 1978.
14. Fantus B: The technic of medication. JAMA 87:563, 1926.
15. Zuntz H: Wiederbelebung durch intracardiale Injektion. Munch Med Wschr 21:562, 1919.
16. Rüdiger G: Die intracardiale Injektion. Wien Med Wochenschr 1916, #4.
17. Bodon C: The intracardiac injection of adrenalin. Lancet 1:586, 1923.
18. Resuscitations and intracardiac injections (editorial). JAMA 94:107, 1930.
19. Hyman AS: Resuscitation of the stopped heart by intracardiac therapy. Arch Intern Med 46:553, 1930.
20. Beecher HK, Linton RR: Epinephrine in cardiac resuscitation. JAMA 135(2):90, 1947.
21. Kay JH: The treatment of cardiac arrest. Surg Gynecol Obstet 93:682, 1951.
22. Gerbode F: The cardiac emergency. Ann Surg 135(3):431, 1952.
23. Lillehei CW, Lavadia PG, Dewall RA, Sellers RD: Four years' experience with external cardiac resuscitation. JAMA 193:651, 1965.
24. Saphir R: External cardiac massage. Medicine 47:73, 1968.
25. Schechter DC: Transthoracic epinephrine injection in heart resuscitation is dangerous. JAMA 234:1184, 1975.
26. Del Guercio LRM, Coomarswamy RP, State D: Cardiac output and other hemodynamic variables during external cardiac massage in man. N Engl J Med 269:1398, 1963.
27. Kuhn GJ, White BC, Swetnam RF, et al: Peripheral versus central circulation times during CPR: A pilot study. Ann Emerg Med 10:417, 1981.
28. Barsan WG, Levy RC, Weir H: Lidocaine levels during CPR: Differences after peripheral venous, central venous, and intracardiac injections. Ann Emerg Med 10:73, 1981.
29. Emerman CL, Pinchak AE, Hagen JF, et al: The effect of injection site on circulation times during CPR. Crit Care Med 17:412, 1988.
30. Iseri LT, Humphrey SB, Siner EJ: Prehospital brady-asystolic cardiac arrest. Ann Intern Med 88:741, 1978.
31. Hurst JW: Cardiopulmonary resuscitation. In Hurst JW (ed): New York, McGraw-Hill Book Co, 1978, pp 734–744.
32. American Heart Association: Standards and guidelines for cardiopulmonary resuscitation (CPR) and emergency cardiac care (ECC). JAMA 244:453, 1980.
33. McIntyre KM, Lewis AJ (eds): Textbook of Advanced Cardiac Life Support. Dallas, American Heart Association, 1981.
34. Riker WL: Cardiac arrest in infants and children. Pediatr Clin North Am 16:661, 1969.
35. Anthony CL Jr, Crawford EW, Morgan BC: Management of cardiac and respiratory arrest in children. Clin Pediatr 8:647, 1969.
36. Scarpelli EM, Auld PAM, Goldman HS: Airway management, mechanical ventilation and cardiopulmonary resuscitation. In Scarpelli EM, et al (eds): Pulmonary Disease of the Fetus, Newborn and Child. Philadelphia, Lea & Febiger, 1978, p 123.
37. Huszar RJ: Emergency Cardiac Care. Bowie, Md, Robert J Brady, 1974, p 200.
38. Pearson JW: Historical and experimental approaches to modern resuscitation. Springfield, Ill, Charles C Thomas, 1965, p 70.
39. Lehman JS, Masser BG, Lykens HD: Cardiac ventriculography. Am J Roentgenol Rad Ther Nuclear Med 77:207, 1957.

40. Brown CG, Gurley HT, Hutchins GM, et al: Injuries associated with percutaneous placement of transthoracic pacemakers. Ann Emerg Med 14:223, 1985.
41. Chen HH: Closed-chest intracardiac injection. Resuscitation 9:103, 1981.
42. Smith PW, Wilson CW, Cregg HA, Klossen KP: Cardioangiography. J Thorac Surg 28:273, 1954.
43. Lehman JS: Cardiac ventriculography: Practical considerations. Prog Cardiovasc Dis 2:52, 1959.
44. Jude JR, Neumaster T, Kfoury E: Vasopressor-cardiotonic drugs in cardiac resuscitation. Acta Anesth Scand 9(Suppl):147, 1968.
45. Sabin HI, Coghill SB, Khunti K, McNeill GO: Accuracy of intracardiac injections determined by a postmortem study. Lancet 2:1054, 1983.
46. Enarson DA, Gracey DR: Complications of cardiopulmonary resuscitation. Heart Lung 5:805, 1976.
47. Bjork VO, Cullhed I, Hallen A, et al: Sequelae of left ventricular puncture with angiocardiography. Circulation 24:204, 1961.
48. McCaughan JJ Jr, Pate JW: Aortography utilizing percutaneous left ventricular puncture. Arch Surg 75:746, 1957.
49. Pondsmenech ER: Heart puncture in man for Diodrast visualization of the ventricular chambers and great arteries. Am Heart J 41:643, 1951.

Chapter **32**

The Clinical Use of Doppler Ultrasound

Thomas Stair

INTRODUCTION

Doppler ultrasound is an indispensable aid in the clinical evaluation of a wide variety of pathologic conditions encountered in the emergency department. Doppler ultrasound is commonly used to measure blood pressure in infants and in patients with low-flow states and to detect fetal heart sounds in utero. With a basic knowledge of waveform analysis and blood flow characteristics, Doppler ultrasound can also help in assessing arterial injury, venous thrombosis, and arterial occlusive disease. The techniques are relatively easy to master, and the equipment is both inexpensive and portable.

PRINCIPLES OF DOPPLER ULTRASOUND

The phenomenon of the Doppler shift was first described by Christian Doppler in 1843, but it was not until the 1960s that the principle was applied to medical diagnosis. The Doppler phenomenon can be stated as follows: when sound waves are transmitted to and then reflected from a moving object, the waves will return to a stationary emitting source at a frequency that is different from the originally transmitted wave. The returning frequency will be higher if the object is moving toward the emitting source and lower if the object is moving away. The change in frequency (Doppler shift) between the transmitted and reflected sound wave can be quantified and expressed as an index of the velocity of the target particle from which the sound wave was reflected. The major clinical application of Doppler ultrasound is the detection of blood flow when the target particle is a moving erythrocyte. The general formula used to determine the Doppler shift is

$$\Delta f = \frac{2f_T \, V \cos \theta}{c}$$

where Δf = frequency shift (Doppler shift); f_T = transmitting frequency (usually 2–10×10^6 cycles per second or 2–10 MHz); V = velocity of reflectors (erythrocytes); θ = angle between the incident/reflected beam and the path of reflectors; and c = velocity of sound in tissue (about 1.5×10^5 cm per second).

Medical Doppler devices couple an energy source to a transmitting piezoelectric crystal and a receiving crystal. Both crystals are placed adjacent to each other at the tip of a probe, which is held against the skin. The processing circuitry of the device transforms the Doppler shift to an audible sound that may be heard with the aid of a speaker or earphones. Some devices are equipped with gauges that quantify the velocity of flow both toward and away from the transmitting crystal and with a chart recorder to permanently record the waveform. Devices that can detect the direction of flow are termed *directional Dopplers*, but an audible pulse may be heard if the flow is either toward or away from the probe.

Figure 32–1 is a diagram of a basic Doppler ultrasound device. Figures 32–2 and 32–3 are two of the nonrecording, nondirectional Dopplers that are popular in the emergency department. Figure 32–4 is a recording directional Doppler. All Doppler devices detect only the *velocity*, not the volume, of blood flow. Therefore, the intensity of the audible signal and the height of the waveform on the printout are representations of velocity, not of flow volume. Although the pitch of the audible signal may change as velocity changes, changes in the volume and clarity of the sound are related to technique, proximity of the artery, and angle at which the vessel is studied. These facts are critical in the interpretation of the results of a Doppler examination.

Blood velocity must be at least 6 cm per second to be detected by currently available Doppler devices. This flow rate is normally found in all arteries and most major peripheral veins, allowing both the arterial and venous systems to be studied.

Smaller piezoelectric crystals are best for measuring flow velocity in small, superficial vessels, whereas larger crystals, approximately a centimeter square, are better for larger vessels and deeper fetal heart sounds. Lower frequency sound waves penetrate deeper tissues with less scatter, whereas higher frequencies provide better resolution of superficial vessels. Frequencies of 2 to 5 MHz are best for fetal heart sounds; 5 to 10 MHz are appropriate for limb arteries and veins; 8 to 10 MHz are best for testicular blood flow assessment; and 10 MHz are used for perivascular intraoperative probes. Doppler instruments are usually supplied with a fixed frequency; however, variable frequency devices are available.

An interface of acoustic gel (not to be confused with abrasive electrical conductive gel or electrocardiographic gel) must be used to couple the piezoelectric crystals to the skin, both to protect the crystals and to reduce attenuation and reflection of the ultrasound signal. At every air-fluid interface, approximately 99.9 per cent of sound will be reflected and 0.1 per cent transmitted, a 30-decibel decrease in sound volume. This attenuation by reflection limits Doppler use in the anterior abdomen, chest, and skull.

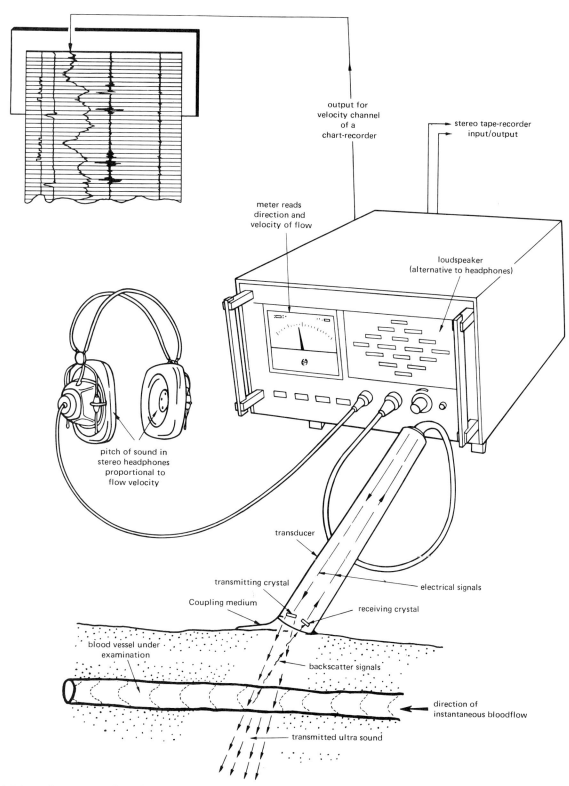

Figure 32–1. Schematic representation of a Doppler ultrasound device. (From Blood velocity waveforms and the physiological interpretation. Sonicaid, Inc., Fredericksburg, Va., p 4. Reproduced by permission.)

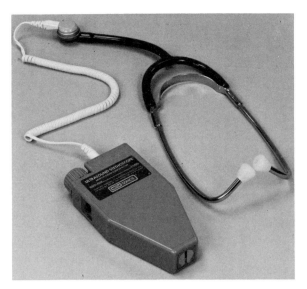

Figure 32–2. Pocket Doppler stethoscope (model BF4A. Medsonics, Inc., Los Altos, Calif.)

After good acoustic contact with the skin has been made, the probe is slowly angled in several directions until an optimum vascular flow signal is received. From the previous equation, because cos θ equals 1, it is evident that frequency shifts will be greatest when the probe is pointed up or down the vessel, using the most acute angle that allows good skin contact. In practice, this is usually about 45 degrees toward the axis of flow. Flow may often be detected by a probe that is held at right angles to the direction of flow; however, the amplitude of the signal will be increased by angling the probe.

Doppler flowmeters that are commonly used in the emergency department have a continuous output of sound waves. Pulsed or electronically gated ultrasound more accurately measures arterial flow velocities, velocity profile, and vessel diameter. Coupled with a position-sensing transducer and a storage oscilloscope, these devices can even produce images of arterial flow in much the same manner as B-mode ultrasound imaging but are specific for moving blood and are comparable to arteriography. The devices that are discussed in this chapter, however, do not display an image on a screen.

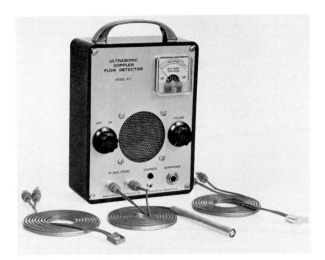

Figure 32–3. Ultrasonic Doppler Flow Detector with speaker and probes (model 811, Parks Electronics Laboratories, Aloha, Ore.)

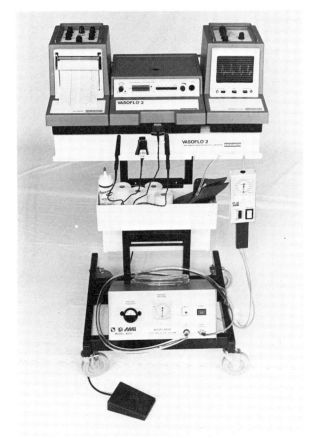

Figure 32–4. A recording directional Doppler device allows sophisticated waveform analysis.

ARTERIAL EVALUATION

Waveforms and Flow Characteristics

The audible signal and graphic waveforms obtained from Doppler devices are subject to analysis and detailed interpretation.[1] If the patient may possibly have arterial disease, from either trauma or occlusive disease, the waveform tracing or sounds from a potentially abnormal vessel, or both, should be compared with data from a normal vessel on the opposite side of the body.

The Doppler waveform of a normal pulse in most peripheral arteries, such as the brachial, femoral, dorsalis pedis, and radial arteries, consists of three components: late systolic forward flow, early diastolic reverse flow, and late diastolic forward flow (also termed *diastolic oscillation*). In a normal artery, one can always hear the first two components and, with practice, the third sound can usually be distinguished. The audible sound wave resembles a double ricochet sound. Various arterial waveforms are shown in Figure 32–5.

In the normal artery, late systolic forward flow is a sharp peak of increased frequency that is damped somewhat distally but remains the most prominent feature of the velocity waveform (Fig. 32–6). This phase is followed immediately by a negative deflection that is not quite as sharp and about half the amplitude, representing early diastolic reverse flow. This reverse flow and subsequent late diastolic oscillation are produced by elastic recoil of the arterial wall and thus are reduced by extensive atherosclerosis, decreased peripheral vascular resistance, or vasodilation.

Reverse flow and velocity oscillations are naturally

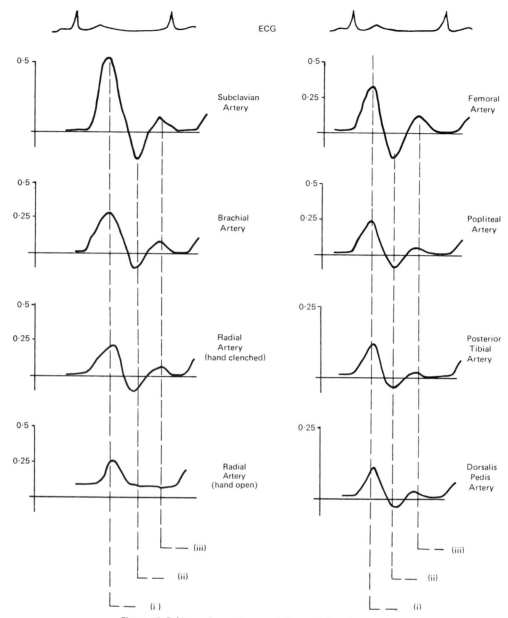

Figure 32–5. Normal waveforms of the peripheral system.

damped distally and may normally be absent in the most distal arteries such as the digital arteries or dorsalis pedis artery (Fig. 32–7). Flow through collateral channels tends to lose the reverse phase, and loss of reverse flow may precede angiographically demonstrable arterial disease (Fig. 32–8).[2, 3]

Arterial Disease

A Doppler device equipped with or without a graphic display can be helpful in the emergency department assessment of a patient with limb trauma by audibly or visually demonstrating the arterial blood flow waveforms of both the injured and uninjured limbs. Much information may be gained by listening to the flow, but to fully evaluate an artery, the printout of the waveform is required. Although significant arterial injury may be present despite good distal pulses, damping of early systolic flow or loss of early diastolic reverse flow and late diastolic oscillations are much more sensitive signs of arterial injury or disease.[1, 2]

To evaluate a peripheral artery, place the probe at various sites over the distal artery and listen for the three-component sound while recording the waveform on the readout device. Arterial injury and disease (such as intimal

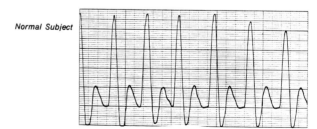

Figure 32–6. Tracing from a femoral artery. Late systolic flow appears as a sharp peak. There is good reverse flow in early diastole. Clear oscillations are seen during diastole. The peak systolic velocity is about 30 cm per second. (From Doppler evaluation of peripheral arterial disease: A clinical handbook. Sonicaid, Inc., Fredericksburg, Va. Reproduced by permission.)

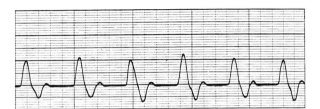

Figure 32–7. Tracing from the dorsalis pedis artery. Although reduced in amplitude at this peripheral site, all characteristics of a healthy waveform persist. The peak systolic velocity is about 12 cm per second. The zero flow at end-diastole is normal in the dorsalis pedis artery. (From Doppler evaluation of peripheral arterial disease: A clinical handbook. Sonicaid, Inc., Fredericksburg, Va. Reproduced by permission.)

damage, thrombosis, stenosis, external compression, and complete disruption) affect the peak velocity of blood flow and modify both the audible sound and the shape of the recorded waveform (Fig. 32–9). A normal Doppler evaluation of an artery is evidence against arterial pathology but is not always conclusive. Pathology should be suspected from even subtle changes in the flow characteristics or waveform analysis, especially if these changes are not seen on the opposite side. It must be stressed that *simply hearing the arterial flow with the Doppler device does not ensure a normal artery.*

Collateral blood flow, although minimal, may be enough to produce an audible pulse that can be detected with sensitive equipment. Collateral flow may even produce a measurable blood pressure despite significant pathology in the proximal artery. The three-component waveform analysis is helpful in such situations. The waveform is also sensitive to vasoconstriction, hypovolemia or vasodilation, temperature changes, and the normal aging process as well as to arterial injury or occlusion (Fig. 32–10). From a technical standpoint, one must keep these variables in mind. In addition, a 45-degree angle must be maintained between the probe and the skin.

Blood Pressure Evaluation

Besides evaluating flow characteristics and waveform analysis of an artery, Doppler-assisted blood pressures should be taken to aid in the evaluation of any extremity.[4]

Because Doppler ultrasound is more sensitive and less suceptible to technical artifacts than auscultation by a stethoscope or detection of a pulse by palpation and because it detects flow rather than turbulence or pulsation, the Doppler device can be used to measure blood pressures that are not accessible for auscultation or palpation. Doppler readings of systolic blood pressure are accurate to as low as 30 mm Hg. (Diastolic pressures cannot be determined.) Such measurements can be of significant clinical value in obese patients, in newborns, and in infants.

The probe is placed over a distal artery, such as the radial or ulnar artery at the wrist or the posterior tibial or dorsalis pedis artery at the ankle or foot, while a sphygmomanometer cuff is inflated proximally and slowly deflated. The pressure at which flow is first heard is recorded as the systolic pressure under the cuff. In addition to blood pressure determinations, segmental blood pressures can be measured to help document the level of arterial disease.[2, 3, 5–7] This is done with the cuff at four sites along each leg.

When evaluating peripheral vascular disease by the use of Doppler-assisted blood pressure determinations, compare the systolic pressure at the ankle and in the brachial artery

(Fig. 32–11). Normally, the ankle systolic pressure (when supine) is higher than the brachial artery systolic pressure and the ankle to brachial index (ratio) is greater than 1. If the index is less than 1, it is suggestive of occlusive peripheral vascular disease in the leg (Fig. 32–12). If segmental pressures are taken, the area of occlusion may be predicted (Fig. 32–13). Ratios between 0.6 and 0.8 are seen with symptoms of claudication; measurements between 0.4 and 0.6 are common with leg pain at rest; and ratios less than 0.5 are frequently seen with gangrene.[8, 9] An exception may occur in diabetic patients who have calcified peripheral arteries. The rigid calcific vessels may be difficult to compress, and a systolic pressure in the range of 250 to 300 mm Hg will be obtained when there is severe vascular insufficiency.

Carotid Vessel Evaluation

Occlusion or stenosis of the internal carotid artery may be assessed with a *directional* Doppler device by noting the direction of flow in the supraorbital artery and by changes in the flow.[10–13] Place the probe over the supraorbital artery, just below the inferior margin of the medial supraorbital ridge, and angle it into the orbit (Fig. 32–14). The direction of flow, either toward or away from the probe, is noted by the waveform recording or by the directional gauges on the directional Doppler device. *Normally blood flow is pulsatile and out of the orbit toward the probe.* Greater than 50 per cent occlusion of the internal carotid artery on one side decreases flow forces enough to leave the supraorbital artery supplied by collaterals from the external carotid and the superficial temporal arteries. The net result is that flow is now *into* the orbit and *away* from the probe. Often damped late diastolic oscillations and other changes in the waveform, which are the result of collateral circulation, can be noted. The opposite side is used for comparison.

Certain compression maneuvers may further elucidate this situation. Normally, compression of the ipsilateral superficial temporal artery will augment flow through the internal carotid system by reducing back pressure of the collaterals, and compression of this artery will increase flow

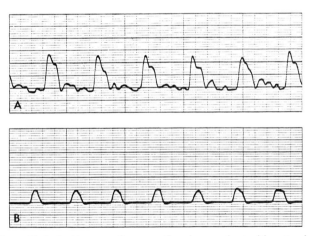

Figure 32–8. *A*, Absence of reverse flow in a patient with extensive occlusions (femoral artery). *B*, Monophasic pulsatility. A monophasic pattern has a readily distinguishable systolic pulse but a lack of oscillatory activity during diastole. Such patterns demonstrate diminished arterial compliance. They may indicate a stenosis proximal to the examination site, a low resistance in distal vessels, or both. (From Doppler evaluation of peripheral arterial disease: A clinical handbook. Sonicaid, Inc., Fredericksburg, Va. Reproduced by permission.)

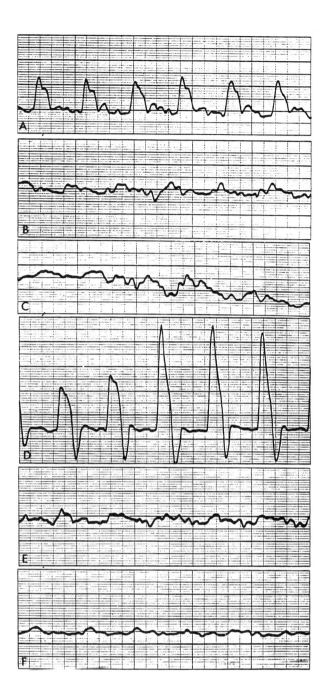

Figure 32–9. Tracings from a patient with severe multilevel disease. This patient, age 64, exhibits symptoms of generalized atherosclerosis and also suffers from polycythemia.

A, Left femoral artery. Pulsatility is adequate, but the peak systolic velocity is only about 7 cm per second. The systolic pulse is wide. There is no reverse flow. The diastolic portion exhibits some oscillation but less than is expected at the femoral site.

B, Left posterior tibial artery. At this level, pulsatility is essentially absent. The maximum velocity is about 7 cm per second, suggesting a patent artery distal to an occlusion in which flow is virtually all derived from collaterals. The left leg ankle to brachial pressure index was determined to be 0.61, also consistent with severe occlusion.

C, Left dorsalis pedis artery. Pulsatility is entirely absent. The velocity is so low that it is at the lower limit of measurability by Doppler techniques. At times, an adjacent venous signal swamps the recording.

D, Right femoral artery. This side yields a much better waveform than that of the left femoral *(A)*. Peak systolic velocity is about 30 cm per second. There is good early diastolic reverse flow. The absence of diastolic oscillations suggests rigid, noncompliant arteries distally.

E, Right posterior tibial artery. The waveform is nonpulsatile, and the maximum velocity is only about 3 cm per second. The right leg ankle to brachial pressure index was 0.58, even lower than that in the left leg.

F, Right dorsalis pedis artery. The completely nonpulsatile appearance of this waveform signifies collateral flow. Again, the maximum forward velocity is a barely measurable 3 cm per second.

(From Doppler evaluation of peripheral arterial disease: A clinical handbook. Sonicaid, Inc., Fredericksburg, Va. Reproduced by permission.)

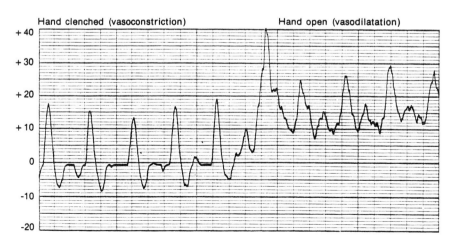

Figure 32–10. Simulated effects of vasoconstriction and vasodilation in the normal radial artery. Vasoconstriction of the lumen can mimic the effect of distal obstructions in the pathway. Vasodilation, on the other hand, can partially mask evidence of occlusion. Therefore, it is necessary for the user of Doppler procedures to be aware of these phenomena. The rather dramatic difference in the patterns obtained during vasoconstriction and vasodilation can be simulated easily in the radial artery by performing the following experiment with a normal subject: Place the transducer over the radial artery and run a waveform with the fist tightly clenched to shut off the network of arteries and capillaries in the hand. As shown in the figure, the pattern obtained changes remarkably, depending on whether vasoconstriction or vasodilation is occurring. (From Doppler evaluation of peripheral arterial disease: A clinical handbook. Sonicaid, Inc., Fredericksburg, Va. Reproduced by permission.)

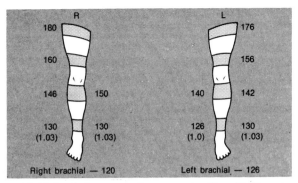

Figure 32–11. Typical pressures in a normal subject. Findings, based on resting pressures, show no evidence of occlusive disease of the large- or medium-sized arteries.

Significant Findings (normal):

1. Ankle to brachial pressure index 1.0 or greater.
2. All pressure gradients less than 30 mm Hg.
3. Upper thigh pressure at least 40 mm Hg above brachial pressure.

(From Doppler evaluation of peripheral arterial disease: A clinical handbook. Sonicaid, Inc., Fredericksburg, Va. Reproduced by permission.)

out of the orbit and toward the probe (Fig. 32–15*A*). If the internal carotid artery is occluded, compression of the superficial temporal artery will decrease or stop flow in the supraorbital artery (Fig. 32–15*B*).[10]

EVALUATION OF THE VENOUS SYSTEM

Although Doppler ultrasound can be used to show varicose veins and postthrombotic valvular incompetency, its greatest clinical value is in demonstrating venous obstruction caused by deep vein thrombophlebitis.[14–18] History and physical examination alone are unreliable means of diagnosing deep venous thrombophlebitis. Iliofemoral thrombi are unlikely to produce clinical signs and symptoms, yet they often embolize to the lung. Other diagnostic tests are time consuming, expensive, or hazardous.

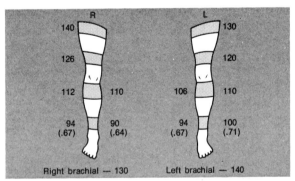

Figure 32–12. Typical pressures in a patient with obstruction of the abdominal aorta or bilateral iliac obstruction.

Significant Findings:

1. Ankle to brachial pressure index less than 1.0.
2. All segmental gradients less than 30 mm Hg.
3. Both upper thigh pressures low with respect to brachial pressure.

Findings are suggestive of severe aorto-iliac occlusive disease. (From Doppler evaluation of peripheral arterial disease: A clinical handbook. Sonicaid, Inc., Fredericksburg, Va. Reproduced by permission.)

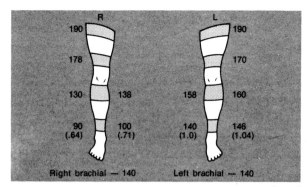

Figure 32–13. Typical pressures in a patient with obstruction of the popliteal or tibial arteries.

Significant Findings:

1. Ankle to brachial pressure index less than 1.0 in right leg.
2. Abnormally high gradient from ankle to below knee and again from below to above knee in right leg.
3. Upper thigh pressures are 50 mm Hg higher than brachial pressures, consistent with normal flow at the aorto-iliac level.

Findings are suggestive of a right popliteal occlusion or an anterior and posterior tibial occlusion, or both. (From Doppler evaluation of peripheral arterial disease: A clinical handbook. Sonicaid, Inc., Fredericksburg, Va. Reproduced by permission.)

Although contrast phlebography or venography is the best technique for revealing deep venous thrombi, it is technically demanding and expensive and involves the risks of radiation exposure and dye allergy and may itself cause thrombophlebitis. Radionuclide scanning with technetium 99m–labeled albumin is technically similar to venography, with less resolution but fewer hazards. Scanning with ^{125}I-labeled fibrinogen is sensitive for active thrombogenesis in the calf but is of little use for detecting established iliofemoral clot. Impedance plethysmography measures the decrease in diameter of the leg after a venous tourniquet is removed and, like Doppler ultrasound, is most sensitive for the iliofemoral thrombi.

Doppler ultrasound and impedance plethysmography share similar (80 to 90 per cent) published sensitivities and specificities in detecting deep venous thrombi. Both techniques can be carried out by a technician, both require calibration and semiportable equipment, and both produce

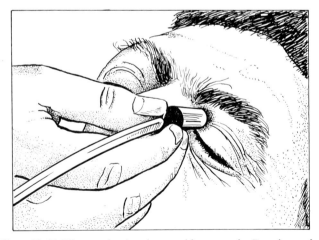

Figure 32–14. When evaluating the carotid system, the Doppler probe is placed on the inferior portion of the medial supraorbital ridge and aimed into the orbit. The probe is moved until a strong supraorbital pulse is noted.

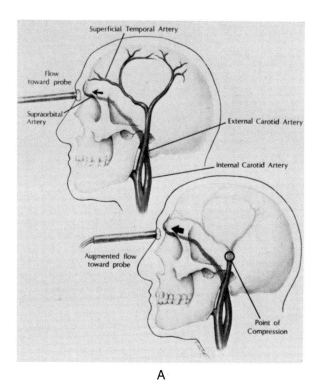

A

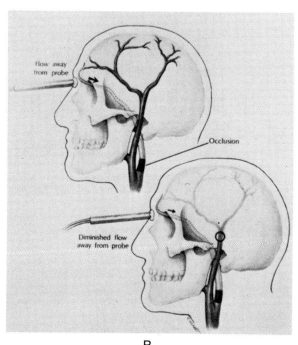

B

Figure 32–15. *A,* The normal direction of blood flow in the supraorbital carotid artery is toward the probe *(top).* With compression of the superficial temporal artery, this flow is augmented *(bottom). B,* With occlusion of the internal carotid artery, flow in the supraorbital artery is away from the probe *(top),* because flow is mainly from the external carotid system. This flow is diminished by compression of the superficial temporal artery *(bottom).* (From LoGerfo FW, Mason GR: Directional Doppler studies of supraorbital artery flow in internal carotid stenosis and occlusion. Surgery 76:724, 1974. Reproduced by permission.)

hard-copy documentation. Doppler ultrasound, however, may also be used in another mode, one that is particularly suited to the emergency department, in the form of a portable, battery-powered device with an audible output (see

Figs. 32–2 and 32–3) to be used by the physician at the bedside to guide immediate clinical decision making.

A patient who has leg pain with swelling, warmth, or discoloration has a differential diagnosis that includes edema, cellulitis, hematoma, and thrombophlebitis. The clinician may, in 5 minutes at the bedside, perform a screening Doppler examination, guiding the subsequent choice of more invasive tests.

In the first 2 years of its use at the University of Iowa, Barnes compared Doppler ultrasound with 122 venograms. The results indicated both a sensitivity and specificity of 94 per cent.[15] Sumner summarized the results of 10 previous studies that had an overall accuracy of 88 per cent, and, in his own study, the results showed an overall accuracy of 94 per cent.[16] In a further study of 156 patients, Doppler evaluation was 94 per cent sensitive and 90 per cent specific in detecting thrombi above the knee and 91 per cent sensitive and 84 per cent specific in detecting thrombi below the knee, with an overall accuracy of 92 per cent.[17] In a review of these and other studies of hand-held Doppler ultrasonography for deep venous thrombi, Turnbull and Dymowski conclude that symptomatic emergency department patients with a positive Doppler study have a high probability of deep venous occlusion (greater than 90 per cent).[19]

Venous Flow Characteristics

Doppler flow characteristics of the venous system differ from those of the arterial system in several important aspects. Flow rates in the peripheral veins may be near the threshold of sensitivity of the instrument and may require various maneuvers to augment the flow velocity. Venous flow does not exhibit arterial-type waveforms, and the flow may be affected by several external variables, leading to false-positive examination results. Some peripheral veins may even be occluded by firm pressure with the Doppler skin probe. Because major arteries and veins often course together but in different directions, one must be able to differentiate flow patterns, either by a trained ear or by the use of directional flowmeters. The most striking difference from the characteristic pulsatile arterial pulse is the low-pitched, soft, blowing, and extended sound of venous flow. The sound of venous flow is best described as a "wind-storm" sound.

When examining the venous system, assess both spontaneous venous flow and augmented venous flow. Spontaneous venous flow sounds can usually be heard in a normal peripheral vein. The absence of spontaneous flow is an indicator of disease, and the presence of spontaneous flow is a sign of a patent vein. Normal spontaneous flow is phasic with respiration and is *not continuous.* Continuous flow in a peripheral vein is a sign of venous disease. Holding one's breath will momentarily stop venous flow in the legs, but even peak normal inspiration will increase the intra-abdominal pressure enough to momentarily decrease (stop) venous flow. Expiration will release the pressure and allow venous flow to increase, producing the characteristic phasic flow during respiration. This phasic flow during respiration can be distinguished in most large peripheral veins, and its presence is a sensitive indicator of a normal vein.

Because spontaneous phasic venous flow is such a sensitive indicator of a normal vein, one must be certain not to produce false-positive examination results owing to technical errors. A false-positive test result may be produced by conditions and situations as subtle as patient anxiety, which tenses muscles; vasoconstriction owing to a cold room; hyperextension of the knee; elevation of the legs; the recent use of elastic support hose; or the patient's raising his head to look at the examiner. Note that if positive-pressure ventilation is used, the respiratory variation of venous flow is reversed.

Venous flow may be augmented both by compression distal to the site being examined and by releasing previous obstructing pressure at a site proximal to the area being examined. As with arterial flow, venous flow may be evaluated by its available characteristics and by the waveforms produced on a recorder (Figs. 32–16 and 32–17).

Venous Examination Technique

In many sites, it is necessary first to locate the arterial flow signal and then the venous sound. Sigel and colleagues termed the spontaneous flow sound, with its respiratory variation, the *S* sound and the brief rush of blood obtained by distal compression and other augmentation maneuvers the *A* sound.[14, 18] Six characteristics of venous flow that should be checked at each examination are patent vein, spontaneous flow, phasic flow (with respiration), augmented flow (with distal compression or release of proximal compression), competence of valves, and nonpulsatile flow.[15]

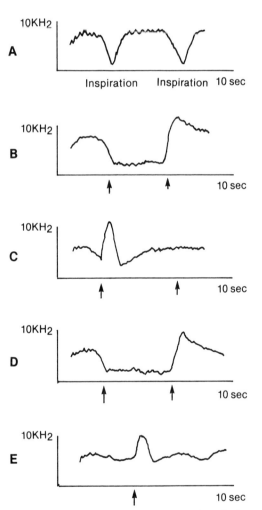

Figure 32–16. Normal Doppler ultrasound recording during examination of the left veins. *A*, Normal respiratory variation at the common femoral vein. Flow decreased with inspiration. *B*, Abolition of femoral vein flow with Valsalva maneuver and return with release. *C*, Augmentation of femoral vein flow with calf compression and no effect of release. *D*, Posterior tibial vein flow slowed by calf compression and augmented by release. *E*, Augmentation of saphenous flow by percussion (note damped respiratory variation).

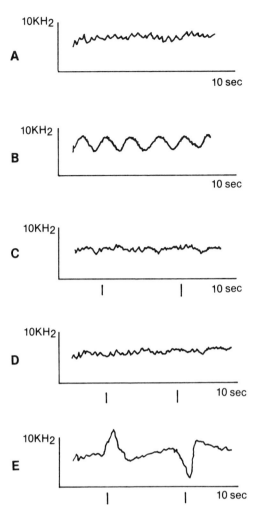

Figure 32–17. Abnormal findings in leg veins. *A*, Lack of respiratory variation. *B*, Pulsatile flow of congestive heart failure (normal in neck and proximal arm veins). *C*, No augmentation with distal compression (suggests obstruction). *D*, No decrease with proximal compression or augmentation with release (obstruction). *E*, Normal augmentation with distal compression, yet retrograde flow with release (suggests incompetent distal valves).

The standardized examination of venous flow in the legs described by Barnes and coworkers[15] is as follows: With the patient in a supine position, the head of the bed should be elevated 30 degrees and the patient's legs should be rotated slightly externally and flexed at the hip and knee. The examiner first locates the flow signal of the posterior tibial vein, posterior to the medial malleolus. After generously applying acoustic gel, the probe is angled at about 45 degrees to the skin, being careful not to press so hard that flow is diminished in the vein. The examiner listens for respiratory variations in the venous flow, if present at this level; compresses the foot, which should augment flow; and then releases the foot, which should not affect flow (Fig. 32–18). Compression should be gentle but brisk. The machine is sensitive enough to identify changes with only light compression. Repeated compressions may drain the leg of blood for a few minutes. It is best to minimize the compressions to avoid false results.

The next site to examine in this position is the common femoral vein, in the femoral triangle, just inferior to the inguinal ligament and medial to the femoral artery, which can be located by palpating the pulse and hearing the characteristic arterial flow. As an aside, congestive heart

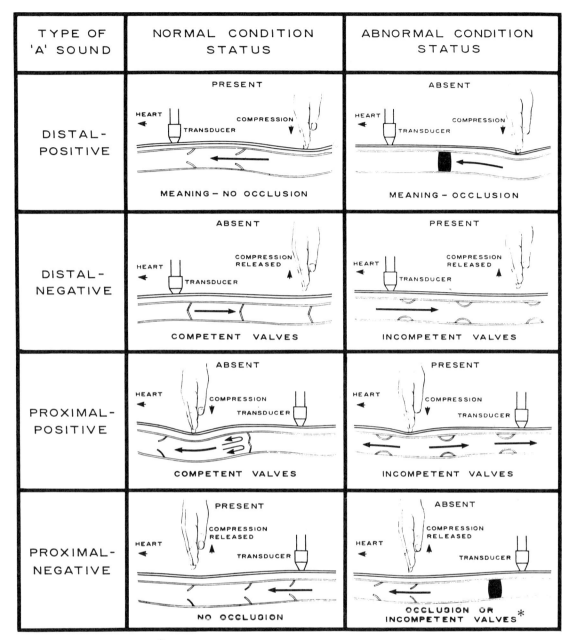

Figure 32–18. The types of *A* sounds and their meaning when present or absent. (From Sigel B, Popky GL, Mapp EM, et al: Evaluation of Doppler ultrasound examination: Its use in diagnosis of lower extremity venous disease. Arch Surg 100:535, 1970. Copyright 1970, American Medical Association.)

failure may produce a pulsatile flow in the common femoral vein. In the femoral vein, there should normally be variations with respiration. Normally inspiration decreases venous flow, whereas expiration increases venous flow, as a result of diaphragmatic movement. A sustained Valsalva maneuver should temporarily stop venous flow and produce an easily identifiable augmentation in flow when it is released. Lack of this augmentation may be a sign of iliofemoral occlusion.

Next, with the probe still over the common femoral vein, the examiner should compress the calf. This should produce augmentation of flow. Subsequent release of the calf should not alter the flow. A lack of augmentation on calf compression or an asymmetric effect suggests occlusion between the calf and the groin. Distal flow on release suggests

incompetent valves. Finally, the thigh should be compressed and released, resulting in the same results and interpretation as calf compression.

The next vein to examine is the superficial femoral vein, in the adductor canal at midthigh, alongside the superficial femoral artery. The examination is the same as that for the common femoral vein except that with the probe at midthigh it is pointless to compress the thigh.

To examine the popliteal vein, the patient must lie in the prone position with a pillow placed under the foot so that the knee is slightly flexed. The popliteal vein is usually best heard just lateral to the popliteal artery. After noting respiratory variations, the examiner can compress and release the thigh, which should slow or stop flow without

Table 32–1. Test Procedure and Interpretation for Deep Venous Thrombosis

Test Procedure Locate vein by using corresponding artery; perform following steps at each examination site*	Findings and Clinical Significance (Sounds usually graded as present, diminished, or absent)			
	Normal		Abnormal	
	FINDING	INTERPRETATION	FINDING	INTERPRETATION
Listen for spontaneous flow sounds	Present (may be absent at ankle)	No significant occlusions	Absent or diminished (at any site above ankle)	Significant occlusions present
Listen for effect of respiration	Sound phasic with respiration	Normal intra-abdominal pressure	Not phasic with respiration	High intra-abdominal pressure
Listen for pulsatility	Sound not pulsatile	Normal venous pressure	Sound pulsates with heart beat	High venous pressure— consider congestive heart failure
Apply compression distal to probe	Augmented sound present	No occlusion between site compressed and probe	Augmented sound diminished or absent	Occlusion between site compressed and probe
Release compression distal to probe	No Doppler sound	Competent valves	Augmented sound present	Incompetent valves
Apply compression proximal to probe	No Doppler sound	Competent valves	Augmented sound present	Incompetent valves
Release compression proximal to probe	Augmented sound present	No occlusion between probe and site compressed	Augmented sound diminished or absent	Occlusion between probe and site compressed

*Posterior tibial, common femoral, and superficial femoral veins normally examined in sequence with patient in a supine position; then popliteal vein is checked with patient in a prone position and with his leg flexed and supported at the calf.

(From Waxham RD: Doppler ultrasound. Radiol Today April/May 1980.)

reversing it and produce a brief augmentation on release of compression. Compression of the calf or dorsiflexion of the foot (as for the Homans sign) should produce an augmentation of flow, and release should not reverse the flow.

The test procedure and interpretation are summarized in Table 32–1. Normal and abnormal venous flows are diagrammed in Figure 32–18. By comparing both legs and noting any asymmetry in spontaneous and augmented flows, the examiner can usually deduce not only the presence but also the level of obstruction, as well as evidence of incompetent deep valves.

Incompetent perforating veins may be revealed by placing a loose venous tourniquet proximal to the probe and showing reverse flow produced by compression of the leg above the tourniquet. Flow and competence in the superficial veins may be tested in a similar manner, but rather than compressing and releasing a segment of leg to augment deep flow, the examiner can simply tap over the saphenous vein to augment superficial flow.

The Doppler device is best suited for an examination of the lower venous sytem, but the veins of the thorax or the veins of the arms and neck may also be assessed. Velocity of blood flow in the internal jugular vein is pulsatile in a way that is approximately inverse to that of the familiar jugular venous pulses. Flow increases with inspiration and decreases but usually does not stop with expiration, although a Valsalva maneuver will stop the flow. Flow in the subclavian, axillary, and brachial veins follows a similar pattern, although in some people, inspiration may compress the subclavian vein and reduce flow. Flow in the brachial vein may also be tested with compression and release of the arm below to augment flow, as in the leg examination.

OTHER APPLICATIONS

Fetal heart sounds may be heard with the Doppler stethoscope as early as the twelfth week of gestation, at a rate of 120 to 140 beats per minute and are audible through the sounds of placental flow. Their presence may aid in the diagnosis of pregnancy and the assessment of fetal distress after abdominal trauma or placental bleeding.

A Doppler probe may be used to provide instantaneous feedback on resuscitation and cardiopulmonary resuscitation, both in the hospital and in the field. A small probe may be taped over a radial artery and attached to a loudspeaker, allowing immediate correction of ineffective cardiopulmonary resuscitation or monitoring of the patient's pulse rather than the cardiac rhythm. In addition to a sphygmomanometer cuff, also left in place for occasional inflation, such a monitoring probe can provide systolic blood pressure measurements without a stethoscope.[20]

A probe taped over the precordium has been described as a sensitive indicator of minute air emboli that may enter the right heart during surgery. The sound reflected by these bubbles has been described as a "squeak" or "chirp."[21]

Doppler ultrasound detection of intravascular bubbles has been suggested as a tool in the diagnosis of bends, or decompression sickness, or in the guidance of hyperbaric therapy. Audible bubbles have been detected in the absence of symptoms and when standard decompression tables have been followed.[22]

Doppler examination may also be used to locate the tip of a catheter within a patient. The flow of intravenous fluid, devoid of cells or bubbles to reflect sound, will not be detectable, but if the examiner withdraws and reinjects a few milliliters of blood or a few *tiny* bubbles, the to-and-fro velocity change along the catheter becomes evident.

Doppler ultrasound is also valuable in the differentiation between epididymitis and testicular torsion. In epididymitis, flow in the affected testicular artery is equal to or greater than that in the unaffected side of the scrotum, whereas in testicular torsion, there is a drop in testicular flow below the torsion. The Doppler evaluation of the acute scrotum is discussed in more detail in Chapter 73.

REFERENCES

1. Felix WR: Doppler ultrasound in the diagnosis of peripheral vascular disease. Semin Roentgenol 10:315, 1975.
2. Strandness DE, Schultz RD, Sumner DS, et al: Ultrasonic flow detection: Am J Surg 113:311, 1967.
3. Strandness DE: The use of ultrasound in the evaluation of peripheral vascular disease. Prog Cardiovasc Dis 20:403, 1978.
4. Felix WR Jr: Ultrasound measurements of arm and leg blood pressures. JAMA 226:1096, 1973.
5. Lennihan R Jr, Mackereth MA: Ankle pressures in vascular insufficiency involving the legs. J Clin Ultrasound 1:120, 1973.
6. Yao ST, Hobbs JT, Irvine WT: Ankle systolic pressure measurements in arterial disease affecting the lower extremity. Br J Surg 56:676, 1969.
7. Lennihan R Jr, Mackereth MA: Ankle pressures in arterial occlusive disease involving the legs. Surg Clin North Am 53:657, 1973.
8. Barnes RW, Wilson MR: Doppler Ultrasonic Evaluation of Peripheral Arterial Disease. Iowa City, University of Iowa Press, 1976, pp 1–23.
9. Bernstein EF, Fronek A: Current status of noninvasive tests in the diagnosis of peripheral arterial disease. Surg Clin North Am 62:473, 1982.
10. Barnes RW, Russell HE, Bone GE, et al: Doppler cerebrovascular examination: Improved results with refinements in technique. Stroke 8:468, 1977.
11. Brodie TE, Ochsner JL: Bilateral carotid stenosis: Diagnosis by Doppler sonography. Vasc Surg 12:53, 1978.
12. Maroon JC, Campbell RL, Dyken M: Internal carotid artery occlusion diagnosed by Doppler ultrasound. Stroke 1:122, 1970.
13. LoGerfo FW, Mason GR: Directional Doppler studies of supraorbital artery flow in internal carotid stenosis and occlusion. Surgery 76:723, 1974.
14. Sigel B, Popky GL, Wagner DK, et al: A Doppler ultrasound method for diagnosing lower extremity venous disease. Surg Gynecol Obstet 127:339, 1968.
15. Barnes RW, Russell HE, Wilson MR: Doppler Ultrasonic Evaluation of Venous Disease. 2nd ed. Iowa City, University of Iowa Press, 1975.
16. Sumner DS: Diagnosis of venous thrombosis by Doppler ultrasound. In Bergan JJ, Yao JS (eds): Venous Problems. Chicago, Year Book Medical Publishers, Inc, 1978, pp 159–185.
17. Sumner DS, Lambeth A: Reliability of Doppler ultrasound in the diagnosis of acute venous thrombosis both above and below the knee. Am J Surg 138:205, 1979.
18. Sigel B, Popky GL, Mapp EM, et al: Evaluation of Doppler ultrasound examination: Its use in diagnosis of lower extremity venous disease. Arch Surg 100:535, 1970.
19. Turnbull TJ, Dymowski JJ: Emergency department use of hand-held Doppler ultrasonography. Am J Emerg Med 7:209, 1989.
20. Grunau CFV: Doppler ultrasound monitoring of systemic blood flow during CPR. JACEP 7:180, 1978.
21. Michenfelder JD, Miller RH, Gronert GA: Evaluation of an ultrasonic device (Doppler) for the diagnosis of venous air embolism. Anesthesiology 36:164, 1972.
22. Gillis MF, Karagianes MT, Peterson PO: Detection of gas emboli associated with decompression using the Doppler flowmeter. J Occup Med 2:245, 1969.

Chapter 33

Transfusion Therapy: Blood and Blood Products

Garrett E. Bergman and Douglas A. Propp

INTRODUCTION

Transfusion of whole blood or its components (red cells, white cells, platelets, whole plasma, or plasma fractions) is indicated to replace certain deficiencies manifested by patients. The indications for the transfusion of *whole* blood have diminished as recent technical advances have made specific component replacement more feasible. Appropriate administration of blood products may be a life-saving procedure in some emergency circumstances but may also be indicated as a prophylactic measure in less urgent situations. By law, transfusions can be given only by a physician; potential life-threatening complications can result, as is true of any intravenous infusion. Almost all physicians have participated in (or independently performed) a blood transfusion *without necessarily knowing* the indications, benefits, proper procedures, risks, or potential complications.

In this chapter, techniques related to transfusion of blood and its components are presented to provide a comprehensive overview of a very common procedure. Equipment is discussed, but commercially available equipment systems are *not* described at length. Representative devices are chosen and described as prototypes; some comparable items produced by other manufacturers are mentioned, and significant differences between or advantages of various devices highlighted. The reader should bear in mind that several manufacturers may produce similar products of similar utility.

BACKGROUND

Blood Groups. In the seventeenth century, radically daring physicians were experimenting with the transfusion of blood from animals into humans to treat a variety of ills.[1, 2] Around the beginning of the century it became obvious that only human blood was fit for humans. Landsteiner found that most human serum contained naturally occurring substances that reacted with the red blood cells of some, but not all, other humans, thereby discovering the ABO red cell antigen-antibody system.

Red Cell Antigens and Antibodies. An integral part of the red blood cell (RBC) membrane is a series of glycoprotein moieties, or antigens, which give the cell an individual identity. Two different genetically determined antigens, type A and type B, occur on the surface of RBCs. The RBCs of any individual may have one, both, or neither of these antigens. Because the type A and type B antigens on the cell surface make the RBC susceptible to agglutination, these antigens are termed *agglutinogens*. The presence or absence of the agglutinogens makes up the ABO blood group classification. If neither the A nor the B agglutinogen is present, the blood group is O. When only type A agglutinogen is present, the blood is group A, and when only type B agglutinogen is present, the blood is group B. When both A and B agglutinogens are present, the blood is group AB. The relative frequencies of the different blood groups are listed in Table 33–1.

Genes on adjacent chromosomes determine the ABO blood group. These allelomorphic genes can be only one of the three different types—that is, A, B, or O—allowing for six possible combinations of genes (OO, OA, OB, AA, BB, and AB). There is no dominance among the three different allelomorphs; however, the type O is basically functionless, in that it causes such weak agglutination that it is normally insignificant. The different combinations of genes signify the individual's genotype, and each person is one of six different genotypes. The resultant blood groups for the various genotypes are listed in Table 33–2.

When type A agglutinogen is *absent* on a person's RBC, antibodies known as anti-A spontaneously develop in the plasma. Likewise, when type B agglutinogen is *absent*, anti-B antibodies develop in the plasma. When the blood is group O, both anti-A and anti-B antibodies develop. These antibodies are termed *agglutinins*. It follows, then, that group AB blood, which contains the agglutinogens A and B, contains no agglutinins at all in the plasma.

Table 33–1. *Frequency of Blood Groups in the General Population*

Type	Per Cent
O	47
A	41
B	9
AB	3
Rh −	15
Rh +	85

(From Guyton AC: Textbook of Medical Physiology. 6th ed. Philadelphia, WB Saunders Co., 1981.)

Immediately after birth, the quantity of agglutinins in the plasma is near zero, but titers begin to develop in the first year of life and reach their maximum titer when the individual is between 8 and 10 years of age. This titer gradually declines throughout the remaining years of life.

The agglutinins are gamma globulins of the IgM and IgG types and are probably produced by exposure to agglutinogens in food, bacteria, or exogenous substances other than blood transfusions. The antibodies (agglutinins) in the plasma of one blood type react with the antigens (agglutinogens) on the RBC of another blood type. This initiates the agglutination and hemolysis that are encountered in a transfusion reaction.

Many other antigenic proteins (as many as 300 of different potency) are present in the RBCs of different persons. Some are of academic or legal importance, whereas others are important for their ability to produce transfusion reactions.

Clinically, the importance of antibodies directed against RBC antigens is determined by their frequency and whether they can cause RBC destruction in the circulation. The ABO system is the most important. With the first transfusion of ABO-*incompatible* blood, severe, potentially fatal reactions can occur. The Rh system is likewise very important, because there is a high likelihood (30 to 50 per cent) that an Rh(D)-negative person will form antibodies after exposure to Rh-positive RBCs; these antibodies are then capable of causing severe hemolysis when RBCs containing the antigen are transfused a second time. Of the 40 antigens in the Rh system, D is the most antigenic, but others can also stimulate the production of antibodies in recipients lacking the antigen (e.g., E), thus complicating future transfusions. Other antigen systems in which antibodies could potentially cause hemolytic reactions are the Kell (K and k alleles), Duffy (Fy^a and Fy^b), Kidd (Jk^a and Jk^b), and MNS (M and N; closely linked S and s) systems. Other antigen systems are very rarely important in transfusion therapy.

Cross-Matching. Compatibility testing, or *cross-matching*, is the procedure by which the RBCs and serum of the donor unit of blood are mixed, respectively, with the serum and RBCs of the recipient to identify the presence of any antibodies and, hence, the potential for a transfusion reaction. These antibodies, after attaching to the appropriate RBC surface antigen, have the potential to cause agglutination and hemolysis of either donor or recipient RBCs. This hemolysis may be immediate or delayed. "Major" and "minor" cross-match procedures are outlined in Table 33–3. The end point of all cross-matches is the presence of RBC agglutination (either gross or microscopic) or hemolysis. Testing is performed immediately after mixing, after incubation at 37° C for varying times, and with and

Table 33–2. *The Blood Groups with Their Genotypes and Their Constituent Agglutinogens and Agglutinins*

Genotypes	Blood Groups	Agglutinogens	Agglutinins
OO	O	—	Anti-A and anti-B
OA or AA	A	A	Anti-B
OB or BB	B	B	Anti-A
AB	AB	A and B	—

(From Guyton AC: Textbook of Medical Physiology. 6th ed. Philadelphia, WB Saunders Co., 1981.)

Table 33–3. *Cross-Match Procedures*

	Major Cross-Match	Minor Cross-Match
Donor	Red cells	Serum
Recipient	Serum	Red cells
End point	Agglutination or hemolysis at 37° C	

without an antiglobulin reagent to identify surface immunoglobulin or complement. Each unit of blood product, when properly cross-matched, can be administered with the expectation of safety.

Transfusion Reactions. When incompatible blood is given, the result to the patient may range from no effect to a fatality. If the recipient does *not* have antibodies (naturally occurring or acquired) directed against the foreign RBC antigen received, there will be no immediate reaction, but within weeks antibodies to the infused blood may develop, which will limit the safety of subsequent transfusions from the same donor or same antigenic type. If the recipient's serum *has* preformed antibodies directed against the donor RBCs (incompatibility in the *major* cross-match), within seconds or minutes the recipient will begin to hemolyze the transfused (donor) cells.

In most cases of major cross-match reactions, RBCs of the *donor* blood are agglutinated and hemolyzed. It is very rare that the transfused blood ever produces agglutination of the recipient's cells. Donor blood is affected because the plasma portion of the donor blood immediately becomes diluted by the plasma of the recipient, thereby diluting the titer of the infused agglutinins to a level too low to cause agglutination. Because the recipient's plasma is not diluted to any significant degree, the recipient's agglutinins can still agglutinate the donor cells. Mismatched blood groups eventually cause hemolysis of the RBCs. Occasionally, antibodies cause immediate hemolysis. More often, the cells first agglutinate, then are trapped in peripheral vessels and, over a period of hours to days, become phagocytized, releasing hemoglobin into the circulatory system.

Clinical manifestations of acute hemolysis are chills, fever, tachycardia, abdominal pain, back pain, hypotension, fainting, and an anxious "feeling of impending doom." From the liberation of intracellular material associated with hemolysis, vasoactive substances may aggravate a preexisting hypotension and cause shock; other substances may precipitate disseminated intravascular coagulation, and high-output cardiac failure or anoxic acute renal failure may result. Hemolytic transfusion reactions are estimated to occur once every 6000 blood units transfused, with a fatality rate of one per every 100,000 units transfused.

An incompatibility in the *minor* cross-match usually causes no serious reaction, although the recipient's (patient's) red cells could be hemolyzed if the titer of the antibody were great. Even when major and minor cross-match compatibility indicates the safety of a transfusion, a delayed hemolytic transfusion reaction can occur days to weeks later. Usually seen in multiply transfused patients (or in multigravidas), these reactions may be unavoidable without complete RBC antigen typing, a procedure occasionally indicated for recipients of numerous repeated transfusions. Fortunately, 90 per cent of transfusions are now given as packed RBCs that contain a small volume of plasma, minimizing the chance for a transfusion reaction due to donor sensitization.

Additional antibodies *not* caused by sensitization from transfused RBCs include autoantibodies (both cold- and warm-reacting) and various agglutinins. Autoantibodies can be "cold," reacting with red cells *more strongly at 4° C* than at 37° C. These antibodies are common and are usually harmless; however, they may be associated with disease states in higher titers (e.g., anti-I in mycoplasma infections). If active at higher temperatures (up to 28 to 32° C), pathologic cold antibodies may cause hemolysis or may even lead to enough RBC agglutination to cause obstruction of blood flow through the small vessels of the hands and the feet on exposure to cold. These would also be present and identifiable at 37° C. The primary significance of cold antibodies stems from their ability to complicate cross-matching procedures in the blood bank.

Warm antibodies, reacting *more strongly at 37° C* than at lower temperatures, can be harmless or can be responsible for a hemolytic anemia of variable severity. Characteristics of the IgG antibody itself determine its significance to the patient. Usually harmless warm autoantibodies that can occasionally cause hemolysis are seen in patients taking α-methyldopa. Harmful warm autoantibodies are encountered in approximately 80 per cent of patients with autoimmune hemolytic anemia.

Additional problems in pretransfusion testing may occur with antibodies directed against various substances that can attach themselves to the RBC surfaces and can cause agglutination of the "innocent bystanders." Examples are the fatty acid–dependent agglutinins; penicillin and cephalosporin antibodies; bacterial polysaccharides; and nonspecific agglutination associated with a high erythrocyte sedimentation rate, caused by high levels of the acute phase reactants: fibrinogen, α-2-macroglobulin, and IgM. A delay in pretransfusion testing may occur when the blood bank has to undertake procedures to identify various proteins on RBC surfaces to ascertain their clinical significance.

Miscellaneous Transfusion Problems. Pyogenic transfusion reactions, such as fever and chills, are rather common and result from the presence in the donor plasma of proteins to which the recipient is allergic. Occasional full-blown anaphylactic reactions can result.

Theoretically, citrate salts, which are the usual anticoagulants in donor blood, may combine with ionized calcium in the plasma, producing hypocalcemia. In clinical practice, the hemodynamic consequences of citrate-induced hypocalcemia are minimal, although the Q-T interval may be prolonged on the electrocardiogram (ECG) with citrate infusion. Supplemental calcium administration is usually not necessary even during massive blood replacement as long as circulating volume is maintained, because the liver is able to remove citrate from the blood within a few minutes. Alterations in this recommendation may be necessary in the presence of severe liver disease.

Crystalloid versus Colloid. In the case of a hypotensive patient suffering from acute hemorrhage, continued debate surfaces regarding whether it is most appropriate to administer crystalloids or colloids before the institution of blood component therapy.[3] Crystalloids are promoted as being the ideal solution to administer to replace the interstitial fluid deficit that occurs during bleeding. Unfortunately, these balanced salt solutions freely cross capillary membranes, thus providing less oncotic pressure and less prolonged plasma volume expansion than is desired. Thus only 10 to 20 per cent of the administered crystalloid remains intravascular, perhaps for only 2 hours.

Colloids are large, oncotically active molecules that remain within the capillary membrane. They are efficient blood volume expanders because fluid deficits can be replaced faster with two to four times less volume than that needed with crystalloids.[4] Unfortunately, colloids cost 20 to 30 times more than a comparable amount of crystalloids.

Three colloid preparations are commercially available. Albumin is manufactured from donor plasma as either 5 per cent or 25 per cent solutions dissolved in normal saline. Volume expansion typically lasts 24 hours. There is a 0.5 per cent incidence of urticaria, fever, or chills when using this fluid. Hetastarch is a synthetic amylopectin available as a 6 per cent solution dissolved in normal saline. It has an osmolality of 310 mOsm and a pH of 5.5. Volume expansion lasts 24 to 36 hours. Minor adverse effects on clotting have been documented. The rate of adverse reactions is the same as that seen with albumin use. Dextrans are high-molecular-weight polysaccharides, which have been known to interfere with typing and crossmatching as well as with platelet function.

There are data to support either viewpoint in the crystalloid versus colloid debate. Unfortunately, the information is confusing and frequently conflicting. Although fluid resuscitation can be adequately accomplished with the use of crystalloids, when severe blood loss is replaced with crystalloids alone, marked overexpansion of the extracellular fluid volume occurs. Although colloids typically offer no obvious clinical advantage and it would be imprudent to use them routinely in hemorrhagic fluid resuscitations, they are more efficient plasma volume expanders.

USE OF BLOOD PRODUCTS

Blood products are divided into components and fractions. Blood components, such as fresh frozen plasma,

packed RBCs, granulocytes, cryoprecipitate, and platelets, are prepared from a single donor and are separated by physical means and transfused as single units. The risk of hepatitis is lower when the blood components are obtained from volunteer donors rather than paid donors.

The availability of autotransfusion devices in most emergency departments provides an opportunity to preserve blood bank resources that might otherwise be needed. The autotransfused blood harvested from the patient's intrathoracic cavity is fresh, warm, compatible, inexpensive, immediately available, and unlikely to cause a transfusion reaction. Once the blood is collected, it is passed through a filter that removes extraneous debris, and then it is reinfused through a standard intravenous line. Although controversial, most authorities recommend administering citrate-phosphate-dextrose (CPD) with the whole blood. Potential complications include air embolization, coagulopathy if large volumes of blood are administered, and sepsis if contaminated blood is disseminated (see Chapter 34).

Although of limited clinical applicability to emergency transfusions, autologous donations are becoming more commonplace. It has been suggested that up to 10 per cent of the blood supply could be provided through this mechanism. Most appropriate applications at this time include elective cardiac, gynecologic, orthopedic, and vascular surgical cases. Benefits of this system include avoidance of exogenous blood-borne disease and sensitization. The individual can donate 1 unit of blood weekly, until 3 days before the surgical need. As blood can be stored up to 35 days, the donations usually begin 5 weeks before they will be needed. The blood donor will require iron supplements and must maintain a hemoglobin of greater than 11 gm.

Albumin, plasma protein fraction, and prothrombin complex concentrate are termed blood fractions (as opposed to components) and are commercially prepared from a plasma pool of multiple donors. Some fractions may be heat-treated to reduce the risk of hepatitis, but because the source of such fractions is largely paid donors, the risk of hepatitis is high with transfusion of blood fractions. Table 33–4 lists some characteristics of blood and its components.

Whole Blood. Individuals normally have 70 to 80 ml/kg of whole blood. Whole blood provides a source of red cells for oxygenation, proteins for coagulation factors and oncotic pressure, and volume for rapid restoration of hypovolemia. Whole blood is indicated only for massive transfusion or exchange transfusion and usually is appropriately used only in treatment of patients with a decreased RBC oxygen-delivering ability and hypovolemic shock, such as after multiple trauma. Whole blood is *not* the indicated treatment for hypovolemic shock that can be treated effectively with crystalloid (e.g., lactated Ringer solution, 0.9 per cent sodium chloride) or colloid (e.g., plasma protein, albumin); it is *not* indicated for correction of thrombocytopenia, replacement of coagulation factors, or treatment of anemia that can be treated with replacement iron, vitamin B_{12}, or folic acid. Most blood banks currently do *not* stock significant quantities of whole blood.

Whole blood is collected from donors into plastic bags containing 63 ml of CPD anticoagulant and preservative in a total volume of 515 ± 50 ml and resultant hematocrit of 35 to 40 per cent. If more than 24 hours old, whole blood is essentially devoid of normally functioning platelets and other clotting factors, especially the labile clotting factors V and VIII. In addition, whole blood contains antigenic leukocytes and serum proteins, which may produce allergic reactions (a risk of 1 per cent).

Because blood products are stored for up to 35 days, various "storage lesions" occur. Cell metabolism continues to occur while blood is being stored, so a small degree of

Table 33–4. **Characteristics of Blood and Its Components**

Component	Volume	Shelf Life	Requirements for Transfusion
Whole blood* ACD CPD CPD-A	450 ml blood 63 ml anticoagulant and preservative 35 to 40% hematocrit	21 days at 4° C 35 days at 4° C	Cross-matched
Packed red cells concentrate washed	280 ml 70% hematocrit 250 ml 70% hematocrit	Same as for whole blood 1 day at 4° C	Cross-matched Cross-matched
Frozen-thawed red cells†	250 ml 70% hematocrit	? years when frozen, 1 day after thawing	Cross-matched
Platelet concentrate	30 ml 10¹⁰ platelets	5 days at 22° C	Type-specific if possible, but not essential, not cross-matched
Fresh frozen plasma	200 to 250 ml	1 year at −18° C, 24 hours after thawing‡	ABO-compatible; random donor, not cross-matched
Cryoprecipitate	10 to 25 ml per bag 60 to 120 units of factor VIII	1 year at −18° C, 6 hours after thawing	ABO-compatible; random donor, not cross-matched
Factor IX or prothrombin concentrate	25 ml per vial	Check label	None required
Granulocyte† concentrate	400 ml 10¹⁰ leukocytes	Transfuse within 24 hours at 22° C	Specific donors for each patient, cross-matched

*ACD, acid-citrate-dextrose; CPD, citrate-phosphate-dextrose; CPD-A, citrate-phosphate-dextrose-adenine.
†Special order—few hospitals have facility inhouse.
‡Use immediately to correct deficiency of coagulation factors.

acidosis commonly develops. However, this acidosis is buffered effectively by the bicarbonate derived from the metabolism of the citrate used as a preservative, assuming normal hepatic function. Even in massive transfusions, acidosis is usually due to the disruption of normal physiologic function rather than the blood products themselves. During storage, levels of 2,3-DPG (diphosphoglyceric acid) also decrease. This decrease results in the shift of the oxygen-hemoglobin dissociation curve to the left. The shift is of small clinical significance, however, because the level soon rises and is usually normal in the recipient within 24 hours of infusion. In addition, potassium commonly leaks out of the cells during storage because of a less efficient sodium-potassium ATPase-dependent pump. Fortunately, most of the potassium is either absorbed by the remaining blood cells, excreted by the kidney, or shifted back into the cells owing to the alkalosis produced by metabolism of the citrate in the preservative. Hyperkalemia is clinically relevant only in newborns and patients with renal impairment.

Sepsis is of theoretic concern in blood component therapy because 0.1 per cent of all transfusions may transmit virulent bacteria. However, sepsis is an uncommon occurrence because both the citrate preservative and the refrigeration kill most organisms. Concern over sepsis has governed the decision to complete transfusions within 4 hours and to return unused blood products to the blood bank refrigerator for future use only if they have been out of the refrigerator for less than 30 minutes. The virulent pathogens involved are most commonly gram-negative organisms.

Most blood products retain the ability to transmit hepatitis. Ninety per cent of the time the etiologic agent is non-A, non-B viral hepatitis. The customary incubation period for this agent following infusion is 2 to 12 weeks, although

80 per cent of patients are anicteric. The likelihood of developing posttransfusion hepatitis ranges from 1 per 100 to 1 per 500 units of blood administered. Up to 20 per cent of patients developing hepatitis ultimately develop cirrhosis. Unfortunately, one of every 3000 to 5000 transfusion recipients dies of hepatitis. One study suggests that pretreatment with immune serum globulin both 24 hours before and 1 week after transfusion of blood may decrease the incidence of posttransfusion non-A, non-B hepatitis.[5] Although syphilis may theoretically be transmitted by transfusion, *Treponema pallidum* does not survive when refrigerated or in a citrated medium. Only fresh blood or platelet transfusions are of concern. The incubation period is 4 weeks to 4 months, and the initial clinical manifestation is a skin rash. Although controversial because of high false-positive and false-negative rates for testing, many blood banks still test for positive *T. pallidum* serology.

Both cytomegalovirus and Epstein-Barr virus can be transmitted through transfusions. A mononucleosis-like syndrome occuring 2 to 6 weeks after a transfusion is suggestive of the presence of either of these agents. Blood products with negative serology for both of these agents should be used for seronegative recipients in high-risk groups such as pregnant females, premature or low-birth-weight newborns, marrow or organ transplant recipients, and immunosuppressed patients.

The likelihood of transmission of malaria through blood products is minimal because of routine preventive measures. Prospective blood product donors who have been to an endemic region within 6 months or treated with malarial prophylaxis within 3 years are not allowed to donate blood products.

The acquired immunodeficiency syndrome (AIDS) epidemic has affected transfusion therapy. In the United States, 3 per cent of AIDS cases have been linked to blood products. In addition, 65 per cent of hemophiliacs in the United States have been exposed to the virus. Voluntary deferment by high-risk groups was encouraged in 1983, and formal screening of all blood products began in 1985. Given that any units that test positive for the human immunodeficiency virus (HIV) antibody are routinely discarded, concern over transmission of the virus centers around the 6- to 8-week "window," during which a donor might be antigen-positive (HIV-infected) but temporarily antibody-negative. It has been estimated that the likelihood of transmitting HIV through blood products is between 1:40,000 and 1:1,000,000 per unit of blood donated. If a blood recipient's antibody level remains negligible 6 months after transfusion, it is extremely unlikely that the disease will develop.

A system of "directed donations" has been proposed to answer the concern over the transmission of HIV. Some believe that the blood products derived from a relative or a friend have a lower likelihood of testing positive for an HIV infection. At this time, directed donation systems have not been widely supported. It is feared that blood products will be less safe because social pressures may result in no self-deferment of high-risk donors and more clerical errors will be made because of the increased complexity of this system. Finally, there is concern that the directed donation plan will disrupt the normal anonymous blood donor system, leaving fewer units available for other needy patients.

The incidence of transfusion reactions following transfusion with whole blood is approximately two and one half times greater than the incidence of reactions following transfusion with packed RBCs.[6] Although it is certainly true that patients bleed whole blood, not packed cells, it is often recommended that even acute blood loss be treated with packed cells as opposed to whole blood; many authorities, however, will defend the continued use of whole blood.[7] One unit of whole blood raises the hematocrit approximately 3 per cent. The plasma of whole blood is no more effective than 5 per cent albumin as a volume expander.

Packed Red Blood Cells. Packed RBCs provide oxygen-carrying capacity and volume expansion. Packed RBCs are prepared by centrifugation and removal of most of the plasma from citrated whole blood. Packed RBCs that have been grouped and have had the Rh factor determined should be the most common blood component used for treating anemia not amenable to nutritional correction. Hazards of metabolic derangements, donor antibodies, volume overload, and (possibly) hepatitis are lessened with packed RBCs as compared with whole blood. Patients with severe or chronic anemia or heart disease or those who otherwise require fluid restriction can receive packed RBCs more safely than whole blood. Furthermore, to prevent circulatory overload in susceptible patients, a rapid-acting diuretic, such as furosemide or ethacrynic acid, can be administered intravenously at the beginning of the transfusion. Criteria for packed RBC transfusion vary. A hemoglobin level less than 10 gm/dl is one criterion commonly suggested for transfusion prior to surgery. The National Institutes of Health suggest that prophylactic transfusion should not be done on anemic patients with a hemoglobin greater than 7 gm/dl (hematocrit 21 per cent). Healthy individuals sustaining acute blood loss may have no significant physiologic impairment with hemoglobin levels as low as 6 to 8 gm/dl (hematocrit 18 to 24 per cent). The patient with circulatory shock and a hemoglobin concentration of 8 gm/dl or greater may not benefit from a transfusion if previously volume-resuscitated.[8]

One unit of packed RBCs contains the same red cell mass as one unit of whole blood at approximately one half the volume and twice the hematocrit (70 to 80 per cent). One unit of packed RBCs raises the hematocrit approximately 3 per cent in an adult or increases the hemoglobin level of a 70-kg individual by 1 gm/dl. In children, there is an approximate rise in hematocrit of 1 per cent for each milliliter per kilogram of packed cells. For example, if 5 ml/kg of packed RBCs is transfused, the hematocrit will rise by approximately 5 per cent. Actual changes are dependent on the state of hydration and the rate of bleeding.

When washed to remove leukocytes, platelets, microaggregates, and plasma proteins, packed RBC transfusions cause fewer transfusion reactions than do whole blood transfusions. RBCs are not routinely washed before transfusion, but washing reduces the titer of anti-A and anti-B, permitting safer transfusion of type O packed RBCs in non-O recipients. Washing does not totally eliminate the risk of hepatitis. Washed RBCs are prepared in the blood bank by centrifugation, filtration, or use of sedimenting agents or by washing the unit of whole blood or packed RBCs.

Frozen deglycerolized RBCs likewise are free of platelets, plasma, and white blood cells, having been washed after an indefinite period of frozen storage in glycerol. Frozen RBCs and fresh RBCs function similarly; frozen RBCs provide normal levels of 2,3-DPG. Washed or frozen preparations should be given to patients who have had febrile (nonhemolytic) reactions to previous transfusions as a result of leukocyte antibodies or IgA sensitization. Blood bank procedures require that these be prepared to order, with routine cross-matching. Considerable delay (6 hours) may occur if the transfusion service does not have the capability of washing RBCs.

Packed RBCs contain less sodium, potassium, ammonia, citrate, and antigenic protein and fewer hydrogen ions than does whole blood. This may offer an advantage in patients with reduced cardiovascular, renal, or hepatic function. The rate of urticaria is still relatively high, at 1 to 3 per cent of transfusions, but the incidence of adverse reactions to packed cells is approximately one third that noted with whole blood.

Many physicians use packed RBCs during surgery and for replacement treatment of acute blood loss of any cause. As is true of whole blood, packed RBCs can be stored up to 21 days by law, although newer preservatives may allow 35-day storage. Red cell viability decreases approximately 1 per cent per day.

Synthetic Blood Substitutes. Techniques are being developed to synthesize an appropriate in vivo oxygen carrier that is readily available, inexpensive, and devoid of complications. Stroma-free hemoglobin is a product derived by chemically processing outdated red blood cells. It has minimal immunogenicity and no hepatitis risk, and it requires no compatibility testing. Because of several problems with the product, it has not been endorsed for routine human use. It has been found to promote nephrotoxicity and coagulopathy. In addition, it has a short circulatory half-life, being cleared by the kidneys in about 4 hours. Furthermore, as oxygen is chemically bound to the product, it does not unload oxygen to the tissues in an ideal fashion. Another product, Perfluorocarbon, is a synthetically produced hydrocarbon. Because it provides physical transport of oxygen, a linear relationship occurs between the fraction of inspiratory oxygen (FI_{O_2}) and the P_{O_2}. Consequently, the patient needs to receive 100 per cent oxygen to use this product in an optimal manner. The inability to maintain a person at a 100 per cent FI_{O_2} for long periods of time limits the usefulness of this agent. Perfluorocarbon is also thought to activate the complement system and cause antigen-antibody accumulations in both the reticulendothelial system and the lungs. Although both products offer theoretic advantages for oxygen-carrying capacity when the risks from blood product administration are high or the availability of blood products is low, neither is at a stage of development for endorsement for clinical use.[9]

Fresh Frozen Plasma. Fresh frozen plasma should be given to patients with a hereditary or acquired deficiency of coagulation factors, provided that a preparation of the specific deficient factor is not available. Each unit has a volume of approximately 200 to 250 ml and is prepared by freezing the plasma separated from single-donor whole blood within 4 to 6 hours of collection. Plasma should be compatible in terms of the recipient's ABO group. Rh compatibility is not considered essential.

Fresh frozen plasma contains all soluble coagulation factors of the intrinsic and extrinsic clotting systems, including the labile factors V and VIII. Fresh frozen plasma also contains fibrinogen, although not as much as does cryoprecipitate. Fresh frozen plasma has a shelf life of up to 1 year, and plasma stored for 3 months retains approximately 60 per cent of the normal factor VIII activity. Fresh frozen plasma contains no platelets.

Fresh frozen plasma is indicated for the clotting factor deficiencies resulting from the diluting effect of massive blood replacement. However, pathologic hemorrhage following massive transfusions is often caused by thrombocytopenia rather than by a depletion of clotting factors. One unit of fresh frozen plasma per 5 units of packed cells or whole blood is a reasonable replacement formula if specific clotting tests are not rapidly available, but plasma replacement is best dictated by evaluation of prothrombin time and partial thromboplastin time. Fresh frozen plasma is indicated for rapid reversal of serious bleeding from warfarin (Coumadin) anticoagulants. In an emergency situation, 5 to 10 ml/kg of fresh frozen plasma will effect a rapid reversal of the vitamin K–dependent factors II, VII, IX, and X. As a rough guide, one unit of fresh frozen plasma increases all coagulation factor levels by 2 to 3 per cent in the average-sized adult. In *life-threatening* hemorrhage from Coumadin excess, factor IX concentrate (Konyne, Proplex) may be used, but such therapy should not be routine because of the high incidence of hepatitis and the possibility of thrombosis with these products. Fresh frozen plasma may be valuable in patients with other clotting abnormalities, such as von Willebrand syndrome, hemophilia A and hemophilia B, or hypofibrinogenemia; however, the effectiveness is limited in severe clotting abnormalities because of the large volume that is generally required. For example, fresh frozen plasma may be successful in the treatment of hemarthrosis or other minor bleeding tendencies in hemophilia, but specific factor replacement is preferred.

Because of the high risk of hepatitis, packed plasma is no longer available. Reactions to fresh frozen plasma include fever, chills, allergic responses, HIV infection, and a risk of hepatitis that is similar to the risk with whole blood.

Fresh frozen plasma should be infused rapidly and given immediately after thawing because of the rapid loss of labile clotting factors.

Cryoprecipitate. Cryoprecipitate is used specifically to correct a deficiency of coagulation factor VIII (in hemophilia A and in von Willebrand syndrome), factor XIII, or fibrinogen. The precipitate is prepared from single-donor plasma by gradual thawing of rapidly frozen plasma, which results in an undissolved protein that is collected and stored at very low temperatures. Cryoprecipitate is a plasma product and as such requires ABO and Rh compatibility, but cross-matching is not necessary.

Cryoprecipitate contains approximately 30 to 50 per cent of the original plasma content of factors VIII and XIII and fibrinogen. Each 15- to 25-ml bag of cryoprecipitate contains 60 to 120 units of factor VIII, 125 to 250 mg of fibrinogen, and an unknown amount of von Willebrand factor. Cryoprecipitate is of no value in the treatment of factor IX deficiency (hemophilia B).

Once spontaneous bleeding has occurred in hemophilia or von Willebrand syndrome, it will usually *not stop until the deficient factor is replaced*. It is best to treat early to prevent minor bleeding from developing into a significant hemorrhage. The goal of therapy is to achieve at least 50 per cent of normal factor VIII activity. In spontaneous intracranial hemorrhage, one should seek 100 per cent activity. The amount of cryoprecipitate required to correct coagulation defects ranges from 10 to 20 units/kg for minor bleeding, such as hemarthrosis, to 50 units/kg for bleeding control in surgery or trauma, but specific replacement should be guided by laboratory assay of factor VIII activity. One bag of cryoprecipitate per 5 kg of body weight will raise the recipient's factor VIII level to approximately 50 per cent of normal. The half-life of factor VIII in plasma is 8 to 12 hours. Mild deficiencies of factor VIII are considered to exist at 10 to 30 per cent of normal, and severe deficiencies exist at less than 3 per cent of normal activity. Many patients know their level of factor VIII, and such levels remain relatively constant.

Rarely, cryoprecipitate may be required to correct significant hypofibrinogenemia (less than 100 mg/dl). Fresh frozen plasma may also be used to treat mild degrees of hypofibrinogenemia.

Factor VIII Concentrate. Factor VIII concentrate is a product for the treatment of classic hemophilia A. It is derived from a large donor pool and can be stored for up to 2 years in a home refrigerator. The product is significantly more concentrated than cryoprecipitate or fresh frozen plasma. The known factor activity is listed on every bottle. Administration of 1 unit per kg of body weight should increase the factor VIII activity by 2 per cent. Minor episodes of bleeding are usually treated with 10 to 20 units/kg, whereas major episodes are treated with 20 to 30 units/kg, with a repeat dose 12 hours later. Antibodies develop in up to 15 per cent of recipients of factor VIII. Various techniques have been used to overcome this problem. Administration of massive doses of factor VIII has been shown to be somewhat beneficial in overwhelming the endogenous antibody response. In addition, immunoadsorbent techniques to remove the antibody have met with some guarded success. The general use of immunosuppressives and plasmapheresis has had limited success. Activated prothrombin complex has been effective, but concern over the cost of preparation, the significant hepatitis risk, and the thrombogenicity associated with its use limits its application.

Because factor VIII concentrate is derived from large donor pools, the likelihood of transmission of hepatitis and HIV infection is higher. Different forms of chemical treatments have been attempted to minimize this threat. These techniques include heat treatment, pasteurization, and use of organic solvents and detergents. The newest preparations use immunoaffinity chromatography to produce a more highly purified factor with higher overall activity. Since the gene for factor VIII production was discovered in 1984, new research into recombinant genetics has been aimed at providing a safer product that theoretically will be more readily available and less expensive to produce.

A synthetic analogue of pituitary vasopressin, 1-deamino-(8-D-arginine)-vasopressin (DDAVP), has been found to stimulate the endogenous production of factor VIII in a subset of mild hemophiliacs. The exact mechanism is unknown, but treatment with 0.3 mg/kg intravenously over 15 minutes has been recommended when avoidance of the inherent risks of the factor VIII concentrate is desired.

Factor IX Concentrate (Prothrombin Complex). Prothrombin complex concentrate, or factor IX concentrate (Konyne or Proplex), is prepared from pooled human plasma and is available as a lyophilized powder. Factor IX concentrate contains the liver-synthesized, vitamin K–dependent factors: II (prothrombin), VII, IX, and X. The actual factor IX activity of each vial is stated on the label. Each vial is reconstituted to a volume of 25 ml and contains approximately 500 units of factor IX, 300 units of factors VII and X, and 200 units of factor II. The use of this product carries a very high risk of hepatitis transmission (almost 100 per cent), and, because of this, it is rarely used. The risk of HIV infection is analogous to that with the use of factor VIII concentrate. Post-treatment hyperthrombosis may also occur.

Factor IX concentrate is used almost exclusively in the treatment of hemophilia B, because cryoprecipitate is effective only for the treatment of hemophilia A (factor VIII deficiency). Patients with hemophilia should always be asked which deficiency they manifest, because the treatment of each type is different. Although factor VIII deficiency is much more common, the routine treatment of all patients with "hemophilia" with cryoprecipitate is not warranted. Factor IX concentrate may theoretically be used instead of fresh frozen plasma in the rare instance in which volume must be kept at a minimum. The use of prothrombin complex is also warranted when there is the possibility of *life-threatening* hemorrhage, such as intracranial bleeding, in patients with *Coumadin-induced* hemorrhage. Vitamin K and fresh frozen plasma, however, are definitely preferred in the noncritical patient with Coumadin-induced bleeding. A new monoclonal antibody purified factor IX preparation, safe from the risks of hepatitis and thrombogenicity is in the final stages of Food and Drug Administration approval.

In hemophilia B, the aim of therapy is to achieve 20 to 30 per cent of normal values of factor IX. Higher levels are desired for the treatment of intracranial bleeding. Most patients know the level of their deficiency, and the deficiency remains relatively constant. Treatment of factor IX–deficient patients with 15 to 30 units of factor IX concentrate per kg of body weight, once or twice a day, usually results in normal hemostasis, but individual responses to therapy may vary. Minor bleeding (soft tissue, joints) may be controlled with 10 to 20 units/kg of body weight. It is a common error to assume that a minor spontaneous bleeding episode will be self-limited in patients with either form of hemophilia. Once spontaneous bleeding occurs, however, it rarely stops spontaneously, and treatment with replacement factors is necessary.

Platelet Concentrates. Platelet concentrates are prepared by rapid centrifugation of platelet-rich plasma, which is obtained by slow centrifugation of freshly collected whole blood to separate the RBCs. Platelet concentrates contain most of the platelets from 1 unit of blood in 30 to 50 ml of plasma; they are given to raise a patient's platelet count and to correct bleeding from thrombocytopenia. One unit (pack) of platelets per 7 kg of body weight will raise the platelet count by 50,000 per mm³ in the absence of antibodies; therefore, 1 unit of platelet concentrate raises the platelet count by 5000 to 10,000 per mm³. The usual adult dose given is 6 to 10 units of platelet concentrate, depending on the clinical condition. This amount should increase the platelet count to more than 50,000 per mm³. Some hospital blood banks prepare platelet concentrates regularly; in some cities a central blood bank service, such as the American Red Cross, prepares platelet concentrates regularly and delivers units on an "as-needed" basis within 1 to 2 hours of the request. Platelet concentrates are viable for 5 days when kept at *room temperature* and gently agitated at intermittent periods or when kept in motion. They should not be refrigerated.

Spontaneous bleeding rarely occurs if the platelet count is above 30,000 per mm³. Even in the event of surgery or trauma, excessive bleeding is uncommon in patients whose platelet count exceeds 50,000 per mm³. It is generally recommended that active hemorrhage be treated with platelet transfusion if the platelet count is below 50,000 per mm³. Patients with idiopathic thrombocytopenia purpura (ITP) should not receive platelets prophylactically but may be transfused if life-threatening bleeding occurs.

Cross-matching is unnecessary for platelet transfusion, but the donor and the recipient should be ABO- and Rh-compatible. Note that platelet concentrates contain enough RBCs to sensitize an Rh-negative individual. There may be a diluting effect to the platelet count that results in thrombocytopenia with massive blood transfusions. When more than 8 to 10 units of blood are transfused, the platelet count must be routinely evaluated, and platelets must be replaced accordingly. Clinically significant platelet depletion rarely occurs if less than 15 units of blood (or 1.5 to 2 times blood volume) have been transfused.

Granulocyte Transfusions. Granulocyte transfusions are given in those unique instances in which a severely neutropenic patient has a suspected or proven bacterial infection not responding to appropriate treatment. They are rarely given in an emergency unit. White blood cell transfusions require prior arrangements with a large blood bank service that has the capabilities of collecting granulocytes from a suitable donor; the collection procedure takes 4 to 6 hours on a continuous-flow cell separator. Transfusions need to be repeated frequently (every 12 hours) to provide a sufficient number of white blood cells to help the patient.

Blood Products for Jehovah's Witnesses. There are more than one and one-half million Jehovah's Witnesses in America. Members of this religion do not accept transfusions of whole blood, packed cells, white blood cells, platelets, or plasma or autotransfusion of predeposited blood. Some may permit infusion of albumin, hemophiliac preparations, or dextran or other plasma expanders and intraoperative autotransfusion.[10] Although no guidelines for administration of blood products to Jehovah's Witnesses are absolute, certain recommendations can be made. It is prudent to administer blood products to patients who either are judged to be incompetent adults or are minors. Although case law often upholds the patient's wishes, pregnant females and significant providers for dependents have been deemed appropriate recipients of blood products against their wishes. Explicit documentation of the intent of the physician to preserve life coupled with an accurate description of the discussion of the issue with the patient and a clarification of the patient's mental capacity is mandatory. Furthermore, emergency legal assistance should be sought immediately with rapid judicial resolution.[11]

Use of Blood Group Dipsticks. The benefit of having type-specific blood immediately available to a patient as on arrival in the emergency department is obvious. The ability to identify the patient's blood group has been faciliated by the introduction of a dipstick that has a high correlation with blood bank–determined blood types. The technique is simple and fast, requiring only 3 minutes to be performed. In addition, the dipsticks are inexpensive and easy to interpret and do not require refrigeration.[12]

Although rapid blood typing to guide administration of un–cross-matched blood may prove to be of value in the future, many emergency departments are using group O un–cross-matched blood for patients in immediate need of a transfusion.[13, 14] Group O Rh(D)-negative blood, when available, is preferred for female patients younger than 40 years old to avoid maternal Rh sensitization.[14, 15]

ADMINISTRATION OF BLOOD COMPONENTS

When it has been decided that a patient needs a transfusion and the patient is stable enough, the physician should question the patient or the patient's relatives concerning any previous transfusion reactions and whether the patient abides by any religious prohibitions to transfusions. A tube of blood (approximately 2 ml for every unit of blood product to be cross-matched) should be drawn from the patient and put into a red-topped, nonanticoagulated tube. The tube must *not* contain a serum separator gel. The label should be signed by the physician. This identifying signature will be used in the blood bank's cross-matching procedures.

Emergency Transfusion. In an emergency or life-threatening situation, three alternatives to fully cross-matched blood exist. The preferred substitute is type-specific blood with an abbreviated cross-match. The abbreviated cross-match includes ABO and Rh compatibility. In addition, the recipient's serum is screened for unexpected antibodies, and an "immediate spin" cross-match is performed at room temperature. This abbreviated cross-match requires approximately 30 minutes, and many institutions are now using this procedure as their standard cross-match for most patients. The safety and utility of the type-specific abbreviated cross-match have been demonstrated repeatedly, and transfusion reactions should occur only rarely.[7, 16]

The second preference for an alternative to fully cross-matched blood is type-specific blood that is only ABO- and Rh-compatible, without screen or immediate spin cross-match. The patient's ABO group and Rh factor can be determined within 2 minutes, and, in an emergency, typing of the blood group and the Rh factor is all that is necessary before transfusion. Type-specific blood that is not cross-matched has been given in numerous military and civilian series without serious consequences.[5, 17] While the type-specific blood is being transfused, the antibody screen and the cross-match are carried out in the laboratory; the transfusion should be stopped if an incompatibility is found to exist.

Ideally, type-specific blood should be similar in Rh factor as well as in ABO group; however, blood with the opposite Rh factor may be used in an extreme emergency or in times of disaster or blood shortage. The patient may develop sensitization to the Rh factor.[15] This may affect a subsequent pregnancy if an Rh-negative woman is given Rh-positive type-specific blood. A male patient may likewise be sensitized to subsequent Rh-incompatible transfusions.

The third preference for an alternative to fully cross-matched blood for an emergency transfusion is group O blood.[13, 14, 17] In general, type-specific blood is preferable to group O blood. There is rarely a situation in which a few minutes cannot safely be expended to allow the blood bank to release type-specific blood. Nevertheless, exceptions may occur, in which case type O blood may be required. Such exceptions would be a trauma victim or a patient with a ruptured aneurysm who has not responded to crystalloid resuscitation in the field.

When type and Rh determination creates an unacceptable delay in transfusion, group O blood (either as whole blood or as packed cells) is transfused. Packed cells are preferred over whole blood. Group O negative *whole* blood was in the past designated the "universal donor" blood, because a recipient's naturally occurring antibodies (anti-A and anti-B) will not react with donor group O RBCs. None-

theless, some donor serum may have a high titer of naturally occurring anti-A and anti-B antibodies capable of hemolyzing the recipient's (patient's) RBCs if large quantities of blood are transfused. True universal donor blood is low in anti-A and anti-B titer. Because group O donors are not regularly screened for unsafe levels of anti-A and anti-B titers, the use of even small amounts of group O *whole blood* that is not cross-matched is potentially dangerous. The significance of varying titers of anti-A and anti-B antibodies in the donor whole blood may be essentially eliminated if *packed cells* are used instead of whole blood. Other RBC antigens on type O RBCs may sensitize the patient or may cause antibody production, complicating future cross-matching or possibly causing future hemolytic transfusion reactions.

Approximately 25 per cent of patients receiving a transfusion of 5 or more units of type O whole blood develop hyperbilirubinemia suggestive of a minor hemolytic reaction. Large amounts of group O whole blood may cause the patient to acquire significant amounts of anti-A and anti-B antibodies that have been passively transfused; hemolysis of RBCs may then occur when the recipient's original blood group is subsequently transfused. In a resuscitation, one should continue to use group O blood if large amounts (more than 2 units) of *whole blood* have already been given.

One may transfuse both Rh-positive and Rh-negative group O packed cells in patients who are in critical condition. It is a common *misconception* that patients who are Rh-negative will have an immediate transfusion reaction if given Rh-positive blood. There is no particular advantage in the Rh factor determination because preformed, naturally occurring anti-Rh antibodies do not exist. Theoretically individuals who are Rh-negative may become sensitized either through pregnancy or by previous transfusions, resulting in a delayed hemolytic transfusion reaction if Rh-positive blood is transfused. However, this scenario is very rare and of no great clinical significance when compared with life-threatening blood loss. Many advise the routine use of *O Rh-positive* packed cells in all patients for whom the Rh factor has not been determined, except in females of childbearing age, for whom future Rh sensitization may be an important consideration.[14] Once resuscitated with Rh-positive blood, patients may receive their own type without a problem developing. Because individuals with O Rh-negative blood represent only 15 per cent of the population and the blood may be in short supply, it is reasonable to save O Rh-negative blood for Rh-negative females of childbearing potential and to use *group O Rh-positive packed cells routinely as the first choice for emergency transfusions.*[13, 14] In a study of emergency blood needs, Schmidt and colleagues reported 601 units of Rh-positive type O blood transfused to 193 patients, including 8 Rh-negative women, before blood type was determined. No acute hemolytic reaction occurred, and no women were sensitized.[14] Rh immune globulin prophylaxis is recommended only for Rh-negative women with childbearing potential receiving Rh-positive blood.

Transfusion Coagulopathy. Within the past 10 years it has been appreciated that pathologic hemostasis occurs following massive blood transfusions.[18–20] The exact cause of the transfusion coagulopathy is poorly defined and poorly understood. Although such abnormalities rarely develop within the time frame of the initial resuscitation in the emergency department, an understanding of the problem leads to a more intelligent approach to transfusion practices and the anticipation of potential problems. The term *massive transfusion* is loosely defined but is usually considered to be the transfusion of more than 10 units of blood to an adult (equivalent to one blood volume) within 24 hours. In patients who are given a transfusion that is equal to two blood volumes, only approximately 10 per cent of the original elements remain. Considering the significant alteration in blood and blood products that occurs during storage, one can readily appreciate the underlying problem associated with such massive transfusions. The development of transfusion coagulopathy is multifactorial and in large part is related to tissue injury and duration of shock.[21-23] Abnormalities in platelets and plasma clotting factors also play a role.

Platelets. Transfusion coagulopathy is related partly to a diluting effect of the transfusion of blood deficient in platelets. Disseminated intravascular coagulopathy plays a secondary role in post-transfusion bleeding.

Banked whole blood and packed cells are devoid of functioning platelets. Dilutional thrombocytopenia is a well-recognized complication of massive transfusion, and a platelet count should be obtained routinely if more than 5 units of blood are transfused. As a general guideline, platelet therapy should be considered after the first 10 units of blood have been given, although the most useful parameter for estimating the need for platelet transfusions is the platelet count.

Plasma Clotting Factors. Factors V and VIII are labile in stored blood and absent in packed cells. Fibrinogen is relatively stable in stored blood but is absent in packed cells. A deficiency of most clotting factors, especially factors V and VIII and fibrinogen, occurs with massive transfusions. This deficiency probably occurs on a "wash-out," or dilutional, basis, although the dynamics are poorly understood. The replacement of these factors may be required. Specific assays for the individual factors are available, but it is more practical to measure activated partial thromboplastin time, prothrombin time, and fibrinogen levels. Fresh frozen plasma has been used to correct clotting factor abnormalities secondary to dilution from massive transfusions, but its effectiveness has not been firmly established. Cryoprecipitate has also been used to replace factor VIII and fibrinogen, but it is rarely required, because fresh frozen plasma contains some fibrinogen. Fresh frozen plasma should be infused to correct the coagulopathy as indicated by clotting studies, but as a general guide, 1 to 2 units of fresh frozen plasma may be given empirically for each 5 to 6 units of blood in the massively traumatized or bleeding patient. Cryoprecipitate may be required if fibrinogen levels fall below 100 mg/dl and are not adequately supplemented with fresh frozen plasma.

ORDERING OF BLOOD

Ordering a type and cross-match procedure on a blood product implies that the decision has already been made to administer a transfusion. A "type and hold" or "type and screen" (no cross-match) request alerts the blood bank to the *possibility* that a blood product will be required for the patient, so appropriate units can be acquired and kept on hand. A type and cross-match procedure takes 45 minutes and restricts a unit of blood to a specific patient. This limits a valuable resource and should not be requested lightly. In the emergency unit, a cross-match procedure should be requested for a blood product only if the adult patient (1) manifests shock, (2) has *symptomatic* anemia (usually associated with a hemoglobin less than 10 gm/dl) in the emergency unit, (3) has a documented loss of 1000 ml of blood, or (4) requires a blood-losing operation immediately (e.g., thoracotomy).[24] A type and hold can safely be requested for all other situations in which a blood transfusion is considered possible during the patient's care; a desirable ratio of units cross-matched to units transfused can thus be achieved.

The number of units to be requested for a cross-match procedure is determined by the size of the patient, the response of the patient to the injury and subsequent emergency treatment, and the presence of ongoing blood losses (e.g., arterial or massive gastrointestinal bleeding). In the majority of fatalities from massive hemorrhage, the patients die from hypovolemia rather than from lack of oxygen-carrying capacity. Specific guidelines for the administration of blood components are given in Table 33–5.

Red blood cell preparations for transfusion are not routinely tested for the presence of sickle hemoglobin. Donors with sickle trait are not excluded, and blood with sickle trait can safely be given to almost every patient, because occlusion of blood flow, caused by intravascular sickling would occur only in extreme conditions of acidity, hypoxia, or hypothermia that are unlikely to be compatible with life. Nonetheless, when transfusion is being performed in infants and patients with known sickle cell anemia, the blood bank should be alerted, and a "sickle prep" should be requested for donor blood to avoid the infusion of sickle-trait blood into such patients. There have been rare instances in which blood from a donor with a mild variant, such as S-C disease, caused massive intravascular sickling and death in a sick, hypoxic, acidotic infant.[25]

Blood Request Forms. The most important part of ordering blood components for a patient is proper identification of the patient and the intended unit of blood. Transfusion of an incorrect unit is a potentially fatal error. Most transfusion mistakes are clerical errors. Several identification systems have been established to minimize the risk of improper transfusions: a prototype is the Typenex Blood Recipient Identification System (Fenwal Laboratories, Inc., Deerfield, Ill.) (Fig. 33–1). A strip of adhesive-backed identically numbered labels is attached to a *second* identically numbered patient identification bracelet. The tube containing a blood sample for cross-match is sent to the blood bank with several adhesive-backed numbered labels attached. These can be removed and affixed to the units of blood prepared for the patient. Just before administering the blood, the nurse or physician checks the identity of the numbered labels. In addition, the blood bank laboratory slip should identify the patient by name and number and should also contain the identification number of the unit of blood. One cannot be overcautious in these identification procedures (Fig. 33–2).

Usual procedures require a separate *blood bank request form* for each unit of RBCs or whole blood that is ordered. A number of units of fresh frozen plasma, cryoprecipitate, and platelet concentrates may be ordered on one form with proper identification (depending on individual blood bank procedures). When the blood bank indicates that the units ordered are ready, the person picking up the blood, along with the blood bank technician, checks the notation on the *blood release form* (transfusion form) to verify the identity of the patient (name, hospital number) and to ensure that the blood unit has been prepared for that patient (blood group and type, unit number). Immediately before administering the blood to the patient, the nurse or physician hanging the unit should check the release form, blood unit, and patient tag for identity as well as the expiration date of the unit (Fig. 33–3).

INTRAVENOUS ADMINISTRATION

One should not open the unit of blood until and unless a free-flowing intravenous access line has been established in a large-bore vein. A 14-gauge intravenous catheter is preferred, both to minimize hemolysis and to ensure rapid

Table 33–5. *Transfusion of Blood Products*

Blood Product	Waiting Time to Receive in Emergency Department	Initial Amount to Transfuse	Expected Response in 70-kg Adult
Un–cross-matched O Rh-positive or -negative red blood cells	5 minutes	2 to 10 units, 10 to 20 ml/kg/hour or as needed based on clinical condition	Stabilize patient in shock
Un–cross-matched type-specific whole blood	15 minutes		Change in hemoglobin/hematocrit depends on hydration and rate of bleeding
Typed and screened whole blood	25 minutes		Approximate rise of 1 gm/dl hemoglobin per unit
Cross-matched whole blood	1¼ hours		
Packed red blood cells	1½ hours		Each unit raises hematocrit 2 to 3 per cent
Frozen red blood cells	4 to 6 hours (if not prepared inhouse)		In children, each ml per kg of packed cells raises hematocrit by 1 per cent
Platelet concentrate†	5 minutes if available	1 unit per 10 kg, usually 6 to 10 units per transfusion in an adult	Rise of 5000 to 10,000 platelets per mm³ per unit; six units usually sufficient to stop bleeding
Cryoprecipitate	20 minutes	1 to 2 bags per 10 kg (7 to 15 bags) 10-minute push, or 20–50 units/kg	Rise of 3 per cent in factor VIII level per bag (40 to 100 per cent activity desired)
Factor IX or prothrombin concentrate	Immediately available (reconstituted powder)	10–50 units/kg	30 to 100 per cent rise in factor IX activity
Fresh frozen plasma	40 minutes	1 bag per 7 kg (4 to 10 bags for adult) 10-minute push,* 3 to 10 ml per kg, depending on clinical condition	Correction in coagulation status; 1 unit raises all coagulation factors by 2 to 3 per cent in average-sized adult

*Administer 1 bag per 4 to 6 units of blood transfused to replace diluted and inactivated coagulation factors.
†Also consider thrombocytopenia as a cause of bleeding from massive transfusion.

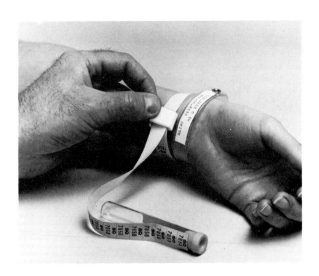

Figure 33–1. The Typenex blood recipient identification system. The identity of the patient and the blood sample are ensured by numbered labels on the tube and on the bracelet. (Courtesy of Fenwal Laboratories, Deerfield, Ill.)

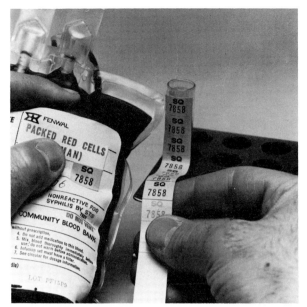

Figure 33–2. In the blood bank, cross-matched units of blood are identified with numbered labels from the patient's blood sample. (Courtesy of Fenwal Laboratories, Deerfield, Ill.)

infusion of fluid for the treatment of hypovolemia or hypotension. When large amounts of blood must be given rapidly, administration by means of a high-flow infusion system is preferred (see Chapter 22). Standard central venous pressure lines are generally too small for adequate volume resuscitation in patients in critical condition. Likewise, the purpose of a large-bore infusion line is defeated if blood is piggybacked with an 18- to 20-gauge needle through a side port in the infusion tubing. For an elective transfusion, however, blood may be given through a smaller needle. No significant hemolysis occurs when small-gauge (21, 23, 25, and 27 gauge) short needles are used for transfusion of fresh blood or packed cells in infants and children and when the maximum rate of infusion is less than 100 ml per hour.[26] For rapid infusion, however, the blood administration tubing is connected directly to the infusion catheter. The infusion

site should be monitored for infiltration, infection, or local reactions. Antiseptic technique is essential.

Each institution has its own preference for establishing an intravenous site for blood infusion. One could follow the same procedures that are used for cleansing the skin before drawing a blood sample for culture. Care should be taken to avoid touching the injection site until the needle is under the skin. The area should be kept clean and dry thereafter. Some practitioners routinely cover the site with topical antibiotic and gauze after securing the needle to the skin.

If the patient already has a suitable intravenous line in place, a solution of 0.9 per cent normal saline only should be used to flush the system before administering the blood. Other intravenous fluids are *not* to be used because of the risks of hemolysis or aggregation (with 5 per cent dextrose in water) or clotting (with lactated Ringer solution).[27] No medications can be placed into the unit of blood or added to the infusion line for the same reasons.

Administration Tubing Sets

Both straight and Y-type tubing sets are commercially available to attach the unit of blood to the needle in the patient. Multi-lead (Y) sets (Figs. 33–4 through 33–8) bearing two hard plastic spikes for entering a blood unit or bottle of intravenous solution are preferred. These provide the option of infusing normal saline while switching blood units or waiting for additional units to be obtained. One should use the sequence in Table 33–6 for flushing the tubing of the blood administration set with normal saline before attaching and administering the unit of blood. Appropriate attention should be paid to the administration set used because new data show marked differences in flow rates and life spans in apparently similar infusion sets provided by different manufacturers.[28]

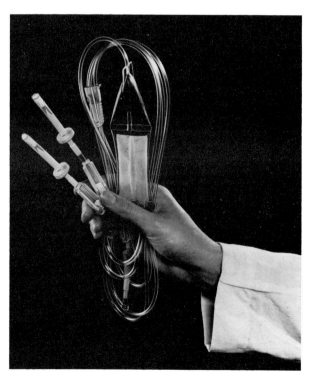

Figure 33–4. An example of a blood administration Y set with two adapters for insertion into a unit of blood or saline; note the in-line filter. (Courtesy of Fenwal Laboratories, Deerfield, Ill.)

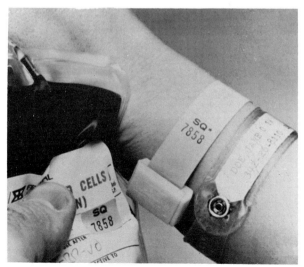

Figure 33–3. Before administration of the blood unit, the numbered labels on the patient's bracelet and on the unit of blood are checked for identity. (Courtesy of Fenwal Laboratories, Deerfield, Ill.)

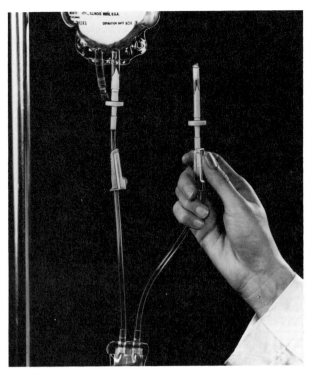

Figure 33–5. One upper adapter has been inserted into a bag containing normal (0.9 per cent) saline. (Courtesy of Fenwal Laboratories, Deerfield, Ill.)

Filters

All blood and blood products should be infused only through an appropriate filter, such as those supplied in-line in the blood administration tubing sets. In the past, filtration was required merely to keep the intravenous line from becoming blocked by clots, but the adverse consequences to the patient that result from infusing unfiltered blood prod-

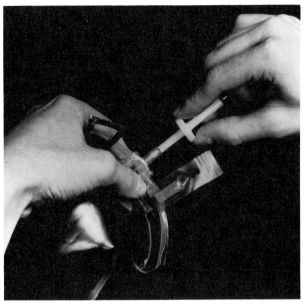

Figure 33–7. Inserting the hard plastic spike of the upper adapter. (Courtesy of Fenwal Laboratories, Deerfield, Ill.)

ucts have now been recognized. Debris consisting of clots and aggregates of fibrin, white blood cells, platelets, and intertwined RBCs (ranging in size from 15 to 200 μ) will accumulate progressively during storage of the blood unit from the first day of collection. The usual filter, made of a single layer of plastic with multiple 170-μ pores, traps larger particles and yet allows for the rapid infusion of blood for 2 to 3 units before flow is greatly obstructed. Purified *components* of blood plasma can be safely administered through a filter with pores as fine as 5 μ.

It has been suggested that microaggregates of debris, which could pass through a 170-μ filter, may in part contribute to the syndrome of "shock lung" seen after transfusions of many units of blood in patients suffering from severe trauma and hemorrhage. Some practitioners there-

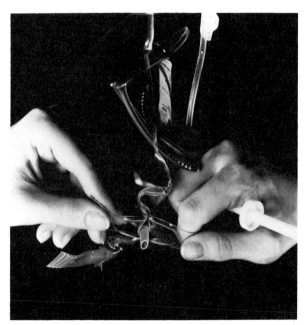

Figure 33–6. The entry site of the unit of blood, into which the other upper adapter of the Y set should be inserted. (Courtesy of Fenwal Laboratories, Deerfield, Ill.)

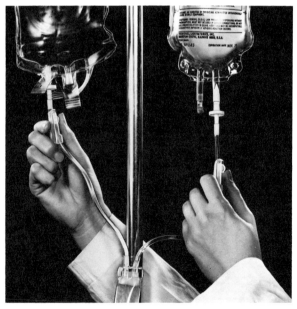

Figure 33–8. After the plastic tubing has been primed with saline, the blood flows through into the patient. (Courtesy of Fenwal Laboratories, Deerfield, Ill.)

Table 33–6. Sequence for Infusing Blood

1. Close the two upper and one lower Flo-trol plastic clamps.
2. Insert one of the upper plastic spikes into a bottle of normal saline (250 ml or more) using standard aseptic technique (see Fig. 33–5).
3. Open both plastic clamps on the upper arms of the Y and allow saline to fill the filter. Saline will also flow back up the second arm (blood port) to the end. Close the clamp on the free, unattached upper tube when this occurs.
4. Open the plastic clamp on the lower, longer tube and allow saline to flow to the end of the infusion line. Close the clamp.
5. Attach the infusion tube to the patient's intravenous site and establish a free flow of saline through the intravenous site.
6. Connect the unit of blood (properly identified) to the short, unattached tubing leading to the filter by finding the portal of entry to the unit. Grasp one plastic tab in each hand and separate them to expose the entry site. With a twisting back-and-forth motion, push the pointed plastic spike of the tubing into the entry site, puncturing it. Use absolute sterile technique (see Figs. 33–6 and 33–7).
7. When ready to transfuse the blood, close off the upper tube leading directly from the saline bottle and open the clamp on the upper tube from the blood. Blood should now be flowing through the upper tubing, the filter, and the lower tubing to the patient (see Fig. 33–8).

fore recommend the use of a microaggregate blood infusion filter with a mesh pore size of 40 μ (Fig. 33–9) when multiple units of blood are administered to a trauma victim, to a patient with compromised pulmonary function, or to a neonate. Filters as small as 20 μ have been suggested.[29] Microaggregate filters tend to become blocked, impeding the rate of infusion more quickly, and are not commonly required in the emergency setting. In addition, whether the infusion of microaggregates (between 40 and 170 μ in size)

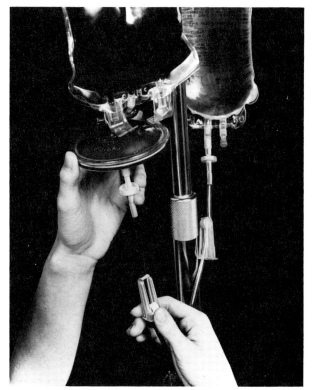

Figure 33–9. Administration of blood through a microaggregate filter attached between the unit of blood and the hard plastic spike of the administration set. (Courtesy of Fenwal Laboratories, Deerfield, Ill.)

is in fact harmful is still an unsettled issue.[30] Standard filters should be replaced after 2 to 3 units of blood product have been administered; most microaggregate filters should be changed after each unit. It is generally agreed that a significant number of platelets are removed by microaggregate filters, and some advise against using these filters when platelet packs are infused. Others believe that, although platelets are removed with the microaggregate filters, the trapped platelets can be removed with saline flush without any significant loss.[31] Table 33–7 lists some available microaggregate filters.

Rate of Infusion

One unit of whole blood can safely be administered to a hypotensive patient at a rate of 20 ml/kg per hour. In the setting of hypovolemic shock and continued hemorrhage, there is no limit to the transfusion rate, and multiple units may be transfused simultaneously, even under pressure. In the stable patient, 1 unit of *whole blood* (500 ml) should be administered over approximately a 2-hour period (3 to 4 ml/kg/hour). After this time, RBCs begin to lose metabolic activity. In addition, the unit of blood, which is an excellent culture medium, is likely to become contaminated if bacteria and fungi are allowed to grow at room temperature. Packed cells should be given at approximately the same rate; plasma products may be given more rapidly. In a patient with a healthy cardiovascular system, one should administer fresh frozen plasma more rapidly (about 15 to 20 minutes per unit) to correct coagulation deficits, because the coagulant activity begins to deteriorate rapidly after 20 to 30 minutes of thawing. In patients with severe anemia and congestive heart failure, a rapidly acting diuretic, such as furosemide, can be given (0.5 mg/kg intravenously) at the onset of transfusion to obviate circulatory overload.

If a transfusion of blood must be interrupted or delayed for some reason, the remainder of the blood unit should be returned to the blood bank. More convenient refrigerators in the emergency unit or on the floor *should not* be used to store blood products unless they are temperature-controlled or continuously monitored.

Patients who are in hemorrhagic shock can receive blood through two large-bore catheters at different sites. Usually, gravity provides a sufficient pressure gradient if the unit is raised higher above the patient to increase the rate of infusion when the clamps are wide open. If a pressure pump is used (e.g., a device made by the Sorenson Research Corp., Salt Lake City, Utah), the infusion can be more rapid (Figs. 33–10 and 33–11).[32] A standard sphygmomanometer cuff should never be wrapped around a unit of blood to create increased infusion pressure, because the nonuniform application of pressure could burst the plastic bag containing the blood component.

One can dilute packed RBCs with normal saline (0.9 per cent) before infusion simply by opening the clamps on the upper tubes of the Y infusion set and leaving the lower (recipient end) clamps closed. Dilution will allow for more rapid infusion by decreasing the blood viscosity, which is dependent on hematocrit, at the risk of increased volume. Alternatively, the direct addition of approximately 200 ml of normal saline to the bag of packed RBCs has been recommended to bring the hematocrit in the blood bag to approximately 45 per cent.

Rewarming

Blood is stored at approximately 4° C to maintain cellular integrity and to prevent the overgrowth of micro-

Table 33-7. In-Line Filters for Blood Transfusion

Filter	Pore Size	Use and Contraindications
Standard		
Fenwal STD Blood Filter	170 μ	All blood components
McGaw STD Blood Filter	170 μ	All blood components
Special Use		
Fenwal 4C2100	170 μ	Platelets, cryoprecipitate, antihemophilic factor concentrates, fresh whole blood
Microaggregate Filters		
Fenwal Microaggregate Blood Filter 4C2423 or 4C2131	20 μ	
Fenwal PDF-10 4C2428		
Intersept Blood Filter (Johnson & Johnson Co., New Brunswick, NJ)	20 μ	Removes most platelets and leukocytes from blood being transfused. Do not use with fresh whole blood or concentrates of platelets or white blood cells. Primarily indicated for use with patients receiving *multiple transfusions* of stored blood and patients with *compromised pulmonary function* and for use in patients undergoing cardiopulmonary bypass. Recommended for use in most newborns.
Alpha Micron-40 (Alpha Therapeutics Corp., Los Angeles, Calif.)	40 μ	
Bentley Disposable Blood Filter PF 127 (Bentley Labs., Inc., Irvine, Calif.)	27 μ	
Hemonate (Gesco Labs., San Antonio, Tex.)	40 μ	
Swank In-Line Blood Filter IL-700 (Pioneer Filters, Inc., Beaverton, Ore.)	20 μ	
Pall Ultipor SQ405 (Pall Biomedical Products Corp., Glen Cove, NY 11542)	40 μ	

organisms. Blood products usually passively warm to 10° C by the time they are administered to the recipient. Adverse effects of hypothermia on cardiac conduction and flow rates are evident when rapid administration of a large volume of blood is performed without prewarming.

Various mechanisms have been used to warm blood to the ideal 35 to 37° C. An ideal blood warmer should allow liberal flow rates while preventing thermal hemolysis of blood cells. Commonly used devices are bath coils that allow a plastic tube to reside in a closely regulated warm water bath, as well as dry heat devices that allow blood to circulate through flat, thin bags sandwiched between aluminum blocks that contain electric heating elements. Both of these devices have relatively low flow rates and suboptimal thermal clearance.[33] Blood bag immersion in warm baths is considered to be an imprecise and a slow method of rewarming. Although much interest surrounds the use of microwave heating devices, concern over hemolysis and lack of proven clinical safety prohibits the recommendation of this technique at this time.

Rapid admixture warming is a promising technique under investigation (see Chapter 22).[34, 35] The unit of whole blood is mixed with an equal amount of normal saline, which has been preheated to between 60 to 70° C. Once mixed, the product is administered to the patient with a resultant delivery temperature of approximately 35° C. This technique combines dilution of blood product and warming into one step. Regardless of the rewarming technique used, warming refrigerated blood to body temperature decreases its viscosity two- to threefold and avoids venous spasm, thus facilitating transfusion.

Monitoring

During the first 5 to 10 minutes and then every 15 minutes during a transfusion of any blood product, the patient must be carefully monitored for evidence of a transfusion reaction. Signs and symptoms that one may encounter are hives, chills, diarrhea, fever, pruritus, flushing, abdominal or back pain, tightness in the chest or the throat, and respiratory distress. A potentially life-threatening acute hemolytic transfusion reaction in a patient who has received prior transfusions may differ clinically from an allergic, nuisance reaction only by its effects on the patient's pulse and blood pressure. One can safely treat an allergic reaction to leukocytes or plasma proteins that cause hives, itching, fever, or chills by administering an antihistamine (but not into the blood infusion line) and stopping the transfusion.

When one encounters an increase in pulse rate, a decrease in blood pressure, respiratory symptoms, chest or abdominal discomfort, or the "sensation of impending doom," one must *stop* the transfusion *immediately* and must infuse normal saline to maintain blood pressure and urine output. Samples of urine and blood should be sent to the laboratory to verify the presence of free hemoglobin. The blood bank should also receive a clotted sample of blood to reassess the presence of any immune reaction. If the conclusion of the blood bank evaluation is that the reaction is a nonhemolytic allergic response, premedication with antihistamines (diphenhydramine or hydroxyzine) and antipyretics is indicated before the next transfusion. Alternatively, washed cells could be used.

The patient in whom a hemolytic transfusion reaction is suspected should be treated vigorously and promptly.[36] Most mortality and morbidity is secondary to hypotension and shock leading to cardiovascular instability, renal insufficiency, respiratory manifestations, or hemorrhagic complications of disseminated intravascular coagulation. The initial treatment is directed toward treating the hypotension by infusion of 5 per cent dextrose in saline or lactated Ringer solution or vasopressors, if required. The volume and rate of infusion are determined by blood pressure response. Symptomatic treatment with acetaminophen, a warming blanket, an inhaled or subcutaneous β-agonist agent for bronchospasm or subglottic edema, or antipruritics or anti-histamines is of secondary importance.

If an acute hemolytic transfusion reaction occurs, there may be some benefit from alkalinization of the urine with intravenous sodium bicarbonate to prevent the precipitation of free hemoglobin. Forced diuresis with mannitol to maintain the urine output at 50 to 100 ml/hour has also been advocated. The benefit from alkalinization and diuresis in the prevention of acute renal shutdown is uncertain, although the use of these techniques is commonly advocated. After shock is controlled, an assessment of hemostasis, respiratory function, renal function, and cardiac function will help direct later therapy of the complications; disseminated intravascular coagulation may call for the administration of plasma, platelets, or fibrinogen, and acute tubular necrosis may dictate careful fluid management. Hemolytic transfusion reactions have become unusual. They are rarely fatal and are usually attributable to an error in identification (such as can result from the treatment of two "John Doe" patients simultaneously).

Delayed, or "late," hemolytic transfusion reactions may occur days, or even weeks, after transfusion of RBCs. They are characterized by dropping hemoglobin levels, jaundice, hemoglobinemia, and indirect hyperbilirubinemia.[37] This complication is usually self-limited and is not life-threatening. Therapy is symptomatic, but future attempts at cross-matching for transfusions may be difficult because of the presence of RBC antibodies. Individuals so affected should wear identification tags or bracelets alerting medical personnel that prior transfusion reactions have occurred.

CONCLUSION

On the completion of a transfusion, an entry in the patient's record should be made to indicate the volume and nature of what was transfused and the presence or absence of any reaction. The

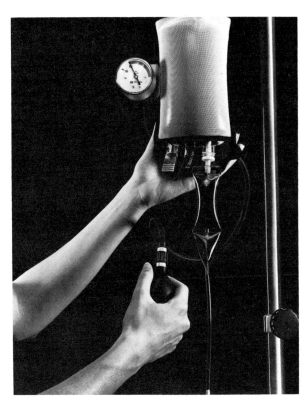

Figure 33–11. A rubber bladder is pumped up, and the blood unit is squeezed uniformly against a reinforced mesh. (Courtesy of Fenwal Laboratories, Deerfield, Ill.)

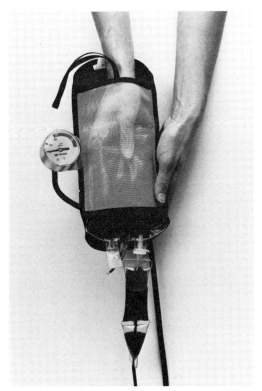

Figure 33–10. A controlled-pressure administration device for rapid infusion of blood products. (Courtesy of Fenwal Laboratories, Deerfield, Ill.)

progress note, the transfusion record sheet, or the transfusion laboratory slip can be used for this purpose and should be signed and dated by the physician or nurse, in accordance with hospital policies. The bag in which the blood was stored might be discarded or returned to the blood bank, as individual policies dictate.

The practitioner should emphasize to the patient and family the critical importance of any blood transfusion in the patient's care. It could then be suggested that the family consider arranging for replacement donations of units of blood to afford future patients the luxury of an ample, available supply of blood products.

REFERENCES

1. Denis J: Philos Proc R Soc No 32, 617, 1667–1668, cited in Mollison PL: Blood Transfusion in Clinical Medicine. 6th ed. Oxford, Blackwell Scientific Publications, 1979, p 1.
2. Cannan RK: Foreword to General Principles of Blood Transfusion. Transfusion 3:304, 1963.
3. Gammage G: Crystalloid versus colloid: Is colloid worth the cost? Internat Anesthesiol Clin 25:37, 1987.
4. Rackow EC, Falk JL, Fein IA, et al: Fluid resuscitation in circulatory shock: A comparison of the cardiorespiratory effects of albumin, hetastarch, and saline solutions in patients with hypovolemic and septic shock. Crit Care Med 11:839, 1983.
5. Sanchez-Quijano A, Lissen E, Diaz-Torres MA, et al: Prevention of post transfusion non-A, non-B hepatitis by non-specific immunoglobulin in heart surgery patients. Lancet 1:1245, 1988.
6. Milner LV, Butcher K: Transfusion reactions reported after transfusions of red blood cells and of whole blood. Transfusion 18:493, 1978.
7. Blumberg N, Bove JR: Un-cross-matched blood for emergency transfusion. JAMA 240:2057, 1978.
8. Dietrich KA, Conrad SA, Herbert CA, et al: Cardiovascular and metabolic response to red blood cell transfusion in critically ill volume-resuscitated nonsurgical patients. Crit Care Med 18:940, 1990.
9. Kahn RA, Allen RW, Baldassare J: Alternate sources and substitutes for theraputic blood components. Blood 66:1, 1985.
10. Dixon JL, Smalley MG: Jehovah's Witnesses: The surgical/ethical challenge. JAMA 246:2471, 1981.
11. Tierney WM, Weinberger M, Greene JY, et al: Jehovah's Witnesses and blood transfusions: Physician's attitude and legal precedence. South Med J 77:473, 1984.

12. Plapp FV, Rachel JM, Sinor LT: Dipsticks for determining ABO blood groups. Lancet 1:1465, 1986.
13. Schmidt PJ, Leparc GF, Smith CT: Use of Rh positive blood in emergency situations. Surg Gynecol Obstet 167:229, 1988.
14. Lefebre J, McLellan BA, Coovadia AS: Seven years experience with Group O unmatched packed red blood cells in a regional trauma unit. Ann Emerg Med 16:1344, 1987.
15. Pollack W, Ascari WQ, Crispen JF, et al: Studies on Rh prophylaxis II: Rh immune prophylaxis after transfusion with Rh-positive blood. Transfusion 11:340, 1971.
16. Boral LI, Henry JB: The type and screen: A safe alternative and supplement in selected surgical procedures. Transfusion 17:163, 1977.
17. Schwab CW, Civil I, Shayne JP: Saline-expanded Group O uncross-matched packed red blood cells as an initial resuscitation fluid in severe shock. Ann Emerg Med 15:1282, 1986.
18. Counts RB, Haisch C, Simon L, et al: Hemostasis in massively transfused trauma patients. Ann Surg 190:91, 1979.
19. Wilson RF, Mammen E, Walt AF: Eight years of experience with massive blood transfusions. J Trauma 11:275, 1971.
20. Shomer PR, Dawson RB: Transfusion therapy in trauma: A review of principles and techniques used in the MIEMS program. Am Surg 45:109, 1979.
21. Hewson JR, Neame PB, Kumar N, et al: Coagulopathy related to dilution and hypotension during massive transfusion. Crit Care Med 13:387, 1985.
22. Harke H, Rahman S: Haemostatic disorders in massive transfusion. Bibl Haematol 46:179, 1980.
23. Harrigan C, Lucas CE, Ledgerwood AM, et al: Primary hemostasis after massive transfusion for injury. Am Surg 48:393, 1982.
24. Clarke JR, Davidson SJ, Bergman GE, Geller NL: Optimal blood ordering for emergency department patients. Ann Emerg Med 9:1, 1980.
25. Murphy RJC, Malhotra C, Sweet AY: Death following an exchange transfusion with hemoglobin SC blood. J Pediatr 96:110, 1980.
26. Herrera AJ, Corless J: Blood transfusions: Effect of speed of infusion and of needle gauge on hemolysis. J Pediatr 99:757, 1981.
27. Ryden SE, Oberman HA: Compatibility of common intravenous solutions with CPD blood. Transfusion 15:250, 1975.
28. Hill RC, Middaugh RE, Menk EJ, et al: Clinical evaluation of commonly used blood administration sets. J Emerg Med 7:103, 1989.
29. Risberg BI, Hurley MJ, Miller E, et al: Filtration characteristics of the polyester fiber micropore blood transfusion filter. South Med J 72:657, 1979.
30. Hassig A: When is the microfiltration of whole blood and red cell concentrates essential? When is it superfluous? Vox Sang 50:54, 1986.
31. Snyder EL, Hezzey A, Cooper-Smith M, et al: Effect of microaggregate blood filtration on platelet concentrates in vitro. Transfusion 21:427, 1981.
32. Ballance JHW: Equipment and methods for rapid blood transfusion. Br J Hosp Med 26:411, 1981.
33. Flancbaum L, Trooskin SZ, Pederson H: Evaluation of blood-warming devices with the apparent thermal clearance. Ann Emerg Med 18:355, 1989.
34. Wilson EB, Iserson KV: Admixture of blood warming: A technique for rapid warming of erythrocytes. Ann Emerg Med 16:413, 1987.
35. Wilson EB, Knauf MA, Donohoe K, et al: Red blood cell survival following admixture with heated saline: Evaluation of a new blood warming method for rapid transfusion. J Trauma 28:1274, 1988.
36. Pineda AA, Brzica SM, Taswell HF: Hemolytic transfusion reaction: Recent experience in a large blood bank. Mayo Clin Proc 53:378, 1978.
37. Pineda AA, Taswell HF, Brzica SM: Delayed hemolytic transfusion reaction: An immunologic hazard of blood transfusion. Transfusion 18:1, 1978.

Chapter **34**

Autotransfusion (Autologous Blood Transfusion)

Thomas B. Purcell

INTRODUCTION

Among the various afflictions that may jeopardize human life and well-being, traumatic injury has, in recent decades, been ravaging an ever-expanding proportion of men and women during their most productive years.[1] This fact, coupled with increasingly efficient and rapid emergency transportation systems, has resulted in growing numbers of these victims arriving at emergency facilities in potentially salvageable condition. The ensuing urgent demand for blood has often exceeded the immediately available supplies of homologous bank blood. Successful approaches to this problem have included earlier hemostasis (i.e., definitive surgery), use of volume expanders (crystalloid, colloid), and autotransfusion.

Autotransfusion may be defined as "collection and reinfusion of the patient's own blood for volume replacement."[2] Emergency autotransfusion most often involves collection of shed blood from a major body cavity, usually the pleural space (hemothorax) and occasionally from the peritoneal space. Autotransfusion in the emergency department is generally limited to acute hemothorax with clinically significant hypovolemia. The following discussion examines the advantages and potential complications of emergency autotransfusion, patient selection, available equipment, and procedural technique for two widely used devices.

BACKGROUND

Autotransfusion has a relatively extended tradition in the Western medical literature. An early report was published in 1818 by Blundell,[3] an English practitioner, who reflected on the possibility of reinfusion of shed blood after witnessing a woman exsanguinate from uterine hemorrhage. His subsequent work with autotransfusion of shed blood in dogs suggested the clinical feasibility of the procedure. Highmore,[4] in 1874, also espoused the use of autotransfusion after recounting his own experience with a patient who succumbed to postpartum hemorrhage. In 1886 Duncan[5] used the technique without notable ill effects while reinfusing blood shed during an amputation. In 1914, the use of the technique in ectopic pregnancies was popularized by Thies,[6] and three years later, Elmendorf[7] published a description of the first case of autotransfusion from traumatic hemothorax. Also in 1917, Lockwood[8] used the procedure for the first time in the United States during a splenectomy performed on a patient with Banti syndrome. By 1922, Burch[9] was able to accumulate 164 cases for review from the world literature.

The discovery of ABO blood typing at the turn of the century and the institution of blood banks in the 1930s led to the almost exclusive use of homologous blood up to and following World War II. Interest in autotransfusion concomitantly declined, and only sporadic reports appeared in the literature during this period. During the 1960s and 1970s, cardiopulmonary bypass surgery generated extensive data regarding intraoperative retrieval of large quantities of blood for reinfusion. Concurrently, the Vietnam War created tremendous new demands for readily available blood in areas remote from conventional reserves of homologous bank blood. Thus revitalized interest, coupled with growing experience, generated the early publications of such investigators as Dyer and associates,[10] Klebanoff and colleagues,[11, 12] and Symbas and co-workers[13, 14] which initiated the "new era" of autotransfusion.

ADVANTAGES

The advantages of autotransfusion over banked blood transfusion in patients who are hypovolemic from traumatic blood loss include the following:

1. Rapid availability to the patient (collection and initiation of reinfusion can be accomplished within minutes).

2. Blood compatibility, avoiding both untoward transfusion reactions and the problem of cross-matching uncommon blood types.

3. Immediate reinfusion of normothermic autologous blood and consequent lessening of life-threatening complications of hypothermia that are created by the administration of room-temperature fluids.[15]

4. Elimination of risk of indirect patient-to-patient transmission of infectious diseases such as hepatitis, malaria, cytomegalovirus, or human immunodeficiency virus.[16]

5. Levels of 2,3-DPG have been found to be significantly higher in autotransfused red blood cells than in stored homologous cells with an average 2,3-DPG shelf life of 4.2 days.[17, 18]

6. No reported direct complications of metabolic acidosis, hypocalcemia, or hyperkalemia.[19–22]

7. Less risk of inadvertent circulatory overload.[23]

8. May be acceptable to those patients whose religious convictions prohibit transfusions with homologous blood.*

9. Allows preservation of limited stores of banked blood, thereby ensuring their availability for other uses.[16]

10. Autotransfusion lowers the cost of medical care.[16] No blood drawing, typing, or cross-matching is required; thus time, money, and personnel expenditures may be conserved. Davidson[25] reported the cost of autologous blood to be $12 per unit for the first three units and $8 per unit thereafter for emergency resuscitation compared with between $25 and $75 per unit of banked blood. Mattox[26] reported the autotransfusion of a total of 134 liters of blood in 69 patients over a 2-year period. The total cost of the disposable equipment used was approximately $1500, which translated to a savings of $13,400 when compared with expenses for similar volumes of banked donor blood. Although the cost of medical care has risen in recent years, these cost differences are expected to remain generally valid today.

INDICATIONS AND CONTRAINDICATIONS

Patient Selection

In general, all victims of severe trauma, whether blunt or penetrating, should be considered potential candidates for autotransfusion. More specifically, Reul and colleagues[22] have described three categories of patients for whom emergency autotransfusion is suitable. First, the ideal candidate is the patient who has sustained blunt or penetrating chest trauma, with an acute chest tube collection of 1500 ml or more of blood. A second category is the patient with less than one whole body blood volume loss for whom no homologous blood, or only limited quantities, are available because of the urgency of the situation, a blood bank shortage, or a difficult cross-match. Under these circumstances, Reul and coworkers used autotransfusion regardless of the type of injury or degree of contamination. A third category is the patient with massive blood loss (over one whole body blood volume) for whom autotransfusion can serve as a supplement to homologous replacement. O'Riordan[20] adds a fourth category: the trauma patient who

urgently requires blood transfusion and whose religious convictions prohibit homologous transfusion. In a broader sense, it seems clinically reasonable to use autotransfusion in all suitable patients who have a hemothorax and require even minimal blood replacement. In situations in which the need for homologous blood transfusion is borderline, autologous blood can be readily reinfused without the risk of complications associated with the use of banked blood.

In our own emergency department, we have simplified the *indications* for initiating collection for possible autotransfusion to the following:

1. Blunt or penetrating chest trauma with significant hemothorax (500 ml or more) as suggested on a chest film.

2. Multiple trauma with shock of uncertain etiology in a patient for whom immediate (prior to chest film) tube thoracotomy is contemplated.

3. Emergency thoracotomy.

4. Hemothorax with an urgent need for blood when the patient's religious beliefs prohibit homologous transfusions.

Reul and coworkers[22] also suggested the following four general *contraindications* to the use of emergency autotransfusion:

1. The presence of malignant lesions in the area of traumatic blood accumulation.

2. Known renal or hepatic insufficiency.

3. Wounds older than 4 to 6 hours (because of the theoretic problem of bacterial overgrowth).

4. Gross contamination of pooled blood, usually as a result of trauma of the gastrointestinal tract.

They added, however, that "the presence of any of these contraindications was occasionally overruled by the lack of available (banked) blood."

Several investigators believe that the reinfusion of possibly contaminated blood from the peritoneal cavity may be accomplished with an acceptable risk,[12, 22, 27–29] but the consensus is that exsanguinating hemorrhage is the only acceptable indication for autotransfusion when there is recognized intestinal contamination. Klebanoff,[30] on the other hand, believes that autotransfusion has "no place" when there is extensive fecal or urinary contamination of the pooled blood. Thus the advisability of autotransfusing possibly contaminated blood from the peritoneal cavity remains controversial (see the section entitled "Complications").

EQUIPMENT AND MATERIALS

Autotransfusion Units

Symbas and associates[13, 31, 32] described a simplified collection system using standard materials available in any emergency department. After insertion of a chest tube, drainage is established into a standard chest tube bottle containing 400 ml of normal saline, maintaining a suction of 12 to 16 mm Hg. (Many of the disposable plastic thoracostomy collection devices now have the ability to act as reservoirs for autotransfusion in case the need arises.) If autotransfusion is required, the collected blood in the chest bottle is reinfused in one of two ways.

1. The chest bottle may be disconnected from the pleural drainage tube and simply inverted on an intravenous stand for reinfusion through a filter into the patient. During infusion, a second sterile chest bottle with saline is connected to the chest tube for continuing collection.

---

*Techniques for intraoperative or extraoperative collection of autologous blood that involve blood storage or reinfusion of shed blood are objectionable to Jehovah's Witnesses. Nonetheless, salvage when extracorporeal circulation is uninterrupted may be acceptable to many members of that religion.[24]

2. After disconnection from the pleural drainage tube, the chest bottle may be connected to a standard blood collection bag and the salvaged blood transferred to this bag for subsequent reinfusion in the conventional manner. Symbas[31] reported on more than 400 patients autotransfused by this method since 1966, with no adverse effects attributable to the procedure.

Von Koch and associates[33] reported their experience with the Sorenson unit in autotransfusing each of 30 trauma patients an average of 1000 ml of salvaged blood. They found this unit could be assembled quickly and was easily operated, and its use resulted in minimal air-blood interfacing (a source of hemolysis). They also described the unit as "efficacious, inexpensive, cost effective and safe." Davidson[25] described in detail the step-by-step use of the Sorenson autotransfusion unit in the emergency department and characterized it as "probably the simplest and most practical device available for the emergency setting." As of December 1988, the cost of this unit remained less than $200. Autotransfusion using this device is explained in the following section.

A unit introduced more recently, the Pleur-evac autotransfusion system (Dehnatel, Inc., Pfizer Hospital Products Group, Inc.), is similar in concept to the Sorenson unit but is designed to be installed directly in series with a standard Pleur-evac underwater seal drainage system. A disadvantage of this unit is the smaller collecting capacity (1200 ml versus 1900 ml in the Sorenson system). Advantages include an overflow accommodation, which sends blood in excess of the 1200-ml collection bag capacity automatically into a spillover collection chamber of the main Pleur-evac unit, and an ability to monitor the patient for air leaks during collection without changing systems.

The Haemonetics Cell Saver (Haemonetics Corp., Natick, Mass.) aspirates the patient's blood into a reservoir and brings the blood, after it has been anticoagulated, through a special suction line to a centrifuge. The centrifuge spins off the supernatant fluid consisting of plasma that contains hemolyzed cells, free hemoglobin, fat cells, electrolytes, anticoagulant, and contaminants. When the hematocrit of the remaining blood approaches 55 to 65 per cent, normal saline washes it clear of hemolyzed cells, and the packed and washed cells are then reinfused. Major disadvantages of the device, in the opinion of Mattox,[34] are its complexity, requiring a specially trained technician for its operation, and its cost (as of December 1988, from $12,000 to $22,000, depending on the model). Use of the Cell Saver system offers the theoretic advantage of avoiding reinfusion of "activated clotting factors." Brewster and colleagues believe that this advantage is achieved "at the expense of an earlier dilutional decrease of coagulation factors, which are totally lost with discarded plasma and wash fluid."[35] Therefore, the system requires the use of fresh frozen plasma as well as additional colloid, such as albumin, to replace the discarded plasma volume.

Two autotransfusion devices that are off the market but may still be found in use are the Bentley ATS-100 (Bentley Laboratories, Inc., Santa Ana, Calif.) and the Pall Autotransfuser (Pall Corp., Glen Cove, NY). The former system consists of an aspirating segment that is activated by a roller pump, a reservoir that may be pressurized to augment return flow, and a delivery system.[30] The requirement of a specially trained technician plus the potential risk of massive air embolism makes this device less useful in the emergency department setting. The Pall autotransfusion device consists of two containers. While aspirating into one container, pressure can be applied on the other, and blood can be given back to the patient. Mattox found "considerable he-

molysis" associated with the device, as well as a filter that required changing after every two units of blood were collected.[34]

Two highly simplified techniques have been described. Schweitzer and coworkers[36] reported successful autotransfusion in dogs by means of a chest tube connected to a Heimlich flutter valve (Bard-Parker, Rutherford, NJ). The valve was connected in turn to a 1900-ml Sorenson blood collection bag. Drainage was entirely by gravity; no suction was applied. Similarly, Barriot and colleagues[37] described the European experience with a device called Hemotraum adapted for prehospital autotransfusion. Blood from the chest tube fills a 750-ml sterile bag by gravity via a 120-μ micropore filter. When full, the bag is clamped, disconnected, and the collected blood is reinfused through a 50-μ micropore filter. While this blood is being transfused, a second sterile bag is connected to the chest tube. No anticoagulant is used. Although neither of these techniques has undergone clinical trials in the United States, they do serve as indications of possible future trends in emergency autotransfusion in the battlefield, the small rural hospital, or the prehospital care setting.

Blood Filters

Some form of in-line filtration is advisable during reinfusion of blood products to reduce the danger of microembolization and resulting pulmonary insufficiency.[26, 38] Drye[39] simply strained aspirated blood through eight layers of gauze into a bottle and reinfused directly into the patient without further filtration. He reported on almost 100 cases, with only one case of morbidity, and in that case, the blood had not been strained. Controversy continues regarding the relationship between the presence of microaggregates and the development of the respiratory distress syndrome[40]; however, most investigators advise some form of micropore filtration during emergency autotransfusion. Pore size seems to be the only issue, and recommendations range from 170 μ[41] to 20 μ.[21] The preponderance of data appears to show that a pore size of 40 μ minimizes the risk of microembolization without undue elevations in filtration pressures.[2, 17, 19, 22, 26, 33, 42, 43]

Vacuum Suction

The amount of vacuum suction used should be limited to minimize red blood cell hemolysis.[35] Reul and colleagues[22] found that 5 to 10 mm Hg was well within the safe range. Von Koch and associates[33] used 10 mm Hg, Davidson[25] used 20 to 40 mm Hg, Noon[41] used 30 to 60 mm Hg, and Brewster and colleagues[35] and Dyer and coworkers[10] found that levels below 100 mm Hg kept hemolysis to a minimum. Suction of 60 mm Hg or less is preferred by most researchers for aspiration of hemothorax or hemoperitoneum,[22, 25, 33, 35, 41] but in the operating room, adequate suction to maintain a bloodless surgical field may require up to 100 mm Hg or more.[10, 21]

Anticoagulation

Anticoagulation of the aspirate during autotransfusion has been ensured using several different methods, including heparin both locally and systemically,[44] acid-citrate-dextrose (ACD),[12, 21] citrate-phosphate-dextrose (CPD),[19, 22, 26, 33, 44] and normal saline.[13, 31, 32] Local heparinization of the tubing and reservoir may lead to the formation of platelet microaggregates on the filter,[13] and systemic heparinization could lead to further life-threatening hemorrhage in an already bleeding patient.[22, 26, 30] Therefore, the use of heparin as an anticoagulant during emergency autotransfusion of the trauma patient is discouraged by most investigators.[13, 17, 41, 45, 46]

In several early studies, ACD was used as an alternative to heparin.[32, 45, 47] Raines and coworkers[21] found no clinical or laboratory evidence of intravascular coagulopathy after autotransfusion using ACD, even in patients who received more than 8000 ml of autologous blood. More recent studies report the use of CPD for extracorporeal anticoagulation. Some advantages of CPD are that it avoids the complications of heparinization,[22] necessitates less volume as an anticoagulant, and results in less acidosis than does ACD.[48] Reul and colleagues[22] found CPD to be well tolerated, even in large amounts.

Although reported volumes of citric acid and sodium citrate solution for each 500 ml of collected blood range up to 700 ml and 1800 ml, respectively,[19, 22, 26, 33, 49] most recent research has recommended lower levels, in the range of 25 to 30 ml, of CPD per 500 ml of collected blood.[19, 22, 26] A ratio of CPD to blood of 1:7 has also been suggested.[46] This level compares favorably with the standard 67 ml of CPD per unit of banked donor blood.[22] Klebanoff[30] believes that CPD is currently the safest method of anticoagulation for autotransfusion and that the use of CPD avoids the problem of clot formation on the blood filter, thus maintaining higher platelet counts in reinfused blood.

Davidson has noted that for the average chest wound, added anticoagulant may not be required,[25] because moderate rates of bleeding allow time for defibrination by contact with serosal surfaces (pleural surfaces) and by mechanical action of the heart. Dog studies have documented pleural deposition of fibrin hemothorax, further substantiating this mechanism as the cause of hypofibrinogenemia in collected blood.[50] Others[11, 13, 37, 42, 51] report the same findings and recommend simple reinfusion through a filter without any anticoagulant. Nonetheless, wounds of the great vessels may bleed at a rate that allows coagulable blood to enter the collection reservoir and clot off the entire system.[25, 33] In such an instance, an anticoagulant, specifically CPD, would be indispensable. Thus accepted procedure includes the use of CPD, which itself undergoes such rapid metabolism that anticoagulation is, to a large degree, confined to blood in the autotransfusion apparatus. Rarely, with excessive use, CPD can cause citrate intoxication because of chelation of calcium and subsequent cardiac dysrhythmias. Use of insufficient or outdated CPD may result in clotting of collected blood.

PROCEDURE

Mattox[34] set forth the properties of the ideal autotransfusion device: (1) easy and quick assemblage, (2) cost effectiveness, (3) easy operation, (4) in-line microfiltration, (5) minimization of air-fluid interfaces, and (6) simple anticoagulation technique. The Sorenson and Pleur-evac devices, both currently in wide use, conform to these specifications and therefore are discussed in detail. The relatively low cost of these collection devices allows one to prepare for possible autotransfusion in all patients who require thoracostomy, with selective use of the system based on the subsequent clinical course.

Sorenson Autotransfusion System

The Sorenson autotransfusion system consists of a closed, rigid, nonsterile plastic canister into which a gas-autoclaved plastic bag is placed for blood collection. The canister is mounted on a movable support device (intravenous pole) and connected to a vacuum regulator valve for control of negative suction pressure. The collection bag is placed in-line with disposable collection tubing, which has a separate inlet valve for admixture of anticoagulant and aspirated blood. This inlet is connected via sterile tubing to a bottle of CPD (Fig. 34–1).

COLLECTION

1. To collect autologous blood from a hemothorax, first open the included "Trauma Drainage Tubing Set" containing one 36 French chest tube, latex drainage tubing (C), and a male-to-male connector (D). While tube thoracostomy is being performed in the usual manner, the burette set (A) is connected to the CPD bottle, and the burette is filled with 150 ml of CPD.

2. Connect the yellow-tipped (E) end of the latex drainage tubing (the end with the side port) to the inlet port (F) of the red liner cap attached to the collection canister (Fig. 34–2). Then remove the protective cap from the side port and connect the anticoagulant (CPD) administration line (Fig. 34–3). Prime the liner with 50 ml of CPD from the burette.

3. Connect the downstream suction hose (H) to wall suction, and turn wall suction to maximum. Be sure that the regulator on the autotransfusion stand does not exceed the preset 60 mm Hg during collection (100 mm Hg in special situations such as thoracotomy); otherwise, excessive hemolysis of red blood cells may result (see Fig. 34–1).

4. When the chest tube is in place, connect the latex drainage tubing and begin collection. During collection, stay ahead of the accumulating blood volume with the CPD in 50-ml increments. Always keep the ratio no less than one part CPD to 10 parts blood (1:7 ratio of CPD to blood is recommended by the manufacturer); otherwise the collected blood may clot, especially with massive ongoing hemorrhage. Do not overfill the liner bag; it will overflow, spilling blood into the regulator valve.

REINFUSION

1. Prepare a standard Y-type blood infusion line with a high-capacity 40-μ in-line filter, prime the line and filter with normal saline, and connect it to a large-bore intravenous access (14 gauge or larger) (see Fig. 34–7).

2. When the liner bag is full, temporarily clamp the chest tube, discontinue suction, and remove the yellow end of the latex drainage tubing (E) from the red liner lid. The liner lid tubing connector (J) is now removed from the canister tee (K) (Fig. 34–4) and connected to the inlet port (F) of the liner cap, thus sealing the top of the collection lid (Fig. 34–5).

3. Remove the liner assembly from the canister by pushing upward on the thumb tab (see Fig. 34–5), lift out the liner bag, invert the bag, and unscrew the protective cap (N) over the bottom stem of the liner. Now insert the free recipient arm (L) of the Y-tube infusion line into the stem of the collection bag (Fig. 34–6), and hang the liner bag on the intravenous stand by the attached tab (M) (Fig. 34–7). Before infusion, briefly disconnect the liner lid tubing connector (J), *vent all air from the bag* (to eliminate the possibility of air embolism), then reconnect it to the inlet port.

4. Gravity flow, manual squeezing of the liner bag, or an in-line roller pump may be used to hasten reinfusion. Although some reports[25, 33] mention the use of encircling pneumatic blood pumps during reinfusion, the Sorenson Company cautions that such devices may damage the pump or rupture the liner bag.

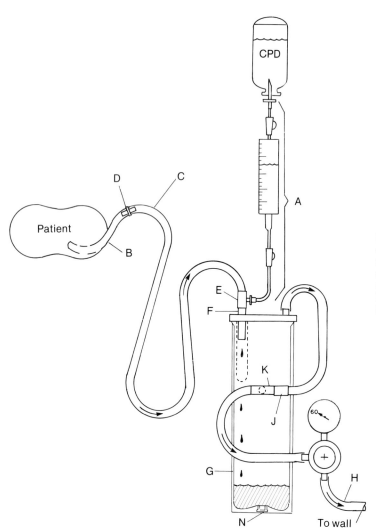

Figure 34–1. Collection apparatus. *A*, Anticoagulant volume control burette; *B*, chest tube; *C*, latex drainage tubing; *D*, male-to-male connector; *E*, end of drainage tubing with side port; *F*, inlet port of red liner cap attached to collection canister; *G*, collection liner bag; *H*, downstream suction hose; *J*, liner lid tubing connector; *K*, canister tee; and *N*, liner stem with protective cap.

Figure 34–2. Collection apparatus. Detail of canister connections before attachment of anticoagulant line. (From Receptal ATS Trauma. Sorenson Research Co, Salt Lake City, Utah, p 5. Reproduced by permission.)

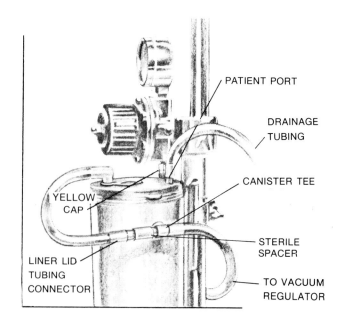

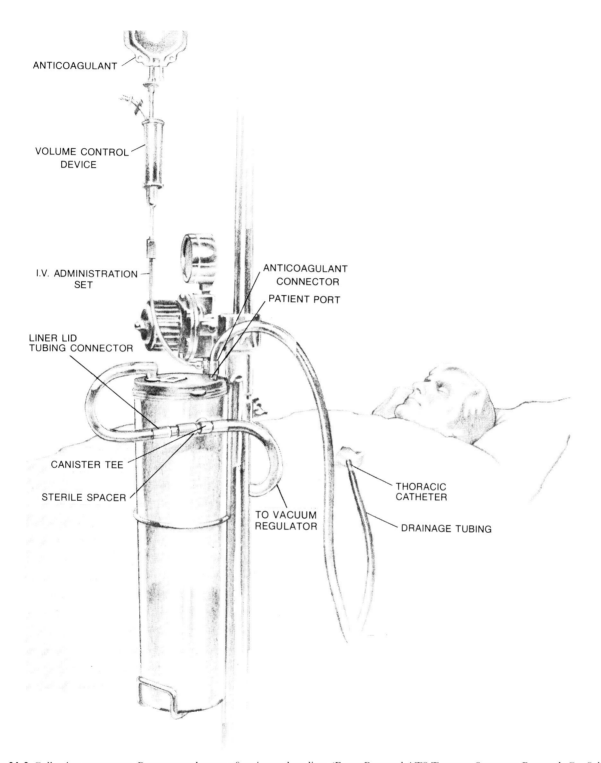

Figure 34–3. Collection apparatus. Proper attachment of anticoagulant line. (From Receptal ATS Trauma. Sorenson Research Co, Salt Lake City, Utah, p 5. Reproduced by permission.)

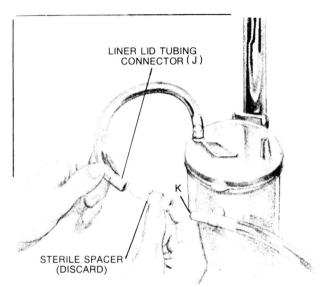

Figure 34–4. Preparation for reinfusion. Removal of liner lid tubing connector (*J*) from canister tee *(K)*. (From Receptal ATS Trauma. Sorenson Research Co, Salt Lake City, Utah, p 5. Reproduced by permission.)

5. During reinfusion, autologous blood collection may be continued with a second liner bag. Be sure that the new liner bag is fully extended before placing it into the canister (Fig. 34–8). If the bag is crumpled at the top of the canister, blood may be sucked directly into the regulator valve. Insert the new liner into the canister, and snap the lid in place with the thumb tab directly over the canister tee (Fig. 34–9). The unit is now ready for collection assembly as previously outlined.

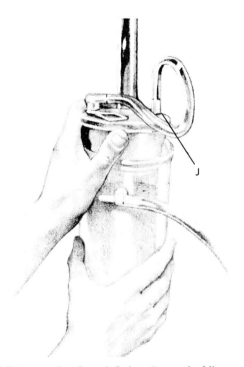

Figure 34–5. Preparation for reinfusion. Removal of liner assembly from the canister after connecting the liner lid tubing connector (*J*) to the inlet port of the liner cap. (From Receptal ATS Trauma. Sorenson Research Co, Salt Lake City, Utah, p 6. Reproduced by permission.)

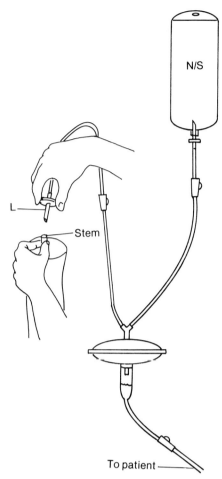

Figure 34–6. Preparation for reinfusion. Inserting the free recipient arm *(L)* of the prepared Y-type infusion line into the stem of the collection bag. (From Receptal ATS Trauma. Sorenson Research Co, Salt Lake City, Utah, p 7. Reproduced by permission.)

Pleur-Evac Autotransfusion System

The Pleur-evac autotransfusion device consists of a sterile, single-use, disposable rectangular-shaped flexible polyvinyl chloride blood collection bag supported by a rigid metal support stand. The bag and support stand are designed to attach in series directly to a standard Pleur-evac underwater seal drainage unit. Inside the collection bag in line with the incoming drainage tube is a 200-μ nylon mesh filter. Attached to the collection bag are two latex tubes, one (red tipped) for collecting shed blood from the drainage site, and one (blue tipped) for connection to the Pleur-evac drainage unit. An injection port is provided on top of the autotransfusion bag for the addition of anticoagulant to collected blood.

COLLECTION

1. The Pleur-evac underwater seal drainage unit (*A*, Fig. 34–10) is first prepared in standard fashion and connected to a source of suction. Slide the metal hanger over the patient drainage tubing port on the right-hand side of the unit (Fig. 34–11), and pull it down flush with the top and side of the Pleur-evac.

2. Unwrap a replacement autotransfusion system (ATS) bag and fit it into the wire frame provided (Fig. 34–12). Close both white clamps on the bag tubing, and place the frame and bag on the wire hanger.

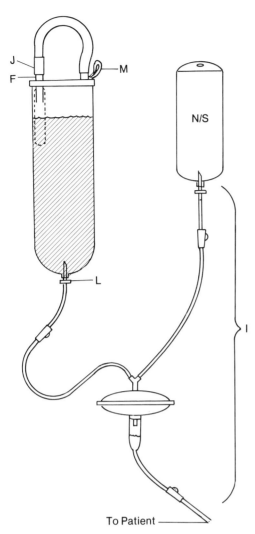

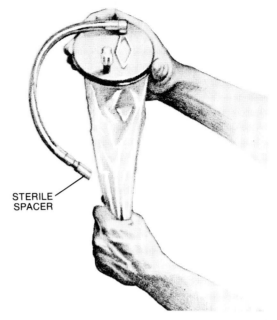

Figure 34–8. Straightening the liner bag before insertion into the canister. (From Receptal ATS Trauma. Sorenson Research Co, Salt Lake City, Utah, p 3. Reproduced by permission.)

and filter with normal saline, and connect it to a large-bore intravenous access (14 gauge or larger) (see Fig. 34–7).

2. When the ATS bag is full, use the negative pressure relief valve (located on top of the drainage unit) (F, see Fig. 34–10) to reduce excessive suction in the unit, and close the white clamps on the chest drainage tubing and ATS bag.

Figure 34–7. Reinfusion apparatus. *F,* Inlet port of liner cap; *I,* Y-type blood infusion line with in-line 40-μ filter; *J,* liner lid tubing connector; *L,* liner bag connection with infusion line; *M,* attached hanger tab at top of liner bag; and *N/S,* normal saline intravenous fluid (for priming and maintaining patency of the system during liner bag changes).

3. Clamp the drainage tubing coming from the patient.

4. Remove the red protective cap from the collection tubing (B, see Fig. 34–10) on the ATS replacement bag and connect it to the patient chest drainage tubing (C, see Fig. 34–10) using the red connector.

5. Remove the blue protective cap from the suction tubing (D, see Fig. 34–10) on the ATS replacement bag and connect to the underwater seal drainage unit using the blue connector.

6. Using a syringe and an 18-gauge (or smaller) needle, inject anticoagulant through the rubber diaphragm (E, see Fig. 34–10) on the ATS bag cap. The manufacturer of the Pleur-evac unit does not offer recommendations regarding specifics of anticoagulation of blood collected in the unit; however, the method outlined for the Sorenson unit may be applied to this unit as well (see step 4 under "Collection—Sorenson Autotransfusion System").

7. Open all clamps; make sure all connections are airtight. The system is now operational.

REINFUSION

1. Prepare a standard Y-type blood infusion line with a high-capacity 40-μ in-line micropore filter, prime the line

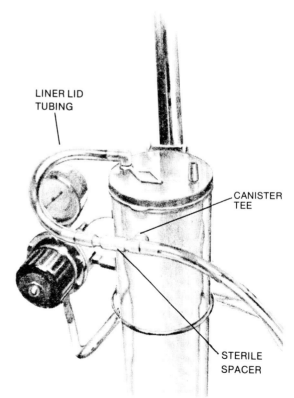

Figure 34–9. Proper placement of the liner bag lid on the canister. (From Receptal ATS Trauma. Sorenson Research Co, Salt Lake City, Utah, p 4. Reproduced by permission.)

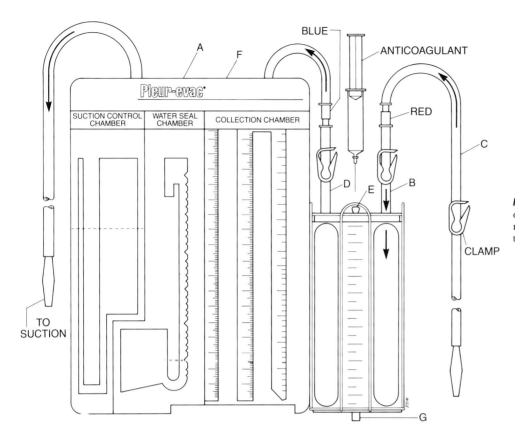

Figure 34–10. The Pleur-evac drainage unit with the replacement autotransfusion bag attached. See text for explanation.

3. Disconnect all connections to the autotransfusion bag.

4. Attach the male (blue) and female (red) connectors on top of the autotransfusion bag to each other, and remove the bag from the drainage unit by spreading and disconnecting each metal support arm.

5. Slide the wire frame off the autotransfusion bag and invert the bag so that the spike port (G, see Fig. 34–10) points upward and remove the protective cap. Insert the

free recipient arm of the Y tube infusion line into the spike port using a constant twisting motion.

6. Invert the autotransfusion bag and suspend it from an intravenous pole (Fig. 34–13).

7. Reinfusion using the Pleur-evac autotransfusion bag may be assisted using a pneumatic pressure blood pump, not to exceed 150 mm Hg infusion pressure. If this is utilized, however, it is of paramount importance that all excess air in the bag be removed before infusion, to minimize

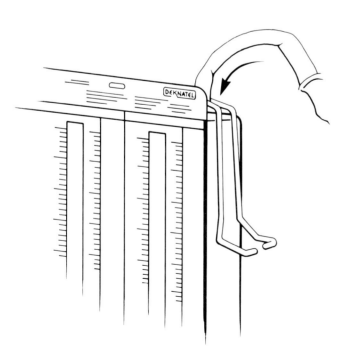

Figure 34–11. Attaching the metal hanger to the Pleur-evac system that will hold the blood collection bag.

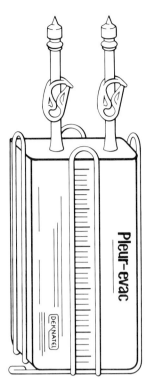

Figure 34–12. The blood collection bag that is attached to the standard Pleur-evac system.

the risk of air embolism. To accomplish this, the red and blue connectors may by disconnected temporarily, one clamp opened, and the bag slowly squeezed until all air is out of the unit. Then the clamp is closed again, and the red-to-blue connection reestablished.

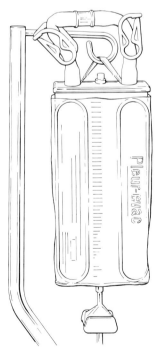

Figure 34–13. Reinfusion of collected blood with the Pleur-evac system. A second collection may be obtained while this blood is infusing.

8. During reinfusion, autologous blood collection may be continued with a second ATS bag, repeating steps 2 through 7 under "Collection."

Additional Information

1. Use each liner bag only once.
2. After reinfusing a total of 3500 ml, or seven units, of autologous blood, one unit of fresh frozen plasma is required, and thereafter, one unit of fresh frozen plasma is required for every two units (1000 ml) of autotransfused blood.[21]
3. To minimize risk from bacterial overgrowth, collected blood must not be allowed to stand for prolonged periods of time before reinfusion.[52] Some authors[46, 53] advise a limit of no more than 4 hours between collection and reinfusion. On the other hand, Mollison[48] believes that "in temperate climates it is not essential to refrigerate blood until at least 8 hours after collection, since this period at room temperature has scarcely any adverse effect on red cell preservation, and partly because during a period of this duration the blood still contains viable phagocytes." The age of collected blood probably should be calculated from the time of injury, and reinfusion of blood older than 4 to 8 hours should be considered hazardous. Because one is performing the procedure for significant hypovolemia in the emergency department, the collected blood is transfused as soon as the collection bag is full.
4. If some or all of the collected blood becomes clotted in the liner bag, the blood should be discarded.
5. The blood filter used during reinfusion is changed as needed (usually after each 1000- to 2000-ml transfusion).

COMPLICATIONS

Complications from autotransfusion are generally clinically insignificant if the proper technique is followed and if less than 3000 ml of blood is reinfused.

Hematologic Complications

The complications of autotransfusion can be categorized as hematologic and nonhematologic (Table 34–1). The most reproducible hematologic consequence is thrombocytopenia (Fig. 34–14). Samples taken from collected autologous blood show low platelet counts; however, the number of platelets found in this blood is significantly greater than that found

Table 34–1. Potential Complications of Autotransfusion
Hematologic
Decreased platelet count
Decreased fibrinogen level
Increased fibrin split products
Prolonged prothrombin time
Prolonged partial thromboplastin time
Red blood cell hemolysis
Elevated plasma-free hemoglobin
Decreased hematocrit
Nonhematologic
Bacteremia
Sepsis?
Microembolism
Air embolism

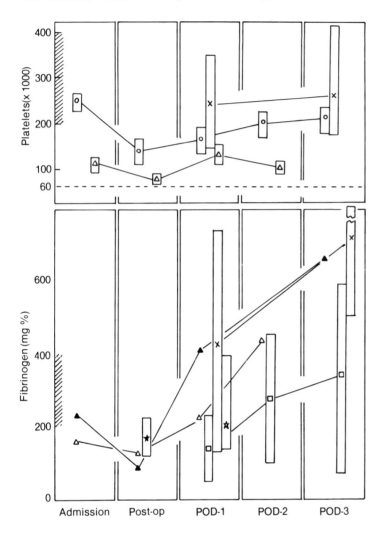

Figure 34–14. Representative platelet counts and serum fibrinogen levels in patients undergoing emergency autotransfusion. Samples were drawn before *(Admission)* and immediately after autotransfusion *(Post-op)* as well as on postoperative days *(POD)* one, two, and three. Normal ranges are represented as shaded areas along the ordinate. Points are coded for source identification (see Key) and designate average or mean values. Bars indicate standard deviations or ranges of reported data.

KEY
△ Broadie[51] 20 Pts—mean vol. 5535 ml
□ Mattox[26] 69 Pts—average vol. 2150 ml
☆ Reul[22] 25 Pts—average vol. 2104 ml
○ O'Riordan[20] 6 Pts—average vol. 4450 ml
x Symbas[13] 11 Pts—average vol. 1800 ml
▲ Stillman[56] (dog study)—150–300 ml/kg
(Sources from which data were extracted. The number of patients studied by each author and the average or mean blood volume autotransfused are noted.)

in banked blood.[42] Until patients receive more than 4000 ml of autologous blood, in vivo platelet counts do not descend below 60,000 per mm³,[3, 19, 21, 25, 31, 35, 37] a level above which trauma surgery can be "performed satisfactorily."[54] Although those platelets collected from autotransfusion reservoirs function abnormally when tested in vitro by aggregation or serotonin uptake and release, postinfusion samples drawn from the patient aggregate normally.[55] However, at least one study conducted with dogs indicates that significant in vivo platelet dysfunction may appear when autotransfused volumes exceed an amount equivalent to one total blood volume.[18] Platelet counts should be followed, and significant thrombocytopenia can be remedied with platelet infusion.

The most common coagulation factor abnormality postautotransfusion is hypofibrinogenemia, especially when the volume of autologous blood used exceeds 4000 ml.[13, 26, 37, 42] Because of the liver's capacity to replenish fibrinogen rapidly (see Fig. 34–14), the low postautotransfusion levels have not proved to be clinically significant.[22, 25, 42] Yet some investigators[22] believe that hepatic insufficiency is a relative contraindication to autotransfusion unless fibrinogen is supplemented.

Symbas and colleagues[13, 14, 31, 32] extended their work with laboratory dogs to the clinical study of 11 victims of traumatic hemothorax. They found no clinical evidence of coagulopathy following autotransfusion in any patient as long as the volume collected and reinfused remained equal to or less than one half the patient's total blood volume. In those few patients who required a larger volume autotransfused, a proportional decrease in platelets and fibrinogen occurred, requiring subsequent correction with fresh frozen plasma and platelet packs. Other investigators[19, 25, 26] have confirmed these findings and have shown that there is a return to normal of both platelet and fibrinogen levels by 48 to 72 hours without replacement therapy. Similarly, elevations in prothrombin and partial thromboplastin times, which were encountered routinely, were not clinically significant. These coagulation abnormalities were self-corrected in 48 to 72 hours (Fig. 34–15).[22, 25, 35]

Raines and associates[21] studied 85 patients receiving autotransfusion and found no clinical or laboratory evidence of intravascular coagulopathy, even in patients receiving blood volumes in excess of 8000 ml. A dilutional coagulopathy was noted when volumes greater than 3500 ml were autotransfused. At least one unit of fresh frozen plasma was given for every two units of autotransfused blood beyond this 3500-ml limit. Silva found that after autotransfusions of massive volumes of blood in dogs, equivalent to twice their total blood volume, there was evidence of a consumptive coagulopathy. Nevertheless, even under these circumstances, levels of clotting factors remained adequate for coagulation.[18]

Red blood cell hemolysis occurs with autotransfusion because of prolonged exposure of the cells to serosal linings of the traumatized body cavities.[56] Hemolysis may also result from mechanical factors during collection and reinfusion, such as high vacuum pressures during aspiration, roller pump trauma, or excess exposure to air-fluid interfaces.[22]

An elevated plasma-free hemoglobin is a consistent finding in patients who have received autotransfusions (see Fig. 34–15).[22, 26, 27, 31, 32] For this reason, any collected blood that clots must be discarded,[22, 51] and pooled blood older than 4 to 6 hours also should not be autotransfused.[20, 22]

Most samples of blood from the autotransfusion reservoir have free hemoglobin levels of less than 100 mg/dl,[22, 31] but some have been reported as high as 1388 mg/dl.[26] Plasma-free hemoglobin values immediately after autotransfusion range from 9 to 110 mg/dl, with most falling between 25 and 80 mg/dl.[22, 26, 27, 31, 32] When the binding capacity of haptoglobin is saturated and the threshold of tubular resorption of hemoglobin is exceeded, hemoglobinuria is seen. This threshold corresponds to a plasma-free hemoglobin concentration of 100 mg/dl.[57] It has been proposed that an

isolated elevation of plasma-free hemoglobin increases the risk of acute tubular necrosis. The presumed nephrotoxicity of plasma-free hemoglobin and tubular obstruction by hemoglobin casts have been refuted by more recent evidence that indicates that acute renal failure following hemolytic transfusion reactions is primarily the result of renal ischemia secondary to antigen-antibody–activated disseminated intravascular coagulation (DIC) and microcirculatory thrombosis.[58] Indeed, it has been shown that "massive hemoglobinuria may follow the transfusion of immunologically compatible hemolyzed RBCs with miminal symptoms and a benign outcome"[59] and that isolated free hemoglobin levels of between 1300 and 1800 mg/dl may be tolerated without renal compromise.[59, 60] Even though renal failure as a direct consequence of autotransfusion has not been reported,[30]

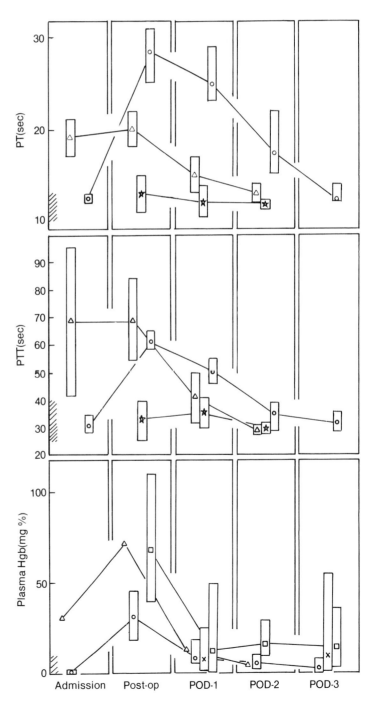

Figure 34–15. Representative prothrombin times *(PT)*, partial thromboplastin times *(PTT)*, and plasma-free hemoglobin levels *(Plasma Hgb)* in patients undergoing emergency autotransfusion. Samples were drawn before *(Admission)* and immediately after autotransfusion *(Post-op)* as well as on postoperative days *(POD)* one, two, and three. Normal ranges are represented as shaded areas along the ordinate. Points are coded for source identification (see Key) and designate average or mean values. Bars indicate standard deviations or ranges of reported data.

KEY
△ Broadie[51] 20 Pts—mean vol. 5535 ml
□ Mattox[26] 69 Pts—average vol. 2150 ml
☆ Reul[22] 25 Pts—average vol. 2104 ml
○ O'Riordan[20] 6 Pts—average vol. 4450 ml
✕ Symbas[13] 11 Pts—average vol. 1800 ml
(Sources from which data were extracted. The number of patients studied by each author and the average or mean blood volume autotransfused are noted.)

transient elevations in serum creatinine do occur,[20] and in the presence of shock and systemic acidosis, acute tubular necrosis remains a potential complication.[57] In fact, some researchers[22] believe that renal insufficiency is only a relative contraindication to autotransfusion unless renal perfusion is at risk.

Finally, the hematocrit falls in direct proportion to the quantity of blood transfused, averaging an approximate drop of 10 to 20 per cent.[13, 22, 27, 31] Raines and associates[21] studied red blood cell mass in each of 15 patients who were receiving an average of six units during autotransfusion and found that red blood cell mass fell by about 50 per cent, apparently as a result of a combination of irretrievable intraoperative losses, hemolysis, and hemodilution with priming solutions and other intravenous solutions. Nontraumatized red blood cell survival has been reported to be normal in all cases studied.[13, 21, 36]

In summary, coagulation problems have not been clinically important when volumes of autotransfused blood remain below 2000 ml in adult patients. However, when reinfused volumes exceed 3500[21] to 4100 ml,[37] laboratory evidence of a dilutional coagulopathy may become evident. Further, when volumes of autotransfused blood are greater than twice the patient's total blood volume, animal studies suggest that there is some risk of a true consumptive coagulopathy.[18]

Recommendations regarding those infused volumes of autologous blood that should trigger replacement therapy of fresh frozen plasma or platelets range from 25 per cent of total blood volume (about 1250 ml in a 70-kg adult)[50] to 2000[46] to 3500 ml.[21] Prudent clinical judgment dictates application of the more liberal guidelines for replacement therapy in those patients with extensive hepatic injury, intractable shock, or ongoing losses requiring immediate surgical intervention.

Nonhematologic Complications

The theoretic risk of sepsis after the administration of potentially contaminated blood exists within the nonsterile surroundings of the typical emergency department resuscitation area. Experience has shown this risk to be minimal after competent autotransfusion of an isolated hemothorax,[12, 13, 19, 20, 30, 61] and there is *no* evidence to suggest that routine prophylaxis with systemic antibiotics is beneficial in this situation.

The issue of whether to autotransfuse shed intraperitoneal blood, however, is somewhat more complex than in the case with hemothorax. Recovery and reinfusion of hemoperitoneum per se has proved to be relatively safe,[12, 19, 20, 28, 29, 61–63] and Klebanoff and associates concluded that "for contaminant-free conditions at least, as in ruptured ectopic pregnancies, ruptured spleen and liver, traumatic hemothorax, and vascular surgery, autotransfusion can be performed readily to reduce the need for homologous blood replacement."[12]

Reinfusion of autologous blood with possible enteric contamination is still considered by most investigators to be ill-advised in all but the most desperate of circumstances, such as in the patient who will exsanguinate *before* homologous blood can be made available. If contaminated blood is infused, systemic antibiotics should be given.[12, 19, 20, 26, 29, 30, 46, 60] Many cases of collection and reinfusion of intestinally contaminated hemoperitoneum have been reported.[19, 28, 29, 61–63] The overall mortality of this selected group was 16 per cent, not unexpectedly high considering the severity of the injuries involved. Experimental studies with dogs also show that autotransfusion of hemoperitoneum contaminated by intes-

tinal contents, urine, or bile is tolerated.[12, 27] Timberlake and McSwain reported autotransfusion of hemoperitoneum in 11 trauma patients using a cell-washing recovery system (Haemonetics Cell Saver). Although the collected blood in all cases had enteric contamination, including gross spillage of fecal material, there followed only minimal infectious complications and no mortality.[29] Nonetheless, when there is confirmed or suspected enteric contamination, autotransfusion should be considered only as a "last-ditch" life-saving option.

Another complication, microemboli secondary to platelet microaggregation or fat emboli, has largely been eliminated by the use of micropore filters.[21, 22, 35] During reinfusion of collected blood, in most instances there is a mild increase in screen filtration pressures, indicating the formation of microemboli trapped by the filter.[35] There has been no clinical evidence of pulmonary insufficiency or unexplained elevation of the alveolar-to-arterial oxygen gradient that might be attributed to the passage of microemboli beyond the micropore filter systems.[22]

Air embolism has been reported sporadically as a complication of autotransfusion.[10, 19, 26, 38, 45, 61, 64] This uncommon but often fatal complication has been associated, in all cases reviewed, with autotransfusion systems using automated roller pump units in which the aspirate reservoir was inadvertently allowed to run dry. Air embolism with gravity or with a manually assisted technique is rare.

Available data indicate that although autotransfusion is not free of complications, the risk-to-benefit ratio weighs heavily in its favor in the resuscitation of selected trauma victims. Klebanoff and coworkers reviewed the evidence as of 1970 and determined that "in over 1000 documented cases of autotransfusion in the Western literature, not a single death or major complication was attributed directly to the transfusion."[12] Symbas[31] reported autotransfusing more than 200 patients with traumatic hemothorax without any significant morbidity related to the procedure. Mattox and associates[19] reported autotransfusing 69 patients an average of 3.9 units each, with only one death (from air embolism) directly attributable to the procedure.

CONCLUSION

Autotransfusion, a technique more than 100 years old, has become a subject of renewed interest in the emergency setting. The previously feared complications of hematologic or metabolic embarrassment and of sepsis have not proved to be of clinical significance when appropriate patient selection and careful technique are followed. In addition, the use of autologous blood has several advantages over the transfusion of stored homologous blood in the emergency patient, including ready availability of compatible blood, homeostasis of core temperature, higher levels of RBC 2,3-DPG, and cost effectiveness. Autotransfusion has been endorsed by the Council on Scientific Affairs of the American Medical Association as a procedure that has been found to be "effective, safe and cost effective for many trauma and surgical patients."[16] A review of the literature reveals that although the technique is not totally free of complications, the benefits to be gained from autotransfusing the selected trauma patient outweigh the relatively limited risks.

REFERENCES

1. Trunkey DD: Trauma. Sci Am 249:28, 1983.
2. Schaff HV, Hauer JM, Brawley RK: Autotransfusion in cardiac surgical patients after operation. Surgery 84:713, 1978.
3. Blundell J: Experiments on the transfusion of blood. Medico Chir Trans 9:56, 1818.
4. Highmore W: Overlooked source of blood supply for transfusion in postpartum haemorrhage. Lancet 1:89, 1874.
5. Duncan J: On reinfusion of blood in primary and other amputations. Br Med J 1:192, 1886.
6. Thies HJ: Zur behandlung der extraurterior graviditar. Zentralbl Bynaek 38:1190, 1914.

7. Elmendorf: Über Wiedeninfusion nach Punktion eines frischern Haemothorax. Munch Med Wochenschr 64:36, 1917.
8. Lockwood CD: Surgical treatment of Banti's disease. Surg Gynecol Obstet 25:188, 1917.
9. Burch LE: Autotransfusion. Trans South Surg Assoc 35:25, 1922.
10. Dyer RH, Alexander JT, Brighton CT: Atraumatic aspiration of whole blood for intraoperative autotransfusion. Am J Surg 123:510, 1972.
11. Klebanoff G: Early clinical experience with a disposable unit for the intraoperative salvage and reinfusion of blood loss. Am J Surg 120:718, 1970.
12. Klebanoff G, Phillips J, Evans W: Use of a disposable autotransfusion unit under varying conditions of contamination. Am J Surg 120:351, 1970.
13. Symbas PN, Levin JM, Ferrier FL, et al: A study on autotransfusion from hemothorax. South Med J 62:671, 1969.
14. Symbas PN, et al: Autotransfusion and its effects upon the blood components and the recipient. Curr Top Surg Res 1:387, 1969.
15. Mattox KL, Espada R, Beall AC, et al: Performing thoracotomy in the emergency center. JACEP 3:13, 1974.
16. Council on Scientific Affairs, American Medical Association: Autologous blood transfusions. JAMA 256:2378, 1986.
17. Orr M: Autotransfusion: The use of washed red cells as an adjunct to component therapy. Surgery 84:728, 1978.
18. Silva R, Moore EE, Bar-Or D, et al: The risk/benefit of autotransfusion: Comparison to banked blood in a canine model. J Trauma 24:557, 1984.
19. Mattox KL, Walker LE, Beall AC, et al: Blood availability for the trauma patient—autotransfusion. J Trauma 15:663, 1975.
20. O'Riordan WD: Autotransfusion in the emergency department of a community hospital. JACEP 6:233, 1977.
21. Raines J, Buth J, Brewster DC, et al: Intraoperative autotransfusion: Equipment, protocols, and guidelines. J Trauma 16:616, 1976.
22. Reul GJ, Solis RT, Greenberg SD, et al: Experience with autotransfusion in the surgical management of trauma. Surgery 76:546, 1974.
23. Rakower SR, Worth MH: Autotransfusion: perspective and critical problems. J Trauma 13:573, 1973.
24. Dixon JL, Smalley MG: Jehovah's Witnesses: The surgical/ethical challenge. JAMA 246:2471, 1981.
25. Davidson SJ: Emergency unit autotransfusion. Surgery 84:703, 1978.
26. Mattox KL: Autotransfusion in the emergency department. JACEP 4:218, 1975.
27. Smith RN, Yaw PB, Glover JL: Autotransfusion of contaminated intraperitoneal blood: An experimental study. J Trauma 18:341, 1978.
28. Glover JL, Smith R, Yaw PB, et al: Autotransfusion of blood contaminated by intestinal contents. JACEP 7:142, 1978.
29. Timberlake GA, McSwain NE Jr: Autotransfusion of blood contaminated by enteric contents: A potentially life-saving measure in the massively hemorrhaging trauma patient? J Trauma 28:855, 1988.
30. Klebanoff G: Intraoperative autotransfusion with the Bentley ATS-100. Surgery 84:708, 1978.
31. Symbas PN: Extraoperative autotransfusion from hemothorax. Surgery 84:722, 1978.
32. Symbas PN: Autotransfusion from hemothorax: Experimental and clinical studies. J Trauma 12:689, 1972.
33. Von Koch L, Defore WW, Mattox KL: A practical method of autotransfusion in the emergency center. Am J Surg 133:770, 1977.
34. Mattox KL: Comparison of techniques of autotransfusion. Surgery 84:700, 1978.
35. Brewster DC, Ambrosino JJ, Darling RC, et al: Intraoperative autotransfusion in major vascular surgery. Am J Surg 137:507, 1979.
36. Schweitzer EJ, Hauer JM, Swan KG, et al: Use of the Heimlich valve in a compact autotransfusion device. J Trauma 27:537, 1987.
37. Barriot P, Riou B, Viars P: Prehospital autotransfusion in life-threatening hemothorax. Chest 93:522, 1988.
38. Dowling J: Autotransfusion: Its use in the severely injured patient. Proceedings of the First Annual Bentley Autotransfusion Seminar. San Francisco, 1972, pp 11–20.
39. Drye JC: Discussion after Mattox KL, et al: Blood availability for the trauma patient—autotransfusion. J Trauma 15:663, 1975.
40. Burch JM: Blood transfusion, microfiltration, and the adult respiratory distress syndrome. Curr Concepts Trauma Care (Fall) 1983, pp 16–21.
41. Noon GP: Intraoperative autotransfusion. Surgery 84:719, 1978.
42. Bell W: The hematology of autotransfusion. Surgery 84:695, 1978.
43. Schaff HV, Hauer JM, Bell WR, et al: Autotransfusion of shed mediastinal blood after cardiac surgery. A prospective study. J Thorac Cardiovasc Surg 75:632, 1978.
44. Second Annual Bentley Autotransfusion Seminar. Chicago, Bentley Laboratories, Inc, 1973.
45. Noon GP, Solis RT, Natelson EA: A simple method of intraoperative autotransfusion. Surg Gynecol Obstet 143:65, 1976.
46. Thurer RL, Hauer JM: Autotransfusion and blood conservation. Curr Probl Surg 19:98, 1982.
47. Oller DW, Rice CL, Herman CM, et al: Heparin versus citrate anticoagulation in autotransfusion. J Surg Res 20:333, 1976.
48. Mollison PL: Blood Transfusion in Clinical Medicine. Oxford, Blackwell Scientific Publications, 1979, pp 69, 638.
49. Johnston B, Kamath BS, McLellan I: An autotransfusion apparatus. Anaesthesia 32:1020, 1977.
50. Napoli VM, Symbas PJ, Vroon DH, Symbas PN: Autotransfusion from experimental hemothorax: Levels of coagulation factors. J Trauma 27:296, 1987.
51. Broadie TA, Glover JL, Bang N, et al: Clotting competence of intracavitary blood in trauma victims. Ann Emerg Med 10:127, 1981.
52. Kluge RM, Calia FM, McLaughlin JS, et al: Sources of contamination in open heart surgery. JAMA 230:1415, 1974.
53. Cowley RA, Dunham CM (ed): Shock Trauma/Critical Care Manual. Baltimore, University Park Press, 1982, p 40.
54. Cowley RA, Dunham CM (ed): Shock Trauma/Critical Care Manual. Baltimore, University Park Press, 1982, p 38.
55. Mollison PL: Blood Transfusion in Clinical Medicine. Oxford, Blackwell Scientific Publications, 1979, p 652.
56. Stillman RM, Wrezlewicz WW, Stanczewski B, et al: The haematological hazards of autotransfusion. Br J Surg 63:651, 1976.
57. Barbanel C: Hemoglobinuria and myoglobinuria. In Hamburger J, Crosnier J, Grünfeld JP (eds): Nephrology. New York, John Wiley & Sons, 1979, pp 185–189.
58. Goldfinger D: Complications of hemolytic transfusion reactions: Pathogenesis and therapy. In Dawson RB (ed): New Approaches to Transfusion Reactions. Washington, DC, American Association of Blood Banks, 1974, pp 15–38.
59. Sandler SG, Berry E, Zlotnick A: Benign hemoglobinuria following transfusion of accidentally frozen blood. JAMA 235:2850, 1976.
60. Relihan M, Litwin MS: Effects of stroma-free hemoglobin solution on clearance rate and renal function. Surgery 71:395, 1972.
61. Duncan SE, Klebanoff G, Rogers W: A clinical experience with intraoperative autotransfusion. Ann Surg 180:296, 1974.
62. Griswold RA, Ortner AB: Use of autotransfusion in surgery of serous cavities. Surg Gynecol Obstet 77:167, 1943.
63. Boudreaux JP, Burnside GH, Cohn I: Emergency autotransfusion: Partial cleansing of bacteria-laden blood by cell washing. J Trauma 23:31, 1983.
64. Bretton P, Reines HD, Sade RM: Air embolization during autotransfusion for abdominal trauma. J Trauma 25:165, 1985.

Chapter 35

Pneumatic Anti-Shock Garment

Robert Norton and Kenneth Frumkin

INTRODUCTION

The pneumatic anti-shock garment (PASG) is widely used, both by emergency medical technicians and paramedics in the prehospital care of hypotensive patients and by hospital emergency departments and critical care personnel. In the commercially available forms—

MAST (David Clark Co., Inc., Worcester, Mass.) and Gladiator Antishock Pants (Jobst Institute, Inc., Toledo, Ohio)[1]—the PASGs resemble a pair of high-waisted men's trousers. The devices are constructed from two layers of an opaque, airtight fabric sewn into three independently inflatable chambers (Figs. 35–1 and 35–2).

The device is easily applied, is considered "essential" equipment on ambulances, and is found in most emergency departments. These devices have been called by many names: MAST (military anti-shock trousers, medical anti-shock trousers), PASG (pneumatic anti-shock garment), circumferential pneumatic compression device, shock pants, external counterpressure suit, air pants, MAST pants, MAST trousers, pressure pants, and G-suit. Other terms have been used to refer to the process of applying external pressure to the body, regardless of the device used. Examples are external (or circumferential) pneumatic compression and external counterpressure.[2] Because some of these names (e.g., MAST) are also registered commercial trademarks and because pneumatic anti-shock garment is the term adopted by the American College of Surgeons for its

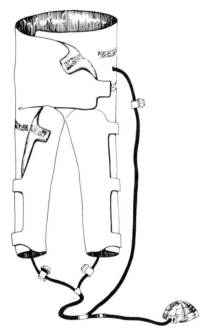

Figure 35–1. Assembled pneumatic anti-shock garment and inflation pump. (Courtesy of the American College of Surgeons, Committee on Trauma.)

Advanced Trauma Life Support course,[3] PASG is used in this chapter to refer to the devices that are currently available.

BACKGROUND

Regardless of the name, the device has changed little in its design or application since 1903, when Crile created a "pneumatic suit" from a double layer of rubber.[4] One or both legs or the abdomen compartment could be inflated separately with a bicycle pump. Designed to manipulate blood pressure during head and neck surgery in the sitting position, the pneumatic suit was subsequently applied to the management of the traumatized patient: "A cut-throat patient was admitted to the wards of Lakeside Hospital, exsanguinated and pulseless. Saline infusions and stimulants had been given in maximum amounts during twelve hours, but the circulation always relapsed, and at the time of the application of the rubber suit the pulse was barely perceptible, the respirations gasping, and the patient unconscious. On applying firm pneumatic pressure up to the costal borders the pulse became immediately better, the blood pressure rising to 110 mm of mercury, and consciousness was regained.[5]" Leaks in the material inhibited wide-

spread use of the device, and the principle of external counterpressure lay dormant until its rediscovery by the military (allegedly at Crile's suggestion) during World War II.[6] Reincarnated as the G-suit, the garment was used to provide momentary compression of up to 100 mm Hg to counteract the cerebral and retinal ischemia (with resultant loss of consciousness or vision) that occurred during certain maneuvers in high-speed aircraft. Medical interest was renewed with investigations performed by Gardner and Dohn in 1956.[7] They used a homemade G-suit in patients who were likely to experience postural hypotension (neurosurgical patients in the sitting position, patients in whom spinal anesthesia had been administered, and those with severe diabetic neuropathy). Their device subsequently became commercially available (Curity) and consisted of a double-layered rectangular blanket wrapped completely around the patient from xiphoid to ankles. For the next decade or more, external counterpressure was used only in the hospital setting and usually as a last resort in cases of uncontrollable postoperative hemorrhage (Table 35–1).

Publication of the military G-suit experience during the Vietnam War was the first recorded routine use of the external counterpressure principle in the preoperative stabilization of trauma patients.[8] The Army continued to develop the device until the current pants-like form (MAST) was achieved.[9] The inventor of the trousers (B. H. Kaplan) became the first to adapt them to their next area of extensive use: civilian prehospital application by paramedics and emergency medical technicians.[10]

In an uncontrolled retrospective review, Pelligra and Sandberg reviewed reported cases (174 over 75 years) in which the application of PASG resulted in elevation of blood pressure and control of bleeding.[2] These patients were reported to show dramatic improvements in blood pressure, pulse, mental status, and decreases in fluid and transfusion requirements. In another retrospective series McSwain evaluated the use of PASG for noncardiogenic shock in 47 patients.[11] In addition to increasing blood pressure, he concluded that MAST use decreased the complications of shock, such as adult respiratory distress syndrome (ARDS) and acute tubular necrosis. In the largest retrospective series, Wayne and MacDonald reviewed the use of PASG for shock in 1120 patients. Of these, 84 per cent responded by an increase in blood pressure greater than 20 mm Hg systolic, a slowing of their heart rate, or evidence of enhanced tissue perfusion.[12]

MECHANISM OF ACTION

The mechanism of action of PASG has been the object of many experimental studies. Interpretation and comparison of results from these studies require attention to several factors: species of subjects, volume status, design of garment, inflation pressures, methods of hemodynamic measurements, and position of subjects (supine or tilted). The increase in blood pressure that results from application of PASG is due to at least three effects: enhanced venous

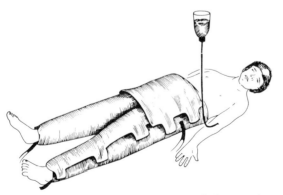

Figure 35–2. Pneumatic anti-shock garment applied to a patient and inflated. (Courtesy of the American College of Surgeons, Committee on Trauma.)

Table 35–1. **Early Uses of the PASG Device**
Retroperitoneal bleeding from massive pelvic trauma
Postoperative bleeding from hypocoagulation
Postural hypotension
Spontaneous rupture of the liver
Postoperative hemorrhage after:
Abdominal procedures
Nephrectomy
Prostatectomy
Renal biopsy
Tubal ligation
Hysterectomy
Leaking and ruptured abdominal aortic aneurysms
Lower extremity fractures
Placenta percreta
Gastrointestinal bleeding
Ruptured ectopic pregnancy

Table 35–2. Pneumatic Anti-Shock Garment: Proposed Mechanisms of Action
Blood pressure elevation
Increased total peripheral resistance
"Autotransfusion"
Control of bleeding
Direct pressure
Fracture stabilization
Effects on bleeding vessels
Decreased transmural pressure

return (autotransfusion); increased total peripheral resistance; and reduced volume loss from control of hemorrhage (Table 35–2).

Enhanced Venous Return

The improvement in blood pressure seen during early PASG device studies was assumed to result from "autotransfusion" of blood from the venous system of the lower extremities and the splanchnic bed to circulation above the diaphragm. Reports stated that this mechanism could account for volumes of transfusion as large as 2 units (1000 ml) of blood.[13, 14] Yet experimental evidence to support such a large volume change has not been found.

Increased central blood volume in humans has been demonstrated in various ways, including changes in calculated pulmonary circulation times,[15] increased lung density on repeated radiographs, and changes in thoracic radioactivity after ^{131}I-labeled albumin injection and PASG application.[16] Redistribution of blood flow centrally after suit application in dogs subjected to phlebotomy was demonstrated by Ferrario and associates.[6] These investigators also found increased carotid blood flow in association with decreased flow in the femoral vessels. Changes in normovolemic subjects are most marked when venous pooling is increased by tilting.[15, 17] Attempts at quantification of "autotransfusion" in humans using displacement of the center of gravity[18] or nuclear scanning after radioactive red blood cell injection[19] have estimated that 150 to 300 ml are actually autotransfused. One study in patients with ARDS being ventilated with positive end-expiratory pressure (PEEP) demonstrated a 22 per cent increase in cardiopulmonary blood volume after PASG inflation, using a measurement of ^{99m}Tc-labeled albumin.[20]

Increased Total Peripheral Resistance

More recent reviews of PASG have focused on the increase in total peripheral resistance as the predominant mechanism of increased blood pressure after PASG application.[21–23] This phenomenon has been well characterized in animal models. Using a hemorrhagic canine model, Niemann and colleagues demonstrated progressive increase in total peripheral resistance, with inflation pressures of 40, 60, and 100 mm Hg.[24] Using both normovolemic and hypovolemic swine, Bellamy and coworkers showed an increased total peripheral resistance in both groups at PASG pressures of 40, 80, and 120 mm Hg.[25] The greater increase in total peripheral resistance occurred in the normovolemic group. Cardiac output increased only in the hemorrhagic hypovolemic group.

Hemodynamic responses to PASG in volunteer subjects are variable and sometimes contradictory. In normovolemic subjects, increases in central venous pressure,[16] intrathoracic blood volume,[16] total peripheral resistance, blood pressure,[15] and cardiac index[15] have been demonstrated following inflation of the PASG. However, Burchard and colleagues reported no change in the cardiac index in ten subjects after coronary artery bypass surgery despite an increase in central venous pressure and left atrial pressure.[26] Using thermal dilution catheters in ten subjects undergoing diagnostic cardiac catheterization, Rubal and associates found no increase in cardiac output or stroke volume despite an increased total peripheral resistance and central venous pressure.[27] Using Doppler measurements of vessel diameter, aortic flow, and cardiac output, Hauswald and Greene reported no change in cardiac output in ten healthy volunteers despite a 75 per cent reduction in aortic flow distal to the superior mesenteric artery and a 10 per cent increase in blood pressure.[28] In a similar study using a head-up tilt to model hypovolemia in healthy volunteers, Mannering and associates found that PASG increased cardiac output and forearm blood flow in tilted patients.[29] Gaffney and colleagues found an elevated blood pressure and peripheral resistance with a decreased cardiac output and stroke volume during supine PASG application, but again when the subjects were tilted 60 degrees (head up), PASG produced a small elevation in stroke volume.[17] Savino and colleagues studied PASG use in elderly, normovolemic patients and demonstrated a progressive decrease in the cardiac index and impairment in left ventricular function with increasing inflation pressures for half their patients.[30] Payen and coworkers demonstrated a significantly increased cardiac index in ventilated patients on PEEP after inflation of PASG using pulmonary artery thermal dilution catheters to measure cardiac output.[20]

The conflicting results seen in animal and human studies can be explained in part by the volume status of subjects before inflation of the PASG and the overall effect of the subjects' homeostatic responses to increased afterload and preload. Young normovolemic volunteers can react to increased afterload rapidly, as manifested by an increased total peripheral resistance, by changing their heart rate or stroke volume so that cardiac output may not change. Also with normovolemia, changes in preload will have little effect on cardiac output.[25] Although no hemodynamic studies have been done on hypotensive, hypovolemic human subjects, the response is expected to be similar to that of the tilted subjects or hypovolemic animals. In that setting, the predominant response is not an increase in afterload but in preload, which results in increased stroke volume and consequently improved cardiac output for a variable duration.[25, 29] The complete explanation for the mechanisms of action of PASG awaits further clinical research.

Control of Hemorrhage

The PASG can serve as a pressure dressing over external bleeding sites. Acting as a pneumatic splint, the device prevents continued bleeding provoked by motion at fracture sites. This is particularly efficacious with long bone fractures and with retroperitoneal bleeding from pelvic fractures. In the management of hemorrhage associated with major pelvic fractures, the use of the PASG has been recommended as part of the initial management to be followed by external fixation, surgery, or selective angiographic embolization.[31] One review of pelvic fractures has demonstrated radiographic realignment of an open-book, diastasis-type pelvic fracture after inflation of the PASG.[32] The PASG combined with other nonsurgical therapy has also been reported to be effective in controlling nontraumatic pelvic hemorrhage in obstetric and gynecologic patients.[33]

$$T = \Delta P \times R$$
$$\Delta P = P_I - P_E$$

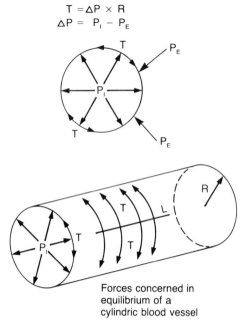

Forces concerned in
equilibrium of a
cylindric blood vessel

Figure 35–3. Diagrammatic expression of Laplace's law. T refers to the wall tension, which is tangential to the circumference of the vessel and acts to pull the edges of a longitudinal laceration (L) apart. Transmural pressure (ΔP) is the difference between the intraluminal (P_I) and extraluminal (P_E) pressures and is decreased by external counterpressure. (Modified from Burton AC: On the physical equilibrium of small blood vessels. Am J Physiol 164:319, 1951.)

The presence of a normal coagulation system contributes strongly to the ability of external counterpressure to control bleeding. Heparinized dogs bleeding from an aortic laceration cannot raise their intra-aortic pressure above the garment-produced intraperitoneal pressure, although nonheparinized animals are able to do so.[34]

One may wonder how external counterpressures that are considerably below the pressure within the bleeding vessel can reduce flow from a sizable vascular defect while still allowing blood to circulate.[28] Much of the explanation derives from the physics involved.

Laplace's law (T = ΔP × R) determines the wall tension (T) for a cylinder (Fig. 35–3). T is the force tangential to the circumference of the vessel that tends to pull apart the edges of a longitudinal laceration (L in Fig. 35–3). Transmural pressure (ΔP) is the difference between the intraluminal (P_I) and extraluminal (P_E) pressures ($\Delta P = P_I - P_E$). Increases in P_E are produced by the PASG, and the tendency

$$\dot{Q} = A \times \sqrt{\frac{\Delta P}{\rho} + V^2}$$

BERNOULLI'S PRINCIPLE

$\dot{Q}$ = RATE OF FLOW FROM INJURED VESSEL
A = SURFACE AREA OF LACERATION
P = TRANSMURAL PRESSURE ($P_I - P_E$)
ρ = DENSITY OF THE FLUID
V = VELOCITY OF THE FLUID IN THE VESSEL

Figure 35–4. Bernoulli's equation quantifies the rate of flow from an injured vessel.

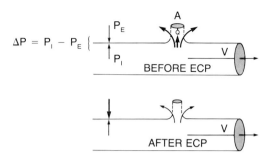

$$\Delta P = P_I - P_E \left\{ \right.$$

Figure 35–5. Representation of the flow through an injured blood vessel (Q) before *(top)* and after *(bottom)* the application of external counterpressure (ECP). (Modified from Hall M, Marshall JR: The gravity suit: A major advance in management of gynecologic blood loss. Obstet Gynecol 53:247, 1979. Reprinted with permission from The American College of Obstetricians and Gynecologists.)

to bleed (ΔP, T) declines. In addition, circumferential pressure causes the radius of the vessel (R) to decrease, limiting both of these contributions to the wall tension.

The Bernoulli principle takes more factors into account (Fig. 35–4). It relates the rate of flow from the injured vessel (Q) to the surface area of the laceration site (A), transmural pressure (ΔP), density of the fluid medium (ρ), and the velocity (V) of the fluid flowing through the vessel. In this model the major action of the external counterpressure suit is to limit transmural pressure along with the surface area of the laceration (Fig. 35–5). Many animal studies have tested these relationships with in vivo, in vitro, and ex vivo models.[34–40] Nearly all models document decreased flow through lacerated vessels with external counterpressure and support one or the other of the equations listed, generally that of Bernoulli.

INDICATIONS (Table 35–3)

The list of clinical applications for the external counterpressure device is modified frequently as new suggestions appear in the literature. Many indications that were controversial in the past have changed as experience with the PASGs increases. There are limited experimental and clinical data to support some suggested indications. Obviously, specific therapy directed at the underlying cause of the patient's illness or injury is the mainstay of successful treatment of any condition that may respond initially to the supportive use of counterpressure.

Table 35–3. Proposed Indications for PASG Application

Hypovolemic shock
Relative hypovolemia and hypotension
    Spinal shock
    Overdose
    Septic shock
    Anaphylaxis
Other uses
    "Prophylactic" use (gastrointestinal bleeding, aortic aneurysm)
    Stabilization of fractures
    Compression of external bleeding
    Postoperative hemorrhage
    Coagulation defects
Investigational uses
    Cardiopulmonary resuscitation
    Paroxysmal supraventricular tachycardia

Hypovolemic Shock

This is the most common indication for the use of PASGs. Several reports from Mattox and colleagues have generated controversy regarding the use of PASG for hypovolemic shock resulting from penetrating trauma.[41–43] In a randomized trial evaluating prehospital trauma scores, fluid administration, emergency department and operative management, and survival, the investigators reported no advantage for use of the PASG in shock due to penetrating abdominal injuries.[42] A subsequent analysis from the same study suggests that the PASG may be harmful when used with hypotensive patients who have penetrating thoracic wounds.[43] The study was conducted in an urban emergency medical services system with mean transport times less than 15 minutes and permitted the concurrent administration of large volumes of prehospital crystalloid fluid. No comparable controlled trials have been done for either rural systems or for blunt abdominal trauma.

In a retrospective study comparing air versus ground transport of patients with primarily blunt multiorgan trauma, Moylan and associates identified use of PASG as one of several interventions in the air-transported group that was associated with improved survival.[44] Until further studies clarify the exact role of PASGs in the management of trauma patients with hypovolemic shock it seems prudent to continue to use them for patients with blunt trauma and hypotension; for patients with penetrating abdominal trauma, hypotension, *and* long transport times when prehospital intravenous fluid therapy is not available; and for patients with signs of shock from other causes of hypovolemia.

There are a number of advantages of the PASG over massive fluid replacement alone for patients with hypovolemic shock. The device is quickly applied and offers some immediate pressor response. Collapsed peripheral veins may become easier to cannulate after inflation. PASGs can be applied by persons without intravenous therapy skills, and the compressive effect may reduce hemorrhage from pelvic and intra-abdominal vessels.[45, 46]

States of Relative Hypovolemia and Hypotension. Other causes of shock in which the pneumatic suit might be helpful, but for which no data currently exist, include neurogenic (spinal) shock, shock secondary to anaphylactic shock,[47, 48] drug overdose,[49] and septic shock.

Other Uses During Hemorrhage. "Prophylactic" application (with or without inflation) may be helpful in potentially hypovolemic or hypotensive patients. Examples are trauma victims who are initially stable at the scene, but who have a potential for developing hypotension, patients with gastrointestinal bleeding, or those with leaking abdominal aortic aneurysms.[50] In patients with leaking aneurysms, one should maintain the systolic blood pressure at approximately 100 mm Hg to avoid contributing to further hemorrhage.[51–54] Pelvic or lower extremity fractures are well stabilized by these devices, adding significantly to the patient's comfort.[31, 32] The PASG may serve as a compression dressing over external bleeding. Controlling postoperative intra-abdominal hemorrhage has been a classic indication.[2] Bleeding aggravated by coagulation defects has also been responsive to external counterpressure.[55]

Other Uses of External Counterpressure

Cardiopulmonary Resuscitation. Interest in the use of external counterpressure devices during cardiopulmonary resuscitation (CPR) is a result of recent changes in the way that blood flow is believed to occur during external chest compression (see Chapter 17).[58, 59] During adult CPR, the heart is no longer thought to act as a pump, propelling blood as it is squeezed between the sternum and the spine. Instead, chest compression serves to raise intrathoracic pressure, and blood flows because of pressure gradients developed between intrathoracic and extrathoracic vessels. External counterpressure from the PASG is believed to augment CPR in two ways: (1) by reducing diaphragmatic excursion and therefore increasing intrathoracic pressures during compression, and (2) by compressing the infradiaphragmatic vascular bed, producing selective perfusion of vital structures above and increased peripheral resistance below the diaphragm.

Animal studies have demonstrated improvements in carotid blood flow and arterial pressures when abdominal compression or the PASG is added to standardized CPR.[60–62] Lilja and coworkers noted that PASG increased systolic blood pressure during CPR in seven of eight patients.[63] However, Mahoney and Murick reported no difference in initial resuscitation or survival between standard CPR and PASG-augmented CPR in a clinical, prehospital study.[64] A review by Niemann and colleagues concluded that the use of PASG as an adjunct to CPR has not been proven to be beneficial and should remain experimental.[65]

Paroxysmal Supraventricular Tachycardia. Case reports have documented cardioversion of paroxysmal supraventricular tachycardia to a sinus rhythm after the application of PASG in adults (with[66] and without[67] Wolff-Parkinson-White syndrome) and in a child.[68] The mechanism for the response has been attributed to reflex vagal excitation from increased aortic and carotid sinus pressure.[69]

CONTRAINDICATIONS (Table 35–4)

Pulmonary edema and congestive heart failure are the only current absolute contraindications to the use of external counterpressure devices. The increased venous return, decreased vital capacity, and elevation in pulmonary wedge pressure produced by these devices serve only to aggravate preexisting pulmonary congestion.

Wayne has advocated the use of the PASG as a quickly "reversible fluid challenge" in patients with cardiogenic shock.[56] The intended use is to identify those patients in cardiogenic shock who might benefit from volume resuscitation and thus guide crystalloid infusion therapy in those individuals. Pressor agents would be reserved for those patients who fail to improve or worsen with inflation. The complete "reversibility" of the effects of the device has not been well documented, particularly in the setting of a poorly functioning cardiovascular system. After 5 minutes of PASG

Table 35–4. Proposed Contraindications to PASG Application

Absolute contraindications
    Congestive heart failure
    Pulmonary edema
Relative contraindications
    Cardiogenic shock
    Penetrating thoracic injuries
    Pregnancy
    Evisceration
    Impaled foreign body
    Lower extremity compartmental injury
    Lumbar spine instability

inflation, central venous pressure, cardiac index, pulse, and central blood volume return to preinflation values. With the release of pressure, the cardiac index increases to compensate for a fall in blood pressure and central venous pressure.[15, 57] The changes after deflation are attributed to unmasking of the compensatory mechanisms (probably vasodilation) that had taken place during external counterpressure to normalize the patient's hemodynamics. Thus mere removal of these devices after application does not necessarily restore the patient's cardiovascular system to a "baseline" state. PASG use for cardiogenic shock is therefore relatively contraindicated.

Other relative contraindications that have been proposed include pregnancy, evisceration of abdominal contents, a foreign body impaled in the abdomen, and lumbar spine injury. For these situations, the leg chambers may be inflated without additional risk, and the relative risks and benefits of inflation of the abdominal binder can then be assessed. Circumferential burns and other injuries that are suggestive of lower extremity compartmental injury also represent significant relative contraindications. The application of external counterpressure elevates the compartment pressure and increases muscle ischemia.

The use of the PASG in the patient with a penetrating thoracic or abdominal injury in the setting of a rapid transport time and concurrent intravenous therapy also should be discouraged.[41–43] Finally, since the hemodynamic response to PASG inflation is quite variable and at times deleterious in the elderly,[30] advanced age represents a relative contraindication to PASG use.

Controversial Applications

There are a number of situations in which the use of PASG devices was discouraged by early writers. Although few data address these circumstances, some general review articles have discussed the judicious use of external counterpressure in these controversial settings.[21–23]

Head Injuries. The only purely intracranial injury that can produce shock is transtentorial herniation. In the absence of this often fatal injury with its unique signs and symptoms, shock is usually the result of associated visceral injuries or spinal cord injury. Yet, fear that the PASG would increase cerebral edema and intracranial pressure has caused the manufacturers to interdict use of the device in head injury. Several animal experiments have found no significant effects of PASG inflation in hypovolemic or normovolemic dogs with or without an experimental intracranial "mass." The studies did document improvement in the cerebral perfusion pressure with PASG use.[70–72] Gardner and colleagues evaluated the use of PASG in 12 patients with severe head injury and an intracranial pressure of less than 20 mm Hg.[73] They found increases in mean arterial pressure and cerebral perfusion pressure without adverse effect on the intracranial pressure as long as the inflation pressure was less than 60 mm Hg. The use of PASG in patients with significant underlying elevations in intracranial pressure has not been studied.

Intrathoracic Injuries. It was initially believed that external pressure applied below the diaphragm would merely increase the rate of blood loss from thoracic injuries. Most authors cite their clinical experience in noting no adverse effects of these devices in thoracic trauma.[11, 14, 74] Ransom and McSwain documented immediate blood pressure increases after PASG application in all eight of their patients with severe hemorrhage above the diaphragm and successful resuscitation in seven.[75] Nonetheless, Mattox and colleagues in a large clinical trial found that PASG use

coupled with aggressive fluid resuscitation in hypotensive patients with penetrating thoracic injury was deleterious.[43]

Cardiac Tamponade and Tension Pneumothorax. Fluid infusion is a standard temporizing measure in cardiac tamponade. In one study of dogs with experimental cardiac tamponade, PASG inflation produced a doubling of mean arterial pressure and temporarily improved cardiac output.[76] Hence, the PASG may be temporizing in this setting when persons skilled in intravenous therapy and subsequent definitive treatment are unavailable. Tension pneumothorax is a similar state of compromised venous return that might also respond temporarily to the redistributed fluid volume resulting from PASG application. Palafox and associates, however, produced cardiac tamponade or tension pneumothorax in hypovolemic dogs and found a *decline* in arterial pressure and a rise in central venous pressure when the abdominal binder was inflated above 80 mm Hg.[72] This deterioration was believed to be caused by PASG-induced diaphragmatic elevation increasing intrathoracic pressures and further compromising venous return. The clinical investigation of Mattox and coworkers suggests that intravenous therapy without PASG is safer in the patient with a penetrating thoracic injury during rapid transport for definitive therapy.[43] Hence, although the cautious use of PASG in hypovolemic patients with cardiac tamponade or tension pneumothorax may be temporizing when other options (including intravenous fluids) are not available, its use is controversial at best.

PROCEDURE

Application of PASG

Before PASG application it is useful to inspect the device and to establish the proper orientation (Fig. 35–6). Many find it helpful to mark the "up" side (inside) with paint or tape to aid in rapid correct application. The patient can be "logrolled" onto the opened trousers. Alternatively, with one person standing on either side and elevating the patient's legs, the trousers can be slid beneath to the buttocks. Then the patient's hips are elevated, and the upper border of the trousers is placed at the costal margin. The cervical spine must be stabilized in those at risk for cervical injury. The medial portion on each leg binder is brought between the legs, and the Velcro fasteners are closed over each leg and over the abdomen.

Many emergency departments prefer to keep the deflated PASG on the resuscitation table at all times. When patients arrive, they are placed on the garment so that it is immediately accessible should its use be required later during treatment. An alternative is to assemble the trousers loosely in advance and slide them over the patient's legs.[77] During application, the operator places his or her own arms through the pants legs from the bottom, sliding the pants legs completely onto the arms. The operator then stands at the patient's feet, grabs the patient's toes, and lifts. An assistant pulls the trousers from the operator's arms and slides them over the patient, and the Velcro straps are retightened.

After device application, the foot-pump hoses are attached to the stopcocks, and the foot-pump is used to inflate the two leg compartments and then the abdomen. The operator can accomplish inflation faster if the compartments are initially filled by blowing into them. The lungs can provide volume more quickly than the pump during initial low-resistance inflation. After resistance to filling is met, the pump becomes more efficient at increasing trouser pressures.[77] Hanke and associates found no difference in redistribution of blood volume between simultaneous and se-

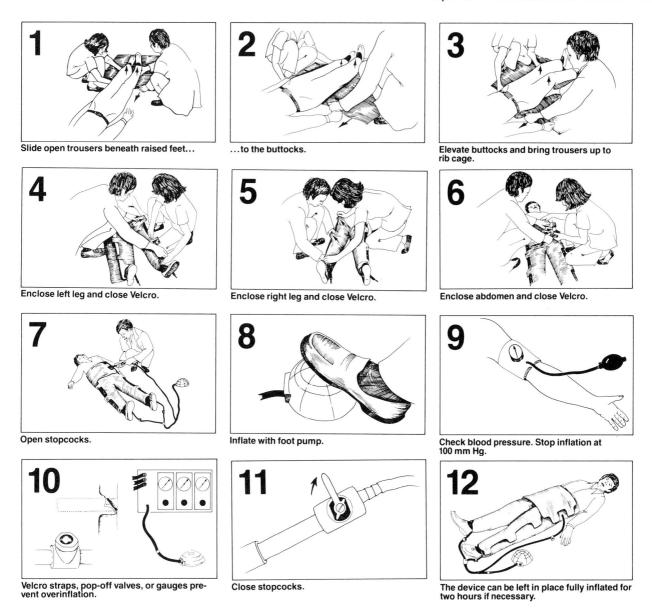

1 Slide open trousers beneath raised feet...

2 ...to the buttocks.

3 Elevate buttocks and bring trousers up to rib cage.

4 Enclose left leg and close Velcro.

5 Enclose right leg and close Velcro.

6 Enclose abdomen and close Velcro.

7 Open stopcocks.

8 Inflate with foot pump.

9 Check blood pressure. Stop inflation at 100 mm Hg.

10 Velcro straps, pop-off valves, or gauges prevent overinflation.

11 Close stopcocks.

12 The device can be left in place fully inflated for two hours if necessary.

Figure 35–6. Pneumatic anti-shock garment application. (Courtesy of the American College of Surgeons, Committee on Trauma.)

quential inflation of the leg and abdominal compartments.[78] Jennings and coworkers similarly found no hemodynamic benefit to simultaneous device inflation.[79] Therefore, it seems prudent when using the device for hypotension to inflate the leg compartments first and then check the blood pressure. If an adequate blood pressure is obtained, the abdominal compartment does not need inflation. If the blood pressure is inadequate, the abdominal compartment is inflated. Blood pressure and pulse should be closely monitored during the procedure, and inflation should be stopped if the systolic blood pressure exceeds 100 mm Hg.

Pediatric devices are available, although they are infrequently used. In the absence of these smaller garments, one can efficiently manage small children by wrapping them in one leg of the adult-sized trousers. A folded sheet or blanket can be placed between the bony prominences of the lower extremities. The inflation pressure should be titrated to a satisfactory pulse and blood pressure response.

The PASG alone can passively splint lower extremity fractures. Of the commonly available traction devices, only the Sager traction splint can be applied after the trousers are in place and inflated. The Sager splint can be used either inside or outside the device to splint one or both legs at the same time. The Hare traction splint and the Thomas splint are significantly more awkward to use with the PASG inflated. The Hare and Thomas splints present some risk of damage to the trousers themselves and result in an uneven application of circumferential pressure (see also Chapter 62). As is discussed later, the application of traction in combination with external counterpressure exacerbates compartmental pressures in the lower extremities.[80]

Inflation Pressure

Of the two major PASG devices that are available, one has a pressure gauge (or gauges) for monitoring pants pressure (Jobst Gladiator). As with any such piece of equipment, gauges should be periodically checked for accuracy. The other device uses pressure-relief ("pop-off") valves that limit inflation pressures to 104 mm Hg. It is reasonable to assume that most side effects and complications of these devices are proportional to the pressure and duration of pressure application. Most animal experiments and some clinical studies have suggested that hemorrhage control (presumably control of venous bleeding) in otherwise stable (often postoperative) patients is often accomplished with less than 40 mm Hg of inflation pressure.[2] "Autotransfusion" and blood pressure elevations may require a higher inflation pressure, although Hanke and colleagues reported a significant increase in central blood volume at 40 mm Hg and only minor progressive increases at 100 mm Hg.[78] Wayne and MacDonald suggest that most prehospital patients in shock will not demonstrate a blood pressure elevation at a 30 mm Hg inflation pressure.[81] One's goal should be to achieve a systolic blood pressure of approximately 100 mm Hg at the lowest inflation pressure possible. Obviously, time constraints may not permit careful titration of inflation pressure to blood pressure response; the patient in extremis may need simultaneous inflation of both leg and abdominal compartments to 100 mm Hg immediately on presentation.

Deflation

When? In the usual case, deflation may be considered when the combination of PASG and other resuscitative measures (e.g., fluids, hemorrhage control) has resulted in restoration of satisfactory vital signs. The gradual deflation procedure to be outlined should be followed. The presence of any contraindications to continued use (e.g., congestive heart failure, renal disease, pulmonary disease) should also be considered. The presence of a coagulopathy may be a relative contraindication to removing the device.

Where? If emergency surgery is indicated, the operating table may be the best place to deflate the PASG. After all monitoring and venous lines have been started, the anesthesiologist is prepared to monitor the patient, and the surgeons are in attendance, the abdominal portion can be deflated (preferably slowly—see "How"). The leg compartments can be left inflated for an abdominal procedure until internal hemorrhage is better controlled. In most situations, following adequate volume resuscitation, PASG deflation can be safely performed in the emergency department.

How? The PASG should be deflated gradually. Rapid deflation of the PASG in the hypovolemic patient can result in a catastrophic drop in blood pressure. The hemodynamic changes seen during deflation result from a rapid reduction in left ventricular afterload followed by a decrease in preload.[82] This process may be exacerbated by the sudden release of lactic acid and other vasoactive chemicals pooled in the abdomen and the lower extremities.[8, 46, 50, 83–85] Hence, deflation particularly in the setting of prolonged PASG use should be approached with caution.

Deflation should begin with the abdominal compartment. Small quantities of air are released, and the patient's blood pressure is rechecked. If no blood pressure drop occurs, more air should be released with repeated blood pressure measurements. If the systolic blood pressure falls more than 5 mm Hg, deflation should be halted and more fluids given until the blood pressure is restored. After the abdominal compartment is deflated, the legs should be deflated in a similar manner.

COMPLICATIONS AND DISADVANTAGES

A number of specific adverse effects have been noted in association with PASG use (Table 35–5). In addition,

Table 35–5. Complications and Disadvantages of PASG Application

Hypotension after removal
Metabolic acidosis
Respiratory compromise
Decreased renal perfusion
Other (infrequent) complications
   Pulmonary edema, congestive heart failure
   Compartment syndromes
   Increased wound bleeding
   Urination, defecation, vomiting
   Skin breakdown
   Lumbar spine movement
Mechanical problems and disadvantages
   Limitation of diagnostic and therapeutic procedures
      Physical examination
      Urinary catheterization
      Peritoneal lavage
      Vascular access
   Environmental influences
      Barometric pressure
      Temperature

patients with penetrating abdominal and thoracic trauma whose management included PASG use in conjunction with vigorous prehospital fluid resuscitation were found to have an increased mortality when compared with patients treated with fluid resuscitation alone in one urban prehospital setting.[42, 43] As noted in the "Indications" and "Contraindications" sections, the use of PASG in patients with penetrating truncal injuries in the setting of rapid transport times or intravenous fluid therapy does not appear to be warranted. Further discussion of other specific complications follows.

Hypotension

Clinical experience has shown that the major life-threatening complication resulting from the use of the PASG in hypovolemic patients has been sudden and severe hypotension due to precipitous removal of the device in the absence of adequate fluid resuscitation.[8, 46, 50, 83–85] Although emergency department physicians and emergency medical technicians are well aware of the problem, many consultants are not. When faced with a patient encased in vinyl from xiphoid to ankles, many have rapidly removed these devices, often with disastrous consequences.

Metabolic Acidosis

Metabolic acidosis has been the most reproducible abnormality after application of external counterpressure. Wangensteen and associates first reported this "detrimental" effect of external counterpressure.[86] They noted acidosis (to a pH of 7.01) and an increased lactate to pyruvate ratio in hyopvolemic dogs after 4 hours of external counterpressure. Hypovolemic dogs without external pressure had less acidosis and lived longer. Ransom and McSwain also found decreased central venous pH and increases in serum lactate and potassium in hypovolemic dogs wearing PASGs; these abnormalities were more pronounced in animals wearing PASGs than those in hypovolemic dogs without counterpressure.[87] Although the treatment of hypovolemia with a PASG alone without concomitant fluid replacement is an unusual situation, these animal studies led to the recommendation to limit PASG application time. Human studies have shown mild metabolic acidosis (pH 7.33 to 7.36), and many reports suggest that the acidosis is not a problem clinically.[50, 75, 88] Although metabolic acidosis may occur, close monitoring of arterial blood gases and correction with bicarbonate as needed should adequately address this potential problem.

Respiratory Compromise

Abdominal binding invariably produces subjective effects on respiration; alert patients frequently complain of shortness of breath when the abdominal compartment is inflated. Espinosa and Updegrove reported an 18 per cent decrease in vital capacity and a slight increase in respiratory rate in volunteers subjected to external counterpressure.[84] However, McCabe and colleagues found no changes in inspiratory and expiratory reserve volumes, maximum breathing capacity, or tidal volume in their volunteers.[89] Similarly Batalden and coworkers found no pulmonary complications in ten patients with external counterpressure garments who underwent positive-pressure ventilation for 24 to 48 hours.[90] Yet, Burdick and colleagues found atelectasis, pulmonary edema, or pneumonia in 14 of 28 similar patients.[88] Cogbill and coworkers[91] demonstrated a mild impairment of pulmonary function in healthy individuals and those with airflow obstruction when the PASG was inflated. The impairment was restrictive rather than obstructive and was not clinically significant with inflation pressures less than 50 mm Hg. In hypotensive patients, Ransom and McSwain[75] failed to demonstrate impaired alveolar ventilation when the PASG was used. McCabe and colleagues suggest that impaired pulmonary function results from mechanical binding of the thorax and decreased excursion of the diaphragm.[89] Newer designs of the device incorporate smaller abdominal compartments, which should not be applied at or above the costal margin and have resulted in less restriction of vital capacity.[89] In general, investigators concerned about respiratory compromise have recommended careful attention to arterial blood gases combined with controlled positive-pressure ventilation in those patients requiring prolonged external counterpressure.[13, 88]

Decreased Renal Perfusion

A number of reversible abnormalities in renal hemodynamics have been reported with external counterpressure. Normovolemic dogs in a PASG undergo a 40 to 50 per cent decline in renal blood flow and an elevation in renal vascular resistance.[92] Ten subjects in PASGs for 4 to 24 hours had no significant alterations in renal blood flow.[93] Normal human subjects experiencing increased abdominal pressure had 24 to 48 per cent declines in effective renal plasma flow and glomerular filtration rate, decreased urine output, elevated renal vein pressures, and increased urine specific gravity.[94] These changes reversed after decompression.

Infrequent Complications

A number of case reports document some infrequent but serious complications of the PASG.

Pulmonary edema and congestive heart failure have been attributed in isolated cases to increased pulmonary venous return and elevated pulmonary capillary wedge pressures.[2, 83, 88, 95]

Lumbar spine instability is another potential complication of the PASG. Older PASG designs included an abdominal bladder that inflated in the back as well as over the abdomen. Rockwell and coworkers[96] reported a case in which a lumbar spine injury was believed to have been aggravated by inflation of a circumferential abdominal bladder. They also demonstrated graphically on a volunteer the marked exaggeration of lumber lordosis that is possible with the older style garment. Newer designs of commercially available suits limit inflation to the anterior aspect of the abdominal compartment. The abdominal portion of all designs of the PASG should be used cautiously in patients at high risk for an unstable lumbar spine injury.

Lower extremity compartment syndromes following use of PASG have been reviewed elsewhere.[97–99] Increased pressure within the limits of a fascial compartment results in impaired microcirculation. The compartment pressure under the PASG is dependent on the PASG inflation pressure,[100, 101] the mean arterial pressure,[100] and the application of passive traction.[80, 100] During hypotension, full PASG inflation compartment pressure is commonly less than the mean arterial pressure.[100] Many factors contribute to the development of a compartment syndrome, including prolonged shock, inflation pressure (and duration of inflation), reperfusion edema, and local tissue injury.[97] It is not completely understood which of the multiple factors are most significant in the compartment syndrome associated with PASG use. Some cases are related to a lower extremity fracture with prolonged application of PASG,[102] but other cases have occurred in the absence of lower extremity injury.[103–105] Improper deflation technique, leaving the abdominal compartment inflated after deflation of the extremity compartments, can cause the syndrome.[106] The overall frequency of this complication seems quite low. In their review of 1120 patients, Wayne and MacDonald reported no cases of compartment syndrome.[12] Mattox and associates found an incidence of anterior compartment syndrome in approximately 1 per cent of their PASG patients and none of the patients without PASG.[41] In addition, reversible peroneal nerve palsy has been reported.[83]

Increased bleeding from lower extremity wounds after suit inflation was attributed in two cases to improvements in blood pressure.[8] The bleeding responded to rebandaging but required temporary deflation of the suit. Such bleeding may be hidden in bandages under the devices and should be considered in the differentiation of persistent hypotension from other conditions.

Stimulation of urination, defecation, and vomiting by suit inflation is noted as a complication in early papers.[45] McLaughlin and coworkers "know of one patient" without a nasogastric tube in place who died of aspirated vomitus after a PASG was applied.[50] Spontaneous defecation "has been a complication" in patients being treated for gastrointestinal bleeding with these devices.[91]

Skin breakdown at pressure points with prolonged use has prompted the suggestion to pad bony prominences.[83, 90, 107]

Diaphragmatic rupture has been reported following PASG inflation.[108] A sudden deterioration in blood pressure or respiratory status following PASG inflation should alert the clinician to this possibility. If significant herniation of abdominal contents into the thoracic space has occurred, deflation of the device may not fully resolve the clinical deterioration.

Mechanical Problems and Disadvantages

Limitation of Diagnostic Evaluation and Therapeutic Procedures. Physical examination of the lower extremities and the abdomen is limited by the PASG. A transparent suit that allows visualization of the lower extremities has been marketed but has had other disadvantages and is not commonly used. For the more common nontransparent device, the examiner must not remove the suit precipitously. In a stable patient, one compartment at a time should be deflated slowly with careful monitoring of vital signs. If necessary for treatment of hypotension, the compartment that has just been deflated may be reinflated. Similar problems exist with performing diagnostic peritoneal lavage. Urinary catheterization is challenging, particularly in female patients, even with the opening provided in the garments.

Vascular access can also be a problem. Lower extremity cutdowns are difficult to perform, and a pressure bag is required to produce flow of intravenous solutions. Animal and clinical investigations[109–111] have confirmed that intravenous fluid infusion beneath inflated PASGs reaches the central circulation promptly and in significant amounts. Access to the femoral artery and vein with the PASG inflated also is severely limited, although newer designs incorporate openings at the inguinal area for better access.

Environmental Influences on Device Pressures. Until recently, little attention had been paid to the role of the important environmental factors of pressure and temperature in modification of PASG inflation pressures.[112, 113] With the current popularity and availability of helicopter ambulance transport, the role of Boyle's law (the volume of the gas is inversely proportional to its pressure) needs to be reemphasized. As the helicopter rises, the air in the suit expands, increasing the trouser pressure. Decreasing altitude has the opposite effect. Similarly, as ambient temperature increases, trouser pressure rises, and vice versa. However, most helicopter transports occur at sufficiently low altitudes that the effects of altitude are not of concern. Nonetheless, when the "optimal" inflation pressure is determined at the scene of the accident, changes produced by movement into the controlled climate of the ambulance or hospital need to be predicted and recognized.

CONCLUSION

The pneumatic anti-shock garment is a useful adjunctive device in the care of the hypotensive patient. When the garment is used, improvements in blood pressure and pulse are often dramatic. In certain situations the device may slow hemorrhage. External counterpressure can "buy time" until definitive therapy is instituted. A major hazard is the profound hypotension that can result from the precipitous removal of the device by those who are unfamiliar with this possibility. Although the device may not be helpful in the urban prehospital setting for management of penetrating trauma when crystalloid therapy is rapidly available, it appears to have a role in other settings.

REFERENCES

1. Anti-shock trousers. Health Devices, vol. 6. Plymouth Meeting, Pa, Emergency Care Research Institutes, 1977, pp 265–277.
2. Pelligra R, Sandberg EC: Control of intractable abdominal bleeding by external counterpressure. JAMA 241:708, 1979.
3. Advanced Trauma Life Support Program: Instructor Manual. American College of Surgeons, Chicago, 1989.
4. Crile GW: Blood Pressure in Surgery: Experimental and Clinical Research. Philadelphia, JB Lippincott Co, 1903, pp 288–291.
5. Crile GW: Hemorrhage and Transfusions: Experimental and Clinical Research. New York, D Appleton and Co, 1909, pp 137–145.
6. Ferrario CM, Nadzam G, Fernandez LA, et al: Effects of pneumatic compression on the cardiovascular dynamics in dogs after hemorrhage. Aerospace Med 41:411, 1970.
7. Gardner WJ, Dohn DF: The antigravity suit (G-suit) in surgery. JAMA 162:274, 1956.
8. Cutler BS, Daggett W: Application of the g-suit to the control of hemorrhage in massive trauma. Ann Surg 173:511, 1971.
9. Kaplan BH: Emergency autotransfusion medical pneumatic trouser. Disclosure of invention, Logbook Entry 21. Ft. Rucker, Ala, US Army Aeromedical Research Laboratory, June 1972, p 6.
10. Kaplan BC, Civetta JM, Nagel EL, et al: The military anti-shock trouser in civilian pre-hospital emergency care. J Trauma 13:843, 1973.
11. McSwain NE Jr: Pneumatic trousers and the management of shock. J Trauma 17:719, 1977.
12. Wayne MA, MacDonald SC: Clinical evaluation of the antishock trouser: Retrospective analysis of five years of experience. Ann Emerg Med 12:342, 1983.
13. Abernathy C, Dickinson TC, Lokey H: A Military Anti-Shock Trousers program in the small hospital. Surg Clin North Am 59:461, 1979.
14. McSwain NE Jr: G-suits and shock: A non-invasive transfusion technique. J Kans Med Soc 77:438, 1976.
15. Gray S, Shaver JA, Kroetz FW, et al: Acute and prolonged effects of g-suit inflation on cardiovascular dynamics. Aerospace Med 40:40, 1969.
16. Bondurant S, Hickam JB, Isley JK: Pulmonary and circulatory effects of acute pulmonary vascular engorgement in normal subjects. J Clin Invest 36:59, 1957.
17. Gaffney FA, Thal ER, Taylor WF, et al: Hemodynamic effects of medical anti-shock trousers (MAST garment). J Trauma 21:931, 1981.
18. Tenney SM, Honig CR: The effect of the anti-g suit on the ballistocardiogram. J Aviat Med 26:194, 1955.
19. Bivins HG, Knopp R, Tiernan C, et al: Blood volume displacement with inflation of antishock trousers. Ann Emerg Med 11:409, 1982.
20. Payen DM, Brun-Buisson CJL, Carli PA, et al: Hemodynamic, gas exchange, and hormonal consequences of LBPP during PEEP ventilation. J Appl Physiol 62:61, 1987.
21. McSwain NE: Pneumatic anti-shock garment: State of the art. Ann Emerg Med 17:121, 1988.
22. Davis SM: Antishock trousers: A collective review. J Emerg Med 4:145, 1986.
23. Randall PE: Medical antishock trouser (MAST): A review. Injury 17:395, 1986.
24. Niemann JT, Stapczynski JS, Rosborough JP, et al: Hemodynamic effects of pneumatic external counterpressure in canine hemorrhagic shock. Ann Emerg Med 12:661, 1983.
25. Bellamy RF, DeGuzman LR, Pedersen DC: Immediate hemodynamic consequences of MAST inflation in normo- and hypovolemic anesthetized swine. J Trauma 24:889, 1984.
26. Burchard KW, Slotman GJ, Jed E, et al: Positive pressure respirations and pneumatic antishock garment application: Hemodynamic response. J Trauma 25:83, 1985.
27. Rubal BJ, Geer MR, Bickell WH, et al: Effects of pneumatic antishock garment inflation in normovolemic subjects. J Appl Physiol 67:339, 1989.
28. Hauswald M, Greene ER: Aortic blood flow during sequential MAST inflation. Ann Emerg Med 15:59, 1986.
29. Mannering D, Bennett ED, Mehta N, et al: Application of the medical anti-shock trouser (MAST) increases cardiac output and tissue perfusion in simulated, mild hypovolemia. Intensive Care Med 12:143, 1986.
30. Savino JA, Jabbour I, Agarwal N, et al: Overinflation of pneumatic antishock garments in the elderly. Am J Surg 55:572, 1989.
31. Moreno C, Moore EE, Rosenberger A, et al: Hemorrhage associated with major pelvic fracture: A multispecialty challenge. J Trauma 26:987, 1986.
32. Mucha P, Welch TJ: Hemorrhage in major pelvic fractures. Surg Clin North Am 68:757, 1988.
33. Mud HJ, Schattenkerk ME, DeVries JE, et al: Nonsurgical treatment of pelvic hemorrhage in obstetric and gynecologic patients. Crit Care Med 15:534, 1987.
34. Wangensteen SL, Ludewig RM, Eddy DW: Effect of external counterpressure on the intact circulation. Surg Gynecol Obstet 127:253, 1968.
35. Eddy DM, Wangensteen SL, Ludewig RM: The kinetics of fluid loss from leaks in arteries tested by an experimental ex vivo preparation and external counterpressure. Surgery 64:451, 1968.
36. Ludewig RM, Wangensteen SL: Effect of external counterpressure on venous bleeding. Surgery 66:515, 1969.
37. Gardner WJ: Hemostasis by pneumatic compression. Am Surg 35:635, 1969.
38. Gardner WJ, Storer J: The use of the g-suit in control of intra-abdominal bleeding. Surg Gynecol Obstet 123:792, 1966.
39. Wangensteen SL, Ludewig RM, Cox JM, et al: The effect of external counterpressure on arterial bleeding. Surgery 64:922, 1968.
40. Low RB, Schmidt C, Wilder RJ, et al: Control of intraabdominal hemorrhage and shock: A comparison of fluid resuscitation, MAST, and balloon occlusion. Ann Emerg Med 14:540, 1985.
41. Mattox KL, Bickell WH, Pepe PE, et al: Prospective randomized evaluation of antishock MAST in post-traumatic hypotension. J Trauma 26:779, 1986.
42. Bickell WH, Pepe PE, Bailey ML, et al: Randomized trial of pneumatic antishock garments in the prehospital management of penetrating abdominal injuries. Ann Emerg Med 16:653, 1987.
43. Mattox KL, Bickell W, Pepe PE, et al: Prospective MAST study in 911 patients. J Trauma 29:1104, 1989.
44. Moylan JA, Fitzpatrick KT, Beyer AJ, et al: Factors improving survival in multisystem trauma patients. Ann Surg 207:679, 1988.
45. Civetta JM, Nussenfeld SR, Row TR, et al: Prehospital use of the military anti-shock trouser (MAST). JACEP 5:581, 1976.
46. Hall M, Marshall JR: The gravity suit: A major advance in management of gynecologic blood loss. Obstet Gynecol 53:247, 1979.
47. Bickell WH, Dice WH: Military antishock trousers in a patient with adrenergic-resistant anaphylaxis. Ann Emerg Med 13:189, 1984.

48. Granata AV, Halickman JF, Borak J: Utility of military anti-shock trousers (MAST) in anaphylactic shock: A case report. J Emerg Med 2:349, 1985.
49. Herrington DM, Insley BM, Weinmann CG, et al: Nifedipine overdose. Am J Med 81:344, 1986.
50. McLaughlin AP III, McCullough DL, Kerr WS Jr, et al: The use of the external counterpressure (g-suit) in management of traumatic retroperitoneal hemorrhage. J Urol 107:940, 1972.
51. Gustafson RA, McDowell DE, Savrin RA: The use of the MAST suit in ruptured abdominal aortic aneurysms. Am Surg 49:454, 1983.
52. Burn N, Lewis DG, MacKenzie A, et al: The g-suit: Its use in emergency surgery for ruptured abdominal aortic aneurysm. Anaesthesia 27:423, 1972.
53. Darling RC: Ruptured arteriosclerotic abdominal aortic aneurysms: A pathologic and clinical study. Am J Surg 119:397, 1970.
54. Abernathy C, Baumgartner R, Butler HG, et al: The management of ruptured abdominal aortic aneurysms in rural Colorado. JAMA 256:597, 1986.
55. Lewis DG, MacKenzie A, McNeill IF: The use of the g-suit in the control of bleeding arising from hypocoagulation. Ann R Coll Surg Engl 52:53, 1973.
56. Wayne MA: The mast suit in the treatment of cardiogenic shock. JACEP 7:107, 1978.
57. Gray S, Shaver JA, Kroetz FW, et al: Acute and prolonged effects of g-suit inflation on cardiovascular dynamics. Circulation (Suppl II) 36:125, 1967.
58. Babbs CF: New versus old theories of blood flow during cardiopulmonary resuscitation. Crit Care Med 8:191, 1980.
59. Luce JM, Cary JM, Ross BK, et al: New developments in cardiopulmonary resuscitation. JAMA 244:1366, 1980.
60. Bircher N, Safer P, Stewart R: A comparison of standard "MAST"-augmented and open-chest CPR in dogs. Crit Care Med 8:147, 1980.
61. Lee HR, Wilder RJ, Dorins P, et al: MAST augmentation of external cardiac compression: Role of changing intrapleural pressure. Ann Emerg Med 10:560, 1981.
62. Rudikoff MT, Maughan WL, Effron M, et al: Mechanisms of blood flow during cardiopulmonary resuscitation. Circulation 61:345, 1980.
63. Lilja GP, Long RS, Ruiz E: Augmentation of systolic blood pressure during external cardiac compression by use of the MAST suit. Ann Emerg Med 10:182, 1981.
64. Mahoney BD, Murick MJ: Pneumatic trousers in refractory prehospital cardiopulmonary arrest. Ann Emerg Med 13:410, 1984.
65. Niemann JT, Rosborough JP, Criley JM: Continuous external counterpressure during closed-chest resuscitation: A critical appraisal of the military antishock trouser garment and abdominal binder. Circulation 74:102, 1986.
66. Tandberg D, Hauswald M, Rusnak R: MAST conversion of paroxysmal supraventricular tachycardia in Wolff-Parkinson-White syndrome. Ann Emerg Med 16:712, 1987.
67. Tandberg D, Rusnak R, Sklar D, et al: Successful treatment of paroxysmal supraventricular tachycardia with MAST. Ann Emerg Med 13:1068, 1984.
68. Walker LA, MacMath TL, Chipman H, et al: MAST application in the treatment of paroxysmal supraventricular tachycardia in a child. Ann Emerg Med 17:529, 1988.
69. Hauswald M, Tandberg D: The effect of patient position and MAST inflation on carotid sinus diameter. Ann Emerg Med 14:1065, 1985.
70. Cram AE, Davis JW, Kealey GP, et al: Effects of pneumatic anti-shock trousers on canine intracranial pressure. Ann Emerg Med 10:28, 1981.
71. Dannewitz SR, Lilja GP, Ruiz E: Effect of pneumatic trousers on intracranial pressure in hypovolemic dogs with an intracranial mass. Ann Emerg Med 10:176, 1981.
72. Palafox BA, Johnson MN, McEwen DK, et al: ICP changes following application of the mast suit. J Trauma 21:55, 1981.
73. Gardner SR, Maull KI, Swensson EE, et al: The effects of pneumatic antishock garment on intracranial pressure in man: A prospective study of 12 patients with severe head injury. J Trauma 24:896, 1984.
74. Lilja GP, Batalden DJ, Adams BE, et al: Value of the counterpressure suit (MAST) in pre-hospital care. Minn Med 58:540, 1975.
75. Ransom K, McSwain NE Jr: Respiratory function following application of MAST trousers. JACEP 7:297, 1978.
76. Davis JW, McKone TK, Cram AE: Hemodynamic effects of military anti-shock trousers (MAST) in experimental cardiac tamponade. Ann Emerg Med 10:185, 1981.
77. Dick T: Putting your pants on using the MAST suit. JEMS 7:22, 1982.
78. Hanke BK, Bivins HG, Knopp R, et al: Antishock trousers: A comparison of inflation techniques and inflation pressures. Ann Emerg Med 14:636, 1985.
79. Jennings TJ, Seaworth JR, Howell LL, et al: The effects of various antishock trouser inflation sequences on hemodynamics in normovolemic subjects. Ann Emerg Med 15:1193, 1986.
80. Aprahamian C, Towne JB, Thompson BM, et al: Effect of circumferential pneumatic compression devices on digital flow. Ann Emerg Med 5:118, 1987.
81. Wayne MA, MacDonald SC: Clinical evaluation of the antishock trouser: Prospective study of low-pressure inflation. Ann Emerg Med 12:285, 1983.
82. Bickell WH, Geer MR, Rubal BJ: Hemodynamic response to rapid pneumatic antishock garment inflation. Ann Emerg Med 15:886, 1986.
83. Bruining HA, Schattenkerk ME, De Vries JE, et al: Clinical experience with the medical anti-shock trousers (MAST) in the treatment of hemorrhage, especially from compound pelvic fracture. Neth J Surg 32–3:102, 1980.
84. Espinosa MH, Updegrove JH: Clinical experience with the g-suit. Arch Surg 101:36, 1970.
85. McSwain NE Jr: MAST pneumatic trousers: A mechanical device to support blood pressure. Med Instrum 11:334, 1977.
86. Wangensteen SL, deHoll JD, Ludewig RM, et al: The detrimental effect of the g-suit in hemorrhagic shock. Ann Surg 170:187, 1969.
87. Ransom KJ, McSwain NE Jr: Metabolic acidosis with pneumatic trousers in hypovolemic dogs. JACEP 8:184, 1979.
88. Burdick JE, Warshaw AL, Abbott WM: External counterpressure to control postoperative intraabdominal hemorrhage. Am J Surg 129:369, 1975.
89. McCabe JB, Seidel DR, Jagger JA: Antishock trouser inflation and pulmonary vital capacity. Ann Emerg Med 12:290, 1983.
90. Batalden DJ, Wickstrom PH, Ruiz E, et al: Value of the g-suit in patients with severe pelvic fracture. Arch Surg 109:326, 1974.
91. Cogbill TH, Good JT, Moore EE, et al: Pulmonary function after military antishock trouser inflation. Surg Forum 32:302, 1981.
92. Shenansky JH II, Gillenwater JY: The effects of external abdominal counterpressure on renal function. Surg Forum 21:528, 1970.
93. Cangiano TL, Kest L: Use of a g-suit for uncontrollable bleeding after percutaneous renal biopsy. J Urol 107:360, 1972.
94. Bradley SE, Bradley GP: The effect of increased intra-abdominal pressure on renal function in man. J Clin Invest 26:1010, 1947.
95. McCullough DL, McLaughlin AP, Warshawsky AB: The gravity suit: A useful device in complicated urologic hemorrhage. Urology 6:468, 1975.
96. Rockwell DD, Butler AB, Keats TE, et al: An improved design of the pneumatic counter-pressure trousers. Am J Surg 143:377, 1982.
97. Kaplan BH, Soderstrom CA: Pneumatic antishock garments and the compartment syndrome. Am J Emerg Med 5:177, 1987.
98. Templeman D, Lange R, Harms B: Lower-extremity compartment syndromes associated with use of pneumatic anti-shock garments. J Trauma 27:79, 1987.
99. Aprahamian C, Gessert G, Bandyk DF, et al: MAST-associated compartment syndrome (MACS): A review. J Trauma 29:549, 1989.
100. Hedges JR, Baker PB, Dalsey WC: Compartmental pressure measurements during application of the pneumatic antishock garment. J Emerg Med 1:377, 1984.
101. Chisholm CD, Clarke DE: Effect of the pneumatic antishock garment on intramuscular pressure. Ann Emerg Med 13:581, 1984.
102. Maull KI, Capehart JE, Cardea JA, et al: Limb loss following military anti-shock trouser (MAST) application. J Trauma 21:60, 1981.
103. Williams TM, Knopp R, Ellyson JH: Compartment syndrome after antishock trouser use without lower-extremity trauma. J Trauma 22:595, 1982.
104. McLellan BA, Phillips JH, Hunter GA, et al: Bilateral lower extremity amputations after prolonged application of the pneumatic antishock garment: Case report. Can J Surg 30:55, 1987.
105. Taylor DC, Salvian AJ, Shackleton CR: Crush syndrome complicating pneumatic antishock garment (PASG) use. Injury 19:43, 1988.
106. Brotman S, Browner BD, Cox EF: MAST trousers improperly applied causing a compartment syndrome in lower extremity. J Trauma 22:598, 1982.
107. Reines HD, Khoury NP: Use of military antishock trousers in the hospital. Am J Surg 139:307, 1980.
108. Hagman J, Iguchi H, Kinsey J, et al: Diaphragmatic rupture following blunt trauma. Ann Emerg Med 13:49, 1984.
109. Joyce SM, Barsan WG, Hedges JR, et al: Effect of a pneumatic antishock garment on drug delivery via distal venous access. Ann Emerg Med 13:885, 1984.
110. Tucker JF, Danzl DF, Teague E, et al: Infusion of intravenous fluid, distal to pneumatic antishock trousers. J Emerg Med 2:79, 1984.
111. Mullen MJ, Krohmer JR, McCabe JB: Intravenous fluid flow beneath inflated antishock trouser in a canine hemorrhagic shock model. Ann Emerg Med 16:153, 1987.
112. Sanders AB, Meislin HW, Daub E: Alterations in MAST suit pressure with changes in ambient temperature. J Emerg Med 1:37, 1983.
113. Sanders AB, Meislin HW: Effect of altitude change on MAST suit pressure. Ann Emerg Med 12:140, 1983.

Vital Sign Measurement

Chapter 36

Determination of Vital Signs

Jody Riva Lewinter and Thomas E. Terndrup

INTRODUCTION

Temperature, pulse, blood pressure, and respirations are the four vital signs that must be determined on every patient who presents to the emergency department. In children, weight should also be obtained. These measurements provide a unique, objective capsule assessment of the patient's clinical status. Vital signs are indicators of the severity of illness and the urgency of intervention. Deteriorating vital signs are frequently the earliest clue to a declining physiologic status, and improvement in these values provides reassurance that an unstable patient is responding to therapy. Despite this, vital signs are frequently taken only once, at triage, when they are perhaps least accurate. When a patient undergoes treatment over an extended time, vital signs should be repeated. Vital signs should be measured and recorded at intervals dictated by the patient's clinical state; before and after fluid resuscitation, invasive procedures, or administration of medications with cardiopulmonary effects; or with any sudden change in the patient's status. In addition, an abnormal vital sign can direct the physician toward a group of diagnoses or a particular organ system for evaluation. An abnormal vital sign may constitute the patient's entire complaint, as in the febrile infant, or be the only indication of the potential for serious illness, as in the patient with a resting tachycardia. For all these reasons, accurate determination and interpretation of vital signs are mandatory in the treatment of every emergency department patient.

In the emergency department, the accurate assessment and management of abnormal vital signs must reflect orderly resuscitation. Determination of airway patency with respiratory rate and pattern assumes first importance. Establishing the presence and quality of an arterial pulse is the second vital sign to be assessed, followed by blood pressure and body temperature. This chapter is organized according to the priorities important to the practice of emergency medicine.

BACKGROUND

Early pulmonary medicine was dominated by the concepts of Herophilus (fourth century B.C.) and Galen (A.D. 131–200), whose belief in the humoral theory of medicine dictated that the lungs functioned as a cooling device and site for generation of body humors. The pulmonary circulation was correctly described in the thirteenth century by Ibnan-Nafis; however, his observations passed unnoticed.

Respiratory physiology did not progress until the significance of the pulmonary circulation was recognized by William Harvey in 1628. His publication, *Anatomica de Motu Cordis et Sanguinis*, described the circulation of blood and recognized the lungs as a conduit for blood flow. It was not until the 1700s that advances in physics and chemistry allowed the identification of the gases involved in respiration.[1]

Sphygmology, or palpation of the pulse, was first appreciated by Herophilus. He believed that interpreting the pulse required a knowledge of both music and geometry and defined the characteristics of the pulse as size, frequency, force, and rhythm. Chinese physicians (second century B.C.) timed the pulse by the respiratory rate of the examiner, believing that four pulsations per respiration was a normal rate for adults. The study of pulses was greatly influenced by Galen, who expanded the subject into a rather complex and obscure art form, writing no fewer than 18 books on the subject.[2]

Blood pressure was first measured directly in 1733 by Stephen Hales, who recorded the arterial pressures in a mare by cannulation with a brass pipe and a blood-filled glass column.[3] Otto Frank used large-bore catheters connected to a rubber membrane in his 1903 manometer description.[4] The invention of inflatable cuff manometers (1896, Riva-Rocci) and the discovery of the arterial phase sounds (1905, Korotkoff) allowed for the development of indirect blood pressure measurement.[3, 4]

The earliest recorded references to fever are from the sixth century B.C. Akkadian cuneiform inscriptions, which appear to have adapted an ancient Sumerian icon of a flaming brazier to denote both fever and the local warmth of inflammation in a single ideogram. Clinical thermometry was introduced by Sanctorius with his publication of *Commentaria in primam fen primi libri canonis Avicennae* in 1625. Air and alcohol thermometers were used by Sanctorius and Galileo. Mercury column thermometers were introduced by Fahrenheit in 1714. Although their routine use was supported by Herman Boerhaave, thermometry was not established as routine clinical practice until the 1870s, following publication of *Das Verhalten der Eigenwärme in Krankheiten*, by Carl Reinhold Wunderlich.[5]

NORMAL VALUES

The range of normal vital signs for specific age groups must be recognized by the clinician to enable identification of abnormal values and their significance. Norms for vital signs may also be influenced by sex, race, pregnancy, and residence in an industrialized nation.

Published vital sign norms for children are incomplete. In Table 36–1, we report normal vital signs for children by age group (0 to 2 months, 3 to 12 months, 1 to 6 years, 7 to 12 years, and 13 to 18 years) as means and standard deviations. The values for pulse, respiration, and blood pressure for 0 to 2 months are adapted from studies of newborn (less than 7 day) populations.[6–8] During this period, systolic blood pressure rises rapidly. Values for pulse and respirations reflect an average of male and female values for 0 to 1-year, 3-year, 9-year, and 16-year-old populations.[9] The values for blood pressure reflect an average of male and female values for the 1- to 6-month and the 3-, 9-, and 16-year-old populations.[8]

For the adult population, normal values for pulse and blood pressure are well established. Normal pulse rate ranges

Table 36–1. *Normal Values for Vital Signs of Infants and Children (Mean ± SD)*

Parameter	0–2 months	3–12 months	1–6 years	7–12 years	13–18 years
Respirations (breaths/minute)	43 ± 6	30.5 ± 7	24 ± 3	19 ± 2	17 ± 2.5
Pulse rate (beats/minute)	126 ± 20	130.5 ± 19.5	88 ± 9	70 ± 7.5	63.5 ± 7
Systolic BP* (mm Hg)	72 ± 9.5	95 ± 15	93 ± 13	100 ± 10	112 ± 12
Diastolic BP (mm Hg)	51 ± 8.7	53 ± 9.8	55 ± 9.6	63 ± 10	67 ± 9.5

*For children (1 to 10 years of age): 2 × age (in years) + 90 = fiftieth percentile for systolic arterial blood pressure.

from 60 to 100 beats per minute. Normal systolic blood pressure is 90 to 140 mm Hg, and normal diastolic blood pressure is 60 to 90 mm Hg. However, there is currently no consensus on what constitutes a normal adult respiratory rate. The majority of studies on respiratory rate support 16 to 24 respirations per minute as the norm for adults.

Pregnancy results in alteration of the normal adult values for pulse and blood pressure. Respiratory rate is unchanged, although the physiologic hyperventilation of pregnancy is well recognized. This is a result of increased tidal volume and decreased residual and expiratory reserve volumes.[10] Resting pulse rate increases through pregnancy to 10 to 15 per cent over baseline values. Norms for systolic and diastolic blood pressure are dependent on patient positioning. When the pregnant patient is sitting or standing, systolic pressures are essentially unchanged. Diastolic pressures decline until approximately 28 weeks gestation and then begin to rise to nonpregnant levels. When the pregnant patient is in the lateral decubitus position, both systolic and diastolic pressures decline until the twenty-eighth week and then begin to rise to nonpregnant levels (Table 36–2).[11]

RESPIRATION

Respiratory frequency must be measured in every emergency department patient. However, the number of respirations per minute reveals only part of the clinical picture. The pattern, effort, and volume of respirations may be more indicative of altered respiratory physiology. An abnormality in respiration may be a primary complaint or a manifestation of other systemic disease.

Physiology

Breathing is initiated and primarily controlled in the medullary respiratory center, a collection of nuclei in the brain stem. The dorsal respiratory nucleus is the best understood and functions as a pacemaker, similar to the sinus node in the heart. In isolation it generates an excitatory signal that lasts for approximately 2 seconds and stimulates the diaphragm via the phrenic nerve. It then becomes quiescent for approximately 3 seconds. The ventral respiratory nucleus is felt to be responsible for stimulating the abdominal and intercostal accessory muscles of respiration. The medullary respiratory center is modulated by the pneumotaxic and apneustic centers in the pons. The pneumotaxic center serves as limiter of length of the inspiratory signal and therefore can greatly increase or decrease respiratory rate.[12]

In addition to being modified by other areas of the brain stem, the medullary respiratory center is modified by voluntary centers in the cerebral cortex; pulmonary stretch receptors of the airways; type J or juxtapulmonary capillary receptors of the pulmonary capillaries; arterial baroreceptors of the carotid sinus; and receptors found in skeletal muscle, tendons, and joints. Central and peripheral chemoreceptors are also powerful influences on respiratory rate. The central chemosensitive area of the medulla responds to acid-base changes of the cerebrospinal fluid. The arterial chemoreceptors of the carotid sinus and aortic bodies respond both to hypoxia and to the acid-base balance of the individual.[13]

Indications and Contraindications

All emergency department patients should have their respiratory rate documented during their emergency department visit. *Repeated assessment and documentation* of the patient's respiratory status is indicated in patients who present with an abnormal respiratory rate or a complaint referable to their airway or breathing.

The only contraindication to a careful measurement of respiratory rate is the setting of respiratory distress that requires immediate therapeutic intervention. A measurement of respiratory rate and effort should be performed as soon as patient care demands permit in these circumstances.

Equipment for Monitoring

Respiratory inductive plethysmography is the technique most frequently used to monitor respiratory frequency and amplitude noninvasively. Placement of two standard chest leads allows measurement of changes in thoracic impedance. Measurement is affected by chest wall expansion, movement, and factors such as pulmonary water content. Validation of the accuracy of direct current–coupled respiratory inductive plethysmography for measuring respiratory frequency has been shown for spontaneously breathing and mechanically ventilated patients. Other methods for monitoring respiratory frequency include the abdominal strain gauge and nasal thermistor.[14]

Limitations of respiratory monitors include falsely negative (nonalarming during apnea), falsely positive (alarming

Table 36–2. *Vital Signs During Pregnancy in the Lateral Decubitus Position (Mean ± SD)*

Parameter	First Trimester	Second Trimester	Third Trimester
Pulse rate (beats/minute)	77 ± 2	85 ± 2	88 ± 2
Systolic BP (mm Hg)	98 ± 2	91 ± 2	95 ± 2
Diastolic BP (mm Hg)	53 ± 2	49 ± 2	50 ± 2

(Adapted from Katz R, Karliner JS, Resnik R: Effects of a natural volume overload state (pregnancy) on left ventricular performance in normal human subjects. Circulation 58:434, 1978. By permission of the American Heart Association, Inc.)

during nasal breathing), and failure to detect airway obstruction while the patient attempts to breathe. Cardiogenic artifact accounts for most false-negative readings, whereas false-positive readings usually result from poorly adjusted sensitivity.[15]

Periodic manual measurements as described later generally suffice for emergency department patients.

Procedure

Respiratory rate is the number of inspirations per minute. Generally, *respiratory rate is best measured with the patient unaware that breathing is being observed*, because awareness makes the patient conscious of the breathing pattern and may alter the rate. Commonly, examiners count respirations while appearing to count the pulse. The respiratory rate is most accurately determined by counting for a full minute. Because the frequency is much less than the pulse, and breathing is less regular, an inaccurate measurement is more likely to occur if a 15-second interval is used. Note that if one chooses to count respirations for 15 seconds, the respiratory rate will be overestimated by 4 respirations per minute unless the count starts with zero.[16]

Respiratory rates in children accurately reflect illness or distress. Infants, in addition to being obligate nose breathers, are primarily diaphragmatic breathers, and their respiratory rate may be more easily determined by observing or palpating excursion of the chest or abdominal wall.[17]

Complications

Problems related to the measurement of respiratory rate are generally due to failure to recognize a patient in obvious respiratory distress or failure to monitor respiratory rate in a patient who may be at risk for respiratory depression (e.g., a sedative-hypnotic or narcotic overdose).

Failure to document respiratory rates or changes in response to therapy may also pose liability risks for emergency physicians when adverse outcomes occur.

Interpretation

RATE

Surprisingly, consensus does not exist regarding what constitutes the range of normal respiratory rate for adults. Hooker and colleagues note that current texts vary considerably in their definitions of a normal respiratory rate and do not support their contentions with scientific literature. These researchers cite published values that range from 8 to 20 breaths per minute.[18]

There are a limited number of studies that examine respiratory rates. In one of the earliest studies of respiratory rates, Hutchinson evaluated respiratory rates in 1897 healthy males at rest and found that 91 per cent had respiratory rates between 16 and 24 breaths per minute.[19] He also noted that 30 per cent had exactly 20 breaths per minute. Mead observed 75 individuals at rest "seated at a public gathering" and observed a mean respiratory frequency of 16 to 18 and a range of 11 to 26 breaths per minute.[20] Bendixen and colleagues studied healthy young adults at rest (16 females and 12 males) and noted a mean respiratory frequency of 19 breaths per minute for females and 16 breaths per minute for males.[21] Gilbert and coworkers studied healthy adults (9 females and 7 males) and reported an average respiratory frequency in breaths per minute of 16.8 for females and

16.3 for males.[22] McFadden and associates studied 142 elderly patients in a long-term care facility and compared them with 60 elderly patients who required hospital admission. They found a respiratory rate of 16 to 25 breaths per minute in the healthy elderly. A respiratory rate greater than 25 breaths per minute was consistently found in patients with respiratory tract infections, frequently predating the clinical illness.[23]

Hooker and associates, in the only study that specifically investigated respiratory rates in an emergency department, measured respiratory rates in 110 afebrile ambulatory patients without respiratory complaints (53 females and 57 males).[18] Medical students measured respiratory rates for a full minute and found a mean rate of 20.1 breaths per minute. Sixty-six patients had their respiratory rates measured again before discharge. There was no significant difference in the pretreatment and posttreatment respiratory rates. When analyzed by sex, females had a mean respiratory rate in breaths per minute of 20.9 and males had a mean respiratory rate of 19.4, a statistically significant difference. The researchers concluded that a normal respiratory rate in their patient population was 16 to 24 breaths per minute.[18]

The value of scientifically determining the range of normal respiratory rates lies in increasing the specificity of the measurement when assessing pathology. Gravelyn and Weg compared changes in respiratory rates with respiratory dysfunction in 46 postoperative patients and found that nine patients had respiratory rates greater than 24 breaths per minute. Of these, five patients had developed infection or congestive heart failure and one patient demonstrated an elevated respiratory rate in response to pain. In the remaining 35 patients, only one had respiratory dysfunction and a normal respiratory rate. They concluded that measurement of respiratory rate is a valuable screening tool.[24] Bell and colleagues, using data from the Urokinase-Streptokinase Pulmonary Embolism Trials, studied the clinical features of pulmonary emboli. Designating a respiratory rate of greater than 16 breaths per minute as abnormal, they report that tachypnea occurs in 92 per cent of patients with pulmonary emboli.[25] Unfortunately, many normal patients have a resting respiratory rate of greater than 16 breaths per minute.

PATTERN AND AMPLITUDE

Abnormal respiratory patterns may be characteristic of metabolic or central nervous system pathology. Hyperventilation and hypoventilation may result from an extensive differential diagnosis including primary pulmonary disorders, such as pneumonia or chest wall pain. Respiratory disturbances also occur secondary to other disease processes. For example, Kussmaul respiration describes the hyperventilation pattern seen in diabetics with ketoacidosis.

Cheyne-Stokes respirations denote an undulating pattern of breathing in which tachypnea alternates with apnea. This pattern results from increased brain stem responsiveness to CO_2, allowing overbreathing when the P_{CO_2} becomes elevated with resultant marked lowering of P_{CO_2}, which then inhibits respirations. Cheyne-Stokes respirations are characteristic of patients with a wide range of central nervous system disease, such as bilateral cerebral infarcts or hypertensive encephalopathy. This pattern may also signal incipient transtentorial herniation.[26] Cheyne-Stokes respirations are found in patients with severe cardiac failure. This results because of delays in the acid-base alterations of the central circulation reaching the chemosensitive area of the brain stem. Corrections in respiratory pattern are therefore delayed, allowing respiratory overcorrection of the P_{CO_2}.[11]

Less common abnormal patterns of respiration include central neurogenic hyperventilation, apneustic, cluster, and

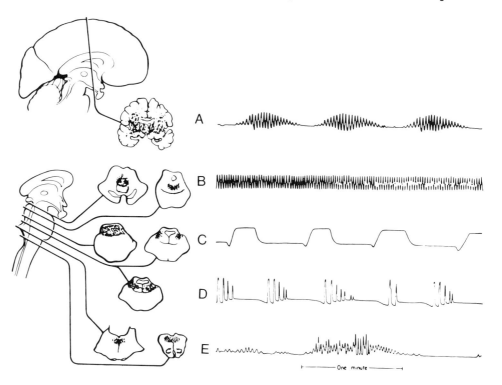

Figure 36-1. Abnormal respiratory patterns associated with pathologic lesions *(shaded areas)* at various levels of the brain. Tracings by chest-abdomen pneumograph, inspiration reads up. *A,* Cheyne-Stokes respiration. *B,* Central neurogenic hyperventilation. *C,* Apneusis. *D,* Cluster breathing. *E,* Ataxic breathing. (From Plum F: The Diagnosis of Stupor and Coma. 3rd ed. Philadelphia, FA Davis Co, 1982. Reproduced by permission.)

One minute

ataxic respirations (Fig. 36–1). *Central neurogenic hyperventilation* describes a pattern of sustained hyperpnea in the face of abnormal blood gases. This pattern is felt to result from destructive lesions extending from the midbrain to the upper third of the pons. *Apneustic breathing* is described as a pattern of respiration in which a pause occurs at end-inspiration. There may be an associated pause at end-expiration. This pattern is associated with lower pontine damage. *Cluster breathing* is associated with lesions in the lower pons or upper medulla and is described as clusters of breaths followed by respiratory pauses. *Ataxic breathing* describes respirations of random pattern and depth. It is associated with injury to the dorsal medullary neurons resulting from ischemia, infection, or posterior fossa processes that impinge on the medulla.[26]

Respiratory patterns in children must be observed carefully. In infants, periodic breathing, which may be normal, must be distinguished from apnea. By definition, *periodic breathing* consists of three or more respiratory pauses greater than 3 seconds in duration, with less than 20 seconds between pauses. There is no associated bradycardia or cyanosis. This contrasts with apnea, which is a particular problem in preterm infants. *Apnea* is defined as a respiratory pause of greater than 20 seconds and is associated with bradycardia and hypoxia.[17] Periodic breathing and apnea are felt to be disorders on a continuum, both stemming from immaturity of the physiologic controls of respiration. However, periodic breathing is felt to be a benign disorder, whereas infants with apneic episodes may be at an increased risk for sudden infant death syndrome.[27]

PULSE

The pulse is examined primarily to establish cardiac rate and rhythm. However, palpation of peripheral pulses to assess both the pulse contour and the pulse amplitude also yields clues to cardiac disease, such as aortic insufficiency, and information about the integrity of the peripheral vascular supply.

Physiology

Blood flowing into the aorta with each cardiac cycle initiates a pressure wave. Blood flows through the vasculature at approximately 0.5 meter per second; however, pressure waves in the aorta move at 3 to 5 meters per second. Thereore, palpated peripheral pulses represent pressure waves, not blood flow. After ventricular depolarization, the pressure pulse is palpated at the carotid, brachial, radial, and femoral arteries at 30, 60, 80, and 75 msec, respectively.[23]

The arterial pulse is initiated by the opening of the aortic valve and the ejection of the stroke volume. Because of the rapidity of ejection, the stroke volume is initially stored in the proximal aorta, causing a large rise in aortic pressure. The aortic pressure curve (Fig. 36–2) begins with the opening of the aortic valve. The initial rise is termed the anacrotic limb and represents the initial distention of the proximal aorta. As the left ventricle relaxes, there is a momentary reversal of proximal aortic blood flow, and the descending limb begins. However, this action snaps the aortic valve closed, and the elastic recoil of the arterial wall and aortic valves causes proximal aortic pressure to briefly rise again. This is represented by a momentary rise in the pressure curve and is responsible for the incisura or notch of the pressure curve. As blood is distributed to the periphery, aortic pressure then gradually falls. The aortic pressure curve is described as having a dicrotic notch because of its distinctive incisura and rebound.[11]

In the peripheral vasculature a normal pulse contour has a rapid, smooth upstroke and a more gradual downstroke. The dicrotic notch should not be palpable. However, changes in the aortic pressure curve, reflecting altered cardiovascular physiology, may result in an abnormal contour of the peripheral pulse.

Pulse amplitude reflects the pulse pressure, which is defined as the difference between the systolic and diastolic pressure. Cardiac output and arterial compliance are the two primary determinants of pulse pressure. Arterial compliance decreases as the pressure wave moves through the

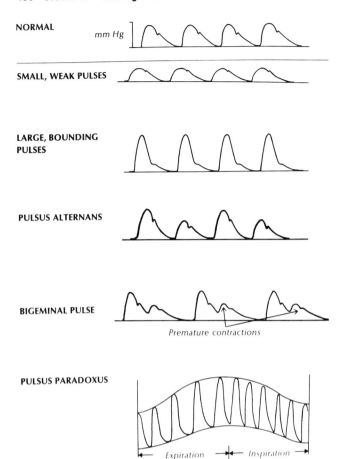

Figure 36–2. Examples of abnormalities of the arterial pulse compared with the normal pulse. The normal pulse pressure is approximately 30 to 40 mm Hg. The pulse contour is smooth and rounded. (The notch on the descending slope of the pulse wave is not palpable.) (From Bates B: A Guide to Physical Examination and History Taking. 4th ed. Philadelphia, JB Lippincott Co, 1987.)

arterial tree. Smaller distal arteries are less compliant than central arteries, causing pressure waves to move faster through these vessels. In addition, pressure waves may be reflected by less compliant distal arteries. If a reflected pressure wave encounters an oncoming wave, the two may summate, augmenting the pulse pressure.[11]

Indications and Contraindications

The evaluation of pulse presence and rate is indicated in every patient who presents to the emergency department. The necessity of repeated evaluations is dictated by the clinical complaint and status of the patient, as is the detailed assessment of pulse contour and amplitude.

There are no contraindications to assessment of pulse, only a few cautionary notes about the examination of the carotid pulse. Bilateral carotid artery palpation should be avoided, as this maneuver could endanger cerebral blood flow. In addition, massage of the carotid sinus, found at the bifurcation of the external and internal carotid arteries at the level of the angle of the mandible, may result in reflexic slowing of the heart rate (see Chapter 10). To avoid inadvertent carotid sinus massage, the pulse should be palpated at or below the level of the thyroid cartilage. There is a risk of precipitating a cerebral vascular event by vigorous palpation of the carotid artery in adults with atherosclerotic disease. This risk may be minimized by prior auscultation of

the carotid artery. If a bruit is present, avoid palpation of the carotid pulse in that patient.

Equipment

Assessment of the pulse should be performed by the clinician at the bedside with any timepiece that has a second hand. This allows simultaneous assessment of all the characteristics of the pulse. If continuous monitoring is deemed necessary, bedside cardiac monitors will constantly monitor pulse rate and rhythm. Pulse oximetry (see Chapter 5), although primarily intended to measure oxygen saturation, may also be used to monitor pulse rate. In a critical care situation more sophisticated invasive monitoring techniques are available (see Chapter 19).

Procedure

Pulses are palpable at numerous sites, although for convenience the radial pulse at the wrist is routinely used. The examiner should use the tips of the first and second fingers to palpate the pulse. There are two advantages to this technique: first, the finger tips are quite sensitive, enabling the pulse to be easily located and counted; second, if one chooses to use the thumb to count the pulse, there is a chance that the palpated pulse will be the examiner's own. Pulses are also easily palpated at the carotid, brachial, femoral, posterior tibial, and dorsalis pedis arteries. Palpation of the pulse at the brachial artery may facilitate the appreciation of pulse contour and amplitude. It is located at the medial aspect of the elbow and is more easily palpated when the elbow is held slightly flexed.[16]

In infants, direct auscultation is the method of choice to determine heart rate. In unstable children, palpation of central arteries is recommended over palpation of peripheral arteries.

Pulse rate is ideally determined by counting the pulse for 1 minute, particularly if there is any abnormality. Note that if the examiner counts the pulse for 15 seconds, the pulse is overestimated by 4 beats per minute unless the count starts with zero.

Pulse rate can also be determined from an electrocardiogram (ECG) strip. Many ECG machines or monitors mark 3-second intervals at the paper edge. The examiner can count the number of beats within a 6-second strip and multiply by 10 for an estimate of beats per minute. Alternately, assuming the paper speed at 25 mm per second, the examiner can count either 1-mm or 5-mm boxes between 2 beats (Fig. 36–3). Dividing the number of boxes into 1500 or 300, respectively, yields beats per minute. If the paper is run at a nonstandard speed, the calculation has to be modified. Obviously, these are less accurate methods than counting the number of beats in a 1-minute strip, and because of the limited sample time these techniques cannot be used for irregular rhythms.[29]

By convention, when assessing the amplitude of peripheral pulses, they are graded from zero to three. Zero designates an absent pulse, one a diminished pulse, two a normal pulse, and three a bounding pulse. However, if an abnormality of the pulse contour is noted, this should also be described.[28]

Interpretation

RATE

Individual physiology must be considered in pulse interpretation. In infants and children, pulse rate must be inter-

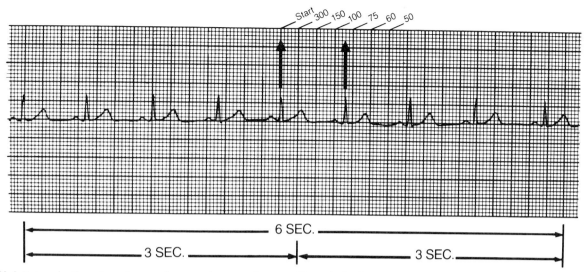

Figure 36–3. Determination of a pulse rate from an electrocardiogram. (From Arrhythmias. In Textbook of Advanced Cardiac Life Support. 2nd ed. American Heart Association, Dallas, 1987. Copyright American Heart Association. Reproduced with permission.)

preted with reference to age. Pulse varies with respirations, increasing with inspiration and slowing with expiration. This is known as a sinus dysrhythmia and is physiologic. Although a bradycardia is defined as a heart rate of less than 60 beats per minute, a well-conditioned athlete may have a normal resting heart rate of 30 to 40 beats per minute.[30] Any abnormal pulse rate or rhythm that is new in onset may indicate a potentially unstable condition and is an indication for obtaining a rhythm strip, 12-lead ECG or for constant monitoring. In particular, resting tachycardia must always be explained.

Consider whether an abnormal pulse rate is a primary or secondary condition. The examination of the entire set of vital signs is instrumental in discerning the cause for the abnormal rate. For example, hyperthermia causes a sinus tachycardia. An increase in heart rate of 10 beats per minute can be expected for every degree Fahrenheit and 18 beats per minute for every degree centigrade of elevated temperature.[11] Drug fever, typhoid fever, and central neurogenic fever are suggested when there is no corresponding tachycardia in a patient with elevated body temperature. Hypothermia, with its reduced metabolic demands, may be associated with a bradycardia. Extreme hypothermia may result in asystole that often prevents successful resuscitation until the patient is warmed.

Clinical evaluation of the patient with an abnormal pulse rate dictates a consideration of medications the patient may be taking or the presence of a mechanical pacemaker. Beta-blockers, digitalis compounds, and antidysrhythmics may alter the "normal" heart rate and the ability of this vital sign to respond to a new physiologic stress. These cardioactive medications may be the cause of the patient's problem.

RHYTHM

In addition to determining the pulse rate, information about the regularity of the pulse is obtained during palpation. If the pulse is found to be variable, the next step is determining whether there is any pattern to the pulse. Occasional ectopic beats, reflecting premature atrial or premature ventricular contractions, may be noted. A pulse may be regularly irregular, that is, a recurring pattern is detected, or it may be irregularly irregular, that is, without discernible pattern. An irregularly irregular pulse suggests atrial fibrillation, and accurate assessment of the pulse should be obtained by auscultation of apical cardiac sounds. The apical pulse is frequently greater than the peripheral pulse, reflecting inadequate filling time and stroke volume, with resultant nontransmitted beats. A greater pulse deficit generally reflects more severe disease.

AMPLITUDE AND CONTOUR

Amplitude of the pulse and contour of the pulse (see Fig. 36–2) are generally assessed simultaneously and provide additional clinical information. Superimposition of one pathophysiologic state on another may modify the pulse. For example, sepsis may manifest with variable pulse amplitude, depending on the stage in the development of the disease at which the patient presents. Early in sepsis there is increased cardiac output and decreased vascular resistance, causing bounding pulses. In advanced sepsis, or septic shock, there is falling cardiac output and increased vascular resistance, and pulses are diminished.[31]

Diminished or weak pulses (pulsus parvus) reflect any condition that decreases cardiac output or results in vascular spasm. For example, a rapid heart rate, with corresponding decreased stroke volume, causes a weak pulse. Conditions that cause increased sympathetic tone, such as hypovolemic shock, also factor into poorly palpable peripheral pulses. Severe aortic stenosis mechanically obstructs blood flow. It is often described as a plateau pulse, slowly rising and leveling off before falling. This delayed peak is also known as pulsus tardus.[12, 16, 17]

Bounding pulses suggest a hypermetabolic state such as fever or hyperthyroidism, abnormal hemodynamics, or the decreased arterial compliance of peripheral atherosclerotic disease. Aortic regurgitation and patent ductus arteriosus both result in bounding peripheral pulses through abnormal hemodynamics. In both conditions, there is rapid run-off of blood from the arterial system and a compensatory increase in stroke volume. In patent ductus arteriosus this results from failure of the ductus arteriosus to close. Blood is then diverted from the proximal aorta into the pulmonary artery. In aortic regurgitation, the diseased aortic valve does not close, and blood flows back into the left ventricle. The term *water-hammer pulse*, or Corrigan pulse, is reserved for description of the bounding pulses of aortic regurgitation.[12, 16, 17]

Pulsus alternans, in which a strong beat alternates with a weak beat, is associated with left heart failure. The physiology of this phenomenon is poorly understood.[12]

Pulsus bigeminus also has a strong beat alternating with a weak beat and therefore can masquerade as pulsus alternans, but it is actually a reflection of a dysrhythmia and should have a regularly irregular pattern. A bigeminal pulse occurs when a regular beat alternates with a premature beat. Decreased filling time on the premature beat results in decreased cardiac output and decreased amplitude.[12, 16, 17]

Pulsus bisferiens is a bifid pulse with two distinct peaks, most readily appreciated at the carotid artery. It is associated with aortic valvular disease and with hypertrophic obstructive cardiomyopathy.[12, 16, 17]

PULSES DURING CARDIOPULMONARY RESUSCITATION

A major factor contributing to forward flow during cardiac massage is the creation of an arteriovenous pressure gradient by competent venous valves at the thoracic outlet. Using cinefluoroscopy, Niemann and colleagues demonstrated that the absence of subdiaphragmatic valves allowed reflux of blood from the right atrium to the inferior vena cava during cardiopulmonary resuscitation (CPR). This suggests that palpated "femoral pulses" during chest compression may represent either forward arterial blood flow or "to-and-fro" movement of blood from the right heart to the venous system. Carotid pulses are the recommended sites to assess the adequacy of chest compressions by palpation during CPR.[32] Other investigators have demonstrated that Doppler ultrasonic flow occurs in peripheral arteries during closed-chest cardiac massage, suggesting femoral arterial flow,[33, 34] although a venous pulse wave may be stronger than the arterial pulse wave in the femoral area during CPR.

ARTERIAL BLOOD PRESSURE

Arterial blood pressure should be measured in all emergency department patients with a pulse. Changes in arterial blood pressure over time are an indication of the success of treatment or the worsening of the patient's overall condition. An abrupt change in the patient's arterial blood pressure is usually an indication of the need for immediate intervention or reconsideration of therapy.

Physiology

The arterial blood pressure indicates the overall state of hemodynamic interaction between cardiac output and peripheral vascular resistance. The arterial blood pressure is the lateral pressure or force exerted by the blood on the vessel wall. The arterial blood pressure indirectly measures perfusion, where blood flow = Δpressure/resistance.[4] However, because peripheral vascular resistance varies, a normal blood pressure does not confirm adequate perfusion.[35] The systolic pressure is determined by the peripheral arteriolar resistance, the volume and velocity of peak left ventricular ejection, the arteriolar distensibility, the end-diastolic volume in the arterial system, and the viscosity of blood. Diastolic pressure is influenced by blood viscosity, arterial distensibility, peripheral resistance to flow, and length of the cardiac cycle. Mean arterial blood pressure can be estimated by adding one third of the pulse pressure to the diastolic pressure.[4, 36]

Indications and Contraindications

Blood pressure measurement and documentation are essential for all adult and most pediatric emergency depart-ment patients seen for the first time. Infants and children with ambulatory complaints not related to the cardiovascular system commonly do not receive blood pressure measurements in the emergency department. Frequent monitoring of the blood pressure is necessary for patients with hemodynamic instability.

Relative contraindications to specific extremity blood pressure measurement include arteriovenous fistula, axillary lymphadenopathy, lymphedema, and circumferential burns over the intended site of cuff application. Placement of a catheter for direct intra-arterial measurement of blood pressure has a higher risk of complications but may be performed safely in the emergency department (see Chapter 19).

Equipment

The equipment required for indirect blood pressure measurement includes a sphygmomanometer (cuff with inflatable bladder, inflating bulb, controlled exhaust for deflation, and manometer) and a stethoscope or Doppler device (for auscultation) or an oscillometric device.[37, 38] To ensure an accurate reading, the sphygmomanometer cuff should be of an appropriate size for the patient. The width of the bladder should be 40 per cent of the distance of the midpoint of the limb (i.e., from the acromion process to the lateral epicondyle). The length of the bladder should be 80 per cent of the midarm circumference or twice the recommended width.[36]

Manometers in common use are either an aneroid or a mercury gravity column. Both types of manometers are convenient for bedside use, although the mercury gravity column must be vertical for accurate measurements. An aneroid manometer uses a metal bellows that elongates with the application of pressure. This elongation is mechanically amplified, transmitting the motion to the indicator needle.

Manometers require annual servicing. Mercury columns may require the addition of mercury to bring the edge of the meniscus to the zero mark. The air vent or filter at the top of the mercury column also should be checked for clogging. The aneroid manometer should be calibrated against a mercury column at least yearly. If the aneroid indicator is not at zero at rest, the device should not be used.[39]

Automatic sphygmomanometers may improve physiologic monitoring with alarm and self-cycling capabilities. They offer indirect arterial blood pressure mesurement with little pain and lack the risks associated with invasive arterial lines.[40] Various manufacturers use oscillometric (Dinamap 845, Applied Medical Research), Korotkoff sound (Pressurometer [Avionics]; Diasyst-T [Siemens Company]), and ultrasonic (Arteriosonde, Hoffmann-LaRoche Company) techniques. Oscillometric blood pressure monitors detect motion of the blood pressure cuff transmitted from the underlying artery. A sudden increase in the amplitude of arterial oscillations occurs at systolic pressure and mean arterial pressure, and an abrupt decrease occurs at diastolic pressure.

Dinamap blood pressures obtained in 29 hemodynamically stable children (mean age 18 months) demonstrated a smaller mean error (systolic −0.24 ± 3.26 mm Hg) than auscultatory measurements in 20 children (systolic −1.65 ± 6.68 mm Hg) using direct radial arterial pressures for comparison.[41] Similarly in adult patients, good correlation was found with mean diastolic and systolic arterial pressures.[42] Ultrasonic arterial wall motion detection uses a combination transmitter-receiver based on the Doppler principle, using a high-frequency (10 MHz) output device.[35, 40] Although these devices are commonly used, their accuracy under various clinical conditions has not been studied in the emergency department. Automatic devices do not provide a continual monitoring of blood pressure, and the static digital readouts may fail to pick up sudden hypotension.

Arterial blood pressure can also be assessed by Doppler technology and by direct arterial cannulation. The principles of Doppler detection of arterial pressure and arterial pressure monitoring are discussed elsewhere (see Chapters 32 and 19, respectively).

Procedure

Indirect blood pressure measurements may be obtained at the patient's bedside by palpation, auscultation, Doppler, or oscillometric methods. The technique is straightforward and accurate when well-maintained, calibrated equipment is utilized by practitioners who follow accepted standards. The patient may be lying or sitting, as long as the site of measurement is at the level of the right atrium and the arm is supported.[36, 37]

Palpation of arterial blood pressure requires cuff inflation to 30 mm Hg above the level at which a palpable pulse disappears. While palpating directly over the artery, deflate the cuff at 2 to 3 mm Hg per second. The initial appearance of arterial pulsations is reported as the palpable blood pressure. The same technique may be used for Doppler blood pressure, with the Doppler auditory signal replacing the palpated pulse. Arterial pressure measurement by palpation and Doppler yields only *systolic* blood pressure estimates. When auscultating the blood pressure at the brachial artery, the blood pressure cuff is applied about 2.5 cm above the antecubital fossa with the center of the bladder over the artery.[37] The bell of the stethoscope is applied directly over the brachial artery but with as little pressure as possible.[43] The systolic arterial blood pressure is defined as the first appearance of faint, clear, tapping sounds that gradually increase in intensity (Korotkoff phase I), whereas the diastolic blood pressure is defined as the point at which sounds disappear (Korotkoff phase V).[36, 37, 43] In children, phase IV defines the diastolic blood pressure (Fig. 36–4).[8] Measurement by auscultation over the brachial artery is preferred because of accepted standardization of measured values. Alternate sites include the radial, popliteal, posterior tibial, or dorsalis pedis arteries, although any fully compressible, noncerebral artery may be used.[36–38, 43, 44]

Direct intra-arterial measurement of blood pressure is used in some circumstances when ongoing, instantaneous results are required. Studies comparing intra-arterial blood pressures in humans at different sites have shown that the femoral systolic blood pressure is a few millimeters of mercury higher and diastolic blood pressure is a few millimeters of mercury lower than simultaneous brachial artery pressures. Studies correlating direct and indirect blood pressure measurements have demonstrated a good correlation between these methods.[45–47]

The accuracy of palpatory, Doppler, and oscillometric methods has also been demonstrated.[46, 48–51] However, when phase I and V Korotkoff sounds are used, indirect methods typically underestimate systolic and diastolic pressure by several millimeters of mercury.[45, 52] In addition, during shock, palpatory and auscultatory methods underestimate simultaneous direct arterial pressure measurements.[53] The flush method, in which return of color after deflation of the cuff is used for estimating blood pressure in infants, may underestimate systolic blood pressure by up to 40 mm Hg.[52] This method is unreliable and is not recommended.

In reference to trauma, the American College of Surgeons previously suggested that the ability to palpate the pulse at various sites provided an indirect assessment of

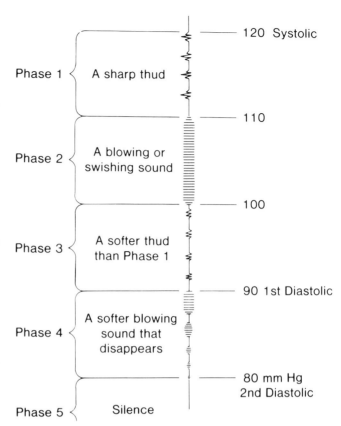

Figure 36–4. Korotkoff sounds. Systole—first audible sound. Diastole—sound disappears. (From Burnside JW, McGlynn TJ: Physical Diagnosis. 17th ed. © 1986, The Williams & Wilkins Co, Baltimore.)

blood pressure in a hypotensive patient. A palpable radial pulse suggested that a systolic pressure of at least 80 mm Hg was present; a palpable femoral pulse suggested that a systolic pressure of at least 70 mm Hg was present; and a palpable carotid pulse suggested that a systolic pressure of at least 60 mm Hg was present.[54] Data supporting the accuracy of this method are lacking, and it is no longer included in the revised edition of the Advanced Trauma Life Support Program.[55]

Complications

Complications of indirect blood pressure measurement are minimal when the proper procedure is followed. Inadvertent prolonged application of an inflated blood pressure cuff may result in false elevation of diastolic pressure and in ischemia distal to the site of application, with its attendant complications.[4, 38]

Invasive blood pressure monitoring is associated with a number of potential problems (see Chapter 19). Complications include damage to nerves or arteries, infection, hemorrhage, thrombosis, and catheter embolus. Recognition of vascular complications occurs by careful inspection of perfusion, sensation, and motor function distal to the catheter site. Immediate removal of the catheter is required for those with recognized ischemia.[56]

Interpretation

Normal blood pressure increases with decreasing distance from the aorta, with age, in males, and in technically developed countries. Individual factors that influence blood pressure include body posture, emotional or painful stimuli, environmental influences, vasoactive foods or medications, and the state of muscular and cerebral activity. Exercise and sustained isometric muscular contraction increase blood pressure in proportion to the strength of the contraction.[4] A normal diurnal pattern of blood pressure consists of an increase throughout the day, with a significant, rapid decline during early, deep sleep.[57] Normal respiration decreases the systolic blood pressure by ≤10 mm Hg during inspiration.

Normal *lower limits* for systolic blood pressure for infants and children can be estimated by adding two times the age (in years) to 70, with the result expressed in mm Hg. The *fiftieth percentile for children's systolic* arterial blood pressure from 1 to 10 years of age can be estimated by adding two times age (in years) to 90. Children older than 2 years of age are considered hypotensive when systolic blood pressure is less than 80 mm Hg.[58] Children, in particular, are able to maintain mean arterial blood pressure until very late during shock.[59] Thus the finding of a normal blood pressure in a child with signs of poor perfusion should not dissuade the emergency physician from appropriate treatment. Adults are considered hypotensive if the systolic blood pressure is less than 90 mm Hg. When accompanied by signs of shock, immediate treatment is indicated.

Adults are hypertensive if either the systolic or diastolic pressure exceeds 140 or 90, respectively.[60] The decision to treat hypertensive emergency department patients must be based on consideration of the overall condition of the patient. Hypertensive emergencies include hypertension in association with myocardial infarction, encephalopathy, aortic dissection, pulmonary edema, cerebral hemorrhage, sympathomimetic drug ingestion, or pheochromocytoma. Hypertensive urgencies occur in hypertensive patients with diastolic pressures greater than 130 mm Hg, or associated with rapidly deteriorating renal function or nasal hemorrhage.[61] Systolic hypertension has recently been demonstrated to be a better predictor of subsequent mortality than diastolic or mean arterial pressure.[62] Borderline hypertension may be unmasked by a static standing assessment of diastolic pressure.[63]

The applicability of population norms for hypertension in a stressful emergency situation is controversial. Patients with hypertension require repeat measurement to assess whether emergency department therapy is required. Because sustained hypertension may be seen in more than one third of initially hypertensive emergency department patients, careful evaluation and follow-up are required.[64]

Erroneous blood pressure measurements may result from several factors. Falsely low blood pressure may be caused by using an overly wide cuff or by rapid cuff deflation.[65] In 470 unselected adults, investigators at Duke University found no spurious effect of cuff size in 350 patients weighing less than 95 kg and with an arm circumference less than 35 cm. However, in 120 patients weighing more than 95 kg and with an arm circumference more than 35 cm, the use of a large cuff reclassified 33 per cent of those with systolic hypertension to borderline, 62 per cent of those with borderline systolic hypertension to normal, and 79 per cent of patients with borderline diastolic hypertension to normal.[66] Forty-one per cent of adults observed at the University of Pittsburgh required nonstandard size cuffs. Undercuffing was associated with a mean error of 8.5 and 4.6 mm Hg in the systolic and diastolic pressures, respectively.[67] Hypotensive patients have unreliable Korotkoff sounds. However, Doppler measurements are well correlated with direct arterial systolic pressure in hypotensive patients.[68]

Falsely high blood pressure may be caused by the use of an overly narrow cuff, anxiety, pain, tobacco, exertion, an unsupported arm, or slow inflation of the cuff. One study of 48 hospitalized patients found that during a physician visit 94 per cent experienced a mean peak increase in systolic pressure (27 ± 2 mm Hg), diastolic pressure (15 ± 2 mm Hg), and heart rate (16 ± 2 beats per minute). The response peaked at approximately 4 minutes and abated at about 10 minutes after initiation.[69] By using noninvasive, ambulatory blood pressure recordings, investigators at New York Hospital found that 21 per cent of 292 patients had "white coat" hypertension. These patients were more likely to be recently diagnosed, female, and younger and to have had their blood pressure measured by a physician.[70]

An auscultatory gap can be appreciated in hypertensive patients and may mislead the examiner. It is heard during the latter part of phase I and should not be confused with diastolic readings. Auscultation until the manometer reading approaches zero should prevent misinterpretation. In patients with aortic insufficiency or hyperthyroidism, after exercise, and in children younger than 5 years of age, the measurement of diastolic blood pressure should occur at Korotkoff phase IV, the period marked by a distinct, abrupt muffling of sound so that a soft, blowing quality is heard.

Irregular heart rates may also interfere with accurate blood pressure determination. A second or third reading, with 2 minutes of deflation between recordings, should be used to obtain an average when premature contractions or atrial fibrillation is present. Ultrasonic methods may be more accurate during shock states and in infants for systolic blood pressure measurement.[68]

Increased pulse pressure (e.g., ≥ 60) is commonly observed in anemia, exercise, hyperthyroidism, arteriovenous fistula, aortic regurgitation, and patent ductus arteriosus. A narrowed pulse pressure (≤ 20) may be a manifestation of hypovolemia, increased peripheral vascular resistance, or decreased stroke volume.

A difference in bilateral brachial artery pressures up to 10 mm Hg may be normal but uncommon. Hashimoto and colleagues found that only 1.4 per cent of elderly patients had a systolic brachial blood pressure difference of more than 10 mm Hg, although 6.5 per cent had a difference exceeding 7.5 mm Hg.[71] Most patients with subclavian steal syndrome, supravalvular aortic stenosis, and aortic dissection have a ≥15 mm Hg difference in contralateral brachial artery systolic pressures.

Pulsus paradoxus occurs when there is a greater than 20 mm Hg decrease in the systolic blood pressure during inspiration. To detect this difference, the blood pressure cuff is deflated until the phase I Korotkoff sound is heard during expiration (see Fig. 36–2). The difference in systolic pressure between this first sound on expiration and the pressure at which sounds are first heard during all phases of respiration is the measurement of pulsus paradoxus. Pulsus paradoxus may occur in patients with chronic obstructive pulmonary disease, pneumothorax, severe asthma, and pericardial tamponade.[72]

TEMPERATURE

Accurate measurement of body temperature is an essential part of clinical medicine. When taken in the context of other vital signs, body temperature is an excellent guide to the severity of illness. In 1797, James Currie, a Fellow of the Royal College of Physicians of Edinburgh in Liverpool, wrote: "If a definition of life were required, it might be most clearly established on that capacity by which the animal preserves its proper heat under the various degrees of temperature in which it lives."[73]

Detection of abnormal body temperature facilitates proper diagnosis and evaluation of presenting complaints.[74–76] The inability of any patient to maintain normal body temperature is indicative of a vast number of potentially serious disorders, including infections, neoplasms, shock, toxic reactions, and environmental exposures. A common example is profound hypoglycemia, a condition that is almost always accompanied by hypothermia. Normalization of body temperature following intervention may have important prognostic and therapeutic implications.[77] Body temperature is useful for assessing patients at the extremes of age as an independent predictor of serious illness.[74, 77] For example, hypothermia may be an initial finding of sepsis in the elderly or the neonate. Fever in neutropenic, immunocompromised, and intravenous drug–abusing patients may be more reliable than laboratory tests or physician assessment in diagnosing serious illness.[77] All emergency department patients with elevated body temperatures should be approached with care, although many may have benign causes for their fever. Patients with hypothermia should be considered seriously ill. Infants are particularly sensitive to thermal stress and may demonstrate lower body temperatures during asphyxia or necrotizing enterocolitis.[78–82]

Physiology

Under normal conditions, the temperature of deep body tissues (i.e., core temperature) remains within ± 0.6° C or ± 1.08° F.[83, 84] Core body temperature can be maintained within a narrow range while environmental temperature varies from 13° C to 60° C (55° F to 140° F).[85] Surface temperature rises and falls with environmental and other influences. Maintenance of normal body temperature requires a balance of heat production and heat loss. Heat loss occurs by radiation, conduction, and evaporation. Approximately 60 per cent, 18 per cent, and 22 per cent of heat loss, respectively, occur by these methods. Heat loss is increased by wind, water, and lack of insulation (e.g., clothing). Sweating, vasodilation, and decreased heat production serve to decrease temperature, whereas piloerection, vasoconstriction, and increased heat production serve to increase body temperature. Heat production is increased by shivering, fat catabolism, and increased thyroid hormone production.[12]

Temperature control occurs by feedback mechanisms operating through the preoptic area of the hypothalamus. Heat-sensitive neurons in this area increase their rate of firing during artificial heating. Receptors in the skin, spinal cord, abdominal viscera, and central veins primarily detect cold and provide feedback to the hypothalamus signaling an increase in heat production. The hypothalamus maintains body temperature at 37.1° C (98.78° F). Stimuli that begin to change the core temperature result in drastic changes in heat loss or production.[12, 86]

Indications and Contraindications

Oral temperature measurement with a digital electronic probe is most commonly used for ambulatory patients.[86] Advantages include convenience, timing, safety, and availability. Disadvantages include accuracy and sensitivity. Electronic temperature probes must be covered with disposable covers, although these have been shown not to be completely effective in preventing probe contamination with microorganisms.[88] Although there are no absolute contraindications for oral temperature assessment, patients with factors shown to produce unreliable results require temperature measurement at other sites.[89–91]

Rectal temperature has been considered the gold standard for ambulatory patients and is routine for children.[87, 92, 93] Advantages include accuracy, sensitivity, and availability. Disadvantages include timing, safety, and convenience. Rectal temperature measurement is contraindicated in patients with neutropenia, recent rectal surgery, and neonates, and possibly during acute myocardial infarction.[94, 95] Complications associated with rectal temperature measurement include rectal perforation, pneumoperitoneum, bacteremia, dysrhythmias, and syncope.[94, 96] Falsely low rectal temperature measurements may be seen during shock.[97]

Body temperature measured as a function of infrared radiation detected from the *tympanic membrane* is easy to use, convenient, and quick. It is accurate over a large temperature range and is unaffected by factors that influence oral measurement.[84, 94, 98, 99]

Axillary and tactile temperature assessment have been demonstrated to be unreliable and insensitive and should not be used in the emergency department, unless other methods are contraindicated.[100–103]

Equipment

Electronic methods of temperature measurement are based on the thermocouple principle, first used experimentally for temperature measurement in 1835. A thermocouple consists of two wires of different metals (e.g., copper and constantan), one wire kept at a certain known low temperature while the other monitors temperature of tissues or sites. The thermoelectric current that is set up between the two electrodes is measured by a potentiometer.[5] Electronic digital thermometers, with continuous or intermittent readout, came into general clinical use in the early 1970s. Modern electronic thermometers signal once equilibration to a steady state (or extrapolation of the temperature-time curve) occurs.[104] Current standards call for an accuracy of ± 0.1° C (0.18° F) over the range of 37 to 39° C (98.6 to 102.2° F).[105]

Thermistor (i.e., small thermocouples with instantaneous readouts) probes for esophageal and vascular temperature measurement were used experimentally in the 1930s. They provide continuous temperature readouts when attached to a potentiometer.[5]

Strips containing plastic-encased thermophototropic detection cells were introduced in the late 1970s. The strips change color in proportion to skin temperature.[106] Temperature screening using liquid crystal strips has been demonstrated to be unreliable. Reisinger and colleagues found that only 45 per cent of 30 febrile children who visited the emergency department were accurately identified by Clinitemp strips.[107] Lewit and coworkers found that fever was detected in only 24 of 56 febrile ambulatory or hospitalized children. The overall sensitivity and specificity were 34 per cent and 99 per cent, respectively, for 624 children.[108] Other investigators have found similar results.[109–111]

Infrared radiation detection devices for temperature measurement from the tympanic membrane were introduced in 1985. Body temperature is measured as a function of infrared radiation detected from the tympanic membrane. Core temperature assessment may be achieved with this method, because the tympanic membrane shares its blood supply with the preoptic hypothalamus, the area recognized as responsible for thermoregulation. The primary determinant of radiation emission is the temperature of blood flowing behind the tympanic membrane. An attached microprocessor (First Temp, Intelligent Medical Systems, Carlsbad, Calif.) computes radiation as a function of temperature and displays the temperature readout on the digital display.[94, 98] Tympanic temperature has been demonstrated to be generally accurate and sensitive, although there has been some concern that this method may fail to detect a fever in infants and children less than 3 years old and may not be as accurate at the extremes of hyper- and hypothermia. Reports in more than 500 adult patients of the correlation between rectal and tympanic membrane temperatures using the First Temp are quite good (r = 0.9).[112] Early emergency department clinical experience with this device is favorable; however, more extensive experience with the device is necessary before it can be recommended for use without substantiation by a secondary temperature system.

Procedure

Temperature measurement begins with site selection. Consideration should be given to accuracy, sensitivity to temperature changes, range of measurement, convenience, timing, safety, and availability in deciding on a site of temperature measurement.[94, 96] Sites used for body temperature measurement include the oral cavity (sublingual), tympanic membranes, skin, axillae, and rectum. Less commonly used sites are the esophagus, blood vessels (peripheral or central veins or arteries), groin, vagina, and bladder. Temperature measurement in a freshly voided urine specimen can validate temperature measurement at other body sites.[96] A nomogram of *expected* urinary temperatures has been derived from measurements of oral and urinary temperatures in 55 subjects (Fig. 36–5).[113]

Tactile temperature assessment is relatively specific, but insensitive.[100, 114] Banco and Veltri found a sensitivity of 74 per cent and a specificity of 86 per cent in 303 ambulatory children. Only 52 per cent of mothers who said their children were febrile were correct.[114]

Oral temperature measurement requires a cooperative adult or child older than 5 years of age. Patients who are grossly uncooperative, hemodynamically unstable, septic, or in respiratory distress require rectal, tympanic membrane, or invasive temperature determination. This group includes children less than 5 years old and children who are intubated.

Axillary temperature may be used for neonatal patients in incubators, but this requires longer equilibration times and is not indicated unless other sites are unavailable.[101, 115] Axillary temperatures obtained in 108 children by Kresch had a sensitivity of only 33 per cent and a specificity of 98 per cent for fever screening.[101] Ogren obtained similar results using an electronic thermometer in the axilla.[115a]

Temperature measurement continues with patient preparation, insertion of temperature probe, and probe equilibration (i.e., a reading is obtained). Proper placement of temperature probes significantly influences results for oral, rectal, esophageal, and vascular temperatures.[83, 116, 117] Sublingual oral temperatures should be obtained in either lateral recess with the mouth closed.[116] The patient should be sitting upright or lying, holding the base of the probe with one hand.[89] Rectal temperatures require removal of clothing, lubrication of the probe, gloving of personnel, and should be obtained with the patient relaxed in the left or right lateral decubitus position. Gentle insertion to 5 cm should ensure accurate, atraumatic results.[83]

Critical core temperatures can be determined instantaneously by measuring esophageal, rectal, bladder, or vascular temperatures. Use of these methods has been reserved for critically ill patients, because the discomfort and complications associated with their use are significant.[94] Vascular temperatures are used to determine cardiac output by thermodilution. These require insertion of a pulmonary artery multilumen catheter with thermistors at ports located in the right atrium and pulmonary artery. Esophageal probes for temperature monitoring require a 30-cm-long naso- or oroesophageal tube equipped with a thermocouple.

Interpretation

Normal values for body temperature vary with the site and methods used for measurement, pregnancy, perfusion, environmental exposure, exercise, and time of day. Although the core body temperature remains nearly constant (37.0 ± 0.6° C or 98.6 ± 0.18° F), the surface temperature rises and falls with changes in ambient temperature, exercise, and time of day.[12] Normal oral temperatures range from 36 to 37.5° C (96.8 to 99.5° F). Normal rectal temperatures range from 36.6 to 38.0° C (97.8 to 100.5° F). Oral temperatures are generally between 0.3° C (0.5° F) and 0.66° C (1.2° F) lower than simultaneously obtained rectal temperatures. Hypothermia is defined as a core body temperature less than 35° C (95° F), whereas hyperthermia is defined as a core body temperature greater than 41° C (105.8° F), with accompanying symptoms and signs.[12, 118]

The interpretation of temperature during clinical assessment must consider the use of antipyretics. The duration of antipyresis with acetaminophen or aspirin is 3.5 to 4 hours. When both drugs are given together, the duration of action may be extended to 6 hours.[119]

Oral temperature measurements may be falsely reduced by probe placement under the tongue, inadequate probe placement time, ingestion of cold liquids, tachypnea, and, possibly, humidified oxygen administration. Erickson, in a study of 100 adult patients, found a 2.7° C (4.9° F) reduction of oral temperature measurement when the probe was placed under the tip of the tongue instead of under the posterior sublingual pocket.[89] When using a mercury-glass thermometer, optimum placement time was found to be 7 and 4 minutes, for oral and rectal temperatures, respectively, in 50 hospitalized children.[92] A series of 237 adults demonstrated similar time requirements. In addition, an extra 60 seconds was required when the ambient temperature was between 18.3 and 21.1° C (65° F to 70° F).[120] Iced-water ingestion significantly reduced oral temperature by up to 4° C (7.2° F) for up to 7 minutes in ambulatory adults.[94] Smoking appears to result in little change in oral temperatures. Woodman and colleagues found a range of ± 0.2° C (± 0.36° F) change in oral temperatures immediately after five cigarette puffs in 66 ambulatory adults.[121] Tandberg and Sklar observed a significant reduction in oral temperature recordings in 192 tachypneic patients. They found that for every increment of 10 in the respiratory rate, the tempera-

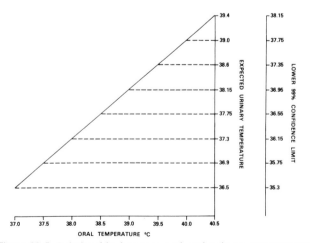

Figure 36–5. Relationship between oral and urinary temperatures constructed as a nomogram. (From Murray HW, Tuazon CU, Guerrero IC, et al: Urinary temperature: A clue to early diagnosis of factitious fever. N Engl J Med 296:23, 1977. Reproduced by permission of the New England Journal of Medicine.)

ture difference between oral and rectal measurements increased by nearly 0.5° C (0.9° F).[87] Several investigators have found little influence of oxygen inhalation on oral temperature assessment and that removal of the oxygen source resulted in hypoxemia in some patients.[109, 122]

Thermometer manipulation and hot-liquid ingestion may falsely elevate oral temperatures. The ingestion of hot liquids may elevate oral temperatures as much as 1.7° C (3.1° F) for as long as 7 minutes following ingestion.[94]

When rapid changes in body temperature are occurring, oral and tympanic temperature measurements appear to be more reliable than rectal temperature. In 20 adults examined during open-heart surgery, tympanic and oral temperatures showed a better correlation with blood temperature during rapid cooling and rewarming.[117] Infrequently, emergency department patients require constant monitoring of temperature (e.g., hypo- or hyperthermia). This can usually be performed using a rectal, bladder, or esophageal probe attached to a potentiometer. Patients with indwelling central venous or arterial catheters may have electronic thermistors inserted into the central circulation to measure "core" body temperature.

Temperature evaluation using skin thermistors may also be useful in assessing emergency department patients.[110, 111, 123] In one study, the difference between core and toe temperatures was found to correlate with the mortality in shock.[124] Although the gradient between core and peripheral temperature (measured with skin thermistors) is a good predictor of mortality in shock, its reliability in assessing peripheral perfusion is still controversial.[125, 126]

CONCLUSION

Vital signs must always be interpreted in relationship to each other to obtain the complete clinical picture. Abnormal vital signs should lead the clinician to a diagnosis or be explained within the context of the patient's illness.

REFERENCES

1. Fishman AP: Pulmonary Diseases and Disorders. 2nd ed. New York, McGraw-Hill Book Co, 1988.
2. Bedford DE: The ancient art of feeling the pulse. Br Heart J 13:423, 1951.
3. Major RH: The history of taking the blood pressure. Ann Med Hist 2(NS):47, 1930.
4. O'Rourke RA: Physical examination of the arteries and veins. In Hurst JW (ed): The Heart. 6th ed. New York, McGraw-Hill Book Co, 1986, pp 138–151.
5. Brock L: The development of clinical thermometry. Guys Hosp Rep 121:307, 1972.
6. Ziegler RF: Electrocardiographic studies in normal infants and children. Springfield, Ill, Charles C Thomas, 1951.
7. Haddad HM, Hsia DY, Gellis SS: Studies on respiratory rate in the newborn: Its use in the evaluation of respiratory distress in infants of diabetic mothers. Pediatrics 17:204, 1956.
8. Report of the Second Task Force on Blood Pressure Control in Children, 1987: Task Force on Blood Pressure Control in Children. Pediatrics 79:1, 1987.
9. Iliff A, Lee VA: Pulse rate, respiratory rate, and body temperature of children between two months and eighteen years of age. Child Dev 23:237, 1952.
10. Key TC, Resnik R: Maternal changes in pregnancy. In Danforth DN, Scott JR (eds): Obstetrics and Gynecology. 5th ed. Philadelphia, JB Lippincott Co, 1986.
11. Katz R, Karliner JS, Resnik R: Effects of a natural volume overload state (pregnancy) on left ventricular performance in normal human subjects. Circulation 58:434, 1978.
12. Guyton AC: Textbook of Medical Physiology. 6th ed. Philadelphia, WB Saunders Co, 1981.
13. Levitsky MG: Pulmonary Physiology. New York, McGraw-Hill Book Co, 1982.
14. Eberhart RC, Weigelt JA: Respiratory monitoring: Current techniques and some new developments. Bull Eur Physiopathol Respir 21:295, 1985.

15. Consensus Statement: National Institutes of Health Consensus Development Conference on Infantile Apnea and Home Monitoring, Sept. 29–Oct. 1, 1986. Pediatrics 79:292, 1987.
16. Burnside JW, McGlynn TJ: Physical Diagnosis. 17th ed. Baltimore, Williams & Wilkins, 1986.
17. Bates B: A Guide to Physical Examination and History Taking. 4th ed. Philadelphia, JB Lippincott Co, 1987.
18. Hooker EA, O'Brien DJ, Danzl DF, et al: Respiratory rates in emergency department patients. J Emerg Med 7:129, 1989.
19. Hutchinson J: Thorax. In Todd RB (ed): Cyclopaedia of Anatomy and Physiology. London, Longman, Brown, Green, Congmans, & Roberts, 1849:IV, pp 1079–1087.
20. Mead J: Control of respiratory frequency. J Appl Physiol 15:325, 1960.
21. Bendixen HH, Smith GM, Mead J: Pattern of ventilation in young adults. J Appl Physiol 19:195, 1964.
22. Gilbert R, Auchincloss JH, Brodsky J, et al: Changes in tidal volume, frequency, and ventilation induced by their measurement. J Appl Physiol 33:252, 1972.
23. McFadden JP, Price RC, Eastwood HD, et al: Raised respiratory rate in elderly patients: A valuable physical sign. Br Med J 284:626, 1982.
24. Gravelyn TR, Weg JG: Respiratory rate as an indicator of acute respiratory dysfunction. JAMA 244:1123, 1980.
25. Bell WR, Simon TL, DeMets DL: The clinical features of submassive and massive pulmonary emboli. Am J Med 62:355, 1977.
26. Plum F: The Diagnosis of Stupor and Coma. 3rd ed. Philadelphia, FA Davis Co, 1982.
27. Rigatto H: Apnea. Pediatr Clin North Am 29:1105, 1982.
28. Marx HJ, Yu PN: Clinical examination of the arterial pulse. Prog Cardiovasc Dis 10:207, 1967.
29. American Heart Association: Textbook of Advanced Cardiac Life Support. 2nd ed. American Heart Association, Dallas, 1987, pp 53–54.
30. Oakley GDG: The athletic heart. Cardiol Clin 5:319, 1987.
31. Harris RL, Musher DM, Bloom K, et al: Manifestations of sepsis. Arch Intern Med 147:1895, 1987.
32. Niemann JT, Rosborough JP, Ung S, et al: Hemodynamic effects of continuous abdominal binding during cardiac arrest and resuscitation. Am J Cardiol 53:269, 1984.
33. Grunau CFV: Doppler ultrasound monitoring of systemic blood flow during CPR. JACEP 7:180, 1978.
34. Lichti EL, Willets P, Turner M, et al: Cardiac massage efficacy monitored by doppler ultrasonic flowmeter: A preliminary report. Mo Med 68:317, 1971.
35. Tabata BK, Kirsch JR, Rogers MC: Diagnostic tests and technology for pediatric intensive care. In Roger MC (ed): Textbook of Pediatric Intensive Care. Baltimore, Williams & Wilkins, 1987, pp 1401–1432.
36. Kirkendall WM, Feinleib M, Freis ED, Mark AL: AHA Committee Report: Recommendations for human blood pressure determination by sphygmomanometers. Circulation 62:1146A, 1980.
37. Petrie JC, O'Brien ET, Littler WA, DeSwiet M: Recommendations on blood pressure measurement. Br Med J 293:611, 1986.
38. Nelson WP, Egbert AM: How to measure blood pressure accurately. Prim Cardiol 10:14, 1984.
39. Perlman LV, Chiang BN, Keller J, Blackburn H: Accuracy of sphygmomanometers in hospital practice. Arch Intern Med 125:1000, 1970.
40. Katona Z, Bolvary G: Automatic sphygmomanometer. Adv Cardiovasc Phys 5:119, 1983.
41. Yelderman M, Ream AK: Indirect measurements of blood pressure in the anesthetized patients. Anesthesiology 50:253, 1979.
42. David RF: Clinical comparison of automated auscultatory and oscillometric and catheter-transducer measurements of arterial pressure. J Clin Monitor 1:114, 1985.
43. Prineas RJ, Jacobs D: Quality of Korotkoff sounds: Bell vs diaphragm, cubital fossa vs brachial artery. Prev Med 12:715, 1983.
44. Webb CH: The measurement of blood pressure and its interpretation. Prim Care 7:637, 1980.
45. Park MK, Guntheroth WG: Direct blood pressure measurements in brachial and femoral arteries in children. Circulation 61:231, 1970.
46. Hartmann AF, Klint R, Hernandez A, Goldring D: Measurement of the blood pressure in the brachial and posterior tibial arteries using the Doppler method. J Pediatr 82:498, 1973.
47. Pascarelli EF, Bertrand CA: Comparison of blood pressures in the arms and legs. N Engl J Med 270:693, 1964.
48. Enselberg CD: Measurement of diastolic blood pressure by palpation. N Engl J Med 265:272, 1961.
49. Reder RF, Dimich I, Cohen ML, Steinfeld L: Evaluating indirect blood pressure measurement techniques: A comparison of three systems in infants and children. Pediatrics 62:326, 1978.
50. Goldring D, Wohltmann H: Flush method for blood pressure determinations in newborn infants. J Pediatr 40:285, 1952.
51. Park MK, Menard SM: Normative oscillometric blood pressure values in the first 5 years in an office setting. Am J Dis Child 143:860, 1989.
52. Elseed AM, Shinebourne EA, Joseph MC: Assessment of techniques for measurement of blood pressure in infants and children. Arch Dis Child 48:932, 1973.
53. Cohn JN: Blood pressure measurement in shock. JAMA 199:118, 1967.
54. American College of Surgeons Committee on Trauma: Advanced

Trauma Life Support Course. Chicago, American College of Surgeons, 1984, p 7.

55. American College of Surgeons Committee on Trauma: Advanced Trauma Life Support Program. Chicago, American College of Surgeons, 1988.
56. Bedford RF, Wollman H: Complications of percutaneous radial-artery cannulation. Anesthesiology 38:228, 1973.
57. Millar-Craig MW, Bishop CN, Raftery EB: Circadian variation of blood-pressure. Lancet 1:795, 1978.
58. American Heart Association: Recognition of respiratory failure and shock: Anticipating cardiopulmonary arrest. In Textbook of Pediatric Advanced Life Support. American Heart Association, Dallas, 1988, pp 1–9.
59. Schwaitzberg SD, Bergman KS, Harris BH: A pediatric trauma model of continuous hemorrhage. J Pediatr Surg 23:605, 1988.
60. The 1988 Report of the Joint National Committee on Detection, Evaluation, and Treatment of High Blood Pressure. Arch Intern Med 148:1023, 1988.
61. Alpert MA, Bauer JH: Hypertensive emergencies: Recognition and pathogenesis. Cardiovasc Rev Rep 6:407, 1985.
62. Menotti A, Seccareccia F, Giampaoli S, Giuli B: The predictive role of systolic, diastolic and mean blood pressures on cardiovascular and all causes of death. J Hypertens 7:595, 1989.
63. Hull DH, Wolthuis RA, Cortese T, Longo MR: Borderline hypertension versus normotension: Differential response to orthostatic stress. Am Heart J 94:414, 1977.
64. Chernow SM, Iserson KV: Use of the emergency department for hypertension screening: A prospective study. Ann Emerg Med 16:180, 1987.
65. Maxwell MH, Waks AU, Schroth PC, Karam M: Error in blood pressure measurement due to incorrect cuff size in obese patients. Lancet 2:33, 1982.
66. Linfors KW, Feussner JR, Blessing CL, et al: Spurious hypertension in the obese patient: Effect of sphygmomanometer cuff size on prevalence of hypertension. Arch Intern Med 144:1482, 1989.
67. Manning DM, Kuchirka C, Kaminski J: Miscuffing: Inappropriate blood pressure cuff application. Circulation 68:763, 1983.
68. Poppers PJ, Epstein RM, Donham RT: Automatic ultrasound monitoring of blood pressure during induced hypotension. Anesthesiology 35:431, 1971.
69. Mancia G, Grassi G, Pomidossi G, et al: Effect of blood pressure measurement by the doctor on patient's blood pressure and heart rate. Lancet 2:695, 1983.
70. Pickering TG, James GD, Boddie C, et al: How common is white coat hypertension? JAMA 259:225, 1988.
71. Hashimoto F, Hunt WC, Hardy L: Differences between right and left arm blood pressures in the elderly. West J Med 141:189, 1984.
72. McGregor M: Pulsus paradoxus. N Engl J Med 301:480, 1979.
73. Ranston WI: Temperature regulation. Br Med J 2:69, 1966.
74. Marantz PR, Linzer M, Feiner CJ, Feinstein SA: Inability to predict diagnosis of febrile intravenous drug abusers. Ann Intern Med 106:823, 1987.
75. Mellors JW, Horwitz RI, Harvey MR, Horwitz SM: A simple index to identify occult bacterial infection in adults with acute unexplained fever. Arch Intern Med 147:666, 1987.
76. Keating HJ, Klimek JJ, Levine DS, Kiernan FJ: Effect of aging on the clinical significance of fever in ambulatory adult patients. J Am Geriatr Soc 32:282, 1984.
77. Baker RC, Tiller T, Bansher JC, et al: Severity of disease correlated with fever reduction in febrile infants. Pediatrics 83:1016, 1989.
78. Scopes JW, Ahmed I: Range of critical temperatures in sick and premature newborn babies. Arch Dis Child 41:417, 1966.
79. Adamsons K, Gandy GM, James LS: The influence of thermal factors upon oxygen consumption of the newborn human infant. J Pediatr 66:495, 1965.
80. Burnard ED, Cross KW: Rectal temperature in the newborn after birth asphyxia. Br Med J 2:1197, 1958.
81. Dahm LS, James LS: Newborn temperature and calculated heat loss in the delivery room. Pediatrics 49:504, 1972.
82. Schneider PA, Hamilton SR, Dudgeon DL: Intestinal ischemic injury following mild hypothermic stress in the neonatal piglet. Pediatr Res 21:422, 1987.
83. Cranston WI, Gerbrandy J, Snell ES: Oral, rectal and oesophageal temperatures and some factors affecting them in man. J Physiol 126:347, 1954.
84. Dubois EF: The many different temperatures of the human body and its parts. West J Surg 59:476, 1951.
85. Goltra ER (Aerospace Medical Research Lab at the Wright-Patterson Air Force Base): Thermal exchanges of the human body in extreme heat. Technical Documentary Report No. AMRL-TDR-63-86; 1963, pp 1–45.
86. Benzinger M: Tympanic thermometry in surgery and anesthesia. JAMA 209:1207, 1969.
87. Tandberg D, Sklar D: Effect of tachypnea on the estimation of body temperature by an oral thermometer. N Engl J Med 308:945, 1983.
88. Litsky BY: A study of temperature taking systems. Supervisor Nurse 7:48, 1976.

89. Erickson R: Oral temperature differences in relation to thermometer and technique. Nurs Res 29:157, 1980.
90. Durham ML, Swanson B, Paulford N: Effect of tachypnea on oral temperature estimation: A replication. Nurs Res 35:211, 1986.
91. Woodman EA, Parry SM, Simms L: Sources of unreliability in oral temperatures. Nurs Res 16:276, 1967.
92. Nichols GA, Kulvi RL, Life HR, Christ NM: Measuring oral and rectal temperatures of febrile children. Nurs Res 21:261, 1972.
93. Dressler DK, Smejkal C, Ruffolo ML: A comparison of oral and rectal temperature measurement on patients receiving oxygen by mask. Nurs Res 32:373, 1983.
94. Terndrup TE, Allegra JR, Kealy JA: A comparison of oral, rectal, and tympanic membrane-derived temperature changes after ingestion of liquids and smoking. Am J Emerg Med 7:15, 1989.
95. Gruber P: Changes in cardiac rate associated with the use of the rectal thermometer in patients with acute myocardial infarction. Heart Lung 3:288, 1974.
96. Blainey CG: Site selection in taking body temperature. Am J Nurs 74:1859, 1974.
97. Buck SH, Zaritsky AL: Occult core hyperthermia complicating cardiogenic shock. Pediatrics 83:782, 1989.
98. Shinozaki T, Deane R, Perkins FM: Infrared tympanic thermometer: Evaluation of a new clinical thermometer. Crit Care Med 16:148, 1988.
99. Nicholson RW, Iserson KV: Core temperature measurement in hypovolemic resuscitation. Ann Emerg Med 18:45, 1989.
100. Bergeson PS, Springfield HJ: How dependable is palpation as a screening method for fever? Clin Pediatr 13:350, 1974.
101. Kresch MJ: Axillary temperature as a screening test for fever in children. J Pediatr 104:596, 1984.
102. Nichols GA, Ruskin MM, Glor BAK, Kelly WH: Oral, axillary, and rectal temperature determinations and relationships. Nurs Res 15:307, 1966.
103. Masters JE: Comparison of axillary, oral, and forehead temperature. Arch Dis Child 55:896, 1980.
104. Anonymous: Intermittent-use electronic thermometers. Health Devices 3, 1982.
105. Abbey JC, Anderson AS, Close EL, et al: How long is that thermometer accurate? Am J Nurs 78:1375, 1978.
106. Lees DE, Schuetta W, Bull JM, et al: An evaluation of liquid crystal thermometry as a screening device for intraoperative hypothermia. Anesth Analg 57:669, 1978.
107. Reisinger KS, Kao J, Grant DM: Inaccuracy of the Clinitemp skin thermometer. Pediatrics 64:4, 1979.
108. Lewit EM, Marshall CL, Salzer JE: An evaluation of a plastic strip thermometer. JAMA 247:321, 1982.
109. Graas S: Thermometer sites and oxygen. Am J Nurs 74:1862, 1974.
110. Scholefield JH, Gerber MA, Dwyer P: Liquid crystal forehead temperature strips. Am J Dis Child 136:198, 1982.
111. David CB: Liquid crystal forehead temperature strips. Am J Dis Child 137:87, 1983.
112. Green MM, Danzl DF, Praszkier H: Infrared tympanic thermography in the emergency department. J Emerg Med 7:437, 1989.
113. Murray HW, Tuazon CU, Guerrero IC, et al: Urinary temperature: A clue to early diagnosis of factitious fever. N Engl J Med 296:23, 1977.
114. Banco L, Veltri D: Ability of mothers to subjectively assess the presence of fever in their children. Am J Dis Child 138:976, 1984.
115. Schiffman RF: Temperature monitoring in the neonate: A comparison of axillary and rectal temperatures. Nurs Res 31:274, 1982.
115a. Ogren JM: The inaccuracy of axillary temperatures measured with an electronic thermometer. Am J Dis Child 144:109, 1990.
116. Erickson R: Thermometer placement for oral temperature measurement in febrile adults. Int J Nurs Stud 15:199, 1976.
117. Molnar G, Read R: Studies during open-heart surgery on the special characteristics of rectal temperature. J Appl Physiol 36:333, 1974.
118. Miller JW, Danzl DF, Thomas DM: Urban accidental hypothermia: 135 cases. Ann Emerg Med 9:456, 1980.
119. Steele RW, Young FSH, Bass JW, et al: Oral antipyretic therapy: Evaluation of aspirin-acetaminophen combination. Am J Dis Child 123:204, 1972.
120. Nichols GA, Kucha DH: Oral measurements. Nurs Res 72:1091, 1972.
121. Woodman EA, Parry SM, Simms L: Sources of unreliability in oral temperatures. Nurs Res 16:276, 1967.
122. Lim-Levy F: The effect of oxygen inhalation on oral temperature. Nurs Res 31:150, 1982.
123. Vaughn SM, Cork RC, Vaughn RW: Inaccuracy of liquid crystal thermometry to identify core temperature trends in postoperative adults. Anesth Analg 61:284, 1982.
124. Henning RJ, Wiener F, Valdes S, et al: Measurement of toe temperature for assessing severity of acute circulatory failure. Surg Gynecol Obstet 149:1, 1979.
125. Joly HR, Weil MH: Temperature of great toe as an indication of the severity of shock. Circulation 39:131, 1969.
126. Woods I, Wilkins RB, Edwards JD, Martin PD, et al: Danger of using core/peripheral temperature gradient as a guide to therapy in shock. Crit Care Med 15:850, 1987.

Chapter 37

The Clinical Use of Orthostatic Vital Signs

Terry M. Williams and Robert Knopp

INTRODUCTION

Orthostatic vital signs are used in the assessment of patients with fluid loss, hemorrhage, syncope, or autonomic dysfunction. The emergency physician is primarily concerned with the accurate detection of acute blood loss or volume depletion. When the clinical syndrome of shock exists, assessment of blood volume deficit poses little difficulty. It is preferable, however, that volume loss be detected before physiologic compensation is overcome and clinical shock occurs. This discussion reviews the utility of orthostatic vital signs in the detection of acute volume depletion.

Many techniques have been advocated to assess volume status. Unfortunately, most of these procedures lack a database on which to judge their reliability. Methods that have been recommended include evaluation of the following parameters: skin color; skin turgor; skin temperature; supine, serial, and orthostatic vital signs; neck vein status; transcutaneous oximetry; and hemodynamic monitoring techniques, such as monitoring of central venous and pulmonary artery pressure. Serial vital signs have been used but do not reliably detect small degrees of blood loss.[1-5] *Up to 15 per cent of the total blood volume can be lost with minimal hemodynamic changes or alteration of the supine vital signs.*[1, 6-8] A decrease in the pulse pressure occurs with acute blood loss,[5, 6, 9] but often the patient's baseline blood pressure values are unknown. Clinical examination of neck veins adds useful information but is less precise than measurement of central venous pressure. Most clinicians use skin color, temperature, and moisture as a reflection of skin perfusion and sympathetic tone but not as an accurate guide to circulatory volume, because the vasomotor tone of the skin is affected by numerous diseases as well as by emotional and environmental factors. Measurement of the urinary output provides an excellent means of monitoring the patient but is not useful in the rapid bedside assessment of acute blood loss or volume depletion.

Central venous pressure and pulmonary artery pressure measurements add useful information in determining volume status but require invasive techniques and are not without complications.[10] The central venous pressure is dependent on four independent variables: intravascular volume, venomotor tone, right ventricular function, and intrathoracic pressure. The complex interaction of these variables can make interpretation of central venous pressure readings difficult. For example, a healthy patient may be able to accept a large intravascular volume overload with little change in the central venous pressure. A patient with isolated left heart failure, however, may have relative volume overload with no elevation in the central venous pressure. Pulmonary artery pressure provides more accurate assessment of left heart function but is usually not practical in the emergency department.[10]

Radionuclide blood volume determinations are accurate but not feasible in the acute setting of the emergency department. Transcutaneous oximetry is noninvasive, but further study is required to determine its merits and limitations during clinical assessment of volume depletion.[11]

The ideal test for determining volume status would rapidly and accurately detect volume depletion of 5 per cent or more using a noninvasive technique. At present, no such test exists. Orthostatic vital signs meet the criteria of being noninvasive and easily used at the bedside. However, in patients with acute blood loss of less than 20 per cent of their total blood volume, orthostatic vital signs lack both sensitivity and specificity.[12]

Orthostatic vital signs tend to be misused in clinical practice, largely because of confusion regarding what constitutes a positive or negative test. Bates[13] and others[14-16] have stated that postural hypotension or postural tachycardia occurs with varying degrees of hypovolemia, but they do not define specific criteria for a positive test. Other sources (without documentation) have perpetuated the notion that relatively small changes in the orthostatic blood pressure or the pulse are reliable in detecting hypovolemia.[17-19] Hayes and Briggs[17] state that a "decrease of 10 mm Hg or more on assuming the sitting position indicates significant hypovolemia." Jacobson[18] notes that "especially upon standing . . . a drop in systolic blood pressure of 10 mm Hg or an increased pulse of 10 beats per minute is consistent with hypovolemia." Watkins[19] states that with a 15-degree tilt, "a pulse increase of more than 10 beats per minute or a drop in blood pressure of more than 10 mm Hg indicates hypovolemia."

In this chapter we discuss the physiologic compensatory mechanisms that are activated by hypovolemia and postural tilting and the clinical use of orthostatic vital signs to accurately detect acute volume loss.

PHYSIOLOGIC RESPONSE TO HYPOVOLEMIA

Acute blood loss decreases the pressure gradient between the venules and the right atrium. A fall in this pressure gradient decreases venous return.[20] As a result, cardiac output falls, and clinical manifestations of shock ensue.[7] Several homeostatic mechanisms are initiated by blood loss (Table 37–1). The dominant compensatory mechanism in shock is a reduction in carotid sinus baroreceptor inhibition of sympathetic outflow to the cardiovascular system.[21] This increased sympathetic outflow results in several effects: (1) an arteriolar vasoconstriction, which greatly increases total peripheral vascular resistance; (2) a constriction of venous capacitance vessels, thereby increasing venous return to the heart; and (3) an increase of heart rate and force of contraction, which helps to maintain cardiac output in spite of significant volume loss.[7] These sympathetic reflexes are geared more for the maintenance of arterial pressure than for the maintenance of cardiac output (Fig. 37–1), because the increase in peripheral vascular resistance has no direct beneficial effect on cardiac output.[7] The value of sympathetic reflex compensation is illustrated by the fact that 30 to 40 per cent of the blood volume can be lost before death occurs while these reflexes are intact.[7] When the sympathetic reflexes are absent, loss of only 15 to 20 per cent of the blood volume may cause death.[7, 8]

Several other reflexes maintain cardiac output in the presence of volume loss. The central nervous system ischemic response elicits a powerful sympathetic stimulation after the arterial pressure falls below 50 mm Hg and is responsible

Table 37–1. Homeostatic Mechanisms in Hemorrhagic Shock

Sympathetic reflex compensation
  Arteriolar vasoconstriction
  Venous capacitance vasoconstriction
  Increased inotropic and chronotropic cardiac activity
  Central nervous system ischemic response
Selective increase in cerebral and coronary perfusion by means of local autoregulation
Increased oxygen unloading in tissues
Restoration of blood volume
  Renin-angiotensin-aldosterone axis activation
  Antidiuretic hormone secretion
  Transcapillary refill
  Increased thirst resulting in increased fluid intake
  Increased erythropoiesis

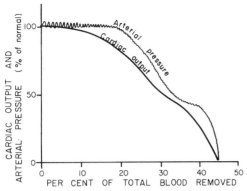

Figure 37–1. The effect of hemorrhage on cardiac output and arterial pressure. (From Guyton AC: Textbook of Medical Physiology. 6th ed. Philadelphia, WB Saunders Co, 1981. Reproduced by permission.)

for the second plateau on the arterial pressure curve (see Fig. 37–1).[7] Other compensatory mechanisms that tend to restore the blood volume to normal include the formation of angiotensin and antidiuretic hormone, which cause arteriolar vasoconstriction and conservation of salt and water by the kidneys.[7, 22] There is also a fluid shift from the interstitium to the intravascular space that helps to restore blood volume over a longer period (1 to 40 hours).[7, 23, 24]

When blood loss results in anemia, part of the loss in oxygen-carrying capacity is countered by an increase in tissue oxygen extraction.[25] Finally, the lost red blood cell mass is slowly replaced by erythropoiesis.

Several investigators examined the changes in blood pressure and pulse that occur with blood loss. Ebert and coworkers[2] acutely removed 15.5 to 19.7 per cent of the total blood volume from six volunteers. Five of the six developed a pulse increase of 14 to 30 beats per minute followed by a fall in arterial pressure and bradycardia (36 to 40 beats per minute). Skillman and associates[3] found that after a loss of 15 per cent of the blood volume there is a modest increase in the pulse (9 beats per minute) and a transient fall in the blood pressure followed by a return of the blood pressure to normal. Others[1, 4, 5] have noted a variable response to blood loss of up to 1 liter. The inability to detect volume loss with supine vital signs and the observation that patients with acute volume loss frequently develop syncope on arising led to the use of orthostatic vital signs. Ironically, few data exist regarding this simple bedside test in our present era of advanced technology and invasive monitoring.

PHYSIOLOGIC RESPONSE TO TILTING

When an individual assumes the upright posture, complex homeostatic mechanisms compensate for the effects of gravity on the circulation in order to maintain cerebral perfusion. These responses include (1) baroreceptor-mediated arteriolar vasoconstriction, (2) venous constriction and increased muscle tone in the legs and the abdomen to augment venous return, (3) sympathetic-mediated inotropic and chronotropic effects on the heart, and (4) activation of the renin-angiotensin-aldosterone system.[26]

These compensatory mechanisms preserve cerebral perfusion in the upright position with minimal changes in vital signs. Currens[27] found that when normal subjects stand, there is an average pulse increase of 13 beats per minute, no change or a small drop in systolic blood pressure, and

either no change or a small rise in diastolic blood pressure. These changes have been confirmed by others.[12, 28, 29]

The Trendelenburg position (head-down tilt) has long been assumed to have beneficial effects on venous return, cardiac output, and cerebral perfusion in hypotensive patients. These effects can be considered the converse of the circulatory changes that occur in the erect position. Unfortunately, few data substantiating a beneficial hemodynamic effect of the Trendelenburg position exist, and the use and actual clinical value of the position have been questioned by some researchers.[30, 31] Bivens and colleagues[30] found that the Trendelenburg position produces only a small (1.8 per cent) autotransfusion of blood volume to the central circulation in normovolemic subjects. Sibbald and coworkers[31] failed to detect any consistent or beneficial effect of the Trendelenburg position in hypotensive patients. The investigators argue against the use of the head-down tilt in critically ill patients because of detrimental effects on pulmonary physiology.[31]

Many conditions affect the compensatory mechanisms that allow us to assume the upright posture (Table 37–2).[26] Because of decreased vasomotor tone, limited chronotropic response, and other factors, the elderly have a higher inci-

Table 37–2. **Classification of Disorders of Postural Blood Pressure Regulation**

I. Poor postural adjustment
    Tall, asthenic habitus
    Advanced age
    Physical exhaustion
    Prolonged recumbency
    Pregnancy
    Gastrectomy
II. Orthostatic hypotension
    A. Secondary orthostatic hypotension
        1. Endocrinologic-metabolic disorders
            Diabetes mellitus
            Primary amyloidosis
            Primary and secondary adrenal insufficiency
            Pheochromocytoma
            Primary aldosteronism with marked hypokalemia
            Porphyria
        2. Central and peripheral nervous system disorders
            Intracranial tumors (parasellar and posterior fossa)
            Idiopathic paralysis agitans
            Wernicke's encephalopathy
            Multiple cerebral infarcts
            Brain stem lesions
            Tabes dorsalis
            Syringomyelia
            Traumatic and inflammatory myelopathies
            Guillain-Barré syndrome
            Chronic inflammatory polyradiculoneuropathy
            Peripheral neuropathies
            Familial dysautonomia (Riley-Day syndrome)
        3. Miscellaneous disorders
            Hypovolemia
            Hypochromic anemia
            Electrolyte disturbance
            Psychotropic and antihypertensive drugs
            Extensive surgical sympathectomy
            Chronic hemodialysis
            Anorexia nervosa
            Hyperbradykininism
    B. Primary or idiopathic orthostatic hypotension
        Idiopathic orthostatic hypotension
        Idiopathic orthostatic hypotension with somatic neurologic deficit (Shy-Drager syndrome)

(From Thomas JE, Schirger A, Fealey RD, et al: Orthostatic hypotension. Mayo Clin Proc 56:117, 1981. Reproduced by permission.)

dence of orthostatic hypotension, which can lead to syncope and fall-related injury.[32] One should note that drugs (such as α-blocking and β-blocking agents and vasodilating drugs) that antagonize the normal autonomic compensatory mechanisms pharmacologically can also produce orthostatic changes. The changes occur often enough to produce frank syncope, especially in the elderly. Even in normal subjects, passive tilting generates a high incidence of orthostatic syncope.[33] Patients with chronic anemia (and a compensated blood volume) seem to have the same postural response as normal subjects.[34, 35] Most of the conditions that affect postural blood pressure regulation have a sympathetic nervous system pathologic condition as a common denominator. Orthostatic hypotension caused by autonomic insufficiency is usually not accompanied by tachycardia, whereas the orthostatic hypotension produced by acute volume depletion is usually accompanied by a pronounced reflex tachycardia.

Few data exist on the effect of acute blood loss on postural vital signs. Shenkin and associates[5] studied 23 young adult volunteers who were bled from 500 to 1200 ml. They found no reliable change in the postural blood pressure but a consistent postural increase in the pulse of 35 to 40 per cent after a 500-ml blood loss was noted. In the six subjects who were bled approximately 1 liter, only two were able to tolerate standing; each of them had a postural increase in pulse of more than 30 beats per minute. The other four subjects experienced severe symptoms on standing, followed by a marked bradycardia and syncope if they were not allowed to lie down.

Green and Metheny[35] studied the effect of passive tilting to 75 degrees in normal subjects and volunteers who were bled 500 to 1500 ml. Before phlebotomy, the pulse increase on tilting never exceeded 25 beats per minute. After a blood loss of 1000 ml, the pulse increase on tilting always exceeded 25 beats per minute. The investigators were unable to detect a blood loss of 500 ml using these criteria and did not find reliable postural blood pressure changes after phlebotomy. These results have limited direct bedside application, because a tilt table was used.

Knopp and colleagues[12] phlebotomized 450 to 1000 ml of blood from healthy volunteers. By using the criterion of a pulse increase of 30 beats per minute or the presence of severe symptoms (syncope or near syncope) during a supine-to-standing test, they were able to distinguish accurately between a 1000-ml blood loss and no blood loss. It should be noted that some patients may become syncopal with a transiently normal blood pressure if vasoconstriction on standing preserves blood pressure at the expense of cerebral blood flow. Changes in blood pressure and pulse were not evaluated in the symptomatic subjects. Most likely, these patients would have had more pronounced blood pressure changes than asymptomatic patients had they not been permitted to lie down immediately. In the study population of 100 normal healthy volunteers with acute blood loss, the sensitivity and specificity using the aforementioned criteria for detecting a 1000-ml blood loss were both 98 per cent, giving an accuracy of 96 per cent (2 per cent false-negative results and 2 per cent false-positive results). The investigators were unable to consistently detect a blood loss of 500 ml by using these criteria.

The utility of orthostatic vital signs in children has been questioned because of reports of a high incidence of false-positive results.[36] Bergman and coworkers[36] found that 25 per cent of clinically normovolemic children had an increase in pulse of greater than 20 beats per minute and 11 per cent had a fall in systolic blood pressure of greater than 20 mm Hg. However, children with fever and diarrhea were included in this "normal" study group. Another study comparing mildly dehydrated children with normal children

found a significant difference in the orthostatic rise in pulse between the two groups.[37] Using near syncope or a change in heart rate of more than 25 beats per minute, orthostatic vital signs have a specificity of 95 per cent, a sensitivity of 75 per cent, and a predictive value of 92 per cent in detecting mild clinical dehydration in children.[37] No difference in orthostatic blood pressure was found between the normal and dehydrated children. Considering resting tachycardia as a positive sign of dehydration increased the predictive value of the test. The investigators concluded that in the appropriate clinical setting, an orthostatic increase in pulse greater than 25 beats per minute is a positive tilt test, and an orthostatic pulse increase of less than 20 beats per minute is a negative test for hypovolemia.[37]

In the elderly, orthostatic vital sign changes in volume-depleted patients are unknown. In one study of *normovolemic* nursing home patients 62 years or older, 39 of 476 (8 per cent) had a drop in systolic blood pressure of more than 20 mm Hg along with a drop in diastolic blood pressure of more than 10 mm Hg.[38] This postural blood pressure change was more common in patients on cardiovascular or psychotropic drugs.

Another complicating factor in interpreting orthostatic vital signs is the development of *paradoxical bradycardia* in the presence of blood loss. Bradycardia in the face of hemorrhage has generally been considered a preterminal finding of irreversible shock, but bradycardia has been documented in hypovolemic, yet conscious, trauma patients. Shenkin and colleagues,[5] Ebert and coworkers,[2] and Green and Metheny[35] noted that when orthostatic syncope occurred, it was accompanied by hypotension and often bradycardia. Many central nervous system factors can contribute to *vagal-mediated* syncope in emergency department patients with acute traumatic blood loss. These factors include pain, the sight of blood, stress, and nausea. Several investigators[39–42] have described women with hemoperitoneum secondary to ruptured ectopic pregnancy who were hypotensive but not tachycardic. The absence of tachycardia persisted with standing, but orthostatic symptoms occurred.[42] Knopp and associates[12] included orthostatic symptoms (syncope or near syncope requiring the patient to lie down) as one of the criteria for a positive tilt test. Jansen[43] reviewed other cases of this "relative bradycardia" that occurred in hypotensive patients with acute intraperitoneal bleeding and postulated a parasympathetic mechanism triggered by the presence of free blood in the peritoneal cavity. This bradycardia may be reversed with atropine,[43] but *aggressive fluid replacement is the treatment of choice* because anecdotal reports mention serious ventricular arrhythmias when atropine was used in this setting.[44] Paradoxical bradycardia has also been described in patients with abdominal or thoracic trauma or arterial bleeding from extremity wounds.[44] The true incidence of bradycardia in the face of hemorrhagic shock is not known, but bradycardia was present in 20 of 273 (7 per cent) patients in one study.[44] In this report by Barriot and Riou[44] the paradoxical bradycardia was associated with rapid and massive bleeding, but those patients with a more gradual blood loss exhibited a typical tachycardic response. *When the patient's clinical presentation is consistent with volume loss or shock, the clinician should not allow the absence of tachycardia to change the assessment.*

CLINICAL USE OF ORTHOSTATIC VITAL SIGNS

Indications and Contraindications

When the volume status of a patient is assessed by use of orthostatic vital signs, several points should be remembered. Many factors influence orthostatic blood pressure, including age, preexisting medical conditions, the use of medication, and idiopathic orthostatic hypotension (see Table 37–2). Data relating the effect of blood loss to orthostatic vital signs are limited to phlebotomized healthy volunteers. These results should be extrapolated with great care to patients with anemia, dehydration, or painful trauma, and the limitations of these studies should be recognized. The clinician must consider the clinical condition of the patient as well as the orthostatic vital signs in evaluating a patient for volume depletion.

Orthostatic vital signs are indicated as part of the evaluation of any patient with known or suspected volume loss or a history of syncope, except in the case of the following contraindications: The use of orthostatic vital signs is unnecessary and dangerous in a patient who manifests the clinical syndrome of shock. Orthostatic vital sign evaluation is also contraindicated in patients with a severely altered mental status, in the setting of possible spinal injuries, and in patients with lower extremity or pelvic fractures.

Technique

Once the decision to obtain orthostatic vital signs has been made, the blood pressure and pulse are recorded after the patient has been in the supine position for 2 to 3 minutes (Table 37–3). The patient should be resting quietly. No painful or invasive procedures should be performed during the test. Anxiety, fever, and other causes of resting tachycardia may make the test uninterpretable.[36] The use of antihypertensive medications may also invalidate the test.

The patient is then asked to stand, and the examiner should be prepared to assist the patient if he or she develops severe symptoms or syncope. A supine-to-standing test is more accurate than a supine-to-sitting evaluation. Knopp and coworkers[12] found that the supine-to-sitting test was not reliable for detecting 1000 ml of blood loss (55 per cent false-negative results). If the patient develops severe symptoms (defined as syncope or extreme dizziness requiring the patient to lie down) on standing, the test is positive and should be terminated. If the patient is not symptomatic, the blood pressure and pulse should be recorded after the patient has been standing for 1 minute. This interval resulted in the greatest difference between the control and 1000-ml phlebotomy groups in the study by Knopp and colleagues.[12]

In the setting of possible blood loss, if the patient has a pulse rise of 30 beats per minute or severe symptoms and if other complicating factors have been excluded, then blood loss is highly likely (2 per cent false-positive rate).[12] The presence of a negative test indicates only that an acute blood loss of 1000 ml is unlikely (2 per cent false-negative rate); a blood loss of 500 ml cannot be excluded (43 per cent false-

negative rate).[12] In children, near syncope or an orthostatic pulse increase of 25 beats per minute may be an accurate predictor of mild dehydration.[37] Further studies are needed to confirm this finding. The presence of resting tachycardia in children may also be an indicator of dehydration in the appropriate clinical setting.[37]

Criteria for significant blood pressure changes cannot be definitive because of the lack of correlation between blood pressure in the phlebotomy and control groups in the study by Knopp and coworkers,[12] but certainly a drop of systolic blood pressure of more than 25 mm Hg should be viewed as suggestive of significant hypovolemia. The medical literature contains varied criteria to define orthostatic hypotension related to medical problems other than hypovolemia.[5, 45] A reasonable criterion would be a decline in the systolic blood pressure of 25 mm Hg or a drop in the diastolic blood pressure of 10 mm Hg that is accompanied by significant symptoms of orthostatic hypotension.

Complication

The possible complications of orthostatic vital sign assessment can be avoided if the aforementioned contraindications and precautions are remembered. Complications include syncope with a resulting fall and injury and the possibility of exacerbating an existing fracture or spinal cord injury.

CONCLUSION

Orthostatic vital signs can provide valuable information in the overall assessment of patients suffering from blood loss or volume depletion. Unfortunately, few studies provide us with an adequate database on which to interpret the results of this test. Orthostatic vital signs are generally *overinterpreted* in clinical medicine. In the setting of acute blood loss in otherwise healthy adult patients, a pulse increase of 30 beats per minute or the occurrence of severe symptoms on standing indicates that blood loss has occurred (96 per cent accuracy). In children a pulse increase of greater than 25 beats per minute suggests clinically significant volume loss. The clinical significance of postural vital sign changes in the elderly remains uncertain.

REFERENCES

1. Burri C, Henkemeyer H, Passler HH, et al: Evaluation of acute blood loss by means of simple hemodynamic parameters. Prog Surg 11:109, 1973.
2. Ebert RV, Stead EA, Gibson JG: Response of normal subjects to acute blood loss. Arch Intern Med 68:578, 1941.
3. Skillman JJ, Olson JE, Lyons JH, Moore FD: The hemodynamic effect of acute blood loss in normal man, with observations on the effect of the Valsalva maneuver and breath holding. Am Surg 166:713, 1967.
4. Shenkin HA, Cheney RH, Govons SR, et al: Effects of acute hemorrhage of known amount on the circulation of essentially normal persons (abstract). Am J Med Sci 206:806, 1943.
5. Shenkin HA, Cheney RH, Govons SR, et al: On the diagnosis of hemorrhage in man: A study of volunteers bled large amounts. Am J Med Sci 208:421, 1944.
6. Walt AJ (ed): Early Care of the Injured Patient. Philadelphia, WB Saunders Co, 1982.
7. Guyton AC: Textbook of Medical Physiology. 6th ed. Philadelphia, WB Saunders Co, 1981.
8. Zuidema GD (ed): The Management of Trauma. 3rd ed. Philadelphia, WB Saunders Co, 1979.
9. American College of Surgeons Committee on Trauma: Advanced Trauma Life Support Course Student Manual. Chicago, American College of Surgeons, 1981.
10. Hartong JM, Dixon RS: Monitoring resuscitation of the injured patient. JAMA 237:242, 1977.
11. Podolsky S, Baraff LJ, Geehr E, et al: Transcutaneous oxymetry measurements during acute blood loss. Ann Emerg Med 11:523, 1982.
12. Knopp R, Claypool R, Leonardi D: Use of the tilt test in measuring acute blood loss. Ann Emerg Med 9:29, 1980.

Table 37–3. Summary of Orthostatic Tilt Testing

1. Blood pressure and pulse are recorded after patient has been supine for 2 to 3 minutes.
2. Blood pressure, pulse, and symptoms are recorded after patient has been standing for 1 minute. The patient should be permitted to resume a supine position immediately should syncope or near syncope develop.

Positive Test

1. Increase in pulse of 30 beats per minute or more in adults.
2. Presence of symptoms of hypovolemia (dizziness, syncope).
3. Drop in systolic blood pressure of greater than 25 mm Hg.*

*See text for explanation.

13. Bates B: A Guide to Physical Examination. Philadelphia, JB Lippincott Co, 1979.
14. Delp MH, Manning RT: Major's Physical Diagnosis: An Introduction to the Clinical Process. 9th ed. Philadelphia, WB Saunders Co, 1981.
15. Prior JA, Silberstein JS, Stang JM: Physical Diagnosis: The History and Examination of the Patient. 6th ed. St. Louis, CV Mosby Co, 1981.
16. Weil MH, Shubin H: Diagnosis and Treatment of Shock. Baltimore, Williams & Wilkins, 1967.
17. Hayes HR, Briggs BA: MGH Textbook of Emergency Medicine. Baltimore, Williams & Wilkins, 1978.
18. Jacobson S: Errors in emergency practice. Emerg Med 10:124, 1978.
19. Watkins GM: Diagnosing multiple trauma, insights into the art of recognizing automobile injuries. Curr Concepts Trauma Care, June, 1978, p 3.
20. Holcroft JW: Impairment of venous return in hemorrhagic shock. Surg Clin North Am 62:17, 1982.
21. Berne RM (ed): Handbook of Physiology. Vol. 1. Bethesda, Md, American Physiological Society, 1979, p 645.
22. Gann DS: Endocrine control of plasma protein and volume. Surg Clin North Am 56:1135, 1976.
23. Drucker WR, Chadwick CDJ, Gann DS: Transcapillary refill in hemorrhage and shock. Arch Surg 116:1344, 1981.
24. Moore FD: The effects of hemorrhage on body composition. N Engl J Med 273:567, 1965.
25. Watkins GM, Rabelo A, Bevilacqua RG, et al: Bodily changes in repeated hemorrhage. Surg Gynecol Obstet 139:161, 1974.
26. Thomas JE, Schirger A, Fealey RD, et al: Orthostatic hypotension. Mayo Clin Proc 56:117, 1981.
27. Currens JH: A comparison of the blood pressure in the lying and standing positions: A study of five hundred men and five hundred women. Am Heart J 35:646, 1948.
28. Hull DH, Wolthius RA, Cortese T, et al: Borderline hypertension versus normotension. Differential response to orthostatic stress. Am Heart J 94:414, 1977.
29. Stair I: Clinical studies in incoordination of the circulation as determined by the response to arising. J Clin Invest 22:813, 1943.
30. Bivens HG, Knopp R, dos Santos PAL: Blood volume distribution in the Trendelenburg position. Ann Emerg Med 14:641, 1985.
31. Sibbald WJ, Paterson NAM, Holliday RL, et al: The Trendelenburg position: Hemodynamic effects in hypotensive and normotensive patients. Crit Care Med 7:218, 1979.
32. Caird FI, Andrews GR, Kennedy RD: Effect of posture on blood pressure in the elderly. Br Heart J 35:527, 1973.
33. Stevens PM: Cardiovascular dynamics during orthostatism and the influence of intravascular instrumentation. Am J Cardiol 17:211, 1966.
34. Duke M, Abelmann WH: The hemodynamic response to chronic anemia. Circulation 39:503, 1969.
35. Green DM, Metheny D: The estimation of acute blood loss by the tilt test. Surg Gynecol Obstet 84:1045, 1947.
36. Bergman GE, Reisner FF, Anwar FAH: Orthostatic changes in normovolemic children: An analysis of the "tilt test." J Emerg Med 1:137, 1983.
37. Fuchs SM, Jaffe DM: Evaluation of the "tilt test" in children. Ann Emerg Med 16:386, 1987.
38. Aronow W, Lee N, Sales F, et al: Prevalence of postural hypotension in elderly patients in a long-term health care facility. Am J Cardiol 62:366, 1988.
39. Stair T: Orthostatic tachycardia and ectopic pregnancy (letter). Ann Emerg Med 11:284, 1982.
40. Cobb TL: Orthostatic tachycardia and ectopic pregnancy. Normal pulse rate in the presence of massive hemorrhage (letter). Ann Emerg Med 11:589, 1982.
41. Adams SL, Greene JS: Absence of a tachycardic response to intraperitoneal hemorrhage. J Emerg Med 4:383, 1986.
42. Stair T: Orthostatic tachycardia and ectopic pregnancy (reply). Ann Emerg Med 11:590, 1982.
43. Jansen RPS: Relative bradycardia: A sign of acute intraperitoneal bleeding. Aust NZ J Obstet Gynaecol 18:206, 1978.
44. Barriot P, Riou B: Hemorrhagic shock with paradoxical bradycardia. Intensive Care Med 13:203, 1987.
45. Kroenke K: Orthostatic hypotension. West J Med 143:253, 1985.

Anesthetic and Analgesic Techniques

Chapter 38

Local and Topical Anesthesia and Nerve Blocks of the Thorax and Extremities

Michael Orlinsky and Edwin Dean

INTRODUCTION

The use of local anesthetic agents is an important aspect of the everyday practice of emergency medicine. This chapter provides an understanding of the mechanism of action; the nuances of clinical use; and the prevention, recognition, and treatment of adverse reactions to commonly used anesthetics. Detailed technical guidance for the performance of local anesthetic procedures is provided.

The first local anesthetic was cocaine, an alkaloid contained in the leaves of the *Erythroxylon coco* shrub from the Andes mountains. Early Incan society used cocaine during the procedure of trephination; the surgeon allowed coca-drenched saliva to drip from his mouth onto the wound to produce local anesthesia.

In 1884, Koller, a colleague of Freud, used cocaine topically in the eye and is credited with the introduction of local anesthesia into clinical practice.[1] In the same year, Zenfel used a topical solution of alcohol and cocaine to anesthetize the eardrum, and Hall introduced the drug into dentistry.[2] In 1885, Halsted demonstrated that cocaine could block nerve transmission and laid the foundation for nerve block anesthesia.[3] The search for alternatives to cocaine led to the synthesis of the benzoic acid ester derivatives and the amide anesthetics.

Although local anesthetics had been used for more than half a century, it was not until the 1960s that a specific understanding of the physiochemical properties, mechanism of action, pharmacokinetics, and toxicity of these agents emerged.

PHARMACOLOGY AND PHYSIOLOGY

Chemical Structure and Physiochemical Properties

Most useful local anesthetic agents share a basic chemical structure:

aromatic segment—intermediate chain—hydrophilic segment

Within this basic structure, each agent's specific chemical composition determines its main physiochemical properties:

negative log of dissociation constant (pKa), partition coefficient (a measurement of lipid solubility), and protein binding. Each property, in turn, is the principal determinant of an agent's pharmacologic activity: onset of action, potency, and duration of action, respectively. In vivo, however, the activity of a given agent may be altered by other factors unrelated to physiochemical properties, and therefore the relationship between physiochemical properties and clinical activity is not exact.

The linkage (intermediate chain) between the aromatic and hydrophilic segments is either an amino-ester or an amino-amide; these two form the basis for the two main classifications of local anesthetics. Ester-type agents include procaine, chloroprocaine, cocaine, and tetracaine, and the amide-type agents include lidocaine, mepivacaine, prilocaine, bupivacaine, and etidocaine. The main difference between esters and amides is their metabolic pathways. Esters are hydrolyzed by plasma pseudocholinesterase, whereas amides are metabolized in the liver through enzymatic degradation. Within the ester or amide group, alterations in chemical structure to either the aromatic or the hydrophilic portion may affect the rate of metabolism and create a different activity profile for each agent within a given group.

Chemically, local anesthetics are poorly soluble weak bases. To be commercially available in solution, an agent is combined with hydrogen chloride to produce the salt of a weak acid. In the resulting acidic solution, salts exist both as uncharged molecules (nonionized) and as positively charged cations (ionized). The uncharged form is lipid soluble, enabling it to diffuse through tissues and across nerve membranes, which the charged form cannot do. The ratio of uncharged to charged forms depends on the pH of the medium (vial solution or tissue milieu) and on the pKa of the specific agent. The pKa is the pH at which 50 per cent of the solution is in the uncharged form and 50 per cent is in the charged form. Because the pKa is constant for a specific agent, the relative proportion of these forms is dependent on the pH of the solution in accordance with the Henderson-Hasselbalch equation:

$$pH = pKa + log \, [uncharged]/[charged]$$

When the pH of the solution or tissue decreases, a given agent exists more in its ionized, charged form; conversely, when a pH increases, the agent exists more in its nonionized, uncharged form. Because the nonionized portion is the form of drug that can diffuse through tissues and nerves, manipulation of the pH of the solution is a useful tool for the physician (see "Factors Affecting Neural Blockade").

Local anesthetic agents are available in plain solution (i.e., without epinephrine), both in single-dose vials or ampules and in multidose vials. For most agents the pH of the solution is greater than 5. Multidose vials contain methylparaben as the antibacterial preservative. Local anesthetics are also available premixed with epinephrine and marketed in single-dose or multidose vials. They contain an antioxidant

Table 38–1. pH and Additives of Amide Local Anesthetics

Solution Content	pH (range)	Preservative (methylparaben)	Antioxidant
Plain—single dose	4.5–6.5	–	–
Plain—multidose	4.5–6.5	+	–
Commercial epinephrine—single dose	3.5–4.0	–	+
Commercial epinephrine—multidose	3.5–4.0	+	+
Prepared epinephrine—single dose	4.5–6.5	–	–

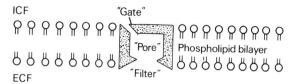

Figure 38–2. Axon membrane. (From Wildsmith JAW: Peripheral nerve and local anesthetic drugs. Br J Anaesth 58:692, 1986.)

(sodium bisulfite or sodium metabisulfite) to prevent deactivation of the vasoconstrictor. These solutions must be adjusted to a more acid pH—approximately 3.5 to 4.0—to maintain the stability of epinephrine and its antioxidant. As with plain solutions, multidose vials also contain methylparaben (Table 38–1).

How an anesthetic is supplied has several implications. First, the lower pH of epinephrine-containing solutions may make the agent more painful on infiltration and may increase its ionized concentration, thereby delaying its onset. Studies of pH measurements have shown adding epinephrine to plain solutions just before use does not change the pH of the solution; this finding has led to the recommendation that when epinephrine is used, it should be added at the bedside.[4, 5] Second, the addition of methylparaben to multidose vials is implicated in many allergic reactions. Understanding this fact helps when dealing with patients who claim to be allergic to local anesthetics.

Nerve Structure and Impulse Transmission

FUNCTIONAL AND STRUCTURAL COMPONENTS OF A PERIPHERAL NERVE

The functional unit is the nerve fiber, which in its practical definition includes the nerve axon and its surrounding Schwann cell sheath. Two distinct arrangements of this nerve sheath are recognized (Fig. 38–1): (1) unmyelinated nerve fibers have a single Schwann cell surrounding several axons; (2) myelinated nerve fibers have a Schwann cell wrapped around a single axon, forming a myelin sheath. Junctions between sheaths along the axon are called *nodes of Ranvier*; they contain sodium channels necessary for depolarization. As myelin sheath thickness increases from autonomic to sensory to motor fibers, the nodes of Ranvier with

their sodium channels are spaced farther apart. This fact is important for differential blockade (see later discussion).

The most important structure affecting nerve impulse transmission is the axon membrane (Fig. 38–2). The membrane is composed of a double layer of phospholipid into which are embedded protein molecules that serve as channels containing pores for the movement of ions into and out of the cell. Most pores have a filter that allows for ion-specific movement, a gate that regulates the passage of ions, and a sensor mechanism that opens or closes the gate.

Bundles of nerve fibers (Fig. 38–3) are embedded in collagen fibrils called *endoneurium* and are surrounded by a cellular layer, the *perineurium*. The perineurium functions as a diffusion barrier and maintains the composition of extracellular fluid around the nerve fibers. Surrounding the entire structure is the outer layer of a peripheral nerve, the *epineurium*, which is composed of areolar connective tissue. The arrangement of fibers within a peripheral nerve is important for the pattern of onset of nerve blockade (see later discussion).

The Nerve Impulse and Its Transmission. At rest, the inside of a nerve fiber, or axoplasm, is negative (−70 mV) compared with the outside. This resting potential is the net result of the marked differences in ionic concentrations on each side of the axonal membrane and the forces that tend to maintain that difference. Specifically, there is a surplus of sodium extracellularly and potassium intracellularly. The sodium channel is closed, preventing these ions from moving along their concentration gradient (out → in). Although potassium can leave the cell to follow its concentration gradient (in → out), it is prevented from doing so completely because of the need to maintain electrical neutrality inside the cell. Potassium reaches an equilibrium between its concentration gradient and the electrochemical gradient, thus creating the negative resting potential.

When a nerve is excited, the sodium channel opens. At first, a slow influx of sodium ions occurs, but after a critical threshold is reached, sodium enters the cell rapidly, following the electrochemical gradients and its own concentration gradient (depolarization). The influx of sodium is halted when the membrane potential reaches +20 mV because the inward concentration gradient for sodium is balanced by the outward electrochemical gradient. The sodium channels then close, but potassium continues to move out until the

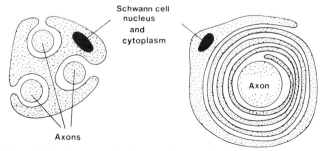

Figure 38–1. Schwann cell sheath of unmyelinated (left) and myelinated (right) nerve fibers. (From Wildsmith JAW: Peripheral nerve and local anesthetic drugs. Br J Anaesth 58:692, 1986.)

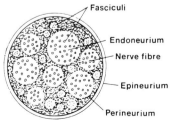

Figure 38–3. Cross section of peripheral nerve. (From Wildsmith JAW: Peripheral nerve and local anesthetic drugs. Br J Anaesth 58:692, 1986.)

resting potential is again achieved (repolarization). When the excitation process has been completed and the nerve cell is electrically quiescent, the relative excess of sodium inside the cell and potassium outside the cell is then readjusted by the adenosine triphosphate (ATP)–dependent sodium-potassium pump.

During the previously discussed process, known as the *action potential*, depolarization of a portion of the nerve causes a current to flow along the adjacent nerve fiber. This current makes the membrane potential less negative and actuates the sensor to open the next sodium channel. The action potential cycle is repeated, thereby propagating the impulse. Nerve conduction is essentially unidirectional because in the segment just depolarized (1) the sodium channel is not only closed but inactivated as well, and (2) delayed closure of specific potassium channels prevents the critical threshold from being reached. In unmyelinated nerve fibers, an impulse spreads continuously down the axon. In myelinated nerve fibers, sodium channels are situated at the nodes of Ranvier, and current flows from node to node, causing intervening segments to depolarize at once. This saltatory conduction accounts for the faster rate of impulse transmission in myelinated fibers.

Mechanism of Action

The way local anesthetic agents produce nerve conduction blockade can be explored practically by discussing three related concepts: (1) the active form of the agent responsible, (2) the physiologic basis for blockade, and (3) the method by which this process is accomplished.

The Active Form. An anesthetic solution exists in uncharged and charged forms with the concentration of the uncharged form increasing in more alkaline milieus. It is only this uncharged (lipid-soluble) form that can cross tissue and membrane barriers. Once the agent is through a barrier, the uncharged form re-equilibrates into uncharged and charged forms, the proportion of which again depends on the prevailing pH.

The finding by Skou in 1954 that local anesthetics were more effective in alkaline solutions led to the conclusion that the uncharged form was responsible for conduction blockade.[6] However, it was also possible that the increased effectiveness of alkaline solutions was solely due to increased penetration through tissue barriers caused by the higher concentration of the uncharged form. The classic experiments of Ritchie, Ritchie, and Greengard in 1965 demonstrated that the cationic charged form was responsible for actual blockade.[7, 8] It is now believed that both the charged and the uncharged forms are responsible for activity, with the charged form predominating for most of the common anesthetic agents.[9]

The Physiologic Basis for Blockade. There is a broad consensus that the prevention of sodium influx across the nerve membrane is the physiologic basis for conduction blockade.[10–12] Local anesthetics decrease sodium influx, which decreases the rate of rise and amplitude of depolarization. When sufficient anesthetic is present, the firing threshold will not be reached, thereby preventing the action potential from forming. With no action potential, no impulse can be transmitted, and conduction blockade is achieved. The end result is local anesthesia.

The Method of Blockade. The means by which anesthetic agents prevent sodium influx is still not completely understood. Strong support for the concept that the uncharged base affects penetration and the cationic charged form produces the anesthetic effect came from several studies.[12–14] It was demonstrated that the cationic charged

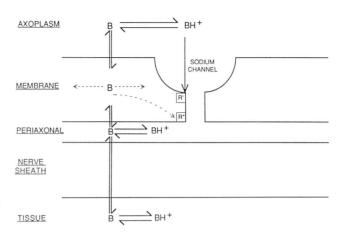

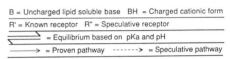

Figure 38–4. Mechanism of action. (Modified from Ritchie JM: Mechanism of action of local anesthetic agents and biotoxins. Br J Anaesth 47:196, 1975.)

form blocks the action potential from inside the membrane, and that the agent enters the sodium channel from the axoplasmic side and binds to a receptor about halfway down the electrical gradient. This so-called specific receptor theory is well accepted and is considered the predominant mechanism in preventing sodium influx. However, this theory cannot account for the action of the benzocaine, the other neutral compounds, or the uncharged base form of the common local anesthetics.

In summary (Fig. 38–4), when a commonly used local anesthetic (other than benzocaine) is applied perineurally, it equilibrates into its uncharged and charged forms based on the tissue pH and agent pKa. The uncharged lipid-soluble form penetrates tissue, nerve sheath, and nerve membrane to gain access to the axoplasm, wherein it re-equilibrates into both forms. The charged form enters the sodium channel to effect blockade by decreasing sodium influx. The uncharged base is also involved with sodium channel blockade, but the exact nature of this mechanism is unknown.

Factors Affecting Neural Blockade

A local anesthetic's activity profile (onset, potency, duration) and its ability to produce a differential blockade in mixed nerves are a function of physiochemical properties, the physiologic environment, and to some extent, manipulation by the physician.

Onset of Action. The pKa of an anesthetic is the primary physiochemical factor that determines onset of action. The lower the pKa, the more lipid-soluble uncharged form is present, which thereby increases the penetrating ability and shortens the onset of action (Tables 38–2 and 38–3). Although in isolated nerve fibers onset of action directly parallels pKa, additional in vivo physiochemical factors exert an influence. For example, prilocaine and lidocaine have the same pKa, but lidocaine's onset is faster because of its enhanced ability to penetrate through nonnervous tissue.

The site of administration has significant influence. As the amount of interspersed tissue or the size of the nerve

Table 38–2. Activity Profile with Primary Physiochemical Determinant

Agent	Onset: pKa	Potency: Lipid Solubility	Duration: Protein Binding
Tetracaine	Slow	8	Long
Procaine	Slow	1	Short
Chloroprocaine	Fast	1	Short
Lidocaine	Fast	2	Moderate
Mepivacaine	Fast	2	Moderate
Prilocaine	Fast	2	Moderate
Bupivacaine	Moderate	8	Long
Etidocaine	Fast	4–6	Long

sheath increases, the onset times are prolonged for all agents because of the greater distance that the agent must travel to reach its receptor. The role of pKa becomes more important as the tissue barrier increases. For example, both lidocaine (pKa 7.9) and bupivacaine (pKa 8.1) have comparably rapid onsets (2 to 5 minutes) with subcutaneous infiltration. However, with brachial plexus block, the onset times are prolonged but less so for lidocaine (15 minutes) than for bupivacaine (25 minutes). The pattern of onset for large nerves is determined by the structural arrangement of fibers. Peripheral fibers (mantle) will be blocked before core fibers. Because mantle fibers innervate more proximal regions, nerve blockade proceeds in a proximal to distal progression.

A faster onset time may be created by the addition of sodium bicarbonate to raise the anesthetic solution's pH, which yields a higher concentration of the uncharged lipid-soluble form more rapidly. Also, the addition of epinephrine just before use results in a higher pH and a faster onset time compared with commercial epinephrine solutions.

Increasing the total dose also shortens onset time. This can be accomplished by increasing the concentration or volume, or both, of the administered drug.

For many years, mixtures of local anesthetics have been compounded to obtain the benefit of the rapid onset of one agent and the longer duration of another. This is no longer necessary, especially for infiltration and minor nerve block procedures, because bupivacaine provides clinically acceptable onsets with prolonged durations.

For most procedures performed in the emergency department, it is unnecessary to choose a local anesthetic (or iatrogenically alter its activity) based on onset time, but one must be cognizant of the normal delays to avoid premature additional doses that might prove toxic.

Potency. The lipid solubility of an anesthetic is the primary physiochemical factor that determines potency, specifically the inherent lipid solubility of an agent as determined by its partition coefficient, as opposed to the concentration of lipid-soluble form that is present (quantitative), which is determined by pKa or pH. Because the nerve

membrane is basically lipid, the more lipophilic an anesthetic, the easier the process of crossing into the cell and the fewer the molecules that are needed for conduction blockade. This results in greater potency (see Tables 38–2 and 38–3).

The relative degree of vasodilation produced by local anesthetics also affects potency. Lidocaine is more lipid-soluble than prilocaine or mepivacaine, but it produces more vasodilation, which leads to more rapid vascular absorption, which decreases the number of molecules available to penetrate the nerve. So although lidocaine is twice as potent in vitro, it is equipotent in vivo to prilocaine or mepivacaine. Another important factor is uptake by adipose tissue. Etidocaine, which in vitro is more potent than bupivacaine, is less so in vivo because its greater absorption by fat results in fewer molecules being available for conduction blockade.

The pH of anesthetic solutions or the tissue pH theoretically can affect potency. For example, the acid pH of an abscess is thought to decrease local anesthetic effectiveness; however, there appear to be few data to support this contention.

Although not a primary reason for its use, epinephrine, by producing vasoconstriction and making more molecules available to the nerve, increases the depth of anesthesia. Agent concentration is also important. By increasing the concentration of the anesthetic agent, potency is enhanced.

Choosing an anesthetic for its inherent potency is usually not necessary for any given site, because the concentration of an agent may be manipulated to make most drugs equianesthetic. For example, lidocaine, being one fourth as potent as bupivacaine, is usually used at four times the concentration (1 to 2 per cent versus 0.25 to 0.5 per cent, respectively). One must be cognizant, however, that for different sites and techniques, different concentrations and volumes of a given agent are needed to produce adequate blockade.

Duration. The protein binding of an anesthetic primarily determines the duration of action. This is because agents that bind more tightly to the protein receptor remain in the sodium channel longer (see Tables 38–2 and 38–3). Similar to potency and for the same reason, vasodilation produced by local anesthetics inversely influences the duration of action. Prilocaine, which is less protein bound than lidocaine, produces, in vivo, a longer duration of action because of its lesser degree of vasoactivity. The duration of action also varies with the mode of administration, being shorter when an agent is applied topically than when it is injected into the tissues.

Physicians may prolong the duration of action by several methods. Increasing the dose, usually by increasing the concentration, prolongs duration but is limited by the possibility of a toxic reaction and the maximum effective concentration of a drug. Although controversial, raising the pH of the anesthetic solution has also been shown to prolong duration.[15, 16]

Table 38–3. Physiochemical Properties of Selected Local Anesthetics

Agent	Type	Site of Metabolism	pKa	Lipid Solubility (Partition Coefficient)	Protein Binding (%)
Tetracaine	Ester	Plasma	8.5	High (4.1)	76
Procaine	Ester	Plasma	8.9	Low (0.02)	6
Chloroprocaine	Ester	Plasma	8.7	Low (0.14)	—
Lidocaine	Amide	Liver	7.9	Med (2.9)	64
Mepivacaine	Amide	Liver	7.6	Med (0.8)	78
Prilocaine	Amide	Liver	7.9	Med (0.9)	55
Bupivacaine	Amide	Liver	8.1	High (27.5)	95
Etidocaine	Amide	Liver	7.7	High (141.0)	94

The most practical way to increase duration is to use solutions that contain epinephrine. Epinephrine causes vasoconstriction, thereby decreasing systemic absorption, which allows more molecules to reach the nerve. The effect of epinephrine varies according to the agent. Anesthetics that produce more vasodilation (e.g., procaine, lidocaine, mepivacaine) are more affected by epinephrine's vasoconstrictive action. The long-acting, highly lipid-soluble agents (e.g., bupivacaine, etidocaine) are less affected because they are substantially taken up by extradural fat and released slowly. In fact, Swerdlow and Jones have shown that for intradermal injections, lidocaine with epinephrine produces almost as long a duration of action as bupivacaine with epinephrine.[17] They also demonstrated that adding epinephrine is more effective than doubling the concentration of a plain solution.

The selection of an agent with a long duration of action should be considered if the procedure is lengthy or if postoperative analgesia is desired. Conversely, a shorter acting agent combined with epinephrine or an alkalinized plain solution could be used. Making a specific choice of agent is discussed with specific applications.

Differential (Motor Versus Sensory) Blockade

Differential blockade in a mixed nerve refers to the different rate of conduction block between sensory and motor fibers. This differential is related to the anatomic structure of these fibers and the physiochemical properties of the agent. Pain fibers have little or no surrounding myelin sheaths and are preferentially blocked before the more moderately covered touch and pressure fibers, which in turn are more readily blocked than the heavily myelinated motor fibers. It is not just the thickness per se of a myelin sheath that is important but also that the nodes of Ranvier (sodium channels) are progressively separated as the diameter of a nerve fiber increases, thus lessening the chance of a favorable drug-receptor interaction. Therefore, penetration and spreadability of an anesthetic determine whether only sensory or both sensory and motor fibers are blocked. Agents with a high pKa and poor lipid solubility do not achieve motor blockade as easily as agents with low pKa and good lipid solubility. Bupivacaine, which provides sensory block without significant impairment of motor function, is especially useful for postoperative analgesia and obstetric deliveries. Etidocaine, on the other hand, produces profound motor block at doses that are needed to provide sensory analgesia, making this agent well suited for procedures that require neuromuscular blockade (e.g., abdominal operations, caesarean section).

Generally, if an anesthetic exhibits slow onset or poor spreadability, ongoing systemic absorption may decrease the number of molecules needed to block the more myelinated fibers (touch, pressure, motor), even though sensory block has been achieved. To decrease this dissociation and provide better sensory or motor block, the physician has several options. The simplest method is to wait a short period for enough anesthetic to spread to effect the blockade. This may be helpful for the patient whose pain sensation is blocked but, who is still aware of touch. Also, increasing the agent's concentration produces an increase in level of blockade, affecting motor more than sensory fibers. Typically, lidocaine 1 per cent is used for anesthesia alone, and lidocaine 2 per cent is used to combine motor with sensory block. Adding epinephrine is the most effective way of increasing block, again motor more so than sensory. As with increased concentration, epinephrine allows more molecules to be presented to the nerve. A practical use of epinephrine would be for an extensive laceration that needs to be anesthetized

when the total dose of lidocaine 1 per cent may approach the toxic range. Combining epinephrine with lidocaine 0.5 per cent would allow for the needed volume at a lower dose and yet would provide adequate analgesia. Other ways to increase spread are to administer an anesthetic rapidly or to use a greater volume of anesthetic (these techniques are also more painful). Increasing volume, even while keeping the total dose the same, causes more spread and achieves block of larger fibers. Thus the physician may use different agents or manipulate a given agent to provide for the appropriate functional method of blockade.

Adverse Effects

LOCAL ANESTHETIC EFFECT ON WOUNDS

In addition to producing neural blockade, local anesthetics also have potential effects on wound healing and wound infection.

Wound Healing. Local anesthetics produce cytotoxic effects on cell structure and function in a dose- and time-related manner. These effects, demonstrated at doses well below those used clinically, involve fibroblasts more than nervous tissue. Collagen synthesis is inhibited by lidocaine and bupivacaine.[18] Morris and Tracey found that lidocaine in increasing concentration progressively reduced the tensile strength of wounds.[19] Epinephrine added to 1 per cent and 2 per cent concentrations of lidocaine further reduced tensile strength, but when epinephrine was added to distilled water or to 0.5 per cent lidocaine it had little effect. Several conclusions appear clinically relevant: (1) although it may delay onset, lidocaine 0.5 per cent solution, without epinephrine if possible, may be best for wound healing; (2) when possible, local anesthetics should be avoided in poorly healing wounds, leg ulcers, or anywhere that fast healing is essential; and (3) local anesthetics in high concentrations might help prevent excessive scarring in patients prone to keloids or hypertrophic scars.

Wound Infection. Although not generally appreciated, it has long been known that local anesthetics possess antimicrobial activity in vitro. Lidocaine and procaine at 2 per cent concentrations, and to a lesser extent at lower concentrations, have been shown to inhibit the culture growth of most gram-negative organisms, with only *Pseudomonas aeruginosa* being particularly resistant.[20] Gram-positive isolates were also significantly affected by lidocaine and to a lesser extent by procaine. Administering anesthetics before obtaining culture material, including injection into a joint prior to arthrocentesis, may give false-negative culture results and should be avoided if possible. This effect may also be significant in obtaining wound cultures when anesthetic ointments have been previously applied.

Although local anesthetics can interfere with culture testing, it may not follow that these agents prevent wound infections. Several studies show that local anesthetics by themselves do not appear to alter the incidence of wound infection.[21–23]

Epinephrine, on the other hand, does appear to exert a deleterious effect on host defenses at least in animal models. Studies with infiltrative and topically applied epinephrine solutions in iatrogenically contaminated animal wounds show an increased potential for infection.[22–24] The proposed mechanism is that epinephrine, by producing vasoconstriction, leads to tissue hypoxia, which has been shown to retard the killing of *Staphylococcus aureus* by leukocytes.[25] A decrease in the total number of leukocytes secondary to vasoconstriction is also likely to play a role. Although it has been recommended that solutions containing epinephrine not be used because of the potential enhancement of wound infection,[22, 23, 26, 27] several clinical studies using TAC (tetracaine, adrenaline, cocaine) or its various components have not demonstrated significantly increased infection rates.[28–35]

LOCAL INJURIES

These injuries may result from the direct application of an anesthetic agent to a nerve or the passage of a needle through tissue. Local reactions are rare, as demonstrated by several large series that listed only three cases of neuropathy in more than 90,000 patients.[36–38] However, local problems can occur from improper technique or lack of due caution. Factors implicated in causing transient or persistent neuropathy include acidic solution pH, additives, the agent itself, needle trauma, compression from hematomas, and accidental injection of neurolytic agents. For example, Born described a series of 49 wrist and metacarpal blocks using bupivacaine in which eight patients developed a significant neuropathy.[39] He postulated that damage occurred from the trapping of the drug in a confined space and recommended cautious use of low concentrations and small quantities whenever bupivacaine is used in this situation. Infection, hematomas, and broken needles are other local problems that can be averted by using proper technique. Erroneous needle placement also can produce complications such as pneumothorax during brachial plexus or intercostal block. In addition, epinephrine-containing solutions, when injected into tissues containing end arteries, can lead to profound ischemia and gangrene. Vasoconstrictors should be avoided when blocking the digits, penis, tip of the nose, or earlobe. The use of vasodilators (e.g., local infiltration with 0.5 to 5.0 mg phentolamine) or sympathetic blocks has been recommended for this complication.[40–41]

SYSTEMIC TOXIC REACTIONS

Although occurring in only 0.1 to 0.4 per cent of local anesthetic administrations, systemic toxic reactions are the most frequent serious adverse reactions encountered (Table 38–4).[37, 42–44] On the administration of a local anesthetic, some of the drug reaches its intended target and some is absorbed quickly into the systemic circulation. Peak blood levels are generally produced within 30 minutes, with levels then falling because of distribution and elimination.

Systemic toxic reactions generally result from high blood levels of local anesthetic agents. The most common way to achieve these toxic levels is by inadvertent intravascular injection. Toxic levels may also be reached with appropriate methods of administration. This is more commonly seen with topical application than with perineural injection (Fig. 38–5). Other factors that produce a higher blood level, thereby enhancing toxicity, include an increased rate of absorption from a more vascular site, a rapid rate of administration, a larger dose or higher concentration, and the absence of a vasoconstrictor.

Factors

Addition of Epinephrine. Although without effect topically on mucosal surfaces, when epinephrine, through its vasoconstrictor action, is infiltrated, it reduces systemic absorption and thereby results in lower peak blood levels.

Specific Drug. When comparing local anesthetics on a milligram-to-milligram basis, the more potent agents are more toxic. Because anesthetics are used in equipotent doses (e.g., 1 mg bupivacaine to 4 mg lidocaine), they are approximately equitoxic. Blood levels achieved by a particular agent depend on its intrinsic absorption into and its distribution and clearance from the circulation. Agents with high lipid solubility and protein binding (etidocaine > bupivacaine > lidocaine > mepivacaine) tend to become sequestered in tissue and have a slower absorption, which produces lower blood levels. Agents with a greater volume of distribution or a faster clearance (etidocaine > lidocaine > mepivacaine > bupivacaine) also produce lower blood levels. These differences produce margins of safety for each anesthetic, with etidocaine having the greatest safety margin followed by bupivacaine, which is equal to or better than lidocaine.

Esters are difficult to measure in the blood because of their rapid hydrolysis by pseudocholinesterase. As a group,

				Excess Catecholamines, Anxiety[1] (endogenous), Vasoconstrictor
Findings	**Toxic Reactions**	**Allergy**	**Vasovagal***	**(exogenous)**
Relatively Specific Signs and Symptoms	Metallic taste Tongue numbness Drowsiness Nystagmus Slurred speech Seizures* Coma Respiratory arrest*	Acute rhinitis Pruritus* Dermatitis Urticaria* Facial swelling Laryngospasm Bronchospasm*	Syncope*[2]	Headache Hypertension* Palpitations Apprehension*[3]
Overlapping Signs and Symptoms	Paresthesia Lightheadedness Tinnitus Tremor Tachypnea Tachycardia (early) Bradycardia* Hypotension* Cardiac arrest	Lightheadedness Tachycardia* Hypotension* Cardiac arrest Nausea and vomiting Dyspnea	Lightheadedness Tinnitus Tachypnea Tachycardia (early) Bradycardia* Hypotension* Diaphoresis	Paresthesia* Lightheadedness* Tremor Tachypnea* Tachycardia* Nausea and vomiting Dyspnea Diaphoresis

Table 38–4. Differentiating Systemic Adverse Reactions

*Denotes common and significant reactions:
1. Anxiety reaction including hyperventilation syndrome.
2. Vasovagal syncope occurs with patient upright; any loss of consciousness in the recumbent position implies a severe toxic or anaphylactic reaction.
3. Although apprehension is classically associated with anxiety and vasoconstrictor reactions, milder toxic and allergic reactions may cause patient apprehension.

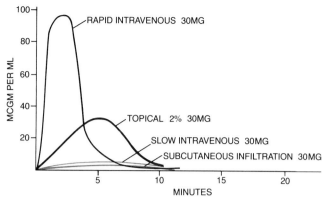

Figure 38–5. Comparison of blood levels obtained after rapid intravenous injection of 30 mg of tetracaine over a 30- to 60-second interval, after application topically to the pharyngeal mucous membranes, after subcutaneous infiltration, and after slow intravenous infusion. (From Adriani J, Campbell D: Fatalities following topical application of local anesthetics to mucous membranes. JAMA 162(17):1528, 1956. Copyright 1956, American Medical Association.)

toxicity is inversely proportional to the rate of hydrolysis, such that tetracaine is slowly hydrolyzed and hence most toxic, chloroprocaine is quickly hydrolyzed and least toxic, and procaine falls between the two.

Clearance. Amides are metabolized by the liver, in which the rate is a function of hepatic blood flow and extraction capacity of the liver. Decreased hepatic flow produced by norepinephrine, propranalol, or general anesthesia slows clearance and potentially raises drug blood levels. Decreased extraction, associated with congestive heart failure, cirrhosis, or hypothermia, likewise may produce a higher blood level. Hypovolemia, which decreases hepatic flow and hence clearance, does not raise blood levels because it causes an offsetting decrease in absorption.

Decreased clearance of esters, hence an increased risk for toxicity, occurs in patients with either low levels of pseudocholinesterase or atypical pseudocholinesterase. Low levels occur in various disease states, including severe liver disease and renal failure, and in pregnancy. Atypical pseudocholinesterase is an inherited trait, and its presence reduces the hydrolysis rate of procaine more than low levels do.

There are significant differences between the pediatric and adult population concerning drug distribution and metabolism. Neonates exhibit both reduced levels of pseudocholinesterase and reduced hepatic metabolism, thus increasing the risk of toxicity. For older children, the effect of an increased hepatic metabolism and a relatively larger volume of distribution increases their tolerance to higher doses.

Maximum Safe Dosage. Before one can appreciate this concept, the principles of dosage calculation must be understood (Table 38–5). The maximum safe dose for a drug may be defined as the dose that produces a blood level of the drug just below the toxic level. Based on the previous discussion, it is obvious that *one* maximum dose for each anesthetic cannot be stated, and that when a dose is given, it must be defined by the conditions under which it is used. There is no justification for basing a maximum safe dose on the weight of a patient. Many studies show that, in an adult, weight does not correlate with peak blood levels because the volume of the drug distribution is relatively constant.[43, 45, 46] However, there must be differences for children, whose body weights, excluding fat, are truly different from adults. Arthur and McNicol have recommended basing maximum dosages for children on weight as the simplest and safest

parameter.[47] Plain lidocaine may be used up to 4.5 mg/kg, whereas the addition of epinephrine allows for a maximum of 7 mg/kg. Bupivacaine is not recommended for children under the age of 12. It is important to modify the dose according to the site and mode of administration.

Maximum safe doses as stated in package inserts should be taken only as guidelines because (1) most of them are derived from animal experiments and are based on absorption data only; (2) they vary with site, use of a vasoconstrictor, and to some extent, with the state of the patient; (3) they can often be exceeded safely when accurately administered (bupivacaine with epinephrine has been shown to be safe in peripheral nerve blocks and local infiltration in doses up to 400 mg); and (4) they may be toxic even within the safe range when inadvertently injected intravenously.

Inadvertent Intravascular Injection. Most toxic reactions are caused by inadvertent intravenous anesthetic injection. In a patient with low cardiac output and hypovolemia, preferential cerebral blood flow can enhance central nervous system toxicity.

Anesthetics that are injected intravenously must pass through the lungs before they reach other organs. Lung tissue sequesters a significant amount of drug, which lowers the arterial blood concentration. Therefore, anesthetics that bypass the lungs—either in cases of inadvertent injection into the carotid or vertebral arteries or in patients with intracardiac right-to-left shunts—can produce central nervous system toxicity at low doses. Similarly, intra-arterial injections about the head or neck are capable of retrograde flow into the cerebral circulation if the injection pressure exceeds the arterial pressure. Because the blood volume in

Table 38–5. *Calculation of Anesthetic Doses*

Anesthetic solutions are marketed with drug concentration expressed as percentages (e.g., bupivacaine 0.25%, lidocaine 1%). To ascertain the strength of a solution, in milligrams per milliliter, consider the following:

A 1% solution is prepared by dissolving 1 gm of drug in 100 ml of solution.

Therefore, 1 gm/100 ml = 1000 mg/100 ml = 10 mg/ml.

To calculate the strength from the per cent quickly, simply move the decimal point one place to the right. Examples:

0.25% = 2.5 mg/ml	(e.g., bupivacaine)
0.5% = 5 mg/ml	(e.g., tetracaine)
1% = 10 mg/ml	(e.g., lidocaine)
2% = 20 mg/ml	(e.g., viscous lidocaine)
4% = 40 mg/ml	(e.g., cocaine)
5% = 50 mg/ml	(e.g., lidocaine ointment)
20% = 200 mg/ml	(e.g., benzocaine)

When combined in an anesthetic solution, epinephrine is usually in a 1:100,000 or 1:200,000 dilution.

1 ml of 1:1000 epinephrine = 1 mg.

0.1 ml of 1:1000 epinephrine in 10 ml anesthetic solution = 1:100,000 dilution = 0.010 mg/ml.

0.1 ml of 1:1000 epinephrine in 20 ml anesthetic solution = 1:200,000 dilution = 0.005 mg/ml.

Some examples of epinephrine content:

	1:100,000	1:200,000
5 ml	0.050 mg	0.025 mg
10 ml	0.100 mg	0.050 mg
20 ml	0.200 mg	0.100 mg

Therefore, 50 ml of 1% lidocaine with epinephrine 1:200,000 contains 500 mg lidocaine and 0.25 mg epinephrine.

the brain is only about 30 ml at any given moment, even 1 mg of lidocaine injected into the carotid artery can produce toxic concentrations.

Other Factors. There are several factors that influence the toxic potential of an anesthetic without increasing the blood levels.

HYPOXIA. In a 1960 review it was postulated that local anesthetic overdose produced central nervous system stimulation and subsequent intracellular hypoxia, which became the key precipitant to all toxic manifestations of the drug.[44] Since then, numerous studies have shown that hypoxia may enhance anesthetic toxicity but that it is not the primary factor.[48-50]

ACID-BASE STATUS. Although studies of metabolic alkalosis have produced conflicting results, acidosis, particularly respiratory, can increase toxicity. The elevated CO_2 produced by respiratory acidosis crosses the blood-brain barrier, where it may act directly on the receptor as well as indirectly by lowering intracellular pH. This latter property causes more drugs to ionize, furthering the block in the sodium channel, and increases toxic potential.

The mechanism whereby metabolic acidosis enhances toxicity is less understood, although it might alter end-organ sensitivity. Clinically, seizures associated with central nervous system toxicity lead to hypoxia, hypercapnia, and acidosis. The resulting cerebral lactic acidosis may affect drug ionization and enhance toxicity.

PROTEIN BINDING. Unbound drug concentration relates more closely to toxic effects than does total drug concentration (bound plus unbound) as measured in the blood. The amount of alpha-acid glycoprotein (AAG), the major plasma protein responsible for binding local anesthetics, is considerably decreased in neonates compared with the amount in adults, thereby allowing for a greater percentage of free drug. Arthur and McNicol imply that low AAG levels in neonates are responsible for an increased toxic potential.[47] Tucker lists several disease states that alter AAG levels and protein binding but questions whether they lead to changes in free drug concentration in vivo.[51]

CONCOMITANT DRUGS. For years, barbiturates were used prophylactically to prevent, and therapeutically to treat, local anesthetic-induced seizures. Although at least the latter purpose proved valid, barbiturates were found to worsen anesthetic-induced apnea and cardiovascular depression. Central nervous system depressants should be used with caution when concern exists for local anesthetic toxicity. Central nervous system stimulants have been shown to increase anesthetic-induced excitability and should be avoided. Mixtures of local anesthetics essentially have an additive effect on toxicity so that if two drugs are used at half strength, they produce the same degree of toxicity as if each was used alone at normal strength.

Recognition of Central Nervous System Toxicity. The earliest manifestation of systemic toxicity is central nervous system stimulation that is due to blockade of inhibitory synapses. Central nervous system depression follows and is produced by direct depression of the medulla, although hypoxia may play a role. Signs and symptoms are dose related, but it is difficult to provide exact correlations between clinical effects and blood levels because plasma or blood, arterial or venous measurements may be used. The increasing order of central nervous system toxicity with a representative plasma lidocaine concentration is numbness of tongue, lightheadedness, tinnitus (4 μg/ml), visual disturbances (6 μg/ml), muscle twitching (8 μg/ml), convulsions (10 μg/ml), coma (15 μg/ml), and apnea (20 μg/ml). Drowsiness, commonly seen at lower doses with lidocaine, is not associated with bupivacaine or etidocaine. Tetracaine may produce apnea or cardiovascular toxicity without central nervous system manifestations.

Recognition of Cardiovascular Toxicity. Moderate blood concentrations (e.g., lidocaine, 3 μg/ml) of local anesthetics produce slight increases in cardiac output, heart rate, and arterial pressure because of the effects of direct peripheral vasodilation and central nervous system stimulation. At concentrations generally well above the central nervous system toxicity levels, local anesthetics cause direct myocardial depression manifesting as hypotension and bradycardia, which can lead to cardiovascular collapse. These effects, like central nervous system toxicity, generally parallel potency, so that equianesthetic doses are approximately equitoxic.

In 1979, Albright brought attention to several cases of sudden cardiac arrest from bupivacaine and etidocaine and questioned whether hypoxia was the cause.[52] This led to a multitude of animal studies that confirmed that depression of myocardial contractility parallels potency but that depression of conduction velocity was disproportionately greater for bupivacaine and etidocaine.[48-50, 53-56] Slowed conduction appears to be responsible for these agents' conduction defects and blocks and, by creating the conditions for reentry, various supraventricular and potentially lethal ventricular dysrhythmias. Clinically, cardiovascular collapse from these effects may occur almost simultaneously with seizures, thereby decreasing the cardiovascular margin of safety for bupivacaine and etidocaine compared with that of lidocaine. Although hypoxia was not found to be the cause, both hypoxia and acidosis enhance this cardiotoxicity.

Prevention. Understanding the causes of a toxic reaction makes preventive measures obvious. Esters should be avoided in patients with an atypical or a quantitative deficiency of pseudocholinesterase. Amides should be used with caution in patients with severe liver disease or congestive heart failure. Maximum safe dosages based on site, technique, epinephrine use, and patient status must be adhered to, and lower doses should be used whenever possible. The addition of epinephrine is useful to decrease the absorption of an anesthetic when a large dose is needed in a highly vascular site, for example, with an intercostal block. Decreasing the drug concentration by adding normal saline may allow for the needed larger volume with multiple or extensive lacerations. Frequent aspiration should be performed in areas of high vascularity or whenever there is a risk of intravascular injection. However, in several series in which an inadvertent intravascular dose led to a toxic reaction, all described cases had negative aspirations before and after injection.[37, 52, 57, 58] Therefore, slow administration is indicated in high-risk situations even if aspiration is negative. Lastly, excessive injection pressures about the face or neck area must be avoided to prevent retrograde flow should an intra-arterial injection occur.

Treatment. No physician should perform local anesthesia without the ability to recognize and treat a toxic reaction; this includes having all necessary equipment and drugs readily available and being knowledgeable in their use. Despite taking all possible precautions, toxic reactions still occur, and maintaining rapport with the patient allows early detection and treatment.

Providing proper oxygenation and ventilation at the earliest sign of a reaction is the cornerstone of treatment. Patients who are alert should be encouraged to hyperventilate to lower the P_{CO_2} and raise the seizure threshold. Likewise, for patients who cannot adequately ventilate, intubation with high-flow oxygen and hyperventilation should be performed. An intravenous line should be started, and vital signs and cardiac rhythm should be monitored closely.

Seizures are generally self-limited but should be treated

if they persist or prevent adequate ventilation. Because respiratory depression secondary to toxicity may follow, low-dose diazepam, 2 to 5 mg, or an ultra–short-acting barbiturate (thiopental or sodium methohexital) is preferred. For seizures that persist, a paralyzing agent is recommended to ensure an effective airway and prevent further lactic acidosis. If toxicity is caused by an ester, especially if there is an associated pseudocholinesterase problem, succinylcholine will compete with the anesthetic and increase the toxicity of both compounds.

Cardiovascular toxicity manifesting as hypotension and bradycardia should be treated with fluids, leg elevation, α and β agonists (epinephrine, ephedrine, or dopamine), or atropine as the need dictates.

Although lidocaine (with diazepam pretreatment) has been shown to be effective for bupivacaine-induced ventricular dysrhythmias, deJong and Davis[59] and Kasten and Martin provide strong theoretic and experimental evidence that bretylium is the drug of choice.[60–61] They also demonstrated that high doses of atropine and epinephrine were successful in correcting pulseless idioventricular rhythm. Cardiopulmonary resuscitation, of course, should be instituted when necessary.

ALLERGIC REACTIONS

Although true allergic reactions amount to only 1 to 2 per cent of all adverse reactions, they are important to recognize because of their serious potential. Esters, specifically the metabolite para-aminobenzoic acid (PABA), account for the great majority of these reactions. Amide solutions are rarely involved, and it is usually the preservative methylparaben (MPB), which is structurally similar to PABA, that is responsible. Hence, although pure esters and pure amides do not cross-react, amides may appear to do so if multidose vials containing MPB are used. Also, patients may manifest an allergic response on first contact to a local anesthetic because of previous sensitization to MPB, which is found in creams, ointments, and various cosmetics, or to PABA, which is an ingredient in many sunscreen preparations.

Although cell-mediated delayed reactions manifesting as dermatitis may occur, it is immediate hypersensitivity that most concerns the emergency physician. A spectrum of signs and symptoms may occur from rhinitis and mild urticaria to bronchospasm and upper airway edema to full-blown anaphylactic shock. Onset may be immediate, at times even occurring during administration of the agent. Diphenhydramine and epinephrine are useful for mild urticaria and bronchospasms, respectively. Intravenous epinephrine, hydrocortisone, and diphenhydramine may be required for more serious reactions.

The more frequent problem facing emergency physicians is the management of the patient who claims to have a past history of local anesthetic allergy. Indeed, most patients, as well as their physicians, tend to blame any adverse reaction to a local anesthetic procedure on an allergy. Because allergy is rarely the cause, a careful history and review of prior records, if available, become crucial in evaluating these patients. The history should attempt to uncover the actual cause of the past reaction and the specific agent involved. Inquiry should be made concerning the exact signs and symptoms, technique of administration, amount of drug used, and how the patient was treated. If an allergic reaction was present or cannot be ruled out and the drug is known, it is often recommended to use an agent from the other class. Lidocaine from a dental cartridge does not contain MPB, and if this were the allergenic source, then an ester could be used. However, if lidocaine from a multidose vial is implicated, one should not use an ester, because

MPB may cross-react with PABA. In this case, it may be safer to use an amide without MPB or to choose an alternative listed later. In most cases, the allergen is an ester, and the patient can safely be given an amide without MPB. Single-dose ampules of lidocaine, readily obtainable from a resuscitation cart, can be used for this purpose.

Usually, however, uncertainty exists regarding the specific agent involved, and the physician must choose an alternative approach to management. If the wounds are extensive and the risk is acceptable, general anesthesia may be used; conversely, if minimal pain is expected and the procedure is short (e.g., one or two sutures or staples in the scalp), no anesthesia may be required. Other alternatives include parenteral narcotics, benzodiazepines, nitrous oxide inhalation, or a combination of these. These methods may be useful, but the degree of anesthesia produced is often not sufficient. Antihistamines injected into a wound have been successfully used for many years and represent a good alternative. Local anesthetic property is found in varying degrees in all antihistamines. Early work showed 1 per cent tripelennamine (Pyribenzamine) to produce a rapid onset, to be of long duration, and, except for occasional local irritation and sedation, to be free of significant systemic toxicity. More potent and longer acting than procaine, it had an excellent success rate with both peripheral nerve blocks and local infiltration. Unfortunately, tripelennamine is no longer marketed in a parenteral form. Although less effective, diphenhydramine (Benadryl) can be used for local infiltration but may be too irritating for peripheral nerve blocks. Importantly, if diphenhydramine is used, the standard 5 per cent parenteral form should be diluted to 1 per cent for subcutaneous injection (1 ml drug:4 ml saline).[62]

Skin testing and progressive subcutaneous challenge doses deserve special mention because they appear to be logical and well-studied approaches. Intradermal skin testing with local anesthetics is, at best, controversial. False-positive results are frequently produced by local histamine release secondary to needle trauma, tissue distention, or preservatives in the solution.[63–66] Considering the high false-positive rate, a negative test may be useful. However, other investigators claim a high incidence of false-negative results and question whether these low-molecular-weight drugs or their allergenic metabolites are ever capable of eliciting positive responses.[67–68] Other disadvantages of skin testing include its time-consuming nature when it is performed properly and its potential hazard when even minute traces of an allergen may precipitate a serious reaction. Subcutaneous challenge testing in graduating doses has been advocated, and it may well eliminate many false responses, but it does not eliminate the problems of time and hazard.[63, 65] Swanson, recognizing that it is extremely rare for allergy to occur to pure lidocaine, recommends 0.1 ml as a one-shot intradermal skin test.[67] Although his approach eliminates the time disadvantage, the intradermal placement can still produce false responses. It would seem more reasonable to give this test dose subcutaneously while exercising due caution in the unlikely event that a patient exhibits a serious reaction.

Practically speaking the optimal approach is to determine the specific anesthetic that caused a definite or presumed allergic reaction and then use a preservative-free agent from the other class (see exception discussed earlier). If the agent is unknown, either use an antihistamine or give 0.1 ml of preservative-free lidocaine as a subcutaneous test dose, proceeding with the full dose if no reaction occurs within 30 minutes.

CATECHOLAMINE REACTIONS

Anxiety and vasoconstrictor (epinephrine) reactions are discussed together because each produces similar manifestations that are related to elevated catecholamine levels. These reactions, which are difficult to distinguish from each other, are relatively common, although generally not serious.

Excess catecholamine levels produce tachycardia, palpitations, hypertension, apprehension, tremulousness, diaphoresis, tachypnea, pallor, and, on occasion, anginal chest pain. Thus catecholamine excess may resemble the central nervous system stimulation phase of local anesthetic toxicity.

Catecholamine reactions are usually not caused solely by exogenous epinephrine, because if it is used in its optimal concentration (1:200,000), the maximum safe dose (0.25 mg) is rarely exceeded. However, many patients produce significant endogenous catecholamines secondary to anxiety about the upcoming procedure. In this case, even the addition of small amounts of epinephrine could trigger a catecholamine reaction. Therefore, patient preparation should include proper explanation and reassurance to decrease anxiety. Caution should also be exercised in patients on monoamine oxidase inhibitors and in those who have hyperthyroidism, hypertension, or atherosclerotic cardiovascular disease.

Treatment includes stopping further drug administration, close observation, and administering α or β antagonists, if necessary, to combat severe reactions.

VASOVAGAL REACTIONS

Vasovagal reactions are not uncommon, especially in dental procedures (reported at 2 to 3 per cent), during which the patient is generally in an upright position. The patient initially experiences anxiety when a triggering event, commonly the sight or sensation of needle insertion, causes a loss of sympathetic tone and an increase in vagal tone. The resultant hypotension and bradycardia may lead to syncope. Preparation to decrease patient anxiety and *administration of injections with the patient recumbent* are useful preventative measures. Concomitant cardiac monitoring may also help identify the onset of vagally induced bradycardia when suggested by past history. Treatment consists of laying the patient flat and elevating the legs. Should a patient lose consciousness while in a recumbent position, a diagnosis other than vasovagal syncope must be considered.

MISCELLANEOUS REACTIONS

Malignant Hyperthermia. There is some concern that amides may produce malignant hyperthermia in susceptible individuals. It is recommended that esters be used in lieu of amides in patients from families with this genetic abnormality.

Methemoglobinemia. Despite an excellent safety margin and the fact that many consider it to be the agent of choice for intravenous regional anesthesia, prilocaine has declined in popularity recently because of its ability to cause methemoglobinemia.[51, 68, 69] The effect is seen when cumulative or single doses exceed 600 mg. In large doses lidocaine may also produce methemoglobinemia.

Benzocaine, a common ingredient in several over-the-counter and prescription topical anesthetics, is well known to produce methemoglobinemia.[70-72] Although this reaction is infrequent and may occur secondary to a heterozygote enzyme deficiency, it is also known to occur with excessive topical or subcutaneous application in normal individuals, especially children.

TOPICAL ANESTHESIA

Local anesthetic agents may be applied topically to mucous membranes, skin, and lacerations. There are sufficient differences among these sites to merit a separate discussion of each. Topical anesthesia of the eye is discussed in Chapter 85.

Mucous Membranes

Effective anesthesia of the intact mucous membranes of the nose, mouth, throat, tracheobronchial tree, esophagus, and genitourinary tract may be provided by several anesthetics, although tetracaine, lidocaine, and cocaine are the most effective and commonly used agents (Table 38-6). For intraoral or pharyngeal anesthesia, benzocaine (14 to 20 per cent) is commonly used. The anesthesia produced is superficial and does not relieve pain that originates from submucosal structures.

Tetracaine solution is a very effective and potent topical agent with a relatively long duration of action. It may be used in concentrations from 0.25 to 1 per cent with a maximum safe dose of 50 mg. However, it has the disadvantage of high toxicity, especially the likelihood of severe cardiovascular toxicity without a warning central nervous system stimulatory phase. Lidocaine is also an effective topical agent that is marketed in a variety of forms (solutions, jelly, ointments) and concentrations (2 to 10 per cent). It is perhaps most familiar to emergency physicians as the 2 per cent viscous solution prescribed for inflamed or irritated mucous membranes of the mouth and pharynx. The advantage of familiarity should not obscure the fact that misuse can lead to serious toxicity (see subsequent discussion). Topical lidocaine provides an adequate duration for most procedures, with a maximum safe dose of 200 to 300 mg.

Cocaine is an effective, albeit potentially toxic topical agent. Its use is limited to mucous membrane anesthesia of the upper respiratory tract. Although it is an ester, hepatic metabolism occurs as well as hydrolysis by plasma pseudocholinesterase. Cocaine is the only anesthetic that produces vasoconstriction at clinically useful concentrations. This major advantage is offset by its susceptibility to abuse and its toxic potential. Absorption is enhanced in the presence of inflammation. Toxicity occurs as a result of both stimulating the central nervous system directly and blocking norepinephrine reuptake in the periphery. It should not be ad-

Table 38-6. Practical Agents for Emergency Department Use—Mucosal Application

Agent	Usual Concentration (%)	Maximum Dosage*		Onset (min)	Duration (min)
		Adult (mg)	Pediatric (mg/kg)		
Tetracaine	0.5	50	0.75	3–8	30–60
Lidocaine	2–10	250–300†	3–4†	2–5	15–45
Cocaine	4	200	2–3†	2–5	30–45

*These are maximum figures; see text for explanations.
†Recommend the lower dosage for a maximum safe dose when feasible.

ministered to patients who are sensitive to exogenous catecholamines. Clinical manifestations include central nervous system excitement that culminates in seizures and hyperthermia plus central and peripheral effects that result in hypertension, tachycardia, and ventricular arrhythmias. Acute myocardial infarction has been reported secondary to topical application.[73] Cocaine is commonly used as a 4 per cent solution with a maximum (though variable and controversial) safe dose of 200 mg (2 to 3 mg/kg). Coronary vasoconstriction may occur with a 2 mg/kg dose applied to the nasal mucosa. Cocaine should not be administered topically in patients with coronary artery disease.

Among other topical anesthetic agents, dyclonine and benzocaine offer distinct advantages. Dyclonine is a ketone derivative without an ester or amide linkage and therefore may be useful in patients who are allergic to the common anesthetics. Extensive experience with the topical preparation has shown it to be effective and safe.[70] Dyclonine is marketed in 0.5 and 1.0 per cent solutions, with maximum safe doses of 300 mg.

Benzocaine is an ester that is marketed only in its neutral form and is available in a 14 to 20 per cent preparation (Cetacaine, Americaine, Hurricaine). Its low water solubility prevents significant penetration of the mucous membranes, making it essentially nontoxic systemically if it is applied to the *intact* mucosa. However, it is not a potent anesthetic; it has a brief duration; and, compared with other topicals, it is more allergenic. Benzocaine is usually dispensed in an admixture with other therapeutic ingredients and is clinically effective only at relatively high (greater than 14 per cent) concentrations. Benzocaine is available as a nonprescription gel and liquid (Anbesol, 6.3 to 20 per cent) and is commonly used topically by dentists to produce mucosal anesthesia before intraoral nerve blocks (see Chapter 39). Adriani and Zepernick recommend this agent for lubricating catheters, airways, endotracheal tubes, and laryngoscopes.[70] In their experience with approximately 150,000 patients, only one adverse reaction occurred: methemoglobinemia.

Similar to reactions to infiltration anesthesia, toxic reactions to topically applied anesthetics correlate with the peak blood levels that were actually achieved and not necessarily the dose that was administered. Compared with infiltration, systemic absorption is more rapid with topical agents (see Fig. 38–5); therefore the total dose for a topical anesthetic should be considerably less than that for infiltration at a given site. Fractionating the total dose into three portions over several minutes effectively reduces peak blood levels.

An important potential adverse reaction with topical anesthesia of the nose, mouth, and pharynx is that inadvertent suppression of the gag reflex combined with difficulty swallowing may lead to aspiration. The danger of infection with the use of solutions from multidose vials when applied to the larynx and trachea has not been substantiated.

Specific Considerations

Oral Lesions and Pharyngitis. Emergency physicians often prescribe 2 per cent viscous lidocaine for patients with pharyngitis, stomatitis, dental pain, or other inflammatory or irritative lesions in the oropharynx. The common misconception that topical anesthesia is relatively innocuous often results in poor patient instruction, which may have serious consequences. Several reports of seizures and death from topical lidocaine exist in the literature.[74–78] Toxic blood levels may occur for several reasons: (1) the anesthetic effect of viscous lidocaine lasts only for 30 to 60 minutes, and patients with recurrent pain may either ignore or be ignorant of the safe dosing interval of 3 hours and medicate themselves more frequently; (2) patients tend to increase each dose to obtain greater relief; and (3) inflammation may increase

systemic absorption. In addition, painful oral lesions may last for several days. Continued medication use allows not only the lidocaine but also its major metabolites monoethylglycinexylidide (MEGX) and glycinexylidide (GX) to accumulate. Both MEGX and GX are produced from hepatic metabolism of lidocaine and are excreted in the urine. They possess anesthetic and antiarrhythmic activity and have central nervous system toxicity potential. Although these metabolites are less potent than lidocaine, their elimination half-lives, especially that of GX, are considerably longer. Therefore, prolonged use of lidocaine, especially in patients with renal dysfunction, may lead to a toxic buildup of these metabolites. In their case reports, several investigators regard MEGX and GX to be the causes of central nervous system toxicity.[76, 77]

The length of time viscous lidocaine is retained in the mouth and whether the excess is expectorated or swallowed also affect the blood level produced. When lidocaine is absorbed through the oral mucosa, it reaches the brain before entering the liver for extraction. If the excess is expectorated, it is reasonable to assume that less agent is absorbed. When swallowed, lidocaine not only is absorbed more slowly from gastric than from oral mucosa but travels directly to the liver for high first-pass extraction and metabolism. Only 30 to 35 per cent is then systemically bioavailable, although one would expect earlier peak levels of metabolites. Greenblatt and colleagues studied plasma concentrations of lidocaine, MEGX, and GX in healthy volunteers who were given maximum safe doses of viscous lidocaine every 3 hours for eight doses.[79] Each participant used the solution three ways: swish and spit, swish and swallow, and swallow. Expectorating the medication produced much lower blood levels than either swallowing method. As expected, swallowing led to higher levels of MEGX than of lidocaine. Each technique produced levels well below the toxic range, but these volunteers did not have any oral lesions, which would enhance absorption. Although not tested, it seems logical that the most hazardous mode of administration would be to retain the solution "until absorbed" in the mouth.

Physicians must explain clearly the proper way to use viscous lidocaine and inform patients *not to dose themselves ad libitum.* The maximum safe dose for most adults is 300 mg (15 ml of a 2 per cent solution) no more frequently than every 3 hours. When possible, the patient should decrease the dose by using direct cotton swab applications. When gargled or swished in the mouth, application time should be limited to 1 to 2 minutes, and the excess solution should be expectorated. It is reasonable to limit use to 2 or 3 days, especially if swallowing the solution is necessary to obtain relief. Lower doses should be prescribed for patients who have risk factors for decreased clearance (see section on systemic toxicity). Doses for children should be based on weight. Because infants cannot expectorate well, *viscous lidocaine should not be given for minor oral irritation and teething.* Because anesthesia of the oropharynx can interfere with swallowing and cause aspiration, it is recommended that no food be eaten for 1 hour after application. Special note should be made of the over-the-counter availability of benzocaine, commonly used for toothaches and teething. A gel or liquid (Anbesol) is available in a 6.3 to 20 per cent formulation. When used repeatedly in the oral cavity on irritated tissue, significant absorption may occur, and systemic toxicity, often in the form of methemoglobinemia, may result.

Skin

Although saturated solutions of the bases of local anesthetics are effective on intact skin, the stratum corneum provides a cutaneous barrier that prevents the commonly marketed aqueous solutions (acid salts) from producing anesthesia.

Acid salt preparations are ineffective in first- and second-degree burns. However, studies show that by stripping the stratum corneum, acid salts can produce anesthesia[80] and that when the skin is abraded or deep burns are exposed by debriding blisters or removing eschars, detectable blood levels of these salts occur.[81] Anesthesia topically applied to abraded skin results in peak blood levels similar to those in infiltration (therefore less than mucosal) in 6 to 10 minutes.

Specific Considerations

Myringotomy and Aural Foreign Bodies. In the emergency department, anesthesia of the external auditory canal and tympanic membrane is indicated for the difficult-to-remove foreign body that is embedded deep in the canal and for the occasional myringotomy. Unattractive options for pain relief are general anesthesia and local infiltration of ear canal skin. General anesthesia may be potentially hazardous, especially in a patient who has just eaten, and local infiltration may prove to be more painful than the procedure to be performed. Many otolaryngologists perform myringotomies on adults or infants without any anesthesia. Fortunately, there are two current methods of topical anesthesia that may be helpful.

PHENOL. Bonain solution (phenol, menthol, cocaine), first introduced in 1898, has been the most commonly used topical anesthesia for the tympanic membrane. Various modifications of the original solution led to the conclusion that phenol was the primary anesthetic in this mixture. Liquified phenol (crystals plus 10 per cent water) is applied in the following manner: a small wisp of cotton attached to a thin metal probe is soaked in the solution, and the excess is squeezed back into a medicine cup; through a speculum, the cotton is gently touched to the proposed incision site; blanching indicates anesthesia.

The major argument against the use of phenol is that it is caustic and might lead to tympanic membrane necrosis with permanent perforation, vestibulocochlear damage, or destructive changes in the middle ear. The very fact that phenol is caustic and alters the intact epithelial surface of the tympanic membrane makes it an effective topical anesthetic. A large amount of clinical experience over many years has shown phenol to be safe if the application technique is performed as described previously. Any excess phenol that enters the middle ear is effectively neutralized by secretory effusions or pus, thereby blocking any destructive action on the mucosa that might occur. Practical drawbacks include pain on application and questioned efficacy in an infected ear. Phenol is not indicated for canal anesthesia. It is contraindicated in nervous patients who cannot tolerate the speculum or the initial pain of application.

TETRACAINE BASE. Tetracaine base is an effective, safe, and practical way to anesthetize the tympanic membrane. Drawbacks include its ineffectiveness in patients with acute otitis media and its relatively long application time of 20 minutes. It is also contraindicated for use in perforated ear drums because of the danger of increased absorption and systemic toxicity. Although the literature describes its use for myringotomy in chronic serous otitis media, it is a good alternative in foreign body removal.

The technique of application involves placing the patient in a supine position and turning the head to the side. The canal is cleared, and the tympanic membrane is inspected to ensure that there is no perforation; 80 mg of tetracaine base powder is dissolved in 8 to 10 drops of 70 per cent isopropyl alcohol, and the solution is placed in the canal to fully cover the tympanic membrane. A cotton plug covered with pet-rolatum jelly is placed in the canal; after 20 minutes, the cotton is removed and the solution is aspirated.

Anesthetic Patch. For many years, Lubens and coworkers have used 30 per cent lidocaine cream, saturated on a gauze pad adherent to an elastic patch, for a myriad of procedures.[82] Both the high concentration of anesthetic and the occlusive nature of the patch are necessary to achieve greater skin penetration. The duration of action varies with the application time. For most procedures, a 45-minute application time is minimum; to achieve a duration of one-half hour, a 2-hour application is necessary. Despite its effectiveness, safety, and painless application, the practicality of use in an emergency setting is doubtful. However, Lubens and colleagues report an impressive list of uses, including minor operative procedures (e.g., excision of lesions, incision and drainage of abscesses), lumbar puncture, venipuncture, and allergy testing.[82] In many of these procedures, duration of effect need not be long, so the shorter application time may be used.

Anesthetic Sprays. Ethyl chloride spray is a commonly used topical agent for abscess incision. It is highly volatile and when sprayed onto skin evaporates with cooling to the point of freezing. Anesthesia is effective and immediate, but drawbacks include duration only up to 1 minute, potential pain on thawing, and possible lowered resistance to infection and delayed healing. Inhalation may produce general anesthesia, coma, or cardiorespiratory arrest. Ethyl chloride is also flammable, which precludes its use with electrocautery. The technique of application is that the inverted bottle is held 25 cm from the skin and a stream of spray is directed along the proposed incision until the area turns white and hard. An incision must be made immediately because the effect may be fleeting.

Lacerations

Topical Anesthesia for Wound Repair—TAC. In 1980, prompted by their experience with a topical anesthetic solution for wound repair and the paucity of literature on the subject, Pryor and colleagues investigated the use of TAC in comparison with lidocaine infiltration.[28] Thus began a decade of controversy concerning the efficacy and safety of this compound. The original formula, used in most subsequent studies, consists of a solution of 0.5 per cent tetracaine, 1:2000 adrenaline, and 11.8 per cent cocaine. Anesthesia is produced by firmly applying a saturated gauze pad or cotton ball directly to the laceration for 10 minutes; the resulting loss of sensation is confined to the area of application.

Anesthetic Effectiveness. Three clinical trials directly compared TAC with infiltrative lidocaine. Without specifying wound location, Pryor's group found equal anesthetic effect.[28] Complete anesthesia produced by TAC ranged from 82 to 86 per cent, compared with 83 to 92 per cent for subcutaneous lidocaine. The remaining patients obtained partial anesthesia. Hegenbarth and coworkers and Anderson and associates demonstrated results similar to those of Pryor and colleagues.[34, 35] However, whereas Anderson's group found no significant difference based on location, Hegenbarth and colleagues found TAC equal to lidocaine only on the face and scalp but inferior at other locations. Although the results are difficult to compare because of different study designs, other investigators who examined TAC demonstrated effectiveness equal to or slightly less than that found by Pryor and associates.[29–33]

Concerned about potential toxic effects and theoretic vasoconstrictor-induced higher infection rates, several investigators compared TAC with its various components.[29, 30, 32, 33]

On the face and scalp, TAC was found to be superior to tetracaine alone, although on nonfacial areas both produced equally poor results. TAC was also shown to be more effective than cocaine alone. Ross and associates believe that tetracaine and adrenaline with a higher concentration of tetracaine may be preferable to TAC because it provides nearly equal efficacy and avoids the high cost and negative public perception of cocaine.[32] Noting that the initial component concentration of TAC was arbitrary, Bonadio and Wagner studied TAC at one half the conventional concentration (0.25 per cent tetracaine, 1:4000 adrenaline, and 5.9 per cent cocaine) and achieved excellent results for dermal lacerations of the face, lip, and scalp.[31]

The clinical experience of some researchers that TAC seemed more effective on the face and scalp than on the extremities or trunk was confirmed by White and colleagues and Hegenbarth and coworkers, although later studies do not support this contention.[30, 33, 34, 35] Results of studies that compared adults with younger age groups support Schaffer's clinical impression that TAC appears to be more effective in children.[28, 29, 30, 32]

Advantages and Disadvantages. Compared with infiltrative anesthesia, advantages of TAC include painless application, no distortion of wound margins, good hemostasis, patient and parental acceptance in the pediatric age group, and a shorter repair time in the 1- to- 5-year-old age group.

As compelling as the case for TAC may appear, some disadvantages have made its acceptance less than unanimous. TAC may be less effective on the trunk and extremities than on the face and scalp and less effective than lidocaine infiltration in these areas. Another drawback to TAC is that several protocols propose wound preparation be done before anesthetic application. Preparation would likely be painful and therefore incomplete. Proper cleansing of traumatic injuries and surgical debridement cannot be accomplished without some form of local anesthesia.

Two other oft-mentioned drawbacks may be more theoretic than real. The previously discussed issue of vasoconstrictor-induced higher infection rates (see "Local Anesthetic Effect on Wounds") has not been borne out clinically. Also, the argument that the necessary 10-minute application period is time consuming and takes valuable nursing time is partially offset by studies that effectively used the child's caretaker or paper tape alone to hold the solution in place.[29, 31, 83]

Precautions. TAC is not an innocuous anesthetic, and specific attention must be paid to technique of application and maximum safe dose. Specifically, mucosal application may lead to significant systemic toxicity. Although blood level studies with TAC have not been done, it is known that anesthetic absorption into the circulation from abraded skin is comparable to that from subcutaneous infiltration, both of which are considerably less than the amount from mucosal absorption. Based on the known maximal safe dose of infiltrative tetracaine and mucosal application of cocaine and an estimate of solution absorption onto the applicator, Hegenbarth's group calculated the maximal safe dose of full-strength TAC to be 0.09 ml/kg.[34] The key to safety is to *avoid TAC on mucosal surfaces or in areas in which sniffing or swallowing may accidentally occur.* A case fatality secondary to mucosal application has been reported.[84]

Ischemic complications from applying vasoconstrictors to tissues containing end arteries may occur. Therefore, TAC should be avoided on the digits, tip of nose, penis, and pinna.

Clinical Use. The use of TAC appears to be most effective for facial and scalp lacerations in children when painless application is desirable. It is necessary to heed the precautions mentioned and to ensure that wound preparation is not more painful than needle infiltration would be.

The half-strength TAC solution and the technique of Bonadio and Wagner[31] seem most appropriate: the wound is placed in a gravity-dependent position, and TAC is instilled to fill the wound cavity; after 3 minutes, a single 2-cm by 2-cm gauze pad or cotton ball saturated with TAC is applied to the wound; the pad should be taped and the caretaker should hold it firmly for 10 to 15 minutes. The average dose needed is 2 ml. Adherence to the volume limit of Hegenbarth and colleagues is recommended.[34]

INFILTRATION ANESTHESIA

Infiltration anesthesia involves injection of an anesthetic agent directly into the tissue to be manipulated surgically. Field block anesthesia may also be considered a form of infiltration anesthesia, particularly because the useful agents, concentrations, and maximum safe dosages are the same. A field block involves a subcutaneous injection of an agent in such a manner as to create a field of anesthesia around the operative site. The injection is made proximal to or surrounding the area to be manipulated.

Infiltration anesthesia is indicated whenever good operative conditions can be obtained by using this technique. It may be used for the majority of minor surgical procedures, such as the excision of tumors, incision of abscesses, and suturing of wounds. It should be avoided for more major procedures in small children and in apprehensive patients, especially those with prior adverse reactions.

An advantage of infiltration over nerve block and general anesthesia is that it is considered both quicker and safer. Local infiltration can also provide hemostasis, both by direct distention of tissue and by the use of epinephrine. The major disadvantage is that compared with nerve blocks, a relatively large dose of drug is needed to anesthetize a relatively small area. For extensive wounds, the amount of anesthetic required may risk systemic toxicity. However, the maximum allowable volume can be increased by adding epinephrine, by using a lower concentration of anesthetic agent, or by doing both (Table 38–7). If anatomically feasible, a nerve block may be preferred.

Choice of Agent

Local anesthetic agents most frequently used for infiltration are 0.5 to 1.0 per cent lidocaine, 0.5 to 1.0 per cent procaine, and 0.25 per cent bupivacaine (Table 38–8). Lidocaine has been the agent most commonly used because of its excellent activity profile, low allergenicity and toxicity, familiarity, and ready availability. Procaine is useful for patients who are allergic to amide anesthetics. Because of its

Table 38–7. *Maximum Allowable Volume (Adults)*

Agent	Concentration (%)	Maximum* Safe Dose (mg)	Maximum Volume (ml)
Lidocaine	0.5	300	60
	1.0	300	30
Bupivacaine	0.25	175	70
Lidocaine-epinephrine	0.5	500	100
	1.0	500	50
Bupivacaine-epinephrine	0.25	225	90
Bupivacaine	0.25	400	160

*Some physicians recommend 400 mg as the maximum safe dose for bupivacaine.

Table 38–8. Practical Agents for Emergency Department Use—Local Infiltration

Agent	Concentration (%)	Maximum Dose*† Adult (mg)	Maximum Dose*† Pediatric (mg/kg)	Onset (min)	Duration‡
Procaine	0.5–1.0	500§ (600)	7 (9)	2–5	15–45 min
Lidocaine	0.5–1.0	300 (500)	4.5 (7)‖	2–5	1–2 hr
Bupivacaine	0.25	175 (225)	2 (3)¶	2–5	4–8 hr

*These are conservative figures; see text for explanation.
†Higher dose for solutions containing epinephrine is in parentheses.
‡These values are for the agent alone; they can be extended considerably with the addition of epinephrine.
§Some authorities recommend up to 1000 mg or 14 mg/kg for procaine.
‖Some authorities recommend up to 7 mg/kg for plain lidocaine in children older than 1 year.
¶Because of lack of experience, drug companies do not recommend the use of bupivacaine in children under the age of 12 years.

prolonged duration, bupivacaine is considered by some physicians to be the preferred anesthetic, especially when postoperative analgesia is desired, for prolonged procedures or even for short procedures that may be interrupted in a busy emergency department.

A comparison of equianesthetic doses of lidocaine and bupivacaine for infiltration anesthesia (Table 38–9) reveals that the duration of action is the major difference between the two agents. For the majority of emergency department procedures, it is not necessary to extend the duration of anesthesia beyond 1 hour. Plain lidocaine would therefore seem to be a logical choice of agent. However, an interesting clinical study of lacerations has shown that after repair, patients do experience a moderate amount of pain after the lidocaine wears off in about 1 hour.[85] Bupivacaine was demonstrated to reduce the pain significantly for at least 6 hours.

Although a prolonged duration of anesthesia may pose hazards of injury to an unprotected limb or be an unwarranted annoyance to patients who have had simple surgical procedures, there are many instances in which such an extended duration is desirable (e.g., abscess drainage). Common methods of providing a prolonged duration of the anesthesia include adding epinephrine, sodium bicarbonate, or both (see section on duration) to lidocaine or by using bupivacaine. Advantages of epinephrine are that it provides excellent wound hemostasis and slows systemic absorption. The resulting decreased peak blood level decreases the potential for a toxic reaction or, conversely, allows a greater volume of agent to be used for extensive lacerations. The major disadvantage of epinephrine is the theoretic damage to host defenses (Table 38–10). Adding bicarbonate decreases the pain of administration, but such an addition entails bedside preparation (see subsequent discussion). Bupivacaine, if used with due caution (see "Adverse Reactions"), is safe and easy to use. The deciding factors are many, but some logical choices would be the following: (1) for a wound with excessive bleeding—lidocaine with epinephrine; (2) for an apprehensive patient—lidocaine with sodium bicarbonate; (3) for anticipated prolonged postprocedure pain—bupivacaine.

Proper Technique

Once an agent has been chosen, proper technique of administration should be used to minimize pain, prevent bacterial spread, and avoid intravascular injection.

Minimizing Pain. For a given anesthetic agent, lowering the pH by adding epinephrine increases pain, whereas raising the pH by adding sodium bicarbonate decreases pain dramatically. However, it is probable that pH per se is not the sole factor. It has been shown that the pain produced by various agents does not correlate strictly with the pH. For instance, although bupivacaine pH 5.5 is more painful than lidocaine pH 6.5, chloroprocaine pH 3.4 is less painful than bupivacaine, and procaine pH 4.3 is less painful than lidocaine. Sodium bicarbonate probably works by increasing the ratio of nonionized to ionized molecules, rendering the pain receptors less sensitive to the solution, or by producing a more rapid inhibition of pain transmission. To use this technique with lidocaine, 1 ml of sodium bicarbonate (8.4 per cent, 1 mEq/ml) is added to every 10 ml of anesthetic solution.[86] The mixture should be prepared immediately before use to avoid the decreased shelf life associated with an increased ratio of nonionized to ionized drug. Bicarbonate in small quantities can cause delayed or rapid precipitation of bupivacaine and should not be used with this anesthetic unless rapid use prior to precipitation can be assured.[86a]

Several aspects of technique should be standard for any infiltration anesthesia. Because the ability to aspirate blood is not dependent on needle gauge size and needle pliability is not critical for infiltration technique, a 30-gauge needle

Table 38–9. Comparison of 1% Lidocaine and 0.25% Bupivacaine—Infiltration Anesthesia

	Lidocaine (L)	Bupivacaine (B)	Advantage
Onset	2–5 min	2–5 min	Equal
Effectiveness (equianesthetic dose)	Excellent	Excellent	Equal
Duration	1–2 hr	4–6 hr	B
Infection potential	No	No	Equal
Administration pain	Less	More	L
Maximum volume*—plain	Less	More	B
Maximum volume—epinephrine	Less	More	B
Toxic potential	Less cardiotoxic; equal CNS	More cardiotoxic; equal CNS	L

*See Table 38–7 for volume and concentration comparison.
CNS, central nervous system.

Table 38–10. Epinephrine Use

Advantages	Disadvantages
1. Prolongs duration	1. Impairs host defenses—increases infection
2. Provides hemostasis	2. Delays wound healing
3. Slows absorption: (A) Decreases agent toxic potential (B) Allows increased dose	3. Do not use for: (A) Areas supplied by end-arteries (B) Patients "sensitive" to catecholamines
4. Increases level of blockade	4. Toxicity—catecholamine reaction

should be used if injection is made through the skin because it produces significantly less pain than a larger size needle. If, as in most cases, injection is made through the cut edges of the wound, a 27-gauge needle should suffice. The rate of injection is also slowed by a smaller gauge needle, which helps prevent the tissue distention that is a factor in pain production. A 10-ml syringe is recommended both for its ease of handling and for the relatively slow rate of injection it allows. Placement of the injection should be subdermal to minimize needle puncture pain and the tissue distention that occurs with intradermal placement. Placing the needle "up to the hub" and injecting while withdrawing along the just-created subdermal tunnel also minimizes distention. After an initial injection, rather than totally withdrawing from the skin, the needle should be redirected along another path, if practical, to lessen the number of punctures. Slowly injecting the smallest volume necessary also helps to reduce pain. Contrary to earlier notions, warming the solution does not seem to affect pain production.

Preventing Bacterial Spread. Because the patient barely feels a needle placed subcutaneously, and skin puncture is quite painful, *all injections should be made through the wound edge and not via a skin puncture.* Concern about spreading infection by passing a needle through a fresh wound edge has not been substantiated clinically. In the case of a grossly contaminated wound, however, it is reasonable to consider injecting the anesthetic through intact skin.

Avoiding Intravascular Injection. Preventing a systemic toxic reaction is best accomplished by avoiding an intravascular injection. However, for infiltration anesthesia with small-gauge needles, aspiration is usually unnecessary unless the injection is deeper than the subcutaneous area or the area to be injected contains many large vessels.

Special Considerations

There are many applications of infiltration anesthesia in the emergency department, but the following special cases deserve separate mention.

Hematoma Block. Hematoma block has been used for many years to provide anesthesia for reduction of fractures, particularly of the distal forearm and hand. Its popularity has waned somewhat because of the fear of introducing infection at the fracture site and its limited efficacy. Although several studies show the hematoma block to be safe, it does not provide as good anesthesia as the Bier block, the brachial plexus block, or general anesthesia.[87–90] However, there are several reasons to retain this technique. The procedure is simple and quick to perform without additional personnel. There is no need to wait for an anesthesiologist or for the patient to digest a meal as when general anesthesia is used. A lower dose of anesthetic agent is required compared with that required for the Bier block (see Chapter 40). Lastly, it

is useful when the Bier block and general anesthesia are contraindicated.

This simple technique involves preparing the skin over the fracture site, inserting the needle into the hematoma (confirmed by aspirating blood), and slowly injecting from 5 to 15 ml of plain 1 per cent lidocaine or 5 to 10 ml of plain 2 per cent lidocaine, depending on the fracture site, into the fracture cavity and around the adjacent periosteum. Onset of adequate anesthesia occurs in about 5 minutes and may last for several hours. This procedure should not be performed through dirty skin, into open fractures, or in small children.

Intra-articular Anesthesia. The history and physical examination of an acutely traumatic knee may underestimate the severity of an injury. Instillation of 5 ml of 1 per cent lidocaine after joint aspiration may help to relieve pain and facilitate examination, but several authorities do not recommend its routine use.[91–92] Spasm and apprehension are often not relieved by local anesthesia, and the occasional knowledge gained usually does not influence the treatment plan. Certain clinical indicators such as immediate joint effusion (hemarthrosis), audible pop, or knee giving way are more predictive of the need to pursue other diagnostic methods such as evaluation under general anesthesia, arthroscopy, or both. A negative exam, even with local or general anesthesia, does not necessarily rule out significant injury since secondary or tertiary knee stabilizers may remain intact. An interesting study by Barrack and coworkers showed that intra-articular anesthesia had no effect on gait pattern nor joint proprioception.[93] Therefore, if otherwise indicated, weight bearing post-procedure may be allowed without fear of producing or increasing injury.

NERVE BLOCKS IN THE EMERGENCY DEPARTMENT

General Considerations

Virtually every peripheral nerve can be blocked at some point along its course from the spine to the periphery. Digital nerve blocks of the fingers and toes are commonly used and are indispensable. The more proximal blocks are seldom used. In a survey of practicing emergency physicians, 99 per cent used digital blocks, 43 per cent used blocks at the wrist, 4 per cent at the elbow, and 4 per cent at the axilla.[94]

For most of the lacerations and injuries seen in the emergency department, local infiltrative anesthesia is adequate and efficient. Typically, the emergency physician repairs injured extremities when (1) tissue distortion from local infiltration anesthesia is minimal and of little consequence during the repair; (2) exploration, irrigation, and a few deep sutures are generally well tolerated using standard periwound local anesthesia; and (3) time is limited. Local infiltration is quick, reliable, and effective compared with many of the nerve blocks, which tend to require a more extensive set-up and have a less reliable and longer onset. Furthermore, those cases that require extensive repair and anesthesia of the entire extremity are often referred to a specialist who may prefer to examine an unanesthetized limb.

Nerve blocks may be underutilized in the emergency department. Potential applications include ankle blocks for foot lacerations, intercostal blocks for rib fractures, supraorbital blocks for foreheads traumatized by contact with the windshield, and ear blocks for ear lacerations. The preparation, technique, choice of anesthesic, precautions, and complications are similar for all nerve blocks and are described in general in the following sections. The clinician is encouraged to use the same basic techniques and precautions for all nerve blocks. Specific precautions unique to a particular nerve block are included with the description of that block; obvious precautions such as aspiration before injection when the needle is in close proximity to a vascular structure are not restated to avoid redundancy.

Indications

The general indication for performing a nerve block is the requirement that it provide anesthesia equal or superior to that offered by other techniques. Scenarios in which this requirement is met are (1) when distortion from local infiltration hampers closure (e.g., face) or compromises blood flow (e.g., finger tip); (2) when anesthesia is required over a large area and multiple injections would be painful, or the large amount of anesthetic needed for local infiltration exceeds the recommended dose; (3) when a nerve block is the most efficacious form of treatment, as in an intercostal block for treating a rib fracture in the patient with chronic obstructive pulmonary disease; and (4) when extensive limb surgery or manipulation is required and other methods or specialists are not available.

Preparation

A brief history from the patient including drug allergies, medications, and systemic illnesses should be taken. Peripheral vascular, heart, and liver disease increase the risk of severe complications. Monoamine oxidase inhibitors preclude the use of epinephrine, which may cause exaggerated cardiac responses in this setting.

Instructions. The procedure should be explained to the patient, including the pain of the needle insertion, paresthesias that may be felt, and possible complications that may occur. The possible need for additional procedures if the nerve block fails should also be discussed.

Equipment. The degree of equipment preparation depends on the extent of the procedure. For a simple digital block, a 10-ml syringe, an 18-gauge needle for drawing the solution from the vial, and a 3.75-cm 25- or 27-gauge needle for the nerve block will suffice. Note that the needle sizes given in the text are general recommendations. For most blocks, a needle two gauges larger or smaller or 1 cm longer or shorter is adequate.

For more elaborate blocks, the necessary equipment is listed in Table 38–11. Use of an extension tubing set between the needle and a stopcock syringe assembly facilitates independent needle placement and syringe manipulation. In addition, standard resuscitation equipment for advanced cardiac life support should be readily available.

Choice of Anesthetic. The factors influencing the choice of anesthetic for nerve block are similar to those for local infiltration. In general, most nerve blocks are done for the repair of painful traumatic injuries that are likely to result in pain for the patient long after the repair is complete. In such cases, anesthetics with the longest duration of action should be selected to maximize the patient's analgesia. For most of the blocks described in this chapter, 0.25 per cent bupivacaine is suggested as the anesthetic of choice, but equal volumes of 1 per cent lidocaine with epinephrine can be substituted. Care must always be taken not to exceed the recommended dosages of anesthetic.

Positioning of the Patient. All nerve blocks should be performed with the patient in the supine position.

Preparation of the Area to Be Blocked. Although the

Table 38–11. Equipment Needed for Proximal Nerve Block Trays
6 gauze sponges
4 towels
1 antiseptic-solution receptacle
1 receptacle for saline flush solution
1 anesthetic-solution receptacle (30-ml capacity)
1 10-ml syringe for local anesthetic injection
1 30-ml syringe for nerve block injection
1 three-way stopcock
1 intravenous extension tubing set
1 18-gauge needle for withdrawing anesthetic from the vial
1 each 3.75-cm 23-, 25-, and 27-gauge needles for nerve blocks

incidence of infection following nerve blocks is minuscule, the field should be prepared in an aseptic fashion before needle puncture. This can be accomplished by swabbing the area with a povidone-iodine solution or alcohol and then using standard aseptic injection technique. Sterile drapes and gloves are recommended in addition to aseptic skin preparation for the initiation of blocks that (1) are close to large joints, vessels, and nerves; (2) are located in inherently dirty areas of the body; or (3) require simultaneous palpation of the underlying structures while injecting.

Choosing the Nerves to Block. Successful anesthesia often requires blocking two or more nerves. When deciding which nerves are involved, two points must be considered. First, the cutaneous distribution of the various peripheral nerves differs slightly from patient to patient, and, second, the sensory innervation of adjacent nerves is overlapping to some degree. A liberal margin of error should be used when determining which nerves supply the desired area of anesthesia.

Locating the Nerve

Inserting the needle in close proximity to the nerve, that is, "next to" small nerves and "into" the nerve sheath of large nerves, is the essential step in a successful block. When searching for the nerve, its anatomic relationship at the block site can be generalized into one of three types. First, are those sites with good structural landmarks (e.g., prominent bones or tendons) immediately next to the nerve. For example, the digital nerves are reliably found at positions 2, 4, 8, and 10 o'clock around and just superficial to the proximal phalanx, and the median nerve lies between the palpable palmaris longus and flexor carpi radialis tendons at the proximal crease of the wrist. Second, are the sites with easily palpable arteries adjacent to the nerves such as in the axilla and groin. Third, are the sites with poor landmarks.

Blocking nerves with good structural or vascular landmarks is straightforward: the landmarks are palpated, the course of the nerve in relation to those landmarks is visualized in the mind's eye, and the needle is inserted in close proximity to the nerve. Paresthesias, as discussed later, may ensure close proximity.

Blocking the nerves with poor landmarks, such as the radial nerve at the elbow, requires skill through practice, some degree of luck, or a nerve stimulator if they are to be blocked consistently.

Nerve Stimulator. Despite its sophisticated name, a nerve stimulator is inexpensive and simple to use. With minimal practice, the needle can be placed easily and reliably within a few millimeters of the nerve. The device is simple, consisting of a battery-operated nerve stimulator that delivers current in the range of 0.1 to 0.5 mA, a disposable Teflon-coated needle, and an electrocardiogram pad. One wire electrode from the nerve stimulator is attached to the electrocardiogram pad, which is placed on the limb approximately 10 to 15 cm from the injection site. The other wire electrode is attached to the Teflon-coated needle at its hub. Once inserted into the tissue, the needle tip is electrically active. When in close proximity to the nerve, electric current stimulates the nerve, producing twitching of the muscles supplied by that nerve. For example, when the ulnar nerve is stimulated, the small and ring fingers flex. Anesthetic solution can then be injected into the area at the stimulation site.

Paresthesia. When a nerve stimulator is not available, another useful technique to ensure that the needle tip is in close proximity to the nerve is to elicit a paresthesia. By touching and mechanically stimulating the nerve with movement of the needle tip, a tingling sensation or jolt known as a paresthesia is felt along the distribution of the nerve.

In practice, the jolt of a true paresthesia is often difficult to distinguish from the "ouch" of a pain-sensitive structure. When blocking proximal nerves of the elbow or axilla, the paresthesia travels far enough away from the injection site that it can be distinguished from locally induced pain. Paresthesias at the level of the hand and wrist are much less reliably distinguished from pain. In both cases, the paresthesia is a subjective feeling that requires intelligent and cooperative patients who understand what they are expected to feel and who remain relaxed and attentive so that they are able to distinguish an ouch from a jolt. All too often, the patient in pain is willing to tell the physician what the physician wants to hear: the sensation that just made the patient jump was a "paresthesia." Before the procedure, a simple explanation of what the patient should or may feel will facilitate cooperation.

Injecting the Anesthetic

Administering the anesthetic requires ensuring that the anesthetic is not inadvertently injected into the vessels or nerve bundle. Before injection, the syringe is aspirated to check for blood. If no blood is aspirated, the anesthetic is injected while the extremity is observed for blanching, which suggests intravascular injection. If blanching occurs, the needle should be repositioned before further injection.

The onset and duration of anesthesia are greatly influenced by the proximity of the injected anesthetic to the nerve. Onset is within a few minutes if the anesthetic is in immediate proximity to the nerve. Onset takes longer or may not occur if the anesthetic must diffuse more than a few millimeters, which underscores the importance of locating the nerve before injection.

More anesthetic is required if it must diffuse a large distance to the nerve. A range of suggested volumes of anesthetic is given with each nerve block description. For blocks in which a definite paresthesia is elicited or a nerve stimulator is used, the minimal recommended amount of anesthetic suffices. For many of the blocks of the smaller nerves, paresthesias are not easily elicited, and the anesthetic is placed in the general vicinity of the nerve. For these blocks, or when doubt exists about proximity of the needle to the nerve, larger amounts of anesthetic are recommended. This point cannot be emphasized strongly enough. The difference between a successful and unsuccessful block may be merely an additional 2 ml of anesthetic. When in doubt, err on the high side of the recommended dosage.

Onset of the anesthesic occurs in 2 to 15 minutes, depending on the distance the anesthetic must diffuse to the nerve. One should wait for 30 minutes before deciding that the block was unsuccessful.

Complications and Precautions

The complications of a peripheral nerve block result from poor technique. General precautions include measures to minimize nerve injury, intravascular injection, and systemic toxicity.

No statistics exist on the complication rate from nerve blocks performed by emergency physicians. Anesthesiologists report rates of less than 1 per cent for blocks of the nerves of the hand and wrist and up to 10 per cent for axillary blocks.[95] There was no breakdown of serious and minor complications, although local complications (hematoma and neuropathy) are most common. Generally, seldomly performed blocks, blocks that require high doses of anesthetic, and blocks close to major vascular structures have the higher rates of problems. The technical ability of the practitioner largely determines the outcome.

Nerve Injury. Neuritis, an inflammation of the nerve, is the most common nerve injury.[96, 97] The patient may complain of pain and various degrees of nerve dysfunction, including paresthesia or motor or sensory deficit. Most cases are transient and resolve completely. Supportive care and close follow-up are the mainstays of treatment.

Nerve injury can occur secondary to (1) direct trauma from the needle, (2) ischemia due to intraneuronal injection, or (3) chemical irritation from the anesthetic. Proper needle style, positioning, and manipulation minimize direct nerve damage. A short bevel needle should be used and maneuvered so that the bevel is parallel to the longitudinal fibers. Sharp pain or paresthesia indicates that the needle is close to or in the nerve. Excessive needle movement should be avoided when the needle tip is contacting a nerve. Attaching the needle to an intravenous extension tube reduces needle movement and subsequent nerve damage as the syringe plunger is manipulated.

Intraneuronal injection may cause nerve ischemia and injury. Eliciting a paresthesia or severe pain suggests that the needle has made contact with the nerve. *When a paresthesia is elicited, the needle must be withdrawn 1 mm before the anesthetic is injected.* If the paresthesia occurs during injection, the needle must be repositioned. Most neurons are surrounded by a strong perineural sheath through which the nutrient arteries run lengthwise. Injection directly into a nerve sheath may increase the pressure within the nerve and compress the nutrient artery. Impaired blood flow results in nerve ischemia and subsequent paralysis. Intraneuronal injection is often heralded by severe pain, which worsens with further injection and may radiate along the course of innervation. The operator may notice difficulty depressing the syringe plunger. If the needle tip is in proper position, slow injection of the anesthetic should be minimally painful, and the anesthetic should go in without resistance.

Concentrated anesthetics can produce a chemical irritation of the nerve. Use only recommended doses and concentrations of anesthetic (Table 38–12).

Intravascular Injection. Intravascular injection results in both systemic and limb toxicity. Inadvertent intravascular injection produces high blood levels of the anesthetic with resultant toxicity, as discussed earlier. Particular care must be taken when administering large amounts of anesthetic in close proximity to large blood vessels.

Intra-arterial injection of anesthetic with epinephrine may cause peripheral vasospasm that further compromises injured tissue. Intravascular anesthetic is not toxic to the limb itself, although it may produce transient blanching of the skin by displacing blood from the vascular tree. Epinephrine, however, can cause a prolonged vasospasm and subsequent ischemia if it is injected into an artery. Severe

Table 38–12. Recommended Volumes of Anesthetic for Various Nerve Blocks

Site	Anesthetic: 1.0% Lidocaine or 0.25% Bupivacaine (Both with Epinephrine) Volume (ml)
Axillary	40–50
Elbow	
Ulnar	5–10
Radial	5–15
Median	5–15
Wrist	
Ulnar	5–15
Radial	5–15
Median	3–5
Hip	
Femoral	10–30
Three-in-one	30–50
Knee	
Tibial	5–15
Peroneal	5–10
Saphenous	5–10
Ankle	
Posterior tibial	5–10
Deep peroneal	3–5
Saphenous, sural, and superficial peroneal	4–10 each
Intercostal	5–15 each

1.0% Lidocaine or 0.25% Bupivacaine (Both Without Epinephrine)

Hand	
Metacarpal and web space	2–4
Finger	1–2
Foot	
Metatarsal	10
Web space	3–5
Toe	2

epinephrine-induced tissue blanching or vasospasm may be reversed with the local or intravascular injection of phentolamine.

Hematoma. Hematoma formation may result from arterial puncture, particularly during axillary and femoral blocks. Direct pressure for 5 to 10 minutes usually controls further bleeding. Using the recommended 23- to 27-gauge needle minimizes bleeding from the punctured artery.

Infection. Infection is rare and can be minimized by following aseptic technique and minimizing the concentration of epinephrine. Injection should be made through noninfected skin that has been antiseptically prepared. Injection through a site of infection may spread the infection to adjacent tissues, fascial planes, and joints. This is particularly a concern in the hand and foot.

Limb Injury. Injury to the anesthetized limb can result if the patient is permitted to use the limb or is advised to use heat or cold application or to perform wound care before the anesthesia has worn off. For major nerve blocks, the patient should not be discharged home until sensation and function have returned. For minor blocks, the patient may be sent home but should be properly cautioned. Care must be taken to avoid ischemia-producing dressings (elastic bandages) because the anesthetized area may not sense impending problems.

Nerve Blocks of the Upper Extremity

The upper extremity is supplied by the brachial plexus, whose branches—primarily the median, radial, ulnar, and musculocutaneous nerves—can be blocked at the axilla, elbow, wrist, hand, or fingers. Nerve blocks at the axilla and elbow are seldom used in the emergency department. Nerve blocks of the wrist are performed occasionally before painful procedures or for repair of injuries to the hand. Metacarpal and digital blocks are used frequently to treat fractures, lacerations, and infections of the fingers.

BRACHIAL PLEXUS BLOCK IN THE AXILLA

Brachial plexus blocks performed correctly provide anesthesia and muscle paralysis to the upper extremity, permitting orthopedic manipulations and surgery. The brachial plexus can be blocked at various sites in the neck and axilla using the interscalene, supraclavicular, subclavian, or axillary approach.

The axillary approach is the safest and has the advantages of (1) easy palpation of the axillary artery, (2) easy compression of any hemorrhage or hematoma, and (3) negligible risk of inadvertent pneumothorax or spinal cord paralysis. Disadvantages of this approach include variable anesthesia to the shoulder, whose innervation branches off the brachial plexus variably at a higher level.

Anatomy. The major nerves of the arm originate from the cervical plexus, C5 to C8 and T1, which forms the brachial plexus from which the median, radial, ulnar, and musculocutaneous nerves originate. Enclosing the nerves and artery, a perivascular sheath extends from the axilla and is continuous with the prevertebral fascia. Clinically this is important because anesthetic injected at the level of the axilla can track proximally and block nerves that exit the sheath at a higher level such as the musculocutaneous nerve and nerves to the shoulder.

Technique. With the patient in the supine position, the arm is abducted 90 degrees and rotated externally (Fig. 38–6). This serves to expose the axilla and axillary artery and to define the border of the pectoralis major, where the artery is stabilized with the nondominant hand. Firm pressure is used to stabilize the artery and is maintained throughout the procedure and for 5 minutes after the injection. This promotes the proximal spread of anesthetic in the nerve sheath and facilitates a successful block.

Proximal to the site at which the artery is stabilized, a 3.75-cm, 23-gauge needle, preferably attached to extension tubing, is inserted over the artery at a 20-degree angle to the skin and directed toward the axilla (see Fig. 38–6). As the needle is advanced, either the patient experiences a paresthesia or the artery is punctured. If a paresthesia is felt, small movements of the needle are used to reproduce the paresthesia, which ensures that the needle tip is in close proximity to the nerve and hence lying within the neurovascular sheath. Once the proper position is confirmed, 40 ml of 0.25 per cent bupivacaine with epinephrine is injected slowly while observations are made for signs of intravascular injection. Subsequent massage at the injection site facilitates the proximal spread of the anesthetic.

If a paresthesia cannot be elicited, the artery is punctured through and through. Angling the needle 90 degrees may make this easier. A blood return signals that the needle tip is in the artery. The needle is further advanced until blood is no longer aspirated, and then it is advanced another couple of millimeters to ensure that the needle tip has passed through the opposite wall of the artery (Fig. 38–7). Occa-

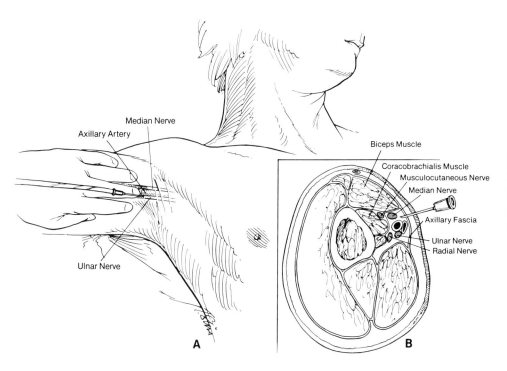

Figure 38–6. Axillary block of the brachial plexus. (Adapted from Rajad P, Pai U: Techniques in nerve blocking. In Raj PP (ed): Handbook of Regional Anesthesia. New York, Churchill Livingstone, 1985, p 180.)

sionally the needle tip becomes blocked with a small blood clot, giving a false "negative blood return." This possibility can be minimized by clearing the tip with small injections of saline. Once reasonably sure of the proper location of the needle tip, the operator injects anesthesia, as discussed previously. Anesthesia begins in 5 to 30 minutes and lasts for 30 minutes to more than 6 hours.

Complications. Partial block of the brachial plexus may occur and require augmentation. Commonly, inadequate proximal spreading of the anesthetic or displacement of the needle outside the sheath is to blame. Even in the properly performed axillary block of the brachial plexus, anomalous anatomy may prevent the normal spread of anesthetic. If

necessary, the spared nerve can be blocked at the level of the elbow or wrist.

Postblock neuritis is reported to occur in 0.3 to 5 per cent of cases and has been attributed to the vigorous exploration for a paresthesia.[96–97] If paresthesia is not elicited after two attempts, the arterial puncture method should be employed. Use of the nerve stimulator greatly facilitates this search.

NERVE BLOCKS AT THE ELBOW

The median, ulnar, and radial nerves can be blocked at the elbow, providing anesthesia to the distal forearm and hand (Fig. 38–8). These nerves are blocked individually to supplement incomplete axillary blocks, or they are blocked together to provide anesthesia to the forearm and hand. For most injuries extensive enough to require nerve block at the elbow, all three nerves must be blocked for successful anesthesia because of the variable and overlapping innervation of the forearm. Furthermore, injuries to the proximal and middle forearm may require an additional circumferential subcutaneous field block of the lateral, medial, and posterior cutaneous nerves.

Ulnar Nerve—Anatomy and Technique. The ulnar nerve can be palpated in the ulnar groove on the posterior medial aspect of the elbow between the olecranon and medial condyle of the humerus (Figs. 38–9 and 38–10). This nerve supplies the innervation to the small finger and ulnar half of the ring finger and the ulnar aspect of the hand (see Fig. 38–8).

With the elbow flexed, the nerve is palpated in the groove. A 3.75-cm, 23- to 25-gauge needle is inserted 1 to 2 cm proximal to the groove and directed toward the groove parallel to the course of the nerve. The needle tip comes to rest close to the proximal end of the groove. Care is taken to avoid blocking the nerve in the groove, where it is prone to damage, between the needle tip and the supporting bony structure. For similar reasons, the paresthesia may be elicited but is not vigorously sought. Once the needle tip is properly positioned, 5 to 10 ml of anesthetic is deposited. If a nerve

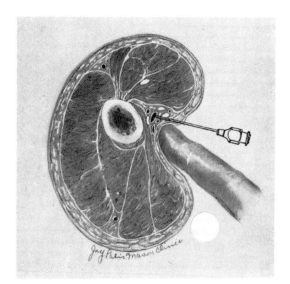

Figure 38–7. Through-and-through needle puncture of the axillary artery. (From Moore DC: Regional Block: A Handbook for Use in the Clinical Practice of Medicine and Surgery. 4th ed. Springfield, Ill, Charles C Thomas, 1971.)

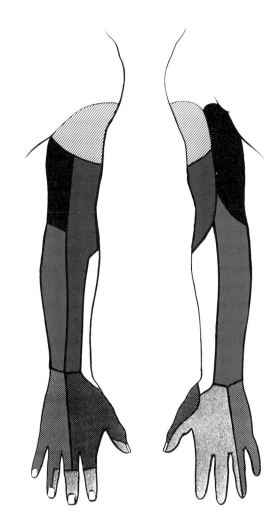

Figure 38–8. Cutaneous nerve supply of the upper limb. (From Bridenbaugh LD: The upper extremity: Somatic blockade. In Cousins M, Bridenbaugh PO (eds): Neural Blockade in Clinical Anesthesia and Management of Pain. 2nd ed. Philadelphia, JB Lippincott Co, 1988, p 412.)

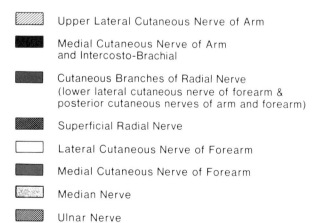

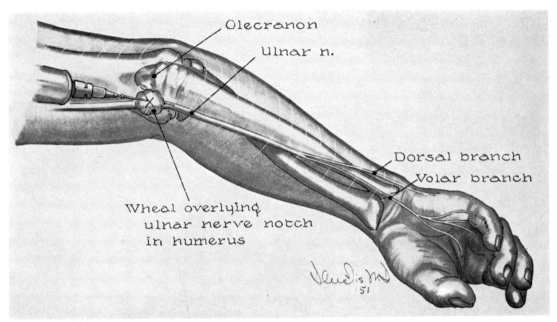

Figure 38–9. Ulnar nerve passing between the olecranon and medial epicondyle of the humerus. (From Moore DC: Regional Block: A Handbook for Use in the Clinical Practice of Medicine and Surgery. 4th ed. Springfield, Ill, Charles C Thomas, 1971, p 271.)

stimulator is used, flexion of the small and ring fingers signals proximity to the nerve.

Radial Nerve—Anatomy and Technique. The radial nerve and sensory branch of the musculocutaneous nerve run together in the sulcus between the biceps and the brachioradialis muscle on the anterolateral aspect of the elbow (Fig. 38–11). The block produces anesthesia to the lateral dorsum of the hand and the lateral aspect of the forearm (see Fig. 38–8).

The sulcus in which the nerve runs is palpated between the sharp border of the biceps muscle and the medial border of the brachioradialis in the antecubital fossa just proximal to the skin crease of the elbow. Palpation is greatly facilitated by having the patient, with the elbow flexed at 90 degrees,

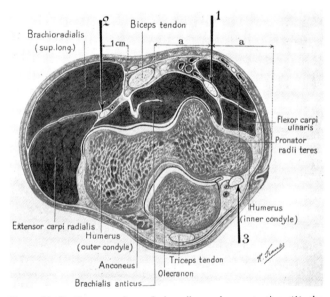

Figure 38–10. Cross section of the elbow, demonstrating (1) the median nerve, (2) the radial nerve, and (3) the ulnar nerve. (From Adriani J: Labat's Regional Anesthesia Techniques and Clinical Applications. 3rd ed. Philadelphia, WB Saunders Co, 1967, p 234.)

contract and relax these muscles isometrically so that their borders are better defined. The skin is punctured with a 3.75-cm, 23- to 25-gauge needle halfway between the muscles, or 1 cm lateral to the biceps tendon, at a point 1 cm proximal to the antecubital crease. A paresthesia is sought at a depth of 2 cm by probing in a fan-like pattern. If one is unsuccessful after a brief search, 5 to 15 ml of anesthetic should be injected at this depth. Because of the depth and poor landmarks of this nerve, the nerve stimulator greatly facilitates the search for the nerve, which, when stimulated, produces extension of the fingers and wrist.

Median Nerve—Anatomy and Technique. The median nerve runs medial to the brachial artery in the anteromedial aspect of the elbow (see Fig. 38–11). The nerve block anesthetizes the index, middle, and radial portion of the ring fingers and the palmar aspect of the thumb and lateral palm (see Fig. 38–8).

The brachial artery is palpated in the flexed arm at the elbow just proximal to the antecubital crease and medial to the prominent biceps tendon. Once the anatomy is defined and marked in the flexed arm, the arm is extended to 30 degrees. A 3.75-cm, 23- to 25-gauge needle is inserted slightly medial to the artery and perpendicular to the skin, to the depth of the artery, about 2 to 3 cm, and 5 to 15 ml of anesthetic is injected. Again, the nerve stimulator facilitates the process and produces flexion of the wrist and index finger.

NERVE BLOCKS AT THE WRIST

The median, ulnar, and radial nerves may be blocked at the wrist, providing anesthesia to the hand. Although 43 per cent of surveyed emergency physicians use this block in their practice, 89 per cent of these stated that they use it rarely.[94]

Most extensive injuries and procedures for which a wrist nerve block could be used can also be managed using local infiltration or a digital block. Compared with direct infiltration, wrist block anesthesia can have a slow and unreliable onset and can require more time to take effect if all three nerves are to be blocked. There are several circumstances, however, in which wrist nerve blocks are more advantageous than other types.

Diffuse lesions that can be difficult to anesthetize with local infiltration can easily be anesthetized with a wrist block. Deep abrasions with embedded debris that are commonly the result of "roadburn" from bike and motorcycle accidents can be cleaned and debrided painlessly after a nerve block at the wrist. In the severely swollen and contused hand, even small amounts of anesthetic injected locally may increase the tissue pressure and produce further pain. Hydrofluoric acid burns, requiring treatment with numerous subcutaneous injections of calcium gluconate, are handled mercifully after a wrist nerve block.

Compared with nerves in the axilla and elbow, the nerves in the wrist are more easily located anatomically and can be blocked more reliably. All three nerves lie in the volar aspect of the wrist near easily palpated tendons. A nerve stimulator is not necessary but may be useful in locating the nerves, particularly when one is learning how to perform these blocks.

The anatomy and technique for blocking each nerve individually follow. Note that the median nerve lies in the midline and deep to the fascia, and the ulnar and radial nerves lie on their respective sides and have branches that wrap around dorsally. To block all three nerves at the wrist requires a block that when viewed end-on roughly resembles a horseshoe straddling a horseshoe stake (Fig. 38–12).

Median Nerve—Anatomy and Technique. In the wrist, the median nerve lies below the palmaris longus or slightly radial to it between the palmaris and the flexor carpi radialis (see Figs. 38–12 and 38–13). Both tendons are easily palpated, but the palmaris may be absent in up to 20 per cent of patients, in which case the nerve is found about 1 cm in the ulnar direction from the flexor carpi radialis. The nerve lies deep to the fascia of the flexor retinaculum at a depth of 1 cm or less.

The palmaris longus is located by having the patient oppose the thumb and small fingers with the wrist flexed against resistance. The site of the nerve block is selected on the radial border of the palmaris tendon just proximal to the proximal wrist crease. A 3.75-cm, 25-gauge needle is inserted perpendicularly and advanced slowly until a slight pop is felt as the needle penetrates the retinaculum and a paresthesia is produced. If no paresthesia ensues, it may be

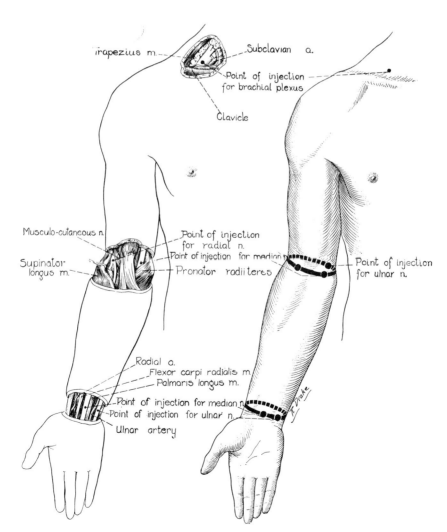

Figure 38–11. Anatomy for nerve blocks at the elbow and wrist. (From Adriani J: Labat's Regional Anesthesia: Techniques and Clinical Applications. 3rd ed. Philadelphia, WB Saunders Co, 1967, p 226.)

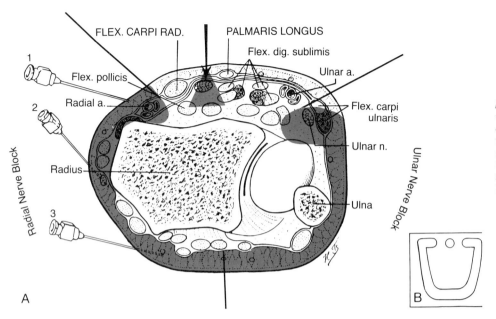

Median Nerve Block

FLEX. CARPI RAD.   PALMARIS LONGUS

Flex. dig. sublimis

Ulnar a.

Flex. pollicis

1

Radial a.

Flex. carpi
ulnaris

Radial Nerve Block

2

Ulnar n.

Radius

Ulnar Nerve Block

Ulna

3

A

B

Figure 38–12. Cross section of the wrist. The arrow points to the median nerve. Shaded region depicts the area infiltrated with anesthetic. (Redrawn from Adriani J: Labat's Regional Anesthesia: Techniques and Clinical Applications. 3rd ed. Philadelphia, WB Saunders Co, 1967, p 234.)

elicited in the ulnar direction under the palmaris tendon. If a paresthesia is still not elicited, 3 to 5 ml of anesthetic are deposited in the proximity of the nerve at a depth of 1 cm under the tendon. It is better to err slightly on the deep side of the retinaculum and continue depositing anesthetic as the needle is withdrawn because the retinaculum is an effective barrier to a successful nerve block from a superficially injected anesthetic.

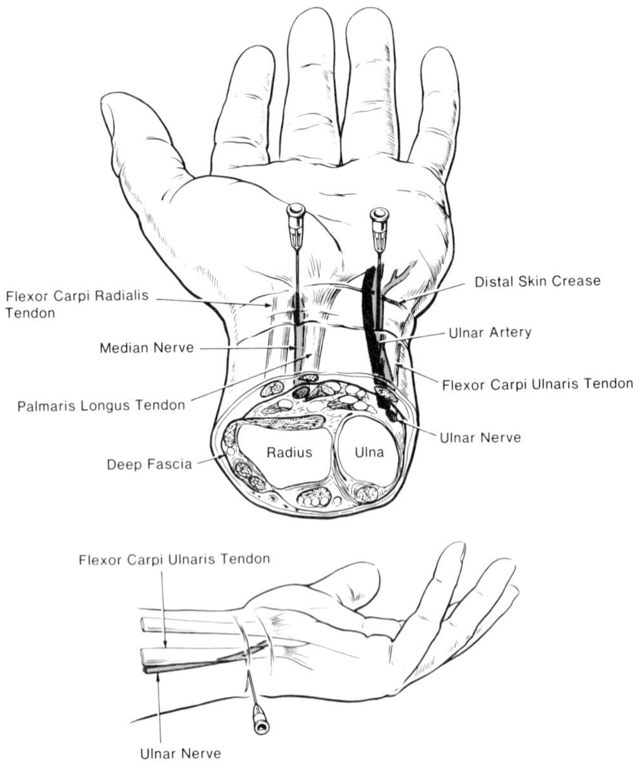

Radial Nerve—Anatomy and Technique. The radial nerve follows the radial artery into the wrist; however, the nerve gives off branches proximal to the wrist. These branches wrap around the wrist and fan out to supply the dorsal radial aspect of the hand (Fig. 38–14).

Nerve block requires an injection in close proximity to the artery and a field block that extends around the dorsal aspect of the wrist. A 3.75-cm, 25-gauge needle is inserted immediately lateral to the palpable artery at the level of the proximal palmar crease. At the depth of the artery 2 to 5 ml of anesthetic is injected. Another 5 to 10 ml is distributed in a subcutaneous field block from the initial point of injection to the dorsal midline. The needle must be withdrawn and repositioned to complete the block. The discomfort of numerous needle sticks is decreased if the needle is repositioned to a site that has been anesthetized previously.

Ulnar Nerve—Anatomy and Technique. The ulnar nerve follows the ulnar artery into the wrist, where they both lie deep to the flexor carpi ulnaris (see Figs. 38–12 and 38–13). The flexor carpi ulnaris tendon is easily palpated just proximal to prominent pisiform bone by having the patient flex the wrist against resistance. At the level of the proximal palmar crease, the artery and the nerve lie just off the radial border of the flexor carpi ulnaris; however, the nerve lies between the tendon and the artery and deep to the artery, making it difficult to approach the nerve from the volar aspect of the wrist without involving the artery.

Nerve block of the ulnar nerve can be carried out by two different approaches: the lateral and the volar (see Fig. 38–13). The lateral approach may be easier because of the reason stated previously. For the lateral approach, a 3.75-cm, 25-gauge needle is inserted on the ulnar aspect of the tendon at the proximal palmar crease and is directed horizontally under the flexor carpi ulnaris for a distance of 1.0 to 1.5 cm. After a paresthesia is elicited, 3 to 5 ml of anesthetic is deposited. It is important to elicit a paresthesia because the nerve lies in a thick neurovascular bundle. If no paresthesia is elicited, the needle can be directed toward the ulnar bone at a point deep to the flexor carpi ulnaris, and the anesthetic can be inserted as the needle is withdrawn.

Distal Skin Crease

Flexor Carpi Radialis
Tendon

Ulnar Artery

Median Nerve

Flexor Carpi Ulnaris Tendon

Palmaris Longus Tendon

Ulnar Nerve

Deep Fascia

Radius   Ulna

Flexor Carpi Ulnaris Tendon

Ulnar Nerve

Figure 38–13. Landmarks and anatomy of the median and ulnar nerves at the wrist. (From Bridenbaugh DC: The upper extremity: Somatic blockade. In Cousins M, Bridenbaugh PO (eds): Neural Blockade in Clinical Anesthesia and Management of Pain. 2nd ed. Philadelphia, JB Lippincott Co, 1988, p 409.)

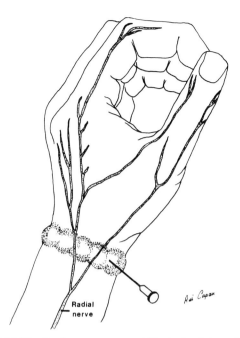

Figure 38–14. Distribution, anatomy, and blockade of the radial nerve at the wrist.

Like the radial nerve, cutaneous nerves branch off the ulnar nerve, wrap around the wrist, and supply the dorsum of the hand. These are blocked with a 5- to 10-ml subcutaneous band of anesthetic from the lateral border of the flexor carpi ulnaris to the dorsal midline (see Fig. 38–12). Another advantage of the lateral approach is that the dorsal branches can be blocked from the same injection site.

NERVE BLOCKS OF THE DIGITS

The digital nerve block is one of the most useful and used blocks in the emergency department. Indications for choosing it include repair of finger lacerations and amputations, reduction of fractures and dislocations, drainage of infections, removal of fingernails, and relief of pain (e.g., from a fracture or burn). Ninety-nine per cent of emergency physicians use this block in their practice; 89 per cent use it frequently.[91]

The digital block is superior to local infiltration in most circumstances. Wound infiltration may be a problem in the finger that has tight skin and can accept only a limited volume of anesthetic. Administration of anesthetic into this restricted space increases the tissue pressure, impairing capillary blood flow and causing pain. Fibrous septa in the finger tip also restrict the space available for the injected substance and even limit the spread of small amounts of anesthetic.

Anatomy. Each finger is supplied by two sets of nerves. These nerves, the dorsal and palmar digital nerves, run alongside the phalanx at positions 2 and 10, and 4 and 8 o'clock, respectively (Fig. 38–15). Most physicians mistakenly believe that all four nerves must always be blocked to obtain adequate anesthesia.

The principal nerves supplying the finger are the palmar digital nerves, also called the common digital nerves. These nerves originate from the deep volar branches of the ulnar and median nerves, where they branch in the wrist. The palmar digital nerves follow the artery along the volar lateral aspects of the bone, one on each side, and supply sensation to the volar skin and interphalangeal joints of all

five fingers. *In the middle three fingers, these nerves also supply the dorsal distal aspect of the finger, including the finger tip and nailbed.* Only the volar branches must be blocked to obtain almost complete anesthesia of these fingers.

The dorsal digital nerves originate from the radial and ulnar nerves, which wrap around to the dorsum of the hand. *They supply the nailbeds of the thumb and small finger* and the dorsal aspect of all five fingers up to the distal interphalangeal joints. Unlike the middle three fingers, all four nerves are usually blocked in the thumb and fifth finger, especially to obtain anesthesia of the finger tip and nailbed.

Technique. The digital nerves can be blocked anywhere in their course, including sites in the finger, in the web space between the fingers, and between the metacarpals in the hand. The technique is similar at each level.

Clinical situations may dictate which site to use; however, given equal circumstances, the preferred site is the web space. Here the nerve's location is more consistent than in the hand, and there is more soft tissue space to accommodate the volume of injected substance than there is in the distal finger.

Digital block requires only aseptic injection technique after the skin is prepared with alcohol or povidone-iodine. Sterile gloves and drapes are not necessary.

Anesthesia is deposited at the positions of the four digital nerves at 2, 4, 8, and 10 o'clock in relationship to the bone, using a 3.75-cm, 27-gauge needle (see Fig. 38–15). The block is performed from the dorsal surface, where the skin is thinner, easier to penetrate, and less sensitive than that of the volar surface. The needle insertion site is at the web space, just distal to the knuckle at the lateral edge of the bone (Fig. 38–16). Once the needle tip is subdermal, it usually contacts the bone. A wheal of 0.5 to 1.0 ml of anesthetic without epinephrine is injected at this level. This serves to block the dorsal digital nerve and provide anesthesia at the injection site. The needle is then passed lateral to the bone and toward the palmar surface until the palmar skin starts to tent slightly. The needle is withdrawn 1 mm and aspirated for checking for an inadvertent intravenous position, and 0.5 to 1.0 ml of anesthetic is injected. This procedure is repeated on the opposite side of the finger. The result is a circumferential band of anesthesia at the base of the finger. Massage of the injected area enhances diffusion of the anesthetic through the tissue to the nerves.

Alternate procedures differ from the technique described previously by the method of injection. In the first alternative, after injecting one side of the finger, the needle

Dorsal surface

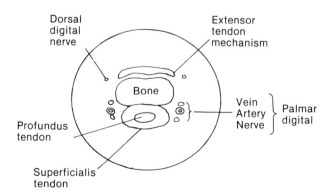

Palmar surface

Figure 38–15. Schematic cross section of the phalanx, demonstrating the relationship of the nerves to the bone. (From Grant's Atlas. 7th ed. Baltimore, Williams & Wilkins, 1978. Reproduced by permission.)

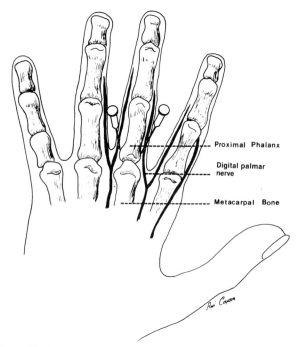

Figure 38–16. Sites of digital nerve blocks at the base of the finger.

the opposite digital nerve (Fig. 38–20). The index finger is used to palpate a fullness as the anesthetic is injected. By redirecting the needle to the adjacent finger without withdrawing it, both fingers may be blocked with a single puncture.

The anesthetic solution should be 2 to 4 ml of anesthetic *without epinephrine*. The total amount is reduced if the block is performed in the finger itself. The injection should go in smoothly without resistance of the syringe plunger. Although the finger is forgiving of transient pressure from excessive anesthetic, if the injection site becomes excessively tense as the volume is injected, the amount injected should be limited.

Onset of anesthesia occurs in 1 to 15 minutes and lasts for 20 minutes to 6 hours (depending on the anesthetic agent used).

Complications and Precautions. The small size of the digital arteries and nerves makes intravascular or intraneural injection less likely, but standard precautions should be taken. Because of the fine needle size, which may limit aspiration, false "negative aspirations" are more likely. Inadvertent intravascular injection may cause digit ischemia from vasospasm or displacement of blood out of the capillary bed by the anesthetic. Blanching of the finger as the anesthetic is injected suggests intravascular injection. If this is observed, the injection should be discontinued. Usually the

is redirected (without removing it) across the top of the digit to anesthetize the skin on the opposite side (Fig. 38–17). The needle is then withdrawn and inserted at the site that was anesthetized, and the block is continued as described earlier. The presumed advantage of this method is that it minimizes the pain of the second skin puncture. This procedure requires that the needle be placed across the dorsal aspect of the finger, allowing the possible disadvantage of extensor tendon puncture and trauma.

Another approach, termed the *volar metacarpal head approach,* can be used most successfully for the middle three fingers. This technique takes advantage of the anatomic fact that only the volar digital nerves must be blocked to obtain anesthesia of the total finger (except the proximal dorsal surface). If the thumb or fifth finger must be anesthetized, the dorsal branches must also be blocked to obtain anesthesia of the finger tip and fingernail area. Both the *palmar* and *web space* approach are available.

A needle insertion in the palm is used with the palmar approach. Although this method is slightly more painful than an injection in the dorsal skin, it provides anesthesia with a single needle puncture. The needle is inserted directly over the center of the metacarpal head, and anesthetic is slowly injected while the needle is advanced to the bone. At this point the needle is withdrawn 3 to 4 mm and angled slightly to the left and right of center to block both digital nerves without withdrawing the needle (Fig. 38–18). To be successful, a palpable soft tissue fullness should be appreciated. The technique requires 4 to 5 ml of anesthetic.

With the web space approach, the patient's hand is held by the physician whereby the physician's thumb and index finger are over the dorsal and volar metacarpal head, respectively. The physician's third finger is used to separate the patient's fingers to expose the web space while the fourth and fifth fingers support the finger being anesthetized (Fig. 38–19). The needle is inserted into the web space, 1 ml of anesthetic is injected, and the needle is slowly advanced until it is next to the lateral volar surface of the metacarpal head. Two milliliters of anesthetic are injected, and the needle is advanced slowly past the midline of the metacarpal head to

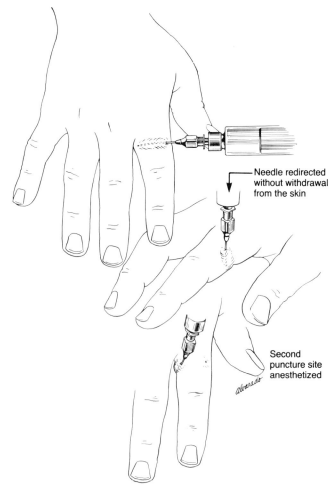

Needle redirected without withdrawal from the skin

Second puncture site anesthetized

Figure 38–17. Technique of anesthetizing the second injection site. (From Adriani J: Labat's Regional Anesthesia Techniques and Clinical Applications. 3rd ed. Philadelphia, WB Saunders Co, 1967, p 445.)

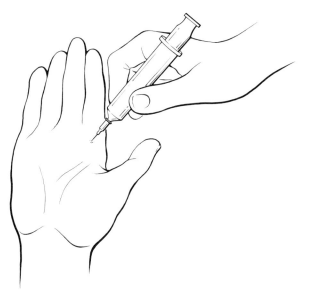

Figure 38–18. Palmar approach to the metacarpal head. After needle puncture in the midline, the needle is directed slightly to the right and left, and anesthetic is deposited along the course of both volar digital nerves. The needle is not withdrawn until both nerves are blocked.

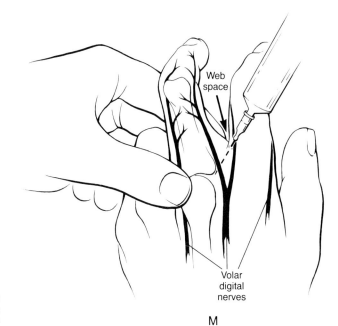

Figure 38–20. After injection of anesthetic into the web space skin, the needle is advanced to the digital nerve where it passes just lateral to the volar metacarpal head. Anesthetic is injected, and the needle is advanced to the opposite digital nerve. This procedure requires about 5 ml of anesthetic. If the index finger also must be blocked, the needle is redirected without withdrawal from the skin. Thus, both fingers are blocked with a single needle puncture.

ischemia is transient and self-resolving, and serious complications are rare. Massage or topical application of nitroglycerin paste may be attempted if ischemia persists. Vasoconstrictors such as epinephrine should not be used when blocking the digital nerves for fear of vasospasm and resultant ischemia. If one mistakenly chooses an epinephrine-containing solution, the ischemia and vasospasm may be relieved with local infiltration of phentolamine.

Commonly the digital nerve is lacerated or damaged by the initial injury to the finger. Careful evaluation using two-

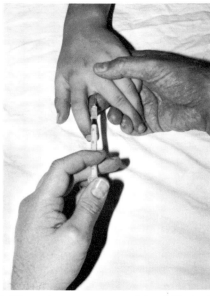

Figure 38–19. The web space metacarpal head block allows two of the three middle fingers to be anesthetized with a single needle puncture. The physician's thumb and index finger palpate the patient's dorsal and palmar metacarpal head, respectively, while the third finger exposes the web space and the fourth and fifth fingers support the finger being blocked. Contrary to the illustration, surgical gloves are recommended.

point discrimination should be able to determine the extent of nerve injury before nerve block. Even if nerve injury is questionable, it should be documented in the chart, and the *patient should be advised of the injury before nerve block.* Careful evaluation and patient education should prevent misconceptions as to the cause of the nerve injury. Although most isolated digital nerve injuries are not debilitating, they heal slowly and can be annoying to the patient. Digital nerve injury proximal to the distal interphalangeal joint may be repaired surgically. Nerve repair may be immediate when specialty consultation is available or delayed following initial simple closure.

Nerve Blocks of the Lower Extremity

The lower extremity is supplied by five nerves whose branches can be blocked at the hip, knee, ankle, foot, or toes. As in the arm, proximal nerve blocks in the leg are seldom used in the emergency department. Nerve blocks at the ankle are used occasionally in the treatment of foot lacerations and to perform otherwise painful procedures on the foot. Metatarsal and digital blocks in the foot are used frequently to treat ingrown toenails, fractures, and lacerations of the forefoot and toes.

NERVE BLOCKS OF THE HIP

Nerve blocks of the femoral, obturator, lateral femoral cutaneous, posterior cutaneous, and sciatic nerves at the hip provide anesthesia and paralysis to the skin and muscles of the leg (Fig. 38–21). Posteriorly, the posterior cutaneous and sciatic nerves can be blocked together with a single injection. Anteriorly, the femoral, obturator, and lateral femoral cutaneous nerves can be blocked by three separate

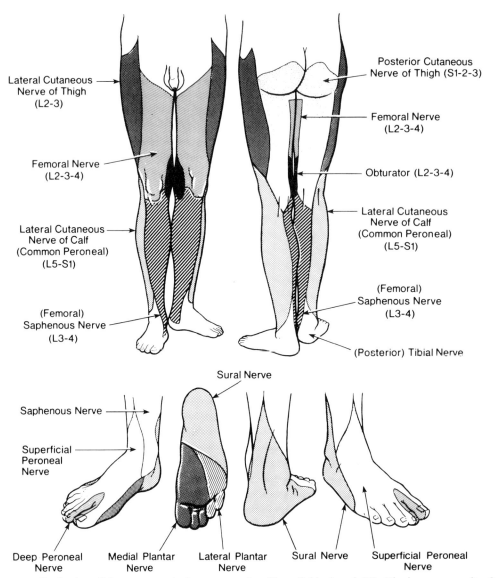

Figure 38–21. Cutaneous distribution of the nerves to the lower extremity. (From Bridenbaugh PO: The lower extremity: Somatic blockade. In Cousins M, Bridenbaugh PO (eds): Neural Blockade in Clinical Anesthesia and Management of Pain. 2nd ed. Philadelphia, JB Lippincott Co, 1988, p 425.)

injections or by a single injection using the three-in-one technique described by Winnie and colleagues,[98] in which a large amount of anesthetic is injected into the femoral nerve sheath and permitted to track into the pelvis to the point at which the anterior nerves run in a common sheath.

Proximal lower extremity nerve blocks are rarely used in the emergency department. Injuries to the thigh and calf that call for extensive repair and anesthesia often require a specialist and repair in the operating room. Injuries to the ankle and foot are more easily anesthetized at that level. Three per cent of emergency physicians use blocks at the hip on occasion.[94]

Femoral nerve blocks alone may be the analgesia of choice for femoral shaft fractures. Studies supporting the femoral block in the treatment of femoral shaft fractures date back to 1940 and continue to appear.[99, 100] In a study by McGlone and colleagues, patients preferred femoral block to narcotic analgesia; however, this means of analgesia has yet to be adopted as routine treatment for femoral shaft fractures.[100] The procedure requires only femoral nerve

blockade and does not rely on the performance of a successful three-in-one block.

Anatomy. The leg is supplied by five nerves. Anteriorly, the femoral, obturator, and lateral femoral cutaneous arise from the lumbar plexus and travel a short distance in a common nerve sheath (Fig. 38–22). In the pelvis, the lateral femoral cutaneous and obturator nerves exit the sheath. The lateral femoral cutaneous nerve supplies the sensory innervation to the lateral thigh. The obturator nerve supplies the sensory innervation to the anterior medial thigh and motor supply to the adductor muscles. The femoral nerve continues as the saphenous nerve, which supplies the sensory innervation to the medial calf and ankle.

Posteriorly, the sciatic and posterior cutaneous nerves arise from the lumbar and sacral plexuses and exit the pelvis together in the sciatic notch. The posterior cutaneous nerve supplies sensory innervation to the posterior thigh and buttocks. The sciatic nerve does not supply the thigh but at the knee divides into the tibial and peroneal nerves and supplies much of the calf and foot. The tibial nerve supplies

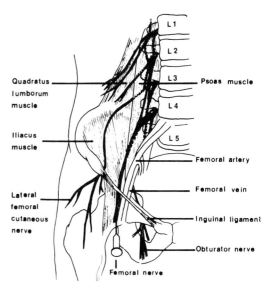

Figure 38–22. Anatomy of the femoral, obturator, and lateral femoral cutaneous nerves and the location of the injection site for the femoral and 3-in-1 nerve blocks. (Adapted from Winnie AP, Ramamurthy S, Durrani Z: The inguinal paravascular technic of lumbar plexus anesthesia: The "3 in 1 block." Anesth Analg 52:989, 1973. Reproduced by permission.)

the muscles of the calf and sensation to the plantar surface of the foot. The peroneal nerve supplies sensation to the lateral aspect of the calf and dorsal and plantar aspects of the foot. Both the tibial and peroneal nerves give off branches that form the sural nerve, which supplies sensation to the lateral aspect of the foot (Fig. 38–23).

Technique for Femoral Nerve Block. With the patient in the supine position, the skin is prepared in an aseptic fashion. The femoral artery is palpated 1 to 2 cm below the

inguinal ligament (see Fig. 38–22), and a wheal of anesthesia is raised immediately lateral to the artery. With the nondominant hand placed firmly on the artery, a 1.25-cm, 22-gauge needle, attached to an extension tube set-up and a 20-ml syringe, is inserted adjacent to the artery at a 90-degree angle to the skin and underlying vessels. The needle is advanced until a paresthesia is elicited or the needle pulsates laterally, indicating a position immediately adjacent to the artery. If a paresthesia is felt or if the needle is assumed to

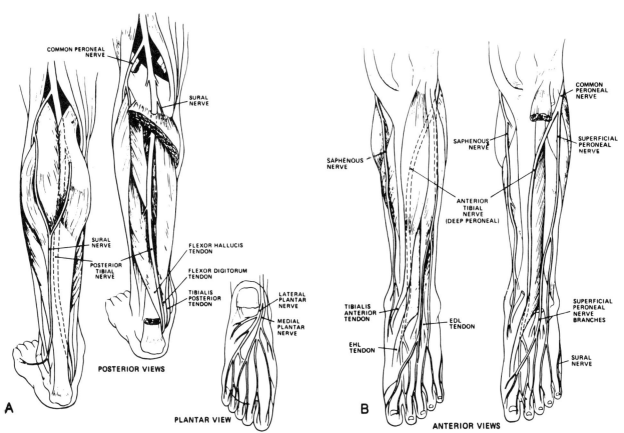

Figure 38–23. *A* and *B*, Anatomy and innervation of the calf and foot. (From Shurman DH: Ankle-block anesthesia for foot surgery. Anesthesiology 44:348, 1976. Reproduced by permission.)

be in the immediate vicinity of the nerve, 10 to 20 ml of anesthetic is injected. If a paresthesia is not elicited, 10 to 20 ml of anesthetic can be injected in a fan-like pattern lateral to the artery in a blind attempt to anesthetize the femoral nerve. The onset of anesthesia should occur in 15 to 30 minutes and should last for 3 to 8 hours.

Technique of the Three-in-One Block. The three-in-one technique differs from the femoral nerve block in that it requires a larger amount of anesthetic solution and compression distal to the injection site. In the thigh, the femoral nerve is sandwiched between the quadratus lumborum and iliopsoas muscles, whose fasciae are continuous with a nerve sheath that contains all three nerves higher in the pelvis. A large amount of anesthetic properly placed next to the femoral nerve tracks back along the sheath and anesthetizes all three nerves.

Blind injections will not produce the three-in-one block, which requires precise injection of the anesthesia into the nerve sheath. In the three-in-one block, once the needle is in the correct position, the fingers palpating the artery are removed and placed gently but firmly distal to the needle while 20 to 30 ml of anesthetic is injected. Distal pressure should be maintained for 5 minutes while the anesthetic diffuses proximally.

A nerve stimulator facilitates the search for the nerve and placement of the needle tip in the fascial sheath. It is particularly useful in the three-in-one block, in which correct needle placement is crucial for a successful block. The nerve is covered by a thick insulating fascia. When the needle punctures this sheath, the nerve is stimulated at currents of 0.5 mA or less.

Precautions. The femoral nerve block requires that large amounts of anesthetic be injected close to large nerves and vessels. Standard precautions should be used to avoid intravascular and intraneuronal injection, and recommended anesthetic dosages should be observed.

Nerve Blocks of the Ankle

Nerve block of the five nerves of the ankle, the deep peroneal (anterior tibial), posterior tibial, saphenous, superficial peroneal (musculocutaneous), and sural nerves, provides anesthesia to the foot. Depending on the desired area of anesthesia, one or more of the five nerves are blocked. These blocks can be used in operative procedures and repair of injuries to the foot. They are particularly useful in providing anesthesia to the sole of the foot for laceration repair and foreign body removal.

Nerve blocks of the ankle appear to be underutilized by emergency physicians. The foot is frequently injured, particularly in warm climates and in summer months when people go barefoot. In one series of 537 patients who required repair of lacerations, 16.5 per cent had a laceration to the toes or feet that required local anesthesia, and 2 per cent of the total of 7627 patients had foot problems for which local anesthesia could have been used.[101] Although some problems that require an ankle block are of a degree that may also require referral to a specialist and repair in the operating room, many problems can be handled in the emergency department. Even minor problems that can be treated using local infiltration may be treated more efficiently and with less discomfort by using a nerve block at the ankle. Only 21 per cent of emergency physicians use this block in their practice.[94]

Nerve block of the foot is better tolerated by the patient than local infiltration in all but the most minor procedures. The skin of the sole is thicker and more tightly bound to the underlying fascia by connective tissue septa than that in other parts of the body. Puncturing this skin can be difficult

and is always quite painful. The fibrous septa can limit the amount and spread of anesthetic. If large amounts of anesthesia are injected, the volume of injected substance quickly exceeds the space available, possibly leading to painful distention of the tissue and circulatory compromise of the microvasculature. Local infiltrative anesthesia is adequate for treating minor injuries in which only small amounts of anesthetic are needed. For treatment of larger injuries, including incision and drainage, extensive wound care, and foreign body removal, the ankle block is better tolerated.

Anatomy. The foot is supplied by the five nerve branches of the principal nerve trunks (see Fig. 38–21). Three nerves are located anteriorly and supply the dorsal aspect of the foot. Two nerves are located posteriorly and supply the volar aspect.

The anteriorly located nerves are the superficial peroneal, deep peroneal, and saphenous nerves. The superficial peroneal nerve (also called the dorsal cutaneous or musculocutaneous nerve) actually consists of multiple branches that supply a large portion of the dorsal aspect of the foot (see Fig. 38–23). These are located superficially between the lateral malleolus and extensor hallucis longus tendon, which is easily palpated by having the patient dorsiflex the big toe. The deep peroneal nerve (also called the anterior tibial nerve) supplies the web space between the big and second toes. In the ankle, it lies under the extensor hallicus longus tendon. The saphenous nerve runs superficially with the saphenous vein between the medial malleolus and tibialis anterior tendon, which is prominent when the patient dorsiflexes the foot. The saphenous nerve supplies the medial aspect of the foot near the arch.

The posteriorly located nerves are the posterior tibial and sural nerves. The sural nerve runs subcutaneously between the lateral malleolus and the Achilles tendon and supplies the lateral border, both volar and dorsal, of the foot (see Fig. 38–23). The posterior tibial nerve runs with the posterior tibial artery, which can be palpated between the medial malleolus and the Achilles tendon. It lies slightly deep and posterior to the artery.

The posterior tibial nerve is one of the major nerve branches to the foot. After passing through the ankle, it branches into the medial and lateral plantar nerves, which supply sensation to most of the volar aspect of the foot and toes and supply motor innervation to the intrinsic muscles of the foot.

Technique. The five nerves of the foot are commonly blocked in combinations of two or more. Small procedures clearly within the distribution of one nerve may require only

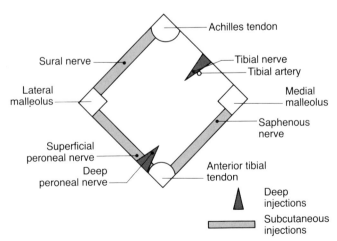

Figure 38–24. Conceptualized figure demonstrating the distribution of anesthetic for a complete nerve block at the ankle.

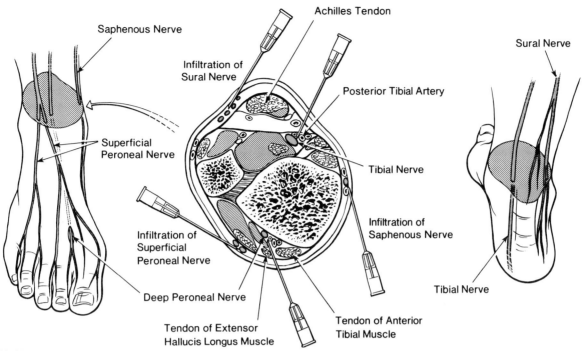

Figure 38–25. Anatomy and injection sites for nerve blocks at the ankle. (From Bridenbaugh PO: The lower extremity: Somatic blockade. In Cousins M, Bridenbaugh PO (eds): Neural Blockade in Clinical Anesthesia and Management of Pain. 2nd ed. Philadelphia, JB Lippincott Co, 1988, p 435.)

a single nerve block; however, overlap of the nerve's sensory distribution frequently necessitates blocking a number of nerves for adequate anesthesia. Nerve block of the sural and posterior tibial nerves together anesthetizes the bottom of the foot and is the most useful combination.

Complete nerve block of the foot requires three subcutaneous and two deep injections. Once familiar with the anatomy, the experienced physician can anesthetize all five nerves quickly, if necessary.

The technique for blocking each nerve individually will be discussed though it may be easier to remember the ankle blocks by conceptualizing the procedure with a schematic anatomic drawing (Figs. 38–24 and 38–25). The shape of the ankle in cross-section is that of a diamond. The lateral points are the malleoli and the inferior and superior points are the anterior tibial and Achilles tendons, respectively. The ankle is blocked by placing subcutaneous band blocks on three of the four sides and two deep injections: one in the remaining quadrant next to the palpable artery and the other in the superior point under the extensor tendon of the big toe.

Posterior Tibial. The posterior tibial nerve is blocked in the medial aspect of the ankle between the medial malleolus and the Achilles tendon. The injection site is determined by palpating the tibial artery just posterior to the medial malleolus. A point 0.5 to 1.0 cm superior to this is marked. If the artery is not palpable, a site 1 cm above the medial malleolus and just anterior to the Achilles tendon is used (Fig. 38–26).

A 3.75-cm, 25-gauge needle is directed at a 45-degree angle to the mediolateral plane (the needle is almost perpendicular to the skin), just posterior to the artery. At the estimated depth of the artery, approximately 0.5 to 1.0 cm deep, the needle is wiggled slightly in an effort to produce a paresthesia. If the paresthesia is elicited, 3 to 5 ml of anesthetic is injected after careful aspiration to check for inadvertent intravascular placement of the needle tip. If no

paresthesia is produced, the needle is advanced inward, again at a 45-degree angle, until it hits the posterior aspect of the tibia. The needle is then withdrawn slightly, about 1 mm, and 5 to 7 ml of anesthetic is injected while the needle

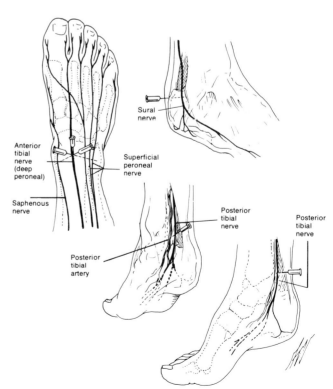

Figure 38–26. Anatomy and injection sites for nerve blocks at the ankle (lateral views). (Adapted from Locke RK, Locke SE: Nerve blocks of the foot. JACEP 4:698, 1976.)

is withdrawn another 1 cm. A rise in temperature of the foot, due to vasodilation from loss of sympathetic tone, may herald a successful block. This finding may be used as an indicator of onset and depth of anesthesia.

Sural Nerve. The sural nerve is blocked on the lateral aspect of the ankle between the Achilles tendon and the lateral malleolus (see Fig. 38–25). It lies superficially and is blocked at a level about 1 cm above the lateral malleolus. A band of anesthesia is injected subcutaneously between the Achilles tendon and the lateral malleolus using 3 to 5 ml of anesthetic.

Superficial Peroneal Nerves. The superficial peroneal nerves are blocked on the anterior aspect of the ankle between the extensor hallucis longus tendon and the lateral malleolus. They lie superficially and are blocked using 4 to 10 ml of anesthetic placed subcutaneously in a band between these landmarks.

Deep Peroneal Nerve. The deep peroneal nerve is blocked anteriorly beneath the extensor hallucis tendon (see Fig. 38–25). It is blocked at a level 1 cm above the base of the medial malleolus and between the extensor hallucis longus and anterior tibial tendons. The tendons are palpated by having the patient dorsiflex the big toe and foot, respectively. After a subcutaneous wheal is placed, the needle is directed about 30 degrees laterally and under the extensor hallucis tendon until it strikes the tibia (at a depth of less than 1 cm). The needle is withdrawn 1 mm, and 1 ml of anesthetic is injected.

Saphenous Nerve. The saphenous nerve is blocked anteriorly between the medial malleolus and the anterior tibial tendon. It lies superficially and is blocked with 3 to 5 ml of anesthetic injected subcutaneously between these landmarks.

NERVE BLOCKS OF THE METATARSALS AND TOES

Like the nerve blocks in the hand and fingers, the nerve blocks in the foot and toes are commonly used in the emergency department. Indications for using these blocks include repair of lacerations, drainage of infections, removal of toenails, manipulation of fractures and dislocations, and otherwise painful procedures requiring anesthesia to the forefoot and toes. Eighty-seven per cent of emergency physicians use this block in their practice.[94]

Digital nerve blocks in the foot and toes are superior to local infiltration anesthesia in all but the most minor procedures. In the toes, the limited subcutaneous space does not accommodate enough injected material for adequate infiltrative anesthesia. Furthermore, the fibrous septa, which attach the volar skin to the underlying fascia and bone, limit the spread and volume of injected substances. On the plantar surface, even small amounts of local infiltrate can cause painful distention and local ischemia of the tissues.

Anatomy. Each toe is supplied by two dorsal and two volar nerves. These nerves are branches of the major nerves of the ankle. The dorsal digital nerves are the terminal branches of the deep and superficial peroneal nerves. The volar nerves are branches of the posterior tibial and sural nerves.

The location of the nerves in relation to the bones varies with the site of the foot. In the toes, the nerves lie at the 2, 4, 8, and 10 o'clock positions in close relationship to the bone. In the proximal foot, the nerves run with the tendons and are not in close relationship to the bones (Fig. 38–27).

Technique. The digital nerves can be blocked at the metatarsals, interdigital web spaces, or toes. The bones of the foot can be palpated easily from the dorsum and are used as the landmarks for estimating the location of the nerves. Proximally, the nerves' relationship to the bones is less consistent, making definitive needle placement and successful block less reliable. In the toes, the position of the nerves is more consistent; however, there is minimal subcutaneous tissue space available for the injected solution. At the web space, the nerves are located in close relationship to the bone, and there is ample space for injecting the anes-

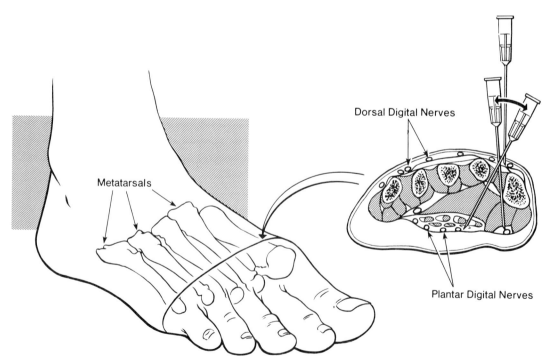

Figure 38–27. Anatomy and technique for digital nerve block at the metatarsals. (From Bridenbaugh PO: The lower extremity: Somatic blockade. In Cousins M, Bridenbaugh PO (eds): Neural Blockade in Clinical Anesthesia and Management of Pain. 2nd ed. Philadelphia, JB Lippincott Co, 1988, p 437.)

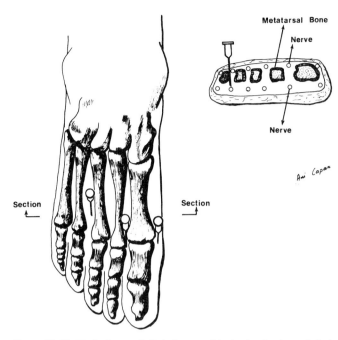

Figure 38–28. Technique of digital nerve blocks in the interdigital web spaces of the foot.

thesia; hence for most procedures, the web space is the preferred site for the digital nerve block.

The technique for toe and metatarsal blocks is similar. All four nerves supplying each toe are usually blocked because of their sensory overlap. The blocks are performed from the dorsal surface, where the skin is thinner and less sensitive than that on the plantar aspect. A total of 5 ml of anesthetic is deposited in a fan-like pattern in the space between the metatarsal bones (see Fig. 38–27). A 1-ml skin wheal is placed dorsally between the metatarsal bones. The needle is then advanced until the volar skin tents slightly, and 2 ml are injected as the needle is withdrawn. Without removing the needle, it is redirected in a different volar direction, and the procedure is repeated. A total of 5 ml is used in each metatarsal space. Again, because of sensory overlap, two or more spaces need to be anesthetized for each toe to be blocked.

For the web space block, a site on the dorsum just proximal to the base of the toe is selected. Using a 10-ml syringe, a 3.75-cm, 27-gauge needle is inserted at the lateral edge of the bone (Fig. 38–28). A wheal is placed subcutaneously between the skin and bone, using 0.5 to 1.0 ml of anesthetic. This serves to block the dorsal nerve and minimize pain at the needle insertion site. The needle is then advanced just lateral to the bone and toward the sole until the needle tents the volar skin slightly. The needle is withdrawn 1 mm, and 0.5 to 1.0 ml is injected. As the needle is withdrawn, another 0.5 ml is injected to ensure a successful block. The procedure is repeated on the opposite side of the toe. In this manner, two columns of anesthesia are placed on each side of the toe in the area through which the four digital nerves run. A total of 2 to 4 ml of anesthetic is used. For blocks done in the toe itself, the procedure is the same, but smaller amounts of anesthetic are used because of the limited subcutaneous space and fear of vascular compression. A total of less than 2 ml is used. Alternate techniques using a single injection site, as described for the finger, can be performed (Fig. 38–29).

Complications and Precautions. The precautions that apply to the hand and fingers apply to the foot and toes.

Ischemic complications can be avoided by paying attention to skin changes during the injection. Blanching heralds possible intravascular injection or vascular compression. If the skin blanches, halt the procedure and reevaluate the position of the needle and the amount and content of the injected solution. The total volume of anesthesia should not exceed the recommended amount. Epinephrine should not be used because of possible vasospasm and ischemia.

Note any neural or vascular injuries before the injection. The close proximity of these structures to the skin and bones means that they are frequently injured. Deficits, even if questionable, should be documented in the records and brought to the attention of the patient before the nerve block.

Intercostal Nerve Block

The blocking of the intercostal nerves produces anesthesia over an area of their cutaneous distribution (Fig. 38–30). It is useful in the emergency department for analgesia of rib fractures.

Rib fractures are typically quite painful, causing the patient to splint respirations to avoid excessive movement of the injured site. The resulting hypoventilation, atelectasis, and poor expectoration may cause hypoxia or lead to pneumonia, particularly in patients with preexisting pulmonary disease and minimal respiratory reserve, in which further impairment of function causes significant respiratory compromise. Anesthetizing the injured rib eases the pain and facilitates deep breathing and coughing.

It is unclear whether intercostal nerve blocks are superior to oral analgesics in the treatment of rib fractures. Current studies suggest that intercostal block may be superior to analgesics in patients who have undergone thoracotomies.[102, 103] Those receiving intercostal nerve blocks had better results on pulmonary function tests, greater oxygenation, and earlier ambulation and discharge than those receiving narcotic analgesics. There are no controlled studies comparing intercostal blocks versus oral analgesics in pa-

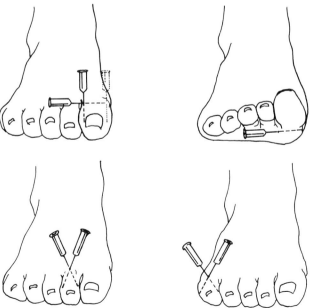

Figure 38–29. Alternative techniques of digital nerve blocks in the toes. (From Locke RK, Locke SE: Nerve blocks of the foot. JACEP 4(9):698, 1976.)

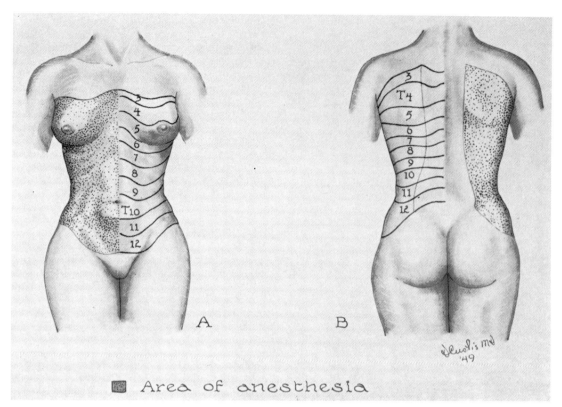

Figure 38–30. Area of anesthesia and cutaneous distribution of the intercostal nerve. (From Moore DC: Regional Block: A Handbook for Use in the Clinical Practice of Medicine and Surgery. 4th ed. Springfield, Ill, Charles C Thomas, 1971, p 159.)

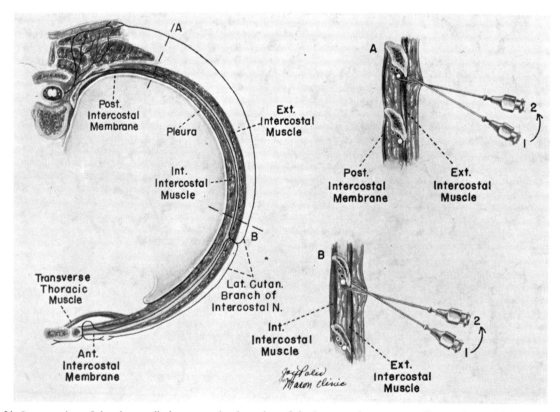

Figure 38–31. Cross section of the chest wall, demonstrating branches of the intercostal nerve, as well as sections of the chest wall at points where intercostal block is usually performed: *A*, at the posterior angle of the ribs, and *B*, at the midaxillary line. (From Moore DC: Regional Block: A Handbook for Use in the Clinical Practice of Medicine and Surgery. 4th ed. Springfield, Ill, Charles C Thomas, 1971, p 146.)

tients with the kind of rib fractures that are commonly seen in the emergency department.

There are several arguments against the routine use of intercostal nerve blocks in the emergency department. Rib fractures are often tolerated well in young patients who usually require minimal oral analgesics. Furthermore, these blocks have a short duration of action. The typical duration of action of a long-acting anesthetic with epinephrine is 8 to 12 hours. Often, the patient receives partial analgesia for up to 3 days, a period of time that cannot be attributed to the direct action of the anesthetic on the nerve. Perhaps the anesthesia reduces muscle spasm and the associated cycle of pain. Further controlled studies would be useful.

The perceived high incidence of pneumothorax and unsuccessful blocks is another reason why intercostal nerve blocks are not used in the emergency department. Yet these fears appear to be unfounded. In more than 10,000 individual rib blocks done by physicians in all stages of training, Moore reported the incidence of pneumothorax was less than 0.1 per cent,[104] and Moore and Bridenbaugh reported a 98 per cent success rate in a series of 5000 intercostal nerve blocks.[105] Only 31 per cent of emergency clinicians use this block, suggesting it may be underutilized.[94]

The suggested approach to administering intercostal blocks is as follows: Patients should be given the facts with regard to duration of analgesia and possible complications and should be allowed to decide on the method for themselves. Often they prefer oral analgesics initially but may return for further relief of pain, at which time they are more amenable to the nerve block.

Anatomy. Each thoracic nerve exits the spine through the intervertebral foramen, which lies midway between adjacent ribs. It immediately gives off the posterior cutaneous branch, which supplies the skin and muscles of the paraspinal area. The intercostal nerve continues and gives off the lateral cutaneous branches at the midaxillary line. These branches are the sensory supply to the anterior and posterior lateral chest wall.

The intercostal nerve runs with the vein and artery in the subcostal groove (Fig. 38–31). Posteriorly, the nerve is separated from the pleura and the lungs by the thin intercostal fascia. Particular care must be taken to avoid puncture of the thin fascia and underlying lung when blocking the nerve in the posterior aspect of the back. Fortunately, most rib fractures occur in the anterior or lateral portion of the ribs and can be blocked in the posterior axillary line, where the internal intercostal muscle lies between the nerve and the lung's pleura and provides a buffer for minor errors in needle placement.

Technique. For adequate analgesia of most rib fractures, the lateral cutaneous branch needs to be anesthetized. Blocks are usually performed between the posterior axillary and midaxillary line at a point proximal to the origin of this branch. Explanation of the procedure, benefits, and risks, including pneumothorax, systemic toxicity, and ineffective block, should be done before proceeding.

A 10-ml syringe with a 3.75-cm, 23- to 25-gauge needle is used. The rib is palpated, and the area is prepared in the usual aseptic manner. The index finger of the nondominant hand is used to retract the skin at the lower edge of the rib cephalad and up over the rib (Fig. 38–32). With the syringe in the opposite hand, the skin is punctured at the tip of the

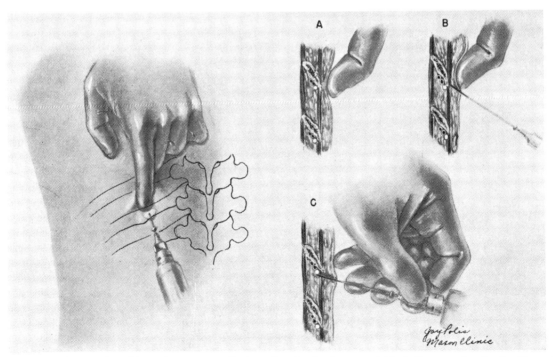

Figure 38–32. Method of retracting skin and proper needle insertion site for intercostal block. See text for details. (From Moore DC: Regional Block: A Handbook for Use in the Clinical Practice of Medicine and Surgery. 4th ed. Springfield, Ill, Charles C Thomas, 1971, p 153.)

finger that is retracting the skin. The syringe is held at an 80-degree angle with the needle pointing cephalad. The hand holding the syringe rests on the chest wall for stability. In this position, the depth of needle penetration is well controlled. The needle is slowly advanced until it comes to rest on the lower border of the rib.

At this point, the skin retraction is released. The skin returning to its natural position moves the needle shaft perpendicular to the chest wall and the needle tip to the inferior margin of the rib. The syringe is shifted from the dominant hand to the index and thumb of the nondominant hand. The middle finger of the same hand rests against the shaft of the needle and, by exerting gentle pressure on the shaft, walks the needle off the lower edge of the rib. Again, the palm of the hand is planted firmly on the chest wall to ensure control of the needle. With the help of the dominant hand, the needle is slowly advanced 3 mm. The needle is aspirated, and then 2 to 5 ml of anesthetic are injected while the needle is carefully moved in and out 1 mm, which ensures that the compartment containing the nerve between the internal and external intercostal muscles is penetrated. This may also serve to minimize intravascular injections. The procedure is repeated on the ribs above and below to ensure that the overlapping innervation from adjacent nerves is blocked.

Although the procedure just discussed seems extensive, it takes a minute or two to perform once the operator is familiar with the technique, and 3 to 5 intercostals can be blocked in 10 minutes' time.

Precautions. The needle must be initially placed at the lower edge of the rib. If it contacts the rib above this point, it cannot be walked off the lower edge of the rib at the proper angle. If it is inserted too low, over the intercostal space, it may be advanced too deep through the pleura and into the lung before the operator realizes the misplacement. Before inserting the needle, the depth of the bone should be estimated. If the bone is not encountered by this depth, reevaluation of the needle position should be made. Even after the needle has been properly walked off the edge of the rib, care must be taken to avoid puncture of the pleura and lung. The depth of the intercostal groove in which the nerve runs is 0.6 cm posteriorly and diminishes to 0.4 cm anteriorly.

Because the incidence of pneumothorax is low, a chest radiograph is not routinely required after this procedure. The asymptomatic patient is observed for 15 to 30 minutes and instructed to return if problems arise. If the patient has symptoms of pneumothorax, such as cough, a change in the nature of the pleuritic pain, or shortness of breath, the patient should have a chest film taken before discharge.

If the physician inadvertently causes a pneumothorax, treatment depends on the size. Many pneumothoraces are small. Those less than 20 per cent may be observed for 6 hours.[105] If the pneumothorax does not grow in size, the patient may be discharged home with arrangements for follow-up. Needle aspiration of larger pneumothoraces may be all that is needed. A chest tube is necessary if this method fails (see Chapters 8 and 9).

Toxicity from the epinephrine and the anesthetic is another complication. The intercostal block is associated with the highest plasma concentrations of anesthetic for a given dose when comparing different sites.[106] The exact reason for the high plasma levels is not entirely clear. Moore suggests this is because the anesthetic is injected close to the intercostal vessels[106]; however, other blocks are also performed close to large vessels without a comparable rise in plasma levels. Regardless, the maximum recommended dose of anesthetic should not be exceeded. Systemic absorption of epinephrine may prove dangerous in patients taking monoamine oxidase inhibitors or with preexisting heart disease of hypertension. Bupivacaine without epinephrine should be used in these patients.

REFERENCES

1. Koller C: On the use of cocaine for producing anaesthesia on the eye. Lancet 2:990, 1884.
2. Hall RJ: Hydrochlorate of cocaine. NY Med J 40:643, 1884.
3. Halsted WS: Practical comments on the use and abuse of cocaine; suggested by its invariably successful employment in more than a thousand minor surgical operations. NY Med J 42:294, 1885.
4. Moore DC: The pH of local anesthetic solutions. Anesth Analg 60:833, 1981.
5. McLeskey CH: pH of local anesthetic solutions (letter). Anesth Analg 59:892, 1980.
6. Skou JC: The blocking potencies of some local anesthetics and of butyl alcohol determined on peripheral nerves. ACTA Pharmacol Et Toxicol 10:281, 1954.
7. Ritchie JM, Ritchie B, Greengard P: The active structure of local anesthetics. J Pharm Exp Ther 150:152, 1965.
8. Ritchie JM, Ritchie B, Greengard P: The effect of the nerve sheath on the action of local anesthetics. J Pharm Exp Ther 150:160, 1965.
9. Strickartz GR, Ritchie JM: Action of local anesthetics on ion channels of excitable tissues. In Strickartz GR (ed): Handbook of Experimental Pharmacology. New York, Springer-Verlag, 1985.
10. Taylor RE: Effect of procaine on electrical properties of squid axon membrane. Am J Physiol 196:1071, 1959.
11. Hille B: Common mode of action of three agents that decrease the transient change in sodium permeability in nerves. Nature 210:1220, 1966.
12. Strichartz GR: The inhibition of sodium currents in myelinated nerve by quaternary derivatives of lidocaine. J Gen Physiol 62:37, 1973.
13. Narahashi T, Frazier DT, Yamada M: The site of action and active form of local anesthetics. I. Theory and pH experiments with tertiary compounds. J Pharm Exp Ther 171:32, 1970.
14. Frazier DT, Narahashi T, Yamada M: The site of action and active form of local anesthetics. II. Experiments with quaternary compounds. J Pharm Exp Ther 171:45, 1970.
15. Galindo A: pH-adjusted local anesthetics: Clinical experience. Regional Anesth 8:35, 1983.
16. Hilgier M: Alkalinization of bupivacaine for brachial plexus block. Regional Anesth 10:59, 1985.
17. Swerdlow M, Jones R: The duration of action of bupivacaine, prilocaine, and lignocaine. Br J Anaesth 42:335, 1970.
18. Chvapil M, Hameroff SR, O'Den K, Peacock E Jr: Local anesthetics and wound healing. J Surg Res 27:267, 1979.
19. Morris T, Tracey J: Lignocaine: Its effect on wound healing. Br J Surg 64:902, 1977.
20. Schmidt RM, Rosenkranz HS: Antimicrobial activity of local anesthetics: Lidocaine and procaine. J Infect Dis 121:597, 1970.
21. Fariss BL, Foresman PA, Rodeheaver GT, et al: Anesthetic properties and toxicity of bupivacaine and lidocaine for infiltration anesthesia. J Emerg Med 5:275, 1987.
22. Barker W, Rodeheaver GT, Edgerton MT, Edlich RF: Damage to tissue defenses by a topical anesthetic agent. Ann Emerg Med 11:307, 1982.
23. Stevenson TR, Rodeheaver GT, Golden GT, et al: Damage to tissue defenses by vasoconstrictors. JACEP 4:532, 1975.
24. Tran D Thao, Miller SH, Buck D, et al: Potentiation of infection by epinephrine. Plast Reconstr Surg 76:933, 1985.
25. Hohn DC, McKay RD, Halliday B, Hunt TK: Effect of O$_2$ tension on microbicidal function of leukocytes in wounds and in vitro. Surg Forum 27:18, 1976.
26. Dronen SC: Complications of TAC (letter). Ann Emerg Med 12:5, 1983.
27. Edlich RF: Complications of TAC (letter). Ann Emerg Med 12:5, 1983.
28. Pryor GJ, Kilpatrick WR, Opp DR: Local anesthesia in minor lacerations: Topical TAC vs. lidocaine infiltration. Ann Emerg Med 9:568, 1980.
29. Schaffer DJ: Comparison of TAC anesthetic solutions with and without cocaine. Ann Emerg Med 14:1077, 1985.
30. White WB, Iserson KV, Criss E: Topical anesthesia for laceration repair: Tetracaine versus TAC (tetracaine, adrenaline, and cocaine). Am J Emerg Med 4:319, 1986.
31. Bonadio WA, Wagner V: Half-strength TAC topical anesthetic. Clin Pediatr 27:495, 1988.
32. Ross DS, Scroggins D, Taylor J, et al: Comparison of topical anesthetic agents in the repair of facial and scalp lacerations in children (abstract). Ann Emerg Med 18:469, 1989.
33. Ernst PA, Crabbe LH, Winsemius DK, et al: Comparison of tetracaine, adrenaline, and cocaine with cocaine alone for topical anesthesia. Ann Emerg Med 19:95, 1990.
34. Hegenbarth MA, Altier MF, Hawk WH, et al: Comparison of topical tetracaine, adrenaline, and cocaine anesthesia with lidocaine infiltration for repair of lacerations in children. Ann Emerg Med 19:111, 1990.
35. Anderson AB, Colecchi C, Baronoski R, et al: Local anesthesia in

pediatric patients: Topical TAC versus lidocaine. Ann Emerg Med 19:519, 1990.

36. Noble AB, Murray JG: A review of the complications of spinal anaesthesia with experiences in Canadian teaching hospitals from 1959 to 1969. Canadian Anaesth Soc J 18:5, 1971.

37. Moore DC, Bridenbaugh LD, Thompson GE, et al: Bupivacaine: A review of 11,080 cases. Anesth Analg 57:42, 1978.

38. Lund PC, Cwick JC, Pagdanganan RT: Etidocaine—a new long-acting local anesthetic agent: A clinical evaluation. Anesth Analg 52:482, 1973.

39. Born G: Neuropathy after bupivacaine (Marcaine) wrist and metacarpal nerve blocks. J Hand Surg 9A:109, 1984.

40. Maguire WM, Reisdorff EJ, Smith D, et al: Epinephrine-induced vasospasm reversed by phentolamine digital block. Am J Emerg Med 8:46, 1990.

41. Gordh T: Complications and their treatment. In Ericksson E (ed): Illustrated Handbook in Local Anaesthesia. 2nd ed. Philadelphia, WB Saunders Co, 1980, p 16.

42. deJong RH: Toxic effects of local anesthetics. JAMA 239:1166, 1978.

43. Scott DB, Jebson PJR, Braid DB, et al: Factors affecting plasma levels of lignocaine and prilocaine. Br J Anaesth 44:1040, 1972.

44. Moore DC, Bridenbaugh LD: Oxygen: The antidote for systemic toxic reactions from local anesthetic drugs. JAMA 174:102, 1960.

45. Tucker GT, Moore DC, Bridenbaugh PO, et al: Systemic absorption of mepivacaine in commonly used regional block procedures. Anesthesiology 37:277, 1972.

46. Moore DC, Mather LE, Bridenbaugh LD, et al: Arterial and venous plasma levels of bupivacaine following peripheral nerve blocks. Anesth Analg 55:763, 1976.

47. Arthur DS, McNicol LR: Local anesthetic techniques in paediatric surgery. Br J Anaesth 58:760, 1986.

48. deJong RH, Ronfeld RA, De Rosa RA: Cardiovascular effects of convulsant and supraconvulsant doses of amide local anesthetics. Anesth Analg 61:3, 1982.

49. Kotelko DM, Shnider SM, Dailey PA, et al: Bupivacaine-induced cardiac arrhythmias in sheep. Anesthesiology 60:10, 1984.

50. Thigpen JW, Kotelko DM, Shnider SM, et al: Bupivacaine cardiotoxicity in hypoxic-acidotic sheep (abstracts). Anesthesiology 59:A204, 1983.

51. Tucker GT: Pharmocokinetics of local anesthesia. Br J Anaesth 58:717, 1986.

52. Albright GA: Cardiac arrest following regional anesthesia with etidocaine or bupivacaine. Anesthesiology 51:285, 1979.

53. Liu P, Feldman HS, Covino BM, et al: Acute cardiovascular toxicity of intravenous amide local anesthetics in anesthetized ventilated dogs. Anesth Analg 61:317, 1982.

54. Crandell JT, Kotelko DM: Cardiotoxicity of local anesthetics during late pregnancy (abstracts). Anesth Analg 64:204, 1985.

55. Morishima HO, Pedersen H, Finster M, et al: Bupivacaine toxicity in pregnant and nonpregnant ewes. Anesthesiology 63:134, 1985.

56. Reiz S, Nath S: Cardiotoxicity of local anesthetic agents. Br J Anaesth 58:736, 1986.

57. Bromage PR, Datta S, Dunford L: Etidocaine: An evaluation in epidural analgesia for obstetrics. Can Anaesth Soc J 21:535, 1974.

58. Moore DC, Crawford RD, Scurlock JE: Severe hypoxia and acidosis following local anesthetic-induced convulsions. Anesthesiology 53:259, 1980.

59. deJong RH, Davis NL: Treating bupivacaine arrhythmias: Preliminary report. Regional Anesth 6:99, 1981.

60. Kasten GW, Martin ST: Bupivacaine cardiovascular toxicity: Comparison of treatment with bretylium and lidocaine. Anesth Analg 64:911, 1985.

61. Kasten GW, Martin ST: Successful cardiovascular resuscitation after massive intravenous bupivacaine overdosage in anesthetized dogs. Anesth Analg 64:491, 1985.

62. Pollack CV, Swindle GM: Use of diphenhydramine for local anesthesia in caine-sensitive patients. J Emerg Med 7:611, 1989.

63. deShazo RD, Nelson HS: An approach to the patient with a history of local anesthetic hypersensitivity: Experience with 90 patients. J Allergy Clin Immunol 63:387, 1979.

64. Aldrete JA, Johnson DA: Evaluation of intracutaneous testing for investigation of allergy to local anesthetic agents. Anesth Analg 49:173, 1970.

65. Incando G, Schatz M, Patterson R, et al: Administration of local anesthetics to patients with a history of prior adverse reaction. J Allergy Clin Immunol 61:339, 1978.

66. Adriani J: Comment in Aldrete JA, Johnson DA: Evaluation of intracutaneous testing for investigation of allergy to local anesthetic agents. Anesth Analg 49:182, 1970.

67. Swanson JG: Assessment of allergy to local anesthetics. Ann Emerg Med 12:316, 1983.

68. Covino BG: Pharmacology of local anesthetic agents. Br J Anaesth 58:701, 1986.

69. Mather LE, Cousins MJ: Local anaesthetics and their current clinical use. Drugs 18:85, 1979.

70. Adriani J, Zepernick R: Clinical effectiveness of drugs used for topical anesthesia. JAMA 188:93, 1964.

71. Gentile DA: Severe methemoglobinemia induced by a topical teething preparation. Pediatr Emerg Care 3:176, 1987.

72. Buckley AB, Newman A: Methemoglobinemia occurring after the use of a 20% benzocaine topical anesthetic prior to gastroscopy (letter). Gastro Endoscopy 33:466, 1987.

73. Chiu YC, Brecht K, DasGupta DS: Myocardial infarction with topical cocaine anesthesia for nasal surgery. Arch Otolaryngol Head Neck Surg 112:988, 1986.

74. Regal RE: Comment: Lidocaine seizures. Drug Intell Clin Pharm 19:680, 1985.

75. Hess GP, Watson PD: Seizures secondary to oral viscous lidocaine. Ann Emerg Med 17:725, 1988.

76. Mofenson HC, Caraccio TR, Miller H, et al: Lidocaine toxicity from topical mucosal application. Clin Pediatr 22:190, 1983.

77. Puczynski MS, Ow EP, Rust C: Cardiopulmonary arrest due to misuse of viscous lidocaine. Arch Otolaryngol 111:768, 1985.

78. Pottage A, Scott DB: Safety of topical lignocaine (letter). Lancet 1:1003, 1988.

79. Greenblatt DJ, Benjamin DM, Willis CR, et al: Lidocaine plasma concentrations following administration of intraoral lidocaine solution. Arch Otolaryngol 111:298, 1985.

80. Monash S: Location of the superficial epithelial barrier to skin penetration. J Invest Derm 29:367, 1957.

81. Campbell D, Adriani J: Absorption of local anesthetics. JAMA 168:873, 1958.

82. Lubens HM, Ausdenmoore RW, Shater AD, et al: Anesthetic patch for painful procedures such as minor operations. Am J Dis Child 128:192, 1974.

83. Lyman JL, McCabe JB: Improving the effectiveness of TAC application (letter). Ann Emerg Med 13:642, 1984.

84. Dailey RH: Fatality secondary to misuse of TAC solution. Ann Emerg Med 17:159, 1988.

85. Spivey WH, McNamura RM, Mackenzie RS, et al: A clinical comparison of lidocaine and bupivacaine. Ann Emerg Med 16:752, 1987.

86. Christoph RA, Buchanan L, Begalla K, Schwartz S: Pain reduction in local anesthetic administration through pH buffering. Ann Emerg Med 17:117, 1988.

86a. Peterfreund RA, Datta S, Ostheimer GW: pH adjustment of local anesthetic solutions with sodium bicarbonate: laboratory evaluation of alkalinization and precipitation. Regional Anesth 14:265, 1989.

87. Dinley RJ, Michelinakis E: Local anesthesia in the reduction of Colles' fracture. Injury 4:345, 1973.

88. Cobb AG, Houghton GR: Local anaesthetic infiltration versus Bier's block for Colles' fractures. Br Med J 291:1683, 1985.

89. Case RD: Haematoma block—a safe method of reducing Colles' fractures. Injury 16:469, 1985.

90. Ericksson E: Infiltration of a fracture haematoma. In Ericksson E (ed): Illustrated Handbook in Local Anesthesia. 2nd ed. Philadelphia, WB Saunders Co, 1980, p 46.

91. Ivey FM: Evaluating acute knee injuries. Am Fam Pract 25:122, 1982.

92. Newman AP: Meniscal and ligamentous injuries of the knee. Top Emerg Med 10:1, 1988.

93. Barrack RL, Skinner HB, Brunet ME, et al: Functional performance of the knee after intraarticular anesthesia. Am J Sports Med 11:258, 1983.

94. Orlinsky M, Dean E: Survey of Anesthesia Use in the Emergency Department, 1990 (unpublished).

95. Swerdlow M: Complications of local anesthetic neural blockade. In Cousins M, Bridenbaugh PO (eds): Neural Blockade in Clinical Anesthesia and Management of Pain. 2nd ed. Philadelphia, JB Lippincott Co, 1988.

96. Selander D, Dhuner KG, Lundberg G: Peripheral nerve injury due to injection needles used for regional anesthesia. An experimental study of the acute effects of needle point trauma. Acta Anaesth Scand 21:182, 1977.

97. Selander D, Edghage S, Wolff T: Paresthesia or no paresthesia? Nerve lesions after axillary blocks. Acta Anaesth Scand 23:27, 1979.

98. Winnie AP, Ramamuthy S, Durrani Z: The inguinal paravascular technique of lumbar plexus anesthesia. The "3 in 1 block." Anesth Analg 52:989, 1973.

99. Berry FR: Analgesia in patients with fractured shaft of femur. Anaesthesia 32:576, 1977.

100. McGlone R, Sadhra K, Hamer DW, Pritty PE: Femoral nerve block in the initial management of femoral shaft fractures. Arch Emerg Med 4:163, 1987.

101. Locke RK, Locke SE: Nerve blocks of the foot. JACEP 4:698, 1976.

102. Bergh WB, Pottori O, Axisonherf B, et al: Effect of intercostal block on lung function after thoracotomy. Acta Anaesth Scand 24:85, 1966.

103. Delikan AE, Lee CK, Young WK, et al: Postoperative local analgesia for thoracotomy with direct bupivacaine intercostal blocks. Anaesthesia 28:561, 1973.

104. Moore DC: Complications of regional anesthesia. Clin Anesth 2:281, 1969.

105. Moore DC, Bridenbaugh LD: Intercostal nerve block in 4333 patients: Indication, technique, and complications. Anesth Analg 41:1, 1962.

106. Moore DC, Mather LE, Bridenbaugh LD, et al: Arterial and venous

plasma levels of bupivacaine following peripheral nerve block. Anesth Analg 55:763, 1976.

SELECTED READINGS

1. Wildsmith JAW: Peripheral nerve and local anesthetic drugs. Br J Anaesth 58:692, 1986.
2. Adriani J, Campbell D: Fatalities following topical application of local anesthetics to mucous membranes. JAMA 162:1527, 1956.
3. Ritchie JM: Mechanism of action of local anesthetic agents and biotoxins. Br J Anaesth 47:191, 1975.
4. Arndt KA, Burton C, Noe JM: Minimizing the pain of local anesthetics. Plast Reconstr Surg 72:676, 1983.
5. Moore DC, Bridenbaugh LD, Thompson GE, et al: Factors determining dosages of amide-type local anesthetic drugs. Anesthesiology 47:263, 1977.
6. Scott DB: Toxic effects of local anesthetic agents on the central nervous system. Br J Anaesth 58:732, 1986.
7. Tucker GT, Mather LE: Pharmacology of local anesthetic agents—pharmacokinetics of local anesthetic agents. Br J Anaesth 47:213, 1975.
8. Aldrete JA, Romo-Salas F, Arora S, et al: Reverse arterial blood flow as a pathway for central nervous system toxic responses following injection of local anesthetics. Anesth Analg 57:428, 1978.
9. Adriani J, Dalili H: Penetration of local anesthetics through epithelial barriers. Anesth Analg 50:834, 1981.
10. Mckay W, Morris R, Mushlin P: Sodium bicarbonate attenuates pain on skin infiltration with lidocaine, with or without epinephrine. Anesth Analg 66:572, 1987.
11. Morris R, McKay W, Mushlin P: Comparison of pain associated with intradermal and subcutaneous infiltration with various local anesthetic solutions. Anesth Analg 66:1180, 1987.

Chapter **39**

Regional Anesthesia of the Head and Neck

James T. Amsterdam

INTRODUCTION

Regional anesthesia of the head and neck involves primarily intraoral and extraoral nerve blocks and anesthesia of the scalp. Such blocks can be used for diagnostic evaluation. Patients with dental pain who do not get relief with a regional dental block most likely do not have pain of dental origin. Regional blocks are also therapeutic for both surgical procedure anesthesia and pain control for dental emergencies such as toothaches and dry sockets (see Chapter 87 on Emergency Dental Procedures). In cases when the patient is thought to be seeking drugs and one wishes to avoid narcotics, a dental anesthetic block is frequently the treatment of choice.

Topical anesthetic solutions such as tetracaine-adrenalin-cocaine (TAC) solution are useful in small lacerations of the scalp and face because of the vascularity of these areas. TAC is not to be used on mucous membranes. Detailed information on the use of TAC appears in Chapter 38. Detailed discussion of the general complications of regional anesthesia is provided in Chapter 38 also.

INTRAORAL AND EXTRAORAL LOCAL ANESTHESIA

The use of intraoral and extraoral regional anesthesia is both simple and convenient.[1-3] Nerve blocks are used to attain anesthesia in areas of broad distribution in the face with a minimal amount of anesthetic and tissue distortion. Local anesthetic blocks are effective for closing facial lacer-

ations, especially those of the lips, the forehead, and the midface, on which the swelling caused by local infiltration is undesirable. Local anesthetic blocks are also effective for the relief of pain, for anesthesia in debridement, and for diagnostic purposes.

The procedures and techniques described here generally carry a low morbidity. The supraperiosteal and mental nerve infiltrations can generally be learned through reading and experimentation; more sophisticated blocks are best learned under the instruction of an experienced physician, a dentist, or an oral and maxillofacial surgeon.

Anatomy of the Fifth, or Trigeminal, Nerve

The fifth cranial nerve (the trigeminal nerve) is the sensory nerve to the face (Fig. 39–1*A*) and is the largest of the cranial nerves. It takes its origin from the midbrain and enlarges into the gasserian, or semilunar, ganglion. One gasserian ganglion supplies each side of the face. The gasserian ganglion is a flat, crescent-shaped structure approximately 10 mm long and 20 mm wide that divides into three branches: the ophthalmic, maxillary, and mandibular nerves (Fig. 39–1*B*).

The first division, the ophthalmic nerve (V-1), is the smallest branch in the gasserian ganglion. It leaves the cranium through the superior orbital fissure and has five cutaneous branches. These branches are:

1. The medial and lateral branches of the supraorbital nerve, which emerge on the face through the supraorbital notch. These two sensory nerves pierce the frontalis muscle and extend to the lambdoid suture on the back of the skull.
2. The supratrochlear nerve, which is sensory to the medial aspect of the forehead just above the glabella.
3. The infratrochlear nerve.
4. The lacrimal nerve.
5. The external nasal nerve.

In addition to being sensory to the forehead, branches of the ophthalmic nerve are sensory to the cornea, the upper eyelid, structures in the orbit, and the frontal sinuses.

The second division, the maxillary nerve (V-2), is sensory to the maxilla and associated structures, such as the teeth, the periosteum and the mucous membranes of the maxillary sinus and the nasal cavity, the soft and hard palate, the lower eyelids, the upper lip, and the side of the nose. The second division exits the cranium from the foramen rotundum and ultimately enters the face through the infraorbital canal; it terminates as the infraorbital nerve. The

---

The material on scalp blocks was originally written by Levon M. Capan, M.D., Katie P. Patel, M.D., and Herman Turndorf, M.D. For ease of organization, this material now appears in this chapter on head and neck anesthesia. The author and the editors appreciate the contribution of the original authors.

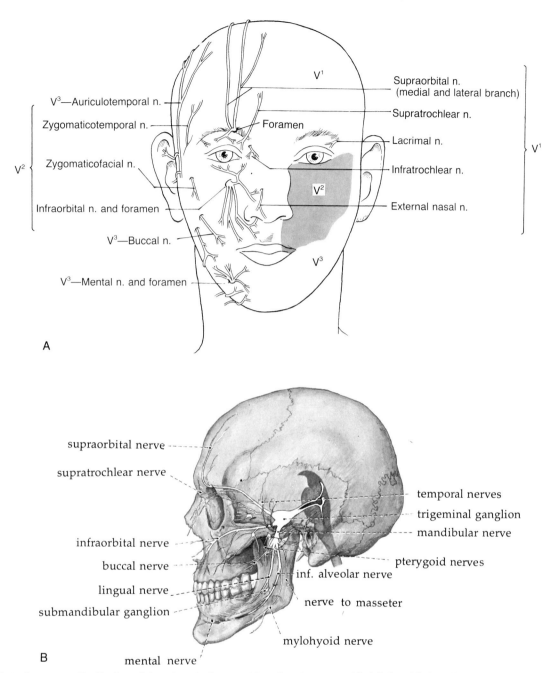

Figure 39–1. *A,* Cutaneous distribution of the trigeminal nerve. Note that the supraorbital, infraorbital, and mental foramina are all in line just medial to the pupil when the person looks straight ahead. *B,* Branches of the trigeminal nerve. (From Langman J, Woerdeman MW: Atlas of Medical Anatomy. Philadelphia, WB Saunders Co, 1978. Reproduced by permission.)

infraorbital nerve gives sensory branches to the lower eyelids, the side of the nose, and the upper lip.

The detailed anatomy of the maxillary nerve is rather complicated, consisting of a number of branches. The first branch comprises two short sphenopalatine nerves to the pterygopalatine ganglion, also called the Meckel ganglion or the sphenopalatine ganglion. The next two branches of clinical importance are the nasopalatine and the greater (anterior) palatine nerves. The nasopalatine nerve arises from the pterygopalatine ganglion, courses down along the nasal septum, and is transmitted through the anterior portion of the hard palate by way of the anterior palatine canal. This canal is located in the midline approximately 10 mm palatally to the maxillary central teeth and immediately

behind the incisors. The nasopalatine nerve is sensory to the most anterior portion of the hard palate and the adjacent gum margins of the upper incisors. This nerve is rarely blocked in clinical practice, except in dental operations (Fig. 39–2A). The anterior, or great palatine, nerve arises from the pterygopalatine ganglion and passes down through the posterior palatine foramen. The posterior palatine foramen is located 10 mm palatally to the third molar and the bicuspid teeth and intermingles with the nasopalatine nerve opposite the cuspid tooth. The greater palatine nerve is sensory to most of the hard palate as well as the palatal aspect of the gingiva. It is rarely blocked in the emergency department (Fig. 39–2B).

The next branch consists of the posterior superior

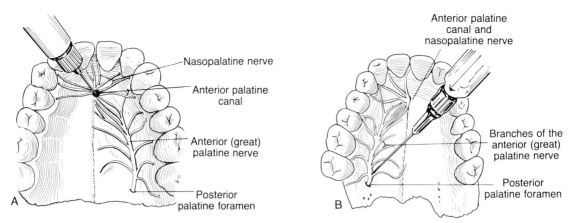

Figure 39–2. *A,* The anterior one third of the palate, from canine to canine, is anesthetized by a local injection near the anterior palatine canal. There may be some overlapping branches of the anterior palatine nerve. *B,* Anesthesia of the posterior two thirds of the palate is obtained by a local injection in the area of the posterior palatine foramen. Note: *Do not enter the foramen itself, because the anesthetic may reach the middle palatine nerve and produce anesthesia of the soft palate, resulting in gagging.*

alveolar nerve, which courses down the posterior surface of the maxilla for approximately 20 mm, at which point it enters one or several small posterior superior dental foramina. This nerve supplies all the roots of the third and second molar teeth and two roots of the first molar tooth. A third branch consists of the middle superior alveolar nerve, which branches off about midway within the infraorbital canal and then courses downward in the outer wall of the maxillary sinus. This nerve supplies the maxillary first and second bicuspid teeth and the mesiobuccal root of the first molar. The last branch consists of the anterior superior alveolar nerve, which branches off into the infraorbital canal approximately 5 mm behind the infraorbital foramen, just before the terminal branches of the infraorbital nerve emerge. This nerve descends in the anterior wall of the maxilla to supply the maxillary central, lateral, and cuspid teeth; the labial mucous membrane; the periosteum; and the alveoli on one side of the median line. There is an intercommunication between the anterior, middle, and posterior superior alveolar nerves.

The third division, the mandibular nerve (V-3), is the largest branch of the trigeminal nerve. It exits from the cranium through the foramen ovale and divides into three principal branches.

1. The long buccal nerve branches off just outside the foramen ovale. It passes between the two heads of the external pterygoid muscle and crosses in front of the ramus to enter the cheek through the buccinator muscle, buccally to the maxillary third molar. The buccal nerve supplies sensory branches to the buccal mucous membrane and the mucoperiosteum over the maxillary and mandibular teeth. The cutaneous branch is the sensory nerve to the cheek.

2. The lingual nerve courses forward toward the midline. The nerve courses downward superficially to the internal pterygoid muscle to pass lingually to the apex of the mandibular third molar. It enters the base of the tongue at this point through the floor of the mouth and supplies the anterior two thirds of the tongue, the lingual mucous membrane, and the mucoperiosteum.

3. The largest of the branches is the inferior alveolar nerve. It is sensory to all of the lower teeth, although the central and lateral incisors and the buccal aspect of the molar teeth may receive additional sensory innervation. The nerve descends, covered by the external pterygoid muscle, and passes between the ramus of the mandible and the sphenomandibular ligament to enter the mandibular canal. It is accompanied by the inferior alveolar artery and vein and proceeds along the mandibular canal, innervating the teeth. At the mental foramen, the nerve bifurcates into an incisive branch, which continues forward to supply the anterior teeth. It gives off a side branch, the mental nerve, which exits from the mental foramen to supply the skin. The mental foramen is located approximately between the apices of the lower first and second bicuspids, or premolar teeth. This is a very useful site, because it is sensory to the integument of the chin and the skin and the mucous membrane of the lower lip.

Equipment for Dental Nerve Blocks

One may easily give extraoral injections with standard injection equipment. Intraoral local anesthesia is conveniently administered with a monojet aspirating dental syringe, which uses Carpule cartridges of anesthetic and disposable needles (Fig. 39–3). A needle not smaller than 27 gauge is recommended for deep block techniques. Generally, a long needle is used for block techniques and a short needle is used for infiltrations. The needle is screwed to the hub of the monojet syringe, which in turn is attached to an adapter; the adapter may be removed for cleaning. When removing the disposable needle, one must take care not to remove and discard the adapter as well; this would render the syringe functionless (Fig. 39–4). One pulls back the end of the syringe on its spring, allowing room for the Carpule of anesthetic to be inserted (Fig. 39–5A). The metal end of the Carpule is inserted, which engages the needle (Fig. 39–5B). The handle of the syringe is then released and tapped to engage a barb into the rubber stopper of the carpule (Fig. 39–5C). One now may perform simple aspiration by retracting the handle, pulling on the rubber stopper within the carpule.

To discard a Carpule, one should leave the needle in place on the syringe. One withdraws the handle of the syringe rapidly, disengaging the barb. If the needle has been removed, great care must be taken, because the negative pressure created in the Carpule upon withdrawal of the barb may cause shattering. Other adjuncts that are helpful in the administration of intraoral anesthesia include topical local anesthetic agents, such as gels or sprays. It should be noted that dental syringes are not mandatory for intraoral local anesthesia but do make the procedure more simple. Reusable glass and disposable plastic aspirating syringes that do not use dental Carpule cartridges are also available.

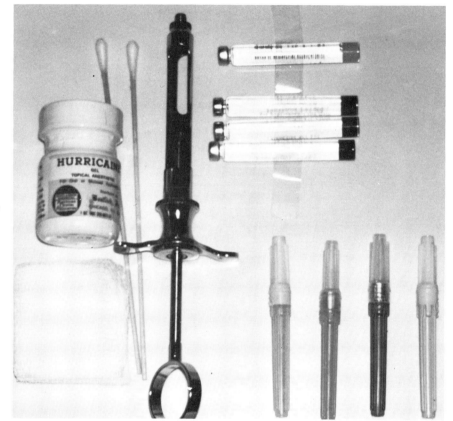

Figure 39–3. Local anesthesia—basic set-up for intraoral application.

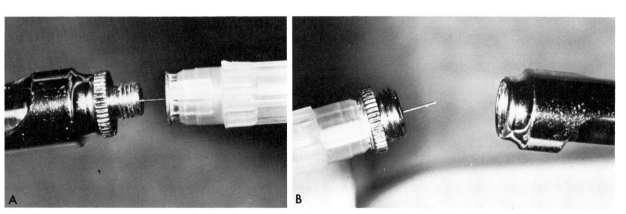

Figure 39–4. *A,* Proper technique for removal of the disposable hypodermic needle from the dental aspirating syringe. *B, Incorrect* technique involves removal of the adapter.

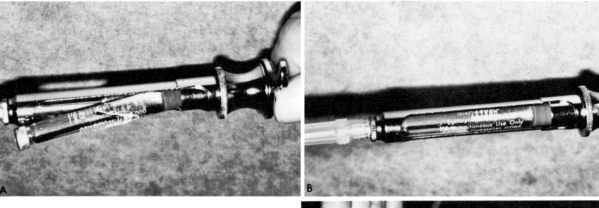

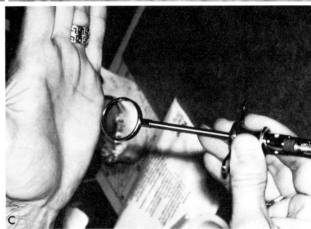

Figure 39–5. Loading the dental aspirating syringe. *A*, The end of the syringe is pulled back. *B*, The Carpule engages the needle. *C*, The barb is snapped into place.

The anesthetic agent most frequently used is 2 per cent lidocaine with a vasoconstrictor, such as 1:100,000 or 1:50,000 epinephrine. Many other anesthetic agents, such as mepivacaine (Carbocaine) and Cetacaine with or without vasoconstrictor agents, are also available. Although available, bupivacaine (Marcaine) is frequently not found in dental Carpules, but this long-acting anesthetic is often ideal for the procedures performed in the emergency department. A Carpule of a different anesthetic may be emptied, however, and bupivacaine may be drawn up in the evacuated Carpule. Because of the rich vascularity of the oral cavity, vasoconstrictors are important in sustaining the duration of anesthesia and should be used wherever possible when no medical contraindications exist.

General Precautions

Needles preferably no smaller than 27 gauge should be used for block techniques, because a higher gauge makes aspiration difficult and may lead to inadvertent intravascular injection. When an intraoral block procedure is performed, the needle should never be inserted to its full length at the hub. Should inadvertent breakage occur in such a situation, needle retrieval may be difficult. Furthermore, the direction of a needle should not be changed while the needle is deep in the tissue. Topical anesthetics can be placed on mucous membranes to make needle puncture painless. One should inject slowly to minimize pain and should always aspirate before injection.

An important precaution for intraoral local anesthesia is that the injection should not be made into or through an infected area. This is especially important in inferior alveolar nerve blocks, in which tracking of an infection can be serious and difficult to treat. Trismus, lack of access, and direct extension to parapharyngeal spaces can result. Therefore, local anesthesia should be only superficial before incision and drainage, unless a block can be performed far proximal to the site of infections.

Topical Anesthesia

Most patients fear dental blocks greatly, and the anxiety and pain may be lessened considerably with the use of topical anesthetics that are applied to the mucous membranes before injection. The area to be injected is first thoroughly dried with gauze. A cotton-tipped applicator is generously coated with 20 per cent benzocaine (Hurricaine, Beutlich, Inc., Niles, Ill.) or 5 to 10 per cent lidocaine. Anesthesia results in 2 to 3 minutes. Note that rather concentrated topical anesthetics must be used, and poor results may be obtained with weaker preparations such as 2 per cent viscous lidocaine.

Infraorbital Nerve Block

INTRAORAL AND EXTRAORAL APPROACH

The infraorbital nerve block injection can be used to anesthetize the midface (Fig. 39–6). A solution of local anesthetic deposited at the infraorbital foramen anesthetizes not only the middle and superior alveolar nerves but also the main trunk of the infraorbital nerve that innervates the skin of the upper lip, the nose, and the lower eyelid. The infraorbital foramen is difficult to palpate extraorally and almost impossible to feel in the presence of facial swelling. It is found on the inferior border of the infraorbital ridge

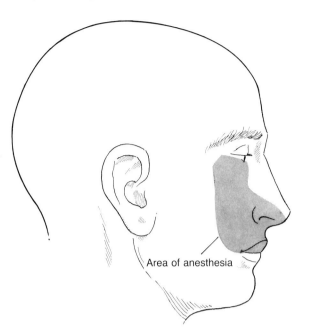

Figure 39–6. Area of anesthesia of a unilateral infraorbital nerve block. Anesthesia includes the lower eyelid and the upper lip. (From Moore D: Regional Block. 4th ed. Springfield, Ill, Charles C Thomas, 1975.)

Area of anesthesia

on a vertical line with the pupil when the patient stares straight ahead.

When performing the intraoral approach, one keeps the palpating finger in place. The cheek is retracted, as in the supraperiosteal injection, and puncture is made in the mucosa opposite the upper second bicuspid (premolar tooth) approximately 0.5 cm from the buccal surface (Fig. 39–7*A*

and *B*). Topical anesthetic applied to the mucosa before injection decreases pain. The needle should be directed parallel with the long axis of the second bicuspid until it is palpated at the foramen, a depth of approximately 2.5 cm. If the entry is too acute initially, one will encounter the malar eminence before approaching the infraorbital foramen. In addition, if the needle is extended too far posteriorly

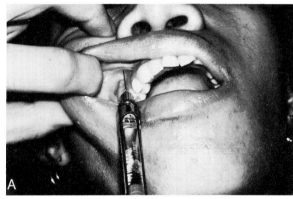

Figure 39–7. *A*, Intraoral approach for infraorbital nerve block. *B*, Note the position of the infraorbital foramen *(arrow)* on the inferior portion of the infraorbital ridge. During infiltration, the needle should be near, but *not* within the foramen, as shown here. *C*, Incorrect infraorbital injection technique may result in needle entry into the orbit.

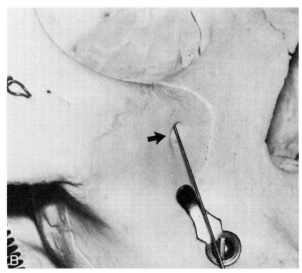

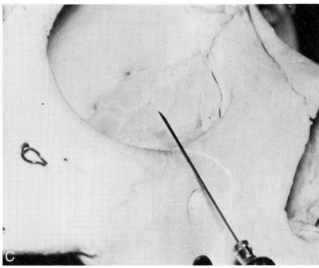

and superiorly, the orbit may be entered (Fig. 39–7C). Therefore, the procedure should be halted if the physician is unsure of the location of the needle or if patient cooperation is unsatisfactory. When the location has been determined and aspiration has been performed, 1 to 2 ml of solution is injected. A finger should be held firmly on the inferior orbital rim to avoid ballooning of the lower eyelid with anesthetic solution. If one is not certain of the exact location of the infraorbital foramen, one may obtain anesthesia by performing a field block. Five ml of the anesthetic solution is infiltrated in a fan-like direction in the upper buccal fold. This technique is not as precise as a discrete nerve block but usually produces the same effect.

The infraorbital foramen may also be approached from an extraoral route (Fig. 39–8). In the extraoral approach, similar landmarks are used to locate the infraorbital foramen. The needle can be felt to pass through the skin, the subcutaneous tissue, and the quadratus labii superioris muscle. Care must be taken not to anesthetize the facial artery and vein, because these may lie on either side of the needle. Vasoconstrictors should not be used in this technique if possible. The extraoral approach, of course, requires external preparation of the skin. If vasoconstrictors are used and severe blanching of the face occurs, warm compresses should be applied to the face immediately.

Inferior Alveolar Nerve Block

In some situations, such as extreme dental pain, the emergency physician may find the use of the inferior alveolar nerve block and the lingual nerve block useful. This injection is somewhat more difficult than the other techniques described, and the emergency physician is advised to view demonstrations of this procedure before attempting it. The inferior alveolar nerve block provides anesthesia of all of the teeth on that side of the mandible and desensitizes the lower lip and the chin along the distribution of the mental nerve. This technique is primarily useful for anesthetizing patients who have sustained severe dentoalveolar trauma; those with complaints of postextraction pain, dry socket, or pulpitis (toothache); or those with periapical abscess.

Anatomy. The anatomy of the region should first be reviewed (Fig. 39–9A). The patient can be seated either in a dental chair or upright with the occiput firmly against the back of the stretcher, so that when the mouth is opened the body of the mandible is parallel to the floor. The physician should be ready for an unexpected quick jerk of the head when the anxious patient first feels the needle despite the use of topical anesthesia. The physician stands on the side *opposite* the one being injected. The technique first involves palpation of the retromolar fossa with the index finger or thumb. With this maneuver, the greatest depth of the anterior border of the ramus of the mandible (the coronoid notch) may be identified (Fig. 39–9B and C). With the thumb in the mouth and the index finger placed externally behind the ramus (Fig. 39–9D and E), the tissues are retracted toward the buccal (cheek) side, and the pterygomandibular triangle is visualized (Fig. 39–9F).

Technique. The mucosa over the area to be injected may be coated with a topical anesthetic. When topical anesthesia has been obtained, the syringe should be held parallel to the occlusal surfaces of the teeth and angled so that the barrel of the syringe lies between the first and second premolars on the opposite side of the mandible (Fig. 39–9G and H). If a large-barrel syringe is used, the corner of the mouth may hamper efforts to obtain the proper angle. The angle is facilitated by carefully bending the 25-gauge needle about 30 degrees. Puncture is made in the triangle, at a point that either bisects the thumbnail or is 1 cm above the occlusal surface of the molars. If the needle enters too low, such as at the level of the teeth, the anesthetic will be deposited over the bony canal that houses the mandibular nerve and not over the nerve itself. The needle should be felt to pass through the ligaments and the muscles covering the internal surface of the mandible. One should stop when the needle has reached bone, signifying contact with the posterior wall of the mandibular sulcus; bone *must* be felt with the needle. Failure to do so generally results from directing the needle toward the parotid gland (too far posteriorly) rather than toward the inner aspect of the mandible. The needle should then be withdrawn slightly and aspirated, and approximately 1 to 2 ml of solution should be deposited. Three to 4 ml may be required if needle positioning is in error. In children, the angulation is not parallel to the occlusal surfaces of the teeth; the barrel of the syringe must be held slightly higher, because the mandibular foramen is lower. One may anesthetize the lingual nerve by placing several drops of anesthetic solution while withdrawing the syringe. Half of the tongue can thus be anesthetized. In actual practice, the lingual nerve is consistently blocked with this procedure owing to the close proximity of both nerves. Following injection, it usually requires 3 to 5 minutes to achieve anesthesia.

Complications include inadvertent administration of anesthetic posteriorly in the region of the parotid gland, which will anesthetize the facial nerves (Fig. 39–9I). This will cause temporary facial paralysis that affects the orbicularis oculi muscle and results in inability to close the eyelid. The eye must be protected until the local anesthetic has worn off (approximately 2 to 3 hours), and the patient must be reassured. Anesthesia with bupivacaine (Marcaine) presents a more significant problem if this complication occurs, because bupivacaine anesthesia lasts from 10 to 18 hours.

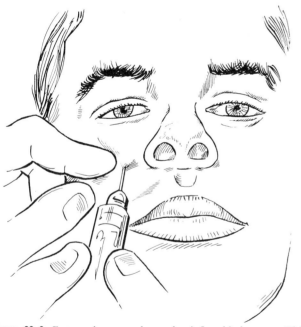

Figure 39–8. Extraoral approach to the infraorbital nerve. This procedure is more difficult than the intraoral approach, especially when attempting to obtain anesthesia of the upper lip. (From Eriksson E: Illustrated Handbook in Local Anesthesia. Philadelphia, WB Saunders Co, 1980.)

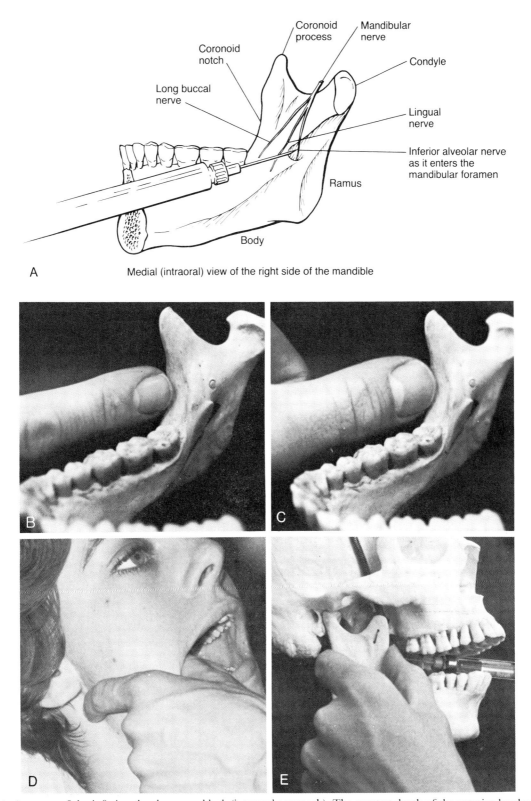

Figure 39–9. *A*, Anatomy of the inferior alveolar nerve block (intraoral approach). The greatest depth of the anterior border of the ramus of the mandible, the coronoid notch, is identified with the left index finger *(B)* or the left thumb *(C)*. *D*, The ramus is grasped between an intraorally placed thumb and extraorally positioned index finger. *E*, Thumb and index finger grasp the ramus and the mandible with the thumb positioned on the coronoid notch. Contrary to the illustration, surgical gloves should be worn.

Illustration continued on following page

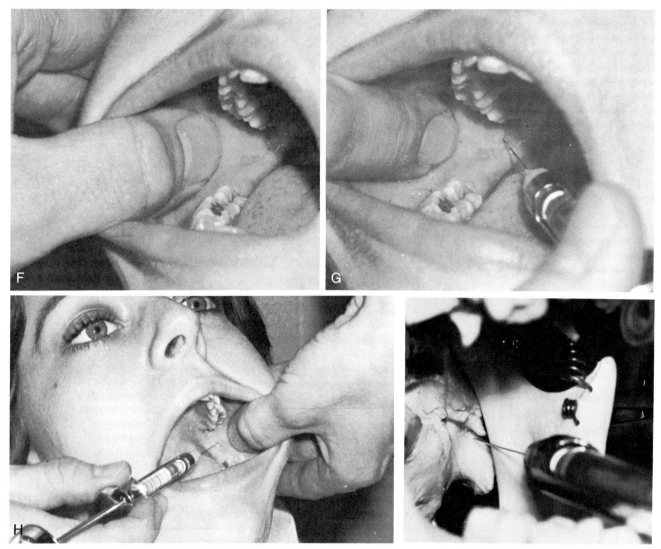

Figure 39–9 *Continued F,* Visualization of the pterygomandibular triangle. Injection location for right *(G)* and left *(H)* inferior alveolar nerve block. *(B, C, D, E, F, G,* and *H* from Bennett CR: Monheim's Local Anesthesia and Pain Control in Dental Practice. St. Louis, CV Mosby Co, 1978.) *I,* Directing the needle too far posteriorly during the inferior alveolar nerve block technique will result in entry into the area of the parotid gland. Anesthesia of the seventh nerve may result. Contrary to the illustration, surgical gloves should be worn.

Supraperiosteal Infiltrations

The most common technique for intraoral local anesthesia of individual teeth is the supraperiosteal infiltration injection. This technique may supply complete relief of a toothache and is a useful emergency department procedure that can provide nonnarcotic analgesia in the middle of the night. The area to be anesthetized is selected and dried with gauze. A topical anesthetic, such as benzocaine (20 per cent) or lidocaine ointment (5 per cent) is applied as before. The mucous membrane of the area is grasped with a piece of gauze; it is pulled downward in the maxilla and upward in the mandible to extend the mucosa fully and to delineate the mucobuccal fold. The mucobuccal fold is then punctured with the bevel of the needle facing the bone. The area is aspirated, and approximately 1 to 2 ml of local anesthetic is deposited at the apex (area of the root tip) of the tooth involved (Fig. 39–10).

The purpose of the injection is to deposit the anesthetic

near the bone that supports the tooth. Because the anesthetic must be absorbed by the bone to reach the nerve of the individual tooth, the injection may fail if the solution is deposited too far from the periosteum, if the needle is passed too far above the roots of the teeth, or if the bone in the area is unusually thick or dense. If anesthesia is unsuccessful, one may also inject the palatal side. It may take 5 to 10 minutes to achieve full anesthesia with this technique, and the procedure may not be as effective for the posterior molars. Infiltration of the area around the maxillary canine and the first premolars will anesthetize the middle and anterior superior alveolar nerves; lacerations of the upper lip can be treated by bilateral injection in the canine fossa areas.

Similarly, infiltration around the mandible and the apices of the first and second premolars provides sufficient anesthesia to block mental nerves that supply the lower lip. This technique is referred to as a *mental nerve infiltration,* as opposed to a *mental nerve block* (Fig. 39–11). A true mental

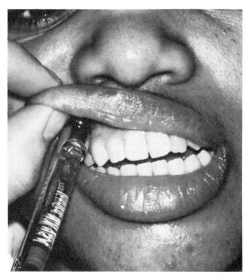

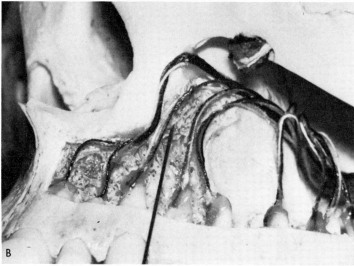

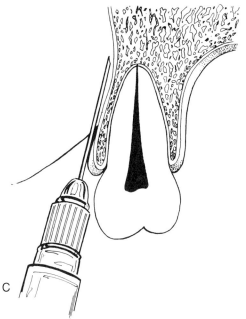

Figure 39–10. *A* and *B*, Supraperiosteal injection technique in maxillary canine fossa for anesthesia of the upper lip or individual teeth. *C*, Schematic illustration of supraperiosteal injection. (From Manual of Local Anesthesia in Dentistry. New York, Cook-Waite Laboratories, Inc. Reprinted courtesy of Eastman Kodak Company.)

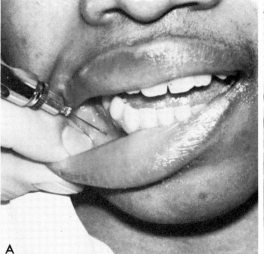

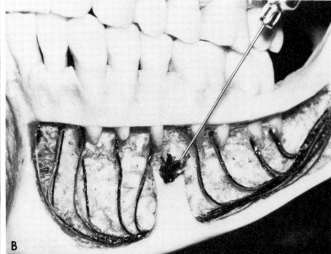

Figure 39–11. Mental infiltration technique. *A*, The correct supraperiosteal approach is an *infiltration* technique; this is all that is required for anesthesia of the lower lip or individual teeth. *B*, Actual introduction of the needle into the mental foramen may produce neurovascular damage, therefore infiltration only is recommended.

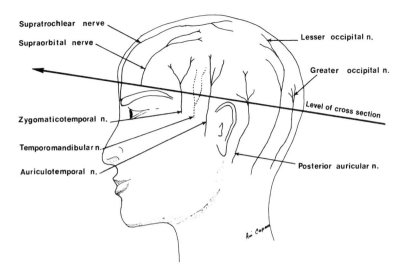

Figure 39–12. The sources of sensory nerve supply to the scalp.

nerve block would involve the introduction of the needle in the mental foramen; this can cause neurovascular damage. Placement of anesthetic only in the region of the mental foramen will provide for anesthesia of the lower lip. Lacerations of the midline of the lips require administration of anesthetic to the side of the midline opposite the site of the attempted block; this location reaches crossing-over fibers. This technique is useful for administering intraoral local anesthesia, especially in children. These blocks are relatively painless if performed after application of a topical anesthetic and if a slow injection technique is used.

BLOCKS OF THE HEAD[4]

Scalp Block

Scalp blocks provide surgical anesthesia for the repair of scalp lacerations and satisfactory anesthesia for surgical decompression of the brain with burr holes.

Anatomy. (Figs. 39–12 and 39–13). The scalp receives its nerve supply from branches of the trigeminal nerve (fifth cranial nerve) and the cervical plexus. The forehead is supplied by the supraorbital and supratrochlear nerves. Both nerves are branches of the ophthalmic division of the trigeminal nerve. The temporal region receives its nerve supply from the zygomaticotemporal (the branch of the second division of the trigeminal nerve), temporomandibular, and auriculotemporal nerves (the branches of the third division of the trigeminal nerve).

The posterior aspect of the scalp is innervated by the greater auricular and the greater, lesser, and least occipital nerves. The nerves that supply the posterior aspect of the scalp originate from the cervical plexus. All the nerves become superficial above a line drawn from the upper border of the external ear to the occiput and the eyebrows and converge toward the vertex of the scalp (see Fig. 39–12).

Topographically, the nerves and vessels of the scalp are located in the subcutaneous tissue above the epicranial aponeurosis. From this level they divide into small branches that extend to the deeper layers (epicranium and periosteum) (see Fig. 39–13).[5]

Techniques. Scalp block can be accomplished by individually blocking each nerve that supplies the scalp, but this approach is time consuming, difficult, and cumbersome. Because the nerves on the scalp are superficially located, the

scalp block can easily be performed by injecting local anesthetic agents into the subcutaneous tissue circumferentially around the area to be blocked. Injection of local anesthetic to the deeper levels is necessary only if bone is to be removed. Note that injection of local anesthetic agents only in the deeper layers without subcutaneous infiltration results in an unsuccessful block and a greater amount of bleeding during surgical intervention.[6]

In preparation for the block, a band of hair may be clipped. (Some physicians prefer to shave the head, but this

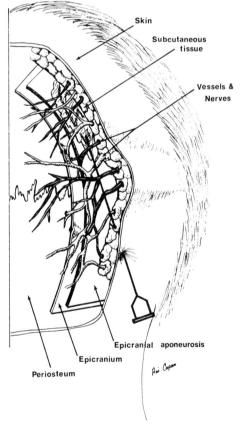

Figure 39–13. Topographic anatomy of the scalp taken above a line drawn from the upper border of the external ear to the occiput and the eyebrows.

procedure is of uncertain benefit.) Local anesthetics are injected in the clipped area. A band 1 cm wide and 3 cm away from the wound can be circumferentially clipped.

The skin is prepared using an antiseptic solution, and a skin wheal is raised at any point of the shaved skin using a ½-inch, 25-gauge needle. A 3-inch, 22-gauge needle is inserted through the skin wheal into the subcutaneous tissue and advanced circumferentially following the previously clipped area. An injection of 0.5 to 1 per cent lidocaine or 0.125 to 0.25 per cent bupivacaine with epinephrine 1:200,000 is used. Epinephrine should be added to the local anesthetic agent to provide vasoconstriction and to prevent excessive blood loss and local anesthetic absorption. The total dose of the local anesthetic agents should not exceed the recommended dose for the particular agent. It may be useful to inject some local anesthetic solution into the temporalis muscle to prevent contraction of the muscle during surgery.

Colley and Heavner demonstrated that when bupivacaine is used, the peak plasma local anesthetic concentrations occur within 10 to 15 minutes after injection.[7] Thus the first 10- to 15-minute period after the injection is the most critical period for the occurrence of local anesthetic toxicity. Colley and Heavner also found that despite the scalp's high vascularity, the absorption of local anesthetics from the scalp is not excessive. Using the upper limit of the recommended dose of bupivacaine without epinephrine (175 mg), they found that peak plasma bupivacaine concentrations were 0.8 μg per ml with a 0.125 per cent solution and 1.2 μg per ml with a 0.25 per cent solution. Considering that the toxic plasma threshold for bupivacaine is 4 μg per ml, these concentrations suggest that a scalp block using bupivacaine has a wide margin of safety even without the use of epinephrine. When epinephrine is used with bupivacaine, its effect on absorption becomes more pronounced with concentrations of 0.125 per cent than with those of 0.25 per cent. This is probably because at low concentrations (0.125 per cent), bupivicaine has a vasoconstrictor property.[8]

Greater and Lesser Occipital Nerve Block

This relatively simple block may be useful in the emergency department for treating occipital neuralgia and tension headaches. For occipital neuritis, a long-acting corticosteroid, such as depomedrol (20 to 40 mg) may be combined with the local anesthetic.

Anatomy. The posterior aspect of the head is supplied by the posterior rami of the cervical nerves. Two important branches of these nerves are the greater and lesser occipital nerves. The greater occipital nerve becomes superficial on each side at the inferior border of the obliquus capitis inferior muscle and runs superiorly toward the vertex over this muscle. The nerve is located medially to the occipital artery. The lesser occipital nerve is located approximately 2.5 to 3.5 cm lateral and 1 to 2 cm caudad to the greater occipital nerve (Fig. 39–14).[9]

Technique. It is not usually necessary to shave or clip the scalp prior to performing greater and lesser occipital nerve blocks. The greater occipital nerve can best be blocked at the nuchal line, which is in the middle of the external occipital protuberance and the mastoid process. The nuchal line is located between the insertion sites of the trapezius muscle and the semispinalis muscles. At this site, the greater occipital nerve is just medial to the occipital artery.

The occipital artery is first palpated, and a 1½-inch, 22-gauge needle connected to a syringe that contains 5 ml of local anesthetic is inserted through the skin (see Fig. 39–14). After obtaining paresthesia at the vertex, 5 ml of local anesthetic solution is injected. The lesser occipital nerve is blocked by a fan-like injection of a local anesthetic solution 2.5 to 3.5 cm lateral and 1 cm caudad to the point described for the greater occipital nerve.[9]

This procedure is not usually associated with any complication; however, intraarterial injections should be avoided by careful aspiration.

Ophthalmic Nerve Block[3]

The lateral and medial branches of the supraorbital nerve, the supratrochlear nerve, and the infratrochlear nerve may be blocked as the nerves emerge from the superior aspect of the orbit by a percutaneous local injection. Anesthesia of the forehead and the scalp is achieved as far posteriorly as the lambdoid suture. Although anesthesia is easily obtained for suturing lacerations of the forehead and the scalp, the nerve block may also be used for débridement or topical treatment of burns or abrasions and for delicate lacerations of the upper eyelid. Such anesthesia is ideal for

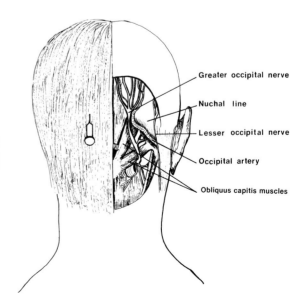

Figure 39–14. The right side of the figure shows the anatomic relationship of the greater and lesser occipital nerves and the adjacent structures at the posterior aspect of the head. The left side of the figure shows the point of entry of the needle for greater occipital nerve block.

Greater occipital nerve

Nuchal line

Lesser occipital nerve

Occipital artery

Obliquus capitis muscles

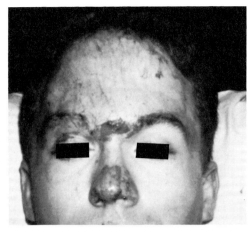

Figure 39–15. This patient had many small pieces of glass embedded in the forehead from a windshield injury. Removal was accomplished painlessly with bilateral supraorbital and supratrochlear nerve blocks.

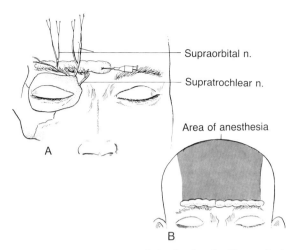

Figure 39–17. *A,* A field block of the forehead will anesthetize the supraorbital and supratrochlear nerves. *B,* Area of anesthesia with a bilateral field block. (From Moore D: Regional Block. 4th ed. Springfield, Ill, Charles C Thomas, 1975.)

removing small pieces of glass that are embedded in the forehead from a windshield injury (Fig. 39–15).

The subtle supraorbital notch, which is in line with the pupil, may be palpated along the superior orbital rim. This landmark is the site of injection for blockage of the supraorbital nerves. The supratrochlear nerve is found 0.5 to 1.0 cm medially to the notch. The infratrochlear nerve is not usually blocked but is found in the most medial aspect of the superior orbital rim. If the anesthetic is placed on the forehead proper, this block may not produce complete anesthesia of the skin of the upper eyelid if the sensory branches to the eyelid are given off before the supraorbital nerve transverses the forehead.

With the patient in the supine position, a skin wheal is raised. Paresthesias in the form of an electric shock sensation over the forehead are sought; these ensure a successful

nerve block. One to 3 ml of the anesthetic is placed in the area of the supraorbital notch. A finger or a roll of gauze should be held firmly under the orbital rim to avoid ballooning of anesthetic into the upper eyelid (Fig. 39–16).

If paresthesias cannot be elicited or if the nerve block is unsuccessful, a line of anesthetic solution placed along the orbital rim from the lateral to the medial aspect will ensure block of all of the branches of the ophthalmic nerve (Fig. 39–17).

Hematoma formation or swelling of the eyelid may occur but requires only local pressure. Occasionally, ecchymosis of the periorbital region will appear the next day, and the patient should be warned of this possibility.

Although this block is infrequently used, it is easily performed and is not associated with serious side effects. Its use should be considered when anesthesia of the forehead or the anterior scalp is desired.

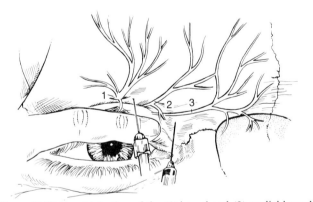

Figure 39–16. Local injection of the *(1)* lateral and *(2)* medial branch of the supraorbital nerve and the *(3)* supratrochlear nerve. It should be noted that a finger is placed on the inferior rim of the infraorbital rim to avoid swelling of the eyelid. (From Eriksson E: Illustrated Handbook in Local Anesthesia. Philadelphia, WB Saunders Co, 1980.)

REFERENCES

1. Manual of Local Anesthesia and General Dentistry. New York, Cook-Waite Laboratories, Inc., 1947.
2. Bennett CR: Manheim's Local Anesthesia and Pain Control in Dental Practice. St. Louis, CV Mosby Co, 1978.
3. Amsterdam J: Anesthetic nerve block. In Tintinnali J et al (eds): Emergency Medicine—A Comprehensive Study Guide. 2nd ed. New York, McGraw-Hill Book Co, 1988, pp 618–620.
4. Capan LM, Patel KP, Turndorf H: Regional anesthesia in the emergency department. In Roberts JR, Hedges JR (eds): Clinical Procedures in Emergency Medicine. 1st ed. Philadelphia, WB Saunders Co, 1985, pp 455–457.
5. Murphy TM: Somatic blockade. In Cousins MJ, Bridenbaugh PO (eds): Neural Blockade in Clinical Anesthesia and Management of Pain. Philadelphia, JB Lippincott Co, 1980, p 410.
6. Bohm E: Local anesthesia of the scalp. In Eriksson E (ed): Illustrated Handbook in Local Anaesthesia. 2nd ed. Philadelphia, WB Saunders Co, 1980, p 25.
7. Colley PS, Heavner JE: Blood levels of bupivacaine after injection into the scalp with and without epinephrine. Anesthesiology 54:81, 1981.
8. Alps C, Reynolds F: The effect of concentration on vasoactivity of bupivacaine and lignocaine. Br J Anaesth 48:1171, 1976.
9. Jenkner FL: Greater (and lesser) occipital nerve block. In Jenkner FL (ed): Peripheral Nerve Block. New York, Springer-Verlag, 1977, p 100.

Chapter 40

Intravenous Regional Anesthesia

James R. Roberts

INTRODUCTION

The clinical use of intravenous regional anesthesia has been well established[1-3] as a safe, quick, and effective alternative to general anesthesia in selected cases requiring surgical manipulation of the upper and lower extremities. Although often relegated to the operating room, the procedure is readily applicable to outpatient use. In the emergency department the technique provides quick and complete anesthesia, along with muscle relaxation and a bloodless operating field. The procedure is free from the troublesome side effects associated with other regional blocks, such as the axillary block. The procedure is easily mastered and has a very low failure rate, and consistently good results can be expected.

The first practical use of analgesia associated with intravenous injection of a local anesthetic agent was described by August Gustav Bier in 1908.[4] Colbern[5] has since proposed the eponym "Bier block." Although the procedure has been in existence for many years, the need for special equipment and a safe anesthetic agent limited its use. However, the Bier block has now gained wide acceptance as a safe and effective procedure, and several papers extol its virtues.[6-9] Although complications do exist, no reported fatalities directly attributed to the use of the Bier block have been reported. In this chapter, the techniques and complications are discussed according to their application in the emergency department.

INDICATIONS AND CONTRAINDICATIONS

Indications for intravenous regional anesthesia include any procedure of the arm or leg that requires operating anesthesia, muscle relaxation, or a bloodless field. I have used the procedure for the reduction of fractures and dislocations, repair of major lacerations, the removal of foreign bodies, the débridement of burns, and the drainage of infection. The procedure may be carried out on a patient of any age who is able to cooperate with the physician.

The only absolute contraindications are an allergy to the anesthetic agent and uncontrolled hypertension. Relative contraindications include an uncooperative patient and the recent ingestion of a large meal, both of which may only delay the procedure rather than contraindicate it.

EQUIPMENT

The equipment required for intravenous regional anesthesia consists of the following:

1 per cent lidocaine (Xylocaine), *without epinephrine*—to be diluted to a 0.5 per cent solution. (*Note:* 1 ml of 1 per cent lidocaine equals 10 mg.)

Sterile saline solution as a diluent
50-ml syringe/18-gauge needle

Pneumatic tourniquet (single or double cuff). (*Note:* Do not use a standard blood pressure cuff.)

Number 18 and number 20 plastic intravenous catheter or a number 21 butterfly needle

Elastic bandage/Webrill padding

500 ml D_5W (5 per cent dextrose in water) and intravenous extension tubing.

PROCEDURE

The procedure should be explained in advance to the patient. If the patient is extremely apprehensive, premedication with midazolam (Versed), diazepam (Valium), or a narcotic may be helpful but need not be routinely used. The only painful portions of the procedure are the establishment of the infusion catheter and the exsanguination procedure. The procedure should not be done on patients who are intoxicated or obtunded or on those with a previous reaction to a local anesthetic.

The patient need not be free of oral intake (NPO) for a specific period of time before the procedure, but it is prudent to delay the procedure if the patient has just eaten a large meal. As a precaution, a large-bore open intravenous line of 5 per cent dextrose in water is established in the unaffected extremity. Resuscitation equipment, including anticonvulsant drugs and oxygen, should be readily available.

The standard dosage of lidocaine is 3 mg/kg, and it is injected as a 0.5 per cent solution (1 per cent lidocaine is mixed with equal parts of sterile saline in a 50-ml syringe). Farrell and associates have described the procedure termed the "minidose Bier block" using 1.5 mg/kg of lidocaine, and they report a 95 per cent success rate.[10] This lower dose may decrease the incidence of central nervous system side effects and is more desirable in the emergency department setting. (Additional lidocaine may be infused if the initial dose is inadequate.) Lidocaine with epinephrine should *not* be used. Plain lidocaine is also available as a 0.5 per cent solution and can be used to avoid the necessity of diluting the stronger solution.

A pneumatic tourniquet with cotton padding to prevent ecchymosis under the cuff is applied proximal to the pathology (Fig. 40–1). *It is strongly advised that one not use a regular blood pressure cuff,* because they often leak or rupture and are not designed to withstand high pressures for any length of time. A specially designed portable double-cuff pneumatic system, such as marketed by OEC Zimmer Corporation, is ideal (Fig. 40–2).

The anesthetic is premixed in the syringe. The tourniquet is inflated and a 20-gauge plastic catheter or a metal butterfly needle is placed in the superficial vein, as close to the pathology as possible, and is securely taped in place (Fig. 40–3). It is usually desirable to use a vein on the dorsum of the hand, but importantly the injection site should be at least 10 cm distal to the tourniquet to avoid injection of anesthetic proximal to the tourniquet. The hub remains on the catheter to avoid back bleeding or the syringe is attached to the butterfly tubing. This catheter will be the route of injection of the anesthetic agent.

The tourniquet is deflated, and the extremity is exsanguinated so that when the anesthetic agent is injected, it will fill the vascular system. Exsanguination may be accomplished by either of two methods. Simple elevation of the extremity for a few minutes may be adequate, but wrapping the extremity in a distal-to-proximal direction with an elastic bandage, being careful not to dislodge the infusion needle, enhances the exsanguination (Fig. 40–4). Wrapping may be painful; this step can be eliminated if it causes too much

Modified with permission from Roberts JR: Intravenous regional anesthesia. JACEP 6:261, 1977.

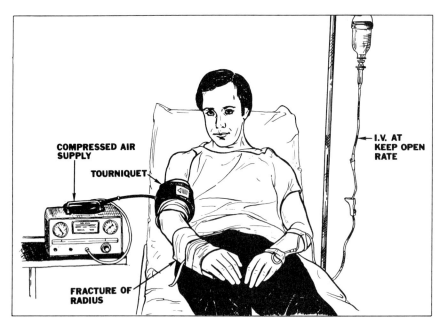

Figure 40–1. Preparation for induction of anesthesia in a patient with a fracture of the right radius. Note precautionary intravenous line and deflated tourniquet in place. The procedure has been explained, and preoperative sedation or analgesia has been given if required. (From Roberts JR: Intravenous regional anesthesia. JACEP 6:263, 1977. Reproduced by permission.)

anxiety to the patient. If the wrapping procedure is not done, the extremity should be elevated for at least 3 minutes. During the wrapping procedure, care must be taken not to dislodge or infiltrate the infusion catheter.

With the extremity still elevated, the tourniquet is inflated to 250 mm Hg, the arm is then placed by the patient's side, and the elastic exsanguination bandage is removed. In a child, the tourniquet is inflated to 50 mm Hg above systolic pressure.

The 0.5 per cent lidocaine solution is then slowly injected into the infusion catheter at the calculated dose. Note that the solution is placed in the arm in which circulation is blocked, *not* in the precautionary keep-open intravenous line on the unaffected side. At this point, blotchy areas of erythema may appear on the skin. This is not an adverse reaction to the anesthetic agent but merely the result of residual blood being displaced from the vascular compartment and it heralds success of the procedure.

In 3 to 5 minutes, the patient will experience paresthesia or warmth, beginning in the fingertips and traveling proximally, with final anesthesia occurring at the elbow. Complete anesthesia ensues in 10 to 20 minutes, followed by muscle relaxation. Note that adequate analgesia may exist even though the patient can still sense touch and position and has some motor function. If the "minidose" technique (1.5 mg/kg of lidocaine) does not provide adequate anesthesia, an additional 0.5 to 1 mg/kg may be infused at this time. Additional lidocaine was required in 7 per cent of cases in one series using the minidose regimen.[10] The physician should be patient, however, and wait a full 15 minutes before infusing additional lidocaine. Alternatively, if analgesia is slow or inadequate an extra 10 to 20 ml of *Saline* solution may be injected to supplement the total volume of solution to enhance the effect. *Do not exceed a 3 mg/kg total dose of lidocaine.* The infusing needle is now withdrawn and the puncture site is tightly taped to prevent extravasation of the anesthetic agent. The surgical procedure or manipulation is performed, including postreduction x-ray films and casting or bandaging (see Fig. 40–5).

Anesthesia from a fingertip-to-elbow direction seems to

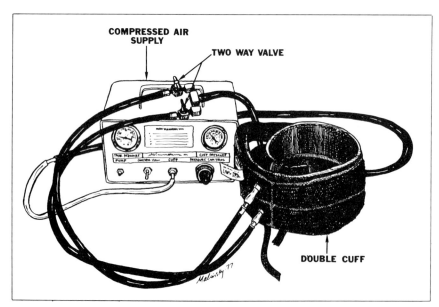

Figure 40–2. Double-cuff apparatus with two-way valves allows longer tourniquet time without pain. A standard blood pressure cuff should never be used. (From Roberts JR: Intravenous regional anesthesia. JACEP 6:263, 1977. Reproduced by permission.)

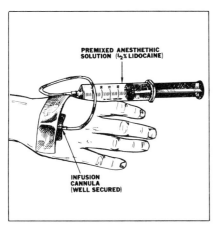

Figure 40–3. Infusion cannula securely taped in dorsum of hand. A butterfly needle is shown here, but a plastic catheter with the hub attached may also be used. (From Roberts JR: Intravenous regional anesthesia. JACEP 6:263, 1977. Reproduced by permission.)

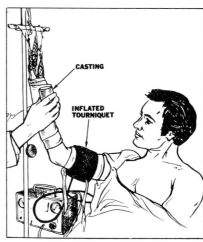

Figure 40–5. Cast is applied under anesthesia. Because the tourniquet is portable, postreduction radiographs may be obtained without losing anesthesia. (From Roberts JR: Intravenous regional anesthesia. JACEP 6:263, 1977. Reproduced by permission.)

occur irrespective of the site of anesthetic infusion, but selecting an injection site near the pathology will provide more rapid anesthesia at a lower dosage.

On completion of the procedure, the deflation of the tourniquet is *cycled* to prevent a bolus effect of the lidocaine that may remain in the intravascular compartment. The cuff is deflated for 5 seconds and reinflated for 1 to 2 minutes. *This action is repeated three or four times.*

If the tourniquet has been in place for *less than 20 to 30 minutes,* it is dangerous to deflate it because adequate tissue fixation of the lidocaine probably has not occurred. This may result in a higher peak plasma lidocaine level with increased side effects. If the surgical procedure is completed rapidly and the 3 mg/kg limit of lidocaine has been infused, *the tourniquet should remain inflated until a full 30 minutes has elapsed, and only then should it be deflated, using the cycling technique.* It is reasonable to use a 20-minute cutoff if the minidose technique is used, because this dose is equal to a commonly administered intravenous bolus.

Sensation returns quickly when the tourniquet is removed, and in 5 to 10 minutes, the extremity returns to its preanesthetic level of sensation and function. After 20 minutes of observation, the patient is released (Table 40–1).

If the procedure takes longer than 20 or 30 minutes, many patients complain of pain from the tourniquet because the tourniquet is not inflated over an anesthetized area. The use of a double-cuff tourniquet alleviates the problem of pain under the cuff.

In the double-cuff system, there are two separate tourniquets placed side by side on the extremity. One is termed the *proximal cuff,* the other is called the *distal cuff.* The proximal cuff is inflated at the beginning of the procedure, and anesthesia is obtained under the deflated distal cuff. When the patient begins to feel pain under the proximal cuff, the distal cuff is first inflated over an already anesthetized area and the pain-producing proximal cuff is then deflated. One must be certain to inflate the distal cuff before the proximal cuff is released; otherwise, the anesthetic will rapidly diffuse into the general circulation.

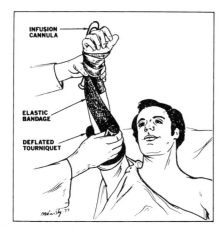

Figure 40–4. Exsanguination by elevation and elastic bandage. The tourniquet has yet to be inflated at this point. Care must be taken not to dislodge the infusion cannula. (From Roberts JR: Intravenous regional anesthesia. JACEP 6:263, 1977. Reproduced by permission.)

Table 40–1. IV Regional Anesthesia—Step-by-Step Procedure

Begin intravenous line in uninvolved extremity.
Draw up 0.5 per cent lidocaine (1.5 to 3.0 mg/kg).
Place padded tourniquet, and inflate upper cuff.
Insert small plastic intravenous cannula near pathologic lesion and secure.
Deflate tourniquet.
Elevate and exsanguinate extremity.
Inflate tourniquet (250 mm Hg), and remove exsanguination device. Inflate the proximal cuff only, if a double-cuff system is used.
Infuse anesthetic solution.
Remove infusion needle, and tape site.
Perform procedure.
If pain is produced by the application of the tourniquet, first inflate the distal cuff, then deflate the proximal cuff.
After the procedure has been carried out, deflate the cuff for a few seconds, then reinflate it for 1 minute. Repeat three times. Do not deflate the cuff if total tourniquet time is less than 30 minutes.
Observe for possible reactions.

(From Roberts JR: Intravenous regional anesthesia. JACEP 6:263, 1977. Reproduced by permission.)

MECHANISM OF ACTION

Some of the anesthesia is undoubtedly related to the ischemia produced by the tourniquet, but most of the anesthesia is secondary to the anesthetic agent itself. Although the exact mechanism by which anesthesia is produced is unknown, the site of action of the anesthetic may be at sensory nerve endings, neuromuscular junctions, or major nerve trunks.[11] Contrast studies have demonstrated that the anesthetic agent does not diffuse throughout the entire arm, yet anesthesia of the entire limb is obtained. For example, when the anesthetic agent is injected into the elbow and kept in that region with both distal and proximal tourniquets, anesthesia of the entire arm develops.[12] Evidence indicates that the local anesthetic does not simply diffuse from the venous system into the tissue but travels via vascular channels directly inside the nerve. Regardless of where the anesthetic is infused, the finger tips are the first area to experience anesthesia, suggesting that the core of the nerve is in contact with the anesthetic agent initially. Following release of the tourniquet, a considerable amount of the drug still remains in the injected limb for at least 1 hour.[13] This would suggest that at least a portion of the anesthetic leaves the vascular compartment and becomes tissue fixed.

PROCEDURAL POINTS

Anesthetic Agent

One-half per cent plain lidocaine at a dose of 1.5 to 3 mg/kg is the agent of choice. Other agents have been used without demonstrable advantage and are not recommended.[14] Bupivacaine (Marcaine, Sensorcaine) is *contraindicated* because of serious cardiovascular and neurologic complications.[15, 16]

Dunbar and Mazze[7] showed that patients with intravenous regional anesthesia actually had significantly lower plasma-lidocaine concentrations than patients with axillary block or lumbar epidural anesthesia for similar procedures. Peak plasma concentrations are reached 2 to 3 minutes after deflation of the tourniquet, and side effects are minimal if the deflation is cycled following the surgical procedure. The plasma half-life of lidocaine is approximately 60 seconds (see the excellent detailed discussion of pharmacokinetics by Covino[17]), but the drug demonstrates a theoretic three-compartment model similar to a direct intravenous infusion once the turniquet is released.[18]

Peak blood levels are related to the duration of vascular occlusion and to the concentration of the anesthetic.[17, 18]

Post release peak plasma lidocaine levels decrease as the time of vascular occlusion (tourniquet time) increases. If the tourniquet is inflated for at least 30 minutes and the deflation-reinflation technique is used when the procedure is finished, plasma concentration of lidocaine should be approximately 2 to 4 μg/ml, below the 5 to 10 μg/ml level at which serious reactions occur.[7] Tucker and Boas demonstrated a peak plasma lidocaine level of 10.3 μg/ml following a 10-minute period of vascular occlusion compared with 2.3 μg/ml if the tourniquet was inflated for 45 minutes.[18]

More dilute solutions of lidocaine are associated with lower peak lidocaine levels. When equal doses of lidocaine are used, the peak arterial plasma levels are 40 per cent lower when the 0.5 per cent solution is used than when the 1 per cent solution is used.[18] For example, following 10 minutes of vascular occlusion, the peak plasma concentration of lidocaine has been demonstrated to reach 10.3 μg/ml with the 1 per cent solution compared with only 5.6 μg/ml when the drug was given under similar circumstances as a 0.5 per cent concentration.[18]

Exsanguination

Exsanguination of the extremity before injection of the anesthetic agent is considered essential for success by many physicians. Others do not believe that it is a critical factor. Exsanguination by simple elevation of the extremity should be done in all cases, but in certain cases, one should consider avoiding the painful wrapping of the extremity with an elastic or Esmarch bandage. (Note that applying an Esmarch wrap over a fracture site is usually quite painful.) A pneumatic splint, such as the type used for prehospital immobilization, is also a reasonable alternative to painful wrapping. The process of exsanguination is believed to allow for better vascular diffusion of the anesthetic.

Site of Injection

Anesthesia is usually obtained no matter where the local anesthetic is injected, but some evidence indicates that the procedure is more successful when the anesthetic is injected distally. Sorbie and Chacho note the following failure rate associated with specific sites of anesthetic injection: antecubital fossa—23 per cent, middle of forearm or leg—18 per cent, and hand, wrist or foot—4 per cent.[3] For most cases, a vein in the dorsum of the hand or foot is most often used. If local pathology precludes the use of the hand, the mid-forearm or antecubital fossa of the elbow are acceptable, albeit less desirable, alternatives as long as the infusion catheter is well below the tourniquet to avoid systemic injection.

Although most of the literature stresses the use of this technique on the upper extremity, it may also be used successfully in the leg. It cannot, however, be used for procedures above the knee. Tourniquet pain appears to be a limiting factor when the procedure is used on the leg. One must be certain to avoid damage to the peroneal nerve by using the tourniquet in the midcalf area only.

COMPLICATIONS

Although intravenous regional anesthesia is both safe and simple, one should not be lulled into complacency, because complications do occur and are usually related to equipment failure or mistakes in the technique.

Anesthetic Agent

Serious complications seldom occur if proper attention is paid to technique. Reactions to lidocaine are rare and are usually systemic reactions from high blood levels.[7, 16, 20] High levels may result from miscalculation of dosages, from too rapid release of the tourniquet before the anesthetic has become tissue-fixed ("bolus effect"), or, rarely, from advancement of the infusion catheter proximal to the tourniquet, resulting in direct intravenous infusion.[19] To emphasize the safety of this procedure it should be noted that the dose of lidocaine used in the "minidose" technique is similar to an intravenous bolus routinely given to patients with significant cardiovascular disease, in the presence of ventricular dysrhythmias.

Generally, the central nervous system (CNS) effects of lidocaine are minor, resulting in mild reactions such as dizziness, lethargy, headache, or blurred vision. This should not occur in more than 2 to 3 per cent of patients and requires no treatment.[7] Convulsions may occur but are extremely rare.

The most common complication relating to the anesthetic agent is rapid systemic vascular infusion, which occurs when a blood pressure cuff explodes or slowly leaks, resulting in both loss of anesthesia and high blood levels.[21] Similar complications may occur if the cuff is deflated before 30 minutes following the induction of anesthesia. Both complications are the result of a bolus effect of the anesthetic, resembling an intravenous injection.

Van Neikerk and Tonkin reported three seizures in a series of 1400 patients.[20] Seizures are generally not recurrent and are treated with oxygen and anticonvulsant drugs. Transient cardiovascular reactions, such as bradycardia and hypotension, are possible with large doses of lidocaine. Vasovagal reactions do occur. If resuscitation equipment is available and a precautionary intravenous line is started in the opposite arm, there should not be any serious sequelae.

One case of cardiac arrest for 15 seconds, following the use of 200 mg of lidocaine was reported, but the actual clinical scenario may have been a vasovagal reaction rather than a true cardiac arrest.[22]

Additional Complications

Thrombophlebitis can occur following intravenous administration of anesthetics, and the formation of insignificant amounts of methemoglobin with the use of prilocaine hydrochloride (Citanest) has been reported.[23] Methemoglobinemia also can theoretically occur with lidocaine but has not been reported.

A particularly bothersome problem has been the infiltration of the infusion catheter during exsanguination, resulting in tissue extravasation of the anesthetic agent. Also, there has been some leakage of anesthetic after the infusion needle has been removed. Both problems may result in poor anesthesia but may be minimized if a small, well-secured plastic infusion needle is used instead of a scalp vein needle and if the puncture site is tightly taped following withdrawal of the catheter.

This procedure cannot be used in manipulations or operations in which the pulse must be monitored as a guide to reduction, such as supracondylar fractures of the humerus, because the tourniquet occludes arterial flow. The use of the Bier block in patients with sickle cell disease is not well documented. It should be used with caution until the ischemic effect of the tourniquet on the red blood cells of such patients has been clarified. In all patients the tourniquet time should not exceed 90 minutes. Ischemia for less than than that amount of time is not associated with serious sequelae.

REFERENCES

1. Holmes CM: Intravenous regional analgesia: A useful method of producing anesthesia of the limbs. Lancet 1:245, 1963.
2. Bell HM, Slater EM, Harris WH: Regional anesthesia with intravenous lidocaine. JAMA 186:544, 1963.
3. Sorbie C, Chacho PB: Regional anesthesia by the intravenous route. Br Med J. 1:957, 1965.
4. Bier A: Ueber einen neuen weg Localanasthesia an den Gleidnassen zu erzevgen. Arch Klin Chir 86:1007, 1908.
5. Colbern EC: Bier block. Anesth Analg 49:935, 1970.
6. Colbern EC: Intravenous regional anesthesia: The perfusion block. Anesth Analg 45:69, 1966.
7. Dunbar RW, Mazze RI: Intravenous regional anesthesia: Experience with 779 cases. Anesth Analg 46:806, 1967.
8. Atkinson PI, Modell J, Moya F: Intravenous regional anesthesia. Anesth Analg 45:313, 1965.
9. Roberts JR: Intravenous regional anesthesia—"Bier Block" Am Fam Phys 17:123, 1978.
10. Farrell RG, Swanson SL, Walter JR: Safe and effective IV regional anesthesia for use in the emergency department. Ann Emerg Med 14:288, 1985.
11. Raj PP: Site of action of intravenous regional anesthesia. Reg Anesth 4:8, 1979.
12. Raj PP, Garcia CE, Burleson JW, et al: The site of action of intravenous regional anesthesia. Anesth Analg 51:776, 1972.
13. Evans CJ, Dewar JA, Boyes RN, et al: Residual nerve block following intravenous regional anesthesia. Br J Anaesth 46:668, 1974.
14. Katz J: Choice of agents for intravenous regional anesthesia. Reg Anesth 4:10, 1979.
15. Albright GA: Cardiac arrest following regional anesthesia with lidocaine or bupivacaine. Anesthesiology 51:285, 1979.
16. Rosenberg PH, Kalso EA, Tuominen MK, et al: Acute bupivacaine toxicity as a result of venous leakage under the tourniquet cuff during a bier block. Anesthesiology 58:95 1983.
17. Covino BG: Pharmacokinetics of intravenous regional anesthesia. Reg Anesth 4:5, 1979.
18. Tucker GT, Boas RA: Pharmacokinetic aspects of intravenous regional anesthesia. Anesthesiology 34:538, 1971.
19. Clinical Anesthesia Conference. NY State J Med 66:1344, 1966.
20. Van Niekerk JP, Tonkin PA: Intravenous regional analgesia. S Afr Med J 40:165, 1966.
21. Roberts JR: Intravenous regional anesthesia. JACEP 6:261, 1977.
22. Kennedy BR, Duthie AM Parbrook GD et al: Intravenous regional anesthesia: an appraisal. Br Med J 5440:954, 1965.
23. Mazze, RI. Methemoglobin concentrations following intravenous regional anesthesia. Anesth Analg 47:122, 1968.

Chapter *41*

Pharmacologic Adjuncts to Painful Procedures

Donald M. Yealy, Susan M. Dunmire, and Paul M. Paris

INTRODUCTION

Pain has been defined as an "unpleasant sensation that is perceived as arising from a specific region of the body and is commonly produced by processes which damage or are capable of damaging bodily tissue."[1] This definition separates pain from generalized moods or emotions referred to as "painful." Often, pain itself is the major motivating factor for the patient to seek emergency medical care. To the clinician, pain often helps identify and guide treatment of a pathologic condition. Numerous studies in inpatient, outpatient, and emergency department settings have documented that *patients with acute pain often receive inadequate analgesic therapy.*[2–6] Undertreatment of pain may result from lack of understanding regarding available agents, undue concern about drug addiction, and inadequate formal and bedside training in acute pain management.

A number of procedures described in this text can produce or increase a patient's pain and anxiety. Although regional and topical anesthesia as described in the preceding chapters is useful for reduction of acute pain associated with a procedure or the condition or conditions necessitating the procedure, other options exist. This chapter addresses the use of pharmacologic adjuncts for reducing anxiety and modifying the psychologic response to procedural pain. Although certain aspects of pain management are addressed in this chapter, the reader is referred elsewhere for a more comprehensive discussion of the management of acute and chronic pain in the emergency setting.[7]

BACKGROUND

Anatomic and Physiologic Considerations. Pain is the result of a noxious stimulus, yet the perception of pain is the result of that stimulus plus the physiologic and psychologic response of the individual to the stimulus. Without the ability to perceive pain, an individual is unable to recognize the need to seek treatment for an injury or painful condition.[8] Although pain leads the patient to seek medical care and to avoid further injury, once care is sought, untreated pain is of little benefit.

Various tissues have nerve endings that are capable of responding to a noxious stimulus that results in the generation of an electrical impulse. The impulse is then transmitted from peripheral sensory nerves through the spinal cord to the brain stem, thalamus, and cortex. The nervous system is capable of modifying the response to painful stimuli at various levels to diminish the perceived pain intensity. Opiate agonists provide analgesia primarily through stimulating specific receptors at the spinal (kappa receptors) and supraspinal (mu receptors) levels. Although sedative agents do not remove the pain stimulus, they may modify the interpretation of that stimulus and in sufficient dosage may produce amnesia for the painful event.

The subjective perception of pain can be quite variable from patient to patient as a result of comorbid medical conditions, previous experiences, and cultural differences. Because pain results from a neuroanatomic process and a cognitive integration of the perceived process, the clinician must rely on the patient to provide information about the location, quality, and intensity of the pain.

Facial expressions, responses, and vital sign changes are of limited value when gauging the degree of pain perceived by an individual.[9] Interestingly, although the minimum stimulus needed to perceive pain among individuals is relatively constant, the amount of the same stimulus necessary to interfere with daily activity or cause alarm varies widely.[10] To treat pain properly, the physician must rely on the verbal or written reports of the patient. "No one feels another's pain and physicians have to believe the patient's words or reactions . . . pain, like disease, is not an abstraction with an existence outside a person."[11]

Misconceptions. One fear voiced by physicians who treat acute pain is that the use of analgesics, particularly narcotic agents, will obscure the diagnosis. *No data support this widely held contention.* Although inappropriately large doses of a narcotic or sedative agent may result in profound sedation and interfere with an abdominal or neurologic exam, such a result is simply a dosing error. In the agitated or hysterical patient who is unable to cooperate because of severe pain (or anxiety), judicious incremental administration of an appropriate analgesic (or sedative) frequently enhances the examination rather than hinders it. Localization of tenderness should be unaffected by this practice, and patient comfort is increased as anxiety is diminished. Although a definitive diagnosis is not mandatory before initiating analgesia in this fashion, examinations before and after treatment are advisable. Should concern be raised that narcotic-induced analgesia or sedation is interfering with physical examination, a titrated reversal of the narcosis using naloxone can be done and followed by reexamination.

Another misconception is that the administration of narcotic analgesics results in addiction. The risk of iatrogenic narcotic addiction as a result of the treatment of acute pain is extremely low.[3, 12] Concern over creating such an addiction should not be used to withhold narcotic analgesia when it is indicated. Furthermore, patients with known narcotic dependence still require appropriate analgesia before undergoing painful procedures.

Practical Considerations. When analgesia is required promptly in the emergency department, narcotic agents are effective and safe. However, the wrong route, dose, and dosing interval are often chosen. *The intramuscular route rarely should be used to provide initial analgesia or pain relief during procedures (e.g., abscess drainage, reduction of dislocations).* Intramuscular administration of any medication is painful and results in erratic serum levels, depending on the site of injection and local perfusion.[13, 14] Individualized titration of analgesia via the intramuscular route is difficult to obtain in a timely fashion, because peak therapeutic effects are delayed (often more than 30 minutes when compared with the time required to use the intravenous route).[13]

The intravenous administration of a narcotic agent results in a more rapid and consistent serum drug level and enables the pain relief to be titrated to the individual's need.[9] Furthermore, individual requirements for pain relief with an agent may vary widely, and incremental intravenous doses at appropriate intervals based on response should be given to provide timely, safe analgesia.

The use of sedative agents, such as the benzodiazepines, can reduce anxiety and serve as a useful adjunct to analgesic agents.[15] Midazolam, given to adults in incremental intravenous doses of 1 to 2 mg until the desired effect is observed, provides short-term (usually less than 30 to 40 minutes) sedation, anxiolysis, and amnesia for many painful procedures. Self-administered nitrous oxide, in a 50 per cent concentration, can provide significant analgesia and anxiolysis in the majority of patients[16, 17] and can augment the effectiveness of analgesic agents (see Chapter 42).

SPECIFIC AGENTS

Narcotic Analgesics

A wide variety of natural and semisynthetic narcotic analgesics have been developed since the original use of opium by the Babylonians in 4000 B.C.. The narcotic analgesics bind to opiate receptors in the central nervous system. Depending on the agent's affinity for different opiate receptors and the location of the opiate receptors in the central nervous system, each analgesic has varying actions and side effects. There are two basic classes of narcotic analgesics:

the pure agonists and the newer mixed agonist-antagonists. The agonist-antagonist analgesics offer the potential advantage of less respiratory depression and more limited abuse potential. Table 41–1 reviews the common dose range and dosing interval for the more popular narcotic analgesics. When these agents are used to permit a specific painful procedure, only a single dose is generally required.

Although the agonist-antagonists are effective analgesics with less sedating properties than the pure agonists, they are not well studied for painful procedures in the emergency department and are not discussed in detail. As experience accumulates, these agents may become attractive alternatives to the pure agonists.

MORPHINE

Pharmacology. Morphine sulfate has a nonselective affinity for central nervous system opiate receptors. The drug is approximately 35 per cent protein bound. It has a rapid onset of action (distribution half-life is 1.6 minutes), making it an attractive analgesic agent for emergency procedures such as joint reduction, fracture relocation, and incision and drainage of abscesses. The major metabolic pathway for morphine is conjugation in the liver with glucuronic acid. This pathway is not significantly affected unless total liver failure is present. The major elimination half-life is 2 to 3 hours in healthy young adults and 4.5 hours in older patients.

Dose. In adults, an initial dose of 2 to 3 mg should be repeated every 10 to 15 minutes intravenously until analgesia is obtained. If there is continued pain, a repeat dose in 1 to 3 hours can be given.

Complications. All narcotic agents can produce nausea and vomiting, constipation, sedation, respiratory depression, biliary spasm, and urinary retention. Morphine use is also associated with histamine release, which may produce hypotension and bronchospasm. Hypotension primarily as a result of venodilation may also result without histamine release. If significant sedation or respiratory depression occurs, these responses are easily reversed with naloxone (0.4 to 0.8 mg intravenously).

MEPERIDINE (DEMEROL)

Pharmacology. The analgesic effects of meperidine are similar to those of morphine. Meperidine has one eighth the potency of morphine and a shorter duration of action (2 to 3 hours). Metabolism occurs mainly in the liver by demethylation and is significantly affected by liver disease. Nor-

meperidine (the active metabolite) is renally excreted and may produce central nervous system toxicity in the setting of renal failure.

Dose. For procedures in the emergency department, a single dose of up to 2 to 3 mg/kg intravenously offers excellent analgesia with limited toxicity. Drug administration should be titrated over 5 to 10 minutes.

Complications. Meperidine depresses respiration to the same degree as morphine in equianalgesic doses and can release histamine as well. Although meperidine was initially thought to offer the advantage of less biliary duct spasm than morphine, the results have not been consistent.[18, 19] Meperidine also has a significant incidence of central nervous system side effects including nervousness, tremors, seizures, disorientation, hallucinations, and psychosis. These effects are believed to result from elevated normeperidine levels with cumulative drug doses.

FENTANYL (SUBLIMAZE)

Pharmacology (see also Chapter 2). Fentanyl is a short-acting parenteral synthetic opiate approximately 50 to 100 times as potent as morphine sulfate. The drug is highly lipophilic and has a rapid serum clearance. It crosses the blood-brain barrier rapidly, producing analgesia in as little as 1.5 minutes. Serum levels decline rapidly as a result of tissue uptake. The duration of action is 30 to 40 minutes, although at high doses a second peak of activity may be seen several hours later during release of the drug from tissue stores.

Dose. For children, a dose of 0.5 to 1.0 μg/kg intravenously should be used initially (infused over 30 to 60 seconds) and titrated until sedation occurs. Generally, a total dose of 2 to 3 μg/kg when administered in a titrated fashion is sufficient for most painful procedures in children. For adults, 75 to 150 μg intravenously is used initially with supplemental drug to produce sedation. Supplemental drug should be given in 0.5 to 1.0 μg/kg increments every 3 to 5 minutes until adequate analgesia and sedation are obtained. Although most adults achieve adequate analgesia at a total dose of 3 to 5 μg/kg, higher doses may occasionally be needed. It must be stressed that further *titrated* doses are safe if continued close observation of patient response, respiratory rate, and oxygen saturation is maintained. Repeat doses may be required in 60 to 90 minutes if continued parenteral analgesia is desired.

Complications. Fentanyl does not stimulate histamine release and therefore rarely produces hypotension. It can produce a vagal effect similar to that of morphine but rarely slows the heart rate. Complications other than sedation and respiratory suppression are rare, although high doses or rapidly infused fentanyl can cause muscle rigidity of the trunk.

Drug Combinations

Frequently subtherapeutic doses of narcotic analgesics are used because of concern regarding potential side effects (respiratory depression, hypotension, nausea and vomiting). Clinicians have long searched for a potentiator of narcotics that would permit smaller narcotic doses and thus minimize the resultant side effects.

PHENOTHIAZINES

Phenothiazines are frequently used in combination with a narcotic to counteract the nausea and vomiting associated with narcotic use. Some of the more popular phenothiazines include promethazine (Phenergan) and prochlorperazine

Name	Dose (IV)*	Dosing Interval
Table 41–1. **Narcotic Analgesics**		
Narcotic Agonists		
Morphine	5–10 mg	3–4 hours
Meperidine (Demerol)	75–150 mg	2–3 hours
Fentanyl (Sublimaze)	0.1–0.2 mg	1–2 hours
Hydromorphone (Dilaudid)	1–3 mg	2–4 hours
Codeine	30–60 mg	3–4 hours
Oxycodone (Percocet, Percodan, Tylox)	—	3–4 hours
Hydrocodone (Vicodin, Hycodan, Lortab)	—	3–4 hours
Methadone	10–30 mg	4–6 hours
Narcotic Agonist-Antagonists		
Pentazocine (Talwin)	30 mg	2–3 hours
Nalbuphine (Nubain)	10–15 mg	3–4 hours
Butorphanol (Stadol)	1–4 mg	2–3 hours
Buprenorphine (Buprenex)	0.3–0.6 mg	5–6 hours

*Average, 70-kg, nontolerant adult.

(Compazine). No analgesic benefit from the combination of a narcotic and phenothiazine over that of a narcotic alone has been shown. Phenothiazines may produce hypotension and extrapyramidal reactions. Thus the combination of phenothiazines with narcotics is not recommended.

One time-honored combination that has been advocated for pediatric procedures is the intramuscular DPT (Demerol, Phenergan, and Thorazine) combination.[20] The combination is administered as 2 mg/kg of meperidine, 1 mg/kg of promethazine, and 1 mg/kg of chlorpromazine. Although this combination may provide reasonable sedation and moderate analgesia for the patient, the onset of effect is delayed and unpredictable. Furthermore, this technique exposes the patient to a painful route of administration and limits the ability to titrate analgesic delivery to need in an expeditious manner.

Hydroxyzine (Vistaril)

Hydroxyzine is a minor sedative with antiemetic, analgesic, and antihistaminic properties. The agent appears to improve analgesia when used in combination with an opiate.[21] One study found that 100 mg of hydroxyzine alone provided analgesia equivalent to 8 mg of morphine.[22] Hydroxyzine also provides a significant anxiolytic effect. One major disadvantage is that hydroxyzine can only be administered intramuscularly. Dosages of 50 to 100 mg are commonly used to augment parenteral narcotic agents.

Other Agents

Ketamine: Dissociative Anesthetic Agent

Pharmacology. Ketamine is a water- and lipid-soluble drug with rapid penetration into the central nervous system (see also Chapter 2). The drug accumulates rapidly in highly vascular organs and then undergoes redistribution. The redistribution half-life from plasma to peripheral tissues is 7 to 11 minutes, and the elimination half-life is 2 to 3 hours.[23, 24] The drug is primarily metabolized in the liver.

Ketamine produces dissociation of the patient from the surroundings (trance-like state), catalepsy, analgesia, amnesia, and nystagmus. Motor reflexes and cardiorespiratory stability are maintained. This agent has been recommended primarily for use with children because of a postemergence delirium noted in adults.[25] Subsequent use of the agent in conjunction with diazepam has limited the emergence problem.[26–29]

Dose. When initiating therapy in the child, 0.5 mg/kg is administered intravenously. Generally the child will become cooperative and sedated in 10 to 15 seconds following this dose. Subsequently 5- to 10-mg doses of ketamine may be administered to sustain the dissociative sedation state. A total dose of 0.01 to 0.20 mg/kg/minute over the course of the procedure is commonly used. Adults may receive 0.5 to 1.0 mg/kg initially with repeat doses used to sustain the dissociative sedation state. Supplemental doses of diazepam (0.08 mg/kg) or midazolam (see later discussion) may be used to minimize postemergence reactions. The benzodiazepine agent should be used after administration of the ketamine so that the cumulative sedation from the drugs can be a guide to benzodiazepine loading.

Complications. Postemergence reactions typically include floating sensations, dizziness, blurred vision, out-of-body experiences, and vivid dreams or nightmares. These reactions may be minimized by the concurrent use of benzodiazepines. Delayed redistribution of the drug from the tissue requires that the patient not drive or operate machinery for at least 12 hours following use of the agent. Other potential complications of ketamine use are discussed in Chapter 2.

Midazolam (Versed)

Pharmacology. Midazolam is a benzodiazepine drug, which in comparison to diazepam (Valium) has a twofold increase in potency, a shorter half-life, and less potential for cardiorespiratory depression. As with other benzodiazepines, the drug has amnestic, sedative, hypnotic, anxiolytic, and anticonvulsant properties. The agent is highly lipophilic, with rapid accumulation in the central nervous system. The onset of sedation may occur in as little as 1 to 2 minutes following intravenous administration. The half-life of elimination is 1 to 4 hours and is dependent on release of the drug from tissue sites. The period of sedation following a single intravenous dose is considerably shorter (generally 15 to 30 minutes).

Dose. For conscious sedation, 0.02 to 0.04 mg/kg is given in 1 mg boluses titrating to effect. No more than 2.5 mg is given over 2 minutes. Although a total dose of up to 0.1 to 0.2 mg/kg may be needed for deep sedation, this amount is seldom required. *It is recommended that a maximum dose of 0.1 mg/kg not be exceeded when the agent is used in conjunction with a narcotic analgesic or ketamine.* When midazolam is used in combination with other drugs, the other agent should be administered first so that supplemental sedation due to midazolam can be monitored closely. Generally one seeks to sedate the patient to the point that speech is slurred or the patient easily looses the order while counting backward. The development of lateral gaze nystagmus also is a helpful sign.

Complications. The primary complications of midazolam use are respiratory depression and hypotension. When used properly in a closely monitored setting, these complications occur in approximately 1 per cent of cases.[30] Older patients are more likely to be sensitive to this agent and hence should receive small doses titrated to effect. Close monitoring of cardiac rhythm, blood pressure, and oxygen saturation also should minimize untoward effects from midazolam. Although a benzodiazepine antagonist (flumazenil, 0.5 to 1.0 mg given intravenously for adults) will soon be available for reversing the effect of benzodiazepines,[31, 32] such an agent is unlikely to be needed for reversal of midazolam. Because of the short duration of action of this agent, supportive care is generally sufficient to reverse any untoward effect.

Sedation for Diagnostic Procedures

Often the emergency physician must sedate a patient before a diagnostic procedure that requires patient compliance (e.g., computed tomography scans, lumbar puncture, and electroencephalographs). A wide variety of agents may be used to produce predominately sedation (Table 41–2). When these agents are used primarily for sedation, close patient monitoring is generally required with particular attention to the patient's airway, ventilatory effort, oxygen saturation, cardiac rhythm, and blood pressure. Sedation is titrated to the degree of cooperation required for the diagnostic procedure.

Combination Analgesia–Sedation: A Suggested Approach

The preceding discussion has addressed the more commonly used pharmacologic adjuncts for ameliorating the anxiety and pain of emergency department procedures.

Table 41–2. Sedation for Diagnostic Procedures

Agent(s)	Initial Dose†	Route
Midazolam	0.03–0.05 mg/kg	IV
	0.2–0.4 mg/kg	Intranasal*
Diazepam	0.05–0.10 mg/kg	IV
Pentobarbital	2.0–6.0 mg/kg	IV
Butorphanol	0.015–0.02 mg/kg	IV
Fentanyl	0.5–1.0 μg/kg	IV
	20–25 μg/kg	Oral transmucosal*
Sufentanil	2 μg/kg	Intranasal*
Meperidine	1.0–2.0 mg/kg	IV, IM
Chloral hydrate	30 mg/kg	Oral*
Droperidol	0.02–0.10 mg/kg	IV, IM
DPT (Demerol/ Phenergan/ Thorazine)	2:1:1 mg/kg (maximum 50:25:25 mg in children)	IM*

*Suggested for pediatric sedation and analgesia.
†Often two doses are needed to obtain adequate sedation in many patients. The use of additional doses should be based on individual responses. In the elderly, smaller doses should be used in an incremental fashion.
IV, intravenously; IM, intramuscularly.

With the current availability of safe and effective analgesics and sedatives, it is barbaric to débride a painful burn or drain a large abscess without the aid of systemic medications. Each physician has his or her own favorite regimen, and it is always best to use a technique with which one is familiar.

The practice of combining an analgesic with a sedative agent to reduce anxiety and pain both before and immediately following the procedure is commonly advocated. The technique preferred by the editors is outlined in Table 41–3 and consists of the combination of intravenous fentanyl and midazolam.[33, 34] In general, intramuscular analgesics are impractical and generally ineffective for painful procedures. Nitrous oxide is an option but is often inadequate when pain is intense. The fentanyl and midazolam combination provides rapid, safe, short-acting, and efficacious analgesia and amnesia. Although these agents are quite powerful, when used with caution and attention to detail, superb results are obtained.

A number of caveats should be emphasized regarding the procedure outlined in Table 41–3. First, the individual response to these drugs is highly variable. Generally patients with a history of alcoholism or long-term narcotic use require careful titration of these agents in higher than usual total doses. Maximal recommended doses should *rarely* be exceeded and *only* in select patients on the basis of close observation of clinical response with attention to detection of side effects. Older patients require smaller doses of both drugs. Although both drugs have a rapid onset of action, it is a common error to attempt to rush the procedure by administering the drug too frequently so that sedation is excessive. The maximum analgesic effect of each dose is reached at 3 to 5 minutes following its infusion. However, the maximum respiratory depression effect occurs 5 to 15 minutes after the last dose. It is recommended that the physician wait at least 5 minutes after the last dose is given before initiating the procedure.

The regimen recommended uses relatively larger (more sedating) doses of fentanyl than of midazolam. This is preferred because the narcotic can be reversed by naloxone. When the benzodiazepine antagonist flumazenil becomes available, a change in this regimen may be warranted. The most common side effects of this drug combination are hypotension or transient respiratory depression, often related to a too rapid drug infusion. One should be careful to avoid bolus injections. Pruritus has been associated with

fentanyl, but it is usually minor. Respiratory depression is easily identified when monitoring with a pulse oximeter and easily treated with naloxone or a few assisted ventilations. Supplemental oxygen should be considered when using these agents in the elderly.

Significant respiratory depression is quite uncommon if the previously discussed precautions are followed. In the series of 841 patients undergoing fentanyl analgesia in the series by Chudnofsky and associates, only six patients experienced transient respiratory depression and no patient required intubation.[35] Doses should be reduced in the elderly and in patients who are on concomitant vasoactive or sedative medications. Caution should be used in the acutely intoxicated patient.

Even after appropriate titrated doses of analgesic agents, a patient may complain of pain at the height of a procedure (e.g., actual abscess incision). When the afore-mentioned combination approach has been used, most will not recall

Table 41–3. Procedure for Providing Analgesia and Amnesia for Painful Emergency Department Procedures (for the average 70-kg adult)

1. Establish an intravenous infusion of normal saline (18-gauge catheter preferred in adults) in the supine patient with the bed rails in the up position.
2. Pulse, respiratory rate, blood pressure, and level of consciousness should be recorded initially, *after every dose of each agent, and every 5 to 10 minutes throughout the procedure.*
3. Continuous monitoring of oxygen saturation with a pulse oximeter probe (to maintain at >95% or no less than 3 to 5 per cent less than the initial value) must be performed. Supplemental oxygen via nasal prongs can be administered based on need. ECG monitoring is optional but suggested in the elderly or those with a cardiac history.
4. A resuscitation cart with a bag-valve mask, oral and nasal airways, endotracheal tubes, and a functioning laryngoscope must be nearby. Suction equipment and naloxone should be at the bedside.
5. Administer 1 mg midazolam over 30 to 60 seconds; if after 3 to 5 minutes there is no evidence of mild sedation (subjective relaxation by the patient with mild drowsiness and normal or minimally altered speech), additional 1-mg doses can be administered in a similar fashion, up to a maximum of 0.1 mg/ kg.* The goal is *mild sedation and anxiolysis*, achievable in most patients with 1 to 2 mg of midazolam.
6. Reassess clinical status (see 2).
7. Administer fentanyl† 100 μg (2 ml) over 60 seconds; this may be repeated in 0.5 to 1.0 μg/kg (50 to 100 μg) increments every 3 to 5 minutes until adequate analgesia and sedation has been obtained (slurred speech, ptosis, drowsy but responsive to painful and verbal stimuli, and good analgesia with initial stages of procedure). The maximal total dose recommended is 5 to 6 μg/kg.*
8. Administer local anesthesia if indicated (this often serves to help gauge effectiveness of systemic analgesia).
9. Perform the procedure. Additional doses of fentanyl may be required based on the response and length of the procedure.
10. If hypoxemia, deep sedation, or slowed respirations unresponsive to external stimuli are seen during or after procedure, ventilation should be assisted with a bag-valve-mask and naloxone (0.4- to 0.8-mg increments) should be administered. Naloxone should not be given routinely at the termination of procedures, since it will abruptly reverse all analgesia.
11. Continue close observation until the patient is awake and alert, and discharge the patient only after a minimum 1 hour of further observation. Instruct the patient not to drive or operate dangerous machinery for at least 6 hours.

*For children, fentanyl alone is suggested in 0.5 μg/kg increments up to a maximum total dose of 2 to 3 μg/kg.
†Sublimaze 50 μg/ml.

the pain because of the amnestic effects of midazolam. However, the physician should not depend on amnesia to supplant inadequate analgesia, and only rarely should this occur. After termination of the procedure, close observation of the patient must continue until the sedative effects have resolved, usually within 15 to 20 minutes. The patient should not be discharged for another hour and should be instructed not to drive or operate any heavy or dangerous machinery for at least 6 hours after release.

REFERENCES

1. Fields HL: Pain. New York, McGraw Hill Book Co, 1987.
2. Marks RD, Sachar EJ: Undertreatment of medical inpatients with narcotic analgesics. Ann Intern Med 78:173, 1973.
3. Perry S, Heidrich G: Management of pain during debridement: A survey of US burn units. Pain 13:267, 1982.
4. Mather L, Mackie J: The incidence of postoperative pain in children. Pain 15:272, 1983.
5. Sirwatanakul K, Weis O, Alloza JL, et al: Analysis of narcotic usage in the treatment of postoperative pain. JAMA 250:926, 1983.
6. Wilson JE, Pendelton JM: Oligoanalgesia in the emergency department. Am J Emerg Med 7:620, 1989.
7. Paris PM, Stewart RD: Pain Management in Emergency Medicine. Norwalk, Conn, Appleton & Lange, 1988.
8. Dyck PJ, Mellinger JF, Reagan TJ, et al: Not "indifference to pain" but varieties of hereditary sensory and autonomic neuropathy. Brain 106:373, 1983.
9. Perry S: Using narcotic analgesics to optimum effect: A modern view. EM Rep 3:91, 1982.
10. Turk DC, Kerns RD: Conceptual issues in the assessment of clinical pain. Int J Psychiatry Med 13:57, 1983.
11. Spiro HM: Visceral viewpoints pain and perfectionism—the physician and the "pain patient." N Engl J Med 294:829, 1976.
12. Porter J, Jick H: Addiction rare in patients treated with narcotics. N Engl J Med 302:123, 1980.
13. Grabinski PY, Kaiko RF, Rogers AG, et al: Plasma levels and analgesia following deltoid and gluteal injections of methadone and morphine. J Clin Pharmacol 23:48, 1983.
14. Abbuhl S, Jacobson S, Murphy JG, et al: Meperidine usage in patients with sickle cell crisis. Ann Emerg Med 15:433, 1986.
15. Geiderman J: Benzodiazepines. In Paris PM, Stewart RD (eds): Pain Management in Emergency Medicine. Norwalk, Conn, Appleton & Lange, 1987.
16. Stewart RD: Nitrous oxide sedation/analgesia in emergency medicine. Ann Emerg Med 14:139, 1985.
17. Sudin RH, Adriani J, Alam S, et al: Anxiolytic effects of low dosage nitrous oxide-oxygen administered continuously in apprehensive subjects. South Med J 74:1489, 1981.
18. Radney PA, Brodman E, Mankikar D, et al: The effect of equianalgesic doses of fentanyl, morphine, meperidine and pentazocine on common bile duct pressure. Anaesthesist 29:26, 1980.
19. Arguelles JE, Frantovic Y, Romo-Salas R, et al: Intrabiliary pressure changes produced by narcotic drugs and inhalation anesthetics in guinea pigs. Anesth Analg 58:120, 1979.
20. Terndrup TE, Cantor RM, Madden CM: Intramuscular meperidine, promethazine, and chlorpromazine: Analysis of use and complications in 487 pediatric emergency department patients. Ann Emerg Med 18:528, 1989.
21. Momose T: Potentiation of postoperative analgesic agents by hydroxyzine. Anesth Analg 59:22, 1980.
22. Hupert C, Yacoub M, Turgeon LR: Effect of hydroxyzine on morphine analgesia for the treatment of postoperative pain. Anesth Analg 59:690, 1980.
23. Wieber J, Gugler R, Hengstmann JH, et al: Pharmacokinetics of ketamine in man. Anaesthesist 24:260, 1975.
24. Zsigmond EK, Domino EF: Ketamine—clinical pharmacology, pharmacokinetics and current clinical uses. Anesth Rev 7:13, 1980.
25. Caro DB: Trial of ketamine in an accident and emergency department. Anaesthesia 29:227, 1974.
26. Vinnik CA: An intravenous dissociative technique for outpatient plastic surgery. Tranquility in the office surgical facility. Plast Reconstr Surg 67:799, 1981.
27. Beekhuis GJ, Klegon RB, Kahn DL: Anesthesia for facial cosmetic surgery: Low dosage ketamine-diazepam anesthesia. Laryngoscope 88:1709, 1978.
28. Tobin HA: Low-dose ketamine and diazepam. Arch Otolaryngol 108:439, 1982.
29. Cartwright PD, Pingel SM: Midazolam and diazepam in ketamine anesthesia. Anaesthesia 39:439, 1984.
30. Wright SW, Chudnofsky CR, Dronen SC, et al: Midazolam use in the emergency department. Am J Emerg Med 8:97, 1990.
31. Ritter JW, Hoshizaki G: Flumazenil antagonizes midazolam induced respiratory rate depression. Anesth Analg 70:S324, 1990.
32. Knudsen L, Lonka L, Sorenson BH, et al: Benzodiazepine intoxication treated with flumazenil (Anexate, RO 15-1788). Anaesthesia 43:274, 1988.
33. Billmire DA, Neale HW, Gregory RO: Use of IV fentanyl in the outpatient treatment of pediatric facial trauma. J Trauma 25:1079, 1985.
34. Miller RI, Bullard DE, Patrissi GA: Duration of amnesia associated with midazolam/fentanyl intravenous sedation. J Oral Maxillofac Surg 47:155, 1989.
35. Chudnofsky CR, Wright SW, Dronen SC, et al: The safety of fentanyl use in the emergency department. Ann Emerg Med 18:635, 1989.

Chapter *42*

Nitrous Oxide Analgesia

David J. Dula

INTRODUCTION

Pain control is an important aspect of emergency medicine. Patients often present to the emergency department because of pain, and many diagnostic and therapeutic maneuvers that are performed in the emergency department cause pain. A wide variety of analgesic agents are available, and the advantages and disadvantages of each agent should be considered. Ideally, an analgesic for emergency department use would be one that has a rapid onset of action and clears quickly when the drug is stopped. The drug should also be safe, effective, easy to use, of low abuse potential, and compatible with other analgesic agents. A drug with these characteristics would have the obvious benefit of relieving a patient's pain during the emergency department encounter while leaving the individual in a suitable state for safe discharge from the department, for signing consent forms for surgery, or for evaluation by other services without obtundation from the analgesic.

An agent that possesses all these characteristics is nitrous oxide.[1] This gas was first described by Humphrey Davey in 1797, who investigated its use for the control of tuberculosis.[2] Since the discovery of the gas, the use of nitrous oxide as an analgesic and anesthetic agent has gained support both in the operating room and in dental suites. Most recently, the gas has been used effectively in emergency departments in Great Britain and the United States as an analgesic agent. Within the last 20 years, nitrous oxide has also become popular in the prehospital care setting for relief of pain.[3] The emergence of nitrous oxide as an effective analgesic agent for use in the emergency department has been a significant advance in pain control.

PHARMACOLOGY

Nitrous oxide has been used in the anesthesia suite for more than 140 years and has proved to be an extremely safe agent. It is a colorless and slightly sweet-smelling gas. Nitrous oxide is highly soluble in plasma, approximately 30 times more soluble than nitrogen. Nitrous oxide does not bind to the hemoglobin molecule and does not produce sickling in sickle cell patients. The gas is not metabolized; it is excreted by the lungs. The effects of nitrous oxide on organ systems other than the central nervous system are quite limited.

The heart and the cardiovascular system are not significantly affected by nitrous oxide analgesia. Data obtained during cardiac catheterization have shown that no clinically significant changes in cardiac output, heart rate, or cardiac rhythm occur during nitrous oxide administration.[4]

In the absence of underlying hypoxemia or hypercarbia, nitrous oxide does not produce any significant change in blood pressure, venous pressure, peripheral vascular resistance, or blood volume. Minor cutaneous venous dilation may occur, producing a flushed appearance.[5, 6]

The respiratory system is not directly affected by nitrous oxide. No change in bronchomotor tone occurs, secretions are not stimulated, and ciliary action is not depressed.

Inhalation of nitrous oxide produces a rapid effect on the central nervous system. Cortical function is rapidly depressed, and all modalities of sensation are affected, as evidenced by a decrease in the senses of hearing, taste, and smell and a decreased sensitivity to touch, temperature, pressure, and pain. Subcortical areas are affected to a less significant degree, and the body is still able to maintain normal temperature control and a normal respiratory drive. The sensitivity of the larynx is not significantly depressed, and the cough and gag reflexes are not notably altered. The risk of regurgitation from stimulation of the vomiting center is not clinically significant. Roberts and Wignall[7] demonstrated that children sedated with nitrous oxide for dental procedures maintained an intact laryngeal reflex and did not demonstrate aspiration during analgesia.

The effects on the central nervous system can vary from euphoria to early levels of anesthesia, depending on the percentage of nitrous oxide delivered. Analgesic effects on skin and bone occur with concentrations of 35 to 80 per cent nitrous oxide.[8] The gas produces an effect on the central nervous system within 1 to 2 minutes.

Inhalation of 50 per cent nitrous oxide and 50 per cent oxygen has been reported to deliver an analgesic effect equal to that of 10 to 20 mg of intravenous morphine, although clinically all patients may not obtain this level of analgesia. Continued administration of the gas does not increase the analgesic effect, and in fact a mild tolerance may develop. Maximal analgesia is obtained within 5 minutes of continuous inhalation. A number of studies have shown that administration of 50 per cent nitrous oxide relieves pain completely 39 to 50 per cent of the time, partially in 35 to 36 per cent of patients, and not at all in 15 to 26 per cent of cases.[1, 5, 9, 10] Because of the subjective nature of pain and accompanying anxiety, nitrous oxide may afford little or no relief in some patients but produce significant analgesia in others.

Nitrous oxide has amnestic as well as analgesic effects. The patient's recollection of pain after nitrous oxide has worn off was found to be significantly less than the amount of pain that was reported by observers. Eighty per cent of patients who had similar procedures using only lidocaine reported the procedure to be much more bearable with the nitrous oxide and lidocaine combination.[1]

Danger to Medical Personnel. Measures to limit contamination of the emergency department with nitrous oxide are in order, because the side effects attributed to *long-term* exposure to nitrous oxide include increased risks of spontaneous abortion, liver ailments, and neurologic problems.[11–15]

For male dentists who were exposed over a long period to low levels of nitrous oxide, the incidence of liver disease in one report[16] was increased 1.7-fold, that of kidney disease was increased 1.2-fold, and that of neurologic disease was elevated 1.9-fold. The incidence of spontaneous abortion was increased 1.5-fold among wives of male dentists exposed to nitrous oxide. In female dental assistants who were exposed to nitrous oxide, the incidence of liver disease was increased 1.6-fold, that of kidney disease was increased 1.7-fold, and that of neurologic disease was elevated 2.8-fold. The incidence of spontaneous abortions among chronically exposed female dental assistants was increased 2.3-fold. Layzer[17] reported a polyneuropathy in 15 patients exposed chronically to nitrous oxide.

Whereas these adverse effects of chronic exposure to low levels of nitrous oxide have been noted in operating room and dental personnel, the incidence of harmful consequences should be lower in emergency department personnel because the gas is used less frequently in the emergency department. At high concentrations, some psychomotor effects may occur in persons administering or working around the gas. These effects are not usually a concern unless high levels of contamination (500 ppm or greater) are experienced by the workers.[18] These side effects have encouraged the National Institute for Occupational Safety and Health (NIOSH) to establish guidelines for the safe use of nitrous oxide in the hospital setting. In the operating room it is recommended that the spillover of the gas not exceed 25 ppm; the recommended limit for dental suites is 50 ppm.[19, 20] Guidelines for emergency department use have not been established; however, levels of 300 to 500 ppm have been noted in emergency department treatment rooms after 4 to 8 minutes of nitrous oxide use (Fig. 42–1).[21] With the current development of the scavenger device (a unit that vents expired nitrous oxide gas to the outside environment), levels in the emergency department can be kept as low as 10 ppm (Fig. 42–2).

Nitrous oxide analgesia during ambulance transport without an exhaust system for the cabin area results in nitrous oxide levels of 650 to 1700 ppm, with a top concentration of 7500 ppm. Use of a local exhaust system to vent expired gases to the outside environment, however, has reduced ambulance levels to less than 25 ppm.[22] Because

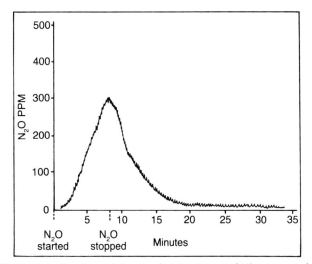

Figure 42–1. Nitrous oxide levels after 8 minutes of Nitronox use in a 16 by 14 by 10-foot room without the scavenger unit in operation.

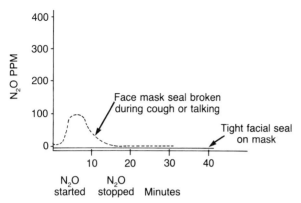

Figure 42–2. Nitrous oxide levels after 8 minutes of Nitronox use with the scavenger unit in operation.

nitrous oxide is heavier than air, it collects near the floor, making it more of a hazard in the ambulance than in a full-sized room.

EQUIPMENT

Two basic units are available for the administration of nitrous oxide analgesia in the emergency department. The Entonox machine (Canadian Oxygen Limited) is designed to administer nitrous oxide and oxygen from a single tank containing an equal mixture of oxygen and nitrous oxide. The concentration that is delivered is 50 per cent nitrous oxide and 50 per cent oxygen. There is one disadvantage to use of the Entonox in ambulances for prehospital care: Nitrous oxide is heavier than oxygen, and when the two gases are mixed in one tank, the nitrous oxide tends to settle at the bottom of the tank, especially in cold temperatures. When this occurs, the potential hazard is that the patient may breathe pure nitrous oxide when the tank is nearly empty. This is of concern only in cold environments and poses no significant threat when the device is used in the emergency department.

The other apparatus used to administer nitrous oxide is the Nitronox unit (Frazer Harlake Inc.—Fig. 42–3). This machine has two separate tanks that contain nitrous oxide and oxygen. The gases are mixed in a 50:50 concentration just before they are inhaled. The mixture can be delivered at up to 140 liters per minute.

The gas mixture in both machines is self-administered. The patient must create a tight seal between the face and the mask while inhaling to cause the demand valve to open and release the gas to the patient. Approximately 2 cm H_2O of negative pressure is required to open the delivery valve; the demand valve prevents continued escape of the gas when the patient is not inhaling. This allows patients who become overly sedated to break the tight seal and thus stop breathing the gas.

In the Nitronox machine, an oxygen fail-safe mechanism automatically stops the flow of nitrous oxide in the system when the oxygen supply is depleted. In the event of nitrous oxide depletion, the unit provides 100 per cent oxygen at a reduced maximum flow rate of 70 liters per minute. Oxygen reference pressure provides automatic enrichment at very shallow breathing rates. Dual diaphragms used throughout the system prevent internal mixing of gas

in the event of diaphragm leakage. Connections for hookups to each gas supply are indexed to prevent improper mixing of oxygen and nitrous oxide tanks. A mixture pressure alarm provides an audible signal in event of valve seat leakage. With the development of a scavenger device, exhaled gases can be vented to the outside atmosphere, preventing the buildup of excessive levels of nitrous oxide in the emergency department (Figs. 42–4 and 42–5).

Both of the units are available in an ambulance model for administration of nitrous oxide gas in the prehospital care setting. The inhospital unit is available either as a portable model, which has a stand on wheels and uses "D"-sized cylinder tanks, or as a wall-mounted unit, which is supplied by standard wall outlets for nitrous oxide and oxygen.

The maximum concentration of nitrous oxide that can be delivered with both Entonox and Nitronox equipment is 50 per cent for the sea level units and 65 per cent for the high-altitude models. At the maximum concentration, the patient may become slightly sedated but does not become unconscious. One must always administer nitrous oxide with at least 30 per cent oxygen to avoid hypoxia. Experience with nitrous oxide administered at higher elevations (specifically 5000 feet above sea level or higher) has indicated that a 50:50 mixture may be inadequate to produce a significant analgesic effect. For this reason, emergency department use at high altitudes may require a higher percentage of nitrous oxide. A 65 per cent nitrous oxide and 35 per cent oxygen mixture has been found to be effective at this higher altitude.[23]

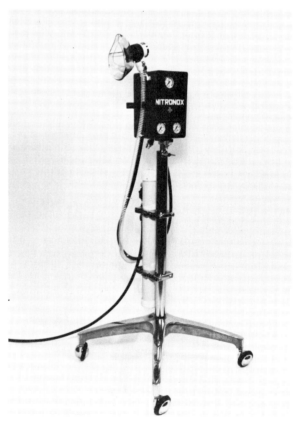

Figure 42–3. Nitronox unit.

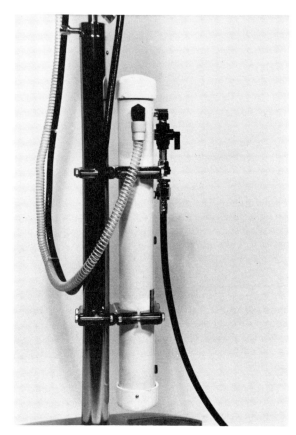

Figure 42-4. Scavenger unit.

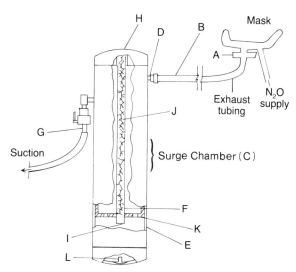

Figure 42-5. Schematic diagram of the Nitronox scavenger.

1. All exhaled gases are diverted to the scavenger system by means of a special collector ring (A) fitted over the Nitronox demand valve.

2. Exhaled gases pass through the scavenger hose (B) and enter the scavenger surge chamber (C) at point D.

3. The surge chamber (C) is composed of a large-diameter outer tube (E) and a smaller diameter inner tube (F).

4. The outer tube (E) is connected at point G to the central suction supply of the hospital.

5. The inner tube (F) is open at one end (H) to the atmosphere, and the other end (I) is open to the outer tube (E). The inner tube is filled with polyurethane cell foam (J) and is separated from the outer tube by a perforated disk (K).

6. In normal operation, exhaled gases enter the outer tube surge chamber at point D and are exhausted through G. The surge chamber has a capacity of 1.6 liters. If the exhaled gas rate is less than the suction rate applied to the surge chamber, atmospheric air will be entrained into the chamber through H. This atmospheric gas path, however, is through the foam (J), through the baffle (K), and then out through the outlet (G). Consequently, the preferential gas passage is always the path from patient inlet point (D) to outlet (G).

7. Any condensed water vapor is eliminated from the surge chamber through a drain valve (L).

INDICATIONS

There are many uses for nitrous oxide in the emergency department (Table 42-1). Any painful procedure or manipulation that requires the use of short-term analgesia is ideal for nitrous oxide administration. Nitrous oxide can be used alone or as an adjunct to standard narcotic analgesics, such as meperidine or morphine, to provide an additive analgesic effect. When multiple analgesics are used, it is best to begin with nitrous oxide alone and judiciously add small increments of intravenous narcotics if necessary. Nitrous oxide may be supplemented with small doses of an intravenous benzodiazepine when relaxation is required, such as for the reduction of a dislocated shoulder or hip. In addition to its use for clinical procedures, nitrous oxide may be administered for its clinical analgesic effect in cases of musculoskeletal trauma, myocardial infarction, or thermal burns.

Nitrous oxide also has been studied clinically as an agent to ameliorate the pain from acute myocardial ischemia. In a double-blind study, patients who suffered chest pain from myocardial ischemia were treated with nitrous oxide.[24] The patients who received nitrous oxide and oxygen had complete or partial relief of pain in 74 per cent of the cases as compared with those who received only oxygen, who had complete or partial relief of pain in only 29 per cent of the cases. The researchers concluded that nitrous oxide for the relief of chest pain from angina or myocardial infarction seems effective and safe and is not accompanied by any significant hemodynamic changes or other serious adverse reactions. Mitchell and colleagues report that nitrous oxide does not induce myocardial ischemia in the setting of poor ventricular function.[24a]

Nitrous oxide is most useful in providing analgesia in clinical situations in which a consistent level of pain is present. The gas is less beneficial in instances in which acute pain is present for a short period. Therefore, the greatest benefit from nitrous oxide is obtained in the relief of pain from dressing changes, burn débridement, myocardial infarction, undiagnosed abdominal pain, skeletal and soft

Table 42-1. Sample Uses of Nitrous Oxide Analgesia
Wound repair
Incision and drainage
Foreign body removal
Removal of ingrown toenails
Burn care
Abrasions
Replacing avulsed teeth
Cardiac chest pain
Labor pain
Removal or insertion of an intrauterine device
Culdocentesis
Extrication
Headache
Incision of hemorrhoids
Reduction of hernia

tissue trauma, thermal burns, and controlled orthopedic reductions. Nitrous oxide is useful, but to a lesser degree, in procedures that inflict acute pain for short periods, such as fracture reduction or abscess incision. The analgesia obtained with the gas is useful for anxiety reduction during culdocentesis, peritoneal lavage, or a painful pelvic examination. The gas is not a substitute for narcotic analgesia in instances such as renal colic or biliary colic, nor is it designed to take the place of local anesthetics in suturing or abscess drainage. Patients may appear to be in pain during the use of nitrous oxide, but often they do not remember the procedure despite complaints of pain at the time.

Nitrous oxide has been used effectively as an analgesic in the prehospital care setting. The effectiveness of this agent has been similar to that noted in the emergency department, with complete to partial pain relief in more than 90 per cent of the cases.[10, 25–27] Its rapid onset of action and short duration of action make it an ideal analgesic for use in prehospital care. It seems to be most beneficial in patients with traumatic injuries, such as fractures, burns, and musculoskeletal injuries, although it can be used for other conditions, such as cardiac chest pain and abdominal pain. Because nitrous oxide settles at the bottom of the tank at colder temperatures, the Nitronox system, which has oxygen and nitrous oxide in separate tanks, is preferable to the Entonox system, which has both gases in a single tank. Both systems pose an occupational hazard, however, because nitrous oxide levels can reach extremely high levels in the cabin of an ambulance. The use of a scavenger system and ventilating system for the ambulance is necessary to eliminate this problem.

CAUTIONS

It is wise to have the nitrous oxide machine periodically inspected for leaks with a nitrous oxide analyzer. Leaking nitrous oxide gas may contaminate the emergency department even though the machine is not in use. Measures to limit the overuse of nitrous oxide in the emergency department are also important, because the longer the gas is administered the more contamination will occur. For this reason, we limit the use of the gas to a short period (10 to 15 minutes) to decrease the contamination of the emergency department.

Diffusion Hypoxia. During general anesthesia with high concentrations of nitrous oxide (greater than 50 per cent), some patients may become relatively hypoxic after the discontinuation of nitrous oxide administration. This is caused by an effect termed *diffusion hypoxemia*. The nitrous oxide diffuses from the blood stream into the alveolar spaces when the gas is discontinued. This results in a dilution of the oxygen content in the alveoli, producing a relative hypoxic alveolar environment, which may be reflected as hypoxemia. In normal patients, this presents no significant hazard; however, in patients with underlying medical conditions that may predispose to a hypoxic state, diffusion hypoxia may be a potential cause of problems. One can prevent this situation from developing by providing 100 per cent oxygen to the high-risk patient for a few minutes after the nitrous oxide is discontinued.

Diffusion hypoxia with a 50:50 mixture of oxygen and nitrous oxide (which is used in the emergency department) may be of theoretic concern only, because 50 per cent oxygen should prevent any significant hypoxemia. Baskett and coworkers[28] demonstrated that the average arterial partial pressure of oxygen (Pa_{O_2}) with the 50:50 mixture is 210 mm Hg. This is significantly higher than the Pa_{O_2} obtained while the patient is breathing room air and even higher than that

Table 42–2. Side Effects of Nitrous Oxide Analgesia
Drowsiness
Giddiness
Nausea
Amnesia
Paresthesias
Dizziness or vertigo
Dysphoria or panic
Voice change
Laughing out loud

routinely obtained while the patient is breathing oxygen at 5 liters per minute through a nasal cannula. In a clinical study to investigate diffusion hypoxia, 20 healthy volunteers had arterial blood gases monitored before, during, and after the self-administration of a 50:50 mixture of nitrous oxide and oxygen for 15 minutes.[29] This study group showed no evidence of diffusion hypoxemia. It was concluded that in patients without respiratory or cardiovascular compromise, administration of nitrous oxide is safe and results in no change in arterial blood gases or vital signs.

Other Side Effects. Other minor side effects of nitrous oxide analgesia experienced by patients are tinnitus and vertigo (Table 42–2). These are self-limiting and resolve once the gas is discontinued. Some of the subjective effects, such as dizziness and paresthesias, may be partially related to hyperventilation. Some patients may experience unpleasant hallucinations, dysphoria, or a panic reaction. The patients with chronic obstructive pulmonary disease, who are carbon dioxide retainers, may experience hypercarbia if their hypoxic drive is diminished by the 50 per cent oxygen concentration delivered with the nitrous oxide. Nausea, giddiness, voice change, and laughing out loud are other minor side effects that are occasionally encountered.

CONTRAINDICATIONS

When used properly, nitrous oxide is safe and is not accompanied by significant complications. In the emergency department, the gas is used in relatively low concentrations and for very short periods when compared with the data for general anesthesia. Many of the contraindications discussed in this section (Table 42–3) are theoretic and have been gleaned from the anesthesia literature. There have been relatively few reports of serious side effects from Nitronox or Entonox in outpatient use.

Nitrous oxide analgesia is contraindicated in patients who are unable to hold the mask to their faces for self-

Table 42–3. Contraindications to Nitrous Oxide Analgesia
Head trauma
Facial trauma
Decreased level of consciousness
Pneumothorax
Intestinal obstruction
Middle ear pathologic condition
Combative patient
Patient too young to self-administer the gas
Significant obstructive lung disease
Pregnant patient or medical personnel
Conditions requiring prolonged or potent analgesia

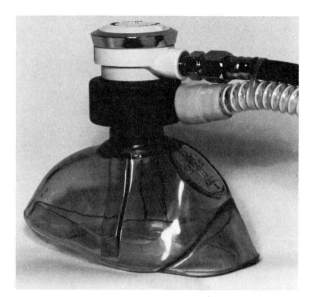

Figure 42–6. Example of a face mask, which must be held in contact with the face by the patient.

administration of the gas because of facial trauma, decreased level of consciousness, or musculoskeletal injury (Fig. 42–6). Patients with head trauma should not receive nitrous oxide, because there may be an increase in intracranial pressure associated with nitrous oxide use in patients with intracranial mass lesions. Furthermore, nitrous oxide should not be used for sedating an unruly patient, because such patients cannot self-administer the gas; hence, they may receive an excessive amount or their underlying injuries may be masked. Intoxicated patients also may become excessively obtunded from the gas.

Because nitrous oxide is so highly soluble, it will diffuse rapidly into any gas-filled structure until it reaches equilibrium with the inspired gas. Therefore, a pneumothorax or an intestinal obstruction may be increased in size if nitrous oxide is administered. It has been estimated that a pneumothorax may double in size in 10 minutes while the patient is breathing 70 per cent nitrous oxide, and intestinal gas may double in volume in 2 hours while the patient is breathing similar concentrations.[30] Reports indicate that the volume of air in a Swan-Ganz catheter balloon may double and predispose to balloon rupture if nitrous oxide is given during anesthesia.[31] Tympanic membranes have been reported to rupture (from a buildup of nitrous oxide in the middle ear with an occluded eustacian tube) following nitrous oxide anesthesia, and the gas should probably not be used in patients with a significant middle ear pathologic condition.[32] The high oxygen content associated with outpatient nitrous oxide analgesia makes significant obstructive lung disease a relative contraindication to its use.

Fetal abnormalities have been detected in animals exposed to nitrous oxide. Although the exact effect on human pregnancy is unknown at this time, it is generally recommended that nitrous oxide not be given to pregnant patients, and pregnant medical personnel should not be exposed to the exhaled gas.

Patients who are too young to self-administer the gas should not be given this form of analgesia in the emergency department without constant physician monitoring. Griffin and associates[33] describe a technique using a nasal inhaler for facilitating minor pediatric surgery. Such a technique requires a more elaborate system and continuous patient monitoring. Gamis and colleagues[34] were able to objectively document pain relief during laceration repair in pediatric emergency patients using such a system.

Although nitrous oxide is useful for supplemental analgesia, in cases of severe clinical pain, such as renal colic, biliary colic, or a fractured hip, it is best to opt for standard narcotic analgesics when the diagnosis is made and the patient is awaiting admission to the hospital or the operating suite.

PROCEDURE

Nitrous oxide may be used routinely without the need for cardiac monitoring or a precautionary intravenous line. If adjunctive narcotics, muscle relaxants, or sedatives are used, resuscitation equipment should be available. The gas should be administered in a well-ventilated room or, preferably, in conjunction with a scavenger device. Both Entonox and Nitronox equipment are applicable to emergency department use. The features of the Nitronox apparatus are detailed here because this device is more popular in the United States.

The Nitronox machine can be set up easily and quickly in the emergency department. The supply tanks of oxygen and nitrous oxide must be turned on (open pressure valve on the tanks) to allow a supply of gas to the machine. After this is done, one should check the pressure gauges to ensure that the nitrous oxide pressure line and the oxygen pressure line are reading in the green bands. This indicates proper pressure in the nitrous and oxygen lines. For models with a scavenger, the vacuum hose should be attached to wall suction.

The patient must be instructed on the use of the device and the effects that will be felt. The need to create and maintain a tight facial seal during both normal inspiration and normal expiration should be emphasized. The patient should be informed that in approximately 2 minutes the effects of the gas will be noticeable. The effects are not unpleasant but make the patient feel a bit drowsy and diminish the pain. One should explain to patients that if at any time they become frightened or feel that they are receiving too much analgesic effect, they should simply remove the mask from the face and breathe room air. Within a minute or so they will begin to "lighten up" and feel normal. When the pain again becomes too severe, the patient should start to breathe the gas again. Thus the patient can titrate the level of analgesia being received from the nitrous oxide. At no time should an assistant hold the mask to the patient's face; *the gas is always self-administered and self-titrated.* The physician or nurse should allow the patient to breathe the gas from approximately 1 to 3 minutes to ensure an appropriate analgesic effect before a clinical procedure is performed. When the procedure is completed, the patient should be instructed to stop breathing the nitrous oxide; within 1 to 3 minutes, the clinical effects of the gas wear off. At this point, additional analgesics may be ordered if necessary.

LIMITATIONS OF NITROUS OXIDE ANALGESIA

Nitrous oxide can induce mild to moderate analgesia in the context of outpatient therapy. The gas does not produce the profound or prolonged analgesia required for pain relief in certain operative conditions or for such conditions as renal colic. The analgesia can be enhanced through the judicious use of adjunctive intravenous narcotics, but the addition of these agents negates some of the advantages of inhalation analgesia. One should not overestimate the analgesic potential of nitrous oxide or eschew the more conventional use of local anesthetics or narcotic analgesics.

The portable machines are convenient, but explanation of the procedure is somewhat time consuming. Reassurance and "verbal anesthesia" are required in many cases to enhance the analgesic effect. Although the gas is self-administered and self-titrated, patients should be kept under observation by emergency department personnel during its use. An empty stomach is not a strict requirement for nitrous oxide use, but the gas should not be given to a patient who has just eaten. Vomiting is an infrequent but well recognized complication of this technique.[33, 34] There is a small but real potential for staff abuse of the gas, but the fact that the machine is kept in full view without the use of keys or storage cabinets minimizes abuse. At this time the actual risk to medical personnel who are subject to long-term low-dose exposure to nitrous oxide in the emergency department is unknown, but it is suggested that reasonable precautions to limit exposure be instituted.

REFERENCES

1. Flomenbaum N, Gallagher EJ: Self administration of nitrous oxide in an analgesic. JACEP 8:95, 1979.
2. Rosenberg H, Orkin FK, Springstead J: Abusive nitrous oxide. Anesth Analg 58:104, 1979.
3. Amey BD, Ballinger JA, Harrison EE: Prehospital administration of nitrous oxide for control of pain. Ann Emerg Med 10:247, 1981.
4. Wynne J, Mann T, Alpert JS, et al: Hemodynamic effects of nitrous oxide administered during cardiac catheterization. JAMA 243:1440, 1980.
5. Churchill-Davidson HC (ed): Wylie and Churchill-Davidson: A Practice of Anesthesia. 4th ed. Philadelphia, WB Saunders Co, 1978, pp 240–247.
6. Collins VJ: Principles of Anesthesiology. 2nd ed. Philadelphia, Lea & Febiger, 1976.
7. Roberts GJ, Wignall BK: Efficacy of the laryngeal reflex during oxygen-nitrous oxide sedation. Br J Anaesth 54:1277, 1982.
8. Allen GD: Dental Anesthesia and Analgesia. 2nd ed. Baltimore, Williams & Wilkins, 1979.
9. Thompson PL, Lawn B: Nitrous oxide as an analgesic in acute myocardial infarction. JAMA 235:924, 1976.
10. Thal ER, Montgomery SJ, Atkins JM, et al: Self-administered analgesia with nitrous oxide. JAMA 242:2418, 1979.
11. Virtue RW, Escobar A, Modell J: Nitrous oxide levels in the operating room air with various gas flows. Can Anaesth Soc J 26:313, 1979.
12. Nitrous oxide hazards. FDA Drug Bulletin 10:15, 1980.
13. Nevins MA: Neuropathy after nitrous oxide abuse. JAMA 244:2264, 1980.
14. Cohen EN, Brown BW, Wu M: Anesthetic health hazards in the dental operatory. Anesthesiology 52:524, 1979.
15. Witcher C, Zimmerman DC, Piziali RL: Control of occupational exposure to nitrous oxide in the oral surgery office. J Oral Surg 36:431, 1978.
16. Cohen EN, et al: Occupational disease in dentistry and chronic exposure to trace anesthetic cases. J Am Dent Assoc 101:21, 1980.
17. Layzer RB: Myeloneuropathy after prolonged exposure to nitrous oxide. Lancet 2:1227, 1978.
18. Ayer WA, Russel EA, Jr, Burge JR: Psychomotor responses of dentists using nitrous oxide-oxygen psychosedation. Anesth Prog 25:85, 1978.
19. Criteria for Recommended Standard, Occupational Exposure to Waste Anesthetic Gases and Vapors. US Department of Health, Education and Welfare, Public Health Service, Centers for Disease Control, National Institute for Occupational Safety and Health, March 1977.
20. Whitcher C: Control of occupational exposure to nitrous oxide in the dental operatory. DHEW Publication 77–171. Cincinnati, US Department of Health, Education and Welfare, Public Health Service, Centers for Disease Control, National Institute for Occupational Safety and Health, Division of Surveillance, Hazard Evaluation and Field Studies, April 1977.
21. Dula DJ, Skiendzielewski JJ, Royko M: Nitrous oxide levels in the emergency department. Ann Emerg Med 10:575, 1981.
22. Aucker K, Halldeni M, Gothe CJ: Nitrous oxide analgesia during ambulance transportation. Acta Anaesthesiol Scand 24:497, 1980.
23. Nieto JM, Rosen P: Nitrous oxide at higher elevations. Ann Emerg Med 9:610, 1980.
24. Thompson PL, Lown D: Nitrous oxide as an analgesic in acute myocardial infarction. JAMA 235:925, 1976.
24a. Mitchell MM, Prokash O, Rulf ENR, et al: Nitrous oxide does not induce myocardial ischemia in patients with ischemic heart disease and poor ventricular function. Anesthesiology 71:526, 1989.
25. Donen N, Tweed WA, White D, et al: Prehospital analgesia with Entonox. Can Anaesth Soc J 29:275, 1982.
26. McKinnon K: Prehospital analgesia with nitrous oxide/oxygen. Can Med Assoc J 125:836, 1981.
27. Stewart RD, Paris PM, Stoy WA, et al: Patient-controlled inhalational analgesia in prehospital care: A study of side-effects and feasibility. Crit Care Med 11:851, 1983.
28. Baskett PJF, Eltringham RJ, Bennett JA: An assessment of the oxygen tensions obtained with premixed 50 per cent nitrous oxide and oxygen mixture used for pain relief. Anaesthesia 28:449, 1973.
29. Stewart RD, Jorayed MJ, Pelton TH: Arterial blood gases before, during and after nitrous oxide oxygen administration. Ann Emerg Med 15:1177, 1986.
30. Eger EJ, Saidman LT: Hazards of nitrous oxide anesthesia in bowel obstruction and pneumothorax. Anesthesiology 26:61, 1965.
31. Eisenkraft JB, Eger EI: Nitrous oxide anesthesia may double the balloon gas volume of Swan-Ganz catheters. Mt Sinai J Med (NY) 49:430, 1982.
32. Perreault L, Normandin N, Plamondon L, et al: Tympanic membrane rupture after anesthesia with nitrous oxide. Anesthesiology 57:325, 1982.
33. Griffin GC, Campbell VD, Jones R: Nitrous oxide–oxygen sedation for minor surgery: Experience in a pediatric setting. JAMA 245:2411, 1981.
34. Gamis AS, Knapp JF, Glenski JA: Nitrous oxide analgesia in a pediatric emergency department. Ann Emerg Med 18:177, 1989.

Soft Tissue Procedures

Chapter **43**

Principles of Wound Management

Richard L. Lammers

INTRODUCTION

Acute, traumatic wound management is one of the most common procedures in the practice of emergency medicine. In the United States, the emergency specialist determines the outcome of wounds for more than 10 million patients every year.[1] There is considerable variation in technique. This is not surprising, because there are also many areas of controversy. Primary wound healing is not an inevitable process. For centuries, victims of wounds commonly experienced inflammation, infection, and extreme scarring; in fact, these processes were considered part of normal wound repair. Only 100 years ago surgeons first realized that sepsis could be separated from healing.[2]

Wound care involves much more than closure of divided skin. The primary goal of wound care is not the technical repair of the wound; it is providing optimal conditions for the natural reparative processes of the wound to proceed.[2] Physicians' attempts to repair the wound can be at odds with the body's attempt to heal the injury. For example, Lister applied phenol to wounds as an antiseptic and in so doing caused extensive tissue necrosis and phenol poisoning.[3] As clinicians identify and abandon practices that retard wound healing, the treatment of traumatic wounds improves. The introduction of antiseptics and antibiotics, refinements in sterile procedure, and improvements in surgical materials and surgical technique have been major advances in the science of wound care.

The primary objectives in wound care are:

1. Preserving viable tissue,
2. Restoring tissue continuity and function,
3. Optimizing conditions for the development of wound strength,
4. Preventing excessive or prolonged inflammation,
5. Avoiding infection and other impediments to healing, and
6. Minimizing scar formation.

This chapter reviews current strategies for achieving these goals.

Wound Healing

A general understanding of the process of wound healing is fundamental to successful management of wounds. Highlights of this complex phenomenon, as they relate to clinical decision making, are reviewed.

Inflammation, epithelialization, fibroplasia, contraction, and scar maturation constitute the stages of scar formation, a nonspecific repair process that occurs in wounds extending beneath the epithelium.[2–7] Most traumatic wounds result in some tissue destruction and hemorrhage and a breach in the epidermis through which bacteria and foreign materials enter. A variety of hemostatic mechanisms control bleeding after the injury; one of these is clot formation. The clot contracts, dehydrates, and forms a scab, which provides some protection from external contamination. Underneath, cells migrate and bring the wound edges together during the process of healing.[8]

Inflammation is a beneficial response that serves to remove the bacteria, foreign debris, and devitalized tissue—a biological débridement. Increased vascular permeability follows hemostasis, with an outpouring of plasma that produces local swelling. Fibrin plugs arising from the plasma occlude lymphatic channels, limiting the spread of bacteria. For some time it was thought that any collection of blood and plasma in a wound was an ideal culture medium for bacteria and therefore must be minimized. Hohn and co-workers demonstrated that humoral factors in this fluid actually provide the wound with some protection against bacteria in the first week following injury.[9] Polymorphonuclear and mononuclear leukocytes concentrate at the site of injury and phagocytose dead and dying tissue, foreign material, and bacteria in the wound. Monocytes (or macrophages) play critical roles in fibroblast replication and angiogenesis.[8]

As the white blood cells die, their intracellular contents are released into the wound. In excessive amounts, they form the purulence characteristic of infected wounds. Some exudate is expected even in the absence of bacterial invasion; however, infection with the accumulation of pus interferes with epithelialization and fibroplasia and impairs wound healing. Wounds contaminated with significant numbers of bacteria or foreign material may undergo a prolonged or persistent inflammatory response and not heal. Granuloma formation surrounding retained sutures is an example of chronic inflammation.[4]

As white blood cells remove debris within the wound, epithelial cells at the surface of the wound begin to cover the tissue defect. In most sutured wounds, the surface of the wound develops an epithelial covering impermeable to water within 24 to 48 hours. Eschar and surface debris impair this process.[10] The epithelium thickens and grows downward into the wound and along the course of skin sutures. Although there is initially some "adhesiveness" to the wound edges during the first few days, this is eliminated by fibrinolysis. By day 4 or 5, newly transformed fibroblasts in the wound begin synthesizing collagen and protein polysaccharides, initiating the stage of scar formation known as fibroplasia.[5] Collagen is the predominant component of scar tissue.[8] In a wound healing by primary intention (following wound closure), the peak rate of collagen synthesis and the

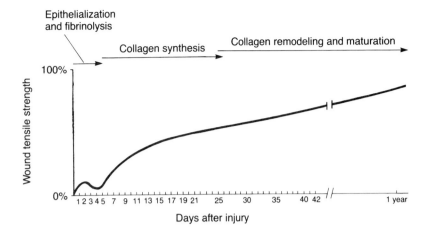

Figure 43–1. Graphic representation of the various phases of wound healing. Note that the tensile strength of scar tissue never reaches that of unwounded skin. Displayed values of tensile strength are *approximate* and demonstrate the general concept of wound healing.

most rapid rate of increase in the tensile strength of the wound begin at approximately 5 to 7 days. The wound gains tensile strength as collagen fibrils are aligned in firm, parallel cords. Wound strength is a balance between the lysis of old collagen and the synthesis of new collagen "welding the wound edges" together.[2] The amount of scar tissue is influenced by physical forces acting across the wound, such as the stresses imposed by movement.[11]

In contrast, contraction is the most important process closing the defect in a wound healing by secondary intention.[8] Contraction is the movement of skin edges toward the center of the defect. For example, a circular defect may contract to form a thin ellipse. Contraction occurs primarily in the direction of underlying muscle.[12]

Significant gains in tensile strength do not begin until approximately the fifth day following the injury. Strength increases rapidly for 6 to 17 days, more slowly for an additional 10 to 14 days, and, almost imperceptibly for as long as 2 years (Fig. 43–1). The strength of scar tissue never quite reaches that of unwounded skin. Although the process of collagen formation is essentially completed within 21 to 28 days, collagen continues to remodel and strengthen the wound for up to 1 year. Scar widening occurs between the twenty-first and forty-ninth days. During the maturation phase of wound healing, collagen fibers reorient into a more organized pattern, and the scar changes in form, bulk, and strength.[2, 4–7]

Decisions regarding the optimal time for suture removal and the need for continued support of the wound with tape are influenced by (1) wound tensile strength, (2) the period of scar widening, and (3) the cosmetically unacceptable effect of epithelialization along suture tracks. Scars are quite red and noticeable at 3 to 8 weeks following closure, but the appearance of a scar should not be judged before the scar is well into its remodeling phase. Therefore, scar revision should be postponed until 6 to 12 months after injury.

Zitelli states that "the most important factor in predicting the cosmetic result is wound location. In general, wounds on concave surfaces heal with better cosmetic results than wounds on convex surfaces.... Besides location, other factors such as *skin color, wound size,* and *wound depth* are helpful in predicting the cosmetic results of wounds healing by secondary intention." Small, superficial wounds in lax, light-colored skin, especially in areas in which the skin is thin, result in less noticeable scars. Wounds on convex surfaces look better with primary closure than following secondary healing. Repigmentation occurs over 3 to 5 years, even in large wounds that heal by secondary intention.[12]

INITIAL EXAMINATION

The approach to the management of a particular wound depends upon information gathered during history taking and on physical examination. The choice of cleaning techniques or the decision to débride a wound is determined by the mechanism of injury; the configuration, extent, and depth of the wound; and the amount and type of contamination present. The decision to close a wound immediately or after a period of observation is based not simply on wound age but on a variety of factors that affect the risk of infection. Identification of injury to underlying structures, such as nerves, vessels, tendons, joints, bones, or ducts, may lead the emergency physician to forgo wound closure and to consult a surgical specialist. It is crucial that the physician recognize wounds that may appear benign but, given the mechanism of injury, belie the extensive and devastating underlying tissue damage. The discovery that an extremity wound was produced by a roller or wringer device, by a high-pressure injection gun, by high-voltage electricity, by heavy and prolonged compressive forces, or by the bite of a human or a potentially rabid animal radically alters the overall management of the affected patient.

History

In the initial evaluation of a wound, the physician should identify all of the extrinsic and intrinsic factors that jeopardize healing and promote infection. These include the mechanism of injury, the time of injury, the environment in which the wound occurred, and the patient's immune status.

WOUND AGE AND THE GOLDEN PERIOD

The likelihood of wound infection is proportional to the time that elapses before definitive wound care.[13, 14] A delay in wound cleaning and closure may allow bacteria contaminating the wound to proliferate. During World War I, French investigators measured the growth of bacteria cultured from battlefield wounds. They determined that approximately 12 hours after wounding, the number of colonies of bacteria on the wound surface doubled. They concluded that wound closure was safe before 12 hours had elapsed but dangerous after that time.[7]

Once the precise number of bacteria necessary to initiate a wound infection was established, investigators were able to demonstrate that a delay in treatment of a contaminated wound for as little as 3 hours could result in infection.[15, 16] Thus the "golden period," the maximum time after injury that a wound may be safely closed without significant risk of infection, *is not a fixed number of hours.*[11] Peacock points out that "a clean razor slice of highly vascular skin of the face might be closed safely 48 hours after injury, whereas a stable-floor-nail penetration of the foot of an elderly person might not be closed safely one minute after injury."[7] There is evidence suggesting that wounds in highly vascular regions (e.g., the scalp) may not be affected by delay in treatment, but this finding requires further study.[17] All of the data accumulated in the initial evaluation, both historical and physical, must be used in the estimation of the golden period for a wound in a particular patient. In addition, the techniques of wound care in themselves may extend the golden period; a skillful clinician can often convert a dangerously contaminated wound into a clean wound that can be safely closed.[7]

OTHER HISTORICAL DATA

Other factors that affect wound healing or the risk of infection include the patient's age and state of health. Patient age appears to be an important factor in host resistance to infection; those individuals at the extremes of age—young children and the elderly—are at greater risk.[18, 19] Infection rates are reported to be higher in patients with medical illnesses (e.g., diabetes mellitus, immunologic deficiencies, malnutrition, anemia, uremia, congestive heart failure, cirrhosis, malignancy, alcoholism, arteriosclerosis, arteritis, collagen vascular disease, chronic granulomatous disease, smoking or chronic hypoxia, or liver failure), in obese patients, and in patients taking steroids or immunosuppressive drugs or those receiving radiation therapy. Shock, remote trauma, distant infection, bacteremia, denervation and peripheral vascular disease also increase wound infection rates and slow the healing process.[8, 20–26]

Additional information pertinent to decision making in wound management includes:

Present medications (specifically, anticoagulants and immunosuppressive drugs),

Allergies (especially to local anesthetics, antiseptics, analgesics, antibiotics, and tape),

Tetanus immunization status,

Potential exposure to rabies (in bite wounds and mucosal exposures),

Potential for foreign bodies embedded in the wound, especially when the mechanism of injury is unknown, was associated with breaking glass or vegetative matter,[27, 28] and

Previous injuries and deformities (especially in extremity and facial injuries).

Physical Examination

All wounds should be examined for amount of tissue destruction, degree of contamination, and damage to underlying structures. A common error in wound management is to assume that a traumatic wound is already contaminated and then, during the examination, to contaminate it further. Despite the fact that all traumatic wounds are contaminated to some degree, these injuries should always be examined using aseptic technique. The examiner must wear sterile gloves and avoid droplet contamination from the mouth by maintaining distance or, preferably, by wearing a mask.[1]

MECHANISM OF INJURY AND CLASSIFICATION OF WOUNDS

The magnitude and direction of the injuring force and the volume of tissue on which the force is dissipated determine the type of wound sustained. Three types of mechanical forces produce soft tissue injury: shear, tension, and compression forces. The resulting disruption or loss of tissue determines the configuration of the wound. Wounds may be classified into six categories:

Abrasions: Wounds caused by forces applied in opposite directions, resulting in the loss of epidermis and possibly dermis (e.g., skin grinding against road surface).

Lacerations: Wounds caused by shear forces that produce a tear in tissues.[18] Tensile and compressive forces also cause separation of tissue. Little energy is required to produce a wound by shear forces (e.g., a knife cutting a finger). Consequently, little tissue damage occurs at the wound edge, the margins are sharp, and the wound appears "tidy." The energy required to disrupt tissue by tensile or compressive forces (e.g., forehead hitting a dashboard) is considerably greater than that required for tissue disruption by shear forces because the energy is distributed over a larger volume. These lacerations have jagged, contused, "untidy" edges.

Crush wounds: Wounds caused by the impact of an object against tissue, particularly over a bony surface, which compresses the tissue. These wounds usually contain contused or partially devitalized tissue.

Puncture wounds: Wounds with a small opening and whose depth cannot be entirely visualized. Puncture wounds are caused by a combination of forces.

Avulsions: Wounds in which a portion of tissue is completely separated from its base and either lost or left with a narrow base of attachment (a flap).[29] Shear and tensile forces cause avulsions.

Combination wounds: Wounds with a combination of configurations. For example, stellate "lacerations" caused by compression of soft tissue against underlying bone create wounds with elements of crush and tissue separation; missile wounds involve a combination of shear, tensile, and compressive forces that puncture, crush, and sometimes avulse tissue.[1, 18]

CONTAMINANTS: BACTERIA AND FOREIGN MATERIAL

Numerous factors affect the risk of wound infection, but the primary determinants of infection are the amount of bacteria and dead tissue remaining in the wound[30] and the presence of local tissue ischemia or hypoxia.[20, 31]

Essentially all traumatic wounds are contaminated with bacteria to some extent. The number of bacteria remaining in the wound at the time of closure is directly related to the risk of infection. A critical number of bacteria must be present in a wound before soft tissue infection develops. In experimental wounds produced by shear forces, an inoculum of $\geq 10^6$ aerobic bacteria per gram of tissue inevitably produces wound infection in time. When the mechanism of injury involves a compressive force, the infective dose of bacteria is $\geq 10^4$ bacteria per gram of tissue. If bacterial counts after injury (or after wound management) are below this level, the wound has a very low probability of becoming infected.[13, 15, 32]

Surgical operations are categorized on the basis of the relative levels of bacterial contamination of the wounds as defined by the Committee on Trauma of the National Academy of Sciences National Research Council. Most traumatic wounds fall into one of two categories:

Contaminated wounds: Traumatic wounds less than 12

hours old (the most common type of wound seen in emergency departments).

Dirty wounds: Wounds heavily contaminated with pathogenic organisms, those with significant numbers of bacteria associated with large amounts of devitalized tissue, or traumatic wounds older than 12 hours.[33]

Infection rates in series of contaminated wounds of all types range from 1.1 to 21 per cent; rates in series of dirty wounds range from 7 to 38 per cent.[19, 21, 34–42]

Most traumatic wounds that fit into the first category are usually described as "clean (traumatic) wounds"; those in the second category are called "heavily contaminated." This distinction between "clean" and "heavily contaminated" wounds is an important one for purposes of management. Any classification system based on wound age alone without consideration of other important factors is misleading.

Haley and colleagues identified four factors that were highly predictive of infections in surgical wounds: anatomic location (abdominal operations were most likely to result in wound infections), length of operation, wound classification (contaminated versus dirty), and number of underlying problems.[40] Similar predictive factors need to be identified for traumatic wounds. The nature and amount of foreign material contaminating the wound often determines the type and quantity of bacteria implanted. The presence of undetected reactive foreign bodies in sutured wounds almost guarantees an infection. Although bullet or glass fragments by themselves rarely produce wound infection, these foreign bodies may carry particles of clothing, gun wadding, or soil into the wound. Minute amounts of organic or vegetative matter, feces, or saliva carry highly infective doses of bacteria. Fecal material contains bacteria in concentrations of 10^{11} bacteria per gram of feces. Bite wounds and intraoral wounds are heavily contaminated with facultative species and obligate anaerobes. Tooth plaque and debris found in gingival recesses also contain bacteria in the range of 10^{11} per gram wet weight.[18] The bacterial inoculum from human bites often contains 100 million or more organisms per milliliter of saliva. At least 42 different bacterial species have been identified in human oral flora.[43]

Soil impairs the ability of a wound to resist infection. Rodeheaver and associates found that adding small quantities of sterile soil to wounds containing subinfective doses of microorganisms leads to infections in those wounds.[44, 45] Inorganic particulate matter, such as sand or road surface grease, usually introduces few bacteria into a wound and has little chemical reactivity; these contaminants are relatively inocuous. Soil containing a large proportion of clay particles readily promotes infection. Presumably because of their marked chemical reactivity, clay particles damage local tissue defenses. These particles also react chemically with amphoteric (e.g., tetracycline) and basic (e.g., gentamicin) antibiotics, limiting their effectiveness in contaminated wounds. In contrast, acidic antibiotics, such as the cephalosporins and the penicillins, do not bind with these soil fractions and so maintain their antibacterial properties.[46] Soils with a high organic content, such as those in swamps, bogs, and marshes, also have a high infection potential.[47]

Most wounds encountered in the practice of emergency medicine have low initial bacterial counts. If wound cleaning and removal of devitalized tissue are instituted before bacteria within the wound enter their accelerated growth phase, 3 to 12 hours following the injury, and if one uses aseptic technique in examining and managing these wounds, bacterial counts will remain below the critical number needed to initiate infection.[13, 15, 18]

WOUND LOCATION

The anatomic location of the wound has considerable importance in the risk of infection. Bacterial densities on the skin surface range from a few thousand to millions per cm^2.[47] Areas with endogenous microflora in numbers sufficient to infect a wound (greater than 10^5 bacteria per cm^2) include the hairy scalp, the forehead, the axilla, the perineum, the foreskin of the penis, the vagina, the mouth, intertriginous areas, and the nails. In other regions, skin bacteria are sparse (10^2 to 10^3 per cm^2) and are not a source of infection.[1] Wounds in regions of high vascularity, such as the scalp and the face, more easily resist bacterial incursions. The high vascularity of the scalp probably accounts for low infection rates with scalp injuries despite the large numbers of endogenous microflora. Distal extremity wounds, in contrast, are more at risk for the development of wound infections than are injuries of most other parts of the body.[18, 19, 45, 48–50] Wounds in ischemic tissue are notoriously susceptible to infection.[51]

DEVITALIZED TISSUE

Identifying devitalized tissue is an important part of the examination of a wound. Tissue damage lowers the resistance of the wound to infection. Devitalized or necrotic tissue enhances the possibility of infection in a wound by providing a culture medium in which bacteria proliferate, by inhibiting leukocyte phagocytosis, and by creating an anaerobic environment suitable for certain bacterial species.[1, 30]

UNDERLYING STRUCTURES

The importance of detecting injury to underlying structures during the examination was mentioned previously. Procedures such as joint space irrigation, reduction and débridement of compound fractures, neurorrhaphy, vascular anastomosis, and flexor tendon repair are best accomplished in the controlled setting of the operating room, in which optimal lighting, proper instruments, and assistance are available.[1]

CLEANING

After the initial evaluation of the wound has been completed, wound management should begin as soon as possible. The cornerstones of wound care are cleaning, débridement, closure, and protection. Although most wounds are contaminated initially with less than an infective dose of bacteria, given time and the appropriate wound environment, bacterial counts may reach infective levels. The goals of wound cleaning and débridement are the same: (1) to remove bacteria and reduce their numbers below the level associated with infection, and (2) to remove particulate matter and tissue debris that would otherwise lengthen the inflammatory stage of healing or allow the growth of bacteria beyond the critical threshold.[24]

Wound Handling

Anyone cleaning, irrigating, or suturing wounds should wear protective eyewear and a mask, because virtually any patient may be seropositive for the human immunodeficiency virus (HIV). Although mucosal exposure to blood or tissue products that are contaminated by the HIV is considered relatively low risk for subsequent infection, universal precautions are currently recommended.

Thorough cleansing of bacteria, soil, and other contaminants from a wound cannot be accomplished without the patient's cooperation. Scrubbing most open wounds is painful, and the patient's natural response is withdrawal. Therefore, local or regional anesthesia often must precede the examination and cleaning of a wound.[18] Approaches to wound anesthesia are discussed in detail in Chapters 38 to 42.

Despite adequate anesthesia, the patient may be unable to cooperate because of apprehension. The physician should explain the wound-cleansing procedure to the patient and should provide the assurance that everything possible will be done to minimize any pain. In the majority of cases, reassurance will not alleviate the fears of young children, and both sedation and physical restraining devices must be used. Approaches to sedation using parenteral sedative-hypnotics and narcotic agents are discussed in detail in Chapter 41. The use of inhaled nitrous oxide is discussed in Chapter 42.

The two primary methods of wound cleaning are mechanical scrubbing and irrigation. The principle of soaking a wound in a saline or antiseptic solution before the arrival of a physician is of little value. The methods of scrubbing and irrigation are reviewed below.

Mechanical Scrubbing

Initially, a wide area of skin surface surrounding the wound should be scrubbed with an antiseptic solution to remove contaminants that in the course of wound management might be carried into the wound by instruments, suture material, dressings, or the physician's gloved hand. Minimal aseptic technique requires the use of gloves during the cleaning procedure. Much controversy surrounds the technique of scrubbing the internal surface of a wound. Scrubbing the wound with an antiseptic-soaked sponge does remove bacteria, debris, and loose devitalized tissue, thus débriding the wound and lessening the need to sacrifice tissue by excision. It is important to remove all nonabsorbable particulate matter; any such material left in the dermis may become impregnated in the healed tissue and result in a disfiguring "tattoo" effect.[4] Rodeheaver and coworkers, however, determined that scrubbing *experimental* wounds with a saline-soaked sponge did not decrease the incidence of infection. They concluded that tissue trauma inflicted by the sponge impairs the ability of that wound to resist infection, allowing residual bacteria to produce inflammation and infection.[52] Custer and associates found that experimental wounds scrubbed with a gauze sponge moistened with saline exhibited as much of an inflammatory response as did untreated wounds.[53] These experimental wounds were surgical incisions contaminated with bacteria rather than traumatic wounds containing particulate matter, cellular debris, and devitalized tissue in addition to bacteria. Other physicians maintain that the importance of eliminating foreign material and nonviable tissue outweighs any concern about destroying viable tissue by excessive scrubbing.[54]

A reasonable compromise between these opposing views is to reserve mechanical scrubbing for "dirty" wounds contaminated with significant amounts of foreign material. If irrigation alone is ineffective in removing contaminants from a wound, the wound should be scrubbed. Because the amount of damage inflicted on tissues by scrubbing is correlated with the porosity of the sponge, a fine-pore sponge (e.g., Optipore sponge, Biosyntek, Inc.—90 pores per linear inch) should be used to minimize tissue abrasion.[52, 55] Detergents have an advantage over saline in that they minimize friction between the sponge and tissue, thereby limiting tissue damage during scrubbing. Detergents also dissolve particles, helping to dislodge them from the wound surface. Unfortunately, many of the available detergents are toxic to tissues.[52, 56]

Antiseptics During Cleaning

For many years, antiseptic solutions have been used for their antimicrobial properties in and around wounds. In the past decade, investigators have begun to consider the effects of these agents not only on the bacteria contaminating the wound but also on the tissues themselves. Intact skin can withstand strong microbicidal agents, whereas leukocytes and the exposed cells of the wound are very susceptible to further damage.[24] Studies of antiseptics in wounds demonstrate that there is a delicate balance between killing bacteria and injuring tissue.[57]

The antiseptic agents most commonly used in wound care at present include:

Povidone-iodine solution (Betadine preparation)—iodine added to the carrier polyvinylpyrrolidone (PVP), a water-soluble organic complex; this combination is called an iodophor. Standard solutions of Betadine preparation are 10 per cent.

Povidone-iodine surgical scrub (Betadine scrub)—the iodophor PVP-I and an anionic detergent (pH 4.5).

pHisoHex—an emulsion of an anionic detergent, entsulfon, lanolin, cholesterols, petrolatum, and hexachlorophene (pH 5.5).

Hibiclens—chlorhexidine gluconate plus a sudsing base (pH 5.1 to 6.5).

Tincture of green soap—potassium oleate, isopropanol, potassium coconut oil, soap.

Dakin's solution—0.2 per cent sodium hypochlorite solution.

Hydrogen peroxide—an oxidizing agent.

Benzalkonium chloride (Zephiran)—a quaternary ammonium compound that works as a cationic surface active agent.[34, 55]

Nonionic surfactants—Pluronic F–68 (Shur-Clens) and Poloxamer–188 (Pharma Clens)—agents that have no antimicrobial activity (pH 7.1).[58]

Edlich and coworkers demonstrated in a 1969 study that *irrigation* of wounds with Betadine *solution* (preparation) provided significant protection against the development of infection in contaminated wounds.[3] In later studies, he and other investigators found that *scrubbing* experimental wounds with the detergents Betadine *scrub* or pHisoHex increased the incidence of infection.[53] They concluded that the deleterious effect of surgical scrub solutions was a consequence of anionic detergent content and advised against the use of these agents inside wounds.[1, 53, 55] By substituting a pluronic polyol for the detergent, they showed that debris in wounds could be dissolved without causing tissue toxicity.[59] In contrast to the povidone-iodine complex, aqueous iodine is irritating and corrosive to tissue, and it should not be used in wounds.[60]

To confirm the toxicity of antiseptic solutions, Faddis and associates injected these agents into the joints of rabbits. Betadine *scrub* and pHisoHex solutions each caused "severe gross and histologic damage to articular cartilage, synovia, and muscle." A 3 per cent hexachlorophene solution caused "moderate histologic damage" and "articular cartilage ground substance loss." Betadine *solution* (preparation) caused "only minimal gross and histologic damage, without any biochemical evidence of articular cartilage damage."[61] In vitro studies by Rodeheaver and colleagues illustrated the toxicity of antiseptics to the cellular components of blood. Exposure to Hibiclens destroyed all white blood cells and, to a lesser extent, red blood cells. Exposure to Betadine surgical scrub destroyed both.[58]

The tissue toxicity of some antiseptic solutions appears to be dependent on their concentrations. Viljanto noted that in surgical (appendectomy) wounds sprayed with a 5 per cent povidone-iodine aerosol, the infection rate doubled—to a rate of 19 per cent compared with an infection rate in control subjects of 8.5 per cent. When a 1 per cent povidone-iodine aerosol was used, the infection rate dropped to 2.6 per cent.[24] Mulliken and coworkers studied the histologic effects of 1 per cent povidone-iodine solution in injuries and found that it did not decrease tensile strength in these healing wounds.[62] Although studies on the efficacy and safety of povidone-iodine solution have shown variable results,[34, 60, 63–80] it appears that povidone-iodine solution in concentrations of less than 1 per cent is both safe and effective for use in contaminated traumatic wounds. The precise concentration that provides the most benefit remains unknown. It should be noted that standard stock solutions of povidone-iodine solution are commonly 10 per cent strength.

Quaternary ammonium compounds are less toxic to tissue but have a limited antimicrobial spectrum; gram-positive organisms are more susceptible to these solutions than are gram-negative bacteria. Benzalkonium chloride is inactivated by anionic compounds, such as soaps and detergents, and by blood and other organic matter. Furthermore, *Pseudomonas* has been known to proliferate in stored solutions. Consequently, use of benzalkonium chloride has fallen into disfavor.[55] Hydrogen peroxide is used by some clinicians for its effervescent effect in cleaning wounds. Gruber and associates found that hydrogen peroxide decreased healing time in experimental wounds, yet it also injured tissue.[65] Lau and colleagues found hydrogen peroxide irrigation of appendectomy wounds to be ineffective in reducing wound infection.[81] Because peroxide is hemolytic, it is best to use it only to clean surrounding skin encrusted with blood and coagulum or to soak off adherent blood-soaked dressings. Peroxide should not be used on granulation tissue, because oxygen bubbles lift newly formed epithelium off the wound surface.[65] Hexachlorophene was used as an antiseptic for a time but was found to be neurotoxic and teratogenic through skin absorption. Its narrow antimicrobial spectrum makes it no more effective than ordinary soap and water.[82]

Another approach to wound cleaning involves the use of a nonantiseptic nonionic surfactant cleaning agent. In contrast to other antiseptic solutions, these preparations cause no tissue or cellular damage, leukocyte inhibition, or impairment in wound healing. The solutions also cause no corneal injury, conjunctival irritation, or pain on contact with the wound.[83] Pluronic F-68 (Shur-Clens—Biosyntec, Inc.) and Poloxamer 188 (Pharma Clens—American Pharmaseal) are nontoxic, even when administered intravenously, and to date are nonallergenic. These pluronic polyols have no antibacterial activity; the infection rate in wounds irrigated with them is equal to the rate in those irrigated with normal saline.[44] Nevertheless, when used on sponges to clean experimental wounds mechanically, Pluronic F-68 has resulted in lower infection rates than those for controls scrubbed with saline solution, proving its ability to cleanse a wound effectively and atraumatically.[52]

Irrigation

Irrigation removes particulate matter, bacteria, and devitalized tissue loosely adherent to the edges of the wound and trapped within the depths of the wound. The effectiveness of irrigation is determined primarily by the hydraulic pressure at which the irrigant fluid is delivered.[84] Rodeheaver and colleagues studied the effect of irrigating experimental wounds contaminated with 20 mg of soil. Irrigating wounds with 400 ml of fluid at 1 pound per square inch (psi) removed 48.6 per cent of the soil, whereas increasing the pressure to 15 psi removed 84.8 per cent, reducing the infection rate from 100 per cent to 7 per cent.[44]

Significantly more force is required to rid the wound of particles with a small surface area (e.g., bacteria) than to remove particles with a large surface area (e.g., dirt, sand, or vegetation).[55] Bulb syringes or gravity flow irrigation devices deliver fluid at low pressures and as such are ineffective in ridding wounds of small particulate matter or in lowering wound bacterial counts. The flow rate of irrigation fluid delivered through intravenous (IV) tubing can be enhanced by inflation of a blood pressure cuff around a collapsible plastic IV bag, although this method provides considerably less irrigation pressure than can be delivered by a syringe. The maximum hydraulic pressure that can be delivered with a syringe varies with the force exerted on the plunger of the syringe and with the internal diameter of the attached needle. The pressure delivered by a simple irrigation assembly consisting of a 19-gauge plastic catheter or needle attached to a 35-ml syringe is 7 to 8 psi. This high-pressure irrigation system is sufficient to remove significant numbers of bacteria and a substantial amount of particulate matter from the wound surface (Fig. 43–2).[1, 55, 85] Commercial irrigation systems with a ring-handled syringe and a one-way valve that connects into a standard intravenous solution are available (Travenol pressure irrigation set, code no. 2D2113, or Irrijet, Ackrad Laboratories, Garwood, NJ).

A number of investigators have compared pulsatile jet irrigation of wounds to wound irrigation with gravity flow and bulb syringe techniques. The pulsatile jet irrigation technique with pressures of 50 to 70 psi is significantly more effective in removing bacteria, foreign contaminants, and tissue fragments and in reducing infection rates.[86–91] Although the irrigation fluid penetrates the wound tissues, predominantly in a lateral direction, high-pressure jet irrigation does not drive significant amounts of bacteria or surface contaminants into the soft tissues of the wound.[92–95] Although jet irrigation can damage tissue defenses,[95] the technique is more effective in cleaning wounds, less traumatic to tissues, and less likely to produce edema than conventional scrubbing with a brush. Pulsatile and continuous irrigation, if delivered at the same pressures, are equally effective in removing bacteria.[44] The jet irrigation system used by these investigators was a Water Pik unit (Teledyne Aquatic Corp.) with a sterile tip nozzle held approximately 4 cm from the wound; the system delivered a 0.9 per cent saline solution at a pressure of approximately 50 psi. The irrigation pressures generated by this unit are considerably greater than those of the syringe system. Thus pulsatile jet irrigation should generally be reserved for use in heavily contaminated wounds in which syringe irrigation proves to be ineffective.[55, 91, 95] Minimum recommended volumes of irrigation fluid vary, but for average-sized wounds, 200 to 300 ml should be used.[54, 55] Greater volumes may be required for larger or heavily contaminated wounds. Irrigation should continue until all visible, loose particulate matter has been removed. Approximately 20 per cent of open, undated bottles of "sterile" saline and water are contaminated; only

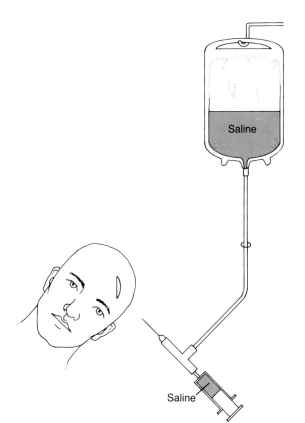

Figure 43–2. An easy method of high-pressure irrigation. Intravenous tubing with an in-line, one-way valve is attached to a bottle of sterile 0.9 per cent saline solution. The other end is connected to a stopcock. Saline solution is aspirated into the syringe. Maximal force is exerted on the plunger of the syringe, delivering the solution in a fine stream through an attached 19-gauge needle held close to the wound.

solutions in bottles opened within the past 24 hours should be used to irrigate wounds.[96, 97]

Antibiotic Solutions for Irrigation

Antibiotic solutions have been instilled directly into wounds or used as irrigation solutions. Halasz reviewed the studies of several investigators who analyzed the technique of irrigating wounds with antibiotic solutions.[98] The antibiotics studied included ampicillin, a neomycin-bacitracin-polymyxin combination, tetracycline, penicillin, kanamycin, and cephalothin. Halasz concluded that "organisms in the wound can be exposed to adequate concentrations of antibiotics, and that the concentration of these drugs in the wound remains in the bactericidal range for long periods of time, far exceeding that obtainable by systemic administration." He recommended placing ampicillin sodium powder, 500 to 1000 mg, or kanamycin, 1 gm, in solutions used to irrigate clean and contaminated wounds.[98] Sher found topical cefazolin to be as effective as systemic cefazolin in preventing infections in wounds contaminated with *Escherichia coli*.[99] Lindsay and associates demonstrated in a clinical trial that flooding traumatic lacerations with 10 ml of 5 per cent sodium benzyl penicillin significantly reduced wound infections when compared with treatment in control subjects, although the overall wound infection rate in this study was high.[100]

The use of antibiotics in irrigant solutions in lieu of antiseptic solutions avoids the tissue destruction of the anti-

septics but theoretically risks the topical sensitization of the patient to the antibiotic, the development of toxic tissue levels of the antibiotic, and the selection of wound-infecting organisms resistant to the antibiotic used. To date, there have been no reports of these complications.[101] Within 3 hours of injury, a proteinaceous coagulum forms within the wound, surrounding the bacteria and probably preventing their contact with topical or systemic antibiotics. Therefore, the wound should be scrubbed before irrigation with an antibiotic solution.[55, 102] Disruption of coagulum and clotted blood by the application of a proteolytic enzyme (e.g., Travase) also has been shown to prolong the effective period of antibiotic action in contaminated wounds when treatment is delayed for as long as 8 hours.[103–106] Because wound coagulum plays a positive role in defense against infection,[3, 48] its removal may not be necessary in injuries for which antibiotics are not indicated.[103, 104] Rodeheaver and associates suggest that using enzymes is more effective than scrubbing the wound, but no comparison study has been performed. They agree that "the mechanism by which trypsin potentiates the effectiveness of antibiotics is, in part, its ability to facilitate removal of bacteria with the gauze sponge." The researchers recommend that for maximum effectiveness the trypsin enzyme be in contact with the wound for a prolonged period (30 minutes). Repeated applications enhance its effectiveness. Proteolytic enzymes are ineffective in decreasing the infection rate if treatment is delayed more than 8 hours.[106] These enzymes also tend to cause considerable bleeding from the wound surface.

Recommendations for Cleaning the Wound

The prerequisites of any wound-cleaning technique are a calm or sedated patient, satisfactory anesthesia, and a thorough scrub of the skin surface adjacent to the wound. The importance of effectively ridding the wound of major contaminants and infective doses of bacteria is unquestionable. Two strategies to accomplish the goals of wound cleaning are apparent from this discussion. The contaminated or "dirty" wound can be irrigated or both scrubbed and irrigated with a 1 per cent povidone-iodine solution (*Betadine preparation,* not scrub). This should be followed by flushing with a 0.9 per cent saline solution. As an alternative, the wound can be scrubbed with pluronic polyols and irrigated with an antibiotic–normal saline solution. Only pluronic polyols should be used near the eyes. All scrubbing should be performed with a fine-pore sponge, and high-pressure techniques should be used for all irrigation. The use of hydrogen peroxide on open wounds is discouraged.

The need for antibiotic solutions in cleaning relatively uncontaminated wounds is not entirely clear, although a decrease in wound infection can be demonstrated.[98–100] Gentle scrubbing with Pluronic F-68 and normal saline high-pressure irrigation both appear to be satisfactory methods for cleaning minimally contaminated wounds.

Preparation for Wound Closure

Before débridement or wound closure, the wound must be prepared and draped. Because of the trauma inflicted on the skin by a razor blade and the resulting dermatitis, the infection rate is greater in wounds that are shaved.[21, 107–109] For wounds in hair-bearing areas, hair should be removed by clipping if the hair interferes with the procedure.[108] Stubborn hairs that continually invade the wound during suturing can be coated with petrolatum jelly or water-soluble ointments to keep them out of the field. Eyebrows should not be shaved, because critical landmarks needed for exact approximation would be lost. Although shaved eyebrows will grow back eventually, shaving produces an undesirable cosmetic effect.

The skin surface adjacent to the wound should be disinfected with a standard 10 per cent povidone-iodine solution. The solution is painted widely on the skin surrounding the wound but should not cover the interior of the wound itself. After brief handwashing, the physician and any assistants involved in the procedure must wear sterile gloves. If talc or other powders are visible on the gloves, they should be rinsed before touching the patient's wound.[47]

Face masks are recommended—they are mandatory for any clinician with a bacterial upper respiratory infection. Because droplets of saliva may leak even from around the edges of a face mask, talking in proximity to the wound must be avoided.[110, 111]

A single fenestrated drape or multiple folded drapes are placed over the wound site. If the wound has not yet been anesthetized, anesthesia can be provided at this time. See Chapters 38 through 42 for details.

The entire depth and the full extent of every wound should be explored in an attempt to locate hidden foreign bodies, particulate matter, bone fragments, and any injuries to underlying structures that may require repair. Lacerations through thick subcutaneous adipose tissue are treacherous because large amounts of particulate matter can be totally obscured in deeper folds of tissue. Unless a careful search is undertaken, these contaminants may be left in the depths of a sutured wound, and infection usually follows. Some physicians are reluctant to extend lacerations to properly clean or explore them; however, opening the wound to permit adequate visualization may be needed for successful wound preparation.

DÉBRIDEMENT

Débridement is of undisputed importance in the management of the contaminated wound. With this technique, the physician can remove tissue impregnated with foreign matter, bacteria, and devitalized tissue that otherwise impairs the ability of the wound to resist infection and prolongs the period of inflammation.[30] Débridement also creates a tidy, sharp wound edge that is easier to repair and results in a more cosmetically acceptable scar. Complete excision of grossly contaminated wounds, such as animal bites, allows primary closure of such wounds with no greater risk of infection than in relatively uncontaminated lacerations.[55]

Irregular wounds have greater surface areas than do linear lacerations. Because skin tension is distributed over a greater length, the scar width is usually less in jagged wounds than if the wound is converted to an elliptical defect with tidy edges. If the edges are devitalized or contaminated, the wound edges must be débrided. To avoid a wide scar in this situation, the wound can be undermined. If the wound is clean and the edges are viable, sharp débridement may not improve the outcome.

Identifying devitalized tissue in a wound remains a challenging problem. Tissue with a narrow pedicle or base, especially distally based flaps on extremities, is unlikely to survive and should be excised. Some practitioners consider muscle to be nonviable if its color and consistency are abnormal; others refer to the absence of bleeding when cut. The most reliable criterion is the inability to contract when electrically stimulated, although rarely is this test necessary or practical in the emergency center setting.[30] Sometimes a sharp line of demarcation distinguishes devitalized skin and

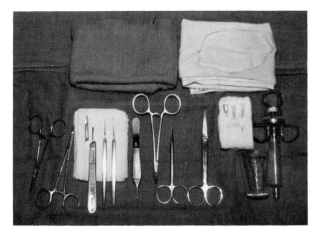

Figure 43–3. Materials for anesthesia and débridement.

viable skin 24 hours after injury.[1] Because most wounds are examined earlier, there is usually only a subtle bluish discoloration. If circulation is adequate, the tissue becomes hyperemic following the release of a proximal tourniquet (unless the tissue is already congested or is blanched by local epinephrine injection). The comparison of capillary refill in wounded tissue with that in adjacent skin is probably the most practical test for tissue viability available to the emergency physician.[112]

Instruments usually required for débridement include two fine single- or double-pronged skin hooks, a scalpel with a number 15 blade, tissue scissors, hemostats, and a small tissue forceps (Fig. 43–3). The jagged wound edges are stabilized with skin hooks or forceps, and the scalpel or scissors are used to cut away devitalized tissue from one end of the wound to the other. After débridement, loose tissue fragments should be irrigated out of the wound.

Certain tissues such as dura, fascia, and tendons perform important functions despite loss of viability. If they can be cleaned adequately, these tissues should not be débrided. They may be left in wounds as free grafts and covered by viable flaps of tissue.[113]

EXCISION

If significant contamination occurs in areas in which there is a redundance or laxity of tissues and if no important structures, such as tendons or nerves, lie within the wound, the entire wound may be excised.[7] This technique is the most effective type of débridement, because it converts the contaminated traumatic wound into a clean surgical wound (Fig. 43–4). Wounds of the trunk, the gluteal region, or the thigh are amenable to this technique. If necessary, the clinician can judge the adequacy of the excision by coloring the wound surface with a vital dye. The clinician would then create a new wound by excising all dyed tissue.[30] Most traumatic wounds can be excised using the elliptic excision technique or a variation thereof. A lenticular configuration should be marked superficially around the wound with the blade of a number 15 scalpel, by cutting only the epidermis. If a puncture wound is being excised, the axis of the excision should parallel a wrinkle, a skin line, or a line of dependency or facial expression, and the long axis should be three to four times as great as the short axis (Fig. 43–5). The clinician may plan this type of excision by premarking the skin with a surgical marking pen. Tension should be placed on the surrounding skin with a finger or a skin hook. With the clinician's hand steadied on the table or on the patient, the

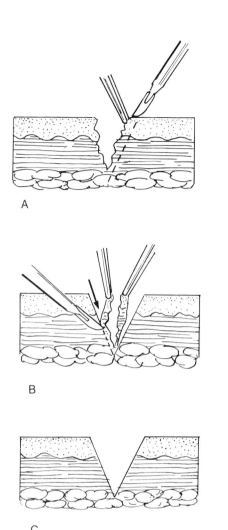

Figure 43–4. *A–C*, Complete excision of a wound. Grossly contaminated wounds may be excised and sutured primarily.

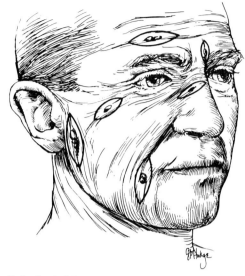

Figure 43–5. If a facial wound is grossly contaminated or too jagged for a cosmetic repair, the wound may be excised. Excisions of small wounds should be lenticular and parallel to skin creases. (From Grabb WC: Basic techniques of plastic surgery. In Grabb WC, Smith JW: Plastic Surgery: A Concise Guide to Clinical Practice. Boston, Little, Brown & Co, 1979. Reproduced by permission.)

SELECTIVE DÉBRIDEMENT

When there is a loss of tissue or an insufficient skin elasticity or when the wound contains structures serving important functions (structures such as dura, fascia, nerves, or tendons), the technique of selective débridement must be used.[7, 30] Complete excision is impossible for most hand wounds. A simple excision of a wound of the palm or the dorsum of the nose would make approximation of the resulting surgical wound edges difficult. Contaminated bone fragments, nerves, and tendons are almost never removed. Every effort should be made to clean these structures and return them to their place of origin, because they may be functional later.[120] Selective débridement is more tedious and time-consuming, but it preserves more surrounding tissue. Stellate wounds and wounds with an irregular, mean-

number 15 blade is used to cut through the skin at right angles or at slightly oblique angles to the skin surface (Fig. 43–6). If complete excision of the entire depth of the wound is not necessary, the tissue scissors may be used to cut the edge of the wound, following the path premarked in the epidermis by the scalpel blade. If a complete excision is desired, the incision on each wound edge should be carried past the deepest part of the wound (see Fig. 43–4). Excision should be done cautiously; excessive removal of tissue can create a defect that is too large to close. In hair-bearing areas of the face, particularly through the eyebrows, the incision should be angled parallel to the angle of hair follicles to avoid linear alopecia (Fig. 43–7). The wedge of excised tissue should be removed carefully, without contaminating the fresh wound surface.[114, 115]

Puncture wounds of the feet frequently contain foreign bodies that are not discovered, or, if found, that are difficult to remove. Contaminated punctures or those likely to contain foreign bodies (such as nail punctures through shoes) should be excised by removing a small cone of surrounding tissue, particularly if the wound extends down to a bone or a joint cavity. Alternatively, the entrance of the wound may be excised with a 4-mm disposable punch biopsy and the wound irrigated a second time.[116–119]

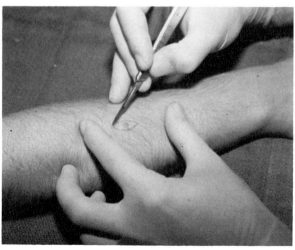

Figure 43–6. Technique of excision.

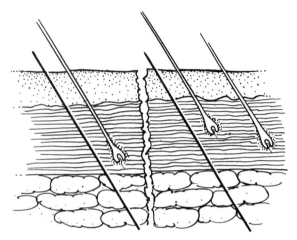

Figure 43–7. Excision through an eyebrow. (From Dushoff IM: A stitch in time. Emerg Med 5(1):2, 1973. Reproduced by permission.)

dering course have greater surface areas and less skin tension per unit length than do linear lacerations. In some cases, excision of an entire wound results in the loss of too much tissue and produces a gaping defect and excessive tension on the the wound edges when closed. This problem can be avoided with selective débridement and approximation of the irregular wound edges.[10] This technique involves sharp débridement of devitalized or heavily contaminated tissue in the wound piece by piece and eventual matching of one edge of the wound with the other.

In heavily contaminated wounds, especially those with abundant adipose tissue, all exposed fat and all fat impregnated with particulate matter should be removed. The subcutaneous adipose tissue attached to large flaps or to avulsed viable skin should be débrided before reapproximation of the wound; removal of this fatty layer allows better perfusion of the flap or the graft.

Following débridement or excision, the wound should be irrigated again to remove any remaining tissue debris.

CONTROL OF HEMORRHAGE

Hemorrhage from a wound may be vigorous, and occasionally it requires control before examination, cleaning, or débridement. If minor bleeding is not a problem before wound débridement, it frequently becomes a complication once the wound edges are excised. Wound exploration or cleaning sometimes induces bleeding. Hemostasis is essential at any stage of wound care. Not only does persistent bleeding obscure the wound and hamper wound exploration and closure, but also hematoma formation in a sutured wound separates wound edges, impairs healing, and risks dehiscence or infection.

Several practical methods of achieving hemostasis are available to the emergency physician. Direct pressure with gloved fingers, gauze sponges, or packing material is always effective in immediately controlling a single bleeding site or a small number of sites. Sustained pressure on the wound for at least 5 minutes can effectively control capillary oozing, by occluding capillaries until coagulation occurs. Arterial and arteriolar bleeding, although brisk initially, frequently subsides within minutes as the cut ends of these vessels constrict. Direct pressure on larger vessels minimizes blood loss until constriction occurs. Direct pressure is most effective when combined with elevation of the bleeding wound above the level of the patient's heart.

In a patient with multiple injuries and several urgent

problems, hemorrhage can be controlled temporarily with a compression dressing. Several absorptive sponges are applied directly over the bleeding site, and these are secured in place with an elastic bandage (e.g., Ace wrap) or elastic adhesive tape (Elastoplast). Pressure is provided by the elasticity of the bandage. The bleeding part should be elevated. Wound care can then be deferred while the physician attends to more pressing matters.

Ligation of blood vessels with fine absorbable suture material is another method of achieving hemostasis. A common error, however, is to spend excessive time attempting to tie off small bleeding vessels while the patient slowly exsanguinates. In highly vascular areas, such as scalp, it is best to suture the laceration following wound exploration and irrigation despite active bleeding; the pressure exerted by the closure will usually stop the bleeding. If bleeding is too brisk to permit adequate wound evaluation and irrigation, hemorrhage can often be controlled by clamping and everting the galea or dermis of each wound edge with hemostats. Lemos and Clark propose the use of scalp clips as an alternative.[121]

Although simply crushing and twisting the end of a vessel with a hemostat avoids the introduction of suture material into the wound, this method provides unreliable hemostasis. Ligation of the vessel is preferred. Bleeding ends of vessels are clamped with fine-point hemostats, effecting immediate hemostasis. Because nerves often course with these vessels, all clamping should be done under direct visualization. The tip of the hemostat should project beyond the vessel to hold a loop of a ligature in place (Fig. 43–8). While an assistant lifts the handle of the hemostat, a synthetic absorbable suture of size 5–0 or 6–0 is passed around the hemostat from one hand to the other (Fig. 43–9). The first knot is tied beyond the tip of the hemostat. Once the suture is securely anchored on the vessel, the hemostat is released.[115, 121]

In practice, the emergency physician seldom has an assistant available to ligate vessels by this method. MacDonald describes a technique that enables a single operator to maintain tension on the ligature while removing the hemostatic clamp. A needle holder is used to grasp one tail of the ligature; the other end is held by the third, fourth, and fifth fingers of the left hand. As the clamp held in the right hand is removed from the vessel, the needle holder is moved away from the left hand by extending the thumb and the index finger, maintaining tension on the ligature. The right hand can discard the clamp, grasp the needle holder, and complete

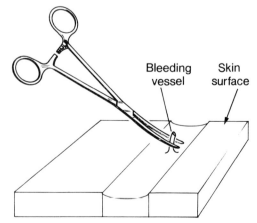

Figure 43–8. When one attempts to tie off a bleeding vessel, the tip of the hemostat should project beyond the clamped vessel.

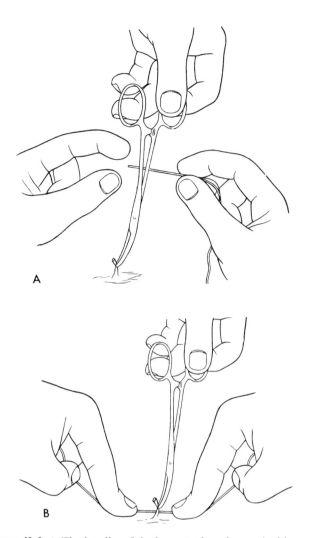

Figure 43–9. *A,* The handles of the hemostat have been raised by an assistant as a ligature is passed under them. *B,* The ligature thread stretched between the index finger tips is carried under the projecting tips of the hemostat. (Modified from Kirk RM: Basic Surgical Techniques. Edinburgh, Churchill Livingstone, 1978, pp 50–51. Reproduced by permission.)

the tie (Fig. 43–10).[123] Three knots are sufficient to hold the ligature in place. The ends of the suture should be cut close to the knot to minimize the amount of suture material that is left in the wound.

Cut vessels that retract into the wall of the wound may frustrate attempts at clamping and ligation. Bleeding should be controlled first by downward compression on the tissue. A suture is passed through the tissue twice, using a figure-of-eight or horizontal mattress stitch, and then tied. The double thread will constrict the tissue containing the cut vessel (Fig. 43–11). The disadvantage of this method is that the tissue constricted by the ligature may necrose and leave devitalized tissue in the wound.

Vessels with diameters greater than 2 mm should be ligated. Those smaller than 2 mm that bleed despite direct pressure can be controlled by pinpoint electrocautery. A dry field is required for an effective electrical current to pass through the tissues; if sponging does not dry the field, a suction-tipped catheter should be used. Trauma is minimized by using fine-tipped electrodes to touch the vessel or by touching the active electrode of the electrocautery unit to a small hemostat or fine-tipped forceps gripping the vessel.[2] The power of the unit should be kept to the minimum level required for vessel thrombosis. Bipolar coagulation (such as that provided by the Bovie Unit) is preferred over monopolar coagulation because it produces approximately one third less tissue necrosis of surrounding tissue.[55] If the amount of tissue cauterized is kept to a minimum, wound healing is no more compromised by this technique than by ligation. Cauterization of medium- and small-sized vessels can quickly provide hemostasis.

Self-contained, sterilizable, battery-powered coagulation units are available. Vessels are cauterized by the direct application of a heated wired filament. These units may damage more surrounding tissue than electrocautery units; however, they are compact and simple and are therefore well suited for use in the emergency center (Fig. 43–12).

Epinephrine is an excellent vasoconstrictor. Topical epinephrine (1:100,000) can be applied to a wound on a moistened sponge to reduce the bleeding from small vessels.[115] Combined with local anesthetics, concentrations of 1:100,000 and 1:200,000 prolong the effect of the anesthetic and provide some hemostasis in highly vascular areas. Epinephrine and other vasoconstrictors used topically or intra-

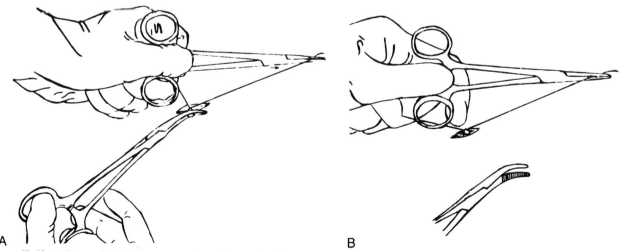

Figure 43–10. *A,* One maintains ligature tension with one hand by grasping one tail of the suture with a clamp and keeping its base between the thumb and the forefinger. *B,* As the pedicle clamp is removed with the other hand, the ligature is tightened by extension of the flexed thumb and index finger to the desired tension. The pedicle clamp is then discarded from the right hand, and further knots are applied in the usual fashion. (Modified from MacDonald RT: Maintenance of ligature tension by a single operator with simultaneous removal of a hemostatic clamp. Am J Surg 143:770, 1982. Reproduced by permission.)

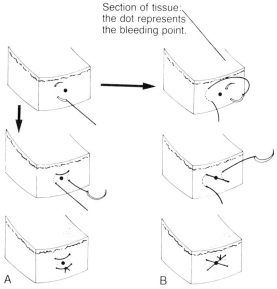

Section of tissue: the dot represents the bleeding point.

A

B

Figure 43–11. Ligation of a retracted, bleeding vessel. *A*, Horizontal mattress technique. *B*, Figure-of-eight technique.

dermally may increase the risk of wound infection. Therefore, use of vasoconstrictors should be restricted to situations in which widespread small vessel and capillary hemorrhage in a wound is not controlled by direct pressure or cauterization.

Fibrin foam, gelatin foam, and microcrystalline collagen may be used as hemostatic agents. Their utility is limited in that vigorous bleeding will wash the agent away from the bleeding site. Their greatest value may be in packing small cavities from which there is a constant oozing of blood.[115] In most simple wounds with persistent but minor capillary bleeding, apposition of the wound edges with sutures provides adequate hemostasis.

TOURNIQUETS

If bleeding from an extremity wound is refractory to direct pressure, electrocauterization, or ligation or if the patient presents with exsanguinating hemorrhage from the wound, a tourniquet can be used to control the bleeding temporarily.

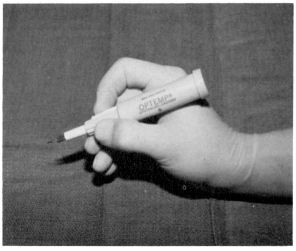

Figure 43–12. Battery-powered cautery.

Tourniquets are also helpful in examining extremity lacerations by providing a bloodless field; a small foreign body or a partially lacerated tendon or joint capsule is easily obscured within a bloody wound.

Tourniquets can cause injury in three ways:

1. They can produce ischemia in an extremity.
2. They can compress and damage underlying blood vessels and nerves.
3. They can jeopardize the survival of marginally viable tissue.

These injuries can be avoided (1) if there is a limit placed on the total amount of time that an extremity is confined by a tourniquet and (2) if excessive tourniquet pressures are avoided.

A single cuff tourniquet (sphygmomanometer cuff) placed around an arm or a leg effectively stops distal venous or arterial bleeding without crushing underlying structures. The length of time that a tourniquet may remain in place is limited by the development of pain underneath and distal to the tourniquet. This occurs within 30 to 45 minutes in a conscious patient, well within the limits of safety.[124, 125]

Before application of the tourniquet, the injured extremity should be elevated and then manually exsanguinated to prevent bothersome venous bleeding. An elastic bandage (e.g., Ace wrap or Esmarch) may be wrapped circumferentially around the extremity, starting distally and moving in a proximal direction. A cuff placed around the arm proximal to the wound should be inflated to 250 to 300 mm Hg and the tubing clamped; the bandage is then removed and the extremity lowered.[125, 126] Other researchers recommend a cuff pressure only slightly higher than the patient's systolic blood pressure.[127] It is recommended that the sphygmomanometer bulb be fully opened after the tube is clamped to permit rapid deflation of the cuff after the procedure. Because tourniquets impair circulation, their use in the emergency department should be limited to a 1 hour maximum.

Tourniquets on digits have a greater potential for complications. The maximum tourniquet time that is safe for a finger may be easily exceeded. Also, finger tourniquets can exert excessive pressures over a small surface area at the base of the finger and injure digital nerves or cause pressure necrosis of digital vessels. For this reason, rubber bands should *not* be used as tourniquets. Tourniquet pressures up to 250 to 300 mm Hg are safe in digits, but pressures of only 150 mm Hg are needed for hemostasis.

Shaw and coworkers studied several common techniques used for hemostasis in fingers. They stretched Penrose drains around fingers to marks corresponding to three quarters, two thirds, one half, and one third of the measured circumference of the digit. Excessively high tissue pressures resulted when a 0.25-inch drain was stretched beyond its one-half fractional circumference mark and a 0.5-inch drain beyond its two-thirds fractional mark. A few millimeters of difference in total stretch made a large difference in the tourniquet pressure applied.[128]

A latex-rubber surgical glove placed over a patient's hand can be used as a finger tourniquet. The appropriate digit is cut from the glove, the tip removed, and the patient's injured digit covered with the glove finger. The latex rubber is then rolled proximally along the patient's finger to form a constricting band at the base. Commercial exsanguinating digit tourniquets are available (Tourni-cot; Mar-Med Co.). There is a danger of forgetting to remove such a small tourniquet and of accidently incorporating it in the dressing. This is less likely if the entire glove is placed over the patient's hand and only the tip of the glove finger removed. The remaining glove finger is rolled to the base of the digit

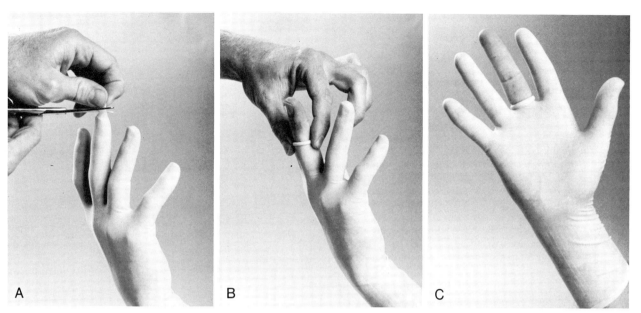

Figure 43–13. Use of a sterile glove to provide a clean field and serve as a finger tourniquet. Distal end of the glove is clipped *(A)* and glove finger rolled proximally over the digit *(B)*. During actual patient care, the physician would use sterile technique.

(Fig. 43–13). Another advantage to covering the entire hand with the sterile glove is that contamination of the wound during closure is less likely.[129] Rolled surgical gloves produce pressures ranging from 113 to 363 mm Hg, depending on the thickness, the amount of glove finger removed, the number of rolls, and the size of the glove in relation to the patient's hand.[128] Lubahn and coworkers calculated pressures under a rolled glove finger ranging between 200 and 1200 mm Hg, and under a Penrose drain tourniquet between 100 and 650 mm Hg. Pressure under a Penrose drain can be more easily controlled.[130]

Some physicians wrap the entire finger with a Penrose drain in the fashion of a miniature Esmarch bandage to exsanguinate the digit. The wrap is unraveled from distal to proximal, leaving two or more turns around the proximal part of the finger to serve as a tourniquet. This technique generates excessive pressures, ranging from a minimum of 300 mm Hg to greater than 800 mm Hg.[128] A finger can be exsanguinated with a Penrose drain, but a separate drain should be used as a tourniquet (Fig. 43–14). Alternatively, a finger can be exsanguinated with a moistened piece of gauze opened to its fullest length, folded in half, and rolled tightly around the elevated finger from tip to base. A Penrose drain is stretched around the base of the finger and secured with a hemostat, and the gauze is removed. The maximum tourniquet time on a finger should not exceed 20 to 30 minutes.[128, 130]

These techniques provide bloodless fields in which to examine, clean, and close extremity wounds. Débridement of questionably devitalized tissue in a wound is best accom-

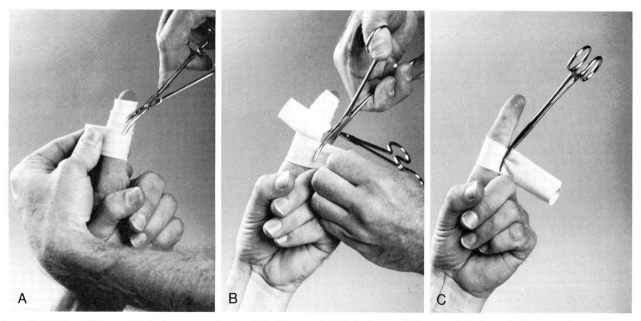

Figure 43–14. Use of Penrose drain for exsanguination *(A)* of a wounded digit. A second Penrose drain is applied *(B)* as a finger tourniquet and the first drain removed *(C)*. During actual patient care, the physician would use sterile technique.

plished *without* a tourniquet or pharmacologic vasoconstriction, because bleeding from tissues is often an indication of their viability.[120]

CLOSURE

Open Versus Closed Wound Management

Two of the objectives of wound care are prevention of excessive or prolonged inflammation and control of scar formation. Wounds that heal spontaneously (by "secondary intention") undergo much more inflammation, fibroplasia, and contraction than those whose edges are reapproximated by wound closure techniques.[4, 131] The process of contraction in wound healing serves to cover the defect of an open wound, yet it may have undesirable consequences—deformity (contracture) or loss of function. Left to itself, the healing process may be unable to close a defect completely in areas in which surrounding skin is immobile, such as on the scalp or in the pretibial area.[4] Exposed tendons, bone, nerves, or vessels may desiccate in an open wound. If the patient is careless with an otherwise adequate dressing that covers an open wound, the wound may be further contaminated.[132] The advantages of surgical closure of wounds are apparent—this procedure minimizes inflammation, fibroplasia, contracture, scar width, and contamination.

On the other hand, risks are incurred when wounds are closed. Closure of contaminated wounds greatly increases the probability of wound infection, with impaired healing, dehiscence, and sepsis as possible complications. After cleaning and débridement, wounds left unsutured appear to have a higher resistance to infection than do closed wounds.[18] Prusak found that inoculation of open wounds with 10^8 *Staphylococcus aureus* organisms resulted in minimal inflammatory response compared with that of uncontaminated wounds left to heal secondarily.[133]

Sutures in themselves are detrimental to healing and increase the risk of infection.[134, 135] Each suture inflicts an intradermal incision, damaging surface epithelium, dermis, subcutaneous fat, blood vessels, small nerves, lymphatics, and epithelial appendages such as hair follicles, sweat glands, and ducts. These appendages, once divided and separated by a stitch, usually undergo inflammation and resorption.[5, 136] Bryant states that "each suture . . . should be regarded as another piece of foreign material that incites an inflammatory response."[4] Furthermore, when a suture is removed, bacteria that have settled on the exposed portion of the suture are pulled into the suture track and deposited there.[5] Raised pretibial flap lacerations in elderly patients often necrose when sutured but survive and heal well by secondary intention if taped back into position (Fig. 43–15).[137]

Guidelines for deciding when to close wounds may be simply stated (but are poorly defined): If the wound is judged to be "clean" or is rendered "clean" by scrubbing, irrigation, and débridement, it may be closed. If the wound remains hopelessly contaminated despite the best of efforts, it must be left open to heal by secondary intention. If the status of the wound is uncertain, the practitioner can base the decision on clinical judgment (an educated guess based on past experience with similar wounds) or on quantitative bacteriologic analysis of the wound. Another option available is delayed primary closure.

Quantitative Bacteriologic Analysis

The primary determinants of wound infection are the level of wound contamination and the amount of residual

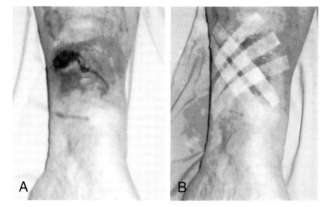

Figure 43–15. Pretibial skin avulsions are common injuries in the elderly (*A*). This thin skin cannot be sutured easily. Good results are usually obtained if the skin is repositioned, the entire flap held in place with SteriStrips (*B*), and a compression dressing, such as an elastic bandage or Dome Paste (Unna boot) dressing applied to minimize flap movement and decrease fluid buildup under the flap. Elevation is key to a successful outcome. This procedure is similar to split-thickness skin grafting.

devitalized tissue. Also of importance is the ability of the patient's immune system to respond to bacterial invasion. Until recently, assessing these factors was a matter of clinical judgment. A number of investigators have demonstrated that quantitative analysis of samples of tissue from wound margins is accurately predictive of subsequent wound infection.

In most studies, 10^5 to 10^6 or more bacteria were needed to cause burn wound sepsis, wound infection, or pustule formation. In the presence of a single silk suture, considerably fewer bacteria were needed to initiate infection in any wound.[132, 138, 139]

A rapid slide technique (available within 20 minutes) has been used with 95 per cent accuracy in determining the safety of wound closure. Edlich and colleagues showed that it was unsafe initially to close experimental wounds contaminated with 10^6 bacteria.[131] Robson and other investigators found that greater than 10^5 bacteria prevented successful delayed surgical wound closure.[51, 140, 141] A quantitative bacteriologic study of a wound thus makes the decision of wound closure a straightforward one. Using this laboratory method, if the number of bacteria per gram of tissue sampled after thorough cleaning and débridement is greater than 10^5, the wound should not be closed at that time.[132, 142] Unfortunately, very few emergency physicians have this test available to them, and it is impractical for routine use.

Delayed Closure

If there is a substantial risk that closure of a particular wound might result in infection, the decision to close or to leave the wound open can be postponed. The condition of the wound after 3 to 5 days will then determine the best strategy. Although cleaning and débridement should be accomplished as rapidly as possible, there is no urgency in closing a wound. Edlich and coworkers point out that "the fundamental basis for delayed primary closure is that the healing open wound gradually gains sufficient resistance to infection to permit an uncomplicated closure."[1] The concept of delayed closure is unfamiliar to many physicians who deal with outpatient wounds. Despite its effectiveness, delayed primary closure is a technique that is underused by most physicians.

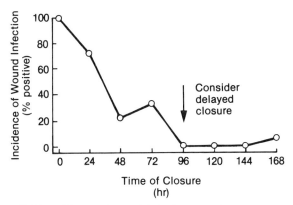

Figure 43–16. Incidence of wound infection over time when delayed closure is performed. Delayed closure is best accomplished on the fourth or fifth day to avoid infection. (From Edlich RF, Thacker JG, Rodeheaver GT, et al: A Manual for Wound Closure. St. Paul, Minn, 3M Medical Surgical Products, 1979. Reproduced by permission of and copyright 1979 by Minnesota Mining and Manufacturing Company.)

Open wound management consists of the usual cleaning and débridement followed by packing of the wound with sterile, saline-moistened fine-mesh gauze. The packed wound is covered by a thick, absorbent, sterile dressing. Unless the patient develops a fever, the wound should not be disturbed for 4 days; unnecessary inspection risks contamination and infection. On the fourth postoperative day, the wound is reevaluated. If no evidence of infection is present, the wound margins can be approximated (delayed primary closure) or the wound can be excised and then sutured (secondary closure) with minimal risk of infection (Fig. 43–16). Because the wound is closed before the proliferative phase of healing, there is no delay in final healing, and the results are indistinguishable from those of primary healing. If available, quantitative microbiology can be used at the time of delayed closure to document further the safety of wound closure.[1, 18, 131, 143]

Certain wounds should almost always be managed open or by delayed closure. These include wounds contaminated by soil or organic matter, purulence, saliva, feces, or vaginal secretions (although primary repair of intraoral lacerations, surgical perineal wounds, and episiotomies is acceptable practice). Also included in this category are wounds associated with extensive tissue damage (e.g., high-velocity missile injuries, explosion injuries of the hand, or complex crush injuries) and most bite wounds. Physicians disagree as to which bite wounds may be closed initially. Most would suture cosmetically deforming injuries, including facial bites, and bite wounds that can be completely excised.[6, 55, 144] Others would suture nonextremity dog bites.[145] In severe soft tissue injuries, delayed closure allows time for nonviable tissue to demarcate from uninjured tissue. Débridement can then be accomplished with maximal preservation of tissue.[132]

Methods

Once the decision to close a wound has been made, the physician must select the closure technique that is best suited for the particular location and configuration of the wound.[18] Available techniques include suturing, taping, and metal stapling.

All emergency physicians should be skilled in the approximation of skin edges with surgical tape (Steri-Strips, Shur-strips, Clearon). Tape is easy to apply and is preferable to sutures when the patient is frightened or uncooperative. Skin tape causes minimal skin reaction, results in no skin suture marks, and is associated with the lowest incidence of infection of any closure technique.[146–149] Although tape will appose the edges of a superficial laceration without difficulty, the subcutaneous layer of a deep laceration must be sutured to prevent inversion of the skin edges by the tape.[114] Metal staples can be applied to approximate a wound rapidly, but their use is limited to easily accessible, linear lacerations in noncosmetic areas.

In most situations, suturing is the method of choice. Detailed discussion of wound closure by tape and staples is provided in Chapter 44. The remaining discussion of wound closure pertains to the use of sutures.

Equipment

INSTRUMENTS

In addition to the instruments used for débridement (see Fig. 43–3), a needle holder and suture scissors are required for suturing. The size of the needle holder that is used should match the size of the needle selected for suturing—the needle holder should be large enough to hold the needle securely as it is passed through tissue, yet not so large that the needle is crushed or bent by the instrument. Instruments used to débride a grossly contaminated wound should be discarded and fresh instruments obtained for the closure of the wound. If the instruments are covered with coagulated blood, they can be cleansed with hydrogen peroxide and then used for suturing.

SUTURE MATERIALS

A wide variety of suture materials are available. For most wounds that require closure of more than one layer of tissue, the physician must choose sutures from two general categories—an absorbable suture for the subcutaneous layer and a nonabsorbable suture for skin closure.

Sutures can be described in terms of four characteristics:

1. chemical and physical properties,
2. handling characteristics and mechanical performance,
3. absorption and reactivity, and
4. size and retention of tensile strength.

Composition. Sutures are made from natural fibers (cotton, silk), from sheep submucosa or beef serosa (plain gut, chromic gut), or from synthetic materials, such as nylon (Dermalon, Ethilon, Nurolon, Surgilon), Dacron (Ethiflex, Mersilene), polyester (TiCron), polyethylene (Ethibond), polypropylene (Prolene, Surgilene), polyglycolic acid (Dexon), and polyglactin (Vicryl, coated Vicryl). Stainless steel sutures are rarely, if ever, useful in wound closure in the emergency center setting because of difficulty in handling, fragmentation, and harmful effects on tissues.[18, 150] Some sutures are made of a single filament (monofilament); others consist of multiple fibers braided together (Table 43–1).[151]

Handling and Performance. Desirable handling characteristics in a suture include smooth passage through tissues, ease in knot tying, and stability of the knot once tied. Smooth types of sutures pull through tissues easily, but knots slip more readily. Conversely, sutures with a high coefficient of friction have better knot-holding capacity, but it is difficult to slide them through tissues. Smooth sutures will loosen after the first throw of a knot is made, and a second throw is needed to secure the first in place. However, the physician may want to tighten a knot further after the first throw is made. This is difficult with rougher types of sutures.

Table 43-1. *Examples of Suture Materials*

Monofilament	
Absorbable Sutures	*Nonabsorbable Sutures*
Plain gut	Dermalon*
Chromic gut	Ethilon*
PDS‡‡	Prolene‖
	Silk
	Steel
	Surgilene‖
	Tevdek††
Multifilament	
Absorbable Sutures	*Nonabsorbable Sutures*
Dexon¶	Ethibond§
Vicryl**	Mersilene†
Coated Vicryl**	Nurolon*
	Surgilon*
	TiCron‡

*Nylon.
†Dacron.
‡Polyester.
§Polyethylene.
‖Polypropylene.
¶Polyglycolic acid.
**Polyglactin.
††Teflon coated.
‡‡Polydioxanone.

Multifilament sutures have the best handling characteristics of all sutures, whereas steel sutures have the worst. In terms of performance and handling, significant improvements have been made in the newer absorbable sutures. Gut sutures have many shortcomings, including relatively low and variable strength, a tendency to fray when handled, and stiffness despite being packaged in a softening fluid.[152, 153] Multifilament synthetic absorbable sutures are soft and easy to tie and have few problems with knot slippage. Polyglactin 910 (coated Vicryl) sutures have been improved with the application of an absorbable lubricant coating. The frictional "drag" of these coated sutures as they are pulled through tissues is less than that of uncoated multifilament materials, and the resetting of knots following the initial throw is much easier. This characteristic allows retightening of a ligature without knotting or breakage, and it allows smooth and even adjustment of suture line tension in running subcuticular stitches.[154] Synthetic monofilament sutures have the troublesome property of "memory"—a tendency of the filament to spring back to its original shape, which causes the knot to slip and unravel. Some nonabsorbable monofilament sutures are coated with polytetrafluorethane (Teflon) or silicone to reduce their friction. This coating improves the handling characteristics of these monofilaments but results in poorer knot security.[150, 153]

Thacker and coworkers found that when sutures were cut 3 mm from the ends of the knot, three square knots are required to secure a silk suture and five are needed for the Teflon-coated synthetic Tevdek.[155] Macht and Krizek warned that an excessive number of throws in a knot weakens the suture at the knot. They recommended three square knots to secure a stitch with silk or other braided, nonabsorbable materials and four knots with synthetic, monofilament absorbable and nonabsorbable sutures.[156] With the use of coated synthetic suture materials, attention to basic principles of knot tying is even more important. If the physician uses square knots (or a surgeon's knot on the initial throw followed by square knots) that lie down flat and are tied securely, knots will rarely unravel.[157]

Absorption and Reactivity. Sutures that are rapidly degraded in tissues are termed "absorbable"; those that maintain their tensile strength for longer than 60 days are considered "nonabsorbable" (see Table 43-1). Plain gut may be digested by white blood cell lysozymes in 10 to 40 days; chromic gut will last 15 to 60 days. Remnants of both types of sutures, however, have been seen in wounds more than 2 years after their placement.[152, 156, 158] A newer type of catgut (Ethicon) is rapidly absorbed within 10 to 14 days but with less inflammation than caused by chromic catgut.[159] Vicryl is absorbed from the wound site within 60 to 90 days[150, 152, 156] and Dexon within 120 to 210 days.[160–162] Wallace and colleagues report that when placed in the oral cavity, plain gut disappears after 3 to 5 days, chromic gut after 7 to 10 days, and polyglycolic acid after 16 to 20 days.[163] In contrast, silk is completely absorbed within the skin in approximately 2 years.[156] The rate of absorption of synthetic absorbable sutures is independent of suture size.[160]

Sutures may lose strength and function before they are completely absorbed from tissues. Braided synthetic absorbable sutures lose nearly all of their strength after about 21 days. In contrast, monofilament absorbable sutures (modified polyglycolic acid [Maxon, Davis & Geck] and polydioxanone [PDS, Ethicon]) retain 60 per cent of their strength after 28 days.[164, 165] Gut sutures treated with chromium salts (chromic gut) have a prolonged tensile strength;[18, 150] however, all gut sutures retain tensile strength erratically.[152, 156] Of the absorbable types of sutures, a wet and knotted polyglycolic acid suture is stronger than a plain or chromic gut suture subjected to the same conditions.[153, 166]

Some researchers claim that silk maintains its tensile strength for approximately 1 year and nylon for greater than a year.[156] Others state that both silk and nylon, although considered nonabsorbable, lose their strength rapidly after the second month in a wound and may disintegrate within 6 months.[18] Polypropylene remains unchanged in tissue for longer than 2 years after implantation.[18, 167] In comparison testing, Hermann found that sutures made of natural fibers, such as silk, cotton, and gut, were the weakest; sutures made of Dacron, nylon, polyethylene, and polypropylene were intermediate in tensile strength; and metallic sutures were the strongest.[153] Kaplan and Hentz use the comparison of suture strength versus wound strength as a measure of the usefulness of a suture. They state that catgut is stronger than the soft tissue of a wound for no more than 7 days; chromic catgut, Dexon, and Vicryl are stronger for 10 to 21 days; and nylon, wire, and silk are stronger for 20 to 30 days.[112]

All sutures placed within tissue will damage host defenses and provoke inflammation. Even the least reactive suture impairs the ability of the wound to resist infection.[167] The magnitude of the reaction provoked by a suture is related to the quantity of suture material (e.g., diameter and total length) placed in the tissue and to the chemical composition of the suture. Among absorbable sutures, polyglycolic acid and polyglactin sutures are least reactive, followed by chromic gut. The nonabsorbable polypropylene is less reactive than nylon or Dacron.[153, 158, 168–170] Significant tissue reaction is associated with catgut, silk, and cotton sutures. Edlich and coworkers advise against the use of these highly reactive materials in contaminated wounds.[18] Adams found the "absorbable" polyglycolic acid sutures less reactive than those of "nonabsorbable" silk.[171]

The chemical composition of sutures is an important determinant of early infection. The infection rate in experimental wounds when polyglycolic acid sutures are used is less than the rate when gut sutures are used. It is surprising that plain gut sutures elicit infection less often in contaminated wounds than do chromic gut sutures.[167] Lubricant coatings on sutures do not alter suture reactivity, absorption characteristics, breaking strength, or the risk of infection.[154, 167] Osterberg and colleagues found that in experimental wounds, multifilament sutures are more likely to produce infection than monofilament sutures if left in place for prolonged periods.[172, 173] Monofilament sutures elicit less tissue reaction than do multifilament sutures, and multifilament materials tend to wick up fluid by capillary action. Bacteria that adhere to and colonize sutures can envelop themselves in a glycocalix that protects them from host defenses,[174] or they can "hide" in the interstices of a multifilament suture and as a result can be inaccessible to leukocytes.[172] Although Edlich and associates found no significant difference in the infective potential of these two configurations of sutures after a period of 4 days,[167] Sharp and colleagues found an increased degree of inflammation in wounds closed with multifilament sutures compared with wounds closed with monofilament sutures.[175] One monofilament absorbable suture, polydioxanone, appears especially promising.[176]

Size and Strength. Size of suture material (thread diameter) is a measure of the tensile strength of the suture; threads of greater diameter are stronger. The strength of the suture is proportional to the square of the diameter of the thread. Therefore, a 4–0 size suture of any type is larger and stronger than a 6–0 suture.[150] The correct suture size for approximation of a layer of tissue depends on the tensile strength of that tissue. The tensile strength of the suture material should be only slightly greater than that of the tissue, because the magnitude of damage to local tissue defenses is proportional to the amount of suture material placed in the wound.[1, 156, 177]

Synthetic absorbable sutures have made the older, natural suture materials obsolete. Polyglycolic acid (Dexon) and polyglactin 910 (coated Vicryl) have improved handling characteristics, knot security, and tensile strength. Their absorption rates are predictable, and tissue reactivity is minimal.[6, 178] The distinct advantages of synthetic nonabsorbable sutures over silk sutures are their greater tensile strength, low coefficient of friction, and minimal tissue reactivity.[6, 167] They are extensible, elongating without breaking as the edges of the wound swell in the early postoperative period.[1, 6] In contrast with silk sutures, synthetics can be easily and painlessly removed once the wound has healed. A new monofilament synthetic suture, Novafil, has elasticity that allows a stitch to enlarge with wound edema and return to its original length once the edema subsides. Stiffer materials lacerate the encircled tissue as the wound swells.[47]

The suture materials most useful to emergency physicians in wound closure are Dexon or coated Vicryl for subcutaneous layers and synthetic nonabsorbable sutures (e.g., nylon or polypropylene) for skin closure. Fascia can be sutured with either absorbable or nonabsorbable materials. In most situations, 3–0 or 4–0 sutures are used in the repair of fascia, 4–0 or 5–0 absorbable sutures in subcutaneous closure, and 4–0 or 5–0 nonabsorbable sutures in skin closure. The skin layer of facial wounds is repaired with 6–0 sutures, whereas 3–0 or 4–0 sutures are used when the skin edges are subjected to considerable dynamic stresses (e.g., wounds overlying joint surfaces) or static stresses (e.g., scalp).

NEEDLES

The eyeless, or "swaged," needle is the type of needle used for wound closure in most emergency centers (Fig. 43–17). The traditional closed-eye needle requires additional handling to enable one to thread the needle with the suture. Because a closed-eye needle must carry a double strand of thread through its eye, it causes more damage in passing through tissue than does a swaged needle, whose diameter is nearly equal to that of the strand it carries.[150]

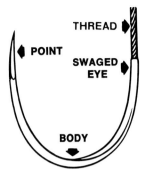

Figure 43–17. The eyeless, or "swaged," needle. (From Suture Use Manual: Use and Handling of Sutures and Needles. Somerville, NJ, Ethicon, Inc, 1977, p 29. Reproduced by permission.)

The selection of the appropriate needle size and curvature is based on the dimensions of the wound and the characteristics of the tissues to be sutured. The needle should be large enough to pass through tissue to the depth desired and to exit the tissue or the skin surface far enough that the needle holder can be repositioned on the distal end of the needle at a safe distance from the point (Fig. 43–18). In wound repair, needles must penetrate tough, fibrous tissues—skin, subcutaneous tissue, and fascia—yet the needles should slice through these tissues with minimal resistance or trauma and without bending. The type of needle best suited for closure of subcutaneous tissue is a conventional cutting needle in a three-eighths or one-half circle (Fig. 43–19). The use of double curvature needles (coated Vicryl with PS–4-C cutting needles, Ethicon) may enhance the physician's ability to maneuver the needle in narrow deep wounds. For percutaneous closure, a conventional cutting-edge needle may permit more precise needle placement and require less penetration force (Fig. 43–20).[179, 180]

Suturing Techniques

SKIN PREPARATION

Before closing the wound, the skin surrounding it is prepared with a povidone-iodine solution and covered with sterile drapes (see the section "Recommendations for Cleaning the Wound"). Some surgeons do not drape the face but prefer to leave facial structures and landmarks adjacent to the wound uncovered and within view. A clear plastic drape

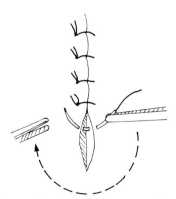

Figure 43–18. The needle should be large enough to pass through tissue and should exit far enough to enable the needle holder to be repositioned on the end of the needle at a safe distance from the point.

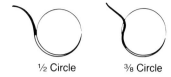

Figure 43–19. One-half and three-eighths circle needles as used for most traumatic wound closures.

(Steri-Drape, 3M) can be used to provide a sterile field and a limited view of the area surrounding the wound. If no drapes are used on the face, the skin surrounding the wound should be widely cleansed and prepared. Wrapping the hair in a sheet prevents stray hair from falling into the operating field (Fig. 43–21).

Four principles apply to the suturing of lacerations in any location: (1) minimize trauma to tissues, (2) relieve tension exerted on the wound edges, (3) close the wound in layers, and (4) accurately realign landmarks and skin edges.

MINIMIZING TISSUE TRAUMA

The importance of careful handling of tissue has been emphasized since the early days of surgery. Skin and subcutaneous tissue that has been stretched, twisted, or crushed by an instrument or strangled by a suture that is tied too tightly may undergo necrosis, and increased scarring and infection may result. When the edges of a wound must be manipulated, the subcutaneous tissues should be grasped gently with a toothed forceps or skin hook, avoiding the skin surface.

When choosing suture sizes, the physician should select the smallest size that will hold the tissues in place. Skin stitches should incorporate no more tissue than needed to coapt the wound edges with little or no tension. Knots should be tied securely enough to approximate the wound edges but without blanching or indenting the skin surface.[114]

RELIEVING TENSION

Many forces can produce tension on the suture line of a reapproximated wound. Static skin forces that stretch the skin over bones cause the edges of a fresh wound to gape and also continuously pull on the edges of the wound once it has been closed. Traumatic loss of tissue or wide excision of a wound may have the same effect. The best cosmetic result occurs when the long axis of a wound happens to be

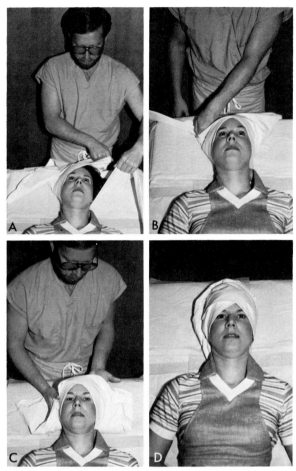

Figure 43–21. *A–D,* Technique for wrapping the scalp to keep stray hair from falling into the operating field.

parallel to the direction of maximal skin tension; this alignment brings the edges of the wound together.[47]

Muscles pulling at right angles to the axis of the wound impose dynamic stresses. Swelling following an injury creates additional tension within the circle of each suture.[18, 114] Skin suture marks result not only from tying sutures too tightly but also from failing to eliminate underlying forces distorting the wound. Tension can be reduced during wound closure in two ways: undermining of the wound edges and layered closure.

UNDERMINING

The force required to reapproximate the wound edges correlates with the subsequent width of the scar.[181] Wounds subject to significant static tension require the undermining of at least one tissue plane on both sides of the wound to achieve a tension-free closure. Undermining involves the creation of a flap of tissue freed from its base at a distance from the wound edge approximately equal to the width of the gap that the laceration presents at its widest point (Fig. 43–22). The depth of the incision can be modified, depending on the orientation of the laceration to skin tension lines and the laxity of skin in the area. A number 15 scalpel blade held parallel to the skin surface is used to incise the adipose layer or the dermal layer of the wound. The clinician can also accomplish this technique by spreading a scissors in the appropriate tissue plane. Undermining allows the skin edges to be lifted and brought together with gentle traction.[136]

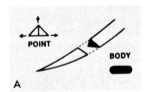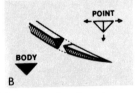

Figure 43–20. Types of needles. *A,* The conventional cutting needle has two opposing cutting edges with a third edge on the inside curvature of the needle. The conventional cutting needle changes in a cross-section shape from a triangular cutting tip to a flattened body. *B,* The reverse cutting needle is used to cut through tough, difficult-to-penetrate tissues, such as fascia and skin. It has two opposing cutting edges, with the third cutting edge on the outer curvature of the needle. The reverse cutting needle is made with the triangular shape extending from the point to the swage area, with only the edges near the tip being sharpened. (From Suture Use Manual: Use and Handling of Sutures and Needles. Somerville, NJ, Ethicon, Inc, 1977, p 31. Reproduced by permission.)

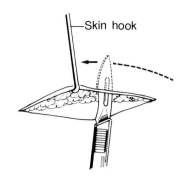

Figure 43–22. The technique of undermining.

Because undermining may harm the underlying blood supply, this technique should be reserved for relatively uncontaminated wounds.[47] Other complications of this procedure may include injury to cutaneous nerves and creation of a hematoma under the flap.[112]

CLOSING THE WOUND IN LAYERS

The structure of skin and soft tissue varies with the location on the body (Fig. 43–23). The majority of wounds handled in an emergency center require approximation of no more than three layers: fascia (and associated muscle), subcutaneous tissue, and skin surface (papillary layer of dermis and epidermis).[177, 182]

Closure of individual layers obliterates "dead space" within the wound that would otherwise fill with blood or exudate. DeHoll and associates demonstrated that the presence of dead space enhances the development of infection; however, it is not necessary to close the adipose layer of soft tissue with a separate stitch. A "fat stitch" is not necessary, because little support is provided by closure of the adipose layer, and the additional suture material that is required may enhance the possibility of infection.[147, 183, 184]

Separate approximation of muscle and subcutaneous layers hastens the healing and return of function to the muscle. *One should suture fascia, not muscle.* A divided muscle should be approximated in a stitch incorporating its fascial covering, because muscle tissue itself is too friable to hold a suture. Layered closure is particularly important in the management of facial wounds; this technique prevents scarring of muscle to the subcutaneous tissue and consequent deformation of the surface of the wound with contraction of the muscle. If a wound is closed without approximation of underlying subcutaneous tissue, a disfiguring depression may develop at the site of the wound. Finally, layered closure provides support to the wound and considerably reduces tension at the skin surface.

There are exceptions to the general rule of multilayered closure. Scalp wounds are generally closed in a single layer. For lacerations penetrating the dermis in fingers, hands, toes, and feet, the amount of subcutaneous tissue is too small to warrant layered closure; in fact, subcutaneous stitches may leave tender nodules in these sensitive locations. In the sebaceous skin of the nasal tip, subcutaneous sutures have a high risk of reaction or infection and should be avoided. Layered closure is not recommended in wounds without tension, those with poor vascularity, and those with moderate infection potential. With single-layer closure, the surface stitch should be placed more deeply.[112]

TECHNIQUES OF SUTURE PLACEMENT

Before suturing, the physician should ensure adequate exposure and illumination of the wound. The physician

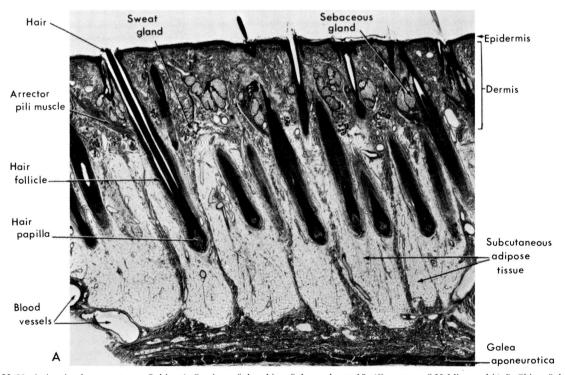

Figure 43–23. Variation in the structure of skin. *A,* Section of the skin of the scalp. ×15. (Courtesy of H Mizoguchi.) *B,* Skin of the human finger tip, illustrating a very thick stratum corneum. Hematoxylin and eosin, ×65. *C,* Section of human sole perpendicular to the free surface. ×100. (After AA Maximow.) *D,* Section through human thigh perpendicular to the surface of the skin. Blood vessels are injected and appear black. Low magnification. (After AA Maximow.) (From Bloom W, Fawcett DW: A Textbook of Histology. 10th ed. Philadelphia, WB Saunders Co, 1975. Reproduced by permission.)

Illustration continued on following page

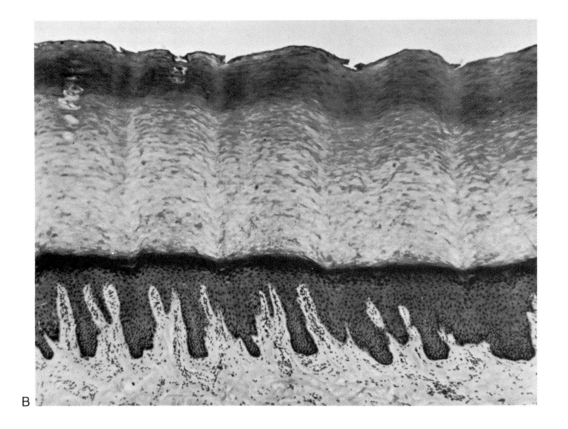

B

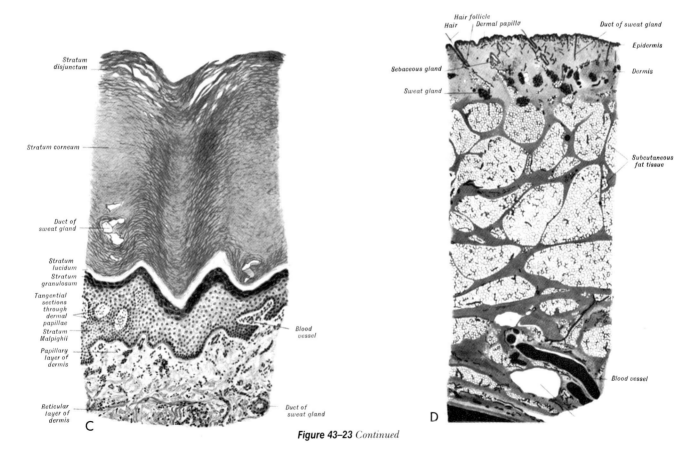

C

Stratum
disjunctum

Stratum corneum

Duct of
sweat gland

Stratum
lucidum
Stratum
granulosum
Tangential
sections
through
dermal
papillae
Stratum
Malpighii
Papillary
layer of
dermis

Reticular
layer of
dermis

Blood
vessel

Duct of
sweat gland

D

Hair follicle
Hair   Dermal papilla
                                        Duct of sweat gland
                                           Epidermis
Sebaceous gland
                                           Dermis
Sweat gland

Subcutaneous
fat tissue

Blood vessel

Figure 43–23 *Continued*

should assume a comfortable standing or sitting position, with the patient placed at an appropriate height. The best position for the physician is at one end of the long axis of the wound.

Subcutaneous Layer Closure. Once fascial structures are reapproximated, the subcutaneous layer is sutured. Although histologically the fatty and fibrous subcutaneous tissue (hypodermis) is an extension of (and is continuous with) the reticular layer of the dermis,[185] suturing of these layers is traditionally referred to as a "subcutaneous" closure. Many researchers recommend closing this layer in segments, placing the first stitch in the middle of the wound and bisecting each subsequent segment until the closure of the layer has been completed.[151] This technique is useful in the closure of wounds that are long or sinuous and is particularly effective in wounds with one elliptic and one linear side. The needle is grasped by the needle holder close to the suture end. Greater facility and speed in suturing is possible if the fingers are placed on the midshaft of the needle holder rather than in the rings of the instrument (Fig. 43–24).

The suture enters the subcutaneous layer at the bottom of the wound (Fig. 43–25A) or, if the wound has been undermined, at the base of the flap (Fig. 43–25B) and exits in the dermis. Once the suture has been placed on one side of the wound, it can be pulled across the wound to the opposite side (or the wound edges pushed together) to determine the matching point on the opposite side. It is at this matching point along the opposite side of the wound that the needle is inserted. The needle should enter the dermis at the same depth as it exited from the opposite side, pass through the tissue, and exit at the bottom of the wound (or the base of the flap). The edges of the wound can be closely apposed by pulling the two tails of the suture in the same direction along the axis of the wound (Fig. 43–26). Some physicians place their subcutaneous suture obliquely rather than vertically to facilitate knot tying. When the knot in this subcutaneous stitch is tied, it will remain inverted, or "buried," at the bottom of the wound. Burying the knot of the subcutaneous stitch avoids a painful, palpable nodule beneath the epidermis and keeps the bulk of this foreign material away from the skin surface. The techniques of tying knots by hand and by instrument are well described and illustrated in various manuals.[18, 115] Once the knot has been secured, the tails of the suture should be pulled taut for cutting. The scissors are held with the index finger on the junction of the two blades. The blade of the scissors is slid down the tail of the suture until the knot is reached. With the cutting edge of the blade tilted away from the knot, the

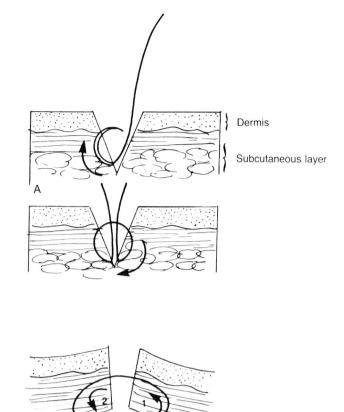

Figure 43–25. A and *B*, Inverted subcutaneous stitches.

tails are cut. This technique prevents the scissors from cutting the knot itself and leaves a tail of 3 mm, which protects the knot from unraveling (Fig. 43–27).[186] The entire subcutaneous layer is sutured in this manner.

After the subcutaneous layer has been closed, the distance between the skin edges indicates the approximate width of the scar in its final form. If this width is acceptable, percutaneous sutures can be inserted.[11] Despite undermining and placement of a sufficient number of subcutaneous sutures, on rare occasions a large gap between the wound

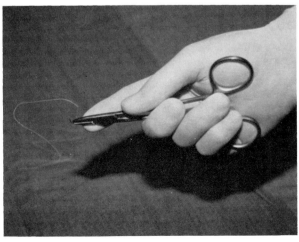

Figure 43–24. Technique of handling the needle holder.

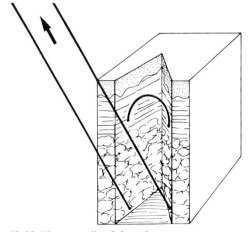

Figure 43–26. The two tails of the subcutaneous suture are pulled in the same direction, tightly apposing the edges of the wound.

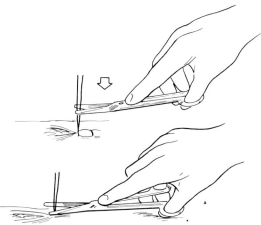

Figure 43–27. Cutting the tails of the suture. (Modified from Anderson CB: Basic surgical techniques. In Klippel AP, Anderson CB: Manual of Outpatient and Emergency Surgical Techniques. Boston, Little, Brown & Co, 1979. Reproduced by permission.)

edges may persist. In such cases, a horizontal dermal stitch may be used to bridge this gap (Fig. 43–28).

Skin Closure. The epidermis and the superficial layer of dermis are sutured with nonabsorbable synthetic sutures. The choice of suture size, the number of sutures used, and the depth of suture placement depend on the amount of skin tension remaining after subcutaneous closure. If the edges of the wound are apposed following closure of deeper layers, small sutures of size 5–0 or 6–0 can be used simply to match the epithelium of each side. If the wound edges remain retracted or if subcutaneous stitches were not used, a larger size of suture may be required. Skin closure may be accomplished with sutures placed in segments (Fig. 43–29) or from end to end. Either technique is acceptable.

"Sutures should be placed in a mirror-image fashion— the same depth and width on both sides of the incision unless uneven edges are encountered."[156] In general, the distance between each suture should be approximately equal to the distance from the exit of the stitch to the wound edge.[115, 151, 187] Grabb suggests that "the number of sutures used in closing any wound will vary with the case, location of the repair, and degree of accuracy required by the physician and patient. In an area such as the face, sutures would probably be placed between 1 and 3 mm apart and 1 to 2 mm from the wound edge."[114] Sutures act as foreign bodies in a wound, and any stitch may damage a blood vessel or strangulate tissue. Therefore, the physician should strive to use the smallest size and the least number of sutures that will adequately close the wound (Fig. 43–30).[4, 19, 167] Wounds with greater tension should have skin stitches placed closer to each other and closer to the wound edge; the technique of layered closure is of great importance in such wounds. If

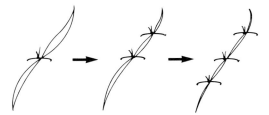

Figure 43–29. Closure of the surface of the wound in segments.

sutures are tied too tightly around wound edges or if individual stitches are under excessive tension, blood supply to the wound may be impeded, increasing the chance of infection, and suture marks may form even after 24 hours.[156, 188, 189]

When suturing the skin, right-handed operators should pass the needle from the right side of the wound to the left.[115] The needle should enter the skin at an oblique angle to produce an everting, bottle-shaped stitch that is deeper than it is wide (Fig. 43–31). If the skin stitch is intended to produce some eversion of the wound edges, the stitch must include a sufficient amount of subcutaneous tissue. Yet encompassing too much tissue with a small needle is a common error. Forcefully pushing or twisting the needle in an effort to bring the point out of the tissue may bend or break the body of the needle. Using a needle of improper size will defeat the best suturing technique. The needle should be driven through tissue by flexing the wrist and supinating the forearm; the course taken by the needle should result in a curve that is identical to the curvature of the needle itself (Fig. 43–32). The angle of exit for the needle should be the same as its angle of entrance so that an identical volume of tissue is contained within the stitch on each side of the wound. Once the needle exits the skin on the opposite side of the wound, it is regrasped by the needle holder and is advanced through the tissue; care should be taken to avoid crushing the point of the needle with the instrument. Forceps are designed for handling tissue and thus should not be used to grasp the needle. The forceps can stabilize the needle by holding the needle within the tissue through which the needle has just passed. Excess thread can be kept clear of the area being sutured by an assistant, or the excess can be looped around the fingers. If the point of the needle becomes dulled before all of the attached thread has been used, the suture should be discarded.[150]

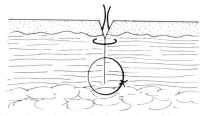

Figure 43–28. Horizontal dermal stitch. (A vertical suture also closes the deep tissue.)

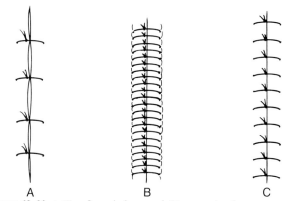

Figure 43–30. *A,* Too few stitches used. Note gaping between sutures. *B,* Too many stitches used. *C,* Correct number of stitches used for a wound under an average amount of tension.

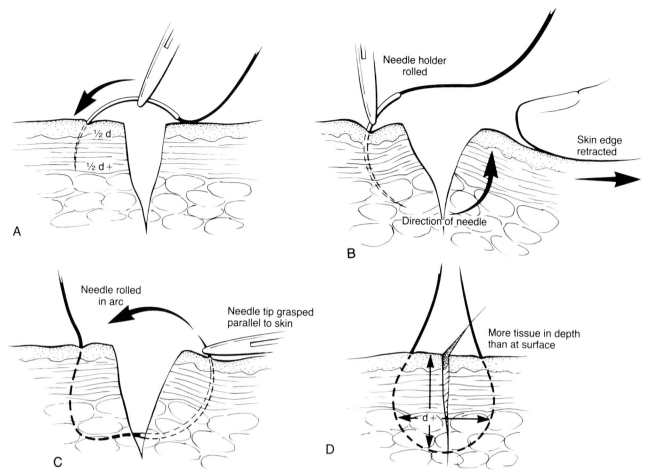

Figure 43–31. The simple suture. *A,* Hold the needle upside down by excessively pronating the wrist, so that the needle tip moves farther from the laceration as the needle penetrates deeper into the skin. Thus there is more dermis in the depth of the wound than at the surface. Drive the needle tip downward and away from the cut edge, into the fat. *B,* Advance the needle into the laceration. The needle tip can be advanced directly into the opposite side. This can be achieved by rolling the needle holder as the needle enters the opposite side at the same level, and the arc pathway of the needle is controlled by retracting the skin edge. This causes more dermis to be incorporated into the depths than at the surface. As an alternative, if a small needle is used in thick skin or the distance across the wound is great, the needle can be removed from the first side, remounted on the needle holder, and advanced to the opposite side. *C,* Advance the needle upward toward the surface so that it exits at the same distance from the wound edge as on the contralateral side of the wound. Grasp the needle behind the tip and roll out in the arc of the needle. *D,* The final position, with more tissue in the depth than the surface. The distance from each suture exit to the laceration is one-half the depth of the dermis. (Redrawn from Kaplan EN, Hentz VR: Emergency Management of Skin and Soft Tissue Wounds: An Illustrated Guide. Boston, Little, Brown & Co, 1984, p 86. Reproduced by permission.)

If these techniques are applied to most wounds, the edges of the wound will be matched precisely in all three dimensions.

Eversion Techniques. If the edges of a wound invert or if one edge rolls under the opposite side, a poorly formed, deep, noticeable scar will result. Excessive eversion that exposes the dermis of both sides will also result in a larger scar than if the skin edges are perfectly apposed, but inversion produces a more visible scar than does eversion. Because most scars undergo some flattening with contraction, optimal results are achieved when the epidermis is very slightly everted without excessive suture tension (Fig. 43–33).[114] Wounds over mobile surfaces, such as the extensor surfaces of joints, should be everted; in time, the scar will be flattened by the dynamic forces acting in the area.

A number of techniques can be used to avoid inversion of the edges of the wound. If the clinician angles the needle away from the laceration, percutaneous stitches can be placed so that their depth is greater than their width.[136] Converse describes this method: "The needle penetrates the skin close to the incision line, diverging from the edge of the wound in order to encircle a larger amount of tissue in the lower depths of the skin than at the periphery."[190] The edge of the wound can be lifted and everted with a skin hook or fine-tooth forceps before insertion of the needle on each side (Fig. 43–34). Eversion can also be obtained simply by slight retraction of the wound with the thumb (Fig. 43–35) or with slight pressure on the wound edge with a closed forceps; each of these two methods also serves to steady the skin against the force of the needle.[115, 190] Vertical mattress sutures are particularly effective in everting the wound edges and can be used exclusively or can be alternated with simple interrupted sutures (Fig. 43–36).[150, 190] Walike states that in the repair of facial lacerations, the subcutaneous (dermal) stitch is a prerequisite to eversion of skin edges with a percutaneous stitch.[136] In wounds that have been undermined, a subcutaneous stitch placed at the base of the flap on each side can in itself evert the wound (Fig. 43–37).

Interrupted Stitch. The simple interrupted stitch is the most frequently used technique in the closure of skin. It

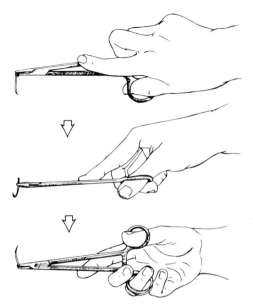

Figure 43–32. Motion of needle holder. (From Anderson CB: Basic surgical techniques. In Klippel AP, Anderson CB: Manual of Outpatient and Emergency Surgical Techniques. Boston, Little, Brown & Co, 1979. Reproduced by permission.)

consists of separate loops of suture individually tied. Although the tying and cutting of each stitch is time consuming, the advantage of this method is that if one stitch in the closure fails, the remaining stitches continue to hold the wound together (Fig. 43–38).[18, 150]

Continuous Stitch. In a continuous, or "running," stitch, the loops are the exposed portions of a helical coil, which is tied at each end of the wound.[18] A continuous suture line can be placed more rapidly than a series of interrupted stitches. The continuous stitch has the additional advantages of strength (with tension being evenly distributed along its entire length), fewer knots (which are the weak points of stitches), and more effective hemostasis.[150] The continuous technique is useful as an epithelial stitch in cosmetic closures; however, if the underlying subcutaneous layer is not stabilized in a separate closure, the continuous surface stitch tends to invert the wound edges.

The continuous suture technique has some disadvantages. This technique cannot be used to close wounds overlying joints. If a loop breaks at one point, the entire stitch may unravel. Likewise, if infection develops and the incision must be opened at one point, cutting a single loop may allow the entire wound to fall open. There is a theoretic problem

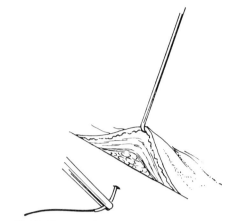

Figure 43–34. The use of a skin hook to evert the wound edge.

of impeded blood supply to the wound edges, particularly if the suture is interlocked.[156] Speer found that wounds closed with an interrupted stitch had 30 to 50 per cent greater tensile strength, less edema and induration, and less impairment in the microcirculation at the wound margin than did wounds closed with a continuous stitch. According to this study, wounds closed with interrupted stitches should have a smaller risk of infection than those closed with the continuous technique.[191] The simple continuous stitch has a tendency to produce suture marks if used in large wound closures and if left in place for more than 5 days.[114] If all tension on the wound can be removed by subcutaneous sutures, stitch marks are seldom a problem.

Among the variations of the continuous technique, the simple continuous stitch is the most useful to emergency physicians (Fig. 43–39). An interrupted stitch is placed at one end of the wound, and only the free tail of the suture is cut. As suturing proceeds, the stitch encircles tissue in a spiral pattern. After each passage of the needle, the loop is tightened slightly and the thread is held taut in the physician's nondominant hand. The needle should travel perpendicularly across the wound on each pass. The last loop is placed just beyond the end of the wound, and the suture is

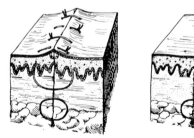

Figure 43–33. Skin edges that are everted will gradually flatten to produce a level wound surface. (From Grabb WC: Basic technique of plastic surgery. In Grabb WC, Smith JW: Plastic Surgery: A Concise Guide to Clinical Practice. Boston, Little, Brown & Co, 1979. Reproduced by permission.)

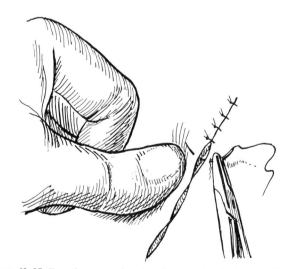

Figure 43–35. Eversion can often be obtained by slight thumb pressure. (From Converse JM: Introduction to plastic surgery. In Converse JM: Reconstructive Plastic Surgery: Principles and Procedures in Correction, Reconstruction, and Transplantation. 2nd ed, vol 1. Philadelphia, WB Saunders Co, 1977. Reproduced by permission.)

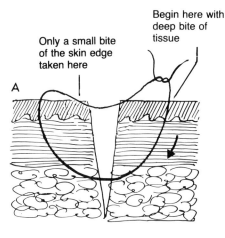

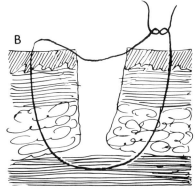

Figure 43–36. The vertical mattress suture is the best technique for producing skin edge eversion. *A,* Usual type of mattress suture for approximating and everting wound edges. *B,* "Tacking" type of vertical mattress suture, extending into deep fascia to obliterate dead space under wound. Note that only a small bite of skin is included on the inner suture. (Modified from Converse, JM: Introduction to plastic surgery. In Converse JM: Reconstructive Plastic Surgery: Principles and Procedures in Correction, Reconstruction, and Transplantation. 2nd ed., vol 1. Philadelphia, WB Saunders Co, 1977. Reproduced by permission.)

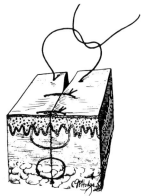

Figure 43–38. Simple interrupted stitch. Additional throws in partially tied knot are not shown. (From Grabb WC: Basic techniques of plastic surgery. In Grabb WC, Smith JW: Plastic Surgery: A Concise Guide to Clinical Practice. Boston, Little, Brown & Co, 1979. Reproduced by permission.)

and are on flat, immobile skin surfaces in patients who have no medical conditions that would impair healing.

Continuous Subcuticular Stitch. Nonabsorbable sutures used in percutaneous skin closure outlast their usefulness and must be removed. On occasion, wounds require an extended period of support, longer than that provided by surface stitches. Some patients with wounds that require skin closure are unlikely or unwilling to return for suture removal. Some sutured wounds are covered by plaster casts. On occasion, the patient (child or adult) is likely to be as frightened and uncooperative for suture removal as for suture placement. The continuous subcuticular (or "dermal") suture technique is ideal for these situations; the wound can be closed with an absorbable subcuticular stitch, obviating the need for later suture removal.[18] In patients prone to keloid formation, the subcuticular technique can be used in lieu of percutaneous stitches, and disfiguring stitch marks can thereby be avoided. (Because children's skin is under greater tension than that of adults, percutaneous sutures are more likely to produce stitch marks in children.) Because stitch marks are avoided, a nonabsorbable subcuticular suture can be left in place for a longer period than a percutaneous suture.[190] Wounds with strong static skin tensions may alternatively benefit from a few interrupted dermal stitches placed horizontal to the skin surface.

Although this technique is commonly used in cosmetic closures, some researchers believe that closure of the sub-

tied with the last loop used as a "tail" in the process of tying the knot (Fig. 43–40). A locking loop may be used in continuous suturing to prevent slippage of loops as the suturing proceeds (Fig. 43–41). The interlocking technique allows the use of the continuous stitch along an irregular laceration.[136]

A continuous stitch is an effective method for closing relatively clean wounds that are under little or no tension

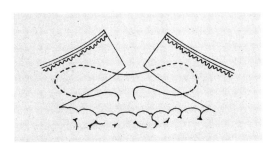

Figure 43–37. Deep dermis suturing technique. Suture enters base of flap, is brought up into dermis, and exits just proximally to wound edge along base of flap to be tied and cut. (From Stuzin J, Engrav LH, Buehler PK: Emergency treatment of facial lacerations. Postgrad Med 71(3):81, 1982. Reproduced by permission.)

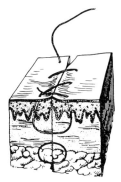

Figure 43–39. Simple continuous stitch. (From Grabb WC: Basic techniques of plastic surgery. In Grabb WC, Smith JW: Plastic Surgery: A Concise Guide to Clinical Practice. Boston, Little, Brown & Co, 1979. Reproduced by permission.)

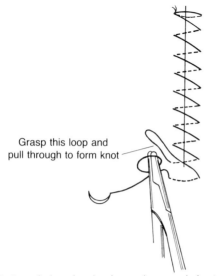

Grasp this loop and
pull through to form knot

Figure 43–40. Completing the simple continuous stitch. A series of square knots are tied with the loop as one of the ties.

cuticular layer alone does not alter the magnitude (width) of scar formation.[192] This technique does not allow for perfect approximation of the vertical heights of the two edges of a wound,[105] and in cosmetic closures it is often followed by a percutaneous stitch. With this technique, the large amount of suture material left in the wound appears to increase the risk of infection and, once infection occurs, allows purulence to spread extensively along the suture line before infection is clinically apparent.[18] Other reports suggest a lower infection rate with the subcuticular technique because the skin microflora are not given an opportunity to invade the deeper tissues along percutaneous suture tracks.[192, 193]

The subcuticular stitch requires a 4–0 or 5–0 suture

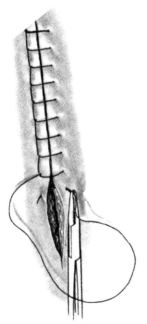

Figure 43–41. Continuous interlocking stitch. (Modified from Suture Use Manual: Use and Handling of Sutures and Needles. Somerville, NJ, Ethicon, Inc, 1977.)

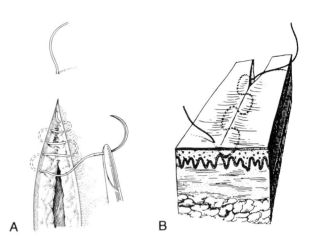

A   B

Figure 43–42. *A,* Pullout subcuticular stitch. The suture is introduced into the skin in line with the incision, approximately 1 to 2 cm away. (From Grimes DW, Garner RW: "Reliefs" in intracuticular sutures. Surgical Rounds 1:46, 1978. Reproduced by permission.) *B,* By backtracking each stitch slightly, one can produce a straight scar. (From Grabb WC: Basic techniques of plastic surgery. In Grabb WC, Smith JW: Plastic Surgery: A Concise Guide to Clinical Practice. Boston, Little, Brown & Co, 1979. Reproduced by permission.)

that either is made of absorbable material or is a nonabsorbable synthetic monofilament suture. An absorbable suture can be "buried" within the wound, whereas a nonabsorbable suture is used for a "pullout" stitch. The absorbable synthetic monofilament suture polydioxanone (PDS, Ethicon) is designed for subcuticular closure. It passes through tissues as easily as nonabsorbable monofilament sutures and is absorbed if left in the wound by accident or by design.

Before the subcuticular stitch is placed, the subcutaneous layer should be approximated with interrupted sutures to minimize tension on the wound. The pullout subcuticular stitch is started at the skin surface approximately 1 to 2 cm away from one end of the wound. The needle enters and exits the dermis at the apices of the wound (Fig. 43–42). Bites through tissue are taken in a horizontal direction with the needle penetrating the dermis 1 to 2 mm from the skin surface. These intradermal bites should be small, of equal proportion, and at the same level on each side of the wound.[6, 190] Accidental interlocking of the stitch should be avoided. Each successive bite should be placed 1 to 2 mm *behind* the exit point on the opposite side of the wound so that when the wound is closed, the entrance and exit points on either side are not directly apposed (see Fig. 43–42). Small bites should be taken to avoid puckering of the skin surface.[114, 194] Some physicians prefer to place a fine (6–0) running skin suture in addition to the subcuticular suture for meticulous skin approximation. The skin suture is removed in 3 to 4 days to avoid suture marks.

If the subcuticular stitch is used on lengthy lacerations, it is difficult to remove the suture. The placement of "reliefs" consisting of periodic loops through the skin during the length of the stitch facilitates later removal (Fig. 43–43). Reliefs should be placed every 4 to 5 cm. The suture is crossed to the opposite side and the needle is passed from subcutaneous tissue to the skin surface. The suture is carried over the surface for approximately 2 cm before reentering the skin and subcutaneous tissue. The subcuticular stitch is then continued at approximately the point at which the next bite would have been placed had the relief not been used.[194]

At the completion of the stitch, the needle is placed through the apex to exit the skin 1 to 2 cm away from the end of the wound. One should tighten the stitch by pulling each end taut. If reliefs have been used, one can take up

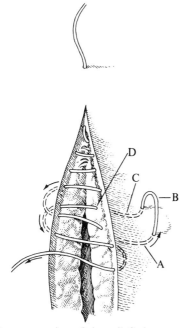

Figure 43–43. In construction of the relief, the suture is crossed to the opposite side, going into the subcuticular area beneath the skin for approximately 2 cm before exiting *(A)*. The suture is then carried over the epidermis for approximately 2 cm *(B)*, and then back under the dermis again *(C)*. Reentry is made into the wound area *(D)* at approximately the same location as the next bite would have been placed had the relief not been used. (From Grimes DW, Garner RW: "Reliefs" in intracuticular sutures. Surgical Rounds 1:47, 1978. Reproduced by permission.)

any slack in the stitch by pulling on the reliefs. The clinician can secure the two ends of the stitch by taping them to the skin surface with wound closure tape,[111] by placing a cluster of knots on each tail close to the skin surface, or by tying the two ends of the suture to each other over a dressing.[194] Laxity of the subcuticular stitch is often noted 48 hours after wound closure with a decrease in tissue swelling. Some physicians will tighten the stitch when they reexamine the wound after 48 hours.

A technique of subcuticular closure using absorbable sutures that do not penetrate the skin is possible. The closure is begun with a dermal or subcutaneous suture placed at one end of the wound and secured with a knot. After placement of the continuous subcuticular stitch from apex

to apex, the suture is pulled taut and a knot is tied using a tail and a loop of suture (Fig. 43–44). The final knot can be buried by insertion of the needle into deeper tissue; the needle exits several millimeters from the wound edge. If one pulls on the needle end, the knot disappears into the wound.[6] The obvious advantage of this technique is that there are no suture marks in the skin. Another method that avoids penetrating the skin is the interrupted subcuticular stitch (Fig. 43–45).[190]

Nonabsorbable sutures can be left in place for 2 to 3 weeks, thus providing a longer period of support than percutaneous sutures without the problem of stitch marks.[114] If skin sutures are used in conjunction with the subcuticular stitch, they are removed in 3 to 4 days. A subcuticular closure in itself is stronger than a tape closure. If the subcuticular technique is used exclusively to approximate the skin surface, it is advisable to apply skin tape to correct surface unevenness and to provide a more accurate apposition of the epidermis.[18]

Mattress Stitch. The various types of mattress stitches are all interrupted stitches. The vertical mattress stitch is an effective method of ensuring eversion of the skin edges (Figs. 43–36 and 43–46). Unfortunately, this stitch causes more ischemia and necrosis inside its loop than either simple or continuous stitches.[195] The horizontal mattress stitch approximates skin edges closely while providing some degree of eversion (Fig. 43–47).[114] The half-buried horizontal mattress stitch, also called a mattress stitch with a dermal component, combines an interrupted skin stitch with a buried intradermal stitch (Fig. 43–48). It is effective in joining the edges of a skin flap to the edges of the "recipient site"; the dermal component is placed through the dermis of the flap.[190] The half-buried horizontal mattress stitch is also useful at the scalp-forehead junction when there is tension on the wound edges. This technique halves the number of suture marks in the skin and avoids necrosis of the edge of a skin flap.

The half-buried horizontal mattress stitch is particularly useful in suturing the easily damaged apex of a V-shaped flap (Fig. 43–49). In the execution of the "corner stitch," the suture needle penetrates the skin at a point beyond the apex of the wound and exits through the dermis. The corner of the flap is elevated, and the suture is passed through the dermis of the flap. The needle is then placed in the dermis of the base of the wound and returned to the surface of the skin. All dermal bites should be placed at the same level. The suture is tied with a tension sufficient to pull the flap snugly into the corner without blanching the flap.[114, 122] If the tip of a large flap with questionable viability may be

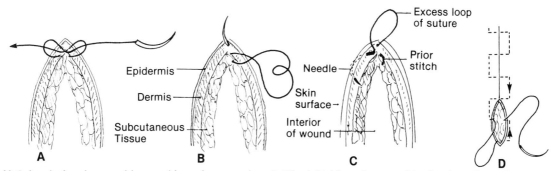

Figure 43–44. Subcuticular closure without epidermal penetration. *A,* The initial knot is secured in the dermal or subcutaneous tissue. *B,* The short strand is cut, and the needle is inserted into the dermis at the apex of the wound. *C,* Needle in dermis, close to the corner of the wound, and exiting the wound at the same horizontal level. *D,* After the subcuticular stitch has been completed, a knot is tied with the tail and the loop of the suture. (Modified from Stillman RM: Wound closure: Choosing optimal materials and methods. ER Reports 2:43, 1981.)

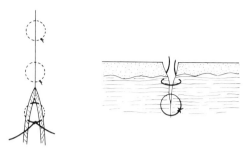

Figure 43–45. Interrupted subcuticular stitch (also called a horizontal dermal stitch). (Deep vertical suture is also shown.)

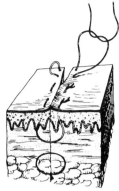

Figure 43–47. Horizontal mattress stitch. (From Grabb WC: Basic techniques of plastic surgery. Grabb WC, Smith JW: Plastic Surgery: A Concise Guide to Clinical Practice. Boston, Little, Brown & Co, 1979. Reproduced by permission.)

further jeopardized by postoperative swelling, a cotton stent can be placed underneath the knot of the corner stitch. The cotton absorbs the tension produced by swelling.

Figure-of-Eight Stitch. The figure-of-eight stitch is useful in wounds with friable tissue, on the eyelids where the skin is too thin for buried sutures, or in areas in which buried sutures are undesirable (Fig. 43–50).[196] This stitch reduces the amount of tension placed on the tissue by the suture, allowing the stitch to hold in place when a simple stitch would tear through the tissue. One disadvantage of this technique is that more suture material is left in the wound. Dushoff recommends the figure-of-eight stitch for approximating muscle and fascial tissue, periosteum, and scalp lacerations.[177] A vertical variation of the figure-of-eight stitch is sometimes used to approximate close, parallel lacerations (Fig. 43–51).[197] Another technique involves a vertical mattress stitch. The central "island" of tissue is secured by passing the superficial portion of the stitch through the island at the subcuticular level (Fig. 43–52).[198] If the viability of the central island is questionable and the surrounding tissue is loose, it can be excised.

Cosmetic Closure of Facial Wounds. The ideal result in the repair of a facial laceration is an extremely narrow, flat, and inapparent scar. In addition to basic wound management, a few additional techniques can be used to achieve this result. One of the factors that contributes to wide scars is necrosis of partially devitalized wound edges. However, skin with apparently marginal circulation may survive because of the excellent vascularity of the face. Subcutaneous fat, which in other locations may be débrided thoroughly, should be preserved if possible in facial wounds to prevent eventual sinking of the scar and to preserve normal facial contours. Therefore, débridement of most facial wounds should be conservative.[182, 199]

Converse pointed out that "precise approximation of skin edges without undue tension ensures primary healing with minimal scarring."[190] A layered closure is essential in the cosmetic repair of a facial wound. Approximation of the dermis with a subcutaneous stitch or a combination of subcutaneous and subcuticular stitches should bring the epithelial edges together or within 1 to 2 mm of apposition—close enough that the use of additional sutures seems unnecessary.[11] If a subcutaneous stitch is the only stitch used to close the deeper layers, it should pass through the dermal-epidermal junction or within 1 to 2 mm of the skin surface. The clinician must tie this stitch snugly, pulling the two ends of the suture in the same direction (see Fig. 43–26). Should the first subcutaneous stitch placed at the midpoint of a wound perfectly appose the skin edges, one can "protect" that stitch from disruption during further suturing by immediately placing a percutaneous stitch in the same location. If there is a slight gap in the wound edges after subcutaneous closure, the skin can be partially approximated with a few guide stitches. The first is placed at the midpoint of the wound, and subsequent stitches bisect the intervening spaces. Guide stitches allow the definitive epithelial sutures to be placed with little strain on each individual stitch, and they protect the subcutaneous stitches from disruption. Once the definitive stitches have been placed, the guide stitches, if slack, can be removed. Because a needle damages tissue with

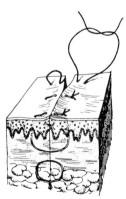

Figure 43–46. Vertical mattress stitch. (From Grabb WC: Basic techniques of plastic surgery. In Grabb WC, Smith JW: Plastic Surgery: A Concise Guide to Clinical Practice. Boston, Little, Brown & Co, 1979. Reproduced by permission.)

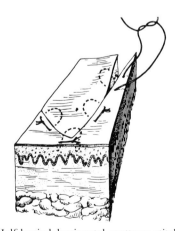

Figure 43–48. Half-buried horizontal mattress stitch. (From Grabb WC: Basic techniques of plastic surgery. In Grabb WC, Smith JW: Plastic Surgery: A Concise Guide to Clinical Practice. Boston, Little, Brown & Co, 1979. Reproduced by permission.)

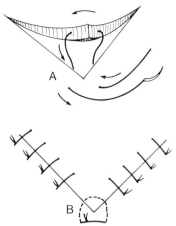

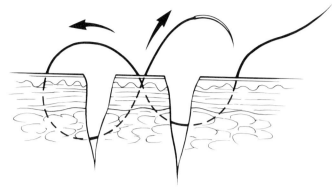

Figure 43–51. Vertical figure-of-eight suture technique.

Figure 43–49. *A* and *B*, Approximation of a corner flap with a half-buried horizontal mattress stitch. Because of its applicability to this closure the stitch is often called a *corner stitch.*

each passage through the skin, guide stitches should be used only when necessary.

The epithelial stitch should never be used to relieve the wound of tension; it serves only to match the epidermal surfaces precisely along the length of the wound. If there is a significant separation of the wound edges after closure of the subcutaneous layer, a 5–0 or 6–0 subcuticular suture can be used to eliminate the tension produced by this separation and to provide prolonged stability. Once the necessary near apposition of skin edges is produced, the epithelial stitch can be used to correct discrepancies in vertical alignment. A 6–0 synthetic nonabsorbable suture is an excellent material for this stitch. A continuous stitch is preferable because it can be placed quickly, but interrupted stitches are acceptable. In a straight laceration, better apposition is achieved if the wound is stretched lengthwise by finger traction or by the use of skin hooks. When the needle is placed on one side of the wound, if that side is higher than the opposite side, a shallow bite is taken. The needle is used to depress the wound edge to the proper height, after

which the needle "follows through" to the other side, "pinning" the two sides together. If the first side entered is lower, the needle is elevated to match the epithelial edges.

Grabb pointed out that "the closer the needle lies to the skin edge, the greater will be its effect in controlling the ultimate position of that edge."[114] Epithelial stitches should be spaced no more than 2 to 3 mm apart and should encompass no more than 2 to 4 mm of tissue.[136] If widely spaced, the sutures will leave marks.[11] Once skin closure is complete, final adjustments in the tension on the continuous suture line are made before the end of the stitch is tied. If any level discrepancies persist, interrupted sutures or tape can be used to flatten these few irregularities.

Surgical tape is useful as a secondary support, protecting the epithelial stitch from stresses produced by normal skin movements (Fig. 43–53). Facial wounds have a tendency to swell and place excessive stretch on an epithelial stitch. This can be minimized by application of a pressure dressing and cold compresses to the wound following closure. Surgical tape can serve to a limited extent as a pressure dressing.

Correction of Dog-Ears. When wound edges are not precisely aligned horizontally, there will be an excess of tissue on one or both ends. This small flap of excess skin that bunches up at the end of a sutured wound is commonly called a dog-ear. This effect also occurs when one side of the wound is more elliptic than the opposite side or when an excision of a wound is not sufficiently elliptic—when it is either too straight or too nearly circular.[151, 190]

If a dog-ear is present, it can be eliminated on one side of the wound in the following manner: The flap of excess skin is elevated with a skin hook; an incision is carried at an oblique angle from the apex of the wound toward the side with the excess skin. The flap is then undermined and laid flat. The resulting triangle of skin is trimmed, and the closure is completed (Fig. 43–54A).[7, 122] An alternative method consists of carrying the incision directly from the apex, in line with the wound. The flap of excess tissue is pulled over the incision while skin hooks retract the extended apex of the wound. Excess tissue is excised, and the remainder of the wound is sutured.[190] If dog-ears are present on *both* sides of one end of the wound, the bulge of excess tissue can be excised in an elliptic fashion and the wound can be closed (Fig. 43–54B).[122]

V-Y Advancement Flap. If a corner stitch produces excessive tension on the tip of the flap, a V-Y closure can be used to approximate the edges without undue tension. An incision carried away from the apex of the wound converts it from a V to a Y configuration (Fig. 43–55). The newly formed wound edges are undermined, and the repair is completed. A half-buried mattress stitch is placed at the fork of the Y.[122]

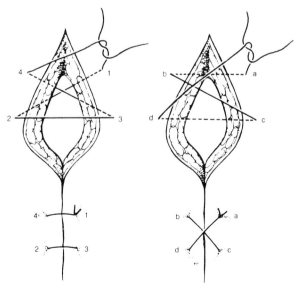

Figure 43–50. Figure-of-eight stitch—two methods. (Modified from Dushoff IM: About face. Emerg Med 6:11:1974. Reproduced by permission.)

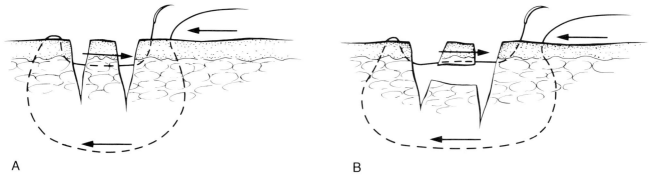

A   B

Figure 43–52. Techniques for closure of parallel lacerations. *A,* Central tissue island with intact base. *B,* Central tissue island shaved from base.

Stellate Lacerations. The repair of a stellate laceration is a challenging problem. Usually a result of compression and shear forces, these injuries contain large amounts of partially devitalized tissue. The surrounding soft tissue is often swollen and contused. Much of this contused tissue cannot be débrided without creating a large tissue defect. Sometimes tissue is lost, yet the amount is not apparent until key sutures are placed. In repairing what often resembles a jigsaw puzzle, the physician can remove small flaps of necrotic tissue with an iris scissors; large, viable flaps can be repositioned in their beds and carefully secured with half-buried mattress stitches. If interrupted stitches are used to approximate a thin flap, small bites should be taken in the flap and larger, deeper bites in the base of the wound. A modification of the corner stitch can be used to approximate multiple flaps to a base (Fig. 43–56). The V-Y advancement flap technique is also useful. Thin flaps of tissue in a stellate laceration with beveled edges are often most easily repositioned and stabilized with a firm dressing.[114] Closure of stellate lacerations cannot always be accomplished immediately, especially if there is considerable soft tissue swelling. It may be best in some instances to consider delayed closure or revision of the scar at a later date. In complicated lacerations, inexact tissue approximation may be all that is possible initially.

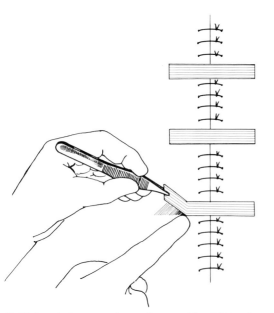

Figure 43–53. Surgical tape can be used to provide additional support while sutures are in place and after they are removed.

Repair of Special Structures

Scalp. The scalp extends from the supraorbital ridges anteriorly to the external occipital protuberances posteriorly and blends with temporalis fascia laterally. There are five anatomic layers of the scalp: skin, superficial fascia, galea aponeurotica, subaponeurotic areolar connective tissue, and periosteum (Fig. 43–57*A*). Surgically, the scalp may be divided into three distinct layers. The outer layer consists of the skin, superficial fascia, and the galea (the aponeurosis of the frontalis and occipitalis muscles). These three layers are firmly adherent and surgically are considered as one layer. The integrity of the outer layers is maintained by inelastic tough fibrous septa, which keep wounds from gaping open unless all three layers have been traversed. Wounds that gape open signify a laceration beneath the galea layer. The galea itself is loosely adherent to the periosteum by means of the slack areolar tissue of the subaponeurotic layer. The periosteum covers the skull. *The periosteum is often mistakenly identified as the galea,* and vain attempts to suture the flimsy periosteum are made in the hope of "closing the galea."[200]

Several unique problems are associated with wounds of the scalp. The presence of a rich vascular network and the fact that severed scalp vessels tend to remain patent are both responsible for the profuse bleeding associated with scalp wounds. The tough, fibrous subcutaneous fascia hinders the normal retraction of blood vessels that have been cut, allowing for persistent or massive hemorrhage in simple lacerations. The subgaleal layer of loose connective tissue contains "emissary veins" that drain through diploic vessels of the skull into the venous sinuses of the cranial hemispheres. In scalp wounds that penetrate this layer, bacteria may be carried by these vessels to the meninges and the intracranial sinuses. Thus a scalp wound infection can result in osteomyelitis, meningitis, or brain abscess.[201, 202] Careful approximation of galeal lacerations not only ensures control of bleeding but also protects against the spread of infection.

Shear-type injuries can cause extensive separation of the superficial layers from the galeal layer (Fig. 43–58). Debris and other contaminants can be deposited several centimeters from the visible laceration.[177] Careful exploration and cleaning of scalp wounds is of obvious importance.

Because the scalp is so vulnerable to blunt trauma and because its superficial fascial layer is inelastic and firmly adherent to the skin, stellate lacerations are common in this region. Stellate lacerations not only pose additional technical problems in closure but also have a greater propensity toward infection. In the patient with multiple injuries, scalp wounds are easily overlooked; they are frequently numerous and hidden by a mat of hair.

When scalp wounds are débrided, obviously devitalized tissue should be removed, but débridement should be con-

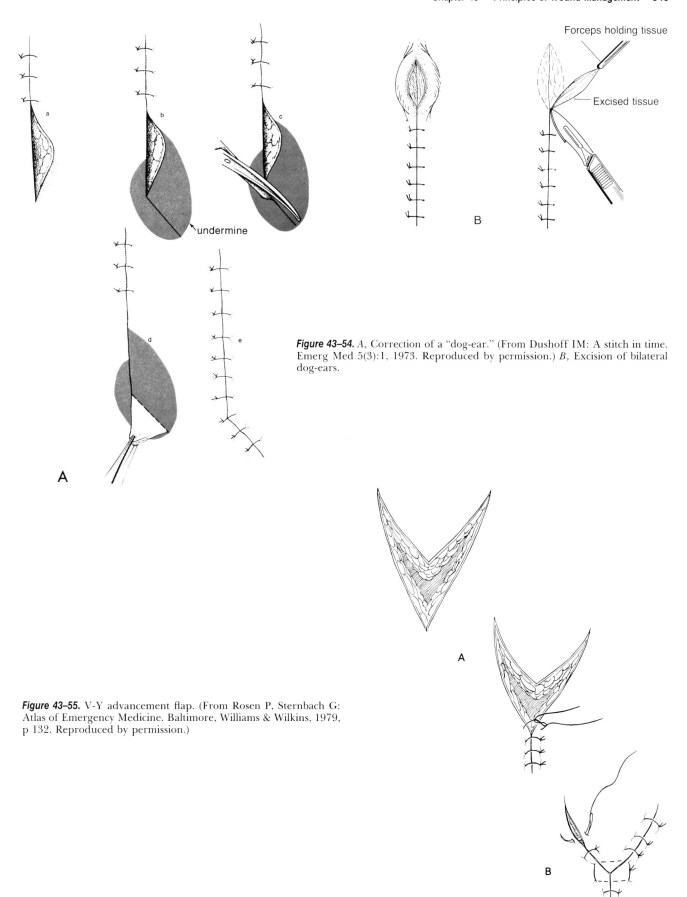

Forceps holding tissue

Excised tissue

Figure 43–54. *A,* Correction of a "dog-ear." (From Dushoff IM: A stitch in time. Emerg Med 5(3):1, 1973. Reproduced by permission.) *B,* Excision of bilateral dog-ears.

undermine

Figure 43–55. V-Y advancement flap. (From Rosen P, Sternbach G: Atlas of Emergency Medicine. Baltimore, Williams & Wilkins, 1979, p 132. Reproduced by permission.)

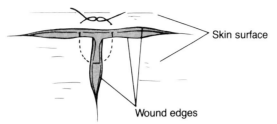

Figure 43–56. View from above stellate laceration, showing closure with half-buried mattress stitches.

servative, because closure of large defects is difficult on the scalp. When facing profuse bleeding, especially from extensive lacerations, the physician should instruct an assistant to maintain compression around the wound during the closure rather than try to tie off bleeding vessels. Unless the vessels are large or few, ligation of individual scalp vessels seldom provides effective hemostasis, and considerable bleeding can occur during the attempt. The bleeding from scalp lacerations is best controlled by expeditious suturing.[122] A simple procedure that often provides hemostasis of scalp wounds is placing a *wide*, tight rubber band around the scalp, from forehead to occiput (Fig. 43–59A). Sterile rubber bands may be kept on the suture cart for this purpose. The clinician also may control bleeding temporarily in some cases by grasping the galea and the dermis with a hemostat and everting the instrument over the skin edge (see Fig. 43–57B). The disadvantage of this technique is that tissue grasped by the hemostat may be crushed and devitalized,[122] and if the subcutaneous tissue is also everted for a prolonged period, necrosis can occur. Without an assistant to apply direct pressure, the use of local anesthetics containing epinephrine is sometimes an effective method of controlling the persistent bleeding from small vessels in scalp wounds. If bleeding from the edge of the scalp wound is vigorous and definitive repair must be postponed while the patient is resuscitated, Raney scalp clips can be applied quickly to the edge of the scalp wound to control the hemorrhage. The applicator is loaded by inserting the tip of the instrument into the back of the clip and then locking the handles. The clip is slid onto the bleeding wound edge and released from the applicator. When the wound is repaired at a later time,

the clip is removed by reversing the procedure. The plastic clips are radiolucent and do not interfere with plain radiography or computed tomography scanning (Fig. 43–59B).[121, 203]

Before wound closure, the underlying skull should be palpated in an attempt to detect fractures. More small skull fractures are detected with the gloved finger than with radiographs. A common error is to mistake a rent in the galea or the periosteum for a fracture during palpation inside the wound. Direct visualization of the area should resolve the issue. In wounds that expose bone but do not penetrate the skull, prolonged exposure may leave a nidus of dead bone that may develop osteomyelitis. Exposed bone that is visibly necrosed should be removed with rongeurs until active bleeding appears.[122] Hair surrounding the scalp wound usually must be clipped far enough from the wound edge so that suturing can proceed without entangling the hair in knots or embedding hair within the wound. If hairs along the wound edges become embedded in the wound, they will stimulate excessive granulation tissue and delay healing.[12] Vaseline or tape may be placed on stubborn hairs that persistently fall into the wound. Although clipping scalp hair is not popular with some patients, failure to expose an area adequately is a common cause of improper preparation and closure of scalp wounds.

Unlike most wounds involving multiple layers of tissue, scalp wounds should be closed with a single layer of sutures that incorporate skin, subcutaneous fascia, and the galea. The periosteum need not be sutured. To minimize the chance of infection, subcutaneous deep sutures generally are avoided. In superficial wounds, skin and subcutaneous tissue should be approximated with simple interrupted or vertical mattress stitches using a nonabsorbable 3–0 nylon or polypropylene suture. Smaller suture material tends to break while firm knots are being tied and should not be used. The ends of the tied scalp sutures should be left at least 2 cm long to facilitate subsequent suture removal. The use of blue nylon, as opposed to black, may make suture removal easier. If the galea is also torn, one should include the galea in the skin stitch.[202] Some investigators recommend a separate closure of the galea with an absorbable 3–0 or 4–0 suture, using an inverted stitch that "buries" the knot beneath the galea.[122] Separate closure of the galea introduces additional suture material into the wound but in some circumstances allows a more secure approximation of this structure.

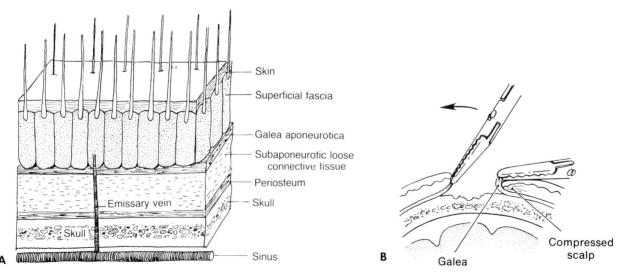

Figure 43–57. *A*, Anatomy of the scalp. *B*, Temporary control of bleeding from scalp lacerations by eversion of galea. (From Rosen P, Sternbach G: Atlas of Emergency Medicine. Baltimore, Williams & Wilkins, 1979, p 128. Reproduced by permission.)

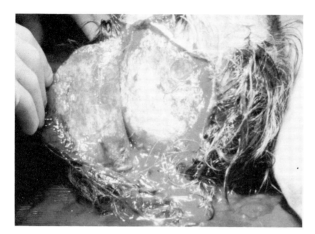

Figure 43–58. Large partial scalp avulsion.

Stellate lacerations or crush lacerations may be excised to produce elliptical incisions if the area involved is not extensive. Large sections of skin avulsed from the scalp can, with microvascular techniques, be reimplanted. The emergency physician should use the same techniques in salvaging avulsed scalp as are used for amputated extremities.[202] (See Chapter 64 for further discussion.)

Because of the extensive collateral blood supply of the scalp, most lacerations in this area heal without problems. Nonetheless, wound care must be careful and thorough if the devastating complication of scalp infection is to be avoided.

Sutured scalp lacerations need not be bandaged, and patients can wash their hair in 24 hours. If bleeding is persistent, an elastic bandage can be used as a compression dressing. Gauze sponges are placed over the laceration to provide direct local pressure beneath the elastic bandage.

Forehead. Although the forehead is actually a part of the scalp, lacerations in this region are treated as facial wounds. Vertical lacerations across the forehead are oriented 90 degrees to skin tension lines, and the resulting scars are more noticeable than are those from horizontal lacerations.

Midline vertical forehead lacerations may result in cosmetically acceptable scars with standard closure techniques; those lacerations that are not centered often require S-plasty or Z-plasty techniques during the initial repair or during later revision of the scar.[177]

Superficial lacerations may be closed with skin stitches alone, but deep forehead lacerations must be closed in layers. The periosteum should be approximated before the closure of more superficial layers. If skin is directly exposed to bone, adhesions may develop that in time may limit the movement of skin during facial expressions. The frontalis muscle fascia and adjacent fibrous tissue should be approximated as a distinct layer; if left unsutured, the retracted ends of this muscle will bulge beneath the skin. If the gap in a muscle belly is later filled with scar tissue, movement of the muscle pulls on the entire scar and makes it more apparent.[177, 182]

A U-shaped flap laceration with a superiorly oriented base poses a difficult problem. Immediate vascular congestion and later scar contraction within the flap produce the "trap-door effect," with the flap becoming prominently elevated (Fig. 43–60). This effect can be minimized by approximation of the bulk of subcutaneous tissue of the flap to a deeper level on the base side of the wound; the skin surfaces of the two sides are apposed at the same level (Fig. 43–61). A firm compression dressing helps eliminate "dead space" and hematoma formation within the wound. Despite these efforts, secondary revision is sometimes necessary.[114] Often, swelling of the flap resolves over a 6- to 12-month period. Because flap elevation can be quite disconcerting, the physician should forewarn the patient and family about a possible "trap-door effect."

When a forehead laceration borders the scalp and the thick scalp tissue must be sutured to thinner forehead skin, a horizontal mattress stitch with an intradermal component can be used (Fig. 43–62).[190]

Eyebrow and Eyelid Lacerations. Jagged lacerations through eyebrows should be managed with little, if any, débridement of untidy but viable edges. The hair shafts of the eyebrow grow at an oblique angle, and vertical excision may produce a linear alopecia in the eyebrow, whereas with simple closure the scar remains hidden within the hair. If partial excision is unavoidable, the scalpel blade should be

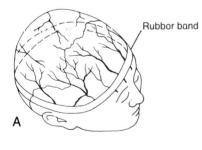

Rubber band

A

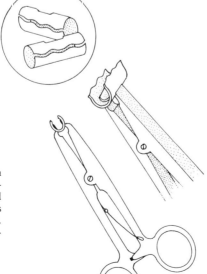

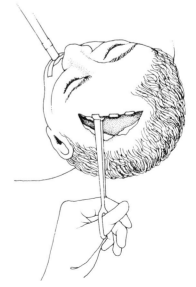

Figure 43–59. *A,* To achieve hemostasis of a scalp laceration, a wide, tight sterilized rubber band or Penrose drain may be placed around the forehead and occiput. This compresses the arterial supply to the scalp. *B,* Raney scalp clips and applier for application to scalp wound edges.

B

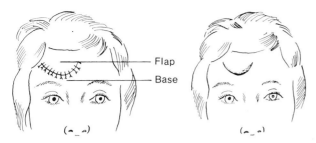

Figure 43–60. Elevation of a forehead flap—the "trap-door effect." (From Grabb WC, Kleinert HE: Technics in Surgery: Facial and Hand Injuries. Somerville, NJ, Ethicon, Inc, 1980. Reproduced by permission.)

angled in a direction parallel to the axis of the hair shaft to minimize damage to hair follicles (see Fig. 43–7).[177]

Points on each side of the lacerated eyebrow should be aligned precisely; a single percutaneous stitch on each margin of the eyebrow should precede subcutaneous closure. The edges of the eyebrow serve as landmarks for reapproximation; therefore, the eyebrow must not be shaved or these landmarks will be lost. Shaved eyebrows grow back slowly and sometimes incompletely, and shaving them often results in more deformity than the injury itself. Care must be taken not to invert hair-bearing skin into the wound.[105]

The thin, flexible skin of the upper eyelid is relatively easy to suture. A soft, size 6–0 suture is recommended for closure of simple lacerations. Traumatized eyelids are susceptible to massive swelling; compression dressings and cool compresses can be used to minimize this problem.

It is essential that the emergency physician recognize complicated lid lacerations that require the expertise of an ophthalmologist. Lacerations that traverse the lid margin require exact realignment to avoid entropion or extropion. Injuries penetrating the tarsal plate frequently cause damage to the globe. A deep horizontal laceration through the upper lid that divides the thin levator palpebrae muscle or its tendinous attachment to the tarsal plate produces ptosis. If this muscle cannot be identified and repaired by the emergency physician, a consultant should repair the injury primarily. A laceration through the portion of the lower lid *medial* to the punctum frequently damages the lacrimal duct or the medial canthal ligament and requires specialized techniques for repair. If adipose tissue is seen within any periorbital laceration, one must assume that the orbital septum has been penetrated and the retrobulbar fat is herniating through the wound. The repair of lid avulsions, extensive lid lacerations with loss of tissue, and any of the

other complex types of lid lacerations mentioned should be left to ophthalmologists.[177, 204]

Ear Lacerations. The primary goal in the management of lacerations of the pinna is expedient coverage of exposed cartilage. Cartilage is an avascular tissue, and when ear cartilage is denuded of its protective, nutrient-providing skin, progressive erosive chondritis ensues. The initial step in the repair of an ear injury involves trimming away jagged or devitalized cartilage and skin. If the skin cannot be stretched to cover the defect, additional cartilage along the wound margin can be removed. Depending on the location, as much as 5 mm of cartilage can be removed without significant deformity. Cartilage should be approximated with 4–0 or 5–0 absorbable sutures initially placed at folds or ridges representing major landmarks. Sutures tear through cartilage; therefore, the anterior and posterior perichondrium should be included in the stitch. No more tension should be applied than is needed to touch the edges together.

In through-and-through ear lacerations, the posterior skin surface should be approximated next, using 5–0 nonabsorbable synthetic sutures. Once closure of the posterior surface is completed, the convoluted anterior surface of the ear can be approximated with 5–0 or 6–0 nonabsorbable synthetic sutures, with landmarks joined point by point. On the free rim, the skin should be everted if later notching is to be avoided. Care should be taken to cover all exposed cartilage. In heavily contaminated wounds of the ear (e.g., bite wounds) that already show evidence of inflammation, the necrotic tissue should be débrided, the cartilage covered by a loose approximation of skin, and the patient placed on antibiotics.[111, 114, 177] After a lacerated ear has been sutured, it should be enclosed in a compression dressing.

Lacerations of the Nose. In the repair of lacerations of the nose, reapproximation of the wound edges is difficult because the skin is inflexible, and even deeply placed stitches will slice through the epidermis and pull out. When the wound edges cannot be coapted easily, 6–0 absorbable sutures can be placed in the fibrofatty junction in a subcutaneous stitch before skin closure. Because it is difficult to approximate gaping wounds in this location, débridement must be kept to a minimum. Nasal cartilage is frequently involved in wounds of the nose, but it is seldom necessary to suture the cartilage itself.

The free rim of the nostril must be aligned precisely to avoid unsightly notching. Many physicians recommend early removal of stitches to avoid stitch marks, yet the oily nature of skin in this area makes it difficult to keep the wound closed with tape. A subcuticular stitch is recommended if the wound is gaping before closure, to provide support for a prolonged period.[177, 201, 205]

Lip and Intraoral Lacerations. Lip lacerations are cosmetically deforming injuries, but if the physician follows a few guidelines, these lacerations usually heal satisfactorily.

The contamination of all intraoral and lip wounds is considerable; they must be thoroughly irrigated. Regional nerve blocks are preferred to local injection, because the latter method distends tissue, distorts the anatomy of the lip, and obscures the vermilion border. Dushoff recommends converting all oblique lacerations through the vermilion border into incisions perpendicular to this line so that the wound remains parallel to skin tension lines (Fig. 43–63).[177] Losses of less than 25 per cent of the lip permit primary closure with little deformity; losses of greater than 25 per cent require a reconstructive procedure. Extensive lacerations directly through the commissure of the mouth also require surgical consultation in most cases.[111, 177] Deep scars in the vermilion of the upper lip may produce a redundancy of tissue that requires later revision.[111, 182, 206]

Through-and-through lacerations of the lip should be

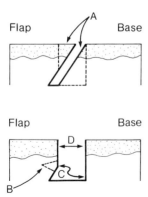

Figure 43–61. Repair of a U-shaped flap laceration with a superiorly oriented base. *A,* Excision of edges. *B,* Undermining. *C,* Approximation of subcutaneous tissue on the flap to subcutaneous tissue at a deeper level on the base. *D,* Skin closure.

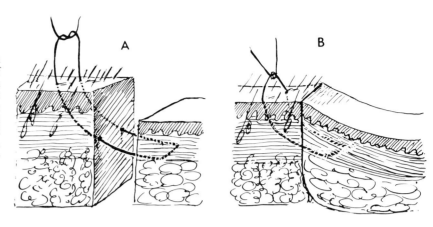

Figure 43–62. Horizontal mattress suture with an intradermal component. *A* and *B,* Eversion of thinner skin to obtain adequate approximation with thicker scalp tissue. (From Converse JM: Introduction to plastic surgery. In Converse JM: Reconstructive Plastic Surgery: Principles and Procedures in Correction, Reconstruction, and Transplantation. 2nd ed, vol 1. Philadelphia, WB Saunders Co, 1977. Reproduced by permission.)

closed in three layers. The muscle layer is approximated with a 4–0 or 5–0 absorbable suture securely anchored in the fibrous tissue located anterior and posterior to the muscle. The vermilion-cutaneous junction of the lip is a critical landmark that, if divided, must be repositioned with precision; a 1-mm "step-off" is apparent and cosmetically unacceptable. The vermilion border should be approximated with a 5–0 or 6–0 nonabsorbable stay suture before any further closure to ensure proper alignment throughout the remainder of the repair (Fig. 43–64). The vermilion surface of the lip and the buccal mucosa are then closed with interrupted stitches using an absorbable 4–0 or 5–0 suture. Finally, the skin is closed with 6–0 nonabsorbable sutures.[207]

Small lacerations of the oral mucosa heal well without sutures. If a mucosal laceration creates a flap of tissue that falls between the occlusal surfaces of the teeth or if a laceration is extensive enough to trap food particles (e.g., a laceration approximately 2 to 3 cm or greater in length), it should be closed. Small flaps may be excised. Closure is easily accomplished with 4–0 Dexon or Vicryl using a simple interrupted suturing technique. These materials are soft and nonabrasive, whereas gut sutures become hard and traumatize adjacent mucosa. Muscle and mucosal layers should be closed separately. Sutures in the oral cavity easily become untied by the constant motion of the tongue. Each suture should be tied with at least four square knots. These sutures need not be removed; they either loosen and fall out within 1 week or are rapidly absorbed.[182, 207, 208]

Tongue Lacerations. There is some controversy regarding when to suture tongue lacerations. Dushoff recommends suturing all lacerations of the tongue to prevent continued bleeding.[177] Snyder suggests that only those lacerations that involve the edge or pass completely through the tongue, flap lacerations, and bleeding lacerations need to be sutured. There is no question that lacerations bisecting the tongue require repair.[201] Small flaps on the edge of the tongue may be excised. Large flaps should be sutured. Small tongue lacerations that are linear, superficial, and involve the central portion of the tongue do well without suturing. Such lacer-

ations are common in falls and during seizures. When peroxide mouth rinses and a soft diet are used for a few days, healing is rapid. Persistent bleeding from minor lacerations brings most patients to the hospital.

The repair of a tongue laceration in any patient is somewhat difficult, but in an uncooperative child the procedure may prove impossible under anything other than general anesthesia. A Denhardt-Dingman side mouth gag aids in keeping the patient's mouth open. A localized area of the tongue may be anesthetized by covering the area with a 4 per cent lidocaine-soaked gauze for 5 minutes. Large lacerations require infiltration anesthesia or a lingual nerve block. If the tip of the tongue has been anesthetized, a towel clip or suture can be used to secure the tongue. Further anesthesia and subsequent wound cleansing and closure are possible while an assistant applies gentle traction to the tongue.

Size 4–0 absorbable or silk sutures should be used to close all three layers—inferior mucosa, muscle, and superior mucosa—in a single stitch or the stitch should include one half of the thickness of the tongue, with sutures placed on the superior and inferior surfaces as well as on the edge of the tongue.[201] Sutures (especially absorbable ones) on the tongue frequently become untied. This problem can be avoided if the stitches are inverted or if silk is used. Do not use nylon sutures in the tongue, because the sharp edges

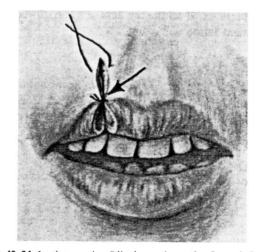

Figure 43–64. In the repair of lip lacerations, the first stitch should be placed at the vermilion-cutaneous border to obtain proper alignment. (From Grabb WC, Kleinert HE: Technics in Surgery: Facial and Hand Injuries. Somerville, NJ, Ethicon, Inc, 1980. Reproduced by permission.)

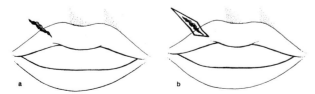

Figure 43–63. Dushoff technique for lip lacerations. (From Dushoff IM: About face. Emerg Med 6(11):25, 1974. Reproduced by permission.)

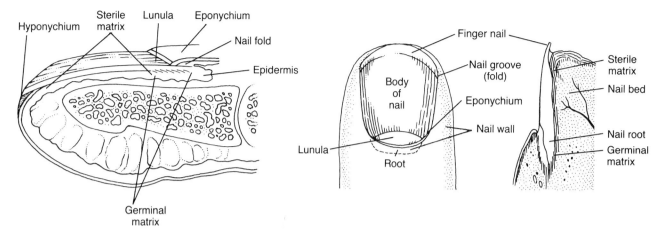

Figure 43–65. Anatomy of the fingernail. The fingernail rests on the nailbed, also termed the matrix. This distal nail covers the sterile matrix; the proximal nail arises from and covers the germinal matrix. The tissue adherent to the proximal dorsal nail is the eponychium (also termed the cuticle), and the potential space between the nail and the eponychium is the nail fold.

are quite uncomfortable.[182] Closure of the lingual muscle layer is usually sufficient to control bleeding and to return motor function to the lacerated tongue. Mucosal healing is rapid, and closure of the muscle layer only with a deep absorbable suture may be desirable when a surface suture is likely to be tugged at—as occurs with small children.

Nail Lacerations. Injuries to the nail and nailbed (also called nail matrix) are common problems in emergency medicine (Fig. 43–65). Although 60 per cent of patients with subungual hematomas greater than one half the size of the nailbed and associated fractures of the distal phalanx have a nailbed laceration, controversy exists over the management of these injuries.[209, 210]

In the case of a simple subungual hematoma (even in the presence of a tuft fracture) in which the nail is firmly adherent and the disruption of the surrounding tissue is minimal, the nail *need not be routinely removed to search for nailbed lacerations.* Despite the presence of a nailbed laceration, a good result can be expected as long as the tissue is held in anatomic approximation by the intact fingernail. Nail trephination is discussed in Chapter 47. If the nail is partly avulsed (especially at the base) or loose, or if there are deep lacerations that involve the nailbed, the nail should be lifted to assess and repair the nailbed. When the integrity of the

fingernail is disrupted and the nailbed is not approximated anatomically, a rippled nail may result as a new nail grows over the rough scarred surface.

If the nailbed is exposed and has been lacerated, it should be approximated with fine absorbable sutures carefully placed using a finger tourniquet to maintain a bloodless field (Fig. 43–66). The exposed nailbed should be protected by reapplying the avulsed nail (best choice) or by applying a nonadherent dressing for approximately 3 weeks. The avulsed nail may be sutured in place or secured with tape.

The replaced nail serves three purposes: (1) it acts as a splint or mold to maintain the normal anatomy of the nailbed; (2) it covers a sensitive area and facilitates dressing changes; and (3) it maintains the fold for new nail growth. Splinting should be maintained for 2 to 3 weeks. If longitudinal scar bands are formed between the proximal nail fold and the matrix, a permanently split or deformed nail may result.

A nail that is partially avulsed distally can be used as a temporary splint or "dressing" that protects and maintains the integrity of the underlying nailbed. When the base of the nail is avulsed from the germinal matrix, its replacement may occasionally result in infection. Some authors advocate trimming the proximal portion of the traumatized nail so

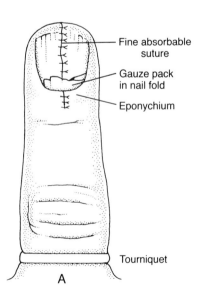

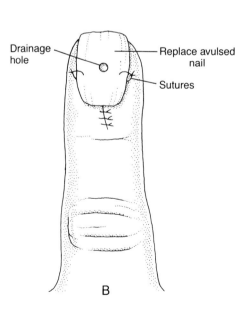

Figure 43–66. A laceration involving the nail bed, germinal matrix, and skin fold must be carefully approximated. First the nail is completely removed. Fine absorbable sutures are placed under a bloodless field provided by a finger tourniquet. The avulsed nail (trimmed at the base) or a gauze pack is gently placed between the matrix and eponychium for 2 to 3 weeks to prevent scar formation *(A).* If the original nail is replaced (the best option), it may be sutured or taped in place *(B).* A large hole in the nail will allow drainage. The old nail is pushed out by a new one. If the nail matrix is replaced quickly and atraumatically, the nail may act as a free graft and grow normally.

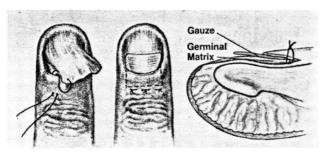

Figure 43–67. Avulsion of the nail leaving the matrix intact requires only a nonadherent dressing to separate the skin fold from the nailbed. If the germinal matrix is avulsed, it should be replaced with 6–0 plain absorbable surgical gut sutures. (From Grabb WC, and Kleinert HE: Technics in Surgery: Facial and Hand Injuries. Somerville, NJ, Ethicon, Inc, 1980. Reproduced by permission.)

that it can be placed more easily in the nail fold.[120] If the *germinal matrix* of the nail is avulsed intact, it should be reimplanted intact, using a 5–0 or 6–0 absorbable suture in a mattress stitch (Fig. 43–67).[182, 211] If the root is not replaced, the space between the proximal nail fold and the nailbed is obliterated within a few days.[212, 213] If an open fracture exists, the matrix must not be allowed to remain trapped in the fracture line.[214] A replaced nail may grow normally, acting as a free graft, but often it is dislodged by a new nail. Nails grow at a rate of 0.1 mm per day, and it requires approximately 6 months for a new nail to reach to the finger tip.

If part of the nailbed has been lost, the patient should be referred to a surgical consultant for a matrix graft.[120, 182, 215] Conservative therapy that allows large portions of an avulsed nailbed to granulate is inadvisable, although this is quite acceptable therapy for a finger tip avulsion that does not involve the nailbed. If a raw nailbed is left open to granulate, it will heal with scar tissue and could produce a distorted and sensitive digit.

Wounds should be rechecked in 3 to 5 days following repair. At that time the nail fold may be repacked if a nonadherent material was used, and the wound is assessed for infection. The use of absorbable suture for nailbed repair negates suture removal. Tape or sutures are removed from any replaced nail in 2 weeks, and the old nail is allowed to fall off as the new nail grows. The value of antibiotics is unproven. All patients with nail injuries should be advised of a possible cosmetic defect in the new nail.

When repairing distal digit lacerations involving a nail, the onychal fold should be approximated first (Fig. 43–68). A sturdy needle attached to a 4–0 thread is recommended for suturing lacerated nails. Needles seem to penetrate nails with the least difficulty when they enter at 90 degrees. The point of the needle carves a rigid path through the nail. Unless the entire length of the needle is allowed to follow this path as it passes through the nail, the needle is likely to bend or break. Alternatively, an electrical cautery instrument or a heated paper clip can be used to perforate the nail, thus permitting easy passage of the needle.

Drains in Sutured Wounds

Drains do not prevent infection; they simply allow wounds to drain any collection of purulence or blood that may develop. When no infection exists and drains are used in soft tissue wounds "prophylactically," they are more harmful than beneficial. Edlich and coworkers state that "drains act as retrograde conduits through which skin contaminants gain entrance into the wound. Furthermore, the presence of a drain impairs the resistance of the tissue to

infection."[1] Magee and colleagues found that drains placed in experimental wounds contaminated with subinfective doses of bacteria greatly enhanced the rate of infection, whether the drain was placed entirely within the wound or was brought out through the wound.[216] Drains behave as foreign bodies, provoking rather than preventing infection. If the wound is considered at high risk for infection, rather than suture the wound with a drain in place (in anticipation of disaster), the physician should leave the wound open and at a later time consider delayed primary closure, when the risk of infection is minimal. Furthermore, drains should not serve as substitutes for other methods of achieving hemostasis in traumatic wounds.

PROTECTION

Dressings

At the conclusion of wound repair, dried blood on the skin surface should be wiped away gently with moistened gauze, and the wound should be covered with a dressing.

Functions of Dressings

Dressings serve a variety of functions. They protect the wound from contamination and trauma, absorb secretions from the wound, immobilize the wound and the surrounding area, exert downward pressure on the wound, and improve the patient's comfort.[11, 217, 218] Occlusive dressings on burns

Suture the nail

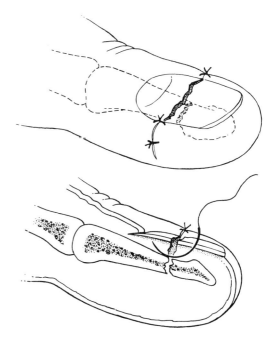

The nail seems to get neglected but it deserves better, particularly when it's cut through. First line up the onychal folds—your landmarks— tack them together, and do the requisite skin closure. Now put a stout reverse-cutting-edge needle, with 4-0 nylon, held halfway down so it doesn't bend, through the distal nail fragment, cross over the bone and up through the proximal nail. Two sutures should do the trick.

Figure 43–68. Repair of distal finger laceration involving the nail and the onychal fold. (From Dushoff IM: Handling the hand. Emerg Med October 1976, p 111. Reproduced by permission.)

Table 43–2. Characteristics of Selected Commercial Dressings[112, 222]

Trade Name	Adherent	Absorptive	Occlusive	Antiseptic	Transparent
Absorptive Dressings					
Cotton gauze	+	+	−	−	−
Nonadherent Dressings					
Adaptic	−	−	−	−	−
Betadine	−	−	±	+	−
Telfa	−	−	+	−	−
Xeroform	−	−	−	+	−
Film Dressings					
Bioclusive	+	−	+	−	+
Op-Site	+	−	+	−	+
Tegaderm	+	−	+	−	+
Foam Dressings					
Epi-Lock	−	+	+	−	−
Hydrocolloid Dressings					
DuoDerm	+	+	+	−	+
Hydrogel Dressings					
Vigilon	−	+	+	−	±

or abrasions prevent painful exposure of the wound to the air and dehydration of the wound surface.[219]

Schauerhamer and coworkers demonstrated that sutured wounds are susceptible to infection from surface contamination during the first 2 days after wound repair. Dressings effectively protect the wound from contamination during this vulnerable period. Taped wounds have a much higher resistance to infection than do sutured wounds.[220]

One of the primary functions of a gauze dressing is to absorb the serosanguineous drainage that exudes from all wounds. Absorbent dressings also minimize the development of stitch abscesses to some extent. Surface sutures produce small indentations at their points of entrance; tiny blood clots and debris overlie these indentations, allowing bacterial growth at the site. Small "stitch abscesses" can develop; these are initially undetectable but are nevertheless destructive to epithelium. Stitch abscesses rarely infect the entire wound but can slightly increase the width of the scar and produce noticeable, punctate suture marks.[11]

The most common type of dressing is constructed in three layers: a nonadherent contact layer, an absorbent layer, and an outer wrap.[221] Ideally, this dressing provides nonadherence without maceration.

CONTACT LAYER: DRY, SEMIOCCLUSIVE, AND OCCLUSIVE DRESSINGS

Petrolatum gauze (e.g., Adaptic, Xeroform, Betadine, Aquaflo) can be applied next to the wound surface to prevent the wound from sticking to the dry gauze in the absorbent layer and to protect the regenerating epithelium (Table 43–2). (Nonadherent material should always be used to cover skin grafts.[143])

Some investigators advise using porous gauze for the contact layer. Coarse weaves of gauze, usually available in the form of multi-layered pads, provide absorbency without occlusion. A dressing will adhere if the interstices of the fabric are relatively large; capillaries and fibrinous and granulation tissue will penetrate and become enmeshed in the material. If the proteinaceous exudate from the wound dries by evaporation, the scab usually clings to the dressing.[221, 222] When the gauze adheres to the wound surface, removal "débrides" the wound. However, it also destroys the healing tissue, particularly the new epithelium. Débridement of the wound with wet-to-dry dressings is quick, but débride-

ment with surgical instruments is more controlled and less traumatic. Adherence to the wound can be avoided if the dressing is nonabsorbent, occlusive, or finely woven. Some physicians use fine mesh gauze (41 to 47 warp threads per square inch) rather than petrolatum gauze on abrasions, especially on those wounds that are heavily contaminated, because removal of this type of dressing débrides only the small tufts of granulation tissue that become fixed in the mesh pores, leaving a clean, even surface. Once a healthy, granulating surface is present and re-epithelialization is proceeding, nonporous dressings can be used.[187] Fine mesh gauze is also used next to exposed tissue in wounds being considered for delayed primary closure; a protective and absorptive bulky dressing is placed on top of the wound.[143]

Wounds covered with permeable dressings such as plain gauze tend to dry out.[218] Drying of the wound surface damages a shallow layer of exposed dermis, which impedes epidermal resurfacing of abrasions, burns, and incisions.[218] Wound desiccation results in further epidermal necrosis, crust formation, and increased inflammation.[223, 224] If the wound is kept moist by covering it with an occlusive film soon after wound management and if the film is left in place for at least 48 hours, the epidermis will migrate over the surface of the dermis up to 100 per cent faster than when a dry scab is allowed to form.[225–229] In one study, the occluded half of a surgical incision produced a more linear, less pigmented scar.[230] Protection of wounds that are healing by secondary intention with occlusive or semiocclusive dressings reduces or eliminates the pain associated with dry healing, increases the rate of healing, and results in fewer wound infections[12] (Table 43–3).

This occlusive effect is achieved with various polyurethane-derived membranes, such as Epi-Lock (Derma-Lock Medical Corp.), Op-Site (Smith and Nephew, Ltd.), Tegaderm (3M), Bioclusive (Johnson & Johnson), and Prima-

Table 43–3. Advantages of Occlusive Dressings[234]

1. More rapid healing
2. Less pain from air exposure
3. Better cosmetic results
4. Fewer dressing changes
5. Better protection from bacteria

derm (ACCO, Inc.); those with soluble collagen or gelatin backing, such as DuoDerm (Convatec) and Biobrane (Woodroof Laboratories); and products with hydrogels, such as Vigilon.[222]

One of the fears of using occlusive dressings is that microorganisms will proliferate in the moist environment beneath the occlusive film and increase wound infection rates.[218, 231] One group tested the abilities of various occlusive dressings to exclude external pathogenic bacteria from experimental wounds and found that DuoDerm prevented inoculation in 100 per cent of cases, although Op-Site and Vigilon provided a less effective barrier.[232] Although *surface* bacteria under occlusive dressings can multiply,[233] chronic wounds, usually contaminated with large numbers of bacteria, are routinely treated with occlusive dressings successfully.[234]

Stillman and associates found that the application of paint-on collodion dressing over a wound closed with a buried subcuticular stitch provided considerable resistance to infection compared with wounds closed by the same technique but with no dressing.[235] The use of collodion obviates the need for a gauze dressing, frequent dressing changes, and uncomfortable dressings in areas such as the groin, the axilla, and the neck.[6] The collodion, however, does not allow drainage of the wound and so is rarely used.

Another concern of physicians is that occlusive dressings will macerate underlying skin. Optimal wound appearance under a dressing is a moist red surface with capillary and epithelial growth. Chvapil and colleagues found that collagen sponge dressings provided this appearance (unless it was accidentally dislodged), whereas both DuoDerm and Op-Site adhered to the wound site, macerated it, and produced a thick eschar that was difficult to remove. However, underneath the eschars of these wounds, the surfaces were epithelialized.[236] To those unfamiliar with these materials, wounds covered with certain occlusive dressings or with silver sulfadiazine (Silvadene, Marion Labs) applications appear to be blanketed with pus; this exudate actually represents the beneficial proliferation of macrophages and polymorphonuclear leukocytes.[229, 237]

Adhesive-backed dressings (e.g., DuoDerm and Op-Site) have a tendency to adhere to and remove new epidermis, and they do not allow exudate to drain out the edges of the dressing. Between dressing changes, the wound should be coated with petrolatum or an antibiotic ointment before these products are applied.[12] Epi-Lock has the advantage of thermally insulating the wound by virtue of its thickness, but unlike Tegaderm and Op-Site, it is opaque and does not allow inspection of the underlying wound surface.[237] Because Epi-Lock allows drainage of exudate, it is better tolerated by patients if the overlying gauze bandage is changed daily.

Other nonadherent-type dressings include Adaptic, Xeroform, Betadine, Dermacell, and the nonabsorbent Telfa. Eaglestein and Mertz found that petrolatum gauze did not enhance epidermal healing.[224]

ABSORBENT LAYER

In dressing wounds with considerable drainage, sufficient gauze should be used to cover the wound and to absorb all of the drainage. Dressings on such wounds can be changed daily, which is frequent enough to avoid bacterial overgrowth beneath the dressing.[4, 187] Once a dressing becomes moist, pathogens can pass through the dressing to the underlying wound.[218] Any dressing should be changed whenever it becomes soiled, wet, or saturated with drainage. Fluid accumulating under an occlusive dressing should be aspirated or the dressing changed every 1 to 2 days during the first week or until the exudate no longer accumulates.[238]

A dressing that is used to absorb exudate or débride the wound must be changed more frequently than one designed to occlude.

OUTER LAYER

Dressings and bandages can serve as surface splints (as can surgical tape) by reducing mechanical stresses on the wound during the early phases of healing. Even when subcuticular stitches have been placed, these "external splints" are useful in relieving tension across the wound. They are most needed between the seventh and forty-second days, the time of collagen synthesis and remodeling.[11] Stronger measures are required for wounds in mobile areas, such as around large joints, where rigid immobilization with plaster splints or braces is needed to protect the wound. Certain chemically treated wide-mesh weaves have the properties of cling and stretch, holding snugly in place but expanding if edema develops.[221]

Compressive dressings may be helpful in preventing hematoma formation and eliminating dead space within a wound. They are particularly useful in wounds that have been undermined extensively and in facial wounds, in which subcutaneous capillary bleeding and swelling can exert tension on fine skin sutures and jeopardize the skin closure (Fig. 43–69). Pressure dressings should be used to immobilize skin grafts. Surgical tape can serve as a pressure dressing in areas such as fingertips, on which bandages cannot be easily applied. Bryant points out that "because it has been amply demonstrated that the pressure beneath a dressing is maintained for only relatively short periods of time . . . a pressure dressing should not be used as a substitute for good hemostasis."[4]

Pressure dressings should be applied to all ear lacerations to prevent hematoma formation and the subsequent deformation and destruction of cartilage. The ear should be enveloped in the dressing so that pressure from the outer bandage is distributed evenly across the irregular surface of the pinna. Moistened cotton is packed into the concavities of the pinna until the cotton is level with the most lateral aspect of the helical rim. Square pieces of gauze cut to fit the curvature of the ear are placed *behind* (medial to) the pinna. Several more gauze squares are placed on the lateral surface of the ear; the packing is then secured in place with a circumferential head bandage. The bandage must not encompass the opposite ear, because it would just as easily cause pressure necrosis of that ear if left unprotected. Application of a pressure dressing for the ear is discussed further in Chapter 86.

Traumatic wounds are bandaged to compress or immobilize the wound or to secure and protect the underlying dressing. Most bandaging is performed on extremities, on which dressings are difficult to secure with tape alone. Rolls of cotton (Kerlix, Kling stretch gauze) are well suited for this purpose. The bandage is wound around the extremity,

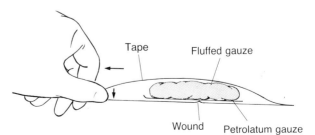

Figure 43–69. Compression dressing on the face. Paper adhesive tape is applied tightly over the dressing.

advancing proximally with circular, overlapping turns. Care should be taken to avoid wrinkles in the bandage that later create pressure points or to make loose turns that "shorten the effective life of the dressing."[187] When joint surfaces are crossed, the cotton is anchored distally with several turns, unrolled obliquely across the joint several times in a figure-of-eight pattern, and anchored proximally by two complete turns. This process is repeated until the bandage is securely in place. The ends of the bandage are fastened to the skin by strips of adhesive tape.

Bandages over the forearm and the lower extremities are particularly prone to slippage because of the constant motion of these parts and because of the marked changes in extremity diameter over a short distance. The roll of bandage can be rotated 180 degrees after each circular turn, producing a reverse spiral and reducing its mobility (Fig. 43–70). A "tube" of elastic cotton netting (e.g., Surgifix, Tubex, Surgitube, Diffuson, Hyginet) pulled over the bandage or unrolled from a metal applicator frame effectively stabilizes the entire dressing in these areas (Fig. 43–71). Another useful technique consists of placing strips of tape on opposite sides of the extremity, leaving the ends free. The bandage is wrapped around the dressing, covering the portions of the tape that are attached to the skin. The free ends of tape are then incorporated in the bandage (Fig. 43–72).[239]

An elastic cotton roll (Kerlix) allows the bandage to conform to body contours, provides some mobility to bandaged joints, and permits the wound to swell without the circumferential bandage constricting the extremity. The inelastic Kling bandage better immobilizes the part.

Most scalp wounds do well when left uncovered. If a dressing is considered to be necessary, it must be held in place by a bandage. There are many techniques of bandaging heads. Stavrakis described the following method:

The assistant tightly holds a strip of bandage three inches wide and three feet long over the patient's head in a frontal plane [Fig. 43–73A]. While one person maintains tension on the first strip of bandage, the second person starts bandaging the head with the main bandage at the forehead level in a horizontal plane, using a full-length gauze bandage [Fig. 43–73B]. (The "Kling"-type bandage is preferred.) After several turns are made to stabilize the main bandage, it is passed near the patient's ear, then wrapped around

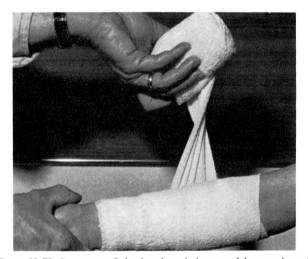

Figure 43–70. Snugness of the bandage is increased by rotation of the bandage roll 180 degrees after each circular turn to effect a reverse spiral. (From Norton LW: Trauma. In Hill GJ II: Outpatient Surgery, 3rd ed. Philadelphia, WB Saunders Co, 1988. Reproduced by permission.)

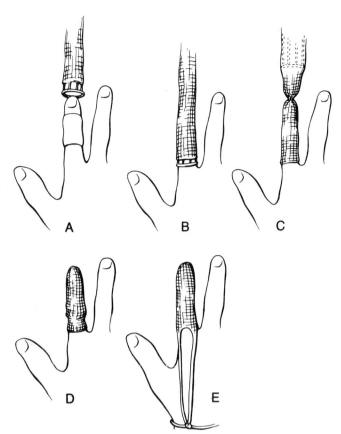

Figure 43–71. Finger dressing. *A,* The inner layer is nonadherent gauze or whatever is required for soft tissue care. The middle layer is 2-inch by 2-inch gauze sponges wrapped circumferentially and held in place with a small strip of tape. *B,* Begin number 2 tube gauze at the base of the finger. It is useful to hold this end with one finger while the tube gauze applicator is pulled toward the finger tip. A twisting motion firms the wrap about the digit—generally about 90 degrees is necessary. Excessive stretch or twisting can compromise circulation. *C,* When the finger tip is reached, make a 360-degree twist. *D,* Pass the applicator toward the finger base with an additional 90-degree twist. Repeat once more; thus three layers are in place. *E,* Cut enough gauze to reach the base of the finger, and tape it there. As an alternative, pull the final layer beyond the tip, leaving it long enough to reach to and around the wrist (about three times the finger length). Split this gauze into two strands; bring them dorsally to the wrist; knot; and loosely wrap around the wrist. (Redrawn from Kaplan EN, Hentz VR: Emergency Management of Skin and Soft Tissue Wounds: An Illustrated Guide. Boston, Little, Brown & Co, 1984, p 86. Reproduced by permission.)

the short strip of bandage in a full turn [Fig. 43–73C]. The main bandage is then taken across the front of the head, wrapped full-turn around the other side of the short bandage, then brought around the back of the head and wrapped around the first side again. This maneuver is repeated, alternating front and back until the head is covered by overlapping passes of bandage [Fig. 43–73D] . . . several turns of the bandage across the forehead in a horizontal plane stabilize the dressing. The dressing is . . . secured by tying the ends of the short strip under the chin [Fig. 43–73E]. Removal of this dressing can be accomplished easily by untying the chin straps and gently pulling both ends upward.[240]

Methods of bandaging wounds in other locations of the body are described in detail in other texts.[112, 217]

Dressings vary in their absorbency, adhesiveness, occlusiveness, opacity, and insulating properties. Further research may identify types of dressings best suited for different phases of the healing wound. Currently, a two- or three-layer dressing is used for most traumatic wounds; the choice

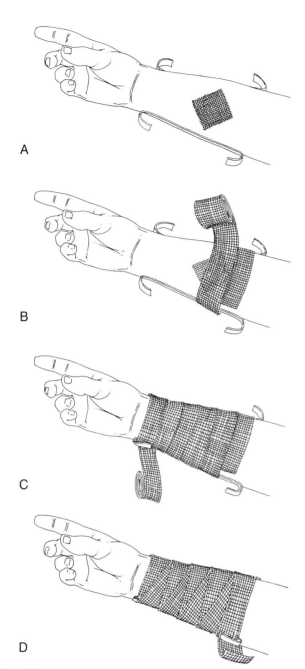

Figure 43–72. *A,* When a Kling or Kerlix wrap must be applied to an area such as the forearm, start by putting a strip of tape on opposite sides of the arm, leaving the ends free. *B,* Wrap the bandage around the arm, covering the portions of the tape that are attached to the skin. *C,* After completing one layer of wrapping, tuck the free ends of the tape down so that the nonadhesive side faces the first layer of wrapping and the sticky side faces out. Place another layer of wrapping around the arm. *D,* After completing a second layer of wrapping, the dressing will not slip because it is adhered to itself as well as to the skin. (From Lazo J: Non-slip dressing technique. Res Staff Phys 22:103, 1976. Reproduced by permission.)

of material for the contact layer is determined by the characteristics of the individual wound.[241]

Splinting and Elevation

Immobilization of an injured extremity promotes healing by protecting the closure and by limiting the spread of

contamination and infection along lymphatic channels. Wounds overlying joints are subjected to repeated stretching and movement, which delays healing, widens the scar, and could possibly disrupt the sutures.[1] Splints are almost always required for lacerations that overlie joints and are frequently necessary for protection of wounds involving fingers, hands, wrists, the volar aspects of forearms, the extensor surface of elbows, the posterior aspect of legs, the plantar surfaces of feet, and on extremities when skin grafts have been applied. Splinting is often underused by the emergency physician in the treatment of lacerations. A reasonable axiom is that all *large* lacerations on the extremity should be splinted for the first few days of healing. Splinting may enhance the healing process and often adds to the comfort of the patient.

A plaster or aluminum splint may be incorporated into a bandage to reduce the mobility of the part. Splinting techniques for extremities are explained more fully in Chapters 65 and 67.

Elevation of injured extremities is important in all but trivial injuries. Elevation serves to limit edema formation, an expected sequela of trauma and inflammation, and allows more rapid healing.[1, 143] Elevation also reduces throbbing pain. Patients given this information are often more motivated to elevate the extremity as instructed. Slings can be used to elevate wounds involving the forearm or the hand.

Ointments

The safety and efficacy of topical antibiotic preparations used on wound surfaces are still being debated. Norton claims that "topical antibiotics are of limited value and in some cases interfere with tissue regeneration."[187] Some investigators warn of skin sensitization by preparations containing neomycin,[136] and others of the emergence of resistant

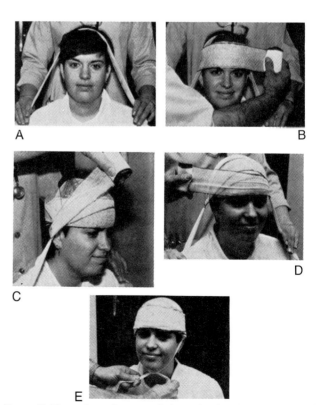

Figure 43–73. *A* through *E,* Technique for bandaging the head. (From Stavrakis P: A better head dressing. Res Staff Phys 26:88, 1980. Reproduced by permission.)

strains of bacteria with any topical antibiotic.[242] Other studies have shown that use of a triple antibiotic preparation containing neomycin, bacitracin, and polymyxin provides a broad spectrum of protection against infection in *abrasions* without systemic absorption and toxicity or the emergence of resistant strains of bacteria. Unless this topical antibiotic ointment is used repeatedly or on inflamed skin, there is a relatively low risk of allergic sensitization.[243] In comparison with controls, the active agents in Neosporin ointment and Silvadene cream as well as their inert bases and vehicles improve wound healing.[219, 244, 245] USP petrolatum has been found both to retard healing[244] and to have no effect on wound healing.[245] The beneficial effect of Silvadene cream placed on healing skin flaps seems to be in its ability to provide a moist environment for the ischemic tissue more than in its antibacterial activity. Knutson and associates reported the use of a granulated sugar (sucrose) povidone-iodine paste in a variety of open wounds. In this uncontrolled series, the combination of this paste, frequent dressing changes, and close follow-up resulted in rapid healing and reduced bacterial proliferation and tissue edema even in contaminated and infected wounds.[246]

Ointments can be used to reduce the formation of a crust that covers and separates the edges of the wound. Lacerations surrounded by abraded skin are especially predisposed to coagulum formation. In such cases the patient can be instructed to cleanse the wound frequently and to follow the cleansing with an application of ointment during the first few days.[1, 136] Ointments also prevent the dressing from adhering to the wound.[7] Some researchers recommend the use of bacitracin applied in a thin coating not for protection against infection but for prevention of these mechanical problems.[136] The stronger topical corticosteroids have detrimental effects on healing. Application of 0.1 per cent triamcinolone acetonide in an ointment retards healing in wounds by as much as 60 per cent, whereas hydrocortisone probably does not interfere with epithelialization.[224, 247] Some physicians believe that single and low doses of oral corticosteroids probably have no effect on wound healing but that repeated, large doses of steroids (≥ 40 mg of prednisone per day) inhibit healing, particularly if used before the injury or during the first 3 days of the healing phase.[248, 249] There is some evidence that topical vitamin A may reverse some of the anti-inflammatory and immunosuppressive effects of corticosteroids.[250] The exact value of ointments in the treatment of lacerations has yet to be determined.

Systemic Antibiotics

Most traumatic soft tissue injuries sustain a low level of bacterial contamination.[132] The standard wound infection rate in unselected emergency department wounds is in the 2 to 3 per cent range. In a number of clinical studies of traumatic wounds, prophylactic antibiotics administered orally[19, 251, 252] and intramuscularly[35, 251, 253–255] in a variety of regimens proved ineffective in reducing the incidence of infection.

In experimental models, antibiotics have no therapeutic value more than 3 hours after the injury.[33, 103, 104, 256] Edlich and coworkers found that delayed treatment with antibiotics was more effective in wounds closed immediately than in wounds closed 3 to 48 hours after injury. They concluded that the exudate filling the wound prevented the antibiotic from reaching the bacteria in the wound.[103]

Most investigations into the use of antibiotics have omitted heavily contaminated wounds in their series. Studies have shown that the therapeutic value of antibiotic treatment decreases as the number of bacteria in the wound increases.

When the wound is contaminated with greater than 10^9 bacteria per gram of tissue, infection will develop despite antibiotic treatment, such as when the wound surface is contacted by either pus or feces.[55]

Studies of antibiotic prophylaxis for animal bite wounds have produced variable results,[257–266] and no large study providing stratification of the many prognostic factors has been done. Antibiotic prophylaxis is unnecessary in small intraoral lacerations that do not require suturing.[267] The effectiveness of systemic antibiotics for bite wounds is still uncertain.[256, 258] Indications for antibiotics vary among physicians, because few conclusions are based on sound, scientific data. Antibiotics are of no benefit in most soft tissue wounds, because the level of bacterial contamination after cleaning and débridement is below that necessary for infection. Antibiotics may be effective (perhaps only marginally effective) when the level of contamination is overwhelming or if the amount of questionably viable tissue left in the wound is considerable. Antibiotics should be considered for extremity bite wounds, puncture-type bite wounds in any location, intraoral lacerations that are sutured, oral-cutaneous lip wounds, wounds that cannot be cleaned or débrided satisfactorily, and highly contaminated wounds (e.g., those contaminated with soil, organic matter, purulence, feces, saliva, or vaginal secretions). They should also be considered for wounds involving tendons, bones, or joints; for wounds requiring extensive débridement in the operating room; for wounds in lymphedematous tissue; for distal extremity wounds when treatment is delayed for 12 to 24 hours; for patients with orthopedic prostheses; and for patients at risk for developing infective endocarditis.[1, 252, 268–269] *If systemic antibiotics are considered necessary, they should be given intravenously or intramuscularly in the earliest stages of wound management.*

The choice of antibiotic, particularly for bite wound prophylaxis, is as controversial as the indications for usage. Many species of bacteria cause bite wound infections, making complete coverage impossible with less than three types of antibiotics.[43, 270–277] Callaham recommends dicloxacillin or cephalexin as economical choices that are effective against the majority of infecting organisms in high-risk dog bite wounds and one of these antistaphylococcal agents plus penicillin for human or cat bite wounds.[270] A single broad-spectrum antibiotic should be used for all other wounds—cephalosporins, penicillinase-resistant penicillins, or, if allergy or cost precludes the use of these two groups, erythromycin.[145] If significant contamination with gram-negative or anaerobic organisms has occurred, an aminoglycoside and clindamycin should be considered.[1] Irrigation with topical antibiotics may be of benefit in these situations. The duration of antibiotic prophylaxis is also in question. It is common practice to provide antibiotics for 72 hours, although data from surgical studies indicate that antibiotics beyond the first postoperative day provide no additional protection.[278] Short courses of antibiotics do not seem to affect the incidence of resistant strains of organisms.[279] In all cases, the use of antibiotics should remain subordinate to careful cleaning and débridement. If the infection risk is high enough to warrant antibiotics, secondary closure should be considered.

Immunoprophylaxis

Recommendations for tetanus prophylaxis have been changing during the past several years. The guidelines published by the Public Health Services Advisory Committee on Immunization Practices (Centers for Disease Control) differ from those of the American College of Surgeons in

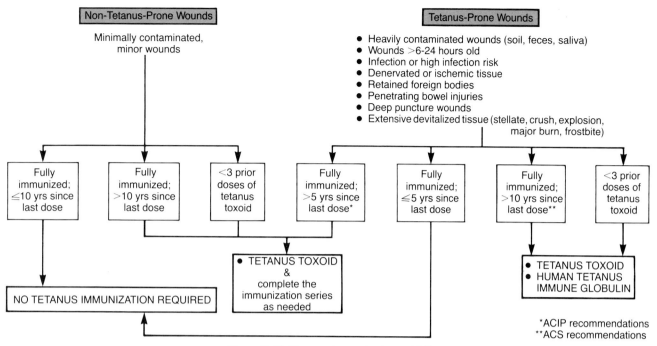

Figure 43–74. Tetanus immunization guidelines.

the use of tetanus immune globulin.[280–282] Many cases of tetanus develop despite prior immunization; tetanus frequently results from minor or clean wounds.[283] Patient's recall of past immunizations is imperfect, and immunity may be inadequate after a complete series of tetanus toxoid.[284] Furthermore, there is no precise consensus on the definition of a "tetanus-prone wound," yet treatment decisions are based on the differentiation between clean and contaminated wounds. Some investigators warn of overtreatment,[281, 285] and others maintain that the risk of therapy is minimal compared with the danger of tetanus.[286, 287] After comparing those risks and benefits, most clinicians would agree that a certain amount of overtreatment is acceptable.

Tetanus-prone wounds include old wounds; those contaminated by feces, saliva, purulent exudate, or soil; those with retained foreign bodies or devitalized or avascular tissue; established wound infections; penetrating abdominal wounds involving bowel; and deep puncture wounds (Fig. 43–74). When questioning patients about their tetanus immunization status, determine whether the patient has completed the primary immunization series, and if not, how many doses have been given.

Patients who have not completed a full primary series of injections may require both tetanus toxoid and passive immunization with tetanus immune globulin. The preferred preparation for active tetanus immunization in patients 7 years of age and older is 0.5 ml of tetanus toxoid (plus the lower, adult dose of diphtheria toxoid); the dose of tetanus immune globulin is 250 to 500 units given intramuscularly.[280] Mild local reactions consisting of erythema and induration are common after tetanus toxoid injections. Some patients with high antibody levels develop a hypersensitivity reaction of tenderness, erythema, and swelling, or serum sickness. Generalized urticarial reactions and peripheral neuropathy have also been reported.

When a wound results from the bite or scratch of a wild or domestic animal, prophylaxis against rabies also must be considered (Table 43–4). Further discussion of the prevention of rabies is provided elsewhere.[288–290] In cases of questionable exposure, consultation with one's state health officer is helpful for therapy selection.

PATIENT INSTRUCTIONS

Successful wound healing is partly dependent on the care given to the wound once the patient leaves the emergency center. "Patient satisfaction depends not only on the cosmetic result, but also on the expectation of that result."[12] Therefore, the patient should receive thorough and understandable instructions.

The patient should be informed that no matter how skillful the repair, any wound of significance produces a scar. Most scars deepen in color and become more prominent before they mature and fade. The final appearance of the scar cannot be judged before 6 to 12 months after the repair.[136]

Patients may experience dysesthesias in or around a scar, particularly about the midface. Rubbing or pressing on the skin may relieve the symptoms, and they usually resolve within 6 months to 1 year. If wounds extending to subcutaneous levels lacerate cutaneous nerves, patients may be bothered by hypoesthesia distal to the wound. Sensation often returns in 6 months to 1 year.[12]

Because the wound edges are rapidly sealed by coagulum and bridged by epithelial cells within 48 hours, the wound is essentially impermeable to bacteria after 2 days.[11, 220, 291] The patient should be instructed to keep the wound protected by leaving the dressing undisturbed, clean, and dry for 24 to 48 hours. In this initial period the dressing should be changed only if it becomes externally soiled or soaked by exudate from the wound. If possible, the injured part should be kept elevated. There is a tendency on the part of most patients to avoid getting sutures wet. *There is no proven harm in exposing sutured wounds to soap and tap water for short periods,* and many physicians routinely allow patients to bathe with sutures in place. Some advise patients to wash

Table 43–4. Rabies Postexposure Prophylaxis Guide—July 1984[290]

The following recommendations are only a guide. In applying them, take into account the animal species involved, the circumstances of the bite or other exposure, the vaccination status of the animal, and presence of rabies in the region. Local or state public health officials should be consulted if questions arise about the need for rabies prophylaxis.

	Animal Species	Condition of Animal at Time of Attack	Treatment of Exposed Person*
DOMESTIC	Dog and cat	Healthy and available for 10 days of observation	None, unless animal develops rabies†
		Rabid or suspected rabid	RIG‡ and HDCV
		Unknown (escaped)	Consult public health officials. If treatment is indicated, give RIG‡ and HDCV
WILD	Skunk, bat, fox, coyote, raccoon, bobcat, and other carnivores	Regard as rabid unless proven negative by laboratory tests§	RIG‡ and HDCV
OTHER	Livestock, rodents, and lagomorphs (rabbits and hares)	Consider individually. Local and state public health officials should be consulted on questions about the need for rabies prophylaxis. Bites of squirrels, hamsters, guinea pigs, gerbils, chipmunks, rats, mice, other rodents, rabbits, and hares almost never call for antirabies prophylaxis.	

*All bites and wounds should immediately be thoroughly cleansed with soap and water. If antirabies treatment is indicated, both rabies immune globulin (RIG) and human diploid cell rabies vaccine (HDCV) should be given as soon as possible, *regardless* of the interval from exposure. Local reactions to vaccines are common and do not contraindicate continuing treatment. Discontinue vaccine if fluorescent antibody tests of the animal are negative.

†During the usual holding period of 10 days, begin treatment with RIG and HDCV at first sign of rabies in a dog or cat that has bitten someone. The symptomatic animal should be killed immediately and tested.

‡If RIG is not available, use antirabies serum, equine (ARS). Do not use more than the recommended dosage.

§The animal should be killed and tested as soon as possible. Holding for observation is not recommended.

(From Leads from the Mortality and Morbidity Weekly Report. JAMA 252:887, 1984.)

wounds daily to remove dried blood and exudate, especially on areas such as the face or the scalp.

After 48 hours, the patient may remove the dressing in uncomplicated wounds and check for evidence of infection—redness, warmth, increasing pain, swelling, purulent drainage, or the "red streaks" of lymphangitis. If there is no sign of infection, the patient can care for the wound until it is time for removal of the sutures. A daily gentle washing with a mild soap and water to remove dried blood and exudate is beneficial.[291, 293] Undiluted hydrogen peroxide may destroy granulation tissue and newly formed epithelium; it is undesirable as a cleaning agent.[65] Generally, a wound should be protected with a dressing during the first week, and the dressing should be changed daily. If the wound is unlikely to be contaminated or traumatized, it may be left uncovered. Although it is generally recommended that uncovered scalp wounds can be washed after 1 to 2 days, a gentle shampoo in the first few hours after wound closure is unlikely to be harmful. Vigorous scrubbing of wounds should be discouraged.

Patients should be informed that sutures themselves do not cause pain. A very painful wound is often a sign of infection or suture reaction, and pain should prompt a wound check.

Some wounds heal with wide, unattractive scars despite the physician's best efforts. These include wounds that cross perpendicular to joints, wrinkle lines, or lines of minimum tension (Kraissel's lines); wounds that retract more than 5 mm; and wounds that are over convexities or in certain anatomic locations (e.g., back, shoulders) where hypertrophic scars are common. A wound crossing a concave surface may result in a bowstring deformity; one crossing a convexity may leave a scar depression. To avoid these complications, a Z-plasty procedure can be done at the time of initial wound management or the scar can be revised later. The patient should be told to expect suboptimal outcomes in these situations.[47, 51]

If an injured extremity or finger is protected by a splint, it should be left undisturbed until the sutures are removed. Patients with intraoral lacerations should be instructed to use warm salt water mouth rinses at least three times a day.

Patients often ask about the efficacy of various creams and lotions (e.g., vitamin E, cocoa butter) in limiting scar formation. At this time there are no data to evaluate the use of these substances. Patients should be told to avoid aspirin. This medication has been shown to decrease the development of tensile strength, and it increases the likelihood of hematoma formation.[293]

SECONDARY WOUND CARE

Reexamination

Wounds should be examined in 2 to 3 days for signs of infection and sooner if the patient experiences increasing discomfort or develops a fever.[217] Bite wounds and other infection-prone wounds should be inspected in 2 days. Wounds being considered for delayed primary closure are evaluated in 4 to 5 days.[131]

Wounds in which extensive dissection of subcutaneous tissue has been performed may develop a low-grade, localized cellulitis. It is rarely necessary to open these wounds. The removal of one or two stitches may relieve some of the tension caused by mild swelling. With daily cleansing using water and a mild soap and with application of warm compresses, this type of wound reaction should subside within 24 to 48 hours.[217]

In most sutured wounds that become infected, the sutures must be removed to allow drainage. The presence of sutures in a contaminated wound considerably limits the activity of various antibiotics.[294] Infection around a suture can lead to the formation of a stitch mark.[114] Infected wounds should be treated with daily cleansing, warm compresses, and antibiotics. They should be left to heal by secondary intention, which involves wound contraction, granulation tissue formation, and epithelialization.[143]

Suture Removal

Because wounds do not heal at a standard rate, no strict guidelines can be set for time of suture removal. The optimal time for suture removal varies with the location of the wound, the rate of wound healing, and the amount of tension on the wound. Certain areas of the body, such as the back of the hand, heal slowly, whereas facial or scalp wounds heal rapidly. Speed of wound healing is affected by systemic factors, such as malnutrition, neoplasia, or immunosuppression. At the time that suture removal is being considered, one or two sutures may be cut to determine if the skin edges are sufficiently adherent to allow removal of all the sutures.[7] Removing sutures too early invites wound dehiscence and widening of the scar, whereas leaving sutures in longer than necessary may result in epithelial tracts, infection, and unsightly scarring.[295, 296]

Small stitch abscesses are common in wounds in which sutures have been left in place for longer than 7 to 10 days. Localized stitch abscesses generally resolve following removal of the suture(s) and with the application of warm compresses. There is usually no need for antibiotic therapy with stitch abscesses.

Stillman warns that "percutaneous sutures . . . provide a nidus for infection, establish a route for the entry of skin and sebaceous bacteria for 5–10 days, and provoke a foreign body reaction. . . . Percutaneous sutures stimulate a granulomatous, then fibrous inflammatory reaction along the suture track."[6] Factors that determine the severity of stitch marks include the length of time skin stitches are left in place, skin tension, the relationship of the suture to the wound edge, the region of the body, infection, and tendency for keloid formation.[114, 297] The skin of the eyelids, palms, and soles, and the mucous membranes seldom show stitch marks, unless the skin of the face is heavy with sebaceous glands (e.g., over the dorsum of the nose or the forehead). In contrast, oily skin and the skin of the back, the sternal area, the upper arms, and the lower extremities are likely to develop the permanent imprints of suture material on the skin surface.[18, 114, 177, 297]

Crikelair found that if sutures are removed within 7 days, no discernible needle puncture or stitch mark will persist.[297] In studying wound tensile strength, Myers and coworkers found that incisions in which sutures were removed on the fourth day were stronger than those in which sutures were removed on the seventh day, suggesting that a moderate amount of tension on wounds enhances healing.[298] Yet at 6 days, the wound is held together by a small amount of fibrin and cells and has minimal strength (see Fig. 43–1).[5] The tensile strength of most wounds at this time is adequate to hold the wound edges together, but only if there are no appreciable dynamic or static skin forces pulling the wound apart.[7] Minimal trauma to an unsupported wound at this point could cause dehiscence. The physician should decide on the proper time of suture removal after weighing these various factors. If early suture removal is necessary, the strength of the closure may be maintained with strips of surgical skin tape. The key to wound tensile strength after suture removal is an adequate deep tissue layer closure.

Helpful general guidelines for suture removal are as follows: Sutures on the face should be removed on the fifth day following the injury, or alternate sutures should be removed on the third day and the remainder on the fifth day. On the extremities and the anterior aspect of the trunk, sutures should be left in place for approximately 7 days to prevent wound disruption. Sutures on the scalp, the back, the feet, and the hands and over the joints must remain in place for 10 to 14 days, even though permanent stitch marks may result.[114] Some physicians recommend the removal of sutures in eyelid lacerations in 48 to 72 hours to avoid epithelialization along the suture tract with subsequent cyst formation.[299]

The technique of removing sutures is relatively simple. The wound should be cleansed, and any remaining crust overlying the wound surface or surrounding the sutures should be removed. The skin is wiped with an alcohol swab. Each stitch is cut with a scissors or the tip of a scalpel blade (number 11 Bard-Parker) at a point close to the skin surface on one side. The suture is grasped on the opposite side with forceps and is pulled across the wound (Fig. 43–75). The amount of exposed suture that is dragged through the suture tract is thereby minimized. It is difficult to remove sutures with very short ends. At the time of suture placement, the length of the suture ends should generally equal the distance between sutures to permit easy grasping of the suture during subsequent removal, yet avoiding entanglement during the knotting of adjacent sutures.

The suture-removal scissors is a cutting instrument with two opposing, shearing blades that grips, cuts, and removes a suture in a single motion. This device facilitates the removal of percutaneous sutures that are tied with limited tension (Fig. 43–76).[300]

Once the skin sutures are removed, the width of the scar increases gradually over the next 3 to 5 weeks unless it is supported. Support is provided by previously placed subcutaneous stitches that brought the skin edges into apposition, by a previously placed subcuticular stitch, or by the application of skin tape (Fig. 43–77). A nonabsorbable subcuticular suture can be left in place for 2 to 3 weeks to provide continued support for the wound. Although complications from prolonged use of this stitch, such as closed epithelial sinuses, cysts, or internal tracts, can occur, they are unusual. These problems can be avoided by the placement of a buried subcuticular stitch using an absorbable suture.[6, 11]

If a subcuticular stitch with reliefs has been used, the suture is cut at the midpoint of the relief. Half of the suture is removed at the original point of entry into the skin and the other half through the original exit point (Fig. 43–78).[194] If a nonabsorbable subcuticular suture cannot be removed or a portion of it ruptures during removal, the protruding end should be grasped with a hemostat, pulled taut, and cut with a scissors as close to the skin as possible so that the end of the suture retracts under the skin.[190]

There are several reasons why wounds fail to heal; some are related to decisions made at the time of wound closure, and others are consequences of later events. Infection is probably the most common cause of dehiscence. If the patient is careless or unlucky, reinjury can reopen a wound

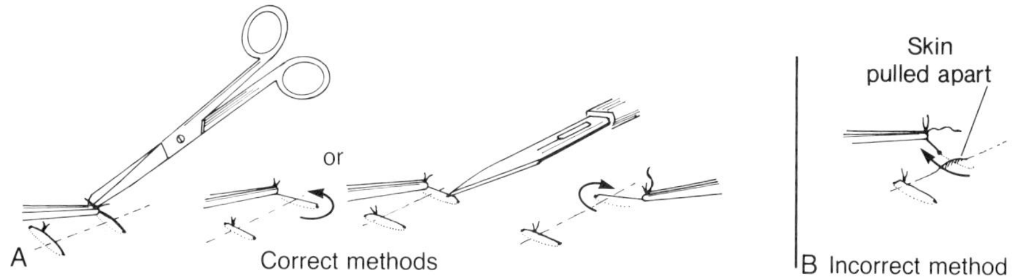

Figure 43–75. Technique for suture removal. Pull should be toward the wound line (A) rather than away from it (B), which causes the skin to tear apart. (Modified from Stuzin J, Engrav LH, Buehler PK: Emergency treatment of facial lacerations. Postgrad Med 71(3): 81, 1982.)

A Correct methods | Skin pulled apart B Incorrect method

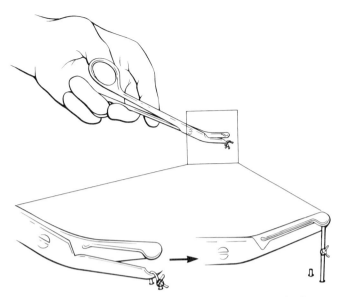

Figure 43–76. Suture removal by means of suture removal scissors. The semilunar tip of one blade is inserted beneath the suture. The flexible spring forceps securely grips the suture, removing it without the need of another instrument.

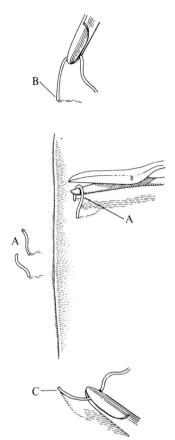

Figure 43–78. At the time of suture removal, the suture is cut at the midpoint of the relief *(A)*. The proximal portion is removed at the point of original entry into the skin *(B)*, and the distal portion is removed through the original exit point *(C)*. (From Grimes DW, Garner RW: "Reliefs" in intracuticular sutures. Surgical Rounds, 1:48, 1978. Reproduced by permission.)

despite the protection of a thick dressing. If the suture size is too small, the stitch may break. A stitch that is too fine or tied too tightly may cut through friable tissue and pull out. Knots that have not been tied carefully may unravel. The suture material may be extruded or absorbed too rapidly. Finally, if a stitch is removed too early before tissues regain adequate tensile strength, the wound loses needed support and falls open.[301] If the wound edges show signs of separating at the time of suture removal, alternate stitches can be left in place and the entire length of the wound supported by strips of adhesive tape.

If time and effort has been invested in a cosmetic closure of the face, the repair should be protected with skin tape after the skin sutures have been removed. Wound contraction and scar widening continue for 42 days after the injury.[5] Because the desired result is a scar of minimal width, the tape should be used for 5 weeks following suture removal. With exposure to sunlight, scars in their first 4 months redden to a greater extent than surrounding skin. This should be prevented in exposed cosmetic areas with the use of a sunscreen containing para-amino benzoic acid (PABA) when prolonged exposure to the sun is anticipated.

CONCLUSION

The objective of traumatic wound management is the restoration of tissue continuity and strength in the least possible time, with maximal preservation of tissues and minimal scar formation, deformity, or loss of function.

Wounds fail to heal for a variety of reasons. Some of the impediments to healing include ischemia or necrosis of tissue, hematoma formation, prolonged inflammation caused by foreign material, excessive tension on skin edges, and immunocompromising systemic factors. In attempting to repair wounds, physicians sometimes inadvertently retard the healing process. Research has identified harmful practices that can be avoided, such as premature closure of contaminated wounds or the use of drains in uninfected wounds. With the development of new methods and solutions for cleansing wounds and the discovery of the optimal concentrations of solutions currently in use, tissue-toxic antiseptic solutions can be abandoned. Better suture materials are replacing reactive sutures that often served as foreign bodies rather than supports. Improved materials used for dressing wounds enhance wound healing.

One of the primary causes of delayed healing is wound infection. Wound cleaning and débridement, atraumatic and aseptic handling of tissues, and the use of protective dressings minimize this complication. All new methods and materials used in wound management must be evaluated with respect to their potential for provoking or preventing infection.

The patient's actions affect wound healing. Delay in seeking treatment for an injury has a significant impact on the ultimate outcome of the wound. In the first few days following an injury, the patient must take responsibility for protecting the wound from contamination, further trauma, and swelling.

The final appearance of a scar is determined by several factors. Infection, tissue necrosis, and keloid formation widen a scar. Wounds located in sebaceous skin or oriented 90 degrees to dynamic or static skin tension lines result in wide scars. Inversion of the edges of a wound during closure produces a more noticeable scar,

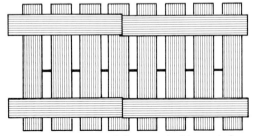

Figure 43–77. Support of the wound with surgical tape.

whereas skillful technique can convert a jagged, contaminated wound into a fine, inapparent scar. There are times when optimal wound management requires that the wound be closed at a later time, when the danger of infection has passed.

It is important that physicians adhere to the established, basic principles of wound care when cleaning, débriding, closing, and protecting wounds and continue to refine their management as further improvements in techniques and materials become available.

REFERENCES

1. Edlich RF, Thacker JG, Buchanan L, Rodeheaver GT: Modern concepts of treatment of traumatic wounds. Adv Surg 13:169, 1979.
2. Hunt, JK, Van Winkle W: Wound Healing: Normal Repair. Fundamentals of Wound Management in Surgery. South Plainfield, NJ, Chirurgecom, Inc, 1976.
3. Edlich RF, Custer J, Madden J, et al: Studies in the management of the contaminated wound III. Assessment of the effectiveness of irrigation with antiseptic agents. Am J Surg 118:21, 1969.
4. Bryant WM: Wound healing. Clin Symp 29:1, 1977.
5. Ordman LJ, Gillman T: Studies in the healing of cutaneous wounds I. The healing of incisions through the skin of pigs. Arch Surg 93:857, 1966.
6. Stillman RM: Wound closure: Choosing optimal materials and methods. ER Reports 2:41, 1981.
7. Peacock EE: Wound healing and wound care. In Schwartz SI (ed): Principles of Surgery. 3rd ed. New York, McGraw-Hill Book Co, 1979.
8. Timberlake GA: Wound healing: The physiology of scar formation. Curr Concepts Wound Care 9:4, 1986.
9. Hohn DC, Granelli SG, Burton RW, et al: Antimicrobial systems of the surgical wounds II. Detection of antimicrobial protein in cell-free wound fluid. Am J Surg 133:601, 1977.
10. Simon B: Treatment of wounds. In Rosen P, Baker FJ, Berkin RM, et al (eds): Emergency Medicine: Concepts and Clinical Practice. 2nd ed. St. Louis, CV Mosby Co, 1988, pp 363–373.
11. Peacock EE, Van Winkle W: Surgery and Biology of Wound Repair. Philadelphia, WB Saunders Co, 1970.
12. Zitelli JA: Secondary intention healing: An alternative to surgical repair. Clin Dermatol 2:92, 1984.
13. Krizek TJ, Robson MC: Evolution of quantitative bacteriology in wound management. Am J Surg 130:579, 1975.
14. Dreyfuss UY, Singer M: Human bites of the hand: A study of one hundred six patients. J Hand Surg 10A:884, 1985.
15. Robson MC, Duke WF, Krizek TJ: Rapid bacterial screening in the treatment of civilian wounds. J Surg Res 14:426, 1973.
16. Ogilvie WH: Prevention and treatment of wound infection. Lancet 2:935, 1940.
17. Berk WA, Osbourne DD, Taylor DD: Evaluation of the "golden period" for wound repair: 204 cases from a third world emergency department. Ann Emerg Med 17:496, 1988.
18. Edlich RF, Thacker JG, Rodeheaver GT, et al: A manual for wound closure. St. Paul, Minn, Surgical Products Division/3M, 1979.
19. Haughey RE, Lammers RL, Wagner DK: Use of antibiotics in the initial management of soft tissue hand wounds. Ann Emerg Med 10:187, 1981.
20. Strauss MB: Wound hypoxia. Curr Concepts Wound Care. 9:16, 1986.
21. Cruse PJE, Foord R: A five-year prospective study of 23,649 surgical wounds. Arch Surg 107:206, 1973.
22. Doig CM, Wilkinson AW: Wound infection in a children's hospital. Br J Surg 63:647, 1976.
23. Fekety RF, Murphy JF: Factors responsible for the development of infections in hospitalized patients. Surg Clin North Am 152:1385, 1972.
24. Viljanto J: Disinfection of surgical wounds without inhibition of normal wound healing. Arch Surg 115:253, 1980.
25. Bierens de Haas B, Ellis H, Wilks M: The role of infection on wound healing. Surg Gynecol Obstet 138:693, 1974.
26. Burke JF: Infection. Fundamentals of Wound Management in Surgery. South Plainfield, NJ, Chirurgecom, Inc, 1977.
27. Craig EV: Delayed laceration of ulnar nerve following hand trauma. JAMA 253:1014, 1985.
28. Lammers RL: Soft tissue foreign bodies. Ann Emerg Med 17:1336, 1988.
29. Trott A: Mechanisms of surface soft tissue trauma. Ann Emerg Med 17:1279, 1988.
30. Haury B, Rodeheaver G, Vensko J Jr, et al: Debridement: An essential component of traumatic wound care. Am J Surg 135:238, 1978.
31. Hunt TK: The physiology of wound healing. Ann Emerg Med 17:1265, 1988.
32. Nylin S, Karlsson B: Time factor, infection frequency and quantitative microbiology in hand injuries. Scand J Plast Reconstr Surg 14:185, 1980.
33. National Academy of Sciences–National Research Council: Post-operative wound infections: The influence of ultraviolet irradiation of the operating room and of various other factors. Ann Surg 160(suppl):1, 1964.
34. Sindelar W, Mason GR: Irrigation of subcutaneous tissue with povidone-

35. Hutton PAN, Jones BM, Low DJW: Depot penicillin as prophylaxis in accidental wounds. Br J Surg 65:549, 1978.
36. Galvin JR, DeSimone D: Infection rate of simple suturing. JACEP 5:332, 1976.
37. Alkan M, Gefen Z, Goldman L: Wound infection after simple suture at the emergency ward. Infect Control 5:562, 1984.
38. Smith MS, Smith D, Mortiere M, et al: Sutured wounds in an urban emergency department (abstract). Ann Emerg Med 14:519, 1985.
39. Rosenberg NM, Debaker K: Incidence of infection in pediatric patients with laceration. Pediatr Emerg Care 3:239, 1987.
40. Haley RW, Culver DH, Morgan WM, et al: Identifying patients at high risk of surgical wound infection: A simple multivariate index of patient susceptibility and wound contamination. Amer J Epidemiol 121:206, 1985.
41. Klimek JJ: Treatment of wound infections. Cutis 36:21, 1985.
42. Gosnold JK: Infection rate of sutured wounds. The Practitioner 218:584, 1977.
43. Mann RJ, Hoffeld TA, Former CB: Human bites of the hand: Twenty years of experience. J Hand Surg 2:97, 1977.
44. Rodeheaver GT, Pettry D, Thacker JG, et al: Wound cleansing in high pressure irrigation. Surg Gynecol Obstet 141:357, 1975.
45. Rodeheaver G, Pettry D, Turnbull V, et al: Identification of the wound infection–potentiating factors in soil. Am J Surg 67:140, 1980.
46. Roberts AH, Rye DG, Edgerton MI, et al: Activity of antibiotics in contaminated wounds containing clay soil. Am J Surg 137:381, 1979.
47. Edlich RF, Rodeheaver GT, Morgan RF, et al: Principles of emergency wound management. Ann Emerg Med 17:1284, 1988.
48. Morgan WJ, Hutchison D, Johnson HM: The delayed treatment of wounds of the hand and forearm under antibiotic cover. Br J Surg 67:140, 1980.
49. Hutton PAN, Jones BM, Law DJW: Depot penicillin as prophylaxis in accidental wounds. Br J Surg 75:549, 1978.
50. Rutherford WH, Spence RA: Infection in wounds sutured in the accident and emergency department. Ann Emerg Med 9:350, 1980.
51. Robson MC: Disturbances of wound healing. Ann Emerg Med 17:1274, 1988.
52. Rodeheaver GT, Smith SL, Thacker JG: Mechanical cleansing of contaminated wounds with a surfactant. Am J Surg 129:241, 1975.
53. Custer J, Edlich RF, Prusak M, et al: Studies in the management of the contaminated wound V. An assessment of the effectiveness of pHisoHex and Betadine surgical scrub solutions. Am J Surg 121:572, 1971.
54. Ervin ME: Minor surgical procedures. In Schwartz GR, et al (eds): Principles and Practice of Emergency Medicine. Philadelphia, WB Saunders Co, 1978, pp 386–398.
55. Edlich RF, Rodeheaver GT, Thacker JG, et al: Technical Factors in Wound Management. Fundamentals of Wound Management in Surgery. South Plainfield, NJ, Chirurgecom, Inc, 1977.
56. Rodeheaver G, Turnbull V, Edgerton MT, et al: Pharmacokinetics of a new skin wound cleanser. Am J Surg 132:67, 1976.
57. Van Den Broek PJ, Buys LFM, Van Furth R: Interaction of povidone-iodine compounds, phagocytic cells, and microorganisms. Antimicrob Agents Chemother 22:593, 1982.
58. Rodeheaver GT, Kurtz L, Kircher BJ, et al: Pluronic F–68: A promising new skin wound cleanser. Ann Emerg Med 9:572, 1980.
59. Edlich RF, Schmolka IR, Prusak MP, et al: The molecular basis for toxicity of surfactants in surgical wounds: 1. EO:PO block polymers. Surg Res 14:277, 1973.
60. Rodeheaver G, Bellamy W, Kody M, et al: Bactericidal activity and toxicity of iodine-containing solutions in wounds. Arch Surg 117:181, 1982.
61. Faddis D, Daniel D, Boyer J: Tissue toxicity of antiseptic solutions: A study of rabbit articular and periarticular tissues. J Trauma 17:895, 1977.
62. Mulliken JB, Healy NA, Glowacki J: Povidone-iodine and tensile strength of wounds in rats. J Trauma 20:323, 1980.
63. Lineaweaver W, McMorris S, Soucy D, et al: Cellular and bacterial toxicities of topical antimicrobials. Plast Reconstr Surg 75:394, 1985.
64. Berkelman RL, Holland BW, Anderson RL: Increased bactericidal activity of dilute preparations of povidone-iodine solutions. J Clin Microbiol 15:635, 1982.
65. Gruber RP, Vistnes L, Pardoe R: The effect of commonly used antiseptics on wound healing. Plast Reconstr Surg 55:472, 1975.
66. Naunton-Morgan TC, Firmin R, Mason B: Prophylactic povidone-iodine in minor wounds. Injury 12:194, 1980.
67. de Jong TE, Vierhout RJ, Van Vroonhoven TJ: Povidone-iodine irrigation of the subcutaneous tissue to prevent surgical wound infections. Surg Gynecol Obstet 155:221, 1982.
68. Lammers RL, Fourré M, Callaham ML, et al: Effect of povidone-iodine and saline soaking on bacterial counts in acute, traumatic contaminated wounds. Ann Emerg Med 19:709, 1990.
69. Rogers DM, Blouin GS, O'Leary JP: Povidone-iodine wound irrigation and wound sepsis. Surg Gynecol Obstet 157:426, 1983.
70. Platt J, Bucknall RA: An experimental evaluation of antiseptic wound irrigation. J Hosp Infect 5:181, 1984.

71. Roberts AHN, Roberts FE, Hall RI: A prospective trial of prophylactic povidone-iodine in lacerations of the hand. J Hand Surg 10:370, 1985.

72. Gravett A, Sterner S, Clinton J, et al: A trial of povidone-iodine in the prevention of infection in sutured lacerations. Ann Emerg Med 16:167, 1987.

73. Oberg MS: Povidone-iodine solutions in traumatic wound preparation. Am J Emerg Med. 5:553, 1987.

74. Branemark PI, Ekholm R, Albrektsson B, et al: Tissue injury caused by wound disinfectants. J Bone Joint Surg 49A:48, 1967.

75. Zamora JL: Povidone-iodine and wound infection. Surgery 95:121, 1984.

76. Walsh JA, Watts JMCK, McDonald PJ, et al: The effect of topical povidone-iodine on the incidence of infection in surgical wounds. Br J Surg 68:185, 1981.

77. Bickerstaff KI, Regnard C: Prophylactic povidone-iodine spray in accidental wounds. J R Coll Surg Edinb 29:234, 1984.

78. Zdeblick TA, Lederman MM, Jacobs MR, et al: Preoperative use of povidone-iodine: A prospective, randomized study. Clin Orthop 213:211, 1986.

79. Tighe B, Anderson M, Dooley C, et al: Betadine irrigation following appendectomy—a randomized prospective trial. Ir Med J 75:96, 1982.

80. Barr LL: Prevention of wound infection by 2-minute lavage with Betadine solution. J Am Osteopath Assoc 77:442, 1978.

81. Lau WY, Wong SH: Randomized, prospective trial of topical hydrogen peroxide in appendectomy wound infection: High risk factors. Am J Surg 142:393, 1981.

82. Sebben JE: Surgical antiseptics. J Am Acad Dermatol 9:759, 1983.

83. Bryant CA, Rodeheaver GT, Reem EM, et al: Search for a nontoxic surgical scrub solution for periorbital lacerations. Ann Emerg Med 13:317, 1984.

84. Madden J, Edlich RF, Schauerhamer R, et al: Application of principles of fluid dynamics to surgical wound irrigation. Curr Top Surg Res 3:85, 1971.

85. Stevenson TR, Thacker JG, Rodeheaver GT, et al: Cleansing the traumatic wound by high pressure syringe irrigation. JACEP 5:17, 1976.

86. Bhaskar SN, Cutright DE, Gross A, et al: Water jet devices in dental practice. J Periodontol 42:658, 1971.

87. Gross A, Bhaskar SN, Cutright DE, et al: The effect of pulsating water jet lavage on experimental contaminated wounds. Oral Surg 29:187, 1971.

88. Gross A, Cutright DE, Bhaskar SN: Effectiveness of pulsating water jet lavage in treatment of contaminated crushed wounds. Am J Surg 124:373, 1972.

89. Grower MF, Bhaskar SN, Horan MJ, et al: Effect of water lavage on removal of tissue fragments from crush wounds. Oral Surg 33:1031, 1972.

90. Hamer ML, Robson MC, Krizek TJ, et al: Quantitative bacterial analysis of comparative wound irrigations. Ann Surg 181:819, 1975.

91. Brown LL, Shelton HT, Bornside GH, et al: Evaluation of wound irrigation by pulsatile jet and conventional methods. Ann Surg 187:170, 1978.

92. Beasley JD: The effect of spherical polymers and water jet lavage on oral mucosa. Oral Surg 32:998, 1971.

93. Gross A, Bhaskar SN, Cutright DE: A study of bacteremia following wound lavage. Oral Surg 31:720, 1971.

94. O'Leary TJ, Shafer WG, Swenson HM, et al: Possible penetration of crevicular tissue from oral hygiene procedures—use of oral irrigating device. J Periodontol 41:158, 1970.

95. Wheeler CB, Rodeheaver GT, Thacker JG, et al: Side effects of high pressure irrigation. Surg Gynecol Obstet 143:775, 1976.

96. Brown DG, Skylis TP, Sulisz CA, et al: Sterile water and saline solution: Potential reservoirs of nosocomial infection. Am J Infect Control 13:35, 1985.

97. Kaczmarek ER, Sula JA, Hutchinson RA: Sterility of partially used irrigating solutions. Am J Hosp Pharm 39:1534, 1982.

98. Halasz NA: Wound infection and topical antibiotics: The surgeon's dilemma. Arch Surg 112:1240, 1977.

99. Sher KS: Prevention of wound infection: The comparative effectiveness of topical and systemic cefazolin and povidone-iodine. Am Surg 48:268, 1982.

100. Lindsay D, Nava C, Marti M: Effectiveness of penicillin irrigation in control of infection in sutured lacerations. J Trauma 22:186, 1982.

101. Benjamin JB: Efficacy of a topical antibiotic irrigant in decreasing or eliminating bacterial contamination in surgical wounds. Clin Orthop 184:114, 1984.

102. Edlich RF, Madden JE, Prusak M, et al: Studies in the management of the contaminated wounds IV: The therapeutic value of gentle scrubbing in prolonging the limited period of effectiveness of antibiotics in contaminated wounds. Am J Surg 121:668, 1971.

103. Edlich RF, Smith OT, Edgerton MT: Resistance of the surgical wound to antimicrobial prophylaxis and its mechanisms of development. Am J Surg 126:583, 1973.

104. Rodeheaver G, Marsh D, Edgerton MT, et al: Proteolytic enzymes as adjuncts to antimicrobial prophylaxis of contaminated wounds. Am J Surg 129:537, 1975.

105. Rodeheaver GT, Rye DG, Rust R, et al: Mechanisms by which proteolytic enzymes prolong the golden period of antibiotic action. Am J Surg 136:379, 1978.

106. Rodeheaver G, Edgerton MT, Elliott MB, et al: Proteolytic enzymes as adjuncts to antibiotics prophylaxis of surgical wounds. Am J Surg 127:564, 1974.

107. Seropian R, Reynolds BM: Wound infections after preoperative depilatory versus razor preparation. Am J Surg 121:251, 1971.

108. Howell JM, Morgan JA: Scalp laceration repair without prior hair removal. Am J Emerg Med 6:7, 1988.

109. Alexander JW, Fischer JE, Boyajian M, et al: The influence of hair-removal methods on wound infections. Arch Surg 118:347, 1983.

110. Haeri GB, et al: The efficacy of standard surgical face masks: An investigation using "tracer particles." Clin Orthop 148:160, 1980.

111. Weatherley-White RCA, Lesavoy MA: The integument. In Hill GJ II (ed): Outpatient Surgery. Philadelphia, WB Saunders Co, 1980, pp 334–346.

112. Kaplan EN, Hentz VR: Emergency Management of Skin and Soft Tissue Wounds: An Illustrated Guide. Boston, Little, Brown & Co, 1984.

113. Westaby S: Wound closure and drainage. In Westaby S (ed): Wound Care. St. Louis, CV Mosby Co, 1986, pp 32–46.

114. Grabb WC: Basic techniques of plastic surgery. In Grabb WC, Smith JW (eds): Plastic Surgery: A Concise Guide to Clinical Practice. Boston, Little, Brown & Co, 1979, pp 3–74.

115. Kirk RM: Basic Surgical Techniques. Edinburgh, Churchill Livingstone, 1978.

116. Edlich RF, Morgan RF, Edlich HS, et al: Puncture wounds. Curr Concepts Wound Care 10:11, 1987.

117. Faust RA, Roy WA, Edwin DM, et al: Management and tetanus prophylaxis in the treatment of puncture wounds. Am Surg 38:198, 1972.

118. Houston AN, Roy WA, Faust RA, et al: Tetanus prophylaxis in the treatment of puncture wounds of patients in the deep south. J Trauma 2:439, 1962.

119. Edlich RF, Rodeheaver GT, Horowitz JH, et al: Emergency department management of puncture wounds and needlestick exposure. Emerg Med Clin North Am 4:581, 1986.

120. Brown PW: The hand. In Hill GJ, II (ed): Outpatient Surgery. Philadelphia, WB Saunders Co, 1980, pp 643–686.

121. Lemos MJ, Clark DE: Scalp lacerations resulting in hemorrhagic shock: Case reports and recommended management. J Emerg Med 6:377, 1988.

122. Rosen P, Sternbach G: Atlas of Emergency Medicine. Baltimore, Williams & Wilkins, 1979, pp 125–133.

123. MacDonald RT: Maintenance of ligature tension by a single operator with simultaneous removal of a hemostatic clamp. Am J Surg 143:770, 1982.

124. Roberts JR: Intravenous regional anesthesia. JACEP 6:261, 1977.

125. Dushoff IM: Handling the hand. Emerg Med 8(10):26, 1976.

126. Wavak P, Zook EG: A simple method of exsanguinating the finger prior to surgery (letter). JACEP 7:124, 1978.

127. Edlich RF, Rodeheaver GT: Scientific basis for emergency wound management. Emerg Med Annu 2:1, 1983.

128. Shaw JA, DeMuth WW, Gillespy AW: Guidelines for the use of digital tourniquets based on physiological pressure measurements. J Bone Joint Surg 67A:1086, 1985.

129. Hoffer EP: To blanch a finger. Emerg Med 15:137, 1983.

130. Lubahn JD, Koeneman J, Kosar K: The digital tourniquet: How safe is it? J Hand Surg. 10A:664, 1985.

131. Edlich RF, Rogers W, Kasper G, et al: Studies in the management of the contaminated wound I. Optimal time for closure of contaminated open wounds II. Comparison of resistance to infection of open and closed wounds during healing. Am J Surg 117:323, 1969.

132. Marshall KA, Edgerton MT, Rodeheaver GT, et al: Quantitative microbiology: Its application to hand injuries. Am J Surg 131:730, 1976.

133. Prusak M, Edlich RF, Payne TJ, et al: Studies in the management of the contaminated wound IX. Quantitation of the Evans Blue Dye content of open and primarily closed surgical wounds. Am J Surg 125:585, 1973.

134. Elek SD: Experimental staphylococcal infections in skin of man. Ann NY Acad Sci 65:85, 1956.

135. Edlich RF, Panek PH, Rodeheaver GT, et al: Physical and chemical configuration of sutures in the development of surgical infection. Ann Surg 177:679, 1973.

136. Walike JW: Suturing technique in facial soft tissue injuries. Otolaryngol Clin North Am 12:425, 1979.

137. Crawford BS, Gipson M: The conservative management of pretibial lacerations in elderly patients. Br J Plast Surg 30:174, 1977.

138. Krizek TJ, Robson MC: Evolution of quantitative bacteriology in wound management. Am J Surg 130:579, 1975.

139. Elek SD: Experimental staphylococcal infections in the skin of man. Ann NY Acad Sci 65:85, 1956.

140. Robson MC, Heggers JP: Delayed wound closures based on bacterial counts. J Surg Oncol 2:379, 1970.

141. Robson MC, Lea CE, Dalton JB, et al: Quantitative bacteriology and delayed wound closure. Surg Forum 19:501, 1968.

142. Magee C, Haury B, Rodeheaver GT, et al: A rapid technique for quantitating wound bacterial count. Am J Surg 133:760, 1977.

143. Herrmann JB: Open wounds. In Wolcott MW (ed): Ferguson's Surgery of the Ambulatory Patient. 5th ed. Philadelphia, JB Lippincott Co, 1974, pp 52–62.

144. Cramer LM, Chase RA: Hand. In Schwartz SI, et al (eds): Principles of Surgery. New York, McGraw-Hill Book Co, 1974, pp 1895–1918.

145. Callaham ML: Human and animal bites. Top Emerg Med 4:1, 1982.

146. Edlich RF, Tsung MS, Rogers W, et al: Studies in management of the contaminated wounds I. Technique of closure of such wounds with a note on a reproducible model. J Surg Res 8:585, 1968.

147. Edlich RF, Rodeheaver GT, Kuphal J, et al: Technique of closure: Contaminated wounds. JACEP 3:375, 1974.

148. Carpendale MTF, Sereda W: The role of percutaneous suture in surgical wound infection. Surgery 58:672, 1965.

149. Conolly WB, Hunt TK, Zederfeldt B, et al: Clinical comparison of surgical wounds closed by suture and adhesive tapes. Am J Surg 117:318, 1969.

150. Suture Use Manual: Use and Handling of Sutures and Needles. Somerville, NJ, Ethicon, Inc, 1977.

151. Grossman JA: The repair of surface trauma. Emerg Med 14:220, 1982.

152. Laufman H, Rubel T: Synthetic absorbable sutures. Surg Gynecol Obstet 145:597, 1977.

153. Herrmann JB: Tensile strength and knot security of surgical suture materials. Am Surg 37:209, 1971.

154. Conn J, Beal JM: Coated Vicryl synthetic absorbable sutures. Surg Gynecol Obstet 150:843, 1980.

155. Thacker JG, Rodeheaver G, Moore JW, et al: Mechanical performance of surgical sutures. Am J Surg 130:374, 1975.

156. Macht SD, Krizek TJ: Sutures and suturing—current concepts. J Oral Surg 36:710, 1978.

157. Westreich M, Kapetansky DI: Avoiding the slippery knot syndrome (letter). JAMA 236:2487, 1976.

158. Postlethwait RW, Willigan DA, Ulin AW: Human tissue reaction to sutures. Ann Surg 181:144, 1975.

159. Webster RC, McCollough G, Giandello PR, et al: Skin wound approximation with new absorbable suture material. Arch Otolaryngol 111:517, 1985.

160. Craig PH, Williams JA, Davis KW, et al: A biologic comparison of polyglactin 910 and polyglycolic acid synthetic absorbable sutures. Surg Gynecol Obstet 141:1, 1975.

161. Postlethwait RW: Further study of polyglycolic acid suture. Am J Surg 127:617, 1974.

162. Katz AR, Mukherjee DP, Kaganov AL, et al: A new synthetic monofilament absorbable suture made from polytrimethylene carbonate. Surg Gynecol Obstet 161:213, 1985.

163. Wallace WR, Maxwell GR, Cavalaris CJ: Comparison of polyglycolic acid suture to black silk, chromic, and plain catgut in human oral tissues. J Oral Surg 28:739, 1970.

164. Rodeheaver GT, Powell TA, Thacker JG, et al: Mechanical performance of monofilament synthetic absorbable sutures. Am J Surg 154:544, 1987.

165. Bourne RB: In-vivo comparison of four absorbable sutures: Vicryl, Dexon Plus, Maxon and PDS. Can J Surg 31:43, 1988.

166. Howes EL: Strength studies of polyglycolic acid versus catgut sutures of the same size. Surg Gynecol Obstet 137:15, 1973.

167. Edlich RF, Panek PH, Rodeheaver GT, et al: Physical and chemical configuration of sutures in the development of surgical infection. Ann Surg 177:679, 1973.

168. Bergman F, Borgstrom SJH, Holmund DEW: Synthetic absorbable surgical suture material (PGA). Acta Chir Scand 137:193, 1971.

169. Filert JG, Binder P, McKinney PW, et al: Polyglycolic acid synthetic absorbable sutures. Am J Surg 121:561, 1971.

170. Stone IK, Von Fraunhofer JA, Masterson BJ: Mechanical properties of coated absorbable multifilament suture materials. Obstet Gynecol 67:737, 1986.

171. Adams IW: A comparative trial of polyglycolic acid and silk as suture materials for accidental wounds. Lancet 2:1216, 1977.

172. Osterberg B, Blomstedt B: Effect of suture materials on bacterial survival in infected wounds: An experimental study. Acta Chir Scand 145:431, 1979.

173. Blomstedt B, Osterberg B, Bergstrand A: Suture material and bacterial transport: An experimental study. Acta Chir Scand 143:71, 1977.

174. Gristina AG, Price JL, Hobgood CD, et al: Bacterial colonization of percutaneous sutures. Surgery 98:12, 1985.

175. Sharp WV, Belden TA, King PH, et al: Suture resistance to infection. Surgery 91:61, 1982.

176. Ray JA, Doddi N, Regula D, et al: Polydioxanone (PDS): a novel monofilament synthetic absorbable suture. Surg Gynecol Obstet 153:497, 1981.

177. Dushoff IM: About face. In Cohen IJ (ed): Back to Basics. New York, EM Books, 1979, pp 341–364.

178. Laufman H: Is catgut obsolete? Surg Gynecol Obstet 145:587, 1977.

179. Towler MA, McGregor W, Rodeheaver GT, et al.: Influence of cutting edge configuration on surgical needle penetration forces. J Emerg Med 6:475, 1988.

180. Bernstein G: Needle basics. J Dermatol Surg Oncol 11:1177, 1985.

181. Wray RC: Force required for wound closure and scar appearance. Plast Reconstr Surg 72:380, 1983.

182. Grabb WC, Klainert HE: Techniques in Surgery: Facial and Hand Injuries. Somerville, NJ, Ethicon, Inc, 1980.

183. DeHoll D, Rodeheaver G, Edgerton MT, et al: Potentiation of infection by suture closure of dead space. Am J Surg 127:716, 1974.

184. Milewaki PJ, Thompson H: Is a fat stitch necessary? Br J Surg 67:393, 1980.

185. Bloom W, Fawcett DW: A Textbook of Histology. 10th ed. Philadelphia, WB Saunders Co, 1975, pp 564–567.

186. Gant TD: Suturing techniques for everyday use. Patient Care 13(14):45, 1979.

187. Norton LW: Trauma. In Hill GJ II (ed): Outpatient Surgery. Philadelphia, WB Saunders Co, 1980, pp 89–133.

188. Stephens FO, Hunt TK, Dunphy JE: Study of traditional methods of care on the tensile strength of skin wounds in rats. Am J Surg 122:78, 1971.

189. Edlich RF, Rodeheaver GT, Thacker JG, et al: Technical factors in wound management. In Hunt TK, Dunphy JE (eds): Fundamentals of Wound Management. New York, Appleton-Century-Crofts, 1979, pp 364–455.

190. Converse JM: Introduction to plastic surgery. In Converse JM (ed): Reconstructive Plastic Surgery: Principles and Procedures in Correction, Reconstruction, and Transplantation. 2nd ed, vol 1. Philadelphia, WB Saunders Co, 1977, pp 3–68.

191. Speer DP: The influence of suture technique on early wound healing. J Surg Res 27:385, 1979.

192. Winn HR, Jane JA, Rodeheaver G: Influence of subcuticular sutures on scar formation. Am J Surg 133:257, 1977.

193. Stillman RM, Bella FJ, Seligman SJ, et al: Skin wound closure: The effect of various wound closure methods on susceptibility to infection. Arch Surg 115:674, 1980.

194. Grimes DW, Garner RW: "Reliefs" in intracuticular sutures. Surgical Rounds 1(12):46, 1978.

195. Myers MB, Cherry G: Functional and angiographic vasculature in healing wounds. Am Surg 36:750, 1970.

196. Bernstein G: The far-near/near-far suture. J Dermatol Surg Oncol 11:470, 1985.

197. Mitchell GC: Repair of parallel lacerations (letter). Ann Emerg Med 16:924, 1987.

198. Samo DG: A technique for parallel lacerations. Ann Emerg Med 17:297, 1988.

199. Ryan AJ: Traumatic injuries: Office treatment of lacerations. Postgrad Med 59:259, 1976.

200. Roberts JR: Pathophysiology, diagnosis and treatment of head trauma. Top Emerg Med 1:41, 1979.

201. Snyder CC: Scalp, face and salivary glands. In Wolcott MW (ed): Ferguson's Surgery of the Ambulatory Patient. 5th ed. Philadelphia, JB Lippincott Co, 1974, pp 153–181.

202. Weinstein PR, Wilson CB: The skull and nervous system. In Hill GJ II (ed): Outpatient Surgery. Philadelphia, WB Saunders Co, 1980, pp 298–302.

203. Kauder DR, Schwab CW: Immediate emergency room control of hemorrhage from severe scalp lacerations. Curr Concepts Wound Care 10:17, 1987.

204. Paton D, Emery J: Injuries of the eye, the lids, and the orbit. In Ballinger WF, Rutherford RB, Zuidema GD (eds): The Management of Trauma. Philadelphia, WB Saunders Co, 1979, pp 254–284.

205. English GM: Ears, nose, throat and sinus. In Hill GJ II (ed): Outpatient Surgery. Philadelphia, WB Saunders Co, 1980, pp 369–459.

206. Edgerton MT: Emergency care of maxilofacial and neck injuries. In Ballinger WF, Rutherford RB, Zuidema GD (eds): The Management of Trauma. Philadelphia, WB Saunders Co, 1979, pp 285–341.

207. Heintz WD: Traumatic injuries: Dealing with dental injuries. Postgrad Med 61:261, 1977.

208. Horton CE, Adamson JE, Mladick RA, et al: Vicryl synthetic absorbable sutures. Am Surg 40:729, 1974.

209. Simon RR, Wolgin M: Subungual hematoma: Association with occult laceration requiring repair. Am J Emerg Med 5:302, 1987.

210. Seaburg DC, Paris PM, Angelos WJ: Treatment of subungual hematomas with nail trephination: a prospective study. (Abstract) Ann Emerg Med 19:472, 1990.

211. Wolcott MW: Hands and fingers: Part I—soft tissues. In Wolcott MW (ed): Ferguson's Surgery of the Ambulatory Patient. 5th ed. Philadelphia, JB Lippincott Co, 1974, pp 396–438.

212. Kleinert HE, Putcha SM, Ashbell TS, et al: The deformed finger nail, a frequent result of failure to repair nail bed injuries. J Trauma 7:177, 1967.

213. Coyle MP, Leddy JP: Injuries of the distal finger. Primary Care 7:245, 1980.

214. Matthews P: A simple method for the treatment of finger tip injuries involving the nail bed. The Hand 14:30, 1982.

215. Shepard GH: Treatment of nail bed avulsions with split-thickness nail bed grafts. J Hand Surg 8:49, 1983.

216. Magee C, Rodeheaver GT, Golden GT, et al: Potentiation of wound infection by surgical drains. Am J Surg 131:547, 1976.

217. Wolcott MW: Dressings and bandages. In Wolcott MW (ed): Ferguson's Surgery of the Ambulatory Patient. 5th ed. Philadelphia, JB Lippincott Co, 1974, pp 35–51.

218. Lawrence JC: What materials for dressings? Injury 13:500, 1982.
219. McGrath MH: How topical dressings salvage "questionable" flaps: Experimental study. Plast Reconstr Surg 67:653, 1981.
220. Schauerhamer RA, Edlich RF, Panek P, et al: Studies in the management of the contaminated wound VI: Susceptibility of surgical wounds to postoperative surface contamination. Am J Surg 122:74, 1971.
221. Noe JM, Kalish S: The problem of adherence in dressed wounds. Surg Gynecol Obstet 147:185, 1978.
222. Eaglstein WH, Mertz PM, Falanga V: Occlusive dressings. Am Fam Phys 35:211, 1987.
223. Rovee DT, Kurowsky CA, Labun J: Local wound environment and epidermal healing: Mitotic response. Arch Dermatol 106:330, 1972.
224. Eaglstein WH, Mertz PM: New method for assessing epidermal wound healing: The effects of triamcinolone acetonide and polyethylene film occlusion. J Invest Dermatol 71:382, 1978.
225. Winter GD: Formation of scab and the rate of epithelialization of superficial wounds in the skin of the young domestic pig. Nature 193:293, 1962.
226. Winter GD, Scales JT: Effect of air drying and dressings on the surface of a wound. Nature 197:91, 1963.
227. Hinman CD, Maibach H: Effect of air exposure and occlusion on experimental human skin wounds. Nature 200:377, 1963.
228. Eaglstein WH, Davis SC, Mehle AL, et al: Optimal use of an occlusive dressing to enhance healing. Arch Dermatol 124:392, 1988.
229. Wayne MA: Clinical evaluation of Epi-Lock—a semiocclusive dressing. Ann Emerg Med 14:20, 1985.
230. Linsky CB, Rovee DT, Dow T: Effect of dressing on wound inflammation and scar tissue, in Hildick-Smith G, Dineen P (eds): The Surgical Wound. Philadelphia, Lea & Febiger, 1981, pp 191–206.
231. Bothwell JW, Rovee DT: The effect of dressings on the repair of cutaneous wounds in humans. In Harkiss KJ (ed): Surgical Dressings and Wound Healing. London, Crosby-Lockwood, 1971, p 78.
232. Mertz PM, Marshall DA, Eaglstein WH: Occlusive wound dressings to prevent bacterial invasion and wound infection. J Am Acad Dermatol 12:662, 1985.
233. Katz S, McGinley K, Leyden JJ: Semipermeable occlusive dressings: Effects on growth of pathogenic bacteria and reepithelialization of superficial wounds. Arch Dermatol 122:58, 1986.
234. Eaglstein WH: Effect of occlusive dressings on wound healing. Clin Dermatol 2:107, 1984.
235. Stillman RM, Bella FJ, Seligman SJ: Skin wound closure: The effect of various closure methods on susceptibility to infection. Arch Surg 115:674, 1980.
236. Chvapil M, Chvapil TA, Owen JA: Comparative study of four wound dressings on epithelialization of partial-thickness wounds in pigs. J Trauma 27:278, 1987.
237. Stair TO, D'Orta J, Altieri MF, et al: Polyurethane and silver sulfadiazene dressings in treatment of partial-thickness burns and abrasions. Am J Emerg Med 4:214, 1986.
238. Falanga V: Occlusive wound dressings: Why, when, which? Arch Dermatol 124:872, 1988.
239. Lazo J: Non-slip dressing technique. Res Staff Phys 22(8):103, 1976.
240. Stavrakis P: A better head dressing. Res Staff Phys 26(9):88, 1980.
241. Turner TD: Which dressings and why? In Westaby S (ed): Wound Care. St. Louis, CV Mosby Co, 1986, pp 58–69.
242. Ayliffe GAJ, Green W, Livingston R, et al: Antibiotic-resistant Staphylococcus aureus in dermatology in burn wounds. J Clin Pharmacol 30:40, 1977.
243. Leydon JJ, Sulzberger MB: Topical antibiotics and minor skin trauma. Am Fam Physician 23:121, 1981.
244. Eaglstein WH, Mertz PM: "Inert" vehicles do affect wound healing. J Invest Dermatol 74:90, 1980.
245. Geronemus R, Mertz PM, Eaglstein WH: Wound healing: The effects of topical antimicrobial agents. Arch Dermatol 115:1311, 1979.
246. Knutson RA, Merbity LA, Creekmore MA, et al: Use of sugar and povidone-iodine to enhance wound healing: Five years' experience. South Med J 74:1329, 1981.
247. Eaglstein WH, Mertz P, Alvarez OM: Effect of topically applied agents on healing wounds. Clin Dermatol 2:112, 1984.
248. Pollack SV: Systemic drugs and nutritional aspects of wound healing. Clin Dermatol 2:68, 1984.
249. DiPasquale G, Steinetz BG: Relationship of food intake to the effect of cortisone acetate on skin wound healing. Proc Soc Exp Biol Med 117: 118, 1964.
250. Hunt TK, Ehrlich HP, Garcia JA, et al: Effect of vitamin A on reversing the inhibitory effect of cortisone on healing of open wounds in animals and man. Ann Surg 170:633, 1969.
251. Grossman JAI, Adams JP, Kunec J: Prophylactic antibiotics in simple hand injuries. JAMA 245:1055, 1981.
252. Thirlby RC, Blair AJ, Thal ER: The value of prophylactic antibiotics for simple lacerations. Surg Gynecol Obstet 156:212, 1983.
253. Day TK: Controlled trial of prophylactic antibiotics in minor wounds requiring suture. Lancet 4:1174, 1975.
254. Morgan WJ, Hutchison D, Johnson HM: The delayed treatment of wounds of the hand and forearm under antibiotic cover. Br J Surg 67:140, 1980.
255. Roberts AHN, Teddy PJ: A prospective trial of prophylactic antibiotics in hand lacerations. Br J Surg 64:394, 1977.
256. Burke JF: The effective period of preventative antibiotic action in experimental incisions and dermal lesions. Surgery 50:161, 1961.
257. Elenbaas RM, McNabney WK, Robinson WA: Prophylactic oxacillin in dog bite wounds. Ann Emerg Med 11:248, 1982.
258. Callaham M: Prophylactic antibiotics in common dog bite wounds: A controlled study. Ann Emerg Med 9:410, 1980.
259. Elenbaas RM, McNabney WK, Robinson WA: Evaluation of prophylactic oxacillin in cat bite wounds. Ann Emerg Med 13:155, 1984.
260. Boenning D, Fleisher G, Campos J: Dog bites in children: Epidemiology, microbiology, and penicillin prophylactic therapy. Am J Emerg Med 1:17, 1983.
261. Rosen RA: The use of antibiotics in the initial management of recent dog-bite wounds. Am J Emerg Med 3:19, 1985.
262. Jones DA, Stanbridge TN: A clinical trial using co-trimoxazole in an attempt to reduce wound infection rates in dog bite wounds. Postgrad Med J 61:593, 1985.
263. Ordog GJ: Cephradine in the prophylactic treatment of dog bites. Can Fam Physician 32:743, 1986.
264. Lindsey D, Christopher M, Hollenbach J, et al: Natural course of the human bite wound: Incidence of infection and complications in 434 bites and 803 lacerations in the same group of patients. J Trauma 27:45, 1987.
265. Schweich P, Fleisher G: Human bites in children. Pediatr Emerg Care 1:51, 1985.
266. Arons MS: Pasteurella multocida: The major cause of hand infections following domestic animal bites. J Hand Surg 47:47, 1982.
267. Altieri M, Brasch L: Antibiotic prophylaxis in intraoral wounds. Am J Emerg Med 4:507, 1986.
268. Edlich RF, Kenney JG, Morgan RF, et al: Antimicrobial treatment of minor soft tissue lacerations: A critical review. Emerg Med Clin North Am 4:561, 1986.
269. Shulman ST, Amren DP, Bisno AL, et al: Prevention of bacterial endocarditis. Am J Dis Child 139:232, 1985.
270. Callaham M: Controversies in antibiotic choices for bite wounds. Ann Emerg Med 17:1321, 1988.
271. Guba AM, Mulliken JB, Hoopes JE: The selection of antibiotics for human bites of the hand. Plast Reconstr Surg 56:538, 1975.
272. Goldstein EJ, Citron DM, Wield B, et al: Bacteriology of human and animal bite wounds. J Clin Microbiol 8:667, 1978.
273. Stevens DL, Higbee JW, Oberhofer TR, et al: Antibiotic susceptibilities of human isolates of Pasteurella multocida. Antimicrob Agents Chemother 16:322, 1979.
274. Goldstein EJC, Citron DM, Finegold SM: Dog bite wounds and infection: A prospective study. Ann Emerg Med 9:508, 1980.
275. Ordog GJ: The bacteriology of dog bite wounds on initial presentation. Ann Emerg Med 15:1324, 1986.
276. Goldstein EJC, Richwald GA: Human and animal bite wounds. Am Fam Phys 36:101, 1987.
277. Goldstein EJC, Citron DM, Yagvolgyi AE, et al: Susceptibility of bite wound bacteria to seven oral antimicrobial agents, including RU–985, a new erythromycin: Considerations in choosing empiric therapy. Antimicrob Agents Chemother 29:556, 1986.
278. Leyden JJ: Effect of bacteria on healing of superficial wounds. Clin Dermatol 2:81, 1984.
279. Oates JA, Wood AJJ: Antimicrobial prophylaxis in surgery. N Engl J Med 315:1129, 1986.
280. Immunization Practices Advisory Committee, Centers for Disease Control: Diphtheria, tetanus, and pertussis: Guidelines for vaccine prophylaxis and other preventive measures. Morbidity and Mortality Weekly Report 30:392–396, 401–407, 1981.
281. Giangrasso J: Misuse of tetanus immunoprophylaxis in wound care. Ann Emerg Med 14:573, 1985.
282. American College of Surgeons, Committee on Trauma: Early Care of the Injured Patient. 2nd ed. Philadelphia, WB Saunders Co, 1982, pp 68–72.
283. Passen EL, Anderson BR: Clinical tetanus despite a 'protective' level of toxin-neutralizing antibody. JAMA 255:1171, 1986.
284. Stair TO, Lippe MA, Russell H, et al: Tetanus immunity in emergency department patients (abstract). Ann Emerg Med 16:1100, 1987.
285. Brand D, Acampora D, Gottlieb LD, et al: Adequacy of antitetanus prophylaxis in six hospital emergency rooms. N Engl J Med 309:636, 1983.
286. White JD, Stair TO: Antitetanus prophylaxis in the emergency department (letter). Am J Emerg Med 2:280, 1984.
287. Lindsey D: Tetanus prophylaxis—Do our guidelines assure protection? J Trauma 24:1063, 1984.
288. Public Health Service Advisory Committee on Immunization Practices: Rabies. Morbidity and Mortality Weekly Report 25:403, 1976.
289. Fishbein DB: Pre-exposure and postexposure immunization against rabies. In Fishbein DB, Sawyer LA, Winkler WG (eds): Rabies Concepts for Medical Professionals. 2nd ed. Miami, Mérieux Institute, Inc, 1986, pp 49–56.
290. Immunization Practices Advisory Committee: Rabies Prevention—United States, 1984. JAMA 252:883, 1984.

291. Goldberg HM, Rosenthal SAE, Nemetz JC: Effect of washing closed head and neck wounds on wound healing and infection. Am J Surg 141:358, 1981.
292. Noe JM, Keller M: Can stitches get wet? Plast Reconstr Surg 81:82, 1988.
293. Lee KH: Studies on the mechanism of action of salicylates. III. Effect of vitamin A on the wound healing retardation action of aspirin. J Pharm Sci 57: 1238, 1968.
294. Rodeheaver G, Edgerton MT, Smith S, et al: Antimicrobial prophylaxis of contaminated tissues containing suture implants. Am J Surg 133:609, 1977.
295. Peacock EE: Control of wound healing and scar formation in surgical patients. Arch Surg 116:1325, 1981.
296. Ordman LJ, Gillman T: Studies in the healing of cutaneous wounds II. The healing of epidermal, appendageal, and dermal injuries inflicted by suture needles and by the suture material in the skin of pigs. Arch Surg 93:883, 1966.
297. Crikelair CT: Skin suture marks. Am J Surg 96:631, 1958.
298. Myers MB, Cherry G, Heinberger S: Augmentation of wound tensile strength by early removal of sutures. Am J Surg 117:338, 1969.
299. Converse JM, Smith B: The eyelids and their adnexa. In Converse JM (ed): Reconstructive Plastic Surgery: Principles and Procedures in Correction, Reconstruction, and Transplantation. 2nd ed, vol 2. Philadelphia, WB Saunders Co, 1977, pp 858–946.
300. Silloway KA, Morgan RF, Kenney JG, et al: Innovations in skin suture removal. Am J Surg 149:799, 1985.
301. Capperauld I: Sutures in wound repair. In Westaby S (ed): Wound Care. St. Louis, CV Mosby Co, 1986, pp 47–57.

Chapter **44**

Alternative Methods of Skin Closure

Alexander Trott

WOUND STAPLES

Introduction

Use of stapling devices dates back to the early part of this century. Several Russian, Hungarian, and Japanese investigators pioneered various instruments, but it was not until the early 1960s that significant interest in the use of these devices developed in the United States.[1, 2] Since that time, there has been a steady improvement in technology, including the introduction of automatic and disposable devices, precocking mechanisms, and optimal staple configurations.

Automatic stapling devices have become commonplace for closure of surgically made incisions. In recent years, they have found increasing acceptance by clinicians for closure of traumatically induced wounds. This acceptance has been facilitated by animal and human studies that have demonstrated similar results using stapling and suturing. In some aspects, stapling may be superior. In animal models, staples have been shown to cause less wound inflammation, to better preserve wound defense mechanisms, and to be more resistant to wound infection in contaminated wounds.[3–5] Wound tensile strength of stapled wounds has been observed to be equal to sutured wounds.[3, 6]

Clinical studies of patients who have stapled surgical incisions have consistently revealed that there is no significant difference between stapling and suturing when infection rates, healing outcome, and patient acceptance are compared.[7–11] Four important studies have demonstrated that some traumatically induced wounds in both adult and pediatric patients can be closed successfully with staples in the emergency department setting.[12–15] Wound stapling and nylon suture closure of skin compared favorably in five different areas: cosmesis, complication rates, patient tolerance, efficiency of closure, and cost. All four studies demonstrated an equivalent cosmetic outcome for stapling and suturing when scar width, color, general appearance, and suture or staple marks were analyzed. In addition, there was no significant difference in infection rates. In one study, two wounds underwent partial dehiscence after staple removal, but the eventual outcome was satisfactory.[15] Patient tolerance and acceptance of staples was noted as being equal to that of sutures.[12, 13, 15] In one study, however, a higher percentage of patients reported that the staples were more uncomfortable to remove when compared with the suture group.[14]

As in the surgical incision studies, the most significant advantage of wound stapling in the traumatic wound studies, when compared with suturing, was speed of closure. On the average, stapling was three to four times faster than suturing traumatic wounds.[12, 14] The time for actual staple application was 30 seconds or less for a laceration 3 to 5 cm in length.[15] Similar findings in comparison studies of wound closure by staples versus by suture have been reported by MacGregor and colleagues[15a] and Ritchie and Rocke.[15b] Cost has been cited as a disadvantage of staple closure, particularly when large, multistaple (25 to 35), surgical units were the only product available.[15] However, with the introduction of smaller devices, which are more appropriate for the average laceration, the cost of stapling devices has been reduced significantly.[15] Retail cost of the Precise 10-shot stapler is close to five dollars, and the cost of a package of nylon suture varies between two and four dollars. When the reduction of closure time by stapling and the reduced need for wound closure instruments are considered, the cost difference is minimal.[12]

Indications and Contraindications

Currently, the indications for stapling are limited to lacerations located on an extremity, the trunk, or the scalp. Selected wounds should have relatively straight, sharp edges. The most efficacious use of staples is in cases of long, linear lacerations, in which the time of closure is a consideration. They may be especially useful for scalp lacerations in the agitated or intoxicated patient. Staples, as they are currently configured and manufactured, *should never be used on the face, neck, hands, or feet.* They are also not to be placed in scalp wounds if computed tomography head scans are to be performed, because the metallic density will produce scan artifacts. Similarly, staples should not be used if the patient is expected to undergo magnetic resonance imaging, because the powerful magnetic fields may avulse the staples from the skin surface.

Equipment

The required equipment consists of standard wound care instruments as previously described in the section on wound preparation (see Chapter 43). In many cases, when débridement and dermal (deep) closures are unnecessary, only tissue forceps are needed to assist in everting wounds. Many stapling devices are commercially available. The most versatile stapler, and least expensive, is the Precise (3M Corporation, St. Paul, Minn.). Different units can be purchased that have between 5 and 25 staples. The 10-staple unit will suffice for most lacerations. Other devices include the Proximate 11 (Ethicon Inc., Sommerville, N.J.), Cricket (US Surgical, Irvine, Calif.), and Appose (Davis & Geck, Columbus, Ohio). These staplers have a minimum of 15 staples and are three to five times more expensive than the Precise.

Procedure

The wound is prepared in the standard manner. Whenever necessary, deep, absorbable sutures are used to close deep fascia and to reduce tension of the superficial fascia and dermal layers. Before stapling, the wound edges should be everted. A second operator can be helpful for assisting in wound edge eversion. This person precedes the operator along the wound and everts the wound edges with forceps ("pickups") or pinches the skin with the thumb and forefinger. This technique allows the staple to be precisely placed. Once the edges are held in eversion, the staple points are gently approximated to the skin surfaces (Fig. 44–1). By squeezing the stapler handle or trigger, the staple is advanced automatically into the wound and bent to the proper configuration (Figs. 44–2 and 44–3). One must take great care not to plunge too deeply, because this error causes excessive wound ischemia. When properly placed, the *crossbar of the staple is elevated a few millimeters above the skin surface* (Fig. 44–4). Enough staples should be placed to provide proper apposition of the edges of the wound along its entire length.

Once the wound is stapled, an antibiotic ointment may be applied to minimize dressing adherence, and a sterile dressing is put in place. If necessary, the patient can remove the dressing and gently clean the wound in 24 to 48 hours. The length of time that staples are kept in place depends on the type and location of the wound and is equivalent to standard suture removal intervals.

Removal of staples requires a special instrument that is made available by each manufacturer of stapling devices. The lower jaw of the staple remover is placed under the

crossbar (Fig. 44–5). One brings down the upper jaw by squeezing the handle (Fig. 44–6). This action compresses the crossbar, thereby releasing the staple points for easy removal (Fig. 44–7). If the patient is referred for office removal of staple, it may be advisable to provide the patient with the staple removal device on emergency department release, because many physicians do not routinely stock the instrument.

Complications

Complications can occur with staple closure wounds, although the incidence is low. In two studies of traumatically induced stapled wounds, the infection rates were reported to be 0 per cent and 5 per cent.[14, 15] Staple acceptance and comfort have been reported to be equal to those of sutures, but in one study, removal of staples was somewhat more uncomfortable than sutures.[14] Wound dehiscence has been reported, but the incidence is not considered significant.[13] A common error is failure to *evert* the skin edges before stapling to avoid the natural tendency of the device to invert the closure. Eversion may be accomplished with forceps or

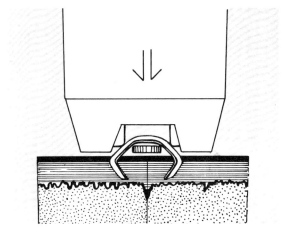

Figure 44–2. By squeezing the stapler handle, a plunger advances one staple into the wound margins. (From Edlich RF: A Manual for Wound Closure. St. Paul, Minn, 3M Medical-Surgical Products, 1979. Reproduced by permission.)

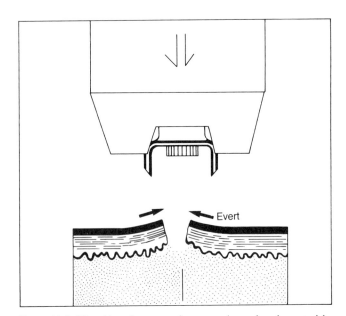

Figure 44–1. The skin edges must be approximated and everted by hand or with forceps before they are secured with staples. Failure to evert the wound edges is a common error that often results in an unacceptable result. (Adapted with permission from Edlich RF: A Manual for Wound Closure. St. Paul, Minn, 3M Medical-Surgical Products, 1979.)

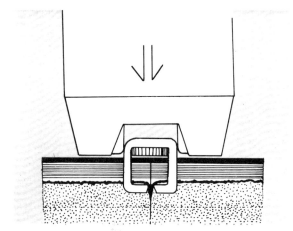

Figure 44–3. An anvil automatically bends the staple to the proper configuration. (From Edlich RF: A Manual for Wound Closure. St. Paul, Minn, 3M Medical-Surgical Products, 1979. Reproduced by permission.)

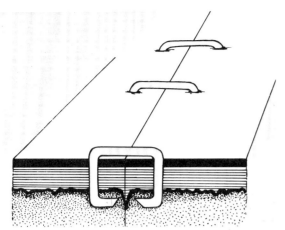

Figure 44–4. Care should be taken to ensure that a space remains between the skin and the crossbar of the staple. Excessive pressure created by placing the staple too deep causes wound edge ischemia as well as pain on removal. Note that the staple bar is 2 to 3 mm above the skin line. (From Edlich RF: A Manual for Wound Closure. St. Paul, Minn, 3M Medical-Surgical Products, 1979. Reproduced by permission.)

by pinching the skin with the thumb and index finger, a procedure that requires some practice.

Conclusion

Overall results are favorable when staples are used for surgical incisions and traumatically induced lacerations of the the scalp, trunk, and extremities. When compared with standard suturing, wound stapling is not significantly different with regard to infection rates, wound healing, and patient acceptance. Stapling is clearly superior in reducing time to closure. With the introduction of new devices, the cost of wound stapling is comparable to that of suturing. Because of the increasing availability and versatility of stapling instruments, increased use of this technique in emergency departments can be anticipated.

WOUND TAPES

Introduction

The use of specially designed tape strips to close simple wounds has become routine in recent years. Tape strips can be applied by

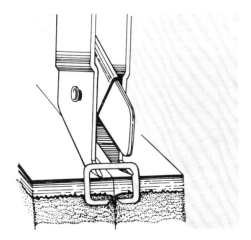

Figure 44–5. The lower jaw of the staple remover is placed under the crossbar of the staple. (From Edlich RF: A Manual for Wound Closure. St. Paul, Minn, 3M Medical-Surgical Products, 1979. Reproduced by permission.)

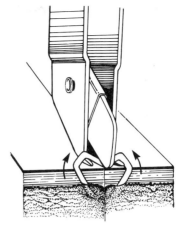

Figure 44–6. By squeezing the handle gently, the upper jaw compresses the staple and allows it to exit the skin. (Adapted with permission from Edlich RF: A Manual for Wound Closure. St. Paul, Minn, 3M Medical-Surgical Products, 1979.)

health care personnel in many settings, including emergency departments, operating rooms, clinics, and first-aid stations. Advantages of tape strips include ease of application, reduced need for local anesthesia, more evenly distributed wound tension, no residual suture marks, no need for suture removal, superiority for some grafts and flaps, and suitability for use under plaster casts. One of the main advantages of wound tapes is their greater resistance to wound infection compared with standard sutures and wound staples.[16–20]

There are also disadvantages to tape closures. Tape does not work well on wounds that are under significant tension or wounds that are very irregular, on concave surfaces, or in areas of marked tissue laxity. In many cases, tape does not provide satisfactory wound edge apposition without underlying deep closures. Tape does not stick well to areas with copious secretions, such as in the axilla, the palms of the hands, the soles of the feet, and the perineum. Tape also has difficulty adhering to wounds that will have copious exudates. Tape strips can also be prematurely removed by young children.

Background

Tape closure of wounds has been reported since 1600 B.C.[21] It was not until the late 1950s, however, with the introduction of woven tapes and nonsensitizing adhesive, that tapes gained widespread acceptance in the United States.[22] Since then, there have

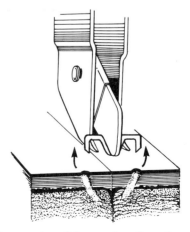

Figure 44–7. Compression of the crossbar allows the staple points to be withdrawn from the wound. (Adapted with permission from Edlich RF: A Manual for Wound Closure. St. Paul, Minn, 3M Medical-Surgical Products, 1979.)

been rapid advances in the manufacture of tapes with increased strength, improved adhesiveness, and presterilized packaging.

Currently, there are several brands of tapes with differing porosity, flexibility, strength, and configuration. Steri-Strips (3M Corporation, St. Paul, Minn.) are microporous tapes with ribbed backing. They are porous to air and water, and the ribbed backing provides extra strength. Cover-Strips (Beiersdorf, South Norwalk, Conn.) are woven in texture and are claimed to have a high degree of porosity. They allow not only air and water but also wound exudates to pass through the tape. Shur-Strip (Deknatel, Inc., Floral Park, N.Y.) is a nonwoven microporous tape, which, like the Cover-Strips and Steri-Strip is designed to permit the passage of gas and water through the tapes. Clearon (Ethicon, Inc., Somerville, N.J.) is a synthetic plastic tape whose backing contains longitudinal parallel serrations to permit gas and fluid permeability. An iodoform-impregnated tape, Steri-Strip (3M Corporation, St. Paul, Minn.), is intended to further retard infection without increased sensitization to iodine.[16] Other tape products include Curi-strip (Kendall, Boston, Mass.), Nichi-Strip (Nichiban Co., Ltd, Tokyo, Japan), Cicagraf (Smith & Nephew, London, England), Suture-Strip (Genetic Laboratories, St. Paul, Minn.), and Suture-Strip Plus.

Scientific studies of the tapes have been limited, and, because of different investigators' choices of products and methods, it is not always easy to interpret the results when comparing study with study. Koehn showed that the Steri-Strip tapes maintained adhesiveness approximately 50 per cent longer than Clearon Tape.[23] Rodeheaver and coworkers compared Shur-Strip, Steri-Strip, and Clearon tape in terms of breaking strength, elongation, shear adhesion, and air porosity.[24] The tapes were tested in both dry and wet conditions. The Steri-Strip tape was found to have approximately twice the breaking strength of the other two tapes in both dry and wet conditions with minimal loss of strength in all tapes when wetted. The Shur-Strip tapes showed approximately two to three times the elongation of the other tapes at the breaking point (whether dry or wet). The shear adhesion (amount of force required to dislodge the tape when a load is applied in the place of contact (angle = 0 degrees) was slightly better for the Shur-Strip tape than for the Steri-Strip tape and approximately 50 per cent better than for the Clearon tape. Of these three wound tapes, Shur-Strips were concluded to be superior for wound closure.

One comprehensive study of wound tapes compared Curi-Strip, Steri-Strip, Nichi-Strip, Cicagraf, Suture-Strip, and Suture-Strip Plus.[25] All tapes were 12 mm wide except for Nichi-Strip, which was 15 mm. Each tape was compared for breaking strength, elongation under stress, air porosity, and adhesiveness. Curi-Strip, Cicagraf, and Steri-Strip exhibited equivalent dry breaking strengths. However, when wet (a condition that can occur in the clinical setting), Cicagraf outperformed all tapes. All of the tested tapes had similar elongation-under-stress profiles with the exception of Suture-Strip Plus. This tape did not resist elongation under low or high forces. Excessive elongation may create a condition under which the wound could be disrupted. Nichi-Strip was the most porous to air, and Cicagraf was close to vapor impermeable. Nichi-Strip and Curi-Strip had the best adherence to untreated skin. When the skin was treated with tincture of benzoin, however, Steri-Strip dramatically outperformed all other products. When all of the study parameters were considered, Nichi-Strip, Curi-Strip, and Steri-Strip achieved the highest overall performance rankings.

Indications

The predominant indication for tape closure is a superficial straight laceration under little tension. If necessary, tension can be reduced by undermining or placing deep closures. Areas particularly suited for tape closure are the forehead, chin, malar eminence, thorax, and nonjoint areas of the extremities. Tape may also be preferred for wounds in children when painful suture placement and removal are not essential. Care must be taken to estimate the potential for premature tape removal by a child.

In an experimental study using guinea pigs, Edlich and colleagues demonstrated that taped wounds inoculated with *Staphylococcus aureus* at various known concentrations resisted

infection better than wounds closed with nylon.[19] Therefore, tape closures can be used on wounds with potential for infection when standard suture closure is not essential. Tape closures work well under plaster casts when superficial suture closures cannot be used. Efron and Ger, in 1968, and Weisman, in 1963, demonstrated the efficacy of using tape to successfully hold flaps and grafts in place.[16, 17] Anatomic areas in which taping of grafts and flaps was useful included the fingers, the flat areas of the extremities, and the trunk. A difficult site to close wounds is the pretibial area. This area is particularly problematic in the elderly because of tissue atrophy. One group has reported that wound tapes outperformed suture closure of the pretibial area with regard to time to healing and complications (Fig. 44–8).[26] Tape closures can be applied to wounds following early suture removal to maintain wound edge approximation while reducing the chance of permanent suture mark scarring. Finally, because of the minimal skin tension created by tapes, they can be used on skin that has been compromised by vascular insufficiency or altered by prolonged use of steroids.

Contraindications

Tape closures are contraindicated in wounds that are irregular or under tension and in those that cannot be

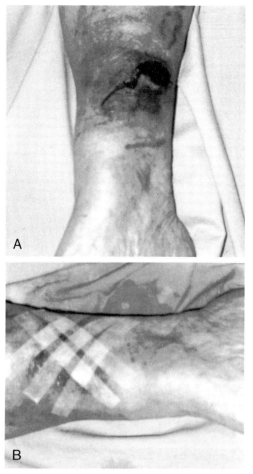

Figure 44–8. *A*, A pretibial skin avulsion is an ideal wound to close with Steri-Strips. *B*, An elderly woman who was on steroids had extremely thin skin that could not be replaced with sutures but healed nicely when Steri-Strips held the skin in place similar to a skin graft.

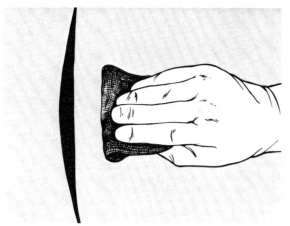

Figure 44–9. After wound preparation (and placement of deep closures, if needed), dry the skin thoroughly at least 2 inches around the wound.

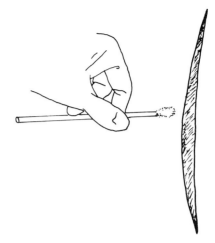

Figure 44–10. If desired, apply a very thin coating of tincture of benzoin around the wound.

appropriately dried of blood or secretions. They are of little value on lax and intertriginous skin, on naturally moist areas, and in the scalp and beard areas.

Tapes should never be placed circumferentially around a digit, because they have no ability to stretch or lengthen. If placed circumferentially, the natural wound edema of an injured digit can make the tape act like a constricting band and can lead to ischemia and possible necrosis of the digit. Semicircular or spiral placement techniques should be used if digits are to be taped.

Equipment

For a simple tape closure, the required equipment includes forceps and tape of the proper size. Most taping can be done in the emergency department with 1/4-inch by 3-inch strips. In wounds larger than 4 cm, however, 1/2-inch wide strips might be desirable. Most companies manufacture strips up to 1 inch wide and up to 4 inches in length. Standard suture instruments should also be available (see Chapter 43).

Procedure

Actual application of the tape must be preceded by proper wound preparation, irrigation, débridement, and hemostasis. The hair is clipped or shaved, and the area of the tape application is thoroughly dried to ensure proper

adhesion. Tincture of benzoin can be applied initially to increase tape adhesion.[19] The physician should use sterile technique at all times. Wound tapes do not adhere unduly to surgical gloves, and sterile glove use allows the operator to maintain proper sterile technique. All tapes come in presterilized packages and can be opened directly onto the operating field.

After the wound has been dried (Fig. 44–9) and tincture of benzoin has been applied (Fig. 44–10), the tapes, with backing attached, are cut to the desired length (Fig. 44–11). Tapes should be long enough to allow for approximately 2 to 3 cm of overlap on each side of the wound. After the tape is cut to length, the end tab is removed (Fig. 44–12). The tape is gently removed from the backing with forceps by pulling straight back (Fig. 44–13). Do not pull to the side, because the tape will curl and be difficult to apply to the wound. One half of the tape is securely placed at the midportion of the wound (Fig. 44–14). The opposite wound edge is gently but firmly apposed to its counterpart (Fig. 44–15). The second half of the tape is then applied. The wound edges should be as close together as possible and at equal height to prevent the development of a linear, pitting scar. Additional tapes are applied by bisecting the remainder of the wound (Fig. 44–16). Enough tapes should be placed so that complete apposition is provided without totally occluding the wound edges (Fig. 44–17). Finally, additional cross tapes are placed to add support as well as to prevent blistering, which may be caused by unsupported tape ends (Fig. 44–18).[18]

Taped wounds are left open, without occlusive dress-

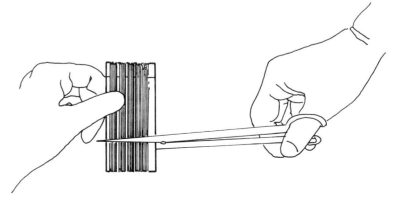

Figure 44–11. Cut the tapes to the desired length before removing from the backing.

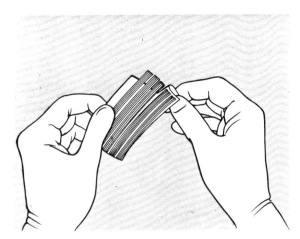

Figure 44–12. The tapes are attached to a card with perforated tabs on both ends. Gently peel the end tab from the tapes.

Figure 44–13. Use forceps to peel the tape off the card backing. Pull directly backward, not to the side.

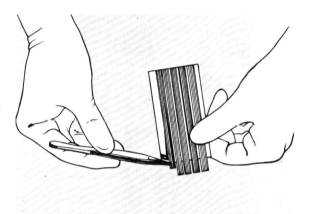

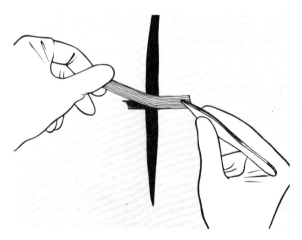

Figure 44–14. Place one half of first tape at the midportion of the wound. Secure firmly in place.

Figure 44–15. Gently but firmly appose the opposite side of the wound, using the free hand or forceps.

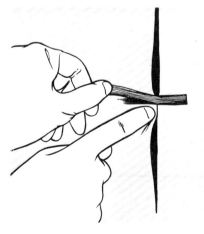

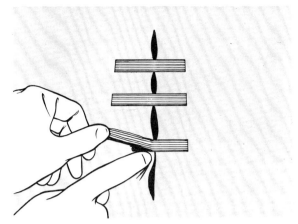

Figure 44–16. The tape should be applied by bisecting the wound until the wound is closed satisfactorily.

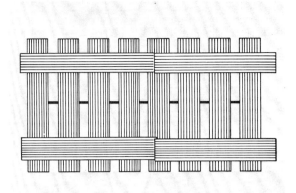

Figure 44–18. Additional supporting tapes are placed approximately 1 inch from the wound and parallel to the wound direction. Taping in this manner prevents skin blistering that may occur at tape ends.

ings. Adhesive bandages (Band-Aids) and other dressings promote excessive moisture, which can lead to premature tape separation from the wound. The Band-Aid also may adhere to the closure tapes, causing separation of the closure tape from the skin at the time of the Band-Aid removal. Tapes may remain in place for approximately 2 weeks and, in some cases, longer. The desired time of application is a decision that varies with the requirements of each wound. The patient can be allowed to clean the taped laceration gently with a moist soft cloth after 24 to 48 hours. If excessive wetting or mechanical force is used, however, premature separation may result. Patients may be instructed to gently trim curled edges of the closure tape with fine scissors to avoid premature avulsion of the tape.

Complications

Complications are uncommon with tape closure. The infection rate is approximately 5 per cent in clean wounds closed with tape.[18] This rate compares favorably with other standard closures. Premature tape separation occurs in approximately 3 percent of cases.[24] Other complications include skin blistering, if the tape is not properly anchored with the cross-stay strip, and wound hematoma, if hemostasis is not accomplished.

When tincture of benzoin is used, it should be applied carefully to the surrounding uninjured skin, because an increased wound infection rate has been noted if spillage

occurs into the raw wound surface.[27] Benzoin vapors have also been known to cause patient discomfort when applied near a wound that has not been anesthetized.

Conclusion

Most investigators believe that the results of proper tape closure are as successful as those of suture closure.[18, 21] Other investigators, however, believe that tape closure leads to inferior cosmetic results.[28] In the aggregate, however, modern tape products and techniques have earned a role in minor wound care management in emergency departments.

HAIR TYING OF SCALP WOUNDS

Introduction

Scalp wounds that gape have traditionally been closed with suture material or more recently with skin staples. One "folk method" of scalp wound closure that has received limited discussion[29] or study[30] is the technique of closing the wound by typing "roped" strands of hair from opposite sides of the wound together.

The advantages of this technique are that no surgical instruments are required, no foreign material is placed in the wound, and it is relatively painless, because a local anesthetic injection is not needed. This technique may be of particular value in wilderness settings, in which wound repair equipment is unavailable and the wound is relatively clean. In certain superficial scalp wounds in children, this technique offers a particularly humane method of wound closure.

Indications and Contraindications

Closure by hair tying is a technique that can be used on small scalp wounds (1 to 2 cm in length). Davies suggests the following criteria for consideration of this technique[30]: (1) the patient's hair must be of adequate length to form "roped" strands that can be tied across the wound, (2) the wound edges should not be contused, (3) there should be no gross wound contamination, (4) there must be good wound hemostasis, (5) the galea (occipitofrontalis aponeurosis) must not be divided, and (6) there must be no underlying skull fracture.

When these conditions cannot be met, the technique should not be undertaken. If local anesthesia must be used to permit evaluation of the deep structures of the wound, it

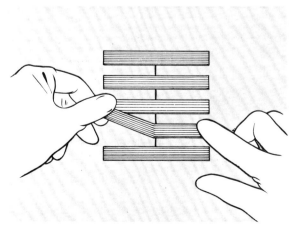

Figure 44–17. Wound margins are completely apposed.

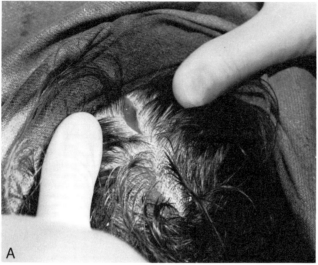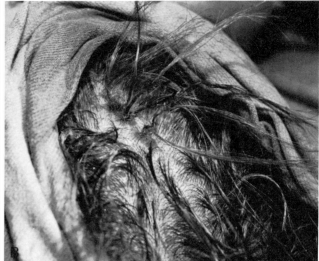

Figure 44–19. *A,* Hair on each side of a laceration is twisted to form "ropes" of hair. *B,* The "roped" strands are tied across the wound in a surgical knot along with additional throws to appose the skin edges.

may be best to simply repair the wound with sutures or staples.

Procedure

When possible, the area surrounding the wound should be cleansed with mild disinfectant, taking care not to place any in the unanesthetized wound. The wound should be irrigated gently but vigorously with normal saline. Exploration of the wound using a gloved hand or cotton-tipped applicator should be gently performed to verify that the galea is not compromised and that no foreign material remains in the wound.

Hair on each side of the laceration is then twisted to form "ropes" of hair (Fig. 44–19A). These "roped" strands are tied across the wound in a surgical knot with several additional throws (Fig. 46–19B) to tightly appose the skin edges. Davies recommends spraying the knot with a plastic sealant to avoid loosening of the knot.[30]

Postclosure wound care is similar to that of routine scalp closure. The patient may gently shampoo the hair, but *vigorous* hair massage or combing in the area should be avoided. The knot is allowed to grow away from the wound edge and can be cut free in 2 to 4 weeks by the parents.

Complications

In one series of 25 children under 8 years of age with scalp wounds closed by hair tying, 48-hour follow-up showed no evidence of wound infection and two cases of mild (2 to 4 mm) wound separation.[30] The investigators noted that some of the children complained of "my hair is being pulled" during wound closure, but all cooperated without restraints or anesthesia. The most common complaint noted at follow-up was that the hair-tie knot was untidy.

Conclusion

The hair tying technique for closure of scalp wounds offers an attractive alternative for small, superficial scalp wounds in children and for scalp wound repair in wilderness settings.

References

1. Cooper P, Christie S: Development of the surgical stapler with emphasis on vascular anastomosis. Trans NY Acad Sci 25:365, 1963.
2. Steichen FM, Ravitch MM: Mechanical sutures in surgery. Br J Surg 60:191, 1973.
3. Windle BH, Roth JH: Comparison of staple-closed and sutured skin incisions in a pig model. Surg Forum 35:546, 1984.
4. Johnson A, Rodeheaver GT, Durand LS, et al: Automatic disposable stapling devices for wound closure. Ann Emerg Med 10:631, 1981.
5. Stillman RM, Marino CA, Seligman SJ: Skin staples in potentially contaminated wounds. Arch Surg 119:821, 1984.
6. Roth JH, Windle BH: Staple versus suture closure of skin incisions in a pig model. Can J Surg 31:19, 1988.
7. Meiring L, Cilliers K, Barry R, et al: A comparison of a disposable skin stapler and nylon sutures for wound closure. South Afr Med J 62:371, 1982.
8. Lennihan R, Macereth M: A comparison of staples and nylon closure in varicose vein surgery. Vasc Surg 9:200, 1975.
9. Steele RJC, Chetty V, Forrest APM: Staples or sutures for mastectomy wounds? A randomized trial. J Roy Coll Surg (Edinb) 28:17, 1983.
10. Nilsson T, Frimødt-Moller C, Jeppensen N: Long-term cosmetic results comparing Proximate with Dermalon skin closure. Ann Chir Gyn 74:30, 1985.
11. Harvey CF, Hume CJ: A prospective trial of skin staples and sutures in skin closure. Ir J Med Sci 155:194, 1986.
12. Shuster M: Comparing skin staples to sutures in an emergency department. Can Fam Phys 35:505, 1989.
13. Dunmire SM, Yealy DM, Karasic R, et al: Staples for wound closure in the pediatric population. Ann Emerg Med 18:448., 1989.
14. George TK, Simpson DC: Skin wound closure with staples in the Accident and Emergency Department. J Roy Coll Surg (Edinb) 30:54, 1985.
15. Brickman KR, Lambert RW: Evaluation of skin stapling for wound closure in the emergency department. Ann Emerg Med 18:1122, 1989.
15a. MacGregor FB, McCombe AW, King PM, et al: Skin stapling of wounds in the accident department. Injury 20:347, 1989.
15b. Ritchie AJ, Rocke LG: Staples versus sutures in the closure of scalp wounds: a prospective, double-blind, randomized trial. Injury 20:217, 1989.
16. Efron G, Ger R: Use of adhesive tape (Steri-Strips) to secure skin grafts. Am J Surg 116:474, 1968.
17. Weisman PA: Microporous surgical tape in wound closure and skin grafting. Br J Plast Surg 16:379, 1963.
18. Connolly WB, Hunt TK, Zederfeldt B, et al: Clinical comparison of surgical wounds closed by suture and adhesive tape. Am J Surg 117:318, 1969.
19. Edlich RF, Rodeheaver GT, Kuphal J, et al: Technique of closure: Contaminated wounds. JACEP 3:375, 1974.
20. Johnson A, Rodeheaver GT, Kuphal J, et al: Automatic disposable stapling device for wound closure. Ann Emerg Med 10:631, 1981.
21. Emmett AJJ, Barron JN: Adhesive suture strip closure of wounds in plastic surgery. Br J Plast Surg 17:175, 1964.
22. Golden T: Nonirritating, multipurpose surgical adhesive tape. Am J Surg 100:789, 1960.

23. Koehn GG: A comparison of the duration of adhesion of Steri-Strips and Clearon. Cutis 26:620, 1980.
24. Rodeheaver GT, Halverson JM, Edlich RF: Mechanical performance of wound closure tapes. Ann Emerg Med 12:203, 1983.
25. Rodeheaver GT, Spengler MD, Edlich RF: Performance of new wound closure tapes. J Emerg Med 5:451, 1987.
26. Sutton R, Pritty P: Use of sutures or adhesive tapes for primary closure of pretibial lacerations. Br Med J 290:1627, 1985.
27. Panek PH, Prusak MP, Bolt D, et al: Potentiation of wound infection by adhesive adjuncts. Am Surg 38:343, 1972.
28. Ellenberg AH: Surgical tape wound closure: A disenchantment. J Plast Reconstr Surg 39:625, 1967.
29. Officer C: Scalp lacerations in children. Aust Fam Physician 10:970, 1981.
30. Davies MJ: Scalp wounds: An alternative to suture. Injury 19:375, 1988.

Chapter **45**

Skin Grafting in the Outpatient

Seung K. Kim and Lars M. Vistnes

INTRODUCTION

Skin grafting allows one to close a clean wound that cannot be closed primarily because of an insufficient skin cover. The wound could be traumatic or secondary to surgical excision or skin loss caused by a burn injury. The skin is a natural barrier between the body and the environment. Early coverage of an open wound and reestablishment of this barrier is essential in the restoration of the internal equilibrium and the prevention of further wound complications. Although uncommonly performed in the emergency department, minor skin grafting can be done easily in the outpatient setting with a minimum of equipment. When recipient site preparation, selection of the skin graft and dressing, and aftercare of the graft are carefully performed with a knowledge of the physiology of skin grafting, the results are excellent.

TYPES OF SKIN GRAFTS

The skin is composed of the epidermis and the dermis. Many of the skin appendages, such as hair follicles, sebaceous glands, and sweat glands, are located within the dermis (Fig. 45–1). A *full-thickness skin graft* contains the entire thickness of the epidermis and the dermis. As a result, if the graft is taken from a hair-bearing area, hair characteristic of the donor site may grow on the transplanted full-thickness skin graft. Other than for occasional use in resurfacing of the palmar aspect of the hand and the fingers, a full-thickness skin graft is rarely indicated in emergency situations.

A *split-thickness skin graft* includes the full thickness of the epidermis and a partial thickness of the dermis (see Fig. 45–1). Depending on the thickness, split-thickness skin grafts can be classified as thin, intermediate, and thick. A thin split-thickness skin graft is roughly 0.008 to 0.010 inches in thickness; an intermediate split-thickness skin graft is 0.012 to 0.014 inches. A thick split-thickness skin graft is usually from 0.015 to 0.025 inches thick. The numeric measurement of thickness is only a guide. The descriptive terminology of thin, intermediate, and thick split-thickness skin grafts is more applicable. Graft thickness can be judged by the appearance of the graft and the donor site. The thicker the grafts, the more opaque they are. The edges of the thicker graft tend to curl up more. The donor site for a thin split-thickness skin graft shows a velvety field of numerous very fine bleeding points. The bleeding pattern of a thick split-thickness skin graft donor site is much coarser. The punctate bleeding points are larger in size and fewer in number.

Once the skin grafts are harvested, they tend to shrink quickly as a result of the inherent elasticity of the dermal element. The thicker the graft, the greater the potential for shrinking. A thin split-thickness skin graft barely shows evidence of shrinking, whereas the full-thickness skin graft shrinks markedly. As the skin grafts heal and undergo maturation, progressive contraction of the skin graft is evident. The degree of contraction again depends on the thickness of the graft. Thin split-thickness skin grafts contract the most, whereas full-thickness skin grafts show minimal evidence of contraction. Skin grafts acquire pigmentation as they mature. The degree of pigmentation is also dependent on the thickness of the skin graft. A thin split-thickness skin graft is more apt to develop a dark pigmentation than is a thicker split-thickness skin graft or a full-thickness skin graft. The problem of pigmentation is worse in skin grafts on sun-exposed areas of the body.

GRAFT REVASCULARIZATION

A skin graft adheres to the recipient bed and is initially held by a fibrin network from the recipient bed. For the first 48 hours, survival of the skin graft is largely dependent on serum imbibition. The endothelial channels of the skin graft become filled with serum-like fluid from the recipient bed. This is thought to be brought about by capillary action and diffusion within the skin graft. The nutritional supply and the metabolic exchange are carried out through this fluid medium.[1] Some believe that the main function of this phase of serum imbibition is to prevent the graft from drying and to keep the vessels open for later communication with the recipient vessels.[2]

During this early phase of serum imbibition, restoration of hemic circulation proceeds concurrently, evidenced by gradual change of the color of the graft from pale white to pink. There are three mechanisms that are believed to be

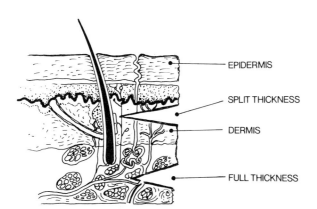

Figure 45–1. A schematic diagram of a cross section of the skin, demonstrating split-thickness and full-thickness skin grafts.

EPIDERMIS

SPLIT THICKNESS

DERMIS

FULL THICKNESS

responsible for revascularization: (1) end-to-end connection of the blood vessels between the recipient bed and the skin graft, known as *inosculation*[3]; (2) ingrowth of vessels from the recipient bed into the preexisting endothelial channels of the skin graft; and (3) ingrowth of endothelial buds into the dermis of the skin graft.[4] Through these mechanisms, normal circulation is restored in the skin graft in anywhere from 4 to 7 days.[5]

The same mechanisms of graft survival and revascularization apply to split-thickness skin grafts and full-thickness skin grafts. A thin split-thickness skin graft, however, can be maintained longer on imbibition alone. This is attributed to the fact that thinner grafts have a shorter distance for diffusion and less cellular mass to be nourished. Revascularization of a thin split-thickness skin graft is also more rapid than revascularization of a thick split-thickness graft or a full-thickness graft for the same reason.[6]

RECIPIENT BED

Skin grafts can be placed on any exposed vascular surface. This includes all the musculoskeletal tissue and all the internal organs. Skin grafts do not survive on nonvascular surfaces, such as bare bone without periosteum, bare cartilage without perichondrium, and bare tendon without paratenon cover. A skin graft can bridge over a nonvascular area by vascularization through the graft edge, however. Up to 5 mm of skin graft from the edge can be vascularized. Hence, theoretically, a maximum of 10 mm of nonvascular area can be covered by bridging, provided that there is an adequate vascular rim of recipient bed at the perimeter of the skin graft.

One can best ensure that the graft will "take" by careful recipient bed preparation. All the nonviable tissue is removed surgically from the wound, creating a well-vascularized surface. Meticulous hemostasis of the recipient bed is also a key to a successful graft.

DONOR SITE HEALING

The surface of the split-thickness graft donor site is a raw dermal surface with multiple openings into the remaining portions of the transected skin appendages, such as sweat ducts and glands, sebaceous glands, and hair shafts and follicles. These appendages are lined with squamous epithelium and are the source of epithelial cells for resurfacing of the exposed dermal surface. The epithelial cells proliferate, migrate out to the dermal surface, and spread radially until they become confluent and cover the entire raw surface. The dermal layer itself may become thicker with scar tissue but does not regenerate. As the thickness of the split-thickness skin graft becomes greater, fewer skin appendages are left in the donor surface. For this reason, the donor site of a thick split-thickness graft takes longer to heal than the donor site of a thinner split-thickness graft. Once the donor site is re-epithelialized, its appearance is again dependent on the graft thickness. A thin split-thickness skin graft donor site containing a thicker residual dermis and more of its skin appendages is closer to its surrounding skin in appearance and is less conspicuous than a thicker split-thickness graft donor site, which has a thin, scarred dermis with fewer remaining skin appendages.

UNFAVORABLE FACTORS

Several factors adversely influence the outcome of skin grafting. They either interfere with the revascularization process or disturb the neovascular network that has already been formed.

1. *Hematoma and seroma.* A hematoma is the most common cause of skin graft failure. A hematoma under the skin graft causes separation of the skin graft from its bed. Consequently, revascularization of the graft is delayed or altogether prevented by the space-occupying effect of this intervening layer of blood or blood clot. The skin graft may survive for a short period on serum imbibition alone. If revascularization is delayed beyond this period of serum imbibition, however, the graft is doomed to fail. To prevent hematoma, one should obtain complete hemostasis of the graft bed prior to application of a skin graft. If complete hemostasis is not possible, the wound should be redressed, and skin grafting should be delayed for one to a few days. A seroma also prevents graft adherence and revascularization through a mechanism similar to that of a hematoma.

2. *Movement.* As discussed before, graft survival depends on reconstitution of the capillary vascular network between the recipient bed and the skin graft. It is easy to see how even the smallest motion of the skin graft relative to the recipient bed could disrupt and interfere with the formation of these fine, early vascular connections. Movement also promotes formation of a seroma or a hematoma. For these reasons, immobilization of the graft to its bed is essential in graft healing.

3. *Necrosis.* Any residual nonviable tissue left in the recipient bed will undergo necrosis and will lead to failure of the overlying graft. In particular, the vascularity of fatty tissue in a traumatic wound is often uncertain. Bits of fat may die and necrose. Again, it is very important to débride all the tissues of questionable vascularity before grafting. If the vascularity of the recipient bed is uncertain, it is best to delay skin grafting.

4. *Infection.* Despite its devastating effect on skin grafting, infection is the least common cause of graft failure. In addition to the obvious space-occupying effect of infection, a purulent collection actively separates the graft from its bed and destroys the newly formed vessels. The abundant proteolytic enzymes from inflammation and from the microorganisms are responsible for the lysis of the fibrin adhesion and the destruction of vascular connections. The most notable virulent organism that affects skin grafting is group A β-hemolytic streptococcus, which rapidly destroys the skin graft and literally melts it away. With prophylactic antibiotic coverage, this complication is seen less often.

INDICATIONS AND CONTRAINDICATIONS FOR SKIN GRAFTING

Whether to close a wound or to leave it open to heal by secondary intention depends on the nature and the history of formation of the wound. Traumatic open wounds may be classified as either clean or contaminated. The majority of traumatic wounds can be considered clean, except for those resulting from bites, those made in a contaminated environment, and those that are 24 or more hours old. Of particular concern is wound contamination by microorganisms. Wounds that contain inorganic material, such as gravel, pieces of broken glass, metal, industrial lubricant, and the like, are not necessarily extensively contaminated. As long as there is no suspicion of major contamination by microorganisms, these wounds can be made clean by débridement and removal of foreign substances. Untidy wounds resulting from tearing, crushing, mangling, or explosive injuries with devitalized tissue debris can also be débrided and converted to clean, tidy wounds. In general, all clean wounds should be closed when possible, and most of the contaminated wounds should be left open.

When there is loss of full thickness of skin and the wound cannot be closed with local tissue alone, closure with a distant tissue is considered. Relatively superficial wounds are most often closed with split-thickness skin grafts. For those wounds in which graft color, texture match, and graft contraction are not of concern, a split-thickness skin graft is an ideal wound cover. In fact, a split-thickness skin graft is often used because of this propensity to undergo contraction. For instance, a split-thickness skin graft on a finger tip wound would contract, pulling the surrounding healthy pulp pad skin over the tissue defect, and would minimize the size of the wound. On the other hand, certain anatomic areas, such as the face and the flexion surface of the hand and the fingers, require coverage that produces minimal contraction. Facial wounds also demand color and texture match. These requirements are best met by full-thickness skin grafts. If deep structures, such as neurovascular bundle, tendon, bone, and joint, are exposed, some other means of distant tissue cover in addition to skin grafting may be considered.

Skin grafting of selected acute wounds in an outpatient setting is beneficial. Grafting affords early closure of the wound and obviates further wound complications, such as desiccation of exposed structures, repeated trauma to tissue, and infection. Grafting may decrease the degree and the length of morbidity significantly. For example, when grafted, a finger tip wound greater than 1 cm² in size would heal much sooner than a wound of equal size that is allowed to close by contraction and epithelialization. Grafted wounds are also more comfortable for the patient than open wounds.

SELECTION OF DONOR SITE

In theory, a skin graft should be able to be taken from anywhere on the body. Indeed, numerous donor sites are necessary when large areas need to be covered, as in a major burn injury. For smaller wounds, the functional and cosmetic quality of the skin graft at the recipient site and the resulting donor site deformity dictates the selection of the donor site.

A full-thickness skin graft is usually taken from a glabrous area of the body. There are many favored areas for taking full-thickness skin grafts. Among them, the hypothenar skin, the antecubital flexion creases, the wrist flexion crease, and the medial arm are most readily accessible and appropriate for emergency outpatient situations.

When a thin split-thickness skin graft is desired (as is the case for most emergency department skin grafting), the anteromedial aspect of the forearm is suitable. Some have expressed objections to this site, claiming obvious scarring in a frequently exposed area. Yet, in experienced hands, a very thin split-thickness skin graft from this area leaves minimal to no appreciable scarring.[7] The posterolateral aspect of the thighs, the buttocks, and the lower abdomen are also available for skin grafting. Relatively thicker skin grafts can be taken safely from these areas. In young women, the graft may be taken within the bikini line to conceal the donor site scar.

EQUIPMENT (DERMATOMES)

There are many different types of dermatomes, varying from simple hand-held instruments to more complex mechanical devices. For outpatient use in an emergency facility, hand-held dermatomes are quite adequate. Only those that are useful for outpatient skin grafting are described here.

Scalpel Blade. A scalpel blade is the simplest dermatome. A number 10 or 20 blade is quite effective for taking a small split-thickness skin graft.

Razor Blade. A sterile, regular double-edged razor blade can be used to take a small skin graft. The razor blade is held with a straight clamp and is used in a freehand manner (Fig. 45–2). Varying thicknesses of split-thickness skin grafts can be cut with this dermatome. The thickness of the skin graft can be judged by the clarity with which the writing on the blade can be read through the skin graft. One can see through the usual thin and intermediate-thickness skin grafts quite readily.

Silver Dermatome. This dermatome consists of a handle and a platform at the opposite end that holds a regular, double-edged razor blade. The razor blade is fixed in place with a cover plate, which is secured with a wing nut. There is a roller just above and parallel to the blade edge. The thickness of the graft can be adjusted by setting the distance between the roller and the blade, which is accomplished by turning the knobs at the ends of the blade (Fig. 45–3). This is only a rough guide; the final product depends on the physician's touch and experience.

Goulian-Weck Knife. This knife is another freehand dermatome. The instrument consists of a handle with a metal slot at one end that holds a safety razor blade measuring 5.5 cm in length. Over this assembly, a blade guard is

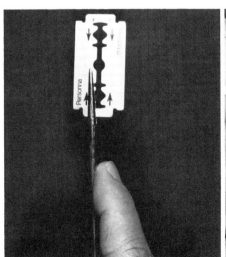
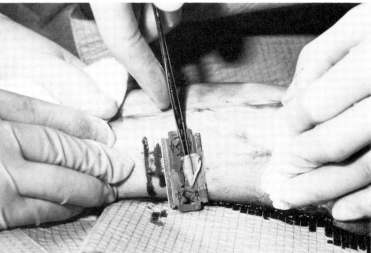

Figure 45–2. A regular double-edged razor blade used as a dermatome.

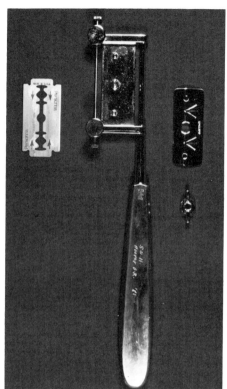

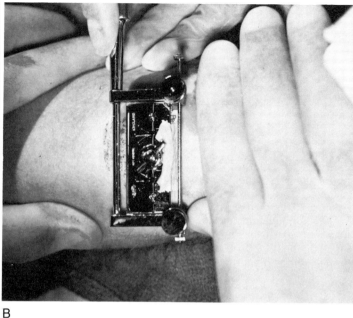

B

Figure 45–3. *A,* Components of the silver dermatome. *B,* The assembled dermatome in use.

A

placed (Fig. 45–4). The blade guard determines the thickness of the skin graft. Three different blade guards with thicknesses of 0.008, 0.010, and 0.012 inches are available. Although these guards are made to cut skin grafts of fixed thicknesses, after repeated use they become sprung and are

not very reliable. These blade guards should be used as rough guides to the thickness of the skin graft. The actual thickness should be controlled visually and by touch.

Humby Knife. This knife is the largest freehand dermatome available. The blade mechanism is similar to that of

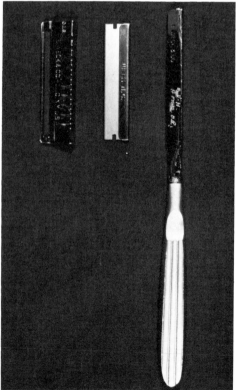

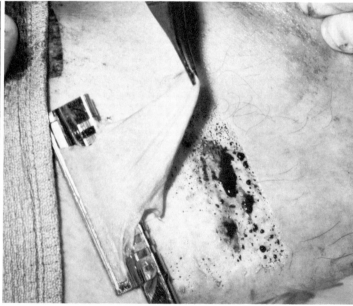

B

Figure 45–4. *A,* Components of the Goulian-Weck dermatome. *B,* The assembled Goulian-Weck dermatome.

A

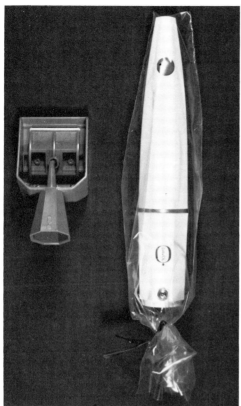

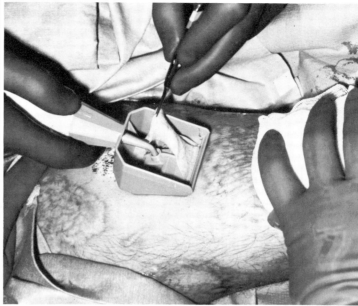

B

Figure 45–5. A Davol disposable dermatome head driven by the battery-operated motor unit in the handle.

A

the Silver dermatome. The device uses a large, single-edged blade that is fixed to a handle. An adjustable roller determines the thickness of the graft.

Davol Disposable Dermatome. A sterile, disposable blade unit that cuts a split-thickness skin graft of intermediate thickness and 3.5 cm in width is available from Davol (Davol Inc., Providence, R.I.). This blade unit is driven by a battery-operated motor in an electric toothbrush handle unit (Fig. 45–5). The handle is placed in a sterile plastic bag. The blade unit is then pushed onto the handle, puncturing the plastic bag, and is attached to the handle. The device is operated by pressure placed on the button switch while the blade unit is kept lightly pressed against the skin with an equally light forward force to advance the dermatome. The battery in the handle is rechargeable through a recharging unit.

HARVESTING OF SKIN GRAFT

The donor site is prepared with any of the number of surgical preparation solutions that are available. Local anesthetic (1 per cent or 0.5 per cent lidocaine [Xylocaine] and 1:100,000 or 1:200,000 epinephrine solution) is used for anesthesia and hemostasis. An area larger than the size of the desired graft is infiltrated. The plane of anesthetic infiltration is in the deep dermis. The anesthetic solution is injected continuously while the needle is being passed back and forth in multiple parallel passes. A 25- or 27-gauge hypodermic needle 1.5 inches in length is used. This results in uniform infiltration of the entire area, forming an evenly elevated plateau (Fig. 45–6).

Full-Thickness Skin Graft. The size and the shape of the wound to be covered are measured on the donor site with a template made of any flat sheet of material that is available, such as glove wrapping paper or a piece of foil

from a suture package. A lenticular pattern of skin that contains the graft pattern is designed. One should plan carefully to orient the long axis of the pattern parallel to the adjacent skin creases; this allows primary closure of the donor defect and produces favorable orientation of the resulting scar. Using a scalpel, a skin incision is made along the lenticular pattern. The full thickness of the skin is removed by running the blade of the scalpel along the junction between the dermis and the subcutaneous fat. Fat is then removed from the graft by stretching it over a finger with the epithelial side down and snipping the bits of fat from the dermal surface with a pair of small scissors. The graft pattern is cut, and the skin graft is then ready for placement.

Often the patient presents to the emergency department with a portion of the finger tip, which has been removed in

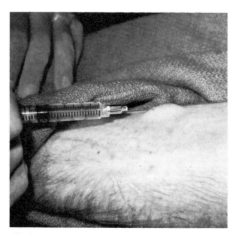

Figure 45–6. The infiltration of anesthetic in the donor site.

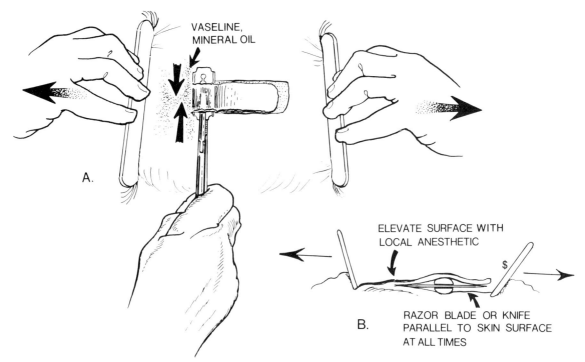

Figure 45–7. *A*, The cutting of a split-thickness skin graft with a double-edged razor blade held in a straight clamp. The skin is held taut by traction and countertraction. *B*, A tangential excision producing a skin graft of uniform thickness.

a slicing injury. The amputated tip, if relatively superficial, can be treated as a full-thickness skin graft. The tissue should be irrigated with saline to remove debris, defatted, and placed in saline-soaked gauze while the recipient bed is being prepared. The thick epidermis of the finger tip is often cut five or six times with a scalpel to avoid separation of the graft and recipient bed as the finger tip dries. The graft is then attached by one of the techniques discussed in the following sections.

Split-Thickness Skin Graft. The skin graft donor site is first lubricated so that the dermatome can glide smoothly. This facilitates taking an even skin graft. Mineral oil, Vaseline, or any of the usual topical ointments can be used. The lubricant is applied thinly over the donor skin surface. The donor skin is stretched manually. The skin is held proximally and distally to the graft donor site by firmly pressing the skin with either a wooden tongue blade or a piece of gauze. Traction is applied by pulling away from the donor site in both directions (Fig. 45–7*A*). This maneuver usually requires two people. The surgeon's free hand should hold the traction toward the direction of the dermatome movement. An assistant applies the countertraction, and the surgeon cuts the skin graft toward the free hand.

The dermatome is held lightly with the fingers and the thumb. The upper extremity is relaxed with the wrist in a relatively fixed position. The motion is mainly at the elbow and the shoulder. The cutting motion consists of frequent to-and-fro strokes with a minimal forward pressure. Too much forward pressure may result in irregular thickness of the graft and possible interruption of graft continuity. The initial contact of the dermatome and the skin should be at an angle when the cut is begun. Once the cut is initiated, the dermatome is flattened out to effect tangential excision of the skin (Fig. 45–7*B*). The downward pressure on the dermatome determines the thickness of the skin graft. For the thin and intermediate-thickness skin grafts, the weight of the dermatome itself, without much additional external

pressure, seems sufficient to cut the desired thickness. With experience, this procedure becomes quite natural.

Once harvested, the skin curls and shrinks immediately. One may think that the graft will not be large enough, because it is now smaller than the area outlined at the donor site. The skin, however, readily stretches when applied to the recipient bed. Uncurling the harvested graft on moist gauze is helpful in keeping the graft flat. Furthermore, the graft should be kept moist between layers of wet gauze if it is not immediately applied to the recipient bed.

APPLICATION OF SKIN GRAFT

Full-Thickness Skin Graft. Following meticulous hemostasis of the recipient bed, the previously cut skin graft is laid on the recipient bed. Because of the inherent shrinkage of the full-thickness skin graft, even if the graft is cut to size, it is usually slightly smaller than the recipient defect. For this reason, the skin graft is sutured to the edge of the defect and is stretched to cover the defect. Several tacking sutures are placed in the periphery for proper fitting. These sutures are left long for a tie-over dressing, although a Tube-gauze dressing is also effective for digits. The remaining edges are sutured with a running circumferential suture. Sutures are easier to place if the needle is driven through the graft first and then through the skin edge of the recipient area.

Split-Thickness Skin Graft. The split-thickness skin graft is placed on the recipient bed with the dermal side down. The dermal side of the split-thickness skin graft is characterized by the wet, glistening sheen as opposed to the relatively dry, dull appearance of the epithelial surface. In addition, the edges tend to curl toward the dermal surface. If the recipient bed is larger than a single sheet of graft, several sheets of graft may be required. Any overlapping of skin grafts does not influence the graft take. On the other hand, it is very important to make sure that the free edges of the graft are fully uncurled so that it is not doubled over on itself. Obviously, any curled portion will not get revascularized, and sectional failure of the graft will result.

The split-thickness skin graft should be laid in such a way that it follows all the hills and valleys of the wound and is in contact with the entire raw surface of the recipient bed. If the skin grafts tend to tent over a deep concavity, it is useful to tack down the tented portion to the base of the concavity using one or two through-and-through stitches; 4–0 or 5–0 chromic sutures can be used. This is supplemented by a conforming dressing. The overhanging edges of the skin graft beyond the wound margin are trimmed. Suturing of the skin graft at the edges is not always necessary but may be desirable to offset the curling of the skin edges. Often adhesive closure tapes are used rather than sutures at the skin graft edge.

DRESSINGS

Full-Thickness Skin Graft. A full-thickness skin graft is classically dressed with a tie-over bolster dressing. This dressing facilitates immobilization and affords moderate, even pressure to prevent collection of blood or serum under the skin graft. The skin graft is fixed in place with several interrupted sutures, usually 4–0 nylon, placed in a relatively evenly spaced pattern around the periphery of the skin graft and the recipient bed. The tails of the sutures are left long. The skin graft is covered with a single layer of nonadherent gauze, such as Xeroform or Vaseline gauze, which is cut larger than the grafted area. A bolster is formed using a wad of cotton, lamb's wool, gauze, or a polyurethane foam pad. The bolster is made to fit the size of the graft. The overhanging edges of the nonadherent gauze dressing are swept up to cover the rough edges of the bolster. The long tails of the sutures are tied, and the bolster is secured in place (Fig. 45–8). An additional soft dressing can be applied to protect the bolster dressing as necessary. Some clinicians prefer to apply a Tube-gauze dressing if the wound is on a distal digit. If the skin graft is on an extremity and motion of the graft bed is a problem, immobilization of the parts involved with a loose plaster cast or a splint may be necessary.

Split-Thickness Skin Graft. There are numerous individual variations among physicians in dressing split-thickness skin grafts. These techniques are all quite functional, as long as they meet several basic requirements. The skin graft dressing should be nonadherent, absorptive, immobilizing, and protective. A split-thickness skin graft on a concave

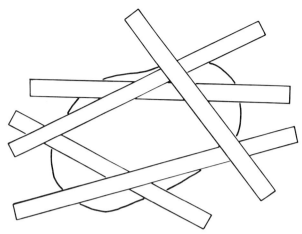

Figure 45–9. A method of graft fixation using multiple adherent, porous wound closure strips.

surface can be effectively immobilized by a tie-over bolster technique, which has been described previously. For uncomplicated small split-thickness skin grafts, there are much simpler and easier methods of applying dressings.

A small split-thickness skin graft on a flat surface can be secured with several strips of adherent porous adhesive closure strips without sutures (Fig. 45–9). The graft is then covered with a nonadherent petrolatum gauze to cover the entire extent of the wound closure strips. If the strips are not covered entirely by the greasy dressing, they may get lifted off as the dressing is removed and, in turn, may disrupt the skin graft. Next, a couple of layers of saline-moistened gauze are applied. This layer of dressing aids in absorption of the early drainage through capillary action of the moist gauze fibers. The entire area is then covered with an oversized, thin sponge with an adhesive backing, such as a Reston pad (Minnesota Mining and Manufacturing [3-M] Co., St. Paul, Minn.). The overhanging portion of the sponge is pressed and is allowed to adhere to the surrounding skin, which has been wiped dry.

If the adhesive sponge dressing is not available, the last step can be modified as follows. A surgical adhesive, such as tincture of benzoin or Aeroplast, is applied to the skin surrounding the moist gauze dressing. An oversized dry gauze is applied over the entire area, and the edges are pressed to stick to the skin, which has been painted with surgical adhesive. The edges of the dressing can be reinforced with tapes if necessary. This last layer of dressing protects the graft from external shearing forces. The entire dressing and the whole graft-recipient unit may move, but the graft is not allowed to move relative to the recipient bed. This layer should not be occlusive. An occlusive layer, such as an adhesive plastic dressing, would prevent evaporation and would allow collection of drainage in the dressing and consequent maceration of the graft.

Contrary to common impression, a split-thickness skin graft on a finger tip wound is quite simple to dress. Fixing the skin graft with sutures is not necessary. This extra step is time consuming and does not add to the outcome of the grafting. The skin graft is simply kept in place with several strips of petrolatum gauze that are placed across the skin graft and the adjacent skin in a criss-cross fashion. The strips should be narrower than the thickness of the finger, so that the gauze strips can be molded to the contour of the finger tip without folding or pleating. A thin layer of moist

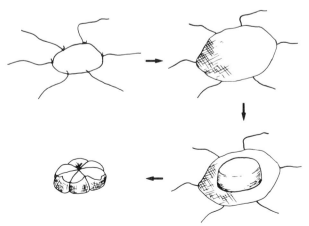

Figure 45–8. A method of tie-over bolster dressing application.

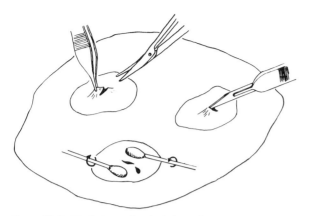

Figure 45–10. Techniques for draining a hematoma or seroma.

dressing gauze cut to size is placed next. Two strips of adhesive sponge foam pad are laid crossing each other over the finger tip. Dry gauze strips could be used in place of the foam pad. The entire assembly of dressing is then covered with a Tube-gauze, if available. No more than two layers of Tube-gauze should be used so that the dressing is not constricting.

The final step of skin graft dressing is immobilization of the graft site. External splinting is important for grafts that are on the parts of the body that normally go through motion, such as the extremities. The best way to splint an extremity with a skin graft is with a plaster cast. Although a cast may appear to be too much for a finger tip graft in the long run, patients are more comfortable and tolerate it well. Small individual finger splints that are taped on are not as reliable. These splints allow much motion and, hence, discomfort and graft disruption. With reinforcing strips of plaster in key areas, a relatively light cast that does the job can be fabricated.

The skin graft on the forearm can be splinted with a long arm cast including the wrist and the elbow. The wrist should be kept in 20 to 30 degrees of extension and the elbow in 90 degrees of flexion. A skin graft on a digit or the hand can be effectively immobilized with a short arm cast or bivalve plaster splint. Even if a single digit is injured, it is advisable to immobilize the fingers in groups, such as the index and middle fingers and the ring and little fingers. The thumb is immobilized with a thumb spica cast. The hand and the fingers are kept in the functional position. All casts should be generously padded with cast padding. The plaster roll should be applied loosely without constriction.

CARE OF SKIN GRAFT

Large split-thickness skin grafts and grafts that are placed on a questionable recipient bed should be examined in 2 days for possible infection, seroma, or hematoma. If no complications are apparent, the graft should be redressed and examined within a week.

Seromas and hematomas are drained by a small stab incision made in the overlying skin graft with a number 11 scalpel blade or a pair of scissors. The incision should be made directly over the center of the fluid collection. One then expresses the fluid by rolling two cotton swabs from the periphery to the center of the collection (Fig. 45–10). Each seroma or hematoma should be drained individually. If an attempt is made to drain a few of them through a single stab incision, the intervening portion of adherent skin

graft may be lifted off the bed and disturbed. Following this, the skin graft is redressed and examined every day or two and is drained if necessary until the graft is fully taken. If there is gross infection, the involved portion of the skin graft is removed and appropriate dressing change is initiated.

Dressings on small split-thickness skin grafts (such as finger tip grafts) and tie-over bolster dressings on full-thickness skin grafts are left undisturbed for 5 to 7 days. Nonetheless, the patient should be seen a couple of days following the operation, and the area of the graft dressing should be examined for signs of infection. If the patient complains of pain and there is tenderness, warmth, and redness around the dressing, the graft should be exposed and examined in its entirety. Prophylactic antibiotics are *not* routinely used with outpatient skin grafts. The pain from a skin graft is usually minor and seldom requires narcotic analgesics.

CARE OF THE SPLIT-THICKNESS DONOR SITE

The donor site is simply dressed with a piece of petrolatum gauze followed by a layer of moist gauze. The wet gauze is for absorption of early wound drainage. A layer or two of dry gauze is placed over this and is secured with tapes. In a day or two, the gauze dressing is removed, leaving the petrolatum gauze that is now adherent to the wound. The wound is then lightly dressed or left open to dry. The petrolatum gauze along with a thin layer of scab is gradually separated from the healed donor site in 10 to 14 days.

The impermeable adhesive plastic dressings (Op-site [T.J. Smith & Nephew Ltd. Welwyn Garden City and Hull, England], Tegaderm [Minnesota Mining and Manufacturing Co., St. Paul, Minn.]) have been used successfully as donor site dressings. A sheet of the adhesive plastic dressing of a size considerably larger than the donor site itself is laid over the donor site area. Care is taken to dry the surrounding skin well so that there is good contact between the adhesive plastic sheet and the skin to form an occlusive dressing. Initially, a moderate amount of serosanguineous drainage may collect over the donor site, forming a blister under the plastic dressing. Although the blister can be drained by sterile aspiration, small blisters (less than 2 cm in diameter) do not require drainage unless there is evidence of infection. With healing, the liquid component of the drainage is reabsorbed, leaving a thin layer of crust under the plastic dressing. The plastic layer is removed in 10 to 14 days when epithelialization is complete. In the case of infection, the plastic dressing is removed and dressing changes are started. Once gross infection is cleared, petrolatum gauze dressings may be applied and cared for as described previously.

REFERENCES

1. Henry L, Marshall DC, Friedman, EA, et al: The rejection of skin hand grafts in the normal human subject. Part II. Histological findings. J Clin Invest 41:420, 1982.
2. Clemensen T: The early circulation in split skin grafts. Acta Chir Scand 124:11, 1982.
3. Thiersch C: Über die feineren anatomischen veranderungen bei Aufheilung von Haut auf Granulationen. Arch Klin Chir 17:318, 1874.
4. Smehel J: The revascularization of a free skin autograft. Acta Chir Plast 9:76, 1967.
5. Converse JM: Reconstructive Plastic Surgery. Vol 1. Philadelphia, WB Saunders Co, 1977, pp 159–162.
6. Mir Y, Mir L: Biology of skin graft: New aspects to consider in its revascularization. Plast Reconstr Surg 8:378, 1951.
7. Newmeyer WL: Primary Care of Hand Injuries. Philadelphia, Lea & Febiger, 1979, p 97.

Chapter 46

Soft Tissue Foreign Body Removal

Richard C. Barnett

INTRODUCTION

Successful removal of a foreign body is one of the most satisfying procedures in medicine. Carried out with skill and a minimum of discomfort to the patient, such a procedure can result in a grateful patient and a satisfied physician. In contrast, the unskillful attempt at removal of foreign material, particularly if the procedure has not been well thought out, may produce considerable discomfort and, occasionally, disastrous results. An extended search for an elusive foreign body may result in frustration to the physician and a dissatisfied patient. Improper setting, improper instrumentation, and insufficient time for the procedure are common pitfalls of foreign body removal.[1]

GUIDELINES FOR APPROACHING FOREIGN BODIES

Initially, the physician should take a history of the method of injury to quickly ascertain the specific characteristics of the foreign material and to formulate the best plan for judicious removal. The history, physical examination, and localization techniques influence decisions about the time and place of foreign body removal. Some material such as wood should be removed immediately, because retained wood will surely lead to inflammation and infection. Other material such as glass or plastic may be removed on an elective basis, whereas innocuous metallic foreign bodies may often be permanently left embedded in soft tissue. If localization is certain and if removal can be easily accomplished under local anesthesia within a manageable period of time (1 hour is usually the upper limit of operative time using local anesthesia), removal is generally indicated on the initial visit. If, in contrast, the material is relatively inert and small (such as a BB) and located near no vital structures but is deeply embedded in the subcutaneous tissues, the time, energy, and effort involved in the removal is probably excessive compared with the possible adverse effects of the foreign material remaining in the soft tissue. The possibility of the foreign body migrating to involve vital structures is remote but should be reviewed in the decision of when and how to remove the foreign body. Cases of reported missile embolization in the vascular system apparently are influenced by the missile caliber, impact velocity, physical wound characteristics, point of vessel entrance, position and movements of the body, and the velocity of blood flow.[2]

All clinical decisions require an evaluation of the possibility of infection. Some foreign bodies produce infection in a few days, whereas with other objects, infection may be delayed for weeks or months, often flaring up for no apparent reason. If the foreign body carries dirt particles, pieces of clothing, or other sources of bacterial contamination with it, expeditious removal of the material may be necessary, even though the foreign body itself is relatively

small and is not likely to cause a reaction. If some time has elapsed since the initial injury, careful review of the history of the type of foreign material and the method of introduction is warranted. One should not attempt a hasty exploration for foreign material that may not exist or that is best left alone. The initial history should also include any unusual medical problem that would preclude the use of adequate local anesthesia, such as allergy to local anesthetics, any bleeding diathesis, or any medical problems, including diabetes mellitus, uremia, or a compromised immune status, that might lead to unusual or more difficult wound management.

It is not uncommon to encounter a soft tissue foreign body even though its presence has not been suggested by the history. Anderson and associates reported that physicians who initially treated a series of hand injuries did not diagnose the presence of a foreign body in 75 of 200 consecutive cases.[3] The patient who experiences a sharp, sudden pain in the foot while walking barefoot across the carpet may have a sewing needle or toothpick embedded in the foot, rather than the "sprained foot," which provoked the initial complaint. A high index of suspicion for retained foreign bodies should be the rule for wounds that are painful or that heal poorly.[4, 5]

An abscess or cellulitis that recurs or does not heal as expected should always be investigated for an unsuspected retained foreign body. Finally, all metallic or foreign bodies that appear on the radiograph of a multiple trauma patient should be proved to be extrinsic to the patient; that is, present on the radiograph table or clothing rather than being embedded in the patient. Foreign objects, such as keys or coins, may be surreptitiously embedded in a trauma patient and may easily be mistaken for artifact.

IMAGING TECHNIQUES

Evidence from radiographs now makes it possible to localize radiopaque foreign bodies and to use the radiographic localization as a guide in the removal of the material. Therefore, it is important to decide whether the material involved is radiopaque. Formerly, it was thought that localization depended upon the lead content of the material, particularly glass. More recent information indicates that the visibility of foreign material in soft tissues is dependent on its composition (relative density), configuration, size, and orientation (Fig. 46–1).

In 1932, Lewis reported that all types of glass can be detected radiographically.[6] In 1977, Pond and Lindsey revealed the ability to localize foreign fragments, including leaded and nonleaded glass, in an experimental phantom.[7] Tandberg subsequently demonstrated that, unless obscured by bone, virtually *all* glass is visible on a standard radiograph.[8] Pieces of glass as small as 0.5 mm may be visible regardless of pigment content or source of the glass, including glass from automobile windshields, light bulbs, and laboratory equipment. In a chicken leg model, Courter found that two-view radiography visualized glass fragments of 0.5, 1.0, and 2.0 mm maximum dimension with a sensitivity of 61, 83, and 99 per cent, respectively.[8a] Because almost all glass may be visible on radiographs, nonvisualization of glass suggests its absence but is not conclusive proof that it is not present if overlying radiopaque structures are visible.

The identification of less dense foreign material such as splinters may be improved by the use of xeroradiography.[9, 10] The presence of some foreign bodies may be suspected by the accompaniment of soft tissue gas, introduced with the foreign body, on the radiograph. It should be noted

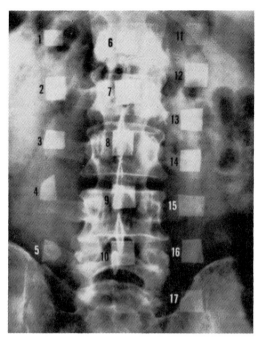

Figure 46–1. Samples of glass superimposed on the abdomen and exposed to x-rays. (Reproduced with permission from Zatzkin HR: *The Roentgen Diagnosis of Trauma.* Copyright © 1965 by Year Book Medical Publishers, Inc., Chicago.)

that even large pieces of wood are notoriously not visible on standard radiographs, although wood that is painted may be seen. Sea urchin spines may or may not be visible on plain radiographs. The use of "soft tissue" (underpenetrated) radiographic films may improve the identification of sea urchin spines.[11] Pieces of cloth or clothing are not visible on radiographs. Fish bones are occasionally visible on radiographs because of their calcium content, but cartilaginous structures, such as spines and fins, are not.

After removing a radiopaque foreign body, it is prudent to take a postoperative radiograph to document that removal was complete (Fig. 46–2). A repeat radiograph may not be needed if the foreign body was a single object, such as a pin or needle, or if there is no evidence of fragmentation.

When a high index of suspicion for a foreign body exists and initial radiographic studies are negative, other imaging methods should be considered. High-resolution ultrasound in the hands of a skilled operator may identify wood splinters, small glass fragments, fish bones, and sea urchin spines.[12-15] Computed tomography and magnetic resonance imaging have the ability to both identify wooden foreign bodies and clarify the surrounding anatomy.[16-17] Although these methods are not commonly used when initial examination (including careful wound exploration) and radiographs are negative for a foreign body, these imaging techniques are of value when complicated wound healing suggests a "radiolucent" retained foreign body (Fig. 46–3).

FOREIGN BODY REACTION

Many soft tissue foreign bodies have to be removed because of either infection or foreign body reaction. A purulent bacterial infection *may* develop in the presence of any foreign body but not in *all* cases. Karpman and associates revealed only a 15 per cent infection rate (*Staphylococcus aureus* and Enterobacteriaceae) in a series of 25 patients treated for cactus thorn injuries of the extremities.[19] Certain

thorns (black thorn, rose thorns), redwood and Northwest cedar splinters, toothpicks, hair, and sea urchin spines are noted for their ability to initiate chronic foreign body reaction. Sea urchin spines are covered with slime, calcareous material, and other debris that may initiate a foreign body granuloma. It has been speculated that the inflammatory reaction seen with cactus thorns may be an allergic reaction to fungus found on the cactus plant. Many foreign body reactions are thought to be due to the inflammatory response to organic material and may not be due to the introduction of bacteria at the time that the wound was incurred. Clinically evident reactions may be delayed for weeks or even years following injury (Fig. 46–4). The chronic infection or inflammatory reaction may not be accompanied by the production of pus, but it may be quite painful and may result in loss of function. Foreign bodies may also be associated with the formation of a chronic pseudotumor, development of a sinus tract, or evidence of osteomyelitis-like lesions of bone and soft tissue.[4] Organic material has also been noted to form a chronic tenosynovitis, chronic monoarticular synovitis, and chronic bursitis.

Rapidly traveling projectiles with considerable inherent heat are less likely to cause infection but are more apt to cause damage in the passage through the tissue. It is obvious, therefore, that one must judiciously evaluate each foreign body injury, and that one should not be dogmatic about exploration or benign neglect policies.

GUIDELINES FOR FOREIGN BODY REMOVAL

Following the initial history, examination, and *preoperative and preanesthetic documentation of the neurovascular status of*

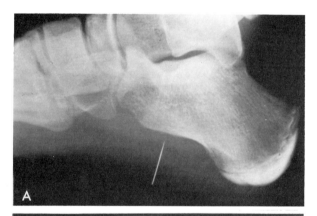

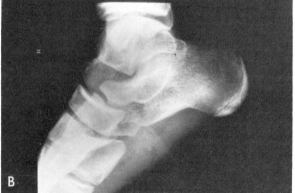

Figure 46–2. Preoperative *(A)* and postoperative *(B)* x-ray demonstrating the complete removal of a metallic foreign body.

Wood   Glass   Plastic

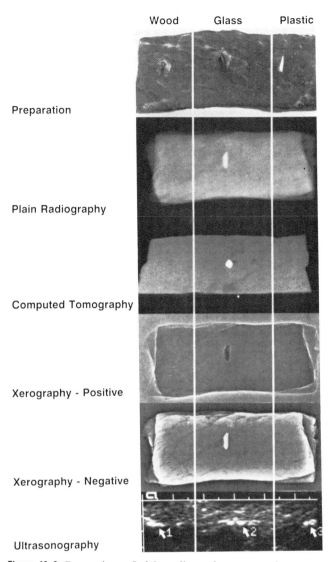

Preparation

Plain Radiography

Computed Tomography

Xerography - Positive

Xerography - Negative

Ultrasonography

Figure 46–3. Comparison of plain radiography, computed tomography, positive and negative xeroradiography, and ultrasonography in imaging wooden, glass, and plastic foreign bodies in an in vitro preparation. (From Ginsburg MJ, Ellis GL, Flom LL: Detection of soft-tissue foreign bodies by plain radiography, xerography, computed tomography, and ultrasonography. Ann Emerg Med 19:701, 1990.)

feel or sound. Glass is difficult to identify by sight in soft tissue but creates a characteristic grating sound when touched with metal. In larger wounds, a gloved finger may be carefully used to probe the wound for the presence of a foreign body.

Radiographs are the best method for estimating the general location, depth, and structure of radiopaque foreign bodies. If one attaches a needle or paper clip to the skin surface at the wound entrance before taking a radiograph, the foreign body will be seen in relation to the entrance wound. This also helps to identify the path that leads to the foreign body and the relative distance from the surface to the foreign body.[20] Needles at two angles may also be passed to help localize the foreign body (Fig. 46–5). A special technique using measurements on anteroposterior and lateral radiographs and a blind dissection method has been advocated to remove needles from the foot.[21] When the material to be detected is suspected of being difficult to visualize on a conventional radiograph, then xeroradiography, high-resolution ultrasound, computed tomography, or magnetic resonance imaging should be considered.[10,12–18]

With the use of fluoroscopic image-intensifying equipment, it may be possible to follow the wound's entrance, to localize the material, and to grasp the foreign body and remove it without making a larger incision. A potential disadvantage of this procedure is the increased amount of radiation that may be required. Ariyan has described a technique in which two needles are placed in the soft tissue from opposite directions toward the foreign body.[22] The extremity is rotated while the physician watches the image under the image intensifier to obtain a three-dimensional effect. An incision is placed perpendicular to the plane of the needles, and the object is removed.

Some researchers have suggested injecting the entrance wound with methylene blue to outline the tract of the foreign body.[23] (Excess methylene blue that spills onto the skin surface may be removed with ether.) The blue line is followed into the deeper tissues. This technique is of limited value, because the tract of the foreign body often closes tightly and does not allow the passage of the methylene blue.

the patient, a decision must be made as to the time and place of removal. If the foreign body is to be removed in the emergency department, it is wise to set a time limit of between 30 minutes and 1 hour and not to exceed that time allotment. Most simple foreign bodies can be successfully removed in 30 minutes to 1 hour, and more difficult procedures should be deferred. Note that many foreign bodies initially appear superficial, and the novice may mistakenly think that removal will be rapid and simple, only to find after prolonged searching that the elusive foreign body is yet to be found.

Localization

Superficial foreign bodies, such as splinters, bullets, or embedded glass may be palpated if they are near the skin surface. Deeper foreign bodies must be localized by other techniques. A metal probe may identify the foreign body by

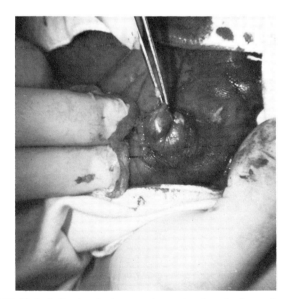

Figure 46–4. A foreign body granuloma developed after a foreign body was stable for 6 months in this laborer's hand. There was no gross infection, but the pain was quite bothersome. The foreign body and reactive tissue were excised under local anesthesia.

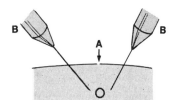

Figure 46–5. When a small entrance wound *(A)* is noted but the foreign body is not seen, noninvasive localization is preferable to blind probing. Metal markers taped to the skin or needles inserted close to the foreign body under local anesthesia *(B)* and radiographed at different angles provide a guide to cutting down and extraction. (Reproduced from Hospital Medicine, © January 1981, with permission of Cahners Publishing Co.)

Equipment

A standard suture tray with a scalpel is usually adequate equipment for removal of most simple foreign bodies. Tissue retractors, special pickups, and loupes may be added as needed. Good direct light is essential for success, and some physicians prefer to use a head lamp.

Local soft tissue injection with lidocaine (1 per cent with epinephrine for other than digital blocks) is the recommended anesthesia for the removal of most soft tissue foreign bodies. Intravenous regional anesthesia or axillary blocks may be useful for foreign body removal in the upper extremity. Children may require general anesthesia or sedation if they are unable to cooperate.

The use of an arterial tourniquet is essential to provide a bloodless field for the removal of a soft tissue foreign body in an extremity. A blood pressure cuff or portable self-contained pneumatic cuff inflated above arterial pressure may be used on the upper arm, forearm, leg, or thigh. To limit back bleeding, the extremity is elevated and wrapped with an elastic bandage to exsanguinate the extremity before the tourniquet is inflated. In the digits, a Penrose drain may be used as a tourniquet at the base of the finger or toes. Most patients can tolerate an ischemic tourniquet for 15 to 30 minutes, and it is safe to stop circulation to an extremity for this time period.

Operative Technique

The specific technique for removal of a foreign body is tailored to each clinical situation. In general, foreign bodies should be removed only under direct vision. *Blind grasping into a wound with a hemostat in an effort to remove a foreign body should be avoided.* Blind grasping is especially dangerous in the hand, foot, or face, where vital structures may be easily damaged.

In most cases, one should *enlarge the entrance wound with an adequate skin incision.* Attempting to remove a foreign body through a puncture wound or an inadequate skin incision is both frustrating and self-defeating. Following a proper skin incision, the wound is explored by carefully spreading the soft tissue with a hemostat (Fig. 46–6). The foreign body can often be felt with an instrument before it can be seen. In an extremity that has been made ischemic by a tourniquet, the tract of the foreign body may be followed, although the tract frequently cannot be identified in muscle or fat.

If the foreign body is difficult to visualize (such as fiberglass or plastic) and if it is located in the superficial soft tissue, excision of a small block of tissue rather than removal of the foreign body alone may be necessary. Block excision

is also required if the foreign body has contaminated the surrounding soft tissue. It must be noted that *excision of a block of tissue is done only under direct vision and after nerves, tendons, and vessels have been identified and excluded from the excision.*

If a foreign body such as a thorn or needle enters the skin perpendicularly, a linear incision may pass to one side of the foreign body and it will be difficult to determine where the foreign body lies in relation to the incision (Fig. 46–7A and B). The search must then be extended into the walls of the incision rather than through the skin.[24] In such cases, it is advisable to excise a small ellipse of skin and undermine the skin for 1/4 to 1/2 inch in all directions (Fig. 46–7C). The tissue is then compressed from the sides in hopes that the foreign body will extrude and can be grasped with an instrument.

Following foreign body removal, the wound is irrigated under pressure with povidone-iodine. If a small incision has been made in a noncosmetic area (such as the bottom of the foot), the incision is left open and is bandaged. The area may be soaked in hot water for a few days, and a return visit is necessary only if signs of infection develop. If a large incision has been created, the skin may be primarily sutured. In cases in which gross contamination has occurred, the wound should not be closed on the initial visit. The wound may be packed open, and the skin should be sutured, if free of signs of inflammation, in 3 to 5 days (delayed closure).

TRAUMATIC TATTOOING

Ground-in foreign material or tattooing of the skin is a troublesome problem, because foreign matter will permanently disfigure the skin. Many cases may be managed with adequate local anesthesia and meticulous débridement with a sponge, a scrub brush, or a toothbrush. If it is impossible to remove all the foreign material with these methods, careful consideration should be given to a secondary excision of the tattooed area, using primary closure and subsequent

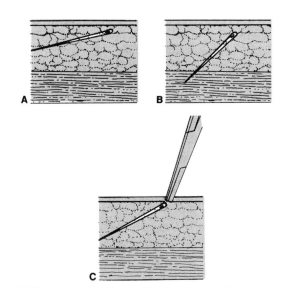

Figure 46–6. A sewing needle completely embedded below the surface *(A, B)* is easily located by a radiograph. Following local anesthesia, a small incision over the superficial end permits removal with a hemostatic forceps *(C)*. The hemostat is introduced through an adequate incision, spread to open the tissue, and is used to "feel" the foreign body as the hemostat is advanced. (Reproduced from Hospital Medicine, © January 1981, with permission of Cahners Publishing Co.)

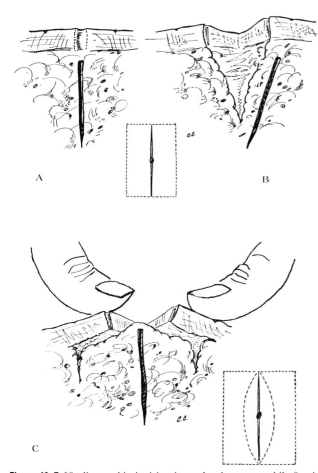

Figure 46–7. If a linear skin incision is used to locate a mobile foreign body that is perpendicular to the skin in the subcutaneous fat *(A)*, the foreign body may be displaced *(B)*. A modified elliptical incision is made *(C)*, and the skin edges are undermined, displacing the foreign body into the middle of the wound. Pressure with the thumbs may be applied to the skin to force the foreign body into view. (From Rees CE: The removal of foreign bodies: A modified incision. JAMA 113:35, 1939. Copyright 1939, American Medical Association.)

plastic surgery to repair the defect. Dermabrasion may be an acceptable late treatment when the tattooing is superficial.[25]

FOREIGN BODIES IN FATTY TISSUE

Foreign bodies located in the fatty tissues may be removed by making an elliptical incision surrounding the entrance wound, grasping the skin of the ellipse loosely with an Allis forceps, undercutting the incision until the foreign body is contacted, and removing the foreign body, skin, and entrance tract in one block (Fig. 46–8). In most instances, a small portion of subcutaneous fat should be removed along with the foreign body to minimize infection. Foreign bodies in fat are very mobile and probing may displace them even more. Foreign bodies that are embedded in fat and that are perpendicular to the skin may also be removed as in Figure 46–7C.

FOREIGN BODIES IN THE SOLE OF THE FOOT

It is reasonable to assume that foreign matter is introduced into many wounds on the sole of the foot. This is particularly true if the wounds are caused by foreign material being driven into the foot such as occurs when one steps on a nail while wearing a shoe with a soft rubber sole. In cases of infected puncture wounds, exploration for a foreign body is mandatory, even when no foreign body is identified on a radiograph.

When exploring lesions on the sole of the foot, foreign material may often be located with the aid of a magnifying device. This enables the location of the sinus tract or the visualization of the tip of a splinter. *An ischemic tourniquet is mandatory when exploring the foot for a foreign body.* The persistence of a mass, a draining sinus, radiographic evidence of an exuberant inflammatory reaction, or a cyst or inflammation of adjacent bony structures should heighten suspicion that a retained foreign body has entered the foot and is now announcing its presence to the patient and physician by the continued efforts of the body to reject the foreign material. Cracchiolo reported three patients who experienced recurrent pain and infection in the foot for a

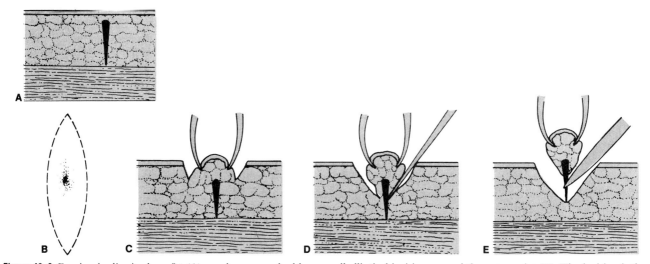

Figure 46–8. Foreign bodies in deep fat *(A)* may be approached by a small elliptical incision around the entry point *(B)*. The incision is then laterally undercut and grasped (without pulling) with an Allis clamp *(C)*. The ellipse is then further undercut until contact with the foreign body is made *(D)*. The foreign body may be grasped and removed along with the entry tract and the soiled local fat *(E)*. (Reproduced from Hospital Medicine, © January 1981, with permission of Cahners Publishing Co.)

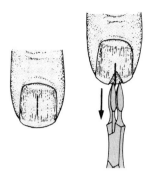

Figure 46–9. For a foreign body deep in the nail bed, take as small a wedge of nail as will allow access to the proximal end of the splinter, then extract with splinter forceps. A digital nerve block may be necessary. (Reproduced from Hospital Medicine, © January 1981, with permission of Cahners Publishing Co.)

number of years.[26] The patients did not respond to antibiotics or to attempts at limited exploration. In each case, a toothpick (not seen radiographically) embedded in the sole of the foot was the cause.

SUBUNGUAL FOREIGN BODIES

Special attention is required for subungual foreign bodies that are deeply embedded in the nail bed.[27] In some instances, this may require removing a small portion of the nail with double-pointed heavy scissors and grasping the foreign material with the splinter forceps (Fig. 46–9). Occasionally, complete removal of the nail may be required. Obviously, a digital block is needed for techniques involving manipulation of the nail or nail bed. An interesting technique has been suggested in which a sterile hypodermic needle, bent at its tip, is slid under the nail and hooks the foreign body, allowing its withdrawal. Alternatively, a 19-gauge hypodermic needle can be slid under the nail to surround a small splinter. The needle tip is then brought against the underside of the nail to secure the splinter. The needle and splinter are then removed as a unit.[28] Wooden splinters are commonly embedded under the fingernail. *Such foreign bodies must be completely removed because infection is certain.* The proximity of the distal phalanx to the subungual area is a constant concern for the development of osteomyelitis.

FISHHOOKS

There are several methods of removing a fishhook. The method that one uses depends on the conditions under which the removal is to take place.[29–33] The traditional manner for removing small fishhooks requires local infiltration with 1 per cent lidocaine, forcing the barb through the

anesthetized skin, clipping off the barb, and removing the rest of the hook along the direction of entry (Fig. 46–10). In the field or stream, removal of a fishhook may be accomplished without local anesthetic by following a technique that enables easy removal. The same technique may be used in the emergency department with 1 per cent lidocaine to facilitate removal. This "stream" technique (Fig. 46–11) is to loop a piece of string or fishing line around the belly of the hook at the point at which it enters the skin. Allow approximately 1 foot of string to be wrapped around the right hand to give strong traction. The shank of the hook should be held parallel to and in approximation with the skin by the index finger of the left hand. The thumb and middle finger of the left hand stabilize and depress the barb, which helps the index finger to disengage the barb from the subcutaneous tissue. When the barb has been disengaged, a *sharp* pull by the right hand removes the hook through the wound of entry. The hook often *flies* out of the patient. Care should be taken to keep bystanders out of the expected path of the hook.

If the hook is large and deeply embedded and if it is not desirable to cause further trauma by pushing the pointed end through the skin, it may be possible to use an 18-gauge needle to cover the barb (Fig. 46–12). After adequate local anesthetic has been administered, the needle should be passed through the entrance wound of the hook parallel to the shank of the hook to sheath the barb and to allow the hook to be backed out while the barb is covered. An alternative to this procedure is to insert a number 11 blade parallel to the shank of the hook down to the barb. Using the point of the blade, free the subcutaneous tissue that is engaged on the barb, sheath the barb with the point of the number 11 blade, and back the hook out, with the blade protecting the barb.

WOODEN SPLINTERS

Because of the potential for inflammation, *pieces of wood must be completely removed from soft tissue.* Simply grasping the end of a superficial protruding splinter may be adequate, but care should be taken not to leave small pieces of the foreign body in the wound (Fig. 46–13). Some splinters cannot be visualized at the point of entry but can be easily and readily palpated beneath the skin. In such cases, it is advisable to cut down on the long axis of the foreign body to remove it via a skin incision rather than through the entrance wound (Fig. 46–14). This method allows for thorough cleaning of the tract and removal of small pieces of the splinter that may otherwise remain. The linear skin incision may then be sutured. Particular mention should be made of certain wood splinters that are reactive and pliable, such as California redwood and Northwest cedar. Any wood that is easily fragmented requires meticulous care to ensure removal of all the material. Wood is generally not visible on a standard radiograph or xeroradiograph unless it is covered

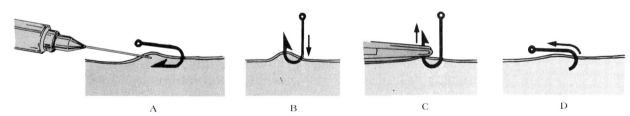

| A | B | C | D |

Figure 46–10. Method of removing an embedded fishhook when anesthesia is available and when the point of the fishhook is close to the skin. *A*, Obtain local anesthesia overlying the point of the hook. *B*, Force the point through the anesthetized skin. *C*, Clip off the barb. *D*, Remove the rest of the hook by reversing the direction of entry. (Reproduced from Hospital Medicine, © July 1980, with permission of Cahners Publishing Co.)

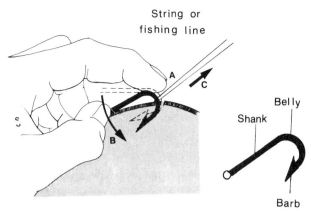

Figure 46–11. Method of removing an embedded fishhook when anesthesia is unavailable or when the barb of the fishhook lies too deep to force it out through a second wound without causing significant additional damage. Loop a piece of string (or thick suture material) around the belly of the hook and hold it down against the skin with the index finger of the left hand (A). Depress the shaft of the hook against the skin with the middle finger and thumb while applying light downward pressure with the index finger of the left hand to disengage the barb from the subcutaneous tissue (B), and pull *sharply* on the ends of the string with the right hand (C) to remove the hook through its entry wound. Bystanders should be out of the expected path of the hook. (Reproduced from Hospital Medicine, © July 1980, with permission of Cahners Publishing Co.)

with lead paint but may be visualized by sonography, computed tomography, or magnetic resonance imaging.

Occasionally, the most expeditious method of removing wooden splinters is complete excision of the entrance tract and the foreign body en bloc, followed by a linear closure, resulting in a more cosmetic wound with less chance for infection.

Pencil Lead

Good judgment must be used in the removal of graphite from pencils when lodged in the skin. Because graphite invariably leaves a pigmented tattooing in the soft tissue, it is preferable to excise the material en bloc when pencil lead is found in a cosmetic area. The graphite specks cannot be irrigated or scrubbed off, and tattooing results if they are not removed.

Metallic Fragments

High-velocity fragments, such as bullets, BBs, chips of wood-splitting mauls, or other metallic particles caused by metal striking metal, are easy to visualize radiographically and relatively simple to remove unless they are embedded in areas that are anatomically difficult to approach. Before removal of the foreign material, the area in which the fragment is embedded should be assessed in order to determine which structures are involved along the wound of entrance, which structures might be encountered in attempting to cut down on the foreign body, and which of those structures can be sacrificed to allow for adequate removal of the foreign material. It is preferable to defer the removal of deeply embedded metallic foreign bodies unless symptoms of infection develop. The extensive treatment of high-velocity foreign bodies, such as modern military or sporting ammunition, is beyond the scope of this discussion, because high-velocity fragments frequently result not only in a foreign body but also cause severe trauma along its path. Retained nonexplosive metallic fragments are inert and rarely cause infection. They usually become encysted after a period of time. Lead toxicity from bullet fragments is rare and generally only of concern when the fragment is in contact with synovium. The value of routine prophylactic antibiotic for metallic foreign bodies left in the soft tissue has not been proved.

Taser darts used for immobilization of violent individuals are like fishhooks and must be removed under local anesthesia after the attached wires have been cut. Backing the dart out as with a fishhook is not possible owing to the dart construction. Cutting down on the dart under local anesthesia is the preferred method of removal.[34, 35]

Sea Urchin Spines

The spines of the sea urchin are often a problem of physicians who treat skin divers or abalone fishermen. Spines are reactive and may be contaminated with slime, debris, and calcareous material initially, causing an intensive foreign body reaction. They are almost colorless and very brittle, so attempts to remove them require the physician's greatest skill and the patient's patience. Retained sea urchin spines may produce significant morbidity and should not be taken lightly. In circumstances in which removal will be difficult, the easiest method may be to allow time for a reaction to take place. The wound is then opened and drained, all the foreign material is removed by curettage, and the wound is allowed to heal by secondary intention.

Cactus Spines

Cactus spines vary considerably in size. The difficulty of removal is generally in inverse proportion to the foreign body size.[36] The larger embedded cactus spines are managed like wood splinter and sea urchin spine foreign bodies. More

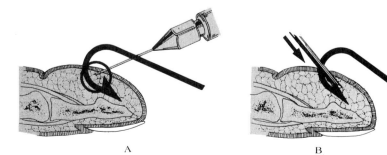

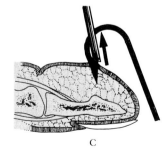

Figure 46–12. Method of removing an embedded fishhook using anesthesia when the hook is large and not too deep in the skin. After anesthetizing the area with 1 per cent lidocaine (A), insert a short-bevel 18-gauge needle through the entry wound of the hook and attempt to sheathe the barb of the hook within the needle (B). If this is done correctly, the hook and needle may then be backed out together (C). (Reproduced from Hospital Medicine, © July 1980, with permission of Cahners Publishing Co.)

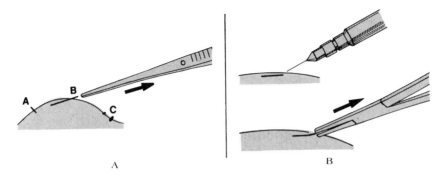

Figure 46–13. *A*, After local cleansing, superficial splinters *(A, B)* and other small foreign bodies *(C)* may be removed with sharp forceps and magnifier, usually without anesthesia. Avoid retention of fragments of long foreign bodies *(B)* by gentle withdrawal in the axis of entry. *B*, In tangentially embedded superficial splinters, careful teasing of the skin over the point of entry with the cutting edge of a fine hypodermic needle often provides access to the proximal end of the foreign body. (Reproduced from Hospital Medicine, © January 1981, with permission of Cahners Publishing Co.)

advanced imaging techniques (xeroradiography, ultrasonography, computed tomography, or magnetic resonance imaging) may be required for localization of deeply embedded spines.

Deeply embedded cactus spines generally produce granulomatous reactions, and infections are rare.[19] Hence, efforts to remove deeply embedded spines should be made after carefully weighing the benefit and potential harm related to a deep exploration, especially in a sensitive location.[36]

Superficially embedded medium- to large-sized cactus spines are best removed by direct axial traction of each spine using forceps. Smaller spines (glochids) may be difficult and tedious to remove individually. Adherent facial mask gel application and removal of spines en masse with the mask is recommended (Fig. 46–15A–E). Depilatory wax melted in a microwave oven and applied warm,[37] commercial facial gels,[36, 38] and household glue (Elmer's Glue-All, Borden Inc., Columbus, Ohio)[39] have recently been recommended for this purpose. The practitioner should be aware that over-the-counter "home-use" facial mask gels are not adherent enough to be effective without multiple applications (up to eight or more).

POSTOPERATIVE FOREIGN BODIES

Foreign bodies in the form of nonabsorbable suture material are frequently encountered in the postoperative period. The characteristic drainage, localized inflammatory reaction along the suture line, and localized pain and tenderness are characteristics of a retained foreign body (suture abscess). In this instance, probing the wound with a sterilized crochet hook or bent needle is frequently rewarding. Hooking the suture material through the sinus tract and removing it allows the wound to heal over the tract.

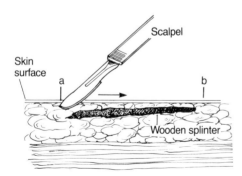

Figure 46–14. An embedded wooden splinter is removed by cutting down on the foreign body from point *a* to point *b*. This allows one to open the tract and remove all pieces of wood. The resultant laceration may be sutured primarily after wound irrigation, if there is no gross infection. (Reproduced from Hospital Medicine, © January 1981, with permission of Cahners Publishing Co.)

RING REMOVAL

Frequently, a ring must be removed to prevent laceration of tissue or vascular compromise. If removal is not possible by thorough lubrication (a water-soluble lubricant, e.g., K-Y jelly) and circular motion with traction on the ring, it may be necessary to either cut the ring off or remove it by the string-wrap method.

String-Wrap Method (Fig. 46–16). A 15- to 20-inch piece of string, umbilical tape, or thick silk suture is passed between the ring and the finger. If there is marked soft tissue swelling, the tip of a hemostat may be passed under the ring to grasp the string and pull it through the ring. The distal end of the string should be 10 to 15 inches long. The distal string is wrapped around the swollen finger (proximal to distal) to include the proximal interphalangeal (PIP) joint and the entire swollen finger. The wrapping is begun next to the ring. The wrap should be snug enough to compress the swollen tissue. The successive loops of the wrap are placed next to each other to keep any swollen tissue from bulging between the strands. When the wrapping has been completed, the proximal end of the string is carefully unwound, forcing the ring over that portion of the finger that has been compressed by the wrap. The PIP joint is the area that is most difficult to maneuver. Occasionally, one must rewrap the finger if it was not carefully wrapped initially. The procedure may be painful and may require a digital block. Some nonanesthetized patients panic during the procedure because of increasing pain due to compression and unwinding.[40]

Ring Cutter. A standard ring cutter should be used if the ring is not of high value or if there is excessive swelling. The ring cutter has a small hook that fits under the ring and serves as a guide to a saw-toothed wheel, which cuts the metal. The cut ends of the ring are spread using large hemostats (e.g., Kelly clamps), and the ring is removed. Cut rings may be repaired by a jeweler.

Obviously, it is preferable to remove all rings before the edema is extensive enough to cause pain or vascular compromise.

TICK REMOVAL

Early removal of ticks is advisable, since the hard tick of the Ixodid family is likely to transmit disease. Rocky Mountain spotted fever, Lyme disease, tularemia, and ascending paralysis have been identified as tick-borne diseases. Tick removal of Ixodid ticks is difficult because the mouth parts are cemented to the skin of the host. Traditional and folk methods of forcing the tick to disengage are ineffectual, and removal by mechanical means is required. Protection by using a hemostat or gloves is advisable to prevent infection of the person removing the tick. The tick is grasped as close to the patient's skin surface as possible and gently pulled

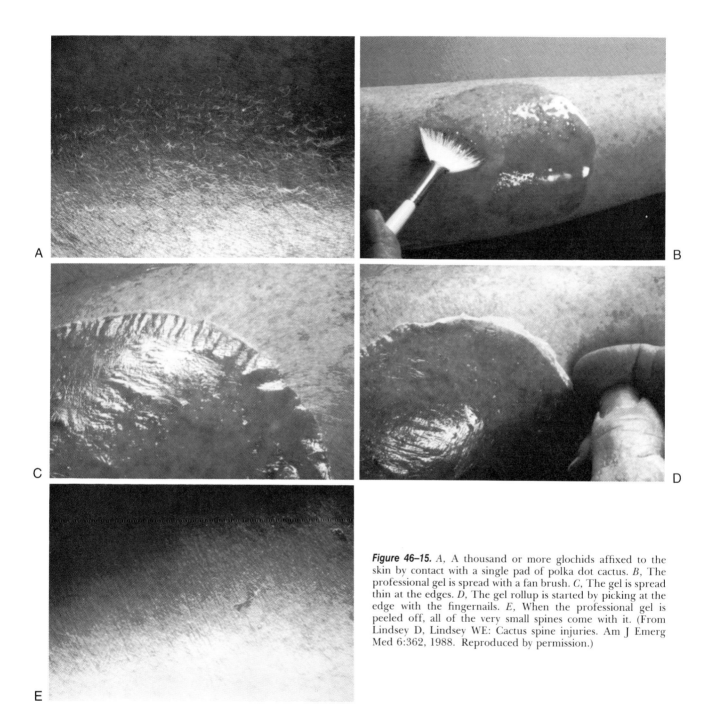

Figure 46–15. *A,* A thousand or more glochids affixed to the skin by contact with a single pad of polka dot cactus. *B,* The professional gel is spread with a fan brush. *C,* The gel is spread thin at the edges. *D,* The gel rollup is started by picking at the edge with the fingernails. *E,* When the professional gel is peeled off, all of the very small spines come with it. (From Lindsey D, Lindsey WE: Cactus spine injuries. Am J Emerg Med 6:362, 1988. Reproduced by permission.)

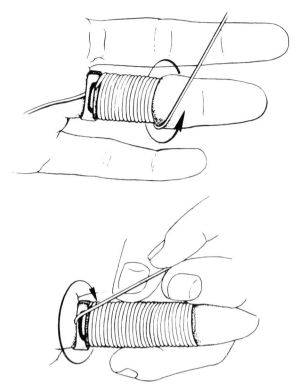

Figure 46–16. Remove a ring from a swollen finger by winding on a bit of string to compress the distal swollen tissues and then unwind the string and ring together. This string is passed under the ring before wrapping the finger. (From Emergency Medicine, September 15, 1982, p 107. Used by permission.)

free with steady axial traction. The tick should not be squeezed, crushed, or punctured. If mouth parts are left behind after removal of the body, excision of remaining parts under local anesthesia is needed to prevent local infection. Since ticks screw themselves into the skin in a clockwise manner, twisting *counter clockwise* is reported to facilitate local mechanical removal.[41]

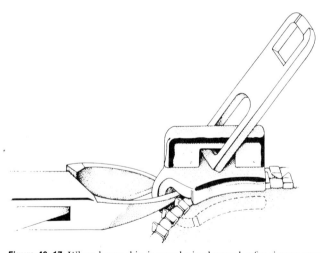

Figure 46–17. When loose skin is caught in the teeth of a zipper, one can release it quickly and without risk to the patient by cutting the diamond that holds the slider together with a bone cutter or a pair of wire clippers. (From Emergency Medicine, October 15, 1982, p. 215. Used by permission.)

ZIPPER INJURIES

The skin of the penis may become painfully entangled in the mechanism of a zipper. Unzipping the zipper frequently lacerates the skin and increases the amount of the tissue caught in the mechanism. Although the physician may anesthetize the skin and excise the entrapped tissue, a less invasive method may be useful.

The interlocking teeth of the zipper fall apart if the median bar (diamond or bridge) of the zipper is cut in half (Fig. 46–17). The skin is subsequently freed. A bone cutter or wire clippers and a moderate amount of force may be required to break the bar.

HAIR-THREAD TOURNIQUET

Hair or thread fibers adherent to infant clothing occasionally become tightly wrapped about the child's digits or genitals. The offending fiber(s) may be difficult to visualize and the child brought for evaluation only after signs of distal ischemia appear. Occasionally the fiber can be grasped with toothless forceps or a small hemostat and unwrapped. More commonly a number 11 blade must be used to cut the constricting bands under a regional nerve block. Because the bands may be quite deep, the incision should avoid known neurovascular tracts. Barton and colleagues[42] recommend a dorsal incision on the digits. One should reexamine the patient within 24 hours to ensure clinical improvement. Generally conservative wound care is sufficient once the band has been removed.

REFERENCES

1. Barnett RC: Removal of cutaneous foreign bodies. J Hosp Med 97:10, 1981.
2. Chapman AJ, McClain J: Wandering missiles: Autopsy study. Trauma 24(2):634, 1984.
3. Anderson A, Newmeyer WL, Kilgore ES: Diagnosis and treatment of retained foreign bodies of the hand. Am J Surg 144:63, 1982.
4. MacDowell RT: Unsuspected foreign bodies in puncture wounds. J Musculoskeletal Med 7:33, 1986.
5. Lammers RL: Soft tissue foreign bodies. Ann Emerg Med 17:1336, 1988.
6. Lewis RW: A roentgenographic study of glass and its visibility as a foreign body. Am J Roentgenol 27:853, 1932.
7. Pond GD, Lindsey D: Localization of cactus, glass, and other foreign bodies in soft tissues. Ariz Med 34:700, 1977.
8. Tandberg D: Glass in the hand and foot: Will an x-ray film show it? JAMA 248:1872, 1982.
8a. Courter BJ: Radiographic screening for glass foreign bodies—what does a "negative" foreign body series really mean? Ann Emerg Med 19:997, 1990.
9. Bowers DG, Lynch JB: Xeroradiography for non-metallic foreign bodies. Plast Reconstr Surg 60:470, 1977.
10. Carneiro RS, Okunski WJ, Heffernan AH: Detection of a relatively radiolucent foreign body in the hand by xeroradiography. Plast Reconstr Surg 59:862, 1977.
11. Newmeyer WL: III: Management of sea urchin spines in the hand. J Hand Surg 13A:455, 1988.
12. Fornage BD, Schernberg FL: Sonographic diagnosis of foreign bodies of the distal extremities. Am J Roentgenol 147:567, 1986.
13. Fornage BD, Schernberg FL: Sonographic preoperative localization of a foreign body in the hand. J Ultrasound Med 6:217, 1987.
14. Gooding GAW: Sonography of the hand and foot in foreign body detection. J Ultrasound Med 6:441, 1987.
15. De Flaviis L: Detection of foreign bodies in soft tissues: Experimental comparison of ultrasonograpy and xeroradiography. J Trauma 28:400, 1988.
16. Bauer AR: Computed tomographic localization of wooden foreign bodies in children's extremities. Arch Surg 118:1084, 1983.
17. Kuhns LR, Borlaza GS, Seigel RS, et al: An in vitro comparison of computed tomography, xeroradiography, and radiography in the detection of soft-tissue foreign bodies. Radiology 132:218, 1979.
18. Bodne D, Quinn SF, Cochran CF: Imaging foreign glass and wooden bodies of the extremities with CT and MR. J Comput Assist Tomogr 9:1135, 1985.
19. Karpman RR, Sparks RP, Fried M: Cactus thorn injuries to the extremities: Their management and etiology. Ariz Med 37:849, 1980.
20. Gahlos F: Embedded objects in perspective. J Trauma 24:340, 1985.

21. Gilsdorf JR: A needle in the sole of the foot. Surg Gynecol Obstet 163:573, 1986.
22. Ariyan S: A simple stereotactic method to isolate and remove foreign bodies. Arch Surg 112:857, 1077.
23. Bhavsar MS: Technique of finding a metallic foreign body. Am J Surg 141:305, 1981.
24. Rees CE: The removal of foreign bodies: A modified incision. JAMA 113:35, 1939.
25. Alt TH: Technical aids for dermabrasion. J Dermatol Surg Oncol 13:638, 1987.
26. Cracchiolo A: Wooden foreign bodies in the foot. Am J Surg 140:585, 1980.
27. Swischuk LE, Jorgenson F, Jorgenson A, et al: Wooden splinter induced pseudo-tumor and osteomyelitis like lesions of bone and soft tissue. Am J Roentgenol Radium Ther Nucl Med 122:176, 1974.
28. Davis LJ: Removal of subungual foreign bodies. J Fam Pract 11:714, 1980.
29. Barnett RC: Removal of fishhooks. J Hosp Med July 1980
30. Barnett RC: Three useful techniques for removing imbedded fishhooks. Hosp Med 72: July 1982.
31. Editorial: A few ways to unsnag a fishhook. Emerg Med 13:22, 1981.
32. Friedenberg S: How to remove an imbedded fishhook in 5 seconds without really trying. N Engl J Med 284:733, 1971.
33. Rose JD: Removing the imbedded fishhook. Austral Fam Phys 10:33, 1981.
34. Koscove EM: The Taser weapon: A new emergency medicine problem. Am J Emerg Med 14:1205, 1985.
35. Ordog GJ: Electronic gun (Taser) injuries. Ann Emerg Med 16:73, 1987.
36. Lindsey D, Lindsey WE: Cactus spine injuries. Am J Emerg Med 6:362, 1988.
37. Schunk JE, Corneli HM: Cactus spine removal. J Pediatr 110:667, 1987.
38. Putnam MH: Simple cactus spine removal. J Pediatr 98:333, 1981.
39. Martinez TT, Jerome M, Barry RC, et al: Removal of cactus spines from the skin: A comparative evaluation of several methods. Am J Dis Child 141:1291, 1987.
40. Mizrahi S, Lunski I: A simplified method for ring removal from an edematous finger. Am J Surg 151:412, 1986.
41. Needham GR: Evaluation of five popular methods for tick removal. Pediatrics 75:997, 1985.
42. Barton DJ, Sloan GM, Nitcher LS, et al: Hair-thread tourniquet syndrome. Pediatrics 82:925, 1988.

Chapter **47**

Incision and Drainage of Cutaneous Abscesses and Soft Tissue Infections

Todd M. Warden and Mark W. Fourré

INTRODUCTION

Cutaneous abscesses are among the soft tissue infections most frequently encountered in the emergency department. Approximately 1 to 2 per cent of patients presenting to the emergency department receive care for cutaneous abscesses.[1, 2] In contrast with most bacterial diseases, which are usually described in terms of their etiologic agent, cutaneous abscesses are best described in terms of their location. There has been little systematic investigation into the bacteriology of simple cutaneous abscesses, and there have been few new recommendations for improved management over the years. The probable reason for this is the predictable and striking recovery of the patient once a mature abscess is incised and drained. The exact reasons for this amelioration of local and constitutional symptoms are unknown, but it is clear that the specific bacteriology of abscesses in the vast majority of cases is unimportant to the outcome.[3]

ETIOLOGY AND PATHOGENESIS

Localized pyogenic infections may develop in any region of the body and usually are initiated by a breakdown in the normal epidermal defense mechanisms, with subsequent tissue invasion by normal resident flora. Thus infection in most areas is likely to be caused by the flora that are indigenous to that area. An exception is direct inoculation of extraneous organisms, such as infections that follow mammalian bite wounds.

Staphylococcal strains, which are normally found on the skin, produce rapid necrosis, early suppuration, and local-ized infections with large amounts of creamy yellow pus. This is the presentation of a typical abscess. Group A β-hemolytic streptococcal infections, on the other hand, tend to spread through tissues, causing a more generalized infection characterized by erythema and edema, a serous exudate, and little or no necrosis. This is the presentation of a typical cellulitis. Anaerobic bacteria proliferate in the oral and perineal regions, produce necrosis with profuse brownish, foul-smelling pus,[3] and may cause both abscess and cellulitis formation.

Normal skin is extremely resistant to bacterial invasion, and few organisms are capable of penetrating the intact epidermis. In the normal host with intact skin, the topical application of even very high concentrations of pathogenic bacteria does not result in infection. The requirements for infection include a high concentration of pathogenic organisms, such as occurs in the hair follicles and their adnexa; occlusion, which prevents desquamation and normal drainage, creating a moist environment; adequate nutrients; and trauma to the corneal layer, which allows organisms to penetrate.[4] This trauma may be the result of abrasions, hematoma, injection of chemical irritants, incision, or occlusive dressings that cause maceration of the skin. Foreign bodies can also potentiate these infections and decrease the number of bacteria necessary for infection. An example of this is the ubiquitous suture abscess, which frequently develops in wounds closed by suture material.

When favorable factors are present, the normal flora of the cutaneous areas can then colonize and infect the skin. The bodily area involved depends primarily on host factors. In persons performing manual labor, the arms and the hands are infected most frequently. In women, the axilla and submammary regions are frequently infected because of minor trauma from shaving and garments and because of the abundance of bacteria in these areas. Intravenous drug users may develop infections anywhere on the body, although the upper extremities are most commonly affected.[5, 6] Deep soft tissue abscesses have also been described following attempts at access to the deep venous structures in addicts who have exhausted all peripheral venous access sites.[7] In addition, areas with compromised blood supply will be more prone to infection, because normal host cell–mediated immunity is not as available.[4] Septic emboli from endocarditis may cause abscess formation by bacteremic migration of infected material into subcutaneous tissue.

Infections in the soft tissue often begin as a cellulitis. Some organisms cause necrosis, liquefaction, and accumulation of leukocytes and debris, followed by loculation and walling off of pus, which result in the formation of one or more abscesses. There may be involvement of the lymph tissues, producing lymphangitis and subsequent bacteremia. As the process progresses, the area of liquefaction increases until it "points" and eventually ruptures into the area of least resistance. This may be toward the skin or the mucous membrane, into surrounding tissue, or into a body cavity. If the abscess is particularly deep-seated, spontaneous drainage may occur with persistence of a fistulous tract and the formation of a chronic draining sinus. This development or the recurrence of an abscess that has been previously drained should always suggest the possibility of osteomyelitis, a retained foreign body, or the presence of unusual organisms, such as *Myocobacterium* or *Actinomyces*.[3]

Bacteriology of Cutaneous Abscesses

Meislin and coworkers[1] cultured abscesses in 135 patients. Their patients received simple incision and drainage, and all subjects were followed as outpatients. Both aerobic and anaerobic cultures were taken. Ninety-six per cent of cultures were positive for bacteria. Four per cent were sterile (Table 47–1).

In this series predominantly mixed aerobic bacteria were isolated in abscesses of the trunk, the axilla, the extremities, and the hand. In the pure cultures, *Staphylococcus aureus* was found in 72 per cent of cases. One third of the cultures from the perianal region contained only anaerobes. Mixed cultures of both aerobic and anaerobic bacteria were obtained from all sites of the body, but there was a 67 per cent incidence of such mixed cultures from the perirectal area. Commonly isolated anaerobes included various *Bacteroides* species, peptococci, peptostreptococci, *Clostridium* species, *Lactobacillus* species, and *Fusobacterium* species.

Bacteria from abscesses in areas remote from the rectum were generally aerobic strains and were primarily indigenous microflora of the skin. *S. aureus* was the most prevalent aerobic organism; it was isolated in 24 per cent of all abscesses.

Gram-negative aerobes were isolated infrequently from cutaneous abscesses. *Escherichia coli*, *Neisseria gonorrhoeae*, and *Pseudomonas* species were rarely found. The most commonly isolated gram-negative organism was *Proteus mirabilis*, and this organism was found almost exclusively in the axilla. This may be related to the use of underarm deodorants.[8]

Brook and associates[9] studied the bacteriology of cuta-

neous abscesses in children. Their results closely correlate with those of Meislin and associates.[1] Brook and colleagues found aerobes (staphylococci and group A β-hemolytic streptococci) to be the most common isolates from abscesses of the head, the neck, the extremities, and the trunk, with anaerobes predominating in abscesses of the buttocks and the perirectal sites. Mixed aerobic and anaerobic flora were found in the perirectal area, the head, and the finger and nail bed area. This study found an unexpectedly high incidence of anaerobes in nonperineal abscesses. Anaerobes were found primarily either in areas adjacent to mucosal membranes, where these organisms tend to thrive (e.g., the mouth), or in areas that are easily contaminated (e.g., by sucking fingers, which causes nail bed and finger infections or bite injuries).

Parenteral drug abusers develop somewhat atypical abscesses. Webb and Thadepalli found anaerobes to be a major pathogen regardless of anatomic location.[10] Because intravenous drug abuse is associated with immunodeficiency syndromes, unusual isolates such as *Candida albicans*[11] and acid-fast bacilli[12] have been obtained.

Special Considerations

Parenteral drug abusers, insulin-dependent diabetics, hemodialysis patients, cancer patients, transplant recipients, and individuals with acute leukemias have an increased frequency of abscess formation. Local symptoms may not be the primary complaint, and, indeed, the patient may present only with an exacerbation of the underlying disease process. These abscesses tend to have exotic or uncommon bacteriologic or fungal causes and typically respond poorly to therapy.[10–12] The diabetic patient in diabetic ketoacidosis should be evaluated extensively for an infectious process; a rectal examination should be included with the physical examination to rule out a perirectal abscess. This also holds true for other patients with abnormal cell-mediated immunity. The increased frequency of abscess formation in these patients and in the parenteral drug abuser is multifactorial. There may be intrinsic immune deficiencies in all these patients; they have an increased incidence of *Staphylococcus* carriage, and they have frequent needle punctures, which allow access of pathogenic bacteria.[13]

It is important to note that a substantial percentage of abscesses in parenteral drug abusers are sterile and are the result of the injection of necrotizing chemical irritants. Drug abusers frequently use veins of the neck and the femoral

Table 47–1. Characterization of 135 Outpatient Abscesses*

Anatomic Areas	Abscesses	Per Cent of Total Cultures	Type of Bacterial Growth (Per Cent from Each Area)				Bacterial Species per Abscess*	
			No Growth	*Aerobes Only*	*Anaerobes Only*	*Aerobes and Anaerobes*	*Aerobes*	*Anaerobes*
	No.						*Average no.*	
Head and neck	25	19	4	28	20	48	1	2
Trunk	11	8	0	45	18	36	1	2
Axilla	22	16	0	55	5	41	1	1
Extremity	16	12	19	44	13	25	1	1
Hand	8	6	25	63	0	13	2	0
Inguinal	7	5	0	29	57	14	0	3
Vulvovaginal	13	10	0	15	46	38	1	3
Buttock	12	9	0	33	33	33	1	3
Perirectal	21	16	0	0	33	67	1	5

*Cultures with no growth were excluded.
(From Meislin HW, et al: Bacterial characterization profile of 135 outpatient abscesses. Ann Intern Med 87:146, 1977. Reproduced by permission.)

areas, producing abscesses and other infectious complications at these sites.[14] Any abscess of the antecubital fossa or the dorsum of the hand should alert the physician to possible intravenous drug abuse.

MANIFESTATIONS OF ABSCESS FORMATION

The diagnosis of cutaneous abscess formation is often straightforward. The presence of a fluctuant mass in an area of induration, erythema, and tenderness is clinical evidence that an abscess exists. An abscess may appear initially as a definite tender soft tissue mass, but in some cases of soft tissue infection, the presence of a distinct abscess may not be readily evident. If the abscess is quite deep, as is true of many perirectal, pilonidal, or breast abscesses, the clinician may be misled by the presence of only a firm, tender, indurated area without a definite mass. Although a localized abscess is present, the uninitiated will frequently diagnose cellulitis in such cases. In borderline cases, one may aspirate the area with a needle and syringe to confirm the presence of pus.[15] Occasionally, one will be misled by a mycotic aneurysm or an inflamed lymph node simulating an abscess. A specific entity that is commonly mistaken for a discrete abscess is the sublingual cellulitis of Ludwig angina. Cellulitis and abscess formation may lead to bacteremia and sepsis, especially in the immunocompromised patient.[10]

LABORATORY FINDINGS

Laboratory tests offer no specific guidelines for therapy and are not generally indicated. An exception would be a blood or urine glucose determination to assess diabetes. The patient may demonstrate a leukocytosis, depending on the severity and duration of the abscess process; however, the majority of patients with an uncomplicated cutaneous abscess will have a normal complete blood count (CBC) and will not experience fever, chills, or malaise.

Gram stain is not indicated in the care of uncomplicated simple abscesses. Patients who are toxic or immunocompromised and those patients who require prophylactic antibiotics (see "Antibiotics") may benefit from Gram stain and cultures. Gram stain results have been shown to correlate well with subsequent culture results and in compromised hosts should be used to direct antibiotic choice.[15, 16] Anaerobic infections should be suspected when multiple organisms are noted on Gram stain, when a foul odor is associated with the pus, when free air is noted on x-ray of the soft tissue, or when cultures are reported as "no growth."[10]

In uncomplicated abscesses, *routine culture is unnecessary* because of the expected prompt response to surgical therapy. However, in complicated cases or in immunosuppressed patients, the pus from an abscess should be cultured. The information obtained from a culture may later be useful if there is poor response to the initial surgical drainage, secondary spread of the infection, or the occurrence of bacteremia.[3] If one takes a culture, it is best to aspirate the pus with a needle and syringe *before* incision and drainage. Material should be cultured for aerobic and anaerobic bacteria. The finding of a "sterile" culture in an abscess that has been cultured with a standard cotton swab *after* incision is frequently the result of improper anaerobic culture techniques. As a side note, there is a general misconception that foul-smelling pus is a result of *E. coli.* This foul odor is actually caused by the presence of anaerobes; the pus of *E. coli* is odorless.

THERAPEUTIC CONSIDERATIONS

Surgical incision and drainage is the *definitive treatment* of a soft-tissue abscess.[16] Antibiotics alone are *ineffective* in the face of a localized collection of pus. The drainage of a suppurative focus results in a marked improvement in symptoms and a rapid resolution of the infection in uncomplicated cases. Premature incision before localization of pus will not be curative and may be deleterious, because extension of the infectious process and bacteremia from manipulation can result. In some cases, the application of heat to an area of inflammation may ease pain, speed resolution of the cellulitis, and facilitate the localization and accumulation of pus. It must be stressed that nonsurgical methods are not a substitute for surgical drainage and should not be continued for more than 24 to 36 hours before the patient is reevaluated for surgical therapy. Diagnostic needle aspiration is recommended if one is unsure of pus localization.

Antibiotics

The use of antibiotics remains controversial for both the prophylaxis and management of cutaneous abscesses. As an overview, there are no data that definitively demonstrate the need for antibiotic therapy in conjunction with incision and drainage of uncomplicated cutaneous abscesses in healthy, immunocompetent patients, without valvular heart disease. The specific value of concomitant antibiotics in the immunocompromised patient is unclear. Patients with risk factors for endocarditis comprise a third group of patients. Because of the concern of inducing a bacteremia by manipulation of infected tissue, parenteral antibiotics are commonly given prior to the incision and drainage procedure in patients at risk from such bacteremia. Transient bacteremia has been documented following manipulation of noninfected tissue (brushing teeth, sigmoidoscopy, rectal examination) and following simple incision and drainage of abscesses. In the report by Fine and colleagues, six of ten patients with cutaneous abscesses were noted to have positive blood cultures immediately following incision and drainage, whereas all cultures were negative before the procedure.[17] Blick and associates evaluated the use of prophylactic antibiotics in abscesses managed in the operating room under general anesthesia. Three of 19 patients developed bacteremia after the procedure. A similar group treated with parenteral antibiotics before the procedure had only one patient with a positive blood culture. That culture yielded an organism resistant to the prophylactic antibiotic used.[18]

PROPHYLACTIC ANTIBIOTICS

The precise risk for endocarditis following incision and drainage of cutaneous abscess is unknown. However, since bacteremia clearly occurs with manipulation of infected tissue, it is generally agreed that those patients at risk for cardiac complications related to transient bacteremia should be treated with appropriate antibiotics within the hour preceding the procedure. The transient bacteremia secondary to abscess drainage is probably of no concern in otherwise healthy, immunocompetent individuals without valvular heart disease.

The Committee on Rheumatic Fever and Infective Endocarditis of the American Heart Association has recommended that prophylactic antibiotics be given prior to incision and drainage of infected tissue of the oral cavity and respiratory tract in patients who have *cardiac lesions that are at high risk for developing endocarditis.* Table 47–2 lists condi-

Endocarditis prophylaxis recommended
   Prosthetic cardiac valves (including biosynthetic valves)
   Most congenital cardiac malformations
   Surgically constructed systemic-pulmonary shunts
   Rheumatic and other acquired valvular dysfunction
   Idiopathic hypertrophic subaortic stenosis
   Previous history of bacterial endocarditis
   Mitral valve prolapse with insufficiency*
Endocarditis prophylaxis not recommended
   Isolated secundum atrial septal defect
   Secundum atrial septal defect repaired without a patch 6 or
     more months earlier
   Patent ductus arteriosus ligated and divided 6 or more months
     earlier
   Postoperatively after coronary artery bypass graft surgery

*Definitive data to provide guidance in management of patients with mitral valve prolapse are particularly limited. In general, such patients are clearly at low risk of development of endocarditis, but the risk-benefit ratio of prophylaxis in mitral valve prolapse is uncertain.
(Adapted from Shulman et al: Circulation 70:1123A, 1984. From Kaye D: Prophylaxis for infective endocarditis: An update. Ann Intern Med 104:419, 1986.)

tions that warrant antibiotic coverage.[19] Although not specifically stated, it makes intuitive sense to provide prophylaxis for all cutaneous abscesses. It should be noted that many of the bacteria found in cutaneous abscesses are not particularly high risk for producing endocarditis, even in the presence of valvular damage. Interestingly, the antibiotic regimen suggested by the AHA (Table 47–3) does not include antibiotics effective against many organisms commonly found in some cutaneous abscesses, specifically *S. aureus*, but is mainly directed against *Streptococcus viridans* and enterococcus. These latter organisms have a predilection for valvular infection.

Two clinical situations deserve special note. Because of the frequent incidence of endocarditis in the patient who abuses drugs intravenously, prophylactic antibiotics may be indicated prior to the incision and drainage of abscesses in these patients. Clearly, any patient with a documented history of endocarditis must receive prophylactic antibiotics prior to the incision and drainage procedure. Because cutaneous abscesses may result from active endocarditis and prophylactic antibiotics may obscure subsequent attempts at identifying an etiologic organism, two or three blood cultures (aerobic and anaerobic) should be obtained from those at risk for endocarditis prior to antibiotic therapy. Patients with the diagnosis of mitral valve prolapse have traditionally been included for treatment with prophylactic antibiotics. The indication for this is unclear. The risk of an allergic reaction may outweigh the benefits of treatment in this group[20] and clinical judgment is required. Kaye[21] suggests prophylaxis only for patients who have a holosystolic murmur secondary to mitral valve prolapse.

Immunocompromised patients have not been adequately studied and may benefit from prophylactic antibiotics. In contrast to the endocarditis risks, they are at risk for developing septicemia secondary to a brief bacteremia. Since intravenous drug users have a high incidence of human immunodeficiency virus (HIV) related disease,[22–24] the treating physician must anticipate varying degrees of immunodeficiency in these patients. Clinical judgment must determine the use of antibiotics in these situations.

No specific guidelines have been offered for the antibiotic regimen used prior to incision and drainage of infected cutaneous tissue in patients at risk for conditions other than endocarditis. Choice of antibiotics is guided by the organism anticipated to cause the bacteremia. Although the location of the abscess will give some clue regarding the organism involved, most abscesses contain multiple strains of bacteria. Since staphylococcus continues to be a significant organism in this setting, a broad-spectrum antistaphylococcal drug is indicated.[5] Prophylaxis should consist of a single *intravenous* dose given one-half hour prior to incision and drainage. A first-generation cephalosporin or penicillinase resistant penicillin is a good initial choice. Vancomycin may also be considered. Based on a recent review of antimicrobial prophylaxis in various surgical procedures (Medical Letter 31(806):105, 1989), cefazolin (Ancef, Kefzol), 1 gm intravenously, may be given one-half hour before surgery. This regimen covers staphylococcal and streptococcal species, many gram-negative organisms, and many anaerobes.

Although not widely used in the United States, parenteral antibiotics have been used to "sterilize" the abscess cavity in Great Britain following curettage. The concentration of clindamycin in the blood that has seeped into the abscess cavity has been shown to have the same concentration of antibiotics as that found in the intravenous circulation.[18] The British literature reports success with "primary closure under antibiotic coverage,"[25–27] although other British reports continue to recommend the traditional procedure.[28, 29] One limitation to the British technique is the need for general anesthesia, since the performance of curettage is extremely painful.

THERAPEUTIC ANTIBIOTICS

In contrast to prophylaxis prior to surgery, the use of oral antibiotics *following* incision and drainage of simple

Standard regimen
   For dental procedures that cause gingival bleeding, and oral or respiratory tract surgery

   Penicillin V, 2.0 gm orally, 1 hour before, then 1.0 gm 6 hours later. For patients unable to take oral medications, 2×10^6 U of aqueous penicillin G intravenously or intramuscularly 30 to 60 minutes before a procedure and 1×10^6 U 6 hours later may be substituted.

Special regimens
   Parenteral regimen for use when maximal protection is desired, for example, for patients with prosthetic valves

   Ampicillin, 1.0 to 2.0 gm intramuscularly or intravenously, plus gentamicin, 1.5 mg/kg body weight intramuscularly or intravenously, 0.5 hour before procedure, followed by 1.0 gm of oral penicillin V 6 hours later. Alternatively, the parenteral regimen may be repeated once 8 hours later.

   Oral regimen for patients allergic to penicillin
   Erythromycin, 1.0 gm orally 1 hour before, then 500 mg 6 hours later.

   Parenteral regimen for patients allergic to penicillin
   Vancomycin, 1.0 gm intravenously, slowly over 1 hour, starting 1 hour before. No repeat dose is necessary.

cutaneous abscesses appears to have less value. Llera and Levy performed a randomized double-blind study to compare outcomes of patients treated with a first-generation cephalosporin following drainage of cutaneous abscesses in the emergency department. They found no significant difference in clinical outcome between the two groups and concluded that antibiotics are unnecessary in individuals with normal host defenses.[2] This confirmed previous less well-controlled studies.[18, 25, 27, 28] It should be noted that high-risk patients were often excluded from these studies. Again, the immunocompromised patient has not been adequately studied in this situation and is therefore often given antibiotics empirically.

Patients with cutaneous abscesses often have concomitant disease processes that may warrant the use of parenteral or oral antibiotics. Cellulitis or lymphangitis often accompany abscesses and the value of therapeutic antibiotics is less well addressed in the literature. Meislin noted that pathogen identification in cases of cellulitis can be difficult and empiric antibiotics may be helpful.[30] Intravenous drug abusers who present with an abscess and fever require parenteral antibiotics after blood cultures have been drawn until such time as subacute bacterial endocarditis can be eliminated as a diagnosis.[31] Obviously, patients who are clinically septic require immediate intravenous antibiotics as well as aggressive surgical drainage of collections of pus.

As a general guideline, therapeutic antibiotics should be given to all immunocompromised patients (e.g., AIDS, diabetes, chemotherapy, steroid use, transplant recipient, alcoholism) and to the immunocompetent patient with "significant" cellulitis, lymphangitis, or systemic symptoms, such as chills or fever. Although it has not been studied, it makes sense to also give *antibiotics prophylactically, before surgery, to all patients who will obviously be given therapeutic antibiotics.* As with prophylactic antibiotics, a first-generation cephalosporin or semisynthetic penicillin is a reasonable therapeutic choice unless the specific abscess site dictates alternative therapy. The ideal duration of therapeutic antibiotics is unknown. As a general guideline immunocompromised patients should receive antibiotics for 5 to 7 days postprocedure and immunocompetent patients for 3 to 5 days, depending on the severity of the condition and clinical response.

INCISION AND DRAINAGE PROCEDURE

Definitive incision and drainage of soft tissue abscesses is performed in either the emergency department or the operating room. The choice of the locale for the procedure depends on a number of important factors. Location of the abscess may dictate management in the operating room. Large abscesses or abscesses located deep in the soft tissues require a procedure involving a great degree of patient cooperation, which may only be possible under general or regional anesthesia. Proximity to major neurovascular structures such as in the axillae or antecubital fossa may necessitate intraoperative management. Infections of the hand (with the exception of distal finger infections) have traditionally been managed in the operating room because of the many important structures involved and the propensity for limb-threatening complications.

Lack of adequate anesthesia is the most common limiting factor in emergency department incision and drainage. If the emergency physician believes the abscess cannot be fully incised and drained because of inadequate anesthesia, the patient should be taken to the operating room for management under general anesthesia.

Some centers prefer to drain all abscesses in a special area of the emergency department, which can subsequently be decontaminated. A standard suture tray provides the adequate instruments if a scalpel and packing material are added. Although sterility is impossible during the procedure, one should avoid contamination of surrounding tissue. Some physicians prefer to use an obligatory skin scrub with an antiseptic solution, but the value of this step is unproved.

It is often quite difficult to obtain local anesthesia in infected tissue because of the poor function of the local anesthetic agents in the low pH of the infected areas. Furthermore, the distention of sensitive structures by a local injection is quite painful and hence poorly tolerated by most patients. Skin anesthesia is usually possible, but total anesthesia of the abscess cavity itself generally cannot be achieved. If a regional block can be performed in the area, this type of anesthesia is preferred. A field block may be used if there is no area of cellulitis surrounding the abscess. It should be noted that infected tissue is very vascular, and local anesthetics are quickly absorbed. Strict adherence to maximum safe doses of a local anesthetic is required.

The skin over the dome of an abscess is often quite thin, making skin anesthesia difficult. If a 25-gauge needle is carefully used, one can often inject the dome of the abscess subcutaneously. The anesthetic solution spreads over the dome through the subcutaneous layers into the surrounding skin and provides excellent skin anesthesia. If the needle is in the proper plane, the skin blanches during infiltration. In the extremely anxious or uncomfortable patient, the judicious use of preoperative intravenous narcotics (such as meperidine), sedatives (such as midazolam),[32] or nitrous

Table 47–3B. Summary of Recommended Antibiotic Regimens for Adults Having Gastrointestinal or Genitourinary Tract Procedures*

Standard regimen	
For genitourinary and gastrointestinal tract procedures	Ampicillin, 2.0 gm intramuscularly or intravenously, plus gentamicin, 1.5 mg/kg body weight intramuscularly or intravenously, given 0.5 to 1 hour before the procedure. One follow-up dose may be given 8 hours later.
Special regimens	
Oral regimen for minor or repetitive procedures in low-risk patients	Amoxicillin, 3.0 gm orally, 1 hour before procedure and 1.5 gm 6 hours later.
Patients allergic to penicillin	Vancomycin, 1.0 gm intravenously, given slowly over 1 hour, plus gentamicin, 1.5 mg/kg body weight intramuscularly or intravenously, given 1 hour before procedure. May be repeated once 8 to 12 hours later.

*Prophylactic antibiotic regimens for various procedures in adults at risk for endocarditis. Although these tables do not specifically address the incision and drainage of cutaneous abscesses, the antibiotics are chosen for their spectrum against organisms known to cause endocarditis and can intuitively be used prior to management of cutaneous abscesses in patients with cardiac conditions listed in Table 47–2.

(Adapted from Shulman et al: Circulation 70:1123A, 1984. From Kaye D: Prophylaxis for infective endocarditis: An update. Ann Intern Med 104:419, 1986.)

oxide makes the procedure easier for both patient and physician.[33] If adequate anesthesia cannot be obtained and pain limits the procedure, the patient should be admitted and treated under general anesthesia.

Some reports recommend the use of topical ethyl chloride spray for the initial skin incision, but the pain relief offered by this agent is variable and fleeting. Ethyl chloride is also highly flammable. Ethyl chloride spray is occasionally useful to provide momentary anesthesia for the initial skin incision if the incision is made while the ethyl chloride is being sprayed. In general this agent is a poor choice of anesthesia for all but the smallest of superficial abscesses (e.g., purulent folliculitis).

One should make all incisions conform with skin creases or natural folds to minimize visible scar formation (Fig. 47–1). Extreme care should be taken in such areas as the groin, the posterior knee, the antecubital fossa, and the neck, so that vascular and neural structures are not damaged.

A number 11 scalpel blade is used to nick the skin over the fluctuant area, and then a simple linear incision is carried the *total length of the abscess cavity* (Fig. 47–2A). This will afford more complete drainage and will facilitate subsequent break-up of loculations. A cruciate incision or an elliptic skin *excision* is to be avoided in the routine treatment of cutaneous abscess. The tips of the flaps of a cruciate incision may necrose, resulting in an unsightly scar. A timid stab incision (the so-called medical incision) is not adequate for proper drainage. An exception to this rule is an abscess in a cosmetic area, where a stab incision may be initially tried to limit scar formation. It should be emphasized that the scalpel is used only to make the skin incision and is never used deep in the abscess cavity.

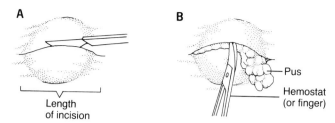

Figure 47–2. *A,* The skin over the abscess is incised the full length of the abscess. A small stab incision does not allow for proper drainage. *B,* A hemostat or a finger is inserted into the abscess cavity to spread the skin, to drain the pus, and to break up loculations.

The physician should probe the depth of an abscess with a gloved finger or a hemostat to assess the extent of the abscess and to ensure proper drainage by breaking open loculations (Fig.49–2B). One is often surprised at the depth or extent of an abscess during probing. Sharp curettage of the abscess cavity is usually not required and may produce bacteremia.[18] Although tissue probing is usually the most painful aspect of the technique, and total local anesthesia is difficult to obtain, this portion of the procedure should not be abbreviated. If the procedure is limited because of pain, the use of an intravenous narcotic should be considered.

Following the break-up of loculations, some physicians advocate copious irrigation with normal saline to ensure adequate removal of excess debris from the wound cavity. Although intuitively helpful, irrigation of the abscess cavity has not been experimentally demonstrated to clearly augment healing or affect outcome. Hyperemic tissue may bleed profusely, but bleeding usually stops in a few minutes if packing is used. Abscesses of the extremities should be drained with the use of a tourniquet to provide a bloodless field. After irrigation, a loose packing of gauze or other material is placed gently into the abscess cavity to prevent the wound margins from closing and to afford continued drainage of any exudative material that may otherwise be trapped. The packing material should make contact with the cavity wall so that upon removal a gentle débridement of necrotic tissue will spontaneously occur. Care must be exercised to ensure that the packing does not exert significant pressure against the exposed tissue and lead to further tissue necrosis. Some prefer to use plain gauze, some use gauze soaked in povidone-iodine, and some use gauze impregnated with iodine (iodoform). For large abscess cavities, 10-cm by 10-cm gauze pads are ideal packing. Thin (0.6 to 1.2 cm) packing strip gauze, either plain or with iodoform, is used for smaller abscesses. The iodoform gauze may sting the patient for a few minutes after it is inserted. The value of antibiotic-impregnated gauze is uncertain. Absorbent gauze dressing should be placed over the packed abscess or, if an extremity is involved, a lightly wrapped circumferential dressing should be used. Generous amounts of dry gauze are used over the packing to soak up any drainage or blood. The affected part should be splinted if possible, and elevation should be routine. Drainage relieves most of the pain of an abscess, but postoperative analgesics may be required.

FOLLOW-UP CARE

Subsequent care of the wound has not been adequately studied. Reevaluation of the wound has occurred anywhere from 24 hours to 5 days following incision and drainage in different study protocols.[18, 28, 32] Hence, follow-up care is dependent on clinical parameters. Most lesions are reevaluated 48 hours following the procedure, with the packing

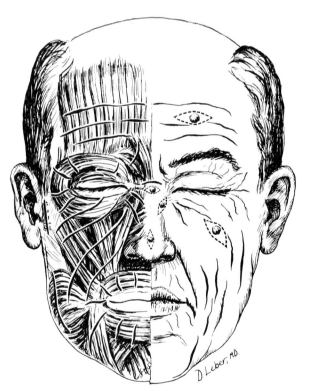

Figure 47–1. The relation of the elective lines of tension in the face to the underlying mimetic musculature. Only in the lower eyelid are these lines not perpendicular to the muscles. The left side of the drawing shows the use of this principle when common facial lesions are excised or a facial abscess is drained. (From Schwartz SI, Lillehei RC: Principles of Surgery. 2nd ed. New York, McGraw-Hill Book Co, 1974. Reproduced by permission.)

being changed at time of reexamination. Many wounds warrant closer monitoring. Diabetic patients or other patients with impaired healing capacities may require admission for more frequent wound care/packing changes or reevaluation within 24 hours. Wounds that are at high risk for complications, such as those about the face or hands, require close follow-up and should ideally be evaluated by the same examiner.

The patient should be instructed to play an active role in wound care. During the first follow-up visit, the patient should be taught to perform packing and dressing changes. If this is anatomically impossible, a friend or family member can be instructed in the technique. If no social support system is available, a home health service can be contacted to aid the patient. In some instances, however, the patient will be unable to receive proper wound care at home and will require admission.

The frequency of packing or dressing changes is also clinically guided. Wounds large enough to require packing should be repacked at least every 48 hours (occasionally daily for the first few visits) until healing continues in a deep to superficial direction. Wounds that are allowed to close superficially will create an unsterile dead space that will potentiate the formation of recurrent abscesses. After the first few days (and in the motivated individual) an alternative to packing is to have the patient swab the base of the abscess three times a day with swabs soaked in peroxide. This promotes drainage, produces gentle débridement, and keeps the incision open. In general, once healthy granulation tissue has developed throughout the wound and a well-established drainage tract is present, the packing may be discontinued. The patient should then be instructed to begin warm soaks of the wound.[32] Gentle hydrostatic débridement may be performed by the patient in the shower at home. With this procedure the patient holds the skin incision open and directs the shower spray into the abscess cavity. Wet to dry normal saline dressing changes should then be performed by the patient or the assistant until healing is completed. When all signs of infection (e.g., erythema, drainage, pain, and induration) have resolved and healthy granulation tissue is present, the patient may be discharged from medical care.

Wounds that require prolonged care are best followed by a single physician and should not be routinely cared for in the emergency department. These patients should receive early referral to their primary care physician or, when appropriate, to a general or plastic surgeon. Wounds in cosmetically important areas may require revision once healing is complete. Patients should be informed of this possibility early on in their care.

An effective alternative to packing the abscess is the catheter system of drainage.[34, 35] In selected cases, in which extensive or prolonged drainage occurs or in patients who are unable to return for proper follow-up care, the catheter system of drainage may be preferred. Following incision, a balloon-tipped or flared-tip catheter is placed into the abscess cavity, and pus is allowed to drain continuously through the catheter lumen. This technique has been most successful in pilonidal and in Bartholin gland abscesses, but the technique is applicable to any abscess *not* on the face.

Facial abscesses should be handled carefully and checked frequently. Any abscess above the upper lip and below the brow may drain into the cavernous sinus, and thus manipulation may predispose to septic thrombophlebitis of this system. Treatment should include antistaphylococcal antibiotics and warm soaks until resolution of the process. Areas *not* in this zone of the face can be treated in a manner similar to that for other cutaneous abscesses. In all facial abscesses, note should be made of the direction of the natural lines of the skin, and the incision over the abscess should be directed along these lines in order to maximize the cosmetic effect (see Fig. 47–1). Because cosmesis is important on the face, the packing should be removed after only 24 hours, at which time warm soaks should be started.

SPECIFIC ABSCESS THERAPY

Staphylococcal Diseases

The *Staphylococcus* is a ubiquitous parasite that frequently colonizes the nose, the skin, the perineum, and the gut. The umbilicus of neonates is also commonly colonized. It grows on the skin and thrives particularly well in hair follicles, causing boils (furuncles), wound infections, and occasionally carbuncles. The pathogenesis of staphylococcal disease is a complex host-bacteria interaction. *S. aureus* invades the skin by way of the hair follicles or an open wound and produces local tissue destruction followed by hyperemia of vessels. Subsequently, an exudative reaction occurs, during which polymorphonuclear cells invade. The process then extends along the path of least resistance. The abscess may "point," or form sinus tracts. The process can disseminate by invasion of vessels and thus can infect other organs. Most cases of staphylococcal osteomyelitis, meningitis, and endocarditis occur by this mechanism.[36, 37]

When a small abscess occurs at the root of a hair, the condition is termed *folliculitis.* Local measures, including warm compresses and antibacterial soaps and ointments, are the usual treatment. Furuncles, or boils, are acute circumscribed abscesses of the skin and subcutaneous tissue that most commonly occur on the face, the neck, the buttocks, the thigh, the perineum, or the breast or in the axilla. The local application of heat and bacitracin ointment is usually adequate until spontaneous drainage occurs,[36, 37] but incision and drainage are occasionally required.

Carbuncles are aggregates of interconnected furuncles that frequently occur on the back of the neck. In this area the skin is thick, and extension therefore occurs laterally rather than toward the skin surface. Carbuncles may attain large size and can cause systemic symptoms and complications. They are found in increased frequency in diabetics. Treatment should consist of surgical drainage and occasionally the administration of systemic antibiotics.[36, 37] Large carbuncles may be impossible to drain adequately in the emergency department. Occasionally, wide excision and skin grafting are required.

Most cases of recurrent staphylococcal skin infections are caused by autoinfection from existing skin lesions or nasal reservoirs. Management is directed at eliminating the organism. This is accomplished by the application of bacitracin to the nares and good hygiene, including frequent cleansing with antibacterial soap. If these measures are unsuccessful, then systemic antistaphylococcal treatment is instituted for 2 to 3 weeks. Detection and treatment of infection in family members may be necessary.[36, 37]

Hidradenitis Suppurativa

Hidradenitis suppurativa (Greek hydros = sweat, aden = gland) is a chronic, relapsing, inflammatory disease process affecting the apocrine gland that primarily involves the axilla or the inguinal region, or both.[38] The condition results from occlusion of the apocrine ducts by keratinatous debris, which leads to ductal dilatation, inflammation, and rupture into the subcutaneous area. Secondary bacterial infection ensues, leading to abscess formation and scarring. This chronic recurring process leads to draining fistulous tracts, which involve large areas and are not amenable to simple incision and drainage procedures.[39]

Genetic factors may play some role in hidradenitis suppurativa. Family history is often significant in these patients. Fitzsimmons has proposed a single dominant gene transmission.[40] Blacks appear to have an increased incidence as compared to whites.

Although certain groups appear to be predisposed to this condition, the precipitating factor for this process is unclear. Because apocrine glands become active during puberty, it is rare to find hidradenitis suppurativa in the pediatric population.[38] Women are affected more frequently than men, for uncertain reasons. Shaving and depilation has frequently been suggested as the cause of this discrepancy; however, this theory was not supported in a study that compared the frequency of these behaviors in patients with hidradenitis suppurativa and a group of controls.[41] Obesity is associated with an increased incidence of the disease.[42] Excessive dermal folds provide dark wet, and warm areas, which are ideal for the proliferation of bacteria that are needed for this infectious process. Antiperspirants and deodorants may decrease wetness and bacterial overgrowth, but they have been known to produce inflammatory responses, which could exacerbate the disease process.

The bacteriology of acute abscess formation in hidradenitis suppurativa reflects organisms seen in other soft tissue abscesses. *Staphylococcus* is the most commonly isolated organism, with *E. coli* and α *Streptococcus* being other important pathogens. In the perineal region, enteric flora are often found. Many of these abscesses have multiple isolates, and anaerobic bacteria are frequently found.

Hidradenitis suppurativa begins as a single inflammatory event involving an apocrine gland, which progresses to frank suppuration and at this stage is no different than a simple furuncle. The clinical entity is only distinguishable in its chronic scarring phase. By then the lesion exhibits multiple foci coupled with areas of induration and inflammation that are in various stages of healing. Progression of the process reveals coalesced areas of firm raised violaceous dermis. The lesion is usually markedly tender. This disease classically involves the axilla and perineal or inguinal region, although multiple sites are often involved.[43]

Emergency department management usually involves intervention in an acute suppurative lesion. Any area of fluctuance requires incision and drainage as described in the section on general abscess management. In cases of extensive cellulitis, a broad-spectrum, antistaphylococcal antibiotic should be used. Unfortunately, hidradenitis suppurativa is not cured with localized incision and drainage. The chronic nature of the disease produces multiple areas of inflammation and subcutaneous fistulous tracts that induce routine recurrences. The patient must be informed of this rather unfavorable prognosis and should be referred to a dermatologist or surgeon for long-term care.

Milder forms of the disease are initially treated with conservative measures. Many different approaches have been tried with numerous case reports and case series noted in the literature. Unfortunately, few controlled studies have been performed. Patients are often counseled to lose weight, refrain from shaving, stop using deodorants, and improve personal hygiene. The benefits of these efforts are unknown. Oral antistaphylococcal antibiotics are most commonly used with varying results.[44] Reports of success with topical clindamycin,[45] isotretinoin,[46, 47] and laser therapy[48] have not been studied in a controlled setting and require further investigation. Dermal infection results from breakdown of the normal host defense mechanism, which occurs with irritation, traumatic injury, or inflammation, coupled with the availability of concentrated opportunistic bacteria. There-

fore, the physician must institute therapies that will decrease bacterial availability without causing further injury to the affected dermis.

Advanced stages of the disease are routinely managed by a surgeon with wide or local excision and primary or delayed closure.[49–51] Despite this radical approach, recurrences do occur.[52] Patients must be counseled about the likelihood of recurrence before the procedure.

Breast Abscess

Postpartum mastitis occurs in 1 to 3 per cent of nursing mothers within the first 2 to 6 weeks after delivery. The infection is usually precipitated by milk stasis following weaning or missed feedings. The cause is usually bacterial invasion through a cracked or abraded nipple by *S. aureus* or streptococci originating from the nursing child. Manifestations are redness, heat, pain, fever, and chills. Treatment consists of antistaphylococcal antibiotics, continued breast emptying with a breast pump, and the application of heat. It is important to encourage continued breast emptying to promote drainage. Nursing can be continued with the non-infected breast, although the passage of the antibiotics through the breast milk may result in some infant diarrhea. Cellulitis may progress to frank abscess formation. These patients may be quite ill and may appear toxic. Abscess formation complicating postpartum mastitis usually necessitates operating room management, because the area is extremely tender and adequate local anesthesia is difficult to obtain. Strict adherence to nipple hygiene to avoid cracks or inflammation is helpful in prophylaxis.

Surprisingly, most breast abscesses occur in women who are not in the puerperium and have been termed *nonpuerperal breast abscesses*.[53] Scholefield reviewed 72 breast abscesses over a 10-year period and noted only 8.5 per cent of patients in the puerperium.[54] These lesions have been divided anatomically.

Peripherally located lesions are most commonly caused by staphylococcus and respond well to traditional conservative incision and drainage.[54] Superficial abscesses in the subcutaneous tissue may be drained under local anesthesia by means of an incision that radiates from the nipple (Fig. 47–3A).

Periareolar abscesses exhibit a more troublesome profile. The microflora often include multiple organisms, and anaerobic bacteria are important isolated pathogens.[53–56] These infections may be the result of occluded and inflamed mammary ducts. Chronic disease may lead to ductal ectasia that provides a nidus for infection. The deeper and more extensive intramammary abscess appears as a generalized swollen, tender breast (Fig. 47–3B). Fluctuance is not always obvious, since the abscess is located in the mammary tissue itself. These intramammary infections are complex and require incision and drainage under general anesthesia.

A retromammary abscess lies in the undersurface of the breast between the breast and the chest wall (Fig. 47–3C). Fluctuance may be difficult to appreciate because of the depth of the infection. Drainage under general anesthesia is required.

Recurrent abscesses are a common, troublesome complication occurring in up to 38 per cent of primary periareolar abscesses treated with standard incision, drainage, and antibiotics.[57] These cases require total excision of the involved area and require the care of a general surgeon and further intraoperative management. It may be difficult to diagnose a breast abscess in the early stages, when cellulitis predominates. In equivocal cases, antibiotics may be curative, but when pus is present, incision and drainage must be performed.

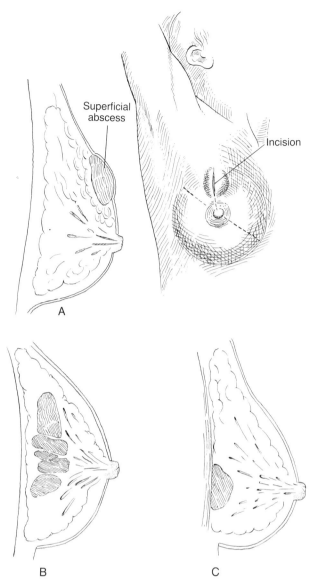

Figure 47–3. *A*, A superficial breast abscess may be drained with a linear incision that radiates from the nipple. *B* and *C*, Diagrams of intramammary abscess *(B)* and retromammary abscess *(C)*. Both require drainage under general anesthesia. The abscess itself may not be fully appreciated if it is deep seated, and the mistaken diagnosis of cellulitis may be made. (Redrawn from Wolcott MW: Ferguson's Surgery of the Ambulatory Patient. 5th ed. Philadelphia, JB Lippincott Co, 1974.)

Bartholin Gland Abscess

The Bartholin glands (vestibular glands) are secretory organs located at the 5 and 7 o'clock positions on each side of the vestibule of the vagina. Asymptomatic cysts frequently occur from duct blockage and retention of secretions. Chronic low-grade inflammation from gonococcal infections has been implicated as an etiologic factor in cyst formation, but occasionally frank abscess formation results. Such patients present with swollen and tender labia and a fluctuant, grape-sized mass that may be palpated between the thumb and the index finger. *N. gonorrhoeae* organisms are infrequently cultured from the abscess cavity, and various anaerobes, especially *Bacteroides* species and other colonic bacteria, are usually found. It is reasonable to take cervical and anal cultures for gonorrhea from patients with Bartholin gland

abscesses because of the association of these infections with venereal disease, but one need not routinely treat patients for gonorrhea.

Word[58] has described an effective treatment of Bartholin gland abscess with a single-barreled, sealed stopper, balloon-tipped catheter that may obviate the need for marsupialization (Fig. 47–4*A* and *B*). In his original description, Word reports only two recurrences in 72 lesions, both of which were successfully treated with a second catheter; no patient required marsupialization. The procedure involves fistulization of the duct cavity by a catheter, which acts as a foreign body. While not a standard incision and drainage procedure, the technique permits continued drainage of the Bartholin gland.

Following a stab incision into the mucosa, a hemostat is used to puncture the abscess cavity proper. It is helpful to stabilize the abscess with the thumb and forefinger to assure

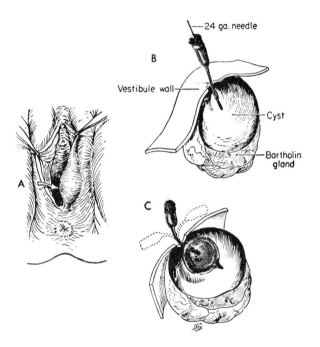

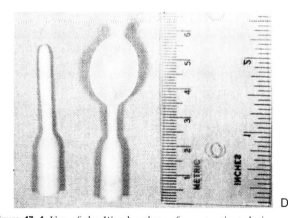

Figure 47–4. Use of the Word catheter for outpatient drainage of a Bartholin gland abscess. This is a fistulization procedure rather than a standard incision and drainage. A stab incision is made on the mucosal surface *(A)*. A catheter is inserted into the cyst cavity *(B)* and filled with 3 to 4 ml of water *(C)*. (From Word B: Office treatment of cyst and abscess of Bartholin gland. JAMA 190:777, 1964. Reproduced by permission.) *D*, Inflatable bulb-tipped catheter. *Left:* uninflated. *Right:* inflated with 4 ml water. (From Word B: Office treatment of cyst and abscess of Batholin's gland duct. South Med J 61:514, 1968. Reproduced by permission.)

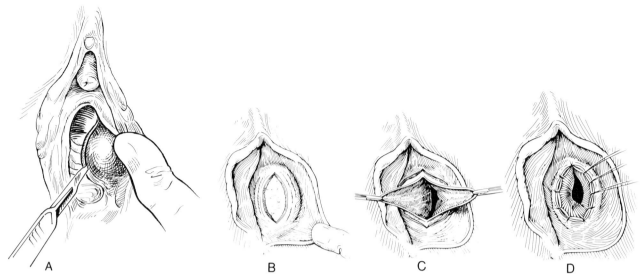

Figure 47–5. *A,* Incision for a Bartholin gland cyst or abscess. The incision should be made over the medial surface of the introitus on a line parallel with the posterior margin of the hymenal ring. At this point, a Bartholin gland cyst or abscess is most superficial. One exposes the incision area by displacing the cyst outward. *B,* Marsupialization of a Bartholin gland cyst: an ellipse is removed from the epithelium. *C,* The cyst wall is incised and everted. *D,* The cyst wall is sutured to the epithelium. (*B, C,* and *D* from Halvorson GD, Halvorson JE, Iserson KV: Abscess incision and drainage in the emergency department. J Emerg Med 3:295, 1985. Reproduced by permission.)

entrance into the abscess. Care is required to make a stab incision only large enough to accommodate the catheter and small enough to prohibit the inflated balloon from being extruded. Once the abscess has been entered (signaled by the free flow of pus), the deflated balloon is placed in the abscess cavity. Using a 25-gauge needle to minimize the hole in the stopper, the balloon is then filled with 2 to 4 ml of water (not air). Persistent pain indicates that too much fluid has been used. The device is left in place for 6 to 8 weeks, so follow-up is required. If the catheter falls out prematurely it should be quickly replaced to fullfil the 6 to 8 week criteria for fistulization. This is an interesting technique that even allows for sexual intercourse with the catheter in place.

The initial treatment of a Bartholin gland abscess may also include simple incision and drainage. The abscess is packed for 24 to 48 hours, and sitz baths are started after the first revisit. Broad-spectrum antibiotics are helpful if there is significant cellulitis or if actual abscess formation has not yet occurred, but these agents are not required following routine incision and drainage.

It is preferable to make the drainage incision on the mucosal surface rather than on the skin surface. The incision is made over the medial surface of the introitus on a line parallel to the posterior margin of the hymenal ring (Fig. 47–5A). The abscess cavity is slightly deeper than most cutaneous abscesses, and one must be certain to enter the actual abscess cavity to achieve complete drainage. This is most easily accomplished if one inserts a hemostat through the mucosal incision and spreads the tips of the instrument in the deeper soft tissue. If the abscess recurs, more definitive therapy in the form of marsupialization (Fig. 47–5B to D) or complete excision of the gland may be required, but these procedures are not performed initially. Because recurrence is common with simple incision and drainage, some authorities suggest definitive surgery routinely following the first infection, whereas others prefer to wait until a recurrence is documented.

Pilonidal Abscess

Pilonidal sinuses are common malformations that occur in the sacrococcygeal area. The etiology of the sinus for-

mation is unclear, but the malformation may occur during embryogenesis. Pilonidal cyst formation is thought to be secondary to blockage of a pilonidal sinus. The result of pilonidal sinus obstruction is repeated soft tissue infection followed by drainage and partial resolution with eventual reaccumulation. The blockage is most commonly the result of hairs in the region, and the lesion may in part be a foreign body (hair) granuloma. Although pilonidal sinuses are present from birth, they usually are not manifested clinically until adolescence or the early adult years and pilonidal abscess formation most commonly affects young (often white) adults. The sinuses and cysts are lined with stratified squamous epithelium and may contain wads of hair and debris when excised. When cultured, pilonidal abscesses generally yield mixed fecal flora with a preponderance of anaerobes.[61]

The patient with a pilonidal abscess will seek care for back pain and local tenderness. On physical examination the area is indurated, but frank abscess formation may not be appreciated. One will usually see barely perceptible dimples or tiny openings at the rostral end of the gluteal crease (Fig. 47–6). A hair or a slight discharge may be noticed at the opening. One may find a more caudal cyst or abscess, possibly with a palpable sinus tract connecting the two. The sinus and cyst may be chronically draining or they may become infected as the size increases and blockage occurs.[62]

Treatment of the acutely infected cyst is the same as previously discussed for any fluctuant abscess; all hair and pus should be removed, and the lesion should be packed. Antibiotic therapy is not usually required. The abscess cavity may become quite large, necessitating a rather lengthy incision to ensure complete drainage. It may take many weeks for the initial incision to heal. The area may be repacked at 2- to 4-day intervals as an outpatient procedure, although some prefer to discontinue packing after the first week. Since simple incision and drainage is often not curative, secondary removal of both the cyst and the sinus should be planned after the inflammatory process has resolved. The elective surgical procedure should be complete and should involve all of the possible arborizations of the sinus.

In a very few cases, recurrence will not take place following simple incision and drainage, especially if the

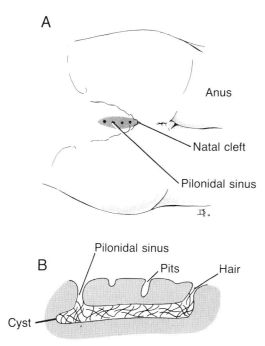

anal crypts. Within these crypts are collections of ducts from anal glands. These glands are believed to be responsible for the genesis of most, if not all, perirectal abscesses. These glands often pass through the internal sphincter but do not penetrate the external sphincter.

The muscular anatomy divides the perirectal area into compartments that may house an abscess, depending on the direction of spread of the foci of the infection (Fig. 47–9).[60, 62] The circular fibers of the intestinal coat thicken at the rectal-anal junction to become the internal anal sphincter. The muscle fibers of the levator ani fuse with those of the outer longitudinal fibers of the intestinal coat as it passes through the pelvic floor. These conjoined fibers then are connected by fibrous tissue to the external sphincter system, which consists of three circular muscle groups.

PATHOPHYSIOLOGY

As described previously, the anal glands are mucus-secreting structures that terminate in the area between the internal and external sphincters. It is believed that most perirectal infections begin in the *intersphincteric* space secondary to blockage and subsequent infection of the anal

Figure 47–6. Pilonidal sinus. *A,* Sinuses occur in midline some 5 cm above the anus in the natal cleft. *B,* Longitudinal section showing sinuses and pits. (From Hill GJ II: Outpatient Surgery. 3rd ed. Philadelphia, WB Saunders Co, 1988. Reproduced by permission.)

incision is wide and adequate drainage is obtained. More commonly, recurrence can be expected unless excision of the sinus tract is performed. Small abscesses may be incised and drained as an outpatient procedure performed under local anesthesia, but the disease process is often extensive, and general anesthesia may be required to complete drainage. One is often surprised by the extent of the cyst cavity and the volume of pus that is encountered when the area is probed during initial incision; because of the degree of these abscesses, only localized infection lends itself to outpatient therapy. A method of catheter drainage for pilonidal abscesses has been described[34, 35] in which a flared-end Pezzer catheter is used for extended periods in the abscess cavity. The catheter allows the patient more freedom from local care and provides continual drainage (Fig. 47–7).

Perirectal Abscesses

Perirectal infections can range from minor irritations to fatal illnesses. Successful management depends on early recognition of the disease process and adequate surgical therapy. Because of the morbidity and mortality associated with inadequate treatment of these conditions, patients with all but the most localized abscesses should be promptly admitted to the hospital for evaluation and treatment under general or spinal anesthesia.

It is important to understand the anatomy of the anal canal and the rectum in order to appreciate the pathophysiology of these abscesses and their treatment (Fig. 47–8). The mucosa of the anal canal is loosely attached to the muscle wall. At the dentate line, where columnar epithelium gives way to squamous epithelium, there are vertical folds of tissue, called the rectal *columns of Morgagni*, which are connected at their lower ends by small semilunar folds, called *anal valves*. Under these valves are invaginations, called

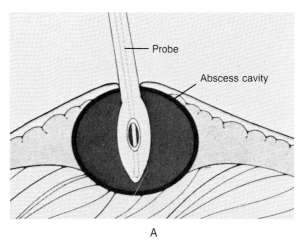

A

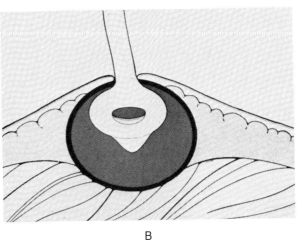

B

Figure 47–7. A method of prolonged drainage of a pilonidal abscess with a flared-end Pezzer catheter. Following a stab incision, a stretched catheter (probe inside lumen) is inserted into the abscess cavity *(A)*. When the probe is removed, the head of the catheter expands and remains in the abscess cavity *(B)*. Drainage is continuous through the lumen of the catheter. (From Phillip RS: A simplified method for the incision and drainage of abscesses. Am J Surg 135:721, 1978. Reproduced by permission.)

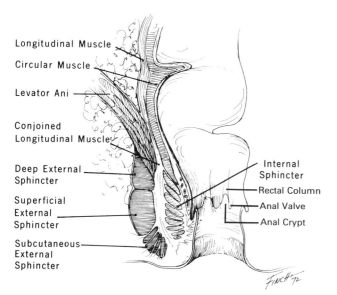

Figure 47–8. Schematic coronal section of the anal canal and the rectum. (From Schwartz SI, Lillehei RC: Principles of Surgery. 2nd ed. New York, McGraw-Hill Book Co, 1974. Reproduced by permission.)

glands. Normal host defense mechanisms then break down, followed by invasion and overgrowth by bowel flora.[63]

If the infection spreads across the external sphincter laterally, an *ischiorectal abscess* is formed. If the infection dissects rostrally, it may continue between the internal and external sphincters, causing a *high intramuscular abscess*. The infection may dissect through the external sphincter over the levator ani to form the *pelvirectal abscess*.[60]

When the infection of an anal crypt extends by way of the perianal lymphatics and continues between the mucous membrane and the anal muscles, a *perianal abscess* forms at the anal orifice. The perianal abscess is the most common variety of perirectal infection. The abscess lies immediately beneath the skin in the perianal region at the lowermost part of the anal canal. It is separated from the ischiorectal space by a fascial septum that extends from the external sphincter and is continuous with the subcutaneous tissue of the buttocks. The infection may be small and localized or may be very large with a wall of necrotic tissue and a

surrounding zone of cellulitis.[36] Perianal abscesses may be associated with fistula in ano. The *fistula in ano* is an inflammatory tract with an external opening in the skin of the perianal area and an internal opening in the mucosa of the anal canal. The fistula in ano is usually formed after partial resolution of a perianal abscess, and its presence is suggested by recurrence of these abscesses with intermittent drainage. The external opening of the fissure is usually a red elevated piece of granulation tissue that may have purulent or sero-sanguineous drainage on compression. Many times the tract may be palpated as a cord. Patients with anal fistulas should be referred for definitive surgical excision.[60]

Ischiorectal abscesses are fairly common. They are bounded superiorly by the levator ani, inferiorly by the fascia over the perianal space, medially by the anal sphincter muscles, and laterally by the obturator internus muscle. These abscesses may commonly be bilateral and, if so, the two cavities communicate by way of a deep postanal space to form a "horseshoe" abscess.[36]

Intersphincteric abscesses are less common. They are bounded by the internal and external sphincters and may extend rostrally into the rectum, thereby separating the circular and longitudinal muscle layers.

The *pelvirectal*, or *supralevator*, *abscess* lies above the levator ani muscle in proximity to the rectal wall and remains extraperitoneal. The etiology of this abscess is controversial.[7] Kovalcik and colleagues[13] suggest that supralevator abscesses are primarily an extension of an intraabdominal process, such as diverticulitis or pelvic inflammatory disease. Read and associates[64] evaluated 474 patients with perirectal abscesses in a prospective study. They found that of the 36 supralevator abscesses, none was caused by an intraabdominal or pelvic pathologic condition. They determined that supralevator abscesses were most commonly associated with ischiorectal abscesses and suggested that these conditions may be an extension of the ischiorectal abscesses through the floor of the levator ani. Nonetheless, the investigators found rare isolated pelvirectal abscesses without intra-abdominal, pelvic, ischiorectal, or perianal infection.

Causes of perirectal abscesses other than the so-called cystoglandular process have been documented but are fairly rare. It is believed that hemorrhoids, anorectal surgery, episiotomies, or local trauma cause abscess formation by altering local anatomy and thus destroy natural tissue barriers to infections.[63–65]

EPIDEMIOLOGY

Anorectal abscesses occur most commonly in healthy adults; they occur more frequently in males, in greater than a 2 to 1 ratio.[63, 64] These abscesses commonly appear during the fourth decade of life. Possible predisposing medical conditions are diabetes mellitus, inflammatory bowel disease, and other immunocompromised states. Thirty per cent of patients have a history of previous perirectal abscess, and 75 per cent of anorectal abscesses occur in the same location as the prior abscesses.[63] Of perirectal abscesses, usually greater than 45 per cent are perianal, 20 per cent are ischiorectal, 12 per cent are intersphincteric, and 7 per cent are pelvirectal.[64]

PHYSICAL AND LABORATORY FINDINGS

The diagnosis of a *perianal abscess* is generally not difficult. The throbbing pain in the perianal region is acute and is aggravated by sitting, coughing, sneezing, and straining. There is swelling, induration, and tenderness, and a small area of cellulitis is present in proximity to the anus. Rectal examination of the patient with a perianal abscess reveals

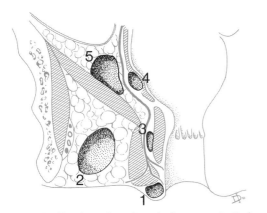

Figure 47–9. Classification of perirectal abscesses: *1*, Perianal. *2*, Ischiorectal. *3*, Intersphincteric. *4*, High intramuscular. *5*, Pelvirectal. (From Hill GJ II: Outpatient Surgery. 3rd ed. Philadelphia, WB Saunders Co, 1988. Reproduced by permission.)

that most of the tenderness and induration is below the level of the anal ring.

Patients with *ischiorectal abscesses* present with fever, chills, and malaise, but at first there is less pain than with the perianal abscess. Initially on physical examination, one will see an asymmetry of the perianal tissue, and later erythema and induration become apparent. Digital examination reveals a large, tense, tender swelling along the anal canal that extends above the anorectal ring. If both ischiorectal spaces are involved, the findings are bilateral.

Patients with *intersphincteric abscesses* usually present with dull, aching pain in the rectum rather than in the perianal region. No external aberrations of the perianal tissues are noted, but tenderness may be present. On digital examination one frequently palpates a soft, tender, sausage-shaped mass above the anorectal ring; if the mass has already ruptured, the patient may give a history of passage of purulent material during defecation.[60, 63, 64]

Diagnosis of the *pelvirectal abscesses* may be very difficult. Usually fever, chills, and malaise are present, but because the abscess is so deeply seated, there are few or no signs or symptoms in the perianal region. Rectal or vaginal examination may reveal a tender swelling that is adherent to the rectal mucosa above the anorectal ring.

Laboratory findings usually do not aid in the diagnosis. Kovalcik[63] found that less than 50 per cent of his patients had a white blood count of greater than 10,000 per cubic millimeter. Cultures of perirectal abscesses usually show mixed infections involving anaerobic bacteria, most commonly *Bacteroides fragilis* and gram-negative enteric bacilli.

TREATMENT

Successful management of perirectal abscesses depends on adequate surgical drainage. Complications from these infections may necessitate multiple surgical procedures, may prolong hospital stay, and may result in sepsis and death. Bevans and associates[65] retrospectively studied the charts of 184 patients who were surgically treated over a 10-year period. These patients were evaluated primarily to identify the factors that contributed to morbidity and mortality. Initial drainage was performed under local anesthesia in 38 per cent of the patients and under spinal or general anesthesia in 62 per cent. The authors identified three key factors in excessive morbidity and mortality: (1) a delay in diagnosis and treatment, (2) inadequate initial examination or treatment, and (3) associated systemic disease. It was their belief that the only way to examine effectively and drain adequately all but the most superficial perirectal abscesses was under spinal or general anesthesia. This was supported by evidence of an increased incidence of recurrence in patients treated with local anesthesia and an increased incidence of sepsis and death. Drainage under local anesthesia simply does not allow drainage of all hidden loculations. In addition, local anesthesia is not adequate for treatment of associated pathologic conditions.

Small, well-defined perianal abscesses are the only perirectal infections that lend themselves to outpatient therapy. The result of incision and drainage is almost immediate relief of pain and rapid resolution of infection. Indications for inpatient drainage are failure to obtain adequate anesthesia, systemic toxicity, extension of the abscess beyond a localized area, or a recurrence of a perianal abscess. Recurrence may be caused by the presence of a *fistula in ano*.

A perianal abscess is drained through a single linear incision over the most fluctuant portion of the abscess in a manner previously described for other cutaneous abscesses. It is extremely painful to probe a perianal abscess and to break up loculations, and liberal analgesia is advised. The patient may begin sitz baths at home 24 hours following surgery. Packing is replaced at 48-hour intervals until the infection has cleared and granulation tissue has appeared. This usually occurs within 4 to 6 days. Antibiotics are generally not required. All other perirectal abscesses require hospitalization for definitive therapy.

Perirectal abscesses are now recognized as a fairly common cause of fever in the granulocytopenic patient. These abscesses have a different bacteriologic profile: *P. aeruginosa* organisms are isolated more frequently. These patients present later because pain develops later in the course, and fever may be the first manifestation. Therefore, any patients who are granulocytopenic with vague anorectal complaints, especially those with fever, should be examined carefully for perirectal abscesses. Any abscess that is found should be drained immediately under appropriate anesthesia, and extensive intravenous antibiotic coverage should be initiated.

Infected Sebaceous Cyst

A very common entity that appears as a cutaneous abscess is the infected sebaceous cyst. Sebaceous cysts may occur throughout the body and result from obstruction of sebaceous gland ducts. The cyst becomes filled with a thick, cheesy sebaceous material, and the contents frequently become infected. Sebaceous cysts may be quite large and may persist for many years before they become infected. When infected, they clinically appear as tender, fluctuant subcutaneous masses, often with overlying erythema.

The initial treatment of an infected sebaceous cyst is simple incision and drainage. The thick sebaceous material must be expressed, since it is too thick to drain spontaneously (Fig. 47–10). A very important difference exists between infected sebaceous cysts and other abscesses. *A sebaceous cyst has a definite pearly white capsule that must be excised to prevent recurrence.* It is preferable to drain the infection initially and to remove the shiny capsule on the first follow-up visit, when it may be more easily identified. At the time of capsule removal, the edges are grasped with clamps or hemostats, and the core is removed by sharp dissection with a scalpel or scissors. Following excision of the capsule, the area is treated in the same manner as a healing abscess cavity.

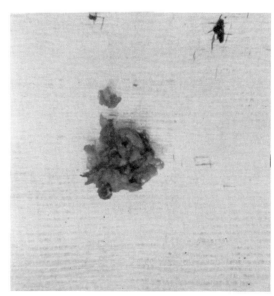

Figure 47–10. The thick, cheesy sebaceous material of a sebaceous cyst must be expressed after incision.

Simple drainage without excision of the capsule often leads to recurrence.

Paronychia

A paronychia is an infection localized to the area around the nail root (Fig. 47–11). Paronychias are common infections probably caused by frequent trauma to the delicate skin around the fingernail and the cuticle. When a minor infection begins, the nail itself may act like a foreign body. Usually the infectious process is limited to the area above the nail base and underneath the eponychium (cuticle), but occasionally it may spread to include some area under the nail as well, forming a subungual abscess. Lymphadenitis and lymphadenopathy are usually not seen. Generally, a paronychia is a mixed infection. *Staphylococcus* is commonly cultured from these lesions; however, anaerobes and numerous gram-negative organisms may be isolated.[66] Paronychias in children are often caused by anaerobes, and it is believed that this is the result of finger sucking and nail biting. Occasionally, a group A β-hemolytic infection will develop in a paronychia if the child with a streptococcal pharyngitis puts his fingers in his mouth.[67]

A paronychia appears as a swelling and tenderness of the soft tissue along the base or the side of a fingernail (Fig. 47–12). Pain, often around a hangnail, usually prompts a visit to the emergency department. The infection begins as a cellulitis, and may form a frank abscess. If the nail bed is mobile, the infectious process has extended under the nail, and a more extensive drainage procedure should be performed. If soft tissue swelling is present without fluctuance, remission may be obtained from frequent hot soaks (six to

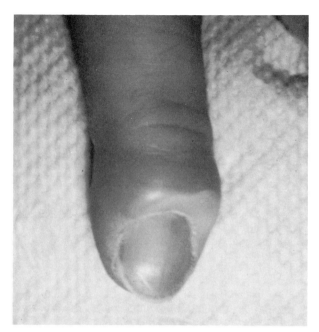

Figure 47–12. A paronychia may occur with obvious pus localization.

eight times a day) and the aid of appropriate antibiotics.[66] Incision will be of no value at this early cellulitic phase. If a significant cellulitis is present, a broad-spectrum antistaphylococcal antibiotic (cephalosporin or semisynthetic penicillin) may be tried. However, plain penicillin or erythromycin are often sufficient for limited inflammation. The digit should be splinted and elevated.[68, 69] One should never rely solely on antibiotic therapy once frank pus has formed.

TECHNIQUE

When a definite abscess has formed, incision and drainage is usually quickly curative. A number of invasive operative approaches have been suggested, but actual skin incision or removal of the nail is rarely required and *need not be the initial form of treatment*. One can obtain adequate drainage by simply lifting the skin edge off the nail to allow the pus to drain. This may be accomplished without anesthesia in selected patients, but it frequently requires a digital nerve block.[68] After softening the eponychium by soaking, a number 11 blade or an 18-gauge needle is advanced parallel to the nail and under the eponychium at the site of maximal swelling (Fig. 47–13).[69, 70] Pus rapidly escapes with immediate relief of pain. A tourniquet placed at the base of the finger may limit bleeding and aid the physician in determining the exact extent of the infection during the drainage procedure.

If more than a tiny pocket of pus is present, one should fan the knife tip or needle under the eponychium, keeping the instrument parallel to the plane of the fingernail. When a large amount of pus is drained, a small piece of packing gauze is slipped under the eponychium for 24 hours to provide continual drainage. Cultures are generally not indicated. Antibiotics are frequently prescribed although not essential if drainage is complete or if the surrounding area of cellulitis is minimal. In 24 hours the patient may be started on frequent soaks in warm tap water at home. The patient may easily remove the packing after the first soak, and the area is covered by a dry, absorbent dressing. An antibiotic ointment may be used on the site for a few days. The benefit of antibiotic ointments in reducing infection is unproved, but instructing the patient concerning the use of the ointment may prompt soaking. In addition, the ointment helps to keep the bandage from sticking.

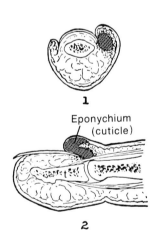

Eponychium
(cuticle)

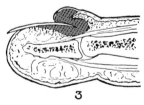

Figure 47–11. Paronychia. *1*, The site of the abscess at the side of the nail. *2*, The infection has extended around the base of the nail. It has raised the eponychium but has not penetrated under the nail. *3*, End stage of paronychia with a subeponychial and subungual abscess. (From Wolcott MW: Ferguson's Surgery of the Ambulatory Patient. 5th ed. Philadelphia, JB Lippincott Co, 1974. Reproduced by permission.)

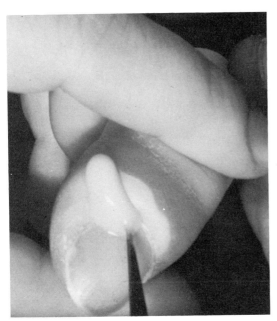

Figure 47–13. An initial treatment method for a well-localized paronychia. The eponychium (cuticle) is elevated at the area of fluctuance. Actual incision or removal of the nail is generally reserved for complicated or resistant infections.

If the infection has produced purulence beneath the dorsal roof of the nail, a portion of the nail must be removed to ensure complete drainage. Most commonly the proximal portion of the nail is involved. This may be treated by bluntly elevating the eponychium to expose the proximal edge of the nail. The proximal one third of the nail is then elevated from the nail bed and resected with a scissors. The distal two thirds of the nail is left in place to act as a physiologic dressing and to decrease postoperative pain (Fig. 47–14). If purulence is found below the lateral edge of the nail, the affected part may be gently elevated and excised longitudinally.[71] Care must be exercised during this procedure to avoid damage to the nail matrix. A wick of gauze should be placed beneath the eponychium for 48 hours to ensure continued drainage. As an alternative to nail removal a hole may be placed in the proximal nail with a hot paperclip. A large opening or multiple holes are required to assure continued drainage.

Most paronychia will resolve in 5 to 10 days and one or two postoperative visits should be scheduled to evaluate healing and reinforce home care. A well-known complication of even a properly drained paronychia is osteomyelitis of the distal phalanx. Clinical infection lasting longer than a few weeks should prompt evaluation for this complication.

Patients will occasionally present to the emergency department complaining of a chronic, indolent infection of the paronychium. These seldom respond to emergency department intervention. Frank purulence is seldom present and conservative treatments are often unsatisfactory. Many etiologies have been described for this frustrating condition including fungal, bacterial, viral, and psoriatic conditions. Treatment modalities are varied and controlled studies evaluating the various techniques are lacking. Meticulous hand care, oral and topical antimicrobial medications, and, occasionally, aggressive surgical intervention have been suggested.[69, 72] These patients should be referred to a dermatologist or hand surgeon because of the prolonged treatment required.

Herpetic Whitlow

Herpetic whitlow is an infection of the distal phalanx caused by the herpes simplex virus. Digital inoculation occurs through a discontinuity of the skin.[71] Health care providers and patients with other herpes infections are most commonly infected.[72, 73] The entity is recognized by the presence of herpetic vesicles, the absence of frank pus, the slow response to treatment, and the tendency to recur. Herpetic lesions are generally quite painful but are self-limited and resolve in 2 to 3 weeks. Surgical intervention is contraindicated as this may potentiate a secondary bacterial infection and delay healing.[76–79] Treatment is symptomatic using splinting, elevation, and analgesia as needed. Consideration must be given to preventing spread of the infection to other individuals. Although an occlusive dressing may lessen the chance for viral transmission, any health care provider with this entity should refrain from patient contact until all lesions have crusted over and viral shedding has stopped.[73] The use of oral acyclovir has been advocated for enhancing resolution of discomfort and viral shedding.

Felon

A felon is an infection of the pulp of the distal finger (Fig. 47–15). The usual cause is trauma with secondary invasion by bacteria. A felon may develop in the presence of a foreign body, such as a thorn or a splinter, but often a precipitating trauma cannot be identified. An important anatomic characteristic of this area is that there are many fibrous septa extending from the volar skin of the fat pad to the periosteum of the phalanx; these subdivide and compartmentalize the pulp area. When an infection occurs in the pulp, these same structures make it a closed space

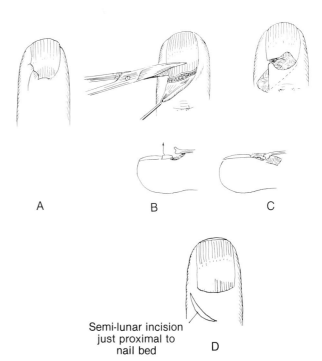

A   B   C

Semi-lunar incision
just proximal to
nail bed   D

Figure 47–14. A–C, Aggressive treatment of recurrent paronychia or subungual abscess includes removal of a portion of the proximal nail and incision of the eponychium. D, Some physicians prefer to use a semilunar incision proximal to the eponychium rather than directly incising and potentially injuring the cuticle permanently. These aggressive therapies are seldom required.

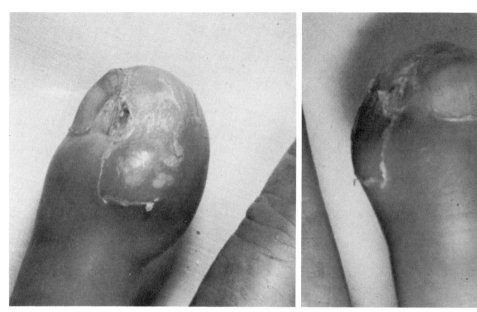

Figure 47–15. A well-developed felon. This advanced case had little pain at the time of presentation, and the distal phalanx was almost completely resorbed owing to the extensive pressure and inflammation.

infection. The septa limit swelling, delay pointing of the abscess, and inhibit drainage after incomplete surgical decompression. Pressure may increase in the closed space, initiating an ischemic process that compounds the infection. The infection can progress readily to osteomyelitis of the distal phalanx. Although the septa may facilitate an infection in the pulp, they provide a barrier that protects the joint space and the tendon sheath by limiting the proximal spread of infection.

The offending organisms are usually *Staphylococcus* or *Streptococcus*, although mixed infections and gram-negative infection may occur. A felon is one of the few soft tissue infections in which a culture should be routinely obtained, since osteomyelitis and prolonged infection may occur. Culture will aid in the subsequent choice of antibiotics for complicated infections.

The patient developing a felon will describe the gradual onset of pain and tenderness of the finger tip. In a few days

the pain may be constant and throbbing and gradually becomes severe. In the initial stages, physical examination may be quite unimpressive, because the fibrous septa limit swelling in the closed pulp space. As the infection progresses, swelling and redness may become obvious. Occasionally, one may elicit point tenderness, but frequently the entire pulp space is extremely tender. The patient characteristically arrives in the emergency department with the hand elevated over the head because pain is so intense in the dependent position. The cessation of pain indicates extensive necrosis and nerve degeneration.

Proper treatment of a well-developed felon consists of early and complete incision and drainage. Antibiotics alone are not curative once suppuration has occurred. Delaying surgery may result in permanent disability and deformity. Most surgeons will routinely administer broad-spectrum antibiotics to the patients for 5 to 7 days following surgical incision.

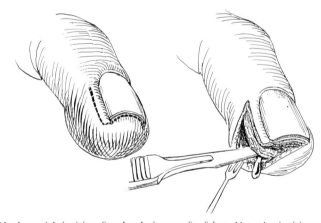
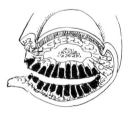

Figure 47–16. Hockey stick incision for the drainage of a felon. *Note:* An incision on the ulnar side of the index, middle, and ring fingers is appropriate. The little finger is best incised on the radial side. The site of the incision on the thumb is also preferably on the radial side, but it may depend on the occupation of the patient. (From Chase RA: Atlas of Hand Surgery. Philadelphia, WB Saunders Co, 1973. Reproduced by permission.)

TECHNIQUE

The surgery can usually be performed as an outpatient procedure using a digital nerve block. A long-acting solution (bupivacaine) will prolong anesthesia. A tourniquet (1.25 cm Penrose drain) should be used to allow digital incision in a bloodless field.

Surgical drainage must be carefully performed to avoid injury to digital nerves, vessels, and flexor tendon mechanisms. Most commonly, a felon can be successfully managed with a limited procedure. The preferred initial treatment is a simple longitudinal incision made over the area of greatest fluctuance,[79] which may occur laterally or along the volar surface. The incision must not extend to the distal interphalangeal crease because of the danger of injuring the flexor tendon mechanism. The subcutaneous tissue is bluntly dissected using a hemostat to provide adequate drainage. A gauze pad may be placed in the wound for 24 to 48 hours to ensure continued drainage.[71]

Recurrent or more severe infections may require a more aggressive approach. The following traditional incisions have a greater propensity for complications such as sloughing of tissue and postoperative fat pad anesthesia or instability,[79] although they may provide for more complete drainage.

The hockey stick incision is a well-accepted drainage procedure (Fig. 47–16). This incision is advantageous if the infection points to one side of the finger. The incision begins in the midline of the tip of the fat pad just under the distal edge of the fingernail. It is extended to the lateral tip of the finger and proximally along the side of the distal phalanx (at the junction of the volar and dorsal skin markings) to a few millimeters distal to the distal interphalangeal joint. The tip of the knife blade is inserted just under the bone to a depth corresponding to the opposite edge of the distal phalanx—slightly more than halfway across the volar surface of the finger. A hemostat is inserted into the incision and is spread in the plane of the fingernail (perpendicular to the septa) to break open remaining septa and loculations. Necrotic tissue or any foreign matter is excised under direct vision and the wound irrigated. A small gauze pack is placed in the incision. Because the incision may produce partial numbness of the finger tip by associated digital nerve injury the incision should *not* be made on the radial aspect of the index finger or the ulnar aspect of the thumb or little finger.

An acceptable alternative to the hockey stick, or median, incision is the through-and-through incision (Fig. 47–17). This is basically a hockey stick–type incision (without the curved distal portion of the hockey stick) that is carried through to the opposite side of the finger. A hemostat is used to break up loculations, and a rubber drain (Penrose) is placed through the incision for continual drainage. The through-and-through incision is probably the easiest procedure for most felons.

The fishmouth, or horseshoe, incision is basically two hockey stick incisions that meet at the tip of the finger. A gauze pack is placed between the flaps and should be removed in a few days. This is a rather radical procedure but allows complete visualization and débridement of necrotic tissue (Fig. 47–18). Some physicians advise against this incision because it is extensive and may take a long time to heal. In addition, it produces a sizable scar and an unstable finger pulp. The fishmouth incision may be used if more conservative incisions are not successful, but it is not recommended for use initially.

No matter which incision is made, it must not be carried proximal to the closed pulp space because of the danger of entrance into the tendon sheath or the joint capsule. The patient should be rechecked in 2 to 3 days. A snug dressing,

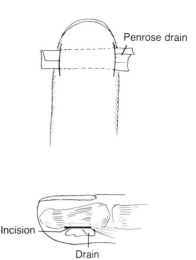

Figure 47–17. Through-and-through incision for a felon. A Penrose drain is placed for a few days to promote the withdrawal of fluid. This is an alternative to the hockey stick incision.

splinting and elevation, and adequate narcotic analgesics are prerequisites for a successful outcome and a happy patient.

On the first postoperative visit, a digital block may again be performed, and any packing removed. The incision is irrigated copiously with saline, and any additional necrotic tissue is removed. At this time, the drain may be replaced for 24 to 48 hours if there is continued drainage, but usually it can be removed and a dressing reapplied. Soaking may be advised. At the first revisit the sensitivities of the bacterial cultures are checked and a decision to continue or change antibiotics is made. Most felons are empirically treated with

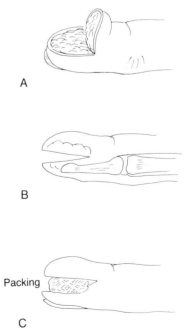

Figure 47–18. Fishmouth incision. This is a rather radical incision that is best reserved for resistant cases. Its advantage is that it allows for complete drainage and visualization of the infection in complicated cases. This incision takes longer to heal than others and may leave a large and sensitive scar. The finger tip may also be left unstable as a result of the lysis of all septa. The incision is seldom used on an outpatient basis for these reasons.

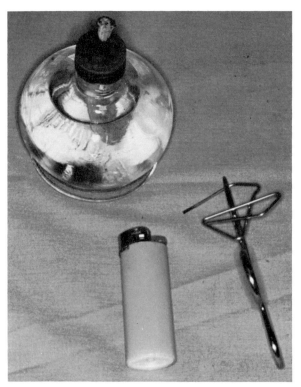

Figure 47–19. An adequately sized drainage hole may be placed in the nail with a heated paper clamp. Small holes, which tend to clog and inhibit drainage, should not be used.

antibiotics for at least 5 days. A broad-spectrum cephalosporin is a reasonable choice, pending cultures.

A few additional points should be emphasized at this time. Frank pus may be encountered during incision, but usually only a few drops are expressed. One more often drains a combination of necrotic tissue and interstitial fluid. A careful search for a foreign body should be made even if the history is not known. Some physicians advocate radiographic evaluation for retained foreign bodies and a baseline evaluation of the bone for subsequent evaluation of osteomyelitis at the initial visit. Other physicians will reserve radiographs for wounds not showing significant improvement in 5 to 7 days. Evidence of osteomyelitis, however, may not be found radiographically for several weeks after the appearance of the lesion. More radical incision and drainage may be required in persistent infections. Following adequate drainage, osteomyelitis may respond surprisingly well to outpatient antibiotic therapy with almost complete regeneration of bone if incision and drainage have been adequate. Persistent cases may require intravenous antibiotics.

Resistant finger tip infections are not uncommon. Difficult or persistent cases require evaluation and care by a hand surgeon. In these cases, early consultation is advisable to avert catastrophic complications such as loss of function or amputation.

Subungual Hematoma

Subungual hematoma is an injury that is frequently seen in the emergency department. Any digit may be affected. The hematoma often results from hitting the finger tip with a hammer. The main concern of the patient is relief of the terrible throbbing pain that accompanies the condition as the pressure of the hematoma increases. Pain relief can be accomplished quickly with nail trephination. Trephination may be performed with a large paper clip that has been heated until red hot. The instrument is applied to burn a hole at the base of the nail (Fig. 47–19). Blood rapidly exits, and the blackened nail regains its normal color (Fig. 47–20*A* and *B*). The blood usually remains fluid for 24 to 36 hours and is easily expressed with slight pressure. Care should be taken to make multiple holes or a single hole large enough to allow continued drainage (Fig. 47–20*C*). An oversized

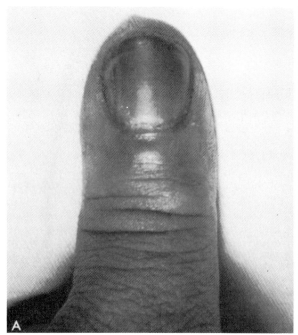
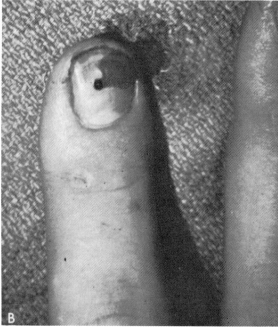

Figure 47–20. *A,* Subungual hematoma with a blackened nail bed. *B,* Following trephination, blood flows freely from the puncture site.

paper clip is the simplest apparatus. Although a portable hot-wire electrocautery unit is available and is frequently recommended, it is difficult to obtain an adequate drainage hole without adapting the instrument and its use. One can modify the electrocautery device to burn a larger hole by "fattening" the end of the wire loop and rotating the device slowly as the nail is penetrated. In addition to being convenient, the cautery device is desirable because the wire stays hotter longer, thus enhancing nail penetration. In the stoic patient no anesthesia may be necessary, but a digital block affords painless trephination, and its routine use is suggested with the anxious patient.

The majority of subungual hematomas are painful but minor injuries. Complicated cases involve fractures of the distal phalanx. When the finger tip is unstable or the mechanism of injury suggests a significant distal phalanx fracture, a radiograph should be obtained. If a significant fracture is present, the digit should be splinted. A distal phalangeal fracture with a subungual hematoma is technically an open (compound) fracture. Such injuries usually heal without problems, although osteomyelitis of the tuft is a theoretical complication. The value of routine antibiotic prophylaxis in such cases is unproved. It is difficult to predict the fate of the fingernail following drainage of a subungual hematoma. Many patients with subungual hematomas will lose the nail. They should be informed of this and should be advised to protect the loosely adherent nail from further trauma. A fractured distal phalanx or a lacerated nail often signifies an underlying nailbed laceration. Further discussion of nailbed injuries is provided in Chapter 43.

REFERENCES

1. Meislin HW, Lerner SA, Graves MH, et al: Cutaneous abscesses: Anaerobic and aerobic bacteriology and outpatient management. Ann Intern Med 87:145, 1977.
2. Llera JL, Levy RC: Treatment of cutaneous abscess: A double-blind clinical study. Ann Emerg Med 14(1):15, 1985.
3. Thorn GW, Adams RD, Braunwald E, et al: Harrison's Principles of Internal Medicine. 8th ed. New York, McGraw-Hill, 1977.
4. Peterson PK, James EC, Ronald AR: The Management of Infectious Diseases in Clinical Practice. New York, Academic Press, 1982.
5. Biderman P, Hiatt JR: Management of soft-tissue infections of the upper extremity in parenteral drug abusers. Am J Surg 154(5):526, 1987.
6. Geelhoed GW, Joseph WL: Surgical sequelae of drug abuse. Surg Gynecol Obstet 139:749, 1974.
7. Merhar GL, Colley DP, Clark RA, et al: Computed tomographic demonstration of cervical abscess and jugular vein thrombosis. Arch Otolaryngol 107:313, 1981.
8. Cutaneous abscesses (editorial). Br Med J 2:1499, 1977.
9. Brook I, Finegold SM: Aerobic and anaerobic bacteriology of cutaneous abscesses in children. Pediatrics 67:891, 1981.
10. Webb D, Thadepalli H: Skin and soft tissue polymicrobial infections from intravenous abuse of drugs. West J Med 130:200, 1979.
11. Podzamczer D, Ribera M, Gudiol F: Skin abscesses caused by Candida albicans in heroin abusers (letter). J Am Acad Dermatol 16(2 pt 1):386, 1987.
12. Boudreau S, Hines HC, Hood AF: Dermal abscesses with Staphylococcus aureus, cytomegalovirus and acid-fast bacilli in a patient with acquired immunodeficiency syndrome (AIDS). J Cutan Pathol 15(1):53, 1988.
13. Floyd JL, Goodman EL: Soft-tissue abscesses in a diabetic patient. JAMA 246:675, 1981.
14. Lewis JW, Groux N, Elliot JP, et al: Complications of attempted central venous injections performed by drug abusers. Chest 79:613, 1980.
15. Meislin HW, McGehee MD: Management and microbiology of cutaneous abscesses. JACEP 7:186, 1978.
16. Ghoneim ATM, McGoldrick J, Blick PWH, et al: Aerobic and anaerobic bacteriology of subcutaneous abscesses. Br J Surg 68:498, 1981.
17. Fine BC, Sheckman PR, Bartlett JC: Incision and drainage of soft-tissue abscesses and bacteremia [letter]. Ann Intern Med 103:645, 1985.
18. Blick PWH, Flowers MW, Marsden AK, et al: Antibiotics in surgical treatment of acute abscesses. Br Med J 281:111, 1980.
19. Schulman ST, et al: Prevention of bacterial endocarditis. Circulation 70:1123A, 1984.
20. Everett ED, Hirschman JV: Transient bacteremia and endocarditis prophylaxis: A review. Medicine 56:61, 1977.
21. Kaye D: Prophylaxis for infective endocarditis: An update. Ann Intern Med 104:419, 1986.
22. Friedland GH, Klein RS: Transmission of the human immunodeficiency virus. N Engl J Med 317:1125, 1987.
23. Robert-Guroff M, et al: Prevalence of antibiotics to HTLV-I, -II, and -III in intravenous drug abusers from an AIDS endemic region. JAMA 255:3133, 1986.
24. Levy N, et al: The prevalence of HTLV-III/LAV antibodies among intravenous drug users attending treatment programs in California. N Engl J Med 314:446, 1986.
25. Ellis M: The use of penicillin and sulphonamides in the treatment of suppuration. Lancet 1:774, 1951.
26. Jones NAG, Wilson DH: The treatment of acute abscesses by incision curettage, and primary suture under antibiotic cover. Br J Surg 63:499, 1976.
27. Rutherford WH, Calderwood JW, Hart D, et al: Antibiotics in surgical treatment of septic lesions. Lancet 1:1077, 1970.
28. Macfie J, Harvey J: The treatment of acute superficial abscesses: A prospective clinical trial. Br J Surg 64:264, 1977.
29. Simms MH, Curran F, Johnson RA, et al: Treatment of acute abscesses in the casualty department. Br Med J 284:1827, 1982.
30. Meislin HW: Pathogen identification of abscesses and cellulitis. Ann Emerg Med 15:329, 1986.
31. Marantz PR, et al: Inability to predict diagnosis in febrile intravenous drug abusers. Ann Intern Med 106:823, 1987.
32. Meislin HW, McGehee MD, Rosen P: Management and microbiology of cutaneous abscesses. JACEP 7:186, 1978.
33. Flomenbaum N, Gallagher EJ, Eagen K, et al: Self administered nitrous oxide: An adjunct analgesic. JACEP 8:95, 1979.
34. Crile GC: A definitive ambulatory treatment for infected pilonidal cysts. Surgery 24:677, 1948.
35. Phillip RS: A simplified method for the incision and drainage of abscesses. Am J Surg 135:721, 1978.
36. Mandell GL, Douglas GR, Bennett JE: Principles and Practice of Infectious Disease. New York, John Wiley and Sons, 1979.
37. Wherle PF, Top FH: Communicable and Infectious Disease. 9th ed. St. Louis, C.V. Mosby Co., 1981
38. Paletta C, Jurkiewicz MJ: Hidradenitis suppurativa. Clin Plast Surg 14(2):383, 1987.
39. Thomas R, Barnhill D, Bibro M, Hoskins W: Hidradenitis suppurativa: A case presentation and review of the literature. Obstet Gynecol 66(4):592, 1985.
40. Fitzsimmons JS: A family study of hidradenitis suppurativa. J Med Genet 22:367, 1985.
41. Morgan WP, Leicester G: The role of depilation and deodorants in hidradenitis suppurativa. Arch Dermatol 118(2):101, 1982.
42. Edlich RF, Silloway KA, Rodeheaver GT, Cooper PH: Epidemiology, pathology, and treatment of axillary hidradenitis suppurativa. J Emerg Med 4(5):369, 1986.
43. Broadwater JR, Bryant RL, Petrino RA, et al: Advanced hidradenitis suppurativa. Review of surgical treatment in 23 patients. Am J Surg 144(6):668, 1982.
44. Highet AS, Warren RE, Weekes AJ: Bacteriology and antibiotic treatment of perineal suppurative hidradenitis. Arch Dermatol 124(7):1047, 1988.
45. Clemmensen OJ: Topical treatment of hidradenitis suppurativa with clindamycin. Int J Dermatol 22(5):325, 1983.
46. Dicken CH, Powell ST, Spear KL: Evaluation of isotretinoin treatment of hidradenitis suppurativa. J Am Acad Dermatol 11(3):500, 1984.
47. Brown CF, Gallup DG, Brown VM: Hidradenitis suppurativa of the anogenital region: Response to isotretinoin. Am J Obstet Gynecol 158(1):12, 1988.
48. Dalrymple JC, Monaghan JM: Treatment of hidradenitis suppurativa with the carbon dioxide laser. Br J Surg 74(5):420, 1987.
49. Jemec GB: Effect of localized surgical excisions in hidradenitis suppurativa. J Am Acad Dermatol 18(5 Pt 1):1103, 1988.
50. Moosa HH, McAuley CE, Rasasastry SS: Surgical management of severe mammary hidradenitis suppurativa. Ann Plast Surg 29(1):82, 1988.
51. Silverberg B, Smoot CE, Landa SJ, Parsons RW: Hidradenitis suppurativa: Patient satisfaction with wound healing by secondary intention. Plast Reconstr Surg 79(4):555, 1987.
52. Harrison BJ, Mudge M, Hughes LE: Recurrence after surgical treatment of hidradenitis suppurativa. Br Med J (Clin Res) 294 (6570):487, 1987.
53. Walker AP, Edmiston CE Jr, Krepel CJ, Condon RE: A prospective study of the microflora of nonpuerperal breast abscess. Arch Surg 123(7):908, 1988.
54. Scholefield JH, Duncan JL, Rogers K: Review of a hospital experience of breast abscesses. Br J Surg 74(6):469, 1987.
55. Brook L: Microbiology of non-puerperal breast abscesses. J Infect Dis 157(2):377, 1988.
56. Leach RD, et al: Anaerobic subareolar breast abscess. Lancet Jan 6, 1979.
57. Watt-Boolsen S, Rasmussen NR, Blichert-Toft M: Primary periareolar abscess in the nonlactating breast: Risk of recurrence. Am J Surg 153(6):571, 1987.
58. Word B: Office treatment of cysts and abscess of Bartholin's gland duct. South Med J 61:514, 1968.
59. Santoro J: Staphylococcal and streptococcal infections in office practice. Curr Top Emerg Med 1(4):1, 1979.
60. Schwartz SI, Lillehei RC, Shires TG, et al: Principles of Surgery. 2nd ed. New York, McGraw-Hill, 1974.

61. Brook I, Anderson KD, Controni G, Rodriguez WJ: Aerobic and anaerobic bacteriology of pilonidal cyst abscess in children. Am J Dis Child 134(7):679, 1980.

62. Arko FR: Anorectal disorders. Am Fam Phys 22:121, 1980.

63. Kovalcik PF, Perriston RL, Cross GH: Anorectal abscess. Surg Gynecol Obstet 149:884, 1979.

64. Read DR, Abcarian H: A prospective surgery of 474 patients with anorectal abscess. Dis Colon Rectum 22:566, 1979.

65. Bevans DW, Westbrook KC, Thompson BW, et al: Perirectal abscesses: A potentially fatal illness. Am J Surg 126:765, 1975.

66. Whitehead SM, Eykyn SJ, Phillips I: Anaerobic paronychia. Br J Surg 68:422, 1981.

67. Brook I: Bacteriologic study of paronychia in children. Am J Surg 141:703, 1981.

68. Neviaser RJ: Infections. In Green DP (ed): Operative Hand Surgery. 2nd ed. New York, Churchill Livingston, 1988.

69. Daniel CR: Paronychia. Dermatol Clin 3:461, 1985.

70. Lee TC: The office treatment of simple paronychias and ganglions. Med Times 109:49, 1981.

71. Zook L: The Paronychium. Green DP (ed): Operative Hand Surgery. 2nd ed. New York, Churchill Livingston, 1988.

72. Baran R, Bureau H: Surgical treatment of recalcitrant chronic paronychias of the fingers. J Dermatol Surg Oncol 7:106, 1981.

73. Palenik CJ, Miller CH: Occupational herpetic whitlow. J Indiana Dent Assoc 61(6):25, 1982.

74. Stern H, Elek SD, Millar DM, et al: Herpetic whitlow: A form of cross-infection in hospitals. Lancet 2:871, 1959.

75. Rosato FE, Rosato EF, Plotkin SA: Herpetic paronychia: An occupational hazard of medical personnel. N Engl J Med 283:804, 1970.

76. Feder HM, Long SS: Herpetic whitlow: Epidemiology, clinical characteristics, diagnosis and treatment. Am J Dis Child 137:861, 1983.

77. Louis DS, Silva J Jr: Herpetic whitlow: Herpetic infections of the digits. J Hand Surg 4:90, 1979.

78. Berkowitz FL, Hentz VR: Herpetic whitlow: A non-surgical infection of the hand. Plast Reconstr Surg 60:125 1977.

79. Polayes IM, Arons MS: The treatment of herpetic whitlow: A new surgical concept. Plast Reconst Surg 65:811, 1980.

80. Kilgore ES, et al: Treatment of felons. Am J Surg 130:194, 1975.

Chapter **48**

Soft Tissue Needle Aspiration

Edward J. Otten

INTRODUCTION

Soft tissue infections, cellulitis, and abscesses are frequent problems encountered in emergency medicine. The management of abscesses is discussed in Chapter 47. Once the diagnosis of abscess has been made, the treatment is surgical incision and drainage. Antibiotics are often used in conjunction with surgical drainage of the abscess but are not a substitute for it. The management of cellulitis is quite different. Although the diagnosis of cellulitis is often obvious, the correct antibiotic treatment may not be as obvious. The goal of treatment is to prevent abscess formation, sepsis, osteomyelitis, and other serious complications. Classically the treatment consists of local wound care, such as cleansing, elevation of an extremity, and warm compresses. Antibiotics are prescribed, and the choice of antibiotics should be based on knowledge of the causative organism. Determination of the causative organism, unfortunately, is often difficult in most cases of simple cellulitis. Many physicians prescribe a broad-spectrum antibiotic such as a first-generation cephalosporin, which will cover some of the common infections. However, most organisms acquired in an aquatic environment, ocean, lake, or swimming pool will be resistant, for example *Mycobacterium marinum, Aeromonas hydrophila,* and *Vibrio* sp. Trimethoprim-sulfamethoxazole, ciprofloxacin, tetracycline, or amoxicillin clavulanate may be more efficacious based on the organism identified. *No single antibiotic is effective against all common cellulitic infections.* In addition, it is often difficult to distinguish other inflammatory soft tissue conditions, such as venous thrombosis, insect bites, tenosynovitis, contusion, or contact dermatitis, from bacterial cellulitis.[1-4]

The site of entry for cellulitis is found in only approximately 50 per cent of clinical cases, and when found, the source is usually a wound, ulcer, injection site, or bite. Although drug addiction, diabetes, alcoholism, and peripheral vascular disease are frequently associated with cellulitis, many patients are healthy, with no obvious underlying diseases. Cellulitis in children is often an indication of an underlying osteomyelitis. Many patients with cellulitis have a normal white blood cell count and normal erythrocyte sedimentation rates, and are afebrile.

Culture isolation of the causative organism using needle aspiration has been variably successful, depending on the area of the body involved and the organism present. The experience of the physician doing the aspiration and the ability of the microbiology laboratory to isolate and identify the organism also are important factors. The current indications and accepted technique for aspiration of cellulitis are discussed.

BACKGROUND

Hughes, in 1912, described a method for diagnosing and treating the offending organism in cellulitis by incising the infected area, inoculating an agar plate with whatever exuded from the incision, and preparing a vaccine against the organism that grew on the agar. Drinker and associates, 1935, found that tissue fluid aspirated from dogs with chronic lymphedema and acute cellulitis was positive for streptococcus if obtained early in the disease (less than 12 hours). He also noted that blood cultures were negative on all occasions when blood samples were drawn concomitantly with the cellulitis cultures. In 1972, Minnefor and Murray found that aspiration of cellulitis in a pediatric patient grew *Haemophilus influenzae* even though the blood culture was negative. Goetz and colleagues, in 1974, found that cultures of facial cellulitis were positive in two of three patients with *H. influenzae* bacteremia. Uman and Kunin, in 1975, described the use of tissue aspiration for seven patients with cellulitis, and their technique subsequently has been advocated. Table 48–1 summarizes several studies that examined the value of aspiration of cellulitis and its correlation with blood cultures.[5-9]

From these results, it can be concluded that aspiration of cellulitis, a procedure with practically zero morbidity, may be helpful in identifying the organism causing the cellulitis, even when blood cultures are negative. *H. influenzae* is the predominant organism cultured from facial cellulitis, whereas *Staphylococcus aureus* and *Streptococcus pyogenes* are the most common extremity pathogens isolated. Although only the predominant organism is listed in Table 48–1, other organisms were occasionally cultured, and mixed infections do occur.[10-13]

INDICATIONS

Because potentially valuable information can be obtained from this procedure with little cost or harm to the patient, it is recommended that needle aspiration be performed on all patients with facial or extensive soft tissue cellulitis. At times, one may be uncertain as to whether the soft tissue infection represents an abscess or cellulitis. Needle aspiration of the central core of the infection should identify abscesses by the aspiration of purulent material. Note that with cellulitis though, tissue fluid from the central portion of the infection may not be adequate for microbiologic

Table 48–1. *Value of Aspiration of Cellulitis and Its Correlation with Blood Cultures*

Author	Number of Patients	Location of Cellulitis	Positive Aspirate	Positive Blood Culture	No Organism Isolated	Predominant Organism
Ho, 1979	76	Various	64	1	12	Staph/Strep
Rudoy, 1979	5	Extremities	3	4	1	*Haemophilus influenzae*
Fleisher, 1980	8	Face	1	3	4	*H. influenzae*
	42	Extremities	20	1	22	Staph/Strep
Fleisher, 1981	5	Face	2	2	2	*H. influenzae*
	23	Extremities	10	1*	11	Staph/Strep
Ginsberg, 1981	16†	Extremities	2	0	41†	Staph/Strep
Szilagyi, 1982	28	Various	12	—	16	Staph/Strep
Liles, 1985	24	Various	8	1	15	Staph/Strep/*Pasteurella*/etc.
Jaffe, 1985	5	Various	2	—	3	Strep/Enterococcus
Hook, 1986	50	Extremities	5	2	27	Staph/Strep
Kielhofner, 1988	87	Various	33	6	54	Staph/Strep

*Blood cultures drawn on only 16 patients.
†Only 16 patients had aspiration, 27 had blood cultures.
Staph, *Staphylococcus;* Strep, *Streptococcus.*

evaluation. The peripheral margin of an area of cellulitis has been recommended as the location for sampling with the best chance of a positive culture. Duvanel and associates have shown that bacterial counts are low throughout the cellulitis area except at the edge of an associated central ulcer.[14] Cultures should be obtained from both sites when a central ulcer exists.

There is no absolute containdication to needle aspiration of cellulitis. Aspiration can be performed in a patient with a coagulopathy or who is immunosuppressed. In fact, Kielhofner and colleagues suggest that the presence of qualitative leukocyte disorders (e.g., diabetes mellitus or malignancy) increases the yield of needle aspiration culture.[15] Sachs noted a correlation of aspiration culture growth with underlying disease and lower temperature.[15a] These are the patients for whom antibiotic selection may be more problematic. One should carefully avoid introducing infection into a joint, tendon sheath, or blood vessel during aspiration.[9–12]

TECHNIQUE

The technique for aspiration of cellulitis is straightforward. An 18-gauge needle (22-gauge is preferred for the face) attached to a 5-ml syringe should be used. The skin should be prepared by wiping with isopropyl alcohol or povidone-iodine solution and allowed to dry. The incorporation of the antiseptic into the culture may affect results. The leading edge of the cellulitis should then be entered to a depth of 1 cm, with the needle bevel pointing downward and the syringe angled approximately 10 to 15 degrees to the skin (Fig. 48–1). The cellulitic area should then be aspirated by pulling back on the plunger. Previous studies have shown that aspiration of the central area of the cellulitis in the absence of a central ulcer does not produce positive cultures.[2] Only a few drops of fluid are usually aspirated. If the initial aspiration fails to produce any material, 0.5 ml of nonbacteriostatic normal saline should be injected and immediately aspirated. The needle should be left in place and a 1-ml syringe with the saline should be used in place of the original syringe. Any material obtained by either method should be inoculated onto sheep blood agar and chocolate agar. If no material is obtained, the needle tip may be used to inoculate the agar or the needle itself cultured by rinsing it in beef infusion broth. Gram stain of aspirated material may be helpful if sufficient material is obtained on initial aspiration; however, in many cases, cultures are positive

when Gram stains have not shown organisms. After aspiration, the puncture site can be covered with a sterile dressing.[8–11, 13, 17, 22]

COMPLICATIONS

Complications of needle aspiration are unusual. The theoretic possibility of extending the cellulitis to deeper structures exists, but the added morbidity associated with this is small. Fistula formation and the possibility of continued bleeding in selected individuals are extremely rare.

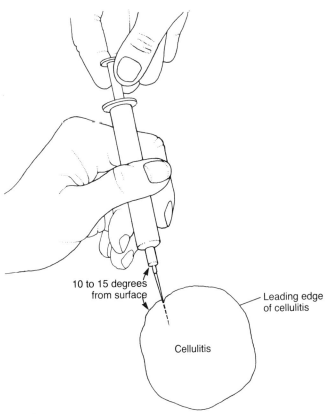

10 to 15 degrees from surface

Leading edge of cellulitis

Cellulitis

Figure 48–1. The technique for the aspiration of cellulitis.

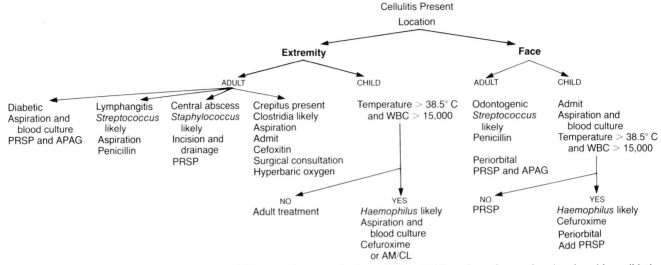

Figure 48–2. Management of cellulitis. *PRSP,* penicillinase-resistant synthetic penicillin; *APAG,* antipseudomonal aminoglycoside antibiotic; *AM/CL,* amoxicillin clavulanate; *WBC,* white blood cell count.

CONCLUSION

Needle aspiration of suspected cellulitis is helpful for microbial isolation and for guiding therapy (Fig. 48–2). The technique described here is rapid and rarely associated with morbidity.[18–21]

REFERENCES

1. Ginsberg MB: Cellulitis: Analysis of 101 cases and a review of the literature. South Med J 74:530, 1981.
2. Szilagyi A, Mendelson J, Portnoy J: Cellulitis of the skin: Clinical observations of 50 cases. Can Fam Phys 28:1399, 1982.
3. Hook EW, Hooton TM, Horton CA, et al: Microbiologic evaluation of cutaneous cellulitis in adults. Arch Intern Med 146:295, 1986.
4. Auerbach PS: Natural microbiological hazards of the aquatic environment. Clin Dermatol 5:52, 1987.
5. Hughes B: The treatment of cellulitis with special reference to the hand and arm. Practitioner 89:142, 1912.
6. Drinker CK, Field ME, Ward HK, Lyons D: Increased susceptibility to local infection following blockage of the lymph drainage. Am J Physiol 112:74, 1935.
7. Minnefor AB, Murray JJ: *Haemophilus influenzae* cellulitis of the lower extremity. Am J Dis Child 124:920, 1972.
8. Goetz JP, Tafari N, Boxerbaum B: Needle aspiration in *Haemophilus influenzae* type B cellulitis. Pediatrics 54:504, 1974.
9. Uman SJ, Kunin CM: Needle aspiration in the diagnosis of soft-tissue infections. Arch Intern Med 135:959, 1975.
10. Fleisher G, Ludwig S, Campos J: Cellulitis: Bacterial etiology, clinical features, and laboratory findings. J Pediatr 97:591, 1980.
11. Fleisher G, Ludwig S, Henretig F, et al: Cellulitis: Initial management. Ann Emerg Med 10:356, 1981.
12. Fleisher G, Ludwig S: Cellulitis: A prospective study. Ann Emerg Med 9:246, 1980.
13. Rudoy RC, Nakashima G: Diagnostic value of needle aspiration in *Haemophilus influenzae* type B cellulitis. J Pediatr 94:924, 1979.
14. Duvanel T, Auckenthaler R, Rohner P, et al: Quantitative cultures of biopsy specimens from cutaneous cellulitis. Arch Intern Med 149:293, 1989.
15. Kielhofner MA, Brown B, Dall L: Influence of underlying disease process on utility of cellulitis needle aspirates. Arch Intern Med 148:2451, 1988.
15a. Sachs MK: The optimum use of needle aspiration in the bacteriologic diagnosis of cellulitis in adults. Arch Intern Med 150:1907, 1990.
16. Ho PWL, Pien FD, Hamburg D: Value of cultures in patients with acute cellulitis. South Med J 72:1402, 1979.
17. Liles DL, Dall LH: Needle aspiration for diagnosis of cellulitis. Cutis 36:63, 1985.
18. Jaffe AC, O'Brien CA, Reed MD, Blumer JL: Randomized comparative evaluation of Augmentin and cefaclor in pediatric skin and soft tissue infections. Curr Therap Res 38:160, 1985.
19. Barkin RM: Facial and periorbital cellulitis in children. J Emerg Med 2:195, 1984.
20. Wheat LJ, Allen SD, Henry M, et al: Diabetic foot infections: Bacteriologic analysis. Arch Intern Med 146:1935, 1986.
21. Middleton DB, Ferrante JA: Periorbital and facial cellulitis. Am Fam Phys 21:98, 1980.
22. Goldgeier MH: The microbial evaluation of acute cellulitis. Cutis 31:649, 1983.

Chapter **49**

The Treatment of Minor Burns and Emergency Escharotomy

Thomas J. Krisanda and Courtney A. Bethel

INTRODUCTION

In the United States each year some 2 million persons suffer burns. Approximately 95 per cent of these burn patients are treated as outpatients, and most complete their treatment course within 2 weeks.

The classification of burns is based on three criteria[1]: depth of skin injury, percentage of body surface area involved, and source of injury (thermal, chemical, electrical, or radiation). The *seriousness* of a burn injury is further defined according to the characteristics and temperature of the burning agent, duration of exposure, location of injury, presence of associated injuries, and age and general health of the victim.

The American Burn Association defines *minor* burns as uncomplicated partial-thickness burns of less than 10 per cent of the total body surface area (TBSA) in children or less than 15 per cent TBSA in adults, or full-thickness burns of less than 2 per cent TBSA.[2] *Serious* burns include injuries that cover a greater surface area as well as burns of the face, hand, feet, perineum, and those with associated inhalation injuries. Percentage of body surface area burned may be calculated in a number of ways. In adults, the "rule of nines" is a useful rule of thumb, but the formula is only a guide and *must be modified for children* who have proportionately larger heads and smaller legs (Fig. 49–1). The Lund and Browder charts are another (more precise) guide to estimating the percentage of TBSA burned (Fig. 49–2). For smaller or multiple burns, one can rapidly estimate the percentage of body surface burned by using the area of the patient's palm as approximately 1.25 per cent TBSA.

Throughout the course of history, physicians have experimented with burn therapies to relieve pain and promote healing. Before the latter half of the nineteenth century, the treatment of burns had little scientific basis. Accepted treatments consisted primarily of bleeding and purging the patient and placing substances on the wound that tended to promote infection or were toxic. Undoubtedly, many of these treatments were recognized as ineffectual, and some were impossibly complex—it being easier for the physician to blame a treatment failure on the patient for not following instructions precisely. Fortunately, the pathophysiology of burn injury and burn healing has gradually been elucidated, and the care of burns has evolved into its present form.

WOUND EVALUATION

Emergency physicians should be aware that the depth of a burn wound cannot always be determined accurately on clinical grounds alone at the time of presentation and that burn injury is a dynamic process that may change over time. It is common, for example, for a seemingly minor or superficial burn to be deeper on the second or third return visit.

First-degree burns involve the epidermis only. The skin is reddened but is intact and not blistered. This injury ranges from mildly irritating to exquisitely painful. Minor edema may be noted. Causes include ultraviolet light (as in sunburn) and brief thermal "flash" burns. First-degree burns frequently blister in 24 to 36 hours; so the patient should be instructed appropriately. Frequently the skin flakes or peels in 5 to 10 days, but no scarring results.

Second-degree burns involve the entire epidermis and extend into the dermis to include sweat glands and hair follicles. *Superficial partial-thickness* burns involve the papillary dermis. These burns are pink, moist, and extremely painful. Blisters may be present or the skin may slough. The burn blanches with pressure, and mild to moderate edema is common. Hair follicles are often noted to be intact. This is the most common depth of minor burns seen in the emergency department. The usual causes are scalds, contact with hot objects, and contact with chemicals. Barring infection, or repeat trauma, these burns heal completely in 10 to 14 days without scarring.

Deep partial-thickness burns extend into the reticular dermis and appear as mottled white or pink. There is obvious edema and sloughing of the skin, and any blisters are usually ruptured. Blanching is absent. These burns are generally not painful initially, but pressure can be perceived. Within a few days these burns can become exquisitely painful. This injury can be converted to a full-thickness burn by further trauma or infection.

In *full-thickness* burns, coagulation necrosis extends into the subcutaneous tissues. These burns may appear a variety of colors but are usually dry, pearly white, or charred. They are initially painless, with a leathery texture. Marked edema and decreased elasticity may necessitate escharotomy when circulation is compromised. Exposure of the skin to temperatures in excess of 77° C for more than 3 to 4 seconds is accompanied by full-thickness injury. Although initially painless, in a few days these deep burns can become painful. Chemical burns often produce full-thickness injuries affect-

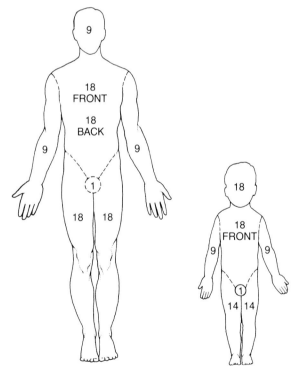

Figure 49–1. The "rule of nines" for estimating percentage of area burned. (As a rough guide, the area covered by the individual's palm is approximately 1.25 per cent of the body surface area.) The rule of nines is a rough estimate of the percentage of body surface burn. Note that adults and children are different. This formula frequently *overestimates* the extent of a burn in clinical practice. See Figure 49–2 for a more accurate method for determining the percentage of body surface burn for children.

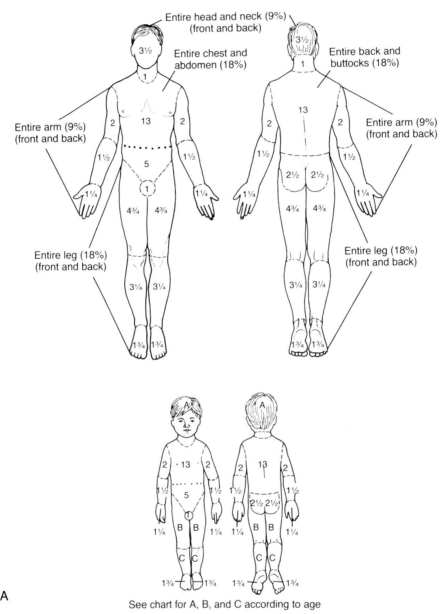

Figure 49–2. *A*, The Lund and Browder charts are somewhat more accurate in estimating percentage of body surface burn than the rule of nines. *B*, Percentage of total body surface area of individual areas, according to age. Compared with adults, children have larger heads and smaller legs. Other areas are relatively equivalent throughout life. The rule of nines is not accurate in determining the percentage of surface area burns in children.

AGE	Birth–1 Yr	1–4 yr	5–9 yr	10–14 yr	15 yr	Adult
Head	19	17	13	11	9	7
Neck	2					
Ant trunk	13					
Post trunk	13					
R buttock	2½					
L buttock	2½					
Genitalia	1					
R U arm	4					
L U arm	4					
R L arm	3					
L L arm	3					
R hand	2½					
L hand	2½					
R thigh	5½	6½	8	8½	9	9½
L thigh	5½	6½	8	8½	9	9½
R leg	5	5	5½	6	6½	7
L leg	5	5	5½	6	6½	7
R foot	3½					
L foot	3½					

B

BODY AREA

Figure 49–2 *Continued*

ing a small surface area. Flame burns produce full-thickness injuries in less than 2 seconds if the temperature of flame exceeds 500° C.

Fourth-degree burns extend deeply into subcutaneous tissue, muscle, fascia, or bone. These may be burns caused by molten metal or severe electrical or flame burns.

HISTOPATHOLOGY OF BURNS

Jackson's thermal wound theory described three zones of injury in burns[3]:

1. Zone of coagulation—dead tissue, which must be débrided.

2. Zone of stasis—less seriously injured tissue, which may or may not necrose.

3. Zone of hyperemia—minimally injured tissue, which will heal.

Histologically, full-thickness burns are characterized by confluent vascular thrombosis involving arterioles, venules, and capillaries. The cellular debris and denatured proteins of the eschar provide a substrate for the proliferation of microorganisms. The devitalized tissue (eschar) sloughs spontaneously, usually as a result of the proteolytic effect of bacterial enzymes. The greater the degree of wound bacteriostasis, the greater the delay to sloughing.

Partial-thickness burns result in incomplete vascular thrombosis, usually limited to the upper dermis. The dermal circulation is gradually restored, usually over several days, resulting in a significant interval of relative ischemia. The eschar in deep partial-thickness burns is thinner than in a full-thickness burn and sloughs as a result of re-epithelialization rather than bacterial proteolysis.

OUTPATIENT VERSUS INPATIENT CARE

One of the first steps in minor burn care is to select patients for whom outpatient care is appropriate. Outpatient candidates are generally adults and children who meet the minor burn criteria as detailed earlier. In addition, patients with the following burn injuries and situations should generally be managed as *inpatients*: persons who have deep burns of the hands, face, feet, neck, or perineum; burns resulting from abuse or attempted suicide; and electrical burns.

Poor candidates for outpatient care of even minor burns include those who have concomitant medical problems such as diabetes mellitus, peripheral vascular disease, congestive heart failure, and end-stage renal disease; patients who are using steroids or other immunosuppressive agents; patients who are very young or very old; those who are mentally retarded; alcoholics; or any individual with a suspect or unacceptable home support system. Inpatient treatment should be considered under these circumstances even though the burn is considered "minor" by TBSA formulas.

PROCEDURE—INITIAL CARE OF THE MINOR BURN VICTIM

Prompt cooling of the burned part is one of the oldest recorded burn treatments, having been recommended by Galen (A.D. 129–199) and Rhazes (A.D. 852–923).[4] Room temperature tap water irrigation, immersion, or compresses (20 to 25° C) are optimal in obtaining pain relief and providing some measure of protection for burned tissues without the problems of hypothermia that iced solutions can cause.[4, 5] First-aid phone advice from the emergency physician includes immediately immersing the wound under room temperature tap water. Packing the wound under ice must be avoided.

Emergency Medical Services (EMS) personnel should have a clear understanding of the proper management of the minor burn victim. The benefits and details of early cooling should be understood and implemented. The victim should first be removed from danger. All involved clothing and jewelry, along with any gross debris, should be removed

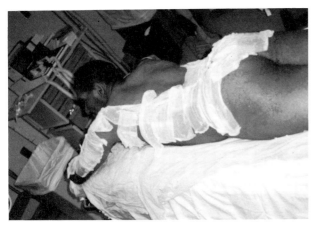

Figure 49–3. To cool a burn that is not easily immersed in water, cover the area with unfolded gauze pads and soak them with room temperature saline. Frequently soak the gauze with cool saline drawn up in a syringe. Towels are generally too bulky to accomplish this procedure.

from the burned area. Chemical burns to the skin or eyes require prolonged tap water irrigation. The burn should be otherwise covered with a moist, sterile dressing—nonmentholated shaving cream makes an excellent temporary covering for prehospital use if a dressing is not available.[6] Home remedies such as butter, grease, or petrolatum should be avoided.

In the emergency department, the burned area should be immediately immersed in room temperature water or covered with gauze pads soaked in room temperature water (Fig. 49–3). The gauze must be kept continually cooled to provide continued pain relief; the patient will quickly let the physician know when additional cooling is required. Burns should be cooled or immersed until supplemental analgesia is effective and dressings are applied. Many physicians use sterile saline for cooling, but it has no proven benefit over tap water, even when the skin is broken. Immersion of burned tissue in ice or ice water should be avoided, because ice immersion increases pain and risks frostbite injury.

The potential benefits of burn cooling are listed in Table 49–1. With the exception of pain relief and removal of debris, the benefits of burn cooling are experienced only if the burn is cooled promptly—within the first 3 minutes after injury.[7]

Prompt burn cooling arrests cell death processes by inhibiting the release of toxic substances by the dying cells. If cooling is not performed, continued cell death results as oxygen free radicals are released, which can cause a "chain reaction" of cell membrane injury, arachidonic acid release, and increased local ischemia.[8]

The threshold temperature for cutaneous pain sensation is approximately 43° C. The prompt alteration in capillary permeability and resultant edema induced by heat has been attributed to histamine release from stimulated or damaged mast cells. The tissue threshold for this phenomenon has been estimated at 52° C. Cooling effects prompt, complete, but reversible inhibition of histamine release.

Table 49–1. Advantages of Prompt Burn Cooling

Reduction or cessation of pain
Elimination of local hyperthermia
Inhibition of postburn tissue destruction
Decreased edema
Reduced metabolism and toxin production

Minor burns are considered tetanus-prone, and tetanus toxoid should be administered when the patient is unsure of his or her tetanus immunization status or when it has been more than 5 years since the last immunization. Nonimmunized patients should receive human tetanus immune globulin, 250 units intramuscularly, along with tetanus toxoid, and should receive a booster injection in 3 weeks.

PROCEDURE—DEFINITIVE CARE OF THE MINOR BURN

Few areas in medicine are fraught with as much mysticism, personal bias, and unscientific dogma as is the care of the minor burn wound. Many physicians are rigidly committed to a specific ritual or approach merely because it is the "way it's done" in a specific institution or because the practitioner has had success with a particular therapy in the past. In reality, the plethora of successful regimens attests to the fact that almost any noninjurious approach results in a favorable outcome. Many misconceptions probably arise because the issues associated with major thermal injury are often erroneously extrapolated to the minor burn wound.

Minor burns are *not* associated with immunosuppression, hypermetabolism, or increased susceptibility to infection.[9] Many complications seen in minor burn care result from *overtreatment* of the injury, rather than from undertreatment. Examples include too-vigorous dressing changes that may peel off newly formed skin and secondary infections or pseudomembrane formation that results from topical or systemic antibiotic use.

Burn Dressings

OPEN VERSUS CLOSED METHOD; SIMPLE DRESSING APPLICATION

Burns are cared for using two general methods: open and closed. In the *open* method, a burn wound dressing is not used. The area is left open to the air and is washed two to three times per day; application of a topical agent usually follows. This is the preferred method of managing burns of the face and neck and is an excellent method of managing hand burns because it allows continuous inspection and range-of-motion exercises. The open method is impractical in young, active persons or in children or other individuals in whom wound contamination is likely. Although many burns may be treated with this method, many patients prefer a dressing over a wound for cosmetic reasons.

The *closed* burn treatment method involves a dressing, of which there are various types. This is the management method of choice for most minor burns treated in the emergency department. Wound preparation and basic bandaging should include the following steps (Fig. 49–4):

1. The hair in the burn itself or around the wound should *not* be shaved. The burn is washed gently with a clean cloth or gauze pads and a mild non–alcohol-based soap or detergent (e.g., Ivory, Dreft, Hibiclens) and then is flushed with normal saline. Adequate wound cleansing prevents further bacterial contamination, promotes early epithelialization in partial-thickness injuries, and aids the development of good granulation tissue in full-thickness injuries.[10]

2. Obviously sloughed skin should be débrided. This may be accomplished with scissors and forceps, but an expeditious and effective (and often painless) method is to use a dry 10-cm by 10-cm gauze pad (Fig. 49–5) to quickly

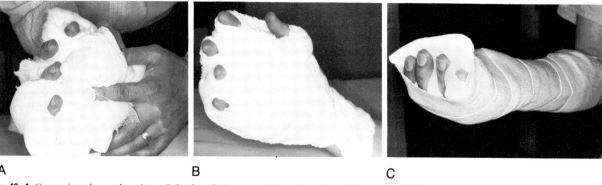

A   B   C

Figure 49–4. Outpatient burn dressing of the hand. Persons with serious hand burns should be admitted to the hospital, but persons with minor burns can be treated in the outpatient setting. Following application of an antibiotic ointment or a dry, nonadherent dressing, the fingers are separated with fluffs *(A)*, and the entire hand is enclosed in a position of function *(B)* (here with the help of a roll of Kerlix). If the wrist is involved, a removable plaster splint may be applied over the dressing *(C)*.

débride loose skin. Meticulous and time-consuming instrument débridement is often quite stressful to the patient. Analgesia should be provided for any painful débridement.

3. Intact blisters are left alone in the absence of infection. Open blisters are débrided (Table 49–2). All sloughed skin and blisters are débrided if infection is present.

4. A fine mesh gauze or a commercial nonadherent

gauze such as Adaptic or Aquaphor is applied to the dry burn wound.

5. The burn is covered with loose gauze fluffs. If fingers and toes are included in the dressing, the digits are padded with strips of gauze.

6. The entire dressing is wrapped snugly (but not tightly) with an absorbent, slightly elastic material such as Kerlix.

7. Antibiotic creams or ointments may be used as an option with this dressing. The topical antibiotic may be applied to the burned skin directly or impregnated into the gauze after step 3.

Burn dressings should enhance healing. *The most important characteristic of a dressing is that it is capable of controlling fluid balance.* To accelerate healing, a burn dressing should be designed to keep the wound surface moist but without pooling of fluids.[11] The best material for this purpose is a generous amount of *simple dry gauze* applied over a nonadherent dressing or topical preparation. The outer dressing layer should be porous, to permit the evaporation of water from the absorbent dressing material.

BIOLOGIC DRESSINGS

Biologic dressings are natural tissues, including skin, consisting of collagen sheets containing elastin and lipid. They are not routinely used in emergency care of minor

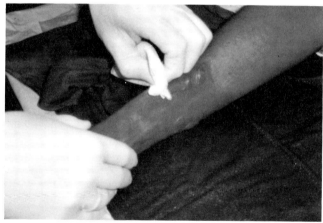

A

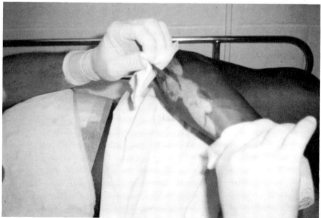

B

Figure 49–5. An expeditious and relatively painless way to débride a burn is to use a dry gauze pad to grasp the dead skin *(A)* and peel it off *(B)*. Meticulous instrument débridement is often time consuming and stressful to the patient.

Table 49–2. General Approach to Blisters in Minor Burns*

If treated less than 48 hours after the burn:
  1. Leave all intact blisters alone.
  2. If blisters have ruptured, treat them as dead skin and débride them completely.
  3. Do not use needle aspiration.
On follow-up or more than 48 to 72 hours after the burn:
  1. Débride large (larger than 5 cm in diameter) intact blisters and all blisters that have ruptured. Large, firm blisters of the palms and soles may be left intact longer. Do not aspirate blisters.
  2. Do not débride small or spotty blisters until they break or until 5 to 7 days after the burn.
Five to 7 days after the burn:
  1. Débride all blisters completely.
Note: Intact blisters provide significant pain relief. Be prepared for an exacerbation of pain immediately after débridement.

*All blisters and burned skin are débrided in the presence of infection.

wounds. Benefits of biologic dressings include a reduction in surface bacterial colonization, diminished fluid and heat loss, prevention of further wound contamination, and prevention of damage to newly developed granulation tissue. Examples of biologic dressings include cadaveric human skin and commercially available porcine xenograft or collagen sheets.

SYNTHETIC DRESSINGS

Synthetic dressings are manufactured in various forms. Film-type dressings have a homogeneous structure and are usually polymers. Because these dressings are nonpermeable, there have been problems with retention of wound exudate. Some second-generation dressings have been developed that address these problems.

1. Tegoderm (3M Inc., St. Paul, Minn.) pouch dressings consist of a thin polyurethane film coated with a water-resistant adhesive. The film is perforated to allow exudate fluid to pass into a pouch. An intact dressing is impermeable to liquids and bacteria. Although this dressing has been used on skin graft donor sites, it has not been studied as a primary burn dressing (C. D. Jones, personal communication).
2. Vigilon (Bard, Inc., Berkeley Heights, N. J.) is a hydrogel formulation of water and polyethylene oxide reinforced with a polyethylene support webbing. It is clear, conformable, and nonadherent and may be used along with topical antibiotic agents. Wound exudate is transmissible through the dressing and is absorbed by an overlying gauze dressing.
3. Duoderm (Convatec, Inc., Arlington Heights, Ill.) is a synthetic hydrocolloid dressing. The outer layer is impermeable to gases, vapor, and fluids. The wound side of the dressing adheres to healthy skin. Wound exudate converts the dressing into a gel, which creates a beneficial moist environment. The dressing may be left in place for up to 5 days.[12] Duoderm is opaque and does not allow for wound inspection. It also has no antibacterial properties and should not be used on infected burns.[12]
4. Biobrane (Winthrop Pharmaceuticals, New York, N.Y.) is a biosynthetic, bilaminar membrane dressing that consists of a knitted nylon fabric mechanically bonded to a thin silicone rubber membrane. Cross-linked collagen peptides coat the membrane and prohibit both desiccation and collection of serum. Biobrane is available with a variety of pore sizes to regulate wound transudation; these pores allow drainage of the exudate, which is absorbed by an overlying gauze dressing.

This dressing is generally well tolerated and permits the transmission of antibacterial activity from topical antimicrobial agents. As long as the wound remains clean and there is no seroma, the collagen side of the dressing adheres to the burn surface, effectively sealing it.[13]

5. OpSite (Smith and Nephew Medical, Massillon, Ohio) is a less than optimal membrane dressing because fluid collections frequently occur beneath the barrier. Because this dressing is clear, however, it allows for ready wound inspection.

USE OF BIOLOGIC AND SYNTHETIC DRESSINGS

All of these dressings are best used on fresh partial-thickness injuries; placement over a contaminated wound often results in nonadherence and infection. Biologic and synthetic dressings are readily available. These dressings provide immediate relief of pain and are the only dressing method that may actually promote faster wound healing.[1] Additionally, these dressings have the potential for a reduced number of dressing changes.

Biologic dressings, such as porcine xenograft, are applied as follows: (1) the dressing is reconstituted as instructed by the manufacturer, (2) the dressing is carefully "fit" to the wound, (3) all fluid and air under the graft are pressed out, (4) the dressing is secured with edge tapes and covered with coarse mesh gauze, and (5) the dressing is wrapped with absorbent gauze and a semielastic wrap. With healing, the biologic dressing dries, curls, and separates from the healed edge underneath. The loose edges should be trimmed frequently and any blisters débrided and fluid accumulations drained.

Synthetic dressings are applied after standard wound cleansing. Blisters must be débrided before application of the synthetic dressings. The thicker membranes are cut to size and applied to the burn surface. The edge of the membrane should extend 2 to 3 cm beyond the burn onto the surrounding unburned tissue. Membranes such as Duoderm can be wrapped about burned digits to permit continued function with limited motion during healing.[12]

Should fluid collect between the débrided burn and the dressing, one attempt at aspiration should be performed. If the fluid reaccumulates beneath the Duoderm or Biobrane membranes after aspiration, the nonadherent portion of the fabric should be removed. The dressing should be checked at least every other day for adherence for the first 5 to 8 days. After epithelialization is complete, the dressing begins to separate spontaneously and may be peeled away.[8]

If infection develops under a synthetic or biologic dressing, the dressing should be removed, the wound cultured, and treatment with topical (and possibly oral) antimicrobials instituted. Xenografts should not be used on superficial partial thickness injuries because the xenograft tissue may become incorporated into the healing burn wound in as many as 35 per cent of patients so treated.[14]

Occasionally, application of a permanent dressing—or skin autograft—is appropriately performed in the outpatient setting. Appropriate patient selection is crucial; patients should be healthy and well-motivated, with small (less than 2 per cent TBSA), noncosmetic deep partial-thickness or full-thickness burns. These burns may initially be treated as outlined previously, with the use of a topical antimicrobial agent recommended. The wound should be reevaluated for excision and grafting within 4 days.

SPECIFIC CLINICAL ISSUES IN MINOR BURN CARE

Analgesia

Pain is a much feared feature of any burn injury. *Pain relief by the appropriate and judicious use of narcotics is of paramount importance in the initial care of burn patients.* Analgesia should be provided *before* extensive examination or débridement is performed. Inadequate analgesia is probably the most common emergency department error in the treatment of burn injuries. Even with minor burns, patients often present with significant pain. Reassurance is important, but adequate analgesia is critical for gaining the patient's cooperation and ensuring comfort. Cooling may dramatically relieve pain temporarily, but parenteral narcotics (meperidine, 1 to 2 mg/kg, or morphine, 0.1 to 0.2 mg/kg) are usually required, especially if painful procedures like débridement and dressing changes are planned. We prefer to use *intravenous* narcotics (occasionally supplemented with a short-acting benzodiazepine such as midazolam) for all painful procedures.

Intramuscular medications following the procedure are helpful for prolonged analgesia. Regional or nerve block anesthesia is an excellent alternative when practical; and when feasible, nitrous oxide analgesia may be used. Oral narcotics are *inappropriate* for initial treatment of significant pain but can be used for continued outpatient analgesia. Local anesthetics may be injected in small quantities when appropriate, such as for the débridement of a deep ulcer or other small burn. Topical analgesics have no role in burn care.

A properly designed dressing will do much toward preventing further discomfort after discharge; however, home burn care and dressing changes may be quite painful. For this reason an adequate supply of an oral narcotic analgesic should be provided, and responsibility should be encouraged in analgesic use.

Edema

Minor burns lead to immediate inflammation mediated by the release of histamine and bradykinins, causing localized derangements in vascular permeability with resultant burn wound edema. This edema is harmful in several ways. First, the increase in interstitial fluid increases the diffusion distance of oxygen from the capillaries to the cells, increasing hypoxia in an already ischemic wound. Second, the edema may have untoward hemodynamic effects on a purely mechanical basis, by compression of vessels in muscular compartments. Third, edema has been associated with the inactivation of streptococcidal skin fatty acids, thus predisposing the patient to burn cellulitis.[15]

The successful management of burn edema hinges on *immobilization* and *elevation*. Most patients are unfamiliar with the medical definition of elevation and are not aware of or convinced of its value. Patient education in this regard is critical; however, certain burns (e.g., burns in dependent body areas) are prone to edema despite everyone's best intentions. It is for this reason that lower extremity burns in general and foot burns in particular are prone to problems.

Use of Topical Antimicrobials

Minor burns result in insignificant impairment of normal host immunologic defenses, and burn wound infection is usually not a significant problem. Topical antimicrobials are often used, however, despite the fact that they may actually impair wound healing.[16] Many physicians routinely use antibiotic creams or ointments on even the most minor burn.

Topical antimicrobials were designed for the prevention and care of burn wound sepsis or wound infection, and there is no convincing evidence that their use alters the course of first-degree burns and superficial partial-thickness injuries. As noted, the burn dressing is the key factor in minimizing complications in all burns. Nonetheless, topical antimicrobials are often soothing to minor burns, and their daily use prompts the patient to look at the wound, assess healing, or otherwise become personally involved in his or her care. Keep in mind that if a topical antimicrobial is used, its effectiveness is decreased in the presence of proteinaceous exudate, necessitating twice-daily dressing changes if the antimicrobial benefit of topical therapy is to be realized. In reality, once-a-day dressing changes are more practical and commonly prescribed; there are no data to indicate that this regimen is inferior.

All *full-thickness* burns should receive topical antimicrobial therapy because the eschar and burn exudate are potentially good bacterial culture media and deep escharotic or subescharotic infections may not be easily detected until further damage is done. All *deep partial-thickness* injuries likewise benefit from the application of a topical antimicrobial. In deep partial-thickness injuries, re-epithelialization occurs from a few remaining deep epidermal appendages whose protection is important. Clinical studies and culture results support the hypothesis of surface destruction of dermal islands by bacterial enzymes and catabolic processes[17] that have the potential to convert a deep partial-thickness injury to a full-thickness injury.

Initial topical therapy is *prophylactic*.[3] A burn wound infection that develops despite this therapy mandates a change to a different agent. Topical therapy, if chosen, should cover the usual bacteria responsible for burn wound infections (see later discussion of burn microbiology). Although topical agents are an important part of a burn treatment program, they are not substitutes for good local wound care or a careful program of management. Their successful use may prevent the conversion of deep thermal burns to deeper injury and allow better wound healing for earlier (and more successful) skin grafting.

Criteria for choosing a specific topical agent include: in vitro and clinical efficacy, toxicity (absorption), superinfection rate, ease and flexibility of use, cost, patient acceptance, and side effects. Note that there are no firm scientific data that convincingly support the use of any specific topical antimicrobial.

SPECIFIC TOPICAL AGENTS

Silver Sulfadiazine (Silvadene). This poorly soluble compound is synthesized by reacting silver nitrate with sodium sulfadiazine. It is the most commonly used topical agent and is well tolerated by most patients. It has virtually no systemic effects.

Silver sulfadiazine is available as a "micronized" mixture with a water-soluble white cream base in a 1 per cent concentration that provides 30 mEq/L of elemental silver. Silvadene does not stain clothes, is nonirritating to mucous membranes, and is easily washed off with water. It may be used on the face but may be cosmetically undesirable for open treatment. The broad gram-positive and gram-negative antimicrobial spectrum includes β-streptococci, *Staphylococcus aureus* and *Staphylococcus epidermidis*, *Pseudomonas*, *Proteus*, *Klebsiella*, *Enterobacteriaceae*, *Escherichia coli*, *Candida albicans*, and possibly Herpesvirus hominis.

Silver sulfadiazine often interacts with wound exudate to form a pseudomembrane over partial thickness injuries. The pseudomembrane is often difficult and painful to remove. Except for term pregnancy and newborns (possible induction of kernicterus), there are no absolute contraindications to the use of Silvadene. Allergy and irritation are unusual, although there is a potential cross-sensitivity between Silvadene and other sulfonamides.

Broad-Spectrum Antibiotic Ointments. Many nonprescription topical antimicrobials are used for minor burn therapy. Included are bacitracin zinc ointment, polymyxin B-bacitracin (Polysporin), triple antibiotic ointments such as Neosporin and nitrofurazone (Furacin). These are all soothing, cosmetically acceptable for open treatment and are effective antiseptics. Some researchers caution against agents containing neomycin because of a potential for sensitization.

Povidone-Iodine. Despite the long record of safety and clinical efficacy this agent enjoys when used on normal skin and mucous membranes, its routine use on burns is not widely accepted. It is available commercially for topical use compounded in a water-miscible cream base. This combination is strongly acidic (pH 2.40), and its use may result in significant systemic absorption of iodine. In short, other safer and more readily available topical antimicrobials should be used routinely.

Gentamicin Sulfate. Gentamicin sulfate is available for topical use as a 0.1 per cent cream or ointment. It is readily absorbed when applied to open wounds and may result in the typical aminoglycoside-induced nephrotoxicity or ototoxicity. Burn specialists eschew its use for fear of the development of resistant strains of *Pseudomonas.*

Chlorhexidine. Chlorhexidine gluconate is widely available commercially in Hibiclens solution. Its prophylactic antibacterial effectiveness is comparable to silver sulfadiazine, but toxicity and absorption characteristics are not fully documented (Stuart Pharmaceuticals, personal communication).

Chlorhexidine phosphanilate differs from other salts of chlorhexidine in that the phosphanilate moiety confers broad gram-negative antibacterial activity to the molecule that is not cross-resistant with silver sulfadiazine.[18]

Aloe Vera Cream. Aloe vera cream is commercially available in a 50 per cent or greater concentration with a preservative. It exhibits antibacterial activity against at least four common burn wound pathogens: *Pseudomonas aeruginosa, Enterobacter aerogenes, S. aureus,* and *Klebsiella pneumoniae.* Heck and colleagues compared a commercial aloe vera cream with Silvadene in 18 patients with minor burns.[19] Healing times were found to be similar, and there was no increase in wound colonization in the aloe vera group as compared with the patients treated with silver sulfadiazine. Aloe vera cream may be a viable, inexpensive option for open, home care of minor burns or skin graft donor sites.

Other Topicals. Silver nitrate and mafenide (Sulfamylon, Winthrop Pharmaceuticals, New York, N.Y.) are two additional topical agents that formerly enjoyed wide clinical usage. Both are excellent antimicrobials, but each has significant disadvantages. Silver nitrate is available commercially as a 0.5 per cent solution, but this is often clinically unavailable, necessitating custom compounding. In addition, silver nitrate is cumbersome to apply and tends to stain clothing and bandages. Mafenide causes considerable discomfort if applied to a sensate burn, but remains clinically useful for its excellent eschar penetration when used on full-thickness injuries.

FOLLOW-UP CARE OF MINOR BURNS

The specifics of outpatient follow-up of minor burns are controversial and often based on physician preference and personal bias rather than on firm scientific data. Follow-up should be individualized for each patient and should be based on the reliability of the patient, the extent of the injury, the frequency and complexity of the dressing changes, and the amount of discomfort anticipated during a dressing change.

If a topical antibiotic agent is used, the dressing should be changed daily at home with reapplication of the antibiotic ointment. The wound should be rechecked by a physician after 2 to 3 days and periodically thereafter, depending on compliance, healing, and other social issues. If a dry dressing is opted for, follow-up every 3 to 5 days is usually adequate. The purpose of any burn dressing changes or home care regimen is defeated if the patient cannot afford the material or is not instructed in the specifics of burn care. Many emergency departments supply burn dressing material on discharge. (A complete pack includes antibiotic cream, gauze pads [fluffs], absorbent gauze roll, sterile tongue blade to apply cream, and tape). Writing a prescription and merely stating that the dressing should be changed daily is often futile.

Daily home care can be performed by the patient with help from a family member or visiting nurse (Table 49–3).

Table 49–3. *How to Change a Burn Dressing at Home: Patient Instructions*

1. Take pain medicine one-half hour before dressing change if you find dressing changes a painful procedure.
2. If the burn is on the hand or foot or other area difficult to reach, have someone else help you.
3. Have all material available. Gloves may be worn.
4. Remove the dressing and rinse off all burn cream or ointment with tap water, under a shower, or in the bathtub. The area can be gently washed with mild soap and a clean cloth or gauze pads.
5. Look at the burn and assess the healing, blistering, and amount of swelling. Note any signs of infection.
6. Gently exercise the area through range of motion.
7. Apply the burn ointment with a sterile tongue blade.
8. Cover the cream with fluffed up gauze.
9. Wrap the area in bulky gauze.
10. Repeat this dressing change daily.

The dressing may be removed each day and gently washed with a clean cloth or a gauze pad with the use of tap water and a bland soap. Sterile saline and expensive prescription soaps are not required. A tub or shower is an ideal place to gently wash off burn cream. The affected area may be put through a gentle range of motion during dressing changes. After the burn is cleaned, it is inspected by the patient. The patient is instructed to return if signs or symptoms of infection develop or if significant blistering or skin slough develops. Following complete removal of the old cream, a new layer is applied with a sterile tongue blade and covered with absorbent gauze.

If the undermost fine mesh gauze of a dry dressing is dry and the coagulum is sealed to the gauze, the patient should simply reapply the overlying gauze dressing. If the wound is macerated, the fine mesh gauze should be removed and the wound cleaned and redressed. The patient is instructed *not to remove a dry adherent fine mesh gauze from the underlying crust.* When epithelialization is complete, the crust will separate and the gauze can be removed at that time. Dryness in healing skin may be treated with mild emollients such as Nivea (Beiersdorf, Inc., Norwalk, Conn.) or Vaseline Intensive Care lotion (Chesebrough Ponds, Inc., Greenwich, Conn.). Natural skin lubrication mechanisms usually return by 6 to 8 weeks.[9] Excessive sun exposure should be avoided during wound maturation as this may lead to hyperpigmentation; a commercially available sun block should be used. Exposure of the recently healed burned area to an otherwise minor trauma (chemicals, heat, sun) may result in an exaggerated skin response. Pruritus may be treated with oral antihistamines or a topical moisturizing cream.

Deep partial-thickness burns take more than 3 weeks to heal and have an unstable epithelium, which often results in late hypertrophic scarring and contractures. These burns are easily converted to full-thickness burns via infection, mechanical trauma, or further thrombosis of the blood supply. These burns, along with small third-degree burns, may be initially managed in the outpatient setting but should be considered for early excision and grafting. Topical antimicrobials are recommended; mafenide (Sulfamylon) cream may be useful in the care of small, full thickness burns because it is capable of penetrating the entire eschar and is present in subjacent tissues at bactericidal levels.[10]

BURN HEALING

Burn healing is different from that of other wounds.[1] The timing is often variable, but it is proportional to burn depth. The inflammatory phase lasts 3 to 7 days (at times longer) and is accompanied by the release of histamine and bradykinins, along with complement degradation. This degradation of complement may lead to immunologic, coagulation, and metabolic aberrations.

Within 1 to 3 weeks, neovascularization of the burn occurs, accompanied by fibroblast migration. Macrophages begin to replace the tissue neutrophils. Collagen production begins but is often laid down in random fashion, leading to a scar. Re-epithelialization follows, but the presence of necrotic tissue and eschar impedes all aspects of wound healing. The amount of scar tissue produced is directly related to healing time. Burns requiring less than 16 days to heal generally do not scar excessively.[1]

Healing in superficial partial-thickness burns occurs within 10 to 14 days. After healing, the new epithelial layer tends to dry easily and crack. Using bland, lanolin-containing creams for 4 to 8 weeks following healing alleviates this problem.

Deep partial-thickness burns heal by re-epithelialization from the wound edge and from residual dermal elements. Healing is slow and often unsatisfactory, frequently taking longer than 3 weeks, producing an unstable epithelium that is prone to hypertrophic scarring and contractures. This is most pronounced in burns that extend across joints. Burns that take longer than 2 to 3 weeks to heal are prone to infection; hence topical antimicrobials should be used. Because these burns often heal in complicated fashion, they should be considered for referral to expedite early excision, grafting, and physical therapy.

Full-thickness burns can only heal by contraction and epithelialization at the wound edge. Burns larger than 2 to 3 cm must be excised and grafted.

Cosmetic and functional recovery follows complete epithelialization of a partial-thickness injury or successful skin grafting of a full-thickness burn. The ultimate goal is to prevent scar thickening, achieve and maintain optimal range of motion, and prevent secondary environmental damage to the skin, particularly from sun exposure.[10] Nonscented skin lotions may be used after epithelialization to keep the burn scar soft. Compression dressings are especially helpful in preventing scar thickening. Repeated evaluations are important because burn contractures can occur up to 12 months after the injury. Nighttime splinting is useful in maintaining full extension of joints.

PROBLEMS IN MINOR BURN CARE

Blisters

The management of blisters in minor burns is controversial. Management arguments are generally theoretic or emotional, because the ultimate outcome of a minor burn is rarely determined by how one deals with blisters. Intact blisters do offer a physiologic dressing that rarely becomes infected; however, most blisters spontaneously rupture after 3 to 5 days and eventually require débridement. When the integrity of the blister is breached, the fluid becomes a potential culture medium. Clinical choices include débridment, aspiration, or simply leaving the blister intact.

Some studies suggest that intact burn blisters may allow for reversal of capillary stasis and less tissue necrosis.[2] Madden and colleagues have shown that burn exudate (as contained within intact blisters) is beneficial for the stimulation of epidermal cell proliferation.[20]

Swain and colleagues demonstrated that the density of wound colonization with microorganisms was much lower in minor burns with blisters left intact.[21] They also found that

37 per cent of patients with aspirated blisters experienced a reduction in pain versus none of those whose blisters were deroofed. Other investigators believe that undressed wounds with débrided blisters have additional necrosis secondary to desiccation, which can convert a partial-thickness burn to a full-thickness injury.[2] Finally, intact blisters clearly provide some pain relief, as evidenced by a sudden increase in pain immediately following débridement. Increased pain should be anticipated and analgesia offered as appropriate when débridement is necessary. We suggest the guidelines in Table 49–2 as a general approach to burn blisters.

Minor Burn Infections

There are bacteria on the skin at all times—normal skin usually harbors nonvirulent pathogens such as *S. epidermidis* and diphtheroids. Therefore, all burns are *contaminated* but not necessarily *infected*. Thermal trauma results in a coagulative necrosis. Burn wounds, therefore, contain a variable amount of necrotic tissue, which, if infected, acts much as an undrained abscess, preventing access of antibiotics and host defensive factors.

The microbial flora of outpatient burns varies with time after the burn. Common organisms seen on days 1 to 3 include *S. epidermidis*, β-hemolytic streptococcus, *Bacillus subtilis*, *S. aureus*, enterococcus, *Mima polymorpha*, *Enterobacter*, *Herellea*, and *C. albicans*. One week after the burn, these organisms may be seen along with *E. coli*, *P. aeruginosa*, *Serratia marcescens*, and *Proteus vulgaris*.

Anaerobic colonization of burn wounds is rare unless there is much devitalized tissue, as would occur in a high-voltage electrical injury.[22] For this reason, routine anaerobic cultures are generally unnecessary in an assessment of infective organisms that produce minor infections.

Most superficial wounds that have been treated properly do not get infected. However, it is sometimes difficult to differentiate wound infection from the normal healing process—both involve pain, edema, and erythema. Early (days 1 to 5) burn infections are generally caused by gram-positive cocci, especially β-hemolytic streptococci. Streptococcal cellulitis is characterized by marked, spreading erythema extending outward from the wound margins. Despite the plethora of organisms and the presence of some gram-negative pathogens noted in superficial burn cultures, first-line treatment is with oral penicillin, 1 to 2 gm/day.

Effective topical treatment at the time of initial burn care and subsequent dressing changes is meant to delay bacterial colonization, maintain the wound bacterial density at low levels, and produce a less diverse wound flora. Because outpatient management of burns should be attempted only when the risk of infection is minimal, the use of systemic antibiotics is generally unnecessary for minor burns even in the setting of delayed treatment, diabetes, and steroid use.[23] Parenteral antibiotics in the management of minor burns have been recommended for patients undergoing an autograft procedure and for patients with a sore throat or other known streptococcal infection in whom penicillin is otherwise indicated.[24]

In minor burn care, wound cultures are not required or recommended. It is useless, for example, to culture blister fluid in the patient who presents for emergency care immediately after a thermal injury. Cultures are necessary only when overt infection develops, especially when this occurs while a topical or systemic antibiotic is being used. Cultures may also be of benefit when the infected wound is old, when hygiene is poor, or when there are old abrasions nearby.[25] Swab surface cultures are generally eschewed. Although they may adequately reflect wound flora, falsely sterile cultures are relatively frequent. These cultures do not reflect deep burn flora and give no quantitative information.

Sterile wound biopsy for culture is most satisfactory for the assessment of intraescharotic, subescharotic, or invasive infections and allows for quantification of bacterial flora. If a wound culture is taken, it should be obtained from the deepest or worst-appearing area of the burn.

Surface bacterial densities of >10⁵/cm² or tissue bacterial densities of $>10^5/gm$ correlate with invasive infection. Surface colonization may be treated with an alternative topical agent, but truly invasive infection warrants the administration of systemic antibiotics. Generally, the infectious process resolves in 24 to 48 hours.

Foot Burns

Despite their relatively small surface area, foot burns are formally categorized as major burns. Foot burns are the most common burn category to fail outpatient therapy and subsequently require admission and inpatient care. Zachary and coworkers[26] reported a series of 104 patients with foot burns. No patient admitted on the day of injury developed burn cellulitis; in contrast, 27 per cent of delayed-admission patients had cellulitis. Their study also noted a higher incidence of hypertrophic scarring and need for skin grafting in the delayed-admission group. Overall, fewer days of hospitalization were required for the initially admitted group.

Specific problems in the care of foot burns include pain, wound drainage, difficulty in changing dressings without help, inability of even motivated patients to comply with requirements for elevation, and prolonged convalescence. Hospital admission allows for splinting, intensive local burn care, physical therapy, and bed rest with elevation, which minimizes edema. For these reasons, initial admission for all but the most minor foot burns is advised.

Facial Burns

Facial burns often result in significant edema, which may compromise vision. Concurrent corneal injury can lead to the development of a purulent conjunctivitis with the risks of corneal ulceration and perforation. Fluorescein staining and slit-lamp examination should be used to confirm the diagnosis of suspected corneal injury. The treatment of a corneal injury involves irrigation, topical ophthalmic antibiotic ointment, and eye patching. Facial burns are otherwise treated with an open technique. Patients are instructed to wash the face 2 to 3 times a day with a mild soap and then apply a thin layer of antibiotic ointment, such as bacitracin zinc. Neck burns are treated similarly. Consideration for inpatient care is given to all facial burns.

Corneal contact burns, as from accidental contact with a curling iron, often present rather dramatically, with opacified, "heaped-up" corneal epithelium. Despite their appearance, the end result is usually excellent. Treatment is as for a corneal abrasion.[27]

Abuse of Children and the Elderly

Recognition of the possibility of deliberate abuse by burning in the pediatric and geriatric populations is essential. Additionally, children under age 2 have a thinner dermis and a less well developed immune system than do adults. Elderly patients older than age 65 likewise tolerate burns poorly, and these two populations are the most prone to

abuse, often by family members. For these reasons, both groups of patients often require inpatient care.[5]

The majority of abused children are 18 to 36 months old, and for unknown reasons the majority are male.[16] Immersion burns are a common type of abuse. These are characterized by circumferential sharply demarcated burns of the hands, feet, buttocks, and perineum. Cigarette burns and burns from hot objects such as irons should be obvious. Contact burns on "nonexploring" parts of the child also warrant suspicion.

Burns in Pregnancy

There is very little information in the literature concerning the special problems of the pregnant burn victim. Ying-bei and Ying-jie reported 24 pregnant burn patients representing a wide range of burn severity.[28] Complications of the burn injuries included abortion and premature labor, although all patients in this series with less than 20 per cent TBSA burns did well and delivered living full-term babies.

As the resistance of pregnant women to infection is lower than that in nonpregnant women, control of burn wound infection is paramount. Gestational age appears to have no direct bearing on prognosis. Silver sulfadiazine cream should be avoided near term because of the potential for kernicterus.

SPECIFIC BURNING AGENTS

Hot Tar Burns

Asphalts are products of the residues of coal tar commonly used in roofing and road repair. These products are kept heated to approximately 450° F. When spilled onto the skin, the tar cools rapidly; but the retained heat is sufficient to produce a partial-thickness burn. Fortunately, full-thickness burns are unusual. Cooled tar is nonirritating and does not promote infection.

When cooled tar is physically removed, adherent skin is usually avulsed (Fig. 49–6). Careless removal of adherent

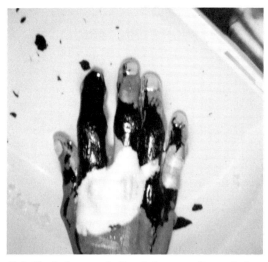

Figure 49–6. Physical removal of cooled tar usually results in avulsion of the underlying skin. Skin that is obviously loose should be débrided, but adherent tar is best liquified with an emulsifying agent. Final removal may be delayed for several days to permit loosening of the tar.

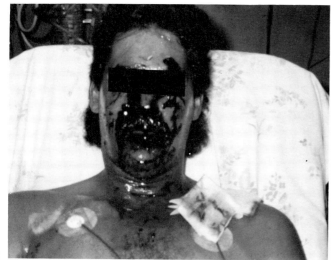

A

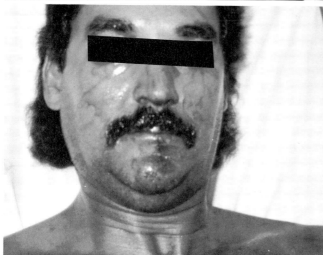

B

Figure 49–7. Tar stuck to the face *(A)* can be emulsified with various agents and a lot of patience and persistence *(B)*. Fortunately, tar burns are usually not full thickness.

tar may inflict further damage on burned tissues. Agents such as alcohol, acetone, kerosene, or gasoline have been used to remove the tar, but these are flammable and may cause additional skin damage or toxicity secondary to absorption.

There is no great need to meticulously remove all tar at the first visit. Obviously devitalized skin can be débrided, but adherent tar should be emulsified or dissolved, rather than manually removed (Fig. 49–7). Polyoxyethylene sorbitan (Tween 80 or polysorbate) is the water-soluble, nontoxic emulsifying agent found in Neosporin and several other topical antibiotic ointments. It is a complex mixture of ethers, esters, and sorbitol anhydrides, which possesses excellent hydrophilic and lyophilic characteristics when used as a nonionic, surface-active emulsifying agent. With persistence, most tar may be removed (emulsified) on the initial visit. However, many physicians prefer to emulsify it on an outpatient basis. A generous layer of polysorbate-based ointment can be applied under a bulky absorbent gauze dressing. The patient is then discharged, and the residual is easily washed off after 24 to 36 hours (Fig. 49–8). Once the residual tar is removed, the wound is treated like any other burn.

Shur-Clens, a nontoxic, nonionic detergent, also works well for tar burn wound cleansing as does mineral oil,

petrolatum, and Medisol (Orange-Sol, Inc., Chandler, Ariz.)—a petroleum-citrus product.

Chemical Burns

Chemical burns usually occur in the workplace, and the offending substance is usually well known. There are more than 25,000 chemicals currently in use that are capable of burning the skin or mucous membranes. Commonly used chemical agents are shown in Table 49–4.

Injury is caused by a chemical reaction, rather than a thermal burn.[29] Reactions are classified as oxidizing, reducing, corrosive, desiccant, or vesicant or as protoplasmic poisoning. The injury to skin continues until the chemical agent is physically removed or it exhausts its inherent destructive capacity. The degree of injury is based on chemical strength, concentration, and quantity; duration of contact; location of contact; extent of tissue penetration; and mechanism of action.

Immediate flushing with water is recommended for all chemical burns, with the exception of those caused by alkali metals. Flushing serves to cleanse the wound of unreacted surface chemical, to dilute the chemical already in contact with tissue, and to restore tissue water lost to the hydroscopic effect of certain agents.

Leonard and colleagues clearly demonstrated that patients receiving immediate copious water irrigation for chemical burns showed less full-thickness burn injury and a greater than 50 per cent reduction in time of hospital stay.[30]

ACID AND ALKALI BURNS

Alkalies cause saponification and liquefactive necrosis of body fats. Alkaline burns are *penetrating* and cause much tissue destruction. With acid burns, tissue coagulation pro-

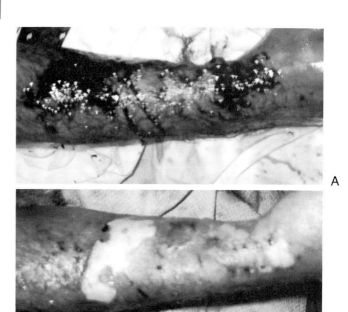

A

B

Figure 49–8. There is no need to remove all the tar on the first visit *(A)*. This extremity was covered with an emulsifying agent and covered with gauze, and the residual tar was washed off easily 36 hours later *(B)*.

Table 49–4. Commonly Used Acids and Alkalies

Acids	Alkalies
Picric	Sodium hydroxide
Tungstic	Ammonium hydroxide
Sulfosalicylic	Lithium hydroxide
Tannic	Barium hydroxide
Trichloroacetic	Calcium hydroxide
Cresylic	Sodium hypochlorite
Acetic	
Formic	
Sulfuric	
Hydrochloric	
Hydrofluoric	
Chromic	

duces a thick eschar that limits the penetration of the agent. Desiccant acids, such as sulfuric acid, create an exothermic reaction with tissue water and can cause both chemical and thermal injury. With extensive immersion injuries, acids may be systemically absorbed, leading to systemic acidosis and coagulation abnormalities.

Chemical burns may be excruciatingly painful for long periods of time. Discomfort can be out of proportion to what one might expect from the depth or extent of the burn.

The emergency care team should remove all potentially contaminated clothing. Any dry (anhydrous) chemical should be brushed off the patient's skin. The involved skin should be irrigated with large amounts of water under low pressure. Any remaining particulate matter should be carefully débrided during irrigation.

Strong alkali burns may require irrigation for 1 to 2 hours before the tissue pH returns to normal. After extensive irrigation, if the burn continues to feel "slippery" or if the tissue pH has not returned to normal, chemical neutralization may be helpful.[31, 32]

WET CEMENT BURNS

Portland cement is a hydroscopic alkaline substance whose major constituent is calcium oxide (64 per cent) combined with oxides of silicon, aluminum, magnesium, sulfur, iron, and potassium. There is considerable variability in the calcium oxide content of different grades of cement—concrete having less and fine-textured masonry cement having more.[30] The addition of water exothermically converts the calcium oxide to calcium hydroxide, a strongly corrosive alkali with a pH of 11 to 13. As the cement hardens, the calcium hydroxide reacts with ambient carbon dioxide and becomes inactive.

Both the heat produced in this exothermic reaction as well as the $Ca(OH)_2$ produced can result in significant burns. Because of its low solubility and consequent low ionic strength, a long exposure to calcium hydroxide is required to produce injury. This usually occurs secondary to a worker's accidentally spilling concrete into boots or kneeling in it for a prolonged period. The burn wound and the resultant protein denaturation of tissues produces a thick, tenacious, ulcerated eschar.

Concrete burns are insidious and progressive. What may appear initially as patchy, superficial burns may in several days become full-thickness burns that require excision and skin grafting.[33] The pain of these burns is often severe and more intense than the appearance of the wound might suggest (Fig. 49–9). Interestingly, many workers are not warned of the dangers of prolonged contact with cement,

and, because initial contact with cement is usually painless, exposure may not be realized until the damage is done.

Treatment is as follows: any loose particulate cement or lime is brushed off, contaminated clothing is removed, the wound is copiously irrigated with tap water (the pH of the effluent is tested and irrigation continued if the effluent is still alkaline), compresses of dilute acetic acid (vinegar) may be applied to neutralize the remaining alkali and provide pain relief after irrigation, and antibiotic ointment is applied to the eschar during the early postburn period.

Sutilains ointment (Travase, Flint Pharmaceuticals, Deerfield, IL) is often recommended because it contains proteolytic enzymes and helps speed eschar separation. The depth of burns from wet cement can be difficult to assess in the first several days. If it becomes apparent that the burns are full-thickness, early excision and skin grafting is recommended.

Cement burns should be differentiated from cement dermatitis, which is far more common. The latter is a contact sensitivity reaction, probably due to the chromates present in cement. The contact dermatitis can initially be treated as a superficial partial-thickness burn.

HYDROCARBON CONTACT BURNS

Hydrocarbons are capable of causing severe contact injuries by virtue of their irritant, fat-dissolving, and dehydrating properties. Cutaneous absorption may cause even more dangerous systemic effects. Gasoline, the usual agent involved, is a complex mixture of C_4–C_{11} alkane hydrocarbons and benzene; the hydrocarbons appear to be the major toxic agent.

Depth of injury is related to the duration of exposure and concentration of the chemical agent. Gasoline immersion injuries resemble scald burns and are usually partial thickness.[34] Occasionally, gasoline-injured skin exhibits a pinkish brown discoloration, possibly related to dye additives. A common source of exposure is a comatose patient from a motor vehicle accident who had been lying in a pool of gasoline.

The lungs are the usual site of systemic absorption and are often the only major route of excretion. The resultant high pulmonary concentrations may lead to pulmonary hemorrhages, atelectasis, and adult respiratory distress syndrome (ARDS). Chlorinated hydrocarbons, such as carburetor cleaner, may cause pulmonary and hepatocellular toxicity. Microscopically, hydrocarbons appear to selectively

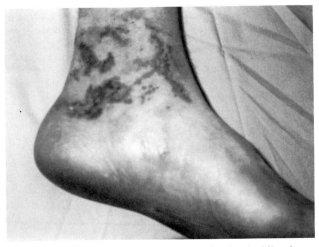

Figure 49–9. Alkali burns from wet cement develop insidiously, are extremely painful, and are frequently full-thickness injuries.

damage vascular endothelium. Renal toxicity is uncommon and usually associated with more extensive systemic absorption. Lipid degenerative changes occur in the glomeruli and proximal convoluted tubules. Neurologic effects range from mild euphoria to a severe toxic encephalopathy and may be related both to any lead compounds present or to the hydrocarbon itself.

Treatment of hydrocarbon burns includes the following: removal of contaminated clothing, prolonged irrigation or soaking of the contaminated skin, early débridement in significant burns caused by lead-containing gasolines (to reduce systemic lead absorption), and use of topical antibiotic ointments.

PHENOL

Phenol is a highly reactive aromatic acid alcohol that acts as a corrosive. Carbolic acid, an earlier term for phenol, was noted to have antiseptic properties and was used as such by Joseph Lister in performing the first antiseptic surgery. Hexylresorcinol, a phenol derivative, is in current use as a bactericidal agent.

Phenols, in strong concentration, cause considerable eschar formation, but skin absorption does occur and can cause systemic effects such as central nervous system depression, hypotension, hemolysis, pulmonary edema, and death. Interestingly, phenol acts differently from other acids, in that it penetrates deeper when in a dilute solution than in a more concentrated form.[29] Therefore, irrigation with water is less than optimal for phenol burns; but because water commonly is readily available, it is frequently used for irrigation.

Full-strength polyethylene glycol (PG 300 or 400) is more effective than water alone in removing phenolic compounds and should be obtained and used after water irrigation has begun. Polyethylene glycol is nontoxic and nonirritating and may be used anywhere on the body. When immediately available, polyethylene glycol can be used to remove the surface chemical before water irrigation (and chemical dilution) is begun.

HYDROFLUORIC ACID

Hydrofluoric acid is a ubiquitous compound used in masonry restoration, glass etching, semiconductor manufacturing, and plastics production and as a catalyst in petroleum alkylating units. It is available in industry as a liquid with varying concentrations up to 70 per cent. It is also found in many home rust-removal products in concentrations of less than 10 per cent.

Fluoride ion is a protoplasmic poison that causes liquefaction necrosis. *It is notorious for its ability to penetrate tissues and cause delayed pain and tissue injury.* With home products, the unwary user does not realize that the substance is caustic until the skin (usually the hands and fingers) is exposed for a few minutes to hours, at which time the burning begins and becomes progressively worse. At this point the damage is done and the absorbed hydrofluoric acid cannot be washed off. With higher-strength industrial products, symptoms are almost immediate.

The initial corrosive burn is due to free hydrogen ions; secondary chemical burning is due to the tissue penetration of fluoride ions. In high concentrations, the fluoride ions may penetrate to the bone and produce demineralization.[35] If the hands are exposed, the acid characteristically penetrates the fingernails and injures the nail bed and cuticle area. As with most caustics, the pain is generally out of proportion to the evident external physical injury. Hydrofluoric acid burns produce variable areas of blanching and

erythema, but rarely are blisters or skin sloughing seen initially. Skin necrosis and cutaneous hemorrhage may be noted in a few days.

Immediate treatment should begin with copious irrigation with water. Another approach is to wash the area with a solution of iced magnesium sulfate (Epsom salts) or a 1:500 solution of a quaternary ammonium compound such as Hibiclens or Zephiran. Magnesium and calcium salts form an insoluble complex with fluoride ions, preventing further tissue diffusion. Unfortunately, topical preparations are often ineffective in limiting injury or controlling pain.

If there is no or minimal visible evidence of skin injury and minimal pain, the burn may be dressed with topical calcium gluconate paste. This is not commercially available but is easily compounded in the pharmacy by pulverizing calcium carbonate or calcium gluconate tablets and mixing in a small aliquot of 10 per cent calcium gluconate solution or a water-soluble gel (such as K-Y jelly) to form a thick paste.

Plastic wrap (e.g., Saran wrap) over a standard dry burn dressing is used to cover the calcium paste on the limbs; a vinyl or rubber glove is used over the paste on the hands. The wound should be rechecked in 24 hours. A digital or regional nerve block with long-acting bupivacaine is an excellent way to provide prolonged pain relief if the hands are involved. Otherwise, oral narcotics are generally required. If bullae or vesicles have formed, these should be débrided to decrease the amount of fluoride present, and the wound should then be treated as any partial-thickness burn. Burns with hydrofluoric acid of less than 10 per cent strength will heal spontaneously, usually without significant tissue loss, but pain and sensitivity of the finger tips may persist for 7 to 10 days. Additionally, the fingernails may become loose.

The presence of significant skin injury or immediate intense pain implies penetration of the skin by fluoride ions. This scenario is particularly common with exposure to hydrofluoric acid solutions in concentrations of 20 per cent or greater, but tissue injury can occur with prolonged exposure to less concentrated products.

Initial treatment of a more concentrated exposure begins as described above and includes immediate wound débridement of necrotic tissue to decontaminate the area of as much fluoride ion as possible. Following this, a 10 per cent solution of calcium gluconate *(note: avoid calcium chloride)* is injected intradermally and subcuticularly (30-gauge needle) about the exposed area using about 0.5 ml per square centimeter of burn. Hydrofluoric acid can penetrate fingernails without damaging them. Soft tissue can be injected without prior anesthesia, but if the nail beds are involved they may be injected via the fat pad under a digital nerve block (Fig. 49–10). Although many investigators recommend that fingernails should be routinely removed, we strongly advise *against* this unless the nails are very loose or there is obvious necrosis of the nail bed.[36] Nails frequently become loose in a few days, but often they return to normal and do not require removal, particularly when lower concentration nonindustrial products are involved.

Several authorities have advocated intra-arterial calcium infusions in the treatment of serious hydrofluoric acid burns of the extremities.[35, 37] This technique is not recommended for burns secondary to dilute hydrofluoric acid (i.e., less than 10 per cent). When using this technique, 10 ml of 10 per cent calcium gluconate is diluted in 50 ml of 5 per cent dextrose and water solution. The dilute solution is given by a slow infusion into an arterial catheter. If only the first three digits are involved, only the radial artery need be cannulated. Otherwise, a percutaneous catheter is inserted into the brachial artery, and the solution is infused over 4

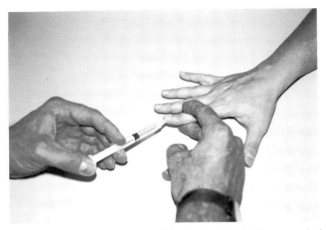

Figure 49–10. In the treatment of hydrofluoric acid burns, topical therapy is often ineffective. Calcium gluconate may be injected into the nail bed via the fat pad under a digital nerve block. Fingernails should not be removed routinely if burns are mild, such as those seen with household products of less than 10 per cent concentration of the acid.

hours. At this point, the catheter is left in place and the patient observed. If pain returns at any time over the next 4 hours, the infusion is repeated. If the patient is pain-free over the 4-hour observation period, the burn is dressed and the patient discharged.

Advantages of the intra-arterial method are elimination of the need for painful subcutaneous injections and avoidance of the volume limitations of the subcutaneous route while providing substantially more calcium to neutralize the fluoride. Both the chloride and gluconate salts of calcium have been used intra-arterially. Ten milliliters of 10 per cent calcium gluconate contain 4.7 mEq of calcium, whereas the same volume of 10 per cent calcium chloride contains 14 mEq of calcium. Thus intra-arterial calcium chloride may provide nearly three times as much neutralizing calcium equivalent as the gluconate salt; however, because calcium chloride can irritate tissues, it is not recommended for subcutaneous use. Disadvantages of intra-arterial calcium therapy include the possibility of local arterial spasm (which can be treated with vasodilators or removal of the catheter), local arterial injury or thrombus, and the long duration of treatment required.

CHROMIC ACID BURNS

Chromium compounds are used extensively in industry, mainly in metallic electroplating. Chromic acid is commonly used in concentrated solutions containing up to 25 per cent sulfuric acid. Chromic acid causes sufficient skin damage to allow the absorption of the toxic chromium ion if intensive irrigation is not undertaken immediately. Heated (60 to 80° C) chromic acid makes the problem of chromium absorption much worse.

Dichromate salts containing hexavalent chromium are the most readily absorbed and the most toxic because they can cross cell membranes. The mortality from these burns is very high if the burn exceeds 10 per cent TBSA. Chromium absorption leads to diarrhea, gastrointestinal bleeding, hemolysis, hepatic and renal damage, coma, encephalopathy, seizures, and disseminated intravascular coagulation.

Treatment includes immediate excision of the burned tissues to lessen the total body dichromate burden. Wounds should be washed with a 1 per cent sodium phosphate or sulfate solution and dressed with bandages soaked in 5 per

cent sodium thiosulfate solution. These actions reduce the hexavalent chromium ion to the less well-absorbed trivalent form.[38]

Chelation therapy with EDTA should be instituted, and intravenous sodium thiosulfate and ascorbic acid given. Hemodialysis, peritoneal dialysis, or exchange transfusion may be indicated.

PHOSPHORUS BURNS

White phosphorus is a translucent, waxy substance that ignites spontaneously on contact with air. As such, it is usually stored under water. It is used primarily in fireworks, insecticides and rodenticides, and military weapons.

Phosphorus causes both thermal burns from the flaming pieces and acid burns, which result from the oxidation of phosphorus to phosphoric acid. The burns classically emit a white vapor with a characteristic garlic odor.[39]

These burns are treated first with immersion in water followed by débridement of any gross debris. The wound is then washed with a 1 per cent copper sulfate solution, which reacts with the residual phosphorus to form copper phosphate; the latter appears as black granules and allows for easy débridement. Following débridement, the residual copper is removed by a thorough water rinse, and the wound is dressed and treated as any other burn.

ELEMENTAL ALKALI METAL BURNS

The commonly encountered alkali metals (sodium, lithium, and potassium) are highly reactive in water and with water vapor in air, producing their respective hydroxide with liberation of hydrogen gas. As such, water should never be used for extinguishing or débridement of the metal. A class D fire extinguisher or plain sand may be used for smothering the fire, followed by the application of mineral or cooking oil to isolate the metal from water, and allowing safe débridement. Then the burn is treated as an alkali burn.

Magnesium burns in a less intense fashion but otherwise acts as do the other alkali metals. These burns may be particularly injurious, however, because if all of the metallic debris is not removed, the small ulcers that form will slowly enlarge until they become quite extensive.

EMERGENCY ESCHAROTOMY

Full-thickness and occasionally extensive partial-thickness circumferential burns may impede peripheral blood flow or chest movement via a tourniquet effect. In such cases, immediate escharotomy may be indicated. During fluid resuscitation and as a direct result of the transcapillary extravasation of fluid from a thermal injury, intracellular and interstitial edema may be progressive. As the soft tissues become edematous and pressure rises under the inelastic eschar, first venous, then arterial flow to the underlying and distal unburned tissue may be compromised. Early elevation of the limb and active range-of-motion exercises every 15 minutes may minimize soft tissue edema; but once signs and symptoms of vascular impairment are present, the clinician must act quickly to prevent tissue hypoxia and cellular death.

Skin temperature and palpation of pulses are *unreliable* and *imprecise* indicators of adequacy of circulation because of peripheral vasoconstriction and local edema. The patient with circulatory embarrassment may complain of deep aching pain, progressive loss of sensation, or paresthesia; but these parameters are difficult to quantitate in the severely burned or mechanically ventilated patient. The best indicators to follow are serial assessment of capillary refill, arterial flow with the use of Doppler technique, and peripheral oximetry.[40, 41] In the fluid-resuscitated patient, absent distal arterial flow as determined with the use of the Doppler ultrasonic flowmeter is an absolute indication for escharotomy. Boardakjian suggests that demonstrating an oxygen saturation below 95 per cent in the distal extremity with pulse oximetry (in the absence of systemic hypoxia) is also a reliable indicator of the need for emergency escharotomy.

Technique of Escharotomy

Because full thickness burns are insensible to pain and involve coagulation of superficial vessels, no general or local anesthesia is necessary, although sedation is highly recommended in the patient who is awake. A properly executed escharotomy releases the eschar to the depth of the subcutaneous fat only. This results in minimal bleeding, which can be controlled by local pressure or electrocautery. These incisions, although limb or life-saving, are potential sources

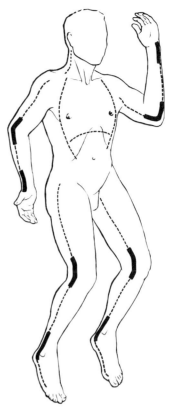

Figure 49–12. Diagram showing preferred sites of escharotomy incisions. (From Davis JH, et al: Clinical Surgery. St. Louis, CV Mosby Co, 1987.)

of infection in the burn patient. The wounds should be loosely packed with sterile gauze impregnated with an appropriate topical antimicrobial. Formal fasciotomy is rarely required in thermal burns, but it may be indicated for high-voltage electrical injuries. If required, fasciotomy should be performed in the operating room.

LIMBS

Under sterile conditions the lateral and medial aspects of the involved extremity are incised with a scalpel, 1 cm proximal to and past the length of the circumferential burn (Fig. 49–11). The incision is carried through the full thickness of skin only and results in immediate separation of the constricting eschar to exposed subcutaneous fat. Because joints are areas of tight skin adherence and potential vascular impingement, incisions should cross these structures (Fig. 49–12). Care must be taken to avoid vital structures, such as the radial nerve at the wrist and the superficial peroneal nerve at the fibular head. The incision should extend to the great toe medially and little toe laterally in circumferential burns of the feet, and to the thenar and hypothenar aspects of the hands as indicated. Improvement in color, Doppler flow signal strength, and oximetry values indicate adequate release.

CHEST

Full-thickness circumferential chest or upper abdominal burns may impair respiration. For release of this eschar, the incision should extend from the clavicle to the costal margin in the anterior axillary line bilaterally and may be joined by

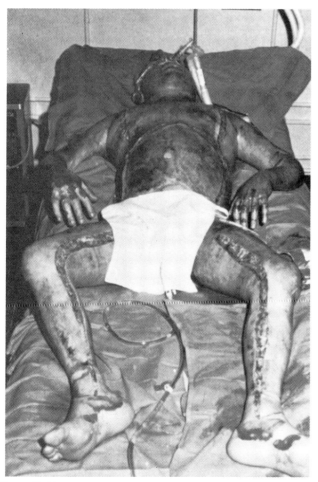

Figure 49–11. The circulatory embarrassment caused by edema beneath the encircling full-thickness burns of the legs of this patient was relieved by escharotomy incisions placed in the midmedial line of each limb. The restriction of the ventilatory excursion of the chest wall caused by the encircling full-thickness truncal burns was relieved by the escharotomies placed in both anterior axillary lines and a costal margin escharotomy. Compression of the abdominal contents and restriction of diaphragmatic excursion by the constricting deep abdominal wall burns was relieved by placement of escharotomy incisions in the lateral abdominal wall bilaterally. (From Davis JH, et al: Clinical Surgery. St. Louis, CV Mosby Co., 1987.)

transverse incisions, which results in a chevron-shaped escharotomy.

Neck escharotomy should be performed laterally, posterior to the carotid and jugular vessels. Penile escharotomy is performed midlaterally for avoidance of the dorsal vein.

REFERENCES

1. Baxter CR, Waeckerle JF: Emergency treatment of burn injury. Ann Emerg Med 17:12, 1988.
2. Alexander JW: Burn care: A specialty in evolution—1985 presidential address, American Burn Association. J Trauma 26:1, 1986.
3. Monafo WW, Ayvazian VH: Topical therapy. Surg Clin North Am 58:1157, 1978.
4. Davies JWL: Prompt cooling of burned areas: A review of benefits and the effector mechanisms. Burns 9:1, 1983.
5. Minor burns. In Trott AT (ed): Principles and Techniques of Minor Wound Care. New York, Medical Examination Publishing Co., 1984, pp 177–187.
6. Yarbrough DR: The history of burn treatment. Emerg Med Serv 17:21, 1988.
7. Demling RH, Mazess RB, Wolbert W: The effect of immediate and delayed cold immersion on burn edema formation and resorption. J Trauma 19:56, 1979.
8. Phillips LG, Robson MC, Heggers JP: Treating minor burns: Ice, grease, or what? Postgrad Med 85:219, 1989.
9. Warden GD: Outpatient care of thermal injuries. Surg Clin North Am 67:147, 1987.
10. Shuck JM: Outpatient management of the burned patient. Surg Clin North Am 58:1107, 1978.
11. Quinn KJ: Design of a burn dressing. Burns 13:377, 1987.
12. Hermans MHE, Hermans RP: Duoderm, an alternative dressing for smaller burns. Burns 12:214, 1986.
13. Gerding RL, Imbembo AL, Fratianne RB: Biosynthetic skin substitute vs 1% silver sulfadiazine for treatment of inpatient partial-thickness thermal burns. J Trauma 28:1265, 1988.
14. Salisbury RE, Wilmore DW, Silverstein P, Pruitt BA Jr: Biological dressings for skin graft donor sites. Arch Surg 106:705, 1973.
15. Ricketts CR, Squires JR, Topley E, Lilly HA: Human skin lipids with particular reference to the self-sterilizing power of the skin. Clin Soc Mol Med 10:89, 1951.
16. Stuart JD, Kenney JG, Morgan RF: Pediatric burns. Am Fam Phys 36:139, 1987.
17. Hunter GR, Chang FC: Outpatient burns: A prospective study. J Trauma 16:191, 1976.
18. Loder JS, Krochmal L: Topical chlorhexidine phosphanilate for prophylactic treatment of burns (letter). N Engl J Med 314:1256, 1986.
19. Heck E, Head M, Nowak D, et al: Aloe vera (gel) cream as a topical treatment for outpatient burns. Burns 7:291, 1980.
20. Madden MR, Nolan E, Finkelstein JL, et al: Comparison of an occlusive and a semi-occlusive dressing and the effect of the wound exudate upon keratinocyte proliferation. J Trauma 29:924, 1989.
21. Swain AH, Azadian BS, Wakeley CJ, Shakespeare PG: Management of blisters in minor burns. Br Med J 295:181, 1987.
22. Monafo WW, Freedman B: Topical therapy for burns. Surg Clin North Am 67:133, 1987.
23. Boss WK, et al: Effectiveness of prophylactic antibiotics in the outpatient treatment of burns. J Trauma 25:224, 1985.
24. O'Neill JA Jr: Burns: Office evaluation and management. Primary Care 3:531, 1976.
25. Shuck JM: Current practices in burn management. Am Surg 40(3):145, 1974.
26. Zachary LS, Heggers JP, Robson MC, et al: Burns of the feet. J Burn Care Rehabil 8:192, 1987.
27. Bloom SM, Gittinger JW Jr, Kazarian EL: Management of corneal contact thermal burns. Am J Ophthalmol 100:536, 1986.
28. Ying-bei Z, Ying-jie Z: Burns during pregnancy: An analysis of 24 cases. Burns 8:286, 1981.
29. Stewart CE: Chemical skin burns. Am Fam Phys 31:149, 1985.
30. Leonard LG, Scheulen JJ, Munster AM: Chemical burns: Effect of prompt first aid. J Trauma 22:420, 1982.
31. Jelenko C III: Chemicals that burn. J Trauma 14:65, 1974.
32. Arena JM: Treatment of caustic alkali poisoning. Mod Treatment 8:613, 1971.
33. Wilson GR, Davidson PM: Full thickness burns from ready-mixed cement. Burns 12:139, 1985.
34. Hausbrough JF, et al: Hydrocarbon contact injuries. J Trauma 25:250, 1985.
35. Vance MV, Curry S, et al: Digital hydrofluoric acid burns: Treatment with intra arterial calcium infusion. Ann Emerg Med 15:890, 1986.
36. Roberts JR, Merigian KM: Acute hydrofluoric acid exposure. Am J Emerg Med 7:125, 1988.
37. Pegg SP, Siu S, Gillett G: Intra-arterial infusions in the treatment of hydrofluoric acid burns. Burns 11:440, 1985.
38. Wang XW, Davies JWL, Zapata Sirvent RL, et al: Chromic acid burns and acute chromium poisoning. Burns 11:181, 1985.
39. Konjoyan TR: White phosphorus burns: Case report and literature review. Milit Med 148:881, 1983.
40. Moylan JA, Wellford WI, Pruitt BA: Circulatory changes following circumferential extremity burns evaluated by the ultrasonic flowmeter: An analysis of 60 thermally injured limbs. J Trauma 11:763, 1971.
41. Bardakjian VB, Kenney JG, Edgerton ML, et al: Pulse oximetry for vascular monitoring in burned upper extremities. J Burn Care Rehabil 9:63, 1988.

Gastrointestinal Procedures

Chapter **50**

Esophageal Foreign Bodies

Gary P. Young and Steven A. Pace

INTRODUCTION

The presentation of a patient with an esophageal foreign body (FB) can range from the adult with dysphagia and a history of acute ingestion to the child with signs mimicking acute epiglottitis or chronic respiratory symptoms such as asthma.[1-12] Three groups of patients are prone to have FBs lodge in the esophagus: older patients with dental prostheses who ingest poorly chewed food and who may have esophageal pathology; small children as a manifestation of oral retentive behavior; and adults with functional or organic impairment, including suicidal, psychotic, mentally retarded, incarcerated, and alcoholic patients. The type of esophageal FB usually depends on the patient's age and underlying condition, for example, coins and food in children, food boluses in the elderly, and almost anything in impaired adults.

The esophagus has three normal anatomic sites of narrowing; in addition, pathologic strictures may develop elsewhere because of intrinsic lesions. Most impactions occur within the upper third of the (cervical) esophagus at the cricopharyngeus muscle. The second site of narrowing occurs where the (cardiac) esophagus crosses the aortic arch. The third site is at the lower esophageal sphincter (LES) also known as the gastroesophageal (GE) junction. Sharp or angulated FBs are prone to remain in the esophagus.

Impacted esophageal FBs must be removed or dislodged. Although the urgency of removal depends on many factors, FBs cannot be left in the esophagus for prolonged periods to "dissolve" or "pass by themselves." This approach courts disaster. After acute airway compromise,[13] esophageal perforation is the most serious complication of esophageal FBs.[14] Blunt objects lodged for any extended period of time can cause pressure necrosis and esophageal perforation. Small button batteries should be removed immediately; they are of special concern because they can cause perforation in as little as 18 hours.[15] Although 80 to 90 per cent of esophageal FBs cause transient symptoms and pass spontaneously, often within minutes,[16] approximately 10 to 20 per cent require endoscopic removal and approximately 1 per cent require surgery.[17] Observation of certain small round FBs or food boluses in the hospital for spontaneous passage should be limited to no longer than 24 hours.[4] Button batteries and sharp, angulated, or large (greater than 2 cm in diameter or longer than 5 cm) FBs are best removed immediately. This chapter focuses on the procedure-oriented issues concerning the diagnosis and management of esophageal FBs.

BACKGROUND

Both the diagnostic work-up and the treatment of esophageal FBs are procedure oriented.[1-12, 17] In 1937, Jackson and Jackson published a classic monograph on the management of FBs of the upper airway and esophagus that was based on the use of the rigid endoscope in 3266 patients.[18] In 1945, Richardson reported the use of papain (a technique currently discouraged) in successfully treating meat obstructions of the esophagus.[19] In 1966, Bigler reported the use of the Foley catheter to extract blunt radiopaque FBs from the upper gastrointestinal tract.[20] More recently, medications and solutions have been used to relax the LES.[16] Although otolaryngologists and thoracic surgeons continue to use the rigid esophagoscope for FB extraction, during the 1970s gastroenterologists began to use the flexible endoscope.[17]

To prevent morbidity and mortality from esophageal FBs, the emergency physician must first rapidly diagnose the presence and site of an FB, often with radiographic assistance.[21] Then the emergency physician must choose the best method of removal, often with the assistance of an otolaryngologist or a gastroenterologist or both.[17] The anesthesiologist, thoracic surgeon, and operating room crew may also be called on to assist in the definitive management of these patients.

Cohen analyzed the reasons for the failure to diagnose esophageal FBs.[22] Among explanations for retained FBs being missed are (1) the absence of a positive history, (2) the omission from diagnostic consideration of the possibility of an FB, and (3) the absence of positive radiologic findings, which may be due to inadequate x-ray studies or to the characteristics of the FB itself. Although definite complications are associated with attempts to remove esophageal FBs,[14] long-term complications are more common with retained esophageal FBs. Children are more prone than adults to such complications.[23-25]

RADIOLOGY OF ESOPHAGEAL FOREIGN BODIES

Background

The radiographic examination of the patient suspected of harboring an esophageal FB is usually straightforward and accurate, assuming proper patient selection. Chaikhouni and colleagues[4] diagnosed esophageal FBs in 67 of 79 patients with standard chest radiographs only. Haglund and coworkers[21] reported a series of 264 patients with suspected esophageal FBs who were studied with plain film x-rays and contrast esophagograms. All patients received esophagoscopy and only one of 195 patients with an FB detected by endoscopy had normal radiographic findings, although 43 patients (18 per cent) had false-positive radiographic findings. Some esophageal FBs are not so readily diagnosable by x-rays (e.g., radiolucent FBs). Wood, plastic, and aluminum cannot be seen on standard radiographs. Occult esophageal FBs can cause chronic respiratory symptoms. Children with previously unrecognized esophageal perforation due to aluminum pop-top cans (radiolucent on plain x-ray) may present in this manner.[26] Unrecognized esophageal FBs may simulate asthma or epiglottitis, and symptoms may even improve when treatment is instituted for the wrong diagnosis.[27]

Indications

Some investigators believe that the concern that an ingested FB may be impacted is often overestimated by physicians, parents, and patients. Boothroyd and coworkers[28] found that if radiographic work-ups were limited to children with a clinical history suggestive of esophageal FB impaction or FB aspiration or following a button battery ingestion, then half their pediatric patients could have been spared the expense of and exposure to x-rays. This is a controversial issue; whereas older patients may be able to localize the hypopharyngeal or esophageal FB by pain, pressure, or FB sensation, preschool children often cannot. Hence, *any child, with or without symptoms, with a history of an FB ingestion should be x-rayed.*

It is axiomatic that a complete radiographic study include the areas from the "nose to the anus." In a small child this is often accomplished with a single x-ray taken with a large cassette. An ingested FB may end up in the nasopharynx of an infant and be missed if only a chest or abdominal film is obtained. Plain films of the neck are indicated in the patient with FB symptoms localized to the hypopharynx or upper chest, unless the hypopharyngeal FB can be visualized directly by the physician or there is a reliable history that a radiolucent FB (e.g., food without bones) was ingested. Plain films of the chest are indicated in the symptomatic patient who has ingested a radiopaque FB. Abdominal radiographs may also be of benefit in locating a radiopaque FB, especially if the neck or chest films are negative and the physician or patient and family would be reassured by finding the FB. Plain radiographs may be necessary even after removal of an FB in an unreliable adult or a child who may have ingested more than one FB. Two ingested coins, for example, may overlap and appear as a single FB if only an anteroposterior film is obtained. Contrast esophagograms may be indicated if an FB ingestion or impaction is suggested by the history or examination but the plain films are negative or equivocal (e.g., radiolucent FBs).

Radiographic studies may also identify complications from esophageal FBs. For example, plain films may identify retropharyngeal air or pneumomediastinum caused by esophageal perforation, and contrast studies can demonstrate the site of perforation or obstruction. Conversely, if the patient just ingested a poorly chewed meat bolus and is now complaining of FB symptoms in the lower chest or epigastrium, then it may be possible to relieve the distal esophageal impaction without benefit of prior x-ray contrast studies. Subsequently, these patients will require either contrast esophagograms or esophagoscopy to rule out any underlying pathology. If the FB has moved into the stomach or is found to be in the stomach, clinical follow-up (such as checking the stools of an infant) should be adequate to verify movement of the FB through the alimentary tract. Follow-up plain x-ray films are indicated after a reasonable period of time (e.g., 4 to 7 days, or sooner when symptoms ensue) if passage cannot be documented. Infrequently, there may also be indications for other radiographic studies, such as computed tomography (CT) and xerograms (described later). The following discussion presents an approach to the use of radiographic studies in patients with presumed esophageal FBs.

Procedures

The diagnostic methods to be discussed include plain film x-rays of the neck and chest, contrast esophagograms, CT, and xeroradiography. In the work-up of a possible esophageal FB, plain roentgenograms begin with anteroposterior and lateral views of the neck, because the majority of foreign objects are located at the level of the cricopharyngeus constrictor muscle (Fig. 50–1).[21] Soft-tissue intensity x-rays

or xeroradiographs enhance the visualization of weakly radiopaque FBs.

Lateral and anteroposterior views of the neck are among the most commonly ordered films to evaluate the presence of FBs of the neck. Soft tissue technique should be routinely requested, and the technician should include the nasopharynx to the seventh cervical vertebra. (Note that FBs of the nose and those ingested and propelled into the nasopharynx are not uncommon and may be missed if only the neck is examined.) If slight hyperextension is performed, the clavicles are projected away from the lower esophagus. Having the patient phonate "Eeeeee" during the exposure traps air in the pharynx to enhance soft tissue landmarks and prevents swallowing, an activity that produces motion and blurs the anatomy. The upper esophagus, vallecula, and retropharyngeal area deserve special attention when reading the film.

Plain radiographs are somewhat difficult to read in the elderly. The physician must be cognizant of the anatomy and be aware that soft tissues (ligaments, glands) and cartilage calcify as aging occurs. It is common to misidentify calcified structures as a possible foreign body (Fig. 50–1A–C).

Posteroanterior and lateral views of the chest are necessary for examination of the remainder of the esophagus. Both projections should be made, because small objects may be visible in only one plane or multiple objects may be recognized in different x-ray planes.[27] Positive radiographic findings include the presence of radiopaque FBs, air-fluid levels, soft tissue swelling, intraesophageal air, subcutaneous emphysema, or free air in the mediastinum. A chest radiograph may reveal infiltrates consistent with aspiration pneumonitis resulting from total esophageal obstruction or a tracheoesophageal fistula.

Contrast esophagograms can be used to pursue the suspicion of an FB in the absence of positive findings on plain x-ray films (Fig. 50–2). The type of FB, its precise location, the degree of obstruction or perforation, and possible underlying anatomic abnormalities can all be delineated by contrast studies. Several controversial choices arise at this point. Should a cotton pledget soaked in contrast agent be used initially? Which contrast agent should be used? Are fluoroscopy and radiologic consultation necessary?

A cotton ball or cotton pledget soaked in contrast can be swallowed, followed by x-ray exposures of the neck and chest during and after the swallow.[29] Total obstruction will impede the cotton, partial obstruction may do the same, and on occasion small pieces of cotton will lodge on irregular or sharp surfaces, thus indicating the presence of an FB. Advantages of this maneuver are that fluoroscopy is not necessary, and it requires very little contrast material, which minimizes interference with follow-up endoscopy should it be required. However, the diagnostic accuracy of this technique is poor,[21] and if negative, this technique does not definitely rule out an FB.

The question of which contrast agent to use is debated among radiologists.[21, 30–32] In general, it is suggested that if a perforation is suspected, a water-soluble material (Gastrografin) should be used because it is less reactive on serosal surfaces than barium. Small perforations, however, may be missed with a Gastrografin study. In all other situations, barium compounds should be chosen because imaging is better and tracheal aspiration of barium is less injurious. Newer nonionic, water-soluble, iodine-containing agents (Amipaque, Hexabrix, Omnipaque) may eventually replace currently used contrast agents.

Fluoroscopy and radiologic consultation are not always necessary. Allen[1] describes excellent results in a series of 22

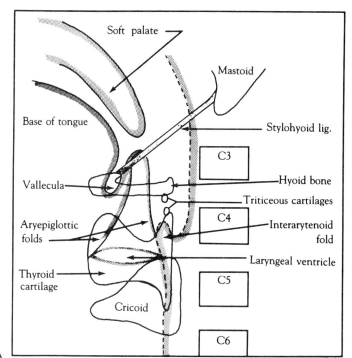

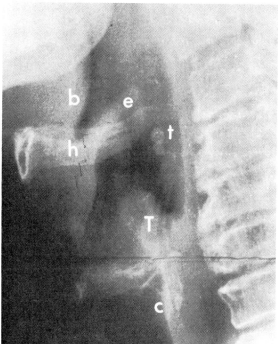

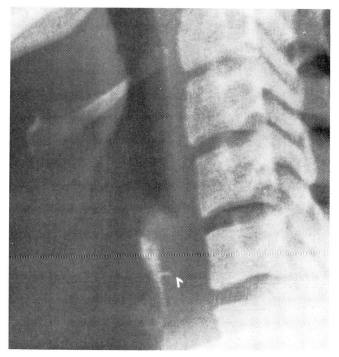

Figure 50–1. *A*, Diagrammatic sketch of a typical soft tissue lateral radiograph of the neck. *B*, Soft tissue lateral radiograph of the neck of an elderly patient with degenerative disc disease and extensive calcification of the neck cartilages. *T*, thyroid cartilage; *t*, triticeous cartilages; *c*, cricoid cartilage; *e*, tip of epiglottis; *h*, hyoid bone; *b*, base of tongue. *C*, The top of the cricoid cartilage is a common area of calcification *(arrowhead)* and should not be confused with a foreign body. (From Hernanz-Schulman M, Naimark A: Avoiding disaster with esophageal foreign bodies. Emergency Medicine Reports. San Francisco, American Health Consultants, 1984.)

patients using barium solutions and spot films. The technique involves asking the patient to swallow the solution and after four to five swallows (approximately 50 ml), frontal, lateral, and perhaps oblique exposures are made. Should total obstruction be suspected despite the absence of an air-fluid level, the patient should be told to ingest only a small amount of barium initially to minimize the risk of aspiration. Positive findings include either positive or negative imaging of the FB in the column of barium and obstruction. In difficult cases, fluoroscopy by a radiologist presumably increases diagnostic accuracy and perhaps precludes the ne-

cessity for further diagnostic evaluation of possible underlying anatomic or motility disorders. Computed tomography is most useful in diagnosing suspected esophageal perforation in which the previously described modalities have been normal or inconclusive.[27, 33] The high resolution of CT may detect small foreign objects not apparent with plain films, barium swallow, or esophagoscopy.[34] Xeroradiography also may have some limited utility in this setting. The technique can identify low-density materials such as aluminum or wood in the cervical esophagus.

In summary, assuming proper patient selection, the

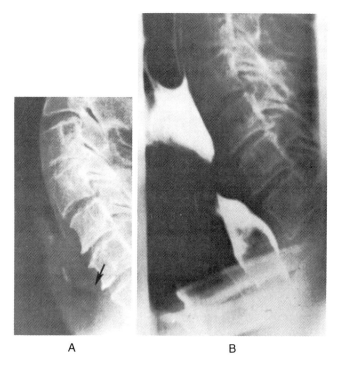

Figure 50–2. Radiographic evolution of an impacted bolus of meat. *A,* The innocuous looking gas density *(arrow)* in the proximal esophagus at the thoracic inlet represents gas around an impacted piece of meat. This is a fortuitous finding. *B,* A barium swallow quickly confirms the diagnosis in the same patient as in *A.* (From Hernanz-Schulman M, Naimark A: Avoiding disaster with esophageal foreign bodies. Emergency Medicine Reports. San Francisco, American Medical Reports, 1984.)

A   B

radiologic diagnosis of esophageal FBs can often be carried out successfully by plain x-rays alone. Contrast esophageal studies can delineate radiolucent objects and define the degree of obstruction. Computed tomography and xeroradiography have limited application in this setting.

ESOPHAGEAL PHARMACOLOGIC MANEUVERS

Unsatisfactory pharmacologic alternatives for removing or resolving esophageal FB impactions include the use of diazepam, meperidine, and atropine.[35] These agents (alone or in combination) have success rates below 10 per cent, no better than observation alone.[4] The pharmacologic alternatives described later (glucagon, nitroglycerin, nifedipine, and gas-forming agents; Table 50–1) are most effective for distal

esophageal food impactions. Most patients with this problem have underlying pathology; a benign fibrotic stricture or Schatzki-type ring is more common than esophagitis with spasm, motility disturbances, or carcinoma.[16]

Glucagon

PHARMACOLOGY

Glucagon is the prototype for the spasmolytic agents.[16, 36, 37] Its use has been advocated for enhancing the passage of esophageal FBs since 1977, and there have been several isolated reports of dramatic relief.[37–40] Glucagon relaxes some esophageal smooth muscle and decreases the LES pressure. It has no effect on the upper third of the esophagus, where

Table 50–1. *Recommended Pharmacologic Therapies for Esophageal Foreign Bodies*

Class and Agents	Site of Action	Dose and Route	Adverse Effects
Spasmolytics			
Glucagon	LES	1–2 mg IV*	Nausea, vomiting, hyperglycemia, hypersensitivity
Nitroglycerin	Body and LES	0.4–0.8 mg SL†	Hypotension, tachycardia or bradycardia
Nifedipine	LES	10 mg SL‡	Hypotension, tachycardia
Gas-forming agents			
Tartaric acid & Sodium bicarbonate	Distal and Proximal	15 ml tartaric acid (18–20 gm/100 ml)§ 15 ml sodium bicarbonate (10 gm/100 ml)§	Vomiting, increased intraesophageal pressure
Carbonated beverage	Distal and Proximal	100 ml PO	Vomiting, increased intraesophageal pressure

*May be repeated once or used in conjunction with nitroglycerin.
†1–2 inches of paste applied under an occlusive dressing may be an alternative.
‡A capsule is punctured, chewed, held in the mouth for 3 minutes, then swallowed.
§Alternatively, dissolve 2 to 3 gm tartaric acid and 2 to 3 gm sodium bicarbonate in 30 ml water.

striated muscle is present and some voluntary control is operative. It only minimally affects the middle third of the esophagus. Peristalsis is not affected by glucagon.

INDICATIONS AND CONTRAINDICATIONS

Glucagon is most useful for meat impactions at the LES that are suspected because of the patient's complaint of pain or "something stuck" in the lower chest or epigastrium. The clinical diagnosis is usually straightforward. Nevertheless, some reports recommend that the FB be localized first by contrast x-rays to establish that the impaction is at the LES and to serve as the baseline study for comparison following glucagon administration.[37] In the case of a classic history and physical examination, most investigators agree that an initial contrast study can be omitted. Glucagon is successful in approximately 30 to 50 per cent of lower esophageal obstructions, although reported case series generally involve small numbers.[37–40] In one study of 19 patients with distal esophageal FBs documented by esophagoscopy, success was noted in 37 per cent.[36] Glucagon is not effective in upper and middle esophageal obstructions, and it is not yet recommended for use in children. Glucagon also is not effective in patients with fixed fibrotic strictures or rings at the GE junction.[16] Glucagon is contraindicated if the patient has an insulinoma, a pheochromocytoma, Zollinger-Ellison syndrome, a hypersensitivity to glucagon, or a sharp esophageal FB.

USE OF GLUCAGON

Some reports recommend a small test dose to check for hypersensitivity to glucagon. The therapeutic dose is 1 to 2 mg intravenously over 1 to 2 minutes in the sitting patient. The patient is given water orally after the injection of glucagon to stimulate normal esophageal peristalsis to help push the food through the relaxed LES into the stomach.[16] Glucagon has a rapid onset of action and a short duration of action. Gastrointestinal smooth muscle relaxes within 45 seconds, and the duration of action is about 25 minutes. If there are no results within 10 to 20 minutes, a second administration of 2 mg may be tried. Some clinicians combine nitroglycerin with glucagon therapy.

COMPLICATIONS

Glucagon is associated with a few minor side effects. If administered too rapidly, glucagon causes nausea and vomiting, so the adult patient must be alert and mobile enough to avoid aspiration. Occasionally the vomiting will dislodge the impacted food bolus. Theoretically, there is a risk of rupture of the obstructed esophagus during induced emesis, so slow injection is preferred.[16] The administration of glucagon is also associated with dizziness, but no fatalities have been reported. Mild elevation of the blood glucose also is common, but it is not of clinical concern.

FURTHER EVALUATION AND THERAPY

If glucagon should fail by lack of symptom relief or absence of resolution of x-ray findings, its use does not preclude another method from being used subsequently. If the patient experiences symptom relief, follow-up contrast x-rays or esophagoscopy at that time or later, depending on the clinical concern for perforation or severe obstruction, should be obtained to rule out coexistent esophageal pathology. Esophageal pathology was demonstrated in all but one such patient in a study of 19 patients.[36]

Nitroglycerin and Nifedipine

PHARMACOLOGY

Both sublingual nitroglycerin and nifedipine have been used in a manner similar to that of glucagon to relieve LES tone to allow the passage of a distal esophageal FB.[41–43] Although these two agents have been used less than glucagon for the treatment of esophageal FBs, both agents are useful for the relief of chest pain associated with esophageal smooth muscle spasm,[42] and may be administered concurrently with glucagon. Manometric and radiographic studies after the administration of nitroglycerin reveal abolition of repetitive high-pressure wave contractions characteristic of esophageal spasm, whereas nifedipine significantly reduces LES pressure without changing contraction amplitudes in the body of the esophagus. Thus nitroglycerin may relieve partial or complete obstruction of the middle or lower esophagus secondary either to intrinsic esophageal disease or to simple FB impaction. However, nifedipine is most likely to succeed when the bolus is lodged at the GE junction.

INDICATIONS AND CONTRAINDICATIONS

As is true for the clinical indications for the use of glucagon, any patient presenting with an impacted esophageal FB, especially a food bolus, may be a candidate for one or both agents. Also similar to the mode of action of glucagon, neither of these agents is expected to relax a fixed fibrotic stricture or ring at the GE junction.[16] Nevertheless, because both agents have a relatively benign side effect profile, if the patient has no contraindication to their use, they may be tried with or without the prior documentation of the distal esophageal obstruction by contrast study. Contraindications to their use include a history of allergic reactions, a sharp esophageal FB, and hypotension.

USE AND COMPLICATIONS

Doses of one to two 0.4-mg sublingual nitroglycerin tablets or 1 to 2 inches of nitroglycerin paste, or one 10 mg of nifedipine (the capsule is punctured, chewed, held in the mouth, then swallowed) have been reported.[41–43] A case report of the administration of one 10-mg dose of sublingual nifedipine to an elderly man with a 3-day history of a distal esophageal FB led to an almost immediate but transient increase in chest pain and pressure followed by the relief of all symptoms. It should be remembered that some patients with esophageal FBs may present with some degree of dehydration due to the inability to swallow liquids or their own saliva. These patients may be prone to hypotension from the vasodilation associated with the use of either agent.

FURTHER EVALUATION AND THERAPY

If treatment is successful, follow-up barium swallow or flexible endoscopy should be performed as mentioned for the use of glucagon. Unsuccessful symptom relief should also be followed up with further study of the distal esophagus.[36] The use of either nitroglycerin or nifedipine does not contraindicate the use of any other method for the treatment of an esophageal FB.[41, 43]

Gas-Forming Agents

PHARMACOLOGY

The use of gas-forming agents for the treatment of distal esophageal food impactions, especially for meat boluses, was first described in 1983.[44] The combination of tartaric acid solution followed immediately by a solution of sodium bicarbonate or even carbonated beverages has been reported. In theory, the use of this acid-base mixture or of a carbonated beverage may produce sufficient carbon dioxide to distend the esophagus, relax the LES, and push impacted food through the GE junction into the stomach.[45, 46] Radiologists use similar gas-forming solutions for upper gastrointestinal contrast studies.[16]

INDICATIONS AND CONTRAINDICATIONS

Gas-forming agents are indicated for the relief of distal esophageal food impactions, with or without prior FB confirmation by a contrast x-ray study. Although gas-forming agents are more likely to work with distal esophageal food impactions, they have also been used successfully in obstructions in the proximal esophagus. One author recommends that this modality be used first when a food bolus impaction is suspected at the GE junction,[16] because a fixed lower esophageal stricture or ring is more common than LES spasm. The concurrent administration of spasmolytic agents may improve the effectiveness of the gas-forming agents, which presumably distend the esophagus and "push" the food into the stomach. In general, nonfood items (especially angulated, abrasive, or sharp FBs) should not be treated with pharmacologic modalities but rather be removed by esophagoscopy.

USE AND COMPLICATIONS

In one study,[44] patients were administered 15 ml of the solution of tartaric acid (18.7 gm/100 ml) followed by 15 ml of a sodium bicarbonate solution (10 gm/100 ml). In this study, Rice and coworkers[44] achieved success in all eight patients. In another study,[45] 1.5 to 3.0 gm of tartaric acid and 2 to 3 gm of sodium bicarbonate were each dissolved in about 15 ml of water. In this study, Zimmers and coworkers[45] observed symptomatic relief in 17 of 26 cases (65 per cent). A study involving the use of carbonated beverages in 28 patients found that eight patients responded to the ingestion of barium sulfate suspension alone and 16 of the remaining 20 patients (or 80 per cent) responded to the ingestion of about 100 ml of a carbonated beverage.[46] Most patients with esophageal FB impactions have been noted to retch after receiving gas-forming agents, which theoretically puts patients with FB impactions at risk for esophageal trauma. The only reported complication with the use of gas-forming agents for this indication was a mucosal tear of the esophagus (requiring surgical exploration to rule out mediastinitis) in a 66-year-old patient with an 18-hour-old esophageal impaction.[45] Because of this complication and the reduced effectiveness in prolonged FB impactions, the investigators recommended that gas-forming agents not be given to patients with impactions of more than 6 hours in duration or to patients with chest pain that might be indicative of an esophageal injury.[45]

FURTHER EVALUATION AND THERAPY

As with the use of glucagon, nitroglycerin, or nifedipine, even if the administration of the gas-forming agent is successful, as judged by the relief of symptoms, further evaluation is necessary for determining the underlying esophageal abnormality that potentially led to the FB impaction. As with the use of the spasmolytic agents, if therapy with gas-forming agents does not relieve the distal esophageal obstruction, the patient remains a candidate for other recommended therapy for the removal of an esophageal FB.

Papain

Papain is *not* a recommended treatment for an esophageal FB. It is a proteolytic enzyme that has been touted for dissolving meat impactions.[47] Papain is available commercially as Adolph's meat tenderizer. This therapy has never been submitted to clinical trial. In vitro studies suggest that the commercial preparation may have no intrinsic proteolytic activity.[48] Although it is harmless when in brief contact with the normal esophagus, if it is left too long in the obstructed esophagus, papain may begin to dissolve the abnormal esophageal mucosa underlying a foreign object.[48, 49] This is likely to occur when the esophageal wall is ischemic due to FB impaction, esophageal injury results from small bony spicules in the FB, or there is an underlying lesion responsible for the obstruction. The subsequent rupture and leakage of the proteolytic enzymes result in a self-perpetuating mediastinitis, which can be followed by great vessel rupture.[45] Patients with esophageal FBs are at increased risk for aspiration; pulmonary aspiration of papain results in acute hemorrhagic pulmonary edema.[46] In general, papain is not currently recommended because of the 2 per cent mortality rate associated with its use and the fact that perforation has occurred in two of 90 cases reported in the literature.

FOLEY CATHETER MANIPULATION OF ESOPHAGEAL FOREIGN BODIES

Introduction

Some esophageal FBs can be safely managed with balloon-tipped catheters (e.g., Foley or Fogarty). Blunt esophageal FBs that are not believed to have resulted in total obstruction, perforation, or other esophageal injury may be amenable to Foley catheter manipulation. The classic patient for this technique is a small child who is brought to the hospital shortly after swallowing a coin. FB extraction or dislodgment into the stomach with this technique are both therapeutic. An 80 per cent or better success rate is expected.[2, 4, 10, 50, 51] No deaths or serious complications have been reported. Emergency physicians, radiologists, otolaryngologists, and surgeons have all described this technique.[10, 50–61] In McGuirt's survey of otolaryngologists, thoracic surgeons, pediatric radiologists, and pediatric surgeons,[37] 50 per cent of the pediatric specialists stated that they use the technique. However, few of the otolaryngologists and thoracic surgeons used this technique, instead preferring endoscopy.[57] Fluoroscopic assistance may be preferable, but it is not essential. Whether the procedure is performed in the emergency department or the radiology department, equipment and personnel capable of emergency pediatric airway management must be present.

Background

In 1966, Bigler[60] first described the use of a Foley catheter for esophageal FB extraction. In 1972, Henry and Chamberlain[62] reported that 14 of 16 children were successfully treated with this technique. Campbell and Foley[53] reported a series of 100 children in which 91 FBs were extracted and seven were dislodged into the stomach. No complications were reported. Nixon[59] reported the successful use of this technique in 12 of 15 patients with radiolucent FBs. The literature abounds with other reports of successful Foley catheter extractions.[51–62]

Indications and Contraindications

It is important that the patient be able to cooperate for the procedure. Some researchers believe that the presence of an uncooperative patient precludes the use of a Foley catheter.[35] Many investigators use various combinations of topical anesthesia and parenteral sedation.[54, 58] Others report restraining children but not sedating them.[10, 51, 56, 61–63]

Recently ingested smooth, blunt objects that are radiographically opaque are the only FBs suited for balloon catheter extraction. Coins are physically amenable to Foley manipulation, and their frequent presentation has resulted in numerous successful reports.[4, 50, 51, 61, 62] Food boluses have also been extracted successfully,[55, 59] as have button batteries.[63] Even patients with preexisting esophageal disease have been treated with Foley catheter manipulation.[59] Recently ingested FBs carry little likelihood of causing pressure necrosis, perforation, or other significant injury. Recommendations for the maximum duration of impaction before treatment range from 24 hours to 2 weeks with inert objects,[4, 52, 53, 64] although most reports cite 48 to 72 hours as the upper limit.[5, 57, 65] However, potentially reactive FBs such as button batteries have caused second-degree mucosal burns in as few as 4 hours[66] and esophageal perforations in less than 24 hours.[15] Animal studies have shown mucosal burns occurring within 1 hour and transmural penetration occurring in as little as 4 hours with button batteries.[15] Sharp or irregular objects with rough edges have not been managed with the balloon catheter technique because esophageal perforation or laceration can result and the balloon may burst during the procedure.

Radiographically opaque objects are most easily located by plain film radiograph. Radiolucent objects can be manipulated,[59] but uncertainties about location mandate contrast esophagograms. Fluoroscopy can be very helpful, and some believe the procedure should not be performed without it.[53, 58, 62] Conversely, many practitioners describe manipulation by traction and tactile stimulation alone.[54, 61, 65] Given the theoretic concern of airway obstruction, it is imperative to perform the procedure with airway equipment and suction available.

Contraindications to catheter removal of esophageal FBs include total esophageal obstruction as manifested by an airfluid level on plain x-ray or by contrast esophagography. The presence of a total obstruction prevents passage of the catheter tip distal to the foreign object. Esophageal perforation as recognized by the usual symptoms and signs of perforation requires immediate surgical consultation and precludes any blind esophageal manipulation. Sharp, irregularly shaped FBs, or those impacted for more than a few hours, should also not be removed with this technique.

Equipment

The equipment necessary is basic and present in most emergency departments (Table 50–2). Although never reported, airway obstruction during the procedure is the most feared potential complication. Thus the proper equipment and personnel capable of managing airway obstruction must

Table 50–2. Equipment for Foley Catheter Extraction of Esophageal Foreign Bodies

Standard resuscitation equipment for advanced
    airway management of children and adults
Foley catheters (10 to 16 French)
*Topical anesthetics
*Parenteral sedatives
*Child restraint device
*Fluoroscope

*Optional equipment

be present, including suction devices. Clamps and forceps (bayonet and Magill) of various sizes should be available to extract the foreign object from the pharynx. Foley catheters ranging in size from 8 French with 3-ml balloons to 26 French with 30-ml balloons have been used.[51, 66] In settings in which both children and adults may be treated, sizes ranging from 10 French to 16 French with 5- to 10-ml balloons should suffice. Child restraint devices (e.g., "papoose board"), topical anesthetics, and parenteral sedation may be used.

Procedure

Every patient should be appropriately coached concerning the procedure and cooperation. Young children must be gently restrained. Light sedation and nasopharyngeal topical anesthesia may be used, although some would argue that the use of topical anesthesia and parenteral sedation depresses physiologic airway reflexes and increases the risk of aspiration.[61] The patient is then placed in a head-down, lateral decubitus or prone position while preparations are made to manage potential complications.

Assuming the procedure is being performed in a young child, a 12 French Foley catheter may be the correct choice. After checking for symmetric balloon inflation, the catheter is most frequently inserted through the nose for patient comfort (Fig. 50–3). Some reports[53] argue that oral insertion is preferred to allow removal of the inflated catheter and foreign object with one smooth, uninterrupted pass. When using fluoroscopy, the catheter is visually passed distal to the FB. If performed without fluoroscopy, the distance from nose or mouth to foreign object is estimated, and the catheter is inserted accordingly. On occasion, the operator feels the catheter tip pass the object. The balloon is slowly filled with saline solution or contrast agent. Balloon inflation should be stopped if the patient complains of increased pain; the catheter should be repositioned before an attempt at reinflation. Fluid is preferable to air as it is less compressible. The catheter is then withdrawn with steady, gentle traction. Contact with the object can be sensed as the friction of withdrawal increases. Significant impedance to traction requires termination of the attempt. Should the catheter slide by the object without dislodging it, the balloon can be enlarged and another attempt made. Often when the object reaches the hypopharynx, the balloon and gravity act in concert to fully externalize the FB, especially if the patient can be instructed to spit it out. The operator can also grasp the object with the fingers, forceps, or a clamp.

A follow-up x-ray may be necessary to exclude the possibility of multiple objects.[56] If fluoroscopy is not used and no foreign object is retrieved, another x-ray should be obtained, because 10 to 20 per cent of the time, the foreign object will pass distally into the stomach.[10] This is considered therapeutic, because once a blunt FB has traversed the esophagus, only rarely will the FB not eventually pass per rectum. Such an occurrence has only been noted with objects longer than 6 to 7 cm. Multiple attempts should not be required if catheter size, placement, and balloon inflation are correct. Failed attempts are best followed by a change in one of the aforementioned parameters or repeat x-ray studies to confirm continued presence of the esophageal FB before esophagoscopy.

Complications

No deaths or serious complications have been reported. Nosebleeds, nasopharyngeal displacement with impaction,

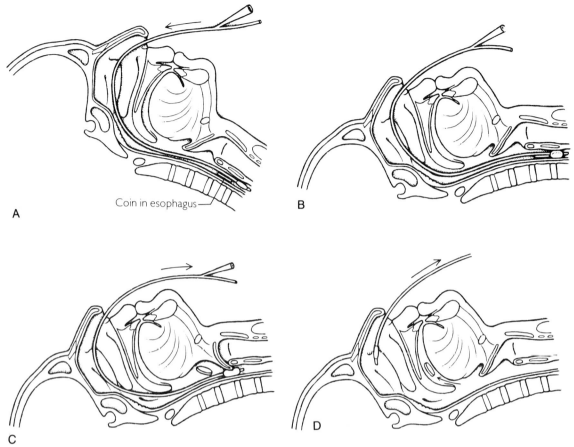

Figure 50–3. Technique of Foley catheter extraction. In children, this procedure is best done with the patient restrained on a papoose board and in the *prone* position. *A,* A catheter is inserted through the nose into the esophagus distal to the coin. *B,* The balloon is inflated. Gentle traction moves the coin proximally through the esophagus. *C,* The coin is moved steadily past the glottis. *D,* The coin is present in the mouth to be expectorated or grabbed. (From McSwain N: Esophageal foreign body. Emerg Med 21:85, 1989.)

and a case of laryngospasm have been described.[57] Failure to move the object at all can be estimated to occur in approximately 15 to 20 per cent of cases.[51, 57, 61, 62] Endoscopists who object to this technique argue that an underlying disease or multiple FBs may be missed; blind manipulation may perforate the esophagus; radiation exposure is prolonged when fluoroscopy is used; and airway obstruction can occur. Although this technique has never been studied with a large, prospective series of patients or with direct comparison with esophagoscopy, none of these objections has been supported in fact.

Disposition

If the extraction was successful or if the foreign object is now in the stomach, the patient may be discharged. If the FB is in the stomach, clinical follow-up (checking the stools) should be adequate to verify movement of gastric FBs through the alimentary tract. Follow-up plain x-ray films are indicated after a reasonable period of time (e.g., 4 to 7 days, or sooner if symptoms ensue) if passage is not documented. Discharge instructions should include warnings about gastrointestinal obstruction, perforation, and hemorrhage. Parents of children who swallow coins can be instructed to watch for "any change in stools." Adults with esophageal FBs that have been removed successfully must be referred for evaluation of possible esophageal pathology. Should an FB

remain lodged in the esophagus, immediate referral to an endoscopist is necessary.

NASOGASTRIC TUBES

Several case reports describe the use of nasogastric (NG) tubes to manage esophageal FBs. Before insertion, the NG tube must be modified by cutting off the end of the tube at the level of the last side hole to allow maximal negative (suction) pressure to be exerted at the tube-FB interface. The initial technique is to place the tip of the catheter just proximal to a totally obstructing object (e.g., a food bolus) to aspirate oropharyngeal secretions. Then maximal suction may be applied directly to the esophageal FB itself in an attempt to lift it out proximally. Other modifications of this technique include the use of larger bore NG tubes or magnets and the insufflation of air above the FB. Although gentle pushing of the FB through the GE junction is a tempting procedure to consider, to prevent esophageal injuries, the technique of blindly pushing an impacted FB distally is strongly discouraged. This technique may be appropriate if performed under direct visualization during endoscopy (see later discussion).

Henry and Chamberlain[62] described the case of a steel ball obstructing the pylorus that was lifted into the esophagus with an NG tube and magnet after which it was removed with a Foley catheter. Jaffe[67] used a similar method to remove button batteries from the stomachs of six patients. The batteries could not be extracted beyond the cricopharyngeus, and Foley catheters were used for ultimate removal. Chaikhouni and colleagues[4] reported a patient who had a needle removed from the lower esophagus under fluoroscopy with an NG tube and a magnet. Kozarek[68] described the use of a 34 French gastric evacuation tube and a syringe to successfully aspirate a meat bolus. Zalev[69] used air insufflation just above a meat impaction to negotiate the esophageal FB through the GE junction in one patient. Binder[2] described one patient whose dysphagia resolved after NG intubation. In summary, NG tubes may have limited usefulness in treating esophageal FBs.

ESOPHAGOSCOPY

Esophagoscopy is the definitive diagnostic and therapeutic procedure for impacted esophageal FBs.[17] With esophagoscopy the physician can document the presence and location of the FB along with any underlying lesion, then remove the object and reevaluate the esophagus after FB removal to rule out perforation or underlying pathology. Although it is not a procedure performed by the emergency physician, its proper role must be understood by the emergency physician (Table 50–3). Esophagoscopy may be necessary even if a radiologic contrast study does not reveal complete obstruction, because x-ray studies are not always conclusive.[70, 71] Esophagoscopy may be necessary to rule out predisposing pathology or resultant perforation even if the symptoms presumed to be due to an esophageal FB resolve.

Indications and Contraindications

Endoscopy is the preferred method for removal of sharp or pointed objects, such as bones, open safety pins, and razors.[70, 71] However, sharp, pointed FBs may require surgery. Toothpicks and bones require surgery more often than nails, needles, pins, blades, and dental prostheses.[70] In the case of sharp objects prone to causing esophageal perforation, intravenous antibiotics should be administered before any removal procedure. It is important to regard button batteries impacted in the esophagus as a true emergency due to their potential to cause perforation secondary to liquefaction necrosis.[15, 63, 67] Once button batteries pass the stomach, surgery may be necessary if serial x-rays indicate that the batteries do not continue to move or if they become symptomatic. In terms of the most common esophageal FBs, coins can cause pressure necrosis and perforate with prolonged impaction. Meat impactions may pass overnight so endoscopy need not be performed immediately in these patients, although it would be necessary eventually to rule out esophageal pathology.

Equipment

The flexible endoscope is now more commonly used than the rigid esophagoscope for several reasons.[17] There are more gastroenterologists and others trained in the use of the flexible endoscope than in the use of the rigid endoscope. The latter remains the tool of surgeons, especially otolaryngologists and thoracic surgeons. Flexible esophagoscopy is easier to use and more mobile, and has magnified visibility. Flexible endoscopic procedures are usually performed without general anesthesia, even in most children.[72] Because of this fact, Webb argued that flexible endoscopy is more cost effective compared with either rigid endoscopy or surgery.[17]

Rigid endoscopy is still favored by some clinicians, because it is superior to flexible endoscopy in containing and removing esophageal FBs.[17] Despite the advantages discussed, some reports contend that flexible endoscopy too often fails to remove the FB. Instead, the FB may become impacted, making subsequent extraction with the rigid endoscope more difficult or impossible. The main danger of flexible endoscopy that is not associated with the use of rigid endoscopy is the accidental loss of the FB into the airway during extraction in the unintubated patient. The requirement for general anesthesia and airway protection is both the main advantage and drawback to rigid endoscopy.

Procedure

Before undertaking the procedure, a "dry run" should first be practiced with a similar foreign object outside the patient. Technology enhances the success of esophagoscopy, including the use of grasping forceps, snares, balloons, and dilators.[73] Overtubes or rubber hoods serve two purposes[73, 74]: to protect the esophageal wall from injury as the

Table 50–3. *Comparison of Rigid and Flexible Esophagoscopy and Laryngoscopy for Esophageal Foreign Bodies (FBs)*

	Flexible Endoscopy	Rigid Endoscopy	Laryngoscopy
Indication	Upper GI tract FB	Esophageal FB	Upper airway FB
Consultant	Gastroenterologist	Otolaryngologist Thoracic surgeon	Otolaryngologist Anesthesiologist Emergency physician
Advantages	Diagnostic Usually effective More available Local anesthesia	Diagnostic Most effective General anesthesia Airway protected	Diagnostic Usually effective Most available Local anesthesia Airway management

Disadvantages	Requires patient
	  cooperation
	Airway unprotected
		Requires general
		  anesthesia
			Requires patient
			  cooperation

Perforation	<0.1%	0.5%	?
Mortality	?	<0.05%*	?

*Mortality is primarily related to the risk of general anesthesia.

object is withdrawn and to prevent the object from being pulled off by the higher pressures present in the upper esophagus. Techniques also enhance the success of esophagoscopy. To prevent the aspiration of the foreign object during removal with a flexible endoscope, the patient should be in the Trendelenburg position, and the object should be removed from the oropharynx with bayonet forceps during exhalation. Meat can be gently pushed through the GE junction with the flexible endoscope after visualization distally to rule out an obstructive lesion or even after dilation of a distal stricture.[70] After the extraction, if the endoscopist is unable to rule out underlying pathology and if the risk of perforation seems negligible, most patients should have a follow-up x-ray contrast study to rule out extrinsic compression.

LARYNGOSCOPY

Immediate laryngoscopy may be necessary in the case of the only immediately life-threatening emergency associated with FB ingestions or aspirations: the "cafe coronary."[70] Diagnostic laryngoscopy may be necessary to visualize objects in the pharynx, hypopharynx, or at the level of the glottis or below. The patient is usually accurate in pointing to the side and to the level of the FB, especially with objects best seen with laryngoscopy rather than with esophagoscopy. The objects are almost always anterior to the epiglottis at the base of the tongue or in the area of the tonsillar pillars.[10, 13, 22, 23, 75] The FB is usually a bone, which can often be felt with the gloved finger. Unfortunately, not all bones are visualized on x-ray, either because they are cartilaginous (fish) or too small (chicken). At times there is no foreign object remaining, but only a residual abrasion causing the sensation of FB.

FBs visible during indirect or direct laryngoscopy can usually be removed with Magill forceps or Kelly clamps. Sedation may be required, but general anesthesia is only necessary if the initial procedure fails to remove the object. In this case, an otolaryngologist should be consulted. If a hypopharyngeal FB is removed, the patient should be told to expect the residual sensation of an FB to last 1 or 2 days and that there may be some expectorated blood. The patient should be told to return immediately if fever, shortness of breath, or progressive pain in the neck or the chest ensue.

Complications of Esophagoscopy and Laryngoscopy

Laryngoscopy and esophagoscopy are not without risk. Complications related to the presence of a hypopharyngeal or esophageal FB or its removal include trauma to the upper airway or the glottic region and the esophagus, including perforation into the mediastinum or retropharyngeal region.[1–14, 17] General anesthesia carries a mortality rate of one out of 10,000 anesthetic procedures and a morbidity rate of almost 0.5 per cent.[76] Rigid esophagoscopy causes perforation in less than 0.5 per cent of cases and death in about 0.05 per cent.[14, 17] Flexible esophagoscopy is associated with perforation in less than 0.1 per cent,[17] and it is safer than rigid esophagoscopy in the hands of the average physician.

Esophageal perforation should be suspected after a difficult extraction in which the endoscopist used force to overcome resistance or pushed the FB distally. Perforation also is more likely following the prolonged presence of any FB, but especially with a button battery or one that is sharp or pointed.[15] Signs and symptoms of a perforation can include fever, tachycardia, dyspnea, chest pain, abdominal pain, neck crepitation, or subcutaneous emphysema.[14] Postprocedure x-ray studies may be helpful in looking for perforation. Soft tissue lateral views of the neck and a chest x-ray may reveal air dissecting through neck soft tissue planes or mediastinal air, respectively. Contrast studies may be necessary to pinpoint the site of perforation, although careful esophagoscopy may be preferable to visualize the extent of the trauma to the esophagus. Outcome is optimized by early diagnosis and prompt surgical repair.

SPECIAL SITUATIONS

Fish Bones in the Throat

It is common to evaluate patients who complain of sharp pain in the throat on swallowing after they have eaten fish. This symptom is perceived by the patient as evidence of a fish bone lodged in the throat.

Because an impacted fish bone can produce serious sequelae if not removed, efforts should be undertaken in the emergency department to diagnose and treat retained bones. It is important to note that a bone is identified in only 20 to 30 per cent of such patients, and symptoms may be due to minor mucosal trauma (abrasion, laceration) simulating the retained foreign body.

A plain radiograph (soft tissue technique, lateral neck projection) may identify some bones in the throat. However, this technique is unreliable in ruling out retained bones, because many commonly eaten fish (e.g., mackerel, trout, salmon) have a radiolucent skeleton.[77] Other radiographic techniques, such as swallowing a contrast-laden cotton ball, are also unreliable in identifying small bones. Although endoscopy is the most accurate method to diagnose a retained fish bone, simply looking in the mouth and pharynx with the use of a tongue blade may identify the majority of impacted bones. Knight and Lesser reported a series of 71 patients who complained of the sensation of a fish bone in the throat and noted that in 56 cases (79 per cent) no bone was ultimately identified after careful follow-up.[78] Of significance, 14 of the 15 retained fish bones (93 per cent) were visible on the initial examination of the oropharynx or hypopharynx. Most commonly the bones were found lodged in the base of the tongue, tonsil, or posterior pharyngeal wall. All were easily removed under direct vision. Saliva strands may mimic or obscure a bone, so care should be taken when extracting possible retained fish bones.

Although any patient persistently complaining of a retained fish bone ultimately should be referred for endoscopy (usually within 48 hours), many patients with the annoying symptoms do not have an esophageal foreign body. If a fish bone is present, however, many may be diagnosed and removed on the initial visit if one merely looks in the mouth and throat with a good light source and a tongue blade or with indirect laryngoscopy. Local anesthetic sprays may aid in the evaluation and removal of a bone or for temporary relief of dysphagia. If a fish bone is not identified, and the patient has no subcutaneous emphysema, soft tissue swelling, hemoptysis, or inability to swallow, referral for follow-up within 24 to 48 hours is acceptable. Note that retained fish bones do not "dissolve" and rarely pass spontaneously once lodged in the mucosa.

Button Battery Ingestion

Small disc batteries, such as those used in cameras, watches, and hearing aids, present a distinct type of esophageal FB because of the potential for serious morbidity and mortality.[79] Batteries range in size from 7 to 25 mm and are

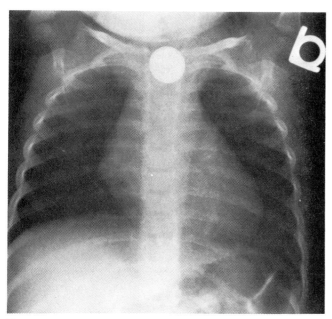

Figure 50–4. Note the battery in the upper esophagus with a typical "double contour." This object may be mistaken for an ingested coin, but the difference is important to note because of the need to remove the battery immediately. (From Kost KM, Shapiro RS: Button battery ingestion: A case report and review of the literature. J Otolaryngol 16:4, 1987.)

radiopaque. Batteries appear as round densities, similar to an impacted coin, but some batteries may demonstrate a "double contour" configuration (Fig. 50–4). The devices consist of two metal plates joined by a plastic seal. Internally the batteries consist of an electrolyte solution (usually concentrated sodium or potassium hydroxide) and a heavy metal, such as mercuric oxide, silver oxide, zinc, or lithium.

If ingested, these batteries often lodge in the esophagus. The mechanisms of injury include electrolyte leakage, injury from an electrical current, heavy metal toxicity, and pressure necrosis. Of particular concern is the development of a corrosive esophagitis (occasionally fatal), or esophageal stricture or perforation due to caustic injury and prolonged mucosal pressure. Although relatively harmless in the stomach and intestines, batteries lodged in the esophagus should be considered an emergency situation, because even new batteries demonstrate corrosion, leakage, and mucosal necrosis within a few hours of contact with the esophagus.

Esophageal impaction mandates immediate removal. The Foley catheter technique may be successful, but it is less ideal than endoscopy. Endoscopy allows for direct esophageal evaluation and a more controlled extraction. In addition, the "invasive" nature of batteries may lead to rapid edema, making the catheter technique technically more difficult. Glucagon or gas-forming agents have no role in the extraction of button batteries. It is particularly dangerous to delay treatment in hopes that the FB will "pass spontaneously." However, when in the stomach, batteries are followed clinically or radiographically, and there seems to be only a theoretic risk of heavy metal poisoning even if the battery disintegrates. Some advise cathartics or metoclopramide (Reglan) if the battery is in the stomach. Ipecac is best avoided.

CONCLUSION

Esophageal FBs should be approached with great clinical respect because their potential to produce serious injury or death is

well recognized. Esophageal FBs can be difficult to diagnose (e.g., in children and impaired adults), difficult to locate (e.g., radiolucent or asymptomatic), and difficult to remove (e.g., requiring the services of radiology and specialty consultation).

REFERENCES

1. Allen T: Suspected esophageal foreign body: Choosing appropriate management. JACEP 8:101, 1979.
2. Binder L: Pediatric gastrointestinal foreign body ingestions. Ann Emerg Med 13:112, 1984.
3. Bloom R, Nakano P, Gray S, Skandalakis J: Foreign bodies of the gastrointestinal tract. Am Surg 52:618, 1986.
4. Chaikhouni A, Kratz J, Crawford F: Foreign bodies of the esophagus. Am Surg 51:173, 1985.
5. Fajolu O, Nigeria L: Foreign body impaction in the esophagus: A review of ten years' experience in a teaching hospital. J Nat Med Assoc 78:987, 1986.
6. Giordano A, Adams G, Boies L, Meyerhoff W: Current management of esophageal foreign bodies. Arch Otolaryngol 107:249, 1981.
7. Keszler P, Buzna E: Surgical conservative management of esophageal perforation. Chest 80:158, 1981.
8. Maitra A: Casualty experience of swallowed foreign body. Br J Clin Pract 15, 1980.
9. Nandi P, Ong G: Foreign body in the oesophagus: Review of 2394 cases. Br J Surg 65:5, 1978.
10. O'Neill J, Holcomb G, Neblett W: Management of tracheobronchial and esophageal foreign bodies in childhood. J Pediatr Surg 18:475, 1983.
11. Phillipps J, Patel P: Swallowed foreign bodies. J Laryngol Otol 102:235, 1988.
12. Selivanov V, Sheldon G, Cello J, Crass R: Management of foreign body ingestion. Ann Surg 199:187, 1984.
13. Blazer S, Naveh Y, Friedman A: Foreign body in the airway. Am J Dis Child 134:68, 1980.
14. Elleson D, Rowley S: Esophageal perforation: Its early diagnosis and treatment. Laryngoscope 92:678, 1982.
15. Maves M, Carithers J, Birck H: Esophageal burns secondary to disc battery ingestion. Ann Otol Rhinol Laryngol 93:364, 1984.
16. Friedland G: The treatment of acute esophageal food impaction. Radiology 149:601, 1983.
17. Webb WA: Management of foreign bodies of the upper gastrointestinal tract. Gastroenterology 94:204, 1988.
18. Jackson C, Jackson CL: Diseases of the Air and Food Passages of Foreign Body Origin. Philadelphia, WB Saunders Co, 1937.
19. Richardson JR: A new treatment for esophageal obstruction due to meat impaction. Ann Otol Rhinol Laryngol 54:328, 1945.
20. Bigler FC: The use of a Foley catheter for removal of blunt foreign bodies from the esophagus. J Thorac Cardiovasc Surg 51:759, 1966.
21. Haglund S, Haverling M, Kuylenstierna R, Lind MG: Radiographic diagnosis of foreign bodies in the esophagus. J Laryngol Otol 92:1117, 1978.
22. Cohen SR: Unusual presentations and problems created by mismanagement of foreign bodies in the aerodigestive tract of the pediatric patient. Ann Otol Rhinol Laryngol 90:316, 1981.
23. Banks W, Potsic WP: Unsuspected foreign bodies of the aerodigestive tract. Ann Otol Rhinol Laryngol 87:515, 1978.
24. Smith P, Swischuk L, Fagan C: An elusive and often unsuspected cause of stridor or pneumonia (the esophageal foreign body). Am J Roentgenol 122:80, 1974.
25. Handler S, Beaugard M, Canalis R, Fee W: Unsuspected esophageal foreign bodies in adults with upper airway obstruction. Chest 80:234, 1981.
26. Newman D: The radiolucent foreign body: An often forgotten cause of respiratory symptoms. J Pediatr 92:60, 1978.
27. Savitt D, Wason S: Delayed diagnosis of coin ingestion in children. Am J Emerg Med 6:378, 1988.
28. Boothroyd AE, Carty H, Robson W: "Hunt the thimble": A study of the radiology of ingested foreign bodies. Arch Emerg Med 4:33, 1987.
29. Zeligman B: Radiology of the hypopharynx and esophagus. Ear Nose Throat J 63:22, 1984.
30. Dodds W, Stewart E, Vlymen W: Appropriate contrast media for evaluation of esophageal disruption. Radiology 144:439, 1982.
31. Hupscher D: Technique of examination of the esophagus. Diagn Imaging Clin Med 55:241, 1986.
32. Ginai A, ten Kate F, ten Berg R, Hoornstra K: Experimental evaluation of various available contrast agents for use in the upper gastro-intestinal tract in cases of suspected leakage: Effects on lungs. Br J Radiol 57:896, 1984.
33. Endicott J, Molony T, Campbell G, Bartels L: Esophageal perforations: The role of computerized tomography in diagnosis and management decisions. Laryngoscope 96:751, 1986.
34. Gamba J, Heaston DK, Ling D, Korobkin M: CT diagnosis of an esophageal foreign body. Am J Radiol 140:289, 1983.
35. Taylor R: Esophageal foreign bodies. Emerg Med Clin North Am 5:301, 1987.

36. Trenkner S, Maglinte D, Lehman G, et al: Esophageal food impaction: Treatment with glucagon. Radiology 149:401, 1983.
37. Ferrucci J, Long J: Radiologic treatment of esophageal food impaction using intravenous glucagon. Radiology 125:25, 1977.
38. Marks H, Lousteau R: Glucagon and esophageal meat impaction. Arch Otolaryngol 105:367, 1979.
39. Glauser J, Lilja P, Greenfeld B, Ruiz E: Intravenous glucagon in the management of esophageal food obstruction. JACEP 8:228, 1979.
40. Handal K, Riordan W, Siese J: The lower esophagus and glucagon. Ann Emerg Med 9:577, 1980.
41. Gibson MS: Nitroglycerin use in esophageal disorders (letter). Ann Emerg Med 9:280, 1980.
42. Goldberg GJ: Emergency department treatment of esophageal obstruction (letter). Ann Emerg Med 9:280, 1980.
43. Bell AF, Eibling DE: Nifedipine in the treatment of distal esophageal food impaction (letter). Arch Otolaryngol Head Neck Surg 114:682, 1988.
44. Rice B, Spiegel P, Dombrowski P: Acute esophageal food impaction treated by gas forming agents. Radiology 146:299, 1983.
45. Zimmers T, Chan SB, Kouchoukos PL, et al: Use of gas forming agents in esophageal food impactions. Ann Emerg Med 17:693, 1988.
46. Mohammed S, Hegedus V: Dislodgement of impacted oesophageal foreign bodies with carbonated beverages. Clin Radiol 37:589, 1986.
47. Cavo J, Koops H, Gryboski R: Use of enzymes for meat impactions in the esophagus. Laryngoscope 87:630, 1977.
48. Goldner F, Danley D: Enzymatic digestion of esophageal meat impaction: A study of Adolph's meat tenderizer. Dig Dis Sci 30:456, 1985.
49. Hall M, Huseby J: Hemorrhagic pulmonary edema associated with meat tenderizer treatment for esophageal meat impaction. Chest 94:640, 1988.
50. Nixon GW: Foley catheter method of esophageal foreign body removal: Expansion of applications. Am J Roentgenol 132:441, 1979.
51. Rubin S, Mueller D: Removal of esophageal foreign bodies with a Foley balloon catheter under fluoroscopic control. Can Med Assoc J 137:125, 1987.
52. Alexander A: Catheter removal of esophageal foreign bodies: Push or pull? Am J Roentgenol 151:835, 1988.
53. Campbell J, Foley C: A safe alternative to endoscopic removal of blunt esophageal foreign bodies. Arch Otolaryngol 109:323, 1983.
54. Dunlap L: Removal of an esophageal foreign body using a Foley catheter. Ann Emerg Med 10:101, 1981.
55. Ginaldi S: Removal of esophageal foreign bodies using a Foley catheter in adults. Am J Emerg Med 3:64, 1985.
56. Mariani P, Wagner DK: Foley catheter extraction of blunt esophageal foreign bodies. J Emerg Med 4:301, 1986.
57. McGuirt W: Use of a Foley catheter for removal of esophageal foreign bodies: A survey. Ann Otol Rhinol Laryngol 91:599, 1982.
58. McSwain N: Esophageal foreign body. Emerg Med 85, 1989.
59. Nixon G: Foley catheter method of esophageal foreign body removal: Extension of applications. Am J Roentgenol 132:441, 1979.
60. Bigler F: The use of a Foley catheter for removal of blunt foreign objects from esophagus. J Thorac Cardiovasc Surg 51:759, 1966.
61. Ong T: Removal of blunt oesophageal foreign bodies in children using a Foley catheter. Aust Pediatr J 18:60, 1982.
62. Henry L, Chamberlain JW: Removal of foreign bodies from esophagus and nose with the use of a Foley catheter. Surgery 71:918, 1972.
63. Rumack B, Rumack C: Disk battery ingestion. JAMA 249:2509, 1983.
64. Binder L: Esophageal foreign body extraction. Am J Emerg Med 3:371, 1985.
65. Jona J, Glicklich M, Cohen R: The contraindications for blind esophageal bouginage for coin ingestion in children. J Pediatr Surg 23:328, 1988.
66. Jones P: Oesophageal bolus extraction by balloon catheter. Br Med J 1(6116):819, 1978.
67. Jaffe R: Fluoroscopic removal of ingested alkaline batteries. Radiology 150:585, 1984.
68. Kozarek R: Esophageal food impaction: Description of a new method for bolus removal. Dig Dis Sci 25:100, 1980.
69. Zalev A: Radiologic treatment of a patient with the "Steakhouse Syndrome": Case report. J Can Assoc Radiol 39:59, 1988.
70. Webb W, McDaniel L, Jones L: Foreign bodies of the upper gastrointestinal tract: Current management. South Med J 77:1083, 1984.
71. Ricote G, Torre LR, De Ayala VP, et al: Fiberendoscopic removal of foreign bodies of the upper part of the gastrointestinal tract. Surg Gynecol Obstet 160:499, 1985.
72. Bending D: Removal of blunt esophageal foreign bodies by flexible endoscopy without general anesthesia. Am J Dis Child 140:789, 1986.
73. Brady P, Johnson W: Removal of foreign bodies: The flexible fiberoptic endoscope. South Med J 70:702, 1977.
74. Rogers G: An improved overtube for therapeutic peroral endoscopy. Gastrointest Endosc 33:374, 1987.
75. Cohen S, Geller K: Anesthesia and pediatric endoscopy: The surgeon's view. Otol Clin North Am 14:705, 1981.
76. Davies JM: Anesthesia in 1984: How safe is it? Can Med Assoc J 131:678, 1982.
77. Carr AJ: Radiology of fish bone foreign bodies in the neck. J Laryngol Otol 101:407, 1987.
78. Knight LC, Lesser THJ: Fish bones in the throat. Arch Emerg Med 6:13, 1989.
79. Kost KM, Shapiro RS: Button battery ingestion: A case report and review of the literature. J Otolaryngol 16:4, 1987.

Chapter **51**

Nasogastric Intubation

Jonathan M. Glauser

INTRODUCTION

The first written account of the use of a stomach tube appeared in a 1790 publication by John Hunter, in which he described the use of a fresh eel skin stretched over a whalebone to feed a patient with paralysis of deglutition. In 1813, a Philadelphia surgeon named Physick described gastric lavage by means of a urethral catheter used to treat a case of morphine poisoning.[1]

In this century, stomach tubes were originally used to treat postoperative ileus and secondary gastric distention. When a patient vomited or when the stomach became distended, a large stomach tube with a metal basket was passed through the mouth, the stomach contents were aspirated, and the tube was then removed. Nasogastric tubes of modern design were first used in the 1920s. In 1921, Dr. Levin described the tube that bears his name, and in 1924 Dr. Matas

introduced the concept of prophylactic nasogastric drainage in prevention of postoperative distention. Paine and Wangensteen popularized this concept in the 1930s.[2] By the mid-1930s, postoperative mortality and morbidity related to gastric distention and perforation were greatly reduced.[3] In 1934, Miller and Abbott introduced the long balloon-tipped intestinal tube that bears their names. The length of the tube made a suction apparatus mandatory. Subsequently, the concept of suction drainage in prevention of gastric distention became widespread.

The first nasogastric tubes were made of soft rubber. More recently, devices made of Silastic and polyethylene compounds have been shown to elicit less of an inflammatory tissue reaction than do soft rubber tubes.[3] Other than the aforementioned change in tube composition from rubber to plastics, little change occurred in the methods of use or design of gastrointestinal suction equipment until the 1960s.

In the early 1960s, manufacturing advances facilitated development of a double-lumen sump tube. The theoretic advantages of this type of tube were the prevention of the gastric mucosal damage and flow blockage that were seen with single-lumen tubes. Today, the two prototypes of nasogastric tubes are the double-lumen Salem sump tube and the single-lumen Levin tube.[2]

TUBE DESIGN

The Levin tube and the Salem sump tube are different in certain fundamental respects (Fig. 51–1). The Levin tube is a single-lumen tube and is not radiopaque. The Salem

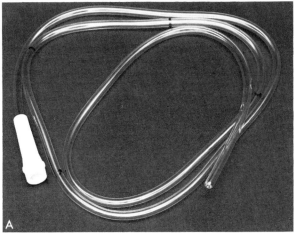

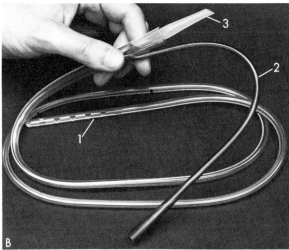

Figure 51–1. A, Standard Levin tube. This tube has a single lumen and is best used for instilling material into the stomach and for diagnostic stomach aspiration. *B,* Salem sump tube. This double-lumen tube is preferred for continuous gastric suction. *1,* Gastric end with suction eyes. *2,* Pigtail extension of the air vent lumen. *3,* "5-in-1" connector.

sump tube is a radiopaque double-lumen tube. In addition to the drainage lumen, it contains a smaller secondary tube that is open to the atmosphere and permits continuous airflow when suction is applied (Fig. 51–2). The Levin tube is adequate for instillation of material into the stomach or for diagnostic aspiration. When continual suction or lavage is desired, the Salem sump tube is preferred.

Both tubes have multiple drainage openings, or eyes, at the distal gastric end. Each tube also has graduated markings so that the length of insertion can be measured.[4] The single lumen of the Levin tube is smaller than the double lumen of the Salem sump. The latter has a blue "pigtail," which is an extension of the vent lumen.

The major advantage of a double-lumen tube is that the constant airflow allows for a controlled suction force at the drainage eyes.[5] Suction applied to a single-lumen tube may pull gastric mucosa into the drainage eyes. The tube may become occluded with tissue, and excessive negative pressure during suctioning may cause ulceration or damage to the gastric mucosa. Development of a suction force above 25 mm Hg, the commonly cited level of capillary fragility, is more apt to occur with Levin tubes for this reason. Suction is inversely proportional to flow, so the less flow through the tube, the higher the level of suction in the tube. If one

end of the tube is blocked, the level of suction inside the tube increases rapidly, even though suction is still being applied at the same level as before. The tube may even collapse if the suction is great enough. As long as flow is maintained, a single-lumen tube can rid the stomach of air, liquid, and small particles. Ultimately, as the stomach is emptied of air and liquid, flow cannot be maintained, and the mobile gastric mucosa is drawn into the drainage eyes of the Levin tube.[2]

Levin tubes are usually attached to intermittent suction pumps. Intermittent suction pumps, such as the Gomco, work in cycles. When an intermittent pump is used at a high setting (usually 120 mm Hg) the initial suction applied is at a safe level, or approximately 20 mm Hg. As the drainage eyes of the Levin tube become invaginated and occluded with tissue, flow stops. The intermittent pump will then move in stages toward successively higher suction settings until full suction is reached (approximately 120 mm Hg). The amount of suction reaching the patient's tissue at the drainage eyes of a Levin tube thus can be unsafe even with an intermittent pump.

When the eyes of a Levin tube are obstructed, flow resumes only when fluid again builds up in the stomach or when tissue is pulled away from the tip of the tube. Although irrigation of the Levin tube will initially correct the problem, occlusion recurs as soon as the irrigant is evacuated from the stomach. Therefore, suction proceeds on a cyclic basis with frequent periods of invagination and possibly harmful suction levels. The fundamental disadvantage of a Levin tube is that there is no way of controlling the amount of suction reaching the gastric mucosa.[2]

The larger lumen of the Salem sump tube is designed for suction drainage, whereas the smaller vent lumen allows outside air to be drawn into the stomach, permitting continuous flow through the tube regardless of the gastric content at the time. This design reduces tissue grabbing and minimizes the suction applied to the mucosa in comparison with the single-lumen tubes. The vent of the double-lumen tube communicates with the suction lumen through a perforation in the septum separating the two lumens at the distal end of the tube (see Fig. 51–2). Ideally, the constant flow of atmospheric air moderates the amount of suction in the tube, keeping it at a maximum of 20 mm Hg (below 25 mm Hg in any case).[2]

In practice, however, vacuum can be applied at levels exceeding the venting capacity of the second lumen. In that case, the sump is overpowered, and the same traumatic suction levels can develop as occur with Levin tubes.[5] Occasionally, personnel who are unfamiliar with the tube may inadvertently clamp the venting pigtail and defeat the purpose of the design of the tube.

INDICATIONS AND CONTRAINDICATIONS

Indications for use of nasogastric tubes fall into two broad categories. The first is aspiration of stomach contents for either diagnostic or therapeutic reasons.[6] Aspiration is mandatory in the assessment and management of upper gastrointestinal bleeding.[5] Nasogastric suction is indicated in the prevention and treatment of paralytic ileus, acute gastric dilation, and intestinal obstruction. Nasogastric tube placement is indicated in management of the patient with multiple injuries to prevent aspiration and in the assessment of possible gastrointestinal trauma. A nasogastric tube should always be used for gastric decompression *before* diagnostic peritoneal lavage. Gastric tubes are also used for gastric lavage in the case of overdose. In general, an orogastric tube

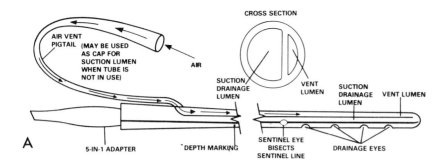

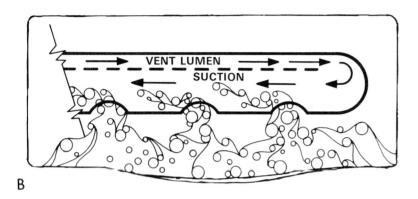

Figure 51–2. Diagram of the Salem sump tube. *A,* General design. *B,* Diagram of double-lumen principle for suction. (Courtesy of the Argyle Division of Sherwood Medical, St. Louis, Mo.)

is used for drug overdose because of the larger bore, which facilitates pill fragment removal (see Chapter 53). The list of nonemergency uses for nasogastric suction is longer yet and includes such procedures as pentagastrin testing and postoperative intubation to protect gastric suture lines.[5]

The second indication for nasogastric tubes is for feedings or for the administration of therapeutic substances, for example, medications, antacids, or activated charcoal in drug overdose patients. For the most part, nasogastric tubes are placed for aspiration, although the emergency physician may be required to replace a feeding tube or to assess tube placement (see Chapter 54).[7]

Contraindications to nasogastric tube placement include the following clinical situations: facial fractures with suspected cribriform plate injuries, which would permit intracranial intubation; esophageal strictures or a history of alkali ingestion, which would increase the possibility of esophageal perforation; comatose state with unprotected airway, which would increase the risk of aspiration; and penetrating cervical wounds in the awake trauma victim, whose gagging efforts could stimulate hemorrhage. Esophageal varices are not a contraindication to nasogastric intubation.

SPECIAL SITUATIONS

Certain presenting complaints occur with such frequency that they are discussed separately. These include pancreatitis, gastrointestinal bleeding, and surgical problems including gallbladder disease.

Pancreatitis

Part of the time-honored therapy for pancreatitis has been nasogastric suction. The rationale for this procedure has been that by preventing gastric juice from emptying into the duodenum, exocrine stimulation is diminished, essentially putting the pancreas "at rest." However, one prospec-

tive study of nasogastric suction in patients with pancreatitis demonstrated no improvement in (1) duration of abdominal pain; (2) interval until bowel sounds returned; (3) need for narcotic administration; (4) length of time that intravenous fluid therapy was needed; or (5) complications, including pseudocyst, abscess, or pulmonary problems.[8] It has been suggested that there is a faster recovery from pain[9] if nasogastric suction is employed, but other reports have not found this to be the case.[10, 11] Unless abdominal distention or persistent nausea and vomiting are present, there is no compelling reason for nasogastric suction to be part of pancreatitis management.

Gastrointestinal Bleeding

Passage of a nasogastric tube is mandatory, however, in the assessment of the patient with melena, hematochezia, or history of hematemesis. If a Levin or Salem sump aspirate indicates the presence of red blood or clots in the stomach, a large (at least a number 30) Ewald or Lavacuator tube should be passed for irrigation if the smaller tube is inadequate for lavage of clots.

The end point of lavage is a matter of some controversy. Removal of blood clots from the stomach has been assumed to be beneficial because it allows the stomach to contract, thereby promoting hemostasis. Clearing the stomach of blood and clots also has been presumed to facilitate endoscopic viewing of the mucosa.[12] However, there has been no evidence that removal of clots decreases hemorrhage.[13, 14]

Generally, 200 ml (10 ml/kg in children) of lavage fluid is instilled into the stomach and then withdrawn. Lavage is continued until the fluid is clear; if the fluid return is still bloody after 30 to 40 minutes, further diagnostic procedures are indicated.[12]

The choice of lavage fluid is a matter of controversy, but either saline or tap water is acceptable in an adult. Because very small amounts of fluid are absorbed from the stomach, there appears to be no danger of electrolyte disturbance from the use of tap water.[15–17] Previously, lavage with iced fluid has been advocated for local vasoconstriction and reduced gastric blood flow. However, iced fluid experimentally offers no advantage over room-temperature fluid and may predispose to gastric ulceration and hypothermia.[18, 19] Lavage with norepinephrine has also been used, generally 8 mg in 100 ml of saline instilled for 30 minutes.[12, 20] This procedure was first described by Le Veen and colleagues in 1972[21] and is controversial and of unproven value.

Historically, caution has been advised in undertaking nasogastric intubation when bleeding esophageal varices are suspected, as when physical signs of cirrhosis are present. Variceal rupture has occurred during the insertion of instruments into the esophagus, and many clinicians are reluctant to place nasogastric tubes in the setting of cirrhosis. However, two studies, one of alcoholic cirrhotics with esophageal varices and recent upper gastrointestinal bleeding,[22] and one of patients with end-stage liver disease undergoing liver transplantation,[23] indicate that blind nasogastric tube placement is safe in patients with suspected or proven varices.

Finally, it must be recalled that 1 to 10 per cent of patients with duodenal bleeding have negative nasogastric aspirates.[24] If bile is present in the gastric return, duodenal bleeding is unlikely. Cuellar and colleagues report that bile acids are more commonly present than suggested by the aspirate color.[24a]

Other Gastrointestinal Settings

Nasogastric intubation is recommended in the emergency management of acute cholecystitis and gallstone ileus.[25] Routine use of nasogastric suction has been challenged in the management of gallbladder and gastrointestinal surgical patients, with a greater number of complications reported with nasogastric intubation.[26] In another prospective study, nasogastric decompression was deemed to be unnecessary in patients undergoing colon operations;[27] no increased incidence of aspiration, wound dehiscence, or abdominal distention was found in patients who had not undergone nasogastric intubation.

The presence of gastric or abdominal distention, or of persistent nausea and vomiting, remain indications for nasogastric intubation. Other "softer" indications must be weighed against the discomfort caused by the tube itself. In addition, no important clinical differences have been shown between Levin and Salem sump nasogastric tubes for postoperative gastrointestinal decompression.[28]

EQUIPMENT

In preparing for nasogastric tube insertion, the following equipment is useful: towel (for covering the patient's gown), tissue, emesis basin, number 14 or 16 nasogastric tube, glass of water with drinking straw, water-soluble jelly, stethoscope, hypoallergenic tape (in strips 4 inches in length), safety pin, rubber band, urethral or bulb syringe, drainage collection bottle, topical anesthetic jelly or ointment, and vasoconstrictor nasal spray.[4, 5, 29]

Depending on the indication, other equipment may be needed (e.g., saline for irrigation or Magill forceps in an uncooperative or anesthestized patient). The equipment in the aforementioned list is adequate for the typical elective intubation in an adult. An antireflux valve (Keith Antireflux Valve, Sherwood Medical Industries, St. Louis, Mo.) is a one-way valve used on the sump port of double lumen tubes.

The device has been found cost-effective by reducing the need for gown and linen change during inpatient nasogastric tube use.[29a]

PREPARATION

In preparing for the insertion, one should observe simple hygiene; nasogastric tube placement, of course, cannot be a sterile procedure. The head of the bed should be raised so that the patient is in a high Fowler position. A towel is placed over the patient's chest to protect the gown, and an emesis basin should be available on the patient's lap.[30]

Generally, the largest possible tube for the nostril size of the patient should be selected. A large tube is less likely to become blocked during use or to curl back on itself during insertion. One should select a 16 French gauge or larger tube for an adult and should curve the end of it by coiling the first 15 cm. The curved end should be pointing down on insertion.

The nasogastric tube should be lubricated with a water-soluble jelly (K-Y or other) for 7 to 10 cm over its distal end. It has been recommended that lidocaine gel (2 per cent) or a similar topical anesthetic be applied to the nose to facilitate passage,[6] especially if the tube does not pass on the first attempt. One way to lubricate the nose is to slowly inject 3 to 5 ml of 2 per cent xylocaine jelly into the nostril with a syringe (needle removed) (Fig. 51–3). The patient is asked to inhale through the nose so that the physician may select the more open passageway. Before passage the more patent nostril should be identified by examination with a flashlight and a nasal speculum or by the gentle exploration of the nares with a lubricated, gloved fifth finger. If significant nasal congestion is present, a spray of a topical vasoconstrictor, such as ephedrine, phenylephrine hydrochloride (Neo-

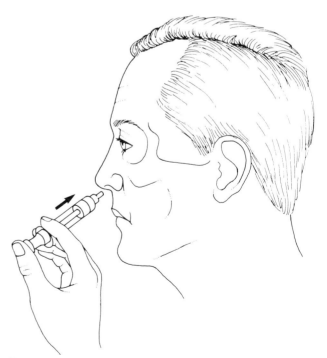

Figure 51–3. One method of instilling lubricant or anesthetic gel into the nose. Fill a syringe barrel with 3 to 5 ml of viscous lidocaine (2 per cent), and, without using a needle, squirt the solution along the floor of the nose and allow it to drip into the nasopharynx and be swallowed. This method works best if the patient is supine.

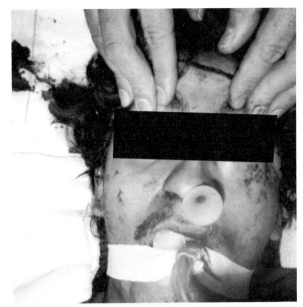

Figure 51–4. A soft rubber nasal airway (trumpet) may serve three useful purposes for the passage of a nasogastric tube. (1) A nasogastric tube smaller in diameter may be passed through the airway, and pain for that part of the procedure is eliminated. (2) The airway may be left in place for 15 minutes to dilate the nasal passage and then be removed. (3) The airway serves as a shield to prevent the inadvertent passage of the nasogastric tube into the brain in cases of fractures of the midface (but not the posterior nasopharynx).

Synephrine), or cocaine should be applied. Cocaine is a good selection because of its additional local anesthetic properties. In addition to nasal anesthesia some prefer to have the patient sip 2 per cent viscous lidocaine (Xylocaine) before tube passage to numb the pharynx and esophagus and thus help prevent gagging. Cetacaine spray applied to the pharynx is another option for anesthetizing the throat and reducing gagging.

In apprehensive patients, patients with facial trauma or those who cannot tolerate nasal passage, some physicians have opted to first pass a soft rubber nasal airway (trumpet). The nasogastric tube may be painlessly passed through the nasal airway or the airway may be kept in place for 10 to 15 minutes to dilate the passage and then be removed (Fig. 51–4).

PROCEDURE

The procedure may be divided into two phases. The first phase involves tube passage into the nasopharynx; the second phase consists of passage down the esophagus. With the patient sitting and the head supported to prevent reflex withdrawal, the lubricated tube is introduced along the *floor* of the nose. *The tube should not be directed toward the bridge of the nose, but rather toward the floor* (Fig. 51–5). If one nostril is narrowed by a deviated septum, the other side may be used, although often even the narrowed side will accommodate the tube below the inferior turbinate along the floor of the nose.[6] If difficulty persists, a smaller tube may be tried. If resistance is severe, the other nostril may again be tried, or insertion may ultimately be attempted through the mouth. At no time should the tube be forced. Failure to advance the tube is more often caused by abutment of the tip against a sensitive structure than by a nasal opening that is too small.

Resistance will be felt as the tip of the tube reaches the nasopharynx; this is the most uncomfortable part of the procedure for the patient and may cause nasal bleeding. Often, the patient can aid this phase of tube passage by taking a sip or two of water through the straw. A slight twisting motion applied to the tube can also be helpful. Once the tube is in the nasopharynx, the physician should pause a few seconds and allow the patient to regain composure. It may help to advise the patient to pant or rapidly mouth breathe at this point.

Reflex gagging may direct the tip of the tube into the mouth as one attempts passage into the esophagus. If this occurs, one of the following may be tried:

1. Repeating the attempt by withdrawing the tip of the tube into the nasopharynx (do not totally remove it) and advancing again until it passes.
2. Removing the tube and cooling the tip for 20 minutes in a container of ice to stiffen it so that it becomes less likely to coil when tube passage is retried.
3. Observing the tube with the aid of a tongue depressor as it passes through the posterior pharynx and then using Magill forceps or a tongue blade to guide the tube down the esophagus.[6, 31]
4. Applying a topical anesthetic to the oropharynx (Cetacaine, viscous lidocaine) and reattempting passage.

There is usually no need to visualize the larynx during the procedure; as long as the tube passes along the posterior pharyngeal wall, it should enter the esophagus. If the tube twists in the mouth or kinks during passage, *it should be withdrawn to the level of the nasopharynx but not completely removed.* Flexion of the patient's neck when cervical injury is not present helps guide the tube into the esophagus.

The cooperation of the patient facilitates passage and should be encouraged by the inserter. The patient should be asked to continue swallowing from a glass of water through a straw once the tube has passed the nasopharynx while the inserter continues to advance the tube.[5] Passage down the esophagus should be accomplished without resistance. If a stricture or a pharyngeal pouch is present, causing obstruction, a general anesthetic and direct visualization of tube passage may be required for tube placement. Once the patient begins to swallow, *the tube should be passed quickly;* hesitation by the inserter serves to increase gagging and prolong the patient's discomfort.[30] Inadvertent intubation of the trachea is usually quickly recognized in the conscious patient by coughing and distress. Inability to speak, another characteristic sign of tracheal passage, is not so easily identified in the unconscious patient, and one must be cognizant

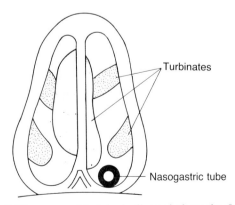

Figure 51–5. The nasogastric tube is directed along the *floor* of the nose, not toward the bridge. The tube often slides through the tunnel beneath the inferior turbinate.

of this fact when passing a nasogastric tube in an obtunded or unconscious individual.

The gastroesophageal junction is reached typically at 40 cm in the adult. If no measurement has been taken beforehand, nasogastric tubes are typically inserted to the second or third black marking in adults. The Salem sump tube is 48 inches long, for example, and has markings at 18, 22, 26, and 30 inches (approximately 45, 55, 65, and 75 cm, respectively).

The desired insertion distance should always be obtained beforehand in the following manner: The tube is placed alongside the patient's nose. The tube is then extended to the tip of the patient's ear lobe on the same side and from there to the end of the xiphoid process. This total distance approximates that required for insertion, and the spot is marked with adhesive tape before the insertion (Fig. 51–6).[5, 30] The nose-ear-xiphoid length (NEX) has been modified to give the following formula for recommended length of insertion (in centimeters):[32]

$$\frac{NEX - 50}{2} + 50$$

Omitting the measurement of needed tube length before tube passage is a common error that may result in esophageal placement or inserting multiple coils of the tube into the stomach.

CONFIRMATION OF TUBE PLACEMENT

Once the tube has been passed, confirmation of correct placement must be obtained as soon as possible. There are several ways of checking tube placement:

1. The suction lumen is aspirated gently. For aspiration, a piston syringe is preferred over the bulb syringe that cannot generate much vacuum. The presence of stomach contents implies that the tube is in the stomach.[29] The patient may have to be placed in a left lateral decubitus position to maximize the return. The aspiration of food may give a false impression of location if lower esophageal obstruction exists. Blue litmus paper may be used to test the aspirate for acid.[6] Fluid has been aspirated from the pleural space and from the lung.[33] Gastric fluid pH should be less than 5 unless the patient is on antacids or H2 antagonists.[34] Duodenal pH approximates 6.5.

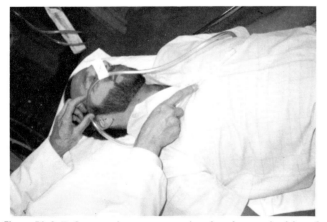

Figure 51–6. Before passing a nasogastric tube, the required length is estimated by placing the tube on the exterior of the patient, and the proper depth is marked with a piece of tape. Failure to premeasure a tube is a common error, resulting in the curling of the tube in the stomach or intubation of the lower esophagus.

2. The patient may be asked to hum or talk. If this is not possible in the awake cooperative patient, the tube should be withdrawn,[35] because it may have passed through the larynx. The mouth should be inspected for coiling of the tube. Coughing, cyanosis, or choking are obvious indications for tube withdrawal.

3. A 60-ml piston syringe filled with air is connected to the suction lumen of the nasogastric tube. The examiner auscultates the stomach while an assistant empties the syringe slowly. A "whooshing" sound of borborygmi is produced by only 10 to 20 ml of air if the tube is in the stomach. The patient may belch on injection of air if the tube is in the esophagus.[29, 30] Alternatively, injection of air in the esophagus may produce typical borborygmi, but in a delayed fashion. Pseudoconfirmatory gurgling in the left upper quadrant may be heard from a tube in the lung, however.

4. The open end of the tube may be placed in a glass of water. Escaping air bubbles imply that the tube is in a bronchus or in the trachea and should be removed immediately.[5] Capnography, if available, is more accurate in proving CO_2 content of the bubbles. Crackling noises heard when the end of the tube is held up to the inserter's ear also suggest location in a bronchus.

5. If the tube is radiopaque, as in the case of a Salem sump, radiographic confirmation of tube location can be obtained.[5, 29] If one is considering films of the abdomen for other diagnostic purposes, it is best to pass the nasogastric tube before obtaining the radiographs so that the position of the tube may be confirmed.

Once again, the neurologically impaired patient is at particularly high risk of tube malposition. Even flexible tubes can pass into the lung past a cuffed endotracheal tube.[34]

SECURING THE TUBE

Once the correct position of the tube is determined, the tube is anchored to the nose with hypoallergenic tape, either in a butterfly fashion around the tube or with vertical taping over the nose and the tube. Tincture of benzoin applied to the dorsum of the nose may help to secure the tape. One should attempt to tape the tube so that it rests in the middle of the nasal opening and does not lie directly in contact with the skin. A rubber band is then looped in a slip knot around the nasogastric tube and is pinned to the patient's gown.[30] This prevents slippage of the tube or tugging on the patient's nose during movement. To prevent pressure necrosis to the nose, the tube should never be taped to the patient's forehead[5] and should not rest against the nostril for long periods.

When a Salem sump tube is used, the blue pigtail should be kept *above the level of fluid in the patient's stomach*. This prevents reflux of gastric contents into the vent lumen. If the pigtail is below the patient's midline, the vent lumen acts as a siphon, allowing gastric contents to flow out the lumen, possibly blocking the sump.[2, 5] When dealing with sump tubes, the collection trap should be placed below the patient's midline to prevent reflux (Fig. 51–7). Otherwise, gastric contents will flow out the vent lumen. Increasing the suction may cause fluids to be lifted the entire length of the tube, but increasing the suction simply for this purpose is ill-advised. Once the tube is devoid of fluid, the full force of suction will be applied to an empty tube and could overpower the sump.[2, 5]

Ambulation is possible with a nasogastric tube in place. The suction-drainage system is disconnected, and, in the case of a Salem sump, the blue pigtail is placed in the connector. Alternatively, for either the Levin tube or the

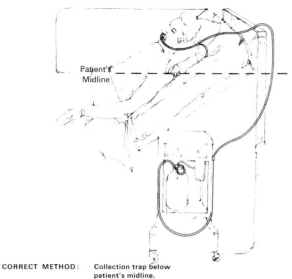

CORRECT METHOD: Collection trap below patient's midline.

Figure 51–7. Correct position of the collection trap below the patient's midline. Note that the pigtail vent lumen is kept above the patient's midline. (Courtesy of the Argyle Division of Sherwood Medical, St. Louis, Mo.)

Salem sump tube, a syringe can be placed into the suction-drainage lumen and taped to the patient's gown so that it does not pull on the tube.

PLACEMENT IN THE UNCONSCIOUS PATIENT

If the patient is intubated, the balloon of the endotracheal tube may be momentarily *deflated* to allow passage of the nasogastric tube. Levin claimed that a nasogastric tube could be easily introduced even when the patient was under anesthesia.[36] This is not always the case, and several methods have been suggested for accomplishing nasogastric intubation in a patient who is unable to swallow.

In an unconscious patient, the nasogastric tube may be placed initially through a nare into the oropharynx. The tip of the tube is then visualized with a laryngoscope, grasped with Magill forceps, and pulled out of the mouth. An endotracheal tube with an internal diameter that is slightly larger than the external diameter of the nasogastric tube is selected and is slit along its lesser curvature from its proximal end to a point 3 cm from its distal end. The slit endotracheal tube is then passed through the mouth into the esophagus.[31] If, instead, the slit endotracheal tube is placed through the nose into the esophagus, a number 7 endotracheal tube is appropriate. If the oral route is used, a number 8 tube will suffice.[37] Passage into the esophagus is facilitated by the stiffness of the larger endotracheal tube and does not require active swallowing. The tip of the nasogastric tube is then threaded into the endotracheal tube and advanced into the stomach (Fig. 51–8). One then removes the slit endotracheal tube from the esophagus. When the distal part of the endotracheal tube is visible, the unslit 3-cm distal part is slit with scissors. The endotracheal tube is removed, and the nasogastric tube remains in place.[38] Alternatively, a nasopharyngeal airway may be passed first, with a well-lubricated nasogastric tube inserted through the airway, if the major problem is in traversing the nose.[39]

Others have advocated simply guiding the nasogastric tube with the fingers once it has been passed through the nose.[40] This has been deemed unreliable by some.[31] Forward displacement of the larynx by manually gripping and lifting

the thyroid cartilage has aided tube insertion,[41] as has simple jaw elevation.

Ultimately, if all other methods fail, a flexible fiberoptic bronchoscope or esophagoscope can be placed under direct vision into and through the esophagus.[42] A guide wire is threaded into the stomach. The nasogastric tube can be placed over the guide wire into the stomach; the guide wire is then removed.[43]

SUCTION SETTINGS

Levin tubes are usually attached to intermittent low-suction or straight-bag drainage. When a Salem sump tube is used, the following guidelines are recommended: If intermittent suction from a pump is used, suction should be set on high (80 to 120 mm Hg). This intermittent suction allows airflow during the closed cycle.[5] Intermittent suction from a central suction source should be set at a low level (30 to 40 mm Hg), and suction should be increased either until there is fluid flow or until bubbling is observed in the Salem sump. When continuous suction is used, it should be set at a low level and increased until fluid flow or bubbling is observed in the Salem sump.[2] At all times, the vent should be kept open; closing the vent of the Salem sump tube may cause mucosal damage similar to that encountered with single-lumen tubes. A functioning Salem sump tube makes a hissing sound, which may be interpreted as an air leak or as a malfunction by those who are not familiar with the design.

USE OF THE TUBE

Nasogastric tubes may be used for feeding or lavage as well as for suction. Anything instilled into a nasogastric tube, such as activated charcoal, antacids, or medications, must be in liquid form. The plug or Hoffman clamp is removed from the nasogastric tube, and the desired material is in-

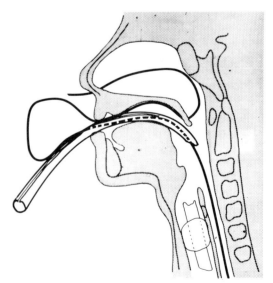

Figure 51–8. Diagrammatic representation of the separation of the nasogastric tube from the endotracheal tube through the slit in the endotracheal tube. The introducing endotracheal tube has been removed from the esophagus before separation from the nasogastric tube. Note the prior placement of an endotracheal tube in the trachea (partially shown). (From Sprague DH, Carter SR: An alternate method for nasogastric tube insertion. Anesthesiology 53:436, 1980. Reproduced by permission.)

stilled with either a bulb syringe or a 50-ml piston syringe. As always, the position of the tube should be confirmed before instillation of liquid. It is preferable to let the medication or charcoal flow by gravity if at all possible rather than by the use of force; the tube may need to be flushed with 30 to 50 ml of water at intervals.[4] After any feeding or administration of antacids or medication, suction should be discontinued for 15 to 20 minutes.

Irrigation of a Salem sump tube may be performed through either the vent lumen or the suction-drainage lumen. When irrigating the pigtail vent lumen, the suction need not be interrupted. Any irrigation should be followed by injection of air through the sump lumen to ensure its patency. During irrigation of the main lumen, the Salem sump tube is disconnected from the suction source, and the connector is removed from the main lumen. An irrigating syringe is inserted and irrigation is carried out with approximately 30 ml of saline. If gastric drainage is particularly viscous, irrigation may have to be carried out at frequent intervals.[2, 4]

COMPLICATIONS

Serious complications from nasogastric tube placement are uncommon, and almost all complications are minor. More serious complications may develop in comatose patients or in those with underlying nasal, cervical, esophageal, or gastric pathologic conditions.

Epistaxis is a frequent occurrence but often can be prevented if the tube is not forced during insertion. Inability to pass the tube is common as well and may be related to the creation of a false passage,[6] the presence of an esopha-geal stricture, a gagging or uncooperative patient, or repetitive coiling of the tube in the mouth or the esophagus.

Perforation of the esophagus has been reported but is rare in the absence of esophageal disease.[6] If choking is noted, the tube should be assumed to be in the trachea until proved otherwise.

Extreme caution should be exercised when passing a nasogastric tube in a patient with suspected or proven facial or skull fracture. Intracranial penetration of nasogastric tubes inserted in patients with head injuries has been reported (Fig. 51–9).[44–46] One can readily appreciate the consequences of suction or irrigation of a tube placed in the cranium. Most reported cases have had a fatal outcome,[47] but intracranial tubes have been surgically removed without increasing the neurologic deficit.[48] Trauma to the cribriform plate of the ethmoid bone is the speculated anatomic injury. Inadvertent central nervous system penetration may be prevented by prior insertion of a lubricated number 34 Davol Silastic nasopharyngeal airway into the nose; the nasogastric tube is subsequently passed through the nasopharyngeal airway. Because of its preformed curve, the Silastic airway is presumably directed away from the cribriform plate.[45] Perhaps it is safer to pass the nasogastric tube through the mouth in such cases or to observe passage of the tube into the pharynx by direct vision with a laryngoscope. Inadvertent passage of a nasogastric tube into the cranium may occur more frequently than previously appreciated.[46]

Hemorrhage from a penetrating neck wound may develop if passage of the nasogastric tube induces gagging in the awake victim of a stab wound. The trauma victim with a cervical spine injury may also be further traumatized if motion of the neck results during tube passage.

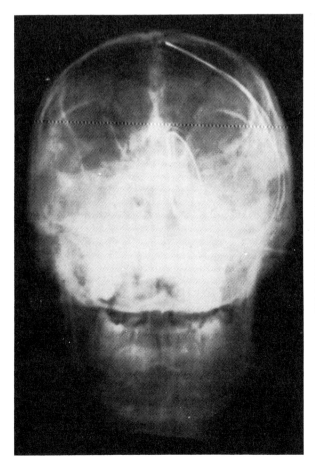

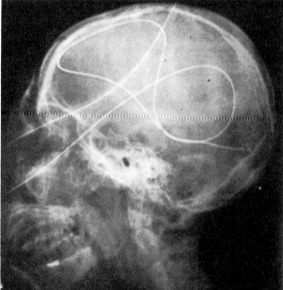

Figure 51–9. Anteroposterior and lateral skull radiographs demonstrating intracranial insertion of a nasogastric tube in a patient with multiple skull fractures. (From Johnson JC: Letter to the editor. Back to basics for morbidity-free nasogastric intubation. JACEP 8:289, 1979. Reproduced by permission.)

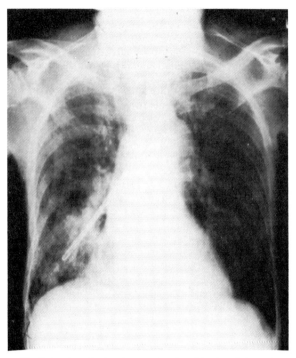

Figure 51–10. Levin tube inadvertently placed in the right main stem bronchus; an alveolar infiltrate consistent with early pneumonia is also shown. (From Johnson JC: Letter to the editor: Back to basics for morbidity-free nasogastric intubation. JACEP 8:289, 1979. Reproduced by permission.)

Several laryngeal injuries have been reported from nasogastric tube usage; often these involve tubes that have been in place for a long time. Hoarseness and pharyngodynia have occurred with long-term use.[1] Cricoid chondritis, arytenoid edema,[49] and bilateral vocal cord paralysis have been reported with long-term use of nasogastric tubes. Airway obstruction may therefore occur even with proper tube placement,[35] and may be related to hypersalivation, depressed cough reflex, or depressed laryngopharyngeal reflexes.

Nasal alar necrosis occurs but should be largely preventable if one does not tape the nasogastric tube to the patient's forehead and if one pins the tube to the patient's gown to prevent pressure necrosis.

A multitude of respiratory tract complications from nasogastric tubes have been reported. Pneumonia has occurred from a tube placement into a patient's right lower lobe bronchus (Fig. 51–10).[45] Hydropneumothorax has resulted from a bronchially placed nasogastric tube.[50] A bronchopleural fistula and empyema also developed in this case. Pleural perforation with pneumothorax,[51–55] usually right-sided, after main stem bronchus placement and even death[55] have been reported often enough to be more than a curiosity. Malpositioned nasogastric tubes in the lung have been described even with cuffed endotracheal tubes in place.[50, 56] In addition, air injected to check the position of the tube may overdistend the alveoli and cause a pneumothorax.[57] One study concluded that routine use of nasogastric tubes postoperatively caused a higher incidence of pneumonia when compared with management without the tubes.[58] The authors of the study postulated that the nasogastric tube may have hindered coughing, causing accumulation of mucous plugs in the bronchial tree. Nasogastric tube use in craniofacial trauma patients with severe multisystem injuries is associated with sinusitis.[59] Gastrointestinal bleeding may oc-

cur from mucosal damage caused by the tube, although this complication is unlikely to be seen immediately after passage of tubes in the emergency department.

Other investigators do not favor routine use of nasogastric tubes because of patient discomfort. Clearly, nasogastric suction has the potential to produce fluid and electrolyte imbalance. There does not seem to be any evidence that increased nasal resistance occurs in adults when a nasogastric tube is in place, but this has been reported in infants.[60]

If Magill forceps are used in nasogastric tube insertion, there is the potential for damage to the uvula, the soft palate, or the pharyngeal mucosa.

As a final note, it should be stressed that a nasogastric tube may inadvertently be passed into a number of undesirable and potentially dangerous places in the unconscious patient. It is incumbent upon the physician to verify the correct passage by direct vision or sequential radiographic studies in all obtunded patients.[52]

REFERENCES

1. Sofferman RA, Hubbell RN: Laryngeal complications of nasogastric tubes. Ann Otol Rhinol Laryngol 90:465, 1981.
2. Clinical Considerations in the Use of the Argyle Salem Sump Tube. St. Louis, Mo., Argyle Division of Sherwood Medical, 1979, pp 1–16.
3. Friedman M, Baim H, Shelton V, et al: Laryngeal injuries secondary to nasogastric tubes. Ann Otol Rhinol Laryngol 90:469, 1981.
4. Jackson EW: Nursing photobooks: Giving medication through a nasogastric tube. Nursing '80 71, 1980.
5. McConnell EA: Ensuring safer stomach suctioning with the salem sump tube. Nursing '77, 1977.
6. Tucker A, Lewis J: Passing a nasogastric tube. Br Med J 10:1128, 1980.
7. McGuirt WF, Strout JJ: Securing of intermediate duration feeding tubes. Laryngoscope 90:2046, 1980.
8. Sarr MG, Sanfey H, Cameron JL: Prospective, randomized trial of nasogastric suction in patients with acute pancreatitis. Surgery 100:500, 1986.
9. Fuller RK, Loveland JP, Frankel MH: An evaluation of the efficacy of nasogastric suction treatment in alcohol pancreatitis. Am J Gastroenterol 75:349, 1981.
10. Field BE, Hepner GW, Shabot MM, et al: Nasogastric suction in alcoholic pancreatitis. Dig Dis Sci 24:339, 1979.
11. Switz DM, Vlahcevic ZR, Farrar JT: The effect of anticholinergic and/or nasogastric suction on the outcome of acute alcoholic pancreatitis: A controlled study. Gastroenterology 68:974, 1975.
12. Bonsan WG, Barker PB: Upper gastrointestinal tract disorders. In Rosen, et al (eds): Emergency Medicine: Concepts and Clinical Practice. St. Louis, CV Mosby, 1988, pp 1428–1429.
13. Larson DE, Farnell MB: Upper gastrointestinal hemorrhage. Mayo Clin Prac 58:371, 1983.
14. Ponsky JL, Hoffman M, Swayngim DS: Saline irrigation in gastric hemorrhage: The effect of temperature. J Surg Res 28:204, 1980.
15. Bryant LR, Mobin-Uddin K, Dillon ML, et al: Comparison of ice water with iced saline solution for gastric lavage in gastroduodenal hemorrhage. Am J Surg 124:570, 1972.
16. Matsumoto T (ed): Current management of acute gastrointestinal hemorrhage. Springfield, Ill, Charles C Thomas, 1977.
17. Rudolph JP: Automated gastric lavage and a comparison of 0.9% normal saline solution and tap water irrigant. Ann Emerg Med 14:1156, 1985.
18. Menguy R, Masters YF: Influence of cold on stress ulceration and on gastric mucosal blood flow and energy metabolism. Ann Surg 194:29, 1981.
19. Gilbert DA, Saunders DR: Iced saline lavage does not slow bleeding from experimental canine ulcers. Dig Dis Sci 26:1065, 1981.
20. Poraicu D: The efficiency of intragastric norepinephrine administration in gastrointestinal bleeding in 50 patients. Resuscitation 11:111, 1984.
21. Le Veen HH, Falk G, Diaz C, et al: Control of gastrointestinal bleeding. Am J Surg 123:154, 1972.
22. Lopez-Torres A, Waye JD: The safety of intubation in patients with esophageal varices. Am J Dig Dis 18:1032, 1973.
23. Ritter DM, Rettke SR, Hughes RW, et al: Placement of nasogastric tubes and esophageal stethoscopes in patients with documented esophageal varices. Anesth Analg 67:283, 1988.
24. Gitrich G (ed): Principles and Practice of Gastroenterology and Hepatology. New York, Elsevier Science Publ Co, 1988, p 1547.
24a. Cuellar RE, Gavaler JS, Alexander JA, et al: Gastrointestinal tract hemorrhage: The value of a nasogastric aspirate. Arch Intern Med 150:1381, 1990.
25. Clark JB Jr: Disorders of the liver, biliary tract, and pancreas. In Rosen

P, et al. (eds): Emergency Medicine: Concepts and Clinical Practice. St. Louis, CV Mosby Co, 1988, pp 1448–1450.

26. Michowitz M, Chen J, Waizbard E, et al: Abdominal operations without nasogastric tube decompression of the gastrointestinal tract. Am Surg 54:672, 1988.

27. Racette DL, Chang FC, Trekell ME, et al: Is nasogastric intubation necessary in colon operations? Am J Surg 154:640, 1987.

28. Ikard RW, Federspiel CF: A comparison of Levin and Sump nasogastric tubes for postoperative gastrointestinal decompression. Am Surg 53:50, 1987.

29. Jackson EW: Performing GI Procedures: Nursing Photobook. Horsham, Pa, Intermed Communications, 1981, pp 44–70.

29a. Shapiro MJ, Minor CB, Keegan M: Usefulness of an antireflux valve in the intensive care unit. Crit Care Med 18:878, 1990.

30. Volden C, Grinde J, Carl D: Taking the trauma out of nasogastric intubation. Nursing '80 64, 1980.

31. Cohen DD, Fox RM: Nasogastric intubation in the anesthetized patient. Anesth Analg 42:578, 1963.

32. Hanson RL: New approach to measuring adult nasogastric tubes for insertion. Am J Nurs 1334, July 1980.

33. Metheny N: Measures to test placement of nasogastric and nasointestinal feeding tubes: A review. Nurs Res 37:324, 1988.

34. Theodore AC, Frank JA, Ende J, et al: Picture a tube gone wrong. Emerg Med 17:45, 1985.

35. May M, Nellis KJ: Nasogastric intubation: Avoiding complications. Resident and Staff Physician 30:60, 1984.

36. Levin AL: A new gastroduodenal catheter. JAMA 76:1007, 1921.

37. Siegel IB, Kahn RC: Insertion of difficult nasogastric tubes through a nasoesophageally placed endotracheal tube. Crit Care Med 15:876, 1987.

38. Sprague DH, Carter SR: An alternate method for nasogastric tube insertion. Anesthesiology 53:436, 1980.

39. Lewis JD: Facilitation of nasogastric and nasotracheal intubation with a nasopharyngeal airway. Am J Emerg Med 4:426, 1986.

40. Rosenberg H: The difficult NG intubation: Tips and techniques. Emerg Med 20:95, 1988.

41. Perel A, Ya'ari Y, Pizov R: Forward displacement of the larynx for nasogastric tube insertion in intubated patients. Crit Care Med 13:204, 1985.

42. Ohn KC, Wu WH: A new method for nasogastric tube insertion. Anesthesiology 51:568, 1979.

43. Lee TS, Wright BD: Flexible fiberoptic bronchoscope for difficult nasogastric intubation. Anesth Analg 60:904, 1981.

44. Seebacher J, Nozik D, Mathieu A: Inadvertent intracranial introduction of a nasogastric tube: A complication of severe maxillofacial trauma. Anesthesiology 42:100, 1975.

45. Johnson JE: Back to basics for morbidity-free nasogastric intubation. JACEP 8:289, 1979.

46. Bouzarth WF: Nasogastric intubation. Ann Emerg Med 9:49, 1980.

47. Tarver RD, Gillespie KR: The misplaced tube. Emerg Med Jan 30:111, 1988.

48. Fletcher SA, Henderson LT, Miner ME, Jones JM: The successful surgical removal of intracranial nasogastric tubes. J Trauma 27:948, 1987.

49. Alessi DM, Berci G: Aspiration and nasogastric intubation. Otolaryngology 94:486, 1986.

50. Culpepper JA, Veremakis C, Guntupalli KK, et al: Malpositioned nasogastric tube causing pneumothorax and bronchopleural fistula. Chest 81:389, 1982.

51. Lie JT: On the positioning (or malpositioning) of a nasogastric tube (correspondence). Am J Med 85:282, 1988.

52. Roubenoff R, Ravich WJ: Pneumothorax due to nasogastric feeding tubes: Report of four cases, review of the literature, and recommendations for prevention. Arch Intern Med 149:184, 1989.

53. Aronchik JM, Epstein DM, Gefter WB, et al: Pneumothorax as a complication of placement of a nasoenteric tube. JAMA 252:3287, 1984.

54. Khan MS, Gross JS: Pneumothorax complicating small-bore nasogastric feeding tube insertion. JAGS 35:1130, 1987.

55. Gough D, Rust D: Nasogastric intubation: Morbidity in an asymptomatic patient. Am J Emerg Med 4:511, 1986.

56. Sweatman AJ, Tomasello PA, Loughhead MG, et al: Misplacement of nasogastric tubes and esophageal monitoring devices. Br J Anaesth 50:389, 1978.

57. Holliman PW, McFee AS: Pneumothorax attributable to nasogastric tube. Arch Surg 116:970, 1981.

58. Argov S, Goldstein I, Barzilai A: Is routine use of the nasogastric tube justified in upper abdominal surgery? Am J Surg 139:849, 1980.

59. Bell RM, Page GV, Bynoe RP, et al: Post-traumatic sinusitis. J Trauma 28:923, 1988.

60. Stocks J: Effect of nasogastric tubes on nasal resistance during infancy. Arch Dis Child 55:17, 1980.

Chapter **52**

Balloon Tamponade of Gastroesophageal Varices

Jonathan M. Glauser

BACKGROUND

The first reported successful control of variceal hemorrhage by tamponade was achieved by Westphal in 1930.[1, 2] He used a Gottstein sound distended with water.[3] In 1950, Sengstaken and Blakemore[4] reported the technique of double-balloon tamponade, a method still widely used. The revised commercially available Sengstaken-Blakemore tube (Davol, Inc.) is a triple-lumen rubber tube (Fig. 52–1). Two of the lumina are used to inflate a gastric balloon and an esophageal balloon, and the third lumen is used for nasogastric suction.

In 1953, a single-balloon tube with only a gastric suction lumen was introduced by Linton; this device was refined in 1955 by Nachlas.[5] The revised commercially available Linton-Nachlas tube contains two lumina for suction—one for the stomach and one for the esophagus.[6] The Linton-Nachlas tube has a single gastric balloon that is larger than the gastric balloon of the Sengstaken-Blakemore tube. The Linton-Nachlas tube probably works through compression of the cardioesophageal junction, cutting off blood flow to the esophageal varices.

In 1962, Boyce introduced a modification of the original Sengstaken-Blakemore tube (Fig. 52–2). The modification consisted of a standard nasogastric tube sutured to the Sengstaken-Blakemore tube, with the tip of the nasogastric tube positioned just proximally to the esophageal balloon.[7] A silk suture was placed through the wall of the nasogastric tube and was tied around the Sengstaken-Blakemore tube. The purpose of the Boyce modification was to enable oropharyngeal secretions to be suctioned from above the balloons, thus reducing in theory the risk of aspiration. Edlich and colleagues have reported on a commercial Sengstaken-Blakemore–type tube with a fourth lumen that is designed to provide suction just proximal to the esophageal balloon, eliminating the need for a separate nasogastric tube.[8] Some believe that the lumen of this device may be too small to permit effective suctioning.[2]

A clear tube has been described that can accommodate a fiberoptic endoscope to permit direct examination of the esophageal and gastric mucosa through the main lumen of the core tube.[9] Lower inflation pressures may be required with this method, if inflation pressures are titrated to control visible bleeding, but this approach is not widely used on an emergency basis. There also are pediatric Blakemore tubes, and modification of the esophageal balloon on an adult tube using heat-contractile tubing has been reported for use in a 14-month-old child.[10] Most clinical situations can be managed with either the Sengstaken-Blakemore tube or the Linton-Nachlas tube. Although these tubes are infrequently used today, they may be life saving, and a thorough knowledge of their structure and function is necessary should the need for their use arise.

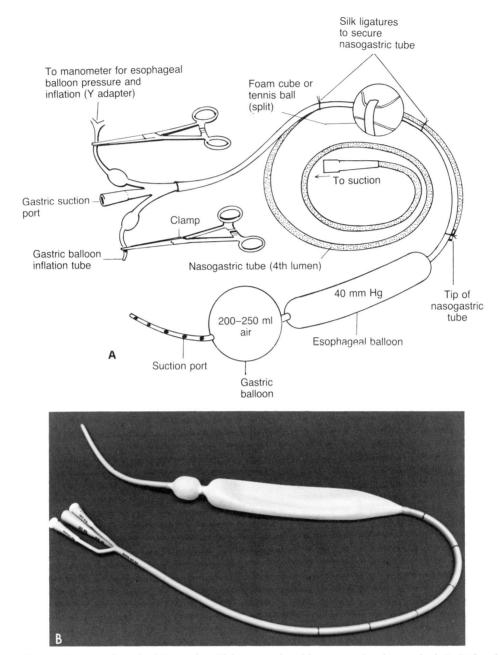

Figure 52–1. *A*, Diagram of standard Sengstaken-Blakemore tube with nasogastric tube attached. *B*, Deflated tube

INDICATIONS

The indications for use of a Sengstaken-Blakemore tube or a Linton-Nachlas tube are not standardized, but in general they include the following:

1. "Severe" variceal bleeding that cannot be controlled with other measures.
2. Moderate or persistent variceal bleeding that requires transfusion of more than 2000 ml of blood over a 24-hour period.[11]
3. Traumatic longitudinal tears of the esophagogastric mucosa (Mallory-Weiss syndrome) that do not stop bleeding spontaneously.

Because the use of balloon tamponade is associated with serious and potentially lethal complications, several caveats are in order. Endoscopy should be performed as soon as possible to document that an episode of upper gastrointestinal bleeding is actually variceal in origin. Endoscopy is most helpful after blood and clots have been evacuated by an Ewald tube.[3, 6, 12–17] Some physicians insist that bleeding varices be endoscopically visualized before a Sengstaken-Blakemore tube is inserted,[18, 19] but in patients with a massive hemorrhage, the endoscopist (if available) may not be able to see the exact source of bleeding. In such cases, angiography or a therapeutic trial with a Sengstaken-Blakemore tube may be necessary.

USE OF BALLOON TAMPONADE

Thirty per cent of patients with cirrhosis of the liver hemorrhage at least once from gastroesophageal varices; the

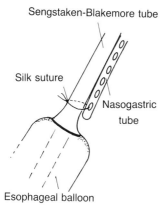

Figure 52–2. The Boyce modification of the original Sengstaken-Blakemore tube is a standard nasogastric tube sutured to secure the tip of the suction tube just proximal to the esophageal balloon.

mortality is 30 to 80 per cent. The initial stabilization of these patients is often complex and difficult and involves more than balloon tamponade. Although definitive treatment is often surgical, it is generally agreed that mortality from any surgical procedure is reduced if the procedure is performed electively,[3, 17, 20] and balloon tamponade may be required to stabilize the patient before elective surgery. The risk of complications from balloon tamponade must be weighed against the chances of death from exsanguination. Because major complications occur with balloon tamponade in up to 10 per cent of patients, the procedure is not usually a first-line treatment. Iced nasogastric lavage,[14, 21] treatment of shock with fluids and fresh blood,[9, 15, 16] intravenous vasopressin,[22–25] central venous pressure monitoring, platelet transfusion,[23, 26] vitamin K replacement,[14, 15] fresh frozen plasma infusion,[22, 23, 25, 26] and methods to lower serum ammonia levels and to prevent hepatic coma (e.g., lactulose, neomycin) may all be used before balloon tamponade. One study reports that it is very unusual for either a Sengstaken-Blakemore or a Linton-Nachlas tube to be inserted within 6 hours of the onset of variceal bleeding.[27]

To reinforce the limits of balloon tamponade, it is emphasized that a Sengstaken-Blakemore tube is used, quite simply, for temporary bleeding control. Balloon tamponade has failed to improve measurably the mortality associated with bleeding esophageal varices in the past three decades.[14] The procedure often does not control hemorrhage definitively. Most studies report that the Sengstaken-Blakemore tube provides initial hemostasis in 80 to 90 per cent of patients who are bleeding from esophageal varices,[2, 5, 29] although rates of initial hemostasis as low as 40 per cent and as high as 95 per cent have been reported.[27, 28] The tube may be used on all patients regardless of the results of hepatic function studies.[21]

Bleeding recurrences after initial balloon tamponade are common. One of the following definitive procedures must be performed after stabilization: sclerotherapy of varices by endoscopic injection,[3, 13, 19, 30–35] percutaneous transhepatic obliteration of varices,[3, 22, 23, 25, 33, 36, 37] laser obliteration of varices,[16] gastroesophageal transection with a staple gun,[24, 33, 34, 37] transthoracic ligation of the esophageal varices,[15, 21, 37] porta-azygous disconnection,[15, 37] emergency or elective portasystemic shunting,[2, 22, 23, 36] or even varix obliteration using electric current passed through longitudinal electrodes placed on a Sengstaken-Blakemore tube.[38]

The Sengstaken-Blakemore tube is used more frequently than the Linton-Nachlas tube. One study has re-

ported that the Sengstaken-Blakemore tube may be more effective than the Linton-Nachlas tube for achieving permanent hemostasis in esophageal bleeding, whereas the Linton-Nachlas tube may be more effective in managing gastric varices.[39] When a hiatal hernia exists, the Sengstaken-Blakemore tube may be more liable to displacement than the Linton-Nachlas tube. Also, if bleeding is from fundic varices, the Sengstaken-Blakemore tube may be less effective than the Linton-Nachlas tube because of the smaller gastric balloon size.

There are generally two sources of blood in bleeding varices. Submucosal vessels of the stomach traverse the cardioesophageal junction and anastomose with periesophageal veins, and periesophageal veins provide perforating branches through the wall of the esophagus. There may also be distinct gastric varices, usually near the cardioesophageal junction or fundus. For these anatomic reasons, bleeding from esophageal varices may often be controlled with inflation of the gastric balloon alone.

It is interesting to question whether it is the pressure transmitted to the esophageal varices by the esophageal balloon that actually stops the hemorrhage. It has been demonstrated that barium freely passes both inflated balloons of a well-positioned and properly inflated Sengstaken-Blakemore tube.[29] The actual transmitted pressure to the esophageal wall is less than one half of the balloon pressure; a balloon inflation pressure of 100 mm Hg maintains an esophageal pressure of 40 mm Hg. A sustained Valsalva maneuver can cause a pressure rise of as much as 195 mm Hg in the varices; this is far greater than any pressure that can be transmitted to the esophageal wall by an intraluminal balloon. At recommended inflation pressures, the average esophageal balloon diameter is 27 mm, and further increases in inflation pressure cause only minor variations in the diameter of the balloon. Although it has been questioned whether the esophageal varices are actually being compressed adequately to control bleeding,[29] in many cases inflation of both balloons does provide more effective hemostasis in bleeding esophageal varices than is provided by a single-balloon Linton-Nachlas tube.[39]

PREPARATIONS AND PRECAUTIONS

The patient must be in an intensive care setting,[11] because patients with a balloon tube in place require considerable nursing care. This includes airway and cardiac monitoring, pharyngeal suctioning,[21, 40] and frequent measurement of vital signs.

Aspiration and airway obstruction from use of the Sengstaken-Blakemore tube have been reported so frequently (especially in obtunded patients) that some physicians favor definitive airway management with either endotracheal intubation, cricothyroidotomy, or tracheotomy before balloon tamponade is used.[6] Although intubation is usually not required in the alert patient, tracheal suction and intubation equipment should be readily available at all times.[2, 41]

Because of the danger of airway occlusion from gastric balloon deflation and slippage of an esophageal balloon forward into the pharynx, scissors should always be available to transect the tube.[33] Cutting the entire tube in cross section ensures balloon deflation for rapid removal.[18] If respiratory distress occurs with the Sengstaken-Blakemore tube in place, the tube should be grasped at the mouth. The tube is cut just above the grasping hand (but below the entrance of the three-channel inlets of the Sengstaken-Blakemore tube) and then is removed immediately.

Only new tubes should be used. One should check all balloons for leakage by inflating them underwater in a basin.[2, 6, 40, 41] In a Sengstaken-Blakemore tube, the esophageal balloon should be tested to a pressure of 50 mm Hg, and the gastric balloon should be tested with 250 ml of air. Patency of all lumina, both for suction and for balloon inflation, should be confirmed before tube insertion.

Local anesthesia of the nose may be appropriate, but the pharynx should not be anesthetized for tube passage so that the patient's gag reflex is preserved.[2] The head of the bed should be raised 6 to 10 inches to prevent hiccups or vomiting.[18] Some very short patients are not suitable for the insertion of a Sengstaken-Blakemore tube, because the esophageal balloon may be inflated in the throat.[40] Although aspiration pneumonia is frequently a complication of balloon tamponade, prophylactic antibiotics are not recommended.

TECHNIQUE

It should be noted that passage of balloon tubes is not a simple procedure. Even under the best circumstances, patient cooperation and passage are difficult to accomplish. In the combative or obtunded patient, the procedure is even more difficult, and in such cases neuromuscular paralysis and tracheal intubation are indicated and are usually a necessity. Importantly, *one must be thoroughly familiar with the function of the various balloons and lumina before passage is attempted.*

Before passage of the Sengstaken-Blakemore tube, a standard nasogastric tube is placed alongside of the Sengstaken-Blakemore tube to premeasure the distance for subsequent insertion of the nasogastric tube. The tip of the nasogastric tube should lie just above the proximal portion of the esophageal balloon. A piece of tape is wrapped around the proximal end of the nasogastric tube as a marker for subsequent proper positioning of the nasogastric tube to evacuate oropharyngeal secretions. Alternatively, a 14- to 16-gauge nasogastric tube can be sutured to the Sengstaken-Blakemore tube with silk sutures before passage, as described by Boyce.[7] Using the method of Boyce, the Sengstaken-Blakemore and nasogastric tubes are passed as a unit rather than sequentially.

Before the procedure, the stomach is emptied of blood and clots with an Ewald tube to decrease the chance of aspiration during passage of the balloon tube. The balloons should be evacuated of all air with a syringe and then twisted around the tube to facilitate passage.[33] The Sengstaken-Blakemore tube is then well lubricated and passed nasally. While the patient swallows some water through a straw, the tube is passed through the esophagus.[2] In some circumstances, it may be necessary to resort to oral passage, although nasal passage is preferred. Flexion of the neck slightly may enhance esophageal entry.

The tube is passed to 50 cm, and the gastric contents are aspirated. It is important to confirm gastric placement to reduce the risk of esophageal perforation by a misplaced balloon. Some clinicians recommend initial inflation of the gastric balloon with only 50 ml of air followed by radiographic confirmation of the position of the balloon below the diaphragm.[3] Once gastric placement of a Sengstaken-Blakemore tube is ensured, the gastric balloon is inflated with 200 to 250 ml of air,[2, 6] and the intake lumen is double-clamped with a rubber-protected surgical clamp. No more than 300 ml of air should be used.[11, 27] It is emphasized that only air should be used to inflate the balloons. If water or contrast material is used, rapid emergency deflation may not be possible. Very gentle hand traction is applied until the gastric balloon is felt to be lodged at the gastroesophageal

junction. It is the pressure of the gastric balloon that produces the majority of the hemostasis.

If a Linton-Nachlas tube is used, the balloon is inflated with 600 ml of air (no more than 750 ml), the intake lumen is double-clamped,[41] and the proximal end of the tube is pulled gently against the gastroesophageal junction. Gentle traction at a maximum of 1 to 2 pounds is applied to produce the tamponade effect. With either tube, a follow-up radiograph is mandatory to verify its position. The radiograph should be portable to avoid disaster in the radiology department.

There are several acceptable ways of providing traction to the tube (Fig. 52–3). Tubes can be taped to the mouthpiece of a football helmet[2, 3, 11] or to eye goggles.[40] Some advocate pulley traction with 1 to 2 pounds of weight,[21] but pulley traction should be avoided in the emergency department because of the higher risk of airway obstruction and aspiration.[3] In addition, disoriented or obtunded patients can become entangled in pulley set-ups. Traction can be maintained with a split tennis ball or a cube of foam rubber. The tube is inserted between the two halves, and the ball or the cube is placed against the nose and firmly strapped to the tube to maintain tamponade at the gastroesophageal junction.[19] Some physicians prefer to avoid traction and simply fix the tube with tape at the corner of the patient's nose.[18]

With the tube in place, the stomach is lavaged with water until the aspirate is clear.[6, 21] If the bleeding is not controlled, the esophageal balloon is inflated to 30 to 40 mm Hg.[2, 41]

The pressure in the esophageal balloon must be calibrated carefully (Fig. 52–4). To inflate the esophageal balloon, the operator inserts one end of a Y connector into the correct lumen opening. A mercury manometer is attached to the other end of the Y connector, and the balloon is inflated until a reading of 30 to 40 mm Hg is attained. The esophageal tubing is then double-clamped.[41]

The pressure in the esophageal balloon varies with respiration. Esophageal spasm and intermittent variations of up to 30 mm Hg above the baseline are acceptable, as long as the pressure returns to 30 to 40 mm Hg in the steady state.

At this point, if the original version of the Sengstaken-Blakemore tube is being used (without the Boyce adaptation) a 14 to 16 French nasogastric tube is passed through the other external nares into the esophagus until it is felt to abut the upper portion of the esophageal balloon.[17] As noted in the preparation section, the nasogastric tube should be measured against the Sengstaken-Blakemore tube before either tube is inserted to ensure that the nasogastric tube is placed above the esophageal balloon.[33] The nasogastric tube is attached to intermittent suction. Oral, nasal, and pharyngeal secretions in excess of 1500 ml per day make suction proximal to the esophageal balloon mandatory to prevent aspiration. The nasogastric tube should be passed even if the esophageal balloon is not inflated, because the inflated gastric balloon does not allow the patient to swallow secretions. Obviously, with either a Linton-Nachlas tube or the Boyce modification of the Sengstaken-Blakemore tube, no extra nasogastric tube is needed.

Once passed, the tube is not disturbed for 24 hours in the absence of complications. During this time, adjunctive therapy and work-up are instituted. If bleeding does not abate, other methods must be considered. It is difficult for most patients to tolerate these tubes for more than a few hours without narcotics or other forms of sedation. Meperidine sedation is acceptable, but one should be careful not to induce respiratory depression. Soft restraints may be needed to prevent the patient from dislodging the tube.

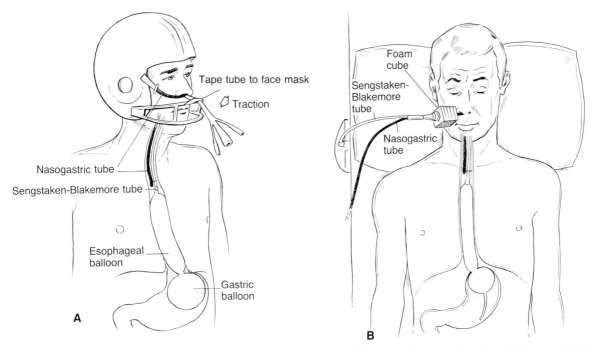

Figure 52–3. *A,* Traction is maintained on the inflated Sengstaken-Blakemore tube by taping the proximal end to the face mask of a football helmet. *B,* An alternative is to split a foam cube in half and run the tube through the center.

COMPLICATIONS

The complications from the use of the Sengstaken-Blakemore and Linton-Nachlas tubes are numerous and are listed as major or minor. Major complications are airway obstruction, aspiration, and esophageal injury. The incidence of major complications from use of the Sengstaken-Blakemore tube generally ranges from 8 to 16 per cent.[2, 15, 21, 27] The mortality directly related to use of the Sengstaken-

Blakemore tube is generally listed at 3 to 3.7 per cent,[15, 21] although one study claims that the tube was a direct cause of death in 22 per cent of the patients on whom it was used.[6] Bleeding from esophageal varices carries a 50 to 80 per cent mortality overall.[3, 23] The best marker of long-term survival seems to be early stabilization.[42] The quality of emergency care is therefore critical in these patients.

Aspiration pneumonitis is the most frequent major complication. Aspiration may result from secretions accu-

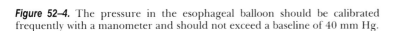

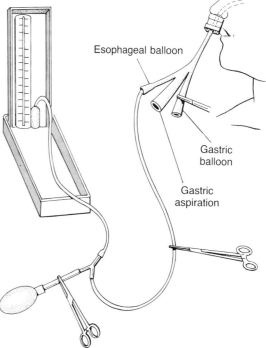

Figure 52–4. The pressure in the esophageal balloon should be calibrated frequently with a manometer and should not exceed a baseline of 40 mm Hg.

mulating in the esophagus or from regurgitation of gastric contents.[2, 11, 21, 27, 30] Death has been reported from aspiration of bloody gastric contents,[2, 18, 40] and the stomach should be emptied before passage of the balloon is attempted.[2, 18] Other major complications include esophageal laceration caused by overinflation of a misplaced gastric balloon[6, 11, 12, 18, 40] (especially in the distal esophagus),[27] esophageal rupture[2, 6] with mediastinitis,[27] and esophageal necrosis caused by excessive or prolonged pressure by the esophageal balloon.[11] One may prevent esophageal necrosis by deflating the balloons intermittently at 6-hour intervals. Death from hemorrhage at the site of esophageal erosion has been reported.[2] Injuries to the esophagus occur more frequently after 24 hours of tamponade.

Airway obstruction can occur with dislodgment of an underinflated gastric balloon and can produce asphyxiation.[2, 16] If this happens, one should divide the tube immediately and extract it. Inadvertent slow deflation or rupture of the gastric balloon may make it possible for the esophageal balloon to slip proximally until it obstructs the airway at the oropharynx or the larynx.[5, 40]

The tubes may fail to control the bleeding.[2] Correctable causes for this include misplaced balloons, inadequate tamponade, and misdiagnosis of the site of bleeding (e.g., duodenal ulcer).[3, 11, 40] Uncommon complications of concern are bilateral hemothorax, jejunal rupture with a Sengstaken-Blakemore tube placed in the efferent jejunal limb of a gastrojejunostomy (rare),[43] innominate vein obstruction by esophageal tamponade,[44] and duodenal perforation due to inadvertent balloon inflation in the duodenum.[45] Tracheoesophageal fistula with fatal hemoptysis has developed following repeated Sengstaken-Blakemore tube insertion.[46]

Minor complications include retrosternal discomfort and chest pain,[27, 31] agitation,[27] gastric erosion, ulcerations at the cardioesophageal junction,[27] epistaxis,[40] deep erosions of the pharynx,[40] and submucosal esophageal hemorrhage. Other minor complications are the inability to pass the Sengstaken-Blakemore tube because of local swelling or muscle spasm or because the patient does not cooperate,[40] coiling of the tube in the stomach or the esophagus,[40] hiccups,[18] and temporary balloon deflation.[18]

The diaphragm may relax following placement, allowing the tube to become dislodged. It is necessary to reassess the position of the tube at frequent intervals to ensure proper and safe use.

CONCLUSION

Gastroesophageal balloon tamponade is an effective way to temporarily control hemorrhage from gastric or esophageal varices. Both single- and double-balloon tubes are useful in conjunction with a method to control oropharyngeal secretions.

Because of the high incidence of serious complications, the procedure should be used only when there is a high risk of exsanguination and when more conservative methods to control hemorrhage have failed.

REFERENCES

1. Westphal K: Über eine Kompressionsbehandlung der Blutungen aus Ösophagusvarizen. Dtsch Med Wochenschr 56:1135, 1930.
2. Bauer JJ, Kreel I, Kark AE: The use of the Sengstaken-Blakemore tube for immediate control of bleeding esophageal varices. Ann Surg 179:273, 1974.
3. Hanna SS, Warren WD, Galambos JT, et al: Bleeding varices: Emergency management. Can Med Assoc J 124:29, 1981.
4. Sengstaken RW, Blakemore AH: Balloon tamponade for the control of hemorrhage from esophageal varices. Ann Surg 131:781, 1950.
5. Burcharth F, Malstrom J: Experiences with the Linton-Nachlas and the Sengstaken-Blakemore tubes for bleeding esophageal varices. Surg Gynecol Obstet 142:529, 1976.
6. Conn HO, Simpson JA: Excessive mortality associated with balloon tamponade of bleeding varices: A critical reappraisal. JAMA 202:587, 1967.
7. Boyce HW Jr: Modification of the Sengstaken-Blakemore balloon tube. N Engl J Med 267:195, 1962.
8. Edlich RF, Lande AJ, Goodale RL, et al: Prevention of aspiration pneumonia by continuous esophageal aspiration during esophagogastric tamponade and gastric cooling. Surgery 64:405, 1968.
9. Idezuki Y, Hagiwara M, Wantanbe H: Endoscopic balloon tamponade for emergency control of bleeding esophageal varices using a new transparent tamponade tube. Am Soc Artif Intern Organs 23:646, 1977.
10. Kline JJ: Modification of the adult Blakemore tube for use in children with bleeding esophageal varices. J Pediatr Gastroenterol Nutr 5:153, 1986.
11. Schwartz GR, Safar P, Stone JH, et al (eds): The Principles and Practice of Emergency Medicine. Philadelphia, WB Saunders Co, 1978, pp 1024–1026.
12. Joelsson B, Borjesson C, Carlsson C, et al: Acute treatment of bleeding oesophageal varices: A retrospective study of 88 patients. Scand J Gastroenterol 16:81, 1981.
13. Johnson AG: Injection sclerotherapy in the emergency and elective treatment of oesophageal varices. Ann R Coll Surg Engl 59:497, 1977.
14. Orloff MJ: Emergency treatment of variceal hemorrhage. Can J Surg 22:550, 1979.
15. Schiff L, Schiff ER: Diseases of the Liver. 5th ed. Philadelphia, JB Lippincott Co, 1982, pp 894–902.
16. Butler ML: Variceal hemorrhage: A review. Milit Med 145:766, 1980.
17. Holman JM, Rikkers LF: Success of medical and surgical management of acute variceal hemorrhage. Am J Surg 140:816, 1980.
18. Pitcher JL: Safety and effectiveness of the modified Sengstaken-Blakemore tube: A prospective study. Gastroenterology 61:291, 1971.
19. Terblanche J: Treatment of Esophageal Varices by Injection Sclerotherapy. Chicago, Year Book Medical Publishers, 1981, pp 257–267.
20. Fischer JE: Portal hypertension and bleeding esophageal varices. Am J Surg 140:337, 1980.
21. Hermann RE, Traul D: Experience with the Sengstaken-Blakemore tube for bleeding esophageal varices. Surg Gynecol Obstet 130:879, 1970.
22. Nabseth DC, Johnson WC, Widrich WC, et al: Bleeding esophageal varices: Treatment by embolization and shunting. Jpn J Surg 11:8, 1981.
23. O'Donnell TF Jr, Gembarowics RM, Callow AD, et al: The economic impact of acute variceal bleeding: Cost-effectiveness implications for medical and surgical therapy. Surgery 88:693, 1980.
24. Sagar S, Harrison ID, Brearley R, et al: Emergency treatment of variceal hemorrhage. Br J Surg 66:824, 1979.
25. Gembarowics RM, Kelly JJ, O'Donnell TF, et al: Management of variceal hemorrhage: Results of a standardized protocol using vasopressin and transhepatic embolization. Arch Surg 115:1160, 1980.
26. Osborn DR, Hobbs KEF: The acute treatment of hemorrhage from oesophageal varices: A comparison of oesophageal transection and staple gun anastomosis with mesocaval shunt. Br J Surg 68:734, 1981.
27. Chojkier M, Conn HO: Esophageal tamponade in the treatment of bleeding varices: A decadal progress report. Dig Dis Sci 25:267, 1980.
28. Feneyrou B, Hanana J, Daures JP, et al: Initial control of bleeding from esophageal varices with the Sengstaken-Blakemore tube. Am J Surg 155:509, 1988.
29. Agger P, Andersen JR, Burcharth F: Does the oesophageal balloon compress oesophageal varices? Scand J Gastroenterol 13:225, 1978.
30. Hennessy TP, Stephens RB, Keane FFB: Acute and chronic management of esophageal varices by injection sclerotherapy. Surg Gynecol Obstet 154:375, 1982.
31. Barsoum MS, Bolous FI, El-Rooby AA, et al: Tamponade and injection sclerotherapy in the management of bleeding oesophageal varices. Br J Surg 69:76, 1982.
32. Terblanche J, Yakoob HI, Bornman PC, et al: Acute bleeding varices: A five-year prospective evaluation of tamponade and sclerotherapy. Ann Surg 194:521, 1981.
33. Jamieson GG, Faris IB, Ludbrook J: A selective approach to bleeding esophageal varices. Henry Ford Hosp Med J 28:210, 1980.
34. Johnston GW: Bleeding oesophageal varices: The management of shunt rejects. Ann R Coll Surg Engl 63:3, 1981.
35. Smith PM, Jones DB: Control of oesophageal variceal bleeding (letter). Lancet 2:747, 1980.
36. Johnson WC, Nabseth DC, Widrich WC, et al: Bleeding esophageal varices: Treatment with vasopressin, transhepatic embolization and selective splenorenal shunting. Ann Surg 195:393, 1982.
37. Matory WE, Sedgwick CE, Rossi RL: Non-shunting procedures in management of bleeding esophageal varices. Surg Clin North Am 60:281, 1980.
38. Taylor TV, Neilson JM: "Currents and clots"—an approach to the problem of acute cariveal bleeding. Br J Surg 68:692, 1981.
39. Teres J, Cecilia A, Bordas JM, et al: Esophageal tamponade for bleeding varices: A controlled trial between the Sengstaken-Blakemore tube and the Linton-Nachlas tube. Gastroenterology 75:566, 1978.

40. Conn HO: Hazards attending the use of esophageal tamponade. N Engl J Med 259:701, 1958.
41. Jackson EW: Nursing Photobook: Performing GI Procedures. Horsham, Pa, Intermed Communications, 1981, pp 33–37.
42. Smith JL, Graham DY: Variceal hemorrhage: A critical evaluation of survival analysis. Gastroenterology 82:968, 1982.
43. Goff JS, Thompson JS, Pratt CF, et al: Jejunal rupture caused by a Sengstaken-Blakemore tube. Gastroenterology 82:573, 1982.
44. Juffe A, Tellez G, Eguaras MG, et al: Unusual complication of the Sengstaken-Blakemore tube. Gastroenterology 72:724, 1977.
45. Kandel G, Gray R, Mackenzie RL, et al: Duodenal perforation by a Linton-Nachlas balloon tube. Am J Gastroenterol 83:492, 1988.
46. Akgun S, Lee DW, Weissman PS, et al: Hemoptysis and tracheoesophageal fistula in a patient with esophageal varices and Sengstaken-Blakemore tube. Am J Med 85:450, 1988.

Chapter 53

Gastric Lavage in the Poisoned Patient

Dan Tandberg and William G. Troutman

INTRODUCTION

At least 2 million cases of accidental and intentional poisoning occur each year in the United States.[1] Some of the patients die, and others who survive are left with permanent disabilities. In one report, approximately 1 per cent of all patients seen in an emergency department were suffering from acute drug overdose[2]; in another series, self-poisoned patients represented 20 per cent of all adult hospital admissions.[3] The diagnosis and management of acute poisoning in children and adults are a common problem and require that physicians caring for these patients be expert in the procedures used in their management.

After initial stabilization of the acutely poisoned patient, an attempt is usually made to diminish further absorption of any ingested toxin from the gastrointestinal tract.[4–10] Methods for accomplishing this include ipecac-induced emesis, gastric lavage, administration of activated charcoal, administration of cathartics, whole bowel irrigation, and rarely, gastrotomy. Although only 3 per cent of reported poisoning cases are managed with gastric lavage, 10 per cent of those patients treated in health care facilities undergo this procedure.[1] This chapter focuses on gastric lavage and discusses its development, its indications and contraindications, the technical aspects of the procedure, and its complications.

BACKGROUND

The use of a hollow tube to evacuate poison from a patient's stomach dates from the early 1800s and has been thoroughly reviewed by Major.[11] In 1810, Dupuytren demonstrated that a rubber tube could be used to remove opium from the stomach of poisoned dogs. Phillip Syng Physick, the father of American surgery, used a long, flexible, hollow tube to remove accidental overdoses of laudanum (opium in alcohol) from the stomach of two infants suffering from whooping cough and reported his results in 1812. A dramatic demonstration of the efficacy of gastric lavage in adults took place in 1822 when Edward Jukes, an English surgeon, tested the procedure on himself after purposefully ingesting a potentially lethal dose of laudanum. He used an elastic gum rubber catheter 25 inches long and one-half inch in diameter attached to an elastic bottle. Warm water was introduced into his stomach and was then removed. Jukes became somewhat nauseated and slept deeply for 3 hours afterward, but suffered no serious after-effects.

Kussmaul, who is commonly credited with inventing gastric lavage for the treatment of poisoning, did much to popularize its use after his 1869 publication.[12] During the next 75 years, gastric lavage was widely held to be the most effective procedure for emptying the stomach of an acutely poisoned patient.

The safety and efficacy of gastric lavage were called into question after the investigative work of Harstad and coworkers was published in 1942.[13] These investigators studied 80 patients suffering from severe poisoning with unknown quantities of phenobarbital or other sedative drugs. They found that in only five of their 80 patients could more than 500 mg of drug be recovered in the gastric washings. In addition, they reported that in some of the patients who died, particles of previously administered activated charcoal could be found in the respiratory tract, suggesting that aspiration of gastric contents had occurred. It was concluded that gastric lavage was relatively ineffective and potentially unsafe. Unfortunately, there were a number of methodologic problems with this study: The size of the stomach tube was not specified, the assay method used (crystallization) was crude and nonquantitative, and the positioning of patients may not have been optimal. In addition, the patients' airways were often unprotected during the procedure. As a result of this study, gastric lavage fell into some disrepute and was thereafter performed less often at many medical centers.[14, 15] This was accompanied by a growing interest in the use of induced emesis as a means of evacuating the stomach in poisoned patients.

Some sources have advocated mechanically induced emesis, but this method was shown to be relatively ineffective by Dabbous and associates.[16] In their study of 30 children poisoned with various substances, gagging the patient with a finger or a tongue blade resulted in emesis in only four of the 30. The use of hypertonic saline to induce emesis fell into disfavor after reports of multiple cases of severe hypernatremia and several deaths in children.[17–21]

Historically, copper sulfate has been advocated as an emetic in poisoning and has been shown to induce vomiting in more than 90 per cent of patients treated.[22] The corrosive complications of this agent together with the possibility of systemic absorption, however, resulted in its being rejected as a clinically useful emetic agent.[23–26]

Parenteral apomorphine has been shown to be an effective emetic in children and adults.[27, 28] MacLean, however, found that many patients treated with apomorphine developed central nervous system depression and concluded that the use of this drug represented an unnecessary risk.[29] This problem, together with the fact that ipecac syrup could be given in the home and did not require parenteral administration, resulted in the widespread acceptance of ipecac syrup as the emetic of choice in acute poisoning.[30–35]

The 1950s saw the beginning of a controversy regarding the relative efficacy of gastric lavage versus ipecac-induced emesis that persists to this day.[36, 37] In 1959, Arnold and his colleagues administered broken sodium salicylate tablets to dogs and found that ipecac-induced emesis produced an average recovery of 45 per cent, whereas gastric lavage recovered only 38 per cent of the administered dose.[38] Unfortunately, lavage was carried out with a 16 French gastric tube, and positioning of the dogs may not have been optimal in this study. Abdallah and Tye carried out a similar experiment in dogs using liquid barium sulfate as a tracer.[39] They found that 62 per cent of the barium could be recovered with immediately administered ipecac, whereas 54 per cent was recovered with immediate lavage. In a third animal study, six mongrel puppies were given 1 gm of barium sulfate in two gelatin capsules and were then treated with gastric lavage, ipecac syrup, or apomorphine on three separate occasions.[40] After a delay of 20 minutes, lavage resulted in a recovery rate averaging 29 per cent compared with a 19 per cent recovery rate in the animals treated with ipecac-induced emesis. Again, the diameter of the tube and the positioning of the dogs impair the usefulness of the study. Furthermore, there is some question whether syrup of ipecac has comparable efficacy in dogs and in humans. Thus animal evidence cannot show conclusively the superiority of one method over the other.

Boxer and colleagues studied the ipecac versus lavage problem in children who had ingested aspirin in unknown amounts.[41] Their 17 patients were randomized to be treated with ipecac-induced emesis followed by gastric lavage or to undergo gastric lavage followed by ipecac-induced emesis. The relative quantities of drug retrieved by each method were then compared for each patient, and a ratio was established. More drug was apparently removed by induced emesis than by lavage, but the precise details of the lavage technique used in this study were not specified. Particularly important omissions from the report included specifications of the gastric tube diameter, the patient's position, the lavage solution volume, and the time delay before instituting treatment. Finally, only negligible amounts of aspirin were removed by either method.

In a series of 259 severely poisoned patients, Matthew and colleagues showed that carefully performed gastric lavage could remove clinically important amounts of ingested drug.[42] Because the actual ingested dose was never known for certain, however, the true efficacy of gastric lavage could not be determined precisely. In another study, Burke performed gastric lavage in ten adult volunteers undergoing general anesthesia for elective bronchoscopy.[43] There is convincing radiographic evidence in this study that water-soluble radiopaque dye can be removed from the stomach if a large gastric tube is used and careful attention is paid to lavage technique and to positioning of the patient. Burke reported an 84 per cent recovery rate but, unfortunately, did not present enough quantitative data to substantiate this figure.

Tandberg and associates attempted to settle this controversy by administering 25 100 μg cyanocobalamin tablets as a tracer to 18 normal adult human volunteers on 2 separate days in a clinical research center.[44] Ipecac-induced emesis was carried out on one occasion and was initiated 10 minutes after ingestion of the tracer. Gastric lavage was carried out on another day, also beginning 10 minutes after tracer ingestion. A modified 32 French orogastric tube, 250-ml aliquots of saline, and a total of 3 liters of lavage fluid was used. Total cobalt recovery from the collected vomitus and lavage returns was measured by atomic adsorption spectrophotometry. A mean of only 28 per cent (6 to 70 per cent) of the administered cobalt tracer was recovered by ipecac-induced emesis, whereas 45 per cent (19 to 68 per cent) was recovered with gastric lavage. (Note the wide range in recovery amount in each group.) These recovery rates are disappointing, especially in view of the short time to the initiation of gastric emptying, the absence of other materials in the stomach, and the optimal circumstances of the procedures.

Auerbach and his colleagues attempted to measure the efficacy of the two procedures using actual patients.[45] In their study, 51 poisoned patients were given liquid thiamine by mouth (mixed with ipecac). Another group of 37 patients was given thiamine by 24 French gastric tube before starting gastric lavage. Thiamine was assayed in the vomitus and lavage specimens by high-performance liquid chromatography. Gastric lavage produced a 90 per cent recovery rate, whereas ipecac yielded only a 50 per cent return rate. A major weakness of this study is that a liquid tracer was used so that these results may not apply to solid ingestants. Furthermore, recovery of more thiamine than was administered in 28 per cent of the patients (and 57 per cent of the lavage patients) suggests that thiamine may not have been an optimal choice as a tracer. Two additional prospective studies in human volunteers have been unable to detect a difference in tracer recovery when 60 minutes were allowed to elapse between tracer administration and commencement of ipecac-induced emesis or gastric lavage.[46, 47]

In summary, the data on gastric emptying are conflicting and difficult to interpret. *In any given circumstance or individual it is probably impossible to predict which procedure will most effectively accomplish gastric decontamination.* However, our interpretation of the currently available evidence in humans is that gastric lavage is more efficient than ipecac-induced emesis for removal of swallowed solid materials but that this advantage only exists if a relatively brief time (less than an hour) has passed since the ingestion. One of the strongest arguments to support lavage over emesis is that the procedure can be done immediately on presentation to the emergency department (negating the 15- to 20-minute delay for ipecac to produce emesis),

and charcoal can be instilled to immediately limit further absorption. This immediacy of emptying may indeed provide a real benefit to patients who have taken a truly lethal overdose.

INDICATIONS AND CONTRAINDICATIONS

The decision to use ipecac-induced emesis, gastric lavage, activated charcoal alone, or other gastrointestinal decontamination procedures in a given instance should be based on the clinical condition of the patient and the history of what was ingested. Ongoing studies are providing evidence that may change the indications for gastric emptying in the future. A number of papers suggest that activated charcoal alone may be equal or superior to ipecac-induced emesis[48–54] and even equal to gastric lavage, especially if there is much delay in therapy.[46, 47, 55] And newer therapies such as whole bowel irrigation,[56, 57] repetitive dose charcoal, and superactivated charcoal[58, 59] may prove equal or superior to traditional gastric emptying methods. Because the topic of gastrointestinal decontamination in the management of acute poisoning has attracted the renewed attention of researchers, it is important that the clinician keep abreast of this evolving literature.

Most experts agree that gastric emptying should be avoided in patients with a clear history of ingestion of an inconsequential amount of toxic substance or ingestion of a nontoxic substance. Attempting to administer ipecac syrup to agitated or uncooperative patients is not likely to be successful and merely delays eventual gastric lavage or charcoal administration. One should not waste valuable time attempting to cajole an uncooperative patient into drinking ipecac.

If the decision is made to empty the patient's stomach by induced emesis or gastric lavage, then the patient's level of consciousness is the most important factor to consider. (It is surprising that normal volunteers who have undergone both induced emesis and gastric lavage in a research setting rate them as equally unpleasant.[60] Thus, anticipated discomfort of the patient should not be a selection criterion.) Patients who are not alert enough to hold the medicine cup unaided should undergo gastric lavage rather than induced emesis. Ipecac-induced emesis should be avoided in patients likely to have diminished airway-protective reflexes; gastric lavage with a cuffed endotracheal tube in place should be carried out instead. Such patients include those with depressed sensorium, diminished gag reflex, absent lid reflex, or seizures.[61] Also, emesis should not be induced in conscious patients who have ingested drugs that are likely to rapidly produce coma or seizures (e.g., sedative-hypnotics, cyclic antidepressants, cyanide, camphor, strychnine). The use of depolarizing or nondepolarizing muscle relaxants may be required to intubate the combative, confused, or obtunded patient.[62]

Traditionally, ipecac-induced emesis has not been recommended in cases of poisoning with phenothiazines or other antiemetics because it was thought that the antiemetic effects of these drugs would make induced emesis ineffective. It has since been shown, however, that approximately 95 per cent of patients treated with ipecac vomit even after antiemetic poisoning.[63, 64] Ipecac-induced emesis should be used cautiously in patients poisoned with phenothiazines, however, because of the risk of dystonic reactions involving the face and neck, which can produce vomiting against a tightly clenched jaw with subsequent pulmonary aspiration of gastric contents. This risk has led one major phenothiazine manufacturer to include a warning against the use of ipecac-induced emesis in its product literature.[65]

The delay between ingestion of the poison and initiation of gastric emptying is also an important consideration. For rapidly absorbed drugs, such as the short-acting barbiturates, older evidence suggests that attempts at gastric emptying more than 4 hours from the time of ingestion are not likely to be of clinical value.[42] More recently, the prospective randomized study of clinical outcome in 592 poisoned patients by Kulig and colleagues showed improved outcome with gastric lavage (compared with that from activated charcoal alone), but only in that subset of patients who were both obtunded and seen within 1 hour of their ingestion.[48] This study and others also suggest that ipecac-induced emesis does not appear to offer any advantage in clinical outcome over activated charcoal alone.[48–50, 55]

Theoretically, many drugs could be retrieved in clinically important amounts more than 1 hour after ingestion. Physiologic gastric emptying is especially likely to be delayed in patients with diminished or absent bowel sounds; with radiographic evidence of poison in the stomach; with a history of ingestion of drugs that have anticholinergic properties (e.g., cyclic antidepressants, antihistamines); or who have ingested large amounts of relatively insoluble drug such as aspirin, ferrous salts, or sustained release preparations.[42, 66] A meal immediately preceding the ingestion may further delay gastric emptying. Finally, the history given by the patient of the time when the ingestion occurred is notoriously inaccurate. Thus many clinicians continue to use gastric lavage in some patients in whom the initial history of the time from ingestion is uncertain.

Another important consideration is the possibility that semisolid masses of drug (bezoars) can form in the stomach and remain there for long periods. These may sometimes be removed by repeated gastric lavage with a large-bore tube following abdominal massage, but in some cases endoscopy, or even gastrotomy, may be required.[67–71]

The possible ingestion of strong alkalis is also a contraindication to both induced emesis and gastric lavage. The esophageal and gastric burns associated with alkali ingestion occur within minutes, and attempts at gastric intubation or the forceful vomiting produced by ipecac syrup may result in serious esophageal injury or even perforation.[72]

The ingestion of strong acids rarely produces severe esophageal injury, however, but subsequently may cause deep burns of the stomach and the duodenum. Continued injury for as long as 90 minutes has been demonstrated in experimental animals[73] and suggests that rapid removal of the ingested acid could be beneficial. Because no esophageal perforation has ever been reported in acid-poisoned patients treated with gastric lavage, this would seem to be the procedure of choice until further evidence is available.[74]

The management of patients who have ingested a hydrocarbon chemical is complicated by the broad range of compounds covered by that label and by the significant controversy that surrounds the selection of a treatment technique. On the one hand, a hydrocarbon product that also contains other toxic chemicals (e.g., pesticides, heavy metals, halogenated aromatic compounds, camphor) must be removed from the gastrointestinal tract promptly. On the other hand, there is no evidence to support the removal of very viscous and relatively nontoxic hydrocarbon products, such as petroleum jelly, grease, paint, or motor oil. Some debate centers on what to do with ingestions of products falling between these two extremes, such as gasoline, kerosene, turpentine, and charcoal lighter fluid.

The most serious complication of hydrocarbon ingestion is the development of a chemical pneumonitis. This complication is much more likely to occur with low-viscosity hydrocarbons. Obviously, one would expect pneumonitis to result from aspiration of the product, but for some time it was believed that hydrocarbons could also produce pulmonary toxicity by reaching the lungs through the blood stream.[75] This assumption placed a high priority on the evacuation of hydrocarbons from the gastrointestinal tract. More recent evidence suggests that pulmonary toxicity is highly unlikely unless aspiration occurs[76] and that aspiration may pose a threat that is more than 100 times greater than that posed by an uncomplicated ingestion.[77–79]

In the past, the decision to remove a hydrocarbon from the stomach was based on an arbitrary cutoff value of 1 ml/kg. This value was established subjectively,[80] and animal data suggest that as much as 20 times this amount can be tolerated safely.[76] Most treatment guidelines have abandoned the arbitrary 1 ml/kg value.[81]

Gastric lavage has long been recognized as having little effect on the clinical outcome in hydrocarbon ingestion cases.[82] Ipecac-induced emesis would be expected to have a comparable lack of impact. Ng and coworkers found a higher incidence of pulmonary radiographic changes in cases of hydrocarbon ingestion treated with gastric lavage than in cases treated with ipecac-induced emesis, but this report lacks certain methodologic details (e.g., efforts that were made to protect the airway) that are necessary to permit the drawing of significant conclusions.[83]

The small quantities of hydrocarbons usually ingested by children[84] do not need to be removed from the stomach unless the product contains a particularly toxic component. In addition, gastric emptying is not recommended for adults who ingest aliphatic hydrocarbons (e.g., gasoline, kerosene, turpentine, mineral spirits, charcoal lighter fluid, trichloroethane), because these substances do not produce serious systemic toxicity even when ingested in large amounts. Pulmonary aspiration of these substances that may occur during gastric emptying can be disastrous. The regional poison center can often be of great help in determining if gastric emptying is indicated, especially when unusual or exotic hydrocarbon products are involved.

EQUIPMENT AND PROCEDURE

If the decision is made to perform gastric lavage, careful attention to the details of the procedure results in increased safety for the patient and more effective removal of the ingested poison.

Before initiation of gastric lavage, the airway should be protected with a cuffed endotracheal tube if the level of consciousness is depressed or the patient's airway-protective reflexes are diminished. The traditional way to test for this is to stimulate the posterior pharynx with a tongue blade or a cotton-tipped applicator. The lack of a grimace or blink reflex after touching the eyelashes is strong evidence for an unprotected airway and the need to intubate the trachea before gastric lavage.[61] A cautious trial of endotracheal intubation may be used in questionable cases; the patient who tolerates the procedure probably needs it. If patients are fully alert and awake, lavage may be done without tracheal intubation. However, if vomiting occurs during lavage, the tube should be withdrawn immediately to allow the patient to protect the airway through normal mechanisms.

The position of the patient during gastric lavage is important. All patients should be placed in the left lateral decubitus position with the head down. This position diminishes the passage of gastric contents into the duodenum during lavage, a fact that has been well documented by fluoroscopy during the procedure[43] (Fig. 53–1). In addition, positioning the patient's body with the head lowered approximately 10 degrees probably decreases the risk of pul-

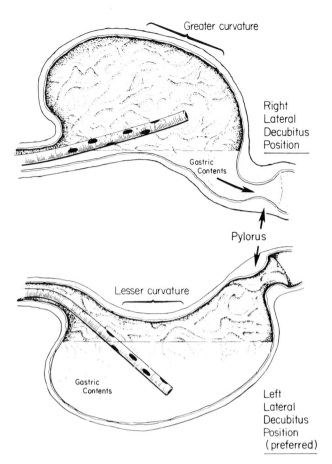

Figure 53–1. The effect of patient positioning on gastric lavage.

monary aspiration of gastric contents should vomiting or retching occur. The uncooperative patient's hands should be restrained to prevent removal of the gastric or endotracheal tube.

Large-diameter gastric hoses with extra holes cut near the tip are recommended for gastric lavage (Fig. 53–2). There are no convincing data on humans to refute or support this recommendation, and one study of a small number of dogs failed to show any difference in efficacy with lavage through a 32 French tube compared with a 16 French lavage tube.[85] It is generally held that large-diameter nasogastric or orogastric tubes (greater than 1 cm) are more likely to retrieve particulate matter successfully. Also,

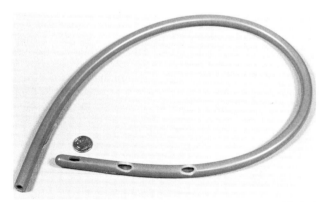

Figure 53–2. A large diameter gastric tube. Note the extra side holes that have been cut near the tip.

smaller, more flexible tubes may kink and are significantly more difficult to pass.[86] A 32 to 50 French tube is usually recommended for adults. Before passage, the length of the tube required to enter the stomach should be estimated by approximating the distance from the nose to the midepigastrium; premeasurement avoids the curling and kinking of excess hose in the stomach. Failure to premeasure a tube before passage is a common error (Fig. 53–3).

The gastric tube should be passed gently to avoid damage to the nose or the posterior pharynx. It may be passed through either the nose or the mouth, although tubes of 36 French size or larger should be passed orally to avoid nasal mucosal or turbinate injury. Passage through the mouth is generally more comfortable for the patient, but the inserter is in danger of being bitten when this technique is used. In addition, orogastric tubes tend to be chewed and occluded by stuporous or combative patients. These problems may be minimized by the concomitant use of a bite block or an oral airway. Elliptically shaped endoscopy bite blocks are recommended.

Nasogastric intubation with larger diameter tubes can be carried out more easily if lubricating or local anesthetic jelly is used; shrinkage of the nasal mucosa with phenylephrine (Neo-Synephrine) is advised. Passage of the tube into the esophagus once the pharynx has been entered can be facilitated by putting the patient's chin on the chest. Should cough, stridor, or cyanosis occur, the tube has entered the trachea; it should be withdrawn immediately and passage reattempted. Once the tube is passed, its intragastric location should be confirmed by auscultation of the stomach during injection of air with a 50-ml syringe. If this step is omitted, the physician may occasionally irrigate the esophagus with a tube that has doubled back on itself during passage or, worse, lavage the patient's lungs.

Before gastric irrigation, a large fraction of the gastric contents can be removed by careful gastric aspiration with repeated repositioning of the tube tip. Only after the stomach has been thoroughly "vacuumed" should gastric lavage be carried out, because aspiration of gastric contents may be the most effective part of the procedure.[42, 43, 66] At this point the tube should be taped in place.

The aliquots of lavage fluid may be introduced using a syringe or a funnel. The use of a Y connector and clamp makes the procedure even easier (Fig. 53–4). This arrangement can be purchased ready-made (Travenol, Ethox, and others) or can be assembled from inexpensive, readily avail-

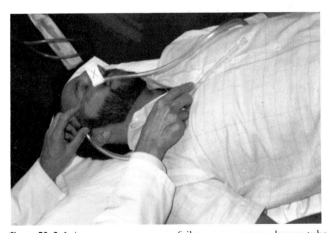

Figure 53–3. It is a common error to fail to premeasure a lavage tube before passage. Here a piece of tape marks the depth of proper passage to ensure that the tip is in the stomach without excess tubing that may hinder fluid egress.

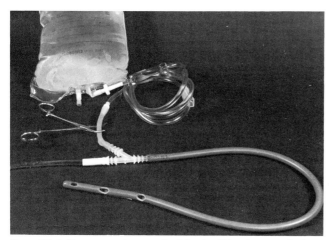

Figure 53–4. One convenient method for instilling lavage solution.

able components. The equipment transforms a messy and difficult task into an efficient procedure that can be performed by one technician or nurse.

Lavage is performed by clamping the drainage arm of the Y adapter and infusing aliquots of fluid into the stomach from a reservoir. The reservoir arm of the Y is then clamped, and the drainage arm is opened to permit gravity drainage of the stomach contents. The procedure is then repeated. Some resistance is produced by the Y connector and tubing. Suction can be applied intermittently to the drainage tubing to enhance stomach emptying. Rudolph has described a device that performs this task automatically.[87]

Severe dilutional hyponatremia has occurred in children lavaged with tap water; physiologic saline is therefore generally recommended.[88] Tap water appears to be a safe lavage solution in adults but may produce measurable decrements in the serum sodium and potassium in some patients.[88] The use of prewarmed (45° C) lavage fluid increases the solubility of most substances, delays gastric emptying, and theoretically should increase the effectiveness of the procedure.[89, 90] In addition, the use of prewarmed fluid diminishes the risk of lowering the patient's body temperature. Small aliquots of lavage solution should be repeatedly introduced into the stomach and removed. The recommended volume of each aliquot is usually 200 ml in adults and 10 ml/kg in children. Larger amounts may increase the risk that the gastric contents will be washed into the duodenum, and much smaller amounts are not clinically practical because of the dead space in the tubing (approximately 50 ml in the 36 French hose) and the increase in time that is required. The amount that is returned is always slightly less than the amount that is introduced. The fluid should flow in freely and drain easily by gravity. If this does not occur, the tube is usually malpositioned or kinked in the stomach, and it should be withdrawn or advanced a few centimeters. Manual agitation

of the patient's stomach before removal of each aliquot may increase recovery and is recommended.[90] This is done by gently "kneading" the stomach with a hand placed on the abdominal wall.

We recommend continuation of lavage for at least 3 liters after the returns are clear by visual inspection. No careful study exists regarding the optimal total volume of lavage solution to be used, and the variation in recommendations regarding this question in the literature is considerable. A minimum volume of 3 liters is a practical compromise.

There is in vitro and some anecdotal clinical evidence supporting the use of specific substances in the solution used to lavage patients who have been poisoned with certain toxins (Table 53–1).[91, 92] These "specific" lavage solutions may convert the poison to an insoluble complex or may change it to a less toxic compound. The clinical efficacy of these modes of therapy is generally unproven, but they are widely used. Perhaps the most common example is the use of 1.5 per cent sodium bicarbonate lavage solution in iron-poisoned patients.[93] Patients poisoned by strong acids or bases should not be lavaged with "neutralizing" solution, because heat is produced and further tissue damage may result.[72, 74, 94]

After gastric aspiration and lavage have been completed, a slurry of activated charcoal (1 gm/kg) should be administered through the gastric tube (Fig. 53–5). The use of newer charcoal products with a larger adsorptive surface, termed superactivated charcoal (Superchar®) may be superior to conventional preparations. Unfortunately, not all substances are well absorbed by activated charcoal; major exceptions include alcohols, hydrocarbons, strong alkalis, boric acid, cyanide, ferrous salts, mineral acids, lithium, and carbamate insecticides.[52, 95] Many clinicians administer charcoal in any case, because of the frequent presence of additional unsuspected ingested substances in patients who have taken an overdose. After adsorption of the poison by activated charcoal, most clinicians administer a cathartic to hasten the elimination of the toxin-laden charcoal, but there is little clinical evidence supporting the efficacy of this practice.[51, 52, 96, 97] The osmotic cathartic, sorbitol (2 ml/kg of a 35 per cent solution) produces the most effective catharsis but this should not be used in small children or hypovolemic adults. Activated charcoal is often withheld in cases of suspected acetaminophen poisoning until the need for N-acetylcysteine therapy is determined; however, if charcoal has already been given, gastric lavage may be used to remove it, or the early doses of N-acetylcysteine may be increased.[98–100]

When no longer needed, the gastric tube should be pinched or clamped during its removal to avoid "dribbling" fluid into the airway. With the increasing use of repetitive doses of activated charcoal, the gastric tube is often left in place after the procedure is completed. However, because this large tube is irritating and may predispose to gagging, drooling, or aspiration, the lavage tube should be removed and a standard nasogastric tube inserted for repeat doses of

Substance Ingested	Special Lavage Solution	Remarks
Ferrous salts	1.5% sodium bicarbonate	Forms insoluble ferrous carbonate complex
		Phosphate lavage is no longer recommended
Fluorides	15–30 gm/L calcium gluconate	Forms insoluble calcium fluoride precipitate
Formaldehyde	10 mg/L ammonium acetate	Forms methenamine (much less toxic)
Iodine	80 gm/L cornstarch	
Oxalic acid	15–30 gm/L calcium gluconate	Forms calcium oxalate precipitate

Table 53–1. Examples of Special Lavage Solutions

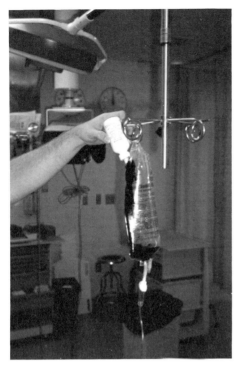

Figure 53–5. A convenient and nonmessy way to administer charcoal through a lavage tube is to cut the end of an empty intravenous infusion bag (used here to provide lavage fluid) and drip it in.

activated charcoal. The endotracheal tube in the intubated patient should not be removed immediately following lavage and charcoal administration; emesis is common after the procedure is finished.

COMPLICATIONS

The complications associated with gastric lavage can be subdivided broadly into those associated with the placement of the tube and those resulting from the lavage fluid itself.

Skillful hands and adequate practice usually allow the physician to place a large gastric tube with minimal trauma. If the nasal route is selected, care must be exercised not to damage the delicate nasal turbinates. We prefer rubber tubes, because they seem to be less traumatic than the harder, stiffer plastic ones. Once the tube has been placed, it is important to make sure that it is in the stomach and not in the lungs, because inadvertent placement of the tube in the lungs can be fatal.[101] A second major concern during gastric lavage is the risk of mucosal injury or perforation of the stomach or lower esophagus.[102–106] This is most commonly encountered in cases in which substantial damage has already been done to these tissues. Alkaline corrosive ingestions represent a situation in which significant esophageal damage can occur, and the risk of perforation is high.[107] Preexisting esophageal stricture or previous gastric bypass surgery also makes tube passage more hazardous.[108]

The lavage fluid itself is a potential but generally inconsequential source of problems. The large amount of fluid used during a lavage procedure has the potential to produce fluid and electrolyte disturbances in the patient; these imbalances have been reported with both hypertonic[109, 110] and hypotonic[88] lavage fluids. These problems appear to be encountered most commonly in children; adults seem to be more resistant to lavage-induced electrolyte disturbances.[88]

Rudolph, however, was unable to document electrolyte changes in 60 patients lavaged with tap water, aged 2 to 94 years.[87] Hypothermia is another possible complication of gastric lavage, leading many pediatricians to warm the lavage fluid after the first liter.

The use of large aliquots of lavage fluid (greater than 300 ml per wash in adults or 10 ml/kg in children) has the potential to force the gastric contents through the pylorus and into the upper small intestine, where more rapid absorption may take place.[111]

Pulmonary aspiration of gastric contents or lavage fluid poses the major potential risk during lavage, although if the lavage is performed properly, this risk should be low. One group reported a 10 per cent incidence of aspiration pneumonia in lavaged patients with careful follow-up.[55] Most of the patients with aspiration pneumonia had been intubated prior to gastric lavage to protect the airway. There were no cases of aspiration in a similar nonlavaged group of overdose patients. It is generally believed that both emesis and gastric lavage increase the incidence of pulmonary radiographic changes in patients who have ingested petroleum distillates or turpentine.[82]

CONCLUSION

Gastric lavage is an old and accepted emergency procedure frequently used by physicians for minimizing the absorption of ingested poisons. A major problem in determining the exact value of gastric lavage in poisoned patients is the difficulty in interpreting the available literature evaluating the efficacy of the procedure compared with alternative therapies. Although the risks associated with properly conducted gastric lavage appear slight, they are measurable, and no patient should undergo gastric lavage unless it is likely that more good than harm will result. These considerations hold true for other gastric emptying procedures as well.

The performance of careful gastric aspiration and lavage requires a great deal more staff and physician time than does ipecac-induced emesis or activated charcoal administration, and in a busy emergency department this consideration often plays a major part in the choice of method. Small children are rarely severely poisoned and are particularly difficult to lavage effectively unless they are obtunded; thus in most instances, ipecac-induced emesis or activated charcoal is used.

REFERENCES

1. Litovitz TL, Schmitz BF, Bailey KM, et al: 1989 annual report of the American Association of Poison Control Centers National Data Collection System. Am J Emerg Med 8:394, 1990.
2. Schernitzki P, Bootman JL, Likes K, et al: Acute drug intoxication at a university hospital: An epidemiological study. Vet Hum Toxicol 22:235, 1980.
3. Smith AJ: Self-poisoning with drugs: A worsening situation. Br Med J 4:157, 1972.
4. Ellenhorn MJ, Barceloux DG: Gut decontamination. In Ellenhorn MJ, Barceloux DG (eds): Medical Toxicology. New York, Elsevier Science Publishing Co, 1988, pp 54–63.
5. Haddad LM, Winchester JF: A general approach to the emergency management of poisoning. In Haddad LM, Winchester JF (eds): Clinical Management of Poisoning and Drug Overdose. Philadelphia, WB Saunders Co, 1983, pp 4–18.
6. Rumack BA, Lovejoy FH: Clinical Toxicology. In Klaassen CD, Amdur MO, Doull J (eds): Casarett and Doull's Toxicology. New York, Macmillan Publishing Co, 1986, pp 879–901.
7. Schwartz GR: Emergency management of the toxicologic patient. In Schwartz GR, Safar P, Stone JH, et al (eds): Principles and Practice of Emergency Medicine. Philadelphia, WB Saunders Co, 1986, pp 1671–1688.
8. Epstein FB, Eilers MA: Poisoning. In Rosen P, Baker FJ, Barkin RM, et al (eds): Emergency Medicine: Concepts and Clinical Practice. St. Louis, CV Mosby Co, 1988, pp 321–362.
9. Hall AH, Rumack BH: Prevention of absorption in overdose. In Calliham ML (ed): Current Therapy in Emergency Medicine. Toronto, Philadelphia, BC Decker Inc, 1987, pp 942–944.
10. Wheeler-Usher DH, Wanke LA, Bayer MJ: Gastric emptying: Risk

versus benefit in the treatment of acute poisoning. Med Toxicol 1:142, 1986.

11. Major RH: History of the stomach tube. Ann Med History 6:500, 1934.
12. Kussmaul A: Über die Behandlung der Magenerweiterung durch eine neue Methode, mittelst der Magenpumpe. Deutsch Arch Klin Med 6:455, 1869.
13. Harstad E, Moller KO, Simesen MH: The value of gastric lavage in the treatment of acute poisoning. Acta Med Scand 112:478, 1942.
14. Value of gastric lavage in treatment of acute poisoning (editorial): JAMA 133:545, 1947.
15. Louw A: Treatment of acute barbituric acid poisoning: Ten years' experience at the centre for the treatment of poisoning in Copenhagen. Dan Med Bull 5:137, 1958.
16. Dabbous IA, Bergman AB, Robertson WO, et al: The ineffectiveness of mechanically induced vomiting. J Pediatr 66:952, 1965.
17. Ward DJ: Fetal hypernatremia after a saline emetic. Br Med J 2:432, 1963.
18. Laurence BH, Hopkins BE: Hypernatremia following a saline emetic. Med J Aust 1:1301, 1969.
19. DeGenaro F, Nyhan WL: Salt—a dangerous antidote. J Pediatr 78:1048, 1971.
20. Robertson WO: A further warning on the use of salt as an emetic agent. J Pediatr 79:877, 1971.
21. Barer J, Hill LL, Hill RM, et al: Fatal poisoning from salt used as an emetic. Am J Dis Child 125:889, 1973.
22. Mellencamp F: Copper sulphate as an emetic. Appl Therap 8:233, 1966.
23. Chuttani HK, et al: Acute copper sulfate poisoning. Am J Med 39:849, 1965.
24. Karlsson B, Noren L: Ipecacuanha and copper sulphate as emetics in intoxications in children. Acta Pediatr Scand 54:331, 1965.
25. Mellencamp F: Copper sulfate as an emetic. Appl Therap 8:233, 1966.
26. Holtzman NA, Haslam RHA: Evaluation of serum copper following copper sulfate as an emetic. Pediatrics 42:189, 1968.
27. Berry FA, Lambdin MA: Apomorphine and levellorphan tartrate in acute poisonings. Am J Dis Child 105:160, 1963.
28. Corby DG, Decker WJ, Moran MJ, et al: Clinical comparison of pharmacologic emetics in children. Pediatrics 42:361, 1968.
29. MacLean WC Jr: A comparison of ipecac syrup and apomorphine in the immediate treatment of ingestion of poisons. J Pediatr 82:121, 1973.
30. Thoman ME: The use of emetics in poison ingestion. Clin Toxicol 3:185, 1970.
31. Shirkey HC: Ipecac syrup. Its use as an emetic in poison control. J Pediatr 69:139, 1966.
32. Abramowicz M: Ipecac syrup and activated charcoal for treatment of poisoning in children. Med Lett Drugs Ther 21:70, 1979.
33. Manno BR, Manno JE: Toxicology of ipecac: A review. Clin Toxicol 10:221, 1977.
34. Robertson WO: Syrup of ipecac—a slow or fast emetic? Am J Dis Child 103:136, 1962.
35. Ilett KF, Gibb GS, Unsworth RW, et al: Syrup of ipecacuanha as an emetic in adults. Med J Aust 2:91, 1977.
36. Matthew H: Gastric aspiration and lavage. Clin Toxicol 3:179, 1970.
37. Meester WD: Emesis and lavage. Vet Hum Toxicol 22:225, 1980.
38. Arnold JA, Hodges JB, Barta RA, et al: Evaluation of the efficacy of lavage and induced emesis in treatment of salicylate poisoning. Pediatrics 23:286, 1959.
39. Abdallah AH, Tye A: A comparison of the efficacy of emetic drugs and stomach lavage. Am J Dis Child 113:571, 1967,
40. Corby DG, Lisciandro RC, Lehman RH, et al: The efficiency of methods used to evacuate the stomach after acute ingestions. Pediatrics 40:871, 1967.
41. Boxer L, Anderson FP, Rowe, DS: Comparison of ipecac-induced emesis with gastric lavage in the treatment of acute salicylate ingestion. J Pediatr 74:800, 1969.
42. Matthew H, Mackintosh TF, Thompsett SL, et al: Gastric aspiration and lavage in acute poisoning. Br Med J 1:1333, 1966.
43. Burke M: Gastric lavage and emesis in the treatment of ingested poisons: A review and a clinical study of lavage in ten adults. Resuscitation 1:91, 1972.
44. Tandberg D, Diven BG, McLeod JW: Ipecac-induced emesis versus gastric lavage: A controlled study in normal adults. Am J Emerg Med 4:205, 1986.
45. Auerbach PS, Osterloh J, Braun O: Efficacy of gastric emptying: Gastric lavage versus emesis induced with ipecac. Ann Emerg Med 15:692, 1986.
46. Tenenbein M, Cohen S, Sitar DS: Efficacy of ipecac-induced emesis, orogastric lavage, and activated charcoal for acute drug overdose. Ann Emerg Med 16:838, 1987.
47. Danel V, Henry JA, Glucksman E: Activated charcoal, emesis, and gastric lavage in aspirin overdose. Br Med J 296:1507, 1988.
48. Kulig K, Bar Or D, Cantrill SV, et al: Management of acutely poisoned patients without gastric emptying. Ann Emerg Med 14:562, 1985.
49. Curtis RA, Barone J, Giacona N: Efficacy of ipecac and activated charcoal/cathartic. Prevention of salicylate absorption in a simulated overdose. Arch Intern Med 144:48, 1984.

50. Tenenbein M: Inefficacy of gastric emptying procedures. J Emerg Med 3:133, 1985.
51. Rosenberg PJ, Livingstone DJ, McLellan BA: Effect of whole-bowel irrigation on the antidotal efficacy of oral activated charcoal. Ann Emerg Med 17:681, 1988.
52. Neuvonen PJ, Olkkola KT: Oral activated charcoal in the treatment of intoxications: Role of single and repeated doses. Med Toxicol 3:33, 1988.
53. Park GD, Spector R, Goldberg MJ, Johnson GF: Expanded role of charcoal therapy in the poisoned and overdosed patient. Arch Intern Med 146:969, 1986.
54. Albertson TE, Derlet RW, Foulke GE, et al: Superiority of activated charcoal alone compared with ipecac and activated charcoal in the treatment of acute toxic ingestions. Ann Emerg Med 18:56, 1989.
55. Merigian KS, Woodard M, Hedges JR, et al: Prospective evaluation of gastric emptying in the self-poisoned patient. Am J Emerg Med 8:479, 1990.
56. Tenenbein M: Whole bowel irrigation in iron poisoning. J Pediatr 111:142, 1987.
57. Tenenbein M: Whole bowel irrigation as a gastrointestinal decontamination procedure after acute poisoning. Med Toxicol 3:77, 1988.
58. Chung DC, Murphy JE, Taylor TW: In-vivo comparison of the adsorption capacity of "superactive charcoal" and fructose with activated charcoal and fructose. J Toxicol Clin Toxicol 19:219, 1982.
59. Jones J, McMullen MJ, Dougherty J, Cannon L: Repetitive doses of activated charcoal in the treatment of poisoning. Am J Emerg Med 5:305, 1987.
60. Tandberg D, Wood DA: Ipecac-induced emesis and gastric lavage are equally unpleasant. Vet Hum Toxicol 30:109, 1988
61. Collins VJ: General anesthesia: Clinical signs. In Collins VJ (ed): Principles of Anesthesiology. 2nd ed. Philadelphia, Lea & Febiger, 1976, pp 253–264.
62. Dronen SC, Merigian KS, Hedges JR, et al: A comparison of blind nasotracheal and succinylcholine assisted intubation in the poisoned patient. Ann Emerg Med 16:650, 1987.
63. Thoman ME: Ipecac syrup in antiemetic ingestion. JAMA 196:147, 1966.
64. Manoguerra AS, Krenzelok EP: Rapid emesis with high-dose ipecac syrup in adults and children intoxicated with antiemetics or other drugs. Am J Hosp Pharm 35:1360, 1978.
65. Thorazine. In Physicians Desk Reference. 36th ed. Oradell, NJ, Medical Economics Co, 1989, pp 2071–2073.
66. Sharman JR, Cretney MJ, Scott RD, et al: Drug overdoses: Is one stomach washing enough? NZ Med J 81:195, 1975.
67. Schwartz HS: Acute meprobamate poisoning with gastrotomy and removal of a drug-containing mass. N Engl J Med 295:1171, 1976.
68. Bartecchi CE: Removal of gastric drug masses. N Engl J Med 296:282, 1977.
69. Sogge MR, Griffith JL, Sinar DR, Mayes GR: Lavage to remove enteric-coated aspirin and gastric outlet obstruction. Ann Intern Med 87:721, 1977.
70. Marsteller HJ, Gugler R: Endoscopic management of toxic masses in the stomach. N Engl J Med 296:1003, 1977.
71. Foxford R: Gastrotomy—a surgical approach to iron overdose. Ann Emerg Med 14:1223, 1985.
72. Kirsh MM, Ritter F: Caustic ingestion and subsequent damage to the oropharyngeal and digestive passages. Ann Thorac Surg 21:74, 1976
73. Ritter FN, Newman MH, Newman DE: A clinical and experimental study of corrosive burns of the stomach. Ann Otol Rhinol Laryngol 77:830, 1968.
74. Penner GE: Acid ingestion: Toxicology and treatment. Ann Emerg Med 9:374, 1980.
75. Diechmann WB, Kitzmiller KV, Witherup BS, Johansmann R: Kerosene intoxication. Ann Intern Med 21:803, 1944.
76. Dice WH, Ward B, Kelley J, Kilpatrick WR: Pulmonary toxicity following gastrointestinal ingestion of kerosene. Ann Emerg Med 11:138, 1982.
77. Richardson JA, Pratt-Thomas HR: Toxic effects of varying doses of kerosene administered by different routes. Am J Med Sci 221:531, 1951.
78. Gerarde HW: Toxicological studies on hydrocarbons. V. Kerosene. Toxicol Appl Pharmacol 1:462, 1959.
79. Gerarde HW: Toxicological studies on hydrocarbons. IX. The aspiration hazard and toxicity of hydrocarbons and hydrocarbon mixtures. Arch Environ Health 6:329, 1963.
80. Mofenson HC, Greensher J: The new correct answer to an old question on kerosene ingestion. Pediatrics 59:788, 1977.
81. Hydrocarbons. In Poisindex. Denver, Colo, Micromedex, 1982.
82. Subcommittee on Accidental Poisoning: Co-operative kerosene poisoning study: Evaluation of gastric lavage and other factors in the treatment of accidental ingestion of petroleum distillate products. Pediatrics 29:648, 1962.
83. Ng RC, Darwish H, Stewart DA: Emergency treatment of petroleum distillate and turpentine ingestion. Can Med Assoc J 111:537, 1974.
84. Watson WA, Bradford DC, Veltri JC: The volume of a swallow: Correlation of deglutition with patient and container parameters. Am J Emerg Med 3:278, 1983.

85. Fane LR, Comba HF, Decker WJ, et al: Physical parameters in gastric lavage. Clin Toxicol 4:389, 1971.
86. Ratzlaff HC, Heaslip JE, Rothwell ES: Factors affecting nasogastric tube insertion. Crit Care Med 12.1:52, 1984.
87. Rudolph JP: Automated gastric lavage and a comparison of 0.9% normal saline solution and tap water irrigant. Ann Emerg Med 14:1156, 1985.
88. Peterson CD: Electrolyte depletion following emergency stomach evacuation. Am J Hosp Pharm 36:1366, 1979.
89. Ritschell WE, Erni W: The influence of temperature of ingested fluid on stomach emptying time. Int J Clin Pharmacol 15:172, 1977.
90. McDougal CB, McLean MA: Modifications in the technique of gastric lavage. Ann Emerg Med 10:514, 1981.
91. Arena JM: Poisoning: Toxicology-Symptoms-Treatments. 3rd ed. Springfield, Ill, Charles C Thomas, 1978, pp 51–54.
92. Skoutakis VA: Clinical Toxicology of Drugs: Principles and Practice. Philadelphia, Lea & Febiger, 1982, p 12.
93. Czajka PA: Iron poisoning: An in vitro comparison of bicarbonate and phosphate lavage solutions. J Pediatr 89:491, 1981.
94. Maull KI, Osmand AP, Maull CD: Liquid caustic ingestions: An in vitro study of the effects of buffer, neutralization, and dilution. Ann Emerg Med 14:1160, 1985.
95. Greensher J, Mofenson HC, Picchioni AL, Fallon P: Activated charcoal update. JACEP 8:761, 1979.
96. Riegel JM, Becker CE: Use of cathartic in toxic ingestions. Ann Emerg Med 10:254, 1981.
97. Krenzelok EP, Keller R, Stewart RD: Gastrointestinal transit times of cathartics combined with charcoal. Ann Emerg Med 14:1152, 1985.
98. Klein-Schwartz W, Oderda GM: Adsorption of oral antidotes for acetaminophen poisoning (Methionine and N-acetylcysteine) by activated charcoal. Clin Toxicol 18:283, 1981.
99. North DS, Peterson RG, Krenzelok EP: Effect of activated charcoal administration on acetylcysteine serum levels in humans. Am J Hosp Pharm 38:1022, 1981.
100. Elkins BR, Ford DC, Thompson MI, et al: The effect of activated charcoal on N-acetylcysteine absorption in normal subjects. Am J Emerg Med 5:483, 1987.
101. Fiori A, Cecchetti G, Giusti FV: A lethal complication to gastric lavage leading to malpractice suit: A case report. Forensic Sci Int 11:47, 1978.
102. Wald P, Stern J, Weiner B, et al: Esophageal tear following forceful removal of an impacted oral gastric lavage tube. Ann Emerg Med 15:80, 1986.
103. Cortesi N, Malagoli M, De Poda D, et al: Iatrogenic ruptures of the stomach. Minerva Chir 35:67, 1980.
104. Coutselinis A, Plulos L, Boukis D, et al: A lethal complication to gastric lavage leading to malpractice suit: A case report. Forensic Sci Int 11:47, 1978.
105. Askenasi R, Abramowicz M, Jeanmart J, et al: Esophageal perforation: An unusual complication of gastric lavage (letter). Ann Emerg Med 13:146, 1984.
106. Calvanese JC: Midesophageal kinking and lodgement of a 34-F gastric lavage tube. Ann Emerg Med 14:1123, 1985.
107. Knopp R: Caustic ingestions. JACEP 8:329, 1979.
108. Rinder HM, Murphy JW, Higgins GL: Impact of unusual gastrointestinal problems on the treatment of tricyclic antidepressant overdose. Ann Emerg Med 17:1079, 1988.
109. Carter RF, Fotheringham BJ: Fatal salt poisoning due to gastric lavage with hypertonic saline. Med J Aust 1:539, 1971.
110. Bachrach L, Correa A, Levin R, et al: Iron poisoning: Complications of hypertonic phosphate lavage therapy. J Pediatr 94:147, 1979.
111. Rumack BH: Management of acute poisoning and overdose. In Rumack BH, Temple AR (eds): Management of the Poisoned Patient. Princeton, NJ, Science Press, 1977, pp 250–280.

Chapter 54

Feeding Tubes: Removal, Replacement, and Unclogging

Leonard Samuels

INTRODUCTION

Although the initial placement of feeding tubes is rarely the province of emergency physicians, patients with feeding tube complications frequently present to the emergency department. The emergency physician thus needs to be familiar with the different kinds of enteral feeding tubes as well as their care, cleansing, and means of replacement.

Material Properties of Feeding Tubes

Enteral feeding tubes are made of various materials. Latex (rubber) tubes are moderately firm, require greater lubrication for passage, are relatively thick-walled, and induce a greater foreign body reaction than tubes of other commonly used materials. *Latex,* and especially latex balloons, deteriorate more rapidly than those made with other materials.[1] *Polypropylene* tubes are the most rigid and are unsuitable for long-term nasogastric use. Although they are less likely to kink than the others, polypropylene tubes are more capable of creating a false passage during placement. *Silicone* tubes are thin-walled, quite pliable, and nonreactive. The walls of silicone tubes are less strong and may rupture if fluid is introduced into a kinked tube.[2] *Polyurethane* tubes are quite nonreactive and relatively durable. Rigidity varies from manufacturer to manufacturer depending on tube thickness. A stylet may aid in the passage of polyurethane tubes, but its use increases their rigidity and capability of tissue dissection, especially in tubes such as the Entriflex that have a small distal end bulb.[3] Some feeding tubes have weights, usually made of tungsten, which are nontoxic if released into the gastrointestinal tract.

Choice of Feeding Tube

Three major classes of enteral feeding tubes are in common use today, classified according to site of insertion. Tubes can enter through the nares, a cervical ostomy, or an abdominal ostomy. The mode of nutritional support is determined by the patient's physiologic requirements and degree of debilitation, the disease process, the anticipated duration of inadequate oral intake, and the facilities and equipment available to initiate and maintain delivery of nutritional support.[4] Tube feeding may be either a temporary or a permanent means of nutritional support and may have supplemental or complete responsibility for providing for the patient's nutritional needs. Enteral nutrition is less expensive and easier to use than total parenteral nutrition[5] and probably safer.[6, 7] Enteral nutrition is indicated when oral intake is less than two thirds of the patient's requirement despite a functioning gastrointestinal system. Nasoenteric feedings are appropriate when less than 4 weeks of feeding are required,[6] although in some cases a pharyngostomy may be preferred because it is less irritating and cosmetically easier to conceal. Cervical or abdominal ostomies are recommended when more than 4 weeks of feeding are necessary.[6] Oral ingestion may continue with gastrostomy tubes and may be possible with nasogastric and cervical ostomy tubes with a gauge of 12 French, or less.[2]

Enteral tubes may terminate in the stomach or the small intestine. Gastric feeding results in better digestion than intestinal feeding. Normally about 20 per cent of gastric antral contents pass into the duodenum, with 80 per cent refluxing back into the body of the stomach for further mixing.[8] If the feeding tube is placed in the antrum of the stomach or in the small bowel, enteral feeding solution passing into the small bowel may not be tolerated, resulting in diarrhea and paradoxical decreased nutrition.[8]

The most common rationale for small intestinal feeding is to reduce regurgitation and aspiration. Disagreement exists concerning the clinical significance and frequency of regurgitation-induced aspiration.[5, 7, 9–12] Nevertheless, the emergency physician should attempt to ensure that the terminal end of a replaced tube is in the same viscus as the original.

Feeding Tube Identification

External inspection may or may not reveal where a feeding tube should terminate. A de Pezzer (mushroom) or Foley gastrostomy tube is designed for intragastric termination. Some tubes have two lumina, one terminating in the stomach for decompression and the other in the small bowel for feeding. These can be confused with tubes that have two entrances to one lumen (one for continuous feeding, the other for medications) and tubes that have a second lumen leading to an inflatable balloon. *Review of the medical record or communication with the surgeon is often necessary when external inspection does not reveal the specific type of feeding tube or indicate where a feeding tube should terminate.*

NASOENTERIC FEEDING TUBES AND THEIR REPLACEMENT

Introduction

Nasoenteric feeding tubes, the oldest form of enteral alimentary support, were first developed in 1790 by John Hunter, who devised rubber tubes similar to those still in use today.[4] Insertion of larger bore, more rigid nasoenteric tubes is discussed in Chapter 51. Smaller diameter, more pliable tubes are more appropriate for feeding because they are less irritating to the nose and throat and less prone to cause erosions, bleeding, cough, and aspiration with prolonged use.[6, 13, 14] A feeding tube whose internal diameter is less than 14 French is unsuitable for stomach irrigation and aspiration or decompression.[15]

Indications and Contraindications

The most common indication for feeding tube replacement in the emergency department is unintentional removal of a preexisting feeding tube. In one prospective study, 38 per cent of tubes were removed unintentionally. Although some of these tubes had fallen out or been coughed out, more than half had been pulled out by the patient.[11] Tube rupture, deterioration, or clogging may also necessitate replacement. Management of the clogged or nonirrigating feeding tube is discussed in the section on "Clogged Feeding Tubes."

Enteric feeding tube replacement is contraindicated in the presence of vomiting, intestinal obstruction, severe ileus, upper gastrointestinal bleeding, distal enteric anastomoses, and conditions in which bowel rest is desired.[6] Occasionally,

the patient does not require nasoenteric feeding tube replacement because oral intake is adequate for nutritional needs. Patients suffering erosions or discomfort may be candidates for *peg* placement (percutaneous endoscopic gastrostomy).

Nasogastric Feeding Tube Lengths and Weights

Nearly all major producers of nasoenteric feeding tubes market polyurethane tubes because of their durability, biocompatibility, and high internal diameter to external diameter ratio (Fig. 54–1). Ross Laboratories makes a polyurethane tube with a 14 French external diameter. Twelve French is the largest polyurethane nasoenteral tube made by most other companies (Ethox Corp., Biosearch Medical Products Inc., Corpak Inc.). Tubes that are 22 inches in length are for pediatric use; these can also be useful for adult gastrostomy tube replacement. Thirty-six-inch tubes are appropriate for nasogastric feeding. Forty-three- or 45-inch tubes are for nasogastric, nasoduodenal, or nasojejunal feeding. Tubes may be unweighted or may have weighted tungsten tips. Weights vary from 1.5 to 7 gm. Tubes with weighted tips of 3 gm or less tend to be narrower at the ends, making them simpler to pass nasally but more capable of pulmonary dissection if they are misplaced into the bronchial tree. The weight and size of the heavier tips may assist in duodenal passage. All major companies produce tubes with and without stylets.

The nasogastric tube *must be premeasured* to estimate how far it should be inserted. Various recommendations for performing this measurement include (1) sum the distances from the nose to the tip of the earlobe and from the tip of the earlobe to the xiphoid, (2) sum the distances from the nose to the tip of the earlobe and from the tip of the earlobe to the umbilicus, and (3) use fixed measurements such as 18 or 22.5 inches (for adults). A high degree of accuracy of length estimation can be obtained with either of the following two methods: (1) nose-to-ear-to-xiphoid distance divided by two, plus 25 cm; or (2) one fifth of the body length plus 18.5 cm.[8] Tubes that should terminate in the duodenum should be inserted 15 to 20 cm further than this. Once measured, the desired length can be easily marked with a piece of tape so the correct length is not forgotten during passage.

Other Equipment

Feeding tube placement can be messy and can be accompanied by coughing, retching, sneezing, bleeding, and spilled water or stomach fluid; both patient and physician should be gowned. The physician requires gloves, a feeding tube

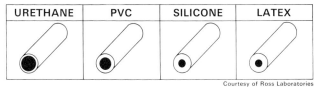

ID/OD Ratio

URETHANE	PVC	SILICONE	LATEX

Courtesy of Ross Laboratories

Stronger material means thinner tube walls, to deliver more flow.

Figure 54–1. Types of nasoenteric feeding tubes. Note that the polyurethane tubes have the highest internal diameter *(ID)* to external diameter *(OD)* ratio.

with stylet, a 50-ml syringe, a penlight, a tongue blade, a stethoscope, a small basin with tap water, and a means of securing the tube to the patient (usually tape and tincture of benzoin). To encourage swallowing, the physician should have a cup of ice chips or water and a straw for the cooperative patient or an additional syringe for the uncooperative patient. Suction apparatus should be immediately available in case the patient regurgitates. Check that the tip of the 50-ml syringe is compatible with the feeding tube. Make sure that the tube is designed for duodenal passage if that is desired. Duodenal tubes are often longer and have a heavier end bulb than nasogastric small-bore tubes.

Procedures and Techniques of Insertion

Nasoenteric feeding tube replacement requires greater time and effort if the patient is uncooperative or has a physically obstructing lesion. Nasoenteric feeding tube migration into the duodenal bulb generally requires about an hour in right decubitus position after successful intragastric passage.[16]

The physician should explain the procedure to the patient before tube passage. The patient's assistance with esophageal passage can be enlisted in two ways. First, the patient can assist with swallowing the tube. Second, the patient can vocalize when requested to confirm that the tube is not passing down the trachea. Many patients find it helpful to develop a signal to indicate to the physician when they need a temporary reprieve and rest. It is generally advisable to restrain the hands of demented, impaired, or otherwise uncooperative patients.

The nares should be prepared before the passage with the generous application of a lubricant and local anesthetic. A local vasoconstrictor will dilate the nasal passages slightly and help prevent bleeding. Mineral oil should not be used as the lubricant because its entry into the trachea or lungs is unusually irritating.[17] Viscous lidocaine or water-soluble jellies (e.g., Surgilube) are probably the best lubricants. A small amount of lidocaine with epinephrine can be squirted from a syringe into the nares a few minutes before lubrication. Application of the lidocaine with epinephrine or the lubricant or both can also be accomplished with soaked cotton-tipped applicators. Alternatively, viscous lidocaine can be introduced into the nose with a gloved finger. The physician should be prepared and garbed for the inevitable sneeze that this will provoke. Patients with a hyperactive gag reflex should gargle with viscous lidocaine or with benzocaine (Cetacaine) before the placement attempt.

The feeding tube stylet should be lubricated and inserted into the feeding tube before the insertion of the feeding tube into the nares. Tube stylets can be lubricated with water-soluble jelly. Dobhoff, Entriflex (Biosearch), and several other tubes have a preapplied lubricant that must be activated with a 5-ml flush of water. Spray kitchen frying lubricant (e.g., Pam) may also work well on the stylet. Other types of lubricants may have greater potential for pulmonary complications or may damage the substance of the tubes. *The stylet should never protrude beyond the end of the feeding tube*, because these stiff, small-diameter wires have the capacity to scratch the esophagus and can encourage the creation of a false passage. The stylet may lock into position on the tube at the proximal end and should be properly secured.

An upright patient position is more comfortable for the physician during nasogastric passage. The distal end of the feeding tube should be moistened or lubricated and then passed down the more patent of the two nasal passages. Most persons' nostrils are fairly symmetric, but in some cases growths or old trauma may narrow the passage. The more

patent nares can be quickly identified by gently exploring the nose with a gloved and lubricated fifth finger. The tube should be inserted into the nostril and then directed toward the ear. A common mistake of the inexperienced practitioner is to continue directing the feeding tube in a cranial direction. If the first nostril is impassable, the opposite side may permit tube passage. In particularly difficult cases, it may be desirable to first pass a lubricated nasal airway (trumpet) and pass the feeding tube through it, reducing nasal and nasopharynx stimulation.

The tube's passage into the nasopharynx can usually be detected by a lessening of resistance. One can then proceed with esophageal passage. Topical anesthesia of the pharynx may be required to ameliorate the excessive gagging that may occur at this point. Cough should warn of incipient respiratory placement of the tube. If the patient can vocalize, the tube has not yet passed through the vocal cords. The patient should bend the head forward if possible. This encourages the tube to pass into the esophagus and aids airway closure. If the patient is gagging or choking, it may be because the tube is beginning to coil in the oropharynx. Look in the mouth with the penlight to see if this is occurring. If the tube is coiled or entering the airway, temporarily pulling the tube back should relieve the problem. When pulling back, some resistance is again felt as the thicker end bulb of the tube begins to enter the posterior nasal passages; at that point, the tube has been pulled back far enough for a fresh try at esophageal intubation. The cooperative patient should swallow ice chips or take small sips of water with a straw. This may greatly facilitate tube passage down the esophagus. In some cases, it may be impossible to avoid coiling when the tube is advanced unless the patient is swallowing. When the patient is uncooperative, the introduction of 5 to 15 ml of water into the mouth or into the proximal end of the feeding tube with a syringe may induce swallowing, facilitating tube passage. Although the patient may not swallow for several minutes, waiting for the swallow may mean the difference between a coiled or pulmonary tube placement and a successful passage.

For some comatose or severely demented patients, Magill forceps and modified endotracheal tube guiding techniques may be helpful (outlined in Chapter 51). Endoscopic placement of the tube under direct vision or fluoroscopic placement are other alternatives.

Another technique for passing soft feeding tubes involves attaching the distal end to a Salem sump tube by means of a gelatin cap (one half of a size 0 gelatin capsule). Lubricate the joined tubes, avoiding lubrication of the soluble capsule. The Salem sump–soft tube complex is passed nasogastrically. Once the tubes are positioned in the stomach, both tubes are irrigated several times with 10 to 20 ml of water. After about 5 minutes the gelatin capsule should have dissolved, allowing independent removal of the Salem sump tube[2] (Fig. 54–2).

Complications of Nasogastric Feeding Tubes

Pulmonary intubation is an uncommon but a well-known and potentially fatal complication of nasal feeding tube insertion. Coughing and respiratory distress are the most common symptoms of respiratory passage of a feeding tube but there may be relatively few symptoms in a demented or comatose patient.[18] Decreased mentation and an absent cough reflex are predisposing factors for unrecognized nasopulmonary intubation with feeding tubes.[3] Frequently a nasogastric tube has previously been passed successfully in the patient who subsequently experiences nasopulmonary intubation.[3] A small end bulb, such as that present on the

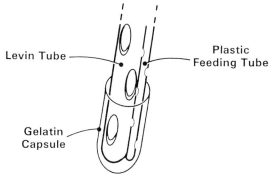

Figure 54–2. To facilitate the passage of a soft or very pliable plastic feeding tube, the tip of the feeding tube is joined to the tip of a stiffer nasogastric tube (such as a Salem sump) with the aid of a gelatin capsule. The capsule dissolves in the stomach in a few minutes, and the companion nasogastric tube separates and is withdrawn, leaving the feeding tube in place.

Entriflex tube made by Biosearch (2.7 mm), can slip past a tracheal high-volume, low-pressure cuff and pass easily to the lung periphery.[3, 18–20] To prevent nasopulmonary feeding tube intubation, one may use the wire stylet only for initial tube passage. This will prevent pulmonary parenchymal penetration but not tracheobronchial intubation. It will also make passage of tubes positioned in the esophagus more difficult.[3] Esophageal entry of the feeding tube can be checked with the use of a laryngoscope. The metal stylet can be left in the tube during esophageal tube passage when an esophageal position is confirmed by laryngoscopy.[21] A stylet should never be reinserted into a tube already in the patient. The stylet may puncture the tube at a kink or exit the side holes and puncture the esophagus.[22]

A pneumothorax may result when a nasogastric tube dissects into or is withdrawn from the pulmonary parenchyma.[22a] Bloody aspirate from a tube should heighten awareness of possible complications.

The end bulb of most nasoduodenal tubes will pass into the duodenum after an hour of right decubitus position. Some researchers recommend pretreatment with metoclopramide to enhance gastric emptying.[5, 23, 24] One investigator found that metoclopramide enhances duodenal passage of nasogastrically placed feeding tubes in diabetics but not in nondiabetics.[16] Gastric antral motility in diabetics is often impaired; metoclopramide helps restore normal synchronized activity in these patients but has little effect on emptying in subjects who have normal antral function. The usual dose of metoclopramide is 10 mg administered intravenously. Endoscopy or fluoroscopy may be necessary if positioning and metoclopramide are not successful.[25]

A clogged or nonfunctional nasogastric tube may prove difficult to remove. Fluoroscopy may allow careful insertion of a guide wire or stylet into an in situ tube to facilitate removal. Fluoroscopy also may identify the mechanical problem interfering with the removal. Bent-double segments are probably the most common; knots are uncommon but do occur. Excessive force should not be used in the removal of a nasogastric tube because serious injury to the patient may result.

Premature removal of the nasogastric tube is the most frequent complication of feeding tube use. To help prevent removal by the uncooperative patient, the nasogastric tube may be secured to a loop anchor passed in the same nares. The anchor works by aversive stimulation of the soft palate and nose with distraction of the nasogastric tube rather than by mechanical stabilization of the tube. Sax and Bower recommend a technique for creating a separate nasogastric

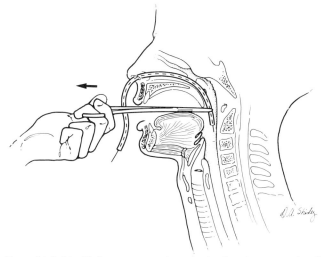

Figure 54–3. Magill forceps grasp the tube in the pharynx and pull it out through the mouth.

tube anchor.[26] A soft weighted nasoenteric tube is cut approximately 12 inches from the top. A heavy (2–0) silk suture is passed through the tube to exit the side hole. The guide wire is inserted with care not to let it protrude from the cut end. Sedation of the uncooperative patient may be necessary. The tube is inserted through the anesthetized nares into the nasopharynx, grasped with Magill forceps, and pulled to exit from the mouth (Fig. 54–3). The excess tube is trimmed without cutting the silk suture. A closed loop is made by tying the silk suture in front of the nose. The loop must be slack enough that it does not apply continuous pressure to the nose or palate at rest. The nasal feeding tube is passed through the same nostril and secured to the loop (Fig. 54–4). This anchor is simpler to construct and more comfortable than anchors passed through the opposite nostril.[26]

Auscultatory confirmation of tube placement can be misleading.[3, 20, 27, 28] The proper technique for auscultation is to inject 20 ml of air into the tube rapidly while listening with a stethoscope in the left upper abdomen. Air insufflation should occur without resistance and without delay in

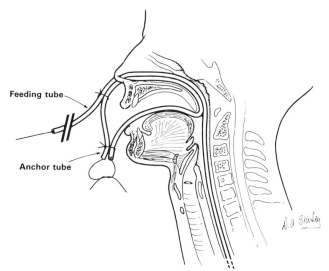

Figure 54–4. One method of securing a nasogastric tube in an uncooperative patient.

borborygmi. If the sound is muffled, faint, or delayed, the physician may reinject another 20 ml of air and listen over the lower lung. If the sound is clearer, the tube may be in the lung. The injected air should be aspirated after placement is confirmed so that the patient is less likely to burp or regurgitate. Air instilled into a feeding tube may generate borborygmi of higher pitch if the end of the tube is in the duodenum. The reliability of this finding has not been checked scientifically.

Proper placement should be confirmed with a radiograph. Tubes should be secured with tape before taking the radiograph. Tincture of benzoin applied to the tube and the patient makes the tape stick better. Commercial tube fixation devices may also be used. The position before and after the radiograph is taken is more likely to be the same if the tube is secured before filming.

Gordon suggests that radiographs are not necessary to check nasogastric feeding tube placement if the following criteria are met *in order*.[2] The tube must be passed beyond the 50-cm mark in a normal-sized adult; palpation and visual inspection confirm that the tube is not coiled in the mouth or oropharynx; air insufflation occurs without resistance and without delay in epigastric borborygmi; 10 ml of water advance through the tube without difficulty; and some water can be retrieved with aspiration. Do *not* inject water into the tube if any of the preceding criteria suggest that placement might not be adequate. A risk exists of delivering water into the airway.[6]

Aspirated pleural or pulmonary fluid contents can be mistaken for return of intragastric fluids.[3] Additionally, radiographic confirmation of tube placement may be misleading. The end of a nasogastric tube may appear to be in the stomach yet be in the left lung behind and below the top of the diaphragm.[20] A nasoenteric tube may lie completely to the left of midline and yet have its tip in the duodenum, or it may have a position entering the right abdomen yet not have entered the duodenum. Contrast study is necessary to ascertain duodenal position.[16, 29] In viewing the radiograph, it is particularly important to study the area around the carina. An esophageal tube shows at most a mild change in course, whereas a tracheally placed tube usually deviates significantly as it travels into the right or left main stem bronchus. When a stylet has been used for passage, the stylet should be left in the feeding tube for the radiograph because the tube's course is not always visible without it. The stylets of most tubes are designed to allow insufflation and aspiration while in place.

The radiograph should also be examined for the presence of mediastinal air and a pneumothorax, which may suggest pulmonary or esophageal puncture. An esophageal puncture should be evaluated with endoscopy and may require surgery, depending on the size of the rent.

Complications of properly placed nasoenteric tubes include nasopharyngeal erosions, esophageal reflux, tracheoesophageal fistulas, gagging, rupture of esophageal varices, and otitis media.[6] One survey of nasogastrically fed patients found that the most distressing features of nasogastric feeding tube use were deprivation of tasting, drinking, and chewing of food; soreness of the nose; rhinitis; esophagitis; mouth breathing; and the sight of other patients who were eating.[14]

Checking feeding tolerance is difficult with small-gauge feeding tubes. Aspiration of tubes to check for residual is not recommended with tubes of 9 French or smaller. Aspiration is likely to clog the tubes because they collapse under pressure and because relatively small particles can occlude the tube. For the same reasons the residual is likely to be inaccurate.[7]

Discharge instructions should include a proscription

against aspiration in small tubes. To maintain catheter patency, small tubes should be flushed with 20 to 30 ml of tap water at least two to three times daily and after administration of medication.[7, 29] Water is a more effective irrigant than cranberry juice.[30] Medications should be in liquid form or be completely dissolved or they may clog the tube. Methods of dealing with a clogged tube are discussed in a later section.

The tube should be anchored to the nose and face in such a way that it is not in contact with the skin at the nasal opening. This reduces tube discomfort and prevents necrosis of the alae nares and distal septum. Patients who exhibit a tendency to pull on their tubes need adequate restraints. Patients receiving tube feedings should have their heads elevated to at least 30 degrees above the horizontal.[7, 31]

PHARYNGOSTOMY AND ESOPHAGOSTOMY FEEDING TUBES

Indications

Cervical pharyngostomy and cervical esophagostomy are both procedures of relatively recent development. Cervical esophagostomy was first described by Klopp in 1951.[32] Cervical pharyngostomy was described in 1967 by Shumrick.[33] Cervical esophagostomies are generally performed at the time of cervical or maxillofacial operations. Malignant growths of the proximal esophagus, head, or neck are the primary indications for esophagostomy. Cervical esophagostomies may eventually evolve a permanent sinus, allowing the feeding tube to be removed between meals.

As with an esophagostomy, a pharyngostomy may be either a simple ostomy or a permanent tract formed by suturing pharyngeal mucosa to the skin.[13, 33, 34] The more common version is a simple opening that closes very rapidly (within a few hours) if it is not stented with a tube (Fig. 54–5). Pharyngostomy is a simple procedure and does not require general anesthesia. It is useful when nasogastric feeding tubes are contraindicated or when prolonged tube feeding is anticipated.[4] Patients with traumatic or congenital anomalies of the maxillofacial region who are undergoing an operation and patients with impaired swallowing from neuromuscular disorders are potential candidates for cer-

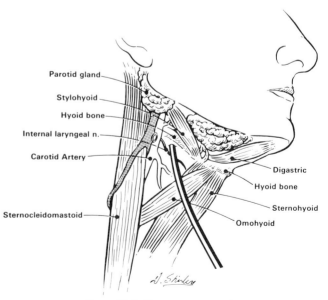

Figure 54–5. Pharyngostomy tube.

vical pharyngostomy.[34] Pharyngostomy is also indicated to bypass obstructing lesions for feeding, to assist healing after head or neck surgery for malignancy, and to feed the unconscious patient. Pharyngostomy can also be used for gastric decompression if it is required for more than 3 days.[13] Cervical pharyngostomy tubes produce only mild discomfort. Patients do not usually complain about pharyngostomy tubes, as they do a nasogastric tube. The additional comfort and ease of productive coughing are especially important in critically ill and elderly patients.

Technique of Esophagostomy and Pharyngostomy Tube Passage

The feeding tubes commonly used for esophagostomy and pharyngostomy feeding are the same as those used for nasogastric feeding. Polyurethane feeding tubes are the most frequently used. The large (more than 3 gm) bolus weights on some feeding tubes may be inconvenient to pass through the ostomy. Tubes that are approximately 90 cm (3 feet) long are appropriate for gastric feeding; tubes that are longer—108 to 112 cm (43 or 45 inches)—are used for duodenal feeding.

The feeding tube replacement technique for pharyngostomy and esophagostomy is the same. The outside of the tube tip can be lubricated with a small amount of water-soluble lubricant jelly. Mineral oil, which irritates the airways if aspirated, should never be used. The tip of the tube is inserted into the ostomy and directed caudally to ensure that it enters the esophagus and does not pass upward into the nasopharynx or mouth (Fig. 54–6). The patient may be able to assist by attempting to swallow. The length of the feeding tube that is required varies depending on the position of the ostomy and is several centimeters longer than the distance from ostomy to xyphoid. For duodenal feeding, the tube should be advanced about 20 cm beyond the distance from ostomy to xyphoid.

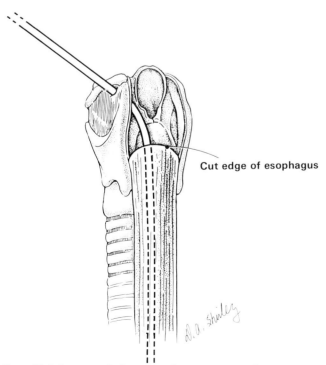

Cut edge of esophagus

Figure 54–6. Proper path for an esophagostomy or a pharyngostomy tube.

If the feeding tube persistently exits the mouth during attempts at passage instead of passing down the esophagus, the following two techniques may prove useful. After insertion of the feeding tube a short distance into the ostomy, a flashlight is used to visualize the tube in the pharynx. The feeding tube is grasped slightly proximal to the end bulb using Magill forceps, and the end bulb is directed toward the esophagus in the posterior inferior pharynx. Once the tube is properly directed, it may be possible to advance the remainder of the tube through the external ostomy. Sometimes it is necessary to use the forceps to advance the entire length of the feeding tube. An alternative method is to allow the feeding tube placed through the ostomy to exit the mouth for the entire distance that must be passed down the esophagus. The end bulb of the tube is then directed into the posterior pharynx, and the patient is directed to swallow as for an orogastric tube. Toward the end of tube passage it may be necessary to use a Magill forcep or to pull back the tube slightly at the ostomy to eliminate a short loop of extra tubing in the oropharynx.

Tube replacement is more difficult in the first week after the creation of a pharyngostomy or an esophagostomy. A tract forms after the first week and helps prevent tissue dissection by the tube. The angle of a well-formed tract also encourages appropriate esophageal passage. A well-formed tract closes more slowly than a new ostomy, although in some people even a long-term ostomy may begin sealing within a few hours. If an ostomy is too narrow for the replacement tube, the ostomy should be stented with a narrower tube and the patient's surgeon contacted.

Complications

Complications of pharyngostomy and esophagostomy include local soft tissue irritation, accidental extubation because of excess length of the external tube, pulmonary aspiration from vomiting, arterial erosion with exsanguination, and esophagitis or stricture of the esophagus from reflux. Accidental pulmonary intubation is less common with cervical ostomy tubes than with nasogastric tubes, at least partially because patients with cervical ostomies are more likely to be alert and have functioning cough reflexes. Auscultation and aspiration are still advisable techniques to check tube placement. Radiographic evaluation may also be necessary and is essential to confirm duodenal feeding.

GASTROSTOMY, GASTROENTEROSTOMY, DUODENOSTOMY, AND JEJUNOSTOMY TUBES

Introduction

The mid–nineteenth-century physician Sedillot described the first functioning gastrostomy, which formed as a complication of a war wound. The gastrostomies performed by Sedillot on two patients resulted in peritonitis and death.[34, 35] The jejunostomy procedure was first performed by Surmay in 1879. It was not until the 1890s that further innovations in surgical technique allowed the gastrostomy to be popularized. The Witzel serosal-lined gastric tunnel technique was developed in 1891 (Fig. 54–7). In 1894 Stamm published his procedure of concentric pursestring sutures around the gastrostomy tube. These two techniques prevent significant intraperitoneal gastric fluid leakage, a complication that had frequently resulted in the deaths of gastrostomy patients. Both Witzel and Stamm gastrostomies tend to close rapidly without a stenting gastrostomy tube. In the early 1900s the tubular gastrostomy (Depage-Janeway) was developed. The Depage-Janeway gastrostomy results in the creation of a permanent mucocutaneous ostomy. Since the turn of the century, more than 30 different operative techniques have been described for tube gastrostomy.[4]

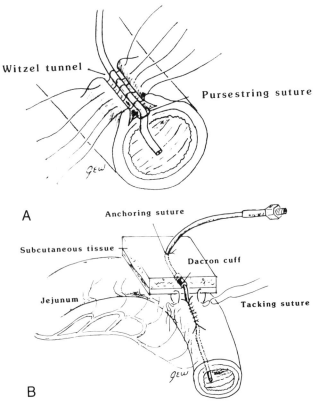

Figure 54–7. *A,* Formation of the Witzel tunnel. *B,* Final catheter placement. (From Wiedeman JE, Smith VC: Use of the Hickman catheter for jejunal feedings in children. Surg Gynecol Obstet 162:69, 1986. Reproduced by permission of Surgery, Gynecology, and Obstetrics.)

Indications

Neurologic diseases constitute the most frequent indication for a gastrostomy tube.[9] Facial fractures, oropharyngeal trauma, and tracheal and laryngeal injuries may be indications for placement of a temporary feeding gastrostomy. Rare indications for gastrostomy include the enhancement of nutrition by continuous feeding in severely debilitated patients who still are capable of oral intake, the provision of a route for bile replacement in patients with an external biliary fistula, and the need for long-term gastric decompression. Indications for gastrostomy tube placement in children include neurologic diseases, facial reconstructive surgery for congenital deformities, and maxillofacial trauma. Young children who require long-term administration of unpalatable medications or dietary components may also require a gastrostomy. Tube duodenostomies are created almost exclusively for duodenal decompression after partial gastrectomy with Billroth II anastomoses.[34] Permanent jejunostomies are rarely used. Tube jejunostomy is indicated when the proximal bowel has a fistula or is obstructed, when recovery of small bowel motility is anticipated long before recovery of gastric motility, and after a gastrectomy.[4, 34]

Contraindications

Contraindications for gastrostomy feeding include severe gastroesophageal reflux, upper gastrointestinal fistulas, repeated aspiration of gastric contents, and intestinal or gastric outlet obstruction.[4] Jejunal feeding is contraindicated

if the highly osmolar feeding solutions required for jejunal feeding are poorly tolerated and cause the patient to experience copious diarrhea.

Ease and safety of transabdominal feeding tube replacement depend on the surgical procedure performed and length of time since placement of the feeding tube. For a simple gastrostomy, the insertion site of the tube through the gastrointestinal wall is sealed by either annular or plication sutures. The gastrointestinal wall is approximated to the peritoneum around the site of penetration to provide a further leakage barrier. The tube is then secured outside the abdominal wall. A Witzel tunnel is a serosal tunnel created when the feeding tube is placed alongside the viscus for a distance after exiting the viscus and the bowel is pulled up over it along this distance and secured with sutures[36, 37] (see Fig. 54–7). In one type of Hickman catheter jejunostomy, the tube passes through a Dacron cuff and a Witzel tunnel.[37] Reinsertion of a Hickman catheter through a tortuous, rough Witzel tunnel is unlikely to be simple.[38] A percutaneous gastrostomy may be placed without any attempt to affix the stomach to the abdominal wall.

Nonoperative tube replacement techniques are safe only through an established tract between the skin and the bowel. Catheter replacement should not be attempted in the immediate postoperative period. A simple gastrostomy takes about a week to form a tract.[13] A Witzel tunnel may take up to 3 weeks after the operation to mature sufficiently for safe nonoperative tube replacement. *A nonfunctional tube can still serve as the stent for the gastrostomy tract and should not be removed if it cannot be promptly and safely replaced.*

Equipment

Gastrostomy tubes come in an unusually varied selection of styles and materials. Rubber, silicone, and polyurethane tubes are all in common use. Many gastrostomy tubes are designed to retain themselves in the stomach once they are placed through the use of a flange. Various flanges are illustrated in Figure 54–8.

Equipment for feeding tube insertion includes gloves, stethoscope, feeding tube, external bolster, lubricant, basin, and a syringe that fits the tube. Tincture of benzoin, tape, and absorbent dressing material may be used to dress the wound, although many are better left undressed.[15] Some feeding tubes require special plugs or connectors. Others need to be pinched with a clamp when not in use to prevent leakage. Some tubes are placed with the aid of accompanying

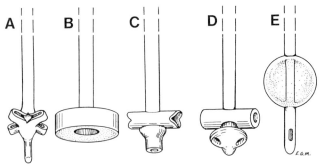

Figure 54–8. Various types of gastrostomy tubes. *A,* Friction-lock catheter (Wilson-Cook Co.). *B,* Silicone catheter (American Endoscopy [Bard]). *C,* Gastrostomy catheter (Ross Laboratories). *D,* Latex catheter with "mushroom" or a de Pezzer-type flange on the end (American Endoscopy [Bard]). *E,* Balloon (Foley) catheter (Wilson-Cook Co.).

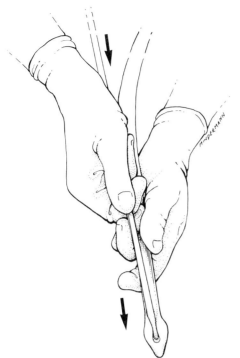

Figure 54–9. An endotracheal tube stylet used to distend the flange of the de Pezzer catheter.

guide wires or stents. For some others it is necessary to use a clamp or hemostat, endotracheal tube stylet, urinary or uterine sound, laryngeal dilator (number 14), guide wire, or other appropriate rod or support as an aid to tube passage (Fig. 54–9). A stylet to assist introduction of de Pezzer catheters can be fashioned by cutting half the stylet from a 9 French pediatric chest tube inserter. The tip can be filed smooth. The device will be 10 to 12 cm long and can be inserted alongside the de Pezzer catheter and into its tip to distend and flatten the mushroom (Fig. 54–10).

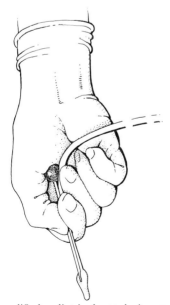

Figure 54–10. A modified pediatric chest tube inserter used to distend the flange of the de Pezzer catheter.

Transabdominal Feeding Tube Removal

A feeding tube may need to be removed because it is irreversibly clogged, leaking or broken, persistently developing kinks, too large or too small, causing a hypersensitivity reaction, associated with an abscess, or not the appropriate length for feeding into the desired viscus. Before a new transabdominal feeding tube is inserted, the old tube must be removed. *Not all tubes can be removed without endoscopy. It is imperative to know whether the tube in place is safe to remove before attempting to remove it.* Standard de Pezzer or mushroom catheters that have been modified with bolsters or rings at the time of endoscopic or surgical insertion may no longer be safe to remove with traction. Occasionally, tubes are secured with sutures. Recently placed feeding tubes may need to be left in until a tract has formed (1 to 2 weeks depending on the procedure) even if the tube is nonfunctional. *The externally visible tube does not always reveal the internal stabilization* (see Fig. 54–8).

A simple Foley catheter gastrostomy is easiest to remove. Once the Foley balloon is deflated the tube should slide right out. If the Foley balloon cannot be deflated, cutting the tube may allow the balloon to deflate. The Foley must not be cut so close to the abdomen that it will be impossible to maintain a grip on it for a traction removal if the balloon still does not deflate. The balloon may also be punctured to cause it to deflate. To puncture a Foley balloon, traction is applied to the catheter to draw the balloon up against the ostomy. Using the taut feeding tube as a guide, an 18- or 19-gauge needle is passed along the tube to puncture the balloon. It may be necessary to try again on the other side of the catheter because the balloon may be asymmetrically inflated and contact with the needle may be established on one side and not the other. The clinician should be careful not to track away from the ostomy into the patient's abdominal wall, or to cause separate punctures of the stomach. The balloon is allowed a minute to deflate before another attempt is made at traction removal. Large balloons should probably be punctured, whereas small balloons may be removed with traction.

Traction is an acceptable removal technique for feeding tubes that are secured by a small mushroom. A towel is placed over the orifice and the physician applies counter-pressure against the abdominal wall as the tube is placed under tension. This causes the tube and end mushroom to narrow, and the tube should come out easily. The inner crossbar, if present, may remain in the stomach when the rest of the feeding tube complex is removed by traction. Obstruction from the crossbar, which will pass in the stool, has yet to be reported for adults. In small children obstruction is a possibility, and the crossbar should be removed by endoscopy.[1, 39]

A local anesthetic may be useful in selected cases of feeding tube removal, especially when the tube is in some way secured subcutaneously, for example, by a Dacron cuff.[37] It may be difficult to remove a catheter accidentally caught by a fascial suture during operative closure.[40]

Removal of gastrostomy tubes with moderate to large mushrooms may be easier if the mushroom is distended with a sound or stylet. The length of the gastrostomy tube should be known so that the sound may be inserted to the correct depth. Firm resistance should be noted at that point. Firm resistance at deeper depths represents pressure on the viscus wall and can result in viscus puncture.[24] The premeasured stylets that come with feeding devices are useful instruments for assisting in device removal. This is particularly true of gastrostomy "buttons," whose ends resemble de Pezzer catheters. Because buttons come in a variety of lengths, it is important to have the proper stylet. Following elective permanent removal of a gastrostomy tube, a pressure dressing should aid in closure of the fistula.[24]

If it is not possible to pull the inner bolster or mushroom out through the ostomy, it may be acceptable to cut the tube at the skin and push the remaining short stump into the stomach and rely on later rectal passage. Although obstruction or impaction is infrequent, it can occur, and this alternative should not be chosen with children or patients who have had previous impaction or stool-passing problems. Rigid or large internal mushrooms and bolsters, the very kind that cause the most difficulty with percutaneous removal, are also more likely to cause difficulty with rectal passage. In no case should a device be released into the gut with a long length of tubing attached. Remember that double-part tubes may have an additional length of tubing for duodenal or jejunal feeding that extends far past the inner bolster. Some physicians and surgeons may strongly condemn cutting off the tube at the skin even when the risks posed by the procedure are very low. It is always advisable to contact the patient's private physician before cutting the tube. In some cases endoscopic retrieval of the tube remnant will be preferred to allowing rectal passage, and the tube should not be cut until just before or during endoscopy to ensure that migration does not occur before endoscopy.

Transabdominal Feeding Tube Replacement

A Foley catheter is a simple gastrostomy tube to replace. After the tract opening and distal Foley are lubricated, the Foley balloon's integrity is checked by inflation. The catheter is then inserted into the tract. Good placement can be recognized by easy passage, prompt borborygmi with 20 ml of air insufflation, and rapid return of stomach juices with aspiration. The balloon is then inflated with saline (30-ml balloons are best), and gentle traction is applied to draw the balloon against the stomach wall. *Always inflate the Foley balloon with saline,* because balloons inflated with air deflate more easily. A bolster should be threaded onto the catheter.

A bolster is a ring or bar of material threaded onto a tube that creates a large bulge on the tube and prevents inappropriate ingress of the tube into the ostomy on the side of the bolster. The anchor must adhere strongly to the tube so that mild stress on the tube does not cause the bolster to migrate up the tube. The bolster can be salvaged from the old tube or constructed in a number of ways. An anchor may be made from the end nipple of a de Pezzer catheter. The ring from a 24 French catheter, taken off at its junction with the end nipple, fits snugly over a 22 French Foley catheter when the balloon is distended slightly. The nipple can be pushed forward to an anchoring position near the stoma. The nipple can be fixed in this position by fully distending the Foley balloon and applying a circle of adhesive tape just adjacent to the nipple on the stem on the side away from the body.[41] Adhesive tape sticks better if the lubricant is removed and the stem is prepared with tincture of benzoin.

An anchor may be made from a segment of tube from a large rubber catheter (Fig. 54–11). A segment approximately 3 cm in length is cut to form the bolster. Two diamond-shaped openings can be formed on both sides of the segment by bending the segment and clipping it with scissors on either side of the bend. The diameter of the holes should be slightly smaller than the catheter (Fig. 54–12). A hemostat or a Kelly clamp can be inserted through both holes to grasp the external end of the gastrostomy tube, which can be bent in half (with some difficulty) to narrow its diameter (Fig. 54–13). The hemostat can then

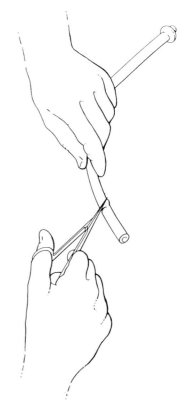

Figure 54–11. A 3-cm segment of thick latex tubing is cut from the proximal segment of a catheter. This segment is used to make a bolster for a feeding tube and anchors the feeding tube, preventing unwanted ingress of the tube into the patient.

pull the tube through the bolster, which can be threaded down the tube and anchored with tape as described previously (Fig. 54–14). The outer crossbar should be located 1 cm away from the skin.[42] Contact between the crossbar and the skin promotes moisture entrapment and maceration. Too much tension on the gastrostomy tube can result in necrosis of the gastric wall where it abuts the inner mushroom or balloon. Proper placement of the external bolster helps avoid this complication.

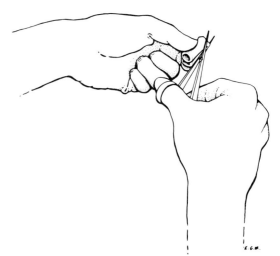

Figure 54–12. A 3-cm segment of latex tubing is bent in half and cut to create a hole on each side of the segment.

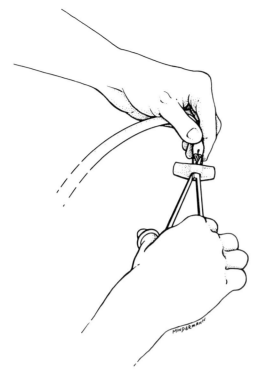

Figure 54–13. A hemostat is inserted through the holes in the completed bolster and grasps the feeding tube. The end of the feeding tube has been folded to reduce its external diameter.

Many physicians prefer mushroom or de Pezzer gastrostomy tubes, which are more difficult to replace than Foley catheters. The advantage of these catheters over Foley catheters is that the mushroom nipple keeps its shape more reliably than the Foley balloon, which tends to deflate.[14]

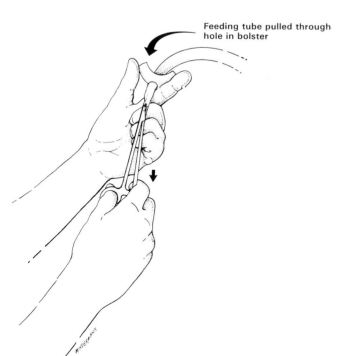

Feeding tube pulled through hole in bolster

Figure 54–14. The feeding tube is pulled through the bolster. The bolster is advanced to 1 cm above the skin of the external abdomen.

Foley catheters also have a greater tendency to migrate internally and block the pylorus.[4] A Kelly clamp or other stylet can be placed through a side hole into the tip of a gastrostomy mushroom and used to elongate the end for easy passage through the gastrostomy (see Figs. 54–9 and 54–10). Lubrication of the mushroom may make it more difficult to maintain the stylet's position in the mushroom. Some stylets are suitable for passage down the catheter lumen to elongate the end. Tubes should never be forced through a stoma for replacement, because this can cause separation of the viscus from the external stoma and lead to viscus leak or tube misplacement.[24]

The replacement tube provided in the emergency department does not have to be, and in a few cases should not be, the same type placed at surgery. The tube needs to be compatible with the feeding system, terminate in the same viscus, and fit through the ostomy. When a Witzel tunnel jejunostomy is created, the catheter most frequently used is a Broviac catheter. An appropriate replacement is a lubricated Entriflex (Biosearch) or other polyurethane tube shortened to a total tube length of 30 to 40 cm. Although the polyurethane tube is strong enough to be used for tube replacement through the Witzel tunnel without a guide wire, Broviac (silicone) catheters are too pliant to be coaxed through the resistive tunnel.[36] Jejunal feeding tubes are generally advanced 20 to 30 cm into the jejunum.

Jejunal feeding tubes may be placed through or alongside a decompressing gastrostomy. Original placement of the jejunal feeding tube is endoscopic. Replacement of these tubes also generally requires endoscopic assistance.[43–45] Fluoroscopic techniques can be used to help guide these tubes; however, these techniques are out of the realm of emergency practice.[6] Occasionally, feeding tubes are placed in the jejunum because of gastric ileus.[4, 46] If gastric ileus is no longer present, a gastrostomy tube may suffice. The rationale for jejunal feeding, risk of aspiration, and acceptability of gastric feeding to the primary physician should be established before changing from a jejunal feeding tube to a feeding gastrostomy tube. Techniques discussed in the nasoenteric feeding section of this chapter (metoclopramide and right decubitus position) may in selected cases coax gastrostomy-placed feeding tubes into the small bowel. Gastric decompression tubes are either clamped or put at continuous drainage.[44]

Complications

If the ostomy is not a mucocutaneous type, it will close rapidly without a stenting tube. Often the stoma begins to contract within hours of feeding tube removal. The physician may be presented with a very narrow ostomy and a tract that is difficult to identify or thread. A sound or blunt stylet can be passed down the tract more easily than a tube. This procedure can identify the opening and direction of the tract for easier tube passage. When a guide wire passes easily down a narrow tract but the needed feeding tube does not, it may be possible to dilate the tract with dilators or a dilation catheter.[47] Viscus puncture, viscus abdominal wall separation, and false tract creation with subsequent tube misplacement are risks of dilation procedures. Such procedures should generally be left to the surgeon. *If tube replacement will be delayed, maintain the narrow tract with the largest available easily placed stent*, usually a Foley catheter. Always secure the stent against internal migration.

The position of the gastrostomy tube should be checked by air insufflation and aspiration of gastric fluid, as is done with nasoenteric tubes. Air should enter the stomach without resistance and with immediate borborygmi. Gastric fluid should return with aspiration. It may be necessary to insert a small volume of water to get good return. Water pooling in the soft tissue may be aspirated back through a misplaced catheter. Good tube placement is indicated when more fluid returns with aspiration than was originally placed into the catheter. If replacement of the gastrostomy or jejunal tube required the overcoming of any resistive force or if either the air or the aspiration tests yield uncertain results, a radiographic study with contrast should be performed. Peritoneal infusion of feeding solution can be fatal.

Complications of gastrostomy include wound infections around the catheter, performance of an unnecessary laparatomy for suspected leakage, gastrocolic fistula, pneumatosis intestinalis, bowel obstruction, peritonitis, and hemorrhage.[39] Jejunostomies can cause most of these complications, as well as other types of fistulas and small bowel obstruction from adhesions or volvulus around the jejunostomy site.[24, 34] The most common complications of gastrostomy and gastroenterostomy are local skin erosions from leakage, wound infections, hemorrhage, and tube dislodgment.[7] Peritonitis and aspiration are the most critical complications of gastrostomy feedings.[7, 34] Jejunostomies are less prone to stomal leakage and cause less nausea, vomiting, bloating, and aspiration than gastrostomies.[4, 48]

Dislodgment of gastrostomy and jejunostomy tubes is most common in the 2 weeks following ostomy creation.[49] Extrusion of the gastrostomy tube is usually caused by excessive tension applied to the tube. Only gentle contact of the gastric and abdominal walls is desirable. Uncooperative patients should be restrained. Mittens are often particularly helpful. Sutures and large mushrooms or balloons are ineffective deterrents to purposeful removal of the gastrostomy tube by the uncooperative patient.

A small amount of drainage is to be expected at the tube entry site. Local leaks of gastric juices may macerate and irritate the skin, predispose to local infections and abscesses, and encourage the development of small granulomas.[4, 36] Granulomas are particularly common in children. They can be treated with silver nitrate at the time of dressing changes. Any dressing used around the entry site of an enteral nutrition tube should absorb fluid and not encourage persistent moisture.[15] An unusually large stoma may promote a leak. Although insertion of a larger tube or firmer traction on the tube may be transiently effective, these measures often result in further stomal enlargement. Rigid gastrostomies promote leakage by widening the stoma as they pivot. Insertion of a soft, pliant feeding tube through the widened stoma is often easy and allows later contraction of the stoma.[1] If these techniques are ineffective, temporary removal of the feeding tube may allow the stoma to shrink. Large amounts of drainage around the stoma site occur with the high residual volumes.[43] The residual should be checked, and feedings withheld until residuals are less than 100 ml. Feeding residual should be checked every 4 hours when a patient is on continuous drip feeding.[46]

Pneumoperitoneum after percutaneous gastrostomy is neither unusual nor dangerous. Benign pneumoperitoneum may be present as long as 5 weeks after percutaneous endoscopic gastrostomy.[39, 43] Pneumatosis intestinalis can occur through the defect in the bowel wall created for the enterostomy tube. Although often insignificant clinically, its occurrence suggests air under pressure in the small bowel. Nasogastric suction and diet change generally permit resolution of the problem. Catheter or feeding tube removal is usually not required.[40]

Clinically significant pulmonary aspiration can occur with gastrostomy feeding. Methods of checking for silent pulmonary aspiration include checking tracheal aspirates with a glucose oxidant reagent strip or placing methylene blue in the formula and monitoring tracheal aspirate for pigmentation.[6, 12, 50]

A Foley balloon accidentally inflated in the small bowel or esophagus can lead to perforation or obstruction.[51] Careful inflation of the balloon soon after it has entered the stomach prevents viscus perforation. A gastrostomy tube may migrate in the stomach and obstruct the gastric outlet. This complication manifests itself clinically with vomiting and high residuals of feeding solution. Volvulus and jaundice may also occur as a result of balloon migration. This problem can be alleviated by gently pulling back the tube. If the balloon of a Foley catheter has migrated into the small bowel, deflation of the balloon before pulling it back further reduces the risk of intussusception. An outer crossbar will prevent distal migration.[1, 43]

Gastrocolic fistula usually manifests itself as copious diarrhea. Once confirmed, treatment consists of removal of the gastrostomy tube. Later creation of a gastrostomy in a different location may be possible. The patient may require hospital admission for nutritional support and monitoring of fluid and electrolyte status.

An external bumper that is snugged down too tightly may result in a short stoma and embedding of the internal bumper into the abdominal wall. An abscess may result. Overly tight external bumpers should be loosened. The correct position is 1 cm from the external abdomen.

Dacron cuffs can serve as the nidus for an abdominal wall abscess. Generally, the cuff can not be removed independently of the tube. A replacement tube without the cuff can be inserted, if one is careful not to dissect the tube into the wall of the abscess. Extensive abscesses may require incision and drainage.

CLOGGED FEEDING TUBES

Clogging is a problem common to all feeding tubes. It is prudent to attempt to unclog a tube before it is replaced, especially if the tube has a complex placement or the physician is unsure of how the tube is secured internally. Large gastrostomy tubes are the least likely to clog. Twenty-eight French gastrostomy tubes can tolerate home-blenderized foods and viscous feeding solutions. Isosmotic feeding solutions are tolerated by fairly narrow tubes and cost one sixth of what elemental feedings cost. Isosmotic feedings will clog needle catheters.[5] When tube lumina are 14 French or smaller, all pills and the contents of all capsules should be dissolved in water to prevent tube obstruction.[15]

Acid precipitation of feeding formulas is an important factor in the occlusion of gastrostomy and nasogastric feeding tubes. Sodium and calcium caseinate and soy protein molecules are most soluble at a pH of 6.3 to 6.6 and least soluble at a pH of approximately 4.7.[52] They are insoluble in nonpolar organic solvents. A study of 14 feeding solutions showed Pulmocare, Ensure Plus, and Osmolite to be the most "clog-prone" on exposure to acidic solutions.[53] Citrotein had the least tendency to clog.

Kinking is a frequent cause of tube blockage during the immediate postreinsertion period. Withdrawing the tube a few centimeters usually relieves the kink and obstruction. A persistently recurring kink requires tube removal and insertion of a fresh tube.

Accumulated feeding solution or medication precipitates are very difficult to clean or remove. Milking a pliant tube backwards may remove some of the cheesy precipitates. Guide wires or stylets may clear the proximal portion of a clogged tube lumen but are unsafe to use in subcutaneous areas of the lumen because they can puncture the tube and injure the patient or create a tube leak.

Fogarty arterial embolectomy catheters can be used to unclog jejunostomy[54] and gastrostomy tubes. The soft tip of the Fogarty catheter is inserted into the feeding tube and advanced while the insertion distance is monitored to avoid penetrating farther than the length of the feeding tube. The allowable length of insertion should be premeasured. A number 4 embolectomy catheter is suitable for a 10 or 12 French tube, whereas a number 5 catheter should be used in 14 French feeding tubes. When the catheter meets an obstruction, the balloon can be inflated, which usually opens the obstruction sufficiently that catheter passage can continue. Once the Fogarty has been manipulated to just proximal to the internal feeding opening, it is withdrawn while the balloon is intermittently inflated and deflated gently. The catheter should not be withdrawn while inflated because it and the feeding tube tend to move as a unit. The procedure may need to be repeated several times. Contrast injection to confirm tube position and integrity should be performed after declogging is completed.[54]

Irrigation with carbonated beverages and high-pressure irrigation with small-volume syringes have also been recommended as techniques for unclogging feeding tubes. Although irrigation seems like a straight forward and simple solution, these techniques are generally ineffective; furthermore, the possibility exists for dangerous tube ruptures with internal leakage. Broviac catheters are especially prone to tube aneurysms that can rupture under pressure.[36] Tubes unclogged by forceful irrigation or by deep luminal probing should be radiographed after injection of contrast to check tube integrity.

Enzymatic declogging of feeding tubes may sometimes be effective. Most enzymatic preparations are insoluble in an acidic environment and require mild alkalinity for effective action. Such precipitates can add to the obstructing material. One study suggested that two enzyme preparations can soften clog consistency sufficiently to enhance tube clearing with insufflation.[52] A crushed chymotrypsin tablet or two papain tablets (effervescent Allergan) can be dissolved in 2 ml of distilled water and irrigated into the drained feeding tube. A 12.5-cm catheter may make such irrigation more effective. The feeding tubes should be closed or clamped and left for 1 to 4 hours. One study only attempted tube insufflation at 4 hours, but clog changes were noted after one-half hour.[52] Insufflation of air with a 50-ml syringe also may clear the tube.

Most clogged tubes should be replaced. Tubes that have been unclogged by using force should be radiographed after contrast injection to check for internal leaks. Regular tap water irrigations and selection of a feeding solution appropriate for the diameter of the feeding tube are vital to prevent tube clogging.

References

1. Gauderer MWL: Methods of gastrostomy tube replacement. In Ponsky JL (ed): Techniques of Percutaneous Gastrostomy. New York, Igaku-Shoin Medical Publishers, 1988, pp 79–90.
2. Gordon AM: Enteral nutritional support. Postgrad Med 70:155, 1981.
3. Sweatman AJ, Tomasello PA, Loughhead MG, et al: Misplacement of nasogastric tubes and oesophageal monitoring devices. Br J Anaesth 50:389, 1978.
4. Meguid MM, Eldor S, Ashe W: The delivery of nutritional support: A potpourri of new devices and methods. Cancer 55:279, 1985.
5. Hinsdale JG, Lipkowitz GS, Pollock TW, et al: Prolonged enteral nutrition in malnourished patients with non-elemental feeding. Am J Surg 149:334, 1985.
6. Korda MJ, Guenter P, Rombeau JL: Enteral nutrition in the critically ill. Crit Care Clin 3:133, 1987.
7. Cataldi-Belcher EL, Seltzer MH, Slocum BA, et al: Complications occur-

8. Hanson L: Predictive criteria for length of nasogastric tube insertion for tube feeding. J Parenter Enter Nutr 3:160, 1977.
9. Baringer DC: Indications for gastrostomy. In Ponsky JL (ed): Techniques of Percutaneous Gastrostomy. New York, Igaku-Shoin Medical Publishers, 1988, pp 5–8.
10. Heynsfield AB, Bethel RA, Amsley JD, et al: Enteral hyperalimentation: An alternative to central venous hyperalimentation. Ann Intern Med 90:63, 1980.
11. Jeffers SL, Dorn LA, Meguid MM: Mechanical complications of enteral nutrition: Prospective study of 109 consecutive patients. Clin Res 32:233A, 1984.
12. Winterhaver RH, Durning RB, Barron E, et al: Aspirated nasogastric feeding solution detected by glucose strips. Ann Intern Med 95:67, 1981.
13. Locker DL, Foster JE, Craun ML, et al: A technique for long term continent gastrostomy. Surg Gynecol Obstet 160:73, 1985.
14. Padilla GV, Grant M, Wong H, et al: Subjective distresses of nasogastric tube feeding. J Parenter Enter Nutr 3:53, 1979.
15. Bruckstein AH: Managing the percutaneous endoscopic gastrostomy tube. Postgrad Med 82:143, 1987.
16. Kittinger JW, Sandler RS, Heizer WD: Efficacy of metoclopramide as an adjunct to duodenal placement of small-bore feeding tubes: A randomized, placebo-controlled, double-blind study. J Parenter Enter Nutr 11:33, 1987.
17. Guiness R: How to use the new small-bore feeding tubes. Nursing 86 16:51, 1986.
18. Lipman TO, Kessler T, Arabian A: Nasopulmonary intubation with feeding tubes: Case reports and review of the literature. J Parenter Enter Nutr 9:618, 1985.
19. Dorsey JS, Cogordan J: Nasotracheal intubation and pulmonary parenchymal perforation. Chest 87:131, 1985.
20. Woodall BH, Winfield DF, Bisset GS III: Inadvertent tracheobronchial placement of feeding tubes. Radiology 165:727, 1987.
21. Hand RW, Kemster M, Levey JH, et al: Inadvertent transbronchial insertion of narrow-bore feeding tubes into the pleural space. JAMA 251:2396, 1984.
22. Cockreel CH, Shao-Ru C: Hazardous use of stiff wire stylet in feeding tube manipulation. AJR 142:1296, 1984. Also, Weyman PJ, Glazer JS: reply.
22a. Roubenoff R, Ravich WJ: Pneumothorax due to nasogastric feeding tubes: Report of four cases, review of the literature, and recommendations for prevention. Arch Intern Med 149:184, 1989.
23. Christie DL, Ament ME: A double blind cross-over study of metoclopramide v. placebo for facilitating passage of multipurpose biopsy tube. Gastroenterology 71:726, 1976.
24. Rombeau JL, Twomey PL, McLean GK, et al: Experience with a new gastrostomy-jejunal feeding tube. Surgery 93:574, 1983.
25. Hatfield DR, Beck JL: An improved technique for feeding tube placement. Radiology 141:823, 1981.
26. Sax HC, Bower RH: A method for securing nasogastric tubes in uncooperative patients. Surg Gynecol Obstet 164:471, 1987.
27. Scholten DC, Wood TL, Thompson DR: Pneumothorax from nasoenteric feeding tube insertion. Am Surg 52:381, 1986.
28. Torrington KG, Bowman MA: Fatal hydrothorax and empyema complicating a malpositioned nasogastric tube. Chest 79:240, 1981.
29. Stogdill BJ, Page CP, Pestana C: Nonoperative replacement of a jejunostomy feeding catheter. Am J Surg 147:280, 1984.
30. Wilson MF, Haynes-Johnson V: Cranberry juice or water?: A comparison of feeding-tube irrigants. Nutr Support Services 7:23, 1987.
31. Steffere WP, Kery SH: Enteral hyperalimentation for patients with head and neck cancer. Otolaryngol Clin North Am 13:437, 1980.
32. Klopp CT: Cervical esophagostomy. J Thorac Cardiovasc Surg 21:490, 1951.
33. Shumrick DA: Pyriformisinusostomy; a useful technique for temporary or permanent tube feeding. Arch Surg 94:277, 1967.
34. Torosian MH, Rohbeau JL: Feeding by tube enterostomy. Surg Gynecol Obstet 150:918, 1980.
35. Stellato TA: Gastrostomy A historical perspective. In Ponsky JL (ed): Techniques of Percutaneous Gastrostomy. New York, Igaku-Shoin Medical Publishers, 1988, pp 1–8.
36. Boland MP, Patrick J, Stoski DS, et al: Permanent enteral feeding in cystic fibrosis: Advantages of a replaceable jejunostomy tube. J Pediatr Surg 22:843, 1987.
37. Wiedeman JE, Smith VC: Use of the Hickman catheter for jejunal feedings in children. Surg Gynecol Obstet 162:69, 1986.
38. Gauderer MWL: Techniques of surgical gastrostomy. In Ponsky JL (ed): Techniques of Percutaneous Gastrostomy. New York, Igaku-Shoin Medical Publishers, 1988, pp 9–20.
39. Ponsky JL, Gaudere MWL, Stellato TA, et al: Percutaneous approaches to enteral alimentation. Am J Surg 149:102, 1985.
40. Cogbill TH, Wolfson RH, Moore EE, et al: Massive pneumatosis intestinalis and subcutaneous emphysema: Complication of needle catheter jejunostomy. J Parenter Enter Nutr 7:171, 1983.
41. Collure DWD: A technique of anchoring a catheter in a feeding gastrostomy. Am J Surg 144:370, 1982.
42. Strodel WE, Ponsky JL: Complications of percutaneous gastrostomy. In

Ponsky JL (ed): Techniques of Percutaneous Gastrostomy. New York, Igaku-Shoin Medical Publishers, 1988, pp 63–78.

43. Kaufman A, Schpitz B, Dinbar A: Reinsertion of a catheter for feeding jejunostomy. Surg Gynecol Obstet 158:293, 1984.
44. Ponsky J, Aszodi A: Percutaneous endoscopic jejunostomy. Am J Gastroenterol 79:113, 1984.
45. Van Stegmann G, Liechty RD: Endoscopic jejunal feeding tube through decompressing gastrostomy. Surg Gynecol Obstet 160:173, 1985.
46. Abbott WC, Echenique MM, Bisman BR, et al: Nutritional care of the trauma patient. Surg Gynecol Obstet 157:585, 1983.
47. Kerlan RK, Pogany AC, Ring EU: A simple method for insertion of large untapered catheters. AJR 141:792, 1983.
48. Heymsfield SB, Horowitz J, Lawson DH: Enteral hyperalimentation. In Berk JE (ed): Developments in Digestive Diseases. Philadelphia, Lea & Febiger, 1980, pp 282–283.

49. Ciocon JO, Silverstone FA, Graves LM, et al: Tube feedings in elderly patients. Arch Intern Med 148:429, 1988.
50. Trebar DM, Stechmiller J: Pulmonary aspiration in tube-fed patients with artificial airways. Heart Lung 13:667, 1984.
51. Chester JF, Turnbull AR: Intestinal obstruction by overdistension of a jejunostomy catheter balloon: A salutary lesson. J Parenter Enter Nutr 12:410, 1988.
52. Nicholson LJ: Declogging small-bore feeding tubes. J Parenter Enter Nutr 11:6, 594, 1987.
53. Marcuard SP, Perkins AM: Clogging of feeding tubes. J Parenter Enter Nutr 12:403, 1988.
54. Bentz ML, Tollett CA, Dempsey DT: Obstructed feeding jejunostomy tube: A new method of salvage. J Parenter Enter Nutr 12:417, 1988.

Chapter **55**

Paracentesis

Jonathan M. Glauser

INTRODUCTION AND BACKGROUND

Diagnostic peritoneal aspiration was originally described by Saloman in 1906.[1, 2] Saloman used a needle with a trocar to place a urethral catheter into the peritoneal cavity.[3] In Saloman's day and until recently, paracentesis was frequently performed for therapeutic reasons (to remove excess peritoneal fluid). This indication has been largely replaced by medical therapy, and paracentesis is now an infrequent procedure because of the potential for rapid fluid shifts from the plasma into the peritoneal cavity, which often leads to vascular collapse, hepatic coma, and renal failure.[4] In cases of tense ascites caused by malignancy, abdominal paracentesis to remove large volumes of ascitic fluid is still useful,[5] and the procedure has been recommended for the emergency relief of massive malignant ascites that may reduce respiratory capacity. Similarly, abdominal paracentesis can be performed in the cirrhotic patient with tense ascites that impairs respirations.

Present-day therapy of ascites consists mainly of medical management with salt and water restriction, diuretic therapy, potassium replacement, and, possibly, the use of LaVeen shunting.[6] Needle paracentesis, or the "four-quadrant tap," was used in the diagnosis of hemoperitoneum before diagnostic peritoneal lavage became popular. It has been demonstrated that 200 ml of free blood in the peritoneal cavity may be detected only 20 per cent of the time with paracentesis, and 500 ml can be detected only 80 per cent of the time.[4] Because of these high false-negative rates, needle aspiration of the abdomen for the diagnosis of hemoperitoneum is currently a technique of mainly historical interest. Abdominal paracentesis is now largely a diagnostic procedure for noninfectious ascites and peritoneal infections.

INDICATIONS

Before elective paracentesis, the presence of peritoneal fluid must be established. The abdominal cavity is divided into compartments according to mesenteric attachments; hence fluid may be localized.[7] These subdivisions are relatively difficult to appreciate by physical examination alone. Ultrasound and roentgenography are the procedures most frequently used in addition to physical examination to diagnose the presence of peritoneal fluid.[8–10] Ultrasonography can detect as little as 100 ml of ascitic fluid and is much more sensitive in diagnosing ascites than physical examination.[11] Many clinicians believe that, unless ascites is unquestionably present on physical examination, an ultrasound of the abdomen should be obtained before proceeding with paracentesis.[12] In fact, ultrasonographic guidance may improve the safety and efficacy of paracentesis, in addition to facilitating the diagnosis.[13, 14] The differential diagnosis of ascites is given in Table 55–1.

When the presence of newly recognized ascites is established, paracentesis is indicated to ascertain its cause. For practical purposes, the most worrisome entities causing ascites and those requiring the most urgent therapy include bacterial peritonitis, tuberculous peritonitis, and pancreatic conditions.[15] For example, in a patient with known cirrhosis who presents with abdominal pain, leukocytosis, fever, hepatic encephalopathy, or rebound tenderness, the presence

---

Table 55–1. Differential Diagnosis of Ascites

Cirrhosis of any cause*
Tuberculosis*
Bacterial peritonitis
Fungal peritonitis
Pancreatic disease
Bile leakage
Congestive heart failure*
Tricuspid insufficiency
Constrictive pericarditis
Nephrotic syndrome, chronic renal disease
Nephrogenic ascites (dialysis related)
Hepatoma*
Myxedema
Vasculitis
Ascites associated with benign tumors of the ovary (Meig syndrome)
Malignant tumor involvement of the liver or peritoneum (ovary, stomach, pancreas, colon, breast, liver, bile duct, testes, various sarcomas, lymphomas)*
Ruptured hollow viscus
Intestinal infarction
Protein-losing gastroenteropathy
Budd-Chiari syndrome
Hepatic vein obstruction
Inferior vena caval obstruction
Portal vein thrombosis
Ventriculoperitoneal shunt
Ureteroperitoneal fistula
Starch reaction (postsurgical)
Lymphatic obstruction with chylous ascites (thoracic duct trauma, filariasis, mediastinal tumors)

*Most common causes of ascites in North America.

of bacterial peritonitis must be established or ruled out quickly. Spontaneous bacterial peritonitis may be very subtle and detectable only by the examination of peritoneal fluid. Paracentesis has been advanced as an aid in the diagnosis of ruptured ectopic pregnancy[4, 16] and bowel perforation,[17] but more accurate diagnostic procedures are currently available. Hemoperitoneum due to trauma[1, 18] is best diagnosed by peritoneal lavage,[3, 19–26] and culdocentesis is accurate in detecting ruptured ectopic pregnancy in up to 95 per cent of cases (see Chapters 56 and 77).

PRECAUTIONS AND CONTRAINDICATIONS

Before performing a diagnostic peritoneal tap, careful preparation is mandatory. This is an invasive procedure, and many complications are preventable. The bladder must be emptied before paracentesis.[15, 27] If the patient is unable to void, a Foley catheter should be placed. Strict aseptic technique should be observed, including shaving, draping, preparation with iodophor or pHisoHex,[3] and the use of sterile gloves and a mask. Because of the risk of hemorrhage and because paracentesis is often performed in alcoholic cirrhosis patients, in whom platelet counts may be reduced and clotting ability may be impaired, one should evaluate and correct the prothrombin time, the partial thromboplastin time, and the platelet count before proceeding with paracentesis.[15] A prothrombin time prolonged more than 6 seconds over control and a platelet count less than 60,000 are relative contraindications to paracentesis.[11] However, some investigators do not believe that a coagulopathy is a contraindication to the procedure if the needle is inserted through the avascular midline.[28]

Some areas are unsuitable for needle insertion. The rectus muscle should be avoided because of the presence of the superior and inferior epigastric vessels.[29] It is also advisable to avoid the upper abdominal quadrants because of the frequency of undetected hepatosplenomegaly in the fluid-filled abdomen.[15] Visible collateral venous channels on the abdominal wall should be avoided. The preferred site is in the midline, a few centimeters below the umbilicus. Entering through the relatively avascular midline (linea alba) lessens the risk of hemorrhage (Fig. 55–1).[10] The right or left lower quadrants lateral to the rectus muscle are alternative sites for paracentesis.

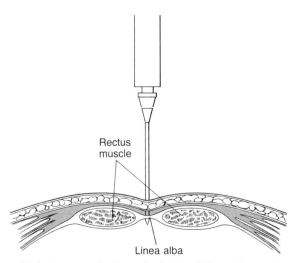

Figure 55–1. The avascular linea alba in the midline, a few centimeters below the umbilicus, is a commonly preferred site for paracentesis.

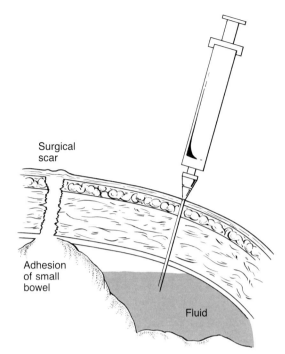

Figure 55–2. Sites of previous surgical incisions must be avoided because adhesions may fix the bowel and predispose to bowel perforation. (Redrawn from Fisher JC: Clinical Procedures: A Concise Guide for Students of Medicine. Baltimore, Williams & Wilkins, 1980. © 1980, Williams & Wilkins.)

There is a risk of intestinal perforation with abdominal paracentesis. Sites of surgical scars and known intra-abdominal adhesions must be avoided (Fig. 55–2).[1] The procedure should be withheld or performed with extreme caution in the presence of a markedly distended bowel (e.g., in cases of bowel obstruction), because abnormally elevated intraluminal pressure may cause leakage of bowel contents following needle puncture.[15, 29] Although it has been shown that mobile loops of bowel are pushed away by the needle during paracentesis and are difficult to penetrate with a needle,[3] adhesions or bowel obstruction may fix the bowel and may predispose to perforation. Mallory[15] reported two cases of bowel perforation that resulted in generalized peritonitis and abscess formation when paracentesis was performed on two patients who had previously undergone abdominal surgery. It is interesting to note that experimentally induced bowel punctures show no leakage until the intraluminal pressure reaches 260 mm Hg,[3] whereas intestinal pressure seldom rises above 20 mm Hg in the nonobstructed small or large bowel.[27] Moretz and Erickson found that bowel in dogs penetrated by a 13- to 20-gauge needle could withstand an intraluminal pressure of 120 mm Hg without leaking.[30] Although the risk of bowel perforation may seem small, areas of possible adhesions should be avoided, and distended bowel is a relative contraindication to performing the procedure.

Pregnancy is also a relative contraindication to paracentesis.[30] If the procedure is deemed necessary, one should choose a site above the umbilicus lateral to the midline. Alternatively, the Seldinger technique of catheter placement could be used. Ascitic fluid from patients whose serum is positive for hepatitis B surface antigen may be infectious and should be processed carefully.[31] Obviously, a needle should not be advanced through unmistakably infected skin or soft tissue. The procedure is more difficult in an uncooperative patient.

PROCEDURE

In general, 50 ml of ascitic fluid is required for adequate study,[10] although larger quantities of fluid (up to 500 ml) may be desired in some instances.[8, 27] In cases of tense ascites that produce respiratory distress, the rapid removal of 1 to 3 liters may be necessary to provide relief of symptoms.

The patient is usually supine during the procedure. Some physicians use the lateral decubitus position or have the patient stand. The hands-knees position may be used if only minimal ascites is present.[28] Standing may predispose to vagal fainting and is not recommended. Theoretically, if the patient is in the lateral decubitus position, the bowel floats upward and away from the midline. Sterile technique should be observed, and 1 per cent lidocaine is infiltrated subcutaneously down to the peritoneum.[3] Differences in technique generally involve location of aspiration and size and type of needle or catheter used. For simple diagnostic paracentesis, a needle and syringe are adequate. Following skin antisepsis, an 18- or 20-gauge short-beveled spinal needle is attached to a syringe and inserted through the abdominal wall. In patients with tense ascites, insertion of the needle at an oblique angle may help seal the needle tract after paracentesis, preventing persistent ascitic fluid drainage.[15] Runyon and associates advise retracting the skin caudad before needle insertion to produce a Z-tract effect when the needle is withdrawn.[28] The needle is advanced while suction is applied until abdominal fluid return is noted; a "pop" may be felt on penetration of the peritoneum when resistance diminishes.[3] If large amounts of fluid are desired, one may use an 18-gauge Intracath or other suitable flexible catheter or a three-way stopcock and drain the fluid into a collection bag.

If fluid is not obtained by suction or if the initial flow stops, the needle or catheter may be advanced slowly with gentle suction. Rotation, angulation, or other manipulation of the needle or catheter may also remedy the problem. Turning the patient to a lateral decubitus position may help if the patient is initially supine.[3] If fluid is not readily obtained, the puncture site may be changed.

A four-quadrant abdominal tap is still recommended by some. The suggested points of entry are in the right and left upper and lower quadrants of the abdomen, equidistant from the midline along the lateral border of the rectus muscle (Fig. 55–3).[29] Obviously, if a satisfactory amount of fluid is obtained at one site, the others need not be used. The four-quadrant method has a theoretic advantage in that the midline is avoided. It is thought that, because air-filled bowel floats upward, the bowel remains in the midline in a supine patient; with the use of physical and roentgenographic diagnosis and localization of ascites, one of the sites in a four-quadrant tap is almost always successful if 200 ml or more exists in the peritoneal cavity. A number of alternative puncture sites have been proposed. The specific site is probably not important if proper attention is paid to technique and contraindications. Most investigators prefer the lower abdominal sites. Aspiration may be successfully performed in either flank midway between the costal margin and the iliac spine.[29] Singh and Kaur[16] used sites approximately 2.5 cm medial to the anterosuperior iliac spines. Rao and Ravikumar[27] used lumbar sites approximately 4 to 5 cm lateral to the lateral border of the rectus muscle in the lumbar region, aspirating with a beveled 20-gauge, 5-cm needle. The lateral edge of either rectus muscle 4 cm below the umbilicus has been used.[22] Others claim that the specific location is not important as long as the site is lateral to the rectus sheath so that the inferior epigastric artery is avoided.[3, 26]

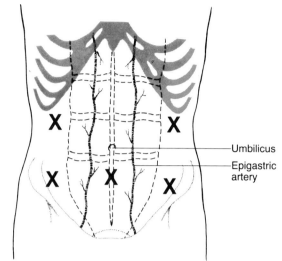

Figure 55–3. Standard landmarks for paracentesis include the four quadrants lateral to the rectus muscle and a few centimeters below the umbilicus in the midline. (Redrawn from Suratt PM, Gibson RS: Manual of Medical Procedures. St. Louis, CV Mosby Co, 1982, p 217.)

Gjessig and colleagues[32] describe a technique similar to that used for peritoneal dialysis. With the patient under local anesthesia, a small skin incision is made 3 to 5 cm below the umbilicus in the midline, and a trocar and a cannula are pushed through the parietal peritoneum (Fig. 55–4). The trocar is then removed, and a soft plastic dialysis catheter is inserted into the peritoneal cavity and gently manipulated into the pouch of Douglas. Fluid is then aspirated for examination. This technique may be preferred if the catheter

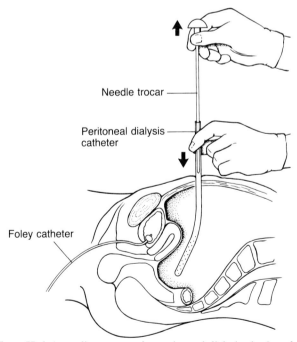

Figure 55–4. A needle trocar and a peritoneal dialysis plastic catheter may be used to perform paracentesis if continued drainage of fluid is required. The bladder *must* be emptied before this procedure is performed. (Redrawn from Suratt PM, Gibson RS: Manual of Medical Procedures. St. Louis, CV Mosby Co, 1982, p 195.)

Table 55–2. Studies to Obtain or Consider in Ascitic Fluid Analysis

Protein concentration
Specific gravity
Gram stain
Acid-fast stain and culture
Culture for bacteria and fungi
Cytology
Amylase concentration
Total fat concentration
Polarized light for double refractile particles (if starch is felt to be the cause)[42]
Sudan stain for fat[16]
Glucose
Ammonia[9]
Lactate dehydrogenase (transudate versus exudate)[43]
pH, lactate levels (consider if bacterial peritonitis suspected)

(Data from Wintrobe MM, Thorn GW, Adams RD, et al [eds]: Harrison's Principles of Internal Medicine. 11th ed. New York, McGraw-Hill Book Co, 1987; Sleisenger MH, Fordtran JS: Gastrointestinal Disease. 3rd ed, vol 1. Philadelphia, WB Saunders Co, 1989.)

is to remain in the peritoneal cavity for continued drainage (see also Chapter 56).

ANALYSIS OF ASCITIC FLUID

A thorough discussion of the evaluation of ascitic fluid is beyond the scope of this chapter. Tables 55–2 through 55–5 offer a summary of characteristics and specific parameters of ascitic fluid. These can be useful in selecting the proper laboratory test. Of note, however, is that ascitic fluid culture may be negative in more than half of all cases of spontaneous bacterial peritonitis. Therefore, a polymorphonuclear (PMN) cell count of more than 250 cells/mm³ warrants therapy.[11, 33] The yield of ascitic fluid cultures may be greatly enhanced if the physician *directly inoculates a standard blood culture bottle with 10 to 15 ml of ascitic fluid at the bedside* rather than sending specimens for culture to the laboratory.[28]

POTENTIAL COMPLICATIONS OF PARACENTESIS

Serious intraperitoneal or abdominal wall hemorrhage has been reported following abdominal paracentesis. Although lacerations of major vessels are occasionally reported,[34] portal hypertension, clotting abnormalities, platelet defects, increased capillary fragility, and clotting factor deficiencies rather than major vessel injury are usually implicated as the cause of hemorrhage.[15, 35]

Table 55–3. Causes of Bloody Ascites

Malignancy, especially hepatoma or ovarian carcinoma
Tuberculous peritonitis
Spontaneous solid viscera injury (e.g., splenic rupture)
Trauma
Leaking ruptured abdominal aneurysm
Ruptured ectopic pregnancy[16, 17]
Strangulating bowel obstruction[17]
Ruptured mesenteric varix in cirrhosis[44]
Perforated duodenal ulcer[45]
Hepatic vein thrombosis[10]
Pancreatitis
Uncomplicated cirrhosis

(Data from Babb RR: Diagnosing ascites—the value of abdominal paracentesis. Postgrad Med 63:219, 1978; Sleisenger MH, Fordtran JS: Gastrointestinal Disease. 3rd ed, vol 1. Philadelphia, WB Saunders Co, 1989.)

Table 55–4. Conditions Causing an Elevated Peritoneal Fluid Amylase (More Than 100 Units/100 ml)

Pancreatitis[1, 10]
Pancreatic pseudocyst[8]
Mesenteric infarction[41]
Pancreatic duct tear
Small bowel perforation[23]
Perforated peptic ulcer

In a retrospective analysis of 242 consecutive diagnostic paracenteses in patients with liver disease,[15] only four cases of significant hemorrhage occurred. It was speculated that clotting abnormalities may have produced hemorrhage in all these patients. In the series of 229 patients reported by Runyon, three patients had bleeding complications (one required transfusion), but Runyon did not routinely measure clotting because coagulopathy was not considered an absolute contraindication.[36]

A precipitous fall in blood pressure and a "shock-like" state may occur following rapid removal of *large* amounts of fluid from the peritoneal cavity. Usually more than 1000 ml must be removed quickly[10] for this to occur. Although as much as 6 to 10 liters have been removed safely over 10 to 15 minutes, the rate should not exceed 1000 ml per 24 hours if more than 1000 ml is to be removed electively.

One report noted that a 5-liter paracentesis over 20 to 40 minutes had a negligible effect on blood volume in 12 nonedematous patients,[37] and another noted that large-volume paracentesis has no immediate hemodynamic effect.[38] However, precipitation or aggravation of fluid or electrolyte imbalance may still follow removal of large amounts of ascitic fluid. Baldus and Summerskill[39] reported the fatal complications of oliguric renal failure, hepatic coma, hyponatremia, and hypotension unresponsive to hypertonic saline infusion in a 56-year-old cirrhotic patient who had 20 liters of ascitic fluid drained over a 36-hour period. Although some cases of hypotension following paracentesis may respond to intravascular fluid replacement, not all of them are reversible. The most commonly precipitated electrolyte disturbance is hyponatremia.

A number of other complications have been reported. Bowel puncture may be innocuous,[40] but perforation of bowel followed by generalized peritonitis and abdominal wall abscess have been reported.[22] Catheter fragments have been sheared off and left in the peritoneal cavity,[15, 19] and mesenteric laceration has been reported.[22] In general, a major complication rate of less than 3 per cent has been reported.[15] Theoretically, paracentesis may cause bacterial peritonitis, but this complication is rare.[36]

Minor complications, which are seldom of clinical importance, include scrotal edema, persistent ascitic fluid leakage,[41] hematoma of the anterior cecal wall and the adjacent mesentery following an iliac fossa tap,[27] and ovarian cyst laceration.[23] Persistent fluid leakage may be remedied by placement of a suture around the puncture site.

CONCLUSION

Simple needle aspiration of ascitic fluid for diagnostic evaluation may be quickly, safely, and easily performed in the emergency department. The procedure is usually an elective one that can be performed at the bedside, but in cases of respiratory compromise or suspected bacterial peritonitis, abdominal paracentesis becomes an urgent or emergency procedure.

The complications of the procedure are usually minor and

Table 55–5. Characteristics of Ascitic Fluid by Etiology

Condition	Appearance	Total Protein	Amylase Concentration	Microscopic Findings (WBCs, RBCs)*	Cytology, Bacteriology, Total Fat
Uncomplicated cirrhosis	Clear, straw-colored	<2.5 gm/dl		Usually <1000 WBCs/mm^3	
Malignant ascites	Bloody, chylous, straw-colored, or mucinous	>2.5 gm/dl		Elevated RBCs >1000/mm^3 in 50%	Malignant cells seen in 60—90%[9, 10]
Tuberculous peritonitis	Fibrin clots, may be bloody, yellow, or chylous	>2.5 gm/dl		Mononuclear leukocytosis (>1000 WBCs/mm^3)	Culture, acid-fast stain
Chylous ascites	Milky, turbid			Variable WBCs with lymphocytes predominating	Sudan stain for fat
Bacterial peritonitis	Thick, cloudy, odoriferous	>2.5 gm/dl	May be high if bowel perforation has occurred	More than 300 WBCs/mm^3 More than 25% polymorphonuclear leukocytes	Culture, Gram stain†
Nephrotic	Clear, straw-colored	Low (<2.5 gm/dl)		Usually <250 WBCs/mm^3; mononuclear, mesothelial	Sudan stain if chylous
Congestive heart failure	Clear, straw-colored	Variable		Usually <300 WBCs/mm^3; mononuclear cells, mesothelial	
Pancreatic ascites	Turbid, chylous or hemorrhagic	>2.5 gm/dl	High	Variable, may be bloody	

(Data from Sleisenger MH, Fordtran JS: Gastrointestinal Disease. 3rd ed, vol 1. Philadelphia, WB Saunders Co, 1989; Cohn EM: Ascites: Pathogenesis and differential diagnosis. In Bockus HL (ed): Gastroenterology. 3rd ed, vol 4. Philadelphia, WB Saunders Co, 1976; Wintrobe MM, Thorn GW, Adams RD, et al (eds): Harrison's Principles of Internal Medicine. 11th ed. New York, McGraw-Hill Book Co, 1987.)

*Only typical figures are given; these vary widely in a given disease state. Use of the corrected WBC is recommended in peritoneal effluent; this figure is more significant in evaluation of bacterial contamination, as from colonic or small bowel rupture. Corrected WBC = total WBC × [peritoneal WBC × circulating RBC/peritoneal RBC].

†Directly inoculate blood culture bottles at the bedside with 10 to 12 ml ascitic fluid.

RBC, red blood cell; WBC, white blood cell.

infrequent. With the availability of the more accurate technique of peritoneal lavage, paracentesis should not be used for the diagnosis of hemoperitoneum.

REFERENCES

1. Brown CH (ed): Diagnostic Procedures in Gastroenterology. St. Louis, CV Mosby Co, 1967, pp 284–286.
2. Saloman H: Die Diagnostische Punktion des Bauches. Berl Klin Wochenschr 43:45, 1906.
3. McCoy J, Wolma FJ: Abdominal tap: Indication, technic, and results. Am J Surg 122:693, 1971.
4. Giacobine JW, Siler VE: Evaluation of diagnostic abdominal paracentesis with experimental and clinical studies. Surg Gynecol Obstet 110:676, 1960.
5. Fischer DS: Abdominal paracentesis for malignant ascites. Arch Intern Med 139:235, 1979.
6. LaVeen HH, Christoudia G, Ip M, et al: Peritoneovenous shunting for ascites. Ann Intern Med 185:580, 1974.
7. Meyers MA: The spread and localization of acute intraperitoneal effusions. Radiology 95:457, 1970.
8. Babb RR: Diagnosing ascites—the value of abdominal paracentesis. Postgrad Med 63:219, 1978.
9. Cohn EM: Ascites: Pathogenesis and differential diagnosis. In Bockus HL (ed): Gastroenterology. 3rd ed, vol 4. Philadelphia, WB Saunders Co, 1976, pp 48–55.
10. Sleisenger MH, Fordtran JS: Gastrointestinal Disease. 3rd ed, vol 1. Philadelphia, WB Saunders Co, 1989.
11. Marshall JB: Finding the cause of ascites. Postgrad Med 83(8):189, 1988.
12. Kandel G, Diamant NE: A clinical view of recent advances in ascites. J Clin Gastroenterol 8:85, 1986.
13. Bard C, Lafortune M, Breton G: Ascites: Ultrasound guidance or blind paracentesis? Can Med Assoc J 135:209, 1986.
14. McGahan JP, Anderson MW, Walter JP: Portable real-time sonographic and needle guidance systems for aspiration and drainage. Am J Roentgenol 147:1241, 1986.
15. Mallory A, Schaefer JW: Complications of diagnostic paracentesis in patients with liver disease. JAMA 239:628, 1978.
16. Singh A, Kaur B: Paracentesis abdominis in ruptured ectopic pregnancy. J Indian Med Assoc 73:54, 1979.
17. Root HD, Hauser CW, McKinley CR, et al: Diagnostic peritoneal lavage. Surgery 57:633, 1965.
18. Manganaro AJ, Pachter HL, Spencer FC: Experience with routine open abdominal paracentesis. Surg Gynecol Obstet 146:795, 1978.
19. Caffee HH, Benfield JR: Is peritoneal lavage for the diagnosis of hemoperitoneum safe? Arch Surg 103:4, 1971.
20. Parvin S, Smith DE, Asher WM, et al: Effectiveness of peritoneal lavage in blunt abdominal trauma. Ann Surg 181:255, 1975.
21. McAlvanah MJ, Shaftan GW: Selective conservatism in penetrating abdominal wounds: A continuing reappraisal. J Trauma 18:206, 1978.
22. Veith FJ, Webber WB, Karl RC, et al: Diagnostic peritoneal lavage in acute abdominal disease: Normal findings in 100 patients. Ann Surg 166:290, 1967.
23. Engrav LH, Benjamin CI, Strate RG, et al: Diagnostic peritoneal lavage in blunt abdominal trauma. J Trauma 15:854, 1971.
24. Olsen WR, Hildreth DH: Abdominal paracentesis and peritoneal lavage in blunt abdominal trauma. J Trauma 11:824, 1971.
25. Lamke L, Varenhorst E: Abdominal paracentesis for early diagnosis of closed abdominal injury. Acta Chir Scand 144:21, 1978.
26. Civetta JM, Williams MJ, Richie RE: Diagnostic peritoneal irrigation—a simple and reliable technique. Surgery 67:874, 1970.
27. Rao RN, Ravikumar TS: Diagnostic peritoneal tap. Int Surg 62:14, 1977.
28. Runyon BA, Umland ET, Merlin T: Inoculation of blood culture bottles with ascitic fluid: Improved detection of spontaneous bacterial peritonitis. Arch Intern Med 147:73, 1987.
29. Schwartz SI, Lillihei RC, Shires GT, et al (eds): Principles of Surgery. 3rd ed. New York, McGraw-Hill Book Co, 1979.
30. Moretz WH, Erickson WG: Peritoneal tap as an aid in the diagnosis of acute abdominal disease. Am Surg 20:363, 1954.
31. Cacciatore L, Molinari V, Guadagnino V, et al: Hepatitis B antigen in ascitic fluid in cirrhosis. Br Med J 3:172, 1973.
32. Gjessing J, Oskarsson BM, Tomlin PJ, et al: Diagnostic abdominal paracentesis. Br Med J 1:617, 1972.
33. Kachintorn U, Chainovati T, Chinapak O, et al: Spontaneous bacterial peritonitis in cirrhotics: Clinical and ascitic fluid findings. Ann Acad Med Singapore 15:221, 1986.

34. Thiel ER, Shires GT: Peritoneal lavage in blunt abdominal trauma. Am J Surg 126:64, 1973.

35. Walls WJ, Losowsky MS: The hemostatic defect of liver disease. Gastroenterology 60:107, 1971.

36. Runyon BA: Paracentesis of ascitic fluid. A safe procedure. Arch Intern Med 146:2259, 1986.

37. Pinto PC, American J, Reynolds TB: Large-volume paracentesis in nonedematous patients with tense ascites: Its effect on intravascular volume. Hepatology 8:207, 1988.

38. Simon DM, McCain JR, Bonkovsky HL, et al: Effects of therapeutic paracentesis on systemic and hepatic hemodynamics and on renal and hormonal function. Hepatology 7:423, 1987.

39. Baldus WP, Summerskill WHJ: The kidney in hepatic disease. Postgrad Med 41:103, 1967.

40. Runyon BA, Hoefs JC, Canawati HN: Polymicrobial bacterial ascites: A unique entity in the spectrum of infected ascitic fluid. Arch Intern Med 146:273, 1986.

41. Ouillen CG, Polk HC Jr: The ascitic leak: A case presentation—management by paracentesis and saline-albumin infusion. Surgery 82:241, 1977.

42. Warshaw AL: Diagnosis of starch peritonitis by paracentesis. Lancet 2:1054, 1972.

43. Bruckstein AH: Management of the patient with ascites. Postgrad Med 82:227, 1987.

44. Rothchild JJ, Gelernt I, Sloan W: Ruptured mesenteric varix in cirrhosis: Unusual cause for hemoperitoneum. N Engl J Med 278:97, 1968.

45. Bristown JD, Medaed NE: Hemorrhagic ascites due to perforated duodenal ulcer: Report of a case. Arch Intern Med 105:105, 1960.

Chapter **56**

Diagnostic Peritoneal Lavage

Samuel Timothy Coleridge and Calvin Bell

INTRODUCTION

The diagnosis of intraperitoneal injury, especially in children, pregnant women, and patients with altered mental status or multiple extra-abdominal injuries, has always been difficult. These clinical situations remain the classic indications for peritoneal lavage.

Clinical signs of serious visceral injury can be notoriously nonspecific, minimal, or absent even when life-threatening injury is present. This is true for both blunt and penetrating abdominal injuries. Likewise, many patients show signs and symptoms suggestive of intraperitoneal injury when none has occurred. The overall accuracy of the *initial* physical examination in diagnosing intraperitoneal injury in the traumatized patient is surprisingly low and has been variously reported to range from 16 to 45 per cent.[1-12] The physical examination is even less helpful in the patient with an altered mental status from head injury, intoxication, drug ingestion, or spinal cord injury.

It is interesting to note that even documented peritoneal penetration may *not* be associated with visceral injury in as many as 53 per cent of cases. Other laboratory tests and organ imaging techniques are generally selective and have been of limited value to the emergency physician. Likewise, if these imaging studies are undertaken in the acute situation to assess intra-abdominal trauma, valuable time may be lost, and the physician may be left with inconclusive results.[3, 7, 9-11] Improvement in computed tomography (CT) scanners in limiting scan time (from 5 to 2 seconds) and commitment by more trauma centers to provide experienced personnel for CT interpretation, patient monitoring, and resuscitation on a 24-hour basis have increased the use of this alternative study for evaluating stable thoracoabdominal trauma patients.[13-23]

Previously, the policy of selective or expectant observation was the rule to minimize the morbidity or mortality associated with negative exploratory laparotomy. Patients without obvious signs and symptoms of intra-abdominal injury were serially and frequently reevaluated. If and when positive signs and symptoms developed, the patients underwent exploration. This delay in diagnosis was also associated with morbidity and mortality because of the development of sepsis or hemorrhagic shock, requiring multiple transfusions and causing prolonged recovery times. Operative delay is reportedly associated with as many as 50 per cent of fatal cases and is directly

---

The opinions or assertions contained herein are the private views of the authors and are not to be construed as official or reflecting the views of the Department of Defense or the Department of the Army.

---

responsible for as many as 17 per cent of these deaths. With combined head and trunk trauma, undiagnosed intra-abdominal injury has been found to be responsible for 20 to 40 per cent of deaths. Several investigators demonstrated that expectant observation not only was significantly less accurate than peritoneal lavage in diagnosing intra-abdominal injury but also led to a delay that increased recovery time or resulted in increased deaths.[2, 4, 8, 11, 24-27] Local wound exploration is an insensitive yet specific method for determining peritoneal penetration. The value of local wound exploration can be further increased when combined with diagnostic peritoneal lavage. Positive local wound exploration followed by positive diagnostic peritoneal lavage suggests the presence of significant injury, and celiotomy is recommended. Positive local wound exploration with a negative diagnostic peritoneal lavage indicates a lower probability of intra-abdominal injury.[28-30]

The use of catheter paracentesis and diagnostic peritoneal lavage as originally described by Root and coworkers in 1965 is now recognized as a rapid, effective means of facilitating diagnosis in problem cases.[61] The procedure can be performed virtually anywhere, is quick, and requires little equipment.

Danto's review of 23 papers published since the initial report of Root and associates describes a total of 9588 documented patients with both blunt and penetrating injuries; 4053 of these patients had a positive test and 5535 had a negative test.[31] The positive test was correct in 97 per cent of cases, resulting in negative celiotomies only 3 per cent of the time (3 per cent false-positive rate). The negative test was correct in 98.7 per cent of cases (1.3 per cent false-negative rate). Subsequent studies continue to emphasize the high accuracy of this test with more false positives than false negatives.[12, 32-35] Controversy continues regarding the criteria for a "positive" lavage for penetrating thoracoabdominal injuries, particularly for injuries that produce minimal hemoperitoneum (hollow viscera and diaphragm). Lowering the criteria increases the rate of unnecessary celiotomies for insignificant, self-limiting injuries (e.g., grade I or II hepatic and splenic lacerations).[27, 34, 36-43]

Peritoneal lavage can be used for other medical and surgical problems (e.g., hypothermia, hyperthermia, and renal failure). The procedure allows retrieval of representative fluid early in the course of disease and offers an access for intraperitoneal fluid therapy or removal of unwanted or toxic chemicals through peritoneal dialysis.[3, 5, 6, 10, 24, 44-52]

Ideally, the surgical consultant managing the trauma patient should perform the diagnostic peritoneal lavage, although often the emergency physician, pending arrival of the consultant, is encouraged to perform this procedure in the multiple trauma patient.[53]

BACKGROUND

In 1906, Saloman in Berlin reported the use of diagnostic paracentesis with a trocar and a urethral catheter to assess disease of the peritoneum.[54] His instrument (Fig. 56–1) was a modification of a device used by Adolf Schmidt, who was performing peritoneal lavage with normal saline or other nutritive substances to increase the resistance of the peritoneum to peritonitis. Fiedler is mentioned as the initiator of the technique. Saloman recognized that diagnostic paracentesis could be valuable in identifying peritonitis caused by gastric perforation or infectious and inflammatory disease as well as hemoperitoneum from a ruptured ectopic pregnancy. He rec-

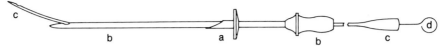

Figure 56–1. Original trocar with urethral catheter used by Saloman in Berlin in 1906 to perform diagnostic abdominal paracentesis: (*a*) outer needle with guard to prevent deep tissue injury; (*b*) streamlined trocar device for penetration of peritoneum and guidance during catheter placement; (*c*) urethral catheter passed through the trocar; (*d*) wire stylet to aid catheter placement. (Modified from Saloman H: Die diagnostische Punktion des Bausches. Berl Klin Wochenschr 43:46, 1906.)

ommended that the technique be used selectively and only to avoid exploratory laparotomy with its higher morbidity.

In 1922, Denzer proposed a method of abdominal puncture in infants and children using a trocar, a cannula, and a glass capillary tube.[55] This technique was improved on by Neuhof and Cohen, who in 1926 used a lumbar puncture needle with stylet to perform paracentesis for diagnosis of acute abdominal conditions, including trauma, pancreatitis, and peritonitis of various causes. Their comprehensive study emphasized the usefulness as well as the limitations of this technique in diagnosing hemoperitoneum.[56] In 1941, Steinberg reported the first complete and organized analysis of peritoneal fluid in various abnormal and normal conditions.[57] Keith and others in 1950 added to this by reporting further peritoneal amylase values in acute pancreatic conditions.[24] Bronfin and coworkers in 1952 used a plastic cannula through their paracentesis needle to gain greater access to potential intra-abdominal fluid accumulations.[58]

In 1954, Thompson and Brown reported 300 cases of abdominal paracentesis used to rule out acute hemoperitoneum in multiple trauma patients, particularly in cases of blunt abdominal trauma associated with head injuries and crushing injuries to the chest. They used a number 22 spinal needle placed approximately 3 cm superior and medial to the anterior superior iliac spine and reported no complications.[59] In 1959, Williams and Zollinger reported a 79 per cent accuracy in diagnosing hemoperitoneum using a short-beveled spinal needle; however, abdominal tenderness was still a more sensitive indicator (86 per cent) in the conscious patient (although the peritoneal tap was more accurate if unconscious patients are included in the assessment).[11]

In 1960, Giacobine and Siler showed with dog studies that the accuracy of needle paracentesis alone is directly related to the amount of fluid in the peritoneal cavity. They commented that large fluid accumulations could exist in the pelvic gutters that are inaccessible to aspiration using the standard midline and four-quadrant approaches.[60] The natural extension of this finding came in 1965, when Root and coworkers reported the use of peritoneal lavage with normal saline to increase the volume of any abnormal intraperitoneal fluids and thus to increase the likelihood of retrieving the irrigant fluid for examination.[61] They introduced an 18 French disposable catheter with multiple side holes overlying a trocar.

Root and associates' initial evaluation of peritoneal lavage in 28 patients with blunt abdominal injury proved very accurate. The diagnosis was correct in all of the 16 cases of significant intraperitoneal injury. The important feature of this new technique was that there were no false-negative as well as no false-positive results. This accuracy in both ruling out and diagnosing injury was supported by numerous subsequent studies using this same technique rather than paracentesis alone.[3, 6, 7, 25, 53, 62–64]

Olsen and colleagues in 1972 established a simple bedside method of measuring the amount of blood in the lavage fluid without the aid of laboratory analysis.[62] Their technique, based on the ability to read newsprint through the intravenous tubing, remains a useful bedside test for distinguishing among patients with minimal or insignificant hemoperitoneum and those requiring prompt celiotomy. Tandberg and colleagues have reported the use of a simple colorimeter for use in the emergency department that allows direct visual comparison of the diagnostic peritoneal lavage sample with known color standards to rapidly and precisely estimate the erythrocyte count.[64a]

Refinements of the blind thrust technique of Root were developed in hopes of minimizing complications and ensuring more meaningful results. These included the open peritoneal lavage technique, or minilap, described by Perry in 1970[65]; the 14-gauge plastic-sheathed needle with side holes cut by a scalpel fashioned by Bivins and coworkers for use in small children in 1976[2]; the periumbilical approach developed by Slavin in 1978[66]; the Lazarus-Nelson guide wire approach, introduced in 1979[67]; the semiopen

technique advanced by Myers and coworkers in 1981[68]; and the percutaneous technique using the Varess spring-loaded, blunt-tipped inner cannula recommended by Lockhart and colleagues in 1987.[69]

PERITONEAL TAP

Special note should be made of the difference between needle aspiration (peritoneal tap) and peritoneal lavage. The peritoneal tap, which uses a large needle on an aspirating syringe, has largely been replaced by the lavage method. A peritoneal tap is notoriously inaccurate in diagnosing hemoperitoneum; there is only a 20 per cent chance that 200 ml of free blood will be detected with needle aspiration and only an 80 per cent chance of detecting as much as 500 ml of intraperitoneal blood.[60] The major problem with needle paracentesis is a false-negative result, which may occur despite a significant hemoperitoneum. The so-called four-quadrant tap may detect a few more cases than a single aspiration attempt; but in general, needle paracentesis for diagnosis of hemoperitoneum is outdated and inferior to the peritoneal lavage procedure. With the peritoneal tap, the return of *any free blood* has classically been termed a positive result and an indication for surgical exploration. A general discussion of abdominal paracentesis for other indications is provided in Chapter 55.

INDICATIONS FOR PERITONEAL LAVAGE

Peritoneal lavage is a diagnostic procedure for recognizing intra-abdominal injury that necessitates immediate celiotomy. There need not be strong physical evidence for abdominal injury, because as many as 40 per cent of patients with unexplained hypotension will have a positive peritoneal lavage. Additionally, in the unconscious patient with head injury or altered mental status secondary to drug or alcohol ingestion, diagnostic peritoneal lavage is indicated to detect hemoperitoneum or other abnormal peritoneal fluid findings. As many as 25 per cent of patients who are unconscious from head injury will have a positive peritoneal lavage. In a patient with recent or preexisting paraplegia, a positive peritoneal lavage may be the only objective finding in intra-abdominal injury. Peritoneal lavage can be diagnostic for intraperitoneal bladder rupture or associated nonurogenital injuries in patients presenting with hematuria after blunt abdominal trauma. In patients with penetrating abdominal injuries, flank or back injuries suspected of penetrating the abdominal peritoneum, or penetrating lower thoracic wounds located between the two anterior axillary lines but below the fifth ribs anteriorly, diagnostic peritoneal lavage is appropriate after aseptic local exploration of the abdominal stab wounds.[3–7, 9, 10, 25, 27, 37, 38, 51, 53, 59, 61, 64, 67, 70–78]

The indications for lavage in children are unexplained shock following trauma, altered sensorium, major thoracic injury, multiple trauma, and major orthopedic injury (such as a fractured pelvis, femur, or hip).[2, 5, 25, 79]

In pregnant patients, the prompt diagnosis and treatment of abdominal injury are critical for fetal survival. The physiologic hypervolemia of pregnancy tends to ameliorate the natural response of the mother to blood loss; in contrast, the fetus suffers early anoxia as uterine flow decreases in response to maternal blood loss. Additionally, abdominal signs and symptoms are often diminished, delayed, or absent in pregnant women who have sustained blunt abdominal trauma.[6, 8] Peritoneal lavage is therefore useful in pregnancy, although the open technique (mini-cutdown) is mandated beyond the first trimester. Some investigators prefer simple culdocentesis to peritoneal lavage in pregnant patients, relying on the presence of free blood to make a positive diagnosis. Another possibility is "culdage," a term applied to peritoneal lavage performed through the cul-de-sac.[80]

Peritoneal lavage has been used to diagnose acute pancreatitis in patients with a normal amylase level, because an elevated amylase concentration may persist in the peritoneal fluid for 3 to 5 days following pancreatitis. Primary peritonitis may also be diagnosed by the finding of pneumococci or staphylococci. Intestinal flora and debris found on Gram stain of lavage sediment may signify perforation of the gastrointestinal tract.[1, 4, 6, 24, 44, 45, 48, 54, 56, 57, 61, 63, 70, 81–83]

Most surgeons would agree that no patient with significant abdominal injury or penetrating lower thoracic injury should be admitted for observation for extra-abdominal surgery under general anesthesia without a negative diagnostic peritoneal lavage.[3, 12, 69, 84]

Role of Computed Tomography

Computed tomography has been suggested as the preferred procedure for evaluation of hemodynamically stable patients with blunt abdominal trauma. These CT scans have permitted conservative management of patients who in the past would have undergone unnecessary or nontherapeutic celiotomy. Furthermore, unsuspected injuries in stable patients frequently can be diagnosed by abdominal CT with or without diagnostic peritoneal lavage. In addition, it is now evident that surgical intervention is no longer mandated in every case of visceral trauma, despite a positive diagnostic peritoneal lavage or a positive CT scan. Some injuries not diagnosed by diagnostic peritoneal lavage (e.g., retroperitoneal hematomas, renal and renovascular injuries) can be identified by CT scan. Minor solid organ injuries (e.g., subcapsular splenic and renal hematomas) that do not require celiotomy can be identified by CT and monitored in the hospital. Computed tomography demonstrates both anatomy and function of the kidney and avoids the performance of multiple single-organ studies, thus saving time, radiation exposure, and cost. Although CT may take longer to perform than diagnostic peritoneal lavage, it can evaluate multiple intra- and extra-abdominal organ systems (e.g., intracranial injuries) at the same time.

Computed tomography is unable to diagnose infarcted or vascularly compromised bowel, intestinal perforations and hematomas, bladder ruptures, and some pancreatic injuries. The major criticism in most studies evaluating CT scans for diagnostic evaluation of blunt abdominal trauma is the relatively high false-negative rate (2 to 25 per cent). Poor quality CT scans (not repeated) or subtle findings not identified by inexperienced radiologists are frequently suggested as causes for the false negatives. Patients also must remain still during a CT scan (many patients require sedation, intubation, and paralysis to obtain scans of high technical quality). Other problems include the following: the 2 to 4 hours delay from contrast administration to scan completion, the additional delays caused by transport to and from CT suites, the expense of equipping CT suites for monitoring and resuscitation of critical patients, the availability of ex-

perienced personnel to monitor the patient and perform the study 24 hours per day, potential aspiration of oral contrast material for enhanced abdominal CT scans, and the need for a radiologist with expertise to interpret the results. Caution is advised in using CT as a primary diagnostic technique until these factors and study reliability are demonstrated at any particular institution.

Both CT and diagnostic peritoneal lavage can miss injuries of the solid and hollow organs as well as the diaphragm. Diagnostic peritoneal lavage has a higher sensitivity, equal specificity, and higher accuracy than CT and is preferred when life-threatening extra-abdominal injuries limit the time for CT scans. Such scans can be a preferred procedure for evaluation of stable patients with blunt abdominal trauma in institutions capable of supporting this modality. Diagnostic peritoneal lavage is indicated in stable abdominal and pelvic trauma when CT scan findings are equivocal, when poor scan quality limits interpretation, or when there is a high index of suspicion of bowel or pancreatic injury despite a negative scan. The complimentary use of CT and diagnostic peritoneal lavage in blunt abdominal trauma can decrease the rate of nontherapeutic celiotomy without resulting in a significant increase in missed injuries and can identify candidates for the nonoperative management of solid organ injuries. CT scanning before diagnostic peritoneal lavage is the preferred sequence, but it is not essential for accurate interpretation of CT scans.

The management of blunt abdominal trauma in children has changed radically over the past decade and remains highly controversial. The sophistication of abdominal pelvic CT scanning (intravenous and intragastric dual contrast) and the recognition of overwhelming postsplenectomy sepsis have been responsible for this strategy. The main weakness in diagnostic peritoneal lavage is its oversensitivity in the face of minor trauma (usually minor lacerations of the spleen, liver, and occasionally with retroperitoneal hematomas). Children are more vulnerable to liver or spleen trauma than adults, and therefore the incidence of nontherapeutic celiotomy due to positive lavage is higher. At this time CT scanning should complement diagnostic peritoneal lavage.[17, 19, 22, 40]

CONTRAINDICATIONS

There are no absolute contraindications for diagnostic peritoneal lavage other than obvious signs of intra-abdominal trauma necessitating celiotomy. Obvious signs of intra-abdominal trauma include blood in the gastrointestinal tract and free air on abdominal radiographs in addition to a distending abdomen or unexplained hypotension.[51, 56] Coagulopathy is not a contraindication to diagnostic peritoneal lavage, and the results are reliable even in these cases.[85]

Relative contraindications to peritoneal lavage include a distended abdomen or scars from multiple previous abdominal surgeries, particularly pelvic surgery, in which one might anticipate adhesions or loculations that make lavage not only dangerous but also more likely to result in false-negative findings. Pregnancy and obesity should prompt consideration of alternative locations and techniques, such as the supraumbilical, periumbilical, and minilap approaches; likewise, inability to catheterize the bladder and distended loops of bowel might cause one to prefer the minilap approach for visualization.[8, 66, 80, 86, 87]

EQUIPMENT

The equipment included in the peritoneal lavage tray (Fig. 56–2) is more than sufficient for the guide wire, or

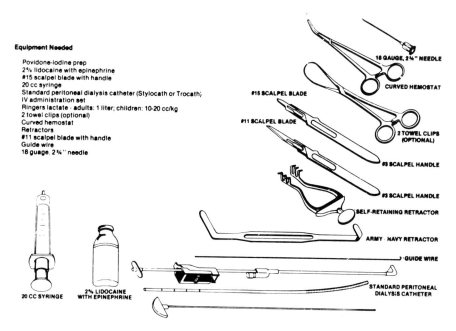

Equipment Needed

Povidone-iodine prep
2% lidocaine with epinephrine
#15 scalpel blade with handle
20 cc syringe
Standard peritoneal dialysis catheter (Stylocath or Trocath)
IV administration set
Ringers lactate - adults: 1 liter; children: 10-20 cc/kg
2 towel clips (optional)
Curved hemostat
Retractors
#11 scalpel blade with handle
Guide wire
18 guage, 2¾" needle

Figure 56–2. Peritoneal lavage tray; standard for all techniques described. Necessary equipment is noted. (From Honigman B, Marx J, Pons P, Rumack BH: Emergindex. Englewood, Colo, Micromedex, Inc, 1983. Reproduced by permission.)

Lazarus-Nelson, technique. The towel clips, number 15 scalpel, and self-retaining and Army-Navy retractors are not needed for this procedure; however, these additional instruments allow adequate resources for all other techniques, including the open minilap and the semiopen, infra- or supraumbilical method as well as the periumbilical and closed percutaneous thrust technique, which is still used in many institutions.[88] Alternatively, all necessary equipment for the guide wire technique, with the exception of the normal saline lavage fluid, is contained in a single, self-contained disposable kit (Arrow Peritoneal lavage kit, product no. AK-09000; Arrow International, Inc., Reading, Pa. Cost of the kit is approximately $20.00).[89]

PROCEDURE

The patient should be counseled regarding the purpose and sensitivity of this procedure and the importance of performing the technique as soon as possible to assess the need for immediate celiotomy or subsequent observation. A consent form should be obtained from the patient if possible, and minimal but specific complications should be discussed (see the section on complications). Allergic reactions to lidocaine should be assessed and documented before the technique is begun.

If the abdomen is distended, lateral abdominal radiographs or, preferably, a left lateral decubitus or an upright chest radiograph may demonstrate free air, thus indicating that immediate celiotomy is mandated; later radiographs may reveal air introduced during the peritoneal procedure. If the abdomen is not distended, the benefits of radiographs are so small that lavage need not be delayed.[2, 7, 11, 31, 90–92]

We recommend the guide wire, or Lazarus-Nelson, approach because of its smaller number of complications; however, each procedure has its advantages and indications.[36, 66–69, 79, 89, 93–99]

Guide Wire Technique

The guide wire approach uses minimal sharp dissection to reach the peritoneal fascia. A relatively small-diameter 18-gauge needle is used to penetrate the peritoneum rather than the larger 9 to 11 French trocar that is normally used. The more time-consuming and meticulous dissection necessary for the infra/supra/periumbilical techniques and, particularly, for the minilap approach is thus avoided.

The site that is generally selected is the abdominal midline in the upper or middle third of the distance between the umbilicus and the symphysis pubis. The midline height can be adjusted upward for smaller patients and downward for larger patients to enable the catheter tip to reach the depth of the pelvic gutters and to minimize complications. The midline supraumbilical location can be used for the patient with a gravid uterus, in cases of lower abdominal surgical scars or lower intra-abdominal known masses, or in children.[5, 87]

The bladder and the stomach are decompressed with a Foley catheter and a nasogastric tube. It should be emphasized that *a Foley catheter and a nasogastric tube should be placed in all patients before lavage is performed* and that recent voiding or vomiting should not be considered an acceptable substitute. The abdomen is shaved and prepared with povidone-iodine solution and then draped with sterile towels. Soft wrist restraints are recommended for keeping the patient's hands to the sides and the surgical field sterile. Lidocaine with epinephrine is infiltrated deeply enough to include the fascia (Fig. 56–3); the anesthesia prevents patient splinting with consequent increase in intra-abdominal pressure, and the epinephrine helps prevent capillary oozing and false-positive results. One minute should pass before a skin incision is made; the delay permits maximum vasoconstriction from the epinephrine.

The skin is then incised vertically with a number 11 blade (Fig. 56–4). The incision is carried through the subcutaneous tissue to the linea alba. The linea alba produces a tough, gritty sensation when scraped with the scalpel. Alternatively, a larger incision (up to 2 to 3 cm) can be made to the linea alba in a search for the decussation of fibers in the avascular midline (Fig. 56–5). A syringe can be attached for support as the 18-gauge, 7-cm needle is used to "pop" through the peritoneum (Fig. 56–6).

The use of a short Angiocath cutting needle containing a spring-loaded blunt-tipped inner cannula (the Varess needle) is recommended by Lockhart and colleagues for percutaneous entry into the abdominal cavity while reducing the risk of bowel or vessel penetration.[69] The blunt tip guards

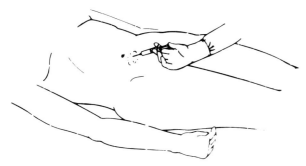

Figure 56–3. Anesthesia and bleeding control. The skin is infiltrated down to and including the fascia with lidocaine *with epinephrine* in the midline. The normal location is approximately 3 cm below or above the umbilicus, as circumstances dictate. (*Note:* The bladder and stomach should be decompressed by a Foley catheter and a nasogastric tube; the abdomen should be prepared from above the umbilicus to the pubis, and the area should be draped.) (From Honigman B, Marx J, Pons P, Rumack BH: Emergindex. Englewood, Colo, Micromedex, Inc, 1983. Reproduced by permission.)

the cutting portion of the needle until resistance is met (i.e., fascia and peritoneum). With resistance, the blunt tip is pushed into the needle shaft, allowing the cutting edge of the outer needle to advance and penetrate the fascia and peritoneum. Once past this point of resistance, the spring-loaded blunt obturator snaps into the previous forward position, protecting viscera from harm.

At this point, the floppy end of the accompanying guide wire is passed through the needle into the peritoneal cavity. If the needle is directed inferiorly, the wire should fall easily into the abdomen toward the pelvis (Fig. 56–7). If this does not occur with ease, the needle should be advanced or redirected to ensure that the guide wire is not subsequently forced into a fascial plane. When approximately one half of the wire is admitted, the needle is removed and replaced with the lavage catheter. *A portion of the guide wire should always be held during its insertion and the subsequent needle removal to prevent inadvertent intra-abdominal wire migration.* The lavage catheter is twisted over the wire through the fascia, eased into the abdominal cavity, and directed toward one of the pelvic gutters (Fig. 56–8). The twisting motion is believed to minimize visceral or omental perforation and to aid in displacing abdominal contents en route to the inferior loca-

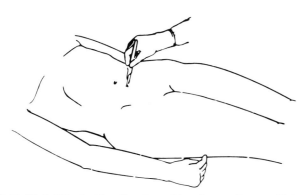

Figure 56–4. Skin incision for the guide wire, or Lazarus-Nelson, technique (also for the blind percutaneous approach). The physician makes a small nick with a number 11 scalpel through the anesthetized skin down to the fascia, palpating the fascia with the point of the scalpel. (From Honigman B, Marx J, Pons P, Rumack BH: Emergindex. Englewood, Colo, Micromedex, Inc, 1983. Reproduced by permission.)

tion of the catheter in the pelvis. Control of the guide wire must also be maintained during catheter placement.

For the blunt thrust, periumbilical, and semi-open techniques, once the trocar is popped through the fascia and the peritoneum, the lavage catheter is similarly advanced and twisted toward the pelvic gutter while the trocar is removed.

The abdominal cavity is next aspirated with a 10-ml syringe (Fig. 56–9). A free return of 10 ml or more of blood is considered a strongly positive result. If this occurs, the catheter can be removed and the area covered, because immediate celiotomy is required. Some investigators view *any free blood return* as a positive tap and forgo lavage in lieu of surgical exploration.

If no blood is aspirated, the peritoneal cavity is lavaged with either lactated Ringer solution or normal saline (Fig. 56–10). A blood pressure cuff or blood infusion pump can be applied to the plastic intravenous (IV) bag to speed the influx (i.e., decrease lavage) time. Large-bore infusion tubing (e.g., urologic irrigation tubing sets; Abbott number 6544 cystoscopy/irrigation set) also shortens fluid influx time.[100] The normal amount is 1 liter in adults or 10 to 20 ml/kg in children. When possible, after infusion the patient is rolled or shifted from side to side to increase mixing. The IV bag or bottle is placed on the floor (or below abdominal level), and the fluid is allowed to return. The fluid may not continue to return because of several factors. Some IV tubing contains a one-way valve; this must be removed, and valveless tubing must be reinserted into the IV bag.[31] Another reason for poor return is inadequate suction. This problem can be corrected by insertion of a needle into the second opening at the bottom of the IV bag or the head of the IV bottle for aspiration of 10 ml of air. Alternatively, the catheter may be adherent to peritoneum. If so, relieving some of the pressure in the IV bottle or wiggling and twisting the catheter as well as applying abdominal pressure may aid flow return.

It is generally accepted that the return of 700 ml or more fluid in the adult is adequate for interpretation of findings. Some state that 10 to 20 per cent fluid return gives a representative sample for both gross and microscopic determinations.[31, 101] The dialysis catheter should be left in place whenever possible until the returned fluid is analyzed. The physician may wish to relavage when the initial results are borderline or an occult bowel perforation is suspected.[94]

Alternative Techniques

The percutaneous thrust technique using the standard 9 French peritoneal lavage catheter and an intraluminal trocar passed through a small 2- to 3-cm incision in the skin (see Fig. 56–4) is similar to the technique discussed previously. The larger caliber stylet and blind penetration of the peritoneum do carry a higher complication rate, making this a less desirable technique, although in experienced hands this technique is more rapid and relatively safe. To decrease the likelihood of penetrating underlying viscera, some operators advocate holding the fingers low on the catheter-trocar instrument such that on entering the abdominal peritoneum the fingers will prevent deep penetration (Fig. 56–11). Excessive pressure during trocar penetration is a common error. Steady "one finger pressure" applied to the handle is sufficient to pop through the fascia and peritoneum with the trocar vertical to the plane of the abdominal wall. After controlled peritoneal penetration of 0.5 to 1.0 cm, the trocar is retracted 1.0 to 2.0 cm, and the catheter is carefully advanced into the right or left lower quadrant as described earlier.

When a larger skin incision is made for the semiopen

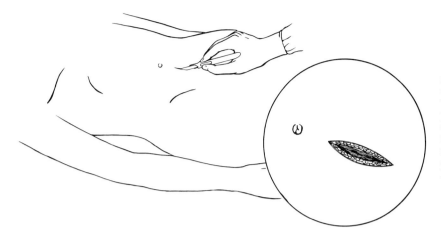

Figure 56–5. Alternative skin incision for the semiopen and minilap approach. The incision that is made is approximately 3 to 8 cm, depending on the abdominal fat pad, down to the decussating fibers of the preperitoneal fascia in the midline linea alba. (Modified from Honigman B, Marx J, Pons P, Rumack BH: Emergindex. Englewood, Colo, Micromedex, Inc, 1983. Reproduced by permission.)

technique and the minilap procedure, the same midline location is used with cautious dissection and meticulous hemostasis through the loose subcutaneous fat until the tough, gritty preperitoneal fascia is reached. This fascia can be grasped and lifted above the underlying viscera with hemostats, towel clips, or self-retaining retractors (Fig. 56–12). The fascia can be either popped through with the trocar or carefully incised under direct visualization. When the latter procedure is performed, a pursestring suture of 0-polypropylene can be placed around the dialysis catheter to ensure hemostasis and, eventually, to close the peritoneum. The skin can likewise be aligned with 3–0 polypropylene suture if the lavage is negative. The direct vision, semiopen technique is quite safe and is the preferred method of some investigators.[68]

The periumbilical technique (Fig. 56–13) is a percutaneous insertion through the inferior portion of the umbilical ring. A gently curved incision is begun to one side of the umbilicus at the level of the infraumbilical ring and is continued over the linea alba for approximately 4 cm. The incision is again extended through the loose subcutaneous tissue, and meticulous hemostasis is obtained. The fascia is elevated from underlying structures with towel clips before a 1-cm vertical incision is made through the linea alba at the

level of the infraumbilical ring, exposing the preperitoneal fat. The pediatric peritoneal dialysis catheter is introduced through the peritoneum with the trocar in place. The trocar is then withdrawn, and the catheter is directed toward the pelvis. The principal advantages of this site are not only its avascularity and absence of subcutaneous fat but also a rigid adherence of the peritoneum to the cicatrical scar of the umbilicus, which expedites entry into the free peritoneal cavity. This technique is particularly useful in the obese patient.[66, 87, 98] Bivins and colleagues suggest cutting side holes in a 14- to 16-gauge Angiocath of appropriate length as another alternative for infants (under 20 kg).[2]

COMPLICATIONS

Serious complications of peritoneal lavage are rare. Of the 9588 diagnostic peritoneal lavages reviewed by Danto,[31] there were only 127 complications, for an overall complication rate of 1.4 per cent. The rate in individual series ranges from 0 to 6 per cent. Minor complications include bleeding within the rectus sheath and at the puncture site with false-positive results, rectus sheath hematomas, retroperitoneal bladder penetrations, laceration of ovarian cysts, lost

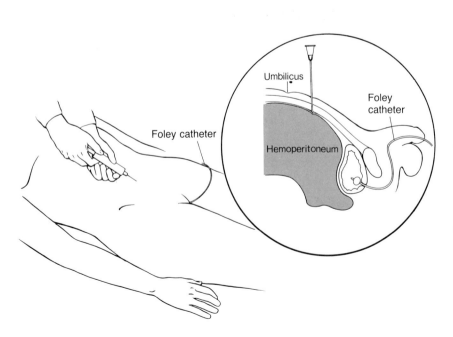

Figure 56–6. Peritoneal penetration. An 18-gauge, 2¾-inch needle is inserted through the fascia into the peritoneum. Note the mandatory Foley catheter in place. (Modified from Honigman B, Marx J, Pons P, Rumack BH: Emergindex. Englewood, Colo, Micromedex, Inc, 1983. Reproduced by permission.)

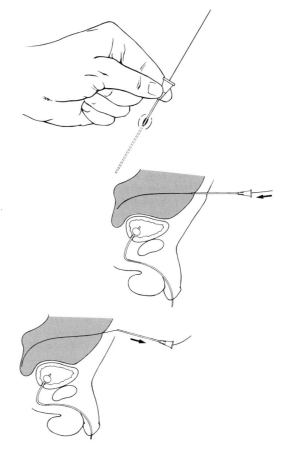

Figure 56–7. Guide wire insertion. The floppy end of the guide wire is inserted through the needle (easy passage suggests peritoneal entry). The needle is then removed, and the guide wire is left in place. A portion of the guide wire should always be held during its use. (Modified from Honigman B, Marx J, Pons P, Rumack BH: Emergindex. Englewood, Colo, Micromedex, Inc, 1983. Reproduced by permission.)

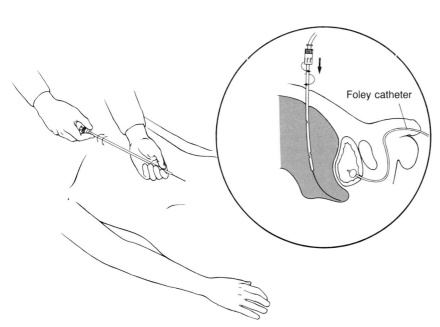

Foley catheter

Figure 56–8. Lavage catheter insertion. A standard 9 French catheter with many side holes is inserted over the guide wire in a twisting and turning fashion and is advanced deeply into the pelvic gutter. The wire is then removed. (Modified from Honigman B, Marx J, Pons P, Rumack BH: Emergindex. Englewood, Colo, Micromedex, Inc, 1983. Reproduced by permission.)

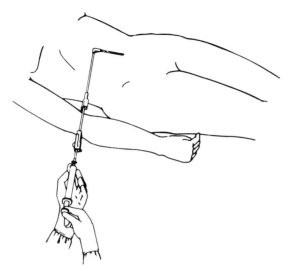

Figure 56–9. Paracentesis (aspiration). The operator attaches the syringe and aspirates for blood. If more than 10 ml of blood is aspirated, the study is positive. (From Honigman B, Marx J, Pons P, Rumack BH: Emergindex. Englewood, Colo, Micromedex, Inc, 1983. Reproduced by permission.)

through-the-needle catheter, incisional hernia, wound infection, wound dehiscence with evisceration, and toxic shock syndrome following diagnostic peritoneal lavage.[3, 7, 9, 64, 66, 69, 86, 87, 96, 102, 103] Mechanical difficulties include lack of fluid return caused by intravenous tubing problems as mentioned in the section on procedure, kinking of the catheter or guide wire, and tearing of the catheter.

Major complications include trocar penetrations of the stomach, the small bowel, the colon, and the mesentery as well as lacerations of the mesenteric vessels and puncture of the abdominal aorta and the iliac artery and vein.[5, 7, 8, 45, 51, 86, 98] Because of these complications, the blind trocar technique is discouraged.

There has been no long-term morbidity associated with these complications, and no complication-related deaths have been reported. Virtually all complications result from errors in technique caused by inexperience or failure of the operators to follow standard precautions.[2, 31]

INTERPRETATION

The main problem in interpretation of lavage aspirate is to decide how much blood indicates a positive lavage. Although some physicians regard the immediate return of any free blood as a positive peritoneal tap, paracentesis is strongly positive for visceral injury if 10 ml or more of nonclotting blood is initially aspirated. This association has not changed since 1906, when it was demonstrated by Saloman.[54] Both quantitative laboratory and visual determinations of lavage effluent have aided the diagnosis of hemoperitoneum and peritonitis of inflammatory and infectious etiology as well as suggested specific organ injury.[47, 54, 104]

Hemoperitoneum. The method reported by Olsen and associates for bedside quantitative determination of hemoperitoneum is a useful screening technique pending the formal cell count.[62] This technique can be performed in the majority of patients and divides them into three groups. In group I patients (clearly positive results), the lavage indicates greater than 25 ml of blood per liter of fluid in the abdomen. This is demonstrated by a bloody lavage aspirate that makes newsprint *unreadable* when IV tubing containing the lavage effluent is placed over newsprint and generally correlates well with the laboratory analysis of greater than 100,000 red blood cells (RBCs) per mm³ of fluid aspirate, a figure that is accepted by most as an *absolute* criterion for exploration. This analysis is dependent on a minimum of 20 per cent fluid return from the lavage.[2, 31] Danto's review of 23 published papers using laboratory analysis as a criterion and documenting results in 9588 patients (both blunt and penetrating cases) revealed the test to be positive in 97 per cent of cases.

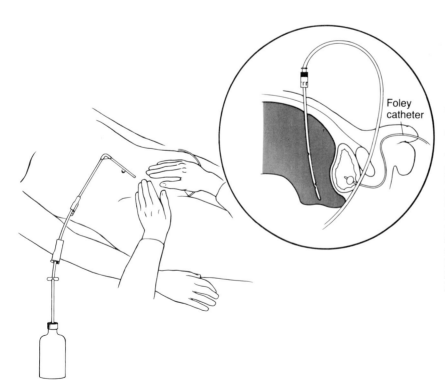

Figure 56–10. Lavage. If no blood is aspirated, the operator attaches intravenous tubing to a connector and runs 1 liter of normal saline (or Ringer's lactate) into the abdominal cavity (10 to 20 ml/kg in children). The operator should gently rock the abdomen to distribute the fluid before lowering the intravenous bottle below the level of the patient to allow fluid to drain into the bottle from the abdominal cavity. Layered skin closure is preferred at the completion of the procedure when the lavage is negative; dressing without repair is preferred when the lavage is positive. (Modified from Honigman B, Marx J, Pons P, Rumack BH: Emergindex. Englewood, Colo, Micromedex, Inc, 1983. Reproduced by permission.)

Foley
catheter

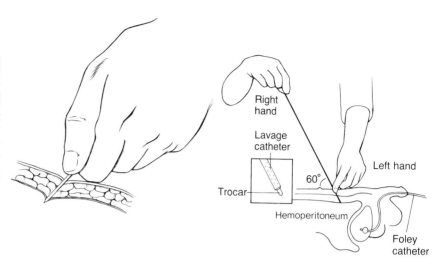

Figure 56–11. Blind percutaneous approach. The index finger and thumb of the left hand hold the trocar and resist the pressure applied by the right hand, thus preventing penetration too deeply into the peritoneal cavity. (Modified from Danto LA: Paracentesis and diagnostic peritoneal lavage. In Blaisdell FW, Trunkey DO: Trauma Management. Vol 1. New York, Thieme-Stratton Inc, 1982; and Simon R, Brenner B: Procedures and Techniques in Emergency Medicine. Baltimore, Williams & Wilkins, 1982. © Williams & Wilkins, Baltimore.)

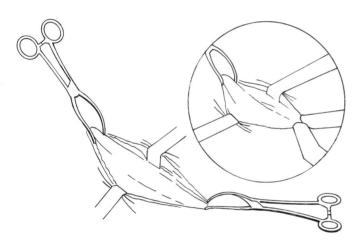

Figure 56–12. Minilap approach. A larger incision is made in the midline, and the fascia is grasped at each end with hemostats or towel clips and is lifted before an incision is made through the peritoneum. (Alternatively, a trocar can be popped through the elevated fascia in the standard approach.) (From Honigman B, Marx J, Pons P, Rumack BH: Emergindex. Englewood, Colo, Micromedex, Inc, 1983. Reproduced by permission.)

Figure 56–13. Periumbilical approach. A percutaneous incision is made through the inferior portion of the umbilical ring. The inset shows the surface anatomy of the umbilicus, with the arrow demonstrating the precise locus of puncture. (From Slavin SA: A new technique for diagnostic peritoneal lavage. Surg Gynecol Obstet 146:446, 1978. Reproduced by permission of Surgery, Gynecology, and Obstetrics.)

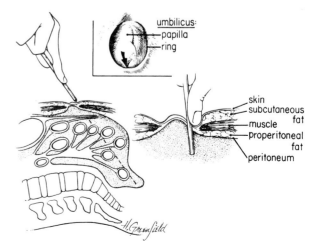

Table 56–1. Criteria for Interpretation of Peritoneal Lavage in Blunt Abdominal Trauma and Penetrating Abdominal Stab Wounds

Positive		
Free aspiration blood*		
Grossly bloody lavage return		
		Greater than
RBCs		100,000/mm³
WBCs		500/mm³
RBCs†		5000/mm³
Negative		*Less Than*
RBCs		50,000/mm³
WBCs		100/mm³
Equivocal		
RBCs‡		50,000–100,000/mm³
WBCs		100–500/mm³

*Some investigators view any free blood as a positive result; others state that from 5 to 10 ml is necessary for surgical exploration.

†Criteria for interpretation of *penetrating wounds to the abdomen and lower chest trauma.*

‡50,000 to 100,000 RBCs/mm³ is an inconclusive lavage for blunt trauma and may be associated with a significant pathologic condition—cases must be handled selectively.

RBC, red blood cell; WBC, white blood cell.

In group II patients (clearly negative results), clear lavage fluid is present in the IV tubing, and newsprint can be read clearly through the effluent. In Danto's review[31] of group II patients, the test was negative in 98.7 per cent of cases. Quantitatively, a negative test is associated with fewer than 50,000 RBCs per mm³ (Table 56–1). Even these low-risk patients should be appropriately observed, however.[8–10, 31, 44, 69, 71, 95, 97, 105, 106]

In group III patients (inconclusive results), the lavage fluid is pink, but newsprint can be read through the IV tubing. The RBC count is between 50,000 and 100,000 per mm³. This generally means that as little as 8 drops to 15 ml of blood per liter of peritoneal fluid may be present. (One milliliter of blood in the peritoneal cavity represents approximately 4500 RBCs per mm³ of lavage effluent.[62, 86])

Some researchers have suggested lowering the criterion for a positive result to 10,000, 20,000, or 50,000 RBCs per mm³, and even less than 5000 RBCs per mm³ has been termed positive if a penetrating injury has occurred.[37–39, 107] There is ample evidence that a small number of significant injuries will be missed if one applies the strict criterion of greater than 100,000 RBCs per mm³ for a positive result. Therefore, patients with an "intermediate," or equivocal, lavage (between 50,000 and 100,000 RBCs per mm³) must be handled selectively. When the patient's condition is unstable as a result of an abdominal injury, celiotomy is obviously indicated, even in the case of an indeterminate RBC analysis. The stable patient should be observed, and a lavage sample should be sent to the laboratory for analysis of RBCs, white blood cells (WBCs), amylase, alkaline phosphatase, and perhaps lavage urea nitrogen and creatinine or for a Gram stain, as desired. Weakly positive results can also be the result of extravasation of RBCs into the abdomen from retroperitoneal and pelvic hematomas as well as from ruptures of the diaphragm and isolated hollow viscus perforations.[10] Computed tomography scanning has generally replaced most other methods for more specific evaluation of the stable patient with an indeterminant lavage.[13, 14, 16, 18, 21, 74, 108, 109] However, repeated lavage with the peritoneal lavage catheter left in place may aid in further diagnosis.[7, 25, 37, 42, 64, 74, 77, 81, 86, 94, 105, 110]

Other Criteria. There is considerable controversy regarding the value of the other quantitative laboratory tests of peritoneal lavage effluent following blunt abdominal trauma. The majority of true-positive tests are based on the presence of grossly bloody fluid. Quantitative cell counts require little time to perform (5 to 10 minutes)[44] and improve the sensitivity of the test, reducing the number of false-negative results.

Patients with a positive WBC count but a negative RBC count normally have sustained injury to the small bowel and, occasionally, to the colon.[4, 34, 37, 38, 41, 44, 53, 105] Isolated small bowel injuries frequently do not produce hemoperitoneum. The contents of a perforated viscus normally produce an intense outpouring of leukocytes into the peritoneal cavity with insignificant hemoperitoneum.[4] *This response is normally delayed for 3 hours after injury,* thus limiting the value of the criterion of greater than 500 WBCs per mm³ for a positive lavage.[37, 53, 61, 72] The lavage WBC count should be "corrected" to distinguish this peritoneal inflammatory response from the contribution of WBCs from peripheral blood secondary to visceral hemorrhage into the peritoneal cavity. This corrected white blood cell count (Cwbc) equals the total lavage white blood cell count (Twbc) minus the WBCs contributed by hemorrhage. (The Twbc is the laboratory WBC per mm³ count report for the peritoneal lavage aliquot.) The Cwbc is calculated by multiplying the peripheral white blood cell count (Pwbc) by the ratio of the lavage red blood cell count (Lrbc) to the peripheral red blood cell count (Prbc) and subtracting this from the total lavage white blood cell count:

$$Cwbc = Twbc - Pwbc \times Lrbc/Prbc$$

The peritoneal lavage is considered positive if the Cwbc is greater than 500 per mm³.[104] A study by some of the same authors, however, questions the results of their earlier quantitative studies on the basis of experimentally induced artifact.[111]

The elevation of amylase and the presence of bile or bacteria are late findings following bowel injury.[72] Most patients with a lavage amylase suggesting a positive result have a WBC count suggesting a positive lavage as well.[44] The measurement of amylase is time-consuming (25 to 45 minutes) and costly ($16 per test versus $9.50 for a WBC/RBC count)[3] and has a low yield.[44, 98] Only rarely is the amylase positive with negative RBC and WBC counts.[4, 24, 53] Nonetheless, when both the examination and laboratory results are equivocal, there is considerable value to these tests in the delayed or repeat lavage at 4 to 6 hours.[4, 7, 72, 105] Elevated amylase levels (greater than serum reference levels) have a high sensitivity for indicating injuries to the pancreas and upper gastrointestinal tract. Additionally, the finding of endotoxin (determination done by Limulus Amoebocyte Lysate assay [LAL] Pyrogent, Mallinckrodt, Inc., St. Louis, Mo.) in the lavage strongly suggests ileocolonic perforation.[41, 81] Marx and coworkers noted an early elevation of lavage alkaline phosphatase (greater than 25 IU versus less than 5 IU) in small bowel injuries when all other quantitative tests are normal.[47] Sensitivity is enhanced by lowering the positive criteria to greater than 3 IU per liter.[110] Megison and Weigelt were unable to demonstrate enhanced sensitivity for diagnosis of hollow viscus injury when lavage alkaline phosphatase levels were obtained in addition to RBC and WBC counts.[111a] Burney and associates noted an elevation of liver enzyme levels in blunt hepatic trauma (but not in penetrating trauma) that appears to correlate with the severity of hepatocellular disruption.[104]

Rubin and colleagues demonstrated in dogs that as little as 15 ml and 50 ml of urine instilled in the peritoneum raises the lavage urea nitrogen and creatinine, respectively, above the serum levels, suggesting intraperitoneal extravasation of urine from a bladder rupture.[77]

False-positive results are usually caused by bleeding at the catheter incision site or by omental or mesenteric laceration from the needle, the trocar, or the catheter. Proper technique with caution taken to elevate the abdominal fascia before puncture into the peritoneum as well as the judicious use of lidocaine with epinephrine in both the conscious and the unconscious patient should help to decrease the number of false-positives.[87] Note should be made of possible false-positive lavages in patients with a pelvic or retroperitoneal hematoma. Operations are generally not performed on such patients, but a lavage catheter inadvertently placed in the hematoma results in a strongly positive (false) lavage.

False-negative results are unusual but can be caused by misplacement of the catheter by the inexperienced operator, compartmentalization by adhesions, and retroperitoneal or bladder placement of the catheter.

CONCLUSION

Diagnostic peritoneal lavage has become one of the most common procedures performed in the emergency department to detect hemoperitoneum in the traumatized patient. Several techniques have been discussed, each involving minimal complications or false results in experienced hands. The results are highly accurate and can demonstrate significant intra-abdominal injury when the clinical examination is negative or equivocal, in the multiply traumatized patient with altered mental status or noncontiguous injuries above and below the abdomen, in penetrating lower thoracic or abdominal injuries, and in the difficult-to-examine traumatized obstetric or pediatric patient.

Peritoneal lavage can likewise prevent unnecessary celiotomy and allow safe observation of the stable patient with clinical signs of intra-abdominal injury. In some instances, serial peritoneal lavage may detect the unusual false-negative initial lavage.[64, 69, 86, 105] Continuing interest in this procedure suggests that it may be useful in differentiating specific organs traumatized in blunt abdominal injuries. Finally, diagnostic peritoneal lavage can be complemented by local wound exploration or CT for stable trauma patients, particularly in the pediatric age group.[19, 21, 112-114]

REFERENCES

1. Baker WNW, Mackie DB, Newcombe JF: Diagnostic paracentesis in the acute abdomen. Br Med J 3:146, 1967.
2. Bivins BA, Jona JZ, Berlin RP: Diagnostic peritoneal lavage in pediatric trauma. J Trauma 16:739, 1976.
3. Danto LA, Thomas CW, Gorenbeim S, Wolfman EF: Penetrating torso injuries: The role of paracentesis and lavage. Am Surg 43:164, 1977.
4. Engrav LH, Benjamin CI, Strate RG, Perry JF: Diagnostic peritoneal lavage in blunt abdominal trauma. J Trauma 15:854, 1975.
5. Fischer RP, Beverlin BC, Engrav LH, Benjamin CI, Perry JF: Diagnostic peritoneal lavage fourteen years and 2,586 patients later. Am J Surg 136:701, 1978.
6. Olsen WR, Hildreth DH: Abdominal paracentesis and peritoneal lavage in blunt abdominal trauma. J Trauma 11:824, 1971.
7. Parvin S, Smith DE, Asher WM, Virgilio RW: Effectiveness of peritoneal lavage in blunt abdominal trauma. Ann Surg 181:255, 1978.
8. Rothenberger DA, Quattebaum FW, Zabel J, Fischer RP: Diagnostic peritoneal lavage for blunt trauma in pregnant women. Am J Obstet 129:479, 1977.
9. Thal ER: Evaluation of peritoneal lavage and local exploration in lower chest and abdominal stab wounds. J Trauma 17:642, 1977.
10. Thompson JS, Moore EE, Van Duzer-Moore S, Moore JB, Galloway AC: The evaluation of abdominal stab wound management. J Trauma 20:478, 1980.
11. Williams RD, Zollinger RM: Diagnosis and prognostic factors in abdominal injury. Am J Surg 97:575, 1959.
12. Rodriguez A, DuPriest RW, Shatney CH: Recognition of intra-abdominal injury in blunt trauma victims: A prospective study comparing physical examination with peritoneal lavage. Am Surg 48:456, 1982.
13. Doris PE: An algorithm for computed tomography and diagnostic peritoneal lavage. Ann Emerg Med 18:592, 1989.
14. Federle MP, Crass RA, Jeffrey RB, Trunkey DD: Computed tomography in blunt abdominal trauma. Arch Surg 117:645, 1982.
15. Frame SB, Browder IW, Lang EK, McSwain NE: Computed tomography versus diagnostic peritoneal lavage and usefulness in immediate diagnosis of blunt abdominal trauma. Ann Emerg Med 18:513, 1989.
16. Goldstein AS, Sclafani SJA, Kupferstein NH, et al: The diagnostic superiority of computerized tomography. J Trauma 25:938, 1985.
17. Haftel AJ, Lev R, Mahour GH, et al: Abdominal CT scanning in pediatric blunt trauma. Ann Emerg Med 17:684, 1988.
18. Kane NM, Dorfman GS, Cronan JJ: Efficacy of CT following peritoneal lavage in abdominal trauma. J Comput Assist Tomogr 11:998, 1987.
19. Karp MP, Cooney DR, Berger PE, et al: The role of computed tomography in the evaluation of blunt abdominal trauma in children. J Pediatr Surg 16:316, 1981.
20. Kearney PA: Blunt trauma to the abdomen. Ann Emerg Med 18:1322, 1989.
21. Kuhn JP, Berger PE: Computed tomography in the evaluation of blunt abdominal trauma in children. Radiol Clin North Am 19:503, 1981.
22. Rothenberg S, Moore EE, Marx JA, et al: Selective management of blunt abdominal trauma in children—the triage role of peritoneal lavage. J Trauma 27:1101, 1987.
23. Sherck JP, McCort JJ, Oakes DD: Computed tomography in thoracoabdominal trauma. J Trauma 24:1015, 1984.
24. Keith LM, Zollinger RM, McCleery RS: Peritoneal fluid amylase determinations as an aid in diagnosis of acute pancreatitis. Arch Surg 61:930, 1950.
25. Powell RW, Smith DE, Zarius CK, et al: Peritoneal lavage in children with blunt abdominal trauma. J Pediatr Surg 11:973, 1976.
26. Perry JF: A five-year survey of 152 acute abdominal injuries. J Trauma 5:53, 1965.
27. Yurko AA, Williams RD: Needle paracentesis in blunt abdominal trauma: A critical analysis. J Trauma 6:194, 1966.
28. Goldberger JH, Bernstein DM, Rodman GH, Suarez CA: Selection of patients with abdominal stab wounds for laparotomy. J Trauma 22:476, 1982.
29. Rosenthal RE, Smith J, Walls RM, et al: Stab wounds to the abdomen: Failure of blunt probing to predict peritoneal penetration. Ann Emerg Med 16:172, 1987.
30. Markovchick VJ, Moore EE, Moore J, Rosen P: Local wound exploration of anterior abdominal stab wounds. J Emerg Med 2:287, 1985.
31. Danto LA: Paracentesis and diagnostic peritoneal lavage. In Blaisdell FW, Trunkey DO: Trauma Management. Vol I. New York, Thieme-Stratton Inc, 1982.
32. Gomez GA, Alvarez R, Plasencia G, et al: Diagnostic peritoneal lavage in the management of blunt abdominal trauma: A reassessment. J Trauma 27:1, 1987.
33. Marx JA, Moore EE, Jordan R, Eule J: Limitations of computed tomography in the evaluation of acute abdominal trauma: A prospective comparison with diagnostic peritoneal lavage. J Trauma 25:933, 1985.
34. Thal ER: Peritoneal lavage: Reliability of RBC count in patients with stab wounds to the chest and abdomen. Arch Surg 119:579, 1984.
35. Trooskin SZ, Boyarsky AH, Greco RS: Peritoneal lavage in patients with normal mentation and hematuria after blunt trauma. Surgery 160:145, 1985.
36. Adkinson C, Roller B, Clinton J, et al: A comparison of open peritoneal lavage with modified closed peritoneal lavage in blunt abdominal trauma. Am J Emerg Med 7:352, 1989.
37. McLellan BA, Hanna SS, Montoya DR, et al: Analysis of peritoneal lavage parameters in blunt abdominal trauma. J Trauma 25:383, 1985.
38. Merlotti GJ, Marcet E, Sheaff CM, et al: Use of peritoneal lavage to evaluate abdominal penetration. J Trauma 25:228, 1985.
39. Merlotti GJ, Dillon BC, Lange DA, et al: Peritoneal lavage in penetrating thoracoabdominal trauma. J Trauma 28:17, 1988.
40. Powell RW, Green JB, Ochsner MG, et al: Peritoneal lavage in pediatric patients sustaining blunt abdominal trauma: A re-appraisal. J Trauma 27:6, 1987.
41. Vij D, Horon DP, Obeid FN, Horst M: The importance of the WBC count in peritoneal lavage. JAMA 249:636, 1983.
42. Obeid FN, Sorensen V, Vincent G, et al: Inaccuracy of diagnostic peritoneal lavage in penetrating colonic trauma. Arch Surg 119:906, 1984.
43. Thal ER, May RA, Beesinger D: Peritoneal lavage: Its unreliability in gunshot wounds of the lower chest and abdomen. Arch Surg 115:430, 1980.
44. Alyono D, Perry JF: Value of quantitative cell count and amylase activity of peritoneal lavage fluid. J Trauma 21:345, 1981.
45. Denzer BS: Abdominal puncture in the diagnosis of peritonitis in childhood. J Pediatr 8:741, 1936.
46. Lucas CE: The role of peritoneal lavage for penetrating abdominal wounds. J Trauma 17:649, 1977.
47. Marx JA, Moore EE, Bar-Or D: Peritoneal lavage in penetrating injuries of the small bowel and colon: Value of enzyme determinations. Ann Emerg Med 12:68, 1983.
48. Maetani S, Tobe T: Open peritoneal drainage as effective treatment of advanced peritonitis. Surgery 90:804, 1981.
49. Press OW, Press NO, Kaufman SD: Evaluation and management of chylous ascites. Ann Intern Med 96:358, 1982.
50. Van Sonnenberg E, Ferrucci JT, Mueller PR, et al: Percutaneous drainage of abscesses and fluid collections: Technique, results and applications. Diagn Radiol 142:1, 1982.

51. Veith FJ, Webber WB, Karl RC, Deysine M: Peritoneal lavage in acute abdominal disease: Normal findings and evaluation in 100 patients. Ann Surg 116:290, 1967.
52. Wright K, Tarr PI, Hickman RO, Gutherie RD: Hyperbilirubinemia secondary to delayed absorption of intraperitoneal blood following intrauterine transfusion. J Pediatr 100:302, 1982.
53. Root HD, Keizer PJ, Perry JF: The clinical and experimental aspects of peritoneal response to injury. Arch Surg 95:531, 1967.
54. Saloman H: Die diagnostische Punktion des Bauches. Berl Klin Wochenschr 43:45, 1906.
55. Denzer BS: Abdominal puncture in the diagnosis of peritonitis in childhood. Am J Med Sci 163:237, 1922.
56. Neuhof H, Cohen I: Abdominal puncture in the diagnosis of acute intraperitoneal disease. Ann Surg 83:454, 1926.
57. Steinberg B: Peritoneal exudate: A guide for the diagnosis and prognosis of peritoneal conditions. JAMA 116:572, 1941.
58. Bronfin GJ, Liebler JF, Katz HM: A new method of abdominal paracentesis. Gastroenterology 21:426, 1952.
59. Thompson CT, Brown DR: Diagnostic paracentesis in the acute abdomen. Surgery 15:916, 1954.
60. Giacobine JW, Siler VE: Evaluation of diagnostic abdominal paracentesis with experimental and clinical studies. Surg Gynecol Obstet 110:676, 1960.
61. Root HD, Hauser CW, McKinley CR, et al: Diagnostic peritoneal lavage. Surgery 57:633, 1965.
62. Olsen WR, Redman HC, Hildreth DH: Quantitative peritoneal lavage in blunt abdominal trauma. Arch Surg 104:536, 1972.
63. Gumbert JL, Froderman SE, Mercho JP: Diagnostic peritoneal lavage in blunt abdominal trauma. Ann Surg 165:70, 1967.
64. Perry JF Jr, Strate RG: Diagnostic peritoneal lavage in blunt abdominal trauma: Indications and results. Surgery 71:898, 1972.
64a. Tandberg D, Reitmeyer ST, Cheney PR: Rapid visual colorimetry of peritoneal lavage fluid. Ann Emerg Med 19:1318, 1990.
65. Perry JF Jr: Blunt and penetrating abdominal injuries. In Saegesser F (ed): Current Problems in Surgery. Chicago, Year Book Medical Publishers, 1970.
66. Slavin SA: A new technique for diagnostic peritoneal lavage. Surg Gynecol Obstet 146:446, 1978.
67. Lazarus HM, Nelson JA: A technique for peritoneal lavage without risk or complication. Surg Gynecol Obstet 149:889, 1979.
68. Myers RAM, Agarwal NN, Cowley RA: A safe, semi-open procedure for diagnostic peritoneal lavage. Surg Gynecol Obstet 153:739, 1981.
69. Lockhart CM, Gerding RL, Imbembo AL, Shuck JM: Percutaneous peritoneal lavage using the Varess needle: A preliminary report. J Trauma 27:1181, 1987.
70. Talbert J, Gruenberg JC, Brown RS: Peritoneal lavage in penetrating thoracic trauma. J Trauma 20:979, 1980.
71. Thal ER: Peritoneal lavage: State of the art. Ann Emerg Med 10:84, 1981.
72. Thompson JS, Moore EE: Peritoneal lavage in the evolution of penetrating abdominal trauma. Surg Gynecol Obstet 153:861, 1981.
73. Wright LT, Prigot A: Traumatic subcutaneous rupture of the normal spleen. Ann Surg 39:551, 1939.
74. Aronoff RJ, Reynolds J, Thal ER: Evaluations of diaphragmatic injuries. Am J Surg 144:671, 1982.
75. Eastman D, Reyna TM: Penetrating wounds of the back and applicable management principles. Milit Med 153:363, 1988.
76. Kearney PA, Rouhana SW, Burney RE: Blunt rupture of the diaphragm: Mechanism, diagnosis, and treatment. Ann Emerg Med 18:1326, 1989.
77. Rubin MJ, Blahd WH, Stanisic TH, Meislin HW: Diagnosis of intraperitoneal extravasation of urine by peritoneal lavage. Ann Emerg Med 14:433, 1985.
78. Stone HH, Strom PR, Mullins RJ: Prospective evaluation of selective laparoscopy for abdominal stabs (abstract). J Trauma 23:666, 1983.
79. Drew R, Perry JF, Fischer RP: The expediency of peritoneal lavage for blunt trauma in children. Surg Gynecol Obstet 145:885, 1977.
80. Cantrill SV: Emergency care records: The use of peritoneal lavage in the evaluation of penetrating abdominal trauma. J Emerg Med 1:73, 1983.
81. Kusminsky RE, Tu KK, Brendemuehl J, et al: The potential value of endotoxin-amylase detection in peritoneal lavage fluid. Am Surg 48:359, 1982.
82. Alverdy JC, Saunders J, Chamberlin WH, Moss GS: Diagnostic peritoneal lavage in intra-abdominal sepsis. Am Surg 54:456, 1988.
83. Glancy KE: Review of pancreatic trauma. West J Med 151:45, 1989.
84. Reiner DS, Hurd R, Smith K, Kaminski DL: Selective peritoneal lavage in the management of comatose blunt trauma patients. J Trauma 26:255, 1986.
85. Berry T, Flynn TC, Miller PW, Fischer RP: Diagnostic peritoneal lavage in trauma patients with coagulopathy. Ann Emerg Med 12:253, 1983.
86. Krausz MM, Manny J, Ultsunomiya T, Hechtman HB: Peritoneal lavage in blunt abdominal trauma. Surg Gynecol Obstet 152:327, 1981.
87. Markovchick VJ, Elerding SC, Moore EE, Rosen P: Diagnostic peritoneal lavage. JACEP 8:326, 1979.
88. Honigman B, Marx J, Pons P, Rumack BH: Emergindex. Englewood, Colo, Micromedex, Inc, 1983.
89. Howdieshell TR, Osler TM, Demarest GB: Open versus closed peritoneal lavage with particular attention to time, accuracy and cost. Am J Emerg Med 7:367, 1989.
90. Kester DE, Andrassy RJ, Aust JB: The value and cost effectiveness of abdominal roentgenograms in the evaluation of stab wounds to the abdomen. Surg Gynecol Obstet 162:337, 1986.
91. Miller RE, Nelson SW: The roentgenologic demonstration of tiny amounts of intraperitoneal gas. Am J Radiol 112:574, 1971.
92. Roh JJ, Thompson JS, Harned RK, Hodgson PE: Value of pneumonperitoneum in the diagnosis of visceral perforation. Am J Surg 146:830, 1983.
93. Wilson WR, Schwarcz TH, Pilcher DB: A prospective randomized trial of the Lazarus-Nelson vs the standard peritoneal dialysis catheter for peritoneal lavage in blunt abdominal trauma. J Trauma 27:1177, 1987.
94. Thompson DC, Pearce WJ, Longerbeam JK: Analytical diagnostic peritoneal lavage in the diagnosis of intra-abdominal injury. J Trauma 25:400, 1985.
95. DuPriest RW, Rodriguez A, Khaneja SC, et al: Open diagnostic peritoneal lavage in blunt trauma victims. Surg Gynecol Obstet 148:890, 1979.
96. Hernandez EH, Stein JM: Comparison of the Lazarus-Nelson peritoneal lavage catheter with the standard peritoneal dialysis catheter in abdominal trauma. J Trauma 22:153, 1982.
97. Moore JB, Moore EE, Markovchick V, Rosen P: Peritoneal lavage in abdominal trauma: A prospective study comparing the peritoneal dialysis catheter with the intracatheter. Ann Emerg Med 9:190, 1980.
98. Moore JB, Moore EE, Markovchick VJ, Rosen P: Diagnostic peritoneal lavage for abdominal trauma: Superiority of the open technique at the infraumbilical ring. J Trauma 21:570, 1981.
99. Roller B, Adkinson C, Bretzke M, Clinton JE: Comparison of open and percutaneous wire guided closed peritoneal lavage. Ann Emerg Med 12:252, 1983.
100. Cotter CP, Hawkins ML, Kent RB, Carraway RP: Ultra rapid diagnostic peritoneal lavage. J Trauma 29:615, 1989.
101. Bivins BA, Sachatello CR, Daugherty ME, et al: Diagnostic peritoneal lavage is superior to clinical evaluation in blunt abdominal trauma. Am Surg 44:637, 1978.
102. Catapano M, Cwinn AA, Marx JA, Moore EE: Toxic shock syndrome following diagnostic peritoneal lavage. Ann Emerg Med 17:736, 1988.
103. Frame SB, Hendrikson MF, Boozer AG, McSwain NE: Dehiscence with evisceration: A rare complication of diagnostic peritoneal lavage. J Emerg Med 7:599, 1989.
104. Burney RE, Mueller GL, Mackenzie JR: Evaluation of experimental blunt and penetrating hepatobiliary trauma by sequential peritoneal lavage. Ann Emerg Med 12:279, 1983.
105. Phillips TF, Brotman S, Cleveland S, Cowley RA: Perforating injuries of the small bowel from blunt abdominal trauma. Ann Emerg Med 12:75, 1983.
106. Ward RE, Miller P, Clark DG, et al: Angiography and peritoneal lavage in blunt abdominal trauma. J Trauma 21:848, 1981.
107. Oreskovich MR, Carrico CJ: Stab wounds of the anterior abdomen: analysis of a management plan using local wound exploration and quantitative peritoneal lavage. Ann Surg 198:411, 1983.
108. Pagliarello G, Hanna SS, Gregory WD, et al: Abdomenopelvic computerized tomography and open peritoneal lavage in patients with blunt abdominal trauma: A prospective study. Can J Surg 30:10, 1987.
109. Mohamed G, Reyes HM, Fantus R, et al: Computed tomography in the assessment of pediatric abdominal trauma. Arch Surg 121:703, 1986.
110. Marx JA, Bar-Or D, Moore EE, Tercier JA: Utility of lavage alkaline phosphatase in detection of isolated small intestinal injury. Ann Emerg Med 14:49, 1985.
111. Mackenzie JR, Gundry SR, Burney RE: Animal model development in peritoneal lavage research: Pitfalls and prerequisites. J Trauma 23:649, 1983.
111a. Megison SM, Weigelt JA: The value of alkaline phosphatase in peritoneal lavage. Ann Emerg Med 19:503, 1990.
112. Davis RA, Shayne JP, Max MH, et al: Computerized axial tomography versus peritoneal lavage in the evaluation of blunt abdominal trauma: A prospective study. Surgery 98:845, 1985.
113. Fabian TC, Mangiante EC, White TJ, et al: A prospective study of 91 patients undergoing both computed tomography and peritoneal lavage following blunt abdominal trauma. J Trauma 26:602, 1986.
114. Sorkey AJ, Farnell MB, Williams HJ, et al: The complementary roles of diagnostic peritoneal lavage and computed tomography in the evaluation of blunt abdominal trauma. Surgery 106:794, 1989.

Chapter 57

Abdominal Hernia Reduction

Jonathan M. Glauser

INTRODUCTION

The emergency physician is often called on to diagnose abdominal hernias. Once the diagnosis has been made, the physician must reduce the hernia sac or properly refer the patient for definitive care. Although by definition a hernia represents a weakness or defect in supporting structures through which an organ may protrude, or herniate, the emergency physician is rarely consulted by the patient unless the hernia is considered irreducible (incarcerated) by the patient or family. The challenge of the emergency physician is thus to differentiate the incarcerated hernia from other forms of swelling and to achieve reduction before ischemia of the incarcerated hernia (strangulation) occurs. Strangulation is believed to result from progressive venous and lymphatic congestion that causes tissue edema and subsequent compromise of perfusion.

Although the exact prevalence of hernias is unknown, Zimmerman and Anson estimate that approximately 5 per cent of the total adult male population is afflicted.[1] Hernias in general are more than five times more common in males. The most common hernia for both sexes is the indirect inguinal hernia. Direct hernias are unusual in women, whereas femoral hernias occur more commonly in women than in men. Indirect inguinal hernias and umbilical hernias are common in children. They occur more frequently in boys than in girls (9:1 ratio) and are often associated with prematurity or developmental defects.

CLASSIFICATION OF ABDOMINAL HERNIAS

Detailed discussions of the historical development of the treatment of hernias, including recognition, preoperative management, and operative repair, can be found elsewhere.[1–3]

A hernia can be defined as a potential weakness in the abdominal wall, and this defect permits protrusion of peritoneum and abdominal contents. If a contained viscus can be returned from the defect in the abdominal wall to the abdominal cavity, the hernia is defined as *reducible*. When the contents of the hernia sac cannot be reduced, the hernia is considered *incarcerated*. For the purposes of this chapter, a hernia is defined as incarcerated when the patient, family, or physician on initial evaluation (before medication and other techniques described later) is unable to reduce the hernia sac. When there is ischemia of the contents of the hernia sac, the herniated tissue is said to be *strangulated*. A *sliding* hernia occurs when a portion of the wall of the hernia sac is composed of an organ (e.g., the cecum). If only a portion of the antimesenteric wall of the bowel is incarcerated or strangulated, the hernia is called a *Richter* hernia.[4, 5]

Groin hernias can be categorized as femoral or inguinal hernias; the inguinal hernias can be either direct or indirect (Figs. 57–1 and 57–2).

Direct Inguinal Hernia. A direct inguinal hernia represents a weakening of the abdominal wall (transversalis fascia) that permits protrusion of peritoneal contents through the Hesselbach triangle. The triangle is bounded laterally by the inferior epigastric artery, inferiorly by the inguinal ligament, and medially by the lateral margin of the rectus muscle sheath. The key to diagnosis of a direct inguinal hernia is the observation that the hernia does not traverse the inguinal canal. In the rare situation in which the hernia sac enters the scrotum, the hernia sac must pass through the external ring separate from and behind the spermatic cord. In contrast with other groin hernias, the direct hernia represents a diffuse weakness of the abdominal wall. The absence of a narrow neck to the direct hernia sac makes incarceration unusual. When incarceration does occur, it is usually associated with the rare entrapment of the hernia sac at the external ring.

Indirect Inguinal Hernia. An indirect inguinal hernia represents the passage of the hernia sac (peritoneum and contents) through the internal ring (because of weakness in the transveralis fascia and the transversus abdominis) a variable distance down the inguinal canal or all the way into the scrotum. The internal ring is defined medially by the inferior epigastric artery. Indirect hernias frequently are associated with scrotal swelling, and incarceration can develop as a result of swelling at either the internal or the external ring.

Femoral Hernia. The weakness in the transversalis fascia that causes a femoral hernia is similar to the weakness that causes a direct inguinal hernia, but it is inferiorly directed rather than anteriorly directed. The peritoneum and contents herniate beneath the inguinal ligament in a small potential space medial to the femoral vein. The resulting hernia sac has a small neck, although once the sac enters the subcutaneous tissue of the thigh, it may enlarge considerably and even double back on top of the external oblique aponeurosis, thus masquerading as an inguinal hernia. The narrow neck makes incarceration common with this type of hernia and makes preoperative reduction unlikely.

Ventral Hernia. Ventral hernias are frequently caused by postincisional weakness of the anterior abdominal wall. Umbilical hernias represent another common ventral hernia and rarely pose a problem. An *epigastric* hernia may penetrate through a defect in the linea alba above the umbilicus. The *Spigelian* hernia is a rare defect located at the inferior one third of the rectus abdominis where the arcuate line meets the lateral border of the rectus muscle.

Other Hernias. Lateral abdominal wall hernias are uncommon but may develop following renal surgery. A rare site of abdominal weakness and herniation is the *Petit* triangle. This triangle is bounded anteriorly by the external oblique muscle, inferiorly by the iliac crest, and posteriorly by the latissimus dorsi muscle. Other hernias that are not discussed further include perineal hernias through the levator ani or through the sciatic foramina, obturator hernias into the medial thigh through the obturator foramen, diaphragmatic hernias, and internal hernias (e.g., bowel herniation through the foramen of Winslow).

Injury to the abdominal wall can cause traumatic hernia, with attendant risk of associated trauma and bowel incarceration.[6]

DIFFERENTIAL DIAGNOSIS OF GROIN MASSES IN CHILDREN

Although groin lumps are often hernias, an inguinal mass may in fact be something else. An enlarged inguinal lymph node, a lipoma, a hydrocele of the cord, a saphenous varix, a psoas abscess, or an incarcerated ovary can appear as a groin mass.[7]

Lymph nodes are usually multiple and are found distal to the groin crease. If a contributory lesion on a lower extremity can be found, differentiation of a lymph node from a hernia is made easier. Ulceration of the urethral

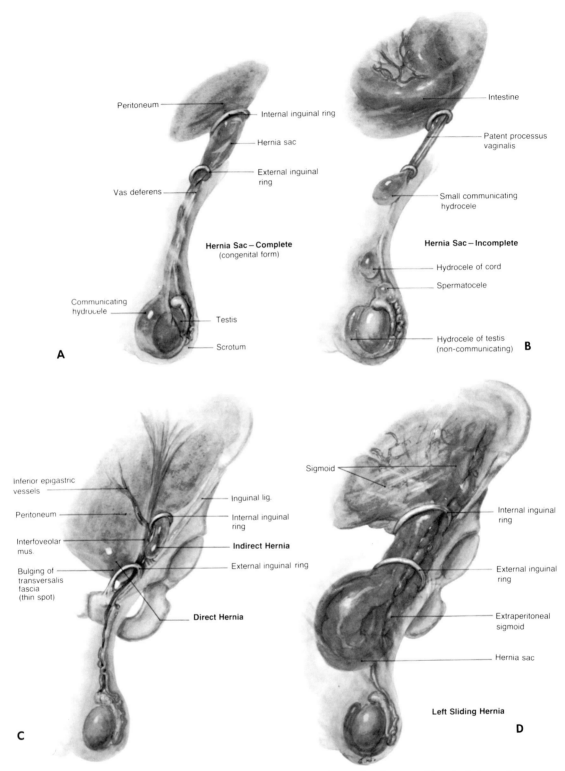

Figure 57–1. *A,* A complete (congenital) hernia sac extending through both the internal and external inguinal rings with communication to a hydrocele in the scrotum. *B,* An incomplete hernia sac with a small communicating hydrocele distal to the external ring. Also shown are noncommunicating hydroceles of the cord and testis and a spermatocele. *C,* Detailed illustration of the anatomic origins of a direct hernia and an indirect hernia. Note the location of the inferior epigastric vessels medial to the internal inguinal ring. *D,* A sliding hernia with the bowel shown traversing both the internal and external rings. (From Schlossberg L, Zuidema GD: Surgical Anatomy of the Abdomen and Pelvis: A Series of Translucent Plates in Color. Philadelphia, WB Saunders Co, 1972. Reproduced by permission.)

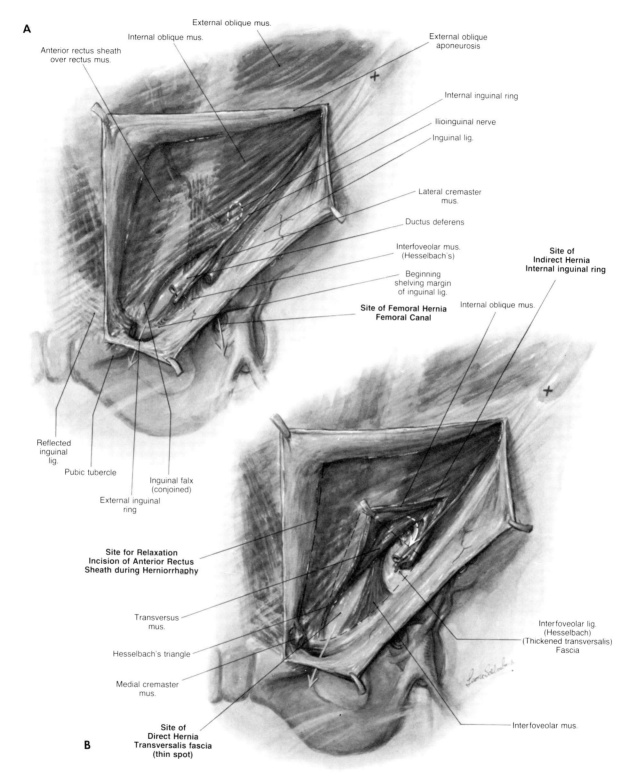

Figure 57–2. *A,* Layers of abdominal wall about the inguinal canal. Note the site of the femoral canal medial to the femoral vessels but lateral to the external inguinal ring. *B,* Hesselbach triangle and sites of direct and indirect herniation. (From Schlossberg L, Zuidema GD: *Surgical Anatomy of the Abdomen and Pelvis: A Series of Translucent Plates in Color.* Philadelphia, WB Saunders Co, 1972. Reproduced by permission.)

meatus can rarely cause adenopathy about the inguinal ligament, so the genitalia must also be examined. Lymphatics in the anal canal below the pectineal line also drain to the superficial inguinal nodes. In most circumstances, however, inguinal nodes are unusual in the anterior abdominal wall immediately superficial to the inguinal ligament. Lymph nodes in general are equally mobile in all directions, unlike (for example) femoral hernias, which tend to have decreased mobility in the transverse direction.

Lipomas in the subcutaneous fat can usually be separated from the underlying fascia and are not associated with a hernia sac neck extending under the inguinal ligament. A saphenous varix may reduce with pressure and may protrude when the patient coughs or stands upright but has a very soft consistency. Furthermore, as the varix enlarges and displaces subcutaneous fat, it appears bluish beneath the skin.

If an infant has a tender, hard bulge at the external ring, to differentiate between incarcerated inguinal hernia and acute hydrocele of the cord may be difficult. The internal inguinal ring can be palpated with an examining finger in the rectum and the other finger over the cord. If the mass is an incarcerated hernia, bowel can be felt entering and exiting the internal ring.

A hydrocele of the cord is not necessarily benign. If the mass is tense and the hydrocele is contained within the rigid walls of the inguinal canal, testicular infarction can occur. This condition can mimic torsion of the testis if the testicle is tender, although the hydrocele may transilluminate. In the case of torsion, the cord should also be shortened on the affected side. Although ultrasound and radionuclide scan examinations may be helpful (see Chapter 73), surgical exploration is often necessary to differentiate among these conditions. In general, an acute hydrocele of the cord should be treated as an incarcerated hernia unless the emergency physician can definitively conclude otherwise by examination. Acute hydroceles within the scrotum rarely become as hard or painful as those within the inguinal canal and can generally be dealt with electively. Psoas abscesses are uncommon and are only rarely confused with a femoral hernia. The margins of the abscess are softer and more ill defined than those of a hernia. Furthermore, psoas abscesses lie in a position lateral to the femoral artery, whereas hernias are medial.

PATIENT PRESENTATION

Incarcerated hernias are common in infancy and are seen most frequently in children under 1 year of age. Usually the hernia has gone unnoticed by the child's parents and is first noted at the time of incarceration. In a small infant, irritability may be the main parental concern, and the physician must be certain to examine the groin to evaluate the child for a potential hernia. Very large infant hernias containing several loops of bowel almost never incarcerate and even more rarely strangulate. Aside from the visible lump, incarceration of the hernia is occasionally associated with discomfort caused by stretching of nerve endings during tissue dissection when the hernia sac first expands.

In female infants, the ovary is the organ most likely to herniate into the inguinal canal. The herniated ovary is usually palpable as a mobile nodule measuring 1 by 2 cm. Although unusual, infarction of the herniated ovary may occur as a result of torsion or compression of the pedicle. This condition may mimic inflamed lymphadenopathy, although the location is atypical for adenopathy. In the case of testicular feminization, the gonad in the inguinal canal is a testicle, although the patient is an "apparent female."

Incarceration occurs in approximately 10 per cent of indirect inguinal hernias and 20 per cent of femoral hernias. Because prolonged incarceration is often associated with intestinal obstruction and strangulation, early attempts at hernia sac reduction are indicated. Another advantage of reduction of an incarcerated hernia is that it permits the inflammatory response in and around the hernia to subside, allowing a delayed, controlled, elective repair.

Incisional hernias infrequently incarcerate and strangulate. Reduction of these hernias is generally routine or spontaneous, although sedation may be required. Incarceration in these cases usually results from adhesions of the contents of the sac either to each other or to the sac itself. Occasionally, feces within the loops of bowel in the hernia prevent reduction. Often, after a reduction attempt, only a small piece of omentum or properitoneal fat remains incarcerated. Although this incarcerated fat is not associated with significant morbidity, pain may be considerable; operative reduction and subsequent repair of the abdominal wall defect may be required.

If strangulation occurs, most commonly the clinical picture is one of intestinal obstruction. The patient experiences severe pain, vomiting, distention, and obstipation. The patient may be febrile and may have a leukocytosis. No impulse may be transmitted to the hernia sac on coughing, and the overlying skin often becomes inflamed and edematous. These features may be less marked if only omentum is contained within the sac. Ultimately gangrene of the bowel or the omentum occurs if strangulation is not relieved and the involved gut perforates into the sac.

The presentation and differential diagnosis of hernias in adults are similar to those of hernias in children, although adults are generally more cooperative in an examination and can provide more extensive historical information. Nonetheless, unusual conditions (e.g., a Richter hernia, which may mimic a groin abscess because of the absence of bowel obstruction symptoms,[8] and traumatic abdominal wall hernias,[9, 10] which may mimic a hematoma following injury[11]) may be confusing. Intra-abdominal hemorrhage and a variety of other more unusual diseases and pathologic conditions can present within an inguinal hernia.[12]

INDICATIONS AND CONTRAINDICATIONS

Whenever possible, incarcerated hernias should be reduced. Reduction minimizes inflammation and tissue edema, thus preventing strangulation. Some clinicians state that it is impossible to reduce a strangulated hernia because of the extensive inflammation, edema, and tenderness. Fortunately, most patients present early after incarceration, and the question of whether strangulation has occurred is rarely an issue. In most cases, the patient presents within hours of the incarceration without fever, leukocytosis, or other evidence of generalized toxicity. In that circumstance, reduction of the hernia is indicated.

A femoral hernia presents a special problem in that the small neck present in the femoral canal and the usual generous overlying subcutaneous tissue make a complete reduction virtually impossible. Therefore, femoral hernias are best referred on an emergency basis to a surgical consultant for evaluation and consideration of operative reduction and simultaneous hernia repair. Attempts at reduction are best deferred until that consultation has been obtained. Similarly, an incarcerated ovary or an undescended testis in an inguinal hernia represents an indication for surgical reduction.

Peritonitis and other clinical evidence of strangulation (e.g., fever, marked leukocytosis, toxic appearance) are contraindications to an attempt at a nonsurgical reduction of an incarcerated hernia. In addition, immediate surgical repair of a traumatic hernia is recommended both for prevention of delayed morbidity from herniation and for evaluation of underlying organ injury.[9]

PROCEDURE

When clinically indicated, gentle reduction of incarcerated hernias should be attempted. Adequate sedation must be given to allay anxiety and to minimize discomfort (see also Chapter 41). For infants, meperidine (Demerol) can be given intramuscularly in the dose of 0.5 mg/kg, whereas for older children morphine sulfate in the dose of 0.05 mg/kg can be administered intramuscularly. Chloral hydrate or phenobarbital may also be effective. Adults often require 50 to 100 mg of meperidine given with 25 to 50 mg of hydroxyzine (Vistaril) to enhance the sedative effects and to reduce the emetic properties of meperidine. The judicious use of analgesia or sedation is the key to successful reduction of an incarcerated hernia.

Following sedation, the patient is placed in a head-down tilt of approximately 20 degrees for groin hernias (no tilt when other hernias are treated). A pillow may be placed under the buttocks. For infants, the legs should be swaddled and secured to prevent slippage. This technique is successful in spontaneously reducing 80 per cent of pediatric incarcerated hernias over a 2-hour period without manipulation. In addition, the light application of a cold pack or a padded ice bag to reduce local blood flow and to diminish intraluminal gas pressure is helpful while the analgesic is taking effect.

If after 20 to 25 minutes spontaneous reduction has not occurred, gentle manipulation can be added to the aforementioned method. For inguinal hernias, the physician positions the thumb and index finger of one hand along the inguinal canal and presses gently on the incarcerated hernia just distal to the external inguinal ring. Simultaneous massage of the inguinal region in the level of the internal and external rings is used as the other thumb and index finger slowly funnel the incarcerated viscera toward the rings. These maneuvers, if successful, often result in a "gurgle" that signifies hernia sac reduction. A slow, steady, atraumatic manipulation is preferred. Repeated forceful attempts at reduction are contraindicated.

Reduced bowel almost certainly will not be strangulated. Rectal examination may confirm reduction. Once reduction occurs, corrective surgery can be performed 1 week later, after local edema has subsided. If reduction cannot be achieved, emergency surgery is indicated after dehydration and electrolyte imbalances are corrected. Nasogastric suction is indicated if obstruction is present. Reduction of other abdominal wall hernias is accomplished in a fashion similar to that described for inguinal hernias.

COMPLICATIONS

An attempt at manual reduction of a hernia may be unsuccessful or only partially successful. The physician must recognize a partial reduction and obtain appropriate consultation. Persistent attempts at reduction produce patient discomfort and may delay operative intervention for relief of bowel obstruction or organ ischemia. Testicular or ovarian rupture may be caused by overzealous attempts to reduce a hernia associated with an undescended or ectopic gonad.

CONCLUSION

By far the greatest challenge in the immediate management of groin lumps is the differential diagnosis of conditions that may mimic a groin hernia. Reduction of groin and other abdominal wall hernias is usually straightforward, as has been discussed. Once the hernia is reduced, the patient and family must be told that straining at stool, urination, or coughing may produce another prolapse of the hernia sac. The patient or family should rapidly reduce any recurrent herniation to avoid recurrent incarceration and the need for a return to the emergency department. A demonstration of the reduction technique to be used by the patient or family usually aids in gaining cooperation. The emergency physician should not overlook the need to evaluate and treat potentially complicating conditions, such as urinary tract infections, bladder outlet obstruction, constipation, and respiratory infections that may increase intra-abdominal pressure and produce recurrent herniation. Appropriate referral for these related problems and subsequent care of the reduced hernia is recommended.

Finally, the emergency physician must be aware that to the patient the development of hernia symptoms is often associated with employment-related activities. Although physical exertion can certainly exacerbate a preexisting weakness in the abdominal wall and can lead to frank herniation, most frequently the abdominal wall defect is congenital in origin. Therefore, to minimize confusion in workmen's compensation cases, the physician should be careful to note that the patient's hernia became symptomatic during an activity rather than stating that the hernia was the result of an activity.

REFERENCES

1. Zimmerman LM, Anson BJ: The Anatomy and Surgery of Hernia. Baltimore, Williams & Wilkins, 1953.
2. Carlson RI: The historical development of the surgical treatment of inguinal hernia. Surgery 39:1031, 1956.
3. Koontz AR: Hernia. New York, Appleton-Century-Crofts, 1963.
4. Gillespie RW, Glas WW, Metz GH, et al: Richter's hernia: Its etiology, recognition, and management. Arch Surg 73:590, 1956.
5. Richter AG: Abhandlung von der Bruchen. Gottingen, Germany, Dietrich, 1785, pp 596–597.
6. Otero C, Fallon WF: Injury to the abdominal wall musculature: The full spectrum of traumatic hernia. South Med J 81:517, 1988.
7. Fallis J: Hernias. In Vaughan BC III, McKay RJ (eds): Nelson Textbook of Pediatrics. 11th ed. Philadelphia, WB Saunders Co, 1979, pp 1107–1109.
8. Doubleday LC: A colocutaneous fistula in the inguinal area. JAMA 247:2407, 1982.
9. Malangoni MA, Condon RE: Traumatic abdominal wall hernia. J Trauma 23:356, 1983.
10. Clain A: Traumatic hernia. Br J Surg 51:549, 1964.
11. Jones TW, Merendino KA: The deep epigastric artery: Rectus muscle syndrome. Am J Surg 103:159, 1962.
12. Sherman HF: The inguinal hernia: Not always straightforward, not always a hernia. J Emerg Med 7:21, 1989.

Chapter 58

Anoscopy and Sigmoidoscopy

Jonathan M. Glauser

ANOSCOPY

Anoscopy is an easily performed outpatient procedure for evaluating the anal orifice and the anal canal. The procedure is not adequate for evaluating all rectal pathologic conditions, because only the most distal portion of the rectum may be visualized with this procedure. The indications for the procedure are the same as for sigmoidoscopy (see the following discussion of sigmoidoscopy), except that the area to be examined is much smaller.[1, 2]

Equipment

The anoscope has two basic designs: (1) a conical tube, and (2) a "slotted" tube with a side opening, or "slot," at the distal end. This latter design allows a portion of the side wall of the anus or the rectum to prolapse within the lumen of the anoscope.[3] Variations affect the length, caliber, and shape (conical versus cylindric) of the tube; the possession of side slits, grooves, or sliding attachments; and the method of illumination.[2] Instruments that incorporate their own light source are very desirable and eliminate the need for an assistant (Fig. 58–1).

For patients with painful anal lesions or with some degree of anal spasm or stenosis, a narrow instrument is necessary. Normally the anal canal of a child is quite distensible and generally is capable of admitting an adult-sized anoscope. A light source is needed. In addition, the examiner

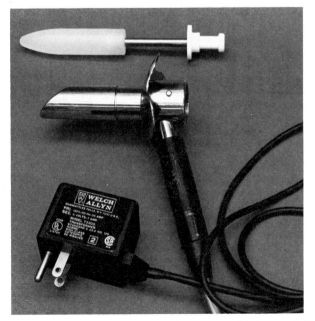

Figure 58–1. Standard anoscope. An instrument with its own light source is preferred.

should have long, nontoothed forceps (such as 20-cm Emmett forceps) and cotton balls for swabbing out the lumen[2, 3] and appropriate culture material, available at the bedside if needed.

Preparation

Anoscopy, like sigmoidoscopy, should be attempted only after digital examination has been performed to detect tenderness or a mass and to determine the axis of the anal canal.[4] No other preparation is necessary.[2, 4]

Positioning

The examination can be performed with the patient in either the Sims lateral decubitus position or the knee-chest position, as described subsequently in the section on sigmoidoscopy. Anal stenosis or severe pain on digital examination is a contraindication to the passage of an anoscope. Some physicians advocate the use of topical anesthetic gels or ointments to produce anesthesia in painful examinations. Others believe that the agents are not needed, because if they are used only as a lubricant they do not produce anesthesia, and they have the potential to cause contact dermatitis or mucosal irritation. Mild pain relief may be afforded if the initial digital examination introduces a generous amount of xylocaine ointment (4 per cent) and the examiner waits 4 to 5 minutes before proceeding with the anoscope. Although the *slow and gentle passage of the instrument is the key to success*, the judicious use of parenteral sedation and analgesia is justified and recommended in selected cases. Midazolam (Versed) is a popular sedative with excellent amnestic properties that can greatly facilitate the examination. It is common for the physician to underestimate the pain produced by simple anoscopy in patients with many anorectal conditions.

Procedure

The instrument is first well lubricated and a digital rectal examination is performed to assess the angle of the anal canal. The obturator is inserted completely in the anoscope, and the device is placed at the anal verge.[2] As the patient bears down, the instrument is advanced initially in line with the axis of the anal canal (in general, with the anoscope pointing toward the umbilicus).[4] The instrument initially follows an inward, downward (anterior), and forward course (Fig. 58–2). The obturator is kept securely in place with the physician's thumb.

Once beyond the level of the sphincter, the anoscope should be directed backward to avoid abutment of the prostate gland and to follow the axis of the rectum along the curve of the sacrum. If the instrument is gripped by the anal sphincters, gentle pressure should be maintained in the long axis of the canal until the muscles gradually relax (generally within 60 seconds).[2] Passage of the instrument to its shoulder is usually accomplished without difficulty until the outer flange impinges against the anal verge.

The obturator must be kept fully engaged in the anoscope during insertion to avoid nipping the anal mucosa and causing pain.[3] For the same reason, the obturator should not be reinserted except when the entire instrument is withdrawn from the patient. Examination of the rectum is performed during gradual *withdrawal of the anoscope*.

The anoscope is then stabilized, and the obturator is removed. A small (1 cm^2) area of ecchymosis or abrasion of

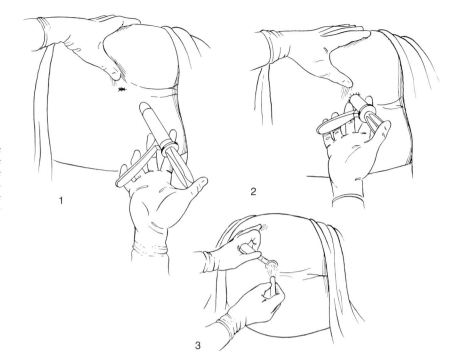

Figure 58–2. Anoscopy. Initially, the anoscope is directed toward the umbilicus, and the obturator is not withdrawn until the scope has been passed to the hilt. Detailed examination is performed on withdrawal of the instrument. A penlight is used in this illustration for illumination.

the mucosa frequently is found where the obturator has rested.[4] The light source is shined into the lumen, and forceps with cotton balls are used as necessary for swabbing to visualize the anorectum.[2] A proper examination cannot be performed without adequate lighting, and anoscopes that incorporate their own fiberoptic light source are preferred.

Normal mucosa is pink and smooth and glistening. The instrument is angled so that the distal lumen of the rectum is seen. The anoscope is then slowly withdrawn, and the lumen is moved in a circular fashion so that the entire wall is inspected.[1, 4]

As the zone above the sphincters is approached, care should be taken to detect the presence of enlarged hemorrhoids.[3] To help demonstrate these structures, the patient is asked to bear down. Enlarged hemorrhoids protrude into the lumen and are easily seen. The Valsalva maneuver should be repeated several times until the instrument passes beyond the pectinate line.[4]

If the patient has much discomfort during the terminal portion of the examination, reflex spasm of the anal sphincter may expel the instrument quickly. For this reason, the examiner may be unable to obtain an adequate view with a single passage. Anoscopy may be repeated several times if necessary.

The following pathologic conditions should also be searched for: anal fistulas and fissures, sentinel tag, thickened or prolapsed anal papillae, tumors and thrombosed or edematous hemorrhoids.[1] The stool should be examined for blood or pus.

The mucous membrane is observed for thickening and granularity. The examiner can check for contact bleeding by rubbing the mucosa gently with a swab or forceps[2]; contact bleeding is an important sign of mucosal inflammation. Pinworms may also be seen writhing in the lower rectum.

SIGMOIDOSCOPY

Desormeaux in 1853 first devised an endoscopic instrument to look into the rectum. He used a reflecting mirror and a lamp burning a mixture of alcohol and turpentine as a light source.[1]

Sigmoidoscopes have classically been subdivided into those with distal lighting and those with proximal lighting. Originally, the devices with distal illumination (e.g., the early Strauss design) used light carried on the distal end of a long wire attachment that projected inside the tube. If either liquid feces or mucus were present in the bowel, the light was submerged, and the instrument had to be removed for cleansing and reinsertion.[2] Sigmoidoscopes with proximal illumination therefore became popular. More recently, sigmoidoscopes have been developed with distal illumination, which is obtained by incorporation of fiberoptic fibers in the wall of the tube to convey light from a bulb at the proximal end.[2, 5] The fiberoptic cold light can be attached proximally to either an anoscope or a rigid sigmoidoscope (Fig. 58–3).

Equipment

The sigmoidoscope itself is a hollow, rigid tube that may be metal or plastic and clear or black.[6] The length may vary but typically is 25 cm. The device can therefore be inserted for a distance of approximately 21 cm above the anal verge. The barrel of the sigmoidoscope is calibrated in centimeters, so that the distance of any lesion from the anal verge can be noted.

The window of the Welch-Allen sigmoidoscope, the most commonly used model, magnifies two times.[2] The internal diameter should be measured before insertion so that the size of any lesions that are seen can be estimated. This diameter typically is 12 to 19 mm and in general can be tolerated by infants and children as well as adults.[1]

The flexible fiberoptic sigmoidoscope is rapidly replacing the rigid sigmoidoscope in screening for colorectal disease.[7] The role of flexible sigmoidoscopy in the practice of emergency medicine has not been defined, although the decrease in patient discomfort[8] as well as its sensitivity when combined with air-contrast barium enema in detection of colonic disease support increased usage. Flexible sigmoidoscopes are either 35 cm or 60 to 65 cm in length.[9]

Accessory materials for proctosigmoidoscopy are listed in Table 58–1.[10]

Indications

It has been claimed that proctosigmoidoscopic examination is indicated in almost all patients with complaints related to bowel.[6] Specifically, the procedure is indicated in the following cases: recent occurrence of constipation or diarrhea or a change in either symptom[5]; bright red blood per rectum or mixed in stool[3, 5, 11]; pain or difficulty in defecation;[3] rectal discomfort; involuntary seepage of stool[5]; pencil-sized stools resulting from a lesion in the anal area or a stenosing process in the rectum[5]; and lesions around the anal opening (characterized by abscesses, fistulas, discharge, ulcers, external piles, or pruritus). The procedure is also indicated in conjunction with examination and specimen collection for suspected parasitic infestation,[3] biopsy of colorectal lesions, and reduction of a sigmoid volvulus.[12] The American Cancer Society has suggested sigmoidoscopy every 3 to 5 years in asymptomatic individuals over the age of 50 as colorectal screening, along with annual stool blood testing.[13] The efficacy of such screening has not been established.[14] Both rigid and flexible fiberoptic sigmoidoscopy has been used in the endoscopic removal of rectal foreign bodies[15] (see also Chapter 60).

Although some physicians suggest using the sigmoidoscope to reduce acute sigmoid volvulus, the procedure is not definitive treatment and is not generally an emergency department practice.

Contraindications

There are few contraindications to the procedure. Imperforate anus is the only absolute contraindication.[6] Various relative contraindications have been reported, including the following: pain on examination (proctosigmoidoscopic examination of some patients with regional enteritis or carcinoma may require general anesthesia), excessive angulation of the rectosigmoid colon, acute peritonitis, rectal abscess, acute inflammatory bowel disease (e.g., toxic megacolon, acute diverticulitis, fulminant ulcerative colitis), and an uncooperative patient.[5] Patients with coronary artery disease can be examined, although caution is advised in these cases, because coronary ischemia or dysrhythmias can be precipitated.[16]

Table 58–1. **Accessory Materials for Proctosigmoidoscopy**
Rectal gloves
Lubricant
Paper towels, sheets
Glass microscope slides and cover slips for examination of stool as indicated
30-cm rectal cotton swabs (alternatively, long 35-cm alligator forceps for gripping absorbent pledgets can be used in swabbing out the bowel lumen)
Suction tube
Waste basket
Guaiac material to test for fecal occult blood
Probes for examination of fistulas

Preparation

Preparation for sigmoidoscopy is often unnecessary, because the rectal ampulla is normally empty.[6] Some recommend a 120- to 140-ml enema 30 to 60 minutes before examination.[4, 17, 18] Plain saline or a commercially available phosphate solution (Fleet enema) in such cases is acceptable and generally cleans to the level of the splenic flexure.

There are drawbacks to enema administration. The enema tube tip may leave a superficial linear abrasion on the anterior rectal wall.[6] The soap in an enema is irritating to the mucosa and causes a discharge of mucus. This mucus, along with the retained enema solution, may interfere with vision and may obscure abnormalities.[5] As a rule, fluid feces are harder to remove for proctoscopic examination than are solid feces.[2] Furthermore, in ulcerative colitis the characteristic bloody purulent mucosa is better recognized without any preparation.[5] Enemas should certainly be avoided if brisk diarrhea is present or if ulcerative colitis is suspected.

Sedation with diazepam (Valium), 5 to 10 mg intravenously, has been recommended by some.[5, 19] Midazolam (Versed) is another popular sedative with excellent amnestic properties. Nitrous oxide analgesia is also appropriate.

In general, no specific bowel preparation is required. Although some researchers recommend bowel preparation for 24 to 48 hours with liquid diet, stool softeners, cathartics, and suppositories,[19, 20] such a regimen is clearly impractical for an emergency procedure.

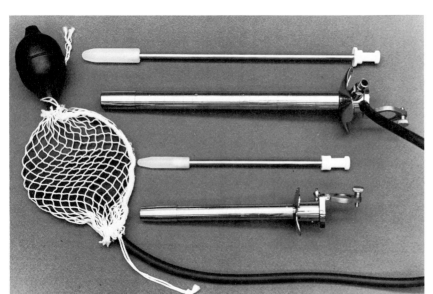

Figure 58–3. Standard rigid sigmoidoscope. Two sizes are shown here, with obturators and an insufflation balloon.

Positioning

Three positions are generally accepted for sigmoidoscopy. These are the lateral decubitus (or Sims) position, the knee-chest position, and the dorsal lithotomy position. All three are described here, although the first two are preferred (Fig. 58–4).

The lateral decubitus position is generally performed with the patient on his or her left side. The lower back is extended, with the buttocks positioned just over the edge of the table or bed.[2, 4, 6] With the lumbar spine extended, the axis of the rectal canal is easier to follow along the rectum. The knees and the hips are flexed, with the patient's trunk obliquely across the table. Optionally, one may move the patient's right shoulder and buttocks slightly forward, perhaps by placing a sandbag under the left hip.

The left lateral decubitus position is preferable for right-handed physicians and is more comfortable for the patient than are the other positions. The major disadvantage is that the examiner's freedom of motion is rather limited; passage of the instrument above the pelvic floor is frequently difficult.

The knee-chest position can be used either on an examination table or, preferably, on a tilt table. If the sigmoidoscopy is performed on an examination table or in bed, the patient is positioned with the knees drawn up, the hips flexed, and the buttocks elevated. The chest is angled down, and the patient lies with the head on upward-folded arms.[7]

If a tilt table is available, the patient is arched with the knees on the step of the table and the chest lying against the flat surface. The platform on which the patient's knees are resting must be kept high enough to extend the lower spine. Flexion of the lumbar spine and resting the abdomen on the table should be avoided.[4] The arms are extended above the head, and the physician then adjusts the forward tilt of the table.[7]

The advantage of this position is that it affords good visualization of the anorectal region. The abdominal contents fall cephalad, the sigmoid colon stretches, and air insufflation is generally unnecessary. The drawbacks to the knee-chest

position concern the patient's discomfort. This position is unacceptable for examinations of long duration and may be unsatisfactory for ill or elderly patients.[5] In experienced hands, sigmoidoscopy takes less than 5 minutes and, if tolerated, the knee-chest position is the one of choice for this procedure.

For completeness, the dorsal lithotomy position is mentioned. This is currently not a popular position for sigmoidoscopy, although it is comfortable for the patient. Another advantage is that a gynecologic examining table, which is necessary for the lithotomy position, is almost always present in physicians' offices, clinics, and emergency departments. The major drawback to the dorsal lithotomy position is that the abdominal contents lie on top of the sigmoid colon and compromise the lumen of the bowel. This necessitates frequent air insufflation to maintain an open lumen.

Anatomy

A general review of the relevant anatomy is suggested for those without extensive experience in sigmoidoscopy (Fig. 58–5).

The distal large bowel is divided into three anatomic areas: the anal canal, the rectum, and the sigmoid colon. As one proceeds proximally from the anus, the first 3 to 4 cm constitute the anal canal. The area 4 to 15 cm proximal to the anus is the rectum. At the junction of the anal canal and the rectum is the pectinate line. At the pectinate line the distal vertical folds of the rectal mucosa form the anal columns, which terminate as the anal valves. The rectum is approximately 12 cm long and has a smooth, plum-colored mucosa. Lateral reflections of the bowel wall in the rectum form the valves of Houston. The rectum is dilated inferiorly to form the ampulla.

At approximately 15 cm in depth, the rectum joins the sigmoid colon at the rectosigmoid. The sigmoid colon is recognized through the sigmoidoscope at this point by its circular mucosal rings.

There are two areas of sharp angulation of the distal

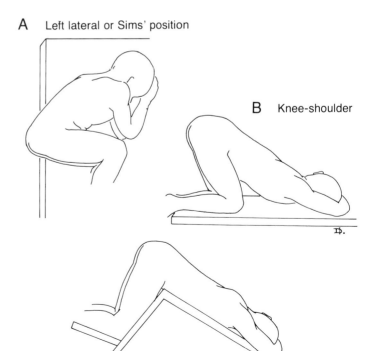

Figure 58–4. Positions for performing sigmoidoscopy or anoscopy. (From Hill GJ II: Outpatient Surgery. 3rd ed. Philadelphia, WB Saunders Co, 1988. Reproduced by permission.)

A Left lateral or Sims' position

B Knee-shoulder

C Prone

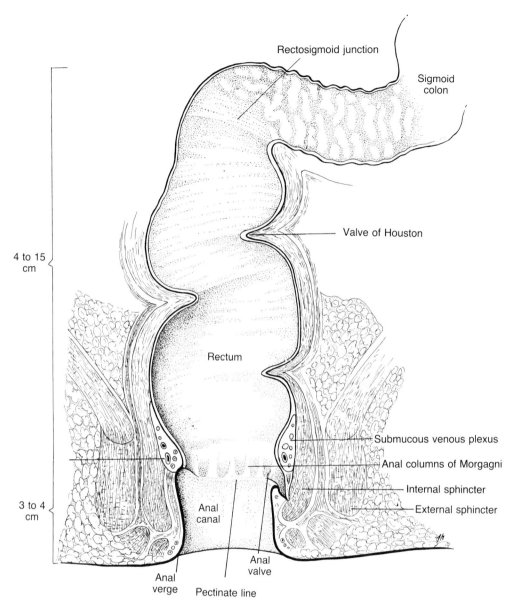

Figure 58–5. Anatomy of sigmoidoscopy. (Redrawn from Abrahams PH, Webb PJ: Clinical Anatomy of Practical Procedures. London, Pitman, 1975. By permission of Churchill Livingstone.)

bowel. As one proceeds with a sigmoidoscopic examination, one encounters the first sharp angle at approximately 15 cm in depth at the rectosigmoid. Here the bowel takes a turn to the patient's left at almost a right angle. The area of extreme angulation is the section that is the most difficult to negotiate with the scope and is the most frequent site of perforation. Four to 8 cm proximal to the rectosigmoid, the colon makes another sharp angle and proceeds cephalad. From this point proximally the anatomy varies considerably.

Procedure

Before insertion of the sigmoidoscope, a rectal examination with a lubricated gloved finger must always be performed.[3] This determines the presence or absence of fecal impaction, rectal tumor, enlarged prostate, or stricture. The angle of the anal canal can also be determined by rectal examination.[6]

The sigmoidoscope, with obturator in place and light source removed, is warmed and extensively lubricated. It is inserted into the anus and passed initially toward the umbilicus. For the first 3 to 4 cm, the initial direction of the tip of the scope is down (anteriorly) and forward into the anal canal (Fig. 58–6). A right-handed examiner holds the head of the sigmoidoscope with the right hand and assists the tip through the anal sphincter with the left hand (Fig. 58–7).[21] A left-handed examiner reverses the hand positions. Insertion is accomplished by gentle pressure; the patient should be warned that there may be a transient sensation of a bowel movement but that this is an artificial sensation.

If the examiner feels muscle spasm of the sphincters, insertion should be delayed until muscle relaxation occurs.[2] A double "give" of both external and internal sphincters may be felt. Asking the patient to "bear down" in a manner similar to a bowel movement helps to relax the sphincter.

Once the sigmoidoscope is within the anal canal, the obturator is removed and the instrument is advanced under direct vision (Fig. 58–8). The obturator is never replaced, and the sigmoidoscope is advanced only under direct visualization of the bowel lumen. The proximal end of the sigmoidoscope carrying the glass window, the light, and the bellows is now firmly attached.[2] After the initial entry into

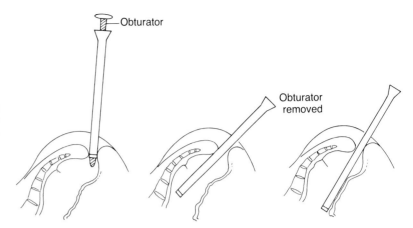

Figure 58–6. Various positions of the sigmoidoscope during examination. Note that the obturator is withdrawn after sigmoidoscope entry into the anal canal.

the anal canal, the tip of the scope is directed posteriorly (the eyepiece is moved anteriorly) to follow the curvature of the sacrum. The scope may be moved from side to side to negotiate the valves of Houston in the rectum. Usually, there is little need for distention of the colon until the instrument nears the sharp turn at the pelvic floor (10 to 12 cm). The hand that is holding the tip of the sigmoidoscope may rest on the patient's buttocks for steadiness. Once the level of the rectosigmoid is reached at approximately 15 cm, the

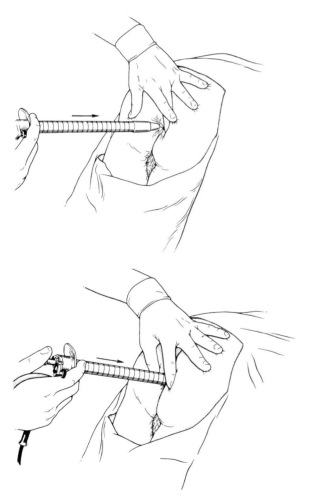

Figure 58–7. Insertion of the sigmoidoscope with obturator in place. The left hand is used to aid in spreading the buttocks and stabilizing the scope. (From Vander Salm TJ, Cutler BS, Wheeler HB: Atlas of Bedside Procedures. Boston, Little, Brown & Co, 1979. Reproduced by permission.)

anterior and leftward curve of the bowel lumen must be followed. The tip of the scope is directed anteriorly and to the patient's left (the eyepiece is swung posteriorly and to the patient's right).[22] If the rectosigmoid is successfully passed, one now simply follows the lumen of the bowel, because the anatomy is variable at this point.

For the beginning examiner, the greatest difficulty is in following the lumen. When a "dead end" or "blind pouch" is reached, the edge of the lumen is inspected in a circumferential manner. In this way, the edge of a valve of Houston may be found to hide a turn in the canal. The free edge should be displaced toward the direction of the lumen, so that the central position is open and passage is continued.[4] If the lumen is lost, it is helpful to withdraw the instrument a few centimeters, because the tip may be in a pouch of bowel.

The sigmoidoscope is advanced gently and slowly. Fine scrutiny of the mucosa is generally left until the withdrawal phase of the examination.[1, 6] Once the device has been inserted 10 cm or more, changes in the axis of the instrument may stretch the peritoneum and cause crampy discomfort. Females may undergo more discomfort than males if the uterus anteriorly increases the leverage necessary for full insertion of the scope.[2] The examiner should anticipate the flexures and should direct the sigmoidoscope accordingly. Major changes in direction and displacement should be made slowly to lessen patient discomfort.

For an adequate study, the sigmoidoscope should be advanced to at least 15 cm. A barium enema is sufficiently accurate to define abnormalities at this level and above. As a rule, the instrument should be inserted as far as possible, with careful scrutiny of each square centimeter of mucosa on withdrawal.[1, 6]

Intermittent insufflation of gas (either air or carbon dioxide) may be essential for effective intubation.[21] Because excessive insufflation of gas is uncomfortable for the patient, use of this technique should be minimized.[2] Insufflation may also stretch adjacent limbs of a redundant loop of sigmoid, causing an unnecessary additional acuteness in the angle to be negotiated.[21] Some physicians are completely against insufflation.[1, 6]

If the lumen cannot be seen easily, the instrument may need to be withdrawn until the examiner can see the lateral wall of the true lumen. Rotation of the leading end of the sigmoidoscope may help locate the lumen. Some side-to-side movement may be necessary for negotiation of the instrument, especially past the lower and middle valves of Houston.

Suction should be provided only with a guarded tube. Pledgets are preferable, either with long, pledget-holding forceps to clean the mucosa[3] or with rectal swabs long enough to extend the length of the sigmoidoscope.[10]

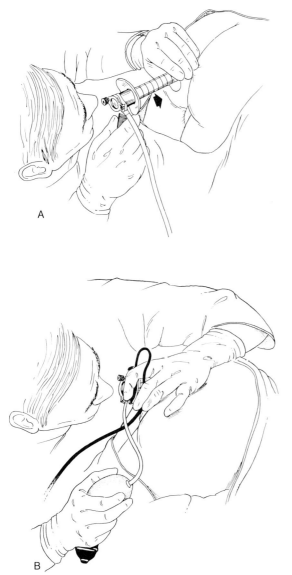

Figure 58–8. The sigmoidoscope is advanced under direct vision *(A)*. Insufflation may be required *(B)*. Detailed examination is performed on withdrawal of the sigmoidoscope. Suction should be available. (From Vander Salm TJ, Cutler BS, Wheeler HB: Atlas of Bedside Procedures. Boston, Little, Brown & Co, 1979. Reproduced by permission.)

The mucous membrane is inspected for color, texture, and mobility. Normal rectosigmoid mucosa is intact, smooth, pink, and glistening. Erosions, ulcers, polyps, blood, pus, or the raised edge of a carcinoma should be sought. The distance in centimeters and the position of any lesions that are found should be noted when findings are reported (e.g., 16-cm level at 10 o'clock position, with 12 o'clock position representing a true dorsal location).[6]

It should be noted that one may see clusters of petechiae on the posterior wall at the rectosigmoid junction where the tip of the sigmoidoscope superficially contused the mucosal membrane as it was impinged on the sacrum. A linear scratch on the anterior rectal wall, caused by an enema tube, may be visible. This minor trauma may also result in a false-positive test for occult blood in the stool.

Some areas are difficult to see, although effort should be made to view them. The examiner may have to describe a wide arc with the proximal end of the sigmoidoscope to see the entire rectal circumference. The upper surfaces of the valves and the posterior rectal wall require special care to visualize.

Full insertion to 25 cm has been reported to be possible in only 42 per cent of patients.[6] In one study, 966 of 1000 sigmoidoscopies were successful in visualizing the sigmoid to 15 cm, the cutoff for accuracy of a barium enema.

Complications

Complications are generally few and minor. Perforation is considered the most catastrophic and was reported as early as 1912.[23] A comprehensive survey performed in 1946 found 46 known cases of perforation. A later study reported a perforation rate from colonoscopy and sigmoidoscopy of 0.2 per cent.[5] Another report claimed a much lower incidence even than this: 5 perforations in 172,351 sigmoidoscopic examinations in one study and 4 perforations in 350,000 cases in another.[6] Perforation of the sigmoid mandates prompt surgical exploration. Perforation usually occurs at 10 to 15 cm on the anterior portion of the bowel, where the sigmoid makes its first sharp turn. This complication is usually quite obvious, but recognition may be delayed, with serious consequences. Rarely, perforation may occur in the rectum, in which case the scope enters the retroperitoneal space. Whitish discoloration of the mucosa (blanching) occurring when the bowel wall slides by and accompanied by patient discomfort should be taken as a warning that excessive pressure is possibly being applied to the wall and that perforation may be imminent. Under these circumstances, the instrument must be withdrawn rapidly. Occasionally, perforation is accompanied by bleeding or the appearance of peritoneal fluid or omentum in the lumen.

Forcible insufflation of air causes abdominal cramping and may be a factor in perforation, especially if diverticulae are present. If there is any question of perforation, one should immediately take an upright chest radiograph following the procedure to look for free air under the diaphragm. If perforation occurs in the rectum, one may see retroperitoneal air along the shadows of the psoas on an abdominal film. Persistent pain, fever, or bleeding after the procedure should raise the possibility of occult perforation. The incidence of deaths attributed to postoperative complications following laparotomy necessitated by perforation is 0.03 per cent.[5]

Proper positioning, a well-cleansed colon, and proper technique should reduce the incidence of perforation. Swabs and suction devices should be used with caution. If unusual angulation of the bowel is present, if the patient is uncooperative, if vision is hampered by stool or blood, or if adhesions from pelvic surgery or past infection make it impossible to negotiate a rectosigmoid angle, the examination should be terminated.

Traumatic insertion may result in anorectal abrasion, ulcerations, and perianal abscess. Insufflation may rupture a diverticulum. Traumatic sequelae and ileus have been noted following sigmoidoscopy, particularly in patients with Crohn's disease or acute ulcerative colitis, making the procedure relatively contraindicated under these circumstances.[24]

Transient bacteremia in as many as 10 per cent of patients (usually enterococcal organisms) has been reported during sigmoidoscopy.[3, 25] In a literature review, the overall frequency of bacteremia following sigmoidoscopy was 4.9 per cent; enterococcus, *Escherichia coli*, and *Klebsiella* were isolated in different cases.[26] This is generally believed to be of no clinical significance. Some physicians have advocated prophylactic antibiotic coverage for patients who have valvular heart disease[27] with past bacterial endocarditis or who have prosthetic heart valves,[26] although there is not agreement on this.

Because transmission of hepatitis B, human immunodeficiency virus, or sexually transmitted diseases such as herpes or condylomata acuminata is a theoretic possibility, mechanical cleansing with 2 per cent chloraldehyde and gas sterilization after each examination has been advocated.[24]

Pain can be severe enough to cause termination of the examination. In one study, 12 per cent of sigmoidoscopies were terminated for this reason,[18] although 88 per cent of patients undergoing the procedure experienced some discomfort.[28]

Sigmoidoscopy has its limitations. The sigmoidoscope does not provide as good a view of the anal canal as does the anoscope.[3, 4] Colonoscopy[29] and flexible sigmoidoscopy provide greater accuracy in diagnosis.[18, 28, 30–33] Furthermore, there is increasing evidence that colonic malignancies today are more proximal than in the past.[11, 28] Although the rigid sigmoidoscope was once thought to be able to diagnose 75 per cent of large bowel malignancies, it cannot reach such a high proportion of colonic malignancies today. The average lengths of insertion in two studies were only 18.6 cm[29] and 20 cm.[28] Neoplasms may be overlooked; conversely, inflammatory polypoid changes or diverticulae have been falsely diagnosed as neoplasm.[24]

References

1. Brown CH (ed): Diagnostic Procedures in Gastroenterology. St Louis, CV Mosby Co, 1967, pp 213–240.
2. Goligher JC, Duthie HL, Nixon HH, et al (eds): Surgery of the Anus, Rectum and Colon. 4th ed. London, Balliere Tindall, 1980, pp 52–68.
3. Ellis DJ, Bevan PG: Proctoscopy and sigmoidoscopy. Br Med J 281:435, 1980.
4. Christian RL: Anorectal disorders. In Branch WT (ed): The Office Practice of Medicine. Philadelphia, WB Saunders Co, 1982, pp 664–678.
5. Otto P, Klaus E: Atlas of Rectoscopy and Colonoscopy. Berlin, Springer-Verlag, 1979, pp 1–16, 23–27.
6. Bockus HL (ed): Gastroenterology. Vol 2. Philadelphia, WB Saunders Co, 1976, pp 836–843.
7. Groveman HD, Sanowski RA, Klauber MR: Training primary care physicians in flexible sigmoidoscopy—performance evaluation of 17,167 procedures. West J Med 148:221, 1988.
8. Winawer SJ, Miller C, Lightdale C, et al: Patient response to sigmoidoscopy: A randomized controlled trial of rigid and flexible sigmoidoscopy. Cancer 60:1905, 1987.
9. Hocutt JE, Hainer BL, Jackson MG: Flexible fiberoptic sigmoidoscopy: Its use in family medicine. J Am Bd Fam Pract 1:189, 1988.
10. Schapiro M, Kuritsky J: The Gastroenterology Assistant: A Lab Manual. Springfield, Ill, Charles C Thomas, 1972, pp 70–73.
11. Leicester RJ, Hunt RH: Letter. Br Med J 283:1607, 1981.
12. O'Connor JJ: Reduction of sigmoid volvulus by flexible sigmoidoscopy (letter). Arch Surg 114:1092, 1979.
13. Winawer SJ, Kerner JF: Sigmoidoscopy: Case finding versus screening (editorial). Gastroenterology 95:527, 1988.
14. Selby JF, Friedman GD: Sigmoidoscopy in the periodic health examination of asymptomatic adults. JAMA 261:595, 1989.
15. Kantarian JC, Riether RD, Sheets JA, et al: Endoscopic retrieval of foreign bodies from the rectum. Dis Colon Rectum 30:902, 1987.
16. Munter DW, Stoner R: Ventricular fibrillation during rectal examination. Am J Emerg Med 7:57, 1989.
17. Marino AWM Jr: Looking ahead: Types of flexible sigmoidoscopes and preparation of the patient. Dis Colon Rectum 20:91, 1977.
18. Marks G, Boggs HW, Castro AF, et al: Sigmoidoscopic examinations with rigid and flexible fiberoptic sigmoidoscopes in the surgeon's office. Dis Colon Rectum 22:162, 1979.
19. Stone RV: Proctoscopy and sigmoidoscopy (letter). Br Med J 281:682, 1980.
20. Devadhar DSC: Preparation for sigmoidoscopy (letter). N Z Med J 93:394, 1981.
21. Coller JA: Technique of flexible fiberoptic sigmoidoscopy. Surg Clin North Am 60:465, 1980.
22. Evans PWG: A sigmoidoscope in the practice. The Practitioner 231:189, 1987.
23. Andresen AFR: Perforations from proctoscopy. Gastroenterology 9:32, 1947.
24. Marks G, Borenstein BD: Complications of flexible fiberoptic sigmoidoscopy: A conceptual approach. Surg Endosc 1:59, 1987.
25. Adami B, Eckhardt VF, Suermann RB, et al: Bacteremia after proctoscopy and hemorrhoidal injection sclerotherapy. Dis Colon Rectum 24:373, 1980.
26. Botoman VA, Surawicz CM: Bacteremia with gastrointestinal endoscopic procedures. Gastrointest Endosc 32:342, 1986.
27. Engeling ER, Eng BF: Bacteremia after sigmoidoscopy: Another view (letter). Ann Intern Med 94:77, 1981.
28. Winnan G, Bergi G, Panish J, et al: Superiority of the flexible to the rigid sigmoidoscope in routine proctosigmoidoscopy. N Engl J Med 302:1011, 1980.
29. Talbott TM: Looking ahead: Evaluation of new flexible sigmoidoscopes. Dis Colon Rectum 20:89, 1977.
30. Foster GE, Vellacott KD, Balfour TW, et al: Outpatient flexible fiberoptic sigmoidoscopy, diagnostic yield, and the value of glucagon. Br J Surg 68:463, 1981.
31. Record O, Bramble MG, Lishman AH, et al: Flexible sigmoidoscopy in outpatients with suspected colonic disease. Br Med J 283:1291, 1981.
32. Bohlman TW, Katon RM, Lipshutz GR, et al: Fiberoptic pansigmoidoscopy: An evaluation and comparison with rigid sigmoidoscopy. Gastroenterology 72:644, 1977.
33. Vallacott KD, Hardcastle JD: An evaluation of flexible fiberoptic sigmoidoscopy. Br Med J 283:1583, 1981.

Chapter 59

Thrombosed External Hemorrhoids

Jonathan M. Glauser

INTRODUCTION

The treatment of hemorrhoids has been of interest to surgeons since Babylonian times.[1] In 1869, Morgan initiated the modern era of hemorrhoid management when he described injection therapy.[2] Whereas recent literature discusses various techniques in the management of internal hemorrhoids, the treatment of thrombosed external hemorrhoids has not changed in recent years.

Hemorrhoids are varicosities of the venous plexus that lie in the wall of the anal canal (Fig. 59–1). The varicosities may be internal or external. *Internal hemorrhoids* lie above the pectinate line in the submucosal space of the upper anal canal and are covered with columnar epithelium. Internal hemorrhoids are usually asymptomatic, but the salient symptoms are bleeding or prolapse. Prolapse out of the rectum may occur during defecation, but when the hemorrhoids are large enough, they may prolapse with coughing or walking. Internal hemorrhoids commonly bleed. With hemorrhage, blood is bright red because of the presence of arterioles, capillaries, and arteriovenous fistulas in the area. Most of the bleeding is not from the hemorrhoid itself but from the traumatized mucous membrane that overlies it. Bleeding may occur during defecation or spontaneously; prolapsed hemorrhoids may produce a mucous discharge. The internal hemorrhoids may be painful when they become thrombosed or remain prolapsed. The treatment of internal hemorrhoids is not covered in this text.

External hemorrhoids may be pruritic or may be noticed by the patient when they become enlarged. When thrombosed, external hemorrhoids become more symptomatic. Thrombosed external hemorrhoids occur in all age groups and are quite common in young adults. A thrombosed external hemorrhoid appears as a purplish mass external to the pectinate line[3] and is usually easily visible when the patient spreads the buttocks (Fig. 59–2). Because it is covered by skin and not colonic mucosa, a thrombosed external hemorrhoid tends to be extremely painful, especially when direct pressure is applied. The bluish color of the contained clot can generally be appreciated through the tense, stretched skin.

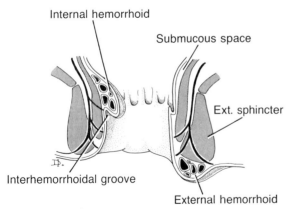

Figure 59–1. Anatomic location of internal and external hemorrhoids. (From Hill GJ II: Outpatient Surgery. 2nd ed. Philadelphia, WB Saunders Co, 1980. Reproduced by permission.)

Labels on figure: Internal hemorrhoid; Submucous space; Ext. sphincter; External hemorrhoid; Interhemorrhoidal groove

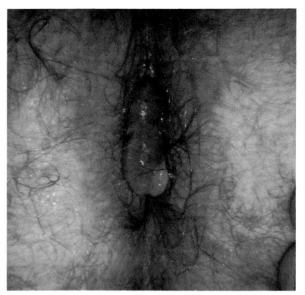

Figure 59–2. Large thrombosed external hemorrhoid.

The patient typically reports the sudden development of a painful lump at the anus, often relating its onset to an episode of constipation or straining at stool.[4] The pain is continuous but is aggravated by defecation and by sitting.[5] The pain and swelling may subside spontaneously, but frequently thrombosis requires surgery. An insignificant amount of bleeding may occur as a result of spontaneous rupture of the hematoma, but simple thrombosed external hemorrhoids do not usually bleed.

The term "thrombosed external hemorrhoid" implies clotted blood in the veins of the subcutaneous external hemorrhoidal plexus. What occurs more commonly is a rupture of one of the external veins during straining at defecation with escape of blood into the subcutaneous tissues, where it clots and forms a tense, painful swelling. This clinical condition is therefore more accurately referred to as anal hematoma[4, 6] or external anal thrombosis.[3]

In the early stages, the swelling is quite tender, but after a few days the tenderness tends to diminish markedly. After 1 week the swelling may be painless.[4] As the process subsides without specific treatment, the overlying skin becomes wrinkled, leaving a residual skin tag when the mass diminishes in size. Spontaneous resolution over the course of weeks generally occurs, with gradual subsiding of pain and swelling.

Spontaneous rupture of the hematoma occasionally occurs and may be followed by complete extrusion of the clot. More often, the clot is only partially extruded through the overlying skin and has to be expressed manually. A residual skin tag frequently remains following rupture. Loculations, tortuous small veins, or multiple hematomas may be present. They can occasionally appear as a conglomerate and cause swelling of most or all of the anal circumference.[4]

Almost immediate relief can be obtained by surgery if the thrombosis is confined to a well-defined mass or masses.[7] Treatment consists of evacuation of the clot under local anesthesia or of excision of the thrombosed segment of vein.

INDICATIONS AND CONTRAINDICATIONS

Although most thrombosed external hemorrhoids resolve spontaneously, many patients cannot tolerate the pain associated with an acute thrombosis, even when oral narcotic analgesia is available. *Incisional* or *excisional* therapy of the thrombosed hemorrhoids should be considered in situations in which the patient is in excruciating pain, although a patient with a small tolerable thrombosed external hemorrhoid or anal hematoma can often be managed satisfactorily with conservative therapy consisting of oral analgesics, sitz baths, and stool softeners.

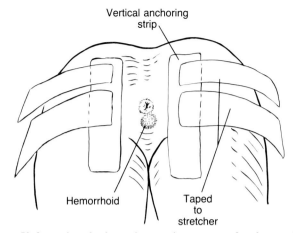

Figure 59–3. Taping the buttocks to gain exposure for the surgical excision of a thrombosed external hemorrhoid.

In healthy, cooperative patients surgical therapy for thrombosed external hemorrhoids is an emergency department or office procedure. Except for the transient pain associated with local anesthesia, the procedure is totally painless with a short and quite mild postoperative course. In the extremely anxious patient, preoperative sedation or analgesia with intravenous narcotics or benzodiazepines, or with both, can be helpful. The judicious use of these agents can markedly decrease the unpleasantness of the surgery.

PROCEDURE

The patient is placed prone on a stretcher, and the buttocks are taped open to expose the anus (Fig. 59–3). Tape adherence is enhanced by the application of benzoin

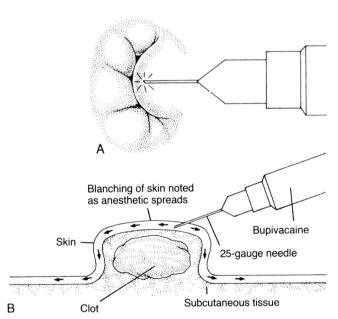

Figure 59–4. Adequate anesthesia often can be obtained by a single injection of long-acting bupivacaine. A, A 25-gauge needle is inserted in the middle of the swollen hemorrhoid, just below the skin surface. B, With the injection, the anesthetic spreads over the surface of the dome and into the surrounding tissue. A field block (Fig. 59–5) about the hemorrhoid can also be used.

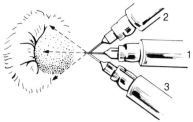

Figure 59–5. The subcutaneous injection of a long-acting local anesthetic using a field block will provide complete anesthesia during clot removal. During tissue infiltration, this technique may be more painful than the method shown in Figure 59–4.

to each buttock followed by a longitudinal anchoring layer of tape. Strips of cloth adhesive tape are subsequently run from the anchoring strips laterally to the sides of the stretcher. A scalpel and a standard suture tray or incision and drainage tray provide sufficient instruments.

Complete anesthesia is often obtained with the injection of only a few milliliters of a local anesthetic. A long-acting preparation such as bupivacaine (Marcaine or Sensorcaine) should be used to produce anesthesia for 4 to 6 hours. A 25-gauge needle is inserted in the middle of the swollen hemorrhoid, just under the skin surface but not into the hemorrhoid itself. This allows the anesthetic to spread over the dome of the hemorrhoid and into the surrounding skin. Blanching should be obvious if the correct tissue plane has been entered (Fig. 59–4A and B). The injection is the only painful part of the procedure. Because the hemorrhoid is covered with skin and not mucosa, topical anesthetics have little ability to decrease the pain from the initial injection. With deep inflammation and tenderness, a field block about the hemorrhoid may be needed (Fig. 59–5).

When anesthesia is achieved, the skin is elevated with forceps, with tension away from the anal orifice. An elliptic incision is made around the clot and is directed radially (Fig. 59–6).[7] The incision can be made either with scissors or with a number 15 scalpel blade. The flap of skin is then picked up and excised to expose the underlying clot or the thrombosed vein. The obvious clots are usually easily removed with forceps or digital pressure (Fig. 59–7A and B). An assistant then spreads the incision, using forceps to expose the base of the hemorrhoid to allow other small clots to be removed with a hemostat (Fig. 59–8). At all times, the incision should not extend under the cutaneous layer; this is a simple unroofing procedure. An alternative to the

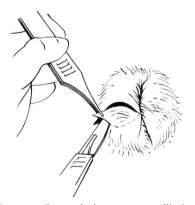

Figure 59–6. An unroofing technique uses an elliptic or triangular incision that removes a piece of the overlying skin. A simple linear incision should not be used.

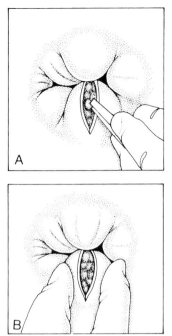

Figure 59–7. Blood clots are removed with forceps *(A)* or expressed with the fingers *(B)*.

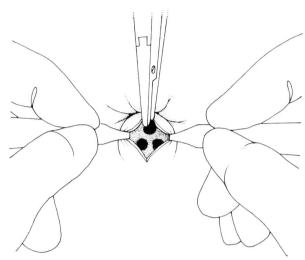

Figure 59–8. After the initial clot is removed, an assistant spreads the incision to expose the base of the hemorrhoid to allow other smaller clots to be removed individually with forceps or with a small hemostat.

elliptical incision is to remove a *triangular* piece of overlying skin. Bleeding is usually minor, and sutures are not required. A small piece of surgical foam (such as Gelfoam) can be placed directly in the wound, and the area is covered with a vaginal pad or sterile gauze. The foam promotes hemostasis; the elliptic or triangular incision reduces pain by eliminating increased tissue pressure during hemostasis. The postoperative dressing need not be elaborate. Folded gauze pads placed in the buttocks with the sides of the buttocks taped together usually suffices.

Small stab-like incisions and squeezing the hemorrhoid to remove the clot through a small opening are to be avoided. It has been claimed that the stablike incision causes a higher incidence of infection than does an unroofing procedure because the skin edges fall together.[7]

When marked edema is present, conservative treatment with hot, moist dressings or sitz baths is preferred until the inflammation has subsided, at which time a definitive procedure, such as wide excision of the hemorrhoidal mass, can be performed. Wide excision is not an emergency department procedure.[7]

POSTOPERATIVE CARE

Postoperative care includes bed rest for a few hours to minimize bleeding. Warm sitz baths[8, 9] at frequent intervals—at least four times a day for 30 minutes during the first 2 days may be initiated as soon as the anesthetic wears off. A dry cotton vaginal pad or rolled gauze dressing may be placed over the anal region for a few days.[4] Bleeding seldom persists for more than a few hours, and many patients do not require a dressing after the first sitz bath. A small amount of spotting for a few days is normal.

The buttocks can be taped together over the vaginal pad or gauze dressing for 6 to 12 hours to apply pressure to the incision site. Pain is usually only mild and is delayed until the patient is home if bupivacaine is used, but the patient should be given adequate oral analgesia, usually

narcotics. Hemorrhoid cream or benzocaine ointment may also be used postoperatively. A stool softener can be prescribed for 3 to 4 days to avoid the constipation associated with narcotic analgesic agents, but it is generally unnecessary in most cases. Diarrhea is to be avoided. Straining at stool can prolong bleeding in the postoperative period. Patients are instructed to avoid prolonged walking or sitting for a few days. Following a bowel movement, the patient is instructed to wash the anal area with soap and water in the shower and to avoid toilet paper for a few days. Antibiotics are not indicated in the absence of an obvious infection following the procedure.

Measures that have been proposed to prevent chronic straining at stool and possible further hemorrhoidal problems generally include the use of stool softeners[8] and a high-residue diet,[5, 9] but these are of questionable value in preventing recurrence.

COMPLICATIONS

Complications of thrombosed external hemorrhoids are rare, although if the clot remains exposed, or even if it is completely evacuated, infection may occur with resulting abscess or fistula formation.[4] Occasionally, a clot may reform in a few days, in which case it may be easily removed under direct vision at the first postoperative visit. Actual bacterial infection is rare. At least one postoperative check is required, preferably within 2 to 4 days. It is possible that the area may become thrombosed again at some future date, and the patient should be warned of possible recurrence. In general, however, the procedure is curative for hemorrhoids in the area in question.

REFERENCES

1. Jeffery PJ, Ritchie SM, Miller W, et al: The treatment of hemorrhoids by rubber band ligation at St. Mark's Hospital. Postgrad Med J 56:847, 1980.
2. Corman ML (ed): Classic articles in colonic and rectal surgery: John Morgan's varicose state and saphena veins, erectile tumour of the forehead,

external haemorrhoids treated successfully by the injection of tincture of persulphate of iron. Dis Colon Rectum 24:491, 1981.

3. Branch WT: Office Practice of Medicine. Philadelphia, WB Saunders Co, 1982, p 671.
4. Goligher JC, Duthie HL, Nixon HH, et al (eds): Surgery of the Anus, Rectum, and Colon. 4th ed. London, Balliere Tindall, 1980, pp 130–131.
5. Dworken HJ: Gastroenterology: Pathophysiology and Clinical Applications. Boston, Butterworth Publishers, 1982, pp 511–513.

6. Kaufman HD: Hemorrhoids. Gastrointest Dis 7:47, 1981.
7. Wolcott MW (ed): Ferguson's Surgery of the Ambulatory Patient. 5th ed. Philadelphia, JB Lippincott Co, 1974, pp 248–250.
8. Medical Letter 17:7, 1975.
9. Dandapat MC: Management of haemorrhoids. J Indian Med Assoc 74:234, 1980.

Chapter 60

Management of Rectal Foreign Bodies

Scott M. Davis

INTRODUCTION

Patients with rectal foreign bodies often seek initial medical care through the emergency department. It is, therefore, imperative that the emergency physician have a basic understanding of the evaluation, treatment, and disposition of these patients.

Reasons that patients with rectal foreign bodies present to an emergency facility include the 24-hour availability of medical care, the patient's perception that the emergency physician is able to treat a wide range of medical problems, and the patient's possible desire for anonymity. The emergency physician should understand that by presenting to a public facility, the patient has already subjected himself or herself to a great deal of embarrassment, and, therefore, the physician should maintain a sense of objectivity and professionalism. A nonjudgmental attitude enhances the physician-patient relationship and the probability of patient cooperation during any subsequent procedure.

Many rectal foreign bodies may be removed successfully in the emergency department. By following appropriate guidelines, treatment in the emergency department can be cost-effective and practical. This chapter details indications for foreign body removal in the emergency department, procedural techniques, potential complications of outpatient management, and indications for inpatient management.

BACKGROUND

Until recently, rectal foreign bodies have been primarily a medical curiosity that warranted only an occasional case report.[1] However, in the last 10 to 15 years, several large series of patients have been reported. Most authorities agree that although rectal foreign bodies were underreported in past years, the recent increase in cases reported likely represents both an increase in reporting and, more important, a true increase in incidence.[1–9] The reasons for this are not certain, but the increase may be associated with relaxed sexual mores of society, leading to an increasing incidence and acceptance of anal autoeroticism.

The etiology of rectal foreign bodies includes (1) autoeroticism (most common), (2) iatrogenic (e.g., thermometer, rectal tube), (3) sexual or criminal assault, (4) self-administered treatment (e.g., enema), (5) accidental ingestion, and (6) concealment (e.g., body packing to conceal cocaine).[10, 11, 12]

The types of foreign bodies seem limited only by the anatomic size of the rectum and the limits of human imagination. Just a few of the foreign bodies described include a vibrator, phallus, spray can, hair pin, pencil, toothpick, chicken bone, corn cob, glass jar, broomstick, candle, flashlight, baseball, cucumber, and an electric lightbulb. Most objects are cylindrical. The largest documented object was a stone that measured 25 cm in diameter. Colorectal foreign bodies constituted 13.3 per cent of all gastrointestinal foreign bodies in one series.[13] Rectal thermometers are the most common object in the pediatric population. Males predominate in most series as much as 28:1.[14]

Older literature on this subject stressed inpatient treatment, and reports were skewed toward complicated cases and resultant complications. Most recent series show that there is a high success rate for the outpatient management of rectal foreign bodies if proper guidelines for evaluation and treatment are followed.[2, 4]

INDICATIONS

Diagnosis of a rectal foreign body can usually be made easily from the history. In unclear cases, digital examination, plain radiographs, or radiography using contrast media may help establish the presence of a foreign body.[1] Once the diagnosis is made, general principles of management include foreign body identification, foreign body removal, and assessment for associated intraperitoneal and extraperitoneal injuries.

All rectal foreign bodies should be removed once they are diagnosed. Although some objects may pass spontaneously, it is safest to assume that extraction is necessary. Delayed removal may lead to obstipation, pain, and infection, with or without rectal perforation. The majority of rectal foreign bodies can be removed successfully and safely in the emergency department.[2, 6, 14, 15] A rational approach in the emergency facility is outlined in Figure 60–1.

If a patient has no signs of perforation and the object is palpable on digital examination, the majority can be removed uneventfully in the emergency department. Radiographs may occasionally be needed to identify the location and type of foreign body or to rule out perforation.[1] The specific technique for removal depends on the size, location, orientation, and composition of a particular foreign body. These techniques are described in the subsequent section.

After removal, sigmoidoscopy or anoscopy to assess mucosal integrity and evaluate for possible perforation is recommended.[1, 6] Patients with normal postextraction examinations without clinical evidence of perforation may be safely discharged home with precautionary instructions.

Indications for hospital admission or outpatient surgery with general anesthesia in certain circumstances include (1) the diagnosis or suspicion of perforation; (2) the presence of a rectal laceration beyond the superficial mucosa, significant bleeding, a nonpalpable foreign body, or broken glass or other extremely fragile foreign material; (3) the need for any procedure that would cause undue patient discomfort; or (4) the failure of emergency department extraction after a reasonable period of time.[1, 2]

Observation in the emergency department for small nonpalpable foreign bodies (above the rectosigmoid junction) to pass into the lower rectum has occasionally been successful.[2] Enemas or cathartics should not be used because

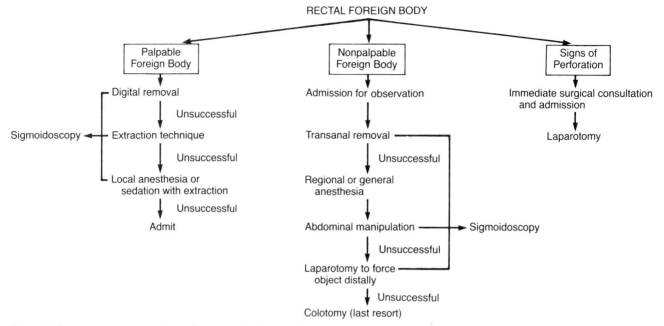

Figure 60–1. Emergency approach to the removal of rectal foreign bodies. Foreign bodies that are fragile or are associated with rectal spasm are generally managed with regional or general anesthesia. The use of supplemental analgesic, anxiolytic, and local anesthetic medications is highly recomended.

they may increase the impaction of a foreign body or may cause it to move higher into the colon.[2, 15]

CONTRAINDICATIONS

As noted previously, admission to the hospital or out-patient surgical unit for removal under general anesthesia or for postremoval care may be recognized before or after attempts at foreign body removal in the emergency department. In general, any attempt at rectal foreign body removal in the emergency department is contraindicated in the following situations: (1) any patient with severe abdominal pain or signs of perforation on presentation, (2) any non-palpable (high-lying) foreign body, or (3) any foreign body that is unusually difficult to remove, in which routine removal could result in perforation or other significant morbidity.

EQUIPMENT

As in any procedure, a private, well-lit room with a comfortable examining table is needed. Equipment that should be available for most extractions includes lubricant, rubber gloves, examining light, anoscope, proctosigmoidoscope, local anesthetic with appropriate syringes and needles, and suitable parenteral narcotics and sedatives.

Other equipment that may be used depends entirely on the specific technique chosen for foreign body removal. Most techniques use some type of speculum to aid in visualization and then some form of clamp or snare to grasp the object. Some of the more common methods of foreign body removal are detailed later and are shown in Table 60–1.

PROCEDURE AND TECHNIQUES

The general principles of management of rectal foreign bodies include proper diagnosis, subsequent removal, as-

sessment for rectal or colonic injury, and recognition and treatment of associated injuries. The indications for radiographs before the extraction procedure are controversial. Some authorities advocate routine radiographs for all patients with rectal foreign bodies. Recent reports that show the safety of outpatient management of uncomplicated foreign bodies suggest that such films only increase the expense and add nothing to patient management. The decision to order films rests on clinical judgment but is clearly indicated when the patient has abdominal pain, peritoneal signs, suspected perforation, or fever or when the patient's clinical history is unclear or unreliable. Once the foreign body is found to be palpable (low-lying) attempts at extraction may be instituted.

The patient may be placed prone or in the Sims position (lying on the side), depending on patient comfort. The knee-chest position can be used but is difficult for the patient to maintain without a proctosigmoidoscopy table with knee support. Specific guidelines for positioning can be found in Chapter 58 on anoscopy and sigmoidoscopy.

If patient discomfort occurs during the procedure, sedation with benzodiazepines or narcotics should be instituted. Analgesia and muscle relaxation are often the key to a successful procedure. A combination of fentanyl and midazolam, as outlined in Chapter 41, is a useful approach when analgesia or muscle relaxation is required. Even with parenteral drugs, supplemental local anesthesia using a field

Table 60–1. Equipment Useful for Rectal Foreign Body Removal

Speculum	Grasping Tool	Example
Operative anoscope	Tenaculum forceps	Cucumber
Operative proctoscope	Ring forceps	Banana
Parks retractor	Tonsil snare	Pencil
Deaver retractor	Obstetric forceps	Apple
Vaginal speculum	Spoons	Vibrator
	Foley catheter	Small ball
	Endotracheal tube	Glass jar
	Suction dart	Light bulb

against the sacrum posteriorly and requires gentle redirection.

If one is unsuccessful at digital extraction, then another technique must be chosen. The specific technique used depends on several factors, including the nature, size, shape, orientation, and composition of the foreign body; the availability of equipment; and the experience and ingenuity of the physician. Numerous techniques have been discussed in the literature. The more commonly accepted techniques are described here. In general, most techniques require adequate visualization, as with a speculum, and the use of a grasping tool.[2]

An operative anoscope, proctoscope, or vaginal speculum may be inserted to allow adequate visualization.[1, 9] The object may then be grasped by a forceps or tenaculum and gentle traction applied to remove both the speculum and grasping clamp simultaneously, because the object often has a greater diameter than the speculum. A Parks retractor has been used successfully to aid in foreign body removal in one series of 100 patients[16] (Figs. 60–2 and 60–3).

A flexible sigmoidoscope with a polypectomy snare has been used for successful foreign body removal.[17] After the tube is inserted, air is gently insufflated to distend the rectum. The object is then grasped with a polypectomy snare. Advantages of this technique include (1) the ability to distend the bowel around the object, (2) the avoidance of sedation, (3) the convenience of outpatient management, and (4) the reported ability of this technique to retrieve high-lying objects.

Other grasping objects that have been used successfully include a suction dart for a glass foreign body,[18] a de Pezzer catheter attached to wall suction to produce a negative-pressure traction,[19] cyanoacrylate (Super-Glue), tonsil snares, surgical instruments such as obstetric forceps, and even spoons (Fig. 60–4). A Sengstaken-Blakemore tube has been inserted into a hollow glass foreign body, inflated, and traction applied, allowing for successful removal.[8]

Glass foreign bodies deserve special mention. Glass may be quite difficult to grasp and, if fragile, may break during attempts at removal. In addition, glass often creates a vacuum effect in the distal colon when traction is applied, making routine removal virtually impossible. To overcome

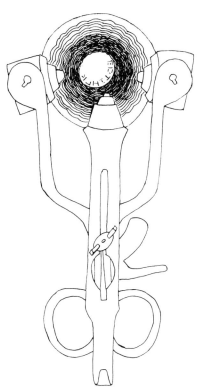

Figure 60–2. A Parks retractor is inserted into the anal canal to visualize the foreign body. (From Sohn N, Weinstein M: Office removal of foreign bodies in the rectum. Surg Gynecol Obstet 146:209, 1978. By permission of Surgery, Gynecology, and Obstetrics.)

block technique may be necessary to achieve optimal dilation of the anal sphincter.[2] After providone-iodine preparation, the perianal tissue can be anesthetized in a radial fashion around the anal sphincter, using 0.5 per cent bupivacaine or 1.0 per cent lidocaine with epinephrine 1:200,000 (unless contraindicated). One then extends the anesthetic submucosally, anteriorly and posteriorly.[16]

Gentle abdominal (suprapubic) pressure often helps deliver the foreign body into the distal rectum, where the examining finger helps the distal end of the foreign body navigate to the anus. Quite often the foreign body lodges

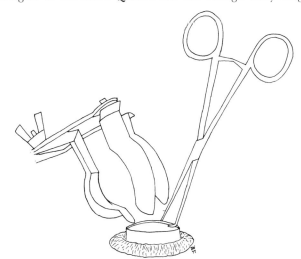

Figure 60–3. The foreign body is grasped with a tenaculum. The foreign body is removed *along with* the Parks retractor. (From Sohn N, Weinstein M: Office removal of foreign bodies in the rectum. Surg Gynecol Obstet 146:209, 1978. By permission of Surgery, Gynecology, and Obstetrics.)

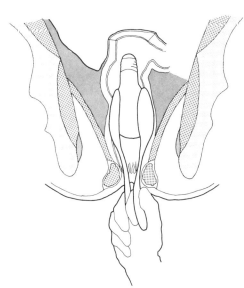

Figure 60–4. Large spoons grasping a fragile foreign body in the rectum. (From Rosen P, Baker FJ, Barkin RM, et al (eds): Emergency Medicine: Concepts and Clinical Practice. St. Louis, CV Mosby Co, 1988. Reproduced by permission.)

this effect, Foley catheters or endotracheal tubes can be inserted past the foreign body to insufflate air and release any suction forces. When the balloons are inflated, traction may be used to allow the foreign body to be removed[1, 18, 20] (Figs. 60–5 and 60–6).

Difficult-to-grasp glass objects have been removed successfully with clamps covered with rubber.[21] Plaster of Paris has been used to fill a hollow object; the plaster is allowed to harden with a handle such as a wooden tongue blade, and then it is removed with traction. Some clinicians frown on using this technique especially with glass objects because, as the plaster hardens, the heat released could cause the glass to break or produce mucosal injury.

The great majority of objects can be removed safely transanally in the emergency department.[1, 2, 6] After removal, proctosigmoidoscopy to evaluate for perforation, bleeding, and mucosal trauma is recommended. Patients with signs of perforation, unstable vital signs, abdominal pain, deep mucosal lacerations, significant bleeding, or suspicion of perforation should be admitted. Perforation commonly occurs at the initial point of rectosigmoid angulation approximately 15 cm from the anal verge. Perforation may occur prior to

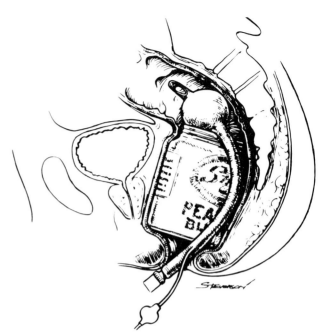

Figure 60–6. Use of an endotracheal tube to remove a foreign body made of glass. (From Garber H, Rubin R, Eisenstat T: Removal of a glass foreign body from the rectum. Dis Colon Rectum 24:323, 1981.)

medical evaluation; thus even atraumatic foreign body removals can be problematic.

The emergency physician should set a realistic time limit, such as 30 minutes, at which time referral to a consultant for treatment or admission to the hospital becomes appropriate if extraction of the foreign body has been unsuccessful.

Once the patient is admitted, a high-lying foreign body may advance over 8 to 12 hours of observation to become a low-lying foreign body that can be removed transanally. If this is unsuccessful, then regional or general anesthesia is used along with abdominal and rectal palpation to maneuver the foreign body.[1] If these attempts fail, then laparotomy should be performed, in which the surgeon "milks" the object in the colon distally. Colotomy is only rarely necessary and is done as a last resort.

Body Packing

With the increase in drug trafficking, the subject of "body packing" should be addressed. Smuggling of illegal drugs by ingestion, especially cocaine and heroin, has become increasingly popular.[22] Objects have been wrapped in various materials such as condoms, plastic wrap, or cellophane. Many times packets are palpated by a digital rectal examination. Some, but not all, ingested packets may be radiopaque, depending on the specific packaging material and whether the packets are surrounded by air. Amazingly, individuals may swallow more than 100 individual packets of illegal drugs. There were initial reports of fragile packets spontaneously rupturing and leading to systemic absorption, acute drug toxicity, and sudden death. Complications of body packing essentially involve bowel obstruction or packet rupture with drug absorption.

Drug smugglers have become more sophisticated in the use of packaging and, therefore, packet rupture is much less common. Early case reports recommended surgical removal of all potentially toxic substances, but currently

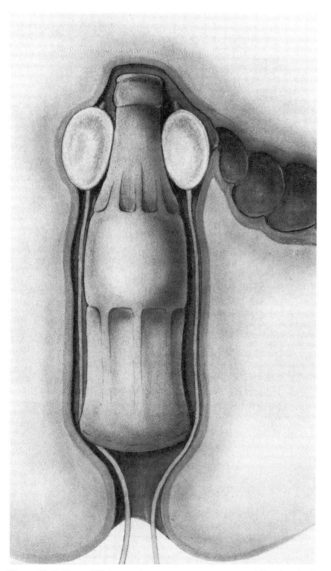

Figure 60–5. Use of Foley catheters to remove a rectal foreign body made of glass. (From Eftaiha M, Hambrick E, Abcarian H: Principles of management of colorectal foreign bodies. Arch Surg 112:693, 1977. Copyright 1977, American Medical Association.)

surgery is rarely performed. Packaging materials have improved, and in a study of 50 patients who had swallowed packets of drugs, Cameron and colleagues were successful in treating 41 of the 50 conservatively with a clear liquid diet and mild laxatives; spontaneous passage of the drug packets occurred in a mean time of 27.7 hours.[23] Six of the 50 patients chose elective surgery, and there were three complications with resultant bowel obstruction that required additional surgery. The patients treated conservatively showed no signs of cocaine toxicity, and there were no deaths. Nonetheless, admission and close clinical monitoring is recommended when treating this special case of colorectal foreign body.

A few additional caveats concerning the approach to ingested packets of drugs should be mentioned. Each package may contain a lethal amount of drug, and if it bursts, serious clinical consequences are possible. In the case of cocaine, death may occur despite aggressive therapy. Because individuals facing imprisonment may be reluctant to be fully truthful with the physician, body packers should be admitted to the hospital for close monitoring.

Most researchers agree that surgery or endoscopy should be avoided in the asymptomatic body packer. Recommendations concerning catharsis are vague and not well studied, but hastening the process of gastrointestinal transport is usually advocated. Recently an approach that uses catharsis with a nonabsorbable polyethylene glycol solution (GoLytely or Colyte) has gained some popularity through anecdotal accounts. With this technique, 2 to 3 liters per hour of solution are instilled in the stomach via a nasogastric tube. This produces a brisk catharsis, the end point of which depends on the specific clinical scenario. It makes sense to add activated charcoal to this regimen to adsorb any free drug, but the effectiveness of this nonspecific antidote in the face of a massive overdose is unknown. Likewise, a contrast material, such as meglumine diatrizoate (Gastrografin), may be added to the electrolyte solution to outline the bowel and identify the number of packets ingested. Mineral oil has also been a suggested cathartic but it may dissolve some forms of rubber and hasten drug release.

COMPLICATIONS

The most feared complication of rectal foreign bodies is bowel perforation. The risk of perforation is related to the force of object introduction and the sharpness of the object. The duration of foreign body impaction may also be a factor for large objects. Perforation may occur during insertion or removal of the object.[2]

Perforation above the peritoneal reflection leads to free air below the diaphragm with signs of an acute abdomen. In suspicious cases, water-soluble contrast material may be used to clarify the diagnosis.[1] If perforation is below the peritoneal reflection, symptoms may be insidious, and patients may present with signs of pelvic abcess or sepsis days after the injury. It is, therefore, recommended that patients treated for foreign body removal undergo proctosigmoidoscopy to rule out associated complications.

Other complications that occur include bleeding, mucosal laceration, torn anal sphincter, or object fragmentation with retention of the foreign body.

When intraperitoneal or retroperitoneal perforation is diagnosed or suspected, the emergency physician should institute appropriate antibiotic coverage. Bowel anaerobes are the primary contaminant; therefore, the choice of antibiotic should reflect an appropriate broad spectrum drug. Currently accepted antibiotic regimens include clindamycin or metronidazole together with an aminoglycoside or, alternatively, ticarcillin-clavulanic acid, imipenem, or cefoxitin.[24]

CONCLUSIONS

The majority of rectal foreign bodies can be removed safely in the emergency department. The emergency physician must be knowledgeable in the evaluation of patients with rectal foreign bodies, the techniques for removal, and the potential for complications. The physician must also be able to determine which patients may be treated safely as outpatients and which patients require admission, referral, or both.

REFERENCES

1. Kingsley A, Abcarian H: Colorectal foreign bodies: Management update. Dis Colon Rectum 28:941, 1985.
2. Wigle R: Emergency department management of retained rectal foreign bodies. Am J Emerg Med 6:385, 1988.
3. Eftaiha M, Hambrick E, Abcarian H: Principles of management of colorectal foreign bodies. Arch Surg 112:691, 1977.
4. Crass RA, Tranbaugh RF, Kudsk KA, et al: Colorectal foreign bodies and perforation. Am J Surg 142:85, 1981.
5. Barone J, Sohn N, Nealon T: Perforations and foreign bodies of the rectum. Ann Surg 184:601, 1976.
6. Barone J, Yee J, Nealon T: Management of foreign bodies and trauma of the rectum. Surg Gynecol Obstet 156:453, 1983.
7. French G, Sherlock D, Holl-Allen R: Problems with rectal foreign bodies. Br J Surg 72:243, 1985.
8. Hughs J, Marice H, Gathwright J: Method of removing a hollow object from the rectum. Dis Colon Rectum 19:44, 1976.
9. Berci G, Morgenstern L: An operative proctoscope for foreign body extraction. Dis Colon Rectum 26:193, 1983.
10. Foreign bodies of the rectum. Br Med J 2:656, 1977.
11. Graves RW, Allison EJ Jr, Bass RR, et al: Anal eroticism: Two unusual rectal foreign bodies and their removal. South Med J 76:677, 1983.
12. Witz M, Shpitz B, Zager M, et al: Anal erotic instrumentation. Dis Colon Rectum 27:331, 1984.
13. Bloom RR, Nakano PH, Gray SW, et al: Foreign bodies of the gastrointestinal tract. Am Surg 52:618, 1986.
14. Busch D, Starling J: Rectal foreign bodies: Case reports and a comprehensive review of the world's literature. Surgery 100:512, 1986.
15. Abcarian H, Lowe R: Colon and rectal trauma. Surg Clin North Am 58:519, 1978.
16. Sohn N, Weinstein M: Office removal of foreign bodies in the rectum. Surg Gynecol Obstet 146:209, 1978.
17. Kantarian JC, Riether RD, Sheets JA, et al: Endoscopic retrieval of foreign bodies from the rectum. Dis Colon Rectum 30:902, 1987.
18. Diwan V: Removal of 100 watt electric bulb from rectum (letter). Ann Emerg Med 11:643, 1982.
19. Steven K, Lykke J, Hansen T: A simple suction device for removing foreign bodies in the rectum. Br J Surg 66:418, 1979.
20. Garber H, Rubin R, Eisenstat T: Removal of a glass foreign body from the rectum. Dis Colon Rectum 24:323, 1981.
21. Siroospour D, Dragstedt L: A large foreign body removed intact through the anus: Report of a case. Dis Colon Rectum 18:616, 1975.
22. Jonsson J, O'Meara M, Young JB: Acute cocaine poisoning: Importance of treating seizures and acidosis. Am J Med 75:1061, 1983.
23. Carvana D, Weinbach B, Goerg D, Gardner L: Cocaine packet ingestion: Diagnosis, management, and natural history. Ann Intern Med 100:73, 1984.
24. Abramowicz M, Rizack MA, Hirsch J, et al (eds): The choice of antimicrobial drugs. Med Lett Drugs Ther 30:35, 1988.

Chapter 61

Rectal Prolapse

Jonathan M. Glauser

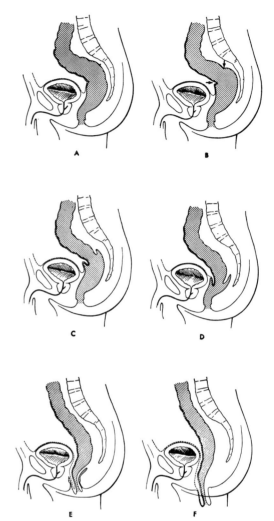

Figure 61–1. *A,* Normal relationship of the rectum to the pelvic structures. *B,* Earliest stage of intussusception (prolapse) just proximal to the uppermost normal fixed point of the rectum. *C,* Fixed point lowers. The upper rectum is separated from the sacrum. Intussusception commencement assumes a lower position. The sigmoid mesentery elongates. A pseudomesorectum may develop. The rectosigmoid begins to straighten. *D,* Further lowering of the fixed point. Previous changes become exaggerated. *E,* The cul-de-sac deepens. The rectum may or may not protrude. *F,* Final stage of intussusception. Commencement occurs at the mucocutaneous border. Deep cul-de-sac (may contain the small bowel). Elongated sigmoid mesentery. Straight rectosigmoid. The rectum and sacrum are separated. The rectum is protruded completely. (From Theuerkauf FJ, Beahrs OH, Hill JR: Rectal prolapse: Causation and surgical treatment. Ann Surg 171:819, 1970. Reproduced by permission.)

INTRODUCTION

Rectal prolapse is a rare condition in which some or all of the layers of the rectum protrude through the external anal sphincter. The definitive treatment of complete prolapse is usually surgical, but the acute prolapse may be reduced in the emergency department. The condition, although not usually serious, is very distressing to the patient or parent and occasionally is painful. Failure to reduce a prolapse may result in eventual gangrene of the bowel. Rectal prolapse may be partial or complete (procidentia).

DIAGNOSIS

The condition is divided into three different types of prolapse. False procidentia, or type 1 prolapse, involves protrusion of redundant colonic mucosa only. The mucosa is seen extruding in radial folds.[1] Generally, this false prolapse is associated with hemorrhoids, and protrusion is only 1 to 3 cm.

Type 2 procidentia is a true intussusception of all layers of the rectum through the anal canal without an associated cul-de-sac sliding hernia (Fig. 61–1). There is no protrusion through the anal orifice. Type 3 prolapse is basically a sliding hernia of the cul-de-sac. The pouch of Douglas is viewed as the hernial sac, which presses on the anterior wall of the rectum and forces the anterior wall into the rectal lumen to produce an intussusception within the rectum and the anal canal with protrusion through the anus (Fig. 61–2).[2] Although there is disagreement among authorities concerning whether procidentia is a sliding hernia or an intussusception, the condition gives the appearance that the rectum has been turned inside out, as is seen when one removes a surgical glove (Fig. 61–3).

In complete or true prolapse, the bowel lumen lies posteriorly because of the greater thickness of the anterior part of the prolapse from the pouch of Douglas. The protrusion is seldom more than 10 cm even in its fully developed form.[3]

The diagnosis of partial (mucosal) prolapse generally can be made by digital examination. A finger is inserted into the lumen of the bowel, and palpation of the prolapse between the examiner's finger and thumb reveals that there is no muscular wall within it.[4, 5] In addition, the presence of prolapse restricted to the left lateral, right anterior, and right posterior positions combined with normal anal sphincter tone is highly suggestive of hemorrhoidal, and not true rectal, prolapse.[6]

Conditions that must be differentiated from true rectal prolapse include a mass of hemorrhoidal tissue, a large rectal or sigmoidal polypoid lesion prolapsing through the anus, and, possibly, a higher intussusception coming through the normally positioned anus. These are each discussed briefly.

Prolapsed hemorrhoidal tissue tends to be lobular, with a definite sulcus between the masses of tissue down to the level of the anal skin. A false impression that the entire rectal wall is protruding may be obtained if such hemorrhoids become thrombosed and the tissue becomes bluish, firm, and edematous. True rectal prolapse occurs with concentric radial folds; a deep sulcus between each tissue mass definitely establishes the diagnosis of hemorrhoids.[7] Polypoid lesions protruding through the anus generally can be diagnosed by digital examination and proctoscopic visualization after replacement of the mass. The mobile mass is felt separately from the lower rectum and the anal canal, which are felt to be in their normal positions. In addition, polypoid tissue appears grossly granular and quite different from rectal mucosa. Finally, the pedicle itself can be visualized endoscopically to confirm the diagnosis.

An intussusception coming through the anus is sug-

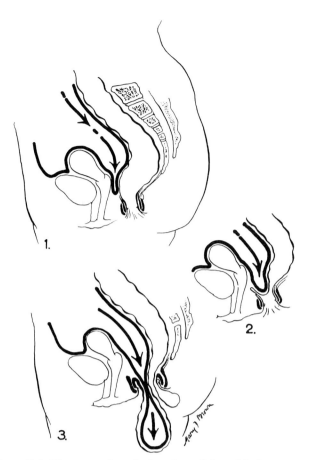

Figure 61–2. Diagrammatic sagittal sections of the pelvis demonstrate the anatomy of complete rectal prolapse conceived as a sliding hernia of the pouch of Douglas. (From Goligher JC: The treatment of complete prolapse of the rectum by the Roscoe Graham operation. Br J Surg 45:323, 1958. Reproduced by permission.)

gested when there is a sulcus around the entire protruding mass. In this case, a finger can be inserted into the anal canal between the wall of the canal and the projecting mucosa-covered swelling, whereas in rectal prolapse no such crevice exists.[3]

In addition to the presence of a protruding mass, the patient with rectal prolapse may present with other complaints. These include a bloody or mucous discharge from the rectum, diarrhea, constipation, fecal incontinence with a patulous anus, or vague perineal pain with a constant urge to defecate.[5, 8]

ETIOLOGY AND EPIDEMIOLOGY

The epidemiology and etiology of rectal prolapse vary with the population studied but deserve some discussion because of related diseases that should be searched for and treated. In Western society the condition is most prevalent in debilitated elderly patients and in young children.[2, 9] Elderly women are affected more than elderly men.[4, 8, 10, 11, 12] In countries with poor sanitation, young men are most frequently afflicted, with amebiases, schistosomiasis, and *Ascaris* infestation noted as inciting factors.[13, 14]

Idiopathic rectal prolapse in developed nations is most common in children aged 1 to 3 years, and it coincides with toilet training. There may be a history of constipation or of prolonged stays on the potty. Occasionally, a child with cystic fibrosis presents with frequent or persistent rectal prolapse. A measurement of sweat chloride confirms the underlying

diagnosis.[15] Prolapse resulting from a severe bout of pertussis generally resolves with conservative treatment.

Children with myelomeningocele or other causes of paraplegia may have rectal prolapse.[14] Various lesions of the cauda equina have been mentioned as causing rectal prolapse as well.[3, 7] Affected patients generally require surgical correction of the problem, unlike most children who have no obvious underlying neurologic cause of rectal procidentia.

Many possible causes and associated factors have been listed for rectal prolapse in adults. The condition has been associated with mental retardation, organic brain syndrome, poliomyelitis, cerebral thrombosis, and tabes dorsalis, among other psychiatric and neurologic conditions.[2, 15] The rate of procidentia is higher among institutionalized patients.[1] Some authorities have postulated other factors predisposing to rectal prolapse, including pregnancy, hemorrhoidal disease, poor bowel habits, diarrhea, and wasting disease in general.[1, 2] Multiparity has been listed as a factor, although rectal prolapse occurs in nulliparous women as well.[6, 17]

Anatomically, it is widely held that intussusception of the rectosigmoid is the true underlying pathologic condition.[6, 10, 18, 19] The intussusception pulls the rectosigmoid from its attachments, and with repeated straining, the rectum pulls away distally. The starting point of the intussusception has been reported from 6 to 8 cm above the anal verge[6] to the rectosigmoid junction.[19] Eventually, the bowel protrudes from the anus, producing stretching and paralysis of the external sphincter.[2, 19]

The concept that rectal prolapse is a sliding hernia was advanced as early as 1912.[7] By this theory, the pouch of Douglas slides through a defect in the pelvic diaphragm, invaginating the anterior wall of the rectum.[1] Today, many doubt that rectal prolapse is a sliding hernia.[11, 20]

INDICATIONS

Cases of rectal prolapse should be referred for surgical evaluation, but the acute prolapse should be reduced in the emergency department. Management of rectal prolapse in children and in adults with type 1 (false) procidentia is generally nonsurgical. Reduction of the acute type 1 prolapse is usually quite easy; the bowel slips back as one starts to examine it,[3] or it may be easily replaced with gentle pressure on the mass.

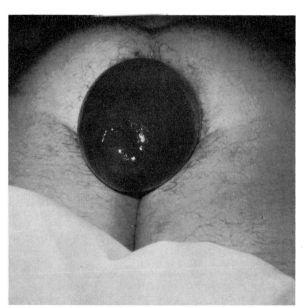

Figure 61–3. Complete rectal prolapse.

PROCEDURE

In children with a prolapse that is difficult to reduce, sedation with chloral hydrate or phenobarbital may be required. Then, with the child prone on the mother's lap, gentle but firm compression is applied to the prolapsed part for 5 to 15 minutes. A gloved finger wrapped in gauze may be placed into the rectal lumen, and gentle force is applied to reverse the direction of the prolapse. Following reduction, a pressure dressing is applied and worn between bowel movements for a day. The child can be sent home with a stool softener prescribed.[9] The condition in children is self-limited as a rule. Increased bulk in the diet may help to prevent constant straining at stool.[4]

There are other adjunctive modes of treatment in children. Defecating in the lateral recumbent position may reduce straining in adults; toilet training may have to be abandoned for several months in children. The parents should be taught to reduce any subsequent prolapse promptly to prevent it from becoming so edematous that replacement is difficult.

For the outpatient management of recurrent prolapse, taping may be useful. First, one should place wide, vertical strips of adhesive tape on both buttocks. A wad of Vaseline-saturated gauze is placed over the anus, and a bulky, dry dressing is placed between the buttocks. The gauze and dressing are then taped securely in place with transverse strips to prevent recurrent rectal prolapse.[15] After each bowel movement, the dressing must be replaced, with the vertical strips of tape left in place on the buttocks. In this way, excoriations from frequent dressing changes are avoided. Later, if necessary, the child can be treated with 5 per cent phenol injected locally as a sclerosant.[7]

Reduction of a complete prolapse in an adult may be more difficult. The patient is placed in bed in a prone position, and moist compresses are applied. Steady, gentle compression to the area is begun, starting at the least prolapsed part.[9] The bowel wall may be slippery and difficult to grasp. It is helpful to place two gauze pads on the prolapsed part at the 3 o'clock and the 9 o'clock positions. The thumbs are placed near the bowel lumen, and the fingers grasp the exterior wall. Then, with pressure placed on the thumbs into the lumen, the sides are gently rolled inward to force the prolapse back through the anus (Fig. 61–4). It may be necessary to sedate the patient for this procedure, because straining hinders reduction. Reduction is best accomplished with a slow and gentle (yet deliberate) approach. Definitive repair may be accomplished at a later date.

Reducible protrusions of less than 3 to 4 cm can be managed on an outpatient basis. For incomplete or mucosal prolapse, treatment can be accomplished either by rubber band ligation or by injection of sclerosing agents, as for internal hemorrhoids.[7, 23]

OPERATIVE MANAGEMENT

Definitive treatment of rectal prolapse in adults is surgical and is not performed as an emergency procedure. Many more than 50 different surgical procedures to cure rectal prolapse have been described since the report of Moschocowitz in 1912.[2, 10, 20] These operations are based on one or more of the following six general principles.[2, 3, 8, 21–25]

1. Resection of the prolapsed and redundant bowel.
2. Reduction of the size of the anus.
3. Plastic reconstruction or reinforcement of the perineal floor.

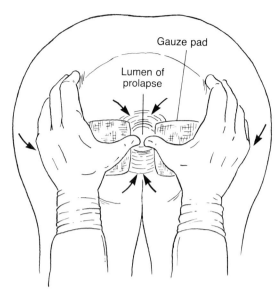

Figure 61–4. Reduction of a complete rectal prolapse.

4. Abdominal suspension or fixation of the prolapsed bowel to the sacrum or to other pelvic structures.
5. Obliteration of the cul-de-sac.
6. Repair of the perineal sliding hernia.

A description of the various fascial or Teflon slings, wire sutures, perineal floor reconstructions, or Marlex mesh or Ivalon-sponge rectopexy is beyond the scope of this text and may be found elsewhere.[1, 2, 5, 7, 10, 13] Surgical complications include fecal impaction, sepsis, pelvic abscess, presacral hemorrhage, fistula, stricture, impotence, and fecal incontinence.[5, 12] Postoperative fecal incontinence and recurrent prolapse are more frequent in those who have undergone repeated operations,[16] although continence may be restored surgically in 40 to 60 per cent of patients who undergo rectopexy.[17]

COMPLICATIONS

Complications of the rectal prolapse itself include ulceration and, rarely, bleeding. Irreducibility occurs as well, with gangrene as a possible complication. If the prolapsed bowel is gangrenous, the patient should be admitted and observed for evidence of intraperitoneal extension of systemic signs. If this appears to be a danger, colostomy may be required with resection of the nonviable tissue. Cineradiography or defecography may demonstrate rectal function either before or after the operation.[21, 22]

REFERENCES

1. Schwartz SI, Lillehei RC, Shires GT, et al (eds): Principles of Surgery. 3rd ed. New York, McGraw Hill Book Co, 1977, pp 1246–1247.
2. Altemeier WA, Culbertson WR, Schowengerdt C, et al: Nineteen years' experience with the one-stage perineal repair of rectal prolapse. Ann Surg 173:993, 1971.
3. Goligher JC: Prolapse of the rectum. In Hyhus L, Condon R: Hernia. 2nd ed. Philadelphia, JB Lippincott Co, 1978, pp 463–477.
4. Ellis H, Calne RY: Lecture Notes in General Surgery. London, Blackwell Scientific Publications, 1977, p 233–234, 253–255.
5. Failes D, Killingback M, Stuart M, et al: Rectal prolapse. Aust N Z J Surg 48:72, 1979.
6. Henry MM: Rectal prolapse. Br J Hosp Med 24: p 302, 1980.
7. Nigro ND: Procidentia of the rectum. Surg Clin North Am 58:539, 1978.
8. Goldberg SM: Procidentia of the rectum: A symposium. Dis Colon Rectum 18:457, 1975.
9. MacLeod JH: A Method of Proctology. New York, Harper & Row, 1979, pp 119–122.

10. Eisenstat TE, Rubin RJ, Salvati EP: Surgical treatment of complete rectal prolapse. Dis Colon Rectum 22:522, 1979.
11. Bates T: Rectal prolapse after anorectal dilatation in the elderly. Br Med J 2:505, 1972.
12. Hughes RG, Holder PD: The management of rectal prolapse in a district general hospital. Br J Clin Practice 42:321, 1988.
13. Aboul-Enein A: Prolapse of the rectum in young men: Treatment with a modified Roscoe Graham operation. Dis Colon Rectum 22:117, 1979.
14. Armstrong AL, Bivins BA, Sachatello CR: Rectal prolapse: A brief review. J Ky Med Assoc 76:329, 1978.
15. Hill GJ II: Outpatient Surgery. 2nd ed. Philadelphia, WB Saunders Co, 1980, pp 1199–1203.
16. Lehtola A, Salo JA, Fraki O, et al: Treatment of rectal prolapse. A clinical study of 50 consecutive patients. Ann Chir Gynaecol 76:150, 1987.
17. Husa A, Sainio P, Smitten K: Abdominal rectopexy and sigmoid resection for rectal prolapse. Acta Clar Scand 154:221, 1988.
18. Miller RL, Thomas JM, O'Leary JP: Ripstein procedure for rectal prolapse. Am Surg 45:531, 1979.
19. Theuerkauf FJ, Beahrs OH, Hill JR: Rectal prolapse: Causation and surgical treatment. Ann Surg 171:819, 1970.
20. Ryan P: Observations upon the etiology and treatment of complete rectal prolapse. Aust N Z J Surg 50:109, 1980.
21. Kuijpers JHC, DeMorree H: Toward a selection of the most appropriate procedure in the treatment of complete rectal prolapse. Dis Colon Rectum 31:355, 1988.
22. Corman ML: Rectal prolapse surgical techniques. Sur Clin North Am 68:1255, 1988.
23. Dutta BN, Das AK: Treatment of prolapsed rectum in children with injections of sclerosing agents. J Indian Med Assoc 69:275, 1977.
24. Uhlig BE, Sullivan ES: The modified Delorme operation: Its place in surgical treatment for massive rectal prolapse. Dis Colon Rectum 22:513, 1979.
25. Moore HD: The results of treatment for complete prolapse of the rectum in the adult patient. Dis Colon Rectum 20:566, 1977.

Musculoskeletal Procedures

Chapter **62**

Prehospital Splinting

Mohamud R. Daya,
Ronald J. Mariani,
and Thom Dick

CERVICAL SPINE

Trauma patients frequently sustain injuries to the cervical spine. These injuries are particularly devastating when associated with injury to the spinal cord. In the United States, there are approximately 12,000 spinal cord injuries per year.[1] The majority of these are a result of motor vehicle accidents. The remainder are due to falls, recreational activities (especially diving), and penetrating trauma. It is estimated that 40 per cent of cervical spine injuries are associated with neurologic deficits and that up to 25 per cent of such deficits are a result of improper handling during evaluation, extrication, and transport of the patient.[2, 3] Therefore it is critically important that the cervical spine be immobilized early and effectively.

Because the minimum degree of motion required to cause spinal cord injury has not been defined, the goal of immobilization is to maintain the head in a neutral position with zero degrees of motion in all directions.[4] To immobilize the entire cervical spine, an orthotic device must fix the head, hold the occiput and mandible, and restrict motion at the cervicothoracic junction.[5] This approach follows the basic orthopedic principle of immobilizing the joint above and below a suspected injury. In addition, to be useful in the prehospital setting, a cervical immobilization device must be portable, be easy to apply, and allow access to the upper airway.

At present, the standard technique of spinal immobilization involves early manual stabilization of the head and neck relative to the long axis of the body. Traction is no longer recommended, because it may aggravate the underlying injury. Manual stabilization is usually followed by the application of a cervical extrication collar. Although its use is controversial, a cervical collar has value as an early adjunct in the sometimes complex process of immobilization and extrication. There are several types of collars, varying in degree of comfort and support, but even the ones with the best combinations of these features provide less than adequate immobilization independently.

The choice of devices used in addition to extrication collars to ensure thorough immobilization depends on the victim's position of origin and the complexity of the disentanglement process. If the victim is found in a sitting position, as in an automobile, some version of the short spine board is commonly used. The most effective of these are wraparound corset-type devices, designed both to immobilize the neck and put handles on the patient.

Following the use of these intermediate short-board immobilizers, the patient is usually fastened to a full-length spine board or a similar rigid appliance for transfer to a litter for transporting. Complete cervical spine immobilization is achieved only when the body is also secured to a rigid device. This full-body immobilization should incorporate lateral immobilization for the head in the form of lightweight bulky objects such as foam blocks, towel rolls, blanket rolls, or cushions and tape.

Background

Since 1965, an entire industry aimed at the prehospital preservation of life and limb has evolved. Specially manufactured spinal immobilizers were developed for field use during the late 1960s and early 1970s. Many variations of these early devices have been further developed to solve specific prehospital problems.

In addition, recent advances have produced more versatile plastics and stronger adhesives. Such materials were not available to the "pioneers" of the 1960s. Medical theory as it applied to spinal protection was also later incorporated into the rescue devices as the medical field became more involved in prehospital care.

It should be stressed that, although there seems to be widespread general agreement about the basic steps of spinal immobilization, prehospital care is a setting for people who can adapt. Because of the variety of circumstances that confront rescuers on a daily basis, there is little room for inflexible rules. An advanced life support unit can carry only a limited number of tools.

The first widely distributed text to devote attention to the role of a cervical extrication collar in early immobilization of the neck after injury was Grant and Murray's *Emergency Care*, first published in 1971. One of its principal contributors was J. D. Farrington, a consultant, whose classic article "Death in a Ditch" was the first widely publicized reference concerning the use of a spine board and undoubtedly influenced rescue training programs worldwide.[6] Farrington emphasized that spinal fractures were frequently mishandled and made worse by rough or hasty movement at the scene. He outlined the use of a backboard, sandbags, and tape for the prehospital extrication and care of patients with suspected spinal injuries. He fashioned extrication collars using universal dressings held in place by soft roller bandages and advocated manual traction during the extrication phase.[7]

Since then, the risks of vigorous manual traction have led to the discouragement of its use in the field.[8] In addition, although sandbags perform adequately in the supine patient, they may cause significant movement of the neck if the board is suddenly tilted, for example, to decrease the risk of aspiration in a vomiting patient. As a result, sandbags have been replaced by more lightweight devices such as foam blocks. Despite these modifications, the original method of splinting the head and torso to a rigid object remains the preferred technique for effective spinal immobilization.

Indications

An extrication collar should be used as a primary adjunct in cases involving trauma to the head and neck. In the absence of obvious trauma, patients should be immobilized if they have a mechanism for a potential cervical spine injury unless this injury can be ruled out by careful questioning of both the victims and the witnesses involved. In any instance of doubt, it is best to immobilize and transport. The most common mechanism for injury is sudden deceleration resulting in hyperflexion and hyperextension forces. Patients under the influence of alcohol or drugs may lack the self-awareness to recognize their own spinal injury and should always be immobilized. Likewise, every unconscious patient should be immobilized to avoid aggravating an underlying spinal injury. Any awake and alert patient who complains of spine pain, paresthesia, weakness, or absent movement should be immobilized carefully to avoid secondary injury to the spinal cord. Documentation of neurologic findings before and after immobilization should also form an important part of the medical record.

It is not uncommon to encounter patients in the field who are both conscious and oriented but unaware of their own neck injuries. The sensory impact of having one's automobile forcibly disassembled by rescue personnel who are using modern tools that produce noise in excess of 80 decibels may result in considerable distraction. In addition, the presence of other painful injuries or concern over other victims may mask the manifestations of an occult cervical spine injury. It also should be remembered that cervical spine injuries can occur in settings not usually associated with trauma.[9] Therefore, a high index of suspicion should always be maintained.

The purpose of an extrication collar is to assist in splinting the head and neck either therapeutically or prophylactically in a neutral position.[5] The collar is useful for the following reasons:

1. It provides substantial protection to the airway by limiting flexion in a patient whose position or mental status threatens airway patency.
2. It relieves stress on the basilar skull and cervical vertebrae when these structures have been injured.
3. It helps reduce cervical spine motion (especially flexion) but also rotation, lateral bending, and extension. In this regard, however, it serves only as an adjunct.
4. If properly chosen it can support the weight of the head while the patient is sitting and help to maintain the alignment of the cervical spine once the patient has been moved to a supine position.
5. An equally important function is to serve as a reminder that the integrity of the basilar skull and cervical spine are suspect because of the patient's mechanism of injury.

Serious cervical cord injuries may occur in the absence of demonstrable fracture, and permanent paralysis may result from spinal cord contusion in an intact bony milieu. Spinal cord injury is common in elderly patients with cervical spondylosis; an arthritic osteophyte may sever a portion of the cord as permanently as a fracture or dislocation. In such cases, there may be little or no subjective pain.

The extrication collar does not constitute complete immobilization of the head and neck, even for the purposes of transportation. The collar was designed as an adjunct and was never intended to provide definitive immobilization in itself. Complete immobilization is not possible until the patient is properly secured to a long backboard-type device. Nonetheless, the collar goes on first and remains in place during this process.

Contraindications

There are few circumstances that contraindicate the use of some type of extrication collar. The presence of a tracheal stoma, which is integral to the management of a patient's airway is a problem with some older collars. With scissors, one can modify these collars to accommodate a stoma hole, although structural support may be compromised. Fortunately, newer devices incorporate a tracheal opening as a consistent feature. Similarly, the presence of an invasive airway (cricothyroidotomy or needle tracheostomy) may necessitate modification of the cervical support.

A second circumstance that might preclude the use of a factory-made collar is cervical dislocation with fixed angulation. This situation is rarely encountered and can be managed with an improvised immobilizer, such as a version of a horse collar or prolonged manual positioning without traction.[10]

A third circumstance that could preclude the use of a collar is massive cervical swelling (e.g., secondary to hemorrhage or tracheal injury). The compressive effect of a collar may impede air exchange, decrease cerebral perfusion, or increase intracranial pressure.[11] A penetrating foreign body such as knife, glass, or metal would also make cervical spine immobilization difficult.

Pediatric collars usually come in limited sizes and may not be well tolerated, in which case manual in-line immobilization becomes necessary.

One must emphasize that the desired effect is the determinant of the type of tool that should be used. Often, an improvised tool works better than one that is manufactured, owing to size and shape of the patient or the special circumstances involved in handling the patient. Adaptability is a trait of well-trained and experienced field personnel.

Equipment

There are two basic types of extrication collars, both of which currently appear in rigid and semirigid designs.[12] Both types rely on the same support structures for the bottom of the collar, namely, the two trapezius muscles posteriorly and the two clavicles anteriorly. These support structures constitute a four-point system. The collar types differ, however, in the way in which they come in contact with the head.

The first type is a relatively short collar that wraps rather tightly around the neck. Depending on the collar's shape (usually fairly straight), it contacts the hyoid, the mastoids, and the occiput (Fig. 62–1). Disadvantages of this type of collar are impingement on the thyroid cartilage and compression of the carotid sinuses and external neck veins. Thyroid cartilage restriction can affect airway management; carotid compression can be expected to decrease cerebral circulation; and jugular compression may increase intracranial pressures.

The second type of collar design for supporting the head incorporates a higher collar with wing-like flaps on its upper posterior edges that engage large areas of soft tissue on the posterior head. Anteriorly, this collar appears to be similar to the lower-type collars, although this flaring design seems to prevent compression of some of the neck structures

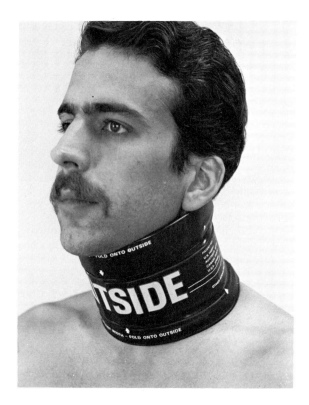

Figure 62–1. Loxley cervical collar. A low-style collar. Note the fact that it fits closer to the neck than other designs. Closer fitting collars tend to be less comfortable than other designs, offering less rotational stability. This one is constructed of plastic over cardboard. (Bound Tree Corporation, 15 Bridge St., P.O. Box 401, Henniker, NH 03242; from Dick T, Land R: Spinal immobilization devices. Part I: Cervical extrication collars. J Emerg Med Serv 7:12, 1982. Reproduced by permission.)

that were mentioned previously, even when the collars are applied firmly (Figs. 62–2, and 62–3).

The higher collars generally provide better rotational stability but allow more extension than those that are tighter fitting. This is a direct consequence of using posterior soft tissues as opposed to bony prominences for support. In addition, some newer collars use the sternum as a fifth thoracic support point[13] (Figs. 62–4 and 62–5).

Soft collars although comfortable have no role in spinal immobilization because they provide minimal support and do not reduce cervical motion to any significant degree.[3, 14] Comfort, however, is extremely important from the standpoint of patient compliance. Some rigid collars, regardless of proper sizing and despite their support characteristics are useless because of patient discomfort.

The bewildering number of devices available on the market makes collar selection a difficult process. Dick and Land, after describing the characteristics of the ideal collar,

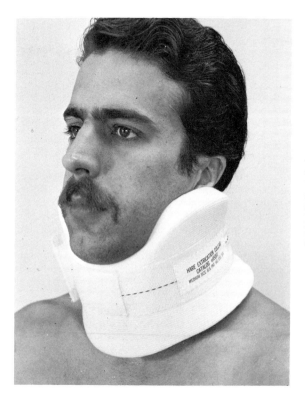

Figure 62–2. Hare cervical extrication collar. One of the earliest forms of extrication collar, this type provides anterior support via the mandible and posterior support by means of wing-like flaps that engage the mastoids but not the occiput in most patients. When properly applied, it provides excellent support. A 5-cm soft insert over the thyroid protects that structure. (Dyna Med/Dyna Industries, 6200 Yarrow Drive, Carlsbad, CA 92008-0996; from Dick T, Land R: Spinal immobilization devices. Part I: Cervical extrication collars. J Emerg Med Serv 7:12, 1982. Reproduced by permission.)

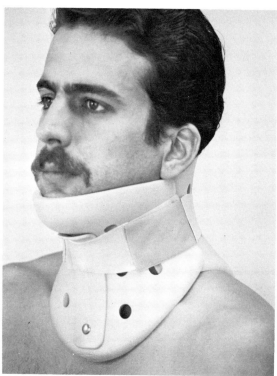

Figure 62–3. Philadelphia collar. This is a two-piece, high-type collar that comes in 17 sizes. The collar supports the head in a dish-shaped contour that is formed when the front and rear halves are joined by Velcro fasteners. When properly sized for a patient, this collar provides excellent support. When applied too tightly, it tends to force the mandible backward and in some patients can cause thyroid compression. It is extremely comfortable. (Armstrong Industries, 575 Knightsbridge Parkway, P.O. Box 700, Lincolnshire, IL 60069-0700; from Dick T, Land R: Spinal immobilization devices. Part I: Cervical extrication collars. J Emerg Med Serv 7:12, 1982. Reproduced by permission.)

published a subjective matrix-type analysis that compared the effectiveness of 13 extrication collars with this ideal model (Table 62–1). Features of the ideal extrication collar included the following:

1. It should support the weight of the head in a neutral position.
2. It should prevent lateral, rotational, and anteroposterior movement of the head.

3. It should be comfortable, translucent on radiographs, and compact enough to fit into a standard paramedic equipment box without undergoing deformity.
4. It should be able to be applied reliably by a single trained technician and an untrained bystander.
5. It should be capable of sustaining repeated sanitation.
6. Its price should be such that it can be carried in sufficient numbers in various sizes by any ambulance.

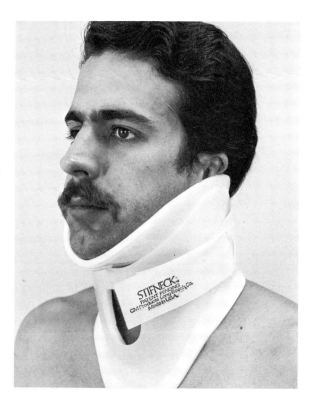

Figure 62–4. Stifneck collar. This collar is a radically different type of high-design collar, made of high-density polyethylene (a hard material) and padded with semiflexible foam margins. It provides probably the best overall support of all field collars, considering the adaptability of a single collar to several patient sizes. Note the low-reaching anterior panel, which contacts the sternum. (California Medical Products, 1901 Obispo Ave, Long Beach, CA 90804; from Dick T, Land R: Spinal immobilization devices. Part I: Cervical extrication collars. J Emerg Med Serv 7:12, 1982. Reproduced by permission.)

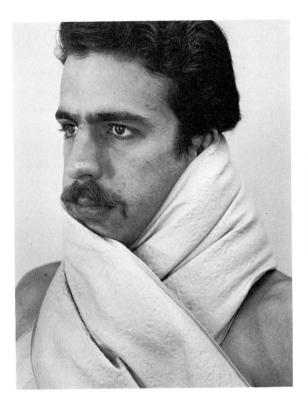

Figure 62–5. Vac-Pac vacuum-type cervical collar. Although expensive, this is a vacuum splint designed for the neck. Vacuum splints are similar to pneumatic devices in their ability to conform to anything while avoiding inward pressure. This device is a phenomenal immobilizer, although it does not maintain traction. The vinyl cover is filled with polystyrene beads, which act as a form when the splint is evacuated with a suction device. (Olympic Medical Corporation, 4400 Seventh Ave South, Seattle WA 98108; from Dick T, Land R: Spinal immobilization devices. Part I: Cervical extrication collars. J Emerg Med Serv 7:12, 1982. Reproduced by permission.)

Table 62–1. Collar Evaluation Chart*

Category	Ferno-Wash-ington	FP Extri-cation	FP Standard	Hare	Immobi-lizer	Loxley	Phila-delphia	Quic-kollar	Rapid-Form	Stif-neck	Stubbs	Thomas	Vac-Pac
Support	+1	+1	−1	+2	+2	+2	+2	0	+1	+2	+2	+2	+2
Lateral	+1	+1	−2	+2	+2	+2	+2	0	+2	+1	+2	+1	+2
Rotational	+1	+1	−2	+1	+2	−2	+2	−2	+2	+2	+1	+2	+2
Flex-extension	+1	+1	+2	+2	−1	+1	+2	+1	+1	+2	+1	+1	+2
Comfort	+2	+2	+1	+1	−2	−2	+2	−1	−2	+2	+1	−2	+2
Compactness	+1	+2	+1	+2	+1	+2	0	+2	+1	0	+1	+2	−1
Simplicity	+2	+2	0	+2	+2	+2	+1	+2	+1	0	+1	0	+1
Cleaning	+2	+2	+2	+2	+2	+2	+2	+2	+1	+2	−2	+2	+2
# Sizes	+1	+1	+2	+1	+1	+2	0	+2	+2	+1	+1	+1	+2
Circulation	+1	+2	+2	+2	−2	−1	+2	0	−2	+2	+2	−1	+2
Ease of application	+2	+2	+1	+2	+2	+2	+1	+2	+1	+2	+1	+1	+1
Airway	+1	+1	−1	+2	+2	0	−1	+1	+1	+2	+2	+2	+2
Price	+2	+1	+2	+2	+2	+2	0	+2	+1	+1	+2	0	−2

*This chart compares 13 collars to an imaginary "perfect" extrication collar. Although x-ray and cold weather performance are important considerations, the collars were not evaluated for these factors. Please note that rigid collar designs are likely to accommodate only narrow ranges of neck sizes, whereas firm but flexible designs tend to be more adaptable while still providing good immobilization.

+2 = Performance is ideal.

+1 = Performance is good, but not ideal.

 0 = Performance is about adequate or marginal.

−1 = Performance is mildly unsatisfactory.

**The collars are presented in alphabetical order.

(Adapted from Dick T, Land R: Spinal immobilization devices, Part I: Cervical extrication collars. J Emerg Med Serv 7:12, 1982. Reproduced by permission.)

7. It should not interfere with the position of function of important airway structures, nor adversely affect cerebral circulation in any way.

8. Simplicity of design should permit its application by two technicians in less than 60 seconds, in darkness, rain, and cold weather, without manipulation of the head or neck.

9. It should be available in the smallest number of sizes (e.g., that adapt to and properly immobilize as many patients) as possible. Proper application is assumed.

Figures 62–1 through 62–6 illustrate the representative devices that are commonly used for prehospital cervical immobilization and the unique features of each.

Other investigators have attempted to evaluate cervical extrication collars objectively. The accepted gold standard for comparison is the Halo brace used in the hospital setting, which restricts motion to 4 per cent flexion-extension, 1 per cent rotation, and 4 per cent lateral bending.[5] The majority of existing studies on extrication collars have used models that do not adequately represent the prehospital setting. Thus the applicability of their findings is often questionable. Podolsky and colleagues[3] compared neck movements in 25 volunteers who were immobilized, wearing various collars, in the supine position. They concluded that of the four collars studied, none was an effective immobilizer alone and that the combination of the Philadelphia collar with lateral support and tape provided the most effective immobilization. Surprisingly, these investigators also found that lateral support and tape alone did more to limit motion than any collar examined (Table 62–2). Aprahamian and coworkers[15] studied the impact of various airway maneuvers with and without collars using a cadaver model for cervical instability. They concluded that the Philadelphia collar does not provide adequate immobilization for airway maneuvers and that the collar's primary value may be only that of a warning device to call attention to a possible cervical spine injury. Cline and coworkers[16] looked at the effectiveness of seven immobilization techniques in 97 normal volunteers. They concluded that no single collar was consistently superior and recommended that the short-board technique (SBT) serve as the gold standard for future evaluations of prehospital spinal immobilization devices (Table 62–3). Unfortunately, the SBT (Fig. 62–7) itself has limited value because it creates hyperextension, is time consuming to apply, and limits access to the airway.[14]

McCabe and colleagues[17] studied the ability of four different extrication collars to immobilize the cervical spine using radiographic studies in seven normal volunteers. Their study demonstrated that the newer polyethylene collars were more effective at reducing flexion and lateral bending than other devices. Graziano and associates[18] radiographically compared three methods of immobilization with the SBT. Their study confirmed the SBT as the gold standard for comparison and established that the Stifneck is one of the best available extrication collars. Solot and Winzelberg[18a] found the Vertebrace (Jobst Institute, Inc., Toledo, OH

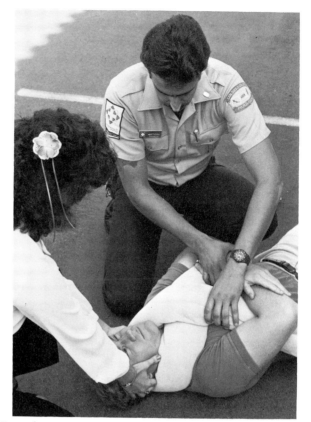

Figure 62–6. Horse collar. Most extrication collars are available in three to five factory sizes. If a collar is not sized properly to fit a particular patient, it performs no function. Patients with extremely long necks or especially short ones can be immobilized by means of a horse collar, fashioned from a bulky rescue blanket. The blanket is rolled to the thickness desired, slid under the patient's neck while a bystander applies traction; the ends of the blanket are then brought across the patient's anterior chest. The patient's forearms are fastened as shown to stabilize the "tails" of the collar. Emergency medical technicians must be able to adapt to a wide range of possible patients and environmental circumstances. (From Dick T: Tricks of the trade: Horse sense, immobilizing necks that don't fit collars. J Emerg Med Serv 7:23, 1982. Reproduced by permission.)

13094) to have similar characteristics. In general these studies merely confirm the fact that extrication collars alone are inadequate to immobilize the cervical spine totally.

At the present time, there is no prehospital device or technique that approaches the Halo in its ability to immobilize the cervical spine, although preliminary data with the TACIT (traction, alignment, cervical immobilization, transport) device appear promising. The TACIT device, which is currently being investigated for interhospital transfers and prehospital use, may someday solve the search for the ideal

Table 62–2. Mean Degrees of Movement ± Standard Deviation of Six Cervical Immobilization Methods and No Immobilization in 25 Normal Volunteers

	No Immobilization	Soft Collar (Howmedica)	Extrication Collar (Hare)	Hard Collar (Orthopedic Systems)	Philadelphia Collar (Philadelphia Collar Company)	Tape and Sandbags	Tape, Sandbags, Philadelphia Collar
Flexion	35.7 ± 5.1	34.2 ± 6.4	26.4 ± 6.4	25.8 ± 6.0	24.2 ± 7.8	0.1 ± 6.0	0.1 ± 0.4
Extension	21.0 ± 5.8	18.1 ± 5.8	16.4 ± 6.7	15.4 ± 5.3	12.0 ± 7.0	15.0 ± 6.9	7.4 ± 5.5
Lateral	21.2 ± 5.4	21.1 ± 4.6	15.4 ± 4.9	14.2 ± 6.3	17.4 ± 5.0	1.8 ± 1.7	1.4 ± 1.5
Rotary	75.8 ± 6.5	67.4 ± 11.7	48.9 ± 11.6	49.9 ± 15.3	49.4 ± 14.2	2.5 ± 2.2	4.0 ± 3.0

(Adapted from Podolsky S, Baraff IJ, Simon RR, et al: Efficacy of cervical spine immobilization methods. J Trauma 23:6, 1983.)

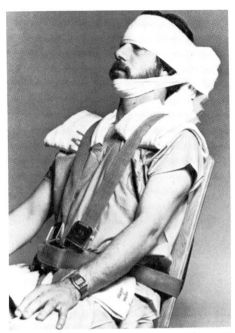

Figure 62–7. Short-board technique. (From Graziano AF, Scheidel EA, Cline JR, et al. Radiographic comparison of prehospital cervical immobilization methods. Ann Emerg Med 16:10, 1987. Reproduced by permission.)

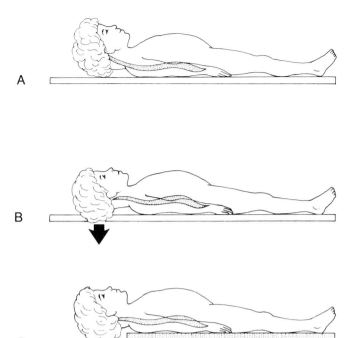

Figure 62–8. *A*, Young child immobilized on a standard backboard (large head forces neck into flexion). Backboards modified by an occiput cutout *(B)* or a double-mattress pad *(C)* to raise chest. (Adapted from Herzenberg JE, Hensinger RN, Dedrick DK, et al. Emergency transport and positioning of young children who have an injury of the cervical spine. J Bone Joint Surg 71A:15, 1989. Reproduced by permission.)

cervical immobilization device. Current data indicate that this device limits motion to 1 to 2 per cent flexion-extension, 1 to 2 per cent rotation, and 1 to 2 per cent lateral bending.[5]

Little information is available regarding the proper selection and application of spinal immobilization devices for children. Half of the total growth in head circumference is achieved by the age of 18 months, giving children a disproportionately large head compared with the rest of the body. Prior to age 8, these anatomic and developmental differences result in a higher incidence of upper cervical spine injuries (C1–C2). Because injuries in this area are frequently unstable, proper cervical immobilization in the neutral position is critically important. Because the head is large, positioning the child's body on a standard backboard may force the neck into flexion or a relative kyphosis. The clinical significance of this is currently unclear, but, theoretically, adult-type immobilization devices may be hazardous for use in a young child. The standard backboard may be modified to accommodate the child's larger head size. As a

rough guide, the external auditory meatus should be on the same level as the midshoulder. Suggested modifications include a cutout in the backboard that accommodates the occiput or a pad under the back at the level of the chest (Fig. 62–8). If not modified, the standard backboard in conjunction with the disproportionately large head of a child may force the neck into hyperflexion, possibly aggravating a cervical spine injury.[19]

Huerta and colleagues[20] have evaluated the performance of commercially available infant and pediatric collars using a mannequin model. They conclude that the high-cut collar (Fig. 62–9) in conjunction with a rigid backboard and lateral neck stabilizers provides the most effective spinal immobilization. In some children, these devices may provoke struggling because of fear, which has the potential to aggra-

Table 62–3. Cervical Immobilization Efficacy

Method	Saggital Plane (Occiput-C7)		Frontal Plane (Lateral Bending)		Horizontal Plane (Axial Rotation)	
	(% Reduction of Control)	*No. of Volunteers*	*(% Reduction of Control)*	*No. of Volunteers*	*(% Reduction of Control)*	*No. of Volunteers*
1. Philadelphia collar	(69)	14	(28)	15	(43)	15
2. Hare extrication collar	(51)	12	(55)	13	(39)	12
3. Rigid plastic collar	(56)	13	(41)	14	(50)	14
4. Philadelphia collar plus short board	(84)	11	(64)	12	(73)	12
5. Hare extrication collar plus short board	(86)	14	(66)	14	(63)	14
6. Rigid plastic collar plus short board	(89)	09	(66)	14	(66)	14
7. Short board only	(88)	13	(64)	14	(71)	14

(Adapted from Cline JR, Scheidel E, Bigsby EF: Comparison of methods of cervical immobilization extrication and transport. J Trauma 25:7, 1985. © Williams & Wilkins, 1985.)

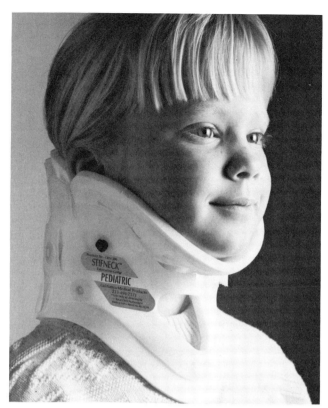

Figure 62–9. Pediatric high-cut extrication collar. (California Medical Products, Long Beach, Calif. Reproduced by permission.)

vate an underlying injury. In these situations, manual immobilization may be more effective and less frightening for the child.[21]

Procedure

Application of an extrication collar is a straightforward procedure (Fig. 62–10). A collar should be treated as a splint. The normal axiom in splinting is to immobilize the joint above and below the area of injury. Because no currently marketed collar performs this function perfectly, a rescuer should be charged with maintaining cervical immobilization in the neutral position until the patient can be fully immobilized in a corset-type immobilizer or on a full backboard. A collar (like any splint) requires one person to stabilize the neck in its position of function and a second person to apply the hardware. The rescuer's intentions should be thoroughly explained to the patient throughout the procedure.

The neck should be examined before application of the collar for swelling, ecchymosis, deformity, or penetrating wounds. Once the collar is in place, a conscious patient should be cautioned repeatedly against movement of the head until all equipment has been removed on arrival at a hospital. Any persistent complaints of pain or dyspnea by the patient should be investigated by removal and possible replacement of the device while manual stabilization is maintained. The collar size should be determined using the manufacturer's suggested guidelines. For example, the Stifneck is available in various sizes and uses the distance from the top of the shoulder to the chin to determine size (Fig. 62–11). The tallest collar that does not cause hyperextension should be used. For extremely short necks, a special extri-

cation collar such as the No-neck is recommended (Fig. 62–12).

In cases in which a factory-manufactured collar of the proper size for a given patient is not available, an improvised device should be made from available materials (see Fig. 62–6). Once the patient is in the supine position on the backboard, lateral stabilization should be added, either by using foam blocks and tape or by adding a factory-made lateral neck stabilizer (Fig. 62–13).

Complications

Improper application of an extrication collar generally occurs in one of two ways: either the wrong size or type of device is used or too little care is exercised in its placement. The best means of preventing either error is strong physician involvement in the training and continuing education of rescue crews, together with vigorous feedback in cases of correct and incorrect application.

A collar that is too small for a patient may be either too tight for the girth of the neck (with obvious complications) or too short to provide adequate immobilization. Too large a collar commonly results in hyperextension, which can exacerbate preexisting injury.

Improper application can result from not removing the patient's shoulder clothing before application of the hardware; when possible this should be done, by cutting if necessary, in every case. Insistence on taking spinal precautions whenever the mechanism of injury even mildly suggests cervical injury ensures high competence levels among rescuers as well as a comfortable margin of safety.

Improper application of an extrication collar may impede venous return and raise intracranial pressure. This is sometimes manifested by facial flushing and is more common with the short collar types.[11]

One final complication should be mentioned. The patient who, for whatever reason, actively resists placement of an extrication collar or other splint should not be forced to wear it. Immobilization of the resisting patient cannot be accomplished without considerable muscular exertion not only by rescuers but also by the patient. If fractures do exist, it is possible that this kind of struggling can cause further damage. If such fractures involve the cervical spine, this could be fatal. If the patient permits manual stabilization, this should be maintained as an alternative.

Conclusion

The competent use of a good cervical extrication collar has proved itself to be important as an early immobilizer in the field, before disentanglement of the traumatized patient, although it is less valuable in a hospital environment. The cervical collar should not be relied on for total immobilization. The latter can be provided in the field only by means of a full backboard and lateral support for immobilization of the head and neck.

THORACOLUMBAR SPINE

Adequate full-body thoracolumbar spinal immobilization in the field, like good cervical spinal immobilization, is probably best done by means of a full-length spine board (also called a *backboard*). Full-body spinal immobilization should incorporate early application of a good extrication collar, lateral immobilization of the head and neck, and ample belting of the entire body. The last measure is important in cases in which the backboard has to be used to

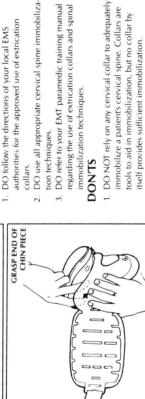

APPLICATION

ALTERNATIVE SUPINE APPLICATION

An alternative is to begin by sliding the back portion of the collar behind the patient's neck. Once the loop velcro is again visible, turn all of your attention to positioning the chin piece and proceed as previously described.

SUPINE APPLICATION

If the patient is supine, position the chin piece as previously described and slide the back portion of the collar behind the patient's neck. Be sure to fold the loop velcro inward on top of the foam padding to prevent it from collecting debris which could limit its gripping ability.

ATTACHING VELCRO

With the patient's chin properly supported, position the back of the collar around the neck and attach the loop velcro so that it mates with, and is parallel to, the hook velcro. Use the trach hole to keep the collar in proper position as you tighten the velcro. BE SURE TO MAINTAIN NEUTRAL ALIGNMENT THROUGH-OUT THIS PROCEDURE.

POSITIONING THE COLLAR

With the patient's head held in neutral alignment, position the chin piece by sliding the collar up the chest wall. Be sure that the chin is well supported by the chin piece and that the chin extends far enough onto the chin piece to at least cover the central fastener. Difficulty in positioning the chin piece may indicate the need for a shorter collar.

DISASSEMBLY

GRASP END OF CHIN PIECE

STIFNECK™ may be disassembled by grasping the end of the chin piece, as shown, with the black fastener between the fingers and working this fastener out of its hole. Do not try to pull the white fastener apart.

APPLICATION

TIGHTENING THE COLLAR

Tighten the collar gently and attach the Velcro so that the two pieces are parallel. Re-check the position of the patient's head and collar for proper alignment. Tighten the collar further until proper support is obtained.

DO'S

1. DO follow the directions of your local EMS authorities for the approved use of extrication collars.
2. DO use all appropriate cervical spine immobilization techniques.
3. DO refer to your EMT paramedic training manual regarding the use of extrication collars and spinal immobilization techniques.

DON'TS

1. DO NOT rely on any cervical collar to adequately immobilize a patient's cervical spine. Collars are tools to aid in immobilization, but no collar by itself provides sufficient immobilization.
2. DO NOT use an improperly sized collar. Too large a collar may hyperextend a patient's cervical spine; too small a collar may not provide appropriate stability.
3. DO NOT hesitate to contact your local EMS dealer or local EMS authority with questions regarding the use of extrication collars.

Figure 62–10. Technique for the application of an extrication collar. (California Medical Products, Long Beach, Calif. Reproduced by permission.)

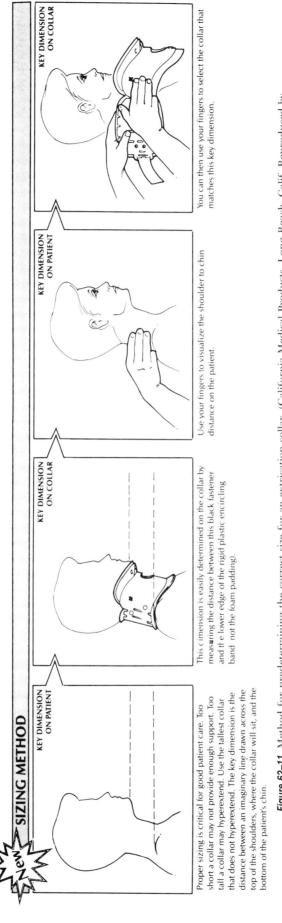

SIZING METHOD

New

KEY DIMENSION ON PATIENT

Proper sizing is critical for good patient care. Too short a collar may not provide enough support. Too tall a collar may hyperextend. Use the tallest collar that does not hyperextend. The key dimension is the distance between an imaginary line drawn across the top of the shoulders, where the collar will sit, and the bottom of the patient's chin.

KEY DIMENSION ON COLLAR

This dimension is easily determined on the collar by measuring the distance between this black fastener and the lower edge of the rigid plastic encircling band not the foam padding).

KEY DIMENSION ON PATIENT

Use your fingers to visualize the shoulder to chin distance on the patient.

KEY DIMENSION ON COLLAR

You can then use your fingers to select the collar that matches this key dimension.

Figure 62–11. Method for predetermining the correct size for an extrication collar. (California Medical Products, Long Beach, Calif. Reproduced by permission.)

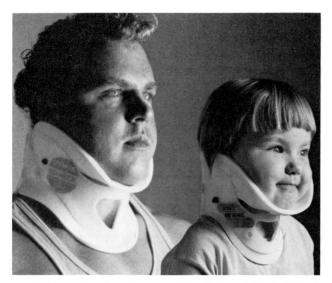

Figure 62–12. No-neck extrication collar. Designed for individuals with extremely short necks. (California Medical Products, Long Beach, Calif. Reproduced by permission.)

carry the patient for any distance or when there is likelihood of emesis, as in the patient with probable head injuries or ingestion of depressants such as alcohol.

Transferring of a victim from a location and position of origin to a backboard may require the use of an intermediate immobilizer. Until recently, this meant using a short spine board to which a patient's head, neck, and torso were fastened by belts. Currently, devices that resemble corsets are preferred. Such devices have extensions that engage the head and neck and are equipped with weight-bearing loops that enable the rescuers to handle the patient more easily. Intermediate immobilizers or extrication splints are indicated either when a patient must be removed from a confined environment in which he or she is found in the sitting position or when circumstances require movement in or from a sitting position.

When extrication is not required by a patient's location, position of origin, or route of egress, the patient is most

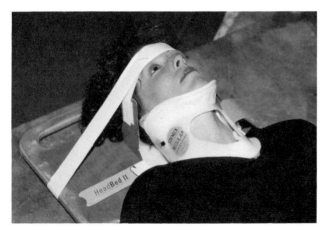

Figure 62–13. Extrication collar combined with a cervical immobilization device. (California Medical Products, Long Beach, Calif. Reproduced by permission.)

often found lying at ground level. With an extrication collar in place and in-line manual immobilization maintained on the neck, the patient may be logrolled onto a backboard. Visual inspection of the back should be carried out during the logrolling process as the body is kept in a single plane.

Although the logrolling technique is routinely used to move patients with suspected thoracolumbar injuries, the potential for movement at an unstable segment always exists. Little research has been done in the past to determine the safety of logrolling.[22] One study[23] evaluated the effect of the logrolling maneuver using three models: a volunteer with a stable spine, a cadaver with a surgically created unstable thoracolumbar injury, and a patient with a T12–L1 fracture dislocation. Radiographic studies on the volunteer demonstrated mild lateral movement when rolled onto the side. The cadaver demonstrated a 2.1-cm anteroposterior displacement and a 5-mm lateral displacement during the logroll. The injured patient demonstrated no anteroposterior displacement but did experience a 7-mm lateral displacement when rolled onto the side. Although the study was small, it does raise concern about the safety of logrolling the trauma patient and suggests caution during any transfer procedure.

An optional but effective means of moving a patient from the ground is provided by a type of stretcher that breaks apart longitudinally and can be slid beneath a victim without disturbing the position. The *scoop stretcher*, as this device is called, facilitates movement and eliminates the need for immediate examination of the back, a factor that should not be considered a limitation of the equipment. One definite advantage to using the scoop stretcher is its shape. Its halves are anatomically contoured, not only enhancing its comfort but also limiting lateral movement of the immobilized patient.

A third means of both immobilizing and moving a trauma victim consists of a specially designed full-body splint, complete with factory-made straps or harnesses. There are several such immobilizers, most of which are highly effective and provide good lateral stability as well as anatomic conformity. The patient must either be logrolled or lifted onto these devices.

Background

As recently as 1965, the principle of "rapid transportation above all" held widespread acceptance among rescuers who had little or no orthopedic training and among physicians whose emergency care experience, by modern standards, was just as limited. The most commonly agreed on means of getting a sitting patient out of a wrecked automobile was to use some version of a chair-carry. If the patient originated in a position other than the sitting position, the patient was first placed into a sitting position and *then* moved by means of a chair-carry or simply dragged out bodily.

In fact, one respectable source of the period stated that rescuers rarely found crash victims in the car unless they were trapped there; civilians had usually dragged them out,[24] or, conditioned by the number of accidents involving higher-octane fuels and the lack of safety-capping systems, victims were just as likely to flee for their lives.[25] A victim may also have been thrown out of the vehicle without the benefit of a safety belt.

Colonel Louis Kossuth, commander of the U.S. Air Force's Medical Service School at Gunter Air Force Base in Alabama, made note of several auto accidents at which he thought patients were handled very roughly by civilians who were trying to be of help. He searched, to no avail, the medical literature of that time for references that might show how these victims should be handled. He questioned several hundred accident victims who had sustained major fractures to determine how they had been removed from their automobiles. Most said that they had been grabbed under the shoulders and dragged, often in terrible pain, from their vehicles.

Kossuth experimented with a torso version of the Timmons splints, a set of canvas splints reinforced with semirigid steel stays as slats, similar to the modern Kendrick extrication device (KED). In addition, Kossuth probably developed the first modern-type spine board.[7]

In 1967 and 1968, Farrington authored two classic articles (filled with detailed illustrations) that showed the use of a type of extrication collar, spinal traction, 9-foot webbing straps, and both long and short spine boards similar to modern designs to remove people in every position from automobiles.[6, 7] Much of today's extrication theory is essentially as Farrington taught it.

In 1967, the Committee on Trauma of the American College of Surgeons listed the minimum amounts and types of equipment that should be carried in an ambulance. The list included both short and long spine boards, with accessories.[26] A similar document published the following year by the National Academy of Science's Division of Medical Sciences also provided a list of medical requirements for ambulance equipment and recommended long and short spine boards.[25]

In 1969, St. Louis surgeons Klippel and Conrad described the use of a full-length spine board that was capable of being broken down into separate components for the upper and lower halves of the body. The lower portion included a simple traction device that could accommodate right- or left-sided lower extremities of various lengths.[27] By 1971, both of the first recognized texts for emergency medical technicians referred to the use of the short spine board as a widespread practice.[28, 29]

Indications

Generally, the application and maintenance of spinal precautions in the field setting depend on the rescuers as well as the receiving emergency physicians being well educated and experienced in the mechanics of injury.

Any mechanism capable of injury to the cervical spine should prompt rescuers to immobilize not only the head and neck but also the entire body. The motion of any vertebral joint is impossible to isolate. To immobilize the head and neck, they both must be fastened into a common plane with the thorax. Extrication devices (such as short spine boards) can be made to do this to an extent, although movement of the lower extremities causes movement of the pelvis, which in turn results in lumbar movement. Movement of the lumbar spine induces some thoracic movement, although the extent has not been quantified. Considering the fact that the most feasible position for transport is the supine position, full-body immobilization is easily achieved on the long spine board. In the absence of deterrent factors, supine full-body immobilization is a reasonable choice.

Mechanisms that arouse suspicion of direct injury to the thoracolumbar spine should also suggest full-body spinal immobilization. Very generally, they include (1) most penetrating injuries to the thorax and abdomen, including all missile-related incidents; (2) blunt trauma involving high-energy impact in any area of the body; (3) blunt trauma involving moderate energy impact to the posterior truncal surfaces; and (4) blunt trauma involving localized impact of any energy level in the posterior thoracic, abdominal, or pelvic spinal areas.

The mechanism of injury should dictate both suspicion of injury and immobilization of potential spinal injuries from a field standpoint, even when no neurologic signs are present, and despite the absence of pain if the mechanism is suggestive enough. In such cases, the possibility of occult fractures is best ruled out by a physician.

In any case in which spinal injury is plausible, rescuers should take vigorous measures to immobilize the spine before transport, leaving diagnosis to the receiving physician. The physician, in turn, should not permit inhospital removal of immobilizers until rescuers have reported on the mechanism of injury.

Contraindications

Essentially, the only known contraindication to the use of commonly recognized means to immobilize the spine of a patient whose mechanism of injury suggests spinal injury, is *the existence of a greater threat*. Recognizing such circumstances and taking appropriate action when they arise are the functions of a competent rescuer. The threat to a patient's life may exceed the threat of *possible* spinal injury under the following circumstances.

Hazards on the Scene. Problems with traffic control in the direct vicinity of the patient's location such that the patient, along with rescuers or other patients, is likely to be further injured suggest urgent extrication. Such hazardous situations include fuel or other flammable substances leaking at the scene (these should be assumed to be in immediate danger of ignition, with possible ensuing explosions); fire on the scene; hostile crowds or persons on the scene; and physically unstable environments, such as partially collapsed structures or unstable vehicles that cannot be stabilized quickly.

Ongoing Gunfire at the Scene. Gunfire is usually considered an indication for rescue personnel to stay away from a scene. Rescuers who find themselves confronted with a patient *and* gunfire are considered fortunate if they can extricate themselves and the victim from such a situation in any way possible.

Overwhelming Casualties. Rescuers may have to improvise in cases in which casualties exceed available resources. In such cases, proper spinal immobilization may merit a lower priority than usual.

Weather Extremes. Under conditions of extremely adverse weather, the urgency of the movement of victims may supersede the priority of normal treatment, including immobilization.

Patient Noncompliance. One cannot overemphasize that if a patient cannot be persuaded to tolerate the placement of any immobilizer it is better not to use the device. A competent rescuer can do much to make a device comfortable by means of padding and reassurance. If this fails, however, immobilization that is applied by force is worse than no immobilization at all.

Equipment

CERVICAL EXTRICATION SPLINTS

There are almost as many variations of short spine boards as there are sizes of victims who will use them. A recently published study analyzed the performance of eight short spine boards and concluded that many were nonanalogous to one another and that strict comparison would be impossible.[30] However, some reasonable expectations of a good cervical extrication (CE) splint, considering its role in the field, can be specified.

During Application. The device should not produce jostling of a patient or change the position of the head, neck, shoulders, or torso during application by two rescuers who are competent in its use.

After Application. Used in conjunction with a good extrication collar that has been properly applied, a CE splint should *immobilize* the head and neck while the patient is being removed from the accident scene and until the patient can be fastened to an auxiliary stretcher, such as a long spine board, for further movement. This immobilization should effectively limit the lateral, flexion and extension, and rotational motions of the head and neck.

Once applied, a CE splint should not cause most patients

to be uncomfortable. An uncomfortable patient is likely to resist its placement, thus defeating its use in the first place. In addition, an extrication device is apt to be left on a patient for up to 2 hours after arrival in an emergency department.

If necessary, a CE splint should be removable from one patient *at the scene* for use in the extrication of another. Properly immobilized by means of a good collar, lateral stabilizers such as foam blocks and tape, and a full-body spine board, a patient should be able to tolerate this procedure in the supine position without adverse changes in position.

The device should be translucent on radiographs, visible but not obstructive. Simplicity of design should allow placement of the device by two technicians in less than 3 minutes in any situation, including darkness and rain, without causing manipulation of the head or neck.

General. The CE splint should take up as little space as possible around a patient, enabling rescuers to apply it in as many types of extrication situations as possible. Cost should be reasonable enough so that at least one device can be carried in every ambulance. Finally, it should be capable of repeated sanitation, whether by wiping the device with a disinfectant or by laundering it in hot water and detergent. Two devices meet all these criteria: the Kendrick extrication device (KED) and the Extrication Plus One (XP-1) (Figs. 62–14 and 62–15).

Kendrick Extrication Device. This snug-fitting, highly adaptable descendant of the military Neil-Robertson stretcher and the Timmons splints is truly designed around the principle of packaging a patient. The KED was developed by EMT-firefighter Rick Kendrick, of El Cajon, California, as a result of the frustration of rescuers with the difficulty of the removal of victims from wrecked race cars.

Properly applied, the KED is a phenomenal immobilizer that can be used under even the most adverse circumstances. Part of its anterior thoracic panels can be folded backward to accommodate the obese, pregnant, or pediatric patient.

The nylon loop behind the patient's head is continuous with the pelvic support straps. All five 5-cm belt buckles are made of polycarbonate plastic. The device is made of two layers of nylon mesh impregnated with plastic; these layers are sewn over 1 cm plywood slats, which act as stays.

Extrication Plus One. The XP-One is very similar to the KED, but it is designed to be used in conjunction with its own two-piece, Philadelphia-type, foam collar. Velcro is used to attach the collar into place by means of a pair of flaps that are part of the splint itself, providing an additional margin of rotational stability. A pair of Velcro shoulder straps engages the top thoracic strap, keeping the thoracic panels snug in the axillae, an important weight-bearing concept, although most of the patient's weight during lifting is borne by the pelvic straps.

The device is slightly more flexible vertically than the KED, to allow easier placement on patients in bucket seats; this flexibility disappears when the splint is wrapped around the patient's thorax. Two layers of ballistic nylon are sewn over an inner layer of 1 cm reinforced polyethylene foam.

FULL-BODY SPINAL IMMOBILIZERS

There are three basic classes of full-body spinal immobilizers, each with advantages and disadvantages.[22] It should be stressed that in the field it is more important for a rescuer to achieve results than to be particular about using one specific piece of equipment to do a given job, such as to immobilize the spine. This flexibility requirement is due to the immense variety of circumstances that can be encountered in the field and demands a rescuer who understands both the anatomy of patients and the capabilities and limitations of rescue equipment.

FULL-BODY SPINE BOARDS (BACKBOARDS)

Basically, backboards (Fig. 62–16) are either rectangular or tapered (like a coffin lid). The tapered, or Ohio type, is preferred by most rescuers, because it takes up less horizon-

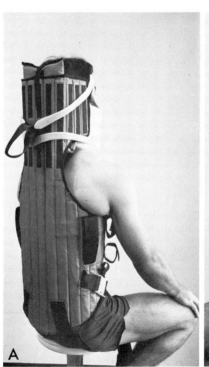
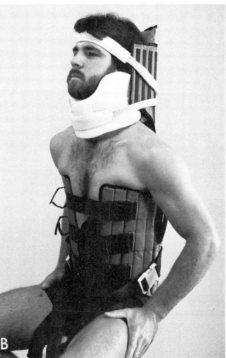

Figure 62–14. The Kendrick extrication device (KED). Note the presence of a cervical collar, applied before the KED (MediX-choice, 1946 John Towers Ave., El Cajon, CA 92020; from Dick T, Land R: Spinal immobilization devices. Part II: Cervical extrication devices. J Emerg Med Serv 8:25, 1983. Reproduced by permission.)

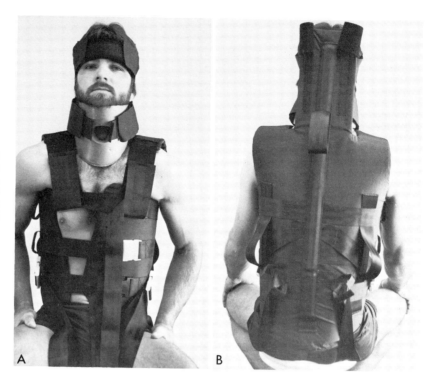

Figure 62–15. The XP-One (Extrication Plus One). The device is designed to be used with its own Philadelphia-type collar. (Med-spec, 4911 Wilmont Road, Charlotte, NC 28208; from Dick T, Land R: Spinal immobilization devices. Part II: Cervical extrication devices. J Emerg Med Serv 8:25, 1983. Reproduced by permission.)

tal room when angled into a narrow doorway (such as that of an automobile). In addition, the slight narrowing of these boards on either end of the recumbent patient tends to enhance the effectiveness of lateral immobilization via strapping.

Many boards also feature hardwood runners, usually about 1 inch thick, on their underside. These serve both as stiffeners and as spacers. They lift the board slightly off the ground so that rescuers can get their fingers under the board during lifting. The runners limit the effectiveness of a board when a patient lying on a hard surface for reason of space must be slid lengthwise onto the board rather than logrolled onto it.

Advantages of boards over full-body immobilizers are their ease of storage, their low cost and ready availability, and their extreme versatility. No single piece of rescue equipment can be used in as many ways. A victim can be slid out of an automobile onto a backboard (its most common application). Also, several boards can be used in conjunction with one another to form a chute to facilitate this process. Boards can be used to protect a victim during removal of a windshield. They can even be used in conjunction with

shoring jacks to help prevent cave-in when the patient is found in a ditch. Boards make good ramps in mud, good insulation against many electrical hazards, and improvised shelter during extrication in bad weather.

Disadvantages of boards as immobilizers are few, but two in particular are important. Board-like splints, as a class, are the least comfortable of all immobilizers. Discomfort can be overcome by means of appropriate use of padding (e.g., small rolled towels), especially in the occipital area. A further disadvantage of the backboard as an immobilizer, ironically, is one of its advantages: it is slippery and by itself provides only one-dimensional immobilization. For this reason, the backboard is an unstable carrying device and must be used cautiously with the addition of lateral support straps. Furthermore, when the immobilized patient must be carried, a backboard is normally used in conjunction with a stretcher.

SCOOP STRETCHERS

If a trauma victim has to be slid out of a tight location, a smooth backboard is probably the best immobilizer. If the victim is not in a tight location, the scoop stretcher is an ideal field immobilizer (Fig. 62–17). The scoop stretcher is comfortable, rigid, adaptable to patients of various lengths, and provides unobstructed radiographic transparency of the entire spine. If necessary, it can be almost instantly applied or removed without disturbing the position of the victim. The stretcher provides good lateral stability owing to the trough-like shape of its top surface. The device is also stable enough to be used for carrying purposes, although for the optimal protection of a potential spinal injury, the scoop stretcher should be placed on a backboard before moving the patient.

The scoop interferes slightly with the ischial ring of a half-ring traction splint but works well in conjunction with the Sager traction splint. The scoop has no adverse effect on any other immobilizers, however, or on cardiopulmonary resuscitation (CPR). In fact, it is probably the best way to move a CPR patient in the field. The Ferno-Washington

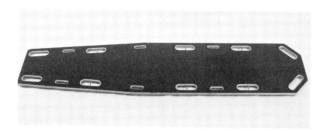

Figure 62–16. The Bound Tree spine board. An example of a commercial plywood backboard. (Bound Tree Corporation, EMS Products Division, 15 Bridge St., P.O. Box 401, Henniker, NH 03242; from Dick T, Land R: Spinal immobilization devices. Part III: Full spinal immobilizers. J Emerg Med Serv 8:34, 1983. Reproduced by permission.)

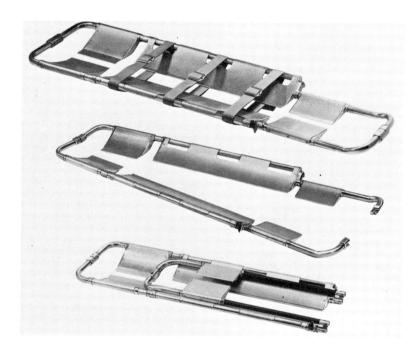

Figure 62–17. The Ferno-Washington Model 65 orthopedic (scoop) stretcher. (Ferno-Washington, Inc, 70 Weil Way, Wilmington, OH 45177-9371; from Dick T, Land R: Spinal immobilization devices. Part III: Full spinal immobilizers. J Emerg Med Serv 8:34, 1983. Reproduced by permission.)

Model 65 Scoop is the most widely accepted stretcher of this type.

FULL-BODY SPLINTS

There are various devices that take the concept of full-body immobilization one step further than the spine board. One such device, designed by Los Angeles County Fire Department paramedic Larry Miller in the mid-1970s, is a narrow spine board shaped like the human body, with handles on both long edges and a system of harnesses to provide immobilization. The Miller body splint, as it is called, consists of a polyethylene shell injected with a closed-cell foam that provides buoyancy in water and also acts as a stiffener (Fig. 62–18). The full-body splint features a removable head harness, a thoracic harness, and pelvic and lower extremity belts, all with ample amounts of Velcro closures. The space between its "lower extremities" facilitates

wrapping with bandage material in the event of fractures. In addition, it is shaped so that it can fit into a basket-type rescue stretcher such as the Stokes.

The Miller body splint is an excellent immobilizer; it is comfortable, firm and adaptable, as well as radiographically translucent. It can also be used as a water-rescue stretcher.

LATERAL NECK STABILIZERS

The Bashaw cervical immobilizer device, or CID, is a lateral neck stabilizer designed to be fastened quickly and easily to a scoop or spine board and then to a patient's head (Fig. 62–19). The CID is made of Herculite nylon and polyethylene foam; its pillows are fastened to a nylon platform by means of large Velcro interfaces. The platform is then fastened to the stretcher, either by elastic belts or by nonelastic belts with buckled closures.

The CID is a superb immobilizer, designed for field

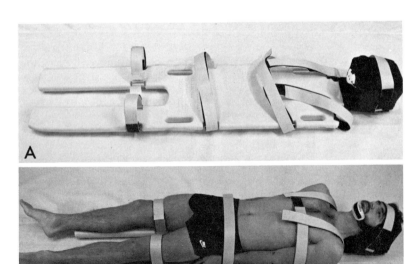

Figure 62–18. The Miller body splint. (Life Support Products, Inc., P.O. Box 19569, Irvine, CA 97213; from Dick T, Land R: Spinal immobilization devices. Part III: Full spinal immobilizers. J Emerg Med Serv 8:34, 1983. Reproduced by permission.)

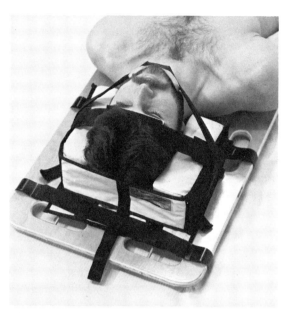

Figure 62–19. The Bashaw cervical immobilizer device (CID). (Bashaw Medical, Inc, 4909-B Mobile Highway, Pensacola, FL 32506; from Dick T, Land R: Spinal immobilization devices. Part III: Full spinal immobilizers. J Emerg Med Serv 8:34, 1983. Reproduced by permission.)

use. Sandbags, which have been used for this purpose for years, are an adaptation of an inhospital immobilizer. They work well on tabletops but, as previously mentioned, are no longer recommended for use in the field. An alternative to sandbags that has become very popular is the foam block. These are made of medium-density rubber, fashioned into 10-cm by 10-cm by 15-cm blocks. They have several advantages over sandbags in that they are lightweight, inexpensive,

disposable, and do not slip on the backboard. An additional advantage is that the patient's hearing is not impaired. More recently, cardboard devices have been developed to provide lateral stabilization (Fig. 62–20). They share the same advantages as the foam block.

Procedure

Once an extrication collar is in place, further spinal immobilization may be either difficult or relatively easy, depending on the situation in which rescuers find the patient and the equipment available. For purposes of discussion, we shall assume ideal circumstances.

Despite the presence of an extrication collar, manual cervical stabilization should be continued until the patient is fully immobilized, either in an extrication splint or on a full-body splint (such as a backboard). The rescue technique used depends on the patient's position of origin.

SITTING POSITION

Sitting patients are placed in an extrication splint by two (or possibly more) rescuers. They are then rotated into a position from which they can be laid in a supine position on a spine board, lateral immobilization can be applied, and they can be slid out of their environment onto a waiting cot that has been elevated to an appropriate level.

The extrication splint should be stored before use in such a way that its straps are secured in their individual retainers. This reduces the likelihood of their becoming tangled during application. When used, the device is opened up, butterfly-style, and gently slid behind the victim, with a rocking motion. If necessary, the patient can be very carefully rocked forward a few degrees, thus facilitating movement of the splint.

Once behind the victim, the splint's pelvic support straps should be freed from their retainers and allowed to dangle

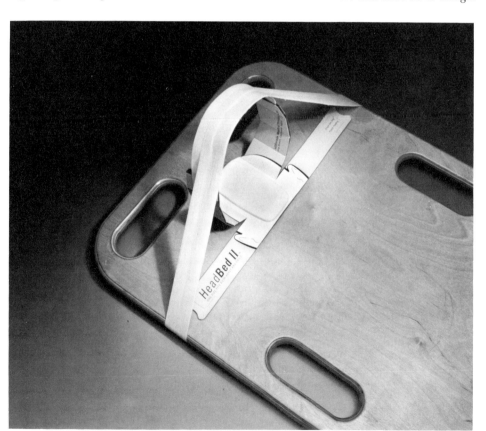

Figure 62–20. The HeadBed: a cervical immobilization device made of a water-resistant corrugated board. (California Medical Products, Long Beach, Calif. Reproduced by permission.)

at the patient's sides. These straps would otherwise be trapped by the splint. Next, the lateral thoracic panels are brought forward beneath the patient's shoulders. While grasping these panels, a rescuer *slides the splint upward until the top edges of the panels firmly engage the patient's axillae.*

Now the thoracic straps can be used to secure the splint, beginning with the middle strap, then the bottom strap, and lastly, the top strap. The straps should be fastened snugly but not tightly; all straps will be tightened slightly before the patient is moved.

In using either device, the pelvic support straps are those that are fastened next. They can be slipped, one at a time, beneath the patient's lower extremities, and *using a back-and-forth motion, they can be brought directly beneath the pelvis.* This is a key point. If the pelvic straps are not applied in this way, they allow considerable slippage when the patient is lifted. The free end of each of these straps mates with a buckle located approximately at the patient's hip on the outside of the splint. Once a strap is ready to be buckled, it can be attached either to the buckle on its own side or moved across the patient's lap and engaged with the opposite buckle. The latter method is preferred by most people, because it allows the patient's knees to remain together without discomfort to the patient. It should be noted that both methods work well.

Next, the head is fastened. When using the KED, the head panels are wrapped snugly around the head and neck by one rescuer while another rescuer applies the diagonal head straps. It may be necessary to place padding behind the head to maintain a neutral position. Care should be taken to not place so much padding as to position the head in front of the panels, rendering them ineffective. The forehead can be used as a point of engagement for one strap, and the cervical collar itself can be used for the other. The XP-One, on the other hand, has broad Velcro straps that are fastened to the splint and are stored rolled up. The bottom pair of straps directly engages the mating Velcro surfaces on the collar; these straps should be secured first. Next, the top pair of straps engages a removable forehead pad, which is secured with Velcro into place.

Lastly, all buckles should be tightened until the entire splint seems to be firmly in place. (It may be necessary to leave the top strap loose if the patient has any respiratory discomfort.)

The patient can now be moved. Neither the KED nor the XP-One is designed specifically for lifting, although lifting is an accepted means of using the splints to get a patient out of a vehicle. If the patient is to be lifted from a vehicle, the ambulance cot, with a spine board on it (all belts and blankets having been removed) is brought as close as possible to the patient. One rescuer then supports the patient by the patient's knees while the other rescuer uses the handholds on the splint, which are located beneath and slightly behind the axillae (on the outside surface of the splint).

It is usually preferable to rotate the patient if possible, and then to lay the patient in a supine position onto a backboard before removing the patient from the vehicle. Before the patient's hips are unflexed, the pelvic straps should be loosened or undone, because they tighten when the patient's thighs return to their anatomic positions.

The patient, who is now in a supine position on a board, can be slid carefully onto a waiting cot. Some type of lateral immobilizer should be applied for the head and neck, and the body should be belted into place on the board.

If for any reason rescuers strongly believe that the patient should be transported in a Fowler position, the long board may be waived and the patient placed on the cot without it. If the extrication splint causes the patient respi-

ratory discomfort, the thoracic straps may be loosened or undone. In addition, if the splint is needed to extricate another patient, it can be removed from the first patient, with manual stabilization applied to the neck until the first patient is fully immobilized on the spine board. Furthermore, if the patient has a flail segment of the chest wall, firm application of the splint may reduce discomfort, although adequate respiration must be ensured. (The splint may be fully unfastened and left beneath a patient to facilitate examination of the chest.)

In the course of any extrication maneuver, special care should be taken to examine the lower extremities to ensure that instability in those areas is not overlooked in the interest of spinal protection.

RECUMBENT POSITION

A patient who is found in a recumbent position should be placed in a supine position, if not already in one. If such repositioning is necessary, it would be worthwhile to examine the back in the process, if possible, which eliminates having to do so at a later time. Generally, having the victim in a supine position makes physical examination easier, makes transport more comfortable, and lends itself well toward the goals of immobilization and airway management.

Patients who are found lying in a supine position generally do not require the use of an intermediate immobilizer for the spine, such as an extrication splint. They should, however, receive initial immobilization by means of manual cervical stabilization and an extrication collar. After that, they are usually fastened to a full-body spinal immobilizer, such as a scoop stretcher, a backboard, or a full-body splint.

Scoop Stretcher. A patient who is in a supine position should be moved by means of a scoop stretcher if one is available and if space is not limited. This device is easily applied, is comfortable once in place, and provides more lateral support for the torso than any other device. Additional means are necessary to immobilize the head laterally. A scoop stretcher may be removed from beneath the patient, without disturbing the patient's position, after transport has taken place.

A scoop is applied as follows: Rescuers first explain to the patient that they are about to apply a scoop-type stretcher beneath his or her body, that the stretcher may be cold to the touch initially, and that it is important that the patient not move. One rescuer applies manual cervical stabilization, even with a collar in place. This stabilization should be maintained until the patient is completely secured to the stretcher. Another rescuer places the scoop on the ground next to the patient and opens the latches that regulate its length. The length should be adjusted so that approximately 2.5 cm or more of space is allowed at the patient's head and feet.

The latches that regulate the length of the device should then be engaged. Two more latches are located at either end of the stretcher; these should be released next, enabling rescuers to separate the two halves of the stretcher. One half is placed on each side of the patient. Next, one rescuer gently pushes half the stretcher under one side of the patient, making allowances at the head and feet, while another rescuer gently rocks the patient, not more than an approximately 1-cm elevation. Then the latch at the head end of the device is engaged. The same procedure takes place with the opposite half of the scoop until both halves are nearly beneath the patient. Now the foot-end latch can be engaged, completing the integrity of the stretcher. The patient can finally be strapped into place and the head immobilized with a pair of foam blocks and tape or any other suitable lateral neck stabilizer. The scoop stretcher is then lifted as a cot is rolled beneath the stretcher.

Whenever possible, a patient should be moved on wheels rather than carried, regardless of whether the patient is in the bed of a pickup truck, on a cot, or in an ambulance. This minimizes the possibility of a rescuer slipping in an oil spot or tripping on glass or other debris commonly found at accident scenes. The scoop stretcher should *not* be used when the patient is in an automobile or other cramped environment.

Full-Body Spine Boards (Backboards). A cramped environment from which the patient must be slid out is precisely the circumstance in which a backboard works best. There are three means of getting a patient onto a spine board; the method used depends on the amount and configuration of space available around the patient.

If movement is only possible lengthwise, as from an automobile seat, the patient may be slid, either footfirst or headfirst. Special care must be taken to ensure that rescuers move the patient by *pulling*, not by *pushing*. Traction minimizes the possibility that a spinal injury will accidentally be compressed.

The procedure should be explained to the patient. A cot is then brought as close to the vehicle as possible, in line with the move, at a level as close to or slightly below that of the patient. Oncoming traffic should be halted or kept at least two lanes away from the scene. One rescuer sits on the cot and keeps the end of the board from moving off the seat or doorsill of the automobile while another rescuer (preferably two rescuers) apply traction on the patient's body and slide the body onto the board. If the patient is being moved feetfirst, a third rescuer should be inside the car directing the rate of movement and managing the head and neck in a neutral position. Once the patient is completely on the board, the board is slid outward until it comes to rest on the cot.

If a patient is recumbent on the ground and a board is chosen as the means of movement, the patient can be logrolled onto it by at least three rescuers. The rescuers decide which way to roll the patient, and one rescuer takes a position at the patient's head. In addition to applying manual cervical stabilization, it will be this person's responsibility to oversee the move, watching the patient's overall body position.

The backboard is positioned next to the body. If one arm is injured, the backboard should be placed against this side, so that the patient can be rolled onto the uninjured extremity. The other rescuers take a position on the side that the patient will be rolled *toward* with one at the midchest and one by the legs. The rescuer at the chest should reach across the victim taking hold of the shoulder and hips while the other rescuer grasps the hips and lower legs. When everyone is ready, the rescuer at the head should give the command to roll the patient. The patient's back should be examined at this point. The backboard is then slid under the patient and when everyone is ready, the rescuer at the head gives the command to lower the patient onto the board. The patient should then be centered and securely strapped to the board. In securing the patient to the board, the body should be secured in place first, using a cross-strapping technique to secure the chest. Another strap is then placed across the legs. After the body has been secured to the board, the head can be secured. Padding should be placed under the occiput to maintain the head in neutral position. The head should then be secured using foam pads and 2-inch cloth tape, one piece across the forehead and one piece across the cervical collar. Note that this method of securing a patient to a backboard is designed for horizontal lifting only.

A patient who is recumbent on the ground can also be slid sideways onto a spine board; this is usually an improvised means and requires three or four rescuers, one of whom can maintain control of the patient's head and neck.

STANDING POSITION

The standing patient with a potential spine injury must be immobilized and placed in the supine position. One technique for placing these patients on a backboard that is quick, safe, and effective is presented here.[31] (Fig. 62–21). The tallest rescuer should be positioned behind the patient to manually stabilize the head while a second rescuer applies an extrication collar. The first rescuer must maintain manual cervical immobilization until the patient is completely secured to the board. The backboard should be centered behind the patient between the arms of the rescuer who is stabilizing the neck. Facing the patient, one rescuer on each side should each reach under the patient's arm and grab the backboard by a handhold at or above the patient's axillae. The patient's elbows are then brought closer to the body. If an additional rescuer is available, this rescuer should be positioned at the feet to prevent the board from sliding out, particularly on slippery floors. The patient should be slowly tilted back by lowering the head of the backboard. The rescuer at the head should step back during this process while maintaining the patient's head and neck in neutral alignment. When the backboard is completely horizontal the patient can be secured to the backboard in the normal fashion.

Complications

In general, complications are more likely to occur as a result of nonimmobilization of spinal injuries before movement than from immobilization. When complications do arise, they may be related to improper choice or use of equipment or ignorance of concomitant problems, or both.

Emergency medical technicians who are trained by qualified instructors to understand the pathophysiology of forces in trauma rather than to memorize rules of treatment are the best guarantee against complications involving equipment. Implicit in the former type of training is a thorough grasp of the capabilities and weaknesses of specific types of rescue equipment rather than an algorithmic approach to treatment, such as is used in cardiac resuscitation. The wide variation of situations that are encountered routinely in the field call for a practical-sense approach to orthopedics, more than in any other branch of field care.

Immobilization of the victim's spine can impair the rescuer's ability to manage or recognize other priorities such as airway patency, respiratory effort, patient comfort, or body position. Bauer and Kowalski[31a] and Walsh and coworkers[31b] report that excessive thoracic immobilization can compromise pulmonary function.

Victims are generally excessively belted in place on a spine board to prevent sliding during transport. If too few straps are used or if the straps are loosely applied, motion during transport becomes a problem. However, patients who are strapped too firmly in place have expressed extreme discomfort and even panic.

Once strapped into place, an unresponsive patient who vomits can be protected from aspiration in one of two ways. The traditional means is to logroll the patient, board and all, onto the left side and suction vigorously. No amount of strapping can keep this patient completely immobilized, however, and what actually takes place is that the spinal precautions are abandoned in favor of the airway. Another

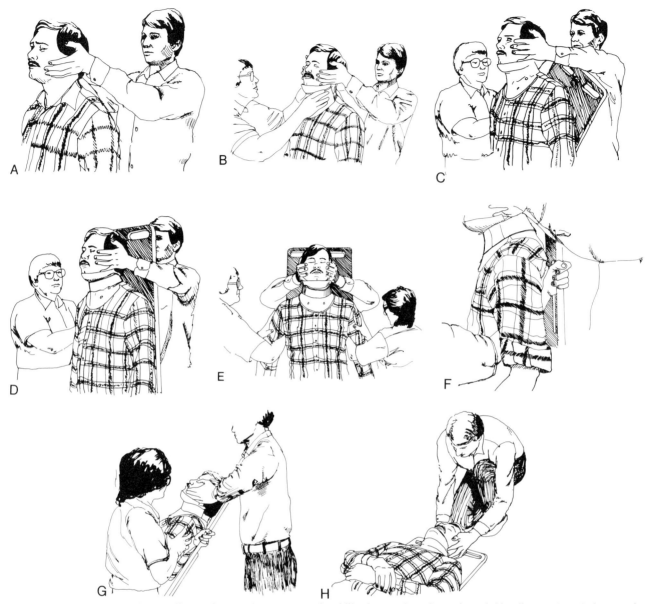

Figure 62–21. Backboarding the standing patient. *A,* Step 1: manual stabilization. *B,* Step 2: apply a rigid collar. *C,* Step 3: insert a long backboard. *D,* Step 4: center the backboard. *E,* Step 5: emergency medical technicians grasp the board. *F,* Use a handle higher than the patient's armpit. *G,* Step 6: slowly lower the patient. *H,* Step 7: fully immobilize the torso, then the head and neck. (From Elling R, Politis J: Backboarding the standing patient. J Emerg Med Serv 12:9, 1987. Reproduced by permission.)

means is to quickly raise the foot end of the board so that vomitus drains into the pharynx. If the patient takes a breath while in this position, assuming incomplete filling of the pharynx, he can inspire without aspirating. Meanwhile, suction can be used to remove any emesis from the pharynx. Spinal precautions are not usually affected with this head-down tilt maneuver.

Conclusion

The wide variety of circumstances in which a traumatized patient is likely to be involved mandates the need for many approaches to full-body spinal immobilization, before and during disentanglement. In general, however, an overall goal of rescuers is to fasten the victim to a board-like full-body immobilizer. After early application of an effective cervical extrication collar, this process involves the following steps:

1. Application of a cervical extrication device that serves to immobilize the cervical and thoracic spine as well as put the patient into a "package" for removal from the scene. This sort of device is used when the patient is first encountered in a confined environment, such as a wrecked automobile or bathtub. The device may have to be used for several patients at the scene.

2. Placement of the patient on a full-body spine board (also called a backboard), a scoop stretcher, or a factory-designed full-body immobilizer.

3. Application of lateral immobilization for the head. Traditionally, this has been done by means of placing sandbags on either side of the head and then taping them in place. Currently, there are factory-manufactured devices that are comfortable, lightweight, and much more effective in the field setting.

4. Use of straps to fasten the patient securely to the stretcher or splint. These straps may best be applied diagonally, rather than transversely, to provide longitudinal immobilization against forces acting on the victim during acceleration and deceleration of the transporting vehicle.

5. Placement of the immobilized patient into a rescue litter, such as a Stokes basket stretcher, if it is necessary to move the patient by foot, helicopter, or other special means before loading in an ambulance.

6. Clear, careful communication by rescuers to the receiving physician about the mechanism of injury, surrounding circumstances, and initial status of the patient, both before and after the disentanglement and immobilization process.

It should be remembered that rescuers may have to improvise or adapt extensively to circumstances that they encounter. The primary measure of success in field orthopedics is, therefore, the overall result, not the choice of equipment used or the rules that are followed in the process.

UPPER EXTREMITY SPLINTING

Fractures and dislocations of the upper extemity are extremely common injuries. A frequent cause of such injuries is a fall broken by landing on the outstretched arm.[32] Although upper extremity injuries are rarely immediately life threatening, it is important to assess and manage these injuries properly. Adequate care of a minor fracture or dislocation in addition to decreasing pain reduces the incidence of serious complications and the risk of permanent disability.

The prehospital care professional must never let obvious injuries to the extremities be a distraction to the care of more life-threatening injuries. In some situations, it may be necessary to rapidly secure the patient to a long backboard that supports and splints every bone and joint in one efficient step.[1] Injuries to nerves or vessels are a frequent complication of upper extremity injuries. It is critically important that circulation, motor function, and sensation distal to the injury be assessed early and monitored closely.

The purpose of splinting is to prevent motion of broken or dislocated bone ends. Carefully applied splints decrease pain while minimizing further damage to muscles, nerves, and blood vessels. Splinting also reduces the risk of converting a closed injury to an open one.[33]

Background

In the past, upper extremity injuries were managed using readily available materials such as wood and pieces of clothing. When possible, immobilization of the extremity to the torso was also used as an effective means of splinting. Although these older techniques have been supplanted by technical advances, the basic principles still apply.

Indications

Indications for splinting an extremity are usually clear. Pain with or without deformity following trauma should arouse suspicion for underlying bone or joint injury. Other signs include swelling, discoloration, deformity, crepitus, or loss of neurovascular function following trauma. The absence of these indications, however, does not always rule out a fracture or dislocation. Whenever a musculoskeletal injury is suspected, a prophylactic splint should be applied and maintained. The old axiom "if in doubt–splint" should always be followed.

Contraindications

There are no contraindications to splinting suspected upper extremity fractures or dislocations. However, in the setting of multisystem trauma with life-threatening injuries, rapid transport may be more important than extremity splinting. Loss of life takes precedence over loss of limb.

Equipment

Various splints are currently available for immobilizing upper extremity injuries. They can be divided into two basic types, rigid and soft.[1]

Rigid splints are made of many different materials including cardboard, plastic, aluminum, wire, and wood. These splints must be fastened to the injured extremity using tape, gauze, cravats, or Velcro straps. They are nonflexible and, when applied, immobilize the limb in a rigid fashion to maintain stability. Although some rigid splints are prepadded, many others require the use of cotton or some other soft material. When applying rigid splints, the fingertips should be left exposed so that circulation can be monitored.

Cardboard splints are excellent for long bone fractures of the upper arm. They can be formed into any desired shape and are inexpensive. Plastic, aluminum, wire, and wood splints, although less malleable, are also good choices.

Vacuum splints are a special type of rigid splint in which the air is evacuated from a closed bag containing tiny foam beads. This compresses the contents into a solid mass resulting in a rigid splint. The injury can be encased and immobilized in the position in which it is found, thereby minimizing patient discomfort. Flexibility of the splint prior to the removal of the air allows molding of the splint to conform to the patient's position. Vacuum splints do not apply pressure to the extremity and are radiolucent.

Soft splints are of two types: air splints and pillows, slings and swaths. Immobilization with pillows, slings, or swaths alone is usually inadequate, because they allow significant flexibility and motion. These splints are therefore most effective when used with some form of rigid device.

Air splints are soft splints that become rigid when inflated. In addition to providing immobilization, they help compress underlying soft tissue to reduce local hemorrhage. These devices are sensitive to differences in atmospheric pressure and temperature. Therefore, their inflation must be constantly monitored to ensure that the underlying tissue is not subject to pressure-induced ischemia. One study suggests a maximum splint pressure of 15 mm Hg to reduce the risk of ischemia.[34] With long ambulance transports, the splint should be deflated for a period of 5 minutes every 1½ hours.[32] A significant disadvantage is that pulses can no longer be monitored once the air splint is in place. Air splints are designed to conform to a specific shape when inflated and should not be used on angulated fractures. In addition to being radiolucent, some types can be inflated with a refrigerant to provide concurrent cooling.

Pillow splints can be fashioned from any soft bulky material and are excellent choices for hand, ankle, or foot injuries. These splints are extremely comfortable and can be easily applied.

Slings and swaths are usually used in combination with a rigid or soft splint. When used alone, they effectively immobilize injuries to the shoulder, clavicle, or humerus.

Procedures

To apply a splint properly to an injured extremity, several general rules must be followed. Communication is important to ensure that the patient understands what is being done at all times. If necessary, clothing should be removed to adequately visualize the injured extremity. Manual stabilization of the fracture site helps prevent further injury and avoid unnecessary movement. The neurovascular status (e.g., pulse, motor, and sensation) should be checked before and after the application of a splint. With a severely angulated extremity, traction, not to exceed 10 pounds of pressure, may be applied to reduce the deformity. If resistance or pain is encountered, the extremity should be splinted in the position found. Open wounds should be covered with a sterile dressing before applying a splint. The splint of choice (Table 62–4) is applied following the orthopedic principle of immobilizing the joint above and below a suspected fracture site. Local cooling and elevation of the injured area help reduce swelling. Following application of the splint, the neurovascular status should be reassessed. Deteriorating function should prompt assessment of the splint to determine if excess pressure is being applied.

RIGID SPLINTS

To apply a rigid splint, an assistant should provide support and gentle traction above and below the injury. The splint is then applied on the side of the extremity away from any open wounds. The splint should be large enough to immobilize the joint above and below a fracture or the bone above and below a dislocation. The splint should be well padded to reduce the risk of pressure necrosis. The splint is then secured to the extremity using gauze or tape (Fig. 62–22).

Vacuum splints are applied in much the same manner as other rigid splints. While an assistant stabilizes the injured site and applies traction, the splint should be wrapped around the extremity and secured with the attached straps. The air is then evacuated from the splint by means of a hand pump until the splint becomes rigid.

SOFT SPLINTS

Air splints are applied in two ways depending on whether the splint is equipped with a zipper. If the splint does not have a zipper, it must first be placed on the rescuer's arm until the bottom edge lies above the wrist. Next, while the rescuer grasps the hand of the patient's injured extremity, the rescuer's free hand provides support and gentle traction above the injury (Fig. 62–23). An assistant should then slide the splint onto the patient's arm (Fig. 62–24).

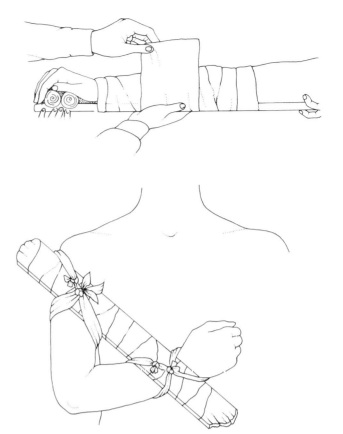

Figure 62–22. Examples of rigid splints.

After making sure that the splint is not wrinkled, it should be inflated until finger pressure makes a slight dent (Fig. 62–25). When using zippered air splints, the zipper should be positioned over the injury and inflation accomplished as discussed previously. With air splints that completely enclose the hand, distal circulation must be assessed by checking capillary refill at the nailbeds.

Pillow splints are applied by encasing the injury in the pillow and securing with tape, cravats, or gauze (Fig. 62–26). If possible, the nailbeds should remain exposed to allow for assessment of circulation.

To apply a sling, an assistant should support the injured arm in a flexed position across the patient's chest. The long edge of the triangular bandage should then be placed lengthwise along the patient's side opposite the injury with its tip over the uninjured shoulder (Fig. 62–27). The other tip is then brought over the injured shoulder to enclose the arm in the sling. The sling should be adjusted so that the arm rests comfortably with the hand higher than the elbow.

Table 62–4. Management of Specific Upper Extremity Orthopedic Injuries		
Site	**Injury**	**Suggested Immobilization Techniques**
Clavicle	Fracture	Sling and swath
Shoulder	Dislocation	Sling and swath, as it lies
Humerus	Fracture	Cardboard or vacuum splint with sling and swath
Elbow	Fracture or dislocation	Cardboard or vacuum splint as it lies
Forearm	Fracture	Cardboard, malleable metal, air, or vacuum splint with sling and swath
Wrist	Fracture	Pillow, cardboard, malleable metal, or vacuum splint applied in position of presentation
Hand	Fracture	Pillow splint in position of function
Finger	Fracture	Tongue depressor or small malleable metal splint

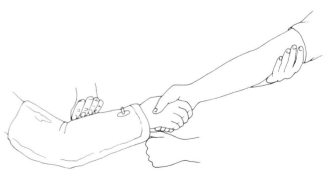

Figure 62–23. Application of an air splint.

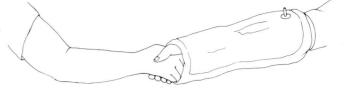

Figure 62–24. Application of an air splint. The assistant slides the splint onto the patient's arm.

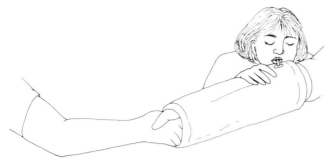

Figure 62–25. Inflating an air splint until finger pressure makes a slight dent.

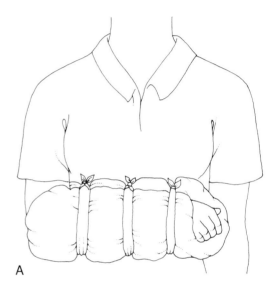

A

Figure 62–26. Hand (A) and foot (B) pillow splints.

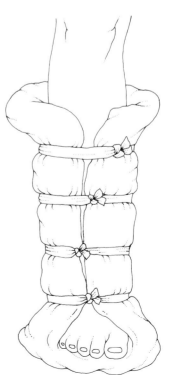

B

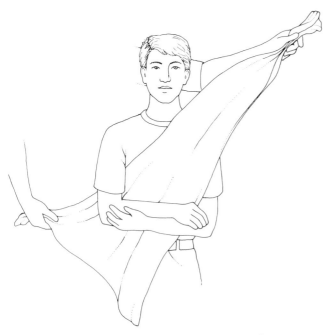

Figure 62–27. Application of a triangular bandage.

The sling is then tied together at the side of the neck, and the knot is padded for patient comfort. The point of the sling at the elbow should be drawn around to the front and pinned. With the sling properly applied, the patient's arm rests comfortably against the chest with the finger tips exposed (Fig. 62–28).

To apply a swath, one or two cravats should be placed under the uninjured arm and over the injured arm at the humerus. This should be done in a circumferential fashion to secure the injured extremity to the chest. The swath should fit snugly and be wide so as not to exert pressure (Fig. 62–29).

Complications

Potential complications of splinting include pressure necrosis, conversion of a closed injury into an open one, and loss of neurovascular function. With the use of air splints,

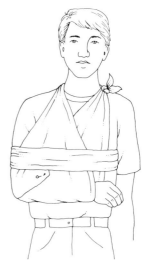

Figure 62–29. Sling with swath.

there is the additional risk of pressure-induced tissue ischemia and possible compartment syndrome.[34]

Conclusion

Injuries to the upper extremities, although not life threatening, can have significant immediate or long-term effects. A high index of suspicion for underlying neurovascular injury should always be maintained. Neurovascular status must be checked before and after application of splints and monitored continuously throughout transport.

LOWER EXTREMITY SPLINTING

Many of the principles and techniques discussed with upper extremity splinting can also be applied to injuries of the lower extremity (Table 62–5). In addition, the pneumatic anti-shock garment (PASG) is an effective splint for such injuries. Prolonged use of this device is discouraged to reduce the risk of developing a compartment syndrome.[35] The following discussion is limited to lower extremity traction splinting.

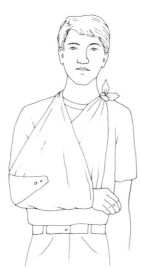

Figure 62–28. Completed triangular bandage.

Table 62–5. *Management of Specific Lower Extremity Orthopedic Injuries*

Site	Injury	Suggested Immobilization Techniques
Pelvis	Fracture	Pneumatic anti-shock garment (PASG), long backboard
Hip	Fracture	Traction splint, long backboard or secure injured leg to uninjured leg
	Dislocation	Long backboard with limb supported by pillows
Femur	Fracture	Traction splint or PASG
Knee	Fracture or dislocation	Cardboard or vaccum splint in position found
Tibia/Fibula	Fractures	Cardboard, air, or vacuum splint
Ankle	Fracture or dislocation	Pillow or air splint
Foot	Fracture	Pillow or air splint
Toe	Fracture	Tape to adjacent toe

Background

Since World War I, when the Thomas full-ring (later to become a half-ring) traction splint was popularized for prehospital use, extremity traction for femur fractures has been an important aspect of prehospital orthopedic care. In fact, the splint devised by Sir Hugh Owen Thomas was credited with decreasing the mortality rate associated with fractures of the femur from 80 to 14 per cent during that period. Since then, several modifications of the traction splints carry the names of their inventors (Glenn Hare, Joseph Sager, Dr. Allen Klippel) and have encouraged further refinements.

Indications and Contraindications

Application of a lower extremity traction splint is indicated whenever a fractured femur is encountered. The use of traction in these injuries helps limit hemorrhage by decreasing the potential space available for accumulation of blood in the thigh.[36] A femur fracture is clinically suspected when there is shortening, angulation, crepitus, swelling, or ecchymosis of the thigh in conjunction with pain.

There is some controversy regarding the merit of applying traction to an open femur fracture. Concern has been expressed that standard traction will retract the bone fragments back into the tissue before adequate operative débridement can be accomplished. One workable compromise is to use the device to apply sufficient traction to provide stabilization without actually retracting the bony fragments into the tissues. Alternatively, a vacuum (beanbag splint) could be substituted to immobilize the bony fragments in the position of presentation. In any case, stabilization of the fracture site to prevent further hemorrhage, neurovascular damage, and soft tissue injury should take precedence over the theoretic risk of increased contamination, which could subsequently be managed surgically.

Equipment

This discussion is limited to several of the popular types of lower extremity traction splints. A comparison of these traction splints is provided in Figure 62–30.[37] With the exception of the Sager splint, the traction splints produce flexion at the hip joint because of their half-ring design. This flexion of up to 30 degrees does not allow complete

Figure 62–30. Comparison of traction splints. (From Dick T: Traction splinting: A comparative look at the tools of the trade. J Emerg Med Serv 6:26, 1981. Reproduced by permission.)

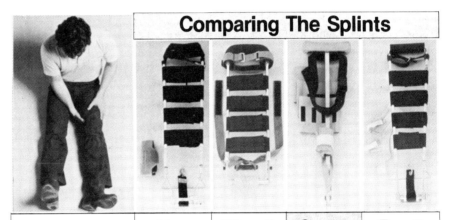

Comparing The Splints

	Hare	Klippell	Sager	Trac 3
1. Weight (± 1 lb.)	7	9	3	6
2. Maximum Extremity Length (measurements in inches)	44½	45	41*	44
3. Minimum Extremity Length	27	31¼	21*	25
4. Maximum Extremity Width	7	7½	Not Limited	4
5. Overhang (Splint past Sole)	7½	1½	7*	9
6. Splint Sizes Avail.	2	1	1	2
7. Harness Sizes Avail. For Ankle	5	1	1	3
8. Ischial Bar Height (Bottom of pad to Top of Bar)	2½	1¼	0	1-5/8
9. Case Provided?	Yes	Yes	Yes	No
10. Pede Version Avail.	Yes	No	(1 size fits all)	Yes
11. Advertised Price	189.00	165.00	185.00	174.95
12. Smallest Stored Size L/W/Thickness	36/15/4	39/12/2	30/11/2	36/9¼ 4¼

*The Sager ankle hitch now in use with the Sager traction splint was not available at the time this study was made. The new adjustable ankle hitch changed the following figures: *Maximum Extremity Length 46" *Minimum Extremity Length 18½" *Overhang of splint past sole, 5½" at 15 lbs. traction.

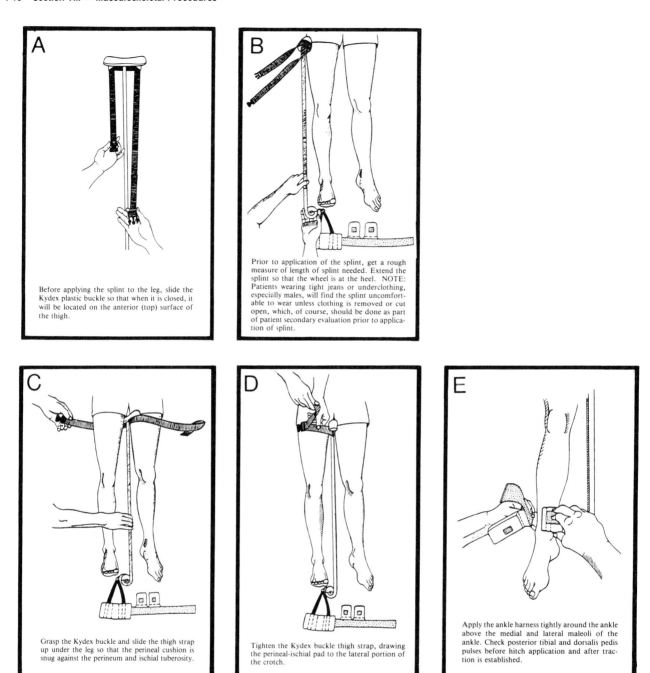

Figure 62–31. Application of the Sager emergency traction splint. *A–J*, Standard application. *K–N*, Application on the outside of the leg. *O–Q*, Application of the bilateral splint.

fracture alignment unless the patient is in a reclining position or the lower extremity is elevated.[38]

Procedure

The application of a traction splint device to an extremity with a femur fracture requires careful attention to associated soft tissue injuries. In particular, the presence of distal pulses and capillary refill must be assessed before and after the application of the device. The loss of pulses with the application of a traction splint requires that the position of strap application and the amount of applied traction be reassessed.

Whenever possible, the splinting procedure should be explained to the patient. There is always pain associated with the application of a traction splint, but the patient should be reassured that the resultant stabilization of the fracture helps to diminish the pain. When possible, the area of injury should be exposed. Open fractures should be managed as discussed previously. If the injured leg is markedly deformed, it should first be straightened using manual traction and maintained in that position by an assistant until mechanical traction has been applied.

If the splint has an adjustable bar, the noninjured extremity can be used for length adjustment. The splint should extend approximately 25 to 30 cm beyond the heel. With the extremity slightly elevated, the half-ring splint is

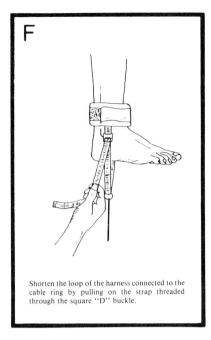

Shorten the loop of the harness connected to the cable ring by pulling on the strap threaded through the square "D" buckle.

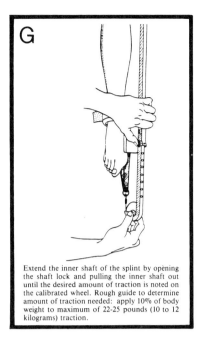

Extend the inner shaft of the splint by opening the shaft lock and pulling the inner shaft out until the desired amount of traction is noted on the calibrated wheel. Rough guide to determine amount of traction needed: apply 10% of body weight to maximum of 22-25 pounds (10 to 12 kilograms) traction.

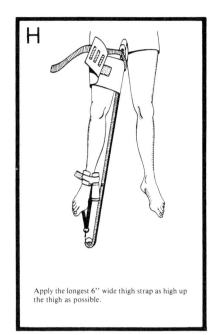

Apply the longest 6'' wide thigh strap as high up the thigh as possible.

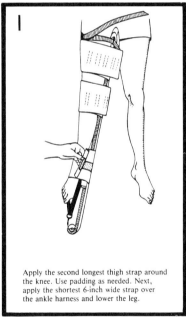

Apply the second longest thigh strap around the knee. Use padding as needed. Next, apply the shortest 6-inch wide strap over the ankle harness and lower the leg.

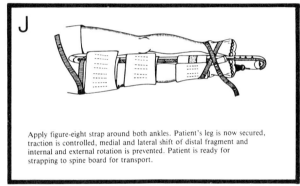

Apply figure-eight strap around both ankles. Patient's leg is now secured, traction is controlled, medial and lateral shift of distal fragment and internal and external rotation is prevented. Patient is ready for strapping to spine board for transport.

Figure 62–31 *Continued*

Illustration continued on following page

placed under the injured leg and brought firmly against the ischial tuberosity. The Sager device is either placed against the symphysis pubis or positioned laterally against the greater trochanter of the femur. When the padded end of the splint is placed in the crotch of male patients, care should be taken to move the genitalia out of the way. The thigh strap is now firmly secured.

An ankle harness is then placed about the ankle above the medial and lateral malleoli. The harness is attached to the distal end of the traction device, and traction is applied gradually. For the Sager device, the inner shaft of the splint is extended by opening the shaft lock and pulling the inner shaft out until the desired amount of traction is noted on the calibrated wheel at the distal end of the splint (Fig. 62–31). Approximately 10 per cent of body weight to a maximum of 22 to 25 pounds (10 to 12 kg) is adequate traction. The Hare traction splint uses a ratchet mechanism to apply traction to the ankle strap. The Klippel pulsion splint uses a foot plate to strap the foot down; traction is applied by adjusting the length of the splint. After application of traction, distal neurovascular status should be rechecked. Before transport, supportive straps about the thigh, knee, and distal leg should be applied to vertically stabilize the extremity.

Removal of a traction splint should be performed in reverse order of application and should follow basic stabilization of the patient. The traction splint should be replaced by definitive stabilization of the fracture at that time.

APPLICATION
ON THE OUTSIDE OF THE LEG

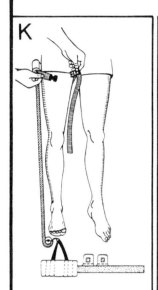

K

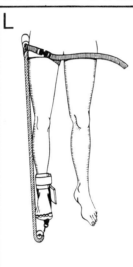

L

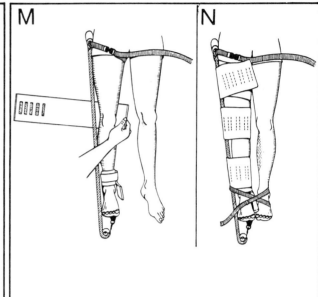

M   **N**

Application of Sager Splint on the outside of thigh is appropriate if perineal injuries or pelvic fractures are encountered. Carry out steps 1 and 2, then apply the splint on the outside of the leg as noted.

Leave the Kydex buckle thigh strap loose so that it makes a sling around the upper thigh and forms an angle of about 55 degrees with the shaft of the splint. Pad the strap as needed.

Apply the thigh straps in sequence, adding figure-eight strap as last step prior to securing the patient on the sping board.

APPLICATION OF THE BILATERAL
SPLINT

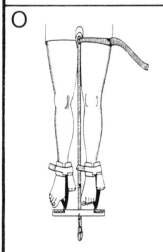

O

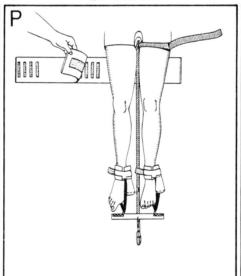

P

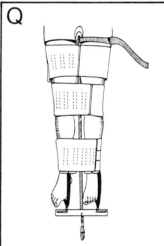

Q

Application of double splint is accomplished in same manner as with the single splint. Modify step 2 by lengthening splint so that the harness bar is adjacent to the patient's heels.

Apply the 6'' wide thigh straps, hooking together more than one thigh strap to give you a proper length to wrap strap around both thighs.

Apply all three sections of leg strapping to secure the legs together. A figure-eight strap may be used around ankles and feet, if needed.

Figure 62–31 *Continued*

Special Considerations

The traction splints in common usage can be applied before application of the PASG. Except for the Sager splint, however, the application of a PASG over a traction splint is awkward and associated with an uneven pressure distribution under the PASG. The Sager splint has the additional advantage that it can be applied *after* application of the PASG as well as before PASG application.

Unless the patient is found in a hazardous environment (e.g., extremely cold surroundings), the shoe on the injured extremity should be removed before splinting so that pulses can be evaluated. Furthermore, change in color, temperature, and pulses distal to the injury can subsequently be monitored en route to the hospital. The shoe can be removed by cutting only the shoelace, then simply pulling forward on the tongue of the shoe. The underlying sock can be removed with scissors. Exposure of the noninjured foot permits comparison of the extremities.

Complications

Complications are generally the result of incorrect application of the device. If the neurovascular status is checked frequently, ischemia should not result from use of the splint. The key to traction application is stabilization of the fracture. Once the fracture site is stabilized, additional traction is unnecessary and potentially dangerous.

REFERENCES

1. Campbell JE (ed): Basic Trauma Life Support. Englewood Cliffs, NJ, Robert J. Brady Co/Prentice-Hall, Inc, 1988, pp 120–132, 151–173.
2. Toscano J: Prevention of neurological deterioration before admission to a spinal cord injury unit. Paraplegia 26:143, 1988.
3. Podolosky S, Baraff LJ, Simon RR, et al: Efficacy of cervical spine immobilization methods. J Trauma 23:461, 1983.
4. Sumchai AP: Prehospital management of cervical spine injuries. CPRT Dispatch 11:5, 1988.
5. Sumchai AP, Sternbach GL, Laufer M: Cervical spine traction and immobilization. Topics Emerg Med 10:9, 1988.
6. Farrington JD: Death in a ditch. Bull Am Coll Surg 52:121, 1967.
7. Farrington JD: Extrication of victims: Surgical principles. J Trauma 8:493, 1968.
8. Bivins HB, Ford S, Bezmalinovic Z, et al: The effect of axial traction during orotracheal intubation of the trauma victim with an unstable cervical spine. Ann Emerg Med 17:25, 1988.
9. Barron MM: Cervical spine injury masquerading as a medical emergency. Am J Emerg Med 7:54, 1988.
10. Dick T: Horse sense: Immobilizing necks that do not fit collars. J Emerg Med Serv 7:23, 1982.
11. Dick T: Are your collars raising intracranial pressure? J Emerg Med Serv 11:28, 1986.
12. Dick T, Land R: Spinal immobilization devices, part 1: Cervical extrication collars. J Emerg Med Serv 7:26, 1982.
13. Dick T: Best in the business: The new StifNeck collar. J Emerg Med Serv 10:51, 1985.
14. Karbi OA, Caspari DA, Tator CH: Extrication, immobilization and radiological investigation of patients with cervical spine injuries. Can Med Assoc J 139:617, 1988.
15. Aprahamian C, Thompson BM, Finger WA, et al: Experimental cervical spine injury model: Evaluation of airway management and splinting techniques. Ann Emerg Med 13:584, 1984.
16. Cline JR, Scheidel E, Bigsby EF: A comparison of methods of cervical immobilization used in patient extrication and transport. J Trauma 25:649, 1985.
17. McCabe JB, Nolan DJ: Comparison of the effectiveness of different cervical immobilization devices. Ann Emerg Med 15:50, 1986.
18. Graziano AF, Scheidel EA, Cline JR, et al: Radiographic comparison of prehospital cervical immobilization methods. Ann Emerg Med 16:1127, 1987.
18a. Solot JA, Winzelberg GG: Clinical and radiological evaluation of Vertebrace extrication collars. J Emerg Med 8:79, 1990.
19. Herzenberg JE, Hensinger RN, Dedrick DK, et al: Emergency transport and positioning of young children who have an injury of the cervical spine. J Bone Joint Surg 71A:15, 1989.
20. Huerta C, Griffith R, Joyce SM: Cervical spine stabilization in pediatric patients: Evaluation of current techniques. Ann Emerg Med 16:1121, 1987.
21. Blum FC: Manual immobilization (letter). Ann Emerg Med 18:427, 1989.
22. Dick T, Land R: Spinal immobilization devices. Part 3: Full spinal immobilizers. J Emerg Med Serv 8:34, 1983.
23. McGuire RA, Neville S, Green BA, et al: Spinal instability and the log-rolling maneuver. J Trauma 27:525, 1987.
24. Kossuth L: The removal of injured personnel from wrecked vehicles. J Trauma 5:703, 1965.
25. Committee on Emergency Medical Services, Division of Medical Sciences, National Academy of Sciences: Medical requirements for ambulance design and equipment. Pamphlet (September 1968).
26. Committee on Trauma, American College of Surgeons: Minimal equipment for ambulances. Bull Am Coll Surg 52:92, 1967.
27. Klippel A, Conrad M: A compact multipurpose spine board. Bull Am Coll Surg 54:362, 1969.
28. Grant H, Murray R, Bergeron DJ: Emergency Care. Bowie, Md, Robert J. Brady Co/Prentice-Hall, Inc, 1971.
29. Committee on Injuries, American Academy of Orthopedic Surgeons: Emergency care and transportation of the sick and injured. Menasha, Wis, George Banta Co, 1971.
30. Dick T, Land R: Spinal immobilization devices. Part 2: Cervical extrication devices. J Emerg Med Serv 8:23, 1983.
31. Elling R, Politis J: Backboarding the standing patient. J Emerg Med Serv 12:64, 1987.
31a. Bauer D, Kowalski R: Effect of spinal immobilization devices on pulmonary function in the healthy, nonsmoking man. Ann Emerg Med 17:915, 1988.
31b. Walsh M, Grant T, Mickey S: Lung function compromised by spinal immobilization. Ann Emerg Med 19:615, 1990.
32. Alvero EM: Life on a limb: Management of upper extremity injuries. J Emerg Serv Med 13:42, 1988.
33. Worsing RA: Principles of prehospital care of musculoskeletal injuries. Emerg Med Clin 2:205, 1984.
34. Christensen KS, Trautner S, Stockel M, et al: Inflatable splints: Do they cause tissue ischemia? Injury 17:167, 1986.
35. Christensen KS: Pneumatic antishock garments (PASG): Do they precipitate lower-extremity compartment syndromes? J Trauma 26:1102, 1986.
36. Borschneck AG: Why traction? J Emerg Med Serv 10:44, 1985.
37. Dick T: Traction splinting: A comparative look at the tools of the trade. J Emerg Med Serv 6:26, 1981.
38. Borschneck AG, Wayne MA: Sager emergency traction splint: A new splinting device for lower limb fractures. Emerg Med Tech J 4:42, 1980.

Chapter 63

Helmet Removal

Jerris R. Hedges

INTRODUCTION

Although originally developed for protection of the head during combat, helmets are most commonly seen on injured football players and motorcyclists. The protective value of a helmet in reducing cerebral injury has been well documented for motorcyclists.[1, 2] The modern helmet is designed to tightly conform to the head. Interestingly, the modern helmet has protected the cranium so well that some football players have adopted the ill-advised technique of "spearing" an opponent with their helmets. This practice has been associated with cervical spine injuries.[3] Increasing use of the helmet in other sports (e.g., ice hockey, kayaking, and lacrosse) and by bicyclists and moped riders will further increase the frequency of appearance and spectrum of injuries that emergency physicians will evaluate in patients with helmets. One report suggests that atlanto-occipital disruptions and C_1-ring fractures are more likely to occur with blows to the head when a motorcycle or moped rider is wearing a helmet.[4]

Careless removal of the helmet may exacerbate a preexisting cervical spine injury. In 1980, the American College of Surgeons endorsed the helmet removal technique that is discussed in this chapter.[5]

INDICATIONS AND CONTRAINDICATIONS

Helmet removal in the prehospital area is rarely needed. Removal *is* indicated when the following conditions cannot be met with the helmet in place: airway control, cervical spine stabilization, and control of hemorrhage. Most motorcycle helmets have detachable or movable face masks that permit airway access in normal situations. Extrication bolt cutters (or preferably a screwdriver, if time permits) can be used to remove the "cage" face guard from football helmets. Cervical spine immobilization can usually be adequately maintained with the helmet in place using tape, lateral foam blocks (or intravenous bags), and a backboard, although some of the newer immobilization devices (e.g., the cervical immobilization device) require prior removal of the helmet. Uncontrollable hemorrhage within the helmet cavity is rarely a problem because of the helmet's intrinsic protection of the cranium.

In the emergency department, removal of the helmet is indicated for a thorough head and neck examination, radiologic (including computed tomography) examination of the head and neck, and application of cervical tongs for traction. Obviously, when the helmet does not interfere with airway management, neck stabilization, or control of hemorrhage, removal of the helmet can be delayed by the emergency physician until the primary trauma survey and initial resuscitative measures have been undertaken.

Contraindications to helmet removal are lack of familiarity with the technique of removal, insufficient assistance (at least two persons are needed), and the need to provide higher priority tasks. As the rapid transport of injured patients from the prehospital phase to the hospital is stressed, the desirability of helmet removal in the prehospital situation will receive greater scrutiny.

PROCEDURE

The key to helmet removal is cervical immobilization.[5] At the outset, before releasing the patient's chin strap, firm in-line axial stabilization should be applied to the neck (Fig. 63–1). Vigorous in-line *traction* is to be avoided, to minimize the risk of subluxation or distraction of the unstable cervical spine.[6] The neck is then further stabilized by an assistant who places one hand on the anterior neck to support the mandible and the other hand posterior to the neck. The assistant can maintain an open airway by using the jaw thrust maneuver. Although a one-person technique of helmet removal has been described,[7] it is best for two people to remove the helmet, especially in the setting of an unconscious or uncooperative patient.

A folded sheet or jacket behind the patient's shoulders helps limit cervical motion during helmet removal.[7] The physician, situated cephalad to the patient, releases the chin strap while applying longitudinal traction on the base of the helmet. The helmet base is simultaneously spread apart, and the lateral aspects are sequentially pulled over each ear to remove the helmet while traction is continued. The helmet may also need to be tilted backward to clear the nose. After helmet removal, the spine is again immobilized while the assistant maintains the manual cervical stabilization.

Aprahamian and coworkers recommend the use of a cast-cutter saw to bivalve the helmet in the coronal plane.[8] Following division of the helmet shell, the foam packing material of the helmet must also be cut with a scalpel or other sharp blade. Although this approach does provide one method of removing the helmet, the potential spinal injury that might result from intense vibrations during use of the cast cutter is unknown. Furthermore, the technique destroys an expensive helmet and dulls the cast-cutter blade, rendering the blade useless for further cast cutting.

COMPLICATIONS

Although no controlled studies have proved this technique of helmet removal to be superior over other techniques, this technique is consistent with the current consensus policy of maintaining continuous in-line cervical stabilization when cervical spine injury is suspected. Furthermore, the lateral flexion and extension motion that is common with patient-initiated helmet removal is minimized.

CONCLUSION

Helmet removal is a skill that is easily learned. As more rapid transport from the prehospital area to the hospital is emphasized, more emergency physicians will be confronted with the helmeted patient. Helmet removal is necessary for a thorough examination, although initial resuscitative measures may take precedence over helmet removal.

REFERENCES

1. Luna GK, Copass MK, Oreskovitch MR, et al: The role of helmets in reducing head injuries from motorcycle accidents: A political or medical issue? West J Med 135:89, 1981.
2. Bachulis BL, Sangster W, Gorrell GW, et al: Patterns of injury in helmeted and nonhelmeted motorcyclists. Am J Surg 155:709, 1988.
3. Torg JS, Vegso JJ, Sennett B, et al: The national football head and neck injury registry: 14-year report on cervical quadriplegia, 1971 through 1984. JAMA 254:3439, 1985.
4. Krantz KPG: Head and neck injuries to motorcycle and moped riders: With special regard to the effect of protective helmets. Injury 16:253, 1985.
5. McSwain NE Jr: Techniques of helmet removal from injured patients. Bull Am Coll Surg 65:20, 1980.
6. Bivins HG, Ford S, Bezmalinovic Z, et al: The effect of axial traction during orotracheal intubation of the trauma victim with an unstable cervical spine. Ann Emerg Med 17:25, 1988.
7. Meyer RD, Daniel WW: The biomechanics of helmets and helmet removal. J Trauma 25:329, 1985.
8. Aprahamian C, Thompson BM, Darin JC: Recommended helmet removal techniques in a cervical spine injured patient. J Trauma 24:841, 1984.

Helmet Removal from Injured Patients

1

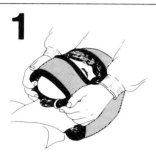

One rescuer applies inline traction by placing his or her hands on each side of the helmet with the fingers on the victim's mandible. This position prevents slippage if the strap is loose.

2

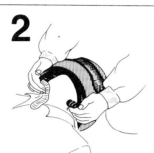

The rescuer cuts or loosens the strap at the D-rings while maintaining inline traction.

3

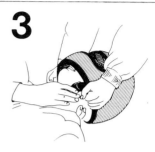

A second rescuer places one hand on the mandible at the angle, the thumb on one side, the long and index fingers on the other. With his other hand, he applies pressure from the occipital region. This maneuver transfers the inline traction responsibility to the second rescuer.

4

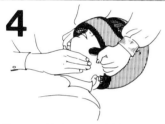

The rescuer at the top removes the helmet. Three factors should be kept in mind.

• The helmet is egg-shaped, and therefore must be expanded laterally to clear the ears.
• If the helmet provides full facial coverage, glasses must be removed first.
• If the helmet provides full facial coverage, the nose will impede removal. To clear the nose, the helmet must be tilted backward and raised over it.

5

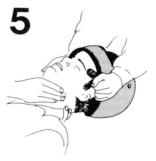

Throughout the removal process, the second rescuer maintains inline traction from below in order to prevent head tilt.

6

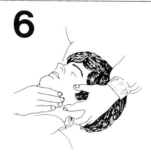

After the helmet has been removed, the rescuer at the top replaces his hands on either side of the victim's head with his palms over the ears.

7

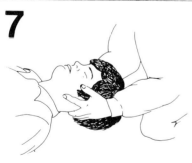

Inline traction is maintained from above until a backboard is in place.

Summary
The helmet must be maneuvered over the nose and ears while the head and neck are held rigid.
• Inline traction is applied from above.
• Inline traction is transferred below with pressure on the jaw and occiput.
• The helmet is removed.
• Inline traction is re-established from above.

American College of Surgeons Committee on Trauma, July 1980

Figure 63–1. Helmet removal technique. (From McSwain N: Techniques of helmet removal from injured patients. Bull Am Coll Surg 65:20, 1980. Reproduced by permission.)

Chapter 64

Management of Amputations

William C. Dalsey

INTRODUCTION

"Injury occurs to the hand more frequently than to any other part of the body and the first person caring for an injured hand will probably determine the ultimate stage of its usefulness."[1] Rapid and appropriate emergency care of a patient with an amputated part is crucial to the salvage and preservation of function. This chapter discusses the acute care of amputated parts before they are replanted and specifically addresses the management of distal digit amputations and dermal "slice" wounds.

Amputation may be partial or complete. Injuries with interconnecting tissue between the distal and proximal portions, even if there is only a small piece of bridging skin, are technically considered incomplete, or partial, amputations. Complete amputations are replanted, whereas partial amputations are revascularized. This distinction is arbitrary; for emergency physicians, treatment for both injuries is very similar. The prognosis and outcome of partial and complete amputations are similar, although partial amputations often have better venous and lymphatic drainage, and functional recovery may be more complete if there is less anatomic damage.

The peak incidence of traumatic amputations occurs between the ages of 20 and 40 years,[2, 3] and men predominate over women at a ratio of 4:1. Local crush injuries are the most common mechanism of injury, and sharp guillotine amputations are the least common.[1-7] Partial amputations occur as often as total amputations.[8] Power saws and lawn mowers are frequently the instruments of destruction.[8] Proximal amputations are less common than distal amputations.

The media have exaggerated somewhat the success of replantation and have often generated unrealistic expectations from the public. The technical limitations of successfully repairing vessels that are less than 0.3 mm in diameter usually preclude replantation of digits distal to the distal interphalangeal joint.[9] Successful revascularization of amputated parts often ensures viability, but neurologic, osseous, and tendinous healing are critical for ultimate function. If there is incomplete neurologic recovery, limited range of motion, and intolerance to cold, the replanted part may have little functional value for the patient. Rehabilitation from replantation surgery may be prolonged, often requiring more than 1 year and repeated surgical procedures. The emergency physician should be aware of limitations of replantation surgery and should not encourage unrealistic expectations in injured patients or their families.

BACKGROUND

The possibility of restoring viability and function to traumatically severed parts has fascinated physicians for centuries. Physicians have attempted to replant parts with little more than a few sutures and secure bandaging and occasionally have had spectacular results. One of the earliest medical reports is by Fiorvanti, who in 1570 reported the successful replantation of a soldier's nose, which was severed by a saber, after first cleansing it with urine and then carefully bandaging it.[10, 11] In 1814, Balfour reported the successful replantation of a finger, which was severed by a hatchet,[12] using only meticulous alignment and secure bandaging. The ability to consistently replant amputated parts awaited the development of modern microvascular surgical techniques. The first reported successful upper limb replantation was by Malt and McKhann in 1962.[13] Later that year, a successful replantation of a hand and arm was reported by Chen Zhang Wei.[14] Developments in microsurgical techniques, advanced optics, and microsurgical instruments have created the ability to consistently replant amputated parts with a high degree of success. Since 1965, when Kleinert and Kasdan reported the first successful microvascular anastomosis of a digital vessel,[15] there have been several large series of replantations, with success rates ranging from 70 to 90 per cent.[4, 8, 16-28] To the original pioneers in replant surgery, survival of the replanted tissue was the criterion for success, but with further refinements, today's surgeons emphasize functional recovery as well as viability. The replantation of a part that is painful or useless or that interferes with function is a disservice to the patient and is less desirable than early restoration of function without replantation.

INDICATIONS

Preservation of the amputated part is generally indicated when replantation or revascularization is a potential therapeutic method for care of the injured part. Revascularization and reanastomosis of partially and completely amputated parts should be provided when there is hope of preservation or restoration of function. Aesthetic considerations, patient avocations, and occasionally religious or social customs may also influence the decision to proceed with surgery.[29-31] Ultimately, the decision must be reached by both the operating microsurgical team and the patient after a rational explanation of potential results and successes.

Indications for replantation of fingers and hands have been proposed and are generally accepted, although they should not be applied rigidly to all circumstances. Successful functional recovery is more likely in distal than in proximal extremity amputations and in multidigit amputations, single-digit thumb amputations, or transmetacarpal amputations.[32, 33] Generally these are indications for replantation (Table 64–1). Single digits proximal to the distal interphalangeal joint and distal to the flexor digitorum superficialis may be replanted successfully with good functional recovery.

Successful replantations have been reported in patients from the ages of 1 to 84 years.[34, 35] There are no fixed age limits for replantation, although particularly good results have been reported in children owing to their regenerative capacity and adaptability to rehabilitation.[3, 36-40] The decision to replant is made on a case-by-case basis by the microsurgical team, which must weigh all the factors involved.

Table 64–1. Replantation of the Amputated Extremity

Indications
Young stable patient
Thumb
Multiple digits
Sharp wounds with little associated damage
Upper extremity (children)

Absolute Contraindications
Associated life threats
Severe crush injuries
Inability to withstand prolonged surgery

Relative Contraindications*
Single digit, unless thumb
Avulsion injury
Prolonged warm ischemia (12 hours or more)
Gross contamination
Prior injury or surgery to part
Emotionally unstable patients
Lower extremity

*If the victim is a child or if there are multiple losses, salvage replantations are attempted and the relative contraindications are ignored.

CONTRAINDICATIONS

There is no contraindication to managing the amputated part and stump as though replantation were going to occur, even when replantation is considered unlikely by the emergency physician. The care of the whole patient must take precedence over that of the amputated part, although the requirements of the amputated part and stump can often be handled by ancillary personnel during resuscitation and transportation of the patient. Contraindications to replantation are listed in Table 64–1 and are discussed in the following sections. Note that even when replantation is contraindicated, tissue (skin, bone, tendon) from the amputated part may be useful in restoring function to other damaged parts. Never discard amputated tissue until all possible uses of the severed parts are considered. For example, even though an amputated finger tip is not suitable for replantation, the skin may be an ideal donor source for a skin graft to the stump.

GENERAL CONSIDERATIONS

Mechanism of Injury

The potential for successful replantation in terms of survival as well as useful function is directly related to the mechanism of injury. Guillotine injuries, which are sharp, are the least common but have the best prognosis owing to the limited area of destruction. Crush injuries, which are the most common, produce more tissue injury and therefore have a poorer prognosis. The avulsion injury has the worst prognosis, because a significant amount of vessel, nerve, tendon, and soft tissue injury invariably occurs.[3, 4, 6–8]

Ischemia Time

The time that an amputated part can survive before replantation has not been determined. After 6 hours, additional delay may decrease the success rate of revascularization and lead to diminished function. Skin, bone, tendons, and ligaments tolerate ischemia much better than do muscle and connective tissue. Therefore, as a general rule, the more proximal the amputation, the less ischemia time the amputated part can tolerate. Attempts to extend viability during ischemia have shown that the most important controllable factor is the *temperature* of the amputated part. Warm ischemia may be tolerated for 6 to 8 hours.[41] When cooled properly to 4° C, 12 to 24 hours of ischemia may be tolerated with distal amputations.[3, 6–8, 16–28, 42] There is a report of a successful digital replantation after 33 hours of cold ischemia.[42] The way in which hypothermia protects tissue from ischemia is currently under investigation. It has been postulated that hypothermia may limit metabolic demand, thereby preserving intracellular energy.[43–46] Other investigations suggest that the effect is due to the retardation in development of an acidotic pH.[47] Hypothermia may also prevent the no-reflow phenomenon that can follow low-flow states.[48]

Delay in replantation of proximal arm and leg amputations containing significant amounts of muscle tissue can lead to the buildup of toxic products. In such cases, when blood supply is restored, the absorbed toxins have been reported to cause respiratory failure, renal failure, cardiovascular collapse, and even death.[49–56]

Perfusion techniques such as those used in organ transplants to extend anoxic time have not yet been developed. In the past, surgical teams used intraoperative perfusion as a technique to help cool the amputated part. The benefits of intraoperative perfusion with cold hypertonic solutions are currently being investigated. Perfusion should not be attempted by emergency physicians. The risk of damage to vessels and the potential delay in care and rapid transport of the patient and the amputated part override the theoretic benefits of emergency department cold perfusion at this time.[49, 57]

SPECIAL CONSIDERATIONS

Hand Function

Hand function is often determined in part by pinch and grasp functions. If the index finger is removed, the pinching function of the index finger is adequately provided by the middle finger. Power in grasping and gripping is mainly considered an ulnar function of the fourth and fifth digits. An effective grip that provides the ability to hold a variety of objects is a central function of the ring and middle fingers. In addition to its function in pinching, the thumb is the major opposing force for successful grip and grasp. The thumb is the most important digit for adequate hand function, and its loss results in 40 to 50 per cent disability. Such disability requires aggressive attempts to replant amputated thumbs. If this is impossible or unsuccessful, pollicization of other digits or toe transfers are secondary alternatives.[38–62]

Lower Extremity Amputations

There are few reports of successful replantation of amputated parts of the lower extremity.[63, 64] Indications for replantation of amputated parts of the lower extremity are different from those for replantation of amputated parts of the upper extremity. The goal of all replantation is restored function. If this cannot be achieved, a patient is substantially better off with a prosthesis.

The lower extremity is primarily used for weight bearing and allows the individual to ambulate. Lower-limb prostheses, especially those used below the knee, are well tolerated and functional. Prostheses provide a secure stance and permit locomotion. Lower-extremity replantation generally requires skeletal shortening, and distal nerve regeneration is often imperfect. Both deficits may produce dysfunction. A patient with a replanted lower extremity with significant shortening and without sensation functions better with a prosthesis. This is not necessarily true of someone with an upper extremity replant. For these reasons, lower limbs are not generally replanted except under ideal circumstances, usually in children, although there are documented cases of successful lower extremity replantation in adults.[63, 64] The final decision regarding replantation should be left to the replantation team.

Finger Tip Amputations and Dermal "Slice" Wounds

Proper treatment of distal finger tip injuries is controversial. Finger tip amputations often heal by normal wound contracture, but occasionally this practice may result in the loss of functional ability to palpate. The basic goals of treatment are to provide tissue coverage, an acceptable cosmetic result, and an early functional recovery. In distal amputations in which the wound area is less than 10 mm², this is not a problem (Fig. 64–1). Larger dorsal wounds also

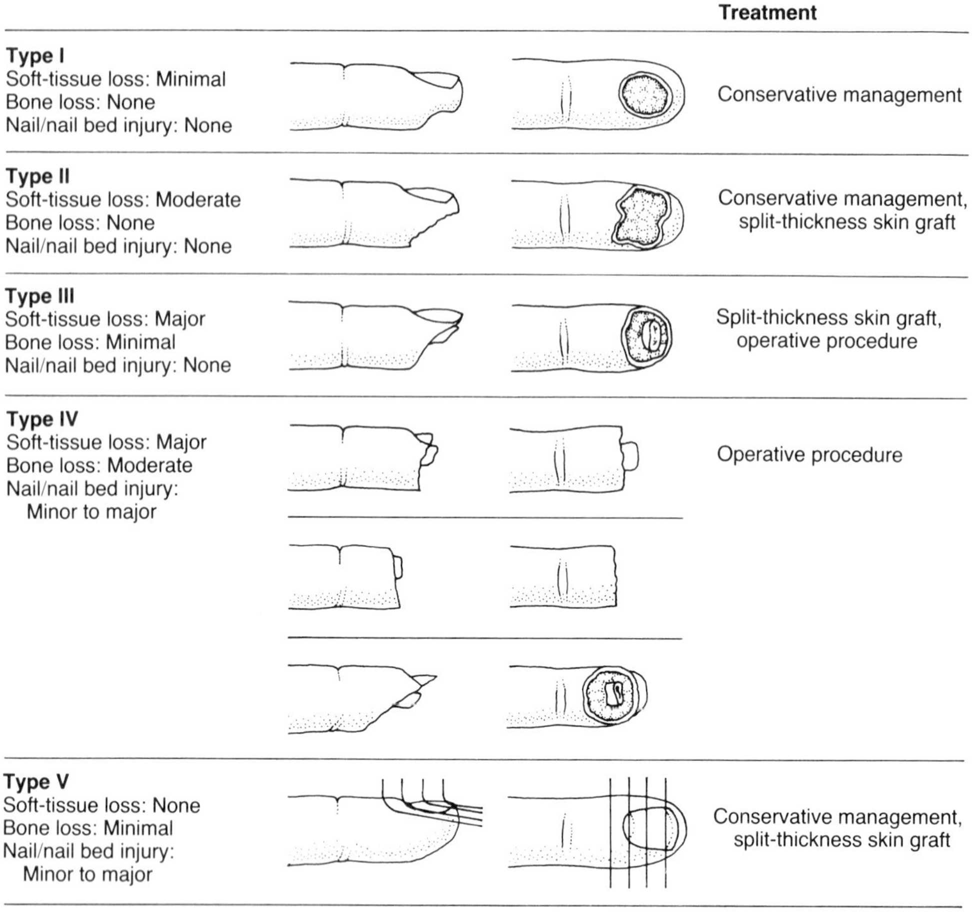

Treatment

Type I
Soft-tissue loss: Minimal
Bone loss: None
Nail/nail bed injury: None

Conservative management

Type II
Soft-tissue loss: Moderate
Bone loss: None
Nail/nail bed injury: None

Conservative management,
split-thickness skin graft

Type III
Soft-tissue loss: Major
Bone loss: Minimal
Nail/nail bed injury: None

Split-thickness skin graft,
operative procedure

Type IV
Soft-tissue loss: Major
Bone loss: Moderate
Nail/nail bed injury:
  Minor to major

Operative procedure

Type V
Soft-tissue loss: None
Bone loss: Minimal
Nail/nail bed injury:
  Minor to major

Conservative management,
split-thickness skin graft

Figure 64–1. Clinical classification of finger tip injuries and treatments for each type. (From Newmeyer WL: Managing fingertip injuries on an outpatient basis. J Musculoskeletal Med 2(2):17, 1985.)

heal well by secondary intention. The challenging problem of finger tip injuries occurs when loss of skin and soft tissue from the fingerpad is significant. Volar skin is unique in its combination of toughness and sensitivity. Wounds with significant volar tissue loss frequently require additional treatment. Children, with their regenerative capacity, often progress very well when significant volar wounds are allowed to heal primarily. For older people and for amputations that involve a more significant amount of the distal digit, a wide variety of techniques for managing the injured finger tip have been advocated, including partial-thickness skin grafts; full-thickness skin grafts; V-Y, Kutler, Kleinert, and island advancement flaps; as well as various local and distal flap-coverage techniques. These procedures are designed to preserve length and to provide soft tissue coverage of exposed bone and sensation to the fingerpad. Each of these procedures has its own indications, complications, and limitations.[65–70] Discussion of these procedures is beyond the scope of this chapter. Most of these techniques are best performed by a specialist in the operating room as primary procedures under ideal circumstances or as delayed procedures when necessary.

In most complete finger tip amputations distal to the distal interphalangeal joint the emergency physician can provide adequate care initially with conservative wound management. Although thinking has changed significantly over the years, many hand surgeons still advise skin grafting to shorten the time for wound healing. Although complete transverse amputations could be handled conservatively, wound healing may take several weeks, and these patients may benefit from operative treatments. Patients with complete transections should be referred for consultation to coordinate their initial care and subsequent follow-up.

Incomplete transections and small distal amputations without significant soft tissue loss may heal well with conservative therapy started by the emergency physician. Nonoperative treatment in selected patients provides excellent functional and cosmetic results, minimizes recovery time, and has few complications.[67–69, 71–74] Children have excellent regenerative capacity and also respond extremely well to conservative treatment. Necrotic or grossly contaminated tissue should be debrided, and the wound should be irrigated thoroughly. If bone is left exposed without soft tissue coverage, the patient will need an operative procedure; alternatively, the bone may be rongeured (shortened) to allow soft tissue coverage and primary healing with better functional recovery. The nailbed tissues should be preserved because the presence of a nail affects the cosmetic result. After cleansing and cautious débridement, an occlusive dressing is placed directly over the wound. Tetanus prophylaxis, wound dressings, and bandages, along with the placement of a protective splint, complete the initial management of these injuries. Amputations that involve the distal phalanx are frequently treated as contaminated open fractures with an initial intravenous drug dose that is followed by an oral course of antibiotics.[75] Wounds managed conservatively need to have serial dressing changes and cleansing. Soaking wounds, cleansing, and replacement of dressings help provide superficial débridement, which may aid healing and minimize the chance of secondary infection. Wound contraction and healing usually result in acceptable cosmetic and functional recovery in 2 to 3 weeks. Patients should have appropriate follow-up to ensure adequate healing and recovery.

Partial finger tip amputations distal to the distal interphalangeal joint can also be managed successfully by the emergency physician. These wounds are treated in a manner similar to that for complete amputations. However, when the amputation has substantial undamaged tissue connecting the finger tip, careful alignment and stabilization is provided by sutures or bandaging and protective splinting. Partially amputated finger tips, especially in children, may occasionally survive and regain vascularization and sensation. If the distal tissue becomes ischemic and necrotic, the amputation becomes complete.

Injury to the nailbed requires special attention to ensure proper alignment. If the nailbed tissues are not aligned properly, permanently disfigured nails may result. Removal of the nail helps provide adequate visualization for the placement of sutures and also minimizes the risk of contamination of the wound.

Dermal "slice" wounds (type 1 in Fig. 64–1) are managed by gentle wound cleansing and application of an antibiotic ointment and a nonadherent dressing, followed by a pressure dressing (e.g., tube gauze). At a dressing change 48 to 72 hours after the initial treatment, the patient can be instructed on daily changes of nonadherent dressings for 10 to 14 days until functional epithelialization of the wound occurs. A protective finger splint or guard also minimizes the risk of further injury and pain from trauma to the sensitive wound area. Protection allows an earlier return to function and employment. Wounds larger than 10 mm^2 and those with deep loss of digit pulp tissue may be candidates for skin grafting (see Chapter 45).

Penis, Ear, and Nose Amputations

Replantation of the penis, ear, and nose generally results in better function and cosmesis than a prosthesis or reconstructive surgery. The amputated parts and wounds should be handled as they are for digital replantations.

Penile amputations are an uncommon problem. Most cases result from self-inflicted trauma in patients who are severely psychologically disturbed. Successful replantation has been reported using microsurgical techniques. Preservation or reconstruction of the urethra to maintain a competent urinary stream is critical for success.[76, 77]

Ears and noses are frequently partially amputated and are occasionally totally amputated. Whenever possible, these body parts should be replanted unless they are severely traumatized and there is gross contamination. These wounds frequently heal well, and patients with such wounds have a high survival rate and a low incidence of total necrosis. Replantation of these parts requires good suture technique and careful placement but does not necessarily require skill in microsurgical techniques.[76, 78, 79]

ASSESSMENT OF THE PATIENT

The initial care and treatment of the patient who has had a body part amputated are the same as those for any trauma patient. The physician must not be distracted by the amputated extremity or the excitement of others from assessing and stabilizing the patient's airway, breathing, and circulation. Amputations are generally not life-threatening injuries, and other potentially more serious injuries must first be assessed and treated. Hemorrhage from amputated limbs is often limited by the retraction and spasm of severed vessels. Therefore, partial amputations may result in more serious hemorrhage than if the vessels were totally severed. Usually, hemorrhage can be controlled adequately with direct pressure and elevation. *Vascular clamps and hemostats have no role in the emergency department management of these injuries and may cause additional injury, which may make replantation impossible.* A proximally placed blood pressure cuff inflated 30 mm Hg above systolic pressure can be used for short periods of time (less than 30 minutes) to control severe bleeding, if necessary.

After the initial primary assessment and treatment and subsequent stabilization of the patient, care of the stump and amputated part can be initiated safely. In addition to the general history obtained from all trauma patients, particular attention should be focused on the exact mechanism of injury, the time and duration of injury, handedness, allergies, medications, illness, prior injury to the affected part, care of the stump and amputated part before arrival in the emergency department, occupation, avocations, and tetanus history.

Tetanus prophylaxis and broad spectrum (e.g., cephalosporins) systemic antibiotic therapy should be initiated. Analgesic medications may be necessary, especially with crushing injuries, for managing patient discomfort. The dose of intravenous narcotics should be titrated to the clinical condition. In finger tip amputations digital or regional nerve blocks are ideal for pain relief but may make functional and neurologic evaluation by a consultant impossible. Some physicians recommend the early use of aspirin or low-molecular-weight dextran, or both, for amputation patients, but such attempts to maintain small-vessel perfusion are controversial and have not proved efficacious in preoperative treatment.

Amputation patients often experience denial, shock, disbelief, and feelings of hopelessness about their injury; some people have even become suicidal. Patients should be treated with supportive and realistic reassurance, but unrealistic medical promises should be avoided. It is important that the emergency physician (or other nonreplantation specialist) not speculate on the specifics of the ultimate prognosis.

Examination of the stump may be brief and should primarily be an assessment of the degree of damage to the surrounding tissue. Gross contamination can be removed by irrigation with normal saline. Local antiseptics, especially hydrogen peroxide or alcohol, *should not be used*, because they may damage viable tissues. Similarly, tissues should not be manipulated, clamped, tagged, or further traumatized in any way. It is important to assess the degree of contamination, the level of injury, and any concomitant injury, such as crushing or multiple levels of injury or amputation. The amputated part should also be examined for the degree of tissue injury, contamination, and possible distal injuries. Radiographs of the amputated part and proximal stump to the level of at least one joint proximal to an extremity injury should be obtained. Preoperative laboratory studies and intravenous access in an uninjured extremity should also be initiated.

The neurologic status of the stump or distal extremity in partial amputations should be assessed by pin prick and two-point discrimination tests. The presence of sweat may indicate autonomic-neurologic functioning. Vascular competence can be assessed by noting the color, temperature, capillary refill, and presence of pulses. An Allen test at the wrist or a modified Allen test at each digit may aid in determining the existence of an arterial injury (see Chapter 19). The neurovascular status should be carefully and clearly documented in the medical record. Motor and tendon function should be evaluated immediately. The regional microvascular resource center should be contacted as soon as possible to arrange transportation and to provide adequate time for mobilization of the replantation team.

CARE OF THE STUMP AND AMPUTATED PART

The stump can be evaluated, and primary care can be rendered during the secondary assessment of the trauma victim (Table 64–2). If replantation is proposed, the goals of initial care include control of hemorrhage and prevention of further injury or contamination. All jewelry should be removed. The stump should be irrigated with normal saline to remove gross contamination. Débridement and dissection should await the specialist. Do not clamp arterial bleeders. The stump wound should then be covered with a *saline-moistened* sterile dressing to prevent further contamination and to limit damage from desiccation. The stump should be splinted for protection and for the prevention of further injury from concomitant fractures or compromise of blood flow owing to change in position. Splinting and elevation may reduce the extent of edema and help control bleeding.

Care of the amputated part follows the same general guidelines as that for the stump. Gross contamination can be eliminated by irrigation with saline. All jewelry should be removed. The amputated part should be handled minimally to prevent further damage and should be wrapped in a saline-moistened sterile dressing. *Direct immersion in saline or hypotonic fluids should be avoided*, because it may cause severe maceration of tissue and may make replantation more difficult technically. The amputated part should be cooled as soon as possible. The ideal temperature is 4° C. Care must be taken to prevent the freezing of tissues. Amputated parts should not be placed directly on ice, because tissue that is in direct contact with the ice may freeze. Currently, the recommended method for cooling amputated parts is to place the part, which is wrapped in saline-moistened gauze, in a water-tight plastic bag and immerse the bag in a container of ice water (Fig. 64–2). A guideline is to use half water and half ice—excessive ice should be avoided. Cooling coils and refrigeration devices have occasionally been used but are generally not available and offer no significant advantages. The tissue containers should be labeled with the patient's name, the amputated part contained within, the time of the original injury, and the time that cooling began.

Treatment for partial amputations with vascular compromise is the same as that just described. Clean the wound with normal saline irrigation. Place a saline-moistened sponge on the open tissue, and wrap the injury in a sterile dressing, incorporating a splint to protect it from further injury. Ice packs or commercial cold packs should be applied over the dressing to cool the devascularized area (Fig. 64–3).

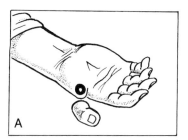

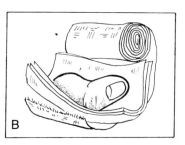

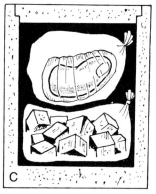

Figure 64–2. Evaluate the patient's condition to ensure that resuscitation is not necessary before transfer. *A*, The wound should be rinsed with saline solution. *Do not scrub or apply antiseptic solution to the wound.* Apply dry sterile dressing, wrap in Kling or Kerlix for pressure, and elevate. *B*, The amputated part should be rinsed with saline. *Do not scrub or apply antiseptic solution to the amputated part.* Wrap it in moist sterile gauze or a towel, depending on its size, and place it in a plastic bag or plastic container. *C*, The part is then put in a container, preferably Styrofoam, and cooled by separate plastic bags containing ice. (Artwork only from Hand Trauma: Emergency Care. Maryland Emergency Services.)

COMPLICATIONS

The care of amputated parts should not lead to avoidable complications if the aforementioned principles are followed. Improper management of the parts or stump with subsequent additional injury of the tissue from overzealous hemostasis or cleansing should be avoided. Furthermore, desiccation, maceration, or freezing of tissue from improper storage should not occur. The physician must consider expediting the preoperative work-up of the patient and immediate notification of the replantation team as crucial factors in the patient's care.

Despite optimal initial care, replantation itself may be associated with acute or long-term complications. There is the usual risk of anesthesia and protracted surgery. Postoperative complications include vascular thrombosis, hemorrhage, infection, and reaction to accumulated toxins. It is not unusual for second and third emergency operations to be required to reestablish adequate blood flow. Patients are often placed on anticoagulants, which create an addition risk. Toxins accumulate in ischemic amputated parts despite cooling. The amount of toxin is directly proportional to the amount of muscle mass and the duration of ischemia. Reports of significant pulmonary failure, electrolyte distur-

Table 64–2. Axioms for Care of Amputations	
Do's	**Don't's**
Splint and elevate	Apply dry ice or freeze tissue
Apply pressure dressing	Place tags on tissue
Protect from further trauma or injury	Place sutures in tissue
Protect from further contamination	Sever skin bridges
Provide analgesia	Initiate perfusion of amputated part
Supply tetanus prophylaxis and antibiotic therapy	Place tissue in formalin or water
Obtain radiographs	

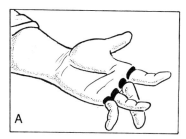

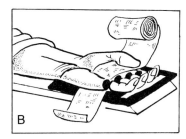

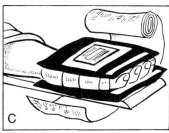

Figure 64–3. For a partial amputation, *(A)* rinse with saline, *(B)* place part(s) in a functional position and apply dry sterile dressing, and splint and elevate. Apply coolant bags to the *outside* of the dressing *(C)*. *Do not scrub or apply antiseptic solution to the wound.* Control any bleeding with pressure. If a tourniquet is necessary, place it close to the amputation site. (Artwork only from Hand Trauma: Emergency Care. Maryland Emergency Services.)

bance, and even death have been reported in replantation efforts.

Later complications include a significant percentage (60 per cent) of patients with cold intolerance, limited function, anesthesia, pain, paresthesias, malunions, and nonunions. Repeated operative procedures may be required to obtain a functionally useful result. To minimize the morbidity from amputations, proper initial care is essential and may be the most important determining factor in the patient's eventual outcome.

References

1. Kleinert HE, Raber RM: Compendium on hand surgery, p 19, 1973.
2. Tamai S: Digit replantation: Analysis of 163 replantations in an 11-year period. Clin Plast Surg 5:195, 1978.
3. May JW, Gallico GG: Upper extremity replantation. Curr Prob Surg 17:634, 1980.
4. Weiland AJ, Villarreal-Rios A, Kleinert HE, et al: Replantation of digits and hands: Analysis of surgical techniques and the fusal results in 71 patients with 86 replantations. J Hand Surg 2:1, 1977.
5. Serafin D, Morris RL, Polack EP (eds): Assessment of viability in transplanted tissue-electromagnetic flowmeter. Microsurgical Composite Tissue Tranplantation. St. Louis, CV Mosby Co, 1979, p 208.
6. Morrison WA, O'Brien BM, MacLeod AM: Evaluation of digital replantation—a review of 100 cases. Orthop Clin North Am 8:295, 1977.
7. Morrison WA, O'Brien BM, MacLeod AM: Digital replantation and revascularization: A long-term review of one hundred cases. Hand 10:125, 1978.
8. Kleinert HE, Juhala CA, Tsai TM, et al: Digital replantation-selection techniques and results. Orthop Clin North Am 8:309, 1977.
9. Kleinert HE, Tsai TM: Microvascular repair in replantation. Clin Orthop 133:205, 1978.
10. Fiorvanti L: In Tesoro della vita Humana. Venetia, Apresso gli heredi di M. Sessa, 1570.
11. Gibson T: Early free grafting: The restitution of parts completely separated from the body. Br J Plast Surg 18:1, 1965.
12. Balfour W: Two cases, with observations, demonstrative of the powers of nature to reunite parts which have been, by accident, totally separated from the animal system. Edinburgh Med Surg J 10:421, 1814.
13. Malt RA, McKhann CE: Replantation of severed arms. JAMA 189:716, 1964.
14. Chen CW, Pao YS: Salvage of the forearm following complete traumatic amputation; report of a case. Clin Med J 82:633, 1963.
15. Kleinert HE, Kasdan MFl: Anastomoses of digital vessels. J Kentucky Med Assoc 63:106, 1965.
16. Yoshizu I, Katsumi M, Tajima T: Replantation of untidily amputated finger, hand, and arm. J Trauma 18:194, 1978.
17. Schlenker JD, Kleinert HE, Tsai TM: Methods and results of replantation following traumatic amputation of the thumb in 64 patients. J Hand Surg 5:63, 1980.
18. O'Brien BM: Replantation surgery. Clin Plast Surg 1:405, 1974.
19. O'Brien BM: Replantation and reconstructive microvascular surgery. Ann R Coll Surg Engl 58:87, 1976.
20. O'Brien BM, MacLeod AM, Miller GD, et al: Clinical replantation of digits. Plast Reconstr Surg 52:490, 1973.
21. O'Brien BM, Miller GD: Digital reattachment and revascularization. J Bone Joint Surg 55A:714, 1973.
22. Tsai TM: Experimental and clinical application of microvascular surgery. Ann Surg 2:169, 1975.
23. Biemer E, et al: Results of 150 replantations on the upper extremity with microvascular surgery. Paper at Third Composium Eur Sect IVPRS. The Hague, Netherlands, May 1977.
24. May JW Jr, Toth BA, Gardner M: Digital replantation distal to the proximal interphalangeal joint. J Hand Surg 7:161, 1982.
25. Urbaniak JR, Kleinert HE, Jablon M, Tsai TM: An overview of replantation and results of 347 replants in 245 patients. J Trauma 20:390, 1980.
26. Urbaniak JR, Soucacos PN, Adelaar RS, et al: Experimental evaluation in microsurgical techniques in small artery anastomosis. Orthop Clin North Am 8:249, 1977.
27. Buncke HJ: Replantation surgery in China. Plast Reconstr Surg 52:476, 1973.
28. Zhong-Wei C, Meyer VE, Kleinert HE, Beasley RW: Present indications and contraindications for replantation as reflected by long-term functional results. Orthop Clin North Am 12:849, 1981.
29. Buncke HJ: Replantation surgery in China. Report of the American Replantation Mission to China. Plast Reconstr Surg 52:476, 1973.
30. Beasley RW: General considerations in managing upper limb amputations. Orthop Clin North Am 12:743, 1981.
31. Wilson CS, Alpert BS, Buncke HJ, Gordon L: Replantation of the upper extremity. Clin Plast Surg 10:85, 1983.
32. Malt RA, Smith RJ: Limb replantation: Selection of patients and technical considerations. In Rutherford RB (ed): Vascular Surgery. Philadelphia, WB Saunders Co, 1978.
33. Lendvay PG: Replacement of the amputated digit. Br J Plast Surg 26:398, 1973.
34. Leung PC: Hand replantation in an 83-year-old woman—the oldest replantation? Plast Reconst Surg 64:416, 1979.
35. Sekiquchi J, Ohmdri K: Youngest replantation with microsurgical anastomosis: A successful replantation of a finger on an infant, aged 12 months and 15 days, by microsurgical repair is reported. Hand 11:64, 1979.
36. Van Beek AL, Wavak PW, Zook EG: Microvascular surgery in young children. Plast Reconst Surg 63:457, 1979.
37. Stelling FH: Surgery of hand in children. J Bone Joint Surg 45A:623, 1963.
38. Wakefield AR: Hand injury in children. J Bone Joint Surg 46A:1226, 1964.
39. Green DP: Hand injury in children. Pediatr Clin North Am 24:4, 1977.
40. Jaegar SH, Tsai TM, Kleinert HE: Upper extremity replantation in children. Orthop Clin North Am 12:897, 1981.
41. Berger A, Millesi H, Mandl H, Frellinger G: Replantation and revascularization of amputated parts of extremities: A three-year report from the Viennese replantation team. Clin Orthop 133:212, 1978.
42. Sixth People's Hospital, Shanghai: Reattachment of traumatic amputations. A summing up of experience. Chinese Med J 1:392, 1967.
43. Hayhurst JW, O'Brien BM, Ishida H, et al: Experimental replantation after prolonged cooling. Hand 6:134, 1974.
44. Lapchinsky AG: Recent results of experimental transplantation of preserved limbs and kidneys and possible use of this technique in clinical practice. Ann NY Acad Sci 87:539, 1960.
45. Levy MN: Oxygen consumption and blood flow in hypothermic perfused kidney. Am J Physiol 197:1111, 1959.
46. Tsai TM, Jupiter JB, Serratoni F, et al: The effect of hypothermia and tissue perfusion on extended myocutaneous flap viability. Plast Reconst Surg 70:444, 1982.
47. Osterman AL, Heppenstall RB, Sapega AA, et al: Muscle ischemia and hypothermia: A bioenergetic study using ^{31}phosphorus nuclear magnetic resonance spectroscopy. J Trauma 24:811, 1984.

48. May JW, Chait LA, O'Brien BM, et al: The no-reflow phenomenon in experimental free flaps. Plast Reconstr Surg 61:256, 1978.
49. Razaboni R, Shaw WW: Preservation of tissues for transplantation and replantation. Clin Plast Surg 7:211, 1980.
50. Wood MB, Cooney WP: Above elbow limb replantation: Functional results. J Hand Surg 11:682, 1986.
51. Ferreira MC, Marques EF, Azze RJ: Limb replantation. Clin Plast Surg 5:211, 1978.
52. Wilson CS, Alpert BS, Buncke JH, Gordon L: Replantation of the upper extremity. Clin Plast Surg 10:85, 1983.
53. Chen CW, Chung Wei C, Yun Qing Q, Zhony Jia Y: Extremity replantation. World J Surg 2:513, 1978.
54. Matsuda M, Shibahara H, Kato N: Long-term results of replantation of 10 upper extremities. World J Surg 2:603, 1978.
55. Tamai S, Hori Y, Tatsumi Y, et al: Major limb, hand, and digital replantation. World J Surg 3:17, 1979.
56. O'Brien BM, MacLeod AM, Hayhurst JW, et al: Major replantation surgery in the upper limb. Hand 6:217, 1974.
57. Harashina T, Buncke HJ: Study of washout solutions for microvascular replantation and transplantation. Plast Reconstr Surg 56:54, 1975.
58. Straunch B: Microsurgical approach to thumb reconstruction. Orthop Clin North Am 8:319, 1987.
59. O'Brien BM, MacLeod AM, Sykes PJ, et al: Hallux to hand transfer. Hand 7:128, 1975.
60. Buck-Gramcko D: Thumb reconstruction by digital transposition. Orthop Clin North Am 8:329, 1977.
61. Bunnel S: Physiologic reconstruction of a thumb after total loss. Surg Gynecol Obstet 52:245, 1931.
62. Little JW: On making a thumb: One hundred years of surgical effort. J Hand Surg 1:35, 1976.
63. Morrison WA, O'Brien BM, MacLeod AM: Major limb replantation. Orthop Clin North Am 8:343, 1977.
64. Jupiter JB: Salvage replantation of lower limb amputation. Plast Reconstr Surg 69:1, 1982.
65. Flatt A: The Care of Minor Hand Injuries. St. Louis, CV Mosby Co, 1959.
66. Illingworth CM: Trapped fingers and amputated fingertips in children. J Pediatr Surg 9:853, 1974.
67. Newmeyer W: Managing fingertip injuries on an outpatient basis. J Musculoskel Med 2:17, 1985.
68. Farrell RG, Rappaport B: Nonoperative management of fingertip amputations. West J Med 142:385, 1985.
69. Massengill JB: Pitfalls in management of fingertip injuries and hand lacerations. Primary Care 7:231, 1980.
70. Schwartz GR, Safar P, Stone J, et al: Principles and Practice of Emergency Medicine. Philadelphia, WB Saunders Co, 1978, pp 208, 725–726, 759–760.
71. Allen MJ: Conservative management of fingertip injuries in adults. Hand 12:257, 1980.
72. Ipsen T, Frandsen PA, Barfred T: Conservative treatment of fingertip injuries. Injury 18:203, 1987.
73. Horner L: Finger tip trauma. Surg Clin North Am 49:1373, 1969.
74. Chow SP, Ho E: Open treatment of fingertip injuries in adults. Hand Surg 7:470, 1982.
75. Sloan JP, Dove AF, Maheson M, et al: Antibiotics in open fractures of the distal phalanx? J Hand Surg 12:123, 1987.
76. Strauch B, Sharzer LA, Petro J, et al: Replantation of amputated parts of the penis, nose, ear, and scalp. Clin Plast Surg 10:115, 1983.
77. Best J, Angelo J: Complete traumatic amputation of the penis. J Urol 87:134, 1962.
78. Grabb WC, Dingman RO: The fate of amputated tissues of the head and neck following replacement. Plast Reconstr Surg 49:28, 1972.
79. Mohler LR, Porterfield HW, Ferraro JW, Drabyn GA: Replantation and revascularization replant potentiality. Ohio State Med J 75:395, 1979.

Chapter **65**

Extensor Tendon Injuries in the Hand and Wrist

William L. Newmeyer

INTRODUCTION

Extensor tendons are more superficial than flexor tendons; they are covered for most of their course by only skin and very thin fascia (Fig. 65–1). The mechanism of action of extensor tendons in the digits is complex and little understood by most physicians. Extensor tendons are more subject to *closed* injury than flexor tendons, and closed injuries are usually more difficult to diagnose than open ones. Extensor tendon injuries can often be definitively treated in a well-equipped outpatient setting if the treating physician is conversant with the pathophysiology involved.

SURGICAL AND FUNCTIONAL ANATOMY[1]

There are 12 extrinsic extensor musculotendinous units, all innervated by the radial nerve in the upper dorsal forearm. Four of these tendons insert at the wrist level. The most radial of these is the abductor pollicis longus (APL) tendon, which arises deep on the lateral side of the forearm from the radius, the interosseous membrane, and the ulna. The APL tendon passes deep to the other extensors and inserts into the base of the first metacarpal. The APL tendon acts as a radial wrist deviator and stabilizes the base of the

first metacarpal. The extensor carpi radialis longus (ECRL) and the extensor carpi radialis brevis (ECRB) arise from the lateral epicondyle and insert into the bases of the second and third metacarpals, respectively. The ECRL is a powerful wrist extensor and, to some extent, a radial wrist deviator, whereas the ECRB is a powerful wrist extensor (Fig. 65–2). The fourth wrist extensor is the extensor carpi ulnaris (ECU), which also arises from the lateral epicondyle and inserts into the base of the fifth metacarpal, acting as a wrist extensor and an ulnar wrist deviator (Fig. 65–3). Wrist extension is critical to hand function because the finger flexors cannot work with force unless the wrist is extended (dorsiflexed).

Fibro-osseous tendon sheaths are present *only* at wrist level on the dorsal or extensor surface (Fig. 65–4). There are six synovial-lined tendon sheaths, some with one or more subdivisions. The APL passes through the first dorsal compartment, the ECRL and ECRB through the second dorsal compartment, and the ECU through the sixth. These sheaths, collectively referred to as the dorsal retinaculum, are necessary to prevent the tendons from bowstringing when the wrist is extended. Distal to the wrist the tendons lie in loose areolar tissue beneath the thin dorsal skin and very thin dorsal fascia.

There are eight digital extensor tendons. The thumb has two, the extensor pollicis brevis (EPB) and the extensor pollicis longus (EPL) (see Fig. 65–2). The EPB arises with the APL and passes through the first dorsal compartment with it. The first dorsal compartment actually has two or more subcompartments for these two tendons. (In fact, the APL may have three or four slips, each with its own compartment.) The EPL passes through the third dorsal compartment, which is just on the ulnar side of Lister's tubercle, a bony prominence on the radial side of the distal dorsal radius. The EPL crosses directly over the two radial wrist extensors and pursues a radial-distal direction to its ultimate insertion on the distal phalanx of the thumb (see Fig. 65–2). The EPB inserts on the proximal phalanx of the thumb.

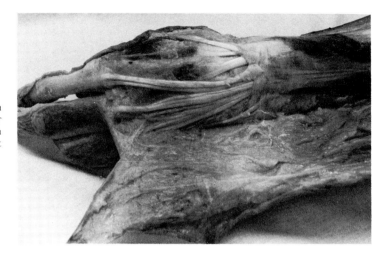

Figure 65–1. The first ten figures show a cadaver dissection of the dorsal hand to illustrate important facets of extensor tendon anatomy. In this figure, the very thin cover of skin and dorsal fascia is demonstrated, and it can be seen that the tendons have sheaths only at wrist level.

The EPL is the only extrinsic digital extensor that has its primary insertion and function on an interphalangeal (IP) joint.

There are six tendons to extend the other four digits; their primary action is at the metacarpal phalangeal (MCP) joints. Each digit has its own extensor digitorum communis (EDC) tendon. The index and little fingers each have an independent extensor, the extensor indicis proprius (EIP) for the index finger and the extensor digiti quinti minimi (EDQM) for the little finger. The four EDC tendons and the EIP pass together through the fourth dorsal compartment, but the EDQM has its own compartment—the fifth (Fig. 65–5A and B).

On the dorsum of the hand at the level of the distal metacarpals the six tendons are interconnected with oblique tendinous bands, called juncturae tendineae (Fig. 65–6). These juncturae can give an examiner a false sense of security because they may allow weak active digital extension even if the main tendon is cut.

The six digital extensors to these four digits (i.e., the second to the fifth digits) have a fibrous insertion distal to the MCP joints and act primarily at this site (Fig. 65–7), but each digit also has a dorsal extension along the proximal phalanges to a final bony insertion on the dorsal proximal lip of the middle phalanx (Fig. 65–8). The central intrinsic muscles (i.e., the four lumbricals and the seven interossei)

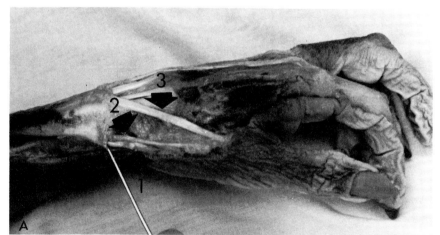

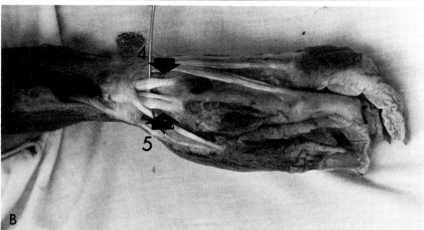

Figure 65–2. A, 1, Abductor pollicis longus; 2, extensor pollicis brevis; 3, extensor pollicis longus. B, 4, extensor carpi radialis brevis; 5, extensor carpi radialis longus. (The extensor carpi radialis longus has one small and one large tendon slip.)

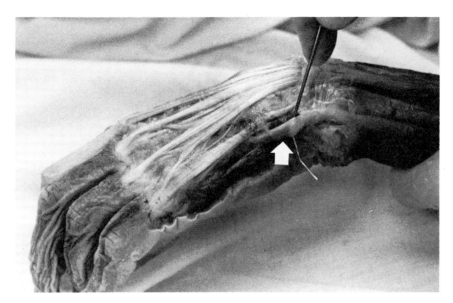

Figure 65-3. The extensor carpi ulnaris tendon *(arrow).*

have tendons known as lateral bands (Fig. 65–9), which act as flexors of the MCP joints but then move dorsally to become extensors of the IP joints. They are connected to the extrinsic extensor tendon by a broad, flat sheet of fascia known as the sagittal fibers. This troika of the central slip and lateral bands is known as the extensor mechanism of the digit. Beyond the level of the proximal interphalangeal (PIP) joint these entities fuse into a tendon known as the terminal extensor mechanism (TEM) (Fig. 65–10). The TEM has its insertion on the dorsal lip of the proximal portion of the distal phalanx. It is very important to understand this mechanism if one is to diagnose and treat extensor tendon injuries—especially in the fingers.

Tendons function by moving. This movement, which varies in degree according to several factors (including how close the tendon is to its insertion), is known as amplitude, or glide. If a tendon is lacerated in an area of large amplitude and it is not otherwise fixed, the proximal (and, to some extent, the distal) ends retract, and retrieval may be a major problem. This may occur on the dorsum of the hand, especially as the site of injury becomes more proximal. This is a significant problem at the wrist level with the complicating factor of having to deal with a synovial-lined sheath (as discussed earlier). Fortunately, on the distal dorsal hand and especially on the fingers not only is the amplitude small but also the extensor mechanism is a broad flat sheet that is

seldom cut in its entirety, and therefore, retrieval is usually not a problem.

It is important to remember that the position of the wrist alters the apparent function of digital flexors and extensors, sometimes very dramatically. For example, if one puts his or her own wrist in maximum flexion and attempts to make a fist, one will note that the resultant fist is both weak and incomplete. This is quite a contrast to what is achieved when the wrist is in maximum extension. Therefore, when examining a hand with a suspected tendon laceration, it is important to examine that hand with the wrist in neutral and at the extremes of flexion and extension.

PATHOPHYSIOLOGY OF EXTENSOR INJURIES

Whereas most (but not all) flexor tendon injuries are open injuries, closed injuries of the extensors, especially in the fingers, are very common. Injuries may occur from closed trauma that may appear to be trivial. One must be aware of this because it is more difficult to diagnose closed injuries than open ones. With injuries at the distal or middle joint level (DIP or PIP), a fracture may be a key part of the problem, and it is usually advisable to obtain a radiograph. This is particularly true of closed injuries.

Extensor tendons of the hand and the wrist are very

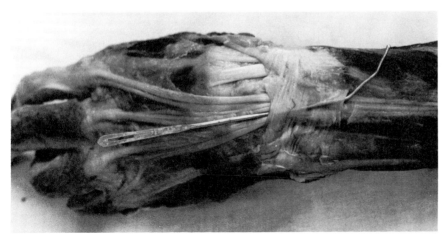

Figure 65-4. The dorsal retinaculum with a probe passing through the fourth dorsal compartment.

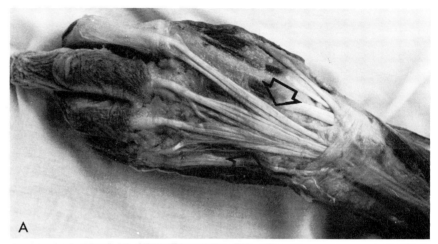

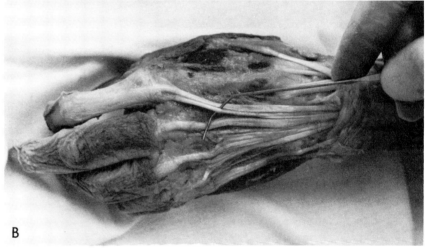

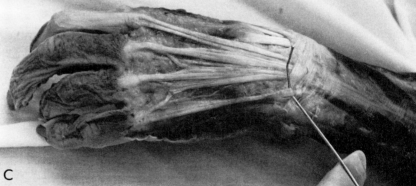

Figure 65–5. *A*, The digital extensor tendons *(between the arrows)*. *B*, The extensor indicis proprius. *C*, The extensor digiti quinti minimi.

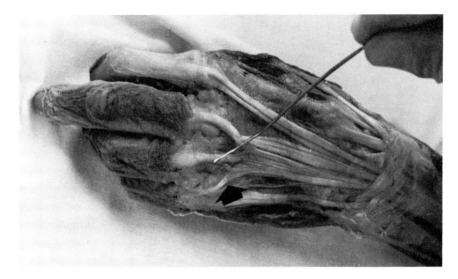

Figure 65–6. The arrow points to an interconnecting band of the extensor tendons on the dorsum of the hand—a juncturae tendineae. The probe is lifting up another such band of tendons.

superficial. Therefore, it is difficult *not* to have at least a partial tendon injury in all but the most superficial wounds in that area. Thus *all dorsal wrist, hand, and digital lacerations should be approached with the thought that there is a partial or total tendon laceration in their depth.* The techniques for determining and repairing these lacerations are outlined in the following sections. Partial tendon lacerations may not be obvious, since function will initially be normal. Therefore, one must inspect all wounds visually and examine the wound while putting the fingers and wrist through a range of motion if partial lacerations are to be discovered. If an injury occurred with the fist closed, the injured area of the tendon may not be visualized in the wound if the hand is examined in full extension. In the case of an open injury, the tendon may be either partially or completely divided. Partial division is the most usual situation on the dorsal finger, whereas on the hand and the wrist, total division is much more common. Completely divided tendons, obviously, must be repaired.

If a tendon is partially lacerated, one must consider the location and extent of the laceration in deciding whether or not to repair it. If the partial laceration is 10 per cent of the total tendon bulk or less, it may be safely left alone. If it is greater than 10 per cent, it should be repaired either with a running (or simple interrupted) 5–0 nylon suture or in a manner similar to that for complete laceration (see later). Because dysfunction may follow repair, some reports advocate nonrepair of partial *flexor* tendon lacerations of up to 50 per cent.[2] The absence of an extensor tendon sheath minimizes the risk of tendon triggering or entrapment with *extensor* repair. Hence, repair of most clean, fresh, and accessible partial extensor tendon lacerations in the hand is prudent.

In the foot, flexor tendons are much more commonly lacerated than extensor tendons because of a greater injury exposure (i.e., we walk on the soles of our feet, not on the dorsum). The diagnosis of a flexor tendon laceration in the foot is made primarily by indirect examination (i.e., loss of flexor function). If the laceration is deep and flexion strength is diminished or if the laceration of a flexor tendon is visualized, the wound is managed conservatively. The wound is cleansed and closed in a single layer. The patient is started on a broad-spectrum antibiotic and specialty follow-up is arranged. When extensor tendon lacerations do occur on the foot (usually as a result of a sharp object falling on the dorsum of the foot), they are generally managed as for similar extensor tendon injuries of the hand.

OPEN INJURY TREATMENT PREREQUISITES

If the repair of open extensor tendon injuries is to be undertaken in the outpatient setting, certain principles must

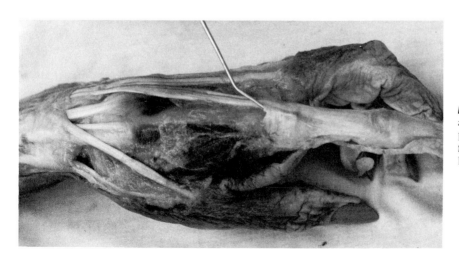

Figure 65–7. The mainly fibrous insertion of an extrinsic extensor tendon on the proximal phalanx just distal to the metacarpal phalangeal joint with a probe inserted under its proximal edge.

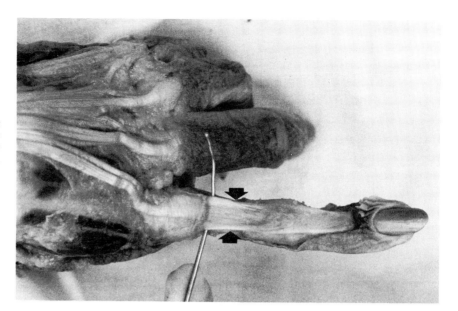

Figure 65–8. The extensor mechanism on the dorsum of a finger. Arrows point to the radial and ulnar lateral band portions of the extensor mechanism. The thinner central portion is the central extensor mechanism, and the probe lifts the entire structure up off the phalanx.

be rigorously adhered to or disaster is sure to follow. These include the following:

1. The procedure must be performed in a relatively clean room with the necessary supplies readily available in the room. This area must be out of the traffic pattern of both hospital personnel and patients.

2. The patient should always be supine on a stretcher or a gurney. The hand should be supported on a firm platform that allows access from either side.

3. There should be good overhead lighting.

4. Plastic surgery–type instruments should be available. These should include a Webster needle holder; two small double-pronged skin hooks; two small right-angled (Ragnell) retractors; one pair of small curved sharp (Iris) scissors (for cutting tissue); one pair of small blunt-nosed scissors (for cutting sutures); several small hemostats, both curved and straight; one pair of small single-toothed (Adson) forceps; and one larger pair of blunt-nosed scissors for cutting the dressings to proper size.

5. Although a variety of suture material can be used, silk suture should be avoided because of its reactivity. Chromic and plain gut also are undesirable because the suture will dissolve before the tendon is healed. Monofilament nylon (Ethilon from Ethicon or Dermalon from Davis & Geck) is an excellent material. Some surgeons like to use a material that is not as slippery as monofilament nylon. Braided nylon (Surgilon), Dacron (Ticron), and polyglycollic acid sutures (Maxon) are satisfactory. The best size is 4–0, although 5–0 may serve in some cases. Plastic needles should be used, such as the P-3 from Ethicon and PRE-2 from Davis & Geck.

6. An arm tourniquet *must* be used. It is not possible to identify and repair small structures in the hand in a pool of blood. An ordinary blood pressure cuff may be used. The cuff is placed on the mid to upper arm with the tube or tubes pointing cephalad. The cuff is wrapped with two or three layers of cast padding after it has been placed on the arm. This is to prevent its unwrapping when the cuff is put to working pressure. Blood pressure cuffs are not designed

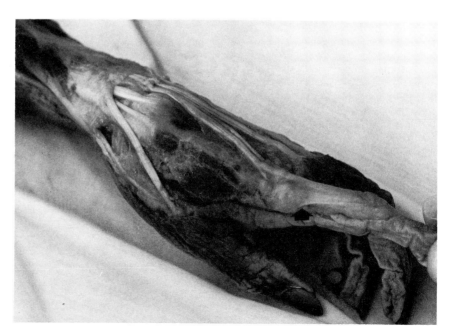

Figure 65–9. The proximal portion of the lateral band *(arrow)*, in this case the one arising from the first dorsal interosseous muscle.

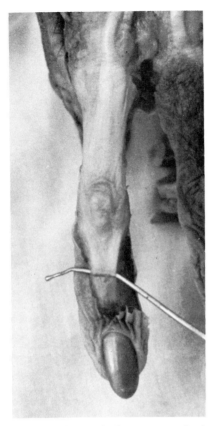

Figure 65–10. The terminal extensor mechanism.

for the pressures used and will unwrap in the middle of the procedure if padding is not used. When all else is ready, the arm is exsanguinated by gravity for 1 minute, the cuff is elevated to 260 to 280 mm Hg, and the tube or tubes are *clamped* to maintain the pressure. If this is not done, the manometer steadily loses its pressure with a resultant venous tourniquet and a very bloody field. After the tubes are clamped the pressure obviously can no longer be monitored. The assistant should be advised of this so that he or she does not fuss with the inflating bulb. In fact, it is advisable to open the bulb screw and to let the monitor go to zero, since it is now separated from the cuff by the clamp. At the conclusion of the procedure, releasing the clamp allows the pressure to go immediately to zero; but if the bulb is still under pressure, a rather awkward situation may result with a persistent venous tourniquet effect until all realize what is going on. This tourniquet is well tolerated by a conscious, alert patient for approximately 15 to 20 minutes. This time duration serves as a good cutoff point, because anything that takes longer than that is probably more than can be comfortably tackled in an outpatient setting. It is a good idea for a physician who is going to be using a tourniquet on conscious patients to try it out on himself or herself for 20 minutes just to see how it feels.

7. Anesthesia must be used when tendons are explored and repaired. The easiest method to use on the dorsum of the hand is a field block of 1 per cent plain lidocaine placed through the already cut skin edges by means of a 3.75-cm number 27 needle. One should always remember to anesthetize not only the area of the wound but also a proximal area if the wound has to be extended. (For further details on local and limited regional anesthesia, consult Chapter 38.) The anesthesia should always be in place and set *before* the tourniquet is inflated. Tourniquet time must be used for

exploration and operating and *not* for ancillary procedures that can be performed without a tourniquet.

8. Exposure must be adequate and can be a problem in the repair of extensor tendon lacerations. One should not hesitate to extend the wound proximally (the usual direction in which more exposure is needed) or distally. An extending transverse incision from each end of a longitudinal laceration (one end directed radially and the other ulnarly) permits the retraction of a flap at each end of the wound for better exposure.

9. The timing of tendon repair depends on several factors, including the time the patient is first seen after the injury, the condition of the wound, the presence or absence of concomitant injuries, and the experience of the potential surgeon. As a general rule only "fresh" (i.e., less than 2 or 3 hours old) extensor tendon injuries should be considered for repair in the emergency department. If the patient does not come in for treatment at the time of injury, the potential for infection is greater and consideration of delayed primary repair should be made. From a technical point of view a delayed primary repair can often be done weeks after the injury if the proximal tendon stump has not retracted, but in general it should be done within about 10 days to maximize the chances for a good functional recovery.

10. The most important principle is that the practitioner must have adequate knowledge. It should be noted that the tendons do not look the same in the living hand as they do in the illustrations.[3] Tendon repair should not be attempted unless the physician performing the repair has had some instruction by a surgeon with hand experience. It is an excellent idea to do a cadaver dissection of the dorsal hand before undertaking repairs on a living hand. The only thing lacking in the cadaver hand is the tendon amplitude, which can stymie the uninitiated. (Also, exposure is easier in cadaver hands.)

EXTENSOR TENDON ZONES

It is helpful to divide extensor tendon injuries into zones (Fig. 65–11) and to consider open and closed injuries in each zone. These zones are somewhat arbitrary but are functionally useful. They are:

Zone I: The area over the DIP joint. An injury at this area is known as a mallet finger.

Zone II: The area over the PIP joint. An injury at this level results in the so-called boutonniere deformity.

Zone III: This is the area on the dorsal finger between the joints. The tendon in this area is a broad, flat sheet of fascia-like tissue and is seldom totally divided.

Zone IV: In this area tendons look like tendons rather than broad bands of fascia. Especially in the proximal part of this zone, retraction of the cut tendon end can be a major problem.

Zone V: This is the area of the dorsal retinaculum. Injuries in this area require treatment in the operating suite under high regional or general anesthesia.

Zone VI: This is above the retinaculum. The problems of exposure and the operative requirements are similar to those for Zone V.

Zone I Injuries

Injuries in Zone I may be the result of closed trauma with attenuation or rupture of the terminal extensor insertion on the distal phalanx, a laceration of the terminal

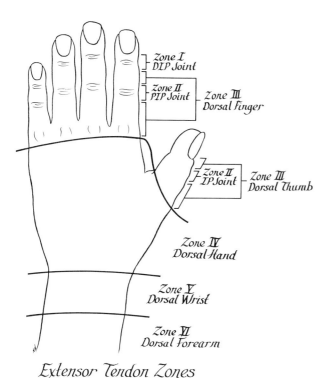

Figure 65–11. Extensor tendon zones. (From Newmeyer WL: Primary Care of Hand Injuries. Philadelphia, Lea & Febiger, 1979. Reproduced by permission.)

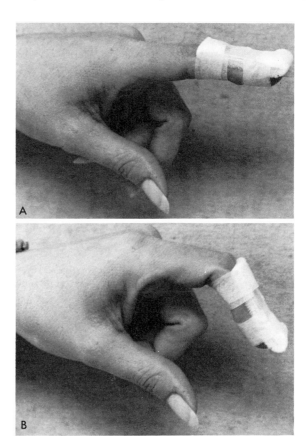

Figure 65–12. A proper mallet finger splint *(A)*. It should allow easy active motion of the proximal interphalangeal joint *(B)*.

extensor tendon, or a fracture avulsion of the bony insertion of the TEM.

The most common injury is the closed avulsion of the tendon. The trauma that causes this is often rather mild. The patient usually complains of a painless droop of the distal phalanx, and a radiograph shows only the flexed distal phalanx. The best treatment for the common condition of mallet finger is splinting in full extension for 8 weeks. The splint should be one that holds the DIP joint in extension while allowing easy motion of the PIP joint (Fig. 65–12). The patient should be advised to change the splint at least once a day to make sure there are no pressure spots under the splint. During the splint change the patient should be advised to avoid flexing the DIP joint and to hold it in full extension either with the other hand or by placing the palmar surface of the finger on a hard table. It is useful to give the patient several extra splints. The patient should be advised to leave the splint in place during bathing and to change the wet splint afterward. In most instances, if the splint is worn faithfully for 8 weeks (and then for 4 more weeks at night) a good result can be expected. If the result is not satisfactory to the patient, there are various tendon reconstructive procedures that can be considered, but none of these is uniformly satisfactory. The joint can always be fused if instability is a major problem.

If the deformity is the result of a fracture, one should consider operative fixation of the fragment if a significant portion of the articular surface is involved (more than 30 to 40 per cent) and especially if there is volar subluxation of the distal phalanx upon the middle phalanx (Fig. 65–13). Unfortunately, operative fixation of this tiny fragment is often quite difficult, and some degree of joint injury often results with less than full restoration of DIP function. If the fracture fragment is small and there is minimal or no distal phalangeal subluxation, treatment is the same as that outlined for the closed mallet deformity.

Open mallet injuries caused by a laceration that severs the TEM should be treated by suture fixation of the tendon. In most instances it is advisable to splint the DIP joint internally with a Kirschner (K) wire (0.088-cm size). The internal splint should be left in place for at least 6 weeks and preferably for 8 weeks. This is a procedure that can be performed in the outpatient setting but is easier if performed in an operating suite, although neither general nor high regional anesthesia is required. Passing a K wire through the distal phalanx and into the middle phalanx is not as easy as it looks. A powered drill simplifies the task. The power may be supplied by either air or electricity; electric drills may be battery powered or wall powered. There are several battery-powered drills on the market that can readily be used in the outpatient setting. Some physicians use a number

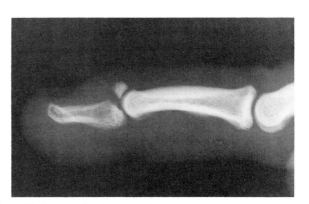

Figure 65–13. A mallet fracture with volar subluxation of the distal phalanx.

19, 3.75-cm disposable needle as a fixation wire. A syringe is used as the "driver." Usually, the top of the needle bends in the course of this maneuver, causing a fair amount of trauma. Although this may be satisfactory in some cases, it is not advised if a more conventional fixation wire is available.

Zone II Injuries

Injuries in Zone II may also be either open or closed. Open injuries are usually straightforward in that they are easy to recognize. Treatment consists of suturing the tendon with a running 4–0 nylon and supporting the joint with an external or internal splint for approximately 4 to 6 weeks. The internal splint, if used, is a K wire or some equivalent (0.088- or 0.113-cm size). The problems of placing this are similar to those outlined in the preceding section for the DIP joint.

The closed injuries cause problems because they are difficult to diagnose, and if they are *not* recognized the so-called boutonniere deformity that results is often difficult to correct surgically. To understand this deformity one has to recall the normal anatomic patterns as discussed previously. If there is an injury to the central extensor mechanism (CEM) over the PIP joint, function may initially be normal, because extension is still possible via the lateral bands. With time the central support for the lateral bands collapses and they sink, lying on the volar side of the axis of flexion of the PIP joint (Fig. 65–14). The joint more or less herniates, or buttonholes, through the extensor mechanism (hence the name of the deformity). It is obvious that the lateral bands are then in the paradoxical position of being flexors of the joint they are supposed to extend. As this occurs they pull on and tighten the *terminal* extensor mechanism, causing the DIP joint to go into hyperextension. If the finger gets fixed in this position, a great deal of function is lost, and it is very difficult to get things back to normal or even back to good function. As with so many other injuries, the best treatment is prevention.

Maneuvers to diagnose an acute boutonniere deformity have been summarized and amplified by Elson.[1] The digit in which this deformity is suspected is placed palm down on a hard table with the PIP flexion crease at the edge of the table. The digit is then passively flexed 90 degrees at this joint. If the CEM is intact, this has the effect of relaxing the lateral bands distal to the joint making the DIP relatively flail. In an attempt to extend the PIP joint against resistance, an examiner can appreciate that force is being exerted at that joint but the distal joint remains flail. However, if the CEM is disrupted, the findings are quite different, with the DIP being under some tension, and an effort to extend the PIP joint against resistance having no effect on that joint but increasing tension at the DIP joint.

When one treats a patient who complains of blunt trauma to a finger and has swelling around the PIP joint, the first step is to obtain a radiograph and rule out a fracture. The patient's usual presenting complaint is, "I jammed my finger." The second step is to assume that there may be at least a potential boutonniere deformity (even if initial function is normal) and to treat accordingly. The treatment consists of splinting the PIP joint in full extension, leaving the MCP and DIP joints free to move (Fig. 65–15). The patient should be followed at fairly frequent intervals in order for the status of the injury to be assessed. Usually, splinting for 4 weeks is sufficient.

Zone III Injuries[5, 6]

Injuries in Zone III, which is the area between the MCP and PIP joints and between the PIP and DIP joints, are

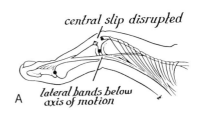

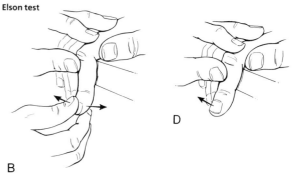

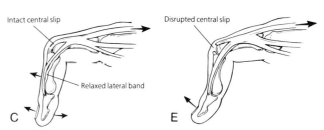

Figure 65–14. *A,* Diagrammatic explanation of a boutonniere deformity. (From Newmeyer WL: Primary Care of Hand Injuries. Philadelphia, Lea & Febiger, 1979. Reproduced by permission.) *B to E,* The Elson test for early diagnosis of an acute rupture of the central slip of the extensor digitorum communis tendon. Such rupture results in boutonniere deformity, in which the proximal interphalangeal joint is flexed, and the distal interphalangeal joint is hyperextended, as shown. With the patient's finger flexed (over a straight edge) at the proximal interphalangeal joint, the examiner palpates the dorsal surface of the middle phalanx *(B).* If the central slip is intact *(C),* proximal interphalangeal joint flexion causes the slip to tighten distally, thereby relaxing the lateral bands and leaving the distal phalanx flail *(arrows).* Thus when the patient is asked to extend the digit, the examiner feels pressure that is necessarily being exerted by an intact central slip. If the central slip is disrupted, however, the examiner feels no pressure on the dorsum of the middle phalanx as the patient tries to extend the digit *(D).* It is possible for the patient to extend the injured finger successfully only by hyperextending (by action of the lateral bands) the distal phalanx *(arrows, D and E).* (From Connolly JF: What to do for a "jammed" finger. J Musculoskeletal Med, May 1988, p 99.)

virtually always open but with only a partial laceration of the tendon. The only way to make the diagnosis is by exploration of the wound. The lacerated tendon should be closed with a running 4–0 or 5–0 suture. The degree of splinting required depends on the amount of the tendon lacerated. If the laceration is a small one, a finger guard (see Chapter 67) for 7 to 10 days is all that is necessary. If the laceration is a large one, a full forearm-hand-wrist-digit splint for 3 weeks is required. When exploring wounds in this area, one should remember that the only thing that can be cut between skin and bone is tendon.

Zone IV Injuries[5, 6]

Zone IV is the area between the distal end of the dorsal retinaculum (the six dorsal sheaths) and the area over the

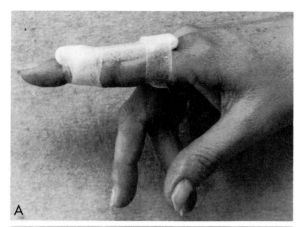

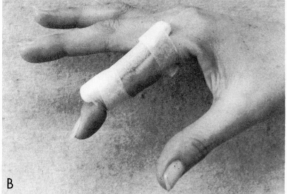

Figure 65–15. *A,* Boutonniere splint. *B,* This splint allows active flexion at the metacarpal phalangeal and distal interphalangeal joints.

MCP joints, where the extensor mechanism of the digits begins. In this area the tendons are discrete structures with interconnecting bands (juncturae tendineae—see earlier). One should assume that any laceration on the dorsum of the hand has a lacerated tendon in its depths; it is up to the treating physician to disprove this thesis. This means that the wound must be explored with tourniquet, anesthesia, and a suitable sterile preparation and field.

The biggest problem in fixing tendons in this zone is retrieving the proximal stump, which almost always retracts to some extent. The more proximal the laceration, the greater the retraction. Recovery of this stump can be quite difficult for the uninitiated, and if the proximal stump cannot be readily found, the attempt should be postponed. The wound should be closed and dressed, and arrangements should be made for repair in an operating suite under high regional or general anesthesia. One can almost always bring the distal stump into view by simply passively bringing the involved digit into full extension.

Because proximal stump retrieval is a problem, it is a good idea to extend the traumatic wound proximally along the course of the divided tendon before even making the effort of locating it. This is done from one corner of the traumatic wound, with care taken to avoid veins and sensory nerves. Often, if the physician lifts up the edge of the skin flap created by wound extension and looks proximally under the flap, a tunnel with blood staining is seen. This is the clue to the location of the proximal stump, and if one carefully puts a small hemostat or tooth forceps up this "canal," the stump can be grasped and drawn into the wound. As will be understood from a reading of the anatomy section, this is not a synovial sheath (unless one is at wrist level) but

rather a pseudocanal. A 4–0 nylon suture should be already loaded, and as one grasps the proximal stump with forceps or clamp tip, the suture is placed as far proximally in the retrieved tendon stump as possible. This acts as a holding suture while the repair is accomplished.

Tendon repairs in this area are performed as shown in Figure 65–16. Basically, these are horizontal mattress sutures placed so that the knot lies between the cut tendon ends. In fair, thin-skinned persons it is a good idea to use clear rather than colored 4–0 nylon, because the colored material may show through the skin and upset the patient, although it does no physical harm. Because there is no tendon sheath on the extensor surface except at the wrist level, there need be no worry about repairing or not repairing the sheath on the dorsal hand and digits. Virtually without exception, extensor tendon lacerations at wrist level require surgical repair in an operating suite under high regional or general anesthesia. The exposure required and the length of time needed for repair at this level are beyond the capacity of local anesthesia.

Following repair, a forearm-wrist-hand-digit splint is used. The wrist is extended 30 degrees, the MCP joints are in approximately 10 to 20 degrees of flexion, and the IP joints are nearly straight. It is wise to splint the adjacent digit or digits, except in the case of the thumb, which is splinted alone. The splint is worn for 3 weeks; however, it may be changed at approximately 10 days for wound inspection and removal of sutures. There is always a question of when to give antibiotics with open trauma. Many hand surgeons (myself included) like to err on the side of giving rather than withholding them. If there is the least suspicion of a contamination from the trauma, antibiotics should be given. Erythromycin, 250 mg every 6 hours, is satisfactory. A penicillinase-resistant penicillin or an oral cephalosporin is also satisfactory. Ampicillin is not a good drug for hand wounds.

Zone V and VI Injuries

Extensor tendon injuries in Zones V and VI are not amenable to repair in the outpatient setting, even by experienced hand surgeons. The structures are too deep and their anatomic arrangement too complex for this. The injury should be diagnosed, the skin closed, and the wound dressed

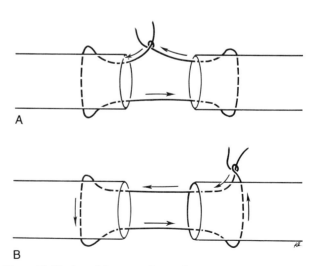

Figure 65–16. A satisfactory scheme for extensor tendon repair. (From Newmeyer WL: Primary Care of Hand Injuries. Philadelphia, Lea & Febiger, 1979. Reproduced by permission.)

and splinted. The patient should be given antibiotics (as noted earlier), and arrangements should be made for surgical repair. This repair need not be performed as an emergency procedure but should be accomplished within a week or so after injury. Management following the repair is similar to that described for Zone IV injuries.

COMPLICATIONS

The problems that may follow treatment of extensor tendon injuries include the general category of wound complications (e.g., infection and wound breakdown with disruption of the repair), disruption of the repair without wound problems, and adhesions at the site of repair that prevent full excursion of the tendon.

Wound infections can be minimized by careful observance of sterile technique at the time of wound treatment and, even more important, by the gentle handling of the tissues. When tissues are not handled gently, there is an increase in posttraumatic swelling, which leads to venous congestion and lowered tissue oxygenation. This is the ideal setup for a wound infection. The principles of wound preparation are discussed in Chapter 43. The use of antibiotics may also lower the incidence of wound infection, but careful tissue handling and wound preparation are by far the most important steps in preventing soft tissue infections following surgical repair of injuries.

Tendon disruption will occur if the sutures are ill placed or if the surgical knot is not well tied. With nylon this means *at least five throws* placed to create *square* knots. If nylon is not laid down flat and squarely, it will untie. Some surgeons prefer to use a less "slippery" material, such as Dacron or braided nylon; this is acceptable, but square knots are still important. The other cause of disruption is inadequate

immobilization. Three weeks of *complete immobilization* followed by another week or two of "protection" are advised. "Protection" means that the patient should not be using the hand with full force. If these steps are observed the incidence of disruption is very low.

Adhesions are fairly common after tendon repair but are less of a problem with extensors than with flexors. Usually, the adhesions loosen up with time. Very occasionally, an extensor tendolysis is required.

AFTERCARE

Usually, the patient can recover good function after extensor tendon injuries by just doing activities of daily living. If the patient is having trouble or needs help, arrangements can be made for hand therapy. Occasionally there may be skin adherence to a tendon repair for months or even permanently. This is of little functional significance, and a lysis can be performed if the condition is very troubling to the patient.

REFERENCES

1. Newmeyer WL: Primary Care of Hand Injuries. Philadelphia, Lea & Febiger, 1979.
2. Cooney WP, Weidman K, Malo D, et al: Management of acute flexor tendon injury in the hand. Instr Course Lect 34:373, 1985
3. Lampe EW: Surgical anatomy of the hand with special reference to infections and trauma. Clin Sympos 21:66, 1969.
4. Elson RA: Rupture of the central slip of the extensor hood of the finger. J Bone Joint Surg [Br] 68:229, 1986.
5. American Society for Surgery of the Hand: The Hand: Examination and Diagnosis. 3rd ed. New York, Churchill, Livingstone, 1989, Chapters 2 and 3.
6. American Society for Surgery of the Hand: The Hand: Primary Care of Common Problems. 2nd ed. New York, Churchill Livingstone, 1989, Chapter 6.

Chapter 66

Management of Common Dislocations

John L. Lyman and
Michael E. Ervin

INTRODUCTION

Joint dislocations are frequent presenting complaints of patients evaluated in emergency departments. At times, a dislocation is seen in association with other more dramatic problems in which case the dislocation may not be the chief complaint. Emergency physicians must be able to recognize, evaluate, and manage appropriately a variety of dislocations.

This chapter addresses the diagnosis and management of common dislocations. For most dislocations, a variety of reduction techniques have been described. This chapter does not attempt to detail all such techniques, but rather to describe a few representative

methods that are relatively safe and easy to perform to accomplish reduction. The emphasis of this chapter is on isolated dislocations, rather than fracture-dislocations. Major fracture-dislocations may require slightly different principles of management, and as a general rule, most fracture-dislocations require prompt orthopedic consultation.

ANALGESIA

Recommendations for types and quantities of analgesics and muscle relaxants vary greatly, and each physician has a favorite regimen. Selection of such agents is based on several factors, including the type of injury, the patient's allergy history, the patient's age and underlying medical condition, and the physician's familiarity with the drugs available. Whereas some dislocations will require high doses of intravenous (IV) analgesic and muscle relaxant agents to facilitate reduction, others require a minimum of such medication or can be reduced with regional anesthesia. See Chapters 40 to 42 for a detailed discussion of anesthesia/analgesia for emergency department procedures.

One key to a successful reduction is adequate analgesia and muscle relaxation. The judicious use of analgesics results in a smooth, less traumatic, and less painful procedure. A variety of narcotic analgesics are available. For most procedures the intravenous route is preferred because it offers so many advantages over the intramuscular route. An option used successfully by some physicians is to administer an intramuscular narcotic while awaiting radiographs and supplement this with intravenous benzodiazepines for the actual reduction. Useful parenteral medications include meperidine (Demerol) 1 to 2 mg/kg (adult and pediatric populations), morphine sulfate 0.1 to 0.2 mg/kg, fentanyl (Sublimaze) titrated IV (2 to 5 µg/kg), and hydromorphone (Dilaudid) 1 to 2 mg (not recommended for the pediatric population). These medications may be readily reversed with naloxone. Titration to effect while observing cardiovascular and respiratory function is mandatory when using these agents (see Chapter 41).

Appropriate drugs for muscle relaxation include the benzodiazepines diazepam and midazolam. Both these benzodiazepines are potent sedatives and can be administered intravenously. Additionally, they are both well tolerated when used appropriately. Midazolam is relatively more potent on a per milligram basis. Its half-life is significantly shorter than that of diazepam, and it provides excellent amnestic effects, both of which are important considerations in the emergency department setting.

A combination of narcotics and benzodiazepines can be used quite effectively. A common pitfall is to underuse analgesics in acute reductions, thereby making the procedure more painful for the patient and more difficult for the physician. A medication that is of particular importance in the pediatric population is ketamine. This dissociative anesthetic agent produces a rapid general anesthetic effect that lasts up to 30 minutes when given intramuscularly. The drug is also effective when given IV. Pharyngeal and laryngeal reflexes are maintained, and airway support generally is not required. The amnestic properties of ketamine are also desirable.

Some joints can be adequately anesthetized with nerve blocks or injection of a local anesthetic. The digits are particularly amenable to nerve blocks; for example, a proximal interphalangeal joint dislocation of the hand can often be reduced after a digital block. A metacarpophalangeal dislocation of the thumb may be reduced more readily with a local lidocaine injection.

In some instances, general anesthesia is required. Those dislocations that may require general anesthesia are indicated.

GENERAL PRINCIPLES OF MANAGEMENT

1. Dislocations are often associated with fractures that may not be evident on physical examination. For this reason, radiographs should be obtained for joint dislocations both prior to and following reduction. Exceptions to this may be made when vascular embarrassment is present and when there may be some delay in obtaining a radiograph. Additionally, children with a history and physical examination classic for radial head subluxation do not always require radiographs before reduction. Some fractures are not evident until a postreduction radiograph has been taken.

2. Joint dislocations are described in terms of where the distal articulating surface is relative to the proximal articulating surface. For example, in an anterior shoulder dislocation, the humeral head (distal articulating surface) takes a position anterior to the glenoid fossa (the proximal articulating surface).

3. A subluxation ("partial dislocation") occurs when there is a joint disruption but the articulating surfaces are maintained in some degree of apposition.

4. Acute dislocations may reduce spontaneously or be reduced by direct patient intervention before presentation in the emergency department. If the physician suspects that a dislocation has been reduced before examination in the emergency department, the joint injury should be treated as if a dislocation or subluxation did in fact occur.

5. Once a dislocation has been reduced, postreduction films should be taken, both to verify and document anatomic reduction and to evaluate for subtle fractures. It is important to immobilize the joint before having radiographs taken, because the joint may be unstable and may redislocate with minimal movement.

6. Inability to relocate a dislocated joint does not necessarily mean that an improper technique has been used. Some dislocations are irreducible by a closed technique, most commonly because of the interposition of soft tissue. Persistent attempts at relocation when soft tissue is interposed may lead to further trauma of the joint and surrounding tissue. After one or two unsuccessful attempts at relocation, appropriate referral for possible open reduction or an attempt at closed reduction under general anesthesia should be made.

7. A properly reduced joint dislocation not only relieves pain but also relieves stress on the surrounding soft tissues. The corollary to this statement is that the sooner a joint is reduced, the sooner the stress on the neurovascular bundles is relieved.

8. The neurovascular and circulatory status of the affected extremity should be checked immediately on the patient's presentation to the emergency department. Any compromise of these structures indicates that prompt action should be taken. The neurovascular status must also be reassessed serially and documented after reduction.

9. Three keys to successful reduction are (1) knowledge of the anatomy and reduction manuever, (2) use of proper analgesia, and (3) proceeding in a slow and gentle manner.

10. The physician should attempt to ascertain the mechanism of injury. Such information provides clues to the type of injury and alerts the physician to the possibility of additional associated injuries.

11. The physician must appreciate common associated musculoskeletal injuries. For example, knee injuries in a motor vehicle accident should alert the physician to the possibility of a posterior hip dislocation. As another example, a fracture of the proximal one third of the ulna should suggest to the physician the possibility of a radial head dislocation (Monteggia fracture).

12. The postreduction treatment is as important as the reduction itself. Following reduction, the joint must be properly splinted. *An acute joint dislocation is not a minor injury.* Because there is always concomitant muscular, ligamentous, or other soft tissue disruption with any dislocation, disability is often the end result. Because soft tissue swelling and muscle spasm may initially obscure joint instability or disability, proper follow-up is mandatory.

13. It is imperative that the physician understand the complications and possible sequelae of the various types of dislocations.

14. Before attempting a reduction, the physician must be properly prepared in terms of adequate assistance.

SHOULDER DISLOCATIONS

The shoulder is designed for a large range of motion, with a large humeral head resting on a shallow glenoid fossa. This anatomic arrangement allows for a wide range of motion, but there is a relative lack of stability. Most shoulder dislocations are anterior, with the humeral head coming to rest in a position anterior to the glenoid fossa. The next most common shoulder dislocation is the posterior dislocation. Inferior (luxatio erecta), superior, and intrathoracic dislocations are rarely seen. Although anterior dislocations are usually relatively apparent on clinical examination, posterior dislocations may be difficult to appreciate clinically and radiographically. Posterior dislocations are the most commonly missed dislocation in the emergency department. Such dislocations may occur during a grand mal seizure or as the result of an electric shock. Shoulder dislocations are uncommon in young children. When dislocations do occur in this age group, the most common major joint dislocation is the elbow.

When a shoulder is dislocated, there is surrounding soft tissue trauma. Despite proper reduction and follow-up care, some people are left with weakness in the surrounding soft tissue of the shoulder, which allows recurrent dislocations. Often these recurrent dislocations follow minor joint position changes, such as raising one's arm over the head to comb the hair or rolling over in bed. Although recurrent dislocations can be reduced by the techniques described, surgical intervention may be needed to prevent subsequent dislocations.

Anterior Shoulder Dislocations

Anterior shoulder dislocations are the most common major joint dislocations in adults. An anterior shoulder dislocation is usually the result of forceful abduction and external rotation of the humerus. A direct blow to the posterior aspect of the humeral head may also result in an anterior dislocation.

There are three subtypes of anterior dislocations that are named according to where the humeral head lies. The humeral head may lie in a position beneath the clavicle (subclavicular), beneath the coracoid process (subcoracoid, most common), or anterior and inferior to the glenoid fossa (subglenoid) (Fig. 66–1). All these anterior dislocations can be reduced in the same manner.

Typically, when presenting, the patient is supporting the injured extremity in some manner and is resisting any movement of the shoulder (Fig. 66–2). The shoulder is usually held in slight abduction. If the trauma was minimal or if the patient has minimal pain in the joint area, the dislocation is probably recurrent rather than an initial injury. Physical examination usually reveals a loss of the deltoid contour of the shoulder when compared with the contralateral side. Although the diagnosis is often straightforward, it can be difficult in heavily muscled, obese, and uncooperative patients. Manipulation of the shoulder is not indicated until radiographs have demonstrated the pathology and associated fractures have been identified. The need for prereduction radiographs in the patient who suffers a *recurrent* dislocation in the *absence* of trauma must be individualized. In all cases, postreduction radiographs are essential.

It is extremely important that the neurovascular status of the affected extremity be assessed early in the evaluation. Circulatory status can be checked quickly by comparing peripheral pulses. The neurologic status should include evaluation of all the major nerves of the arm. The axillary nerve is the most commonly injured nerve in anterior shoulder dislocations. Injury of this nerve may produce an area of anesthesia on the upper lateral aspects of the arm (Fig. 66–3) and can result in paralysis of the deltoid muscle. Deltoid function is often difficult to evaluate in the acutely painful shoulder, but sensory evaluation can be accomplished without difficulty. Usually axillary nerve injuries are transient and resolve with time. The presence of an axillary nerve injury does not change the initial treatment of an anterior shoulder dislocation.

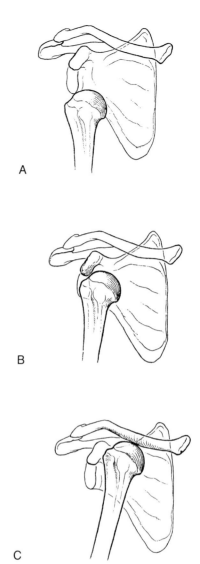

Figure 66–1. Types of anterior dislocations. These types of anterior dislocations should receive the same treatment. *A*, Subglenoid dislocation (rare type). *B*, Subcoracoid dislocation (most common type). *C*, Subclavicular dislocation (rare type). (From DePalma AF: Management of Fractures and Dislocations: An Atlas. Philadelphia, WB Saunders Co, 1970, p 617. Reproduced by permission.)

RADIOGRAPHS

Radiographic evaluation of suspected shoulder dislocations should include at least two views of the shoulder. True anteroposterior (AP) views of the shoulder and true lateral radiographs of the scapula (also called the scapular "Y" view) are the films of choice in shoulder trauma (Figs. 66–4 and 66–5). The true AP view is shot at a right angle to the scapula, not at a right angle to the coronal plane. This requires the rotation of the patient 30 to 40 degrees as shown in Figure 66–4. The true lateral scapular view is shot tangential to the scapula. The resultant radiograph clearly delineates the relation of the humeral head to the glenoid fossa and is the best view to demonstrate a posterior dislocation (see Fig. 66–5).

Postreduction radiographs should include a true AP view, the true lateral scapular view, and preferably an axillary view. The internal rotation view may reveal an impaction fracture of the humeral head, known as *Hill-Sachs*

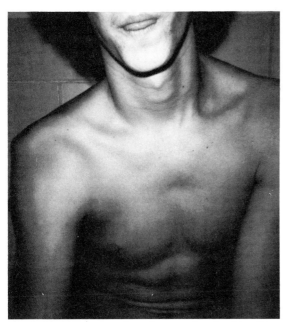

Figure 66–2. Typical presentation of an anterior shoulder dislocation. The shoulder is very painful; thus, the patient resists movement. The outer round contour of the shoulder is flattened, and the displaced humeral head may be appreciated in the subcoracoid area. Often the patient will abduct the arm slightly, bend the torso toward the injured side, and support the flexed elbow on the injured side with the other hand.

lesion. When the patient is sent for postreduction radiographs, the shoulder should be properly immobilized. To prevent redislocation, manipulation of the shoulder should be gentle and minimal.

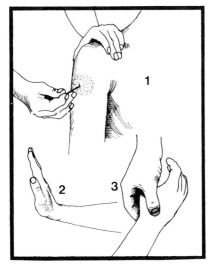

Figure 66–3. Evaluation of the upper extremity with a shoulder dislocation. Axillary (circumflex) nerve palsy is the most common neurologic complication. Test for integrity of the nerve by assessing sensation to pin prick *(1)* in its distribution over the "regimental badge" area. (The shoulder is usually too painful to assess deltoid activity with certainty.) Look for other (rare) involvement of the radial portion of the posterior cord *(2)* and involvement of the axillary artery *(3)*. (From McRae R: Practical Fracture Treatment. Edinburgh, Churchill Livingstone, 1981, p 84. Reproduced by permission.)

REDUCTION

Many methods have been proposed for reducing anterior shoulder dislocations. Successful reduction is usually quite obvious, as indicated by a marked reduction in pain, by the practitioner or patient feeling the shoulder slip back into place, and by the return of the normal contour of the shoulder. Following reduction, the shoulder may be gently manipulated through a small 10- to 15-degree range of motion to ensure that anatomic alignment has been achieved. The palm of the injured arm may be easily placed on the opposite shoulder after reduction. If reduction has been successful, such passive range of motion is not particularly painful or dangerous and it ensures proper reduction.

In this section, a number of methods that are relatively safe, atraumatic, and easy to master are discussed. The key to a successful shoulder reduction is a slow, yet steady, approach with adequate analgesia and muscle relaxation. Most physicians prefer less traumatic traction methods of reduction to leverage techniques, such as the Kocher method, which can produce soft tissue injuries.

Stimson Maneuver (Fig. 66–6). In this classic technique, the patient is placed in the prone position on a bed or cart with the affected shoulder toward one side. The arm should hang down but not touch the floor. A small weight (10 to 20 pounds) is strapped to the wrist or attached above the elbow to produce steady traction. A bucket of water or a sand bag may also be used. The weight is left in place for 20 to 30 minutes or until the shoulder is reduced. This is not a particularly painful reduction, but some analgesia is recommended. The scapula may be rotated with the patient in this position (see "Scapular Rotation") or gentle internal or external humeral rotation may be performed. With physician patience, this method is often successful because it allows gravity, with the help of weights, to gradually overcome the associated muscle spasm and permit reduction without the use of excessive analgesics. Care must be taken to secure the patient to the stretcher, especially if the patient is intoxicated or sedated.

Scapular Rotation or Manipulation. For this reduction the patient is placed and secured in a prone position on a cart, in the same manner as for the Stimson technique (Fig. 66–7). Alternatively this technique may be performed with the patient sitting. For traction, 5 to 15 pounds of force are applied to the forearm by an assistant or by a hanging weight applied in the same manner as in the Stimson maneuver. After appropriate relaxation or analgesia, the interior tip of the scapula is rotated medially by applying pressure with one hand. At the same time, the superior aspect of the scapula is rotated laterally with the other hand. Successful reduction is signified by a palpable, and often audible, clunk. This method is touted as having a high degree of success (greater than 90 per cent), often without the use of adjunct sedation.

External Rotation Method. With this technique, the patient is placed in a supine position and the affected arm is adducted to the side (Fig. 66–8). The elbow on the affected side is flexed to 90 degrees, and then, slowly, the physician externally rotates the arm using the forearm as a lever. The external rotation should be slow and gentle. No traction is applied, and the rotation is periodically halted as pain is produced. It requires about 10 minutes for the forearm to go from a sagittal plane to a coronal plane. Usually the shoulder is reduced by the time the coronal plane is reached. This method is often successful and requires only one physician and little exertion or strength. If reduction has not occurred by the time the coronal plane is reached, gentle traction or countertraction is applied.

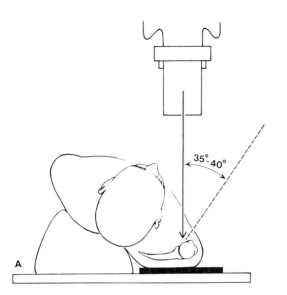

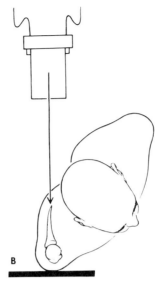

Figure 66–4. *A* and *B*, Trauma series includes two views of the shoulder made perpendicular and parallel to the scapular plane. The advantage is that roentgenograms may be obtained without moving the patient or removing the arm from the sling. (From Heppenstall RB: Fracture Treatment and Healing. Philadelphia, WB Saunders Co, 1980, p 374. Reproduced by permission.)

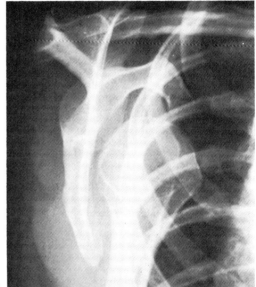

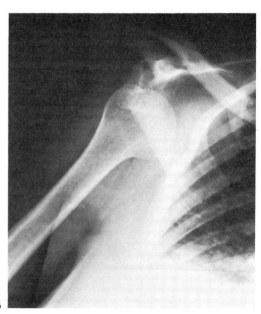

Figure 66–5. In the trauma series, a lateral view of the scapula (also called scapular Y view) demonstrates the head of the humerus displaced inferiorly and medially, the most common position for an anterior dislocation *(A)*. If this were a posterior dislocation (see Fig. 66–13), the humeral head would be displaced laterally. The same anterior dislocation is shown on the anteroposterior projection *(B)*. (From Heppenstall RB: Fracture Treatment and Healing. Philadelphia, WB Saunders Co, 1980, p 392. Reproduced by permission.)

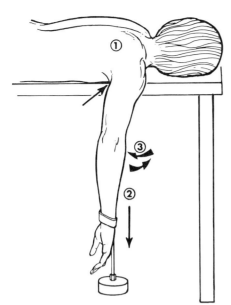

Figure 66–6. Stimson technique. This technique should be tried first, because it is the least traumatic if the patient can relax the shoulder muscles. *1*, The patient is lying prone on the edge of the table. One must be careful that the drugged or intoxicated patient does not fall off the table. Belts or sheets can be used to secure the patient to the stretcher. *2*, 10-kg weights are attached to the arm, and the patient maintains this position for 20 to 30 minutes, if necessary. *3*, Occasionally, gentle external and internal rotation of the shoulder with manual traction aids reduction. (From DePalma AF: Management of Fractures and Dislocations: An Atlas. Philadelphia, WB Saunders Co, 1970, p 618. Reproduced by permission.)

Traction–Countertraction. With this method, the patient is placed in a supine position on a cart and a sheet or a strap is wrapped around the upper chest and under the axilla of the affected shoulder (Fig. 66–9). An assistant holds the ends of this sheet and applies countertraction. Alternatively the strap may be attached to the stretcher itself. The physician then flexes the elbow of the injured extremity and places a second sheet or strap about the patient's forearm, just distal to the flexed elbow. The sheet is securely fastened behind the physician's back. In-line traction is applied by the physician, who gently and steadily leans back. Such steady in-line traction helps overcome the associated muscle

spasm and dislodges the humeral head. (One must be careful not to produce a friction burn of the skin of the forearm or axilla with the sheet, a particularly common event in the elderly patient with thin or fragile skin.) The forearm and hand are held in neutral position by the physician. Gentle external rotation of the forearm may be needed if in-line traction alone does not effect reduction.

As an alternative, the physician applies in-line traction to the affected extremity with the elbow in complete extension by holding the extremity at the wrist or elbow with both hands. Slight external rotation can be helpful after the application of traction although the application of rotation with traction has been associated with humeral neck fractures in the elderly. If relocation does not occur, slight lateral traction may be applied by another sheet placed on the upper arm by an assistant. If necessary, the physician can adduct the arm across the midline while maintaining traction. It is best if the physician holds the patient's upper extremity and leans backward, using the body to give continuous traction rather than attempting to pull on the patient's arm using the power of biceps.

Other Methods. The use of the Hippocratic technique (physician's foot placed on the chest wall to provide countertraction) is discouraged. Although the Hippocratic technique is often successful, it is dangerous and is associated with neurovascular complications. Uncomplicated dislocations should be easily reduced with the aforementioned methods.

A rather unique method suggested by Poulsen is the "Eskimo technique."[1] This maneuver may be performed in the field and may be taught to individuals with chronic dislocations or to nonmedical personnel. With this technique the patient is placed on the floor, lying on the nondislocated shoulder. Two persons lift the patient up by the abducted dislocated arm, keeping the opposite shoulder suspended a few inches off the ground, using the patient's body weight for countertraction (Fig. 66–10). This procedure has the potential to place the brachial plexus or axillary nerve under undue stretch, but in the small series by Poulsen (23 patients) such complications were not observed. Another technique for the application of countertraction outside the hospital has been described by Dutky.[2] If the patient is wearing a flotation device, the clinician sits facing the supine patient's injured shoulder. The clinician's leg cephalad to the patient is placed through the flotation device's arm opening, under the patient's neck, and against the opposite inner wall of the device. Alternatively a strap of clothing or cravat can be

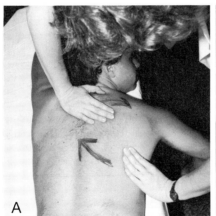

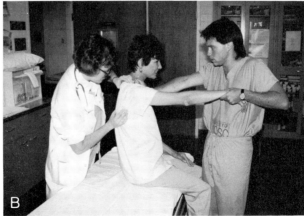

Figure 66–7. Scapular rotation method for reducing an anterior shoulder dislocation. With the patient prone *(A)* and traction or weights applied to the wrist, the physician rotates the inferior tip of the scapula medially (toward the midline) and the superior portion laterally. With the patient seated *(B)*, an assistant provides traction-countertraction, and the physician rotates the scapula in the same manner.

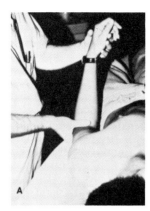
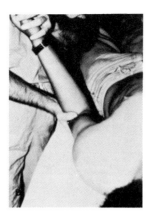
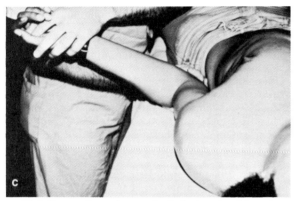

Figure 66–8. External rotation method. *A,* Arm is adducted to the patient's side. In one hand, the elbow is held flexed at 90 degrees while other hand grasps the wrist. *B,* Slowly and gently, the forearm is used as a lever to rotate the arm externally. *C,* Usually by the time the forearm has reached the coronal plane, the shoulder will have been reduced. (From Mirick MJ, Clinton J, Ruiz E: External rotation method of shoulder dislocation reduction. JACEP 8:529, 1979. Reproduced by permission.)

looped around the patient's upper thorax and similarly held by the clinician's leg.

If standard techniques coupled with appropriate analgesic and muscle relaxant medication are unsuccessful, orthopedic consultation is recommended. General anesthesia for closed or open reduction may be required in complicated cases.

POSTREDUCTION CARE

Following reduction, the shoulder should be immobilized with a sling and swath or shoulder immobilizer. The patient must avoid abduction and external rotation of the arm. This activity is best explained to the patient by demonstrating that combing the hair with the affected arm simulates abduction and external rotation. The circulatory status of the shoulder should be reassessed, and the integrity of the axillary nerve should be rechecked and documented. Postreduction radiographs should be taken. If relocation has occurred and if no fractures are noted on the postreduction film, the patient can be discharged with a shoulder immobilizer or a similar immobilization device. The patient should be given instructions for follow-up but generally does not have to be seen for 5 to 7 days. If any fractures are noted on the postreduction radiograph, orthopedic consultation is suggested. The length of time that the uncomplicated anteriorly dislocated shoulder is immobilized depends on the age of the patient as well as associated injuries. Generally,

the shoulder is immobilized for 3 weeks in younger patients, followed by 3 weeks of gentle, active range-of-motion exercises. Older patients may have considerable stiffness and other disabilities following dislocation; thus, mobilization may be begun sooner to avoid complications such as a frozen shoulder. Orthopedic follow-up is recommended in all such cases.

Posterior Shoulder Dislocations

Posterior shoulder dislocations account for a small percentage of all acute shoulder dislocations and can be very difficult to diagnose both clinically and radiographically. Posterior dislocations are encountered most commonly after seizures or electric shock accidents, and the pathology may be bilateral in such cases. The causal mechanism for posterior dislocations is usually abduction and internal rotation, although occasionally posterior dislocations result from direct anterior forces.

The patient may present with complaints of shoulder pain, having sustained a mechanism of injury compatible with posterior dislocation. The arm will be adducted and internally rotated, and resistance to any movement will be noted. Physical examination may reveal a shoulder that has a loss of contour compared with the other shoulder (beware of a bilateral dislocation), and passive or active external rotation is usually not possible. Neurovascular deficits are infrequent following posterior dislocations.

RADIOGRAPHS

As with anterior dislocations, a true AP and a true lateral shoulder radiograph should be obtained. The AP view may appear deceptively normal, although close examination usually reveals a slight distortion of the normal elliptical overlap of the humeral head on the glenoid rim (Figs. 66–11 and 66–12). A true lateral (transscapular, or Y) view reveals the humeral head to be located posterior to the glenoid fossa (Fig. 66–13).

TREATMENT

Posterior dislocations can usually be reduced with gentle in-line traction as described previously for anterior shoulder dislocations. With the patient in a supine position, in-line traction is applied to the arm. Countertraction is supplied in the same manner as described for anterior dislocations. The physician should maintain gentle in-line traction for 10 to 15 minutes. If the humeral head does not relocate with in-line traction, the physician may apply direct pressure over the humeral head to gently manipulate the head around the glenoid rim and into the glenoid fossa. After the shoulder has been reduced, the arm can be gently internally and externally rotated without difficulty.

POSTREDUCTION CARE

Following shoulder reduction, the neurovascular status should be reassessed and postreduction films should be taken. If the shoulder joint is grossly stable, a shoulder immobilizer may be used to immobilize the shoulder. If the shoulder appears to be grossly unstable, a spica cast with the humerus in external rotation is usually required. Such unstable shoulder dislocations should be promptly referred to an orthopedist.

Because posterior dislocations are uncommon injuries, early orthopedic consultation and referral are suggested.

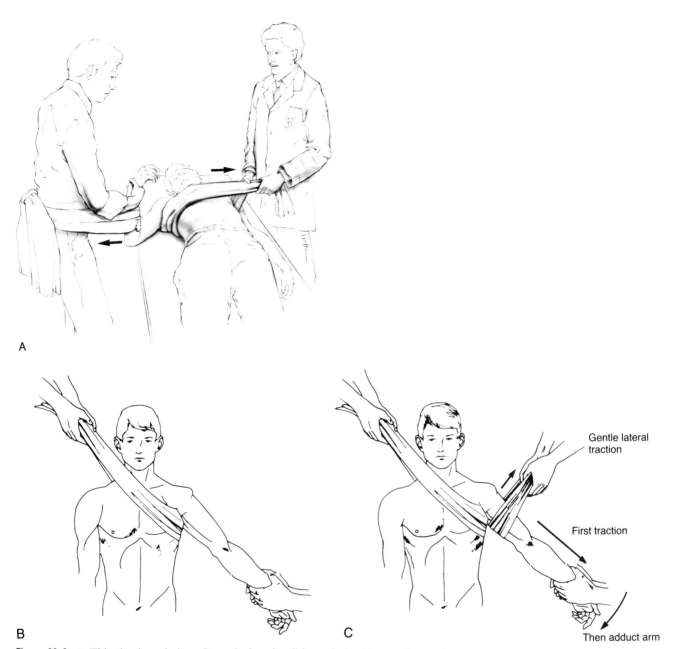

A

B

C

Gentle lateral traction

First traction

Then adduct arm

Figure 66–9. *A,* This simple technique for reducing the dislocated shoulder applies gradual and steady traction along the axis of the dislocated limb. A bedsheet, wrapped around the supine patient's upper chest wall and over the unaffected shoulder, is either tied or held by an assistant and acts as a fixed counterforce. A second bedsheet is placed around the patient's flexed forearm, just distal to the flexed elbow, and securely tied behind the physician's back. Note that a significant skin avulsion or friction burn may occur if there is excessive motion of the sheets, especially in the elderly patient with thin, delicate skin. With the patient's forearm held in a neutral rotation and the hand in a vertical position, the physician applies traction by leaning back. (From Respet PB: A practical technique for reducing shoulder dislocations. J Musculoskel Med 5:29, 1988.) *B,* Traction-countertraction technique for reducing anterior shoulder dislocations. *C,* Traction–lateral traction technique for reducing anterior shoulder dislocations. An additional sheet should be wrapped around the upper arm *(B),* and lateral traction should be applied. If traction in this line is not successful, slowly bring (adduct) the extended arm across the abdomen while maintaining traction. (From Simon R, Koenigsknecht S: Orthopedics in Emergency Medicine. New York, Appleton-Century-Crofts, 1982, p 343. Reproduced by permission.)

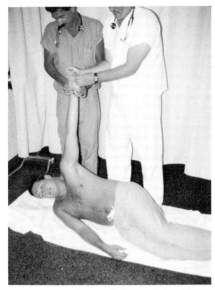

Figure 66–10. With the Eskimo technique of shoulder reduction, the patient is literally picked up and suspended by the affected arm.

Conclusions

1. The neurovascular status must be checked both before and after reduction.

2. Failure to reduce a dislocation may indicate entrapment of soft tissue or a fracture fragment in the joint space. If the dislocation does not reduce readily, it should not be assumed that it is because the wrong technique is being used or that not enough force is being applied, or both.

3. The shoulder should be immobilized when postreduction radiographs are being taken.

4. Posterior dislocations can occur bilaterally, especially when the etiology is a major motor seizure.

5. Although recurrent dislocations can be reduced by the aforementioned methods, surgical intervention may eventually be necessary and early orthopedic referral is strongly recommended.

6. Usually successful reduction is obvious to both the patient and the physician, but before the patient is discharged from the hospital, it should be ascertained that anatomic reduction has been achieved. The physician may be misled by a partial reduction if reliance is placed on feeling motion during the reduction maneuver.

ACROMIOCLAVICULAR SUBLUXATIONS AND DISLOCATIONS

The acromioclavicular joint can be injured either indirectly, such as can occur during a fall on an adducted arm, or directly, such as can occur from a direct blow to the shoulder during a fall. Although the acromioclavicular ligament directly attaches the acromion and the clavicle, two other ligaments help to maintain the integrity of this joint by attaching the clavicle and the coracoid process of the scapula. These two ligaments are the conoid and the trapezoid ligaments.

Acromioclavicular joint subluxations and dislocations are classified by the degree of ligamentous damage and consequent joint disruption. *First-degree* injuries involve a partial tear of the acromioclavicular ligament. Clinical examination reveals point tenderness and pain with movement of the shoulder, although no radiographic abnormalities are seen. Treatment consists of 2 to 3 weeks of sling immobilization, ice packs for 24 hours and analgesics, and nonemergency referral.

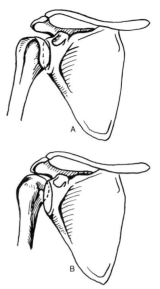

Figure 66–11. *A*, Note the normal elliptical pattern of overlap produced by the head of the humerus and the glenoid fossa. *B*, In the patient with a posterior dislocation, this pattern is lost and there is also internal rotation of the greater tuberosity. (From Simon R, Koenigsknecht S: Orthopedics in Emergency Medicine. New York, Appleton-Century-Crofts, 1982, p 344. Reproduced by permission.)

Second-degree injuries involve a disruption of the acromioclavicular ligament and a partial disruption of the conoid and trapezoid ligaments. Point tenderness and pain with shoulder movement are seen, often with moderate edema. Radiographs are often normal, although stress radiographs (with the patient standing and holding approximately 10 pounds of weight in each hand) *may* reveal a subluxation of the clavicle relative to the acromion. This subluxation is indicated by a separation of the clavicle from the acromion of up to 50 per cent of the clavicle's diameter. Treatment is similar to that described for first-degree injuries, with referral to an orthopedist.

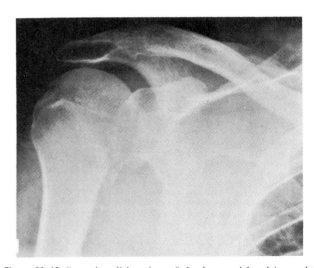

Figure 66–12. Posterior dislocation of the humeral head is a subtle finding on the anteroposterior view. This film shows a medial displacement of the humeral head and an abnormal overlap with the glenoid rim. A fracture fragment of the lesser tuberosity is superimposed on the inferior rim of the glenoid. (From Greenbaum E (ed): Radiology of the Emergency Patient. New York, John Wiley & Sons, Inc, 1982, p 511. Reproduced by permission.)

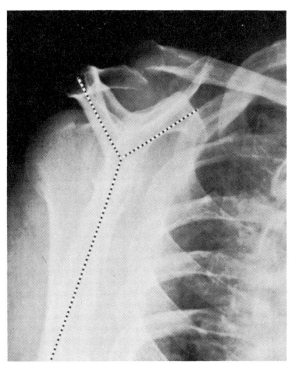

Figure 66–13. Transscapular projection showing the dislocated humeral head, posterior in relationship to the intersecting limbs of the Y. Note that in a posterior dislocation, the humeral head lies lateral to the scapular Y. (From Greenbaum E (ed): Radiology of the Emergency Patient. New York, John Wiley & Sons, Inc, 1982, p 512. Reproduced by permission.)

Third-degree injuries involve a complete disruption of the acromioclavicular, conoid, and trapezoid ligaments, with a consequent upward displacement of the distal clavicle. Tenderness, pain with movement, and edema are present. Radiographs confirm the upward displacement of the distal clavicle (as in all suspected acromioclavicular joint injuries, radiographs should be made with the patient standing, if possible, as spontaneous reductions tend to occur in recumbency). Prompt orthopedic referral is indicated for these injuries, with sling immobilization in the interim.

Radiographs

Radiographs are usually obtained in cases of suspected acromioclavicular injuries to rule out fractures and to assess the degree of separation. Ideally, simultaneous views of both shoulders are obtained, and measurements are compared between the injured and normal sides. Traditionally, "weighted films" have been performed with the patient holding on to a weight with the arms at the side to distract the acromioclavicular joint. It has been suggested that splinting or muscle spasm may mask a third-degree injury on the unstressed film. Such evidence is anecdotal, and the routine use of weighted radiographs has been questioned, because of their lack of proven benefit, increased pain, radiation exposure, and expense to the patient. Bossart and associates advocate that routine additional weighted radiographs be abandoned because in their prospective study of 84 patients the stress films provided additional diagnostic information in only three cases.[3] Additionally, in some cases the weighted films themselves caused the acromioclavicular injury to appear less obvious. It is noted that surgery is rarely performed for even a third-degree acromioclavicular separation; hence the routine use of weighted radiographs in the emergency department is not justified.

ELBOW DISLOCATIONS

The elbow is the second most frequently dislocated joint in adults and is the most commonly dislocated joint in children younger than 10 years of age. As the elbow is a relatively stable joint, dislocation often involves severe disruption of associated ligaments and surrounding soft tissues. Fractures frequently accompany elbow dislocations, especially those involving the coronoid process, radial head, capitellum, or olecranon. An avulsion fracture of the medial epicondyle of the humerus may be seen in children with elbow dislocations. The radius and ulna frequently displace as a unit, and elbow dislocations are classified according to the relationship between the proximal ulna and radius and the distal humerus. For example, in a posterior dislocation, the ulna and radius are displaced backward and lie behind the humerus (Fig. 66–14).

One of the feared consequences of elbow dislocations is damage to the neurovascular bundles that traverse the elbow. The various forces applied to the elbow during dislocation can cause severe damage to the brachial artery or to the ulnar and median nerves. It is vitally important that an adequate neurologic assessment of the major nerve trunks distal to the elbow be carried out before and after reduction. The same is true for the circulatory status of the forearm. Compromise of the vascular status of the forearm demands immediate radiographic assessment and urgent reduction of the elbow. Elbow dislocations may result in marked soft tissue swelling of the elbow and forearm even after reduc-

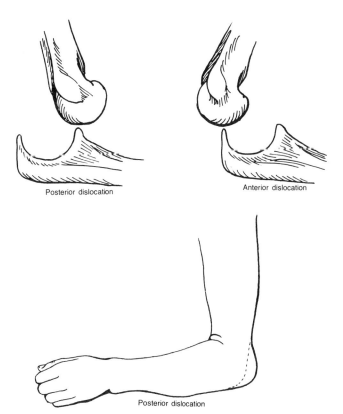

Figure 66–14. Classification of elbow dislocations. (From Simon R, Koenigsknecht S: Orthopedics in Emergency Medicine. New York, Appleton-Century-Crofts, 1982, p 333. Reproduced by permission.)

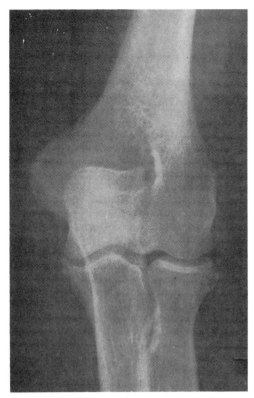
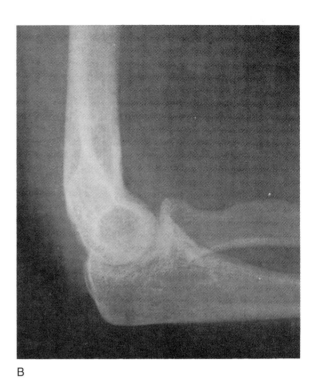

Figure 66–15. Routine anteroposterior *(A)* and lateral *(B)* radiographs of a normal adult elbow. In the frontal projection, note the relationship between the articulating surface of the radius and the capitellum and the articulating surface of the coronoid process and the trochlea. Note, also, in the frontal projection, the normal smooth concave cortical sweep from the radial neck to the radial head. In the lateral projection *(B)*, note that the image of the coronoid process is superimposed on the image of the radial head and that the soft-tissue density around the elbow is homogeneous. (From Harris JH Jr, Harris WH: Radiology of Emergency Medicine. 2nd ed. Baltimore, Williams & Wilkins, 1981, p 203. Reproduced by permission.)

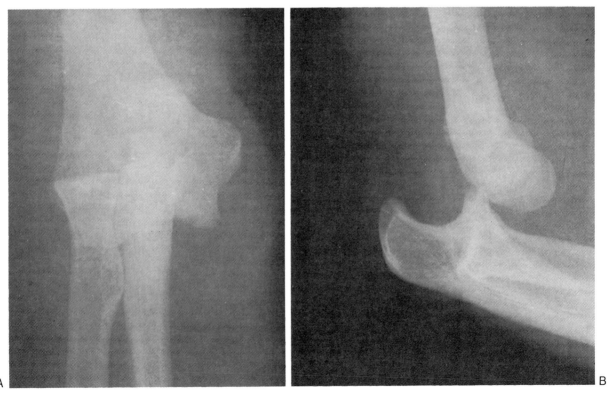

Figure 66–16. *A* and *B,* Complete posterior dislocation of the elbow. (From Harris JH Jr, Harris WH: Radiology of Emergency Medicine. 2nd ed. Baltimore, Williams & Wilkins, 1981, p 208. Reproduced by permission.)

tion. The swelling itself may cause embarrassment of the neurovascular bundles of the forearm, a type of compartment syndrome. For this reason, it is advised that all patients with elbow dislocations be admitted to the hospital for ongoing evaluation of the neurovascular status of the forearm for a period of 24 hours. Traumatic myositis ossificans of the brachialis muscle or ossification of a subperiosteal hematoma may be seen following an elbow dislocation. Stiffness, especially in elderly patients, is also a common sequela.

Analgesia

Elbow dislocations are usually quite painful, and inadequate analgesia will make reduction difficult. Intramuscular and intravenous regimens of analgesia and muscle relaxant agents as described previously can be used. Nitrous oxide may also be helpful. Axillary blocks or intravenous regional anesthesia (see Chapters 38 and 41) may also be used.

If none of these methods is applicable or available, general anesthesia may be necessary.

Radiographs

Two radiographic views, including a lateral and an AP view (Fig. 66–15), should be obtained.

Posterior Dislocations

A posterior dislocation is the most common type of elbow dislocation. In a posterior dislocation, the olecranon assumes a position posterior to the distal humerus (Fig. 66–16). The usual mechanism of injury is a fall on an outstretched arm held in extension. The patient usually presents with the arm held to the side with the elbow in moderate flexion of about 30 to 40 degrees. Physical examination reveals an unusually prominent olecranon process, although the severe swelling sometimes seen with elbow dislocations may make palpation of the olecranon difficult.

REDUCTION OF POSTERIOR DISLOCATIONS OF THE ELBOW

Reduction of a posterior elbow dislocation can be a relatively simple procedure (Fig. 66–17). When extremity muscle spasm is severe, an axillary nerve block may be needed to obtain adequate muscle relaxation. Once muscle relaxation is attained, the patient is placed in a supine position. An assistant then stabilizes the humerus by holding it with both hands. The physician holds the wrist of the affected extremity with one hand and applies slow and gentle, yet steady, in-line traction. It is important to supinate the patient's wrist and to maintain the elbow in slight flexion, avoiding hyperextension. A clunk can be heard or felt as the elbow is reduced. The forearm may be flexed gently as traction is maintained if reduction is not easily achieved by traction alone.

If the elbow does not reduce with this technique, the physician may need to apply downward pressure at the proximal forearm or apply pressure behind the olecranon while, at the same time, maintaining in-line traction. This downward force may help to "unlock" the coronoid process, which may be trapped in the olecranon fossa. At times, reduction can be best accomplished with the shoulder abducted and the distal humerus resting on the back of a chair. In this position, the olecranon can be pushed up and away from the distal humerus by the physician while an assistant applies gentle longitudinal downward traction on the flexed forearm. When reduction does occur, gentle flexion and extension of the elbow will be possible and should be performed to confirm anatomic reduction and stability.

Anterior Dislocations

Although uncommon, anterior dislocations are the second most common elbow dislocations seen in the emergency department. The mechanism of injury is a fall on the flexed elbow with a direct force displacing the olecranon anteriorly so that it assumes a position anterior to the distal humerus. Great forces are required to cause such a dislocation, and

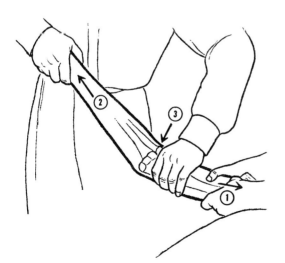 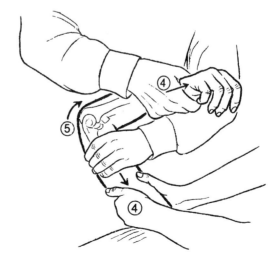

Figure 66–17. Manipulative reduction of posterior elbow dislocation. While an assistant holds the arm and makes steady countertraction *(1)*, grasp the wrist with one hand, and apply steady traction on the forearm in the position in which it lies *(2)*. While traction is maintained, correct any lateral displacement with the other hand *(3)*. While traction is maintained *(4)*, gently flex the forearm *(5)*. *Note* that with reduction, a click is usually felt and heard as the olecranon engages the articular surface of the humerus. (From DePalma AF: Management of Fractures and Dislocations: An Atlas. Philadelphia, WB Saunders Co, 1970, pp 793 and 794. Reproduced by permission.)

consequently such dislocations are often associated with fractures, especially about the olecranon process.

Injuries to the neurovascular bundles are seen more frequently with anterior dislocations than with posterior dislocations. Again, it is imperative that the neurovascular status of the forearm be adequately assessed as soon as possible during the evaluation process.

On physical examination, the elbow joint will be markedly disrupted. Because there is nothing overlying the elbow except skin, one may be able to palpate the olecranon anterior to the distal humerus. The elbow itself is generally held in full extension, and the patient usually resists any attempt at flexion or extension of the elbow.

Reduction of Anterior Dislocation of the Elbow

After adequate analgesia, the patient is placed in a supine position (Fig. 66–18). An assistant stabilizes the humerus with two hands while the physician applies steady inline traction by holding the wrist with one hand while the second hand applies a downward force at the proximal radius and ulna. This downward force helps to lift the olecranon process over the distal humerus.

Postreduction Care

Patients with anterior or posterior elbow dislocations (except radial head subluxation in children) are generally admitted to the hospital for 24 hours for elevation of the injured extremity and neurovascular monitoring. Splints should be used as follows: Posterior dislocations should be splinted with a posterior splint to include the wrist with the elbow in 90 degrees of flexion and the wrist in neutral position. Anterior dislocations should be splinted with a

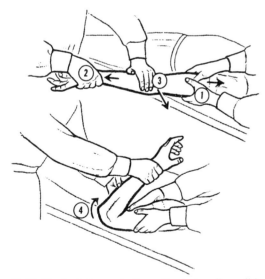

Figure 66–18. Manipulative reduction of anterior elbow dislocation. Reduction is performed with the patient under local or general anesthesia. *1,* An assistant grasps the arm and provides countertraction. *2,* The operator grasps the wrist with one hand and applies traction in the line of the arm, and with the other hand applies firm, steady pressure downward and backward on the upper end of the forearm *(3).* A click usually indicates that reduction is achieved. *4,* The arm is flexed to 45 degrees beyond a right angle. (From DePalma AF: Management of Fractures and Dislocations: An Atlas. Philadelphia, WB Saunders Co, 1970, p 796. Reproduced by permission.)

posterior splint with the elbow in 45 degrees of flexion. As noted previously, radial head subluxations do not usually require splinting, but if splinting is required, a posterior splint with the elbow in 90 degrees of flexion can be applied.

It should be emphasized that elbow injuries can result in marked swelling of the elbow and the forearm. For this reason, circumferential casts are contraindicated initially.

Significant Follow-up Points

1. The physician must have a high index of suspicion of associated fractures.
2. Circulatory compromise can occur by direct injuries to the brachial artery as well as secondary to posttraumatic swelling.
3. Compartment syndrome can develop secondary to elbow dislocations. The physician must have a high index of suspicion to diagnose and prevent progression of this dreaded complication. The classic end result of this syndrome, if untreated, is development of forearm ischemic contracture (Volkmann contracture).
4. Another known complication of elbow dislocations is traumatic myositis ossificans. This is a localized intramuscular ossification that develops secondary to a hematoma in an injured muscle. The most common ossifying muscle involved in an elbow injury is the brachial muscle.

Radial Head Subluxation

This is a common elbow subluxation seen in children between the ages of 1 and 4 years. It accounts for one fifth of all upper extremity injuries in children. The injury is commonly referred to as a *pulled elbow* and *Nursemaid's elbow.*

The proximal head of the radius articulates with the proximal ulna, and this joint is stabilized by the annular ligament. In children, the lip of the radial head is not fully developed and sudden traction may cause the radial head to slip out from the confines of the annular ligament. The mechanism of injury for this radial head subluxation is generally sudden traction of the forearm that extends and pronates the elbow. Such sudden traction often occurs when a child is pulled up by the wrist.

A child usually presents with the elbow in slight flexion with the forearm pronated and hanging to the side and refuses to use the arm. As long as the arm is not being used or moved, there is minimal pain, but as soon as any attempt is made to flex the elbow or supinate the arm, the child expresses pain and displeasure. Parents often think that the elbow is sprained and may delay medical care for 24 to 36 hours. There is no associated soft tissue swelling, ecchymosis, or neurovascular deficit.

Radiographs

Radiographic findings of the radial head subluxation are generally normal but are occasionally required to rule out any associated fractures. Ossification of the radial head does not occur until age 3 or 4 years. Joint fluid is not excessive with a subluxation, and therefore no positive fat pad signs are evident. With a straightforward history and clinical presentation or with recurrences, the physician may wish to treat the patient without radiographic films. If radiographs are obtained, a standard AP and lateral radiograph are sufficient. Some investigators have reported a measurable malalignment of the proximal radius and the capitellum.[1]

REDUCTION

Reduction can usually be accomplished without anesthesia. The physician sits facing the child and cups the affected elbow with the opposite hand (e.g., using the left hand if the right elbow is injured). The physician then places the thumb of the supporting hand over the radial head area. The forearm is flexed or extended and *supinated* with the physician's other arm, using the supporting thumb as a fulcrum. Slight longitudinal traction is often helpful before and during elbow extension (Fig. 66–19). A palpable click is usually noted, although the child may continue to refuse to use the elbow for a few minutes and may continue to cry until the physician leaves the room. Giving the child a popsicle or a balloon to play with usually confirms the success of the reduction. No immobilization is required if the child is able to use the arm without pain. If the child does not use the arm in a normal manner within 10 to 15 minutes, it should be suspected that reduction was not accomplished or that the diagnosis was in error. Delays in use of greater than 10 minutes may be seen in up to 23 per cent of children, postreduction.[4a] Delayed use is more common in children under 24 months of age. If the physician is assured that reduction has occurred on the basis of active use of the arm but pain persists, a posterior splint and sling are indicated, with instruction to have the child rechecked within 24 hours.

HAND INJURIES

Hand injuries can be particularly debilitating, and hand injuries that are improperly managed initially may become chronically disabling. Cursory examination of an injured hand may lead to incomplete or erroneous diagnoses, as subtle structural abnormalities may be overlooked. As a general rule, generic diagnoses (e.g., sprained thumb) should be avoided, and the specific tissue injured indicated (e.g., lateral collateral ligament tear).

Dislocations of the digits of the foot should generally be evaluated and managed according to the principles outlined below for the hand. Specific discussion of toe dislocations will not be provided.

Thumb Dislocations

The thumb is involved in many hand functions. This activity, in conjunction with the fact that the thumb is the first digit of the hand, makes it particularly susceptible to joint injuries. Dislocations and subluxations of the thumb joints are commonly seen in the emergency department. These injuries occur in spite of the strong ligamentous support of the thumb.

METACARPOPHALANGEAL JOINT INJURIES OF THE THUMB

One of two mechanisms usually serve to subluxate or dislocate this joint. With marked hyperextension of the metacarpophalangeal (MCP) joint, dorsal dislocation may result. In this most common type of dislocation, the proximal phalanx takes the position dorsal to the first metacarpal (Fig. 66–20). The second mechanism that may cause subluxation or dislocation of the MCP is severe valgus strain, resulting in a rupture of the ulnar collateral ligament (Fig. 66–21).

The MCP and interphalangeal joints are stabilized by a joint capsule comprising a collateral ligament–volar plate apparatus (Fig. 66–22). On the lateral surfaces, the two collateral ligaments span each side of the joint space to provide stability. The dorsal surface has no collateral liga-

ments, and on the volar (anterior) surface, the collateral ligament is replaced by a fibrocartilaginous (hence radiolucent) volar plate.

When a joint becomes completely dislocated, at least two of the three supporting structures (two collateral ligaments, one volar plate) tear. The clinical significance of this anatomic disruption is twofold. First, the volar plate may become interposed in the joint space and prevent reduction. Second, a complete tear of the capsule means that the joint is unstable, requiring prolonged immobilization or surgery to mend. In the thumb, the volar plate is attached more firmly to the base of the phalanx, and more loosely to the base of the metacarpal. Thus in a dorsal dislocation, the volar plate may become avulsed from the metacarpal and dislocate with the phalanx, and hence become interposed in the MCP joint space (Fig. 66–23).

There are primarily two types of dorsal dislocations of the thumbs: simple and complex. The importance of distinguishing between these two types of dislocations is that a simple dislocation can be reduced with a closed technique, whereas a complex dislocation can be reduced only with an open technique. In a complex MCP dislocation, the volar plate is avulsed during the dislocation and becomes interposed between the articulating surfaces of the joint. The volar plate is not visible on a radiograph, but the presence of a sesamoid bone, which dislocates with the volar plate in the joint space, may indicate volar plate interposition between the two bones (Fig. 66–24). Closed reduction of this dislocation is impossible. If the dislocation is complex, repeated attempts at reduction of the MCP can lead only to discomfort for the patient as well as an increased risk of damage to the surrounding soft tissue and the neurovascular bundles.

In simple dislocations, the volar plate is not entrapped in the joint space. Because there is no tissue interposition, closed reduction is usually possible in these injuries.

It may be difficult to differentiate the complex from the simple dislocation on clinical grounds. In the complex dislocation, the proximal phalanx often lies parallel to the metacarpal, whereas in the simple dislocation, the proximal phalanx usually sits at a right angle to the metacarpal (see Fig. 66–23). If it is not possible to reduce a supposed simple dislocation in one or two attempts, a presumptive diagnosis of a complex dislocation should be made and the patient should be referred appropriately.

The second most common injury to the thumb MCP joint is a *rupture of the ulnar collateral ligament* (see Fig. 66–21). Years ago, this type of injury was most commonly seen in gamekeepers as a result of breaking rabbits' necks with the webbed space between the thumb and index finger and acquired the interesting name of *gamekeeper's thumb*. Today, the injury most commonly results from catching one's thumb on a ski pole and therefore is known as *skier's thumb*.

The diagnosis of this injury requires a high degree of suspicion. The patient usually presents with pain and soft-tissue swelling at the base of the thumb, especially at the ulnar side of the MCP joint, without obvious bony deformity. The ulnar collateral ligament itself may rupture, or the ligament may remain intact while the ligament avulses a small fragment of bone. Standard radiographic findings will be normal unless there is an associated avulsion fracture. The diagnosis of this injury requires an understanding of the mechanism of injury and the proper use of stress radiographs (see subsequent discussion). An improperly treated ulnar collateral ligament injury may lead to significant dysfunction of the thumb and may especially compromise one's strength for pinching with the thumb and index finger.

Radiographs. A true AP view, a true lateral view, and

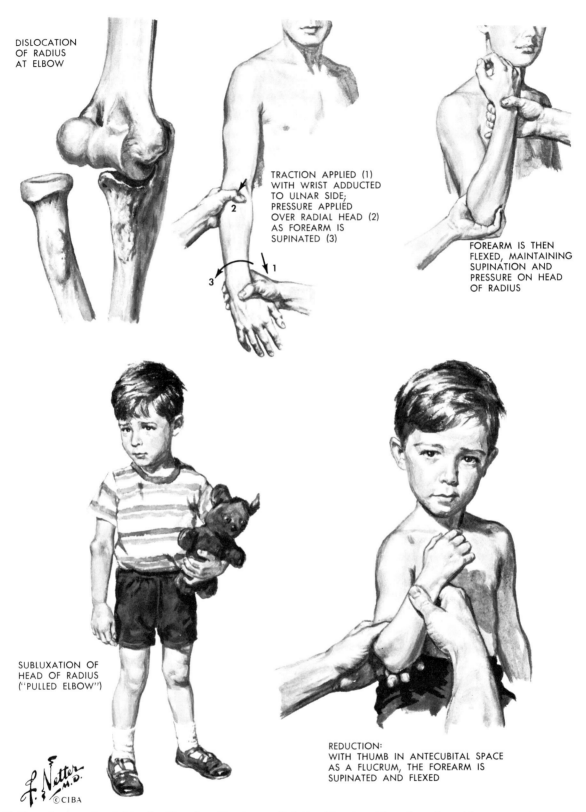

Figure 66–19. Reduction of radial head subluxation. Traction applied *(1)* with wrist adducted to ulnar side. Pressure is applied over the radial head *(2)* as the forearm is supinated *(3)*. The forearm is then flexed, maintaining supination and pressure on the head of the radius. (Copyright 1969, CIBA Pharmaceutical Company, Division of CIBA–GEIGY Corporation. Reprinted with permission from Clinical Symposia, illustrated by Frank H. Netter, M.D. All rights reserved. Legend adapted.)

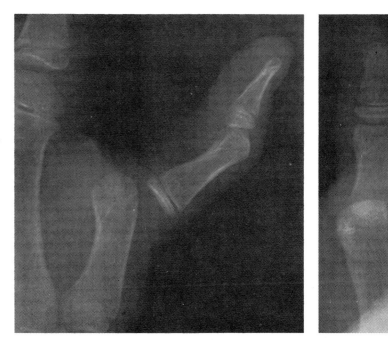

Figure 66–20. Complete dorsal dislocation at the metacarpophalangeal joint of the thumb. There is neither associated fracture nor epiphyseal separation. (From Harris JH Jr, Harris WH: Radiology of Emergency Medicine. 2nd ed. Baltimore, Williams & Wilkins, 1981, p 239. Reproduced by permission.)

one oblique view should be obtained in MCP joint injuries (Fig. 66–25). The fingernail can be used as a guide to proper positioning. It is important that the radiology technician obtain a true lateral film and be instructed to cone down on the injured joint.

To properly identify an ulnar collateral injury, stress radiographs of the thumb must be obtained. It is difficult to document instability by clinical examination alone. Following anesthesia, the stability of the ulnar ligament is checked with the thumb in full extension (Fig. 66–26). If the joint "opens," it may be compared with the other hand, both clinically and with stress radiographs (Fig. 66–27). If there is greater than 20 degrees instability when compared with the other hand

a presumptive diagnosis of ulnar collateral ligament tear may be made.

Anesthesia. Proper anesthesia for MCP joint injury is local infiltration or a combined median and radial nerve block at the wrist.

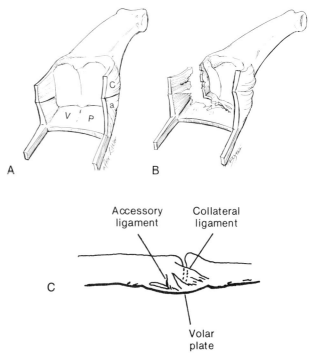

Figure 66–22. *A* and *B*, The collateral ligament–volar plate relationship. The metacarpophalangeal and interphalangeal joints derive their strength from a combination of the two collateral ligaments and the volar plate. Dislocations of these joints require tearing of at least two parts of this three-part structure. (From Carter P (ed): Common Hand Injuries and Infections. Philadelphia, WB Saunders Co, 1983, p 114. Reproduced by permission.) *C*, Lateral view, demonstrating collateral ligament–volar plate relationship. (Redrawn from Eaton RG: Joint Injuries of the Hand. Springfield, Ill, Charles C Thomas, 1972.)

Figure 66–21. Rupture of the ulnar collateral ligament (gamekeeper's thumb). *1,* This injury is caused by forcible abduction. If unrecognized and untreated, there may be progressive metacarpophalangeal subluxation *(2)* with interference during grasp, causing significant permanent disability. Suspect this injury when there is complaint of pain in this region. Look for tenderness on the medial side of the metacarpophalangeal joint. (From McRae R: Practical Fracture Treatment. Edinburgh, Churchill Livingstone, 1981, p 162. Reproduced by permission.)

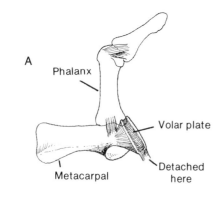

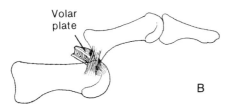

Figure 66–23. *A,* In a simple dorsal metacarpophalangeal joint dislocation (note right angle between phalanx and metacarpal), the volar plate remains in front of the metacarpal head, although it is detached from its weaker metacarpal insertion. *B,* In a complex dislocation (note more parallel alignment between phalanx and metacarpal), the volar plate becomes entrapped in the joint and results in an irreducible reduction by closed methods. (From DePalma AF: Management of Fractures and Dislocations: An Atlas. Philadelphia, WB Saunders Co, 1970, p 1177. Reproduced by permission.)

Reduction. A simple dorsal dislocation of the thumb usually reduces quite easily. If the reduction is not done in the proper manner, however, a simple dislocation may be converted to a complex dislocation. To facilitate reduction, the thumb of the patient and the hand of the physician are wrapped with gauze, thereby increasing the gripping

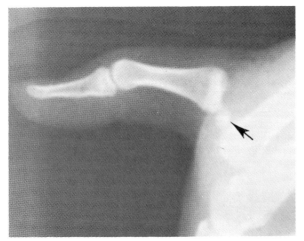

Figure 66–24. Irreducible metacarpophalangeal joint dislocation of the thumb. Note the sesamoid bone *(arrow)* indicating volar plate interposition between the two bone ends, which may prevent reduction. (From Carter P (ed): Common Hand Injuries and Infections. Philadelphia, WB Saunders Co, 1983, p 115. Reproduced by permission.)

strength and decreasing the risk of the hand slipping off the thumb. Wearing dry surgical gloves is also helpful for maintaining a good grip. The phalanx is then hyperextended on the metacarpal bone to greater than 90 degrees. As the phalanx is gently hyperextended, in-line traction is applied to the phalanx. While hyperextending the phalanx and applying in-line traction, pressure can be applied to the dorsal surface of the proximal phalanx, in a sense "pushing" rather than "pulling" the joint to a reduced position. The MCP can then be gently flexed as reduction occurs (Fig. 66–28).

Postreduction Care. Following reduction, ligamentous stability of the joint must be assessed with stress testing, as noted previously. The thumb should then be splinted in a position of function, with the MCP and the IP joints flexed at approximately 45 degrees. The thumb is usually splinted or placed in a cast for 3 to 4 weeks. Unstable injuries after reduction or complex dislocations should be considered for surgical treatment.

Minor strains of the ulnar collateral ligament should be splinted with a plaster splint or thumb spica cast for 3 to 4 weeks and reexamined for stability. Unstable sprains or complete ruptures of the ulnar collateral ligament often require surgery and should be referred to an orthopedic surgeon. One should be cautious of making the diagnosis of a simple sprain of the thumb, and the splinting of even minor soft-tissue injuries of the thumb should be routine.

INTERPHALANGEAL JOINT DISLOCATION OF THE THUMB

Interphalangeal joint dislocations are less common than MCP dislocations of the thumb. When they do occur, they are often open. Most commonly, the distal phalanx is dislocated dorsally with respect to the proximal phalanx, although lateral dislocations do occur.

The joint capsule of the interphalangeal joint is relatively strong and resistant to rupture. Although the avulsion of the volar plate on the distal phalanx can occur, it is rare. When it does occur, it is the result of an open injury, and it can become interposed in the joint space. The reduction of such a joint dislocation is impossible by the closed technique.

Radiographs. An AP view, a lateral view, and an oblique view usually reveal any associated fractures or other bony injuries.

Anesthesia. A digital block is usually sufficient.

Reduction. The thumb of the patient and the hand of the physician should be wrapped with gauze to prevent slippage. With mild hyperextension of the distal phalanx and in-line traction, the joint should reduce easily. If it does not reduce easily, the volar plate may be interposed and further attempts should not be made.

Postreduction Care. Following reduction, ligamentous stability of the joint should be assessed and postreduction films should be obtained. The joint should be splinted in slight flexion of 30 to 45 degrees for a minimum of three weeks. Follow-up examination is required.

Finger Dislocations

Dislocations of the fingers are relatively common injuries seen in the emergency department. Most finger dislocations involve the proximal interphalangeal joint, followed in frequency by dislocations of the distal interphalangeal joint and then the relatively rare MCP joint dislocations. When MCP joint dislocations do occur, they often occur en bloc and are complex dislocations that require open reduction.

Most often proximal interphalangeal dislocations are posterior (dorsal), with the middle phalanx taking a position

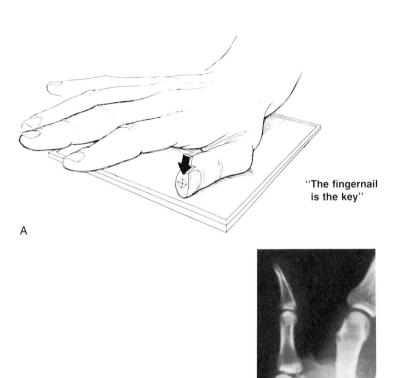

"The fingernail is the key"

A

B

Figure 66–25. *A* and *B*, Thumb lateral radiograph. Use the thumbnail as a landmark. Do not take an anteroposterior film of the hand and expect a lateral of the thumb. *C* and *D*, Thumb anteroposterior radiograph. Use the thumbnail as a landmark. (From Carter P (ed): Common Hand Injuries and Infections. Philadelphia, WB Saunders Co, 1983, p 79. Reproduced by permission.)

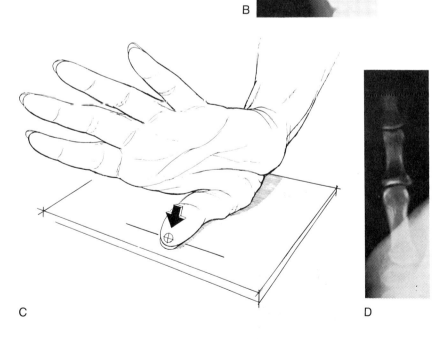

C

D

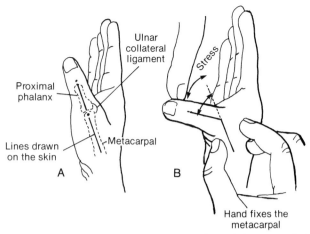

Figure 66–26. Stress testing of the ulnar collateral ligament of the thumb. This is done both clinically and with an anteroposterior radiograph. A line is drawn on the skin with a pen *(A)*. The line is along the long axis of the metacarpal and the proximal phalanx. Deviation of the straight line during stress indicates instability *(B)*. The metacarpal is fixed with the physician's other hand.

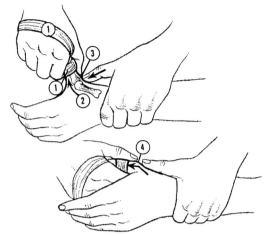

Figure 66–28. If a simple thumb metacarpophalangeal dislocation is treated with traction alone, the forces will often interpose the volar plate and result in a nonreducible complex dislocation. The proper technique for reduction includes *(1)* a good hold on the patient's distal thumb, *(2)* initial hyperextension of the dislocated phalanx, *(3)* pushing the base of the dislocated phalanx rather than traction alone, and *(4)* flexing of the thumb. (From DePalma AF: Management of Fractures and Dislocations: An Atlas. Philadelphia, WB Saunders Co, 1970, p 1178. Reproduced by permission.)

dorsal to the proximal phalanx. The mechanism of injury is usually hyperextension of the proximal interphalangeal joint. Because of the hyperextension, there is either simple rupture of the junction between the volar plate and the middle phalanx or avulsion of a small bone fragment together with the volar plate (Fig. 66–29). Usually the volar plate does not interpose in the joint space, and therefore closed reduction is possible.

Lateral dislocations can also occur secondary to adduction or abduction stress at the joint. Complete lateral dislocation is not possible unless both the volar plate and one of the collateral ligaments are torn. Volar dislocations are rare but are associated with either extensor tendon rupture (leading to a later boutonniere deformity) or an irreducible dislocation, because the condyle of the proximal phalanx "buttonholes" itself through the extensor mechanisms and becomes trapped.

Distal interphalangeal joint injuries, although less common than proximal interphalangeal joint injuries, are frequently seen in the emergency department. In distal interphalangeal dislocations, the direction of the dislocation is usually volar and the mechanism of injury is usually hyperflexion of the distal phalanx. If there is an avulsion of the

extensor tendon and it is not treated appropriately, the distal phalanx will be pulled in an unopposed direction by the flexor tendon. The long-term consequences will be a distal phalanx that cannot be extended and must be held in a stance of continuous flexion. This is known as a *mallet* or *baseball finger* (Fig. 66–30). Extensor tendon injuries are discussed in detail in Chapter 65.

Radiographs. Three views of all joint injuries of the fingers should be obtained: a true AP view, a true lateral

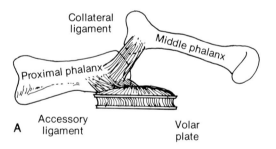

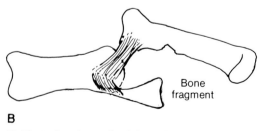

Figure 66–29. A dorsal proximal interphalangeal joint dislocation may involve rupture of the volar plate itself *(A)* or may involve an avulsion of varying amounts of bone from the middle phalanx *(B)*. If a large fragment of bone is avulsed from the base of the phalanx, the dislocation is unstable after reduction. The collateral ligaments will tear in varying degrees and should be assessed with stress testing following reduction.

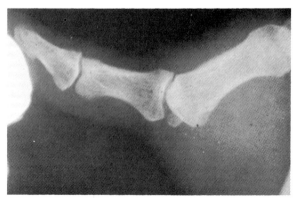

Figure 66–27. Radiograph demonstrating ulnar collateral ligament instability of greater than 45 degrees. (From Heppenstall RB: Fracture Treatment and Healing. Philadelphia, WB Saunders Co, 1980, p 573. Reproduced by permission.)

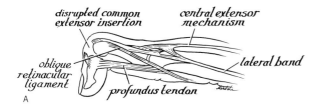

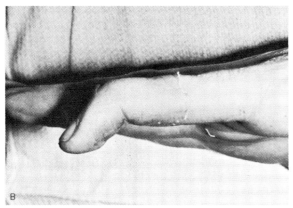

Figure 66–30. *A,* The mallet finger injury. *B,* This mallet deformity was caused by a laceration, but the appearance in profile is the same as that of a closed mallet injury. (From Newmeyer WL: Primary Care of Hand Injuries. Philadelphia, Lea & Febiger, 1979, p 142. Reproduced by permission.)

view, and an oblique view. A radiograph of the injured joint should be ordered, not simply a radiograph of "the hand." If a general hand radiograph or insufficient views are ordered, the extent of joint injury may be difficult to discern secondary to overlapping structures (Fig. 66–31). Additionally, small avulsion fractures are often not seen until the postreduction film has been taken (Fig. 66–32).

Anesthesia. Joint injuries to the fingers are particularly amenable to digital blocks (see Chapter 38).

PROXIMAL INTERPHALANGEAL DISLOCATIONS

Proximal interphalangeal joint dislocations usually reduce quite easily unless a complex dislocation is present, in

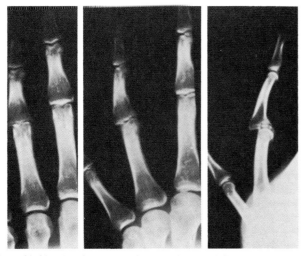

Figure 66–31. This fracture dislocation is only fully appreciated on the true lateral film. (From Carter P (ed): Common Hand Injuries and Infections. Philadelphia, WB Saunders Co, 1983, p 113. Reproduced by permission.)

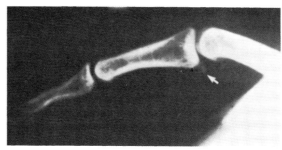

Figure 66–32. A small fragment of bone was avulsed with the volar plate. This frequently is appreciated only with the postreduction film in a true lateral projection. (From Carter P (ed): Common Hand Injuries and Infections. Philadelphia, WB Saunders Co, 1983, p 113. Reproduced by permission.)

which case they do not reduce at all. After a digital block has been administered and the injured digit of the patient and the hand of the physician have been wrapped with gauze (as pictured in Fig. 66–28), gentle in-line traction should be applied to the digit with slight hyperextension of the joint (Fig. 66–33). The injured hand should be held by the physician's other hand for countertraction. As noted for thumb reductions, it is best to exert a minimal amount of traction sufficient to permit the distal digit to be gently pushed into proper articulation. If the dislocation does not easily reduce, it should be assumed that it is a complex dislocation and proper orthopedic referral should be initiated.

Postreduction Care. Following reduction, the proximal interphalangeal joint should be examined for instability in extension, indicating a volar plate tear (Fig. 66–34). Lateral instability is also tested to document collateral ligament integrity. Inability to fully extend the proximal interphalangeal joint may indicate an extensor tendon avulsion. One cannot adequately test a proximal interphalangeal joint that is acutely painful; thus a digital block is usually required. Instability of a proximal interphalangeal joint following reduction mandates orthopedic referral.

If there are no associated fractures or instability, simple proximal interphalangeal joint dislocations that have been adequately reduced should be splinted with the proximal interphalangeal joint in flexion of 15 to 20 degrees for 7 to 10 days. A dorsal foam-padded splint is preferred to a volar splint, because it affords better immobilization and patient acceptance. "Buddy taping" may also be done in simple dislocations (see illustrations in Chapter 67). Gentle range-of-motion exercises can usually be initiated 7 days after injury.

All complicated proximal interphalangeal joint dislocations, or those associated with even small avulsion fractures, should be considered complex injuries and require proper referral. Even seemingly minor proximal interphalangeal (PIP) joint injuries may produce significant or permanent disability, and *injuries to this joint should not be taken lightly.* Lateral and volar dislocations should be considered complicated.

DISTAL INTERPHALANGEAL DISLOCATIONS

Distal interphalangeal joint dislocations usually reduce easily with inline traction. The hand of the physician and the fingertip of the patient should be wrapped with gauze to reduce slippage. The injured hand should be stabilized by the physician's other hand. Occasionally, soft tissue interposition in the joint space will not allow proper reduction and an open technique is required. In any case, orthopedic

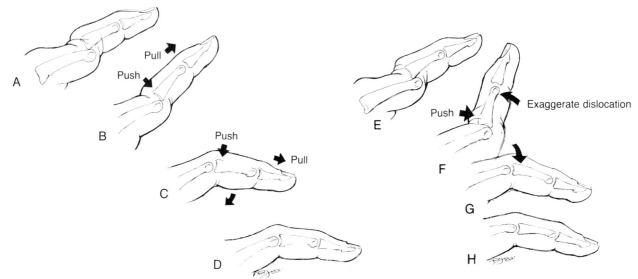

Figure 66–33. *A–D,* Traction method of joint reduction. Complete anesthesia using a regional block should precede reduction attempts. *E–H,* Exaggeration of existing deformity method. First, exaggerate the deformity that is present, then in addition to steady traction, push the joint back into position. (From Carter P (ed): Common Hand Injuries and Infections. Philadelphia, WB Saunders Co, 1983, pp 109 and 110. Reproduced by permission.)

referral is suggested for all distal interphalangeal joint dislocations and is a necessity if there is any avulsion fracture associated with the dislocation.

Postreduction Care. Distal interphalangeal joint dislocations may be splinted with a splint that holds the joint in full extension (Fig. 66–35). Splints should be designed to hold the distal interphalangeal joint in full extension while allowing full range of motion in the proximal interphalangeal joint; padded dorsal splints are also used (see Fig. 65–12).

Conclusions

1. If dislocations in the digits are not reduced easily, there may be interposition of soft tissue in the joint. Repeated attempts at

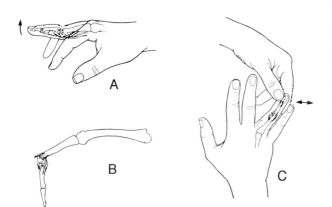

Figure 66–34. Postreduction stress of proximal interphalangeal dislocation. *A,* If the volar plate has been completely disrupted, the proximal interphalangeal joint will hyperextend with both passive and active motion. *B,* An inability to actively extend the proximal interphalangeal joint indicates a rupture of the central slip of the extensor tendon. *C,* Passive lateral stress is performed to check integrity of collateral ligaments. (From DePalma AF: Management of Fractures and Dislocations: An Atlas. Philadelphia, WB Saunders Co, 1970, pp 1203 and 1204. Reproduced by permission.)

relocation are not indicated and may increase the amount of damage already done to the joint.

2. Injuries at the proximal interphalangeal joint can result in damage to the extensor mechanism at this joint. If the extensor mechanism is damaged, the lateral bands may stretch to a position that is volar to the axis of the proximal interphalangeal joint. These lateral bands, which are normally extensors of the proximal interphalangeal joint, then become flexors of this joint. The result is a digit that is hyperflexed at the proximal interphalangeal joint and hyperextended at the distal interphalangeal joint. This is referred to as a *boutonniere deformity* and is not always obvious on initial examination. All proximal interphalangeal joint injuries require proper orthopedic referral.

HIP DISLOCATIONS

The hip is generally a stable joint. The head of the femur fits deeply into the hip socket and is well supported by the surrounding ligaments and muscular attachments. Because of this inherent stability of the hip, dislocations are rare and when they do occur they are the result of major forces. Because great forces are involved in traumatic hip dislocations, associated fractures are common.

The blood supply to the femoral head is rather tenuous and is often disrupted with hip dislocations. For this reason a dislocated hip should be reduced as soon as possible. One of the feared complications of hip dislocations is avascular necrosis of the femoral head. Even with early reduction and proper management, this complication is seen. With delayed reduction, the incidence of avascular necrosis increases significantly.

As might be expected, sciatic nerve injuries are also seen with hip dislocations, especially posterior hip dislocations. Although early reduction does not repair damage that has already been done to the sciatic nerve, such action prevents further damage from occurring by minimizing traction or compression of the nerve.

Most hip dislocations seen in the emergency department are of the posterior variety. In this injury, the femoral head comes to rest in a position posterior to the acetabulum (Fig. 66–36). A small percentage of hip dislocations are anterior, wherein the femoral head comes to rest in a position anterior

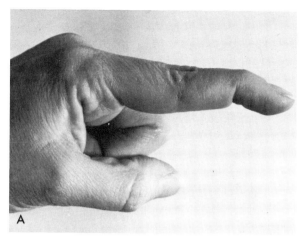

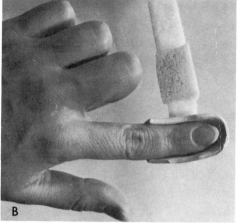

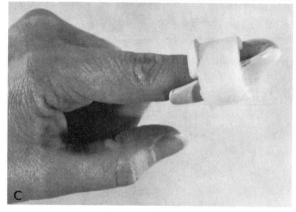

Figure 66–35. *A,* Mallet finger. *B* and *C,* Conservative treatment of mallet finger splint, with distal interphalangeal joint held straight. (From Heppenstall RB: Fracture Treatment and Healing. Philadelphia, WB Saunders Co, 1980, p 567. Reproduced by permission.)

to the acetabulum. In an anterior dislocation, the femoral head usually comes to rest in one of three locations: within the obturator canal, in front of the pubic symphysis, or beside the iliac bone (Fig. 66–37).

Hip dislocations are often associated with other major trauma and, as a result, are sometimes overlooked, because attention is focused on more critical aspects of the patient's

management. The physician must maintain a high index of suspicion for hip injuries in major trauma; it is recommended that pelvic films be taken of all seriously injured patients. Although hip dislocations are not life-threatening entities, delay in reduction or delay in proper management greatly increases the morbidity.

RADIOGRAPHS

The suspected hip injury should be assessed radiographically with at least two different views. A standard AP view, as well as an oblique view, is required. Both of these film views can be obtained without moving the patient by placing a cassette under the patient and rotating the x-ray machine from an anterior to an oblique position.

ANALGESIA

An attempt often can be made in the emergency department to relocate the dislocated hip. Depending upon the condition of the patient and associated injuries, parenteral narcotics and benzodiazepines, either alone or in combination, may be used. If emergency department reduction is not successful, it is recommended that spinal anesthesia or general anesthesia be used in the reduction of hip dislocations.

Posterior Dislocations

A posterior hip dislocation is usually the result of forces applied to a flexed knee with the hip in flexion, such as seen in a motor vehicle crash when the knee strikes the dashboard during deceleration. Forces are transmitted down the femur

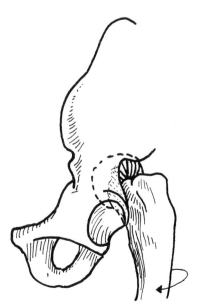

Figure 66–36. Posterior dislocation of the hip. (From Simon R, Koenigsknecht S: Orthopedics in Emergency Medicine. New York, Appleton-Century-Crofts, 1982, p 366. Reproduced by permission.)

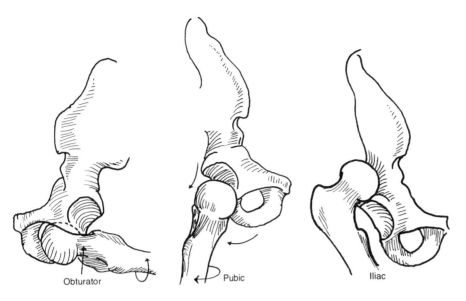

Figure 66–37. Anterior dislocations of the hip: obturator, pubic, and iliac. (From Simon R, Koenigsknecht S: Orthopedics in Emergency Medicine. New York, Appleton-Century-Crofts, 1982, p 367. Reproduced by permission.)

to the hip joint, and the femoral head is forced out of the acetabulum. The femoral head comes to rest in a position posterior to the acetabulum. Such dislocations are commonly associated with a fracture of the acetabulum (Fig. 66–38).

REDUCTION

There are two methods of reduction of posterior dislocations. The first is the Stimson technique, in which the patient is placed in a prone position on the table with his hips at the edge and the affected extremity hanging over the edge of the table. While an assistant stabilizes the pelvis, the knee of the affected extremity is flexed at 90 degrees and the physician applies steady downward traction at the proximal calf for 10 to 15 minutes (Fig. 66–39). While this downward traction is maintained, an assistant may apply pressure over the greater trocanter and gently push it into the acetabulum.

The second method of reduction is the Allis technique. With the patient in the supine position, the pelvis is again stabilized by an assistant (Fig. 66–40). The hip and knee of the affected extremity are flexed at 90 degrees, maintaining the extremity in adduction with slight internal rotation. Upward traction is then applied at the proximal calf, thereby lifting the head of the femur into the acetabulum. During this maneuver, the physician may stand on the stretcher above the patient. Forceful rotation should be avoided, because it may result in a fracture of the femoral neck.

After reduction has been accomplished, the leg should be placed in longitudinal traction, such as Buck traction (Fig. 66–41). The leg should be maintained in slight abduction and slight external rotation. Alternatively, a pillow may be placed between the knees to prevent adduction, and the legs may be tied together. As with other dislocations, postreduction radiographs are needed to ensure proper reduction and anatomic realignment and to rule out associated fractures.

Anterior Dislocations

Anterior hip dislocations are usually the result of forced abduction such as may occur in a fall or a motor vehicle crash. The forced abduction results in a levering of the femoral head out of the acetabulum and through a rent in the anterior capsule. If the hip is in flexion when the forced

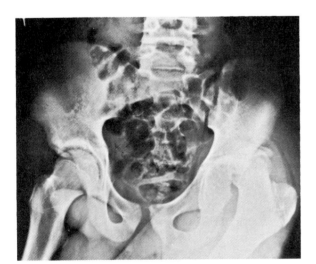

Figure 66–38. Posterior dislocation of the hip. The femur is adducted, internally rotated, and superiorly displaced, with an associated posterior acetabular fracture. A Malgaigne fracture of the pelvis is also present, with diastasis of the pubic symphysis and left sacroiliac joint. (From Greenbaum E: Radiology of the Emergency Patient. New York, John Wiley & Sons, Inc, 1982, p 563. Reproduced by permission.)

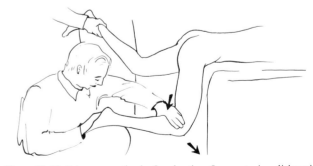

Figure 66–39. Stimson method of reduction for posterior dislocation of the hip (see text for description). This is the preferred method. (From Heppenstall RB: Fracture Treatment and Healing. Philadelphia, WB Saunders Co, 1980, p 672. Reproduced by permission.)

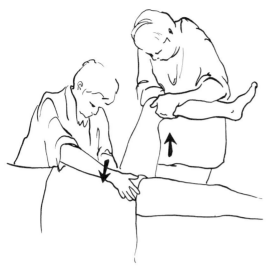

Figure 66–40. Allis method of reducing posterior dislocation of the hip (see text for description). (From Heppenstall RB: Fracture Treatment and Healing. Philadelphia, WB Saunders Co, 1980, p 672. Reproduced by permission.)

abduction occurs, the femoral head comes to rest in the obturator canal. If the hip is in extension, the femoral head comes to rest anterior to the pubic symphysis or iliac spine. Obturator dislocations are slightly more common than the other two types of anterior hip dislocations. These three types of anterior dislocations can be managed in the same way.

REDUCTION

For reduction of anterior dislocations, the patient should be placed in a supine position and the pelvis should be stabilized by an assitant putting pressure on the iliac spine (Fig. 66–42). The hip and knee should be gently flexed to 90 degrees and the femur should be rotated to a neutral position. The physician should then apply steady in-line traction while applying upward traction at the proximal calf, which lifts the femoral head into the acetabulum. Gentle internal rotation may aid in this reduction. Do not forcefully adduct the femur, because this may fracture the femoral

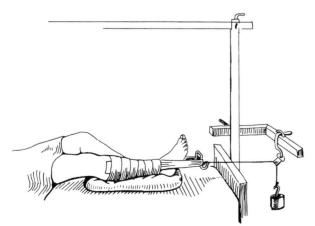

Figure 66–41. Buck skin traction. (From Simon R, Koenigsknecht S: Orthopedics in Emergency Medicine. New York, Appleton-Century-Crofts, 1982, p 369. Reproduced by permission.)

head or neck. Postreduction treatment includes the application of in-line traction with Buck's traction as well as obtaining postreduction radiographs.

Conclusions

1. Hip dislocations are usually caused by great forces and as such are often associated with fractures or severe trauma of soft tissue.

2. If attempts at closed reduction are not successful, open reduction is mandatory.

3. All hip dislocations require hospitalization with bed rest and traction.

KNEE DISLOCATIONS

Dislocations of the knee (with the exception of patellar dislocations) are rare and require a great deal of force in order to occur. This force may be of either a direct or an indirect nature. The knee is a stable joint, the stability being enhanced by strong ligaments. For knee dislocations to occur, these ligamentous attachments must be disrupted by varying degrees. For complete dislocation, both the anterior and posterior cruciate ligaments must be ruptured.

The incidence of damage to the neurovascular structures that cross the knee as a result of dislocation is high. Dislocations may produce both neurologic and vascular embarrassment. For this reason, a knee dislocation must be reduced as soon as possible and, once reduced, continuous observation is essential.

Dislocations of the knee are classified with respect to the position of the tibia in relation to the femur. The most common dislocation is anterior, in which the tibia takes the position anterior to the distal femur. Knee dislocations can also be posterior, lateral, medial, or rotary (Fig. 66–43). Any of these dislocations implies severe damage to the knee joint, and although definitive therapy requires surgical intervention, immediate therapy involves reduction of the dislocation. Often, the extensive ligamentous damage accompanying the dislocation renders the knee extremely unstable. Frequently, prehospital personnel will have reduced the dislocation during the process of splint application. This reduction is obviously unstable.

The patient with a knee dislocation will usually present to the emergency department with a grossly deformed knee. As with any joint injury, distal neurovascular bundles must be assessed immediately and subsequently at appropriate intervals.

Radiographs

Anteroposterior and lateral views are necessary, with additional views as required for clarification. Radiographs of the pelvis and hip should also be considered to rule out the possibility of associated injuries.

Analgesia

General anesthesia may be required for reduction of a knee dislocation when the knee is fixed in the dislocated position. If general anesthesia is not available, contraindications prohibit its use, or the dislocation is to be reduced in the emergency department, analgesia with parenteral narcotics and muscle relaxant agents should be used.

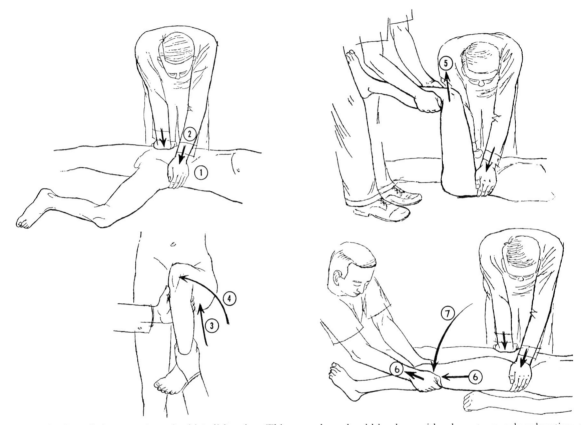

Figure 66–42. Reduction of obturator (anterior hip) dislocation. This procedure should be done with adequate muscle relaxation, although occasionally simply positioning the hip for radiographs will reduce the dislocation. *1*, The patient is placed on the floor in a supine position. *2*, An assistant puts downward pressure on the anterosuperior iliac spines. *3*, Grasp the affected limb and flex the hip and knee to a right angle. *4*, Rotate the limb to a neutral position. (This position converts an anterior dislocation to a posterior dislocation.) *5*, Make steady traction on the leg directly upward, lifting the head of the femur into the acetabulum. *Note:* Do not adduct the hip until it is reduced in the acetabulum; otherwise, a fracture of the femoral head or neck may occur. *6*, While upward traction is maintained, lower the thigh to the floor to the extended position *(7)*. (From DePalma AF: Management of Fractures and Dislocations: An Atlas. Philadelphia, WB Saunders Co, 1970, p 1319. Reproduced by permission.)

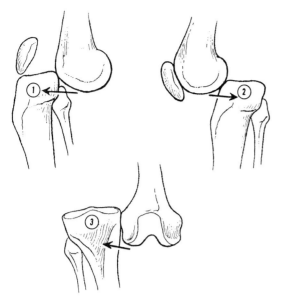

Figure 66–43. Types of dislocations. *1*, Anterior, *2*, posterior, and *3*, lateral. (From DePalma AF: Management of Fractures and Dislocations: An Atlas. Philadelphia, WB Saunders Co, 1970, p 1621. Reproduced by permission.)

Reduction

Reduction of a rigidly fixed dislocated knee is probably best accomplished with a closed technique under general anesthesia. Attempts at reduction in the emergency department may prove to be unrewarding and, for this reason, should not be undertaken unless there is vascular compromise or if no immediate orthopedic provider is available. In this instance, an attempt at reduction is warranted.

As with other dislocations, traction, countertraction, and manipulation (and at least two persons) are required if reduction is to be attempted. While an assistant stabilizes the distal femur, in-line traction is applied by the physician with the knee in extension (Fig. 66–44). For anterior dislocations, in which the proximal tibia lies anterior to the distal femur, the assistant attempts to lift the distal femur into a reduced position while in-line traction is applied by the physician. This lifting of the distal femur into position should not occur with pressure over the popliteal space, because such pressure would increase the chance of injury to the structures that traverse this space. For posterior knee dislocations in which the tibia is located posterior to the distal femur, the tibia is gently lifted into a reduced position while in-line traction is maintained. Again, avoidance of pressure over the popliteal fossa is indicated.

Lateral and medial dislocations can also be reduced with stabilization of the distal femur and in-line traction. Lateral dislocations may benefit from flexion of the knee approximately 90 degrees to relax the hamstrings.

Postreduction Care

After the knee has been relocated, the neurovascular status of the lower extremity must be serially reassessed at appropriate time intervals. Any vascular compromise following reduction demands further evaluation, including arteriography. If the neurovascular status appears to be intact, the knee should be immobilized and postreduction radiographs should be taken. Following reduction of a dislocated knee and after postreduction films have indicated proper

alignment without fractures, the stability of the knee joint must be evaluated. This is best accomplished while the patient is under general anesthesia, because this allows for the evaluation of the ligamentous structures of the knee without resistance from the patient.

All patients with dislocated knees should be hospitalized. Evidence of vascular compromise may be delayed, and close observation and immediate vascular evaluation at the first sign of vascular compromise are indicated.[5, 6] The knee should be immobilized in a slight flexion of approximately 20 to 30 degrees. No weight bearing is allowed initially. Surgical intervention is eventually required for repair of the damaged ligamentous structures and other associated knee injuries.

Conclusions

1. Knee dislocations require a great deal of force.
2. There is a high incidence of associated neurologic and/or vascular embarrassment.
3. If vascular embarrassment is present, attempts at reduction in the emergency department are warranted. When immediate orthopedic consultation is available, generally the knee should be reduced in the operating room under general or spinal anesthesia.
4. Hospitalization is required for reduced knee dislocations.

PATELLAR DISLOCATIONS

Patellar dislocations are relatively common injuries, especially in adolescents, particularly in adolescent girls. Patellar dislocations occasionally result from direct trauma to the patella, although more commonly the mechanism of dislocation is sudden flexion and external rotation of the tibia on the femur with concomitant contraction of the quadriceps, as might occur with the twisting of the knee in a golf swing or certain dance moves. These indirect forces cause the patella to ride over the lateral condyle of the femur.

Patellar dislocations are described by indicating where the patella is located in relation to the knee joint. By far, the most common dislocation is a lateral dislocation, with

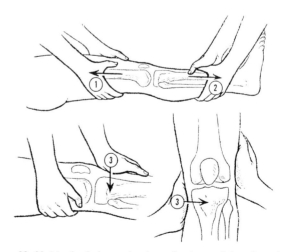

Figure 66–44. Manipulative reduction of a knee dislocation. *1*, An assistant fixes and provides countertraction on the thigh. *2*, Another assistant provides straight traction on the leg (this usually reduces the dislocation). *3*, The physician puts direct pressure over the displaced bones. (From DePalma AF: Management of Fractures and Dislocations: An Atlas. Philadelphia, WB Saunders Co, 1970, p 1623. Reproduced by permission.)

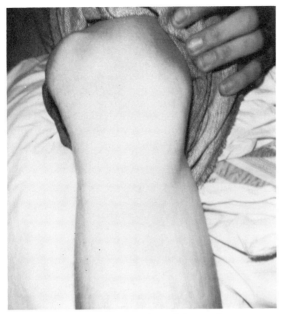

Figure 66–45. Lateral dislocation of the patella.

usually exhibits some mild apprehension when examination of the patella is attempted, especially lateral movement. Any lateral motion of the patella generally elicits a reaction (apprehension sign) from the patient, such as a grasp for the examiner's hand and stating that it feels as if the patella is going to dislocate again.

Radiographs

Initially, AP and lateral views of the knee are sufficient to indicate the type of dislocation as well as to rule out the possibility of associated fractures. Postreduction radiographs should again include AP and lateral views (see Fig. 66–46) as well as a sunrise view, that is, a view in which the patella is isolated on the radiograph, allowing the under surface of the patella to be examined (Fig. 66–47).

Analgesia

In most instances, the patella may be reduced without parenteral analgesia, especially if the reduction is slow and deliberate, and adequate explanation is given to the patient. Occasionally however, parenteral analgesia is required.

Reduction

the patella lateral to the knee joint (Figs. 66–45 and 66–46). Uncommon patellar dislocations include superior, medial, and the very rare intra-articular[7] dislocations.

Patellar dislocations often reduce spontaneously, and the physician may not note any obvious abnormalities of the knee when the patient presents to the emergency department. In such a case, when the patient's history is consistent with a patellar dislocation, radiographs should be obtained and the knee should be treated as if a patellar dislocation did in fact occur. Patients with recurrent dislocations usually know their diagnosis.

The patient with a dislocated patella is unable to bear weight and usually presents with the affected knee held in slight flexion. Pain is a significant element of this injury, and there may be some associated swelling or mild hemarthrosis. Even if the patella has reduced spontaneously, the patient

Lateral dislocations are usually easily reduced using a closed technique. The patient should be placed in a supine position, and the knee should be gently flexed and supported, followed by gentle extension of the knee to 180 degrees. Extension alone may suffice to reduce the patella. If the knee is fully extended and the patella does not reduce, slight anteriorly directed pressure over the lateral aspect of the patella aids in moving the patella over the lateral condyle and back into its normal anatomic position (Fig. 66–48).

The other types of patellar dislocations (superior, medial, and intra-articular) are usually resistant to reduction with closed techniques. For this reason, orthopedic consultation is recommended and no attempt at closed reduction is made in the emergency department.

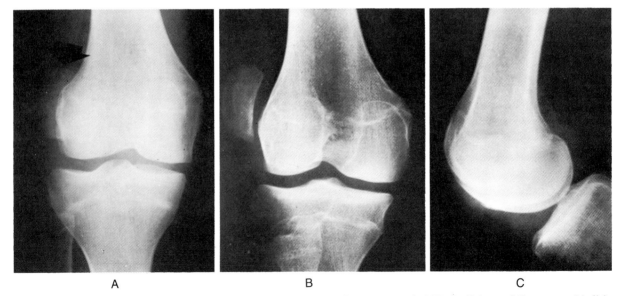

A   B   C

Figure 66–46. *A–C,* Complete lateral dislocation of the patella. (From Harris JH Jr, Harris WH: Radiology of Emergency Medicine. 2nd ed. Baltimore, Williams & Wilkins, 1981, p 575. Reproduced by permission.)

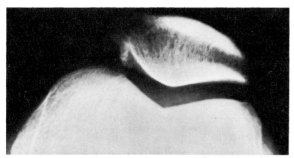

Figure 66–47. Dislocated patella. The fracture of the medial aspect of the patella, seen with this "skyline" or "sunrise" view, was the only evidence of a previous traumatic patellar dislocation. (From Greenbaum E: Radiology of the Emergency Patient. New York, John Wiley & Sons, Inc, 1982, p 575. Reproduced by permission.)

Postreduction Care

Postreduction care for lateral displacements includes postreduction radiographs and the placement of the knee in a knee immobilizer. The patient should be instructed not to bear weight, and orthopedic referral is made for 1 to 2 days after the reduction. Hospitalization is not usually required for lateral dislocations.

ANKLE DISLOCATIONS

The ankle joint comprises the distal fibula and tibia, which are firmly attached to one another by the interosseous membrane, and the talus bone of the foot. The ankle is a stable joint with strong ligamentous support. Dislocations of the ankle are the result of great forces applied to the ankle, and they are often associated with fractures.

Dislocations are classified according to the description of the talus in relation to the distal tibia and fibula. In a posterior dislocation, the talus is found in a position posterior to the distal tibia and fibula. An anterior dislocation places the talus in a position anterior to the distal tibia and fibula (Fig. 66–49).

Posterior dislocations are the most common type of ankle dislocations. They are most often the result of a forced

plantar flexion, which might be seen with a fall on a plantar-flexed foot. Such dislocations are often accompanied by malleolar fractures or fractures of the posterior tibia (Fig. 66–50). The patient usually presents with a markedly swollen ankle that is unable to bear weight and resistant to any attempt at dorsiflexion. Although the fact that the patient has had a serious ankle injury will be obvious to the examiner, clinical diagnosis without radiologic confirmation of a dislocation is rather difficult. Attempts at manipulation of the ankle should be kept to a minimum until radiographic films are obtained. Neurovascular injury to the foot should be ascertained prior to the taking of radiographs.

Anterior dislocations of the ankle are usually the result of forced dorsiflexion of the foot, although a direct blow to the heel with the foot in dorsiflexion may also produce an anterior dislocation. The most common causes of such dislocations are the deceleration injuries seen in motor vehicle accidents with forced dorsiflexion. Anterior dislocations are also associated with malleolar fractures (Fig. 66–51). The

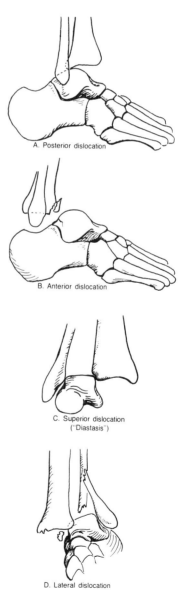

Figure 66–49. The types of dislocations of the ankle. (From Simon R, Koenigsknecht S: Orthopedics in Emergency Medicine. New York, Appleton-Century-Crofts, 1982, p 419. Reproduced by permission.)

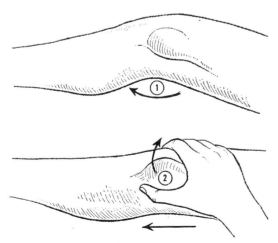

Figure 66–48. Manipulative reduction. *1,* Extend the knee gradually while medially directed pressure is applied on the patella *(2),* pushing it over the lateral femoral condyle. (From DePalma AF: Management of Fractures and Dislocations. Philadelphia, WB Saunders Co, 1970, p 1665. Reproduced by permission.)

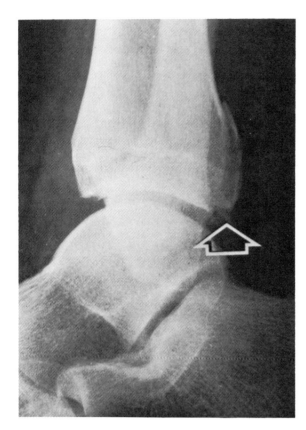

Figure 66–50. Isolated posterior tibial lip fracture *(open arrow)*, seen after reduction of posterior ankle dislocation. (From Harris JH Jr, Harris WH: Radiology of Emergency Medicine. 2nd ed. Baltimore, Williams & Wilkins, 1981, p 629. Reproduced by permission.)

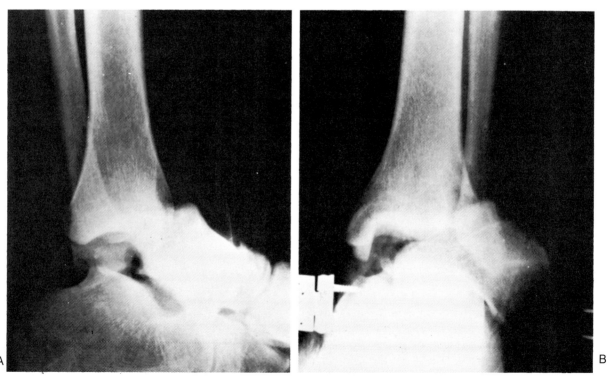

Figure 66–51. *A* and *B*, Anterior dislocation of the talus. (From Harris JH Jr, Harris WH: Radiology of Emergency Medicine. 2nd ed. Baltimore, Williams & Wilkins, 1981, p 629. Reproduced by permission.)

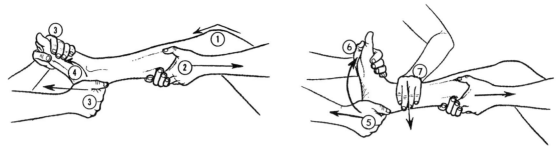

Figure 66–52. Manipulative reduction of a posterior ankle dislocation. *1,* The knee is flexed. *2,* The assistant provides countertraction on the leg. *3,* The forefoot is grasped with one hand and the heel with the other hand. *4,* The foot is flexed slightly plantar. *5,* Apply straight downward traction on the plantar-flexed foot, then pull the foot forward *(6)* while a second assistant provides counter pressure on the front of the lower leg *(7).* (From DePalma AF: Management of Fractures and Dislocations. Philadelphia, WB Saunders Co, 1970, pp 1916 and 1917. Reproduced by permission.)

third type of dislocation of the ankle is an upward dislocation of the talus. In this type of dislocation, the talus is driven upward, disrupting the syndesmotic tibiofibular joint (Fig. 66–49). This type of injury most commonly results when a person falls from a distance and lands on his feet. The force is directed upward and drives the talus into the tibiofibular joint. This type of dislocation requires open reduction and internal fixation. Lateral dislocations of the joint can also occur and are most often the result of marked inversion of the foot. Lateral dislocations are always associated with fractures of the malleoli and are often open and require surgical correction.

Any indication of vascular compromise demands expeditious reduction. One complication of dislocations of the ankle is avascular necrosis of the talus, and a delay in reduction increases the risk of this complication.

Radiographs

The minimal radiographs required for evaluation of an ankle injury are AP, lateral, and oblique views. Additional views may be obtained as needed to more clearly delineate fractures and anatomic relationships.

Analgesia

Although most reductions can be performed using parenteral analgesia and muscle relaxants, especially when vascular compromise is evident, general anesthesia or spinal anesthesia is occasionally required.

Reduction

For posterior dislocations, the patient is placed in supine position and the knee of the affected extremity is flexed 30 to 45 degrees. The physician should than grasp the foot with both hands, one hand holding the heel and the other hand holding the forefoot. While traction is applied to the foot, an assistant should hold the calf and apply countertraction (Fig. 66–52). While traction and countertraction are being steadily maintained, a second assistant should apply downward pressure on the distal calf. At the same time, the physician should lift the foot anteriorly and gently dorsiflex the foot. When the relocation occurs, dorsiflexion will be accomplished without resistance.

For anterior dislocations, the patient is placed in a

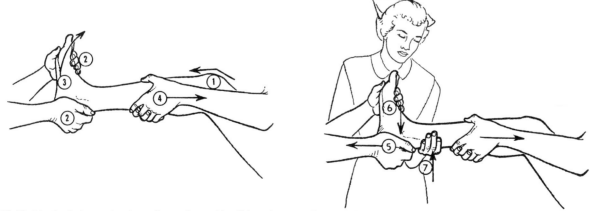

Figure 66–53. Manipulative reduction of anterior ankle dislocation. *1,* The knee is flexed. *2,* The physician grasps the forefoot with one hand and the heel with the other hand. *3,* Dorsiflexion of the foot is slightly increased (to disengage the talus). *4,* An assistant provides countertraction on the leg. *5,* Straight longitudinal traction is applied, then the foot is pushed directly backward *(6)* while a second assistant provides countertraction on the back of the lower leg *(7).* (From DePalma AF: Management of Fractures and Dislocations. Philadelphia, WB Saunders Co, 1970, pp 1918 and 1919. Reproduced by permission.)

supine position and the knee is slightly flexed. While an assistant applies countertraction to the calf, the physician should grasp the foot with both hands as previously described and apply traction to the foot. The foot, which is in mild dorsiflexion secondary to the dislocation, may need to be dorsiflexed to a greater degree in order to disengage the talus. With traction being maintained on the foot, a second assistant should apply pressure in an anterior direction at the posterior calf at the same time that the physician pushes the foot in a posterior direction (Fig. 66–53). It is important that in-line traction be maintained during this maneuver. When the ankle is reduced, gentle plantar flexion is possible without resistance.

Postreduction Care

Postreduction care includes hospitalization for 24 to 48 hours, with the ankle splinted in a neutral position. In 24 to 48 hours, the splint can be replaced with a circular plaster cast below the knee. No weight bearing should be allowed for at least 6 weeks.

Conclusions

1. The ankle joint has strong ligamentous support; thus, dislocations are usually the result of great forces.
2. Reductions of ankle dislocations that cannot be easily reduced in the emergency department are best carried out under general or spinal anesthesia.
3. All patients with ankle dislocations require hospitalization.

References

1. Poulsen S: Reduction of acute shoulder dislocations using the Eskimo technique: A study of 23 cases. J Trauma 28:1383, 1988.
2. Dutky P: A simple method of treating shoulder dislocations for the white water enthusiast (and others). Wilderness Medicine 5:9, 1988.
3. Bossart P, Joyce S, Manaster B, et al: Lack of efficacy of "weighted" radiographs in diagnosing acute acromioclavicular separation. Ann Emerg Med 17:20, 1988.
4. Snyder HS: Radiographic changes in radial head subluxation in children. J Emerg Med 8:265, 1990.
4a. Schunk JE: Radial head subluxation: Epidemiology and treatment of 87 episodes. Ann Emerg Med 19:1019, 1990.
5. Lefrak EA: Knee dislocation: An illusive cause of critical arterial occlusion. Arch Surg 111:1021, 1976.
6. Dart CH, Braitman HE: Popliteal artery injury following fracture or dislocation at the knee: Diagnosis and management. Arch Surg 112:969, 1977.
7. Nsouli AZ, Nahabedian A: Intra-articular dislocation of the patella. J Trauma 28:256, 1988.
8. Carter P: Common Hand Injuries and Infections. A Practical Approach to Early Treatment. Philadelphia, W. B. Saunders Company, 1983.
9. Connolly J: DePalma's The Management of Fractures and Dislocations 3rd ed. Philadelphia, WB Saunders Co, 1981.
10. Conwell H: Injuries to the elbow. Clin Symp 21:35, 1969.
11. Greenbaum E (ed): Radiology of the Emergency Patient. An Atlas Approach. New York, John Wiley & Sons, Inc, 1982.
12. Harris J, Harris W: The Radiology of Emergency Medicine. 3rd ed. Baltimore, Williams & Wilkins, 1990.
13. Heppenstall R: Fracture Treatment and Healing. Philadelphia WB Saunders Co, 1980.
14. McRae R: Practical Fracture Treatment. New York, Churchill Livingstone, 1989.
15. Mirick M, Clinton J, Ruiz E: External rotation method of shoulder dislocation reduction. JACEP 8:528, 1979.
16. Newmeyer W: Primary Care of Hand Injuries. Philadelphia, Lea & Febiger, 1979.
17. Rockwood C: Fractures. Philadelphia, JB Lippincott Co, 1984.
18. Simon R, Koeningsknecht S: Orthopedics in Emergency Medicine. The Extremities. New York, Appleton-Century-Crofts, 1987.
19. Wilson J (ed): Fracture and Joint Injuries. New York, Churchill Livingstone, 1982.

Chapter 67

Splinting Techniques

Carl R. Chudnofsky, Edward J. Otten, and William L. Newmeyer

INTRODUCTION

Splints are frequently used in the emergency department for temporary immobilization of fractures and for definitive therapy of soft tissue injuries.[1, 2] Immobilization is the mainstay of fracture therapy, but it is difficult to find firm scientific data that support the use of splinting for soft tissue injuries.[3, 4] Although the general principle of immobilizing sprains and contusions is strongly supported by custom and personal preference, its exact influence on healing, number of complications, and ultimate return to normal activity is not known. In most studies of ankle sprains, for example, the function and pain of the injured joint are similar at 6 weeks' follow-up, regardless of whether treatment consisted of ad lib walking, a simple elastic bandage, a posterior splint, or a formal cast.[5, 6]

Most splinting techniques are handed down from house staff or experienced physicians, but the procedure is often suboptimal and haphazard.[7] In this chapter we present guidelines for the adequate immobilization of injuries that are commonly encountered by emergency physicians.

Patients routinely present to the emergency department with injuries that are amenable to splinting to relieve pain and to augment healing (Table 67–1). Emergency physicians have virtually abandoned the use of circumferential casts in favor of premade commercial immobilizing devices or plaster of Paris splints. The impetus for this change is primarily related to the complications frequently associated with circumferential casts, liability issues, and ease of application brought about by new technology. In most instances, splints provide short-term immobilization equal to that of casts, while allowing for continued swelling, thus reducing the risk of ischemic injury. Other obvious advantages of splints are that patients

Table 67–1. *Conditions That Benefit from Immobilization*

Acute arthritis
Severe contusions and abrasions
Skin lacerations that cross joints
Tendon lacerations
Tenosynovitis
Puncture wounds to the hands, feet, and joints
Animal bites to the hands or feet
Deep space infections of the hands and feet
Joint infections
Fractures and sprains

can take them off when immobilization is no longer needed or remove them temporarily to bathe, exercise the injured part, or perform wound care.

INDICATIONS

Theoretically, immobilization facilitates the healing process by decreasing pain and protecting the extremity from further injury. Other benefits of splinting are specific to the particular injury or the problem that is being treated. For example, in the treatment of fractures, splinting helps maintain bony alignment. Splinting deep lacerations that cross joints reduces tension on the wound and helps prevent wound dehiscence. Immobilizing tendon lacerations may facilitate the healing process by relieving stress on the repaired tendon. The discomfort of inflammatory disorders such as tenosynovitis or acute gout is greatly reduced by immobilization. Deep space infections of the hands or feet as well as cellulitis over any joint should similarly be immobilized for comfort. Limiting early motion also may reduce edema and improve the immune system's ability to combat infection. Hence, selected puncture wounds and mammalian bites of the hands and feet may be immobilized until the risk of infection has passed. Splinting large abrasions that cross joint surfaces prevents movement of the injured extremity and reduces the pain that is produced when the injured skin is stretched. Finally, multiple trauma patients should have fractures and reduced dislocations adequately splinted while other diagnostic and therapeutic procedures (e.g., peritoneal lavage, computed tomography scan) are completed. Immobilization decreases blood loss, minimizes the potential for further neurovascular injury, decreases the need for narcotic analgesia, and may decrease the risk of fat emboli from long bone fractures.

EQUIPMENT

Plaster of Paris. Plaster of Paris is the most widely used material for emergency department splinting.[8] Its name originated from the fact that it was first prepared from the gypsum of Paris, France. When gypsum is heated to approximately 128° C, most of the water of crystallization is driven off, leaving behind a fine white powder—plaster of Paris. When water is added to plaster, the reaction is reversed, and the plaster recrystallizes or *sets* by incorporating water molecules into the crystalline lattice of the calcium sulfate dihydrate molecules.

Today, plaster is impregnated into strips or rolls (2-, 3-, 4-, or 6-inch widths) of a crinoline-type material. The crinoline allows for easy application, helps keep the plaster molded to the proper form during the setting process, and adds support to the finished splint. Plaster rolls and sheets are available in a variety of setting times and widths. The distinct advantage of plaster over commercially available, premade splints is that plaster can be molded and tailored to the individual's anatomy, negating the "one size fits all" approach. Also, plaster is generally less expensive than premade splints.

Prefabricated Splint Rolls. The use of plaster splints in the form of prefabricated splint rolls (OCL, specialist J-Splint) have gained popularity among emergency physicians. These splint rolls have 10 to 20 sheets of plaster enclosed between a thick layer of foam padding on one side, and a thin layer of cloth on the other side. Like custom constructed splints they are secured to the extremity with an elastic bandage. The major advantage of prefabricated splint rolls

is that significant time is saved because the splint and padding come ready to apply. In addition, prefabricated splint rolls are ideal for intermittent splinting and can be removed and reapplied by the patient as needed. However, prefabricated plaster splint rolls are more expensive than simple plaster rolls, and they lack some of the versatility and custom-fit qualities of self-made plaster splints.

Stockinette. A single layer of stockinette is commonly used under circumferential casts and splints. It protects the skin and, when folded back over the ends of the plaster, creates a smooth, professional-looking, padded rim. It may also be used as a sling for upper extremity injuries. Stockinette is available in 2-, 3-, 4-, 8-, 10-, and 12-inch widths.

Padding. Padding under the splint protects the skin and bony prominences and allows for swelling of the injured extremity. In general, the older thin cotton padding known as sheet wadding has been replaced by newer materials such as Webril (Curity). Webril is soft cotton that has a much coarser weave than sheet wadding and consequently has greater tensile strength, adheres better, and can be applied more evenly.

Elastic Bandages. Elastic bandages are used to secure the splint in place. Elastic bandages are available in 2-, 3-, 4-, and 6-inch widths.

Orthopedic Felt. Half-inch-thick felt may be used to pad bony prominences.

Adhesive Tape. Adhesive tape is used to prevent slippage of the elastic bandages, to line the cut edges of a bivalved cast, and to buddy tape digits.

Utility Knife and Plaster Scissors. A utility knife, a number 10 scalpel blade, or plaster scissors can be used to cut and shape dry plaster.

Bucket. A large bucket (preferably stainless steel) is used for wetting plaster. Plaster should not be prepared in the sink because the residue quickly clogs the drain. A special drain is required to accept plaster residue.

Protective Clothing. Gowns or sheets prevent soilage of the both the patient's and the physician's clothing.

Gloves and Safety Glasses. Gloves and safety glasses are recommended to prevent skin or eye damage from plaster dust and wet plaster. Wearing gloves also decreases clean-up time for the physician.

GENERAL PROCEDURE OF SPLINT APPLICATION (Fig. 67–1A–D)

The following section refers to the application of custom-made plaster splints unless otherwise stated. If periodic wound care is required, a more easily removable splint (e.g., an OCL or a Velcro-type splint) should be applied in lieu of the standard splint to be described. The issue of removability should be addressed before the splint is applied.

Patient Preparation

If the clinical situation permits, the patient should be covered with a sheet or gown to protect the clothing and the surrounding area from water and plaster. Nursing staff and housekeeping also appreciate this courtesy. The involved extremity should be inspected carefully before splinting. All skin lesions and soft tissue injuries should be examined and documented clearly on the emergency department record. All wounds should be cleaned, repaired, and dressed in the usual manner. When immobilizing open fractures or joints, the soft tissue defect should be covered with saline-moistened sterile gauze.

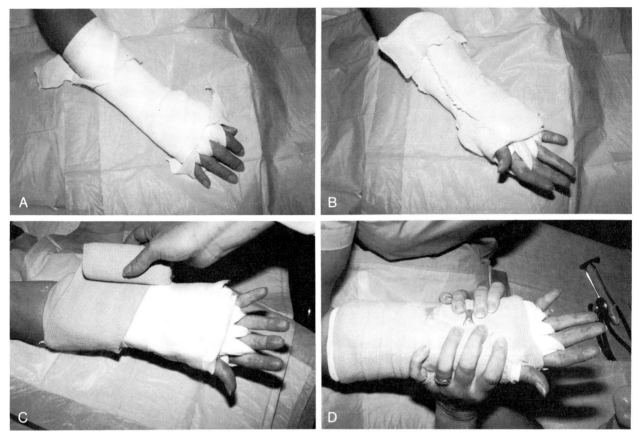

Figure 67–1. Principles of splint application. *A*, The fingers (or toes) are padded with Webril, the stockinette is applied to extend 3 to 4 inches beyond the plaster, and two to three layers of Webril are evenly and smoothly applied over the area to be splinted. *B*, The plaster slab is applied and the stockinette is folded back to secure the slab and to make smooth rounded ends. *C*, The elastic bandage is applied over the splint. Note that a single layer of Webril is placed over the plaster so the elastic bandage is not incorporated into the splint by the drying plaster. *D*, The metal clips are applied and secured with tape. While still wet, the plaster is molded to conform to the shape of the extremity. This is an important step that is often overlooked.

Padding

When the splint involves the digits, padding must be placed between the fingers and toes to prevent maceration of the skin. This can be done with pieces of Webril or gauze cut to the appropriate length.

Following placement of padding between the fingers and toes, stockinette is often used as the next protective layer in self-made splints. The stockinette should extend at least 10 to 15 cm beyond the area to be splinted at both ends of the extremity. Later, after plaster has been applied, the stockinette can be folded back over the ends of the splint to create smooth, padded rims. Folding back the stockinette can also help hold the splint in place when applying elastic bandages. Care is needed to avoid pressure damage from pulling the stockinette too tightly over bony prominences, such as the heel. Wrinkling over flexion creases should also be avoided by slitting and overlapping the stockinette at bony prominences. One may also use two separate pieces of stockinette (one at each end of the splint) to produce the smooth padded rims. As a general rule, 3-inch-wide stockinette is used for the upper extremity, whereas 4-inch-wide is used for the lower extremity.

After the stockinette has been properly positioned, Webril should be wrapped around the entire area that will be exposed to plaster. The Webril should extend 2.5 to 5.0 cm beyond the ends of the splint so it too can be folded back over the splint to help create smooth, well-padded edges. The Webril should overlap by 25 to 50 per cent of its width and should be at least 2 to 3 layers thick. Extra padding should be placed over areas of bony prominence, such as the radial condyle or the malleoli (Table 67–2). If significant swelling is anticipated, 3 to 4 layers of Webril should be applied as padding. Care should be taken to avoid wrinkling because it can result in significant skin pressure when a tight splint is used for a long period of time. Wrinkles can be eliminated by proportionately stretching or even tearing the side of the Webril that must wrap around the

Table 67–2. Bony Prominences of the Upper and Lower Extremity That Require Additional Padding

Upper Extremity
Olecranon
Radial styloid
Ulnar styloid
Lower Extremity
Upper portion of the inner thigh
Patella
Fibular head
Achilles tendon
Medial and lateral malleoli

bigger portion of an extremity. Joints that must be immobilized in a 90-degree position, such as the ankle, make continuous Webril wrapping difficult. To avoid wrinkles in the area of the ankle, the joint should be placed in the proper position before padding. Webril is then wrapped around the malleolar and midtarsal regions first. The bare calcaneal region can then be covered with overlapping vertical and horizontal Webril strips until the entire heel region is evenly padded. The same approach can be used in similar areas such as the elbow. The width of Webril that should be used varies depending on the extremity to be splinted. In general, the 2-inch width should be used for hands and feet, the 3- to 4-inch width for the upper extremity, and the 4- to 6-inch width for the lower extremity.

A final caveat when using Webril is to be aware of the potential for ischemic injury. This rare complication is most likely to occur in an extremity that continues to have significant swelling after the patient is released from the emergency department. Ischemia may result because the concentrically placed Webril can become a constricting band. If this situation is anticipated, it can be prevented easily by cutting through the Webril along the side of the extremity opposite to the plaster splint. The splint is then secured to the extremity in the usual manner.

Plaster Preparation

The choice of plaster setting time depends on the nature of the injury and the expertise of the physician. Extra-fast-setting plaster is typically used when rapid hardening is desired to help maintain an acutely reduced fracture. However, for the majority of emergency department splints, plaster with slower setting times is recommended.[9] Plaster that sets more slowly is easier for some physicians to use because the longer setting times allow more leeway in applying and molding the splint. Importantly, plaster with a longer setting time produces less heat, thus reducing both patient discomfort and the risk of serious burns.[10] Table 67–3 lists the setting times for commonly used plaster. These setting times are created by adding different substances to the plaster during the production process (Table 67–4). Given plaster with equal setting times, the most important variable affecting the rate of crystallization is water temperature. *Hot water hardens a splint faster than cold water* and should not be used when extra time is needed for splint application.

The ideal length and width of plaster depends on the body part to be splinted and the amount of immobilization required. The best way to estimate length is to lay the dry splint next to the area to be splinted. It is best to use a generous length, because if the wet splint is too long, the ends can be folded back easily. In addition, wet plaster shrinks slightly from its dry length. The plaster width varies according to the type of splint being made and the body part that is injured, but generally it should be slightly greater than the diameter of the limb to be splinted. Specific rec-

ommendations regarding splint length and width are made in sections describing individual splints.

The thickness of a splint depends on the size of the patient, the extremity that is injured, and the desired strength of the final product. An ankle splint may crack quickly and become useless if only eight layers are used, but this thickness may be ideal for a wrist splint. In general it is best to use the minimum number of layers that are necessary to achieve adequate strength. Thicker splints are heavier and more uncomfortable. Importantly, plaster thickness is a major determinant of the amount of heat given off during the setting process. With more than 12 sheets of plaster, there is an increased risk of significant burns, especially when using extra-fast-drying plaster, dipping water with a temperature greater than 24° C, or placing a pillow under or around the extremity for support during the setting process (Table 67–5). In an average-sized adult, upper extremities should be splinted with 8 sheets of plaster, whereas lower extremity injuries generally require 12 to 15 sheets. This layering usually gives the strength necessary for adequate immobilization while reducing the patient's discomfort and the risk of significant burns. In a 300-pound patient, however, up to 20 layers may be required to make a durable ankle splint.

The dipping water should be kept clean and fresh. The use of water that has been used previously for wetting plaster increases the amount of heat given off during crystallization and causes plaster to set more quickly. As a rule of thumb, the temperature of the water should be kept around 24° C. This temperature allows for a workable setting time and has not been associated with an increased risk of significant burns. As the temperature of the dipping water approaches 40° C, the potential for serious burns increases, even at splint thicknesses of less than 12 plies. Interestingly, water temperature has been shown to be only a minor consideration in heat production in some studies (see Table 67–5).

Table 67–4. *Effect of Water Temperature and Different Additives on Setting Time of Plaster*

Accelerates Setting Time	Slows Setting Time
Reusing dip water	Cool dip water
Higher dip water temperature	Glue
Salicylic acid	Gum
Zinc	Borax
Magnesium	
Copper	
Iron	
Aluminum	
Salt	
Alum	

Table 67–3. *Setting Times of Fast- and Extra-Fast-Drying Plaster*

Plaster	Setting Time (min)
Fast-drying	5–8
Extra-fast-drying	2–4

Table 67–5. *Variables That Increase Heat Production During Crystallization*

Major	Minor
Increased splint thickness	High humidity
Setting time*	High ambient temperature
High dip water temperature†	Reusing dip water
Wrapping the extremity for support while drying	

*Faster setting times produce more heat.
†Dip water temperature has been a minor determinant of heat production in some studies.

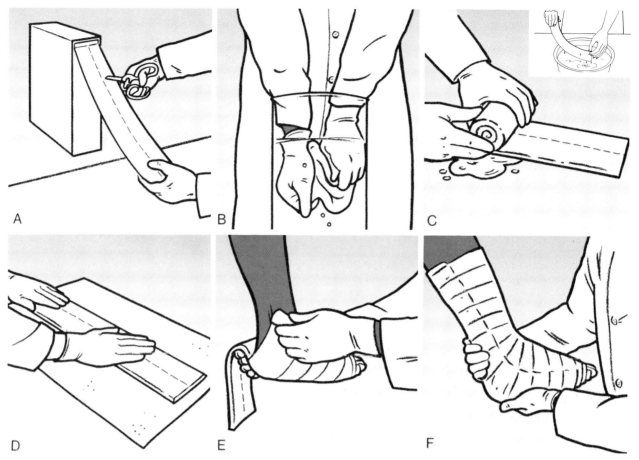

Figure 67–2. Application of plaster. *A,* Measure appropriate length. (Note that plain plaster slabs shrink a few inches when wet. Measure the length slightly longer because the excess may be folded back on itself if necessary). *B,* Submerge until bubbles stop (do not oversoak). *C,* Roll and squeeze excess water from the premade splint. *Inset,* If using plain plaster slabs, allow the water to drip off. *D,* Smooth the sheets to remove wrinkles, and mix the plaster throughout the layers. *E,* Apply the splint and secure it with an elastic bandage. *F,* Mold the splint to fit the contour of the extremity—a very important step. (Specialist J-Splint. Drawings courtesy of Johnson & Johnson Products, Inc., New Brunswick, N. J.)

Splint Application (Fig. 67–2)

The dry splint should be completely submerged in the water until bubbling stops. The splint is removed and excess water is gently squeezed out until the plaster has a wet and sloppy consistency. The splint is placed on a hard table or counter top (a protective covering is recommended to prevent water or plaster damage) and smoothed out to remove any wrinkles and to ensure uniform lamination of all layers. Lamination helps to increase the final strength of the splint. The splint is placed over the Webril and gently smoothed over the extremity. Plaster is usually somewhat adherent to Webril, but an assistant may be required to hold the splint in place. Once the splint has been properly positioned over the extremity, folding back the underlying stockinette and Webril also helps hold it in place. The splint is secured with an appropriately sized elastic bandage by wrapping in a distal to proximal direction. Finally, the extremity is placed in the desired position and the wet plaster is molded to the contour of the extremity using *only the palms of the hand.* Finger indentations may cause a ridge that will produce a pressure point.

Molding the wet splint to conform to the body's anatomy is probably the most important, yet the most frequently overlooked step to ensure adequate immobilization. Molding itself may cause some pain, and the patient should be forewarned. All manipulation of the wet plaster should be completed before it reaches a thick creamy consistency. Any movement after this time, also known as the *critical period,* results in an imperfect crystalline network of calcium sulfate molecules and greatly weakens the ultimate strength of the splint. While the plaster is setting, *a pillow or blanket should not be wrapped around the extremity for support.* This leads to inadequate ventilation around the splint and greatly increases the amount of heat produced (see Table 67–5).

If an elastic bandage is applied directly over wet plaster, the elastic bandage may be incorporated into the drying plaster, making subsequent removal of the bandage difficult. To make it easier for patients to remove and reapply the splint, a single layer of Webril or roll gauze can be wrapped around the wet plaster loosely before application of the elastic bandage. This prevents the wet plaster from becoming stuck to the elastic bandage. Only one layer of Webril should be used over the plaster because multiple layers have been associated with high drying temperatures.

Before discharge, the splint should be checked for adequate immobilization, and the patient should be observed for any evidence of vascular compromise or significant discomfort. If either occurs, the elastic bandage should be loosened. If the discomfort persists, additional padding should be placed over the painful areas. If this measure too is unsuccessful, a new splint should be made, and special attention should be paid to proper molding so that the wet plaster does not become indented. By resting tender tissue,

Table 67–6. *Suggested Length of Immobilization for Conditions That Frequently Require Splinting*

Condition	Length of Immobilization (Days)
Contusions	1–3
Abrasions	1–3
Soft tissue lacerations	5–7
Tendon lacerations	Variable*
Tendonitis	5–7
Puncture wounds and bites	3–4
Deep space infections and cellulitis	3–5
Mild sprains	5–7
Fractures and severe sprains	Variable†

*There is considerable controversy surrounding the length of immobilization for tendon lacerations, and duration therefore is best left to the orthopedic or plastic surgeon.

†Usually requires prolonged immobilization; best determined by an orthopedic surgeon.

splinting usually relieves discomfort quickly, and patients generally say that they feel better immediately after the splint has been applied. Never discharge a patient who complains of *increased* pain after a splint has been placed.

After a proper-fitting, comfortable splint has been applied, one may place two strips of tape along each side of the splint to prevent the elastic bandage from slipping. Tape should always be applied over the metal fasteners used to secure the elastic bandages. Note that these objects can be easily swallowed or aspirated by infants and small children. Finally, a sling should be provided for upper extremity injuries, and, if required, crutches should be dispensed (and instructions given for their proper use) for lower extremity injuries.

Discharge Instructions

All patients should receive both verbal and written instructions on splint care and precautions (Table 67–6). The importance of elevation to help decrease pain and swelling should be stressed and *demonstrated* (most patients do not understand the medical definition of elevation). If the injury is less than 24 hours old, the application of ice bags or cold packs should also be encouraged. It is useless to apply ice over plaster, but it can be beneficial if it is applied over Webril and an elastic bandage or directly over an injury if the splint is removed. Cold therapy stiffens collagen and thus reduces the tendency for ligaments and tendons to deform. Cold therapy also decreases muscle spasm and excitability, decreases blood flow (thus limiting hemorrhage and edema), increases the pain threshold, and decreases inflammation. Because the thermal conductivity of subcutaneous tissue is poor, ice packs should be applied for at least 30 minutes at a time. This guideline is in contrast to the popular recommendation of "ice 20 minutes on, 20 minutes off," which does nothing more than cool the skin. Ice packs should not be applied for more than the first 24 to 48 hours because cold can interfere with wound healing. The patient should be instructed not to stress the splint for at least 24 hours because plaster does not approach optimal strength until evaporation has reduced the water content of the plaster to approximately 21 per cent of its initial hydrated level. This process of removing excess water by evaporation is called *curing* and generally takes several days to be completed. However, by 24 hours the water content of the plaster has usually been reduced enough to produce a strong resilient splint. In addition, because the chemical process involved in the formation of plaster is reversible, the patient

should avoid getting the splint wet. However, if the injury permits, the splint can be removed for showering and then reapplied. Alternatively one or more plastic bags may be placed over a splint before showering.

Splints may crack, break, or disintegrate with wear, and a useless splint should be removed or replaced. Patients should be given general guidelines for length of immobilization and appropriate follow-up care. Long-term immobilization, particularly in the elderly, can produce permanent disability.

After discharge it is extremely important for the patient to continue to check for signs of vascular compromise. If the patient experiences a significant increase in pain, any numbness or tingling of the digits, pallor of the distal extremity, decreased capillary refill, or weakness, he or she should be instructed to return to the emergency department or to see the primary physician without delay. As with casting, increased pain after splinting is a warning sign that should prompt a return visit—*not telephone advice*. Strong narcotics should be avoided during the first 2 to 3 days after splinting to allow pain to prompt a follow-up visit.

UPPER EXTREMITY SPLINTS

General Considerations

Upper extremity splints are used primarily to immobilize reduced dislocations of the elbow, radial head fractures, hemarthrosis of the elbow, midshaft forearm fractures, wrist sprains and fractures, carpal bone fractures, finger sprains and fractures, tendon repairs, acute gouty arthritis, and any soft tissue injury or laceration that may benefit from rest. Commonly applied splints are the long arm posterior splint, the short arm volar splint, and the single or double sugar tong. Splints of the arm are usually used in conjunction with a sling. A full arm splint extends from the proximal humerus to include the wrist and metacarpals. Sugar tong splints and posterior arm splints prevent pronation and supination of the forearm. A forearm splint allows motion at the elbow and extends from the proximal forearm to the base of the fingers, allowing free movement of the thumb and fingers. The thumb and fingers are immobilized with gutter splints, and individual fingers may require specialized splints.

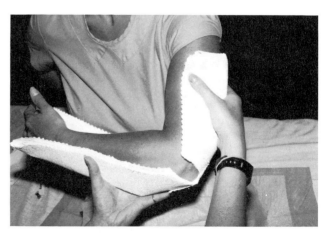

Figure 67–3. Fitting a long arm posterior splint. The 6-inch-wide splint begins at the proximal humerus and extends to the distal metacarpals. The elbow is flexed at a 90-degree angle, the forearm is in neutral (thumb up) position, and the wrist is in a neutral position or slightly dorsiflexed. A notch has been cut out of the plaster to ensure a smooth fit around the elbow.

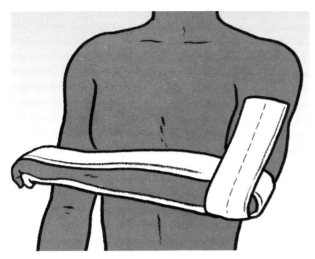

Figure 67–4. An alternative to the full arm posterior splint is a double sugar tong. This splint extends from the proximal humerus to the distal metacarpals with the elbow at a 90-degree angle and the forearm in a neutral (thumb up) position or slightly pronated (shown). A sling is used for support. (Specialist J-Splint. Drawing courtesy of Johnson & Johnson Products, Inc., New Brunswick, NJ.)

Long Arm Splint. This splint immobilizes injuries of the elbow, forearm, or wrist. The elbow is flexed at the 90-degree position for a posterior splint (Fig. 67–3) or a double sugar tong (Fig. 67–4). It is generally safe to place the wrist in slight extension (10 to 20 degrees), with the forearm in a neutral position (thumb upward), avoiding extremes in supination or pronation. Four- or 6-inch plaster is used for the posterior splint with the sides folded up to make a gutter. Three- or 4-inch plaster is used for a double sugar tong. It is important to extend the splint to the metacarpals to immobilize the wrist, but the thumb and fingers should remain free.

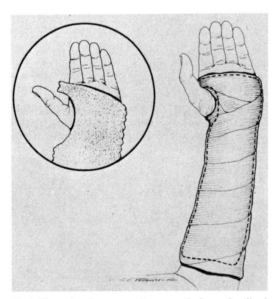

Figure 67–5. The volar forearm splint extends from the distal metacarpals to the proximal forearm and allows the thumb and fingers to remain free. For fractures an additional dorsal slab may be used to create a bivalve splint. The wrist is placed in slight (10- to 20-degree) extension. A thumb spica is added to immobilize a navicular fracture. (From Howes DS, Kaufman JJ: Plaster splints: Techniques and indications. Am Fam Physician 30:215, 1984. Reproduced by permission.)

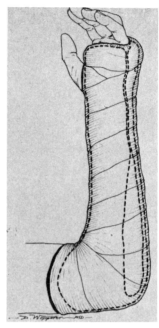

Figure 67–6. The sugar tong forearm splint immobilizes the forearm and wrist and eliminates pronation or supination. The elbow is placed in a 90-degree angle, and the forearm is in a neutral (thumb up) position. The splint extends to the distal metacarpals (volar and palmar), and the thumb and fingers have normal movement. (From Howes DS, Kaufman JJ: Plaster splints: Techniques and indications. Am Fam Physician 30:215, 1984. Reproduced by permission.)

Forearm Splint. A volar forearm (Fig. 67–5) or volar-dorsal bivalve splint immobilizes the wrist and carpal bones. A single sugar tong immobilizes the forearm in addition (Fig. 67–6). With fractures of the wrist, it is desirable also to immobilize the elbow for the first few days, so often a sugar tong is the best choice. Ulna or radial shaft fractures should be immobilized with the single sugar tong splint. For sprains of the wrist or for soft tissue injuries, the simple volar splint suffices. Some prefer to use a bivalve splint when a fracture is immobilized because it is more stable than a simple volar splint. Forearm splints should include the metacarpals but should leave the thumb and finger free.

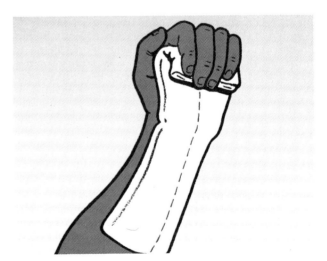

Figure 67–7. Plaster may be folded back on itself to give the fingers something to rest on or grasp yet still be free enough to prohibit stiffness. The elastic bandage applied to this splint extends only as far as the metacarpal heads. (Specialist J-Splint. Drawing courtesy of Johnson & Johnson Products, Inc., New Brunswick, NJ.)

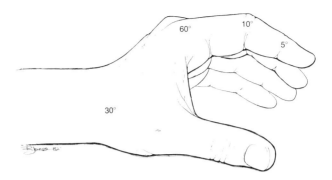

Figure 67–8. A safe splint position for the hand. The wrist should allow alignment of the thumb with the forearm, the metacarpophalangeal joint should be moderately flexed, and the interphalangeal joints should be only slightly flexed. The thumb should be abducted away from the palm. Consider this position similar to grasping a softball or holding the bowl of a large wine glass. (From Carter P: Common Hand Injuries and Infections. Philadelphia, WB Saunders Co, 1983.)

The distal end of the splint may be folded back to allow the finger to remain free yet "grasp" the rounded distal end when at rest (Fig. 67–7).

The forearm is placed in a neutral position (thumb upward) with the wrist slightly extended (cocked up). Wrist flexion should be avoided. After the splint is applied but with the plaster still wet, it is desirable to mold the splint to conform to the contours of the palm and wrist.

Hand Splints. The hand is splinted for carpal or metacarpal fractures, hand infections, burns, lacerations, or contusions. The hand is immobilized by splinting the wrist and fingers. When more than one finger is included, Webril or gauze should be placed between the digits, or the fingers should be wrapped individually. The hand is splinted in either the safe or the intrinsic position (Figs. 67–8 and 67–9).

When splinting injured hands, one should avoid the rest-injury position, the posture reflexly assumed following an injury, because if the hand becomes stiff in this position, little or no function can be salvaged (Fig. 67–10). Elderly patients should never be splinted for more than 2 weeks without reevaluation because stiffness is common with prolonged immobilization.

The ulnar gutter splint is used to immobilize fractures of the metacarpals and phalanges of the fourth and fifth fingers (Fig. 67–11). A thumb spica or gutter splint immobilizes the sprained or fractured thumb or de Quervain tenosynovitis (Fig. 67–12). For navicular fractures a volar splint with a thumb spica is required (Fig. 67–13).

Finger Splints. Fingers are splinted following sprains, fractures, tendon repair, or infection. Specific conditions, such as a mallet finger, require a specialized splint (Fig. 67–14). Many sprained fingers can be managed with buddy taping (Fig. 67–15), but fractures, tendon repairs, and some soft tissue injuries benefit from formal splinting. In certain finger injuries it is not necessary to apply a hand-wrist-forearm splint, and mallet fingers, potential boutonnière

fingers, finger tip injuries, and some local wounds are well treated by a splint limited to the finger alone (Fig. 67–16).

"One-surface splints" are commercially available foam splints with aluminum backing. Splints with numerous fancy curves are expensive, excessively elaborate, and generally not appropriate. One device that is particularly to be discouraged is the "Freddy the frog" splint (Fig. 67–17). This splint is designed to hold the distal interphalangeal joint hyperextended while holding the proximal interphalangeal joint flexed. This is an almost intolerable position even in a normal finger, and the patient will take it off or loosen it, which negates its purpose. Specific fingers can be splinted with an apparatus that incorporates an aluminum splint into a plaster splint—the "outrigger splint" (Fig. 67–18A and B). With this splint, the proximal and distal ends of the metal splint must be padded and trimmed carefully to avoid injury to the palm or adjacent fingers.

ELEVATION OF THE INJURED EXTREMITY

It is important that the injured extremity be kept elevated. Patients usually learn that an elevated hand hurts less than a dependent one. It is important to emphasize this to patients and to assist them with elevation. A variety of slings are available. Many of these are elaborate yet do not allow adequate elevation of the hand, that is, at or above heart level. The old-fashioned muslin triangular sling is effective, but the hand must be elevated to the shoulder (Fig. 67–19). At night a pillow wrapped around the hand helps the patient keep it satisfactorily elevated (Fig. 67–20).

PITFALLS OF HAND DRESSINGS AND SPLINTS

The two most common problems with hand dressings are putting them on too tightly and leaving them on too long (Table 67–7). One must be especially careful to avoid wrapping elastic bandages too snugly. The patient should be instructed to loosen an elastic bandage if it feels too tight.

Figure 67–9. The intrinsic plus position (also known as the protected position or position of safety). Note that the wrist is slightly extended (dorsiflexed), the metacarpophalangeal joints are flexed to approximately a 90-degree angle, the interphalangeal joints are in nearly full extension, and the thumb web is open (abducted). This position maximally relieves tension on intrinsic muscles. This is the best position from which stiffness can be treated and should be used for long-term splinting (more than 2 weeks) or for splinting extensor tendon repairs.

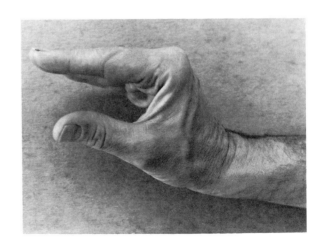

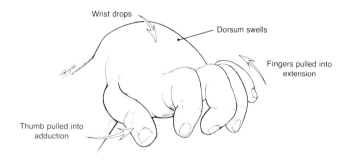

Figure 67–10. A sequence to loss of function occurs if the rest-injury posture, the one patients usually assume after a hand injury, is allowed to persist. Wrist flexion leads to dorsal swelling that leads to metacarpophalangeal hyperextension and thumb adduction. This position is a nonfunctional one if the hand becomes stiff. It can be avoided by proper splinting of the wrist in extension. (From Carter P: Common Hand Injuries and Infections. Philadelphia, WB Saunders Co, 1983.)

Figure 67–11. Gutter-type splints are used to immobilize second to third (*A*, radial gutter splint) and fourth to fifth fingers (*B*, ulnar gutter splint). Four-inch plaster is used. The two fingers are separated with gauze or cotton wadding. The metacarpophalangeal joint is at 90 degrees' flexion, and the interphalangeal joints are placed in slight flexion. Generally two fingers are immobilized. (From Howes DS, Kaufman JJ: Plaster splints: Techniques and indications. Am Fam Physician 30:215, 1984. Reproduced by permission.)

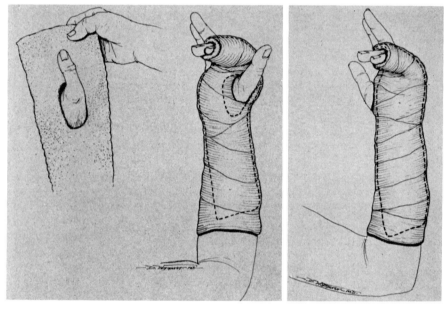

A

B

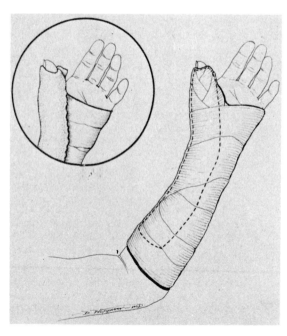

Figure 67–12. The thumb spica (gutter) splint extends from the thumbnail to the mid forearm. The thumb is held in abduction with 4-inch plaster. (From Howes DS, Kaufman JJ: Plaster splints: Techniques and indications. Am Fam Physician 30:215, 1984. Reproduced by permission.)

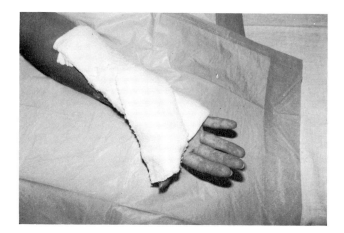

Figure 67–13. To immobilize a navicular or thumb fracture, a thumb spica extension is added to a volar short arm splint.

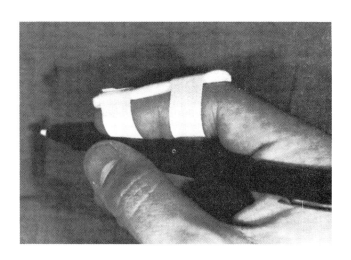

Figure 67–14. In splinting a mallet finger the dorsal splint immobolizes only the distal interphalangeal joint. This allows the patient use of the finger. Hyperextension of this joint predisposes to skin slough and should be avoided. The patient should be advised not to flex the joint during splint changes. (From Carter P: Common Hand Injuries and Infections. Philadelphia, WB Saunders Co, 1983.)

Figure 67–15. Buddy tape technique. Taping between the digital joints allows the normal neighboring finger to protect the collateral ligament of its injured neighbor. (From Carter P. Common Hand Injuries and Infections. Philadelphia, WB Saunders Co, 1983.)

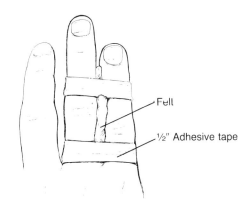

Felt

½" Adhesive tape

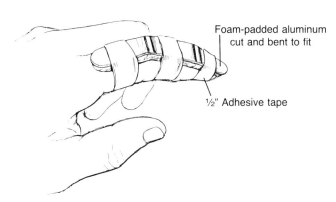

Foam-padded aluminum cut and bent to fit

½" Adhesive tape

Figure 67–16. Dorsal aluminum foam splint. The bone is subcutaneous dorsally, and splints here afford better immobilization of the digit. The dorsal splint also allows preservation and use of the tactile sense, which encourages function and better splint acceptance on the part of the patient. (From Carter P: Common Hand Injuries and Infections. Philadelphia, WB Saunders Co, 1983.)

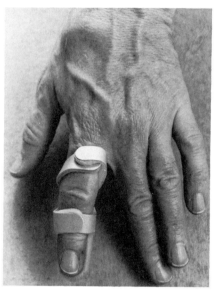

Figure 67–17. A "Freddy the frog" splint, which is considered suboptimal by the authors.

Table 67–7. Useful Estimates of Splint Times for Various Hand Problems

Injury	Splint Type	Immobilization Time*
Mallet finger	FIN†	8 weeks
Boutonniere deformity	FIN	6 weeks
Distal phalanx—soft tissue	FIN	2 to 2 weeks
Extensor tendon	DHWF‡	3 weeks
Sprain-strain§		
Interphalangeal joint	FIN	1 to 2 weeks
Wrist	DHWF	1 to 2 weeks
Hand burn	DHWF	5 to 7 weeks
Infection		
Digit	DHWF	5 to 7 days
Hand	DHWF	5 to 7 days
Severe hand contusion	DHWF	5 to 7 days
Fracture		
Distal phalanx	FIN	2 to 3 weeks
Middle phalanx	FIN	2 to 3 weeks
Proximal phalanx	DHWF	2 to 3 weeks
Metacarpal	DHWF	2 to 3 weeks
Carpal tunnel	DHWF	Night only
De Quervain disease	DHWF	2 to 3 weeks
Trigger finger	FIN	Night only

*These are average times only. Every patient is treated as an individual when a splint is used. Clinical judgment is critical.
†Finger splint.
‡Digit-hand-wrist-forearm splint.
§The diagnosis of a sprain should be made only after a thorough effort has been made to rule out a fracture or a dislocation. This is particularly true in the wrist.

The patient should always have access to emergency follow-up care. It is often advisable to start patients on early protected motion. This means that the patient removes the splint for a specified period, does a prescribed exercise, and then replaces the splint. A splint is not an all-or-none device, and generally the patient is weaned slowly from it before it is discarded entirely. A stiff hand is a nonfunctional one, and stiffness is often a consequence of overlong immobilization. It is important for the patient to be made aware of his or her responsibility for the injured hand.

Sling, Swathe and Sling, and Shoulder Immobilizer

INDICATIONS

The sling, a combination of the swathe and sling, and the shoulder immobilizer are the most common ways of immobilizing the upper extremity without plaster (Fig. 67–21). Although many types of commercial slings are available, these expensive devices do not allow the versatility of a simple, inexpensive triangular muslin bandage and stockinette. The sling should be used to elevate and immobilize the hand or forearm, the elbow, and the shoulder. The sling is often used in conjunction with a plaster splint or cast. The swathe and sling (or the commercially available "shoulder immobilizer") is the treatment of choice for most proximal humerus fractures and shoulder injuries, such as reduced dislocations. The sling supports the weight of the arm, and the swathe immobilizes the arm against the chest wall to minimize shoulder motion. If used for more than a few days the axilla should be padded to absorb moisture and decrease skin chafing. The shoulder immobilizer has virtually replaced the standard swathe and sling. Its advantage is that it may be removed for showering and range-of-motion exercises and is easily reapplied by the patient (a desirable option in the care of a shoulder dislocation).

The Velpeau bandage is a sling and swathe device that positions the forearm diagonally rather than horizontally across the chest with the hand elevated to the level of the

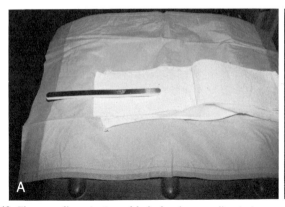
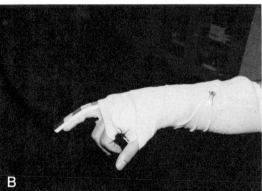

Figure 67–18. Finger splint. *A,* A padded aluminum splint is incorporated into the middle of a plaster splint, forming an outrigger configuration. *B,* This is applied to the dorsum of the finger with an elastic bandage, and the finger is taped to the aluminum splint.

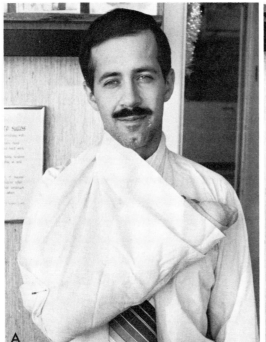
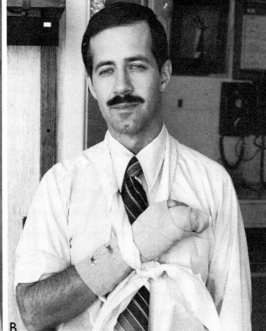
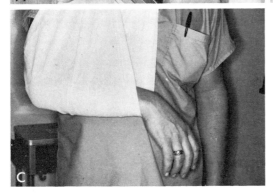

Figure 67–19. A triangular muslin sling can be used either as shown in *A* or as seen in *B*. The sling shown in *C* is *too low*, and the hand is hanging out—a *poor arrangement*. Wrist flexion kinks venous flow in the dorsum of the hand and promotes edema.

shoulder. This offers no particular advantage over a standard sling and swathe, is difficult to apply, cannot be removed easily, and is not tolerated for prolonged immobilization.

Figure-of-Eight Clavicle Straps. Clavicle fractures have been traditionally treated with an uncomfortable and complex figure-of-eight bandage. Despite its widespread use, this device has never been proved superior to a simple sling.[11, 12] We advise that the figure-of-eight dressing be abandoned because it may actually promote nonunion or increase the deformity at the fracture site; it prohibits bathing, often causes chafing and discomfort in the axilla, and may predispose to axillary vein thrombosis.

LOWER EXTREMITY SPLINTS

Knee Splints

KNEE IMMOBILIZER

Indications. The knee immobilizer (AOA and others) is commonly used for mild to moderate ligamentous and soft tissue injuries of the knee. It is removable and extremely easy to apply, making it very popular among patients and physicians alike (Fig. 67–22). In many emergency departments it has almost totally replaced the more bulky plaster splint. Its use should be restricted to injuries that do not

require immediate surgical intervention, traction, or casting. For these injuries, in which temporary but more complete immobilization is needed, a plaster knee splint can be used because it provides better stabilization and costs much less than a knee immobilizer. The exact scientific benefit of the knee immobilizer is poorly studied and difficult to document. However, it clearly helps relieve pain and, at least theoretically, hastens healing.

Application. The knee immobilizer is available in small, medium, large, and extra-large sizes. To choose the appropriate size, the knee immobilizer is placed next to the injured leg so that the tapered end lies distally and the cutout patellar area on the anterior aspect of the splint lies adjacent to the patient's knee. In this position, the splint should extend distally to within a few inches of the malleoli and proximally to just below the buttocks crease. To apply the knee immobilizer, the open splint is slid under the injured extremity so that when wrapped around the leg, the cutout area is over the knee. The splint is firmly secured in place using the Velcro straps. The knee immobilizer can be applied directly over clothing, obviating the need to remove or cut the patient's pants.

POSTERIOR KNEE SPLINT

Indications. In many emergency departments, the knee immobilizer has virtually replaced the plaster knee splint for

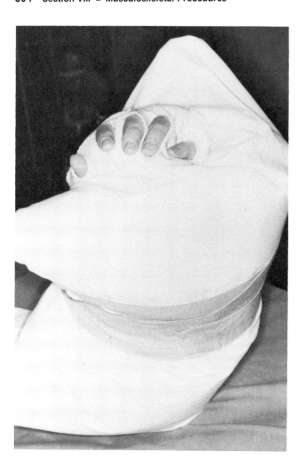

Figure 67–20. The "pillow" method of elevation for use while in bed. This can be set up easily by the patient and family and is very useful.

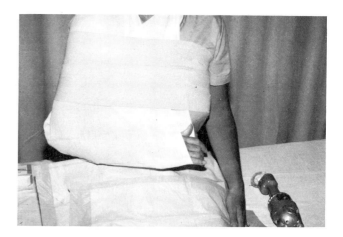

Figure 67–21. A sling and swathe are applied to immobilize the shoulder. A premade shoulder immobilizer accomplishes the same effect and can be removed for showering and range-of-motion exercises and reapplied by the patient.

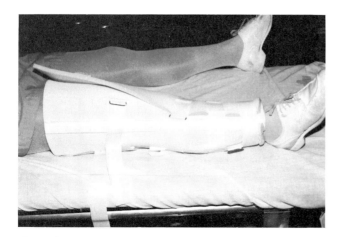

Figure 67–22. The Velcro strap bulky knee immobilizer is easily removed and reapplied by the patient. It can be worn over clothes.

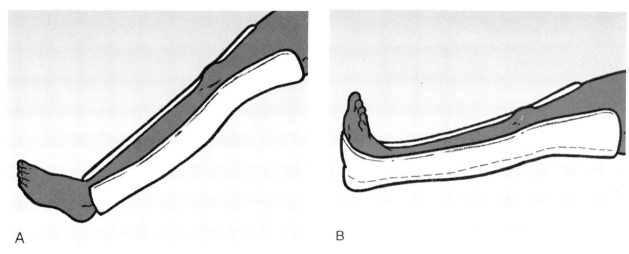

Figure 67–23. *A*, Posterior gutter. The knee is immobilized with either a long leg posterior gutter splint or parallel lateral slabs from the proximal thigh to the distal leg. Many prefer to use the easily removable Velcro knee immobilizer as an alternative. *B*, Fractures of the knee or leg may be immobilized with the long leg sugar tong. This splint eliminates inversion or eversion of the ankle. (Specialist J-Splint. Drawing courtesy of Johnson & Johnson Products, Inc., New Brunswick, NJ.)

mild to moderate injuries to the knee. However, the plaster knee splint can be particularly useful in patients whose extremities are too large for the knee immobilizer, in the treatment of angulated fractures, or for temporarily immobilizing other knee injuries that require immediate operative intervention or orthopedic referral. The posterior (gutter) knee splint is the type most commonly applied, but as an alternative, two parallel splints can be placed along each side of the leg and foreleg, creating a bivalve effect, or a long leg sugar tong can be applied (Fig. 67–23*A* and *B*). The bilateral knee splint is slightly more difficult to apply than the posterior knee splint, but it may provide better immobilization of the lateral and medial collateral ligaments and can be used for injuries to these structures.

Construction. The knee splint is made with eight to ten layers of 6-inch plaster. It should run from just below the buttocks crease to approximately 2 to 3 inches above the malleoli. The sides of the splint are folded upward to form a gutter configuration.

Application. A stockinette should be placed in the usual manner, and the leg should be well padded with 4- to 6-inch Webril. If available, an assistant can help elevate the leg and hold the splint in place while it is being secured with 4- or 6-inch elastic bandages. If there is no aide available, the patient can be placed in the prone position. The splint can now be laid on the posterior surface of the extremity without needing to be held in place. Also, the patient's toes will keep the lower part of the leg off the bed, allowing sufficient room to wrap the Webril and elastic bandages around the injured extremity.

JONES COMPRESSION DRESSING

Indications. A Jones compression dressing is commonly used for short-term immobilization of soft tissue injuries of the knee. It immobilizes and compresses the knee, reducing both pain and swelling. However, because it does allow slight flexion and extension of the knee, it should not be used for injuries that require strict immobilization. In addition, it is difficult to maintain the splint for more than a few days.

Construction. A Jones dressing is made using 6-inch Webril and elastic bandages.

Application. To apply a Jones dressing, the patient is placed on a stretcher lying on the back. If available, an

assistant can elevate the patient's leg to facilitate wrapping. If no help is available, a pillow placed under the patient's heel should suffice. Webril is then wrapped around the extremity from the groin to a few inches above the malleoli. Two or three layers of Webril can be used, and each turn should overlap the previous turn by 25 to 50 per cent. The elastic bandage (two are usually required) is then wrapped around the Webril. If more support is required, the process can be repeated with another two to three layers of Webril held in place by a second elastic bandage.

Ankle Splints

POSTERIOR SPLINT

Indications. The posterior ankle splint is one of the most common splints applied in the emergency department (Fig. 67–24). It is used primarily to immobilize second- and third-degree ankle sprains, fractures of the distal fibula and tibia, and reduced ankle dislocations. It can also be used for fractures of the tarsal and metatarsal bones or for other foot

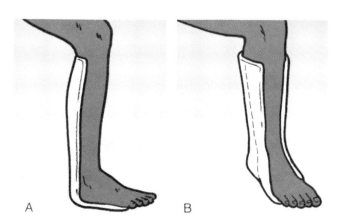

Figure 67–24. *A*, The short leg posterior splint is used alone or in conjunction with a stirrup splint. *B*, The posterior splint should extend far enough on the foot to support the distal metacarpal heads. (Specialist J-Splint. Drawing courtesy of Johnson & Johnson Products, Inc., New Brunswick, NJ.)

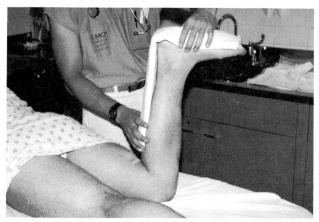

Figure 67–25. The most convenient way to apply an ankle splint is to have the patient lie prone and bend the knee to a 90-degree angle, thereby relaxing the calf muscles. The ankle should be at a 90-degree angle so that the foot is flat for partial weight bearing.

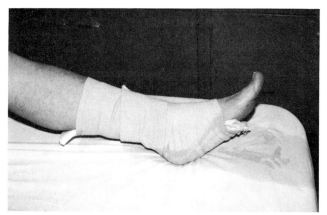

Figure 67–26. There are three things wrong with this splint: (1) It does not extend distally enough to support the entire foot. (2) The ankle is not maintained at a 90-degree angle. (3) The edges and ankle area are not molded, which gives an overall sloppy appearance.

conditions that require immobilization. In particularly severe or unstable injuries, an additional anterior splint may be used to provide extra immobilization resembling that of a formal cast. For severe lateral or bilateral ligamentous injuries, a sugar tong or stirrup splint (see following section) may be added to the posterior splint for increased immobilization. With minor soft tissue injuries, patients may have partial weight bearing on ankle splints after 24 hours. If the patient will be bearing weight, a cast shoe over the splint makes it easier to walk. In addition, a cast shoe increases the longevity of the splint because walking on an unprotected splint quickly destroys the device. Generally, walking on the splint is prohibited if immobilization for more than 2 or 3 days is desired.

Construction. The posterior splint is made using 4-inch-wide plaster strips. It should extend from the plantar surface of the great toe or metatarsal heads along the posterior surface of the foreleg to the level of the fibular head. If it hurts to move the toes, they should be incorporated into the splint (after padding is placed between the digits). It is a common mistake to apply a posterior splint that does not extend far enough to support the ball of the foot. Fifteen to 20 layers should be used if partial weight bearing is allowed because this splint frequently breaks or cracks when walked on.[13]

Application. The easiest way to apply a posterior splint is to place the patient in the prone position with the knee and ankle flexed at a 90-degree angle (Fig. 67–25). Failure to place the ankle in a 90-degree angle results in a plantar-flexed splint. The supine patient may help maintain the ankle in a 90-degree angle by pulling up on the foot with a wide stockinette stirrup. Flexing the knee to a 90-degree angle relaxes the gastrocnemius muscle and facilitates ankle motion. With the knee and ankle in the proper position, stockinette may be applied and the foot and leg padded with Webril as described earlier. Extra padding is used over bony prominences, particularly the malleoli. Again, Webril or gauze is placed between the toes if they are to be included in the splint. The wet plaster is then laid over the plantar surface of the foot and secured in place by folding back the ends of the stockinette and wrapping with one or two 4-inch-wide elastic bandages. The wet plaster is carefully molded around the malleoli and instep to ensure maximum comfort and immobilization. The toes should be left partially exposed for later examination of color and capillary refill. Three common application errors are shown in Fig. 67–26.

SUGAR TONG (STIRRUP) SPLINT

Indications. The sugar tong or stirrup splint is used primarily for injuries to the ankle (Fig. 67–27). It functions like the posterior splint, and either of the two provides satisfactory ankle immobilization. In one study that compared these splints in normal volunteers, the sugar tong splint allowed less plantar flexion and broke less often with plantar flexion than the posterior splint.[13] Also, because it actually covers the malleoli, the sugar tong splint may protect the medial and lateral ligamentous area from further injury better than the posterior splint.

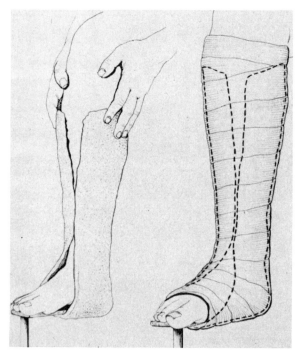

Figure 67–27. The short leg stirrup (sugar tong) may be used alone or in conjunction with a posterior short leg splint. The stirrup prevents inversion or eversion at the ankle and is ideal for medial or lateral ligamentous injuries. (From Howes DS, Kaufman JJ: Plaster splints: Techniques and indications. Am Fam Physician 30:215, 1984. Reproduced by permission.)

Construction. The sugar tong splint is made using 4- or 6-inch-wide plaster strips. The splint passes under the plantar surface of the foot from the calcaneus to the metatarsal heads and extends up the medial and lateral sides of the foreleg just below the level of the fibular head.

Application. The patient is positioned, and the extremity is padded as described for the posterior splint. If both posterior and sugar tong splints are used, the posterior splint is applied first. The wet plaster is laid across the plantar surface of the foot between the calcaneus and metatarsal heads with the sides extending up the lateral and medial aspects of the foreleg. The plaster is secured in place with 4-inch elastic bandages. The elastic bandage should be wrapped around the extremity starting at the metatarsal heads and continuing around the ankle using a figure-of-eight configuration. Once the ankle has been wrapped, a 4- or 6-inch elastic bandage can be used to secure the remainder of the splint in place. The splint should be carefully molded around the malleoli. The plaster may overlap on the anterior aspect of the ankle; this overlap does not interfere with the splint's ability to accommodate further swelling.

ANTERIOR SPLINT

Indications. The anterior splint is never used by itself, but it can augment a posterior splint, creating a bivalve effect. It is used for serious fractures and soft tissue injuries.

Construction. A piece of plaster should be cut several centimeters shorter than the one used for the posterior splint, but because this splint does not bear weight, only eight to ten layers are required.

Application. The patient should be positioned and padded as for the posterior splint. After the wet posterior splint has been applied, the anterior splint is placed over the anterior aspect of the ankle and foreleg parallel to the posterior splint. The two are then held in place with elastic bandages as described earlier for the posterior splint alone. An assistant is necessary to apply the anterior-posterior splint because it is extremely difficult to hold both splints in place while wrapping the elastic bandages. Once secured, both splints are carefully molded over the instep and ankle joint.

SEMIRIGID ORTHOSIS

Indications. Patients with minor ankle sprains seen initially or patients recovering from more severe strains are often able to return to function more quickly with the use of an ankle or leg orthosis.[13a, 13b]

Application. The Air-Stirrup braces (Aircast, Inc., Summit, NJ 07902) resemble a sugar tong splint with air bladders for cushioning the malleoli. After partial inflation of the air bladders, the braces are secured about the ankle by Velcro straps. The device is worn within the patient's shoe over a sock and appears to eliminate ankle instability.[13c]

HARD SHOE (CAST OR REESE SHOE)

Indications. A hard shoe can help reduce the pain associated with ambulation in patients with fractures or soft tissue injuries to the foot. This device can also be used over a splint or cast to allow partial weight bearing.

Application. If the cast shoe is going to be used by a patient with a fractured toe, the injured digit should first be buddy taped to the one next to it. After this is done, the patient merely slips on the hard shoe like a sandal or loafer. The shoe is then fastened with ties or Velcro straps.

SOFT CAST

Indications. A "soft cast" is basically a modified Jones compression dressing. It is useful for minor ligamentous and soft tissue injuries of the foot and ankle that do not require prolonged or complete immobilization. A soft cast can help reduce the pain and swelling often associated with mild ankle sprains and gives support for early weight bearing.

Construction. A soft cast is made using 3- or 4-inch Webril and elastic bandages.

Application. A soft cast is as simple to apply as the Jones compression dressing. To begin, the patient is placed in a supine position with the foot and ankle extending off the end of the stretcher. Alternatively, the leg can be elevated by an assistant or by placing pillows under the knee and foreleg. The ankle and foot are then wrapped with two to three layers of Webril, starting at the metatarsal heads and continuing around the ankle in a figure-of-eight configuration. The Webril should extend 5 to 7 cm above the malleoli and, as discussed earlier, should overlap by 25 to 50 per cent of its width. After the Webril is in place, an elastic bandage is wrapped around the foot and ankle in a similar fashion. Additional layers of Webril and elastic bandages are seldom required.

UNNA BOOT DRESSING

Ligamentous injuries of the ankle may be treated with a cloth dressing impregnated with calamine gelatin–zinc oxide (Dome-Paste or Unna Boot).[14] This moist dressing is applied like that for a rolled cast in a figure-of-eight design, from the metatarsal heads to the distal leg (Fig. 67–28). This dressing remains moist for a few days (it should be covered with a gauze roll or an elastic bandage) and dries to a

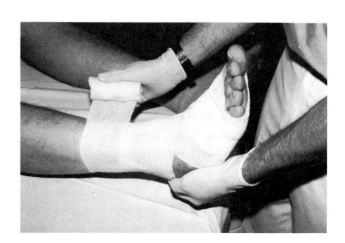

Figure 67–28. Unna Boot provides simple, effective immobilization of an ankle soft tissue injury. It is applied from a semisolid paste roll, is covered with gauze or an elastic bandage, and can be cut off by the patient at home.

leathery consistency. It requires minimal maintenance or patient compliance, is lightweight, can be worn under a shoe, and is associated with few complications. It is cut off with scissors by the patient after 5 to 10 days, depending on symptoms. This dressing is nonyielding; hence evaluation for ischemia is essential in the edema-prone extremity.

COMPLICATIONS OF SPLINTS

Ischemia

A compartment syndrome leading to ischemic injury and ultimately to a Volkmann ischemic contracture is the most worrisome complication of cylindric casts. Although the risk of ischemia is drastically reduced with splinting, Webril or elastic bandages can cause significant constriction. To reduce the likelihood of this occurring, the elastic bandage should not be excessively tight. If the patient has a high-risk injury, the Webril may be cut lengthwise before the plaster is applied. Elevation, no weight bearing, and application of cold packs should be stressed to each patient. Furthermore, signs and symptoms of vascular compromise should be explained carefully, and all patients whose injuries have the potential for significant swelling or loss of vascular integrity should receive follow-up in the first 24 to 48 hours. Complaints of increasing pain under a splint should not be ignored by the patient or physician and should not be treated with a telephone prescription for narcotics.

Plaster Burns

Many physicians are unaware of the potential for drying plaster to produce second-degree burns.[15] Thermal injury can occur with both cylindric casts and plaster splints. Some physicians have reported a higher incidence of burns with the use of plaster splints, although the reasons for this are unclear.[15, 16] Table 67–5 lists those factors that can increase the amount of heat that is produced during plaster recrystallization. Their effects are additive, and this fact should be taken into account when applying a splint. For example, if 15 sheets of plaster are needed for strength in a particular splint, one should not increase the heat production further by using extra-fast-drying plaster or by reusing the warm dip water. To avoid plaster burns it is prudent to use only 8 to 12 sheets of plaster when possible, to use fresh dip water with a temperature near 24° C, and never to wrap the extremity in a sheet or pillow during the setting process. Peak temperatures usually occur between 5 and 15 minutes after plaster wetting. The patient should be warned that the hardening process produces warmth. If the patient complains of significant burning while the plaster is drying, *do not ignore this complaint!* Immediately remove the splint, and promptly cool the area with saline or tap water. Patients with vascular insufficiency or sensory deficits (e.g., diabetic neuropathy, stroke) are at high risk for plaster burns and require close observation during the drying process.

Pressure Sores

Pressure sores are an uncommon complication of short-term splinting.[17] They can result from stockinette wrinkles, irregular wadding of Webril, incorrectly padded or unpadded bony prominences, irregular splint ends, plaster ridges, or indentations produced from using the fingers rather than the palms to smooth and mold the wet plaster. Attention to detail during padding and splinting reduces the incidence of pressure sores. However, whenever a patient complains of a persistent pain or burning sensation under any part of a splint, the splint should be removed and the symptomatic area inspected closely.

Infection

Bacterial and fungal infections can occur under a splint.[18, 19] Infection is more common in the presence of an open wound but may occur despite intact skin. The moist, warm, and dark environment created by the splint is an excellent nidus for infection. Also, it has been shown that bacteria can multiply in slowly drying plaster. To avoid infection, all wounds should be cleaned and débrided before splint application, and clean, fresh tap water should be used for plaster wetting. In some instances, it is preferable to apply a removable splint that allows for periodic wound inspection or local wound care.

Dermatitis

Occasionally patients develop a rash under a cast or splint.[20–23] Allergy to plaster is exceedingly rare, but there are several reports of contact dermatitis when formaldehyde and melamine resins are added to the plaster.[20, 21] The rash is usually pruritic, with weeping papular or vesicular lesions. Because these resins are unnecessary for emergency department splints, their use should be avoided whenever possible.

Joint Stiffness

Some degree of joint stiffness is an invariable consequence of immobilization. It can range in severity from mild to incapacitating and can result in transient, prolonged, or, in some cases, permanant loss of function. Stiffness appears to be worse with prolonged periods of immobilization, in elderly patients, and in patients with preexisting joint diseases such as rheumatoid or osteoarthritis. Thus splints should be left on only for that period of time necessary for adequate healing. Table 67–6 lists several injuries that commonly require splinting, along with some suggestions for length of immobilization. Fractures, dislocations, or other conditions that require prolonged immobilization (more than 7 days) should have orthopedic follow-up. Patients must be told that a splint is only a short-term device and that prolonged immobilization can be detrimental. For minor injuries, the physician can suggest that the patient use his or her own judgment about when to remove the splint, but a definite end point should be set.

CAST PAIN

Cast-related pain is a common complaint that brings patients to the emergency department. Because of the potential for ischemia with circumferential casts, all complaints should be fully investigated, and vascular compromise must be ruled out. A detailed history and physical examination should be performed on all such patients. The nature and onset of the pain is of particular importance. A dull, nonspecific pain that has worsened gradually since the time of injury may be the only clue to an early compartment syndrome (see Chapter 72). The sudden onset of throbbing pain associated with swelling and redness suggests a possible

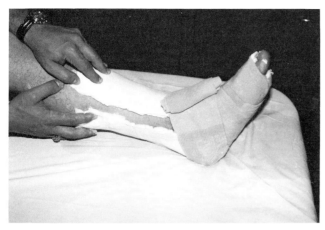

Figure 67–29. This cast felt tight to the patient, and so it was bivalved with a cast saw and secured into place with an elastic bandage. Note that the Webril was cut to relieve the pressure but that it was not removed. A bivalved cast provides temporary immobilization equal to that of an intact cast.

deep venous thrombosis. In both these cases, rapid intervention is the key to decreasing morbidity and mortality. The physical examination should pay particular attention to the areas of tenderness and the effect of active and passive movement on the severity of pain. With a compartmental syndrome, tenderness over the involved compartment is a common finding; stretching or contracting ischemic muscle also elicits significant pain. The examination should also evaluate the presence and quality of distal pulses, amount of edema fluid present, distal sensation, capillary refill, and color and temperature of the digits. The finding of pain, pallor, parasthesias, paralysis, and pulselessness (the five P's) are said to be pathognomonic for ischemia. Unfortunately, they seldom occur simultaneously, and their presence all together is usually a late finding that carries a poor prognosis. Hence, the emergency physician must maintain a high index of suspicion for possible ischemia and *remove the cast if any possibility of vascular compromise exists.* Almost any cast can be bivalved and reapplied after inspection without significant loss of short-term immobilization.

To loosen a cast, an oscillating cast saw is used to cut along the medial and lateral aspects of the cast. This is called *bivalving the cast,* and it allows the halves to be spread and reapplied in a less constricting manner while still maintaining proper immobilization (Fig. 67–29). To use the oscillating power saw, proceed in a series of downward cutting movements, removing the blade between cuts (Fig. 67–30). The blade is removed between cuts to prevent it from getting hot enough to burn the skin. This is particularly important if synthetic materials have been used in the cast. Also, the blade should not be allowed to slide along the skin, and the saw should never be used on unpadded plaster. In the apprehensive patient, the physician can demonstrate that the cast saw blade only vibrates (it does not turn) and that it does not cut the skin. After completely cutting through the medial and lateral sides of the cast, the two halves are separated using a cast spreader, and the padding is cut lengthwise with scissors. This may be sufficient to relieve early ischemia if the problem is simple posttrauma swelling, but both the padding and cast can be removed totally to inspect the injured area if necessary. If ischemia cannot be ruled out, compartment pressures should be measured, and an orthopedic consultation should be obtained. If vascular integrity is established and no other problems are found, the bivalved cast can be replaced. The extremity should first be padded in the usual manner using fresh Webril. The cut ends of the bivalved cast are then lined with white adhesive tape, and the cast is replaced around the extremity. Finally, the cast is secured in place using elastic bandages.

If plaster sores are the cause of the patient's discomfort, the physician who placed the cast should be consulted. In some cases, additional padding is all that is needed, but in others a window should be cut out over the problem area. Because pressure sores can lead to significant tissue necrosis, the patient should receive follow-up care within 24 hours.

If the patient's problem is plaster (or more likely, resin) dermatitis, treatment generally consists of topical or oral steroids and antihistamines. Therapy should be done in concert with an orthopedic surgeon because the patient may require admission for other forms of immobilization until the cast can be replaced. With mild cases, changing the cast or splint and using antihistamines for symptomatic relief may suffice. All of these patients should receive close follow-up, and if the condition does not improve, the cast must be removed.

REFERENCES

1. Howes DS, Kaufman JJ: Plaster splints: Techniques and indications. Am Fam Physician 30:215, 1984.
2. Wu KK: Techniques in Surgical Casting and Splinting. Philadelphia, Lea & Febiger, 1987.
3. Simon RR, Koenigsknecht SJ: Emergency Orthopedics. The Extremities. 2nd ed. Norfolk, Conn, Appleton & Lange, 1987.
4. Rockwood CA, Green DP: Fractures in Adults. 2nd ed. Philadelphia, JB Lippincott Co, 1984.
5. Brackenbury PH: A comparative study of the management of ankle sprains. Br J Clin Pract 37:181, 1983.
6. Hedges JR, Anwar RA: Management of ankle sprains. Ann Emerg Med 9:298, 1980.
7. Wehbe MA: Plaster uses and misuses. Clin Orthop 167:242, 1982.
8. Luck JV: Plaster of Paris casts: An experimental and clinical analysis. JAMA 124:23, 1944.
9. Lavalette R, Pope MH, Dickstein H: Setting temperatures of plaster casts. J Bone Joint Surg 64A:907, 1982.
10. Gannaway JK, Hunter JR: Thermal effects of casting materials. Clin Orthop 181:191, 1983.
11. Stanley D, Norris SH: Recovery following fractures of the clavicle treated conservatively. Injury 19:162, 1988.
12. Andersen K, Jensen PO, Lauritzen J: Treatment of clavicular fractures: Figure-of-eight bandage versus a simple sling. Acta Ortho Scand 58:71, 1987.
13. Halvorson G, Iserson KV: Comparison of four ankle splint designs. Ann Emerg Med 16:1249, 1987.
13a. Bergfeld JA, Cox JS, Drez D, et al: Symposium: Management of acute ankle sprains. Contemp Orthop 13:83, 1986.

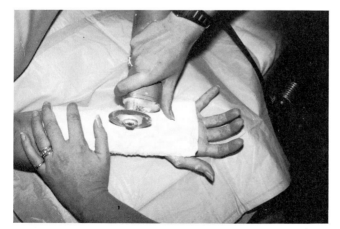

Figure 67–30. The cast saw vibrates; it does not rotate. The blade is controlled by placing the thumb on the splint and lowering the saw to the plaster. The blade is raised and lowered for each cut; it is not drawn across the plaster like a knife.

13b. Gross MT, Bradshaw MK, Ventry LC, et al: Comparison of support provided by ankle taping and semirigid orthosis. J Orthop Sports Phys Ther 9:33, 1987.

13c. Friden T, Zatterstrom R, Lindstrand A, et al: A stabilometric technique for evaluation of lower limb instabilities. Am J Sports Med 17:118, 1989.

14. Pointer J: Using an Unna's boot in treating ligamentous ankle injuries. West J Med 139:257, 1983.

15. Kaplan SS: Burns following application of plaster splint dressings. Report of two cases. J Bone Joint Surg 63A:670, 1981.

16. Becker DW Jr: Danger of burns from fresh plaster splints surrounded by too much cotton. Plast Reconstr Surg 62:436, 1978.

17. Beidler JG: Skin complications following cast applications. Report of a case. Arch Derm 98:159, 1968.

18. Houang ET, Buckley R, Williams RJ, et al: Outbreak of plaster-associated pseudomonas infection. Lancet 1:728, 1981.

19. Houang ET, Buckley R, Smith M, et al: Survival of *Pseudomonas aeruginosa* in plaster of Paris. J Hosp Inf 2:231, 1981.

20. Conrad AH, Ford LT: Allergic contact dermatitis caused by Melmac orthopedic composition. JAMA 153:557, 1953.

21. Logan WS, Perry HO: Cast dermatitis due to formaldehyde sensitivity. Arch Derm 106:717, 1972.

22. Lovell CR, Staniforth P: Contact allergy to benzalkonium chloride in plaster of Paris. Contact Derm 7–8:343, 1981–1982.

23. Logan WS, Perry HO: Contact dermatitis to resin-containing casts. Clin Orthop 90:150, 1973.

Chapter **68**

Podiatric Procedures

Lancing P. Malusky

INTRODUCTION

The painful foot frequently motivates a person to seek professional medical care more readily than other limited musculoskeletal conditions, because mobility is compromised. This chapter addresses some common presentations of and procedures for the painful foot. A number of procedures (e.g., local and regional anesthesia, foreign body removal, soft tissue injections) are addressed in detail elsewhere in the text. These procedures are also discussed here in a limited fashion when they are relevant to the unique anatomy or function of the foot. The management of a paronychia, felon, and subungual hematoma is discussed in Chapter 47. Joint aspiration for synovial fluid analysis is discussed in Chapter 71. Lower extremity splinting techniques are discussed in Chapter 67. Joint reduction techniques for digital and ankle dislocations are discussed in Chapter 66.

LOCAL AND REGIONAL ANESTHESIA

Most invasive podiatric procedures require local or regional anesthesia. A digital or metatarsal block is administered in the same fashion as that for anesthesia of the hand (see Chapter 38). Because the digital arteries are end arteries, anesthesic agents without epinephrine are recommended.[1]

Although field blocks and local infiltration are generally adequate for anesthesia of the dorsal surface of the foot, regional nerve blocks at the ankle are preferred for anesthesia of the volar (plantar) surface (see Chapter 38). The plantar surface is thickly calloused, but it is also exquisitely sensitive. Distention of the tissues by local infiltration on the plantar surface can be quite painful.

A device that has been used to facilitate placement of a skin wheal before deeper soft tissue infiltration is the MadaJet (Gill Podiatry Supply Co., Middleburg Heights, Ohio) (Fig. 68–1). The device mechanically injects a skin wheal using 0.1 ml of anesthetic without a needle. The device should be loaded daily with fresh anesthetic. After cocking the MadaJet, the aperture is placed about 1 cm from the skin site for anesthetic placement. The patient is warned about feeling a momentary sensation like a rubber band snap. The raised wheal area is instantly numbed and injection of the remainder of the anesthesia using a standard needle and syringe technique can be begun immediately. The MadaJet is not recommended for the thicker adult plantar skin.

The physician who intends to use a jet injector should review and practice current disinfection recommendations. These devices have been linked with hepatitis B[2] and *Mycobacterium chelonei*[3] spread.

SHAVING OF PLANTAR LESIONS

The plantar skin is the thickest skin of the entire body and is specially designed to adapt to environmental influences in its effort to protect the foot's internal structures. Shearing forces and high pressure points will create hyperkeratoses on the plantar skin. These hyperkeratotic areas further focus weight-bearing forces in the foot, hence producing discomfort.

When the verruca virus is introduced to the plantar skin, its presence also frequently induces a hyperkeratotic response. Unfortunately, *the definitive treatment methods for a wart are at odds with the appropriate regimen for a callus.* The wart should be treated with some form of epidermal eradication (see section on verruca curettage), whereas the hyperkeratosis requires simple débridement with podiatric rebalancing of the weight-bearing surface.

Most hyperkeratoses occur directly over an area of focal friction or pressure, such as beneath a metatarsal head, on the ridge of the calcaneal skin, or adjacent to a digital bony prominence that is experiencing excessive shoe pressure. Verrucae may occur on any site in the plantar skin; they are less likely to occur on the digits and are rare on the dorsal skin.

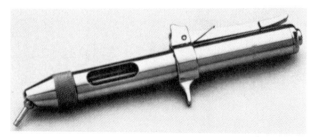

Figure 68–1. MadaJet needleless anesthetic injector. (Courtesy of Gill Podiatry Supply Co., 7803 Freeway Circle, Middleburg Heights, OH 44130.)

Other, less common skin lesions can mimic the wart. A common error is to assume that a macerated lesion between two digits, especially at the crease between the fourth and fifth toes, is a verruca. This lesion is more likely a "soft corn" (heloma molle) discussed later. Another common misdiagnosis is the porokeratosis plantaris discretia ("poro"), which is a small cyst-like lesion found in plantar locations and is histologically a sweat duct filled with a cone of keratin. This lesion often has been given the misnomer of "seed wart."

A "hard corn" (heloma duru, hammertoe, clavus) is a hyperkeratosis that occurs adjacent to a bony prominence on a digit. Hammertoes occur when the intrinsic (foot) muscles lose their stabilizing influence on the interphalangeal joints. The extrinsic (leg) muscles then overpower, producing flexion at the interphalangeal joints. Friction and pressure over the bony prominence, usually the proximal phalangeal head, cause a keratinization process that attempts to protect the dermis from penetration. The heloma durum may become macerated when it occurs between the toes, therefore becoming a heloma molle (soft corn), which may even perforate to the fascia. The heloma durum may become so chronically inflamed from recurrent friction or infection that a small sensitive neurovascular bundle (heloma milliare) may form amidst the keratosis.

The application of alcohol to the lesion enhances skin line visibility. The skin lines of a hyperkeratosis should pass through the lesion or, in the case of severe pressure or scarring, may flow into and disappear in the lesion. In contrast, the skin lines should pass around a verruca, which has a cystic capsule. A plantar verruca frequently has a coexistent surrounding hyperkeratosis, a response to the additional friction from the foreign mass. The differential diagnosis between a plantar verruca and plantar hyperkeratosis also may be enhanced by observing the patient's response to pressure on the lesion. Direct pressure on a keratosis often elicits a more painful response than will a squeezing maneuver of similar force. The reverse is true for a verruca.

Indications

The lesion type may be more definitively determined by débriding the keratinized layers of skin. The clinician examines the shaved surface seeking specific diagnostic signs of verrucae. Warts display the minicauliflower-like appearance of the papillomatous formation and the small capillary ends, which appear as black dots in the lesion. The process of débridement also affords a measure of temporary relief from the discomfort of the lesion. Should the shaving reveal a keratosis, more definitive shaving should be performed. If a wart is found, definitive curettage or podiatric referral should be provided.

Equipment

Although a number 10 or 15 Bard Parker blade on a handle may be used for débridement, these instruments are frequently difficult to handle when trying to débride thin layers of tissue from an oblique angle. Safer, more convenient instruments are the Beaver miniblades and the Gill chisel blades numbers 312 and 313 with appropriate handles (Gill Podiatry Supply Co., Middleburg Heights, Ohio) (Fig. 68–2). When these instruments are held like a pencil, the physician can achieve a cutting angle more parallel to the skin.

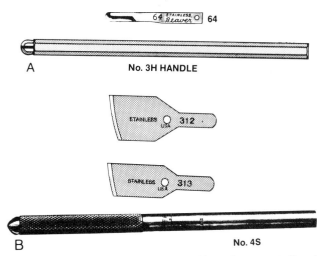

Figure 68–2. Equipment for débridement of hyperkeratoses (calluses). *A,* Beaver miniblade and handle. *B,* Gill chisel blades, numbers 312 and 313 with handle. (Courtesy of Gill Podiatry Supply Co., 7803 Freeway Circle, Middleburg Heights, OH 44130.)

Technique

After softening the hyperkeratotic area in warm tap water for 10 to 15 minutes, the patient is placed in a chair, and the patient's foot is elevated to a comfortable eye level for the clinician. Heel lesions are often débrided with the patient in the prone position. After appropriate anesthesia for very sensitive lesions, the lesions are shaved under a bright examination light. A fresh sharp blade is used for each patient.

The lesion is further moistened with an alcohol swab, and the skin is grasped above the area to be débrided using the fingers and below the area with the thumb of the nondominant hand. With the skin under traction, the beaver blade handle is held like a pencil and placed at a 10- to 40-degree angle to the skin surface. The clinician rests or presses the knuckles or fingers of the dominant hand on the patient's foot and begins débridement tangential to the area of skin traction (Fig. 68–3). The rhomboid-shaped blade is held so that the end of the cutting edge distal to the clinician is wider than the proximal edge. Short, superficial strokes toward the clinician are used until a feel for the tissue and a feel for the patient's reactions are established. This hand placement technique provides a safety buffer for the patient, because if the patient jumps, all materials move with him.

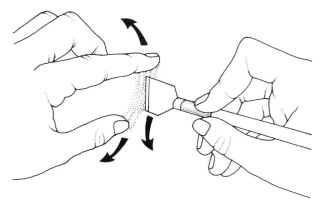

Figure 68–3. Technique for using chisel blades to shave hyperkeratosis. See text for details. (Courtesy of Kenneth R. Walker, D.P.M.)

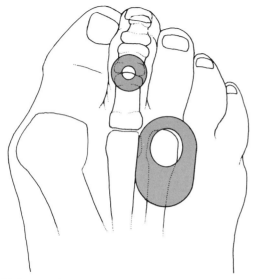

Figure 68–4. Use of aperture pads to redistribute pressure from a bony prominence following shaving procedures. Self-adherent foam or felt pads are used. Pad protecting the interphalangeal prominence is placed on the dorsal surface. Pad protecting the metatarsal head is placed on the plantar surface. (Courtesy of Kenneth R. Walker, D.P.M.)

The skin surface to be pared should buckle outward to some extent. Using only the middle two thirds of the cutting edge, the layers are pared, and the site is repeatedly examined. A fresh swipe of an alcohol swab aids inspection. The clear, plastic-like appearance of keratinized skin over or around the shaved area identifies the safe débridement zone. No nerves or capillaries should exist in this tissue. However, even an experienced clinician occasionally inadvertently opens an end capillary, which bleeds into the field and obscures the diagnosis. The topical astringent Lumicaine (Gill Podiatry Supply Co., Middleburg Heights, Ohio) seals these bleeders off, but its application may be momentarily uncomfortable for the patient who has not had the lesion anesthetized before shaving. After initial shaving, the lesion should be more easily identified.

When the plantar skin thickens beneath the palpably prominent metatarsal head or heads, it is termed a callus. When this occurs in combination with a discrete, centrally bruised plug of keratin, it is called an intractable plantar keratosis. These lesions may require periodic podiatric evaluation for débridement, protective padding, and balancing of the weight-bearing surface with orthotics.

The routine corn is treated by periodic débridement and felt corn pads with an aperture to transfer pressure to the surrounding healthy skin (Fig. 68–4). The perforated soft corn is frequently misdiagnosed as an interdigital verruca by visual inspection. After a regional block, the lesion should be débrided with a mini-Beaver knife and a number 64 blade for clearer diagnosis and relief of pain. Subsequent home care for this lesion includes astringent boric acid soaks twice daily, antibiotic ointment topically, and a small, opened gauze pad laid into the web crease. The toes should be separated during healing with a cotton ball or small gauze pad taped in place. The soft corn may later require a foam interdigital cushion. All of these hyperkeratotic lesions are candidates for podiatric referral for bony correction if conservative care does not relieve pain adequately.

Definitive management of verrucae and "poro" requires treatment by curettage, acid, or freezing. Considerable com-

fort before podiatric referral can be obtained, however, by débridement under regional anesthesia.

CURETTAGE OF VERRUCA AND POROKERATOSIS

Indications

The preferred treatment regimen for the common verruca plantaris (plantar wart) varies among physicians and specialties, but all procedures concentrate on separating the verruca and epidermis from the basement membrane. Salicylic acid lyses the tissue interface, liquid nitrogen blisters it with cold, and the hyfercator and the low-dose CO_2 laser blister it with heat. The curet mechanically separates the two skin layers. When the pain of a wart is severe because of its prominence, curettement may provide definitive therapy.

Technique

After placement of a regional nerve block, several sterile curets (Fig. 68–5), tissue nippers, and a hyfercator needle are readied. An oval curet with a more pointed end is initially chosen. The skin distal to the site of the verruca is stretched taut with the physician's nondominant hand, and the handle of the curet is rested in the palm of the dominant hand. The dominant hand index finger guides the curet in a sweeping motion, directed opposite to the skin stretching vector of the stabilizing hand (Fig. 68–6).

If the skin surrounding the verruca is still thick, the curet may face too much resistance, and the clinician may wish to give the curet a head start by making a snip 2 or 3 mm deep in the skin, just distal to the lesion in normal epidermis, using tissue nippers (see Fig. 68–5B). Larger lesions may require larger curets; choosing the right size curet initially will simplify the process. Warts are cystic in structure and generally separate easily from normal tissue once the lesion begins to break away (Fig. 68–7). The clinician will appreciate the basement membrane when the

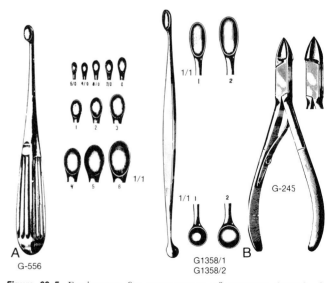

Figure 68–5. Equipment for curettement of verrucae (warts). *A,* Various curets. *B,* Tissue nipper with convex jaw. (Courtesy of Gill Podiatry Supply Co., 7803 Freeway Circle, Middleburg Heights, OH 44130.)

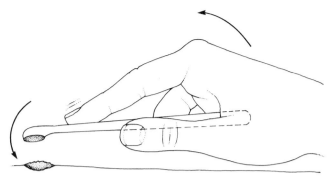

Figure 68–6. Technique of curettement of a verruca. The verruca is scooped out using a curet. See text for details. (Courtesy of Kenneth R. Walker, D.P.M.)

curet scrapes on the skin lines. This process may mimic a metallic chime when encountered. The basement membrane is the protective layer of the dermis, and by design, the normal curet does not penetrate this zone unless undue force is used.

Some clinicians hyfercate the lesion first to blister the wart and make curettement through the epidermis easier. Once the verruca has been thoroughly curetted with the various curets, the hyfercator may be used to sweep the area to loosen or destroy adjacent skin to discourage regrowth. If any purulence is uncovered, the base of the lesion should be inspected for the existence of a foreign body, which may have originally implanted the virus.

Postoperatively, the treated area looks and feels like a blister to the patient, and 2 to 4 weeks of topical antibiotics and a gauze pad are commonly prescribed. Periodic débridement of the eschar may be needed to assist wound drying and resist plug formation. Recurrences rates are about 25 per cent for most verruca procedures, and the patient should be warned to watch for regrowth.

The *porokeratosis* curettement process is similar to that of the verruca process, but a sharper, smaller curet is needed. Whereas the verruca provides a relatively mild, broad-based pressure on the basement membrane, the porokeratosis creates a narrower, deeper pressure that may depress, scar, or even obliterate the dermis. The porokeratosis excision is

begun with the same hand motions, but the narrow, cone-shaped lesion is found and followed into the basement membrane. The base appears bruised, and no hyfercation is needed. A recurrence rate of 30 to 40 per cent is common and more frequent if the lesion is over a weight-bearing metatarsal head. Many podiatrists use a CO_2 laser on this lesion with reported recurrence rates of less than 15 per cent. The postoperative care is similar to that for a wart curettage, but postoperative débridement of the eschar plug may be needed during follow-up care.

FOOT PAD USE

Foot pads are applied to redistribute pressure applied to a tender, inflamed area of the foot. The type of pad used and its placement are dependent on the underlying problem. A number of commercial aperture pads are available for protection of bony prominences (Fig. 68–8). These pads are helpful for management of corns and hyperkeratoses secondary to hammertoe deformities (Figs. 68–4 and 68–9). The use of these shields for management of bunions is discussed subsequently.

Metatarsalgia

Firm palpation that elicits pain directly beneath the metatarsal head can be diagnosed as a metatarsal bruise or

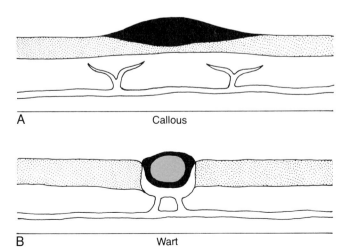

Figure 68–7. Structural differences between a callus *(A)* and a wart *(B).* Warts are cystic in structure and generally separate easily from normal tissue at the basement membrane once the lesion begins to break away. (Courtesy of Kenneth R. Walker, D.P.M.)

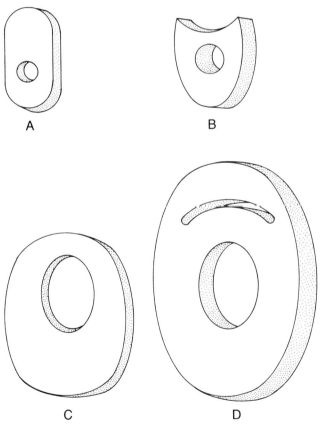

Figure 68–8. Various commercial aperture pads for areas of bony prominence. *A,* One-eighth-inch self-adherent felt corn pad. *B,* One-fourth-inch nonadhesive foam soft corn pads. *C,* One-eighth-inch self-adherent felt bunion shield. *D,* One-fourth-inch felt slip-on bunion shield. Note that the slit may be used for passage of the great toe and the bunion is set in the large oval opening in the shield. Paper tape may be used to further secure the shield.

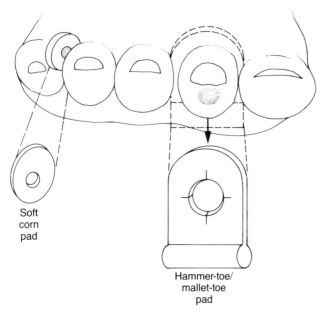

Figure 68–9. Application of soft corn and slip-on hammertoe pads. (Courtesy of Kenneth R. Walker, D.P.M.)

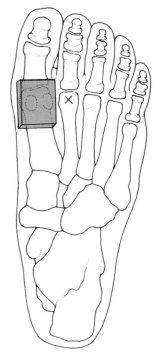

Figure 68–10. Use of a sub first metatarsal head raise of about 1 cm thickness pad placed beneath an innersole (rectangular area) to protect the second metatarsal head (marked *X*). (Courtesy of Kenneth R. Walker, D.P.M.)

contusion if it involves one head, or metatarsalgia if it involves more than one head. The metatarsalgia patient will complain of discomfort that comes on during walking and becomes progressively worse during the day and is relieved only by rest. The patient can often identify the painful spot for the clinician. Frequently the pain is felt beneath the second or the second and third metatarsal heads.

The physician palpates each of the lesser metatarsal heads and identifies the site of pain under the metatarsal head or heads. A hyperkeratosis may be associated with this condition, either diffusely under the central lesser metatarsus, or discretely beneath a metatarsal head. Débridement of the hyperkeratosis (as discussed earlier) is important for diagnosis and treatment. A discrete lesion may be the real origin for discomfort, and adequate débridement and podiatric follow-up to address the source of the hyperkeratotic reaction may be sufficient emergency department therapy.

Therapy

Any hyperkeratosis should be cushioned with a pad (e.g., Spenco [Gill Podiatry Supply Co., Middleburg Heights, Ohio] or PPT [Langer Biomechanics Group, Inc., Wheeling, Ill.]). For discrete pain beneath the second metatarsal head, a sub first metatarsal head raise of about 1 cm thickness PPT can be placed beneath an innersole (Fig. 68–10). Nonsteroidal anti-inflammatory drugs and a quality athletic or walking shoe should also be recommended. Continued symptoms require podiatric follow-up.

Hallux Abducto Valgus (Bunion)

The basis for a bunion is complex and represents a dynamic imbalance between the structures on the lateral side of the metatarsophalangeal (MTP) joint and the medial side of the MTP joint[4, 5] (Fig. 68–11). When there is lateral displacement of the distal hallux, a bunion begins to form. A number of anatomic, physiologic, and footwear elements contribute to bunion development.

The typical bunion deformity develops in a woman wearing heels occupationally. She may state she has numbness on the distal medial aspect of the hallux (from compression of the terminal branch of the medial dorsal cutaneous nerve). She may recall a time when the intermetatarsal space was tender, or the area of the fibular sesamoid was

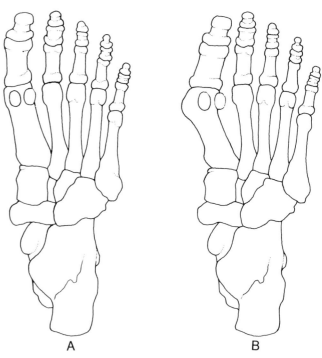

Figure 68–11. Illustration of a normal *(A)* and a pathologic *(B)* (bunion) bony alignment of first metatarsophalangeal joint. (Courtesy of Kenneth R. Walker, D.P.M.)

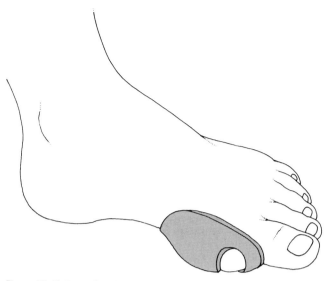

Figure 68–12. Use of self-adherent commercial bunion shield. (Courtesy of Kenneth R. Walker, D.P.M.)

tender for a short time. Other foot complaints such as lesser metatarsalgia, intermetatarsal neuroma, ingrown toenails, and corns and callus may be common. First MTP joint bursitis commonly occurs over the medial bunion bump.

THERAPY

Removal of the offending footgear is advised, or a hole may be cut in the shoe to allow the sensitive area freedom from pressure. A precut bunion shield (Figs. 68–8C and D and 68–12) may be dispensed or constructed from 1-cm-thick felt. Nonsteroidal anti-inflammatory drugs are also commonly used. When inflammation is severe, aspiration of the bursal fluid with a 20-gauge needle followed by instillation of 0.5 ml of a local anesthetic and a short-acting steroid (e.g., 5 mg methylprednisolone) can be performed.

Heel Pain Syndromes

In-depth discussion of the multiple causes of heel pain is beyond the scope of this text. The use of foot pads as adjunctive therapy for these conditions is addressed later. Other supportive therapies for most of the entities include modification of physical activity, use of nonsteroidal anti-inflammatory drugs, local injection of anesthetic and steroid agents, and use of orthotic foot wear.

HEEL SPUR SYNDROME

The patient presents with gradually worsening heel pain over several months. Palpation elicits pain about the medial border of the calcaneus, possibly extending distally at the radiographic site of a bony spur ledge (Fig. 68–13). Supportive therapy is helpful, including a local steroid injection (e.g., 10 to 20 mg methylprednisolone). Injections are performed from the medial aspect of the calcaneal spur, thus avoiding the sensitive plantar area. The medication is distributed along both the medial calcaneal tubercle and the central plantar calcaneus at the spur fascia junction. Shoe support in the form of a heel raise of 1.25 cm bilaterally reduces heel weight bearing. A temporary donut-shaped heel cushion cut from 1 cm PPT or a similar high-density foam rubber also suffices for this purpose.

RETROCALCANEAL BURSITIS

With this condition, pain is present at the specific site of achilles tendon insertion. Either or both bursae may be sensitive, and the clinician can palpate for either (see Fig. 68–13) by relaxing the achilles tendon with plantar flexion of the foot. A squeezing force applied anterior to the tendon displays inflammation of the retrocalcaneal bursae in the depression above the calcaneus, and thumb pressure on the back of the insertion of the tendon behind the calcaneus checks the status of the postcalcaneal bursa. Treatment is as for the heel spur syndrome with the exception that injection of steroids, when used, is into the inflamed bursae. A PPT heel pad lift or varus pad in the shoe is also helpful. All shoes worn (at home and work) by the patient should have a uniform heel height with a nylon cleat on the lateral side.

CALCANEAL APOPHYSITIS (SEVER DISEASE)

This condition commonly occurs in active children between the ages of 8 and 14 years old. The incomplete fusion of the apophysis at the plantar posterior aspect of the juvenile's heel is stressed at its cartilaginous connection by the achilles tendon. The clinician palpates great tenderness directly over the apophysis. There should be no significant tenderness of the achilles tendon, and there is usually no edema. Treatment is as for the heel spur syndrome with the exception that steroid injections are not recommended.

OTHER CONDITIONS

A painful heel may be due to other conditions including a partially ruptured achilles tendon, gouty and psoriatic arthritis, and calcaneal stress fractures. These conditions are generally identified by history and physical examination; specific therapies for these entities are discussed in standard orthopedic references.

INJECTION THERAPY FOR A NEUROMA

The neuroma, also known as the Morton neuroma, is a painful forefoot condition most likely to affect the female

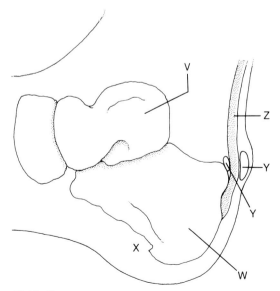

Figure 68–13. Illustration of potential sites of heel pain: *(V)* talus, *(W)* calcaneus, *(X)* calcaneal bone spur, *(Y)* calcaneal bursae, *(Z)* achilles tendon. (Courtesy of Kenneth R. Walker, D.P.M.)

adult, especially if she wears heels occupationally. The neuroma is usually unilateral, but it may occur bilaterally. This lesion frequently occurs in the third intermetatarsal space but may occur in the second interspace; it rarely occurs in the first or fourth interspace. Its preponderance for the third space is thought to be due to a dual innervation of the lateral plantar nerve and the medial plantar nerve to this interspace and to the fact that the fourth metatarsal is the most mobile. An intermetatarsal ligament (deep plantar aponeurosis) connects each metatarsal head on its plantar aspect, and the sensory nerve passes beneath this ligament (Fig. 68–14).

In high heels, the sensory nerve is forced to bend around this ligament and is compressed against it during weight bearing. The perineural covering becomes fibrotic from chronic irritation. Although the normal sensory nerve is the size of a pencil lead, the neuroma is the size of a pencil. The damaged nerve trunk no longer conducts normal impulses, and a burning pain or numbness is reported in the third or fourth toes.

The condition is diagnosed with careful forefoot palpation, ruling out arthritis, metatarsalgia, capsulitis, ganglion, or stress fracture. The space between and just proximal to the metatarsal heads is squeezed, and the resultant pain suggests a neuroma. A tender spot may be noted in the depression just behind and between the involved metatarsal necks, where the nerve first encounters the intermetatarsal ligament. Pain distally in the intermetatarsal sulcus also suggests the neuroma. The pain is reproduced by squeezing the metatarsal heads together. The differential diagnosis includes ganglion, metatarsal phalangeal joint capsulitis, and stress fracture.

Therapy

A serial treatment plan may include a reduction in heel height, a sub fourth metatarsal shaft raise (Fig. 68–15), and local injection. After skin preparation, the tender neuroma is injected with a 1- to 2-ml mixture of a long-acting local anesthetic (e.g., 0.5 per cent marcaine) and steroid (e.g., 5 to 10 mg methylprednisolone). Podiatric follow-up for additional care is warranted.

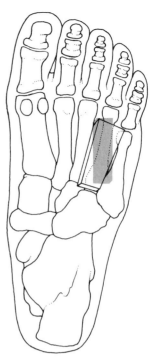

Figure 68 15. Use of a felt foot pad for a sub fourth metatarsal shaft raise to reduce pressure on a neuroma. (Courtesy of Kenneth R. Walker, D.P.M.)

ASPIRATION AND INJECTION OF A GANGLION

A ganglion is histologically similar to a synovial sheath and frequently contains synovial fluid. The ganglion is considered traumatic in origin and usually has a stalk traceable to a tendon sheath or joint capsule. Although the ganglion is easily diagnosed when it occurs over a tendon on the dorsum of the foot, it can be a challenging diagnosis when present among the compact forefoot structures. This lesion may mimic the neuroma or MTP joint capsulitis.

When the clinician finds edema in the forefoot, the location of this swelling is a key diagnostic consideration. A neuroma usually does not cause edema of the intermetatarsal space unless it is unusually large. An MTP joint capsulitis causes swelling at the MTP joint, perhaps brawny in nature, but careful palpation confirms its location. A small ganglion causes swelling directly beneath the flexor apparatus of the involved digit or perhaps directly beneath a metatarsal head or the tibial sesamoid. The larger ganglion grows in the path of least resistance, which is to an available intermetatarsal space. If painful, a ganglion associated with the lesser metatarsus structures should provide a localized stinging or burning sensation on palpation, whereas the neuroma's pain travels out into the involved toes. The ganglion should roll under the examiner's fingers. If the lesion is painless and nonmovable, other soft tissue neoplasms should be considered.

Therapy

When the clinician is suspicious that the lesion is a ganglion, the diagnosis may be confirmed and treatment begun by the aspiration of synovial fluid. The physician, with local or regional anesthesia, blocks the tender area and anticipated skin penetration site. After skin preparation, a 20-gauge needle is inserted, and under negative pressure,

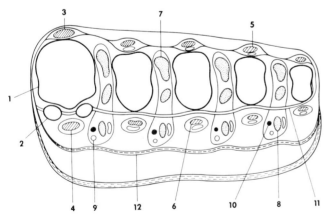

Figure 68–14. Topographic anatomy of the foot: *(1)* the metatarsals; *(2)* sesamoids; *(3)* extensor hallucis longus tendon; *(4)* flexor hallucis longus tendon; *(5)* extensor tendon of the toe; *(6)* flexor tendon of the toe; *(7)* interosseous muscles; *(8)* lumbricals; *(9)* blood vessels; *(10)* nerves; *(11)* deep plantar aponeurosis, intermetatarsal ligament; and *(12)* superficial plantar aponeurosis. (From Jahss MH [ed]: Disorders of the Foot. Vol 1. Philadelphia, WB Saunders Co, 1982, p 664. Reproduced by permission.)

the suspected ganglionic structure is explored for fluid. When fluid is encountered, the lesion should be drained. The fluid should have a yellow, thick, gelatinous character. Further aspiration and exploration with rotation of the bevel of the needle should be performed; infiltration with a steroid solution and local anesthetic is appropriate to enhance resolution. Although a small volume (<0.5 ml) will reexpand the cyst somewhat, the medication is generally absorbed within 24 hours. Fluid is not always found, but if the clinician is certain of the diagnosis, the steroid infiltration may still be entertained. The ganglion frequently remains deflated and asymptomatic, although recurrences are common and warrant specialist follow-up.

SPLINTING TOE FRACTURES

Although many clinicians and laypersons shrug their shoulders at a fracture of a toe and state that nothing can be done, something can and should be done to relieve the pain and encourage healing. As with any other fracture, attention should be paid to the possibility of breach of joint cartilage, hypermobility of fracture segments, and malposition and malunion of the fracture segments.

Aggressive fracture reduction is indicated for the great toe, as it represents the main propulsive segment of the forefoot. A plaster cast is *insufficient* treatment in all cases except the simple nondisplaced fracture through the body of a great toe phalanx. Any displacement should raise concern regarding the possibility of an axial rotation or a deviation in the way the hallux interacts biomechanically within its own interphalangeal or MTP joint. In the acute setting, a non–weight-bearing ankle splint with attached plantar component extending beyond the great toe provides protection until the patient with a complicated great toe fracture can obtain follow-up. Open fractures obviously need immediate referral for débridement and continued antibiotic therapy.

A fracture of the first MTP joint *sesamoid* bone may result from a jump from a height. The great toe sesamoid bones lie in grooves on the bottom of the metatarsal head. Each bone lies within the tendon of its respective flexor hallucis brevis muscle belly. With a sesamoid bone fracture, there is localized pain on the plantar aspect of the first metatarsal head. Bipartate sesamoids (tibial more frequently than fibular) are common and bilateral radiographs are helpful.

Fractures of the lesser toes usually result from jamming the toe into a night stand or bed post while barefoot. Radiographs of the phalanges will confirm the clinical suspicion.

Therapy

For a tibial sesamoid injury, an aperture bunion-type pad, reinforced medially, of 0.5- to 0.75-cm-thick felt protects the sesamoid and transfers weight bearing to the surrounding structures (Fig. 68–16). A Reese shoe and nonsteroidal anti-inflammatory drugs are also prescribed.

The treatment of closed lesser phalangeal fractures is "immobilization" for 6 weeks. The patient is put in a less restrictive, stiff-soled shoe, or a Reese orthopedic shoe. The injured toe is folded toward an adjacent noninjured toe. A "soft corn" pad is placed between the toes, and the toes are held together with an adherent wrap around both digits (Fig. 68–17). Thus the normal toe splints the injured toe. The procedure is demonstrated to the patient or family and

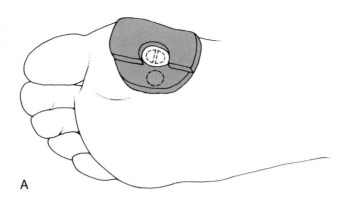

A

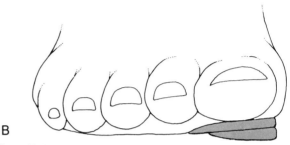

B

Figure 68–16. Use of bunion shields to redistribute pressure away from a sesamoid bone fracture. (Courtesy of Kenneth R. Walker, D.P.M.)

materials dispensed so that the splint can be changed every 2 to 3 days at home.

MANAGEMENT OF FUNGUS TOENAILS (ONYCHOMYCOSIS)

The mycotic toenail can occur at any age group, but occurs more frequently with increasing age. The condition is caused by the usual tineal fungi, most frequently of the *Trichophyton* species. Onychomycosis can also occur posttraumatically and is more frequently seen in the hallux and fifth toenails, where the greatest shoe friction occurs. Spontaneous resolution is rare and is less likely as the nail plate becomes more extensively involved and thickened. Occasionally a traumatic avulsion leaves an individual free of the hypertrophic mycotic toenail temporarily, but the matrix retains its acquired predilection for growing a hypertrophied toenail. A new tinea subsequently colonizes the nail in most cases.

The tinea is contained in the nail plate, and the body usually maintains the integrity of the viable dermis of the nailbed (Fig. 68–18). The fungus feeds on the nail plate, and deposits its waste products within the nail plate, and on the nailbed. The dusty, brownish-yellow debris encountered in the mycotic nail consists of fungus spores and hyphae, desiccated toenail, and desquamated skin from above the nailbed. During the initial stages of the fungus infection, only the free edge or the surface of the nail plate is involved. As time proceeds, the fungus extends proximally and more deeply into the nail plate along longitudinal lines of stress. Once the entire free edge of the toenail is mycotic, the fungus works its way back to the central nailbed in a series of striations (see Fig. 68–18).

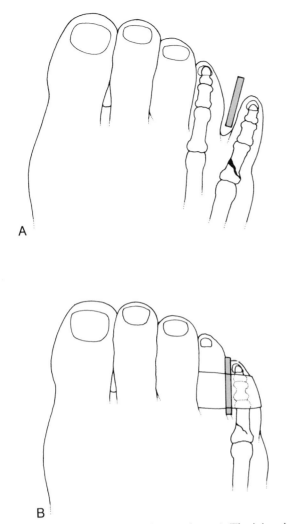

Figure 68–17. "Buddy-taping" of a fractured toe. *A,* The injured toe is folded toward an adjacent noninjured toe after placement of a "soft corn" pad between the toes. *B,* The toes are held together with an adherent wrap placed around both digits. (Courtesy of Kenneth R. Walker, D.P.M.)

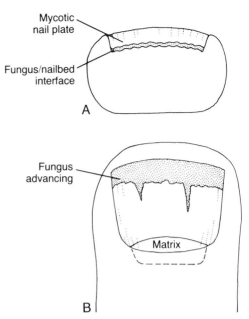

Figure 68–18. Mycotic nail disease. *A,* Tangenital "end-on" view. *B,* Dorsal view showing advancement of fungus toward the growing nail matrix. (Courtesy of Kenneth R. Walker, D.P.M.)

Any mechanical or shearing force causes microtrauma to the invaginated nailbed folds, and a resultant lysis of the nailbed–nail plate interface occurs. A local, transient primary fungal infection of the nailbed may be followed by a secondary bacterial infection. Eventually the fungus reaches the nail matrix, which in turn responds by growing a hypertrophic nail plate. The mycotic nail subsequently causes greater friction or pressure on the nailbed, and recurrent inflammation and infection may occur.

Therapy

When the fungal infection is limited to the distal nail, simple surface nail plate filing with topical antitinea therapy is often effective. When the involvement is more extensive, avulsion of the nail plate and an oral antifungal agent for 1 month are prescribed, along with local wound care. Topical antifungal therapy is applied twice daily as the new nail plate develops. Therapy of secondary bacterial infections should incorporate broad-spectrum antibiotics (e.g., second-generation cephalosporin agents).

Once the fungus reaches the level of the nail matrix as

visualized by obliteration of the lunula, the hypertrophy becomes fixed, and the condition is usually irreversible. Surgical approaches to treatment of chronic onychomycosis include nail plate avulsion with nailbed débridement (with or without phenol nail matrix destruction (described later) and periodic limited débridement of the involved nail using a dremel tool (Gill Podiatry Supply Co., Middleburg Heights, Ohio) and nail burs (Fig. 68–19).

PLANTAR PUNCTURE WOUNDS

Plantar puncture wounds often present a diagnostic and therapeutic dilemma to the clinician.[6] Considerable controversy exists regarding the proper initial management of these wounds. Although up to 98 per cent of such wounds are produced by nails,[7] various other objects have been reported as causing these wounds, including other metal objects, wood, and glass. The host response to the injury is dependent on the penetrating material, location of the wound, depth of penetration, footwear, time from injury until presentation, and underlying health. Because superficial puncture wounds generally do well, the depth of penetration may be a primary determinant of outcome. This may in part explain why distal wounds in the metatarsal-phalangeal joint area that are associated with increased weight bearing during ambulation are often more serious.[8]

Because most minor puncture wounds are not seen in the emergency department, the true risk of infection and in particular osteomyelitis remains speculative. One review of these wounds suggests that no more than 2 to 8 per cent of puncture wounds become infected, and only a small percentage of these go on to develop osteomyelitis.[6] The retention of foreign material (e.g., a portion of a tennis shoe sole) in the wound is an important factor in persistent infection.

Therapy

The approach to the patient is dependent on several factors including the time from wounding to presentation,

FINE CUT

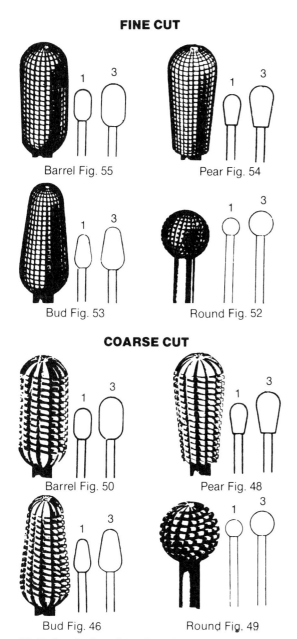

Barrel Fig. 55   Pear Fig. 54

Bud Fig. 53   Round Fig. 52

COARSE CUT

Barrel Fig. 50   Pear Fig. 48

Bud Fig. 46   Round Fig. 49

Figure 68–19. Standard podiatry burs for débriding mycotic nails. (Courtesy of Gill Podiatry Supply Co., 7803 Freeway Circle, Middleburg Heights, OH 44130.)

the suspicion regarding a foreign body, and the presence of infection (Fig. 68–20).

Patients presenting within 24 hours and without signs of infection generally require only simple wound care. Although irrigation of all exposed dermal tissue is recommended, high-pressure irrigation of deep tissues with distention of soft tissue is unlikely to be helpful.

The extent to which a foreign body work-up is pursued depends on the history and physical findings. When a patient clearly states that the puncture was produced by a new nail that was removed intact, a radiographic series or local wound exploration for a retained metallic foreign body is not needed. When the wound is large and the patient was wearing rubber-soled shoes, however, local wound exploration may be warranted to exclude the possibility of a retained portion of the shoe. Exploration should be performed under a regional anesthetic block after an ellipse of tissue has been

removed from around the puncture site. Blunt probes should be used. General discussion of the management of suspected foreign bodies is discussed in further detail in Chapter 46.

Patients who delay presentation for medical attention have an increased risk for a retained foreign body. Unless the patient presents without infection or with a clearly superficial cellulitis expected to respond to simple oral antibiotics, local wound exploration is warranted as discussed earlier. Recurrent infections, deep soft tissue tenderness, and increasing soft tissue swelling raise the probability of a retained foreign body or deep space infection. Such patients require prompt specialty referral. Consideration of the need for additional diagnostic studies (e.g., wound cultures, ultrasonography, or computed tomography of the puncture area) should be made.

DIABETIC FOOT CARE

The diabetic patient is at special risk for serious cutaneous injury and infection as a result of microcirculatory insufficiency and neuropathic changes. The diabetic often does not appreciate the development of pathologic conditions such as hyperkeratotic lesions, corns, ingrown toenails, and ulcers. Often these conditions are exacerbated by the patient's choice of footwear and activities.

Therapy

In general, the diabetic patient with foot lesions is instructed not to stand for longer than 20 minutes at a stretch. The patient is also cautioned to avoid extreme temperatures when cleansing the feet.

A hole or slit may be cut in the shoe over any obvious non–weight-bearing prominence. Hyperkeratotic lesions should be shaved and shielded with an aperture pad (see Fig. 68–9). For a hammertoe lesion, the toe is covered with the aperture pad. For the bunion area, a large commercial adhesive bunion pad or bunion shield cut from felt may be applied.

Ingrown toenails and mycotic toenails can be managed as for nondiabetic patients. The only caveat is that these conditions can become serious for the patient before the patient is aware of the problem. The diabetic with advanced disease who has an infected or progressive lesion should also have differential blood pressures checked in all four extremities to assess large artery patency. Evidence of large artery insufficiency requires urgent vascular referral. The diabetic patient's metabolic status should also be closely monitored.

When ulcers develop, the necrotic rim should be débrided. Antibiotic ointments or biologic membranes as used for burn patients (see Chapter 49) are also helpful. These lesions should be shielded with aperture pads, and the patient should be followed closely. A pillow placed under the patient's calf that allows the heel to overhang permits heel ulcers to repair (Fig. 68–21).

INGROWN TOENAIL (ONYCHOCRYPTOSIS)

The ingrown toenail represents a progressive nail curvature or static widening of the lateral sides of the toenail such that the nail impinges on the skin of the nail groove. Normally, the cuticle and periungual nail structures undergo a progressive maturation and sloughing process that permits the nail to slide forward easily as it grows anteriorly from the nail matrix. Additional frictional forces are present in

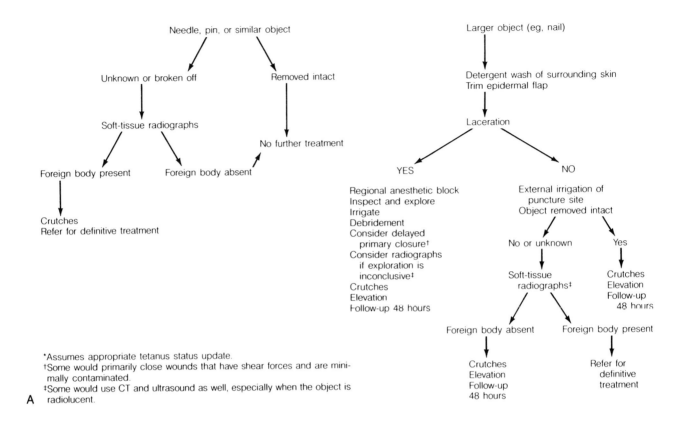

*Assumes appropriate tetanus status update.
†Some would primarily close wounds that have shear forces and are minimally contaminated.
‡Some would use CT and ultrasound as well, especially when the object is radiolucent.

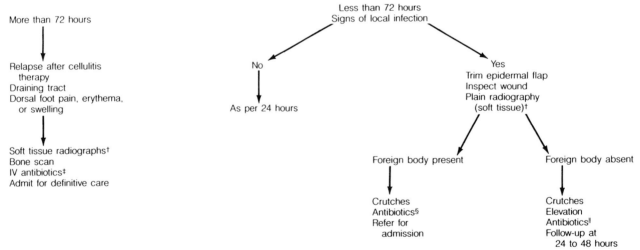

*Assumes appropriate tetanus update.
†Add CT or ultrasound if high suspicion of radiolucent retained foreign body.
‡Include *Pseudomonas* coverage.
§IV, antistaphylococcal.
‖Orally, antistaphylococcal.

Figure 68–20. *A,* Plantar puncture wound management—presentation within 24 hours of wounding. *B,* Plantar puncture wound management—presentation 24 hours after wounding. (From Chisholm CD, Schlesser JF: Plantar puncture wounds: Controversies and treatment recommendations. Ann Emerg Med 18:1352, 1989. Reproduced by permission.)

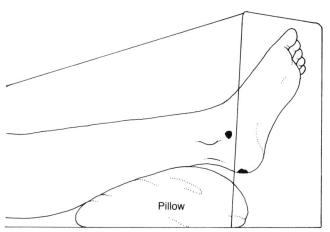

Figure 68–21. Use of a pillow placed under the calf to remove pressure on heel ulcer. Also note the use of a bed sheet cradle to maximize air contact with healing ulcers. (Courtesy of Kenneth R. Walker, D.P.M.)

the nail groove when the nail is severely incurvated or hypertrophic, when the patient habitually wears tight shoes, or when the patient has a digit that is axially rotated against an adjacent digit or the bottom of the shoe. These frictional forces may stimulate a hyperkeratotic response in the nail groove.

The vast majority of ingrown toenails occur in the halluces. Discomfort occurs when the nail impingement causes a hyperkeratosis of the nail groove with localized nerve irritation or when a foreign body reaction is generated. The foreign body response may be simply a mild erythema and edema of the nail fold, or it may progress to a purulent granulomatous formation. If the patient cuts his nails in a curved, rather than transverse, manner, there is also the potential for a spicule of nail remaining in the nail fold to impinge upon the hyperkeratosis (Fig. 68–22).

Evaluation

In the presence of the predisposing nail changes, the decision to treat is primarily based on the subjective complaints of the patient. The offending margin in the non-granulomatous ingrown toenail must be examined closely for determination of the exact location of the problem. With this condition, the patient will complain of pain reproduced by fingertip pressure over the nail groove. The clinician also should apply pressure to the central portion of the nail plate, proximal cuticle, and opposite nail margin to rule out other potential sources of pain. Other causes for discomfort include stress fracture of the distal phalanx and subungual exostosis, a proximal bony bump on the dorsum of the distal phalanx that can produce central nail bed pain. Other considerations producing referred pain include diabetic neuropathy and shoe pressure–induced neuritis of the dorsal medial cutaneous nerve.

The clinician should continue diagnosis and treatment by cleaning the nail groove with an alcohol pad. Hyperkeratosis, mycotic debris, and impacted periungual debris can be visualized with this technique. The nail groove should be inspected with a minicuret. The free edge of the nail should have a clear path to exit the nail groove. The clinician should curet the extraneous periungual debris with the minicuret until the nail and nail groove are separate and visible. The physician must be careful not to put a great amount of

pressure directly on the nail groove with the sharp edge of the curet, because the area is quite sensitive. The blunt curve of the back of the minicuret can be used for gentle probing of the nail groove for locating the hyperkeratotic plug. This plug will elicit tenderness and will be visible as a yellowish to gray translucent tissue after being cleansed with alcohol.

Further treatment will generally involve a digital block (see Chapter 38). At this point, the clinician's options are to offer temporary removal of the presumed nail spicule and/or débridement of the periungual hyperkeratotic plug versus permanent correction of the toenail deformity by the phenol technique (see below). The decision is primarily based upon the chronicity of the complaint, the degree of nail curvature, the subjective discomfort of the patient (without a concurrent desensitizing neuropathy), and the history of infection or current infection. The clinician will also need to factor concurrent patient care demands in the emergency department.

Removal of Nail Spicule and Débridement of Hyperkeratosis

This procedure is primarily reserved for those ingrown toenails with minimal inflammation, a small amount of incurvation, no concurrent infection, and limited discomfort. Spicule removal can also be used where the nail is loosely adherent to the nail groove and can be freed without causing any capillary bleeding.

Following a digital block, the toe is cleansed with a standard skin preparation. An oblique portion of the offending nail (about one third to two thirds of the way back to the posterior nail fold) is removed (Fig. 68–23). Ideally, an English anvil nail splitter or nail forceps is used (Fig. 68–24). If the nail is found to be spiculated more than two thirds of the way back, the clinician can switch to the permanent phenol correction technique described below.

Following removal of the oblique nail portion, the free edge of the remaining nail should be smoothed so that it will glide freely out of the nail groove as it grows. Loose keratinized debris exposed beneath the removed side of the nail plate can be curetted off the nailbed. Next, the keratotic

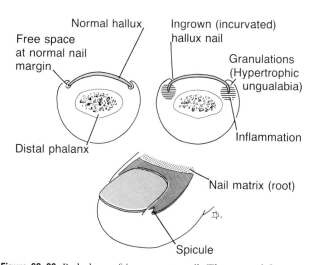

Figure 68–22. Pathology of ingrown toenail. The normal free space at the nail margin is obliterated by inflammation and granulation tissue, which is caused by improper nail trimming, trauma to the matrix, and faulty foot gear. (From Hill GJ II: Outpatient Surgery. 3rd ed. Philadelphia, WB Saunders Co, 1988. Reproduced by permission.)

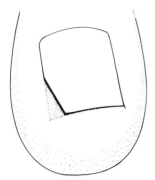

Figure 68–23. An oblique wedge of nail is trimmed from the lateral margin of the nail to free the nail from the hyperkeratotic area. This technique is less definitive than removal of the entire lateral margin of the nail with subsequent phenol treatment. (Courtesy of Kenneth R. Walker, D.P.M.)

plug in the nail groove is débrided (preferably with a mini-Beaver handle and blade number 64 or 67). The blade should be sharp to facilitate débridement and to reduce the risk of trauma, with resultant scarring of the nail groove. The nondominant hand should firmly grasp the toe while the clinician's thumb or index finger plantarly rotates the nail groove open. The keratotic plug is débrided down to normal epidermis or dermis, which may be ecchymotic in character. The clinician should attempt to prevent the patient's bleeding during the procedure. Should bleeding occur, a digital tourniquet (see Chapter 43) can be used for maintaining a dry field during the procedure. The area is then dressed with antibiotic ointment, Adaptic (or similar nonadherent material), and a dry dressing. A dressing change should occur at 48 hours with nail fold reevaluation. Follow-up podiatric care with consideration for permanent correction should be advised.

Technique of Partial Toenail Removal

The decision to permanently remove a portion of a toenail is based on the following criteria. Ingrown toenails associated with chronic inflammation, severe pain, or infection (with the exception of paronychia—without a hyperkeratotic reaction) should be considered for nail removal. Phenol is applied to the exposed nailbed to produce neurolysis of nerve endings and necrosis of the germinal matrix.

After a digital block on the involved hallux or toe (see Chapter 38), the digit is squeezed or wrapped for exsanguination of the blood currently in the toe, and a digital tourniquet is applied (see Chapter 43). Hemostasis is mandatory for subsequent phenol application.

While stabilizing the toe in the nondominant hand, one uses English nail nippers to clip the involved lateral quarter of the nail approximately one half to two thirds of the way back to the cuticle, following the longitudinal lines of the nail (Fig. 68–25). Care must be used to avoid cutting or tearing the nail further, because the danger of phenol seepage onto the desired remaining portion of nail matrix exists. The clinician proceeds by splitting the nail the rest of the way back with a mini-beaver number 61 blade; an 11 or 15 scalpel blade on a handle can also be used but is less effective. An angulated nail splitter (or straight scissors, less desirable) may be used for thicker toenails. The end of the chosen instrument is placed in the palm of the clinician's pronated dominant hand for stability. The blade is placed into the formerly created nail defect. The index finger of the dominant hand guides the blade as the palm forces it into the defect. Any residual blood pooled in the toe now appears in the wound; the blood should be removed by daubing with dried gauze. If minor hemorrhage persists, the toe tourniquet should be reapplied and tightened. The index finger of the dominant hand should press against the patient's toe or the clinician's opposite index finger to pro-

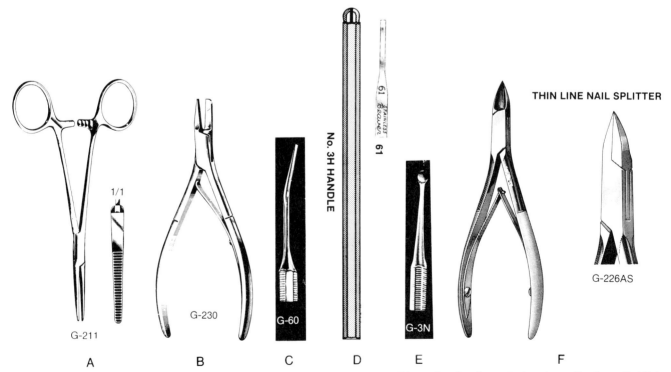

Figure 68–24. Instruments for nail procedures. *A,* Kelly hemostat, straight. *B,* English anvil nail splitter. *C,* Angular nail splitter. *D,* Mini-Beaver handle and number 61 blade. *E,* Nail curet. *F,* Thin line nail splitter. (Courtesy of Gill Podiatry Supply Co., 7803 Freeway Circle, Middleburg Heights, OH 44130).

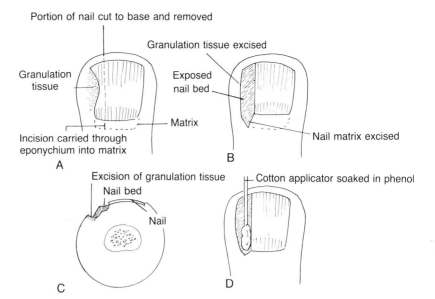

Figure 68–25. The nail ablation technique for the treatment of an ingrown toenail. The lateral portion of the nail is cut and removed *(A)*, exposing the nailbed. The matrix is excised. Granulation tissue is excised in a V-shaped wedge *(B and C)*, and the nail matrix is cauterized with absolute phenol *(D)* (see text).

vide a stabilizing counterpressure as the blade is slowly forced into the nail and beneath the cuticle. One should gently rock the splitter to ease it proximally. The nail is cut until the sensation of resistance is gone after passing several millimeters beneath the posterior nail fold. Care must be taken to keep the blade directed slightly downward and perpendicular to the nail plate, or the cut may angle obliquely into the corner of the posterior nail fold. If this happens, a portion of toenail may remain directly over the unwanted matrix, thus blocking the phenol cautery and reducing the correction.

Once the nail is split, a blunt angulated nail splitter is then used to separate the unwanted toenail from the nail groove, nailbed, and posterior nail fold. The nail remnant is then grasped with a small straight hemostat and removed from the wound by rolling (twisting) the hemostat overhand toward the remaining nail plate. The clinician inspects the remnant to ensure that all of the desired nail is removed. The exposed nail groove is then inspected for the keratotic plug; the lateral nail groove is curetted or sharply débrided down to the vascular nonsquamous epidermis. The cuticle that is tucked back under the exposed posterior nail fold also should be curetted with counterpressure on the skin above; this tissue may not initially yield to curettement until it has been exposed to phenol lysis, but removal should be attempted before dressing the operative site to prevent a possible foreign body reaction postoperatively. Some clinicians prefer to sharply débride the lateral nail matrix prior to phenol treatment.

The wound must be freed of hemorrhage or pooled blood by daubing the area with gauze or a dry cotton-tipped applicator. Again, if even minor hemorrhage persists, the toe tourniquet must be tightened. The wound is now ready for phenol cautery. The 88 per cent phenol solution is applied by means of cotton-tipped applicators. If the cotton-tipped applicators are too bulky to fit into the nail defect, they should be debulked prior to use. The applicators should be thoroughly moistened, but not saturated, with phenol solution, and one should make three 30-second applications to the nail groove, concentrating on the matrix beneath the posterior nail fold. For small toes in children, a reduced dosage of three 20-second applications by means of a cotton wisp on a toothpick should be used. The applicator is rolled

counterclockwise if the remaining nail is to the left of the applicator and is rolled clockwise if the remaining nail is to the right of the applicator. One uses this technique to avoid forcing phenol under the remaining nail plate.

The chemical cautery should turn the nail groove tissue to a brown-tinged grayish color. If fluid should drip from the wound or migrate along the posterior nail fold, it must be daubed quickly with gauze to prevent it from lysing normal tissue. Upon completion of the third phenol application, the wound is lavaged with a small stream of sterile water. While the stream is flowing over the defect, the clinician rubs his or her latex-gloved finger over the wound until a greasy feeling is replaced by a squeaky friction sensation, indicating removal of the phenol. There should be no gross loss of nail groove tissue or matrix observed after the cautery; the tissue will merely appear gray and dry. Some clinicians will use silver nitrate sticks rather than phenol to destroy the nail matrix. The silver nitrate sticks should be left in place for only 1 minute.

After chemical treatment, the area is inspected for any remaining cauterized cuticle or dead skin, which is snipped away with tissue scissors. The wound is dressed with an antibiotic ointment, Adaptic (or other nonadherent dressing), small gauze pads, and tape or Kling wrap. A wound check is appropriate in 24 to 48 hours when significant underlying infection is present.

Postoperative care includes twice-daily scrubs, antibiotic ointment, and dry dressing changes for several weeks. Oral antibiotics generally are not required unless the patient is immunocompromised. The early wound will display red, moist granulation tissue. Wound drainage is often present for the first two weeks and appears clear and straw colored. A dry scab will remain in the wound of the uneventful phenol correction for 1 month and may need to be débrided if there is a complaint of tenderness persisting in the former ingrown corner of the nail fold.

The surgery is approximately 90 to 95 per cent successful in preventing lateral nail regrowth after partial removal.[7–13] In addition to nail regrowth, infection and postsurgical foreign body reaction to remaining cuticle or nail may occur. An inclusion cyst may also form around the nail remnants, and curettement of the nail groove and posterior nail fold may be necessary.

Total Toenail Removal

The entire nail is sometimes removed when there is extensive infection and bilateral symptoms. If infection has been present for greater than 1 month, osteomyelitis should be considered and digit radiographs obtained. Periosteal abnormalities limited to the affected digit suggest concurrent osteomyelitis and warrant consultation with an orthopedist or podiatrist. The presence of osteomyelitis is not a contraindication to nail removal when removal is otherwise indicated. The patient should be warned that osteomyelitis is possible despite normal radiographs, especially if the toe still has a generalized achiness or swelling after the nail procedure is healed. With significant evidence of infection or in an immunocompromised patient, a wound culture and sensitivity should be obtained from the nail fold after nail removal.

The digit is prepared in a fashion similar to that of partial nail removal. Rather than splitting the nail, the open arm of a small hemostat is placed under the nail with the toothed surface upward toward the nail. The hemostat is pushed straight back toward the proximal nail fold while an elevating pressure is kept on the arm of the hemostat for avoidance of tearing of the nail bed as the instrument is forced proximally. The hemostat is similarly inserted in bordering zones beneath the nail plate until the toenail is completely loosened from side to side. An alternative method is to insert a small straight hemostat sideways beneath the central nail plate and open the hemostat repeatedly. After the nail is removed, all debris is curetted and the entire nail bed treated with phenol as outlined above. The phenol solution is flushed from the wound after the third treatment as previously discussed. Postoperative care and complications are similar to those of partial nail removal.

REFERENCES

1. McGlamry D (ed): Fundamentals of Foot Surgery. Baltimore, Williams & Wilkins, 1987, p 331.
2. Canter J, Mackey K, Good LS, et al: An outbreak of hepatitis B associated with jet injections in a weight reduction clinic. Arch Intern Med 150:1923, 1990.
3. Wenger JD, Spika JS, Smithwick RS, et al: Outbreak of *Mycobacterium chelonae* infection associated with use of jet injectors. JAMA 264:373, 1990.
4. McGlamry ED (ed): Comprehensive Textbook of Foot Surgery. Vols 1 and 2. Baltimore, Williams & Wilkins, 1987.
5. Hallux valgus and allied deformities. Clin Podiatr Med Surg 6:1–213, 1989.
6. Chisholm CD, Schlesser JF: Plantar puncture wounds: Controversies and treatment recommendations. Ann Emerg Med 18:1352, 1989.
7. Fitzgerald RH Jr, Cowan JD: Puncture wounds of the foot. Orthop Clin North Am 6:965, 1975.
8. Patzakis MJ, Wilkins J, Brien W, et al: Wound site as a predictor of complications following deep nail punctures of the foot. West J Med 150:545, 1989.
9. Palmer BV, Jones A: Ingrowing toenails: The results of treatment. Br J Surg 66:575, 1979.
10. Cameron PF: Ingrowing toenails: An evaluation of two treatments. Br Med J 283:821, 1981.
11. Wallace WA, Milne DD, Andrew T: Gutter treatment for ingrowing toenails. Br Med J 2:168, 1979.
12. Brown FO: Chemocautery for ingrowing toenails. J Dermatol Surg Oncol 7:331, 1981.
13. Lathrup R: Ingrown toenails: Cause and treatment. Cutis 20:119, 1977.
14. Murray WR, Robb JE: Soft-tissue resection for ingrowing toenails. J Dermatol Surg Oncol 7:157, 1981.
15. Leahy AL, Timon CI, Craig A, et al: Ingrowing toenails: Improving treatment. Surgery 107:566, 1990.

Chapter 69

Trigger Point Therapy

Anders E. Sola

INTRODUCTION

Myofascial pain is probably the most common pain problem faced by physicians.[1] It may be the primary complaint or may be a crippling adjunct to any number of other problems and is often accompanied by either local or generalized fatigue. Unless properly diagnosed and treated, persistent symptoms haunt patients and often result in misdiagnoses, unnecessary pain, and debilitation.

Treatment of myofascial pain is an effective way of sorting out pain problems. Elimination or reduction of myofascial pain often unmasks other painful disorders and therefore is useful in differential diagnosis. Myofascial pain is a very common complaint in the emergency department, and affected patients often present with torticollis, headache, or lower back pain. For many years, highly localized, exquisitely sensitive areas that are found usually within or near the painful region have been recognized as a common feature of myofascial pain. Pressure on these areas, known as trigger points, causes local pain, referred pain, or both.[1–9]

The local or referred pain associated with trigger points may not follow segmental neurologic patterns and therefore may not occur with a well-defined dermatome distribution. Actions taken at the trigger points, such as application of heat or cold, electrical stimulation, injection with local anesthetic or saline, or simply stimulation of the sensitive point with a needle, have proved the trigger points to be, in many cases, the key to control of the painful experience. A somewhat similar needling effect is associated with acupuncture points (many of which are located in areas in which trigger points are commonly found).[10–12] The exact mechanisms by which trigger points are involved in and contribute to myofascial pain, as well as the response to intervention at trigger points, indicate a continuous, cyclic relationship between trigger point activity and the pain phenomenon.

BACKGROUND

The trigger point phenomenon has its western origin in Germany, the Scandinavian countries, and Great Britain (the "rheumatic" countries).[3, 4] The Germans first reported on these painful muscular problems (*Muskel schmerzen*) and "hard" muscles in the mid-nineteenth century. Most of the investigations were directed at the microscopic findings of these "hard nodules," or so-called rheumatic lesions of muscle. These sensitive areas in muscle caused local pain or tenderness on palpation with or without a predictable pain reference away from the local point of maximal tenderness. The British followed with similar studies and failed to determine the faulty microanatomy and pathophysiology of these elusive pain problems—these conditions were referred to as fibrositis, myalgia, and nonarticular rheumatism. Gower introduced the term *fibrositis* at the turn of the century, and it became fixed in the English literature when Llewellyn and Jones's massive text was published in 1915.[13, 14] Despite intensive investigation, no satisfactory explanation of the mechanisms of (muscular) pain was discovered to resolve the controversy.

Kraus published an innovative study on the use of the ethyl

chloride spray technique to relieve myofascial pain in 1937.[15] This was followed by the studies of Travell, who has done extensive research and has published works on the trigger point problem over many years. She has carefully plotted the pain patterns most commonly encountered and has emphasized the use of procaine injections and the coolant spray, Flouri-Methane (Gebaur Chemical Co., Cleveland, Ohio), instead of the more dangerous ethyl chloride.

Travell has described a trigger point caused by acute or chronic overload of a muscle as a palpable, firm, tense band in the muscle. The trigger point is characterized by a local twitch response to tapping of the muscle, restricted range of motion, weakness without atrophy, and no neurologic deficit. Subjectively, the patients complain of pain in a predictable pattern, stiffness and fatigue, and deep tenderness at the trigger point.[9]

In addition to muscular overload, a variety of stress-inducing stimuli—emotional or physical—may be implicated in the onset of myofascial pain (Fig. 69–1). The power of these stressors to induce pain in a particular individual is moderated by the genetics, personality, conditioning, and physiologic state of that individual. Once established, however, a painful event may sustain itself in spite of control or elimination of the initiating stimuli through a characteristic internal cyclic process of self-stimulus and response. Furthermore, the painful trigger point itself may become the stressor that involves other muscles in the event. Thus trigger points may act both as translators of stress to pain and, secondarily, as stressors that perpetuate pain.[16]

Trigger points can occur in any muscle or muscle group in the body. Since the stresses involved in the onset of myofascial pain can commonly affect not only single muscles but also whole muscle groups, trigger points tend to cluster. In the upper trunk, a common trigger point cluster involves the muscles of the neck and the shoulder area—the trapezius, the levator scapulae, and the infraspinatus. In the lower trunk, a group of muscles that is often involved includes the quadratus lumborum, the gluteus medius, and the tensor fasciae latae. As individuals age there is an increase in the potential for nerve root irritation problems and subsequent pain as suggested by Gunn.[17] Although nerve root irritation cannot be alleviated by treatment of trigger points, myofascial disturbances that may arise as a result of the irritation may be reduced through such treatment.

Painful trigger points in a given muscle often affect all other muscles innervated from the same spinal segments, and treatment is usually directed at those muscles innervated by both the *posterior* branch of the spinal nerve(s) and the *anterior* spinal branch (Fig. 69–2). Therefore, the search for trigger points and subsequent treatment should be directed at both spinal nerve divisions. Pain may be felt in a muscle innervated by an anterior spinal nerve, whereas little or no pain may be initially felt in muscles innervated by the posterior branch of the same spinal nerves. Palpation of the muscles innervated by the posterior branch, however, may reveal

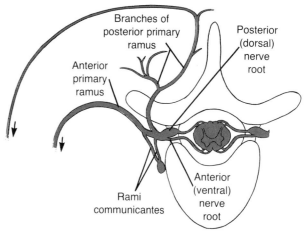

Figure 69–2. Cross section of a typical spinal nerve, showing the anterior and posterior divisions. The posterior segment innervates the erector spinae, whereas the anterior segment innervates the remaining muscles supplied by the spinal nerves.

evidence of active trigger points: hypersensitive areas, or, more important, a tight band-like local spasm plus hypersensitivity.

Trigger points in a given muscle may affect not only the anterior and posterior branches of the specific segmental spinal nerve but also the spinal nerves related by common musculature for several segments above and below the major trigger point. Thus muscles in the erector group in the cervical area can be the source of noxious impulses that can cause pain to be transmitted as far as the midthoracic area (Fig. 69–3).[18]

Trigger points abound in the lower trunk, gluteal muscles, abductors and adductors of the thigh. Their presence in the gluteal or lumbar muscles may often be related to hypersensitivity in the muscles of the upper trunk group. Therefore, a patient who is suffering muscle tension headaches on one side should be checked not only for trigger points in the ipsilateral upper trunk muscles but also for hypersensitive areas (trigger points) in the gluteal and

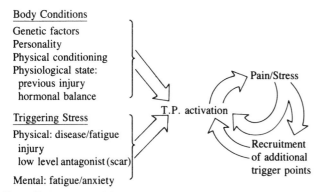

Figure 69–1. Stress and body conditions. A variety of stress-inducing stimuli may be implicated in the onset of myofascial pain. The power of these stimuli to induce pain in a particular individual is moderated by the genetics, personality, conditioning, and physiologic state of that individual. Once established, however, a painful event may sustain itself in spite of control or elimination of the initiating stimuli. (From Sola AE: Myofascial trigger point therapy. Resident and Staff Physician 27(8):44, 1981. Reproduced by permission.)

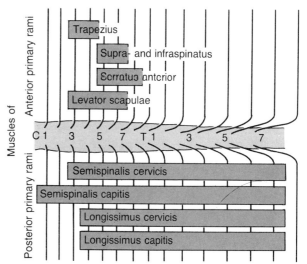

Figure 69–3. This schematic illustration gives examples of upper extremity muscles supplied by the anterior primary rami of the cervical spine. Note the length of the muscles supplied by the posterior rami shown for the same cervical region. Activation of trigger points that exist along the entire length of a muscle can cause or intensify pain felt in muscles supplied by any common nerve segment. Therefore, pain experienced along a muscle such as the semispinalis capitis can contribute to shoulder pain. Injection treatment of posterior primary rami muscles beginning at T-6 is indicated if hypersensitive trigger points are found in the muscles.

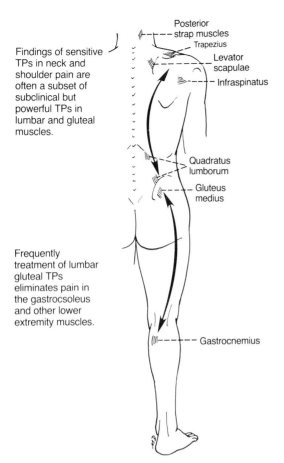

Figure 69–4. Ipsilateral pain, a diagnostic key to treatment of refractory local pain. An ipsilateral pattern of pain is very common, with simultaneously active painful trigger points in the neck and shoulder, quadratus lumborum and gluteal muscles, and frequently in the calf muscles. The patient may not be aware of pain in the lumbar gluteal region or lower extremity but may confirm achiness or stiffness in the hip area, sciatica-like pain, or fatigue in the lower back and extremities. Hyperactive trigger points in the lumbar gluteal muscles must be treated before positive results can be expected from treatment of trigger points in head, neck, or extremities. *TP*, trigger point.

lumbar musculature (Fig. 69–4). If trigger points are found, they should be treated to reduce both the hyperactivity in the lower segment and the sensitivity of the upper muscle group. If hyperactive trigger points are ignored in the lumbar and (especially) the gluteal region, treating only the cervical trigger points can precipitate a painful low back spasm. This may be severe enough to cause another trip to the emergency department.

Both the longevity and the spread of myofascial pain may be caused by cycles of physiologic responses that involve one or more trigger points. These may include such well-defined pathways as motor reflexes, less well-known autonomic feedback cycles, and, quite probably, a number of as yet ill-defined interrelationships that include changes in the microenvironment of the tissues in the area. Frequently seen autonomic concomitants of trigger points include decreased electrical skin resistance, pilomotor reactions in the reference area, and vasodilation with dermatographia and skin temperature changes.[9] I have also noted hypoesthesia in the involved extremity (and, when upper and lower muscle groups are involved, in the affected side), local and general fatigue, fine tremor, and weakness.

The exact physiologic mechanism of trigger points has not been defined. Trigger points may be considered as "weak points" within the muscle or fascia that are particularly sensitive to stress-induced change. In the absence of stress, the trigger point may remain quiescent, only to become activated by a number of positive-feedback cycles that involve sensory motor reflexes, autonomic responses,

vascular changes, and numerous other ill-defined events ultimately leading to muscle tension, fatigue, and pain.

The initiating stress may also be soft tissue trauma, such as a muscular strain or contusion, causing prolonged pain that is more intense, out of proportion, or of excessively long duration, given the initial injury. Such may be the case with a worker who suffers a relatively minor injury on the job but has persistent disability or impairment long beyond the expected period of disability for that particular injury (Fig. 69–5).

PATIENT PROFILE

All parts of the musculoskeletal system are susceptible to myofascial pain syndromes. The patient presents with

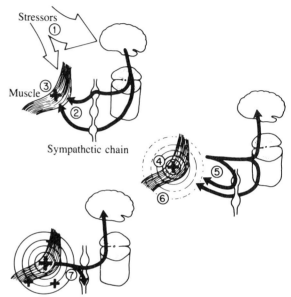

Figure 69–5. When stressed *(1)*, the individual responds with defense mechanisms that include various physiologic changes, such as splinting and bracing of muscles, vasomotor changes, increased sympathetic discharge, and hormonal and other humoral changes in the plasma and extracellular fluids *(2)*. A particular point in a braced, stressed muscle or fascia that is more sensitive than the surrounding tissue—perhaps because of previous injury or genetic mandate—fatigues and begins to signal its distress to the central nervous system *(3)*. A number of responses may result. The most readily understood involves the motor reflexes. Various muscles associated with the trigger point become more tense and begin to fatigue. Sympathetic responses lead to vasomotor changes within and around the trigger point. Local ischemia following vasoconstriction or increased vascular permeability following vasodilation may lead to changes in the extracellular environment of the affected cells, release of algesic agents (bradykinins, prostaglandins), osmotic changes, and pH changes, all of which may increase the sensitivity or activity of nociceptors in the area. Sympathetic activity may also cause smooth muscle contraction in the vicinity of nociceptors, thus increasing their activity *(4)*. Increased nociceptor input contributes to the cycle by increasing motor and sympathetic activity, which in turn leads to increased pain *(5)*. The pain is shadowed by growing fatigue, which adds an overall mood of distress to the patient's situation and feeds back to the cycle *(6)*. As tense muscles in the affected area begin to fatigue in an environment of sympathetic stimulation and local biochemical change, latent trigger points within these muscles may also begin to fire, thus adding to the positive feedback cycle and spreading the pain to these adjacent muscle groups. Finally, the stress of pain and fatigue, coupled with both increased muscle tension and sympathetic tone throughout the body (conceivably with ipsilateral emphasis through the sympathetic chain), may lead to flare-ups or trigger points in other muscles remote from the initial area of pain *(7)*. (From Sola AE: Myofascial trigger point therapy. Resident and Staff Physician 27(8):39, 1981. Reproduced by permission.)

localized or diffuse pain, ranging from intense, "burning," and debilitating to dull and bothersome. The affected areas are often described as stiff, heavy, or numb. The pain frequently affects a joint, and range of motion may be inhibited. The chronic fatigue associated with myofascial pain may be exacerbated by disturbed sleep patterns.

Many patients attribute their symptoms to overuse of muscles, sitting in drafts, or a "cold" in the muscle. Physical examination fails to elicit any neurologic deficits or atrophy, although there may be some weakness of involved muscle groups. Thorough examination of the affected areas may reveal edema, coolness in an affected extremity, or exaggerated pilomotor reflexes.

Patients with prolonged or complicated myofascial pain syndromes may present to the emergency department after becoming frustrated with unsuccessful attempts to achieve relief from their symptoms. They may have consulted numerous physicians, chiropractors, or both; tried home remedies or vitamin therapy; or received treatment with a variety of muscle relaxants, anti-inflammatory medications, or potent analgesics. Their symptoms may have been diagnosed vaguely as overuse injuries, chronic bursitis, arthritis, or sciatica; or they may have been dismissed because there were no radiographic or laboratory confirmations of their complaints. Many patients labeled "chronic complainers" have myofascial syndromes that can be treated, which eliminates or reduces their symptoms.

EXAMINATION FOR TRIGGER POINTS

Any treatment of myofascial syndromes must be preceded by a history and physical examination to rule out other causes of apparent myofascial pain. Once this is accomplished, a systematic search for trigger points is carried out, with special emphasis placed on the painful muscles and their segmental associates. Trigger point areas should be compared with the contralateral counterparts as a guide to their relative sensitivity. The most reliable method of locating trigger points is by searching in the painful area with the tip of the finger. Pressure applied to the hypersensitive area in the muscle reproduces or accentuates the pain. This is usually accompanied by an involuntary "wince" by the patient. The hypersensitive area may feel rope-like, indurated, or tight, depending on which muscle is examined. The muscles should be examined in both relaxed and stretched positions. Although there may be a halo area or a surrounding zone of tenderness, one should search for the area of maximal tenderness or response.

In sedentary populations, trigger points are common and are usually associated with chronic strain and stress. They tend to occur with great regularity in the same areas. In my clinical experience, trigger points are less common in laborers and athletes and, when present, are usually the result of overuse or injury rather than chronic strain or stress. This suggests that regular exercise is of therapeutic value in prevention, as well as treatment, of myofascial syndromes, which start at an early age. Conversely, the presence of trigger points inhibits the effectiveness of a well-designed exercise program.

Although the pain reference pattern may help to isolate the hypersensitive area, one should remember that the pattern differs according to severity and longevity of the trigger point injury, body build, state of health, gender, and degree of injury or weakness (Table 69–1).

When searching for trigger points, one should carefully examine the entire area of all muscles that may be involved. For example, in treating torticollis, one should check the levator scapulae, trapezius, sternocleidomastoid, and posterior strap muscles (supplied by the posterior spinal ramus),

Table 69–1. **Clinical Features of Myofascial Pain**
Continuous, dull, deep, aching pain
Pressure on tender spots or bands (trigger areas) in muscles reproduces pain
Pain relieved by inactivating trigger points
Restricted range of movement (ROM) in affected muscle (Full ROM does not rule out presence of trigger points)
Local muscle twitch produced by trigger point stimulation
Patient startle or jump sign with trigger point pressure

(Adapted from Fields HL: Pain. New York, McGraw-Hill Book Co, 1987, p 213.)

especially the splenius and semispinalis muscles. The muscles are often innervated from many vertebral segments—for instance, innervation of the splenius starts at the C2 vertebral level and reaches to the midthoracic level. Thus hypersensitivity at one level may readily involve other muscles with overlapping segmental innervation. When treating neck pain problems, one must look for tender trigger points along the entire spinal insertion of these muscles. The same principle of extended search is also important in the treatment of myofascial shoulder pain and headache pain (Fig. 69–6). A common finding is an ipsilateral pattern, involving cervical shoulder, lumbar, and gluteal muscles. The patient frequently complains of numbness on one entire side of the body. When headache or neck pain is severe, often the patient is aware of stiffness, discomfort, or pain in the hip area.

INDICATIONS

Treatment of sensitive trigger points by injection is often quite effective for pain relief when the trigger point is the

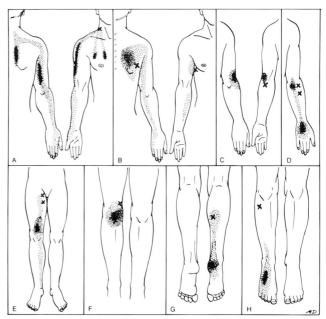

Figure 69–6. Typical locations of trigger points with pain reference patterns in the extremities. *A*, Scaleni. *B*, Latissimus dorsi. *C*, Supinator. *D*, Extensor carpi radialis. *E*, Adductor longus and adductor brevis. *F*, Vastus medialis. *G*, Soleus. *H*, Extensors digitorum longus and hallucis longus. (*A* to *D* adapted from Travell JG, Simons DG: Myofascial Pain and Dysfunction: The Trigger Point Manual. Baltimore, Williams & Wilkins, 1983. *E* to *F* adapted from Simons DG: Myofascial pain syndromes and their treatment. In Basmajian JV, Kirby RL: Medical Rehabilitation: A Student's Textbook. Baltimore, Williams & Wilkins, 1984. © Williams & Wilkins, 1984.)

primary source of myofascial pain. Such treatment may reduce pain and may speed recovery at sites of trauma in the same segment. Treatment of trigger points that flare up secondarily to other painful stimuli, such as nerve root lesions and nerve compression, is never more than moderately successful in relieving pain. Nonetheless, it is often difficult to ascertain the source of the stress that leads to the myofascial involvement until trigger point injection has been tried. Therefore, in many cases, the response to injection treatment may also be an element of the diagnosis.

Under certain conditions, injection treatment not only may be ineffective but also may precipitate a medical or emotional crisis. Contraindications to injection treatment include the presence of a systemic illness (especially with fever), high anxiety or emotional stress levels (including "needle" anxiety, manifestations of psychosis, and abuse of drugs or alcohol), and a history of hypersensitive or syncopal reactions to injections. If there is doubt concerning the diagnosis of myofascial pain caused by trigger point involvement as opposed to such possible causes as a nerve root lesion, one should not inject the patient but should have the patient return for further studies. Although the possibility of injection treatment may discourage some malingerers, it is less effective as a screening tool than is acute observation of the "too-perfect" account of symptoms often given by these patients.

EQUIPMENT

Little equipment is necessary for the injection procedure. A simple tray may contain a 5-ml syringe, a 25- or 27-gauge needle, an antiseptic preparation, and a local anesthetic (1 per cent lidocaine, 0.25 per cent bupivacaine, or 1 per cent procaine hydrochloride) or physiologic saline for injection. Some physicians use a repository corticosteroid preparation, such as hydrocortisone or prednisolone tebutate, methylprednisolone acetate, or triamcinolone acetonide or hexacetonide (see Chapter 70, Table 70–3).

GENERAL PROCEDURE

Injection of the hypersensitive trigger point often provides dramatic pain relief. A body of evidence indicates that at least a portion of the benefit is derived from the stimulation of the trigger point by the needle regardless of the substances injected. Although local anesthetics are often used, I have used normal physiologic saline for many years with good results.[20–23] In one controlled study, Frost and coworkers[21] actually demonstrated better results when plain saline was used in comparison with the local anesthetic mepivacaine.

When injection therapy is performed in patients with moderate to severe pain in the emergency department, the supplemental use of a local anesthetic is advised for immediate relief, although good results have been obtained even in severe pain with saline injection alone. Local injection should be used in conjunction with appropriate oral analgesics and muscle relaxants. Some clinicians routinely inject small doses of a long-acting steroid preparation into painful trigger points in conjunction with saline or a local anesthetic. Although steroids are of proven value in the treatment of inflammatory conditions, their usefulness in trigger point therapy is unknown. A therapeutic trial of steroids may be warranted if proper precautions concerning the side effects are observed.

It is wise to inject patients placed in a supine position in order to minimize syncopal reactions. If the upper back,

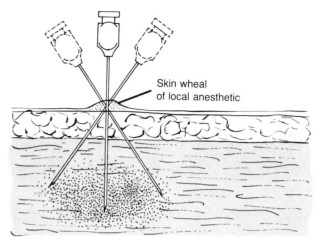

Figure 69–7. The needle is used in a fan-like motion to distribute the solution throughout the trigger point.

the neck, or the shoulder is being injected, a pillow is placed under the hips.

The hypersensitive point is located by palpation, and the area for injection is prepared in the usual manner. The point of entry should be in the area of maximal tenderness. One inserts the needle and injects 0.5 to 2 ml of fluid using a "fanning" technique, in which the needle is repeatedly withdrawn part of the way and redirected (Fig. 69–7). This ensures maximal coverage of the area of the trigger point. In most cases, a short series of two to five injections over a period of days to weeks is enough to rule out myofascial pain caused by muscle strain or injury. After injection, a moist pack applied to the area relieves the temporary discomfort of the injection. It has been my experience that younger patients are more responsive to trigger point injection than older individuals. In younger patients, trigger points are more easily located and are less complicated in their pain reference patterns. As people age, muscle weakness and shortening and the effects of degenerative processes frequently confuse the pain reference pattern.

Follow-up treatment for patients with myofascial pain may include one or more of the following: repeated injection therapy; adjunctive physical therapy; and special techniques, including intermittent cervical or lumbar traction, relaxation techniques, ultrasound, electrical stimulation, massage (especially deep friction) and application of coolant sprays or ice packs, and, routinely, therapeutic exercise.

COMPLICATIONS

Some patients are hyperreactors. These individuals may respond to even an injection of saline by fainting if sitting upright and may have an excessive flare-up of pain after treatment (that night). I always ask about an allergic history (e.g., allergies to foods and drugs and sensitivity to the sun). It has been my experience that patients with red or auburn-colored hair and certain fair-skinned, blue-eyed blondes are more likely to faint. I also monitor patients with the back of my hand, touching their skin to detect excessive sweating.

If complications occur, one should stop injecting. Some physicians inject as much as 5 to 10 ml of fluid at a given trigger point. I have found that this is excessive. The patient frequently develops a flu-like syndrome, characterized by malaise and myalgias, the next day. I have experienced few complications using saline with a normal pH. Some patients have fainted, but these individuals were seated rather than supine. The use of local anesthetics, a standard procedure in emergency departments, increases the risk very little if "caine" allergies, excessive drug quantities, and intravenous injections are avoided.

Particular care must be used in injecting the neck, the intercostal muscles, and the periscapular area, because these areas contain many large vessels and nerves and the pleura is in close proximity to the injection sites. This is complicated if the patient is agitated or young or is in a state of confusion.

EMERGENCY DEPARTMENT TREATMENT OF COMMON PRESENTATIONS OF MYOFASCIAL PAIN

Shoulder Disorders

A painful shoulder will frequently have trigger points located in the posterior scapular muscles. Other muscles that are often involved include the supraspinatus, the infraspinatus, and the pectoralis major. Less commonly, the teres, the deltoid, and the triceps are involved. Trigger points in the splenius, the semispinalis, and the gluteal muscles may also contribute to shoulder pain and should be treated if found in conjunction with myofascial shoulder pain. Such pain often prompts the diagnosis of bursitis, which is usually a catchall or insurance diagnosis and is often not correct. Patients may have had numerous unsuccessful treatments with muscle relaxants and potent anti-inflammatory medications.

When injecting the scapular and periscapular muscles, one should take extreme care to stabilize the scapula. The patient should lie on a bed with his arms along his sides and a pillow under his chest to round the shoulders and to facilitate injection. A small pillow may be used to rest the forehead. The boundaries (borders) should be noted before injection, and the patient should be warned not to move his shoulder. If the lower portion of the scapula moves, one can easily miss the muscle and pierce the pleura. Therefore, one should "fix the scapula" before injecting and should always double-check. I frequently hook my thumb on the medial border while injecting trigger points in the infraspinatus muscle.

Myofascial pain is commonly associated with a number of muscles at the medial border of the scapula. These include the rhomboids, the serratus anterior, the subscapular muscles and, at the superior edge, the levator scapulae muscle. It is best to inject the levator at an oblique angle to the muscle, because patients frequently flinch during injection, and the needle could puncture the pleura.

If the painful areas are on the lower medial border, then the patient should place the hand behind the back. This causes a winging of the scapula, allowing easier and safer injection. A tangential laterally directed needle reaches much of the scapular undersurface (Fig. 69–8). The rhomboids and the serratus anterior are easily treatable with this maneuver. On occasion, the subscapularis muscle is involved, and the only complaint besides poorly localized scapular pain may be a sensation of "sleeping on a marble." When injecting along the lateral border (teres major and minor and lateral dorsi), one should fix the scapula and should warn the patient not to move.

Headaches

Trigger points are a frequent cause of the muscle component of any type of headache. These are usually found

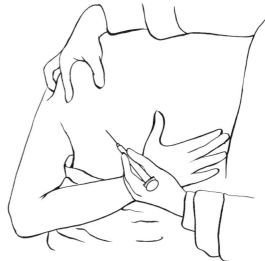

Figure 69–8. Surface view of serratus anterior muscle. The internally rotated arm is slid across the back toward the midline, bringing the inferior angle of the scapula into a "winged" position. The needle is slipped in anteriorly to the edge of the angle of the bone.

in the sternocleidomastoid, levator scapulae, and trapezius muscles and, not infrequently, in the scalp and facial muscles. In addition, the posterior strap muscles are often involved, particularly the semispinalis and splenius muscles (Fig. 69–9). When preparing to treat a patient with headache, one should carefully examine the entire back for hypersensitive areas, paying special attention to the paraspinal muscle group. As previously discussed, trigger points located in the quadratus lumborum and the gluteus medius may contribute to headache problems. These muscles seem to have particular significance if the headache is unilateral.

Back Pain

Unilateral back pain is usually responsive to trigger point injection. The trigger points are most commonly found in the quadratus lumborum, gluteus medius, and tensor fasciae latae muscles. Hip pain caused by gluteal trigger points may mimic trochanteric bursitis, and by far the most frequently diagnosed syndrome, sciatica, is often caused by gluteal trigger points (Fig. 69–10).

The lumbosacral muscles are commonly involved in lower back pain. Here the trigger points are frequently secondary to vertebral or nerve root irritation, and treatment may be of only temporary benefit. Affected patients, if no better after treatment, should be referred for further evaluation and treatment.

Torticollis

Torticollis usually is a simple problem involving one to three muscles. The trapezius, sternocleidomastoid, and levator scapulae are the main offenders. A careful search of the posterior strap muscles, however, may reveal exquisite tenderness of the splenius and the semispinalis muscles. If the trapezius is involved, particular care must be taken with the injection technique (Fig. 69–11).

The apical pleura in some individuals is much higher than normal. If there is a sudden upward flinch of the shoulder during injection, the pleura could be punctured.

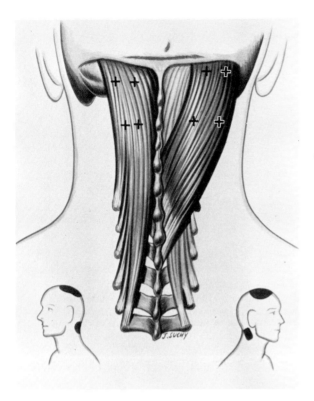

Figure 69–9. Splenius and semispinalis capitis. Pain resulting from involvement of these muscles may be located over the muscles themselves. Both the splenius and the semispinalis can mediate pain to the head and the face, and both are commonly involved in headache. Occasionally, dizziness will accompany involvement of these muscles. Because trigger points are difficult to pinpoint in these muscles, patient cooperation in pointing out positions of maximal tenderness is extremely helpful. (From Sola AE: Myofascial trigger point therapy. Resident and Staff Physician 27(8):44, 1981. Reproduced by permission.)

If possible, one should inject transversely with the trigger point located between index finger and thumb.

Reflex Dystrophy Syndrome

Reflex dystrophy–like symptoms are often alleviated with trigger point therapy directed primarily toward the infraspinatus and gluteus medius.

SPECIFIC MUSCLE SYNDROMES

Some of the muscles that are commonly involved in pain problems are listed in the following paragraphs. Although the pain reference sites are fairly consistent, they may differ because of involvement of more than one muscle.

Infraspinatus. Because of its multiple functions, this muscle is subject to earlier degeneration than other muscles of the rotator cuff and therefore is more vulnerable to

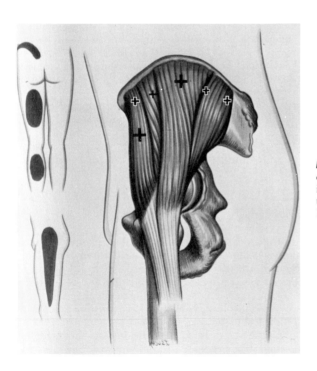

Figure 69–10. Trigger points about the hip. These muscles are easy to examine, and it is easy to locate the common trigger points that are present in the muscle bellies. Pain is usually referred to the lateral aspect of the thigh as far as the knee. (From Sola AE: Myofascial trigger point therapy. Resident and Staff Physician 27(8):44, 1981. Reproduced by permission.)

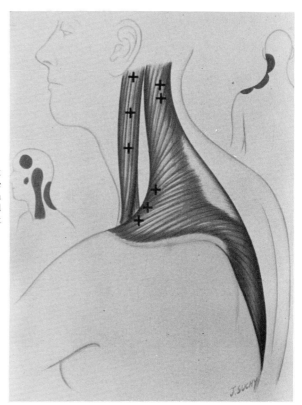

Figure 69–11. Trapezius and sternocleidomastoid. Trigger points are most commonly located at the occiput insertion in the upper two thirds of the muscle and frequently on its sternal and clavicular origins. The pain pattern may involve the muscle or may be referred to the ear region, the face, and the frontal area. (From Sola AE: Myofascial trigger point therapy. Resident and Staff Physician 27(8):45, 1981. Reproduced by permission.)

trigger points in association with many types of shoulder lesions. Trigger points in the infraspinatus invariably cause sympathetic hyperactivity and may be a major contributor to dystrophy-like syndromes of the upper extremity (Fig. 69–12). Careful palpation is necessary to locate trigger areas. It is useful to search the entire muscle along the length of the muscle bundles as well as across the "grain" of the muscle. Related pain is usually located on the posterior and

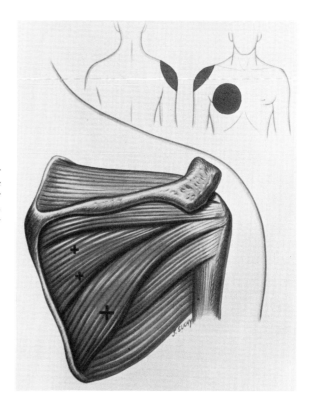

Figure 69–12. Infraspinatus. Careful palpation is necessary to locate trigger areas. It is useful to search the entire muscle along the length of the muscle bundles as well as across the "grain" of the muscle. All of the scapular muscles are frequently involved, either singly or in concert with each other. (From Sola AE: Myofascial trigger point therapy. Resident and Staff Physician 27(8):43, 1981. Reproduced by permission.)

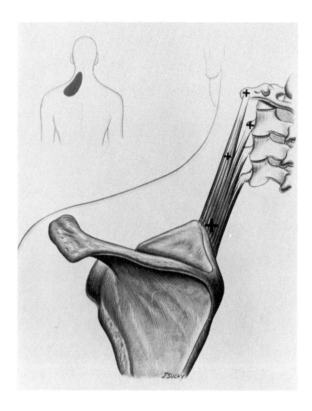

Figure 69–13. Levator scapulae. Painful, sensitive foci may occur at the origin of the superior medial aspect of the scapula, along the entire flat muscle belly, or on the insertions on the transverse processes of the first four cervical vertebrae. (From Sola AE: Myofascial trigger point therapy. Resident and Staff Physician 27(8):43, 1981. Reproduced by permission.)

lateral aspect of the shoulder and, occasionally, may return to the anterior chest. All of the scapular muscles are frequently involved either singly or in concert with each other.

Levator Scapulae. Painful sensitive foci may occur at the origin on the superior medial aspect of the scapula, along the entire flat muscle belly, or on the insertions on the transverse processes of the first four cervical vertebrae

(Fig. 69–13). Invariably, the levator scapulae muscle is involved in chronic cervical conditions as well as in torticollis. The pain is usually referred to the posterior cervical region, the posterior scalp, and the area around the ear.

Quadratus Lumborum. Travell has referred to this muscle as "the joker" in the lower back syndrome, and it deserves this title.[24] It is a hip hiker and a lateral flexor of

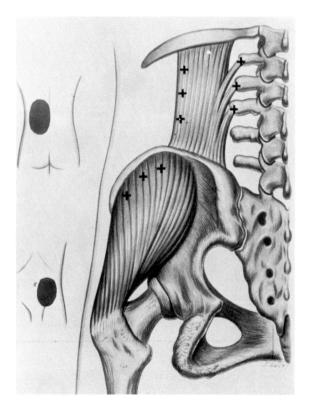

Figure 69–14. Quadratus lumborum and gluteus medius. Trigger points occur on the twelfth rib and the iliac crest and along the lateral border of the entire muscle. The trigger points of the gluteus medius most commonly are found along the iliac shelf, and with extensive involvement the entire gluteal ridge, including the gluteal minimus and maximus muscles from the sacroiliac joint to the anterior superior spine, may contain painful trigger points. (From Sola AE: Myofascial trigger point therapy. Resident and Staff Physician 27(8):43, 1981. Reproduced by permission.)

the spine, and in addition it assists respiratory function by anchoring the twelfth rib for the pull of the diaphragm. It frequently signals its distress on deep inspiration with twelfth-rib pain. Pain can be local or it can be referred to the anterior abdominal wall. This may accentuate postoperative pain or painful abdominal scars over the lower quadrant. Trigger points occur on the twelfth rib, on the iliac crest, and along the lateral border of the entire muscle (Fig. 69–14).

Gluteus Medius. The trigger points in the gluteus medius may well be the most critical in the lower extremity. Like the infraspinatus, this muscle is associated with sympathetic hyperactivity. Activity of these trigger points often involves activation of trigger points in the quadratus lumborum, the tensor fasciae latae, and the other gluteal muscles, thus inducing widespread lower back discomfort (see Figs. 69–10 and 69–16). There is also an interaction between the trigger points of the gluteus medius and those in the cervical area, sometimes involving this remote muscle in cervical pain and headache. Although this muscle seldom causes pain without involving other muscles, the pain pattern most often attributed to the gluteus medius is along the iliac crest and into the posterior thigh and calf. It is a frequent cause of hip pain in the later stages of pregnancy and simulates sciatica. The trigger points most commonly are found along the iliac shelf and, with extensive involvement, the entire gluteal ridge (including also the gluteus minimus and maximus muscles from the sacroiliac joint to the anterior superior spine) may contain painful trigger points. It is

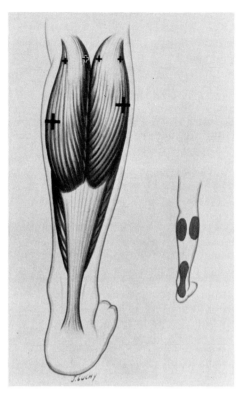

Figure 69–16. Gastrocnemius/soleus. Trigger points are usually found on the medial and lateral margins of the muscle group and along the midline of the group. (From Sola AE: Myofascial trigger point therapy. Resident and Staff Physician 27(8):44, 1981. Reproduced by permission.)

estimated that 10 per cent of the population have legs that differ in length by at least 1 cm. This difference can cause unilateral back pain and trigger points of the gluteus, erector spinae, and quadratus lumborum muscles.

Tensor Fasciae Latae. This muscle is easy to examine, and it is also easy to locate the common trigger points that are present in the muscle belly. Pain is usually referred to the lateral aspects of the thigh as far as the knee (see Fig. 69–10).

Anterior Tibialis. Pain in the anterior ankle is usually experienced when the trigger points of this muscle flare up, although in severe cases the entire muscle may be painful. Trigger points are most commonly found in the upper one third of the muscle, and pain is referred to the anterior portion of the leg and into the dorsal portion of the ankle (Fig. 69–15).

Gastrocnemius/Soleus. Myofascial pain related to this muscle group is felt behind the knee, over the muscle bellies, and along the achilles tendon near the heel. Trigger points are usually found on the medial and lateral margins of the muscle group and along the midline of the group. These trigger points often flare up when a patient is experiencing vascular problems of the lower extremities. One report has suggested injecting these trigger points for the relief of pain associated with intermittent claudication.[25] The pain is referred to the achilles tendon and the heel (Fig. 69–16).

Splenius Capitis/Semispinalis Capitis. Pain resulting from involvement of these muscles may be located over the muscles themselves. Both the splenius and the semispinalis can mediate pain to the head and the face, however, and both are commonly involved in headache. Occasionally, dizziness accompanies involvement of these muscles. Because trigger points are difficult to pinpoint in these muscles,

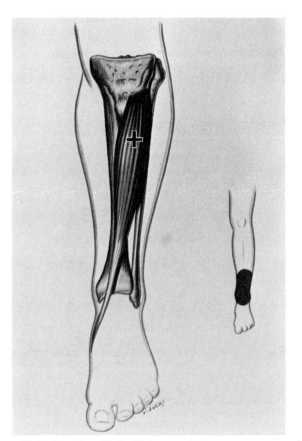

Figure 69–15. Anterior tibialis. Trigger points are most commonly found in the upper one third of the muscle, and pain is referred to the anterior portion of the leg and into the dorsal portion of the ankle. (From Sola AE: Myofascial trigger point therapy. Resident and Staff Physician 27(8):44, 1981. Reproduced by permission.)

patient cooperation in pointing out positions of maximal tenderness is extremely helpful (see Fig. 69–9).

Rectus Abdominis. These muscles are frequent sites of anterior abdominal wall pain. The trigger points are best located with the patient in the supine position and with his head and neck flexed so his abdominal rectus muscles are under tension. These trigger points frequently flare up after abdominal surgery and can be one of the chief constituents of postoperative pain. The trigger points are most commonly found in the upper three segments of abdominal rectus muscle, and the pain is usually localized over the muscle (Fig. 69–17).

Pectoralis Major/Pectoralis Minor. The pectoralis major muscles are a frequent site of myofascial pain in the area of the muscle insertion on the anterior medial shoulder. The inferior belly of the muscle is a common area of trigger points; however, the entire muscle must be searched diligently. The clavicular portion of this muscle usually refers pain to the uppermost part of the muscle. On occasion, there is some referral into the arm (Figs. 69–17 and 69–18).

Intercostals. One should examine the intercostals for chest pain routinely by palpating the intercostal spaces with the fingers. The intercostals are frequently involved after any chest surgery or trauma. In treating chest pain when intercostal blocks are not successful, one must take care on injection to avoid entry into the pleural space. Pain from the exterior intercostal muscle is usually localized near the site of the trigger point and is emphasized during inspiration (see Fig. 69–18).

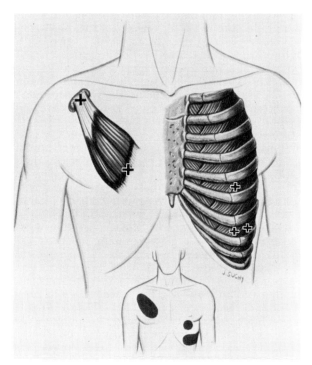

Figure 69–18. Pectoralis minor and intercostal muscles. In the pectoralis minor, pain is usually deep and sharply circumscribed over the outline of the muscle when involved. Trigger points are most commonly found near the origin and insertion of the muscle. (From Sola AE: Myofascial trigger point therapy. Resident and Staff Physician 27(8):45, 1981. Reproduced by permission.)

Trapezius. The trapezius is a frequent source of muscle pain and headache, especially at the angle of the neck or at the occipital insertions of the muscle, where trigger points are most commonly located. When injecting trigger points at the angle of the neck, one must take care to avoid the apical pleura (see Fig. 69–11).

Sternocleidomastoid. This muscle is often the source of neck pain and headache. In addition, dizziness and ipsilateral ptosis, lacrimation, and reddening of the conjunctiva have been reported in association with the involvement of these muscles.[26] Trigger points are most commonly located at occiput insertion in the upper two thirds of the muscle and frequently on its sternal and clavicular origins. The pain pattern may involve the muscle or may refer to the ear region, the face, and the frontal area (see Fig. 69–11).

CONCLUSION

In summary, trigger points may be involved in any painful event. They may play either a primary role (translating stress to pain) or a secondary role (supporting and intensifying a painful stimulus). They can complicate any type of pain and may mimic underlying visceral disorders. Obviously, interventions that directly affect the trigger point have a much greater chance for complete pain control if the trigger point is acting in the primary role of translator than if it is acting in the secondary role of pain intensifier. Even in the secondary role, however, there is the potential for benefit from properly administered treatment. Treatment considerations in addition to trigger point injection include administration of muscle relaxants, anesthetics, and analgesics; referral for physical therapy; reduction of stress; and prescription of therapeutic exercise following resolution of the event. The importance of trigger point therapy for differential diagnosis cannot be overemphasized.

Injections of local anesthetics, injection of saline solution, and dry needling are all effective in treating trigger point pain syn-

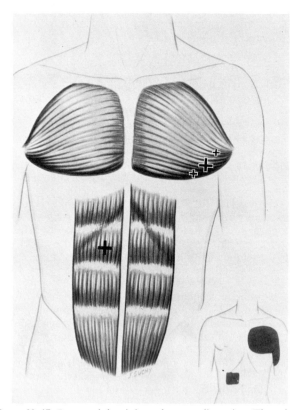

Figure 69–17. Rectus abdominis and pectoralis major. The trigger points are commonly found in all segments of the abdominal rectus muscle, and the pain is usually localized over the involved site of the muscle. The inferior belly of the muscle is a common area of trigger points; however, the entire muscle must be searched diligently. The clavicular portion of this muscle usually refers pain to the uppermost part of the muscle. (From Sola AE: Myofascial trigger point therapy. Resident and Staff Physician 27(8):45, 1981. Reproduced by permission.)

dromes; however, use of local anesthetics is most appropriate when immediate reduction of severe pain is called for.

REFERENCES

1. Skootsky SA, Jaeger B, Oye RK: Prevalence of myofascial pain in general internal medicine practice. West J Med 151:157, 1989.
1a. Bonica JJ: Management of myofascial pain syndromes in general practice. JAMA 164:732, 1957.
2. Cooper AL: Trigger point injection: Its place in physical medicine. Arch Phys Med 43:704, 1961.
3. Simons DG: Muscle pain syndromes: Part I. Am J Phys Med 54:289, 1975.
4. Simons DG: Muscle pain syndromes: Part II. Am J Phys Med 55:15, 1976.
5. Sola AE, Kuitert JH: Quadratus lumborum myofascitis. Northwest Med 53:1003, 1954.
6. Sola AE, Kuitert JH: Myofascial trigger point in the neck and shoulder girdle. Northwest Med 54:980, 1955.
7. Travell J: Myofascial pain syndrome masquerading as temporomandibular joint pain. Oral Surg 43:11, 1977.
8. Travell J: Myofascial trigger points. *In* Advances in Pain Research and Therapy. New York, Raven Press, 1976.
9. Travell J, Rinzler SH: The myofascial genesis of pain. Postgrad Med 11:425, 1952.
10. Melzack R, Stillwell DM, Fox EJ: Trigger points and acupuncture points for pain: Correlations and implications. Pain 3:2, 1977.
11. Lawrence RM: New approach to the treatment of chronic pain: Combination therapy. Am J Acupuncture 6:59, 1978.
12. Gunn CC: Prespondylosis and some pain syndromes following denervation supersensitivity. Spine 5:185, 1980.
13. Gower WR: Lumbago: Its lesions and analogues. Br Med J 1:117, 1904.
14. Llewellyn LJ, Jones AB: Fibrositis. London, Heinemann, 1915.
15. Kraus H: Behandlung akuter Muskelharten. Wien Klin Wochenschr 50:1356, 1937.
16. Sola AE: Myofascial trigger point therapy. Resident and Staff Physician 27:38 August, 1981.
17. Gunn CC: Early and subtle signs in low-back sprain. Spine 3:267, 1978.
18. Edagawa N, Friedmann LW: The Treatment of Disordered Function. Smithtown, NY, Exposition Press, 1981.
19. Fields HL: Pain. New York, McGraw-Hill Book Co, 1987.
20. Sola AE, Williams RL: Myofascial pain syndromes. Neurology 6:91, 1956.
21. Frost FA, Jeason B, Siggaard-Anderson J: A controlled, double-blind comparison of mepivacaine injection versus saline injection for myofascial pain. Lancet 1:499, 1980.
22. Tfelt-Hansen P, et al: Lignocaine versus saline in migraine pain. Lancet 1:1140, 1980.
23. Bray EA, Sigmond H: The local and regional injection treatment of low back pain and sciatica. Ann Intern Med 15:840, 1941.
24. Travell J: Personal correspondence, 1955.
25. Dorigo B, Swintak EF, Schriver WR, et al: Fibrositic myofascial pain in intermittent claudication effect of anesthetic block of trigger points on exercise tolerance. Pain 6:183, 1979.
26. Travell J: Referred pain from skeletal muscle. NY State J Med 55:331, 1955.

Recommended Reading

Travell JG, Simons DG: Myofascial Pain and Dysfunction: The Trigger Point Manual. Baltimore, Williams & Wilkins, 1983.
Sola AE: Upper extremity pain. Wall PD, Melzack R (eds): Textbook of Pain. Edinburgh, Churchill Livingstone, 1990.
Sola AE: Treatment of myofascial pain syndromes. In Benedetti C, et al (eds): Advances in Pain Research. Vol 7. New York, Raven Press, 1984.
Bonica JJ: Management of Pain. 2nd ed. Philadelphia, Lea & Febiger, 1990. Chapters on myofascial pain by AE Sola and JJ Bonica.
Fields HL: Pain. New York, McGraw-Hill Book Co, 1987.

Chapter 70

Injection Therapy of Bursitis and Tendinitis

David H. Neustadt

INTRODUCTION

Bursitis and *tendinitis* are terms frequently used to describe a variety of regional musculoskeletal conditions that are characterized chiefly by pain and disability at the site involved. Bursitis of the shoulder may be considered as the prototypical disorder. All too often in ill-defined regional soft tissue rheumatic problems, the designation *bursitis* or *tendinitis* is used as a "wastebasket" diagnosis. For purposes of this chapter, in consideration of the accurate diagnosis that is necessary to institute appropriate therapy, the terms are reserved for well-defined specific clinical entities.

GENERAL ANATOMIC CONSIDERATIONS OF BURSAE AND TENDON SHEATHS

Bursae are potential spaces or sacs, subcutaneous or deep, that develop in relation to friction and are provided to facilitate the gliding motion of tendons and muscles. There are approximately 78 bursae on each side of the body. These were well described in the classic atlas of anatomy by Monro[1] in 1788 and were later elaborated in greater detail in the atlas of Spalteholz.[2]

The normal bursal wall is lined with a thin layer of synovial cells that appear to be similar to those of joint synovial membrane when examined by electron microscopy.[3] When a bursa becomes subacutely or chronically inflamed, the normally thin surface of sparse cells may become thickened to 1 to 2 mm. The cause of bursitis may be trauma, infection, crystal deposition, chronic friction, or a systemic inflammatory arthropathy. In addition, so-called adventitial bursae may form in response to abnormal shearing stress at sites subjected to chronic pressure, such as the "bunion" over the head of the metatarsal bone of the great toe.

Involvement of the synovial lining of bursae and tendon sheaths may also result from underlying systemic diseases, including rheumatoid arthritis, ankylosing spondylitis, psoriatic arthropathy, and gout. The most common bursal lesions in these systemic inflammatory arthropathies involve the olecranon at the elbow and the trochanter region of the hip. Smaller bursae, especially those around the Achilles tendon, also may be affected.

Septic bursitis usually affects the superficial bursae, such as the olecranon and the prepatellar regions.[4] Factors that predispose to infected bursae include trauma, steroid therapy, uremia, diabetes mellitus, and alcoholism.[5] Tuberculosis may affect any bursa but is rare, whereas other types of mycobacteria, such as *Mycobacterium kansasii*, are occasionally reported.[6] Another uncommon cause of involvement of superficial bursae and tendon sheaths is sporotrichosis, which can be contracted by gardeners and farmers. In addition, tendon sheaths at the hands, the wrists, and the ankles may be affected by acute bacterial infections, such as gonorrhea.

Tendinitis and *tenosynovitis* are useful terms that describe inflammatory reactions in tendons and tendon sheaths. Tendon sheaths are relatively long and tubular, whereas bursae

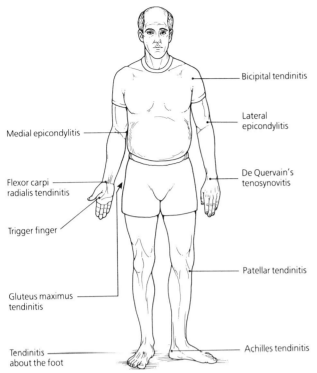

Figure 70–1. Common sites of tendinitis. (From Walker LG, Meals RM: Tendinitis: A practical approach to diagnosis and management. J Musculoskel Med 6(5):24, 1989.)

are round and flat. Except for their shape, however, the structures are similar. Common sites of tendinitis in the body are depicted in Figure 70–1.

Flexor tenosynovitis, ("trigger," or "snapping," finger) is a frequent extra-articular manifestation of rheumatoid arthritis and occasionally may be the presenting symptom.

In *calcareous* (or calcific) tendinitis of the shoulder, there is a calcific deposit in and about one of the rotator cuff tendons (commonly the supraspinatus). The musculotendinous rotator cuff is composed of the supraspinatus, infraspinatus, teres minor, and subscapularis muscles, which insert as the conjoined tendon into the greater tuberosity of the humerus. The bursae in relation to the greater tuberosity and the subdeltoid (subacromial) bursa are the most common sites of calcific deposits. The nidus of the pathologic process is considered to be the calcific deposit (hydroxyapatite) within the substance of one or more of the involved tendons. The process has been likened to a chemical furuncle, or the so-called calcium boil. Calcific tendinitis may be hyperacute or acute, and release of the pressure from the inflammatory edema with rupture into the contiguous bursa (for example, the subacromial bursae) provides prompt relief.

Bursitis and tendinitis embrace a variety of conditions that may be grouped together on a regional basis for the sake of a simple and convenient classification (Table 70–1).

RATIONALE FOR STEROID INJECTIONS

The management of pain resulting from bursitis and tendinitis may be greatly enhanced by the proper selection and administration of local injections. The successful application of local injection and intrasynovial therapy requires an understanding of the diagnosis, accurate localization of the pathologic condition, and the choice of suitable injection

techniques. Not infrequently, injections of lidocaine or corticosteroid preparations provide the additional aid that alone or as an adjunct to the management program overcomes the refractory pain.

Although local injection intrasynovial therapy is essentially palliative, it may provide striking and lasting relief. Restoration of function may follow a single injection, especially in a self-limited painful soft tissue condition. The precise mechanism of the lasting analgesia and the beneficial therapeutic effects have not been clarified. Explanations that have been considered include induction of local hyperemia, relaxation of reflex muscle spasm, generalized response from systemic absorption, pain relief allowing controlled activity or rest, favorable influence on local tissue metabolism, and mechanical benefit. The increased mobility permitted as a result of pain relief certainly accelerates recovery and restoration of function. Finally, the "power of suggestion" of the needle must not be underestimated (placebo therapy). Some observers believe the pain relief may result from stimulation and release of the patient's endorphins.

Some physicians prefer to follow local injection with a short course of salicylates, oral corticosteroids, or nonsteroidal anti-inflammatory medications. Others prefer to prescribe simple analgesics and to evaluate the response to injection. Cases must be individualized according to the specific pathologic condition and patient variables.

INDICATIONS FOR AND CONTRAINDICATIONS TO INJECTION THERAPY

Local injection therapy with corticosteroids or local anesthetics may provide valuable aid in a variety of acute or subacute bursitides and other painful soft tissue conditions. Abolition of symptoms would confirm the localization of the involved site or structure even if the response were not lasting. Visceral disease must be ruled out as a source of referred pain. Appropriate injection therapy is indicated when there are local accessible signs that are likely to respond to direct therapeutic infiltration. Acute localized bursitis or tendinitis warrants immediate direct injection for rapid relief.[7, 8]

Contraindications are relative and include infections, either local or in the vicinity of the site of involvement, and hypersensitivity to any preparation or substance that might be injected. The procedure is also contraindicated in patients receiving anticoagulants or those with any bleeding disorder.

Table 70–1 *Classification of Bursitis and Tendinitis (Regional)*

Upper Extremity Disorders
Elbow
　Radiohumeral bursitis, olecranon bursitis, epicondylitis
Shoulder
　Bicipital tendinitis, calcareous tendinitis (subacromial, subdeltoid bursitis), rotator cuff tendinitis
Wrist and Hand
　Stenosing tenosynovitis ("trigger" finger syndrome), de Quervain syndrome
Lower Extremity Disorders
Hip
　Trochanteric bursitis, ischiogluteal bursitis
Knee
　Prepatellar, suprapatellar, and anserine bursitis
Ankle, Foot, and Heel
　Ankle tendinitis, bunion bursitis, calcaneal bursitis (with heel spur)

The patient with a preexisting tendon injury may be subject to tendon rupture that can inhibit full activity when the corticosteroid injection removes pain. Hence, partial tendon rupture is a relative contraindication.[9] Poorly motivated "needle-shy" and severely neurotic patients obviously are considered poor subjects for this type of treatment. Active herpes simplex infection and tuberculosis are generally considered contraindications.

HAZARDS AND COMPLICATIONS

Local anesthetics are often mixed with a corticosteroid preparation to increase volume, to decrease postinjection pain, and to assess the accuracy of the injection. Local anesthetics may also be used before injection of the corticosteroid. The major hazards in the use of local anesthetics are hypersensitivity and accidental intravenous or intra-arterial introduction. Serious (possibly even fatal) hypersensitivity to procaine and other regional anesthetic compounds is encountered very rarely; the possibility is usually suggested by a history of previous reactions. Lidocaine or one of the newer "caine" derivatives may be used to avoid sensitivity reactions to procaine. If a past history of a reaction is suggested, one should proceed cautiously and use small dilute anesthetic solutions. When there is a definite history of sensitivity, it is wise to avoid the use of anesthetic agents during injection therapy.

In the event of accidental intravenous injection of a "caine" drug or if symptoms of hypersensitivity arise from these compounds (a significant slowing of the pulse rate, or even a seizure, is an indication of a major reaction to intravenous administration), one of the soluble barbiturate preparations, such as sodium pentothal or the anticonvulsant diazepam, should be readily available and should be given promptly in accordance with the reaction and response. In addition, a clear airway should be maintained and oxygen should be administered.[10] Severe reactions from accidental vascular injection of these drugs in the doses usually given are very rare.

A repository corticosteroid given intravenously by accident has been reported but has not been observed by us.[11] To my knowledge, no serious reaction to a depot corticosteroid preparation given intravenously has been reported. The possibility of an allergic reaction caused by corticosteroids is highly unlikely. A report, however, has described an unusual skin rash following an intra-articular methylprednisolone injection that appears to be consistent with a delayed type of hypersensitivity.[12]

Minor reactions occasionally seen after injection of "caine" preparations include lightheadedness or dizziness, pallor, weakness, sweating, nausea, and (rarely) fainting and tachycardia. These symptoms usually disappear within a few minutes after the injection and rarely require any treatment except reassurance and a cold compress to the forehead of the patient. Often it is difficult to decide whether the symptoms are the result of sensitivity to the drug or a fright reaction (vasovagal). The patient should always be supine, prone, or seated in a reclining position during the injection to minimize the effect of any vasovagal reaction.

The obvious precautions against entering a blood vessel are for the physician to be aware of the local anatomy and to aspirate after every 1 to 2 ml of solution is injected. Penetration into or striking a nerve may cause sharp pain or paresthesias, and the patient should be warned of this possibility in advance.

Complications are listed in Table 70–2. Although the possibility of introducing infection is the most serious potential complication, in a review of our extensive experience

Table 70–2. **Complications of Injection Therapy**
Infection
Postinjection flare
After-pain
Bleeding (local)
Cutaneous atrophy (local)
Tendon rupture

and that of others we have found that infections occurring as an aftermath of intrasynovial injections are extremely rare.[13–16] I do not recommend routine prophylactic antibiotic administration unless the patient has had a significant recent systemic infection. Although with meticulous attention to aseptic technique the problem of infection is usually avoided, the patient should be cautioned to report the development of any significant pain, redness, or swelling after any local injection.

Local undesirable reactions are usually minor and reversible. A postinjection "flare" may begin within a few hours after steroid injection and usually tends to subside spontaneously in up to 24 hours. Rarely, it can continue for as long as 72 hours. This transient increase in inflammation is considered to represent a true "crystal-induced synovitis" caused by precipitation of the microcrystalline steroid ester suspension.[17] Usually, the reaction is mild and adequately controlled with application of ice or cold compresses and analgesics as needed. Rarely, "after-pain" lasting for a few to several hours may occur following injections. Although the cause is obscure, this phenomenon may result from the trauma of needle insertion, penetration of inflamed tissue, or pressure on adjacent nerves from local swelling or bleeding. After-pain usually is relieved by application of moist or dry heat and analgesics until the pain abates but is best handled by mixing a long-acting anesthetic, such as bupivacaine, with the steroid preparation.

Occasional subcutaneous bleeding at the site of injection may occur with penetration of a venule, an arteriole, or a capillary. The patient should be warned that this may occur and should be reassured that the discoloration or hematoma will disappear spontaneously. Ice packs or cold compresses to the involved area for the first 24 hours are commonly advised.

Another relatively minor complication is localized subcutaneous or cutaneous atrophy at the site of the injection.[8, 18] This problem is chiefly of cosmetic concern and is recognized as a small depression in the skin frequently associated with depigmentation, transparency, and, occasionally, the formation of telangiectasia. These changes in the skin occur when injections are made near the surface and some of the injected steroid leaks back along the needle track. The depression usually recedes and the skin returns to normal with time when the crystals of the steroid have been completely absorbed. Careful technique (avoiding the leaking of the steroid suspension to the skin surface) prevents this complication. A small amount of lidocaine or normal saline can be used to flush the needle of the suspension before removal of the needle.

The potential danger of "spontaneous" tendon rupture (especially of Achilles tendons) following local corticosteroid injections in the Achilles bursal area must be given serious consideration. Cautious administration with infiltrations around and beneath the tendons to keep any of the material from entering the substance of the tendon minimizes the occurrence of this complication.[9, 19] In general, *the injection of major stress-bearing tendons,* such as the Achilles and patellar tendons, *should be avoided in the emergency department.* Treat-

Table 70–3. Injectable Corticosteroids

Intrasynovial Preparations	Trade Name	Strength per ml	Range of Usual Dosage
Hydrocortisone tebutate	Hydrocortisone TBA	50 mg	12.5–75 mg
Prednisolone tebutate	Hydeltra TBA	20 mg	5.0–30 mg
Methylprednisolone acetate	Depo-Medrol*	20 mg	4.0–30 mg
Triamcinolone acetonide	Kenalog-40	40 mg	4.0–40 mg
Triamcinolone diacetate	Aristocort Forte	40 mg	4.0–40 mg
Triamcinolone hexacetonide	Aristospan	20 mg	4.0–25 mg
Betamethasone acetate and disodium phosphatate	Celestone Soluspan	6 mg†	1.5–6.0 mg
Dexamethasone acetate	Decadron-La	8 mg	0.8–4.0 mg

*Supplied in 20 mg per ml, 40 mg per ml, and 80 mg per ml preparations.
†Available as 3 mg acetate, 3 mg phosphate.

ment with oral anti-inflammatory medications and splinting is preferred.

AVAILABLE PREPARATIONS AND CHOICE OF COMPOUND

Hydrocortisone and a variety of available corticosteroid repository preparations are described in Table 70–3. Local anesthetics, such as lidocaine or bupivacaine, can be mixed with the corticosteroid preparation in the same syringe. All corticosteroid suspensions, with the exception of cortisone and prednisone, can produce a significant and rapid anti-inflammatory effect (in synovial spaces). Unfortunately, soluble corticosteroids are absorbed and dispersed too rapidly, having only a brief duration of action locally. The tertiary butyl acetate (TBA) ester prolongs the duration of local tissue effect because of decreased solubility. The decreased solubility probably causes dissociation of the corticosteroid by enzymes to proceed at a delayed rate.

No single steroid agent has demonstrated a convincing margin of superiority, with the exception of triamcinolone hexacetonide.[20, 21] Prednisolone tebutate, however, simply by virtue of price advantage and long-term usage, is generally the drug of choice. Triamcinolone hexacetonide is the least water-soluble preparation currently available. Triamcinolone hexacetonide is two and one half times less soluble in water than prednisolone tebutate, providing the longest duration of action. There is minimal systemic absorption, or "spillover," with this preparation, but because of its high potency and higher cost it is usually reserved for use in conditions in which prednisolone tebutate or one of the other compounds has shown an inadequate response.

DOSAGE AND ADMINISTRATION

The dose of any corticosteroid suspension used for intrasynovial injection must be arbitrarily selected. Factors that influence the dosage and expected response include the size of the affected area, the presence or absence of synovial fluid or edema, the severity and extent of any synovitis, and the steroid preparation selected for injection.

A useful guideline for estimating dosage follows: For relatively large spaces, such as subacromial, olecranon, and trochanteric bursae, 20 to 30 mg of prednisolone tebutate or equivalent; for medium- or intermediate-sized bursae and ganglia formation at the wrists, the knees, and the heels, 10 to 20 mg; for tendon sheaths, such as flexor tenosynovitis of digits and the abductor tendon of the thumb (de Quervain disease), 5 to 15 mg. Sometimes it may be necessary to give larger doses for optimal response. Intrabursal therapy of the elbow (olecranon) or knee (prepatellar) bursae containing considerable fluid may require 30- to 40-mg doses.

Unlike intra-articular injections for synovitis in chronic joint disease, repeat infiltrations for soft tissue conditions, such as bursitis and tendinitis, frequently are not required. If only a partial response occurs or if recurrence develops, however, a single repeat injection can be given; the length of the interval between injections should not be a source of undue concern. In contrast with intra-articular injections, in which the hazard of "overworking" an injected joint is usually not a problem, following intrasynovial injection we recommend a reduction in activity with rest or splinting of the involved extremity. Limiting motion also delays somewhat the systemic absorption of the steroid. Anecdotal evidence suggests that those patients with inflammatory soft tissue lesions who follow a postinjection modified rest regimen obtain a more rapid and lasting resolution of the painful disorder. Frequency of injections is considered further in the discussion of techniques for the specific entities.

PREPARATION OF THE SITE

Preparation of the site before injection requires meticulous adherence to aseptic technique. Anatomic "landmarks" are outlined with a black or red skin pencil. Tincture of iodine or Merthiolate applied with a sterile swab can be used in place of the skin pencil. The point of entry is cleansed with povidone-iodine (Betadine) and alcohol. Sterile drapes and gloves are not generally considered necessary, especially after sufficient skill and experience with the procedure has been acquired.

TECHNIQUES

General Considerations

Materials required for local injection procedures include needles, syringes, and items for preparation of the injection site. Disposable needles and syringes are convenient and adequate for emergency department use. Special trays may also be stocked for this purpose. The usual sizes of needles for various approaches are as follows:

Intracutaneous skin wheal	0.5 inch, 25 gauge
Tendinitis in elbow and shoulder inflammation	1.5 to 2.0 inches, 22 or 25 gauge
Digital tenosynovitis	7⁄8 inch, 25 gauge
Bursitis with fluid	1.0 to 1.5 inches, 20 gauge
Deep gluteal bursitis	3.0 to 4.0 inches, 20 gauge

Table 70–4. A Guide for Needle Size and Dosage for Injection of Common Regional Disorders

Disorder or Injection Site	Needle Size	Usual Dosage of Prednisolone Tebutate
Bicipital tendinitis	1.5–2.0 inches, 22–23 gauge	20–30 mg
Calcareous tendinitis / Subacromial bursitis	1.5–2.0 inches, 22–23 gauge	20–40 mg
Radiohumeral bursitis / Epicondylitis	1.5 inch, 22–23 gauge	20–30 mg
Olecranon bursitis	1.0–1.5 inches, 20 gauge	15–30 mg
Ganglia on wrist	1.0 inch, 18–20 gauge	10–15 mg
de Quervain syndrome	7/8 inch, 22–23 gauge	10–20 mg
Carpal tunnel syndrome	1.0–1.5 inches, 22 gauge	20–40 mg
Digital flexor tenosynovitis	7/8 inch, 22–23 gauge	5 mg
Trochanteric bursitis	1.5–2.0 inches, 22–23 gauge	20–40 mg
Prepatellar bursitis	1.0–1.5 inches, 22–23 gauge	15–20 mg
Anserine bursitis	1.0–1.5 inches, 22–23 gauge	20–40 mg
Bunion bursitis	1.0 inch, 22 gauge	5–10 mg
Calcaneal bursitis	1.0 inch, 22–23 gauge	10–20 mg

Table 70–4 lists appropriately sized needles for various injection sites.

Once the point of entry has been determined and the site is prepared, either a superficial skin wheal is made with 1 per cent lidocaine (Xylocaine) or 0.25 per cent bupivacaine (Marcaine, Sensoricaine) or the skin is sprayed with a refrigerant, such as Frigiderm. Some physicians do not use a skin wheal when the steroid is mixed with a rapid-acting local anesthetic. Ordinarily, preanesthesia is not necessary, but occasionally in highly nervous or agitated individuals, it may be advisable to give narcotics or benzodiazepines intravenously, or to administer a nitrous oxide–oxygen mixture before beginning the procedure. Thus an anxiety-provoking injection can be carried out with patient cooperation.

Local injections can be administered with corticosteroids and local anesthetics mixed together in the same syringe, or the local anesthetic can be given alone. Generally, when injecting synovial spaces the steroid is introduced without anesthetic, but often syringes are changed and lidocaine is used to flush out the needle, frequently injecting and depositing several milliliters of the local anesthetic. When injecting a painful soft tissue structure directly, it is best to administer a mixture of corticosteroid and anesthetic. This both relieves pain immediately and confirms the accuracy of the injection. The duration of action of lidocaine is approximately 100 minutes, whereas bupivacaine may last for a few hours. The patient should be cautioned that the local anesthetic effect may "wear off" within a couple of hours and that the beneficial effects of the corticosteroid may be delayed.

The most important aspect of a successful technique is accurate positioning of the needle. The needle must "hit the mark" or the results are disappointing. Injecting an inflamed synovial space, such as a bursitis-containing fluid, may be as simple as puncturing a balloon. Aspiration of the fluid confirms that the needle has correctly entered the sac. On the other hand, injecting directly into a painful soft tissue lesion requires additional skill that can be acquired only with experience. When a bursa is injected, as much fluid as possible is aspirated before instillation of the corticosteroid suspension to reduce the dilution factor. Sometimes it is advisable to reaspirate and reinject several times within the barrel of the syringe, so-called *barbotage*, to obtain heterogeneous mixing and maximal dispersion of the steroid throughout the synovial cavity.

Specific Regions and Clinical Entities

Table 70–1 and Figure 70–1 list the areas of involvement by region. In addition, certain nonarticular disorders that may require local injection are included.

UPPER EXTREMITY REGIONS

The Shoulder Region. Pain associated with disability may result from any of the intrinsic shoulder disorders, including bicipital tendinitis, calcareous tendinitis, and subacromial bursitis (Fig. 70–2). These areas are frequently injected because of the consistently good response to therapy and the danger of persistent inflammation resulting in a "frozen shoulder."

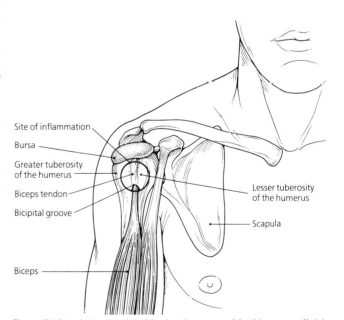

Figure 70–2. Pain in the shoulder is often caused by biceps tendinitis or subacromial bursitis. (From Walker LG, Meals RM: Tendinitis: A practical approach to diagnosis and management. J Musculoskel Med 6(5):24, 1989.)

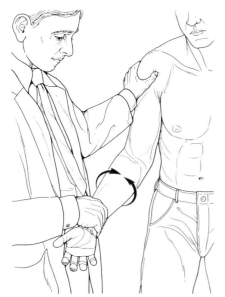

Figure 70–3. The Yergason test helps determine the stability of the long head of the biceps tendon in the bicipital groove. This test, which involves resisted supination of the forearm with the elbow flexed to 90 degrees, may accurately reproduce symptoms of bicipital tendinitis. (From Walker LG, Meals RM: Tendinitis: A practical approach to diagnosis and management. J Musculoskel Med 6(5):24, 1989.)

Bicipital Tendinitis (Tenosynovitis). This is a nonspecific low-grade inflammation or irritation of the long head of the biceps tendon sheath.[22] The tendon courses through the joint and along the bicipital (intertubercular) groove. Pain at the shoulder is accompanied by restricted motion and disturbed scapulohumeral rhythm. Efforts to elevate the shoulder, reach the hip pocket, or pull a back zipper all aggravate the symptoms. "Rolling" the bicipital tendon produces localized tenderness (Lipman test), and the Yergason test may be positive. The Yergason test elicits pain along the bicipital groove when the patient attempts supination of the forearm against resistance, holding the elbow flexed at a 90-degree angle against the side of the body (Fig. 70–3). Radiographs are normal.

TECHNIQUE. The point of maximal tenderness of the bicipital tendon is located. Entry is made with a 22- or 25-gauge, 1.5- to 2.0-inch needle through a lidocaine skin wheal (Fig. 70–4). The needle is brought in along the side of the tendon aimed at one border of the bicipital groove to give a peritendinous infiltration. One third of the injection is administered at this point. The needle is then withdrawn slightly but is kept subcutaneous. It is redirected upward approximately 1 inch for another one third of the injection, withdrawn again, and redirected downward, touching the bicipital border gently; the remainder of the drug is deposited at this point. Usually the corticosteroid suspension, 1 to 1.5 ml of prednisolone tebutate, is instilled at the maximum area of tenderness and the lidocaine is injected along the upper and lower borders of the tendon. Two to four repeat injections may be required at 1- to 2-week intervals.

Calcareous Tendinitis, Supraspinatus Tendinitis, and Subacromial Bursitis. These inflammations are so similar that their symptoms and signs are difficult to distinguish. The acute irritative inflammation of the bursa is a secondary reaction produced by the calcific tendinitis of the supraspinatus or one of the other rotator cuff tendons. After the calcific material ruptures into the subdeltoid bursa, spontaneous relief usually is obtained within a few days. During the acute or hyperacute stage, the patient holds the arm in a protective fashion against the chest wall. Pain may be incapacitating, and all ranges of motion are disturbed, with internal rotation markedly limited. Tenderness is often diffuse over the perihumeral region. Constitutional symptoms are rare, but sometimes in the hyperacute form actual swelling may be visible, and even fever and an accelerated sedimentation rate may develop. When shoulder radiographs demonstrate a calcific deposit, the shadow appears "hazy" with lightening of the periphery caused by the pres-

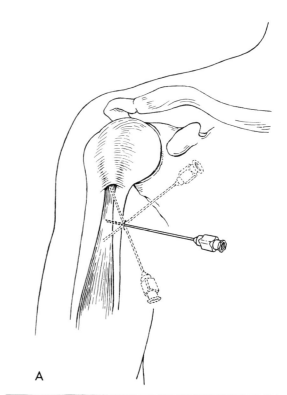

A

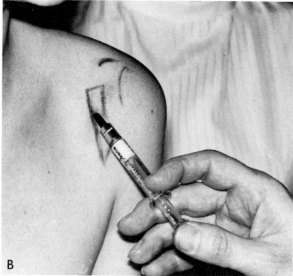

B

Figure 70–4. *A,* Fan-wise method of infiltration of bicipital tendon sheath. *B,* Actual injection of bicipital tendinitis: patient seated with arm in lap and externally rotated. (From Steinbrocker O, Neustadt DH: Aspiration and Injection Therapy in Arthritis and Musculoskeletal Disorders: A Handbook on Technique and Management. Hagerstown, Md, Harper & Row, 1972. Reproduced by permission.)

sure of inflammatory edema. Night pain may be intolerable, requiring narcotics for control.

TECHNIQUE (ANTERIOR APPROACH). In calcific tendinitis or supraspinatus tendinitis without calcification, the injection is given by the anterior (subcoracoid) or lateral approach, below the acromion (Fig. 70–5). If the tenderness is not localized, a point is selected over the depression that is palpable between the anterolateral or anteromedial border of the acromion and the head of the humerus.

ANOTHER TECHNIQUE (POSTERIOR APPROACH). With the patient sitting and the lower part of the extremity resting on the lap, a lidocaine skin wheal is made at a posterolateral point under the acromion. A 1.5- to 2.0-inch, 22- or 21-gauge needle is then directed toward the center of the head of the humerus upward at an angle of approximately 10 degrees. After the site has been penetrated 0.75 to 1.25 inches, aspiration is carried out for any fluid or calcific material. The syringe is then removed, leaving the needle in position. Another syringe containing 20 to 40 mg of prednisolone suspension or equivalent is attached, and the medication is instilled. This injection can be followed with 1 to 5 ml of 1 per cent lidocaine, or 1 to 2 ml of lidocaine can be given combined with the steroid in the same syringe. A single treatment relieves the majority of acute disorders, but occasionally it may have to be repeated once or twice.

Sometimes a painful reaction may follow when the analgesic has worn off. To avoid severe pain the patient

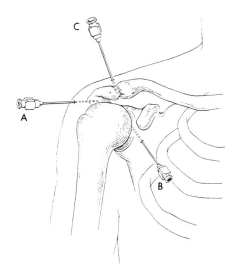

Figure 70–6. Injections at the shoulder. *A*, Lateral approach to the subacromial bursa or supraspinatus tendon. *B*, Anterior approach to the glenohumeral joint (see Chapter 71). *C*, Approach to the acromioclavicular joint. (From Steinbrocker O, Neustadt DH: Aspiration and Injection Therapy in Arthritis and Musculoskeletal Disorders: A Handbook on Technique and Management. Hagerstown, Md, Harper & Row, 1972. Reproduced by permission.)

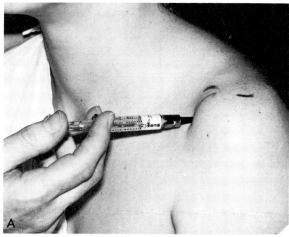

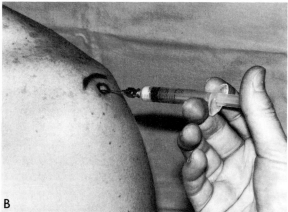

Figure 70–5. *A*, Anterior approach to subacromial bursa or supraspinatus tendon. *B*, Lateral approach to subacromial bursa or supraspinatus tendon. (From Steinbrocker O, Neustadt DH: Aspiration and Injection Therapy in Arthritis and Musculoskeletal Disorders: A Handbook on Technique and Management. Hagerstown, Md, Harper & Row, 1972. Reproduced by permission.)

should be warned about this possibility and given appropriate analgesia.

Acromioclavicular Joint Inflammation. Pain arising in the acromioclavicular joint is frequently an aftermath of an acute injury. With this injury, all ranges of motion of the shoulder cause pain, and the joint is tender and rarely swollen.

TECHNIQUE. Entry is made through a cutaneous lidocaine wheal over the interosseous groove at the point of greatest tenderness (Fig. 70–6). The joint line is relatively superficial, and a ⅞-inch or 1-inch, 22- or 25-gauge needle is adequate. One to 1.5 ml of lidocaine and 5 to 10 mg of a prednisolone suspension are injected. It is not necessary to advance the needle beyond the proximal margin of the joint surface.

The Elbow Region. The elbow is subject to frequently occurring characteristic extra-articular disorders. These include radiohumeral bursitis, epicondylitis ("tennis" and "golfer's" elbow), and olecranon bursitis ("barfly's" elbow).

Radiohumeral Bursitis. This occurs at the juncture of the radial head and the lateral epicondyle of the elbow. Radiohumeral bursitis is commonly found in combination with lateral epicondylitis. The symptoms of the two adjacent problems are indistinguishable, but tenderness in bursitis overlies the site of the radiohumeral groove, whereas tenderness in tennis elbow occurs chiefly at the lateral epicondyle (Fig. 70–7). A clinical sign supporting the diagnosis of tennis elbow is the provocation of pain when the patient attempts elevation of the middle finger against resistance with the wrist and the elbow held in extension.

TECHNIQUE. The entry site is the point of maximal tenderness, usually found at a point slightly distal to the lateral epicondyle. The radial head can be palpated and confirmed by rotation of the patient's forearm (Fig. 70–8). The injection enters through a skin wheal with a 1.5-inch, 22-gauge needle, depositing 20 to 30 mg of prednisolone mixed with lidocaine. Alternatively, the steroid is followed with 1 to 3 ml of the local anesthetic. Part of the repository preparation may be instilled into the radiohumeral bursa and part at the lateral epicondyle (Fig. 70–9). Generally, it

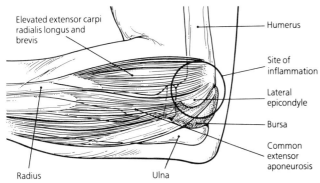

Figure 70–7. Lateral epicondylitis—commonly known as "tennis elbow"—is the result of microscopic rupture and incomplete tendinous repair of the extensor carpi radialis brevis origin on the lateral epicondyle of the humerus. Pain usually occurs over the lateral humeral epicondyle during work or recreation. (From Walker LG, Meals RM: Tendinitis. A practical approach to diagnosis and management. J Musculoskel Med 6(5):24, 1989.)

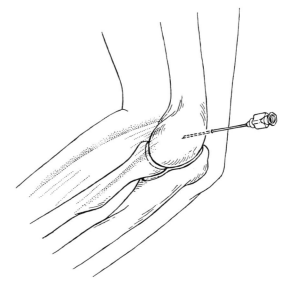

Figure 70–9. Injection at lateral epicondyle. (Redrawn from Steinbrocker O, Neustadt DH: Aspiration and Injection Therapy in Arthritis and Musculoskeletal Disorders: A Handbook on Technique and Management. Hagerstown, Md, Harper & Row, 1972. Reproduced by permission.)

is wise to limit repeat injection attempts to two or three. In medial epicondylitis (golfer's elbow), a similar technique can be used, but it is important to remember to avoid the ulnar nerve, which lies in a groove behind the medial epicondyle.

Olecranon Bursitis. "Student's" elbow, or "miner's beat" elbow, is a common condition that is frequently idiopathic or provoked by minor trauma (Fig. 70–10).[4, 23] The bursa also can be involved in rheumatoid arthritis and gout. Although most cases of olecranon bursitis are sterile, the olecranon bursa is the most frequent site of septic bursitis. The diagnosis of olecranon bursitis is obvious when the elbow is inspected and examined during flexion and extension. Occasionally in rheumatoid arthritis and gout, nodules, or tophi, may be readily palpated within the bursal sac. The olecranon bursa that is most commonly involved lies between the skin and the olecranon process. Motion at the elbow joint remains complete and painless unless there is also "true" elbow joint involvement. Olecranon bursitis is both-

ersome to the patient but often does not cause discomfort and may resolve spontaneously unless there has been bleeding into the bursa or the effusion is extremely tense. When the bursa is large and subject to trauma or is tender and inflamed, provided that infection is excluded, aspiration and a steroid injection will expedite resolution (Fig. 70–11). Smith and associates demonstrated the superiority of intrabursal methylprednisolone acetate over oral naproxen or placebo at 6 months, noting faster resolution and less reaccumulation of fluid with the steroid injection.[24] The addition of a nonsteroidal drug after steroid injection did not affect the outcome. Aspiration without injection is often followed by recurrence in a few days or weeks.

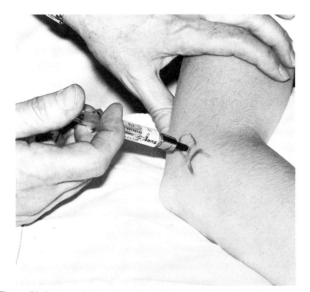

Figure 70–8. Actual injection of radiohumeral bursitis. (From Steinbrocker O, Neustadt DH: Aspiration and Injection Therapy in Arthritis and Musculoskeletal Disorders: A Handbook on Technique and Management. Hagerstown, Md, Harper & Row, 1972. Reproduced by permission.)

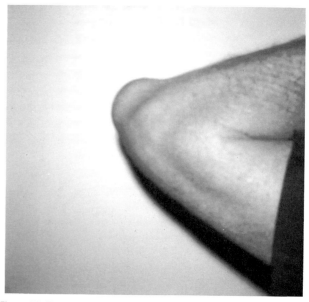

Figure 70–10. Atraumatic painless swelling over the elbow, characteristic of nonseptic olecranon bursitis. This mass is soft and fluctuant, usually filled with a serosanguinous fluid. Initial treatment includes aspiration with sterile technique; if infection can be ruled out clinically, injection with a corticosteroid is indicated.

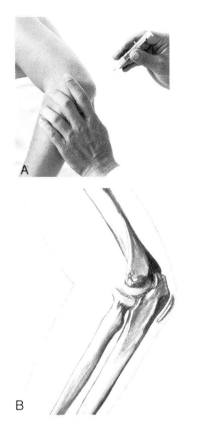

Figure 70–11. Procedure for draining olecranon bursitis.

Fluid may be aspirated for analysis and culture to help distinguish a noninflammatory process from an inflammatory or septic bursitis. Clear or serosanguineous fluid is seen with a sterile bursitis, whereas cloudy fluid should suggest a septic process. It is usually easy to detect a septic bursitis by physical examination. The bursal area is red, hot, swollen, and painful. Fever and leukocytosis are not generally sensitive or specific findings. Smith and associates reported that the surface temperature of the skin overlying the olecranon bursa may be a very sensitive and specific indicator that can differentiate septic from nonseptic cases.[25] In their study, using an electronic temperature probe attached to the skin, the mean temperature difference uniformly between the affected and contralateral elbow was 3.7° C (2.2° C or greater) in cases of septic olecranon bursitis versus 0.7° C in nonseptic bursitis. This finding (sensitivity 100 per cent, specificity 94 per cent) was more helpful than bursal fluid leukocyte count, cell differential, or Gram stain. This study suggests a possible role for the recently marketed infrared thermometer that detects surface temperatures.

Initial treatment of a septic bursitis includes aspiration of all fluid, appropriate culturing, and antibiotic therapy. Corticosteroid injections should not be used for cases of clinically apparent septic bursitis.[26] Antibiotics directed against penicillin-resistant *Staphylococcus aureus* are indicated, either orally or parenterally dependent on the extent of infection. In frank septic bursitis, especially with thickening of the bursal wall or cases resistant to antibiotic therapy, open incision with drainage may be required, with possible subsequent excision of the bursa. Rarely, acute gout or a cholesterol crystal synovitis develops, and this may mimic a suppurative bursitis.

TECHNIQUE. A 1.0- to 1.5-inch, 20-gauge needle is introduced at a dependent aspect of the bursal sac through a skin wheal, Frigiderm spray, or unanesthetized skin. After

all the fluid is aspirated, 15 to 30 mg of prednisolone tebutate or equivalent preparation is injected. The elbow is wrapped with an elastic compression bandage for 5 to 7 days following aspiration and injection. If infected or inspissated fluid is anticipated, a 16- to 18-gauge needle may be necessary for aspiration of the viscous contents.

The Wrist and Hand

Ganglia. These are cystic swellings occurring frequently on the hands and the feet, especially on the dorsal aspect of the wrist. The cystic structures are attached or may arise from tendon sheaths or near the joint capsule. They contain a clear gelatinous or mucoid fluid of great density. The material in the cyst may sometimes represent almost pure hyaluronic acid. Spontaneous regression is common. When the ganglion is painful or tender, aspiration with a 1-inch, relatively large-gauge needle (17 to 18 gauge) and introduction of 10 to 15 mg of corticosteroid suspension is generally a satisfactory approach. Surgical excision may become necessary if this technique is unsuccessful.

de Quervain Disease. This disease is a stenosing tenosynovitis of the short extensor (extensor pollicis brevis) and long abductor tendon (abductor pollicis longus) of the thumb. Although occasionally associated with rheumatoid arthritis, the disorder more often occurs following repetitive use of the wrist, especially with a wringing motion. The syndrome has been called "washerwoman's sprain." Tenderness and, occasionally, palpable crepitation is elicited just distal to the radial styloid process. A useful specific clinical examination is the Finkelstein test (Fig. 70–12). The test is conducted by adducting the patient's thumb into the palm of the hand and folding the fingers over the thumb. Forcible ulnar deviation at the wrist is then carried out, provoking severe pain at the site of the affected tendon sheaths when the test is positive. It should be noted that gonococcal tenosynovitis of the wrist may mimic de Quervain disease.

TECHNIQUE. A ⅞-inch, 25-gauge needle is introduced at the most tender point (just distal to the radial styloid) through a skin wheal, and 10 to 20 mg of prednisolone suspension is deposited in the tendon sheath with or followed

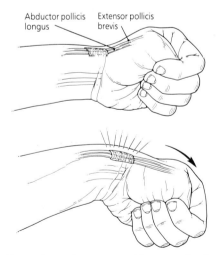

Figure 70–12. De Quervain tenosynovitis occurs in the first dorsal compartment of the wrist secondary to tenosynovitis of the abductor pollicis longus and extensor pollicis brevis tendons. Symptoms, which include pain over the radial styloid, are generally caused by overuse. The Finkelstein test is positive when pain is reproduced by ulnar deviation of the wrist while the patient grasps the thumb with the fingers. (From Walker LG, Meals RM: Tendinitis: A practical approach to diagnosis and management. J Musculoskel Med 6(5):24, 1989.)

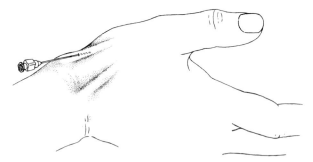

Figure 70–13. Injection of abductor tendon sheath (de Quervain disease). (From Steinbrocker O, Neustadt DH: Aspiration and Injection Therapy in Arthritis and Musculoskeletal Disorders: A Handbook on Technique and Management. Hagerstown, Md, Harper & Row, 1972. Reproduced by permission.)

by lidocaine (Fig. 70–13). The injection may be repeated one or two times at 7- to 14-day intervals if needed. A lightweight splint for wrist support and protection may be used at night for several weeks after the injection.

Carpal Tunnel Syndrome. Carpal tunnel syndrome is a common nerve entrapment caused by median nerve compression. It is characterized by pain at the wrist that sometimes radiates upward into the forearm and is associated with tingling and paresthesias of the palmar side of the index and middle fingers and the radial half of the ring finger. Typically, the patient wakes during the night with burning or aching pain, numbness, and tingling and shakes the hand outside the bed in order to try to obtain relief and restore sensation. Occasionally the discomfort is extremely severe, causing the patient to seek emergency aid. Clinical signs supporting the diagnosis include a positive Tinel sign, in which one reproduces the tingling and paresthesias by tapping (with a reflex hammer) over the median nerve at the volar crease of the wrist.[27] Additionally, one can perform wrist flexion maneuvers (Phalen sign) in an effort to provoke the symptoms in the median nerve distribution.[28] Severe muscle atrophy of the thenar eminence may develop in advanced or neglected cases. Causes of carpal tunnel syndrome include rheumatoid arthritis (sometimes as the presenting manifestation), pregnancy, hypothyroidism, diabetes, and acromegaly, but in many cases the disturbance is idiopathic without a recognizable underlying cause.

TECHNIQUE. When injecting the carpal canal, one should insert the needle through a skin wheal at a site just medial or ulnar to the palmaris longus tendon and proximal to the distal crease at the wrist (Fig. 70–14). Injecting medial to the palmaris longus is preferred because it avoids direct injection of the median nerve and superficial veins. A 1.0- to 1.5-inch, 22-gauge needle is directed at an angle of approximately 60 degrees to the skin surface, pointing toward the palm. The needle is advanced 1 to 2 cm, and 20 to 40 mg of prednisolone suspension with or without lidocaine is injected along the track and into the tissue space. Up to 2 weeks may be required for the symptoms to abate significantly. A lightweight wrist splint may hasten recovery. Repeat injections may be given, but if response is not successful or lasting after two or three injections, decompressive surgery should be considered. Nerve compression should be confirmed by nerve conduction studies before surgery.[29]

Digital Flexor Tenosynovitis. A "trigger," or "snapping," finger is characterized by a stenosed tendon sheath on the palmar surface over the base of the metacarpal head. Tenderness is usually confined to this site. The area of stenosis leads to intermittent catching of the enclosed tendon. Lock-

ing occurs when the offending digit is in flexion and is especially bothersome when the patient awakens in the morning. The common causes are trauma and rheumatoid arthritis. A nodule or fibrinous deposit may form at a point in the tendon sheath at the site where the snapping occurs.

TECHNIQUE. The technique for injecting flexor tenosynovitis includes locating and marking the tendon point at the involved metacarpal base and instilling 0.25 ml of any corticosteroid suspension subcutaneously with a ⅞-inch, 25-gauge needle into the involved tendon sheath (Fig. 70–15). Frigiderm can be used to numb the skin before entry of the needle. Resistance should not be encountered on injecting. Similar injections can be administered to the base of the thumb metacarpal for a "snapping" thumb. Up to four

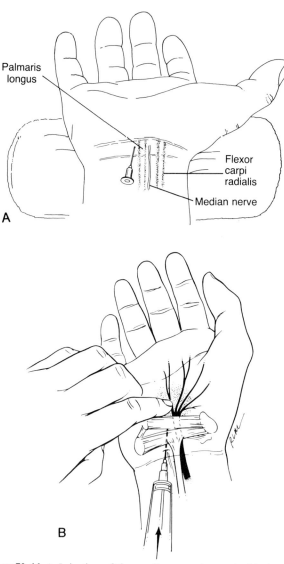

Figure 70–14. *A,* Injection of the median carpal tunnel with the wrist dorsiflexed over a rolled towel. To avoid direct injection of the median nerve, the needle is introduced just medial (ulnar) to the palmaris longus tendon. (Redrawn from Steinbrocker O, and Neustadt DH: Aspiration and Injection Therapy in Arthritis and Musculoskeletal Disorders: A Handbook on Technique and Management. Hagerstown, Md, Harper & Row, 1972. Reproduced by permission.) *B,* A palpable bulge at the distal edge of this ligament indicates correct placement of the injection. Direct injection into the median or ulnar nerve is to be avoided. (From Dehaan MR, Wilson RL: Diagnosis and management of carpal tunnel syndrome. J Musculoskel Med 6(2):47, 1989.)

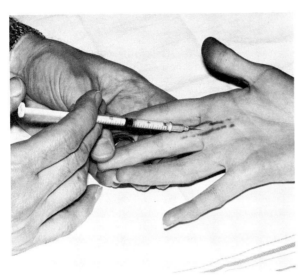

Figure 70–15. Injection of flexor tendon sheath in digital tenosynovitis. (From Steinbrocker O, Neustadt DH: Aspiration and Injection Therapy in Arthritis and Musculoskeletal Disorders: A Handbook on Technique and Management. Hagerstown, Md, Harper & Row, 1972. Reproduced by permission.)

repeat injections may be given at 6- to 8-week intervals. If relapses are frequent or the clinical response is not satisfactory, then surgical release is indicated.

LOWER EXTREMITY REGIONS

Painful lower extremity disorders that deserve consideration for local injection procedures include affected bursae at the hip, knee, and heel regions.

The Hip Region

Trochanteric Bursitis. Trochanteric bursitis may simulate hip joint disease and sciatica.[30] The principal bursa lies between the gluteus maximus and the posterolateral prominence of the greater trochanter. The chief locus of the pathologic condition is in the abductor mechanism of the hip. Pain occurs near the greater trochanter and may radiate down the lateral or posterolateral aspect of the thigh. Pain is provoked by lying on the side of the hip, stepping from curbs, and descending steps. Tenderness may be elicited over and adjacent to the greater trochanter. In contrast with true hip involvement, the Patrick (fabere) sign may be negative, and there is a relatively painless complete passive range of motion. Active abduction when the patient lies on the opposite side typically intensifies the discomfort, and sharp external rotation may accentuate the symptoms. Hip radiographs may demonstrate a calcific deposit adjacent to the trochanter.[30] Trochanteric bursitis is a fairly frequent complication in rheumatoid arthritis.[31]

TECHNIQUE. Intrabursal injection uses the site of maximum tenderness for the entry point. A 1.5- to 2.0-inch, 20- or 21-gauge needle is advanced until the needle tip reaches the trochanter. The needle is then withdrawn slightly, and the site is infiltrated fairly widely with 3 to 10 ml of lidocaine and 20 to 40 mg of prednisolone tebutate or equivalent. The condition usually improves following one or two local injections.

Ischiogluteal Bursitis. "Weaver's bottom" is a painful disorder characterized by pain over the center of the buttocks with radiation down the back of the leg.[32] This condition is rarely diagnosed, but when recognized a skillful intrabursal injection coupled with a few days' rest usually

relieves the extreme pain. The bursa is adjacent to the ischial tuberosity and overlies the sciatic and posterior femoral cutaneous nerves. Pain is provoked by sitting on hard surfaces. Tenderness is present over the ischial tuberosity.

TECHNIQUE. The usual technique for injection requires that the patient lie in a prone position. A 2-inch, 20- to 22-gauge needle is inserted through a skin wheal and is advanced cautiously in an effort to avoid the sciatic nerve, which lies at a depth of approximately 2.5 to 3 inches. Paresthesias occur on striking the nerve, and if this occurs the needle should be withdrawn from the nerve. Generally, 5 to 10 ml of lidocaine and 20 to 40 mg of prednisolone suspension are introduced into the bursa.

The Knee Region. Of the numerous bursae in the region of the knee, only the prepatellar, suprapatellar, and anserine commonly are considered for injection.

Prepatellar Bursitis. "Housemaid's," or "nun's," knee is characterized by swelling with effusion of the superficial bursa overlying the lower pole of the patella. Passive motion is fully preserved, and pain is generally mild, except during extreme knee flexion or direct pressure. Although the disorder is usually caused by pressure from repetitive kneeling on a firm surface ("rug cutter's" knee), rarely it can develop after direct trauma and occasionally is a manifestation of rheumatoid arthritis. The prepatellar bursa is also a common site of septic bursitis.

TECHNIQUE. Aspiration often yields a surprisingly scant amount of clear, serous fluid, owing to the fact that the prepatellar bursa is a multilocular structure rather than the usual single cavity. The instillation of 1 to 2 ml of lidocaine with 15 to 20 mg of a prednisolone suspension with a 1-inch 20- to 21-gauge needle is usually sufficient to cause the swelling to abate. In some cases the procedure may need to be repeated several times to obtain a lasting result. The provocative activity should be discontinued.

Suprapatellar Bursitis. Suprapatellar bursitis usually is associated with synovitis of the knees. On occasion the bursa is largely separated from the synovial cavity with only a very minor communication, and the swelling and effusion are chiefly confined to the suprapatellar area. This may be traumatic in origin or may be an associated manifestation of an inflammatory arthropathy.

TECHNIQUE. The procedure for aspiration and injection of the suprapatellar area is similar to that for the knee (see Chapter 71).

Anserine Bursitis. "Cavalryman's" disease now mainly occurs in heavy women with disproportionately large thighs in association with osteoarthritis of the knee. The bursa is on the anteromedial side of the knee, inferior to the joint line at the site of the insertion of the conjoined tendons of the sartorius, semitendinosus, and gracilis and superficial to the medial collateral ligament. The entity is characterized by a relatively abrupt onset of knee pain with localized tenderness and a puffy sensation in the vicinity of the anserine bursa.

TECHNIQUE. An injection of 2 to 4 ml of lidocaine with or followed by approximately 20 to 40 mg of a corticosteroid suspension is given at the point of greatest tenderness from an anterior or medial approach with a 1.0- to 1.5-inch, 22-gauge needle. Prompt symptomatic relief frequently is obtained, but the duration of benefit is variable and probably correlates with the patient's weight-bearing activities.

The Ankle, Foot, and Heel Region

Ankle Tendinitis. This is a relatively uncommon condition. It may result from unusual repetitive activity or, rarely, from acute trauma. Crepitant swollen tendon sheaths commonly occur in rheumatoid arthritis. The disorder is differentiated from ankle joint involvement by the lack of pain or restricted motion during passive flexion and extension of the ankle. Active flexion and extension of the toes does produce pain. Local tenderness is elicited along the flexor and extensor tendons. Injection of the tendon sheaths is useful, producing considerable relief of symptoms.

TECHNIQUE. A 1.0- to 1.5-inch, 22- or 25-gauge needle is used. One makes a tangential entry to the enlarged tendon sheath, distending the sheath with approximately 2 to 4 ml of a mixture of corticosteroid and lidocaine and instilling 20 to 40 mg of prednisolone tebutate. It may be necessary to repeat the injection after several months.

"Bunion" Bursitis. A common condition is "bunion" bursitis overlying the first metatarsophalangeal joint at its medial surface on the great toe. On occasion, tense swelling occurs and decompression is required. Aspiration with culture of the fluid should be performed.

TECHNIQUE. If no infection is present, the bursa is injected with 5 to 10 mg of prednisolone suspension with a 1-inch, 20-gauge needle. Special shoes or an orthopedic correction will be needed if the swelling recurs.

Heel Pain. "Talalgia" may be caused by Achilles tendinitis, calcaneal bursitis, or plantar fasciitis. The bursae of clinical significance around the heel include the space between the skin and the Achilles tendon, the retrocalcaneal bursa, and the subcalcaneal bursa. Achilles tendinitis or bursitis may be traumatic in origin but is more apt to be part of a systemic disease, such as rheumatoid or gouty arthritis. Although the normal Achilles tendon is thick and strong, when affected by an inflammatory arthropathy it is predisposed to degeneration, and since the Achilles tendon is not invested by a full synovial sheath, it is more vulnerable to intratendon instillation. *Because of the potential hazard of tendon rupture after local steroid injection, it is wise to avoid infiltration of steroids into this area.*[33] It is preferable to treat Achilles tendinitis with rest, splinting, and oral medication. The major injectable condition in this region is calcaneal bursitis (plantar fasciitis), which is frequently associated with painful heel spurs ("policeman's," or "soldier's," heel). If orthopedic shoe corrections and aids are not effective, injection of the painful heel is sometimes beneficial.

TECHNIQUE. At the spot of maximal tenderness a 1.0-inch, 22- to 24-gauge needle enters the plantar surface at 90 degrees, sliding into the space at the midpoint of the calcaneus. The tip of the needle lies in the aponeurosis of the attachment to the os calcis (Fig. 70–16). One ml of lidocaine and 10 to 20 mg of prednisolone tebutate are instilled. The injection may need to be repeated once or twice at an interval of 6 to 8 weeks.

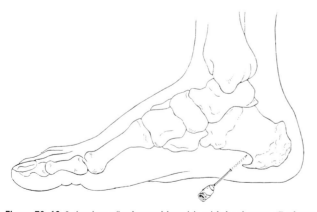

Figure 70–16. Injection of calcaneal bursitis with heel spur. (Redrawn from Steinbrocker O, Neustadt DH: Aspiration and Injection Therapy in Arthritis and Musculoskeletal Disorders: A Handbook on Technique and Management. Hagerstown, Md, Harper & Row, 1972. Reproduced by permission.)

SEPTIC BURSITIS

Occasionally, bursitis may be caused by an acute bacterial infection of the bursal fluid and surrounding soft tissue.[5, 34] Septic bursitis is most common in the olecranon and prepatellar bursae, whereas infection of other bursae is exceedingly rare.[34] The infection is probably secondary to acute trauma that results in direct penetration of the bursa by common skin pathogens rather than by hematogenous spread. The patient frequently reports a history of minor trauma or is engaged in an occupation associated with sustained pressure on the knees or the elbows.

Septic bursitis is not associated with septic arthritis of the underlying joint, although rarely, adjacent bone may become involved.[35] Many patients have an underlying predisposition to infection (e.g., diabetes mellitus, alcoholism, uremia, or gout). Rarely, an infection may follow a bursal injection of corticosteroids.

In most cases, the diagnosis of septic bursitis is obvious. The onset of pain and swelling may be quite rapid (over 8 to 24 hours) as compared with the more prolonged onset of aseptic bursitis. The bursa is tense and swollen and is very painful. Pitting edema and classic cellulitis of the peribursal soft tissue may be present. In some cases it may be difficult to distinguish septic bursitis from trauma or other acute inflammatory disorders, such as acute gout or tenosynovitis. In questionable cases it is prudent to aspirate and culture the fluid and to treat with antibiotics and oral nonsteroidal antiinflammatory medications. Corticosteroid injection is withheld pending negative bacteriologic findings.

The diagnosis is confirmed by culturing bacteria from the bursal aspirate. Fluid is usually easily obtained from the tense bursa and (in the case of an advanced infection) is cloudy or grossly purulent. The white blood cell count of the fluid is 50,000 to 100,000 cells per mm[3] or greater, and polymorphonuclear cells usually exceed 90 per cent. Gram-positive organisms may be seen on Gram stain. The infecting organism is usually penicillin-resistant *S. aureus*, but streptococcal organisms may be isolated. The treatment of septic bursitis includes the use of antibiotics directed against penicillinase-producing staphylococcus, splinting, hot soaks, and drainage of the bursa. Drainage may be adequately performed with one or more needle aspirations, but open incision and drainage may be required. Corticosteroid injections should not be performed in infected tissue. Outpatient therapy with oral antibiotics is generally acceptable.

CONCLUSION

Local injection therapy for painful nonarticular rheumatic disorders is a relatively simple, safe, and effective form of treatment. The patient may experience rapid relief of pain and swelling, and on occasion may return to work after a single injection. The response may be long lasting as well as very gratifying. An additional benefit of injection therapy is that it may avoid surgical intervention in such soft tissue problems as carpal tunnel syndrome, digital tenosynovitis (de Quervain disease and trigger finger), and ganglia.

The local introduction of a corticosteroid suspension should be carried out with due regard for any coexisting disease, such as diabetes mellitus and peptic ulcer. It is highly unlikely that these diseases would be provoked or aggravated after a single intrasynovial injection in usual therapeutic dosage. However, systemic "spillover" and absorption may occur, depending on the size of the dose and the solubility of the preparation injected. Transient adrenal suppression may develop but rarely lasts longer than a few days.

REFERENCES

1. Monro AS: A Description of All the Bursae Mucosae of the Human Body. Edinburgh, Elliott, 1788.

2. Spalteholz W: Hand Atlas of Human Anatomy. Vol 2, 6th ed. Philadelphia, JB Lippincott Co, 1932.

3. Bywaters EGL: Lesions of bursae, tendons and tendon sheaths. Clin Rheum Dis 5:883, 1979.

4. Neustadt DH: Bursitis and tendinitis. In Conn HF, Conn RB (eds): Current Diagnosis. Philadelphia, WB Saunders Co, 1980, p 964.

5. Canoso JJ, Sheckman PR: Septic subcutaneous bursitis. J Rheumatol 6:96, 1979.

6. Parker MD, Irwin RS: Tendinitis due to *Mycobacterium kansasii*. J Bone Joint Surg 57A:557, 1975.

7. Finder JC, Post M: Local injection therapy for rheumatic diseases. JAMA 172:2021, 1960.

8. Steinbrocker O, Neustadt DH: Aspiration and Injection Therapy in Arthritis and Musculoskeletal Disorders: A Handbook on Technique and Management. Hagerstown, Md, Harper & Row, 1972, p 16.

9. Halpern AA, Horowitz BG, Nagel DA: Tendon ruptures associated with corticosteroid therapy. West J Med 127:378, 1977.

10. Bonica JJ: The Management of Pain. Philadelphia, Lea & Febiger, 1953, p 234.

11. Murnagham GF, McIntosh D: Hydrocortisone in painful shoulder. A controlled trial. Lancet 2:798, 1955.

12. Konttinen YT, Friman C, Tolvanen E, et al: Local skin rash after intraarticular methylprednisolone acetate injection in a patient with rheumatoid arthritis. Arthritis Rheum 26:231, 1983.

13. Hollander JL: Intrasynovial corticosteroid therapy in arthritis. Md State Med J 19:62, 1972.

14. Gray RG, Tenenbaum J, Gottlieb NL: Local corticosteroid injection treatment in rheumatic disorders. Semin Arthritis Rheum 10:231, 1981.

15. Fitzgerald RH: Intrasynovial injection of steroids. Uses and abuses. Mayo Clin Proc 51:655, 1976.

16. Gottlieb NL, Riskin WG: Complications of local corticosteroid injections. JAMA 243:1547, 1980.

17. McCarty DJ, Hogan JM: Inflammatory reaction after intrasynovial injection of microcrystalline adrenocorticosteroid esters. Arthritis Rheum 7:359, 1964.

18. Cassidy JT, Bole GG: Cutaneous atrophy secondary to intra-articular corticosteroid administration. Ann Intern Med 65:1008, 1966.

19. Neustadt DH: Tendon rupture and steroid therapy (letter to the editor). South Med J 73:271, 1980.

20. Neustadt DH: Chemistry and Therapy of Collagen Diseases. Springfield, Ill, Charles C Thomas, 1963, p 52.

21. Bain LS, Baleh HW, Wetherly JMR, et al: Intraarticular triamcinoline hexacetonide: Double-blind comparison with methylprednisolone. Br J Clin Pract 26:559, 1972.

22. Steinbrocker O, Neustadt DH, Bosch SJ: Painful shoulder syndromes. Med Clin North Am 39:1, 1955.

23. Thompson M: Joints and their diseases. The elbow. Br Med J 3:399, 1969.

24. Smith DL, McAfee JH, Lucas LM, et al: Treatment of nonseptic olecranon bursitis: A controlled, blinded prospective trial. Arch Intern Med 149:2527, 1989.

25. Smith DL, McAfee JH, Lucas LM, et al: Septic and nonseptic olecranon bursitis: Utility of the surface temperature probe in the early differentiation of septic and nonseptic cases. Arch Intern Med 149:1581, 1989.

26. Ho G, Tice AD: Comparison of nonseptic and septic bursitis: Further observations on the treatment of septic bursitis. Arch Intern Med 139:1269, 1979.

27. Sonntag VKH: Tinel's sign. N Engl J Med 291:263, 1974.

28. Sheon RP, Moskowitz RW, Goldberg V: Soft Tissue Rheumatic Pain: Recognition, Management and Prevention. Philadelphia, Lea & Febiger, 1982, p 107.

29. Wakefield G: The entrapment neuropathies. Clin Rheum Dis 5:941, 1979.

30. Leonard MH: Trochanteric syndrome. JAMA 168:175, 1958.

31. Raman D, Haslock I: Trochanteric bursitus: A frequent cause of "hip" pain in rheumatoid arthritis. Ann Rheum Dis 41:602, 1982.

32. Swartout R, Compere EL: Ischiogluteal bursitis. JAMA 227:551, 1974.

33. Neustadt DH: Complications of local corticosteroid injections (letter to the editor). JAMA 246:835, 1981.

34. Ho G, Tice AD, Kaplan SR: Septic bursitis in the prepatellar and olecranon bursae. Ann Intern Med 89:21, 1978.

35. Simonelli C, Zoschke D, Bankhurst A, et al: Septic arthritis. Ann Intern Med 89:575, 1978.

Chapter 71

Arthrocentesis

Sandra L. Ezell, Marc E. Kobernick, and Georges C. Benjamin

INTRODUCTION

Arthrocentesis, the puncture and aspiration of a joint, is an acknowledged, useful procedure that is easily performed in the emergency department. It has been established as both a diagnostic and a therapeutic tool for a variety of clinical situations. Many physicians are wary of joint fluid aspiration because of a lack of experience and because of the fear of introducing infection. When performed properly, however, the procedure offers a wealth of clinical information and is associated with very few complications. In the emergency department it is almost impossible to make an accurate assessment of an acutely painful, hot, and swollen joint without performing arthrocentesis.

INDICATIONS AND CONTRAINDICATIONS

The indications for arthrocentesis include:[1]

1. Diagnosis of nontraumatic joint disease by synovial fluid analysis (septic joint or crystal-induced arthritis).

2. Diagnosis of ligamentous or bony injury by confirmation of the presence of blood in the joint. Arthrocentesis may be required to differentiate a traumatic joint effusion from an inflammatory process.

3. Establishment of the existence of an intra-articular fracture by the presence of blood with fat globules in the joint.

4. Relief of the pain of an acute hemarthrosis or a tense effusion. Although a minor hemarthrosis need not be drained, arthrocentesis not only reduces pain in large effusions but also facilitates examination of an injured joint.

5. Local instillation of medications in acute and chronic inflammatory arthritides. The instillation of lidocaine into an injured joint also makes the initial examination of a traumatic injury much easier.

6. Obtaining of fluid for culture, Gram stain, immunologic studies, and cell count in cases of suspected joint infection.

The most important contraindication to arthrocentesis is the presence of infection in the tissue overlying the site to be punctured, for example, an abscess or a frank cellulitis. Inflammation with warmth, swelling, and tenderness may overlie an acutely arthritic joint, and this may mimic a soft tissue infection. Once convinced that a cellulitis does not exist, one should not hesitate to obtain the necessary diagnostic joint fluid. A relative contraindication to joint puncture is the presence of a bacteremia. Not all joint infections following arthrocentesis are the result of poor antiseptic technique, because the hematogenous spread of bacteria into the joint, with or without hemorrhage, in a bacteremic patient may also lead to infection.

Bleeding diatheses may at times be a relative contraindication, but arthrocentesis to relieve a tense hemarthrosis in bleeding disorders, such as hemophilia, is an accepted practice following infusion of the appropriate clotting factors. Arthrocentesis is also relatively contraindicated in a patient receiving anticoagulants or in the presence of a joint prosthesis, unless the procedure is being performed to rule out infection.

Articular Versus Periarticular Disease

Periarticular disease such as tendinitis, bursitis, contusion, cellulitis, or phlebitis may mimic articular disease and suggest the need for arthrocentesis. Therefore, administration of the correct therapy for acute joint disease requires that the physician first determine whether the patient's constellation of signs and symptoms derives from the joint itself and not from some other musculoskeletal or periarticular structure.

If swelling is secondary to joint effusion or inflammation, the entire articular capsule is inflamed and distended, and fluid can often be palpated within the joint. In the knee, this condition must be differentiated from effusion into the prepatellar bursa, where swelling distends the bursa that lies mainly over the lower portion of the patella, between it and the skin. Effusion into the joint occurs posterior to the patella, whereas bursal swelling occurs anterior to it. When there is considerable articular effusion the capsule of the joint is distended, and an inverted U-shaped swelling of the joint occurs. This characteristic shape occurs because the dense patellar ligament prevents distention of the capsule along its inferior border. Also, with the knee extended, a large effusion causes the patella to "float" or lift away from the femoral condyles. A sharp thrust of the fingers makes the patella click against the condyles, confirming the effusion.[2] Complete extension and flexion are often impossible because of the joint tension produced by the effusion.

Joint effusion causes limited movement of the joint in all directions with active and passive motion producing pain. The pain arising from a pathologic condition involving a joint may be diffuse, clearly localized to the joint, or it may radiate. Hip pain, for example, frequently radiates into the groin or down the front of the thigh into the knee. Shoulder joint pain also commonly radiates into the elbow or the neck. Because of this, complete examination of contiguous structures is essential for adequate diagnosis.

In contrast, pain from a periarticular process is often more localized, and tenderness can be elicited only with certain specific movements or at specific points around the joint. In periarticular inflammation one can often passively lead a joint through a range of motion with minimal discomfort, yet pain is significant when the patient attempts active motion. Crepitus may be elicited in tendinitis, or the pain may be traced along the course of a specific tendon.

Septic Arthritis

Acute monoarticular arthritis is a common problem in emergency medicine. Although there are many causes of acute monoarticular arthritis, the one most requiring urgent diagnosis and treatment is septic arthritis. Infectious arthritis is still relatively frequent, and suspicion of a septic process in the joint is the first step in appropriate management; confirmation requires arthrocentesis and synovial fluid culture. Although repeated arthrocentesis may be needed when treating a septic joint, such therapy is usually performed on an inpatient basis.

Infection of a joint occurs by one of four mechanisms: hematogenous spread, spread from a contiguous source of infection, direct implantation, or postoperative contamination. The joint distribution of septic arthritis is typically monoarticular with a swollen, erythematous, and painful joint. Radiographically the differential diagnosis includes limited rheumatoid arthritis, gout, synovial osteochondromatosis, and pigmented villonodular synovitis. Early diagnosis is essential to prevent complications such as growth impairment, articular destruction with ankylosis, osteomyelitis, or soft tissue extension.[3]

Because an acutely swollen joint may be indicative of a number of disease entities, a thorough history and physical examination are the cornerstones of evaluation followed by arthrocentesis. Laboratory findings can be useful in diagnosis, as can response to therapy (e.g., response to penicillin in gonococcal arthritis is often the only criterion for diagnosis, as the organism is difficult to culture). Patients with malignancy (especially leukemia) or who are immunosuppressed or otherwise debilitated are at particular risk for a septic etiology. Infectious arthritis should be the first potential cause looked for in these patients as well as in patients with such preexisting joint diseases as rheumatoid arthritis. In no case should a swollen joint be injected with corticosteroids until the possibility of infection has been eliminated.[4]

Gonococcus, staphylococcus, and streptococcus are the most frequently identified etiologic agents.[3] Gonococcus is the most common organism causing septic arthritis among adolescents and young adults.[5] Patients over 40 and those with other medical illnesses are more likely to have staphylococcus joint infection, whereas infants aged 6 months to 2 years show a higher incidence of *Haemophilus influenzae*. In neonates, staphylococci and *Escherichia coli* predominate.[6] Intravenous drug abusers may develop staphylococcal or *Pseudomonas* infections.

Although precise incidences for nongonococcal septic arthritis have not been established, predisposing factors have been described. These include chronic debilitating disease; prior antibiotic or immunosuppressive medications; a previous history of joint damage, such as from rheumatoid arthritis or degenerative joint disease; and prosthetic joints.[7-9] In a study by Sharp and coworkers, 19 per cent (22 of 113) of patients with septic arthritis had other arthritides, the most common being rheumatoid arthritis.[3] Elderly patients with a debilitating arthritis and minor skin infections seem to be the most susceptible; the infection may be overlooked and the patient's findings thought to be an exacerbation of the rheumatoid arthritis.[10]

The simultaneous occurrence of gout and septic arthritis may be more common than generally recognized. One should not allow the establishment of a diagnosis of crystal-induced disease to shut off a thorough search for infection.[11]

Because gonococcus is the most common organism causing septic arthritis, gonococcal arthritis deserves special mention. The incidence in men is increasing, but the majority of disseminated gonococcal infections occur in women with asymptomatic anogenital infections. Dissemination usually occurs during menstruation or pregnancy.[12, 13]

A useful context in which to view gonococcal arthritis was presented by Gelfand and coworkers.[14] Three *sequential stages* with associated clinical subgroups have been described, although in practice fewer than 50 per cent of patients will fit classically into one of the three stages. Patients in the first group (hematogenous phase) have constitutional symptoms (high fever and chills), polyarthralgias-polyarthritis (but with very little effusion), tenosynovitis, and dermatitis. They then enter a second transitional phase with skin lesions, positive blood cultures, and, occasionally, positive joint fluid cultures in a developing arthritis with effusion. Those in the third stage (joint localization phase) do not have systemic symptoms or skin lesions. The infection settles into one or two large joints, yielding a purulent arthritis.[14]

Whereas gonococcus-infected joint fluid is usually "septic" in character, the yield of positive synovial fluid cultures has ranged from 25 to 60 per cent.[15] It is rare to find simultaneously positive joint fluid cultures and blood cultures.[5] A positive Gram stain is immediately diagnostic of septic arthritis. A Gram stain is positive in approximately 65 per cent of cases of septic arthritis. Certainly a negative Gram stain does not rule out an infectious process. A white blood cell count and a synovial fluid glucose reduction may give confirmatory data. Counterimmunoelectrophoresis and latex agglutination have been evaluated for early identification of infection.[16]

Hemarthrosis

Isolated nontraumatic hemarthrosis may occasionally be seen by the emergency physician. An inflammatory reaction may follow an intracapsular bleed, and the proliferative reaction and hyperplastic synovium formed may predispose to recurrent hemorrhage in that joint, especially in patients with bleeding diatheses. The knee is the most commonly affected joint (whether the cause is hemophilia or oral anticoagulants), followed by the foot and the ankle.[17]

The most common cause of intra-articular hemorrhage in the setting of no trauma or minor trauma is a hereditary clotting factor deficiency, as in hemophilia. Hemarthrosis is an infrequent complication of oral anticoagulant therapy but may occur even with prothrombin times within the normal range.[18] Chronic arthritis does not appear to be a long-term complication in patients with intra-articular bleeds from oral anticoagulant therapy. Hemarthrosis may also be a complication of sickle cell anemia, pseudogout, amyloidosis, pigmented villonodular synovitis, synovial hemangioma, rheumatoid arthritis, and infection.[17]

Management of acute hemarthrosis depends on the cause. Studies by Jaffer and Schmid and Wild and Zvaifler showed that the synovitis associated with oral anticoagulant therapy improves only after the oral anticoagulant is discontinued and the prothrombin time returns to normal.[18, 19]

Hemarthrosis following trauma is a frequent occurrence. It is most common in the knee and often denotes significant internal damage.

Distention of the joint by effusion or hemorrhage causes considerable pain and disability. If the exudate or the blood is not removed, it is partly absorbed, but part of it may undergo organization, resulting in formation of adhesions or bands in the joint. This is one argument for drainage of the joint.[2] Some believe that in an otherwise healthy joint that is subjected to a single traumatic event, even a relatively large hemarthrosis will be spontaneously resorbed without significant sequelae and therefore presents no pressing need to drain.[18, 19] This remains an area of controversy.

Nonetheless, a large, tense traumatic effusion is quite painful, and its presence precludes proper evaluation of an injured joint. Therapeutic arthrocentesis to drain a symptomatic traumatic effusion is a well-accepted practice.[20] The source of blood following trauma is frequently a tear in a ligamentous structure, knee capsule, or synovium or a fracture. Cruciate (especially anterior) ligament injury is the most common cause of significant hemarthrosis following trauma to the knee.[21] A joint effusion that develops 1 to 5 days following trauma may be secondary to a slow hemorrhage or a reinjury, but the swelling is often caused by a nonhemorrhagic irritative synovial effusion.

Occasionally, one will diagnose an occult fracture by the presence of fat globules in the arthrocentesis blood. If a history of trauma is vague, arthrocentesis may be required to differentiate hemorrhage from other causes of joint effusion. Following therapeutic arthrocentesis for a hemarthrosis, it may be desirable to inject 2 to 15 ml of a local anesthetic, depending on joint size, into the joint to facilitate examination or to provide temporary symptomatic relief.[20]

Intra-articular Corticosteroid Injections

Hollander and coworkers in 1951 first demonstrated that intra-articular corticosteroid injections were useful for symptomatic relief in patients with severe rheumatoid arthritis.[22] The use of steroids has proved to be a dependable method for providing rapid relief from pain and swelling of inflamed joints, although it is strictly local, usually temporary, and rarely curative.[23, 24]

Corticosteroid injections are most helpful when only a few of a patient's joints are actively inflamed. The most frequently used corticosteroids for intra-articular injection are shown in Table 71–1.[12] Diminution of joint pain, swelling, effusion, and warmth is usually evident within 6 to 12 hours after injection.

The most serious complication of this practice is intra-articular infection. Therefore, steroids should never be injected into a joint if there is any suspicion of a joint space infection. Repeated injections into one joint carry the risk of necrosis of juxta-articular bone with subsequent joint destruction and instability. Other complications include local soft tissue atrophy and calcification, tendon rupture, intra-articular bleeding, and transient nerve palsy.[24] Deposition of steroid crystals on the synovium may give rise to a transient, self-limited flare-up of a synovitis.[25]

It is always important to ascertain if local corticosteroid therapy has been used previously, not only to consider the array of clinical conditions associated with steroid use but also because crystalline corticosteroid material can hinder proper interpretation of crystals found in synovial fluid.[25]

EQUIPMENT

Necessary materials for arthrocentesis include skin preparation solutions (usually povidone-iodine followed by alcohol), sterile gloves and drapes, local or topical anesthetics, a syringe, and various sized needles (Table 71–2). Fluid for cell count should be collected in a lavender-topped tube with EDTA anticoagulant; however, glucose and viscosity determinations do not require anticoagulants. One should immediately examine fresh synovial fluid in its unadulterated form for crystals. Calcium oxalate and lithium

Table 71–1. Intrasynovial Corticosteroid Preparations*

Preparation	Large-Joint Dose (mg)	Small-Joint Dose (mg)†
Triamcinolone hexacetonide	20	2–6
Triamcinolone acetonide	20	2–6
Prednisolone tebutate	25	2.5–7.5
Betamethasone sodium phosphate/acetate	1 ml	0.25–0.5 ml
Methylprednisolone acetate	35	3.5–10.5
Triamcinolone diacetate	20	2–6
Prednisolone acetate	30	3–9
Dexamethasone acetate	5	0.5–1.5

*Listed in approximate descending order of duration of action.
†Dose will depend on joint size, capsular distensibility, and degree of inflammation.
(From Gray RG, Gottlieb NL: Corticosteroid injections in RA: Appraisal of a neglected therapy. J Musculoskeletal Med 7(10):53, 1990. Used with permission.)

Table 71–2. *Emergency Department Arthrocentesis Tray*

Standard shave kit
Sterile gloves
Surgical scrub or plain green soap
Povidone-iodine solution
Alcohol sponges
Sterile towel (with center perforation)
Vapor coolant (e.g., fluoromethane solution)
1% or 2% lidocaine
Sterile saline for injection
Sterile gauze dressings (2 inch by 2 inch)
Sterile syringes (2 ml, 10 ml, 20 ml) Luer-Lok
Needles (18, 20, 22, and 25 gauge) or over-the-needle intravenous
  catheters
Hemostat
Three-way stopcock (optional)
Plastic adhesive bandages
Sterile basin
Plain test tubes
Test tubes with liquid anticoagulant
Microscope slides and coverslips
Clear nail polish (to seal coverslip over material)

heparin anticoagulants have been reported to introduce artifactual crystals into the fluid. Joint fluid to be analyzed for crystals should be collected in a green-topped tube containing sodium heparin. If one is culturing for *Neisseria gonorrhoeae*, the fluid should be immediately placed on proper medium and stored in a low oxygen environment in the emergency department.

GENERAL ARTHROCENTESIS TECHNIQUE

Joint fluid may be obtained even when there is little clinical evidence of an effusion. Although one may successfully aspirate where the joint bulges maximally, certain landmarks are important. The most crucial part of arthrocentesis is spending adequate time in defining the joint anatomy by palpating the bony landmarks as a guide. These are described in detail later in this chapter. A puncture site and an approach to the joint should be selected; tendons, major vessels, and major nerve branches should be avoided. In most instances, the approach is via the extensor surfaces of joints, because most major vessels and nerves are found in flexor surfaces. Also, the synovial pouch is usually more superficial on the extensor side of a joint.

Aseptic technique is essential to avoid infection. Only sterile instruments should be used. Arthrocentesis should never be attempted if the skin or subcutaneous tissue overlying the joint is infected. Any thick hair in the area around the joint should be shaved or clipped. Sterile gloves should be worn for the remainder of the preparation. The skin is thoroughly scrubbed with a surgical scrub, such as povidone-iodine scrub, and the skin is painted with an iodinated solution, such as povidone-iodine (Betadine). This antiseptic solution should be applied three times, allowing it to dry for several minutes, because the bactericidal effects of iodine are both concentration and time dependent. The iodine solution is then removed with an alcohol sponge to prevent transference of iodine into the joint space with a resultant inflammatory process. Gloves should be changed after preparing the skin and a sterile perforated drape placed over the joint.

With appropriate local anesthesia arthrocentesis should be a relatively painless procedure; without anesthesia it may be quite painful and distressing to the patient. The synovial membrane itself has pain fibers associated with blood vessels, and the articular capsule and bone periosteum are richly supplied with nerve fibers and are very sensitive. The articular cartilage has no intrinsic pain fibers. It is important to have the patient relax during the procedure. Tense muscles narrow joint spaces and make the procedure more difficult, requiring repeated attempts at aspiration, or result in inadequate drainage. Distraction of the joint may enhance the target area, especially in areas such as the wrist and the finger joints. Traction not only increases the chance of entering the joint but also lessens the chance of scoring the articular cartilage with the needle.

Using a vapor coolant topically and then rapidly inserting the needle through the skin minimizes patient discomfort. Alternatively, one can infiltrate the skin down to the area of the joint capsule using a local anesthetic agent such as 1 or 2 per cent lidocaine (Xylocaine) with a 22- or 25-gauge needle before performing arthrocentesis.

The landmarks described under "Specific Procedures" should be used and care should be taken not to bounce the needle off bony structures as a means of finding the joint space because this may damage the cartilage.[26] An 18- to 22-gauge needle or intravenous catheter and needle set of appropriate length attached to a syringe is inserted at the desired anatomic point through the skin and subcutaneous tissue into the joint space. The largest needle that is practical is used to avoid obstructing the lumen with debris or clot. In large joints such as the knee, which can accommodate large effusions, it is suggested that one use a 30- to 55-ml syringe, because it may be difficult to change a syringe when the needle is within the joint cavity. A three-way stopcock placed between the needle and syringe is an option for draining large effusions. If the syringe must be changed during the procedure, the hub of the needle should be grasped with a hemostat and held tightly while the syringe is removed. If the intravenous catheter and needle set is used, the needle is removed leaving the outer atraumatic plastic catheter in the joint space. The syringe is now attached to the catheter for aspiration. Now manipulation of the joint or catheter can occur with little threat of injury.

Aspiration of synovial fluid and the easy injection and return of fluid indicate intra-articular placement of the needle tip. As a general rule, *one should completely remove all fluid or blood*. If the fluid stops flowing, this is a sign that the joint has been drained completely, the needle tip has become dislodged, or debris or clot is obstructing the needle. One should slightly advance or retract the tip of the needle, rotate the bevel, or ease up on the force of aspiration. Occasionally, reinjecting a small amount of fluid back into the joint space confirms the needle placement and may clear the needle. If fluid flows freely back into the joint and is easily reaspirated, one has probably removed all the fluid. If resistance is met, the needle has probably been jarred from the joint space and is lodged in the soft tissue. In some instances minor changes in the flexion or extension of the joint may allow the fluid to flow more freely. Scraping or shearing the articular cartilage with the needle should be avoided, since this may produce permanent cartilage damage. One should enter the joint in a straight line and avoid unnecessary side-to-side motion of the syringe. After aspiration, the needle is removed and a sterile dressing is applied over the puncture site.

Synovial fluid should be sent for studies as indicated by the clinical situation. Studies usually obtained include cell count with differential, crystal analysis, Gram stain, bacterial culture and sensitivity analysis, and synovial fluid sugar measurement. Less frequently obtained studies include synovial fluid protein measurement, rheumatoid factor analysis, lupus erythematosus (LE) cell preparation, viscosity analysis, mucin clot, fibrin clot, fungal and acid-fast stains, fungal and tuberculous culture, and synovial fluid complement analysis. If the arthrocentesis is performed for the relief of a hemarthrosis, the fluid need not be sent for analysis. One should be selective in ordering tests. There is no need to order a large battery of tests routinely on all fluids.

If the volume of fluid collected is low, culture and examination of the "wet prep" under regular and polarizing microscopy have the highest priority.

To avoid misdiagnosing borderline inflammatory fluids, missing crystals that dissolve with time, or overinterpreting the findings because of new artifactual crystals that appear over prolonged time, prompt examination of synovial fluid specimens should be performed.[27]

COMPLICATIONS

Significant complications are rare with arthrocentesis. They include:

1. *Infection.* Skin bacteria may be introduced into the joint space during needle puncture. One can, of course, prevent this complication by maintaining rigorous sterile technique and avoiding inserting the needle through obviously infected skin or subcutaneous tissue. The chance of introducing infection with arthrocentesis through a noninfected area is minimal if proper attention is paid to technique. Various studies report the incidence of infection following routine arthrocentesis to be in the range of 1 per 10,000 aspirations.[28] Joint aspiration in the presence of a bacteremia has been discussed previously.

2. *Bleeding.* Bleeding with subsequent hemarthrosis is rarely a complication, except in the patient with a bleeding diathesis. If a patient has a bleeding diathesis, such as hemophilia, arthrocentesis should be delayed until clotting competence has been enhanced by the infusion of specific clotting factors.

Occasionally, a small quantity of blood may be aspirated along with the synovial fluid. This happens most often when the joint is nearly emptied. A small amount of blood-tinged fluid is generally the result of nicking a small synovial blood vessel; this is usually inconsequential. A grossly bloody effusion must be investigated.[4]

3. *Allergic reaction.* Hypersensitivity to the local anesthetic that is used can usually be prevented by thorough history taking. Fainting during the procedure is not uncommon and is the result of vasovagal influences.

4. *Corticosteroid-induced complications.* (See section on intra-articular corticosteroid injections.)

SPECIFIC ARTHROCENTESIS TECHNIQUES

First Carpometacarpal Joint (Fig. 71–1)

Landmarks: The radial aspect of the proximal end of the first metacarpal is the arthrocentesis landmark for this joint. The abductor pollicis longus tendon is located by active extension of the tendon.

Position: The thumb is opposed against the little finger so that the proximal end of the first metacarpal is palpable. Traction is applied to the thumb in order to widen the joint space between the first metacarpal and the greater multangular.

Needle insertion: A 22-gauge needle is inserted at a point proximal to the prominence at the base of the first metacarpal, on the palmar side of the abductor pollicis longus tendon.

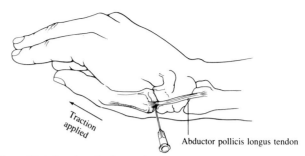

Figure 71–1. Landmarks for arthrocentesis of first carpometacarpal joint (see text). (From Akins CM: Aspiration and injection of joints, bursae, and tendons. In Vander Salm TJ, Cutler BS, Wheeler HB: Atlas of Bedside Procedures. Boston, Little, Brown & Co, 1979. Reproduced by permission.)

Comments: Degenerative arthritis commonly affects this joint. Arthrocentesis is of moderate difficulty. The anatomic "snuff box" (located more proximally and on the dorsal side of the abductor pollicis longus tendon) should be avoided, because it contains the radial artery and superficial radial nerve. A more dorsal approach may also be used.

Interphalangeal and Metacarpophalangeal Joints (Fig. 71–2)

Landmarks: The landmarks are on the dorsal surface— the prominence at the proximal end of the proximal phalanx for metacarpophalangeal joints and the prominence at the proximal end of the middle or distal phalanx for interphalangeal joints. The extensor tendon runs down the midline.

Position: The fingers are flexed to approximately 15 to 20 degrees and *traction is applied.*

Needle insertion: A 22-gauge needle is inserted into the joint space dorsally, just medial or lateral to the central slip of the extensor tendon.

Comments: Synovitis causes these joints to bulge dorsally. Normally, it is unusual to obtain fluid in the absence of a significant pathologic condition.

Radiocarpal Joint (Wrist) (Fig. 71–3)

Landmarks: The dorsal radial tubercle (Lister tubercle) is an elevation found in the center of the dorsal aspect of

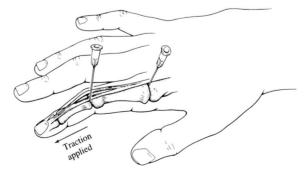

Figure 71–2. Landmarks for arthrocentesis of interphalangeal and metacarpophalangeal joints (see text). (From Akins CM: Aspiration and injection of joints, bursae, and tendons. In Vander Salm TJ, Cutler BS, Wheeler HB: Atlas of Bedside Procedures. Boston, Little, Brown & Co, 1979. Reproduced by permission.)

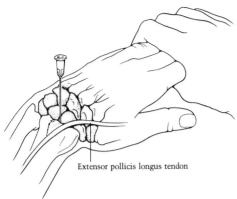

Figure 71–3. Landmarks for arthrocentesis of the radiocarpal joint (see text). (From Akins CM: Aspiration and injection of joints, bursae, and tendons. In Vander Salm TJ, Cutler BS, Wheeler HB: Atlas of Bedside Procedures. Boston, Little, Brown & Co, 1979. Reproduced by permission.)

the distal end of the radius. The extensor pollicis longus tendon runs in a groove on the radial side of the tubercle. The tendon can be palpated by active extension of the wrist and thumb.

Position: The wrist should be positioned in approximately 20 to 30 degrees of flexion. *Traction is applied to the hand*.

Needle insertion: A 22-gauge needle is inserted dorsally, just distal to the dorsal tubercle and on the ulnar side of the extensor pollicis longus tendon. The anatomic "snuff box" located more radially should be avoided.

Radiohumeral Joint (Elbow) (Fig. 71–4)

Landmarks: The lateral epicondyle of the humerus and the head of the radius are the arthrocentesis landmarks for the radiohumeral joint. With the elbow extended, the depression between the radial head and the lateral epicondyle of the humerus is palpated.

Position: With the palpating finger still touching the radial head, the elbow is flexed to 90 degrees. The forearm is pronated and the palm is placed down flat on a table.

Needle insertion: A 22-gauge needle is inserted from the

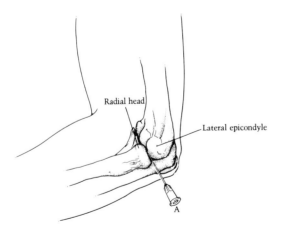

Figure 71–4. Landmarks for arthrocentesis of the radiohumeral joint (see text). (From Akins CM: Aspiration and injection of joints, bursae, and tendons. In Vander Salm TJ, Cutler BS, Wheeler HB: Atlas of Bedside Procedures. Boston, Little, Brown & Co, 1979. Reproduced by permission.)

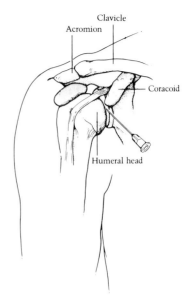

Figure 71–5. Landmarks for arthrocentesis of glenohumeral joint (see text). (From Akins CM: Aspiration and injection of joints, bursae, and tendons. In Vander Salm TJ, Cutler BS, Wheeler HB: Atlas of Bedside Procedures. Boston, Little, Brown & Co, 1979. Reproduced by permission.)

lateral aspect just distal to the lateral epicondyle and is directed medially.

Comments: Effusions in the elbow joint may bulge and be readily palpated. Often the effusion appears inferior to the lateral epicondyle. The bulge can then be aspirated from a posterior approach on the lateral side. A medial approach should not be used, because the ulnar nerve and the superior ulnar collateral artery may be damaged. This is a common joint for gout or septic arthritis. A small hemarthrosis need not be aspirated.

Glenohumeral Joint (Shoulder)

Anterior Approach (Fig. 71–5)
Landmarks: The coracoid process medially and the proximal humerus laterally are palpated anteriorly.

Position: The patient should sit upright with his arm at his side and his hand in his lap.

Needle insertion: A 20-gauge needle is inserted at a point inferior and lateral to the coracoid process and is directed posteriorly toward the glenoid rim.

Comments: Arthrocentesis of this joint is of moderate difficulty. Other approaches have been suggested but are less well accepted.

Knee Joint

Anteromedial Approach (Fig. 71–6)
Landmarks: The medial surface of the patella at the middle or superior portion of the patella is the landmark for the knee joint.

Position: The knee is fully extended as far as possible. Relaxation of the quadriceps muscle greatly facilitates needle placement.

Needle insertion: An 18-gauge needle or catheter and needle set is inserted at the midpoint or superior portion of the patella approximately 1 cm medial to the anteromedial patellar edge. The needle is directed between the posterior

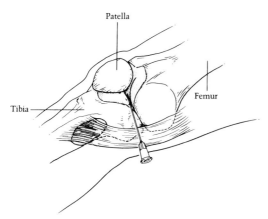

Figure 71–6. Landmarks for arthrocentesis of the knee joint (see text). (From Akins CM: Aspiration and injection of joints, bursae, and tendons. In Vander Salm TJ, Cutler BS, Wheeler HB: Atlas of Bedside Procedures. Boston, Little, Brown & Co, 1979. Reproduced by permission.)

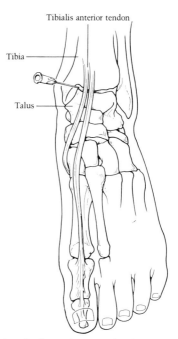

Figure 71–7. Landmarks for arthrocentesis of the tibiotalar joint (see text). (From Akins CM: Aspiration and injection of joints, bursae, and tendons. In Vander Salm TJ, Cutler BS, Wheeler HB: Atlas of Bedside Procedures. Boston, Little, Brown & Co, 1979. Reproduced by permission.)

surface of the patella and the intercondylar femoral notch. The patella may be grasped with the hand and elevated.

Comments: If the patient is tense, contraction of the quadriceps will greatly hinder entering the joint. The knee is probably the easiest joint to enter, however. Removal of a tense hemarthrosis will relieve pain and facilitate examination for ligamentous injury. If fluid stops flowing, one should *squeeze the soft tissue area of the suprapatellar region to "milk" the suprapatellar pouch of fluid*. The knee can easily accommodate 50 to 70 ml of fluid, and the clinician should therefore be prepared to change syringes during the procedure. The knee is a common site for septic arthritis (especially gonococcal) and various inflammatory or degenerative diseases. An anterolateral approach can be accomplished in a similar manner if the patella is approached laterally.

Tibiotalar Joint (Ankle) (Fig. 71–7)

Landmarks: The medial malleolar sulcus is bordered medially by the medial malleolus and laterally by the anterior tibial tendon. The tendon can be easily identified by active dorsiflexion of the foot.

Position: With the patient lying supine on the table, the foot is plantar flexed.

Needle insertion: A 20-gauge needle is inserted at a point just medial to the anterior tibial tendon and is directed into the hollow at the anterior edge of the medial malleolus. The needle has to be inserted 2 to 3 cm to penetrate the joint space.

Comments: If the joint bulges medially, one may use an approach that is more medial than anterior, entering at a point just anterior to the medial malleolus. The needle may have to be advanced 1 to 1.5 inches with this approach.

Metatarsophalangeal and Interphalangeal Joints (Fig. 71–8)

Landmarks: For the first digit, landmarks are the distal metatarsal head and the proximal base of the first phalanx. For the other toes, the landmarks are the prominences at the proximal interphalangeal and distal interphalangeal joints. The extensor tendon of the great toe can be located by active extension of the toe.

Position: With the patient supine on the table, the toes should be flexed 15 to 20 degrees. *Traction is then applied.*

Needle insertion: A 22-gauge needle is inserted on the dorsal surface at a point just medial or lateral to the central slip of the extensor tendon.

SYNOVIAL FLUID INTERPRETATION

Synovial fluid examination is essential for the diagnosis of septic arthritis, gout, and pseudogout. Inflammatory joint disease of previously unknown etiology can often be diagnosed precisely by synovial fluid studies. Joint fluid is a dialysate of plasma that contains protein and hyaluronic acid. Normal fluid is clear enough to allow newsprint to be read through it and will not clot. Normal fluid is straw

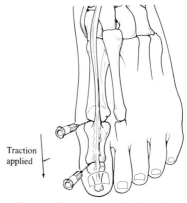

Figure 71–8. Landmarks for metatarsophalangeal and interphalangeal joints (see text). (From Akins CM: Aspiration and injection of joints, bursae, and tendons. In Vander Salm TJ, Cutler BS, Wheeler HB: Atlas of Bedside Procedures. Boston, Little, Brown & Co, 1979. Reproduced by permission.)

colored and flows freely with the consistency of motor oil. Normal fluid produces a good mucin clot and gives a positive "string" sign (see later). The uric acid level of joint fluid approaches that of serum, and the glucose concentration is normally at least 80 per cent that of serum. A normal joint contains only a few milliliters of fluid. Clarity of fluid reflects the leukocyte count. High leukocyte counts result in opacity, the degree of which generally correlates with the degree of elevated synovial fluid leukocytes.

String Sign

Viscosity correlates with the concentration of hyaluronate in the synovial fluid. Any inflammation degrades hyaluronate, characteristically resulting in low-viscosity synovial fluids. The "string" sign is a simple test for assessing viscosity. The practitioner measures the length of the "string" formed by a falling drop extruded from a syringe of synovial fluid. Normal joint fluid produces a string of 5 to 10 cm (Fig. 71–9). If viscosity is reduced, as in inflammatory conditions, the synovial fluid forms a shorter string or falls in drops.

Mucin Clot Test

The mucin clot test also corresponds to viscosity and inflammation. Therefore, the greater the inflammatory response, the poorer the mucin clot and the lower the viscosity. The mucin clot test is useful to define the degree of polymerization of hyaluronate. Mucin clots are produced by mixing 1 part joint fluid with 4 parts 2 per cent acetic acid. A good clot indicates a high degree of polymerization and correlates with normal high viscosity. In inflammatory synovial fluid such as with osteoarthritis and rheumatoid arthritis–related effusions, the mucin clot is poor.[29]

Cell Count and Glucose

A leukocytosis consisting predominantly of neutrophils is usually seen with inflammatory arthritides; a white blood cell count greater than 50,000/mm³ is highly suggestive of a septic joint. Joint fluid glucose usually decreases as inflammation increases, but a proper interpretation requires a simultaneous blood glucose evaluation. A ratio of joint fluid to serum glucose of less than 50 per cent suggests a septic joint. Shmerling and coworkers[29a] have found a white blood cell count of >2000/mm³ to be 84 per cent sensitive and specific for *all* inflammatory arthritides. Thirty-seven per cent of their septic arthritis patients had a total white blood cell count less than 50,000/mm³. However, 89 per cent of their patients with a total white blood cell count greater than 50,000/mm³ had a septic joint.

Serology

The detection of succinic acid is helpful in identifying patients with septic arthritis who have received antibiotic treatment before arthrocentesis.[30] Gas-liquid chromatography, a rapid and sensitive method for the detection of short-chain fatty acids, may complement the currently available methods used to diagnose septic arthritis of synovial fluid.[31] Counterimmunoelectrophoresis and latex agglutination also are useful and are available in some centers on an emergency basis. Other immunologic markers such as complement, rheumatoid factor, and antinuclear antibodies have little diagnostic value in the acute setting but may be useful when compared to serum levels.

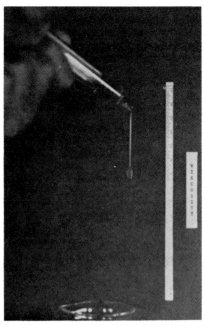

Figure 71–9. Ability of normal synovial fluid to form a long tenacious string. (From Schmid FR, Ogata RI: Synovial fluid evaluation in joint disease. Med Clin North Am 49:165, 1965. Reproduced by permission.)

Fluid Processing

Proper collection of the joint fluid is essential for examination and testing. Tests for viscosity, serology, and chemistries are done on fluid collected in a red top (clot) tube, whereas cytology samples are collected in tubes with an anticoagulant (purple top). One should always transfer the fluid for crystal examination into a tube with liquid heparin (green top), because undissolved heparin crystals from powdered anticoagulant tubes can be seen on microscopy. Early transfer of synovial fluid to this green tube is essential to prevent clotting. Culture requirements for transport and processing should be accessed before the procedure to ensure appropriate processing or plating of specimens. A useful data form and summary of specimens developed by Alexander Trott of the University of Cincinnati is shown in Figure 71–10.

Polarizing Microscope

No synovial fluid analysis is complete until the fluid has been examined under a polarizing light microscope for crystals. Microscopic analysis requires a compensated polarized light microscope with 10×, 40×, and 100× (oil immersion) objectives; a phase condenser and an oil immersion phase objective are highly recommended (Fig. 71–11). The polarizing microscope used for crystal identification differs from the ordinary light microscope because it contains two identical polarizing prisms or filters.[32] One filter, called the polarizer, is positioned below the condenser. The other filter is called the analyzer and is inserted at some point above the objective. In some instruments these filters are mounted to permit horizontal rotation of the polarizer and analyzer. The mechanical stage of the polarizing microscope is mounted on a circular stage that rotates on a vertical axis coinciding with the center of the field; this allows the objective lens to be centered, keeping the specimen in the field of view. A removable first-order red compensator is

JOINT FLUID EXAMINATION

DATE: PHYSICIAN:

TIME: A.M.   P.M.   JOINT:

AMOUNT OBTAINED: AMOUNT SAVED FOR CONSULT:

APPEARANCE: COLOR:

TEST	LABORATORY	CONTAINER	VOLUME	RESULTS
1. Viscosity	Hematology	1. Red Top Tube	1.5 ml	Good
Drop Test				Fair
Stringing				Poor
Mucin Clot				
2. Cell Count	Hematology	2. Lavender (EDTA)	Need half of	Cell Count:
and		or	tube filled;	RBC_____
Crystals		Green (heparin)	if 7 ml tube,	WBC_____
			need 3 ml; if	Diff _____
			ped. tube	Other_____
			need 1.5 ml	Crystal Type_____
3. Glucose	Chemistry	3. Red Top Tube	1 ml	Serum Glucose_____
and				Joint Glucose_____
Protein				Protein_____
4. Bacteriology	Bacteriology	4. Syringe (air	Ideally 5 ml	Gram Stain_____
		removed and		Cultures Sent_____
		syringe capped)		(mark those sent)
				Aerobic
				Anaerobic
				GC (Choc. Agar)
				Fungal

OPTIONAL

5. Immunology	Immunology	5. Red Top Tube	1 ml	
RF				
ANA				
Complement				

PRIORITY OF TESTS FOR VERY SMALL AMOUNTS OF FLUID ASPIRATED

1. First drop: slide, coverslip, and examine for crystals, then Gram stain if possible.

2. Second drop: Gram stain

3. Third drop: culture

Signed: _____ M.D.

Figure 71–10. Data form and summary of specimens needed for joint fluid examination. (Courtesy of Alexander Trott, M.D.)

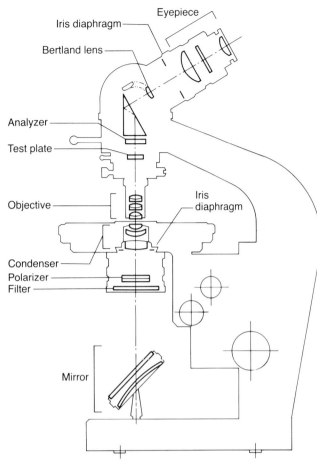

Figure 71–11. Polarizing light microscope.

located between the objective and the analyzer. All lenses and objectives are of "strain free" (nonpolarizing) glass. Although these microscopes can be expensive, relatively inexpensive ones can be used and are quite adequate.[33]

One can also obtain polarizing filters for insertion in a regular light microscope. One filter is placed between the light source and condenser; another is placed above the objective or in the eyepiece. The filters are rotated until a black field is obtained. This produces the white birefringence that shows crystals more easily than ordinary light but cannot separate positive and negative birefringence.

An effect similar to that obtained with a commercial compensated polarizing microscope can be achieved by applying two layers of clear cellophane tape to the top of a clean glass slide and placing this over the polarizing filter above the light source.[34] The long axis of the slide is then substituted for the axis of slow vibration of the first-order red compensator. Some variation has been noted with different tapes, and newer tapes that appear semiopaque before use do not work. Before clinically using such a set-up, the technique should be compared with a commercial compensator using sample crystals.

POLARIZATION PHYSICS

The polarizer allows passage of light in only one specific orientation. The analyzer acts as a crossed filter, removing all light in the light path unless the material being examined rotates the beam from the polarizer into the plane of the analyzer. The compensator functions by imparting color of a certain wavelength (red at about 550 nm). Birefringent materials change the wavelength to blue or yellow depending on the direction (negative or positive) of refringence.

PREPARATION OF "WET PREP"

To prepare the "wet prep" for polarized microscopy, a drop of fluid is put on a clean slide and a small coverslip placed over the fluid. Sedimented or centrifuged "button" material is best, although any part of the specimen that ensures the drop contains cells, cellular debris, or unidentified material likely to contain crystals may be used. Liquid heparin should be the anticoagulant used, because undissolved powdered (crystalline) anticoagulants may appear as crystals under the microscope. Clear nail polish can be used to seal the coverslip over a specimen used for crystal analysis. This procedure preserves the slide and arrests fluid motion. The specimen is examined as noted subsequently and repeated once if no crystals are seen.

VIEWING TECHNIQUES

Long periods of scanning can cause fatigue, frustration, and inaccurate observations. This can be prevented by appropriate viewing techniques. The most effective initial approach to a slide is scanning under low power ($10\times$) with compensated polarized light. One should vary the light intensity and adjust the condenser iris for better vision. The field should not be too light, because this will cause the crystals to be "washed out." With the naked eye, the test material or a bubble is placed on the stage in the center of the light path. If a small amount of specimen is present, this may be difficult to do. One approach is to place an ink dot on the underside of the slide and focus on this first, then focus on the test material. If focusing to the correct depth is still difficult, one can focus on the edge of the coverslip. Frequently, trapped air bubbles, streaming cells, areas of increased cell concentration, or precipitated nail polish that is refractile along this edge will be of assistance with focusing.

Once focused on the slide's upper surface, scanning is performed under low power looking for a cluster of cells and fibrils. Areas of clumping are scrutinized for regularly shaped material in or about the cells by rotating the microscope stage 90 degrees back and forth while fine focusing slightly up and down. The crystal length may be up to one tenth the diameter of a white blood cell. Thinking small will help identify crystals promptly.

To use the polarizer for crystal identification one must use the compensator and adjust the light source and mirror to maximum light intensity. Both the polarizer and analyzer are then engaged by pulling to the far right and adjusting both to 90 degrees. The slide to be examined is placed on the stage and focused as noted earlier. The background should now be dark and the crystals bright white. If the

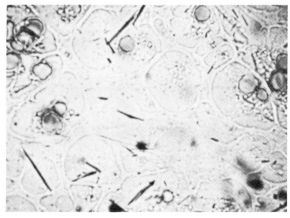

Figure 71–12. Synovial fluid with uric acid crystals. (From Schumacher HR, Finkinson CA, Weiss JJ: Guidelines for obtaining and analyzing synovial fluid. ER Reports 4:40, 1983. Reproduced by permission.)

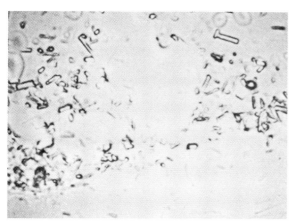

Figure 71–13. Synovial fluid with calcium pyrophosphate crystals. (From Schumacher HR, Finkinson CA, Weiss JJ: Guidelines for obtaining and analyzing synovial fluid. ER Reports 4:40, 1983. Reproduced by permission.)

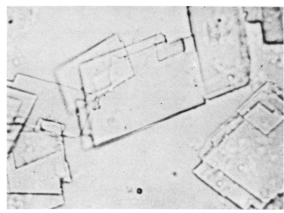

Figure 71–15. Appearance of cholesterol crystals. (From Schumacher HR, Finkinson CA, Weiss JJ: Guidelines for obtaining and analyzing synovial fluid. ER Reports 4:40, 1983. Reproduced by permission.)

background is not dark, the polarizer and the analyzer are adjusted as before. Crystals (preferably ones within leukocytes) are centered on the crosshairs. The compensator is engaged with lettering up. The background should now be red. Note that the X and Z axis are marked on the compensator. The stage is rotated so that the long axis of the crystal is parallel to the Z axis (the axis of slow vibration of the compensator). The color of the crystal is noted; the stage is rotated 90 degrees, and the change in color of the crystal is again noted.

Although high dry magnification (40×) may confirm crystal identification, a complete examination should include evaluation under oil immersion (100×). A 10× to 12.5× eyepiece or a total of 100× to 1250× will achieve an optimal two-point discrimination of 0.5 to 1.0 μ. Often a fluid that initially appears to have only a few crystals or none at all is found to have a large population of small crystals or a second, different crystal population.

Thorough searching of many cellular clumps with variation of light and condenser settings may be needed to find the thin, flat crystals of intracellular calcium pyrophosphate. A phase oil immersion objective (100×) is helpful in this situation. Once one crystal is identified, others are sought to confirm the findings. One should estimate the number of crystals of each type that are present as "few," "moderate," or "many," and estimate what percentage are intracellular and extracellular. A systematic scan is necessary for this until

one is satisfied that a fair estimate is possible. These data are helpful and relate to the acuteness of the arthritic process. Occasionally, a joint fluid has so few cells and such sparse extracellular material that centrifugation of the fluid and microscopic examination of the button are necessary. When these are done, one must record that the results were obtained from a concentrated specimen to avoid confusion.

INTERPRETATION

If the long axis of the crystals is blue when parallel to the Z axis and yellow when perpendicular to it, it is calcium pyrophosphate and is termed *positively birefringent*. If the long axis of the crystal is yellow when parallel to the Z axis and blue when perpendicular to it, it is monosodium urate and is termed *negatively birefringent*. Urate crystals are 2 μ to 10 μ, and are usually needle shaped. Calcium pyrophosphate crystals range from 10 μ down to tiny crystals that have to be examined with the oil objective; they appear as rods, rhomboids, plates, or needle-like forms and are weakly birefringent. Cholesterol crystals are sometimes seen and are large, very bright, square, or rectangular plates with broken corners.

Items found in synovial fluid that can be confused with sodium urate (Fig. 71–12) or calcium pyrophosphate crystals (Fig. 71–13) include collagen fibrils, cartilage fragments (Fig. 71–14), cholesterol crystals (Fig. 71–15), metallic fragments

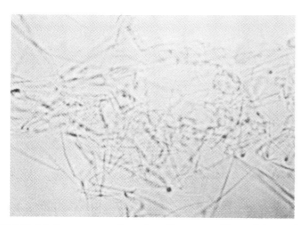

Figure 71–14. Appearance of cartilage fragments. (From Schumacher HR, Finkinson CA, Weiss JJ: Guidelines for obtaining and analyzing synovial fluid. ER Reports 4:40, 1983. Reproduced by permission.)

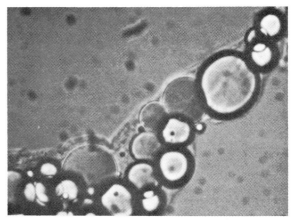

Figure 71–16. Appearance of fat globules in synovial fluid. (From Schumacher HR, Finkinson CA, Weiss JJ: Guidelines for obtaining and analyzing synovial fluid. ER Reports 4:40, 1983. Reproduced by permission.)

Table 71–3. *Synovial Fluid Interpretation*

Diagnosis	Appearance	WBCs/mm³	Polymorphonuclear Leukocytes	Glucose: % Blood Level	Crystals Under Polarized Light	Culture
Normal	Clear	<200	<25	95 to 100	None	Negative
Degenerative joint disease	Clear	<4000	<25	95 to 100	None	Negative
Traumatic arthritis	Straw-colored, bloody, xanthochromic, occasionally with fat droplets	<4000	<25	95 to 100	None	Negative
Acute gout	Turbid	2000 to 50,000	>75	80 to 100	Negative birefringence;* needle-like crystals	Negative†
Pseudogout	Turbid	2000 to 50,000	>75	80 to 100	Positive birefringence;* rhomboid crystals	Negative
Septic arthritis	Purulent/turbid	5000 to >50,000	>75	<50	None	Positive (usually)
Rheumatoid arthritis/ seronegative arthritis (Reiter disease, psoriatic arthritis, ankylosing spondylitis, inflammatory bowel disease)	Turbid	2000 to 50,000	50 to 75	~75	None	Negative†

*Negative birefringence means that crystals appear yellow when lying parallel to the axis of the slow vibration of light of the first-order red compensator. With the same orientation to the compensator, positive birefringence crystals appear blue. When the crystals lie perpendicular to the axis, the opposite is true; that is, negative birefringence crystals are blue, positive ones are yellow. A polarizing microscope is necessary for this distinction to be made.
†May be coexisting infection.

from prosthetic arthroplasty, and corticosteroid esters.[31] One may also identify fat globules (Fig. 71–16). Note that rare cases of uric acid spherulites in gouty synovia have been reported.[35] The spherulites are birefringent and do not take up fat stains.

Table 71–3 summarizes synovial fluid features for the joint diseases commonly encountered and studies commonly performed in the emergency department.

CONCLUSION

When performed correctly, arthrocentesis is a relatively safe procedure that is used to obtain valuable diagnostic information as well as to provide therapy for acute joint disease. The key to success is strict adherence to sterile technique, observance of anatomic landmarks, and proper preparation of the synovial fluid for examination.

REFERENCES

1. Gilliand BC, Mannik M: Approach to disorders of the joints. In Isselbacher K (ed): Harrison's Principles of Internal Medicine. New York, McGraw-Hill Book Co, 1980.
2. Ruoff A III, Martin A: Lower extremity. In Wolcott M (ed): Ambulatory Surgery and the Basics of Emergency Surgical Care. Philadelphia, JB Lippincott Co, 1981, pp 607–608.
3. Sharp JT, Lidsky MD, Duffy J, Duncan MW: Infectious arthritis. Arch Intern Med 139:1125, 1979.
4. Gray RG, Gottlieb NL: Corticosteroid injections in RA: How to get best results. J Musculoskeletal Med 1:54, 1984.
5. Brandt KD, Cathcart ES, Cohen AS: Gonococcal arthritis: Clinical features correlated with blood, synovial fluid, genitourinary cultures. Arthritis Rheum 17:503, 1974.
6. Wolski KP: Staphylococcal and other Gram-positive coccal arthritides. Clin Rheum Dis 4:181, 1978.
7. Berg E: The acutely swollen joint. First impressions may mislead. Postgrad Med 75(1):69, 73, 1984.
8. Goldenberg DL, Cohen AS: Acute infectious arthritis. Am J Med 60:369, 1976.
9. Goldenberg DL, Brandt KD, Cathcart MD, et al: Acute arthritis caused by gram-negative bacilli: A clinical characterization. Medicine 53:197, 1974.
10. Rimoin DL, Wennberg JE: Acute septic arthritis complicating chronic rheumatoid arthritis. JAMA 196:109, 1966.
11. Hamilton ME, Parris TM, Gibson RS, Davis JS: Simultaneous gout and pyarthrosis. Arch Intern Med 140:917, 1980.
12. Masi AT, Eisenstein BI: Disseminated gonococcal infection (DGI) and gonococcal arthritis (GCA). Clinical manifestations, diagnosis, complications, treatment and prevention. Semin Arthritis Rheum 70:173, 1981.
13. Holmes KK, Counts GW, Beaty HN: Disseminated gonococcal infection. Ann Intern Med 74:979, 1971.
14. Gelfand SG, Masi AT, Garcia-Kutzbach A: Spectrum of gonococcal arthritis: Evidence for sequential stages and clinical subgroups. J Rheumatol 2:83, 1975.
15. Rodnan GP, McEwan C, Wallace SL: Primer on the rheumatic diseases. JAMA 224(Suppl.):661, 1973.
16. Deluca PA, Gutman LT, Ruderman RJ: J Pediatr Orthop 5:167, 1985.
17. Hume RL, Short LA, Gudas CJ: Hemarthrosis: A review of the literature. J Podiatry Assoc 70:283, 1980.
18. Jaffer AM, Schmid R: Hemarthrosis associated with sodium warfarin. J Rheumatol 4:215, 1977.
19. Wild JJ, Zvaifler NJ: Hemarthrosis associated with sodium warfarin therapy. Arthritis Rheum 19:98, 1976.
20. Holdsworth BJ, Clement DA, Rothwell PNR: Fractures of the radial head—the benefit of aspiration: A prospective controlled trial. Injury 18:44, 1987.
21. Castelyn PP, Handelberg F, Opdecam P: Traumatic hemarthrosis of the knee. J Bone Joint Surg [Br] 70B:404, 1988.
22. Hollander JL, Brown EM, Jessar RA, et al: Hydrocortisone and cortisone injected into arthritic joints: Comparative effects of and use of hydrocortisone as a local antiarthritic agent. JAMA 147:1629, 1951.
23. Anastassiades TP, Dwosh IL, Ford PM: Intra-articular steroid injections: A benefit or a hazard? CMA J 122:389, 1980.
24. Cohen SH: Regional corticosteroid therapy. In Katz WA (ed): Rheumatic Diseases: Diagnosis and Management. Philadelphia, JB Lippincott Co, 1977, p 910.
25. Kahn CB, Hollander JL, Schamacher HR: Corticosteroid crystals in synovial fluid. JAMA 211:807, 1970.
26. Rosen P, Sternbach G: Atlas of Emergency Medicine. Baltimore, Williams & Wilkins, 1979.
27. Kerolous G, Clayburne G, Schumacher HR Jr: Is it mandatory to examine synovial fluids promptly after arthrocentesis? Arthritis Rheum 32:271, 1989.
28. Katz WA: Diagnosis of monoarthritis, polyarthritis and monoarticular rheumatic disorders. In Katz WA (ed): Rheumatic Diseases, Diagnosis and Treatment. Philadelphia, JB Lippincott Co, 1977, pp 192–197.

29. Hogan DB, Pritzker KPH: Synovial fluid analysis: Another look at the mucin clot test. J Rheumatol 12:242, 1985.
29a. Shmerling RH, Delbanco TL, Tosteson ANA, et al: Synovial fluid tests: Which should be ordered? JAMA 264:1009, 1990.
30. Borenstein DG, Gibbs CA, Jacobs RP: Gas-liquid chromatographic analysis of synovial fluid. Succinic acid and lactic acid as markers for septic arthritis. Arthritis Rheum 25(8):947, 1982.
31. Brooks I: Abnormalities in synovial fluid of patients with septic arthritis detected by gas-liquid chromatography. Ann Rheum Dis 39, 168, 1980.
32. Phelps P, Strole AD, McCarty D Jr: Compensated polarized light microscopy. JAMA 203:167, 1968.
33. Owens DS: A cheap and useful compensated polarizing microscope. N Engl J Med 285:115, 1971.
34. Fagen TJ, Lidsky MD: Compensated polarized light microscopy using cellophane adhesive tape. Arthritis Rheum 17:256, 1974.
35. Fiechtner JJ, Simkin PA: Urate spherulites in gouty synovia. JAMA 245:1533, 1981.

Chapter 72

Compartmental Syndrome

David E. Van Ryn

INTRODUCTION

A compartmental syndrome requires prompt recognition and treatment. The syndrome may be defined as a condition of increased tissue pressure within an enclosing envelope, resulting in compromised local circulation and subsequent dysfunction of contained myoneural elements. Despite this specific definition, the syndrome is poorly understood. The point at which significant microcirculatory compromise occurs remains a matter of conjecture. Although the syndrome is still relatively uncommon, its incidence is increasing as physicians become more aware of the problem. Recognized etiologies include an increasing number of traumatic, surgical, and ischemic conditions as well as toxic etiologies (e.g., carbon monoxide poisoning).[1] If acute muscle ischemia is extensive enough, a progression to myoglobinuric renal failure and shock may occur.[2] If the syndrome is not treated, the long-term sequelae of loss of function of the involved myoneural elements can be devastating. Because clinical signs are easily misinterpreted, the diagnosis is often unclear even to physicians who are experienced with the problem. In this potentially disastrous condition with its complicated clinical picture, any tool that aids in the early recognition of the problem is invaluable. Compartmental pressure measurement can serve as that tool. The purpose of this chapter is to describe the various techniques for compartmental pressure measurement and to discuss their usefulness to the practitioner.

BACKGROUND

Postischemic myoneural dysfunction and contractures were first described in the 1870s by Von Volkmann.[3] In 1935, Henderson and associates developed an open-needle technique for measuring "muscle tonus."[4] Their method consisted of the three-way connection of a syringe, a manometer, and a needle placed into the muscle itself. In the 1960s, the technique was applied to muscle compartmental pressure measurement. In 1975, Whitesides and colleagues refined the technique and described its ability to accurately reflect muscle compartmental pressures.[5] They also related elevated pressures to a need for fasciotomy to relieve a compartmental syndrome.

Other investigators were less comfortable with the reproducibility of the intermittent readings. In 1976, Matsen and coworkers modified the technique to include a constant infusion pump that allowed for prolonged, continuous monitoring.[6] Mubarek and associates objected to the modification made by Matsen and coworkers, because the continuous infusion method injected more fluid into a compartment with increased pressure.[7] Modifying a technique developed by Scholander and colleagues[8] for fluid monitoring in

plants, Mubarek and associates showed that a "wick" catheter accurately reflected compartmental pressures in humans.[7, 9] This method proved as reproducible as the infusion technique. Objections subsequently arose to the degeneration of the biodegradable wick as a source of error and to the potential for retaining the wick on removal of the catheter. Rorabeck and colleagues developed a "slit" catheter to replace the wick.[10] Accuracy and reproducibility of the wick and the slit catheter techniques have been very similar.[11, 12] In the mid 1980s, development of solid-state electronic transducers (intracompartmental and otherwise) has allowed more accurate measurement and less dependance on catheter design.[13]

PATHOPHYSIOLOGY OF COMPARTMENTAL SYNDROME

Pressure studies clearly show a linear relationship between increased tissue pressure and decreased blood flow.[1] These data argue against a "critical closure" pressure of compartmental vessels or a microvascular occlusion mechanism. The most acceptable theory for the reduced perfusion relates local blood flow to the arteriovenous pressure gradient: the greater the gradient, the greater the blood flow.[1, 14] In this model, veins are easily collapsed and therefore venous pressure can be no lower than tissue pressure. As tissue pressure increases, venous pressure increases. Without a concomitant increase in arterial pressure, the arteriovenous gradient and, hence, local blood flow decreases. When local blood flow fails to meet metabolic needs, ischemia causes tissue dysfunction, and a compartmental syndrome follows. This theory accounts for observed exacerbations of compartmental syndromes by decreased arterial pressure such as that occurring with systemic hypotension or elevation of a limb. These relationships have been explored and upheld in several pressure studies.[15–17] In an elegant evaluation by Heppenstall and colleagues, nuclear magnetic resonance analysis of muscle cell phosphorus metabolism confirmed the relationship between arteriovenous gradient (perfusion pressure) and cellular ischemia.[18]

Early in the syndrome, the dysfunction is reversible if conditions are changed. Histologic studies have shown that as ischemia continues, degeneration and necrosis occur.[19] As cell death occurs, edema may further exacerbate the pressure problem, and the entire process may become worse. If the situation has progressed to this point, some permanent dysfunction is inevitable. Early attention to ischemic symptoms coupled with pressure measurements helps identify this syndrome and leads to early therapy, which means the potential avoidance of these sequelae.

CLINICAL PRESENTATION

Even experienced personnel may find it difficult to evaluate a potential compartmental syndrome, because the time of onset is extremely variable. Matsen and Clawson have found the onset of symptoms to range from 2 hours to 6 days after the insult.[20] The peak time seems to be 15 to 30 hours.

The limiting envelope required to produce a compartmental syndrome may include fascia, skin, casts, external dressings, or even epimysium alone.[1] General categories for the many etiologies of increased pressure within these envelopes include decreased compartmental volume, increased compartmental contents, and externally applied pressure. Table 72–1 lists the reported etiologies in each category. Because of the nature of the limiting envelopes and the acknowledged etiologies, compartmental syndromes are most commonly seen in the extremities. The lower leg is at

---

Table 72–1. Etiologies of Compartmental Syndrome

Decreased Compartmental Volume
  Closure of fascial defects
  Application of excessive traction to fractured limbs

Increased Compartmental Content
  Bleeding
    Major vascular injury
    Coagulation defect
      Bleeding disorder
      Anticoagulation therapy
    Postarterial line placement
  Increased capillary filtration
    Reperfusion after ischemia
      Arterial bypass grafting
      Embolectomy
      Ergotamine ingestion
      Cardiac catheterization
      Lying on limb
    Trauma
      Fracture
      Contusion
    Intensive use of muscles
      Exercise
      Seizures
      Eclampsia
      Tetany
    Burns
      Thermal
      Electric
    Intra-arterial drug injection
    Cold
    Orthopedic surgery
      Tibial osteotomy
      Hauser procedure
      Reduction and internal fixation of fractures
    Snakebite
  Increased capillary pressure
    Intensive use of muscles
    Venous obstruction
      Phlegmasia cerulea dolens
      Ill-fitting leg brace
      Venous ligation
  Diminished serum osmolarity, nephrotic syndrome
  Other causes of increased compartmental content
    Infiltrated infusion
    Pressure transfusion
    Leaky dialysis cannula
    Muscle hypertrophy
    Popliteal cyst
    Carbon monoxide poisoning

Externally Applied Pressure
  Tight casts, dressings, or air splints
  Lying on limb
  Pneumatic anti-shock garment
  Congenital bands

(Modified from Matsen FA: Compartmental Syndromes. New York, Grune & Stratton, 1980.)

---

high risk because of its propensity for injury and the existence of several low-volume compartments. Interestingly, lumbar paraspinal compartmental syndrome may represent an unusual presentation of low back pain.[21]

Clinical examination is the first step in the evaluation of an injury at risk for a compartmental syndrome. Signs and symptoms resulting from locally decreased tissue perfusion are pain and neurologic dysfunction. Evidence of dysfunction forms the basis for the physical diagnosis.

Often the first symptom described by the patient is pain greater than expected for a given clinical situation. There is often increased pain with the passive stretching of muscles in the involved compartment. The muscles may also be weak in comparison to normal. There may be hypesthesia in the distribution of nerves and palpable tenseness in the involved compartment. Decreased vibratory sensation may be one of the earliest sensory findings.[22] These findings usually progress during a period of observation. As a rule, *the presence or absence of arterial pulsation is not an accurate indicator of increased pressure;* pulses may be present in a severely compromised compartment.[23] When pulses are obliterated distally, irreversible damage has often occurred. Table 72–2 provides a summary of the signs and symptoms of compartmental syndrome according to compartment.

Patients who have an altered mental status and younger, uncooperative patients may make the interpretation of neuromuscular signs difficult. In addition, casts or bulky dressings may make careful examination impossible. Attributing the signs and symptoms to other pathologic entities is also a problem. Primary nerve and muscle injuries can produce similar findings, but the deficit should be maximal initially and should not progress. Arterial injuries and subsequent ischemia may produce pain and dysfunction, although neurologic changes may be less pronounced unless secondary edema produces a compartmental syndrome. Thrombophlebitis[24] and cellulitis[20] must also be considered in the differential diagnosis.

INDICATIONS FOR MONITORING

The diagnosis of compartmental syndrome must be made early if serious sequelae are to be avoided. Permanent damage may occur within 6 to 12 hours of the onset of elevated pressure. In cases of high clinical suspicion or when bulky dressings or poor cooperation make evaluation difficult, pressure measurement is warranted. Furthermore, in high-risk injuries, such as severe lower leg fractures, long-term prophylactic monitoring may be desired.

PRESSURE MEASUREMENT TECHNIQUES

The pressure measuring techniques described in this chapter include the needle-manometer, wick catheter, slit catheter, and needle-direct solid-state transducer techniques. All of the techniques are based on the premise that pressures are equal in an open system. All of the methods provide rapid pressure measurement with acceptable accuracy. The needle-manometer or direct solid-state techniques are the easiest to perform.[5, 13] The required equipment for the needle-manometer technique is the most readily available and the least expensive, although this technique is also least accurate and the least reproducible.[1, 7, 12] After they have been properly set up, the wick and slit catheter methods allow automatic prolonged continuous pressure reading.

Before attempting to measure compartmental pressure, the physician should review the regional anatomy. To accurately reflect compartmental pressure, the probe must be

Table 72–2. Compartmental Syndromes and Associated Physical Signs

Compartment	Sensory Loss	Muscles Weakened	Painful Passive Motion	Tenseness Location
Forearm				
Dorsal	—	Digital extensors	Digital flexion	Dorsal forearm
Volar	Ulnar/median nerves	Digital flexors	Digital extension	Volar forearm
Hand				
Interosseus		Interosseus	Abduct/adduct (metacarpophalangeal joints)	Dorsum hand between metacarpals
Leg				
Anterior	Deep peroneal nerve	Toe extensors Tibialis anterior	Toe flexion	Anterior aspect leg
Superficial posterior	—	Soleus and gastrocnemius	Foot dorsiflexion	Calf
Deep posterior	Posterior tibial nerve	Toe flexors Tibialis posterior	Toe extension	Distal medial leg between Achilles tendon and tibia
Gluteal	(Rarely sciatic)	Gluteals, piriformis, or tensor fascia lata	Hip flexion	Buttock
Upper arm				
Flexor	Ulnar/median nerves	Biceps and distal flexors	Elbow extension	Anterior upper arm
Extensor	Radial nerves	Triceps and forearm extensors	Elbow flexion	Posterior upper arm
Foot	Digital nerves	Foot intrinsics	Toe flexion/extension	Dorsal/plantar foot
Lumbar	—	Erector spinae	Lumbar flexion	Paraspinous

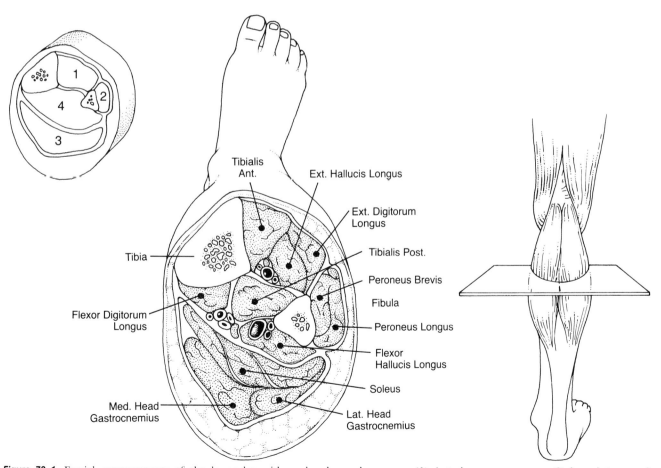

Figure 72–1. Fascial compartments of the lower leg with enclosed muscle groups. *(1)* Anterior compartment; *(2)* lateral (peroneal) compartment; *(3)* superficial posterior compartment; *(4)* deep posterior compartment.

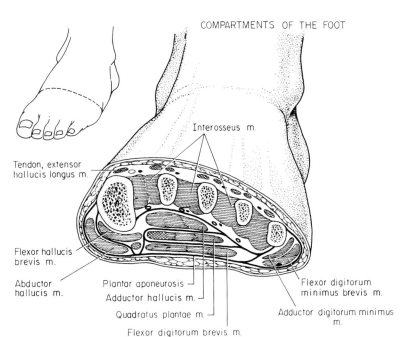

Figure 72–2. The compartments of the foot. (From Mubarak SJ, Hargens AR: Compartment Syndromes and Volkmann's Contracture. Philadelphia, WB Saunders Co, 1981.)

in the correct compartment. Published investigations provide little specific advice for probe placement. Reference to a gross anatomy text and to Figures 72–1 through 72–4 help the physician identify landmarks and permit entry into the desired compartment while avoiding penetration of neurovascular structures. Most compartments are superficial. The deep posterior compartment of the leg and the gluteal compartments of the hip may require deeper placement (spinal needle). The open needle is generally placed perpendicular to the skin, whereas wick and slit catheters are placed and anchored at an angle. Adequate sterile preparations and anesthesia are common to all methods and should be meticulously observed. Equipment listings that follow are suggestions only; alternatives are listed wherever possible.

Needle-Manometer Technique[5]

EQUIPMENT

Intravenous extension tubing (2)
18-gauge needles (2)
20-ml syringe
Three-way stopcock
Bacteriostatic normal saline
Column-type mercury manometer
Skin preparation equipment
Anesthetic equipment
Dressing equipment

PROCEDURE

The needle technique is based on the premise that the pressure required to inject a small amount of saline into a compartment should be equal to the pressure of the compartment. This pressure is quantified by elevation of a mercury column that is also open to the system.

The syringe, stopcock, extension tubing, and 18-gauge needle are assembled as shown in Figure 72–5. The needle is inserted into the vented vial of saline. A column of saline is carefully aspirated into the tubing approximately halfway to the stopcock, avoiding bubble formation. The stopcock is closed to avoid loss of saline during transfer.

The compartment to be entered is selected by testing for paresthesias and pain (during passive or active muscle stressing), representing myoneuronal dysfunction within the compartment. An area overlying the compartment to be entered is prepared as for any sterile procedure. When an overlying cast is present, a window can be cut from it. The skin may be anesthetized with a small amount of local anesthetic. During placement of the anesthetic, care should be taken to avoid deep injection into the muscle or surround-

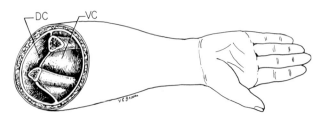

Figure 72–3. Two compartments of the forearm: the volar compartment *(VC)* and the dorsal compartment *(DC)*. (From Matsen FA: Compartmental Syndromes. New York, Grune & Stratton, 1980.)

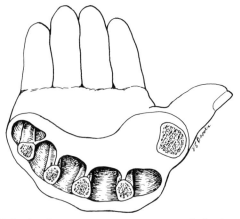

Figure 72–4. Five interosseous compartments of the hand. (From Matsen FA: Compartmental Syndromes. New York, Grune & Stratton, 1980.)

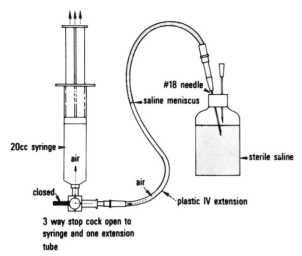

Figure 72–5. Needle technique for measurement of compartmental pressure. The syringe is used to aspirate a column of saline approximately halfway up the tubing. The stopcock is then closed to the tubing to avoid loss of saline during transfer of the needle to the tissue compartment. (From Whitesides TE, Haney TC, Morimoto K, et al: Tissue pressure measurements as a determinant for the need of fasciotomy. Clin Orthop 113:43, 1975. Reproduced by permission.)

ing fascia, which could elevate the pressure obtained. The needle is carefully inserted into the compartment. Entry into *deep* compartments may require an 18-gauge spinal needle. A second extension tubing is connected between the third port of the stopcock and the manometer. The stopcock is turned to create an open system as shown in Figure 72–6. The syringe plunger is slowly depressed to increase the pressure in the system. When the system pressure just equals the tissue pressure, a small amount of saline is injected into the compartment, and the saline column moves toward the patient. Just as the air-fluid meniscus moves toward the needle, the pressure is read from the manometer. At least two readings should be made. A third reading may be required to get two that are in agreement. Rapid depression of the syringe may cause rapid fluctuations of the mercury column and less accurate readings. The needle should be checked between readings for tissue plugs or blood clots.

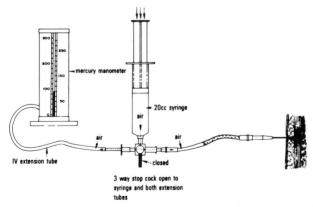

Figure 72–6. Needle technique for measurement of compartmental pressure. The stopcock is turned to create an open system. The syringe is depressed to slowly increase the pressure in the system. When the system pressure equals the tissue pressure, the saline column begins to move, and the pressure may be read from the manometer. (From Whitesides TE, Haney TC, Morimoto K, et al: Tissue pressure measurements as a determinant for the need of fasciotomy. Clin Orthop 113:43, 1975. Reproduced by permission.)

Wick Catheter Technique[7]

EQUIPMENT

Wick catheter
Low-pressure transducer (e.g., Statham P-23 transducer)
Low-pressure monitor or recorder
High-pressure connector tubing (intravenous connector tubing can also be used)
Three-way stopcock
20-cm epidural catheter
1–0 Dexon suture
6–0 nylon suture
20-ml syringe
Heparinized sterile saline (20 units/ml)
Skin preparation equipment
Anesthetic equipment
Dressing equipment
16-gauge intravenous catheter

PROCEDURE

This method uses a wick in the tissue catheter orifice to prevent blockage of the catheter tip. A low-pressure transducer is coupled to an electronic monitor to read equilibrium compartmental pressures. Essentially, any pressure monitor available for measuring arterial pressure can be connected to a wick catheter with saline-filled connector tubing for the determination of compartmental pressure.

The wick catheter may be constructed by tying two 3.5-cm lengths of 1–0 Dexon at their midpoint to a 25-cm length of 6–0 nylon. The nylon suture is passed through the distal end of the epidural catheter until it protrudes from the other end. The nylon suture is used to pull the Dexon suture pieces about 1 cm into the end of the catheter. The nylon is then cut off inside the Luer-Lok adapter on the epidural catheter (Fig. 72–7). This entire assembly is sterilized by the ethylene oxide technique.

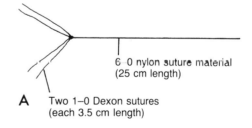

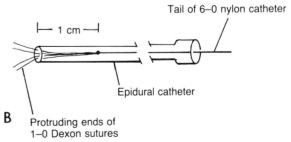

Figure 72–7. Assembly of wick catheter for pressure measurement. *A,* Nylon suture is used to tie two Dexon sutures at their midpoint. *B,* Nylon suture is drawn through the epidural catheter so that the knotted end extends approximately 1 cm into the distal end of the catheter. The nylon suture is then cut off inside the Luer-Lok adapter.

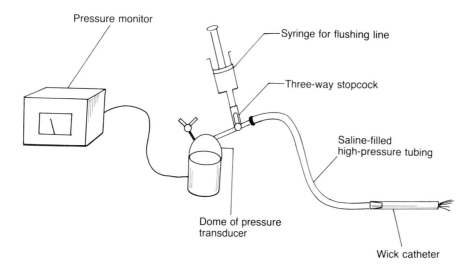

Figure 72–8. Arrangement of equipment for use of wick catheter. Note that the dome of the pressure transducer is zeroed at the same elevation as the compartment is entered with the wick catheter. The equipment is arranged similarly for the slit catheter with the substitution of the slit catheter for the wick catheter.

The catheter, high-pressure connector tubing, transducer, and monitor are assembled as shown in Figure 72–8. The entire system is filled with heparinized saline, which expels any residual air in the system. The transducer and catheter are immobilized at the level of the compartment to be measured. The catheter is wiped of excess saline, and the monitor is set to zero.

The overlying skin is prepared and anesthetized as in the needle technique. The 16-gauge intravenous catheter is introduced into the compartment at an angle (30 to 45 degrees) to the skin. The introducer needle is removed, and the wick catheter is inserted through the 16-gauge catheter until resistance is met. The catheter is secured, and a dressing is placed over the site. Pressure readings may begin after a 5-minute equilibration period. Confirmation of catheter position may be obtained by digital pressure over the compartment or muscular motion, which should produce transient pressure elevations.

Slit Catheter Technique[10]

EQUIPMENT

Slit catheter (PE-60 tubing)
Low-pressure transducer
Low-pressure monitor
14-gauge intravenous catheter
20-gauge blunt-tipped needle
High-pressure connector tubing (intravenous connector tubing can be substituted)
Three-way stopcock
Skin preparation equipment
Anesthetic equipment
Heparinized normal saline (20 U/ml)

PROCEDURE

With this method, a modified catheter is slit several times up the end to help prevent tissue obstruction. An electronic transducer–monitor system detects changes in pressure through a continuous saline column, without repeated infusion.

The slit catheter is constructed from a 20-cm length of PE-60 tubing slit five times approximately 2 mm up the end, as shown in Figure 72–9. A 20-gauge needle is inserted into the opposite end of the tubing to provide an adapter for the pressure tubing. Before clinical use, the slit catheter is gas sterilized. The high-pressure connector tubing is con-

nected between the catheter and the transducer. The transducer is connected to the monitor as in the wick catheter technique. The syringe is filled with saline and connected to the other transducer port by the stopcock. The monitoring set-up is the same as for the wick catheter technique as depicted in Figure 72–8. Using the 20-ml syringe, the transducer, pressure tubing, and catheter are filled with saline. Care must be taken to avoid bubbles. The monitor is set at zero by holding the catheter tip at the level of the transducer and adjusting the monitor to zero.

The overlying skin is prepared and anesthetized as in the previously described techniques. The limb is immobilized at the level of the transducer. A 14-gauge intravenous catheter is inserted at an angle (30 to 45 degrees) to the skin. The needle is withdrawn, and the slit catheter is inserted into the catheter until resistance is met. The catheter sheath is removed. Care must be taken not to move the slit catheter. A small amount of saline should be injected with the syringe to expel any air at the tip of the catheter. Pressure introduced in the system can be removed by temporarily decompressing the transducer dome. The catheter is secured, and a dressing is placed. Readings may begin after a 5-minute equilibration period. The system is checked by direct digital pressure over the compartment or by muscular motion, as described previously.

Solid-State Needle Technique

EQUIPMENT

Solid-state pressure monitor (e.g., Hewlett Packard)
18-gauge spinal needle
High-pressure connector tubing (intravenous tubing can be substituted)

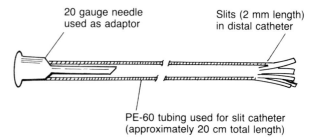

Figure 72–9. Assembly of slit catheter.

Skin preparation equipment
Anesthetic equipment
Heparinized normal saline (20 U/ml)

PROCEDURE

For the solid-state needle technique, a spinal needle is connected by saline-filled tubing to a sensitive solid-state pressure monitor for quick, accurate, episodic measurements. The set-up is similar to that depicted in Figure 72–8 for the wick catheter method.

A 20-ml syringe filled with heparinized saline is used to fill the pressure tubing and needle while care is taken to avoid bubble formation. The overlying skin is prepared and anesthetized as before. The needle is inserted into the appropriate compartment, and the tubing is attached to the monitor system. After a 5-minute equilibration period, a pressure measurement can be read from the monitor. The system may be checked by pressure over the compartment or by movement of compartmental muscle groups as previously described.

Stryker System. A convenient adaption of wick catheter and solid-state techniques is contained in the Stryker S.T.I.C. hand-held monitor system. This commercial product simplifies the equipment to a one-piece system. Prefabricated slit catheters are available for continuous monitoring although side-ported noncoring needles are generally used with the technique for single-use pressure measurements.[25] Setting the level of the transducer to zero at the level of the needle is simplified because of its small size and self-contained transducer.

COMPLICATIONS

All the procedures described have a similar risk of infection, both local and systemic; exact risk figures are unavailable. Strict adherence to aseptic technique, careful sterilization of catheters, and use of sterile, disposable components whenever possible helps to minimize this risk.

All monitoring procedures cause some pain. The pain associated with the actual insertion of needles and catheters may be reduced by local anesthesia. Caution is advised to avoid intracompartmental injections, which might result in inaccurate readings or actually increase tissue pressure. Once inserted and secured, the wick or slit catheters should produce only minimal discomfort. The needle technique may cause increased pain by injection of saline into an already tense compartment. Reassurance and systemic analgesia may be required to gain the cooperation necessary for accurate readings. Technically, the injection of fluid may actually exacerbate a compartmental syndrome. Whitesides and colleagues found an increase in compartmental pressure of 1 mm Hg for each 1 ml of saline infused into human anterior leg compartments.[5] It is difficult to assess the relevance of this problem, but recognition of the potential is important.

The wick catheter also has the potential for retained wick on removal. Wick and slit catheters require the use of a 14- to 16-gauge needle for placement. This factor, combined with the use of heparinized saline for these techniques, may lead to an increased risk of bleeding. These larger needles may also cause slightly more pain on insertion.

INTERPRETATION

When properly performed, each method has an acceptable accuracy in the clinical setting. Investigators report standard deviations from 2 to 6 mm Hg with any of the techniques.[1, 7, 11, 12] It is generally agreed that the needle-manometer technique is the least accurate. The solid-state monitor in a simple needle set-up provides a high degree of accuracy for simple, episodic readings. For research, the infusion (described elsewhere[1, 6]), wick, or slit techniques offer increased accuracy and continuous readings. Reports of normal human compartmental pressures vary in the literature. In comparing several techniques, Shakespeare and associates found an average pressure of 8.5 mm Hg.[11] Other investigators have found similar pressures with a range from 0 to 16.[1, 7, 19, 24] Shakespeare and associates found higher pressures in individuals who were physically fit.

Hargens and coworkers found dog muscle capillary pressures to be 20 to 30 mm Hg.[17] Whitesides and associates showed a significant decrease in tissue perfusion when compartmental pressures rose to 10 to 30 mm Hg below diastolic blood pressure.[5] Mubarak and colleagues showed that tissue pressures of 30 mm Hg closely corresponded to the onset of pain and paresthesias.[9] Therefore, a tissue pressure of 25 to 30 mm Hg is abnormal but does not necessarily precipitate a compartmental syndrome in the absence of other factors.

There seems to be some variability among patients for tolerance of increased pressures. Matsen found that no patients with pressures of less than 45 mm Hg had symptoms of compartmental syndrome, whereas all patients with pressures greater than 60 mm Hg had symptoms.[1] Heppenstall and colleagues used phosphorus metabolism to study perfusion pressures and anaerobic metabolism in skeletal muscle. Cellular injury was confirmed by electron microscopy. Their results confirm that cellular perfusion is dependent on the pressure differential (ΔP). This value is obtained by subtracting the compartmental tissue pressure from the mean arterial blood pressure. Anaerobic metabolism became significant in normal muscle when the ΔP was 30 mm Hg or less. More important, in traumatized muscle (in which metabolic demands are greater), the critical ΔP was 40 mm Hg.[18] Factors other than compartment pressure alone may become important. Situations lowering the mean arterial pressure may compromise a patient's ability to tolerate even mildly elevated compartment pressures. Zweifach and associates showed that there is significant muscle damage with tissue pressure at 20 mm Hg in the presence of a systemic blood pressure at 65 mm Hg.[16] Duration of increased pressure is also important. Matsen found that 12 hours of increased pressure reliably produces deficits.[1] One series showed that none of the patients undergoing fasciotomy for compartmental syndrome before the passage of 12 hours had residual deficits. In another Matsen series, 3 of 18 compartments decompressed before 12 hours, and 22 of 24 of those decompressed after 12 hours had residual deficits.

As always, all data, including symptoms, physical examinations, and pressures must be considered before a decision to treat can be made. Falsely elevated pressures may be a result of needles placed into tendons or fascia, plugged catheters, or faulty electronic systems. Falsely low readings may result from bubbles in the lines or transducer, plugged catheters, or faulty electronic systems. One must carefully troubleshoot the system before making a decision to treat a presumed compartmental syndrome.

Actual treatment consists of improving the perfusion pressure gradient. Support of arterial pressures in hypotensive patients can prevent ischemia in marginal compartments. If external pressure is at fault, removal of pneumatic anti-shock garments, casts, or dressings may be therapeutic. Interstitial edema may be a factor in increased tissue pressure as well.

Significant reduction of tissue pressure, resulting in an improved perfusion gradient, has been observed after the use of systemic diuretics[26] and intracompartmental hyaluronidase. If noninvasive therapies fail, fasciotomy, which involves opening the skin and muscle fascia at key points overlying the involved compartments, should be considered. The escape of enclosed muscles causes a decrease in compartmental pressure, thereby improving blood flow to the tissues. This procedure is best left to personnel who are experienced in the problem and who will subsequently manage the patient. Details of fasciotomy technique may be found in surgical or orthopedic texts.

CONCLUSION

A compartmental syndrome is a challenging problem for all physicians. If untreated, the sequelae can be devastating. There are a myriad potential causes. Appropriate management requires rapid assessment and treatment. Because of a variety of factors, clinical examination may be equivocal. Pressure readings can be an objective aid to prompt recognition of this problem. All the techniques outlined in this chapter are clinically acceptable. Whether using a solid-state transducer or a basic manometer set-up, placement of a needle into the compartment for a pressure reading appears to be the technique best suited to episodic emergency department evaluation of acute compartmental syndromes.

For more prolonged inhospital monitoring or research, a technique with reliable serial measurement capability is needed. For these applications, the wick or slit catheter techniques (or the continuous infusion technique, discussed elsewhere[1]) may be preferable. The complications from all these procedures are negligible.

The information presented in this chapter should aid in the evaluation of a patient with a potential compartmental syndrome. Once the decision is made to measure compartmental pressures, these techniques should provide sufficient information to guide decisions regarding treatment management.

REFERENCES

1. Matsen FA: Compartmental syndromes. New York, Grune & Stratton, 1980.
2. Mubarak SJ, Owen CA: Compartment syndrome and its relation to the crush syndrome: A spectrum of disease. Clin Orthop 113:81, 1975.
3. VonVolkmann R: Verletzingon und Krankheiten der Beuengungsorgane. Hanbude der Allgemeinen und Speciellen Chirurgie, 1872.
4. Henderson Y, Oughterson AW, Greenberg LA, et al: Muscle tonus, intramuscular pressure, and the venopressor mechanism. Am J Physiol 114:261, 1935–1936.
5. Whitesides TE, Haney TC, Morimoto K, et al: Tissue pressure measurements. A determinant for the need of fasciotomy. Clin Orthop 113:43, 1975.
6. Matsen FA, Mayo KA, Sheriden GW, et al: Monitoring of intramuscular pressure. Surgery 79:702, 1976.
7. Mubarak SJ, Hargens AR, Owen CA, et al: The wick catheter technique for measurement of intramuscular pressure. A new research and clinical tool. J Bone Joint Surg 58:1016, 1976.
8. Scholander PF, Hargens AR, Miller SC: Negative pressure in the interstitial fluid of animals. Science 161:321, 1968.
9. Mubarak SJ, Owen CA, Hargens AR, et al: Acute compartment syndromes: Diagnosis and treatment with the aid of a wick catheter. J Bone Joint Surg [Am] 60:1091, 1978.
10. Rorabeck CH, Castle GS, Hardie R, et al: The slit catheter: A new device for measuring intracompartmental pressure. Am Coll Surg Surgical Forum 31:513, 1980.
11. Shakespeare DT, Henderson NJ, Clough G: The slit catheter: A comparison with the wick catheter in the measurement of compartment pressures. Injury 13:404, 1981.
12. Rorabeck CH, Castle GS, Hardie R, et al: Compartmental pressure measurements: An experimental investigation using the slit catheter. J Trauma 21:446, 1981.
13. McDermott AGP, Marble AE, Yabsley RH: Monitoring acute compartment pressures with the S.T.I.C. catheter. Clin Orthop 190:192, 1984.
14. Matsen FA: Compartmental syndrome: A unified concept. Clin Orthop 113:8, 1975.
15. Matsen FA, Krugmire RB, King RU: Increased tissue pressure and its effects on muscle oxygenation in level and elevated human limbs. Clin Orthop 144:311, 1979.
16. Zweifach SS, Hargens AR, Evans KL, et al: Skeletal muscle necrosis in pressurized compartments associated with hemorrhagic hypotension. J Trauma 20:941, 1980.
17. Hargens AR, Akeson WH, Mubarak SJ, et al: Fluid balance within canine anterolateral compartment and its relationship to compartment syndromes. J Bone Joint Surg 60:499, 1978.
18. Heppenstall RB, Sapega AA, Scott R, et al: The compartment syndrome. An experimental and clinical study of muscular energy metabolism. Clin Orthop 226:138, 1988.
19. Sanderson RA, Foley RK, McIvor GW, et al: Histological response of skeletal muscle to ischemia. Clin Orthop 113:27, 1975.
20. Matsen FA, Clawson DK: The deep posterior compartment syndrome of the leg. J Bone Joint Surg 57A:34, 1975.
21. Carr D, Gilbertson L, Frymoyer J, et al: Lumbar paraspinal compartment syndrome. Spine 10:816, 1985.
22. Phillips JH, Mackinnon SE, Beatty SE, et al: Vibratory sensory testing in acute compartment syndrome: A clinical and experimental study. Plast Reconstr Surg 5:796, 1987.
23. Matsen FA, Mayo KA, Krugmire RB Jr, et al: A model compartmental syndrome in man with particular reference to quantification of nerve function. J Bone Joint Surg 59:648, 1977.
24. Gelberman RH, Garfin SR, et al: Compartment syndromes of the forearm: Diagnosis and treatment. Clin Orthop 161:252, 1981.
25. Stryker: S.T.I.C. Monitor Operating Manual. Kalamazoo, Mich, Stryker Surgical, 1989.
26. Christenson JT, Wulff K: Compartment pressure following leg injury: The effect of diuretic treatment. Injury 16:591, 1985.
27. Owen CA, Moody PR, Mubarek SJ, et al: Gluteal compartment syndromes. Clin Orthop 132:57, 1978.
28. Starosta D, Sacchetti AD, Sharkey P: Calcaneal fracture with compartment syndrome of the foot. Ann Emerg Med 17:856, 1988.

Section IX

Genitourinary Procedures

Chapter 73

Emergency Urologic Procedures

Ivan Zbaraschuk, Richard E. Berger, and Jerris R. Hedges

URETHRAL CATHETERIZATION

Introduction

Urethral catheterization seems a simple task—insertion of a tube into a larger tube. Nonetheless, many difficulties may arise. Patients often remember catheterization—either painfully, as a reflection on the institution's personnel, or with admiration for the fine coordination of expertise, confidence, and gentleness that marks a skilled catheterist.

Patients are often apprehensive about catheterization. If the physician shows concern regarding position and exposure, the patient will be reassured of the competence and kindness of the catheterist. A moment should be spent in making sure a patient is positioned comfortably and appropriately for the procedure. Although adequate exposure may be obtained from a frog-legged position, the use of a table with stirrups may be helpful with female catheterization. Support under the knees makes the patient (male or female) more comfortable.

Preparation of all materials necessary for a smooth catheterization reassures the patient that he or she is in the hands of a competent person. It is frustrating for the catheterist to hunt for a missing item and upsetting to the patient to be told "not to move or touch anything" while the search is made. Most catheterizations are performed with the use of a "cath tray." The trays usually contain most of the needed equipment. Our uniform practice is to go through the tray with sterile gloves and to arrange every item from the tray on the sterile paper around it. Only when every item has been considered and the tray is empty is the preparation complete. When a tray is not used, catheterists should go through the procedure mentally, trying to visualize all the items they will need and then make them available before starting.

Background

Catheterization of the bladder has been widely practiced at least since the time of Hippocrates. Paul of Aegina (A.D. 625–690) described in detail the mechanics of male catheterization, which are largely used today. Phazes (c. A.D. 850–923) described malleable catheters made of lead as well as the first catheter guide and stylet. In 1853, Reybards invented the self-retaining catheter, which is the prototype of today's Foley catheter.

Indications and Contraindications

Urinary catheterization and instrumentation can be a direct cause of urinary infection. Therefore, catheterization needs to be limited only to clinical situations in which the benefits outweigh the risk. The following are usually considered to be indications for urinary catheterization:

1. Acute urinary retention with inability to void.
2. Urethral or prostatic obstruction leading to hydronephrosis and decreased renal function.
3. Urine output monitoring in the critically ill, unstable patient.
4. Collection of an uncontaminated urine specimen for diagnostic purposes.
5. Intermittent bladder decompression in patients with neurogenic bladders.
6. Urologic study of the anatomy of the urinary tract.

Although there are few absolute contraindications to urethral catheterization, the procedure should be avoided when other less invasive methods may obtain the same information. The only absolute contraindication to urethral catheterization is in the case of the trauma patient with suspected urethral injury as evidenced by blood at the ureteral meatus, prostatic displacement on rectal examination, or perineal hematoma.

Equipment

The equipment listed in Table 73–1 must be at hand before catheterization attempts. Most of this equipment is available in prepackaged catheterization kits. The catheterist should check the list of contents on the kit *before* catheterization, however, because some kits do not include certain items. For most routine adult catheterizations, an 18 French Foley device is adequate. In infants or neonates, a 5 French feeding tube taped in place produces the least ureteral trauma. In older boys, a 5 to 12 French retention catheter may be used. An 18 French Coudé catheter should be used

Table 73–1. Sterile Equipment Required for Urethral Catheterization

Sterile tray
Sterile drapes
Sterile gloves
Sponges (5 to 10)
Antiseptic solution
Water-soluble lubricant for catheter
Sterile specimen cup with lid
Forceps
Foley catheter of appropriate size
10-ml syringe of sterile water
Sterile drainage bag with tubing

in a male patient with a known enlarged median lobe of the prostate or after unsuccessful passage of a straight retention catheter in such a patient. If a Coudé catheter is not available, a 22 to 24 French catheter should be used. In a male patient with a urethral stricture, insertion of a silicone catheter of 12 to 14 French may be attempted before the use of filiforms and followers.

Anatomic Considerations

FEMALE CATHETERIZATION

The female urethra is short (approximately 4 cm), straight, and usually of wide caliber. Yet this urethra must be approached between double labia, and its meatus is often not obvious (in contradistinction to that of most males). If the patient nervously adducts her legs, success is most uncertain (Fig. 73–1).

Because the urethra is so short, urine may start to come through the catheter before the balloon has disappeared into the meatus. Because the female urethra is approximately 4 cm in length and the balloon and tip portions of the catheter add up to another 4 cm, it is clear that approximately half the total length of the catheter has to be inserted before it is safe to inflate the balloon.

The urethral meatus may be difficult to find. If uncertain of its location, the catheterist may resort to hunting for the meatus with the catheter tip—an unsettling experience for both the patient and the catheterist. The urethra is a narrow tube lying on top of a larger tube—the vagina. The urethral meatus is an anteroposterior slit with rather prominent margins that is situated directly anterior to the opening of the vagina and approximately 2.5 cm posterior to the glans clitoris.[1] Occasionally, the meatus has receded into the vagina either because of surgical procedures or for other reasons and is not immediately visible. In such cases, if the index finger is gently advanced into the vagina in the superior midline, the meatus can usually be found as a soft center surrounded by a firmer ring of supporting tissue. Rarely, the meatus will have receded so far that it cannot be visualized at all, and the catheterization must be carried out in conjunction with a speculum examination or by palpation

alone. From the meatus (if the patient assumes a supine position), the urethra proceeds slightly upward as it advances toward the bladder just behind the symphysis pubis. Trying to push the catheter down forces the tip into the sensitive wall of the floor of the urethra. In women with a urethrocele in whom the urethra or the bladder sags into the vagina, the course is more posterior, but the relationship of urethra to vagina does not change. If the anterior vaginal wall bulges into the introitus, the catheter must be proportionately redirected according to the degree of prolapse.

MALE CATHETERIZATION

In males, because the urethral meatus is usually evident, it may seem a simple matter to insert a catheter.[2] Yet catheterization of the male involves more hazards than does catheterization of the female. The normal male urethra is approximately 20 cm long from the external meatus to the internal meatus at the bladder neck (Fig. 73–2). The prostatic urethra is approximately 3.5 cm long, and the external sphincter is 4 cm from the bladder neck. The catheter must be inserted at least 24 cm in males before it is safe to inflate the balloon. At the first return of urine from the catheter, the balloon is just passing through the membranous portion of the urethra. The catheter still has 3 cm or more to go before clearing the bladder neck. In practice, it is customary to insert the catheter to the "hilt" (balloon-inflating sidearm channel) before inflating the balloon.[3]

The male urethra is relatively fixed at the level of the symphysis pubis; traction downward kinks the urethra at the level of the penile suspensory ligament and creates a point of obstruction, through which the catheterist has to pass the catheter (Fig. 73–2B). One should place the distal urethra on a slight stretch straight up to straighten the urethra. The catheter then needs to make only a single curve rather than a complex S curve on its way into the bladder.

General Procedure

Following exposure of the external urethra in the female and the penile urethra in the male, an antiseptic solution

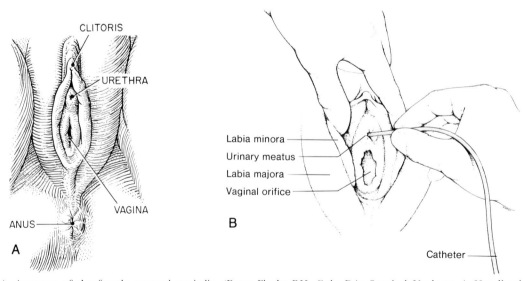

Figure 73–1. *A,* Anatomy of the female external genitalia. (From Flocks RH, Culp DA: Surgical Urology: A Handbook of Operative Surgery. 4th ed. Chicago, Yearbook Medical Publishers, Inc, 1975, p 357. Reproduced by permission.) *B,* Uncomplicated catheterization in the female. (From Brunner LS, Suddarth DS: Lippincott Manual of Nursing Practice. Philadelphia, JB Lippincott Co, 1974, p 465. Reproduced by permission.)

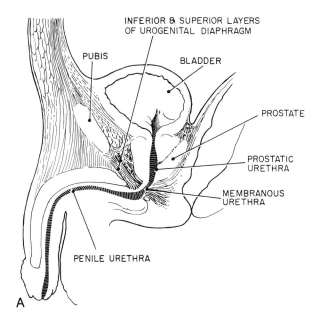

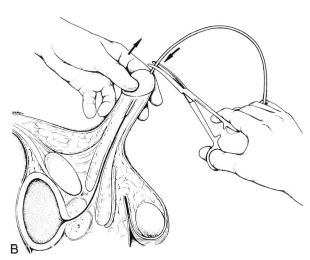

Figure 73–2. *A*, Anatomy of the male urethra. (From Flocks RH, Culp DA: Surgical Urology: A Handbook of Operative Surgery. 4th ed. Chicago, Year Book Medical Publishers, Inc, 1975, p 359. Reproduced by permission.) *B*, Proper uncomplicated male catheterization with upward traction on the penis. (From Brunner LS, Suddarth DS: Lippincott Manual of Nursing Practice. Philadelphia, JB Lippincott Co, 1974, p 465. Reproduced by permission.)

(e.g., povidone-iodine) is used to cleanse the exposed urethra and the surrounding tissue. An appropriately sized catheter (10 French is adequate for small children, whereas 18 French is commonly used in adults) that has been prelubricated is gently passed into the urethra using sterile technique. Injection of the male urethra with 5 ml of lidocaine jelly squirted through a syringe can be helpful for urethral distension and topical anesthesia. Nonetheless, the patient should be forewarned of urethral discomfort and the urge to void. During passage, one should be aware of the anatomic considerations, as discussed previously. A catheter that inadvertently enters the vagina should not be reused. After passage into the bladder, the balloon should be *gradually* inflated with 5 ml

of saline. Resistance or the complaint of discomfort on balloon inflation should signal incomplete passage of the catheter. If resistance is met or pain is felt, the balloon should be immediately deflated, and passage of the catheter "to the hilt" should again be assessed prior to reinflation. After successful passage and inflation of the balloon, one gently pulls the catheter distally until the balloon contacts the bladder neck. The catheter is connected to a sterile closed-drainage system. The catheter is secured to the thigh or the abdomen (preferred with males) with adhesive tape.

The use of antibiotics before catheterization is uncommon. However, patients with known valvular heart disease or fever and a tender prostate are reasonable candidates for prophylactic parenteral therapy.

Difficulties in Catheterization of Males

Phimosis. The foreskin, especially in diabetics, is susceptible to recurrent infections and inflammation. A scarred, contracted ring of foreskin may result and may be difficult to retract. Inability to retract the foreskin because of a narrowed ring of foreskin is termed *phimosis*. Phimosis precludes optimal cleansing, resulting in a consequent increased risk of infection. Occasionally, the phimotic ring is so tight that the meatus cannot be visualized, even for a nonsterile catheterization. If the patient truly needs to have a catheter, it will probably be necessary to make a dorsal slit in the foreskin to expose the glans sufficiently for cleansing and for catheterization. This procedure is discussed elsewhere in this chapter. Physiologic inability to retract the foreskin is commonly seen in children and should be distinguished from phimosis due to recurrent inflammation and scarring.[1] At birth the foreskin is retractable in only 4 per cent of boys. Sufficient foreskin retraction to visualize even the external meatus is possible in only half of newborn boys. Although the foreskin can be retracted completely in only 20 per cent of 6-month-old boys, 90 per cent of 3-year-old boys have a fully retractable prepuce. By 17 years of age, the foreskin should be fully retractable for all boys. Although it is not essential to retract the foreskin in uncircumcised boys at the time of catheterization if the meatus otherwise can be visualized, skin cleansing is optimal if the glans is exposed.

Edema of the Foreskin. Patients with anasarca or with significant lymphatic obstruction from irradiation or cancer may have marked edema of the foreskin, so that the glans is totally buried in several centimeters of boggy foreskin. Because these patients often require careful fluid monitoring, they may need a catheter. The physician's problem is to retract enough foreskin to enable location of the meatus.

Two separate methods of visualizing the glans are available to the physician.[5] The simplest method is to compress the foreskin between opposing cold packs or with the hand in an attempt to reduce the amount of edema. Snugly wrapping the penis distally with a 5-cm elastic wrap for 10 minutes may also be helpful. In less severe cases, compression is often successful, and no further maneuvers are required. In the more severe cases, the foreskin may be swollen to several inches in diameter. In such cases, the least traumatic way to visualize the glans is to use a pediatric-sized vaginal speculum. The outer surfaces of the speculum are lubricated, and the speculum is inserted into the edematous foreskin. It is possible to tell when the glans has been reached by palpation. The operator then opens the speculum gently and visualizes the glans as a cervix is visualized between the leaves of the speculum. Cleansing and catheterization must be performed with instruments. A ring forceps is a helpful tool for advancing the catheter, although we have accomplished catheterization with only the plastic forceps in the catheterization tray.

Meatal Stenosis. The meatus may be either congenitally or secondarily narrowed by scarring. The narrowing may prevent a normal-sized catheter from being introduced. If the meatus admits a small-caliber tube (i.e., 5 French pediatric feeding tube or larger), this may be all that is required for short-term use. It should be remembered that the inner diameter of the drainage tube is the effective diameter for drainage. A smaller, single-lumen tube may provide better drainage than will a larger, double-lumen tube.

If a larger-caliber catheter or a self-retaining catheter is required, a meatotomy or meatal dilation may be performed.[6] Meatal dilation is accomplished by the use of progressively larger meatal dilators or urethral sounds. This procedure should be performed with local or topical anesthesia.

A meatotomy may be performed in men in whom long-term catheterization is required. Using a 27-gauge needle, one infiltrates the ventral midline of the glans with local anesthesia from the corona to the edge of the meatus. A straight hemostatic clamp is then gently applied, with one jaw inside the meatus and the other on the anesthetized midline of the glans. After the hemostat has been applied for 1 or 2 minutes, it is removed. The crushed tissue is then cut with scissors. Some physicians place a chromic 4–0 suture through the apices of the skin and urethral incisions to prevent re-formation of the stricture. A catheter left indwelling for several days may also prevent re-formation of the stenosis.

Urethral Stricture. Obstruction met proximal to the prostate (less than 20 cm) during catheterization may be a result of urethral strictures.[6] *Force should never be used to bypass strictures.* Force merely causes false passages, bleeding, and increased difficulty in subsequent catheterization.

Stricture that cannot be easily passed with the catheter may require dilation with filiforms and followers. Filiforms are very narrow, flexible, solid catheters usually not exceeding 4 French in caliber. Each filiform has a female-threaded coupling into which a male follower may be threaded. Under topical anesthesia with the penis stretched upward, the filiform is passed through the narrow strictured portion of the urethra (Fig. 73–3A). Filiforms are *not* dilators and have the sole function of finding the true urethral passage through the stricture. Filiforms should not be used to overcome any resistance as they are advanced into the urethra. Resistance represents the edge of the stricture or a fold of urethral mucosa. Any undue pressure on the filiform may result in perforation of the urethra and creation of a false passage along the urethra and under the bladder. Our practice, therefore, is to advance the filiform with the gentlest of pressure. If the filiform meets resistance, it is partially withdrawn, rotated slightly, and advanced again. If resistance is met at the same location again, the first filiform is left in place (to block that particular obstructing point) and a second is advanced alongside it. A third and a fourth may be necessary before one of them slips easily through the narrowed stricture into normal urethra and bladder (see Fig. 73–3B–D). The sine qua non of success is *effortless passage of the filiform* into the bladder. Pigtail filiforms (with a corkscrew-shaped tip) may be helpful in advancing over an abrupt urethral edge (Fig. 73–3E). Once through the stricture, the filiform is advanced until the tip is in the bladder or until the threaded coupling is near the glans. Because filiforms are very pliable, they must be held securely in place. One can accomplish this best by stabilizing the penis just proximal to the glans between the fourth and ring fingers and holding the filiform at the glans with the index finger and the thumb.

A follower of the smallest caliber (usually 8 French) is selected, lubricated, and threaded onto the filiform. When it has been threaded on completely (no threads showing), it is advanced into the urethra with the penis on stretch to straighten the urethra (Fig. 73–3F and G). Stretching the penis prevents kinking of the filiform in a telescoped urethra. The follower is advanced into the bladder until some urine escapes through the inner channel, guaranteeing the successful passage of the follower through the stricture and into the bladder. The same procedure is repeated with larger followers until one size larger than the catheter proposed for retention is introduced. Occasionally, the urethral course is so irregular that it is not possible to pass a catheter, even after dilation. The filiform with follower may be then left in place to provide bladder drainage. Occasionally, a stricture may be so dense that only a single follower can be introduced. The follower may be taped in place for 1 or 2 days until the stricture "softens" enough for a larger tube to be passed.

The following procedure is used to secure the follower in place. After wiping excess lubricant from the tube and from the penile glans and shaft, one may apply tincture of benzoin to the tube and to the unbroken skin of the penile shaft (not to the glans). When the benzoin is dry, strips of paper tape 1.25 cm in width are placed on the penile shaft without overlapping and then are wrapped around the tube. These longitudinal strips will securely keep the tube in place. It is important not to have a circumferential strip of tape over the penis, because the tape may constrict venous and lymphatic return sufficiently to produce a paraphimosis.

Dilation with filiforms and followers should be neither bloody nor excessively uncomfortable for the patient. Should the procedure be bloody or uncomfortable or should no urine be returned despite advancement of the follower for at least 24 cm, the physician should consider that the filiform may not be in the urethra, but instead be in a false passage. In such a situation, it may be better to place a suprapubic cystostomy tube rather than persist with an unsuccessful dilation.

Spasm in External Urethral Sphincter. The male patient may voluntarily or involuntarily contract the striated urethral sphincter at the apex of the prostate. (This is especially true of men with neurologic dysfunction and pelvic floor spasms.) The catheterist will meet a resistance at approximately 16 cm. Because increased abdominal pressure causes reflex contraction of the external sphincter, the patient should be encouraged to lie flat and to take slow, deep breaths through his mouth. Plantar flexing of the toes also aids in relaxation of the pelvic floor. Because the external sphincter is composed of striated muscle and will fatigue within a few minutes, gentle but steady pressure should be exerted on the catheter. If these maneuvers do not result in passage of the catheter, the catheterist may be confronting a rigid stricture that will require dilation.

High Bladder Neck. Occasionally, when a man has an enlarged prostate with a high bladder neck, the tip of the catheter hits against the posterior lobe of the prostate and does not slip up through the bladder neck. Resistance is usually encountered after the catheter has been passed 16 to 20 cm into the urethra. Slow injection of 20 to 30 ml of sterile lubricating jelly by syringe into the urethra may allow the catheter to slip over the prostate and into the bladder. If this fails, a coudé catheter (elbow catheter) may be inserted. This catheter has a bend in the tip, and one will almost always be able to maneuver it gently into the bladder (Fig. 73–4). Passage of the Coudé catheter may be enhanced by digital guidance of the catheter tip superiorly using a gloved finger placed in the patient's rectum. Use of a stylet is generally not necessary and may encourage creation of a false passage. If the Coudé catheter cannot be advanced, a scarred, fixed narrowing at the bladder neck may be present.

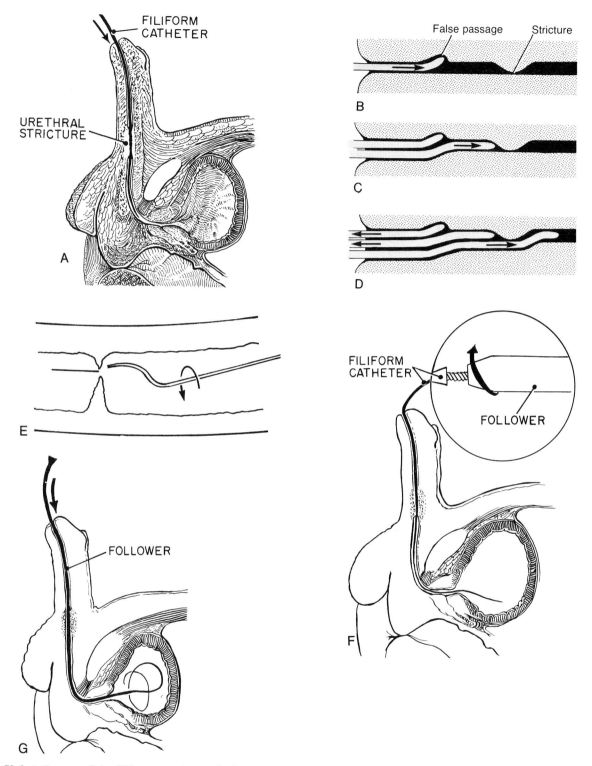

Figure 73–3. *A,* Passage of the filiform past the urethral structure. *B,* Sequential passage of filiforms, with entry of the first catheter into the false passage. *C,* Advancement of the second filiform to the stricture site. *D,* Passage of the third filiform past the stricture. Following passage of the filiform into the bladder, redundant catheters are removed. *E,* Pigtail filiform passing through the stricture. *F,* Attaching a follower to the filiform. *G,* Dilation of the stricture with a follower. (*E* from Blandy J: Operative Urology. Oxford, Blackwell Scientific Publications, 1978, p 204. Reproduced by permission. *B, C, D* from Hill GJ: Outpatient Surgery. Philadelphia, WB Saunders Co, 1973. Reproduced by permission.)

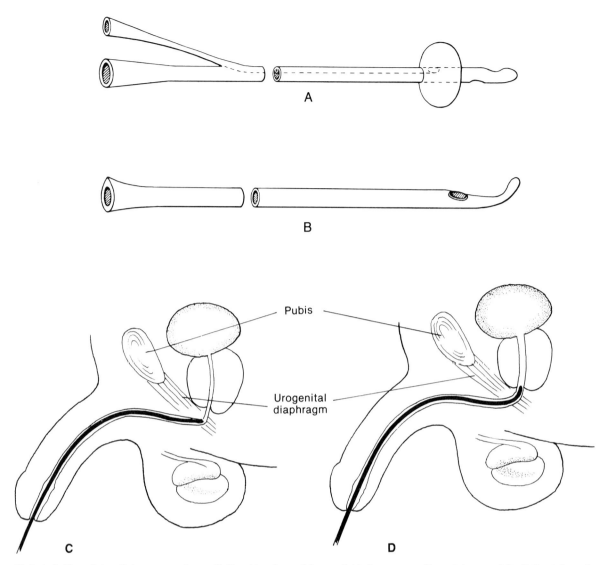

Figure 73–4. *A*, Self-retaining Foley-type catheter. *B*, Coudé catheter (also available in a non–self-retaining model). *C*, Straight catheter may not pass over the rise in the prostate. *D*, Coudé catheter passes more easily over the enlarged median lobe.

Such a contracture is usually secondary to scarring from a previous prostatectomy and is often very difficult to pass. The insertion of a suprapubic catheter or direct visualization of the obstruction by a urologist may be required.

Catheterization in the Patient with Pelvic Trauma

The patient with pelvic trauma or a straddle injury presents special problems in urinary management. The patient may often be in shock from blood loss into the pelvis or from associated injuries. Accurate minute-to-minute monitoring of urinary output, requiring bladder catheterization, may be of assistance in the initial resuscitation. Furthermore, radiographic evaluation of the degree of urinary injury requires a cystogram, which usually necessitates catheterization.

The hazard of catheterization in the patient with pelvic trauma is the potential exacerbation of urethral injuries that are often associated with such trauma. The crucial finding on physical examination suggesting such an injury is *blood at the urethral meatus*. This most often results from injury of the membranous urethra just above the pelvic diaphragm, where the prostate is displaced from its attachments to the pubic bone (puboprostatic ligaments) during the pelvic fracture. A partial urethral disruption may heal with little or no scarring. On the other hand, a complete disruption of the urethra usually results in a significant urethral stricture. The danger of urethral catheterization in this situation therefore is that a partial injury may be converted to a complete injury, which results in a stricture that requires extensive surgical repair. Successful atraumatic placement of a urethral catheter, however, could obviate the need for open cystostomy placement in the patient who does not otherwise require laparotomy.

Prior to bladder catheterization all patients with significant abdominal or pelvic trauma should be examined for blood at the urinary meatus. Blood present at the urinary meatus and a "high-riding" or absent prostate on rectal examination almost always indicate complete urethral disruption and are a contraindication to blind catheterization. In such cases a retrograde cystourethrogram (see Chapter 74) should be performed before catheterization and, preferably, prior to an excretory urogram. In the unlikely event that contrast flows easily from the urethra into the bladder with little or no extravasation, an attempt to pass an 18 French Foley catheter should be made. If *any* resistance to passage is encountered, the attempt should be immediately aborted. If passage is successful, relatively clear urine will usually be found in the patient's bladder. A cystogram can now be performed to rule out bladder rupture (see Chapter 74). If required, an excretory urogram can also be performed to rule out renal or ureteral injury. If the urethrogram shows extravasation, no further attempt at urethral catheterization should be made. If possible, an excretory urogram should be performed to identify renal or ureteral injuries and to identify the condition and the position of the bladder. In total disruption, the bladder is often higher than usual in the abdomen and may be laterally placed because of an asymmetrically expanded hematoma. Once identified, the position of the bladder may be confirmed by placement of a 22-gauge spinal needle into it. Further contrast may be introduced through the needle. Once the bladder is identified and is adequately filled, a Cystocath may be placed into the bladder alongside the spinal needle. Clear urine is obtained if no damage to the bladder or the kidneys has occurred. (The Cystocath can later be exchanged for a larger tube after the patient's condition has clinically stabilized.) Alternatively, a small catheter can be placed using the guide wire technique described elsewhere for vascular access. A patient who is not stable enough to undergo an excretory urogram will probably require exploratory laparotomy, and an open cystostomy tube may be placed at that time.

Complications of Urethral Catheterization

Although urethral catheterization performed by skilled personnel in appropriate circumstances has an acceptable complication rate, untoward sequelae of catheterization are not unusual.

The frequency of bacteriuria after a single catheterization in a healthy outpatient population is probably less than 1 per cent.[7] On the other hand, in hospitalized, elderly, debilitated, or postpartum patients, the rate may be considerably higher. Urinary catheterization is the leading cause of nosocomial urinary tract infections. The mortality in patients with nosocomial urinary tract infection is approximately three times that in patients not acquiring infection.[8] Of patients catheterized for 2 to 7 days with a closed system, 8 to 10 per cent will have significant bacteriuria once the catheter is removed.[9] Patients with catheters in place longer than 10 days almost always acquire an infection. Infection from the urethra and the bladder may spread to cause epididymitis, pyelonephritis, and sepsis. Although the use of a povidone-iodine lubricating gel has been shown to reduce the inoculation of bacteria into the bladder at the time of catheterization,[10] further study will be needed to determine if this antiseptic lubricant reduces infectious complications.

In addition, complications may occur during the act of catheterization. False channels may be established even with soft latex catheters in either the pendulous urethra or the posterior urethra when force is placed on the catheter. In an uncircumcised patient, negligence in replacing the retracted foreskin over the glans penis after catheterization may lead to painful paraphimosis and even gangrene of the penis.

Leaving a catheter in place too long or using a catheter that is too large leads to poor drainage of the periurethral glands and to urethritis and periureteral abscess, which in time may lead to urethral stricture. Likewise, in chronic catheterization concretions may form around a catheter balloon and may lead to the formation of bladder stones, which require removal.

The use of silicone catheters rather than latex catheters for postoperative catheterization in adult males undergoing cardiac surgery has been shown to reduce the incidence of subsequent urethral stricture.[11] Although these men were catheterized less than 48 hours, there was a 2 per cent incidence of urethral stricture at 1 year and a 5 per cent incidence at 2 years for those catheterized with latex catheters. None of the patients catheterized with silicone catheters developed a stricture.

Hematuria has long been assumed to be common immediately following even an atraumatic catheterization. Although Sklar and colleagues found a small increase in urinary red blood cell count with catheterization, only one in 47 patients had an increase of more than four cells per high power field attributable to the procedure.[12] They suggest that more than four cells per high power field following catheterization is unlikely to be due to the procedure and is, in fact, evidence of preexisting hematuria.

Retained catheters are an uncommon but frustrating problem. Catheters may be retained because of balloons that do not deflate (see following section) or because of a knot tied in the catheter. Catheter knotting has been associated with the insertion of a highly flexible catheter far into the bladder.[13] A guide wire passed up the catheter may be successful in manipulating some knots free, but urethral dilation with progressively larger catheters adjacent to the retained catheter may be needed to permit urethral passage of the knot. This complication can be avoided during intermittent catheterization, by passage of the catheter only as far as necessary to obtain urine.

With long-term catheterization, bacteriuria is invariable. Although episodes of high temperature ($\geq 38.8°$ C) due to urinary tract infection in patients with long-term catheterizations are rare (2 per 1000 patient days), these episodes are associated with bacteremia and patient death.[14] Use of a condom catheter in men or an external urine collection device in women[15] represents noninvasive alternatives to long-term catheterization in nonambulatory incontinent individuals. Other rare complications of long-term urethral catheterization include bladder perforation[16] and urethral erosion by a penile prosthesis.[17]

REMOVING THE NONDEFLATING CATHETER

Introduction

The self-retaining balloon of the Foley-type catheter obviates cumbersome taping or suturing of the catheter to keep it in place. Occasionally, however, a self-retaining balloon does not deflate. Needless to say, this problem has challenged and frustrated physicians who encounter it and has produced a number of solutions. The usual cause of the nondeflating catheter balloon is the presence of a flap-type valve in the inflating lumen of the catheter, which allows fluid to enter the balloon of the catheter but prevents fluid removal (Fig. 73–5).[18] The ideal solution is one that resolves the problem—getting the balloon to deflate—without creating a second problem (e.g., unnecessary irritation of the bladder or fragmentation of the balloon). Of the methods used to deflate catheter balloons, the only technique that approaches the ideal is treatment of this flap valve deformity. Other methods of deflation often produce secondary problems and therefore should be avoided when possible.

Techniques

One method of catheter removal is inflation of the catheter balloon with water or air until the balloon is over-

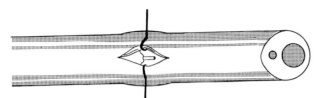

Figure 73–5. A flap-like defect in the inflating channel of a balloon catheter being raised by a wire stylet passed down the inflating channel to deflate the balloon. (From Eichenberg HA, Amin M, Clark J: Non-deflating Foley catheters. Intern Urol Nephrol 8:171, 1976. Reproduced by permission.)

stretched to the point of rupture. Up to 200 ml of fluid can be injected before a 5-ml balloon will rupture.[18, 19] Adding volume to the empty bladder may not be a problem. Unfortunately, this solution may produce unacceptably painful bladder distention for the patient whose catheter is blocked and whose bladder is distended to the point of discomfort. An even more compelling reason not to use this method of balloon deflation is the disconcerting frequency of balloon fragmentation. In an experimental study of 100 catheters (50 of which were overdistended with water and 50 of which were overdistended with air), all 100 catheter balloons ruptured into fragments.[18] Consequently, fragments of balloon may be left in the bladder to become nidi for calculus formation. Cystoscopy to inspect the bladder and to remove any fragments is indicated if this method of balloon deflation is used.

A second method of balloon deflation involves injecting an erosive substance into the balloon. This causes the balloon to deflate after part of the wall has been eroded. Organic compounds that attack the latex polymers are often used. Ether, acetone, mineral oil, and even petrolatum ointment have been used. In general, the more volatile the substance, the more rapidly it ruptures the balloon. Rupture of the balloon may be partly a result of the rapid expansion that some of these volatile substances—especially ether—undergo at body temperature. Ether was reported to rupture 58 of 60 catheter balloons within 2 minutes of injection into the balloon. Unfortunately, in 56 of the catheters, a free fragment of the balloon was ruptured off. Mineral oil, which works more slowly, was associated with fragment production in 95 of 100 catheters tested.[18] When released into the bladder, organic substances often produce a very symptomatic chemical cystitis.

A third method of deflating the balloon is to pierce it with a sharp instrument. With gentle traction, the balloon is drawn against the bladder neck and is punctured with a thin spinal needle suprapubically (transvesically), transvaginally, or transperineally. This may be done either blindly[20] or with the help of some system of visualization. Fluoroscopy with the balloon or bladder filled with contrast media, ultrasonography, and cystoscopy have been used. In women, the spinal needle may be gently introduced along the catheter transurethrally. Fragmentation during rupture can occur.

The most rational way to deflate a nondeflating balloon is to attack the valve-like defect in the inflate-deflate channel that prevents the removal of the inflating fluid. Cutting the catheter may result in rapid deflation if the valve-like defect happens to be present in the part of the catheter that is cut off. A cut catheter with a more proximal valve-like defect can often be left for 24 hours with frequent slow deflation, but this maneuver leaves the problem of managing an unconnected catheter. Devising a waterproof and aseptic method of collecting urine from the cut balloon may require use of a ureteral catheter drainage bag or another ingenious invention.

It is often helpful to insert a very thin, rigid item into the lumen of the inflating channel in an effort to deform the valve defect sufficiently to allow the inflating fluid to escape from the balloon. A stainless steel wire suture of 3–0 or 4–0 gauge is the thinnest suitable material. The wire stylet from an angiographic catheter, stylets from ureteral catheters, and very small, well-lubricated ureteral catheters have all been reported to achieve success. When a ureteral catheter stylet was used in one series, 34 of 39 balloons were deflated without fragmentation. In the five unsuccessful cases, a needle rupture was required.[21]

Our recommended method is to use a stepwise series of maneuvers. If the balloon does not deflate, we remove the syringe adaptor plug from the inflating channel. This rules out a malfunction of the adaptor. If the inflating water does not escape, we next insert one angiographic catheter stylet into the inflating channel and rotate it. Usually, the water from the balloon flows along the wire. If it does not, we cut the catheter short and wait for 24 hours before trying to puncture the balloon. The shortened catheter is firmly attached to a drainage system to avoid intravesicular migration and to collect drained urine. If deflation must occur more urgently, transcatheter puncture of the balloon using a steel wire suture or metal stylet passed down the balloon channel is recommended.[22]

Once a problem balloon has been deflated, it is mandatory to inspect the balloon portion carefully for missing fragments. If a piece of the balloon is missing, it is necessary to arrange for cystoscopy to remove the fragment. Pretesting Foley catheter balloons by trial inflation and deflation before insertion may minimize this complication.

SUPRAPUBIC ASPIRATION OF THE BLADDER

Introduction

One of the problems of interpreting voided urine samples is that the urine from the bladder passes through a progressively more contaminated urethral conduit. In the female, the perineum is a site where bacteria are seemingly eager to be swept along into the sterile cup and onto the agar plate. To avoid this dilemma of interpretation, physicians have devised maneuvers to minimize contaminating organisms. Male patients are instructed to retract the foreskin, cleanse the meatus, discard the first portion of urine, and catch the midstream urine. Female patients are asked to perform even more difficult maneuvers to avoid the bacterial contamination: hold the labia apart with one hand, cleanse the periurethral skin blindly with the other, then reach for the cup, initiate voiding, and catch the midstream urine—all the while holding the labia apart and maintaining a precarious position on the commode. Some experts[23] have women void in the lithotomy position while an assistant retracts the labia, cleanses the perineum, and then catches the midstream urine.

In transurethral bladder catheterization, even with sterile materials, the catheter must traverse the contaminated urethra and may introduce contaminating bacteria into the specimen and into the bladder of the patients, resulting in infection. In addition, the procedure is often uncomfortable.

Suprapubic aspiration of the bladder, first reported as a method of collecting urine for bacteriologic study in 1956,[24] offers the physician a relatively simple means for obtaining uncontaminated bladder urine. Urethral contamination is successfully avoided, and positive results always represent true bacteriuria.

Indications

In the neonate or the young child who cannot collect a reliably clean-catch urinary specimen, suprapubic aspiration can provide the physician with a sample that is useful for bacteriologic interpretation.[24-26] This is not a dangerous procedure and the reliability of the urine obtained approaches 100 per cent. For children above the age of 2 years urine should be collected by urethral catheterization.

For adult patients, the indications for suprapubic aspiration are more limited, because these patients usually can cooperate with the physician. Men with condom catheters or phimosis, however, may require suprapubic aspirate to minimize contamination. Aspirate cultures may be needed to rule out contamination in patients with asymptomatic bacteriuria on routine urine collection. In infections caused by organisms that in other circumstances are often discounted as contaminants (e.g., staphylococci or *Candida albicans*) suprapubic aspiration may be required in order to confirm the significance of such pathogens.

In patients in whom the possibility of infravesicular infection must be evaluated (e.g., in those with chronic infections of the urethra or the periurethral glands), suprapubic aspiration helps to separate "bladder urine" from "urethral urine."

Procedure

The physician should first locate the bladder. A full, palpable, percussable bladder is most helpful, but even a partially filled bladder may be aspirated. The point of entry in the skin should be 1 to 2 cm cephalad to the upper edge of the symphysis. The angle of needle advancement toward the bladder through the intervening tissues is perpendicular to the abdominal wall, (usually 10 to 20 degrees from the true vertical) in children and somewhat caudad in adults (Figs. 73–6A and B and Fig. 73–7). Note that the bladder of a newborn is an abdominal organ and will be missed if the needle is inserted too close to the pubis or is angled toward the feet.

The child is placed supine and restrained with the legs in a frog-legged position. Once the prepared skin has been draped and the point of entry has been chosen, a skin wheal of local anesthetic agent is raised to reduce discomfort. When the skin has been anesthetized, a longer, larger-caliber needle (usually 22 gauge, 3.75 to 8.75 cm in length) is advanced in the midline through the skin and quickly into the bladder. We prefer to advance the needle attached to a syringe, with minimal aspiration during advancement. As soon as the bladder is entered, urine enters the syringe. A short needle is adequate for virtually all pediatric patients. Aspiration is commenced as soon as the bladder is entered. If urine is not obtained, the needle is not removed but withdrawn slightly and redirected at another angle. A child may start voiding as soon as the bladder is irritated by the needle. An assistant may prevent urination by occluding the penile urethra in the male infant or by applying pressure to the anterior aspect of the rectum (with a finger tip in the rectum) in the female. Prior placement of a perineal collection bag may assist urine collection. After the urine has been collected, the syringe and the needle are withdrawn. Usually, no further care is needed. Microscopic hematuria virtually always occurs after the procedure but gross hematuria is uncommon.

In most patients, a urine sample can be obtained with the first needle pass. If the needle points too caudad, to avoid entering the peritoneum, it is possible to enter the retropubic space, skimming the bladder muscle and never penetrating the bladder mucosa. After the urine has been collected, the syringe and the needle are withdrawn. Usually, no further care is needed.

Complications

Stamey has performed several thousand aspirations without complications.[23] Bacteremia does not result from the procedure.[27] Bowel penetration has occurred in children who had "distended" abdomens from gastrointestinal disturbances.[28] The combination of gaseous distention of bowel and relative hypovolemia may displace and flatten the relatively empty bladder against the pelvic floor. Even when the large bowel has been penetrated, the patient has recovered uneventfully. Pathologic examination of a clinically penetrated bowel wall was performed in a single postmortem case (the patient died of an already established peritonitis); no entry "needle track" could be found in the deceased. A simple penetration of the bowel with a needle is considered an innocuous event and requires no specific treatment.

PERCUTANEOUS SUPRAPUBIC CYSTOSTOMY

Background

Although suprapubic cystostomy was described as early as four centuries ago, the safety of the procedure was first demonstrated by Garson and Peterson in 1888. The first modern method was the Campbell trocar set, described in 1951.[29, 30] Campbell used a sharp trocar passing through a sheath. The sheath had a longitudinal portion of its wall missing to permit a balloon-type retention catheter to be passed into the bladder. The Campbell trocar is a large-diameter instrument, accepting up to a 20 French catheter. It is thus probably unsuitable for use under local anesthesia in a nonsurgical suite setting.

Subsequently, a wide variety of smaller suprapubic cystostomy devices were reported: large-gauge intravenous Teflon catheters,[31-33] thin polyethylene catheters inserted through large-gauge needles,[34] and spinal needles.[35] Although it is true that all of these may have a useful role in the management of bladder and urethral problems, their small caliber makes them prone to obstruction and applicable only for short-term use.

The development of punch thoracostomy tube sets suggested their use as modified cystostomy tubes. This led to the invention of medium-caliber cystostomy tubes, which were easier to insert than the Campbell trocar but provided more satisfactory drainage than adaptations of intravenous infusion sets.[36-38] Ingram's trocar catheter is perhaps the best known of these tubes. It has three lumina: one for inflating the retention balloon and the other two for drainage or irrigation. The Ingram catheter is available in a 12 or 16 French size. The Stamey suprapubic catheter is another variation of this type, but it uses a four-wing Malecot-type retention device rather than an inflatable balloon.

Perhaps the most widely known and frequently used trocar cystostomy tube is the Cystocath.[39] It is available in 8 and 12 French sizes. The latter is more commonly used for adult patients. The Cystocath is packaged as a self-contained set supplying virtually everything needed for insertion. The device is easy to insert and may be satisfactory for relatively long periods of trouble-free use if the patient is given conscientious nursing care.

A major difficulty with cystostomy tubes of all designs has been securing them to the patient's skin. Those with retention balloons, such as the regular Foley urethral catheter or the Ingram catheter, are most secure and need tape only to provide a "safety factor" security. Virtually all other systems depend on tape or skin adhesive to hold either the tube or the appliance in place. With the development of newer adhesives and secure taping of the tubing to the urinary drainage bag, these devices may also be securely maintained. As with all tubing, these urinary drainage devices require awareness and care on the part of all personnel involved.

Indications

In general, any patient who would require a urethral catheter but in whom a catheter cannot be passed needs a

A

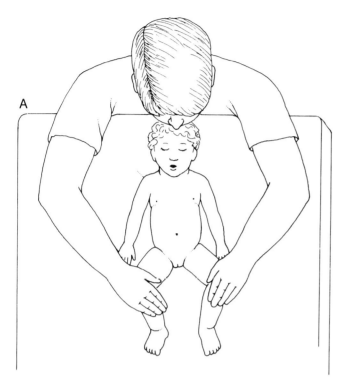

B

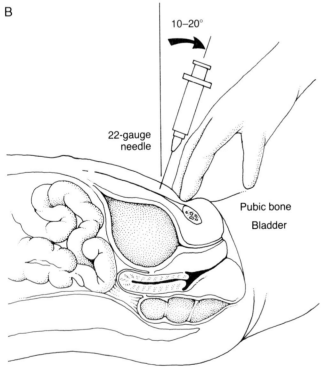

10–20°

22-gauge
needle

Pubic bone

Bladder

Figure 73–6. A, For a suprapubic bladder tap, the infant is restrained
and placed in a frog-legged position. *B,* A 22-gauge needle punctures the abdominal wall in the midline approximately 1 to 2 cm
cephalad to the superior border of the pubic bone. The syringe is
perpendicular to the plane of the abdominal wall (usually 10 to 20
degrees from the true vertical). In infants the bladder is an abdominal organ, and placing the needle too close to the pubic bone or
angling toward the feet may miss the bladder.

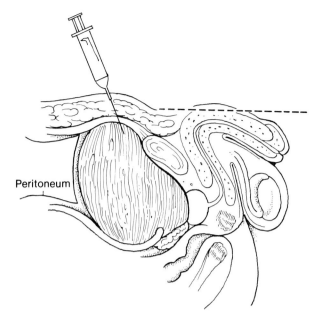

Figure 73–7. The peritoneum is pushed cephalad by the filled bladder during suprapubic aspiration in an adult. The needle is directed slightly caudad.

suprapubic cystostomy tube. In emergency situations, the majority of these patients are men with urethral or prostatic disease. Dilation can usually be performed in patients with urethral strictures using filiforms and followers. If there is any difficulty with the passage of either filiforms or followers, a cystostomy tube is prudent and prevents further injury to an already diseased urethra. Patients who present with acute urethral trauma may also need a cystostomy tube either to prevent further trauma to the urethra or to bypass a completely transected urethra. Complete urethral transection associated with a pelvic fracture is an indication for emergent suprapubic cystostomy. Many affected patients need laparotomy because of associated injuries, and a large tube can be placed at surgery. On the other hand, if the patient does not require laparotomy, a percutaneous urinary diversion allows urologic surgery to be delayed until the patient is clinically stable.

Patients with lower genitourinary infection deserve special care before urethral instrumentation. The risk of inciting an episode of sepsis with urethral catheterization is considerable. Suprapubic drainage should be considered in these patients. In men with acute prostatitis or epididymitis who require drainage, a suprapubic catheter allows both urinary drainage and unobstructed drainage of prostatic, seminal vesicular, and urethral secretions.

Neurologically disabled patients (e.g., quadriplegics or paraplegics) who have been maintained on a program of intermittent catheterization occasionally have difficulties with urethral catheter passage. In such patients, especially high paraplegics and quadriplegics, suprapubic cystostomy can be a rapidly effective method of relieving bladder distention. Catheter passage in the dysreflexic, profusely perspiring, hypertensive quadriplegic in "sympathetic crisis" or "autonomic dysreflexia" is perhaps the most dramatic example of suprapubic cystostomy tube placement as a truly emergency procedure.

Suprapubic catheterization is *not* recommended for a patient who is merely voiding poorly from lower tract obstruction. Such a person, although symptomatic, is better off without instrumentation. Patients with uninfected chronic retention should not be introduced to the hazards of catheter drainage before definitive surgical correction. A sterile residual urine is less of a hazard to the patient than an offense to the physician. Patients with idiopathic retention, typically young females with psychosocial or emotional problems, can often be managed by intermittent urethral self-catheterization.

Contraindications

Because placement of a suprapubic tube involves some risk, patient selection is important. The procedure should not be performed in a patient whose bladder is not definable. Although no absolute reported minimum bladder volume has ever been established, there must be enough urine in the bladder to allow the trocar to penetrate the bladder dome fully without immediately exiting through the base. There also must be enough urine in the bladder to push the bowels free from the anterior surface of the bladder and the entrance of the trocar (Fig. 73–8). If there is doubt

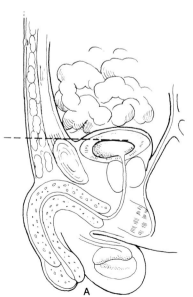
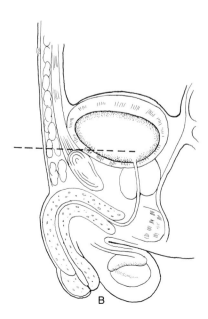

Figure 73–8. Cystostomy tube placement. Relation of peritoneum to bladder with bladder empty and full. *A,* With an empty bladder or a peritoneum scarred down into the pelvis from previous surgery or radiation, the peritoneal reflection may descend below the top of the symphysis pubis and thus "close the window" for passing the trocar along the dotted line. *B,* As the bladder fills, it lifts the peritoneum above the symphysis pubis and "opens the window" for safe trocar insertion.

about the bladder limits, ultrasound guidance may be used to place the catheter.

Individuals who have a lower abdominal scar and a history of intraperitoneal surgery or irradiation may have adhesions of bowel to the anterior bladder and are at risk for bowel injury during percutaneous cystostomy tube placement. Blind suprapubic cystostomy tube placement in these patients should be avoided. The absence of a lower abdominal scar or irradiation history unfortunately does not totally protect the patient from the risk of bowel or intraperitoneal injury.

Patients with bleeding disorders are at relatively greater risk for postinsertion bleeding either into the bladder or into the retropubic space.

Equipment

The items of equipment needed for Cystocath placement are listed in Table 73–2.

Procedure

The comments that follow describe the use of the Cystocath set. With modifications, they are applicable for any type of suprapubic tube.

PREPARING THE PATIENT

Having decided that a particular patient is a suitable candidate for the procedure, we prepare him for placement of the device. If necessary, the lower abdomen is shaved. Povidone-iodine skin preparation or another suitable bactericide is used to cleanse the area. The extra liquid is then wiped off, and the skin is allowed to dry. Next, a 1-ml syringe is half filled with 1 per cent lidocaine, and a 22-gauge, 7.75 cm spinal needle is attached. A skin wheal in the proposed site (approximately 2 to 3 cm above the pubic symphysis) is raised, and the subcutaneous tissue and the fascia of the rectus abdominis muscle are infiltrated at a 10- to 20-degree angle toward the pelvis. By the time the rectus fascia has been infiltrated, the syringe is empty (Fig. 73–9).

With the same needle, an attempt is next made to *find* the bladder. Our experience has been that when one can find the bladder with the smaller needle rather than the trocar, success is virtually assured and complications of placement are eliminated. Placement of the patient in a 10-degree head-down (Trendelenburg) position is believed to aid in movement of bowel away from the pelvis and bladder.[40, 41] Filling of the bladder is also recommended to minimize catheter misplacement.[41]

One finds the bladder by advancing the needle in the prescribed direction while pulling back on the syringe plunger. When the bladder is entered, urine is easily aspi-

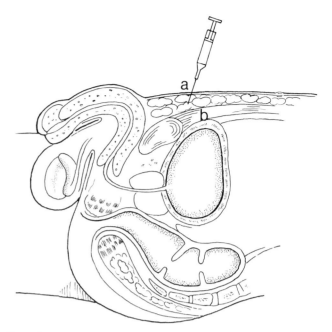

Figure 73–9. Cystostomy tube placement. Anesthetizing the trocar tract. After the skin wheal *(a)* is raised, the suprapubic tract for the trocar is anesthetized, including the rectus fascia *(b)*. Anesthetizing until the bladder is penetrated ensures total comfort for the patient during trocar insertion.

rated. The operator should then make a mental note of the angle and the depth of entry. The needle may be left in place. Care should be taken not to advance the needle into the prostatic fossa under the pubis in the male with a large prostate.

PLACING THE TUBE

Having found the bladder, the operator now makes final preparation of the Cystocath apparatus. First, the face plate is inspected and the central hole is enlarged with a scalpel or a scissors. We have found that this is necessary because the trocar insertion is restrained by the small hole in the face plate and increases the pressure required to advance the trocar. Enlarging the opening also facilitates cleaning of the entry site.

Next, if the patient's pubic hair line (even after shaving) interferes with satisfactory placement of the face plate hole over the anesthetized skin wheal, part of the lower half of the face plate may be trimmed off. The adhesive bottle is opened, and both the face plate and the patient's skin are covered with adhesive and allowed to dry.

While the adhesive is drying, the tubing is "customized." The bladder end of the tubing has only two side openings supplied by the manufacturer. We always make four or five extra side openings using a scalpel or a scissors. This reduces the possibility of blockage of the tube.

By the time the tubing has been prepared, the face plate is ready for positioning. We position the face plate with the flanges at the 10 and 4 o'clock positions rather than at 9 and 3 o'clock (Fig. 73–10). Positioned in this manner, the tubing approaches the face plate from above the iliac crest, not over it, and is much more comfortable for the patient (see Fig. 73–14). In addition, the iliac crest will "protect" the tubing if the patient turns on his side.

The faceplate is then carefully placed on the skin with the central opening over the skin wheal. When the faceplate is well adhesed, we use the scalpel to make a stab wound in

Table 73–2. Materials for Cystocath Placement (Authors' Method)

Cystocath set
Urinary cath tray (without catheter)
1 per cent lidocaine (Xylocaine)
10-ml syringe with 22-gauge, 1½″ or 22-gauge, 3½″ spinal needle
Scalpel blade (number 11)
Urinary collection bag
Cloth or plastic tape
Benzoin (for increasing tape adherence)

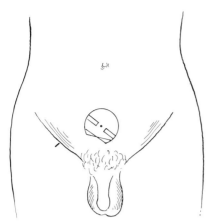

Figure 73–10. Cystostomy tube placement. Faceplate orientation. If the faceplate is rotated with the flange in the 10:00 to 4:00 o'clock position, the tubing passes above the iliac crest and is protected by it. We also trim the lower edge of the faceplate to permit placement lower on the abdomen.

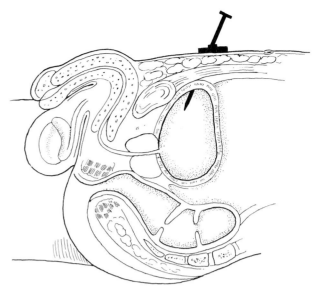

Figure 73–12. Cystostomy tube placement. Trocar position. The trocar should be advanced until the sheath, as well as the point, is fully in the bladder.

the skin at the entry site. In thin patients, we also incise the previously anesthetized rectus fascia. Incising the skin and the fascia with the scalpel reduces the resistance to the trocar and allows the operator's fingers to sense the layers of the abdominal wall and the bladder without having to "discount" the resistance of the skin and the rectus fascia.

Using the angle of approach and depth of penetration already known from the earlier needle search, one advances the trocar into the bladder (Fig. 73–11). The characteristic release of resistance when the trocar penetrates the bladder muscle and mucosa is an indication of success, but the sine qua non is return of urine through the trocar sheath. After urine is obtained, we advance the trocar another 2 to 3 cm to make sure that the trocar *sheath* as well as the trocar *point* is in the bladder, because urine may escape along the trocar point and into the sheath even if the sheath is not well into the bladder (Fig. 73–12).

The trocar is then withdrawn. Escape of urine is pre-

vented by a finger over the trocar sheath end, and tubing is advanced into the sheath. We always advance the tubing until the black midway mark is inside the trocar sheath. Then the trocar sheath is withdrawn while the tubing is gently advanced. The soft Silastic tubing easily coils in the bladder (Fig. 73–13).

With the trocar sheath withdrawn, the tubing is connected to the three-way urine bag adapter. The *adapter* is then positioned in the groove of the face plate flange.

After the urine collection bag has been attached and the three-way stopcock has been opened, the urine may be allowed to drain freely. The puncture site is cleaned, and antimicrobial ointment is placed over the tube entry site. The face plate adhesive may be reinforced with tape at this time.

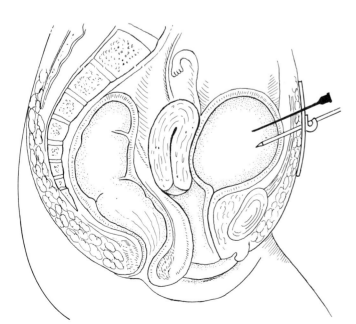

Figure 73–11. Cystostomy tube placement. Needle localization of the bladder. A spinal needle may be used even during trocar insertion to locate the bladder.

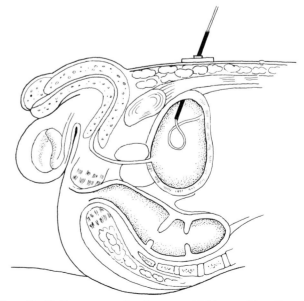

Figure 73–13. Cystostomy tube placement. Tubing position. Enough tubing should be inserted so that it does not pull out of the bladder when the bladder empties.

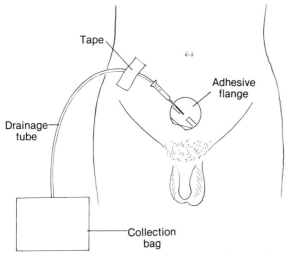

Figure 73–14. Cystostomy tube placement. The urine bag is taped firmly to the patient.

The tubing of the urine bag *must* be taped to the patient so that the flange and the adapter do not hold the urine bag up, because they are not designed for this purpose (Fig. 73–14).

Complications

A wide variety of complications have been reported and serve as reminders that suprapubic cystostomy is not innocuous. Occasionally, despite the best intentions, the tube cannot be positioned or maintained successfully without untoward sequelae (Table 73–3).

The most serious complications involve perforation of the peritoneum or the intraperitoneal contents. Any condition that might fix the anterior peritoneum so low that the filled bladder cannot lift the peritoneum cephalad may result in either transperitoneal bladder puncture or possible perforation of the small or large bowel (Fig. 73–15).[40–42]

The cystostomy tube that merely traverses the peritoneum may produce a mild ileus, serve as a route for peritoneal infection, or drain the bladder contents into the peritoneum. The last situation should be expected if one of the extra holes of the tubing opens into the peritoneal cavity. Through-and-through bladder penetration with associated rectal, vaginal, or uterine injury is also possible, although the consistent use of small-gauge bladder needles and the judicious advancement of the trocar should reduce the incidence.

Table 73–3. Reported Complications of Suprapubic Cystostomy
Bowel perforation
Intraperitoneal extravasation (without a prior history of surgery)
Extraperitoneal extravasation
Infection of space of Retzius
Ureteral catheterization
Obstruction of tubing by blood, mucus, or kinking
Tubing comes out
Faceplate not secure
Hematuria

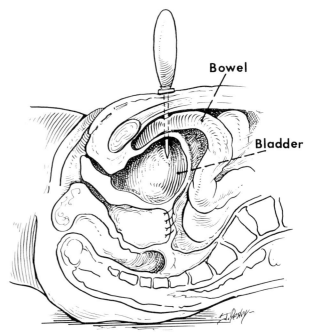

Figure 73–15. Bowel injury in suprapubic cystostomy. Previous injury, radiation, or even an empty bladder may result in the peritoneal reflection dipping below the symphysis pubis and allowing the intraperitoneal contents to be interposed into the trocar tract. (From Noller KL, Pratt JH, Symmonds RE: Bowel perforation with suprapubic cystostomy. Obstet Gynecol 48:695, 1976. Reproduced by permission.)

We believe that our practice of finding the bladder with a small-gauge needle helps to reduce bowel injury, but we are cognizant of the fact that even in the most apparently successful bladder punctures a complication may result.

Occasionally, the physician is tempted to continue with suprapubic cystostomy when the bladder is not palpable and has not been found with the needle. Injury of adjacent organs is much more frequent in such circumstances. If physicians remind themselves that the bladder eventually refills, they will find waiting much more tolerable. If the bladder cannot be found with the trocar at the first pass, one should resist the inclination to "look for" it with the trocar. It is better to backtrack, using the small-gauge needle to find the bladder again, and then to advance the trocar alongside the spinal needle (see Fig. 73–11). If one finds a small bladder with the needle only, one may fill it by putting saline into the bladder through the needle. If a catheter can be passed, the bladder may be filled by way of the catheter. Rarely, the Cystocath tubing ends up in a ureteral orifice or in the urethra.[43] By aspirating on the tubing gently while retracting it, one can usually reposition it correctly. Fluoroscopy may be helpful in such circumstances. Because the Cystocath tubing comes coiled up and may still be slightly curled, inserting the tube with the coil pointing posteriorly or laterally allows the tube to enter the bladder away from the urethra.

Tube drainage may cease for several reasons. A small blood clot or mucus may obstruct the tubing. The tubing may kink in or outside of the bladder. When kinked, the tube can be irrigated easily, although no fluid can be aspirated.

The catheter tubing may be inadvertently pulled partially out of the bladder, causing extravasation out of one of the tubing holes. One can often prevent this problem by inserting enough tubing into the bladder so that minor dislocation will not alter drainage. One catheter system has had catheter breakage occur below the surface of the skin, resulting in leakage and separation.[44]

Infection may occur at the skin puncture site or anywhere along the course of the tube.[45] Use of antimicrobial ointment daily with cleaning of the tube entry site reduces purulence around the tube. Deeper infections may result from infected urine or from a superficial infection spreading along the tube to a hematoma at the bladder, rectal, or fascial level. Parenteral antibiotics may be required, although open drainage is rarely needed.

Hematuria is rarely more than a temporary problem.[46] After insertion, bladder irrigation may occasionally be required.

PHIMOSIS AND DORSAL SLIT

Introduction and Background

Subsequent to injury, the foreskin reacts (as do other tissues) by forming scar tissue. The normally highly pliable foreskin can therefore develop sufficient scar tissue to make retraction difficult. This is especially true if the end of the foreskin is injured, such as in zipper injuries, in toilet seat or other crush injuries (known as the Tristram Shandy syndrome, named after the well-known literary character who had a window sash fall on him while he was urinating out of the window), or in chronic irritation and superficial infection, such as often occurs in diabetes.[47] Occasionally, a tight phimosis and accompanying poor hygiene can lead to abscesses of the foreskin, which may result in further contracture.

Asymptomatic phimosis does not ordinarily call for any emergency treatment but may prevent sterile (or even unsterile) catheterization. In such situations, the phimosis may be relaxed by a dorsal slit of the foreskin. This minor operative procedure is similar to the relaxing incision in treating irreducible paraphimosis and can be performed with local anesthesia in the cooperative patient.

Phimosis has existed since ancient times. Models of phimotic foreskin have been found near the altars of Hygeia and Aesendopius in ancient Greece. Orikosius (A.D. 325–403) was the first to describe the treatment of phimosis by incision.

Indications and Contraindications

The dorsal slit is used to allow urethral catheterization in an emergency situation in which phimosis is present. The technique should not be used in a nonemergency situation in which circumcision could be performed.

Procedure

The items of equipment needed are listed in Table 73–4. After cleansing the penis using sterile technique and

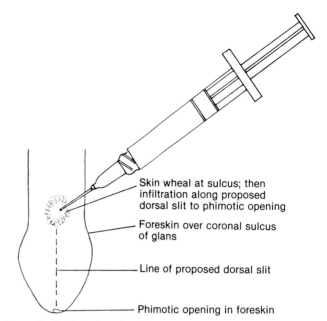

Figure 73–16. Technique for obtaining anesthesia before performing a dorsal slit.

Skin wheal at sulcus; then infiltration along proposed dorsal slit to phimotic opening

Foreskin over coronal sulcus of glans

Line of proposed dorsal slit

Phimotic opening in foreskin

draping it with sterile towels, one infiltrates 1 per cent local anesthetic *without* epinephrine into the dorsal midline of the foreskin along the course of the proposed slit, starting proximally and proceeding distally (Fig. 73–16). After an appropriate duration, the foreskin is tested for anesthesia with a forceps. The operator should be certain that the inner surface of the foreskin is also anesthetized. If it is not, a more circumferential infiltration of the skin around the base of the penis may need to be made (Fig. 73–17).[48, 49]

After adequate anesthesia, the operator takes a straight hemostatic or Crile forceps and advances one jaw carefully under the foreskin but *not* into the glans or the urethra (Fig. 73–18). After the forceps has been positioned correctly, the instrument is closed. The forceps is allowed to remain in place for a few minutes. When the forceps is removed, the serrated, crushed skin should be cut lengthwise with scissors. Normally little bleeding occurs, and often there is no separation of the skin edges. Nonetheless, to prevent bleeding and to keep the cut edges of the foreskin from separating, a 4–0 chromic suture is used to close the edge of the incision (Fig. 73–19A and B).

After suturing the slit open, the operator may retract the foreskin for cleansing and for completing the procedure that necessitated the dorsal slit.

After a dorsal slit procedure, a delayed elective circumcision is often required. A dorsal slit alone produces a "beagle-eared" deformity by transposing all the foreskin to a ventral position. The patient may complain about the appearance and the inconvenience during urination (Fig. 73–19C).

Complications

Injury to the meatus and the glans penis may occur if the hemostat or scissors are introduced into the urethra. Bleeding may occur if the hemostat has not adequately crushed the tissue or the incision made was lateral to the crushed area.

Table 73–4. Equipment Needed to Perform Dorsal Slit for the Emergency Treatment of Phimosis
1 per cent lidocaine (Xylocaine) without epinephrine
5-ml syringe
27-gauge needle
1 straight Crile clamp
1 straight scissors
1 needle holder
4–0 chromic catgut suture

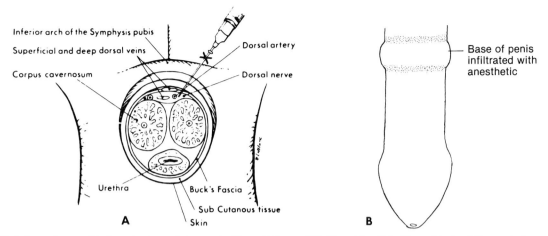

Figure 73–17. *A,* Dorsal nerve block at the base of the penis. (From Soliman MG, Tremblay NA: Nerve block of the penis for postoperative pain relief in children. Anesth Analg 57:495, 1978. Reproduced by permission.) *B,* Subcutaneous infiltration for a field block at the base of the penis, providing anesthesia to the entire distal penis.

PARAPHIMOSIS

Introduction and Background

Paraphimosis is secondary retraction of a phimotic foreskin causing painful swelling in the glans penis. In the obtunded or demented patient, pain is not a voiced symptom. Paraphimosis has probably existed ever since the first retraction of the foreskin. Today, the most common cause is iatrogenic—the catheterist forgets to replace the foreskin after urethral instrumentation. The condition may be misinterpreted as an allergic reaction or a penile trauma or infection by those unfamiliar with the condition (Fig. 73–20A). The constricting ring interferes with venous and lymphatic return, precipitating swelling. The swelling then prevents reduction of the retracted foreskin. When left untreated, a paraphimosis may progress from tissue anoxia to skin ulceration and infection or penile gangrene.[50] Paraphimosis may occur if the foreskin is left retracted proximal to the glans after the patient has cleansed under the foreskin (even in as benign a procedure as penile cleaning).

Reduction of the edematous foreskin is a temporary measure to relieve discomfort and edema and to permit resolution of more serious effects—skin ulceration and infection—until a definitive treatment (circumcision) can be performed.

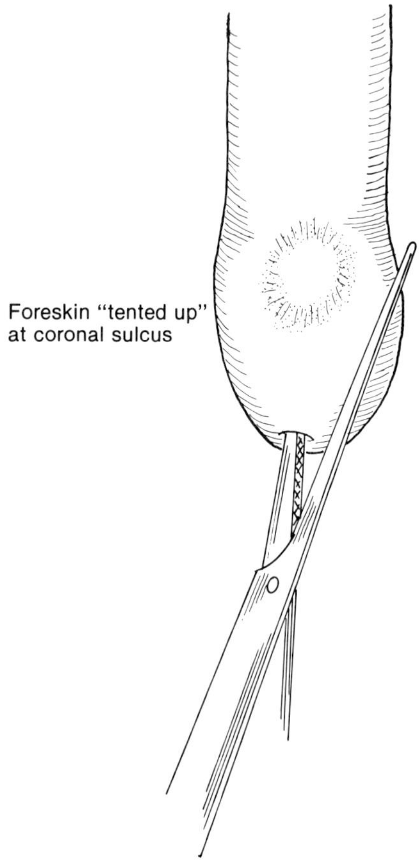

Foreskin "tented up" at coronal sulcus

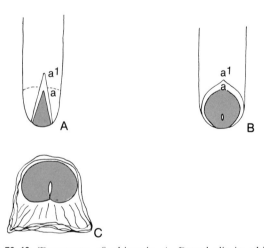

Figure 73–19. Treatment of phimosis. *A,* Dorsal slit in phimotic foreskin. Exposed glans is shaded. A single (dorsal) lengthwise incision has been made through crushed tissue. a^1, outer layer of foreskin; a, inner layer of foreskin. *B,* Cut edges of foreskin drawn back around glans penis. First, a^1 is sutured to a, then the remainder of the cut edges are sewn together for hemostasis. *C,* Final "beagle-ear" deformity of ventral transposed foreskin after the dorsal slit procedure has been completed.

Figure 73–18. Placement of forceps for treatment of phimosis. The foreskin "tented up" in this manner proves that the tip of the forceps is not in the urethra or under the glans.

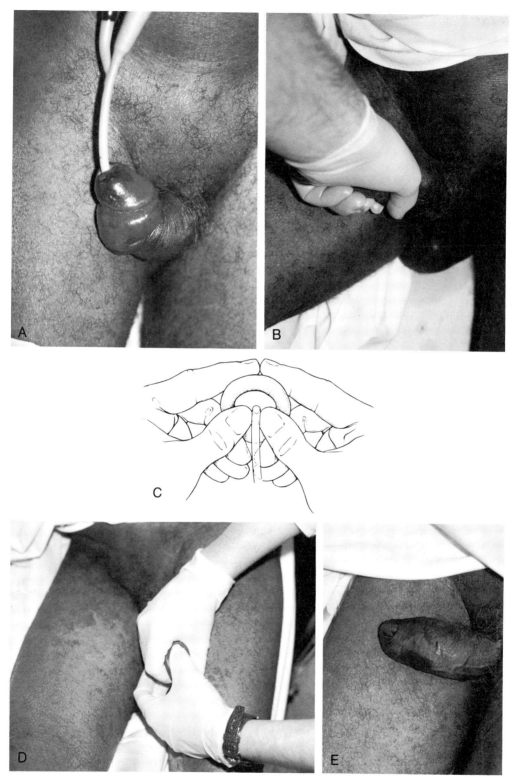

Figure 73–20. *A,* Paraphimosis, pictured here, may be mistaken for penile trauma, angioedema, or infection. The cause of paraphimosis in this case was failure to replace the foreskin following a catheter change in a demented nursing home patient. *B,* Manual compression of the foreskin may reduce edema before attempting a reduction of the paraphimosis. *C,* Technique for reduction of paraphimosis. Gentle, steady pressure is placed on the glans with the tips of the thumbs while gentle traction is applied to the foreskin. If replacement is difficult, the Foley catheter should be removed. *D,* In a manner reminiscent of removing a rubber glove, the thumb forces the glans through the foreskin that is encircled by the entire palm to achieve final reduction *(E).* *(C* from Neuwirth H, et al: Genitourinary imaging and procedures by the emergency physician. Emerg Med Clin North Am 7:1, 1989.)

Indications

Reduction of a paraphimotic foreskin is indicated whenever the condition is present. There are no contraindications.

Methods of Reduction

The items of equipment needed for reduction of paraphimotic foreskin are listed in Table 73–5.

Manual Reduction.[50, 51] A nonirritating lubricant is applied to the undersurface of the foreskin (not to the shaft of the penis) and the glans to reduce friction. A topical anesthetic lubricant jelly decreases the considerable discomfort of the procedure. A penile block may be performed if required. The foreskin is then manually compressed for several minutes to reduce edema as much as possible (Fig. 73–20B). Snugly wrapping the distal penis in a 5-cm piece of elastic wrap for 10 minutes may also be useful.[52] Injection of hyaluronidase[53] has also been reported to reduce edema but is unnecessary. If the patient is catheterized, *the catheter is removed to be replaced later.*

The glans penis is then gently but persistently pressed through the phimotic constricting ring with both thumbs until it slips through (Fig. 73–20C). At the same time, an attempt is made to draw the foreskin back down over the glans with the index and middle fingers. The physician must determine that the glans has truly passed through the ring, since the proximal foreskin may easily hide the glans and may give a false appearance of reduction. Alternatively, the thumb may be used to push the glans through the foreskin that has been encircled by the entire palm—in a maneuver similar to taking off a rubber glove (Fig. 73–20D and E). The key to success in both of these maneuvers is the application of slow, steady pressure.

Assisted Manual Reduction ("Iced-Glove" Method[54] or Babcock Clamp Method[55]). If the constricting ring cannot be brought down over the glans easily, additional measures may be tried. In the "iced-glove" method,[54] cold compression is used to reduce foreskin swelling and to induce vasoconstriction in the glans. A large latex glove is half filled with crushed ice and water, and the cuff end is securely tied. The thumb of the glove is invaginated by the operator and then is drawn over the lubricated paraphimotic penis. The thumb of the glove is held securely in place over the penis for 5 to 10 minutes. The combination of cooling and compression usually decreases the edema sufficiently to permit full reduction of the foreskin. If the constricting ring cannot be brought down over the glans after this maneuver, it may be necessary to be more forcible. Six or eight Babcock clamps (*not* Allis clamps, which are serrated and intolerably painful

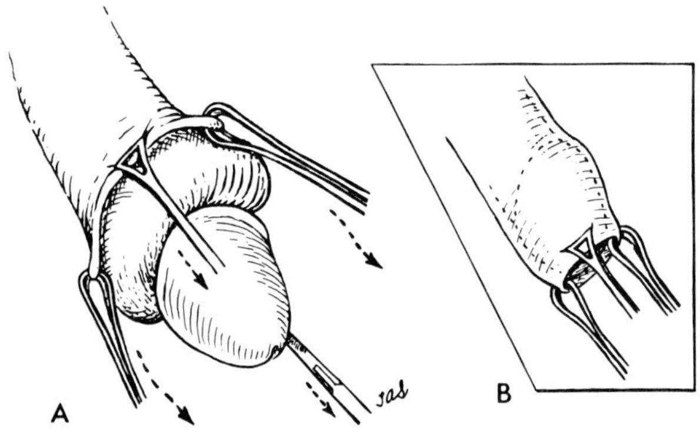

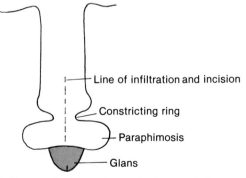

Figure 73–21. *A,* Application of Babcock clamps to reduce paraphimosis. *B,* Foreskin reduced. (From Skoglund RW, Chapman WH: Reduction of paraphimosis. J Urol 104:137, 1970. Reproduced by permission. © Williams & Wilkins, 1970.)

for the patient) are used to grasp the phimotic ring circumferentially.[55] The clamps are then slowly levered forward over the glans. With gentle, slow traction, the ring is brought over the glans (Fig. 73–21).

Dorsal Slit.[48] This procedure is indicated when other methods are not successful or when skin ulceration and infection are present. Should manual or assisted reduction not be successful, a dorsal slit may be required.[56–58] Although it is usually recommended that this procedure be performed in the operating suite, it may be undertaken with local anesthesia in the emergency department.

The penis is cleansed and draped with sterile towels. Using a 1 per cent solution of local anesthetic *without epinephrine,* one infiltrates the foreskin at the 12 o'clock position, making sure to infiltrate proximally and distally as well as into the constricted ring (Figs. 73–22 and 73–23).

The skin, the edematous subcutaneous layer, and the constricting ring are then incised with a knife. One should take care not to injure the penile shaft below the dartos fascia or the glans. The skin on the penile shaft should not be incised too proximally, because a tethered or hidden penis may result. When the constricting ring is incised completely, the foreskin edges will relax laterally and produce a diamond-shaped defect, which is then ready for suturing.

Using 3–0 or 4–0 chromic sutures, the two apices of the dorsal slit (labeled *a* and *b* in Fig. 73–23) are approximated. The two wings of the slit are then sutured in interrupted or continuous fashion to ensure hemostasis and rapid healing.

Table 73–5. Equipment Needed for Reduction of Paraphimosis

For Nonoperative Emergency Reduction of Paraphimosis
1 per cent lidocaine (Xylocaine) jelly
Crushed ice
Size 8 latex surgical glove
Babcock clamps (6 to 8)

For Operative Reduction of Paraphimosis
Sterile preparation solution
1 per cent lidocaine (Xylocaine) without epinephrine
5-ml syringe
27-gauge needle
Number 15 surgical knife with handle
Needle holder
4–0 chromic catgut suture

Line of infiltration and incision

Constricting ring

Paraphimosis

Glans

Figure 73–22. Anesthetizing the penis for surgical treatment of paraphimosis. Line of infiltration of local anesthesia used before performing dorsal slit.

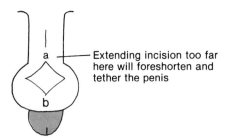

Figure 73–23. Incision for paraphimosis. Diamond-shaped defect resulting from incision of foreskin. The two apices of the dorsal slit (*a* and *b*) are approximated.

Few patients with a dorsal slit will be satisfied with the "beagle-eared" appearance of their foreskin after the edema resolves, and a circumcision will be needed to complete the treatment of the paraphimosis. (Circumcision is elective, however, and should be delayed until edema, inflammation, and ulceration have cleared.)

Complications

In reduction of paraphimosis with Babcock clamps, if traction is applied asymmetrically or too vigorously, tearing of the skin may result. If tearing occurs, operative reduction using a dorsal slit should be performed.

PENILE ASPIRATION FOR PRIAPISM
Introduction

Priapism is a painful, persistent, purposeless, penile erection. Although reported for most age groups, the condition is most common between the ages of 30 and 50 years. Priapism may be secondary to a number of medical (e.g., hematologic, neoplastic, and drug-related) conditions, but approximately 35 to 50 per cent of cases are idiopathic. Of note is the recent practice of using vasoactive substances (e.g., papaverine and phentolamine) to induce a penile erection in impotent males. These substances, which promote engorgement of the corpora cavernosum, have been associated with priapism.[59-61]

Dilation of the cavernosal arteries with relaxation of the cavernosal tissue and constriction of the emissary veins lead to engorgement of the corpora cavernosum with blood during an erection. When the cavernosal pressure approaches the arterial pressure, blood flow is markedly reduced. Ischemia results after several hours of continuous erection. Ischemia acutely results in acidosis and sludging of blood with subsequent thrombosis of the cavernosal arteries, fibrosis of the corporal tissue, and impotence.

Therapeutic Concepts

The emergency physician should attempt to identify etiologic factors contributing to the patient's priapism and initiate specific corrective therapy when available. Analgesia, sedation, hydration, and supplemental oxygen are often helpful, especially for the sickle cell patient. Subcutaneous or oral β-agonist therapy (e.g., terbutaline 0.25 mg subcutaneously or 5 mg orally) has been recommended to improve venous outflow from the corpora and can be safely administered in the emergency department.[62]

Indications

More aggressive therapy should be considered in the patient whose priapism does not respond to drug therapy or has persisted for longer than 2 hours. Lue and associates suggest that therapy should be guided by cavernosal blood gas and pressure measurements.[63] When urologic evaluation is delayed, the emergency physician should consider diagnostic and therapeutic corporal aspiration. Whenever possible, invasive therapy should be done after discussion of treatment alternatives with the urologic consultant. Priapism that has persisted for more than 24 hours is unlikely to respond to aspiration alone.

Equipment

The items of equipment needed for aspiration and injection of the corpus cavernosum are listed in Table 73–6.

Procedure

The patient is placed supine in a private setting and made comfortable. Following local anesthesia with 1 per cent lidocaine (plain) or placement of a penile block (see Fig. 73–17), the penis is sterilely prepared and draped. When standing to the right of the patient, the clinician grasps the shaft of the penis with the left hand. The thumb is placed over the dorsal surface and the index finger volarly over the urethra. An engorged corpus cavernosum is palpated laterally and the 19-gauge butterfly needle is inserted through the glans into the distal end of the corpus cavernosum.[64] While a corpus cavernosum may be entered over the shaft of the penis at approximately the 2 o'clock position dorsally, hematomas are more common from the lateral approach.

Blood is aspirated and sent for blood gas analysis. From 5 to 100 ml of additional blood is aspirated while milking the corpus with the left hand until bright red arterial blood is obtained. A second blood gas can be obtained to verify that arterial blood is obtained. Because multiple anastomoses exist between the two corpora, bilateral aspiration is not indicated.

If tumescence returns, one of the α-agonist agents should be injected through the butterfly needle. The use of β agonists for corporal injection or irrigation has also been reported and the advantage of α agonists over β agonists is a subject of debate. O'Brien and associates recommend a 1:100,000 solution of epinephrine (1 mg/100 ml saline), irrigating with 2 to 3 ml at a time to a maximum dose of 0.1 mg (10 ml).[64] Some clinicians wrap the penis snugly in an elastic wrap with the needle securely in place following aspiration to discourage tumescence.

Table 73–6. Equipment Needed for Aspiration of Corpus Cavernosum for Priapism

27-gauge needle (for penile block)
One 12-ml syringe (for local anesthetic)
1 per cent lidocaine without epinephrine (for penile block)
Sterile drapes
Gauze sponges
Povidone-iodine (or alternative) preparation solution
19-gauge butterfly needles (for aspiration)
Two 30-ml syringes (for aspiration and injection)
Sterile basin for aspirated blood
Blood gas syringe with cap
Injection fluid (one of the following diluted with normal saline to
   10 ml volume)
    Phenylephrine 0.2 mg
    Norepinephrine 0.02 mg
    Metaraminol 2–4 mg

Complications

Although hematoma and infection can occur with properly performed aspiration, these complications are infrequent. Adverse hemodynamic effects have occurred with systemic delivery following the use of α-agonist drugs.[63] Blood pressure and cardiac rhythm should be closely monitored during the procedure and following drug delivery. Supplemental oxygen also should be considered in the patient with underlying respiratory or cardiac disease. Because impotence may result following priapism regardless of the cause or promptness of therapeutic intervention, the patient should be cautioned that the clinician cannot guarantee potency following therapy.

Interpretation

The initial corporal blood gas results are believed to reflect the degree of ischemia present in the penis with priapism. Sequential blood gas analysis showing an initial acidosis (pH ≤ 7.10) that does not reverse with the above therapy suggests that a more aggressive shunting procedure may be needed and urgent urologic intervention should be sought. A corpus cavernosum–spongiosum shunt can be created so that blood may drain out of the corpus spongiosum. The corporal needle may also be used for measurement of intracorporal pressures similar to the approach outlined for muscular compartment pressures (see Chapter 72).[63]

DOPPLER DIAGNOSIS OF TESTICULAR BLOOD FLOW

Introduction

Diagnosis in the patient with acute scrotum can at times be difficult. The condition most easily confused with acute epididymitis is torsion of the testicle. The prompt diagnosis and differentiation of this condition is crucial to the patient's care. The treatment of acute epididymitis requires appropriate antimicrobial and supportive therapy. On the other hand, treatment of torsion of the testicle requires that detorsion be performed within 4 to 6 hours to obtain an acceptable testicular salvage rate.[65]

Torsion of the testicle is the most frequent cause of acute testicular pain in boys and in men under the age of 30. In men over the age of 30, torsion is less common, although it may occur into the seventh decade.[66] In contrast, epididymitis is an *uncommon* condition in children and a frequently occurring problem in older men.[67] One pediatric series reported a prevalence of 15 per cent for epididymitis in patients with a painful scrotum versus 45 per cent for testicular torsion and 40 per cent for torsion of the appendix testis and other causes.[68] Interestingly, pyuria was seen in only 24 per cent of the children with epididymitis and in 4 per cent of the patients with testicular torsion. In men under the age of 30, epididymitis is commonly associated with either coliform urinary tract infections or gonococcal or nongonococcal (e.g., chlamydial) urethritis; signs and symptoms of infection may be minimal when the patient is first examined.[69] Because urethritis may easily go unnoticed if the patient has urinated recently, evidence of infection may be lacking. The presence of genitourinary infection may, however, provide an important clue to the diagnosis of epididymitis. Furthermore, if one makes the clinical diagnosis of epididymitis, one should have some objective confirmation, since the misdiagnosis of torsion as epididymitis means the destruction of the testicle.

The "gold standards" for the diagnosis of torsion are the testicular scan or operation. However, because blood flow to the testicle is increased with the inflammation of epididymitis and decreased in torsion of the testicle, the Doppler ultrasound stethoscope can provide objective information that may aid in the differential diagnosis. Although the accuracy of the Doppler examination has been challenged and there have been reports of both false-negative and false-positive results, the advantage of Doppler ultrasound examination is that it can be performed (in the outpatient setting) by anyone familiar with its use. In any questionable case, however, a testicular scan or scrotal exploration should be performed.

Background

In 1974, Milleret and Liaras reported the use of the Doppler ultrasound stethoscope in two cases of torsion of the testicle.[70] Levy[71] in 1975 reported seven more cases. Pederson and coworkers in 1975 used the Doppler stethoscope to examine 45 patients. Levy,[71] Perri and colleagues[72] and Pederson and associates[73] reported 100 per cent accuracy in the diagnosis of torsion of the testicle. Caution was, however, advised by Perri and coworkers,[74] Thompson and colleagues,[75] Rodriquez and coworkers,[76] and Brereton,[77] who found false-positive and false-negative results. The most common error was the false impression of blood flow in the twisted testicle. Haynes reported the results of Doppler ultrasound in the evaluation of 80 adults with scrotal pain and noted that the procedure was accurate in diagnosing torsion in only 7 of 16 (44 per cent) patients. In this series the ultrasound test was indeterminate in 25 per cent and falsely negative in 31 per cent.[78] However, in a review of the Haynes study and other literature, Hardwick notes that no study has reported a false-negative Doppler examination when used within the first 10 hours of pain.[79] Therefore, time of examination may be the cortical factor affecting accuracy of Doppler ultrasound.

Indications and Contraindications

Testicular blood flow determination by Doppler ultrasonography should be used to *confirm* the diagnosis of epididymitis in men of the age group in which torsion may commonly occur. This would include any male under the age of 30. Because epididymitis is uncommon in children, the diagnosis of torsion in boys with acute scrotum should be presumed, and surgical exploration for detorsion should be undertaken. In postpubertal men in the absence of convincing evidence of urethritis or urinary tract infection, torsion should also be presumed and exploration should be performed promptly. Radioisotope scans are also useful for the differential diagnosis but are beyond the scope of this chapter.[74, 76, 80] In young men in whom the diagnosis of epididymitis is suggested both by findings on physical examination and by the presence of genitourinary inflammation (pyuria), Doppler ultrasound may be used to confirm the diagnosis by showing that there is blood flow to the testicle. Doppler ultrasound should not be relied upon as the sole diagnostic indicator in the differentiation of torsion from acute epididymitis. Clinical history, physical signs, and examinations of the genitourinary tract for signs of infection should be used to suggest the diagnosis and Doppler used to confirm it. Most errors in diagnosis could have been prevented if the physicians had not overrelied on the Doppler technique. As discussed later, the Doppler also can be used to monitor testicular perfusion during manual detorsion.

Equipment

The directional Doppler operating on a 5.3- to 10-mHz transducer is often used. See Chapter 32 for a detailed discussion of Doppler ultrasound physics. A pencil transducer is the most appropriate; the Model 806 Directional 10-mHz Doppler (Park Electronics Laboratory, Beaverton, Oreg.) and the Medtronics 8-mHz Model BF5A are acceptable devices. The Doppler response may be transmitted over

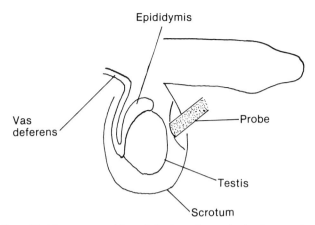

Figure 73–24. Proper position of the Doppler probe in the examination of the acute scrotum. Note caudal orientation of the probe.

a loudspeaker, copied on a measuring device, or transmitted through a stethoscope to the physician. The higher the megahertz, the narrower the beam and the less distance of transmission through the tissues. In this respect, a 10-mHz transducer may be more appropriate for examination of the testicle.

Procedure

Because scrotal tenderness often precludes adequate examination, proper anesthesia must be obtained. We perform a cord block using 1 per cent lidocaine (Xylocaine) at the external ring.[81] The skin is first prepared with an iodophor solution. The cord can usually be grasped between thumb and forefinger, and 10 ml of 1 per cent lidocaine can be directly injected. If the cord is also swollen or if the testicle is very high in the scrotum (so as to preclude grasping), the cord may be palpated as it passes over the pubis and the lidocaine injected at this point. The patient often thanks the physician for this anesthetic procedure after the pain in his testicle acutely subsides.

At this time, adequate examination of the testicle may be performed and the area of maximum swelling determined. An aqueous transmission gel is then placed over the scrotum. Holding the testicle in one hand and the Doppler probe in the other, one displaces as much of the scrotal wall as possible between the skin and the underlying testicle. The Doppler probe should be placed in the center of the testicle, pointing slightly caudally so that one does not pick up pulsations in the cord (Fig. 73–24). (Firm probe pressure "focuses" the ultrasound waves deep to the scrotum into the testis.) The pulsation in the ipsilateral testicle is then compared with that in the contralateral testicle. Decreased or absent flow to the ipsilateral testicle is most surely a result of torsion. Increased flow to the ipsilateral testicle may be a result of epididymitis, inflamed scrotal tissue, a false signal from either the cord or the examiner's fingers,[76] or a false comparison with a contralateral partial torsion of the testis.[74–77, 80]

The *funicular compression test* as described by Pederson and associates[73] is then performed. If the increased signal lessens on compression of the patient's spermatic cord, then the signal is most probably coming from the patient's testicle and not from inflamed scrotal tissues. If there is no change in the signal on adequate cord compression, the increased flow may be originating in inflamed scrotal tissue, and torsion should still be suspected.

TESTICULAR DETORSION

If the diagnosis of torsion is made, the Doppler stethoscope may be used to monitor *manual detorsion* of the testicle.[82–84] Lee and colleagues[85] were able to perform manual detorsion with local anesthesia in 70 per cent of their adult cases of torsion. Kresling and associates[86] had success in 15 of 16 patients and noted that torsion usually resulted from an initial lateral to medial rotation (Fig. 73–25*A*). They also noted an element of caudal to cranial rotation and cremasteric muscle spasm that must be relieved.

Before detorsion, one must ensure that the spermatic cord block is effective and that the patient is in a comfortable reclining or supine position. Some prefer to use intravenous narcotics instead of a block and use relief of pain as an indication of successful detorsion. During detorsion the testis is moved through two planes (Fig. 73–25*B*). Initially an attempt is made to rotate the testicle in a caudal to cranial direction to release the testicle. The testicle is then simultaneously rotated in a medial to lateral direction. With successful detorsion, the testicle returns to its anatomic location, and there is rapid resolution of induration and swelling of the spermatic cord. Occasionally the testis rotates in the opposite direction or has multiple twists. The clinician must assess the results of the procedure by palpation, relief of edema, and return of Doppler tones. After the testicle has been untwisted, the evaluation of the Doppler will show that blood flow has been reestablished. Manual detorsion may save valuable time while the operating suite is being prepared for the patient. *It should not be allowed to delay operative preparations.*

Sources of Error

There are several sources of error in the performance and interpretation of Doppler ultrasound of the testicle. An understanding of these errors will lead to better use and assessment of the procedure. Errors include failing to detect blood flow when it is present and falsely attributing flow from vessels other than the testicular artery as testicular perfusion.

The use of Doppler probes with low-megahertz transducers (less than 10 mHz), which are used for large arteries, is not proper for medium-sized arteries, such as are found in the testes. These probes are able to pick up adjacent arteries in the cord or in the examiner's finger, which may produce positive flow signals.[80] False-positive signals from secondarily inflamed scrotal vessels may be heard. This results from inadequate compression of the skin of the scrotum with the transducer because of pain in an inadequately anesthetized testis. Failure to perform the funicular compression test may lead to the mistaking of scrotal blood flow for testicular blood flow. As the testis liquefies, it may act as a blob of tissue-sonic jelly, and a false-positive signal may be heard from the opposing examining finger. With a partial twist of the testicle, one may also hear an arterial pulse in the testicle with an early partial torsion. For these reasons, it should be evident that one cannot rely entirely on the Doppler ultrasound examination.[77] False-positive flow signals may also be heard if the Doppler is directed upward instead of slightly downward, thus picking up a pulse in the cord above the testicle. A partial twist of the contralateral testicle may also serve as a falsely low standard for arterial blood flow in the rare patient with bilateral torsion.[77]

A false-negative signal may be obtained if the testicular artery in the cord is inadvertently manually compressed by the examiner while he holds the testicle.[77] Hydroceles may also create false-negative results. If these pitfalls are kept in

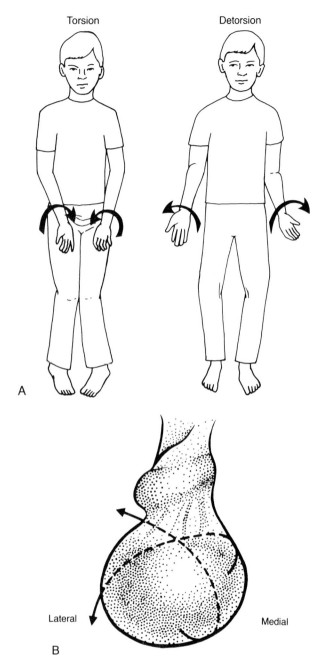

Figure 73–25. *A,* Testicular torsion usually occurs in a medial direction. Detorsion should be attempted initially by rotating the testis outward toward the thigh. This is most successful if attempted within the first few hours of torsion, before the onset of significant scrotal swelling. Intravenous narcotics (such as fentanyl) or a cord block should be administered before attempting detorsion. *B,* Detorsion of the testicle usually requires testicular rotation through two planes. To release the cremasteric muscle, the testis is rotated in a caudal to cranial direction simultaneously with medial to lateral rotation. The right testis is shown. (*B* from Freeman S, et al: Urologic procedures. Emerg Med Clin North Am 4:543, 1986.)

mind and the Doppler ultrasound examination of testicular blood flow used only as one clinical parameter in the management of patients with acute scrotal pain, many errors in diagnosis may be avoided.

REFERENCES

1. Warwick R, William PL: Gray's Anatomy. 35th British Edition. Philadelphia, WB Saunders Co, 1973, p 1336.
2. Blandy JP: Acute retention of urine. Br J Hosp Med 19:109, 1978.
3. Sellett T: Iatrogenic urethral rupture due to preinflation of a urethral catheter. JAMA 21:1548, 1971.
4. Kaplan GW: Complications of circumcision. Urol Clin North Am 10:543, 1983.
5. Walden TB: Urethral catheterization in anasarca. Urology 13:82, 1979.
6. Blandy JP: Urethral stricture. Postgrad Med J 56:383, 1980.
7. Turck M, Goffe B, Petersdorf RG: The urethral catheter and urinary tract infections. J Urol 88:834, 1962.
8. Platt R, Polk BF, Murdock BS, Rosner B: Mortality associated with nosocomial urinary tract infection. N Engl J Med 357:637, 1982.
9. Gulhan PD, Bayley BC, Metzger W, et al: The case against the Foley catheter. Initial report. J Urol 101:909, 1969.
10. Cohen A: A microbiological comparison of a povidone-iodine lubricating gel and a control as catheter lubricants. J Hosp Infect 6(Suppl):155, 1985.
11. Ferrie BG, Groome J, Kirk D: Comparison of silicone and latex catheters in the development of urethral stricture after cardiac surgery. J Urol 58:549, 1986.
12. Sklar DP, Diven B, Jones J: Incidence and magnitude of catheter-induced hematuria. Am J Emerg Med 4:14, 1986.
13. Klein EA, Wood DP, Kay R: Retained straight catheter: Complication of clean intermittent catheterization. J Urol 135:780, 1986.
14. Warren JW, Damron D, Tenney JH, et al: Fever, bacteremia, and death as complications of bacteriuria in women with long-term urethral catheters. J Infect Dis 155:1151, 1987.
15. Johnson DE, O'Reilly JL, Warren JW: Clinical evaluation of an external urine collection device for nonambulatory incontinent women. J Urol 141:535, 1989.
16. Merguerian PA, Erturk E, Hulbert WC, et al: Peritonitis and abdominal free air due to intraperitoneal bladder perforation associated with indwelling urethral catheter drainage. J Urol 134:747, 1985.
17. Steidle CP, Mulcahy JJ: Erosion of penile prostheses: A complication of urethral catheterization. J Urol 142:737, 1989.
18. Eichenberg HA, Amin M, Clark J: Non-deflating Foley catheters. Int Urol Nephrol 8:171, 1976.
19. Moisey CA, Williams LA: Self-retained balloon catheter—a safe method for removal. Br J Urol 52:67, 1980.
20. Reammon RO: Balloon catheters which will not deflate: Simple method of puncturing balloon. J Urol 84:438, 1960.
21. Sood SC, Sahota H: Removing obstructed balloon catheter. Br Med J 4:735, 1972.
22. Browning GG, Barr L, Horsburg AG: Management of obstructed balloon catheters. Br Med J 289:89, 1984.
23. Stamey TA: Pathogenesis and Treatment of Urinary Tract Infections. Baltimore, Williams & Wilkins, 1980.
24. Huze LB, Beeson PB: Observations on the reliability and safety of bladder catheterization for bacteriologic study of the urine. N Engl J Med 255:474, 1956.
25. Pryles PV: Percutaneous bladder aspiration and other methods of urine collection for bacteriologic study. Pediatrics 36:128, 1965.
26. Nelson JD, Peters PC: Suprapubic aspiration of urine in term infants. Pediatrics 36:132, 1965.
27. Mustonen A, Uhari M: Is there bacteremia after suprapubic aspiration in children with urinary tract infection? J Urol 119:822, 1978.
28. Weuthers WT, Wenzl JE: Suprapubic aspiration. Perforation of the viscus other than the bladder. Am J Dis Child 117:590, 1969.
29. Campbell M: A new fenestrated trocar for introduction of balloon catheter in cystostomy, nephrostomy and pyelostomy. J Urol 65:160, 1951.
30. Hodgkinson CP, Hodari H: Trocar suprapubic cystostomy for postoperative bladder drainage in the female. Am J Obstet Gynecol 96:773, 1966.
31. Simon G, Berdon WE: Suprapubic bladder puncture for voiding cystourethrography. J Pediatr 81:555, 1972.
32. Cameron E: Urinary retention managed without urethral catheterization. Lancet 2:606, 1963.
33. Sinha AK: Intracath in suprapubic cystostomy. Lancet 2:1160, 1971.
34. Mattingly R: Commentary on #51. Am J Obstet Gynecol 96:782, 1966.
35. Hey HW: Asepsis in prostatectomy. Br J Surg 33:415, 1945.
36. Ingram JM: Suprapubic cystostomy by trocar catheter. Am J Obstet Gynecol 113:1108, 1972.
37. Tinckler LF: Intracath in suprapubic cystostomy. Lancet 2:206, 1971.
38. Mitchell JP, Gingell JC: Intracath in suprapubic cystostomy. Lancet 1:206, 1972.
39. Greene WR, McLeod DG, Mittemeyer BR: Nonoperative suprapubic urinary drainage. Am Fam Physician 16:136, 1977.
40. Moody TE, Howards SS, Schneider JA, et al: Intestinal obstruction: A complication of percutaneous cystotomy. A case report. J Urol 118:680, 1977.
41. Herbert DB, Mitchell GW Jr: Perforation of the ileum as a complication of suprapubic catheterization. Obstet Gynecol 62:663, 1983.
42. Noller KL, Pratt JH, Symonds RE: Bowel perforation with suprapubic cystostomy. Obstet Gynecol 48(Suppl. 1):67s, 1976.
43. McLeod WL: Commentary on #57. Am J Obstet Gynecol 113:1112, 1972.

44. Drutz HP, Khosid HI: Complications with Bonanno suprapubic catheters. Am J Obstet Gynecol 149:685, 1984.
45. Langley II: Suprapubic cystostomy. Postgrad Med 50:171, 1972.
46. Wolf H, Olsen S, Madsen PO: Suprapubic trocar cystostomy with balloon catheter. Scand J Urol Nephrol 1:66, 1967.
47. Chapra R, Fisher RD, French R: Phimosis and diabetes mellitus. J Urol 127:1101, 1982.
48. Goulding FJ: Penile block for postoperative pain relief in penile surgery. J Urol 126:337, 1981.
49. Soliman MG, Trumble NA: Nerve block of the penis for postoperative pain relief in children. Anesth Analg 57:495, 1978.
50. Campbell M, Harrison JH (eds): Urology. Vol 3, 2nd ed. Philadelphia, WB Saunders Co, 1963.
51. Schenck GF: The treatment of paraphimosis. Am J Surg 8:329, 1930.
52. Ganti SU, Sayegh N, Addonizio JC: Simple method for reduction of paraphimosis. Urology 25:77, 1985.
53. Ratcliff RK: Hyaluronidase in treatment of paraphimosis. JAMA 156:746, 1954.
54. Houghton GR: The "iced-gloved" method of treatment of paraphimosis. Br J Surg 60:876, 1973.
55. Skoglund RW, Chapman WH: Reduction of paraphimosis. J Urol 104:137, 1970.
56. Cletsoway RW, Lewis EL: Treatment of paraphimosis. US Armed Forces J 8:361, 1957.
57. Cumston CG: The correct operation for paraphimosis. Int Clinic 2:47, 1920.
58. Barry CN: A simple method for reduction of paraphimosis. J Urol 71:450, 1954.
59. Kursh ED, Bodner DR, Resnick MI, et al: Injection therapy for impotence. Urol Clin North Am 15:625, 1988.
60. Fernandez JA, Basha MA, Wilson GC: Emergency treatment of papaverine priapism. J Emerg Med 5:289, 1987.
61. O'Brien WM, O'Connor KP, Lynch JH: Priapism: Current concepts. Ann Emerg Med 18:980, 1989.
62. Shantha TR, Finnerty DP, Rodriguez AP: Treatment of persistent penile erection and priapism using terbutaline. J Urol 141:1427, 1989.
63. Lue TF, Helstrom WJ, McAninch JW, et al: Priapism: A refined approach to diagnosis and treatment. J Urol 136:104, 1986.
64. O'Brien WM, O'Connor KP, Lynch JH: Priapism: Current concepts. Ann Emerg Med 18:980, 1989.
65. Deluillar RG, Ireland GW, Cass AS: Early exploration in acute testicular conditions. J Urol 108:887, 1972.
66. Barker K, Raper RP: Torsion of the testis. Br J Urol 36:35, 1964.
67. Dolittle KH, Smith JP, Saylor MI: Epididymitis in the prepubertal boy. J Urol 108:987, 1972.
68. Anderson PAM, Giacomantonio JM: The acutely painful scrotum in children: Review of 113 consecutive cases. Can Med Assoc J 132:1153, 1985.
69. Berger RE, Alexander ER, Harnisch JP, et al: Etiology, manifestations, and therapy of acute epididymitis: Prospective study of 50 cases. J Urol 121:750, 1979.
70. Milleret R, Liaras H: Ultrasonic diagnosis and therapy of torsion of the testes. J Urol 107:35, 1974.
71. Levy B: The diagnosis of torsion of the testicle using the Doppler stethoscope. J Urol 113:63, 1975.
72. Perri A, Slacha G, Feldman A, Kendall AR, Karafin L: The Doppler stethoscope and the diagnosis of the acute scrotum. J Urol 116:598, 1976.
73. Pedersen JF, Holm HH, Huld T: Torsion of the testes diagnosed by ultrasound. J Urol 113:66, 1975.
74. Perri AJ, Rose J, Feldman AE, et al: An evaluation of the role of the Doppler stethoscope and the testicular scan in the diagnosis of torsion of the spermatic cord. Invest Urol 15:275, 1978.
75. Thompson I, LaTourette H, Chadwick S, et al: Diagnosis of testicular torsion using Doppler ultrasonic flowmeter. Urology 6:706, 1975.
76. Rodriguez DD, Rodriguez WC, Rivera JJ, et al: Doppler ultrasound versus testicular scanning in the evaluation of the acute scrotum. J Urol 125:343, 1981.
77. Brereton RJ: Limitation of the Doppler flow meter in the diagnosis of the "acute scrotum" in boys. Br J Urol 53:380, 1981.
78. Haynes BE: Doppler ultrasound failure in testicular torsion. Ann Emerg Med 13:1103, 1984.
79. Hardwick WC: Doppler ultrasound failure. Ann Emerg Med 14:1243, 1985.
80. Blackshear WM, Phillips DJ, Strandness DE: Pulsed Doppler assessment of normal human femoral artery velocity patterns. J Surg Res 27:73, 1979.
81. Smith DP: Treatment of epididymitis by infiltration at spermatic cord with procaine hydrochloride. J Urol 46:74, 1941.
82. Nazrallah PF, Murzone D, King LR: Falsely negative Doppler examinations in testicular torsion. J Urol 118:194, 1977.
83. King LM, Sekasan SK, Schwantker FN: Untwisting in delayed treatment of torsion of the spermatic cord. J Urol 112:217, 1974.
84. Frazier WJ, Bucy JG: Manipulation of torsion of the testicle. J Urol 114:415, 1975.
85. Lee LM, Wright JE, McLoughlin MG: Testicular torsion in the adult. J Urol 130:93, 1983.
86. Kresling V, Schroeder D, Panljev P, et al: Spermatic cord block and manual reduction: Primary treatment for spermatic cord torsion. J Urol 132:921, 1984.

Chapter 74

Radiologic Procedures for the Evaluation of Urinary Tract Trauma

Martin Schiff, Jr., Morton G. Glickman, and Geoffrey E. Herter

Trauma to the urinary tract is frequently seen in emergency departments. The signs of genitourinary (GU) trauma are not usually subtle, and the injury can often be thoroughly evaluated in the emergency department setting. Radiologic imaging of the entire urinary tract can be performed quickly and easily, yielding valuable information to the physician prior to any surgical intervention. The timing of the radiologic evaluation may be challenging to the emergency physician when faced with a critically ill patient with multiple systems trauma. Nonetheless, rarely during resuscitation is a patient not in the emergency department long enough for at least a minimal but critical diagnostic GU evaluation. The extent of such an evaluation, of course, must be determined by the physicians involved in each situation.

INDICATIONS FOR EVALUATION

The urinary tract includes the kidneys, ureters, bladder, and urethra. The primary indications for radiologic evaluation of these structures after trauma are hematuria, blood at the urethral meatus, pelvic fracture, and a high index of suspicion. Approximately 8 to 10 per cent of *blunt* abdominal trauma is associated with injuries to the urinary tract.[1] Seven per cent of gunshot wounds and 5.9 per cent of stab wounds to the abdomen resulted in *penetrating* wounds to the kidney in one large series.[2]

Controversy has arisen regarding the particular type of renal diagnostic imaging that should be performed initially, with advocates for both ultrasound[3] and computed tomography (CT)[4, 5] as opposed to intravenous pyelogram (IVP). Renal ultrasound provides easy accessibility on a 24-hour basis, is portable, repeatable, and inexpensive. However, injuries to the renal pelvis, ureter, and renal pedicle are not reliably diagnosed with this method, and even definition of the renal parenchyma may prove difficult in the presence of large amounts of abdominal gas, a frequent finding in patients with blunt abdominal trauma.

Computed tomography provides greater resolution and sensitivity than intravenous urography and has the advantage of looking at other intra-abdominal structures. However, it is expensive and may not be available on a 24-hour basis in many institutions. A reasonable course of action would seem to be to continue to use IVP as the first imaging method, being prepared to investigate further with CT if an ill-defined or poorly visualizing kidney is seen on IVP. Furthermore, CT may be performed primarily if thoracic or intra-abdominal injuries are present or suspected or if one is concerned about an injury to the renal pedicle.

Hematuria

Gross hematuria is an *absolute* indication for diagnostic evaluation. Renal imaging with an IVP or CT is definitely indicated, and retrograde cystourethrography should also be considered when significant pelvic or lower abdominal trauma is present.

The necessity for undertaking uroradiographic evaluation in the presence of only microhematuria* following blunt abdominal trauma has been questioned by several studies. Nicolaisen and associates[6] studied 359 consecutive patients with renal trauma of whom 221 sustained blunt trauma, had only microhematuria, and were hemodynamically stable. All patients in this group were found to have either a completely normal IVP or only a renal contusion on arteriography or CT; all were managed nonoperatively with no complications. Kisa and Schenk[7] found no significant abnormalities on IVP in 48 consecutive patients who sustained blunt abdominal trauma and had only microscopic hematuria, and Demetriades and coworkers[8] in a similar study found only one abnormal IVP in 47 patients with microscopic hematuria and a normal abdominal examination; the one patient had an associated head injury that made abdominal examination unreliable. In a review of 234 patients with traumatic pelvic fractures, no single major lower tract injury was found in the absence of gross hematuria.[9] A more conservative approach has been recommended by Guice and associates[10] and Levitt and colleagues,[11] who suggest obtaining IVPs if microhematuria is quantitatively greater than 4+ on dipstick or greater than 50 RBC/hpf. Other investigators have suggested 20 to 30 RBC/hpf on the basis of similar findings.[12, 13]

It is important to remember that patients with significant urinary tract trauma can present without *any* red blood cells in the urine. Approximately 25 per cent of renal pedicle disruptions may not have even microhematuria, and complete ureteral transection may also be present without hematuria.[14] These injuries are generally associated with *major* forces directed to the flank and are usually accompanied by hemodynamic instability. Hence, although these injuries should always be considered in the setting of flank contusion, transverse process, or lower rib fractures, and penetrating

flank trauma in the absence of hematuria, they are relatively rare. Therefore, in alert, cooperative patients sustaining blunt trauma who have only microhematuria, are hemodynamically stable, and have no other associated abdominal or pelvic injuries, uroradiographic imaging can be safely omitted from the initial emergency evaluation. However, the persistence of hematuria or the development of flank pain or hemodynamic instability suggests reconsideration of urologic imaging for the blunt trauma patient with initial microscopic hematuria.

It should be emphasized that microscopic hematuria is also an early sign of urinary tract malignancy. Patients (especially the elderly) evaluated in the emergency department for minor trauma who have microscopic hematuria may, in fact, have an occult malignancy that was serendipitously discovered by routine urinalysis. Therefore, it is imperative that *all patients with microscopic hematuria be followed until the urine is completely free of blood or otherwise appropriately evaluated.* It should be stressed that the presence of microhematuria of any significant degree (greater than 3 RBC/hpf) should *never be assumed to be due to the process of catheterization* since this procedure almost never results in such a finding.[15, 16]

Management of patients in these circumstances or of patients with a greater degree of hematuria in whom a normal IVP or CT is obtained consists of decreased activity at home with follow-up urine microscopy in 3 to 5 days. Patients managed in this fashion are usually completely free of microscopic hematuria within 2 to 3 weeks of the injury, and initial or repeat renal imaging studies should be considered if clearing of the urine does not occur within this time frame.

Blood at the Urethral Meatus (Urethral Injury)

When there is evidence of major trauma, placement of a Foley catheter has become the standard method of monitoring urinary output. Blood at the urethral meatus, however, may mean partial or complete urethral disruption. Great care should be taken in this situation before proceeding with any urethral instrumentation. We believe that monitoring urine output during *initial* resuscitation of the critically injured patient is rarely useful clinically, and that the hemodynamic stability of the patient can readily be ascertained by monitoring vital signs and central venous pressure until a retrograde urethrogram can be performed. This study can easily be done in the emergency department or on the operating room table if the patient needs immediate surgical intervention for other life-threatening injuries. The patient may suffer if a partial urethral tear is converted to a complete disruption of the urethra by the attempted passage of a catheter. Therefore, we consider urethral instrumentation to be *contraindicated* if blood is seen at the meatus before retrograde urethrography. If the patient is able to void easily, it is unlikely that he has a urethral injury, but the presence of blood at the meatus still mandates urethrography before catheterization. Patients should not be forced to void, however, because extravasation of urine is undesirable.

The posterior male urethra, which includes the membranous portion and the prostatic urethra, is injured more frequently than the anterior urethra. The urogenital diaphragm fixes the membranous urethra; the prostate and prostatic urethra are firmly attached to the posterior surface of the symphysis pubis by the puboprostatic ligaments. Blunt trauma and pelvic fractures, especially in the presence of a full bladder, may result in shearing forces that partially or completely avulse portions of the firmly attached posterior

---

*Microhematuria is defined as "trace" or greater reading on a urine dipstick or greater than 3 red blood cells per high power field (RBC/hpf) on the microscopic analysis, in the presence of a clear urine. Note that both myoglobinuria (common in blunt muscle trauma) and hemoglobinuria (secondary to red blood cell lysis) produce a positive dipstick reading and a *negative* microscopic analysis. The absolute number of red blood cells present on microscopic analysis is dependent on urine flow, fluid resuscitation, time of centrifugation, volume of supernatant, etc. Therefore, 20 RBC/hpf has the same diagnostic significance as 100 RBC/hpf.

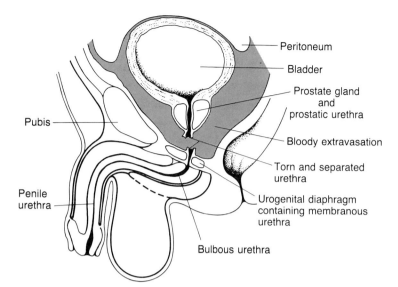

Figure 74–1. A common posterior urethral injury is a disruption of the membranous urethra. In this case, a distended bladder and attached prostate gland are sheared from the fixed membranous urethra. Note the development of a perivesical hematoma and the presence of a "high-riding" prostate gland.

urethra. Usually the bladder and prostate gland are sheared from the membranous urethra, resulting in a complete urethral disruption (Fig. 74–1). The female urethra is short and relatively mobile and generally escapes injury in blunt trauma. Occasionally, a significant pelvic fracture will result in avulsion of the female urethra at the bladder neck. Direct injuries to the female urethra may also occur secondary to penetrating trauma of the vagina or perineum.

Contusions or lacerations of the anterior male urethra occur when the bulbous urethra is compressed against the inferior surface of the symphysis pubis. This happens most commonly as a result of straddle injuries in males but may result from any blunt perineal trauma. Significant trauma to the penile urethra is rare when there are no penetrating injuries or urethral instrumentation. Anterior urethral injuries may result in extravasation of blood or urine into the penis, scrotum, perineum, or anterior abdominal wall. This

is in contrast to posterior urethral injuries, in which blood and urine extravasate into the pelvis (Fig. 74–2).

The rectal examination is used by some physicians for the evaluation of urethral disruption. If the prostate is clearly high riding or if a hematoma can be palpated, one should be suspicious of a posterior urethral injury, and a retrograde urethrogram should be performed before attempted catheterization. A normal rectal examination alone, however, *should never be considered definitive evidence of an intact urethra* when other clinical signs indicate that additional evaluation is necessary.

Pelvic Fracture in the Male

Pelvic fracture in the male is an indication for retrograde urethrography with cystography. Urethral injuries resulting

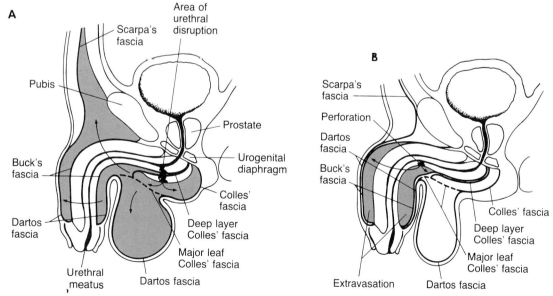

Figure 74–2. *A,* Disruption of the anterior urethra (bulbous urethra) occurs with straddle-type injuries in the male. There may be extravasation of urine and blood into the perineum, scrotum, or anterior abdominal wall. Note that in this diagram Buck's fascia has been penetrated. *B,* Anterior urethral injury in which Buck's fascia remains intact. In this diagram, extravasation results in a swollen and ecchymotic penis. Such an injury may occur with instrumentation of the anterior urethra.

from pelvic fractures in the female are extremely rare and thus are seldom of concern. The incidence of lower-tract injuries in males with pelvic fractures ranges from 7.5 to 25 per cent. Approximately 80 per cent of all urethral injuries are associated with pelvic fractures.[9] Because of the severity of late complications, especially severe stricturing that requires difficult surgical repair, it is paramount that these injuries are not overlooked initially.

High Index of Suspicion

A high index of suspicion of urinary tract injury is an indication in itself for further diagnostic study. Flank tenderness, abrasions, hematoma of the flank or upper quadrant, hypotension without obvious cause, penetrating flank trauma, or external genitalia trauma should lead one to suspect urinary tract injury. We believe that erring on the side of excessive diagnostic tests is preferable to overlooking a significant injury.

RADIOGRAPHIC CONTRAST MATERIAL

Radiographic contrast material is used to fill vessels and other structures to render them diagnostically radiopaque. To evaluate the urinary tract, contrast material is injected as a bolus into the venous system and is excreted unchanged in the urine or it is retrogradely placed into the urethra or bladder. Three types of contrast material are currently available (Table 74–1). All contain iodine, and all are hyperosmolar with respect to blood. Conventional agents, such as Hypaque and Renografin, are tri-iodinated water-soluble agents (ionic monoacetic monomers) that completely dissociate into anion and cation moieties upon intravascular injection. Osmolality is quite high, ranging from 1200 to 2000 mOsm/kg. Many of the toxic effects of contrast material have been attributed to the large osmotic load associated with intravascular injection. Although iodine concentrations do determine the quality of the radiographic image, iodine itself is not thought to play a major role in toxic reactions.[17]

Two new classes of contrast material are loxagiate (Hexabrix), an ionic monoacetic dimer, and nonionic (nondissociating) agents, such as iopamidol (Isovue) and iohexol (Omnipaque). The newer agents have twice the iodine atoms per particle in solution as conventional agents and therefore provide significantly higher urinary iodine concentration, offering better diagnostic quality to radiographic studies. The osmolality of the newer agents is markedly lower, ranging from 600 to 700 mOsm/kg. The lower osmolality and improved chemical structure may be associated with fewer adverse side effects and have been better tolerated by patients in some studies.[18, 19] These new agents are promising, but there is still some skepticism that they will truly limit major or clinically significant hypersensitive reactions.[20] These nonionic agents have not been associated with a lower incidence of contrast-induced nephropathy.

TECHNIQUE

Kidney, Ureter, and Bladder

The plain film of the abdomen taken in such a way as to include the kidneys, ureters, bladder, and full pelvis is essential for diagnostic purposes as well as for comparison of all future contrast films. Important diagnostic signs that may alert the physician to the possibility of urinary tract injury include the following:

1. Loss of one or both psoas shadows secondary to blood in the retroperitoneum.
2. Spinal curvature secondary to splinting—concave to the side of the injury.
3. Lower rib or transverse process fractures, both of which may be close to the kidney.
4. Pelvic fracture. The KUB should always precede an IVP because radiopaque shadows seen on the plain film must be differentiated from extravasation on later contrast films.

Intravenous Pyelography

Although formal IVP with or without CT can and should be performed in the radiology department on stable trauma patients, valuable time should not be lost if the patient is unstable and likely to require immediate surgery. We have found that an abbreviated IVP with one or two postcontrast injection films can provide critical information concerning the kidneys and ureters and can be performed with ease in the emergency department. As part of the resuscitation room equipment, two 50-ml syringes filled with contrast material are always ready for injection. These syringes are kept available in a designated location to save time during resuscitation of the critically injured patient. As soon as plain films have been taken, contrast material (e.g., 100 ml of 60 per cent Renografin in adults) is injected intravenously through either a central or peripheral line. The injection should be performed quickly over 30 to 60 seconds. The physicians may continue with other resuscitative measures while the radiology technicians prepare for additional films. We routinely take a single 10-minute film initially, followed by a 30-minute film if necessary and if the patient is still in the emergency department. These films are examined for the following:

1. Bilateral and symmetric nephrograms indicating the integrity of the renal pedicles.
2. Evidence of major parenchymal disruption (Fig. 74–3).
3. Evidence of major urinary extravasation (Fig. 74–4).
4. Presence of two kidneys and their position within the retroperitoneum. There may indeed be contrast outlining the bladder at the time of the 10-minute or 30-minute film. This abbreviated IVP should never be used as the definitive examination of the bladder. A formal cystogram should be performed if bladder injury is suspected.

Urethrogram

Several techniques have been used to perform the retrograde urethrogram, two of which will be described. The choice of technique is not as important as attention to a few critical details. First, a plain film must be taken before injection of contrast material. For the injection film, we prefer to oblique the patient's pelvis slightly on a foam wedge placed under one hip. This position produces a better view of the entire urethra and prevents the double image of the proximal penile and bulbous urethra from being superimposed. Second, after sterile preparation, an 8 French Foley catheter is placed into the urethral meatus and the balloon is inflated in the fossa navicularis or further up the penile urethra with approximately 2 to 3 ml of sterile water or saline. Inflation of the balloon in this position, when performed slowly, causes minimal discomfort to the patient. Third, approximately 10 to 15 ml of suitable contrast material is then *slowly* injected into the Foley catheter (Fig. 74–

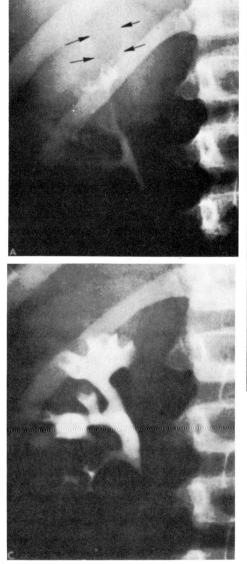

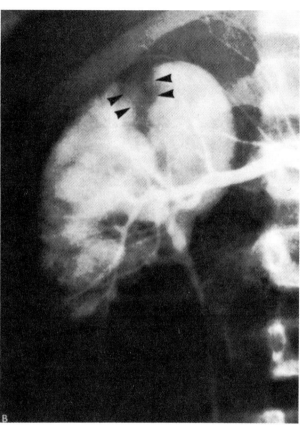

Figure 74–3. *A,* An intravenous pyelogram delineates a defect on a nephrogram in the right superior pole *(arrows)* of the kidney in an 11-year-old boy who fell from a tree. *B,* An arteriogram substantiates a sharply demarcated laceration *(between arrows). C,* A delayed film taken after the arteriogram shows an intact pelvicalyceal system. (From Richter MW, Lytton B, Myerson D, Grnja V: Radiology of genitourinary trauma. Radiol Clin North Am 11(3):600, 1973.)

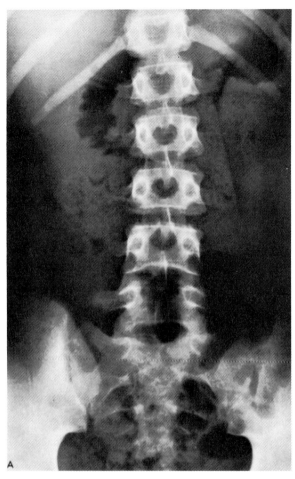

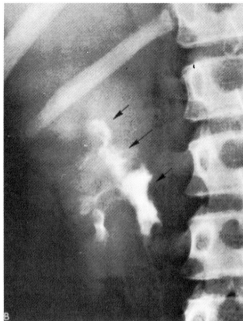

Figure 74–4. Radiograph of a 15-year-old girl who presented with right flank pain and gross hematuria after falling down a flight of stairs. *A,* Scout film shows scoliosis, concavity toward the injured kidney, and loss of psoas and renal outlines. *B,* Excretory urography shows extravasation of the contrast material *(arrows)* from a tear in the pelvicalyceal system.

5). Forceful injection may cause intravasation of contrast material into the venous drainage of the urethra. We routinely use solutions of either Hypaque (50 per cent), Cystografin 40, or Renografin 60, diluted to less than a 10 per cent solution using sterile saline for the diluent (see Table 74–1). Fourth, during the injection, a film is taken.

The alternative to this method is to take a sterile irrigating-tipped piston syringe with the contrast material drawn up and place the lubricated tip directly into the urethral meatus. A tight seal is made by compression of the glans around the tip of the syringe with one hand, while injection is accomplished with the other (Fig. 74–6).

The extravasation of contrast material from a tear in the urethra appears as a flame-like area outside the urethral contour. Figure 74–7A–C shows examples of urethral injuries diagnosed by urethrography. If contrast material is seen within the bladder along with extravasation, it is said that the urethral injury may be partial in nature rather than a complete disruption. Occasionally, contrast material can be seen in the venous drainage of the periurethral area (Fig.

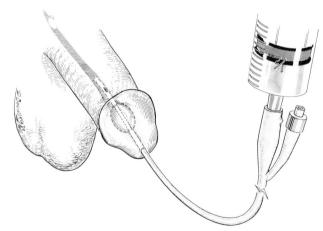

Figure 74–5. Urethrogram using a Foley catheter (8 French). Slowly inflate the balloon with 2 ml of sterile fluid; then slowly inject 10 ml of a 10 per cent solution of contrast material through the catheter lumen (see text).

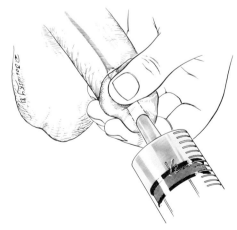

Figure 74–6. An alternate method of injecting contrast material before performing a urethrogram.

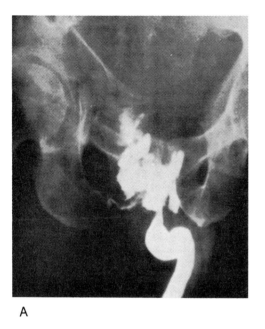

A

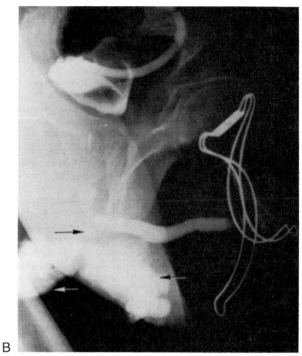

B

Figure 74–7. *A,* Retrograde urethrogram. Urethrogram in case of supramembranous rupture. Dye extravasation is typical of that seen with this type of injury. (From Morehouse DD, MacKinnon KJ: Posterior urethral injury: Etiology, diagnosis, initial management. Urol Clin North Am 4(3):74, 1977.) *B,* A rupture at the proximal bulbous urethra into the scrotum *(arrows). C,* Residual contrast material within perineum and scrotum. (From Richter MW, Lytton B, Myerson D, Grnja V: Radiology of genitourinary trauma. Radiol Clin North Am 11(3):627, 1973.)

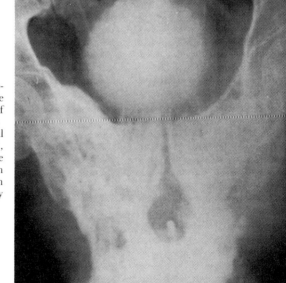

C

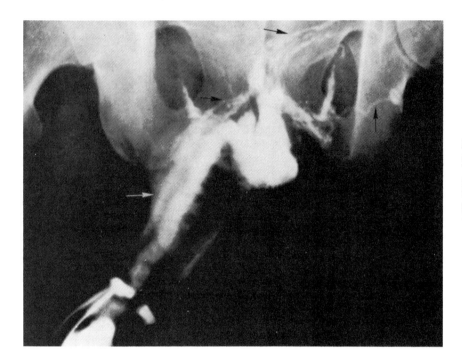

Figure 74–8. Venous intravasation *(arrows)* during a forceful retrograde urethrogram. This may mimic a urethral injury, but its presence is benign. (From Richter MW, Lytton B, Myerson D, Grnja V: Radiology of genitourinary trauma. Radiol Clin North Am 11(3):626, 1973.)

74–8). Sometimes it is mistaken for extravasation; however, it is of no consequence.

If a Foley catheter has been successfully placed into the bladder and yet a partial urethral injury is still suspected, such an injury can be demonstrated easily without removing the catheter. The lubricated end of a pediatric feeding tube is placed into the penile urethra alongside the existing Foley catheter. A seal can be obtained with compression of the glans using one hand and injecting contrast material via a Luer-Lok syringe with the other (Fig. 74–9). In this way, extravasation can be detected. It should be noted, however, that successful placement of a Foley catheter obviates the need for further work-up of a possible urethral tear in the emergency setting, because an indwelling catheter alone is appropriate initial management for this type of injury.

Cystogram

A cystogram is performed with a Foley catheter in place. Again, a plain film is taken so that it can be used as a comparison for all further films. Following this, films are obtained after the bladder has been filled with contrast material. Anteroposterior and both oblique projections are usually taken. A final film is obtained after contrast material is allowed to drain out via the Foley catheter.

The technique involves allowing the bladder to fill with contrast material by means of gravity drainage, performed by attaching a 60-ml catheter-tip syringe to the Foley catheter and holding it above the level of the patient's bladder. The contrast material is then poured into the syringe and allowed to drain by gravity into the bladder. Again, a *dilute solution of contrast material* (see Table 74–1) is used in case there is extravasation. It has been our policy when performing both urethrograms and cystograms to use this dilute solution of contrast material (10 per cent or less) because extravasation into periurethral or perivesical tissues may cause considerable inflammatory reaction at higher concentrations. We have never found that this dilute solution compromises the quality of the study.

Optimally, the bladder should be filled to approximately 400 ml and the catheter should then be occluded with a

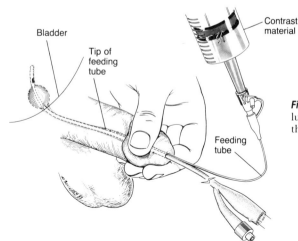

Figure 74–9. Evaluation of a urethral injury with a Foley catheter in place. A lubricated pediatric feeding tube has been advanced into the urethra beside the indwelling Foley catheter.

Table 74–1. *Clinical Use of Radiographic Contrast Material (RCM) for Intravenous Pyelogram (IVP)*

	Iodine Content (mgI/ml)	Osmolality (mOsm/kg) (H₂O)	Average Volume For IVP
Conventional Ionic RCM			
Renografin 60 (sodium diatrizoate)	288	1511	Adult: 100 ml over 30–60 seconds* Child: 1.5 ml/kg‡
Hypaque 50% (sodium diatrizoate)	300	1500	Adult: 100 ml over 30–60 seconds* Child: 1.5 ml/kg‡
Conray (methyl glucamine iothalamate)	282	1217	Adult: 100 ml over 30–60 seconds* Child: 1.5 ml/kg‡
New Nonionic RCM			
Isovue (iopamidol)	300	616	Adult: 50 ml over 30–60 seconds† Child: 1–1.5 ml/kg‡
Omnipaque 300 (iohexol)	300	672	Adult: 50 ml over 30–60 seconds† Child: 1–1.5 ml/kg‡

*Average dose of iodine for IVP with ionic RCM: 350–400 mgI/kg or 1.5 ml/kg

Adult: Low dose: 10 gm
      Intermediate dose: 30 gm
      High dose: 60 gm

†Because the ratio of iodine atoms to dissolved particles is 1.5 with conventional ionic agents and 3.0 with the nonionic agents, less volume is required with the new agents. Average dose is 200–350 mgI/kg.
‡Do not exceed 3 ml/kg total dose.

Use of RCM for Retrograde Studies

RCM	Use	Procedure
Renografin 60 or Hypaque 50%	Dilute stock solutions with saline 1:10 (10% solution)	Urethrogram: 10–15 ml of dilute solution injected slowly through urethral meatus. Children: 0.2 ml/kg Cystogram: after plain film and with Foley catheter in place, fill bladder of adult with 400 ml dilute contrast material, introduced under gravity. Children: 5 ml/kg

Kelly clamp. Volumes of 250 ml or less have been associated with false-negative retrograde cystograms.[21] At times, the patient may have difficulty cooperating because of head injuries or pain, and, if severely injured, may have involuntary bladder contractions, causing contrast material to back up into the syringe. If this is the case, one may have to manage with somewhat less than optimum films. Care must be taken to ensure that the contrast material is not spilled on the patient during the procedure. Spilled contrast can lead to spurious findings on the fill-up films. Once the fill-up films have been obtained, the Foley catheter is unclamped and the contrast material is allowed to drain out of the bladder. The drain-out film is then obtained in order to visualize any posterior extravasation that may have been hidden by the distended bladder during the fill-up phase.

Extravasation from an injured bladder may be intraperitoneal, extraperitoneal, or both. Extraperitoneal extravasation is usually seen as flame-like areas of contrast material projecting lateral to the bladder into the pelvis (Fig. 74–10). If the contrast material extravasates intraperitoneally, there is usually an outline of intraperitoneal structures, particularly the bowel, by the contrast material (Fig. 74–11).

CONTRAST MEDIUM REACTIONS AND TOXICITY

The introduction of a new generation of contrast media (United States Food and Drug Administration approval in 1986) has once again stimulated publicity, research, and controversy over the problem of contrast medium reactions.

It is important, however, to maintain this issue in perspective. While the topic has occupied thousands of pages of published material and has caused great anxiety among patients and their physicians, the frequency of contrast medium reactions of sufficient severity to require medical intervention is low, between 1:1000 and 1:10,000. In fact, one review stated that IVP contrast material is "among the most innocuous of injectable drugs."[17]

The mechanism of contrast medium reactions is not yet understood, but high osmolarity is believed to be at least one of the factors responsible. In the new generation of contrast media, osmolarity is 50 per cent of the level in the traditional contrast media. These have been called "low osmolarity contrast media," although their osmolarity remains considerably higher than most injected substances. The new contrast media are also called "nonionic contrast media" in some literature. This is also a misnomer, because at least one of the new media separates into positive and negative ions in solution.

Many claims have been made about the safety and efficacy of the low osmolar media based on in vitro, animal, and human studies. Because the data are not conclusive and the pathophysiologic mechanisms remain elusive, the clinical problem of how to determine which contrast medium to use in a given patient should be made on the basis of clinical judgment and institutional experience, taking into consideration legal and financial realities. The problem of how to handle patients at risk for contrast medium reactions also has many unknowns and requires individual consideration and judgment.

Contrast medium reactions are of two types: reactions

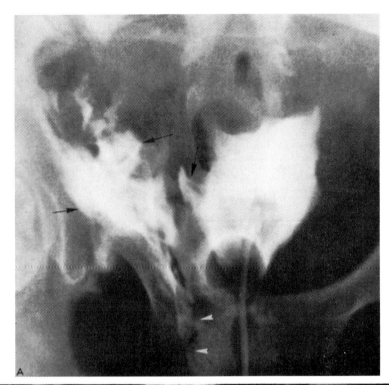

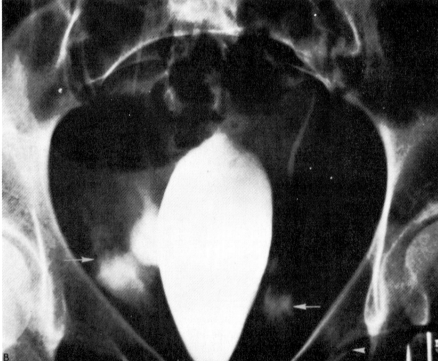

Figure 74–10. Examples of extraperitoneal bladder rupture. *A,* Note the amorphous extravasation of contrast material within the perivesical space *(arrows)* in a patient with a right pelvic fracture *(arrowheads). B,* A second patient with a pelvic fracture *(arrowhead)* and perivesical hematoma shows the teardrop shape of a deformed bladder and an extraperitoneal extravasation *(arrows).* (From Richter MW, Lytton B, Myerson D, Grnja V: Radiology of genitourinary trauma. Radiol Clin North Am 11(3):623, 1973.)

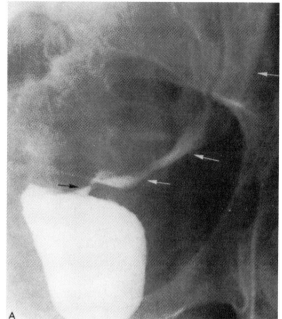

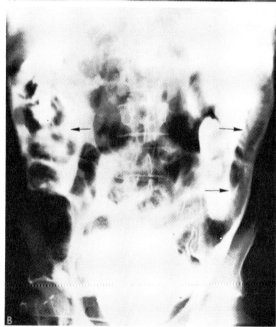

Figure 74–11. Intraperitoneal bladder rupture. *A,* A 22-year-old pedestrian hit by an automobile. Note extravasation of contrast material beginning at the dome and tracking up the left paracolic gutter *(arrows). B,* This 57-year-old man had exfulguration of a tumor at the bladder dome and sustained perforation. A cystogram dramatically demonstrates the extravasation of contrast material that outlines the bowel loops *(arrows)* and the paracolic gutters. (Courtesy of Morton A, Bosniak MD, New York, New York.) (From Richter MW, Lytton B, Myerson D, Grnja V: Radiology of genitourinary trauma. Radiol Clin North Am 11(3):623, 1973.)

that are directly toxic to the kidney and idiosyncratic systemic reactions. These two types must be considered separately since prophylaxis and treatment are different.

Renal Toxicity

Risk factors for renal toxicity include preexisting renal insufficiency, diabetes, severe congestive heart failure, hyperuricemia, and myeloma.

Renal toxicity is manifest first by creatinine elevation. (Contrast-induced renal failure is clinically defined as a rise in serum creatinine of at least 50 per cent of baseline or 1.0 mg/dl within 48 hours after administration of contrast material.) Mild cases are asymptomatic. Severe cases may result in oliguria or, in the extreme, anuria. Renal toxicity is usually self-limited and reversible. Even patients that require dialysis usually return their serum creatinine to baseline within a few days. Irreversible renal failure occurs rarely.[22]

The severity of renal toxicity is probably related to the dose of contrast medium and in patients with known risk factors the dose administered should be limited. Angiographic studies, for example, should be performed with digital subtraction angiography whenever possible.[23] Both the concentration of contrast medium and the contact time within the renal tubules are reduced if the patient is well hydrated. Consequently, intravenous hydration and administration of diuretics such as mannitol and furosemide are prudent measures in patients at risk who must undergo contrast studies.[22] Patients with hyperuricemia and myeloma are particularly likely to benefit from these protective measures.[22, 24] It has not been established that the low osmolar contrast media reduce the incidence of renal toxicity.[20, 23] Elevated preprocedure serum creatinine, diabetes, myeloma, and hyperuricemia are not in themselves indications to use low osmolar contrast media. In severe congestive heart failure, the low osmolar media should be used in order to minimize the volume impact on cardiac function. Conventional contrast material may increase blood volume acutely by 15 per cent.

The incidence of postprocedure serum creatinine elevation is negligible in patients without preexisting renal insufficiency, even in the presence of other risk factors. The incidence and severity of renal toxicity increases with the degree of preexisting renal insufficiency. Diabetes does not appear to be a risk factor independent of renal function. In one study neither renal insufficiency nor diabetes alone increased the likelihood of renal failure following contrast medium administration, although diabetics with renal insufficiency were found to be at increased risk.[25]

Idiosyncratic Reactions

Idiosyncratic reactions to contrast material are of two types: anaphylactoid and vagal. Serious acute reactions, occurring immediately or within 30 minutes of injection, are not truly anaphylactic in nature and have been termed "anaphylactoid." The reaction consists of hypotension, tachycardia, atrial and ventricular dysrhythmias, urticaria, wheezing, angioedema, and dyspnea. Myocardial infarction, pulmonary edema, airway obstruction, seizures, and cardiac arrest have been reported. The exact biochemical and pathophysiologic nature of the reaction is not known. IgE antibodies to the contrast material have not been consistently demonstrated, rechallenge results in a similar reaction in only about one third of patients, and subsequent reactions are not progressively worse as seen with true anaphylaxis. The test administration of a few milliliters of contrast material is not a reliable method to determine sensitivity.

Risk factors for an anaphylactoid reaction include an allergic history and a prior reaction to contrast medium. The notion that idiosyncratic reactions result from a specific allergy to seafood and other iodine-containing materials should be relegated to the status of myth. The incidence of idiosyncratic reactions is doubled in patients with a strong allergic history compared to the nonallergic population, but this increased incidence is nonspecific.[23] The stronger the allergic history the more likely that patient is to have a reaction to contrast medium, regardless of the allergen to which the patient has proven sensitive in the past.

Once again, however, it is useful to keep the incidence in perspective. The incidence of fatal contrast medium reactions is approximately 1:12,000 to 1:75,000 patients. Even though the incidence in patients with a strong allergic history is doubled, severe reactions and fatal outcomes even in this population remain rare. Although it is prudent to consider carefully whether an alternative diagnostic examination might solve the problem, an allergic history should not deprive a patient of the benefit of an important and necessary diagnostic procedure.

Vagal reactions are also seen following injection of contrast material and are manifested by bradycardia, hypotension, and diaphoresis. Initially a vagal reaction may be misinterpreted as an anaphylactoid reaction but a helpful distinguishing feature is bradycardia with a rapid response to supportive care. Vagal reactions may be more common in patients with significant pain, preexisting nausea, or anxiety.

The significance of anxiety as an independent variable for idiosyncratic reactions is unclear, but some evidence suggests that if the patient can be relaxed by thorough discussion and reassurance or by antianxiety medication, the

likelihood of a contrast medium reaction is reduced.[26] Discussion of contrast medium reactions with a patient should be careful, thoughtful, and fully informed.

It is common for patients to experience warmth, tingling, mild pruritus, pain at the injection site, and nausea immediately following injection of contrast material. This is not an allergic reaction, per se, but the exact nature of the reaction is not known. Many researchers attribute these symptoms to the hyperosmolality of the dye and these symptoms seem to be lessened with the use of the lower osmolar agents. These reactions generally do not progress and usually do not require treatment.

Informed Consent for Contrast Media

The need for written informed consent before administration of contrast media is controversial.[27] One patient survey found that 90 per cent of patients preferred receiving a written description of the risks of contrast media.[28] One report suggests that the legal necessity of a written informed consent statement has been further complicated by the availability of the low osmolar contrast media, which may not be covered by the patient's medical insurance.[29] Bush's consent form (Fig. 74–12) was associated with questions in less than 5 per cent of patients, examination refusal in less than 1 per cent, and a request for low osmolar contrast media in less than 1 per cent. Written informed consent is commonly impractical in the multiple system trauma patient and should be considered only in the clearly stable, alert patient.

Prophylaxis

To date, it has not been *conclusively* established that severe idiosyncratic reactions occur less frequently with low osmolar contrast media than with the older media. Patients are, however, more comfortable when low osmolar media are used. These media cause less pain on injection into muscular arteries during arteriography than the traditional media and should be used for abdominal aortography and extremity angiography. They also result in a reduced incidence of minor reactions, such as nausea and vomiting, during intravenous injections. Each facility must establish its own policy regarding whether this level of patient protection justifies the increased cost.

Patients with a prior contrast medium reaction or a strong allergic history have in the past been treated prophylactically with antihistamines and corticosteroids, on the assumption that idiosyncratic contrast medium reactions are allergic reactions. One multiinstitutional study suggests that a *two-dose regimen* of the corticosteroid methylprednisolone prior to intravenous contrast medium administration may afford protection in patients at risk for contrast reaction.[17] The doses in this study were 32 mg methylprednisolone orally 12 hours and again 2 hours before the examination.

In a small study addressing this issue, Greenberger and coworkers[30] gave 200 mg of hydrocortisone intravenously and 50 mg of diphenhydramine intramuscularly immediately before contrast material injection to ten patients with previous reactions who required an emergency procedure with intravascular dye. No patient developed a reaction. This study is small (only ten subjects) and no patient had prior cardiac arrest, but it does lend some credence to immediate prophylaxis. Nonetheless, there is no clear evidence that any steroid or antihistamine pretreatment regimen provides effective prophylaxis against a life-threatening contrast medium reaction.

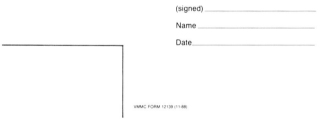

Figure 74–12. An informed consent form. (From Bush WH: Informed consent for contrast media. AJR 152:867, 1989. © by American Roentgen Ray Society. Reprinted by permission.)

The most important protection from contrast medium reactions is the availability of instruments, medication, and personnel for rapid treatment. Facilities that inject radiographic contrast media should have emergency medication such as epinephrine, intravenous fluids, tubing, needles, endotracheal intubation apparatus, and an EKG machine immediately at hand. Contrast media should be given by or under the supervision of an individual who knows how to administer cardiopulmonary resuscitation and whose medical background permits rapid evaluation and treatment.

Treatment

While an allergic history or a documented prior contrast medium reaction increases the likelihood of a subsequent reaction in any individual patient, idiosyncratic reactions most commonly occur in patients without such risk factors. It is therefore necessary to be prepared for a reaction in every patient to whom contrast medium is administered for any examination.[31] The most important measures are careful observation of the patient especially within the first 5 minutes after injection, and an open intravenous access. As a precaution, the infusion fluid should be normal saline. At least an 18-gauge intravenous catheter should be used for adults. Intravenous tubing compatible with high flow infusion techniques should also be chosen. After intravenous injection of contrast medium the intravenous infusion should be maintained ("kept open") for 30 minutes until the danger of an acute reaction has passed. If a reaction occurs, vital signs should be checked immediately, cardiac monitoring instituted, the patency of the intravenous line assured, and fluid and oxygen administration begun.

Idiosyncratic reactions to contrast medium may be categorized as mild, moderate, or severe. Mild reactions include nausea, vomiting, itching, flushing, or other symptoms that do not require treatment. Moderate reactions, such as urticaria, wheezing, or vasovagal reaction may require treatment depending on their severity. Diphenhydramine, 50 mg intramuscularly or 25 mg intravenously, may be useful for urticaria. If wheezing is severe, inhaled β-agonist therapy should be used (see Chapter 5).

Vasovagal reactions, consisting of hypotension and bradycardia, are fairly common. The hypotension may be severe enough that pulses may not be palpable and blood pressure may be unobtainable. These reactions may be accompanied radiographically by a prolonged nephrogram on IVP or CT scan with little or no progression of contrast medium down the tubules to form urine in the collecting system, as a result of markedly reduced renal arterial flow. Vasovagal reactions are usually self-limited, seldom need therapy other than elevation of the legs, and clinically significant sequelae are rare. If prolonged, a vasovagal reaction is potentially life threatening and should be treated with atropine and intravenous fluids.

The hypotension accompanying anaphylactoid reactions may be severe and resistant to treatment. Therapy consists of the rapid infusion of intravenous crystalloid and pharmacologic agents. VanSonnenberg and colleagues[32] note that intravenous fluids are superior to drug therapy alone, and, in fact, agents commonly used to treat allergic reactions may be ineffective for the reversal of the hypotension and possibly may precipitate hypotension or cardiac dysrhythmias unless supplemented with fluid resuscitation. Although epinephrine, antihistamines, and perhaps corticosteroids should be used in severe anaphylactoid reactions, aggressive fluid therapy is first line treatment. In severe cases of laryngospasm or respiratory distress, tracheal intubation may be required.

In the absence of cardiac arrest, epinephrine should be administered as intravenous boluses of no more than 0.1 to 0.2 mg (1 to 2 ml of 1:10,000). Alternatively 1 mg of epinephrine may be added to 500 ml saline and titrated as a continual infusion. Intravenous epinephrine may cause ventricular dysrhythmias and severe hypertension and should only be used with continuous electrocardiographic and blood pressure monitoring.

COMPLICATIONS

Several potential problems in the diagnosis of urinary tract injury deserve to be emphasized. First, the IVP cystogram should never be used as the definitive examination for a suspected bladder injury. One can easily be misled by accepting the normal-appearing cystogram on the IVP, only to discover extreme trauma to the bladder wall at the time of laparotomy performed because of other injuries. Second, occasionally, during vigorous fluid administration for hypotension, or after mannitol administration for head injury, a brisk diuresis may ensue. This can occasionally cause nonvisualization of both kidneys on a 10- and 30-minute IVP film, but later the patient is found to have normal renal arteriograms. This phenomenon is probably due to extreme dilution of contrast material in the former instance or to the rapid clearance of contrast material in the latter. Third, the importance of performing all uroradiographic diagnostic studies in the emergency department when possible cannot be overemphasized. Although such studies can be obtained intraoperatively, they are often inadequate and much more difficult to interpret.

CONCLUSION

Trauma to the GU tract is commonly seen in the emergency department. The kidneys, ureters, bladder, and urethra may be involved. By performing any or all three of the basic uroradiologic studies—the IVP, cystogram, and retrograde urethrogram—the physician can simply, quickly, and accurately assess the status of the urinary tract.

REFERENCES

1. McAninch JW: The injured kidney. Monogr Urol 4:46, 1983.
2. Carlton CE, Scott R Jr, Goldman M: The management of penetrating injuries of the kidney. J Trauma 8:1071, 1968.
3. Jakse G, Furtschegger A, Egender G: Ultrasound in patients with blunt renal trauma. J Urol 138:21, 1987.
4. McAninch JW, Fedeele MP: Evaluation of renal injuries with computerized tomography. J Urol 128:456, 1982.
5. Erturk E, Sheinfeld J, DiMarco PL, Cockett ATK: Renal trauma: Evaluation by computerized tomography. J Urol 133:946, 1985.
6. Nicolaisen GS, McAninch JW, Marshall GA, et al: Renal trauma: Re-evaluation of the indications for radiographic assessment. J Urol 133:183, 1985.
7. Kisa E, Schenk WG III: Indications for emergency intravenous pyelography (IVP) in blunt abdominal trauma: A reappraisal. J Trauma 26:1086, 1986.
8. Demetriades D, Rabinowitz B, Sofianos C, Landau A: Haematuria after blunt trauma: The role of pyelography. Br J Surg 72:745, 1985.
9. Antoci JP, Schiff M Jr: Bladder and urethral injuries with pelvic fractures. J Urol 128:25, 1982.
10. Guice K, Oldham K, Eide B, Johasen K: Hematuria after blunt trauma: When is pyelography useful? J Trauma 23:305, 1983.
11. Levitt MA, Criss E, Kobernick M: Should the emergency IVP be used more selectively in blunt renal trauma? Ann Emerg Med 14:959, 1985.
12. Lieu TA, Fleisher GR, Mohboubi S, et al: Hematuria and clinical findings as indications for intravenous pyelography in pediatric blunt renal trauma. Pediatrics 82:216, 1988.
13. Klein S, Johs S, Fujitani R, et al: Hematuria following blunt abdominal trauma: The utility of intravenous pyelography. Arch Surg 123:1173, 1988.
14. Stables DP: Traumatic renal artery occlusion. J Urol 115:229, 1976.
15. Sklar DP, Diven B, Jones J: Incidence and magnitude of catheter-induced hematuria. Am J Emerg Med 4:14, 1986.
16. Hockberger RS, Schwartz B, Connor J: Hematuria induced by urethral catheterization. Ann Emerg Med 16:550, 1987.
17. Lasser EC, Berry CC, Talner LB, et al: Pretreatment with corticosteroids to alleviate reactions to intravenous contrast material. N Engl J Med 317:849, 1987.
18. Spartaro RF: New and old contrast agents: Pharmacology, tissue opacification, and excretory urography. Urol Radiol 10:2, 1988.
19. Katzberg RW: New and old contrast agents: Physiology and nephrotoxicity. Urol Radiol 10:6, 1988.
20. Schwab SJ, Hlatky MA, Pieper KS, et al: Contrast nephrotoxicity: A randomized controlled trial of a nonionic and an ionic radiographic contrast agent. N Engl J Med 320:149, 1989.
21. Cass AS: False-negative retrograde cystography with bladder rupture owing to external trauma. J Trauma 24:168, 1984.
22. Bettmann MA: Radiographic contrast agents: A prospective. N Engl J Med 317:891, 1987.
23. Berkeseth RO, Kjellstrand CM: Radiologic contrast-induced nephropathy. Med Clin North Am 68:351, 1984.
24. Brezis M, Epstein FH: A closer look at radio contrast-induced nephropathy. N Engl J Med 320:179, 1989.
25. Parfrey PS, Griffiths SM, Barrett BJ, et al: Contrast material-induced renal failure in patients with diabetes mellitus, renal insufficiency, or both. N Engl J Med 320:143, 1989.
26. Lalli A: Urography, shock reaction, and repeated urography. Am J Roentgenol 125:264, 1975.
27. Spring DB, Akin JR, Margulis AR: Informed consent for intravenous contrast-enhanced radiography: A national survey of practice and opinion. Radiology 152:609, 1984.
28. Spring DB, Winfield AC, Friedland GW, et al: Written informed consent for IV contrast-enhanced radiography: Patient's attitudes and common limitations. Am J Radiol 151:1243, 1988.
29. Bush WH: Informed consent for contrast media. AJR 152:867, 1989.
30. Greenberger PA, Halwig JM, Patterson R, et al: Emergency administration of radiocontrast media in high risk patients. J Allergy Clin Immunol 77(4):630, 1986.
31. Bettmann MA, Kandarpa K: Angiographic contrast media. In Krishna K (ed): Handbook of Cardiovascular and Interventional Radiologic Procedures. Toronto, Little, Brown & Co, 1989.
32. VanSonnenberg E, Neff CC, Pfister RC: Life threatening hypotensive reactions to contrast media administration: Comparison of pharmacologic and fluid therapy. Radiology 162:15, 1987.

Obstetric and Gynecologic Procedures

Chapter 75

Emergency Childbirth

Lynnette Doan-Wiggins

INTRODUCTION

Since ancient times, midwives, specialists of the obstetric art, have supervised the labor of women and the delivery of babies. Physicians did not become involved in this practice until the end of the eighteenth century.

With improved prenatal and obstetric care, the perinatal death rate has fallen by almost 50 per cent in the past 25 years; the maternal death rate has decreased from 582 per 100,000 live births in 1935 to 7.2 per 100,000 live births in 1986.[1, 2]

From the viewpoint of safer care during labor, the outstanding advance of the past 40 years has been the great increase in the proportion of inhospital deliveries. As recently as 1940, less than 60 per cent of births took place in hospitals. For those women in the middle and upper socioeconomic classes, this figure now exceeds 99 per cent.[1] Inhospital births have not only the advantage of better facilities but also care by individuals who are specially trained in obstetrics and perinatology.

The degree to which the emergency physician interacts in the process of labor and delivery varies among institutions, depending on the availability and readiness of inpatient obstetric services. The role of the emergency physician may be only to determine that the patient is indeed in active labor and to order transport directly to the labor and delivery area. In a hospital with little or no obstetric services, the emergency physician may alternatively be called on to manage a complicated delivery and neonatal resuscitation until transfer to another hospital is possible.

To this end the emergency physician must be able to assess the stage and timing of labor, aid the mother in delivery of the infant, and provide initial stabilization of the neonate.

LABOR

Labor is defined as the coordinated effective sequence of involuntary uterine contractions that result in progressive effacement and dilation of the cervix. This, coupled with the voluntary bearing-down efforts of the mother, terminates in delivery, the actual expulsion of the products of conception.

Labor is normally divided into three stages. The first stage begins when uterine contractions reach sufficient force to cause cervical effacement and dilation and ends when the cervix is completely dilated. The average duration of the first stage of labor is 6 to 8 hours in multiparous patients and is 8 to 12 hours in primiparous patients.[3] The second stage of labor begins when dilation of the cervix is complete and ends with delivery of the infant. This stage varies from several minutes to 2 hours. In general, if the second stage lasts more than 2 hours, abnormal labor has developed.[1, 3] The third stage of labor begins after delivery of the infant and ends after delivery of the placenta. Infrequently, a fourth stage of labor is described as that period during which myometrial contractions and vessel thrombosis occur (usually lasting approximately 1 hour), effectively controlling bleeding from the former placental implantation site.[1, 3]

Identification of Labor

TRUE VERSUS FALSE LABOR

Before the establishment of true or effective labor, women may experience so-called false labor. Quite common in late pregnancy, false labor is characterized by irregular, brief contractions of the uterus, usually with discomfort confined to the lower abdomen and groin. The contractions, commonly referred to as *Braxton Hicks contractions*, are typically irregular in timing and strength; there is no change in the cervix and no descent of the fetus.

True labor, on the other hand, is characterized by a regular sequence of uterine contractions, with progressively increasing intensity and decreasing intervals between contractions. The discomfort produced by the uterine contractions of true labor begins in the fundal region and radiates over the uterus into the lower back. The uterine contractions of true labor are accompanied by effacement and dilation of the cervix, with descent of the presenting part of the fetus.

False labor is most common in late pregnancy and in parous women. Although false labor usually stops spontaneously, it may convert rapidly to the effective contractions of true labor (Table 75–1). True labor contractions generally

Table 75–1. Characteristics of Contractions of True Versus False Labor

False Labor	True Labor
Occur at irregular intervals	Occur at regular intervals
Intervals remain long	Intervals gradually shorten
Intensity remains same	Intensity gradually increases
Discomfort mainly in lower abdomen	Discomfort in back and upper to midabdomen
Cervix does not dilate	Cervix dilates
Usually relieved by sedation	Not stopped by sedation

(Adapted from Taylor ES: Obstetrics and Fetal Medicine. 2nd ed. Baltimore, Williams & Wilkins, 1977. Reproduced by permission.)

occur at intervals of 10 minutes or less following the onset of labor.[4]

SHOW

A rather dependable sign of the approach of labor is the "show" or "bloody show." Occasionally preceding the onset of labor by as much as 72 hours, show consists of a small amount of blood-tinged mucus discharged from the vagina. Show represents extrusion of the mucus plug that filled the cervical canal during pregnancy and is evidence of cervical dilation and effacement.[1, 3, 4] *Bloody show must be distinguished from more active third trimester bleeding*, which is classified as a true emergency and in which vaginal examination is *contraindicated*.

RUPTURE OF THE MEMBRANES

Spontaneous rupture of the membranes usually occurs during the course of active labor, although it may occur before the onset of labor in approximately 10 per cent of cases.[3] Rupture of the membranes is typically manifested by a sudden gush of a variable amount of clear or slightly turbid fluid. Rupture of the membranes can be verified if amniotic fluid is extruding from the cervical os or is found in the vaginal fornix on sterile speculum examination.

Differentiation of amniotic fluid from vaginal fluid may be made by testing a drop of the fluid with *nitrazine paper*. Amniotic fluid has a pH of 7.0 to 7.5 and turns the paper blue-green to deep blue. In the presence of vaginal secretions only, with a pH of 4.5 to 5.5, nitrazine paper remains yellow.[1, 5, 6]

Because of its neutral pH, blood may cause a false-positive nitrazine reading in women who have intact membranes and an unusually large amount of bloody show.[1, 6] Abe found the nitrazine test to be positive in 98.9 per cent of women with known rupture of the membranes and negative in 96.2 per cent of women with intact membranes.[5] In clinical practice, however, the test is less reliable, because it is frequently used in cases of questionable rupture in which the amount of amniotic fluid is small and therefore more subject to pH changes from admixed blood and vaginal secretions.[1]

A less frequently used method to test for amniotic fluid is *ferning*. A drop of fluid from the cervical os or vaginal fornix is placed on a clean glass slide. Owing to the high sodium-chloride content of amniotic fluid, a fern pattern is seen through the microscope as amniotic fluid dries. Blood may interfere with ferning, causing a false-negative result.[4]

A new test to determine the presence of ruptured membranes makes use of amniotic fluid's reaction to heat. A Pasteur pipette is used to gently collect a small amount of material from just inside the cervical os. The material is then spread on a glass slide and heated on an alcohol burner for 1 minute. Material containing amniotic fluid turns white; endocervical mucus alone turns brown.[7]

Documentation of rupture of the membranes is significant for three reasons. First, if the presenting part is not already fixed in the pelvis, the possibility of prolapse of the cord with cord compression and subsequent fetal distress is increased. Second, labor may be imminent. Finally, if labor does not begin within 24 hours after rupture of the membranes, the pregnancy must be considered to be complicated by prolonged premature rupture of the membranes with an increased chance of intrauterine infection.[1, 3] If rupture of the membranes is documented in the emergency department, the patient's obstetrician should be notified and hospital admission of the patient should be considered.

Evaluation of Labor

When a woman presents in labor, the general condition of the fetus and mother must be quickly ascertained by means of the patient history and physical examination. Inquiry is made as to the onset and frequency of contractions, the presence or absence of bleeding, the possible loss of amniotic fluid, and the prenatal care and condition of the mother and fetus. In the absence of active vaginal bleeding, the position, presentation, and lie of the fetus are determined by abdominal palpation and sterile vaginal examination. Staging of labor is assessed by vaginal examination. Fetal well-being is monitored by auscultation of fetal heart tones, particularly immediately following a uterine contraction.

LIE, PRESENTATION, AND POSITION

In the latter months of pregnancy, the fetus assumes a characteristic posture within the uterus, usually forming an ovoid mass that corresponds roughly to the shape of the uterine cavity. Typically, the fetus becomes folded or bent on itself in such a way that the back becomes markedly convex, with the head, thighs, and knees being sharply flexed. Usually the arms are crossed over the thorax and are parallel to the sides of the body. The umbilical cord lies in the space between the arms and the lower extremities. This characteristic posture is due in part to the mode of growth of the fetus and is also a result of accommodation to the uterine cavity.

Lie refers to the relation of the long axis of the fetus to that of the mother. Lie is either longitudinal or transverse (Fig. 75–1). Longitudinal lies occur in more than 99 per cent of pregnancies at term.[1]

The *presentation*, or presenting part, refers to that portion of the body of the fetus that is nearest to or foremost in the birth canal. The presenting part is felt through the cervix on sterile vaginal examination. In longitudinal lies, the presenting part is either the fetal head or the buttocks or the feet. In transverse lie, the shoulder is the presenting part.

Cephalic presentations are classified by the relation of the fetal head to the body of the fetus (Fig. 75–2). Ordinarily, the head is sharply flexed so that the occipital fontanel is the presenting part. This is referred to as the *vertex* or *occiput presentation*. Less commonly, the neck is fully extended and the face is foremost in the birth canal; this is termed *face presentation*. Occasionally the fetal head assumes a partially

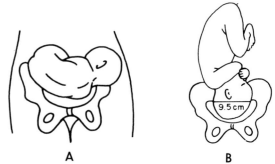

Figure 75–1. *A,* Transverse lie with shoulder presentation. *B,* Longitudinal lie with vertex presentation. (From Romney S, Gray MK, Little AB, et al (eds): Gynecology and Obstetrics: The Health Care of Women. New York, McGraw-Hill Book Co, 1975. Reproduced by permission.)

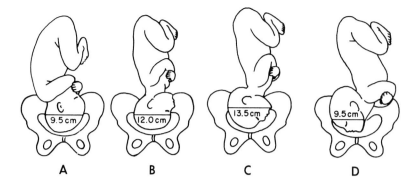

Figure 75–2. Cephalic presentations—deflexion attitude of fetal head. *A,* Vertex. *B,* Sinciput. *C,* Brow. *D,* Face. Diameter of the presenting fetal head is shown for each of the attitudes. (From Romney S, Gray MK, Little AB, et al (eds): Gynecology and Obstetrics: The Health Care of Women. New York, McGraw-Hill Book Co, 1975. Reproduced by permission.)

flexed or partially extended position, resulting in sinciput and brow presentations, respectively. Sinciput and brow presentations, associated with preterm infants, are almost always unstable and convert to either the occiput or face presentation as labor progresses.

Breech presentations are classified as frank, complete, and footling or incomplete (Fig. 75–3). When the fetus presents with the hips flexed and the legs extended over the anterior surfaces of the body, this is termed *frank breech.* Flexion of the fetal hips and knees results in complete breech presentation. When one or both of the feet or knees are lowermost in the canal, an incomplete or footling breech results.

At or near term, the incidence of the various presentations is approximately 96 per cent for vertex, 3.5 per cent for breech, 0.3 per cent for face, and 0.4 per cent for shoulder.[1]

Position refers to the relation of the presenting part to the birth canal and may be either left or right. The occiput, chin, and sacrum are the determining parts in vertex, face, and breech presentations, respectively. The presentation and position of the fetus are initially determined by abdominal palpation using Leopold maneuvers.

Abdominal Palpation (Leopold Maneuvers). Abdominal palpation may be performed throughout the latter months of pregnancy and during labor in the intervals between contractions. The findings from abdominal palpation provide information about the presentation and position of the fetus and the extent to which the presenting part has descended into the pelvis (Fig. 75–4). The mother should be placed on a firm bed or examining table with her abdomen bared. For the first three of the four maneuvers, the examiner stands at the side of the bed facing the patient. During the first maneuver (Fig. 75–4A), the upper abdomen is gently palpated with the finger tips of both hands to determine which fetal pole is present in the uterine fundus. The fetal breech gives the sensation of a large, nodular

body, whereas the fetal head is hard, round, and freely movable.

During the second maneuver, the examiner places his hands on either side of the abdomen, exerting deep, gentle pressure (Fig. 75–4B). On one side, the hard, resistant back is felt; on the other side, the fetal extremities or small parts are felt. By noting whether the back is directed anteriorly, posteriorly, or transversely, fetal orientation or lie is determined.

The third maneuver is performed by grasping the lower portion of the maternal abdomen just above the symphysis pubis with the thumb and forefinger of one hand (Fig. 75–4C). If the presenting part is not engaged, the position of the head in relation to the back and extremities is ascertained. If the cephalic prominence is palpated on the same side as the small parts, the head must be flexed and therefore a vertex or occiput presentation exists. If the cephalic prominence is on the same side as the back, the head must be extended. If the presenting part is deeply engaged in the pelvis, the findings from this maneuver indicate that the lower pole of the fetus is fixed in the pelvis. The details of presentation and position are then defined by the fourth maneuver.

To perform the fourth maneuver, the examiner changes position and faces the mother's feet. With the tips of the first three fingers of each hand, the examiner exerts deep, gentle pressure in the direction of the axis of the pelvic inlet (Fig. 75–4D). When the head is the presenting part, one examining hand will be stopped sooner than the other by a rounded body, the cephalic prominence, while the other hand continues more deeply into the pelvis. The cephalic prominence is felt on the same side as the small parts in vertex presentations and on the same side as the back in face presentations. In breech presentations, the information obtained from this maneuver is less precise.[1]

Vaginal Examination. Unless there has been bleeding in excess of a bloody show, a manual (not speculum) vaginal

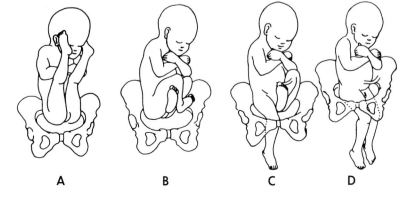

Figure 75–3. Fetal attitude in breech presentations. *A,* Frank. *B,* Complete. *C,* Single footling—incomplete. *D,* Double footling—incomplete. (From Romney S, Gray MK, Little AB, et al (eds): Gynecology and Obstetrics: The Health Care of Women. New York, McGraw-Hill Book Co, 1975. Reproduced by permission.)

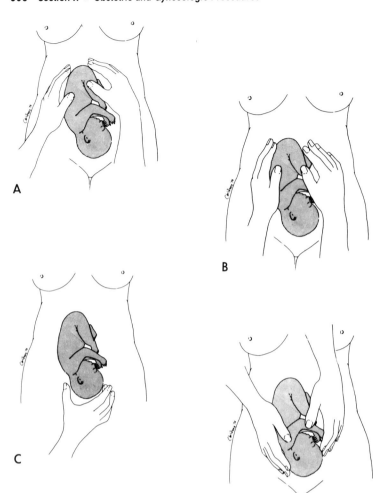

Figure 75–4. Abdominal palpation (four maneuvers of Leopold). *A,* Determination of the fetal part occupying the uterine fundus. *B,* Palpation of fetal small parts and back. *C,* Determination of the part occupying the lower uterine segment. *D,* Determination of the cephalic prominence. (From Romney S, Gray MK, Little AB, et al (eds): Gynecology and Obstetrics: The Health Care of Women. New York, McGraw-Hill Book Co, 1975. Reproduced by permission.)

examination should be performed to identify fetal presentation and position and to assess the progress of labor.

First the vulva and perineal area are prepared with an antiseptic solution such as povidone-iodine. The woman is placed on a bedpan with her legs widely separated. Scrubbing is directed from anterior to posterior and away from the vaginal introitus; each sponge should be discarded after it passes over the anal region. A dry sponge placed on the introitus prevents contaminated solution from running into the vagina.

Following preparation of the vulvar and perineal regions, the examiner uses the thumb and forefinger of a sterile-gloved hand to widely separate the labia to expose the vaginal opening; this prevents the examining fingers from coming into contact with the inner surfaces of the labia. The index and second fingers of the other hand are then introduced into the vagina to perform the examination. Cervical effacement, dilation, and fetal station are assessed. Fetal presentation and position are confirmed.[1]

Effacement of the cervix is the process of cervical thinning that occurs before and during the first stage of labor (Fig. 75–5). The degree of cervical effacement is assessed by palpation and is determined by the palpated length of the cervical canal compared with that of the uneffaced, or normal, cervical canal. Effacement is expressed as a percentage from 0 per cent, or totally uneffaced, to 100 per cent, or completely effaced. The completely effaced cervix is usually less than 0.25 cm thick.[3]

Cervical dilation is determined by estimating the average

diameter of the cervical os. The examining finger is swept from the cervical margin on one side across the cervical os to the opposite margin. The diameter transversed is expressed in centimeters. Ten cm constitutes full cervical dilation. A diameter of less than 6 cm can be measured directly. For a diameter greater than 6 cm, it is frequently easier to determine the width of the remaining cervical rim and subtract twice that measurement from 10 cm. For example, if a 1-cm rim is felt, dilation is 8 cm.

Station refers to the level of the presenting fetal part in the birth canal (Fig. 75–6). The ischial spines are used as the reference point. Zero station is used to denote that the presenting part is at the level of the ischial spines. When the presenting part lies above the spines, the distances are stated in negative figures, for example, −1 cm, −2 cm, −3 cm, and floating. If the presenting part is below the spines, the distances are stated in positive figures, for examples, +1 cm, +2 cm, and +3 cm. Determination is made by simple palpation.

Progressive cervical dilation with no change in fetal station suggests fetopelvic disproportion.[1, 8]

Position and presentation of the fetus may be inconclusive before labor, because the presenting parts must be palpated through the lower uterine segment. After dilation and effacement of the cervix, however, further delineation of presentation and position of the fetus may be made by vaginal examination.

After the perineal area has been appropriately prepared, as described previously, three maneuvers are used to

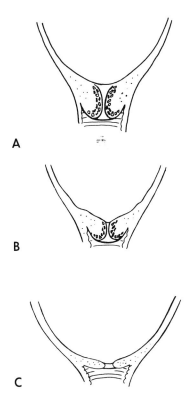

Figure 75–5. Effacement of the cervix. *A*, None. *B*, Partial. *C*, Complete. (From Romney S, Gray MK, Little AB, et al (eds): Gynecology and Obstetrics: The Health Care of Women. New York, McGraw-Hill Book Co, 1975. Reproduced by permission.)

determine fetal presentation and position. In the first maneuver, two fingers of the examiner's gloved hand are introduced into the vagina and advanced to the presenting part, differentiating face, vertex, and breech presentations. In vertex presentations, the examiner's fingers are carried up behind the symphysis pubis and then swept posteriorly over the fetal head toward the maternal sacrum, identifying the course of the sagittal suture. The positions of the two fontanels, located at opposite ends of the sagittal sutures, are then defined by palpation. The anterior fontanel is

diamond shaped; the posterior fontanel is triangular in shape (Fig. 75–7).

In face and breech presentations, the various parts are more readily distinguished. In breech presentations, the fetal sacrum is the point of reference; in face presentations, the easily identifiable fetal chin is used.

Auscultation. Auscultation of fetal heart tones is necessary to determine fetal well-being. The heart rate of the fetus can be identified with a stethoscope, a fetoscope, or preferably a Doppler placed firmly on the maternal abdominal wall overlying the fetal thorax and repositioned until fetal heart tones are heard. When a Doppler is used, a conducting gel should be applied to the abdominal wall, interfacing with the Doppler receiver. To avoid confusion of maternal and fetal heart sounds, the maternal pulse should be palpated as the fetal heart rate is auscultated.

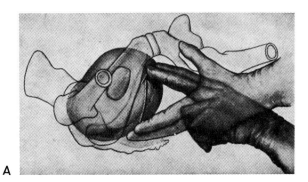

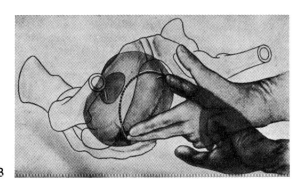

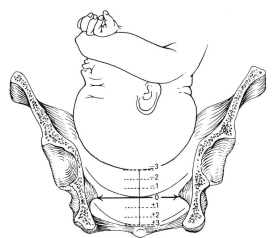

Figure 75–6. Station of the fetal head. (From Bensón RC (ed): Current Obstetric and Gynecologic Diagnosis and Treatment. 3rd ed. Los Altos, Calif, Lange Medical Publications, 1980. Reproduced by permission.)

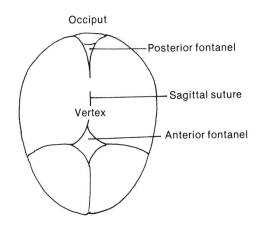

Figure 75–7. Locating the sagittal suture *(A)* and fontanels *(B)* on vaginal examination. *C*, Diagram of the fontanels and sutures. (From Pritchard JA, MacDonald PC: William's Obstetrics. 16th ed. New York, Appleton-Century-Crofts, 1980. Reproduced by permission.)

Normal baseline fetal heart rate is 120 to 160 beats per minute. Changes in the fetal heart rate that are indicative of fetal distress are usually evident immediately after a uterine contraction. During labor, fetal distress is suspected if the fetal heart rate repeatedly drops below 120 beats per minute immediately following a contraction. If prolonged monitoring of labor is necessary in the emergency department, fetal heart sounds should be assessed immediately after a contraction at 15-minute intervals during the first stage of labor and at 5-minute intervals during the second stage of labor.[1, 9] If trained personnel and equipment are available, an external fetal monitor provides a noninvasive method for continuous assessment of fetal heart rate and maternal uterine contractions.

Management of Fetal Distress. If fetal distress is suspected on the basis of resting fetal heart rate or changes after contractions, changing of maternal position, typically into the left lateral recumbent position, may be beneficial. Maternal oxygen should be administered to improve fetal oxygenation. In the absence of bleeding, a vaginal examination should be performed to rule out the possibility of prolapse of the umbilical cord. If immediate obstetric services are not available, consideration should be given to tocolytic therapy to improve fetoplacental blood flow until delivery can be accomplished. By stopping uterine contractions a more sustained placental blood flow is maintained and, in the case of cord prolapse, intermittent pressure on a compromised umbilical cord may be averted.[10] The definitive therapy for fetal distress is delivery of the infant, either vaginally or by cesarean section.[3, 4]

Cord prolapse usually occurs at the same time as rupture of the membranes and is diagnosed by palpation of the umbilical cord on vaginal examination or by visualization of the cord protruding through the introitus. The incidence of cord prolapse in labor is approximately 0.5 per cent and most often occurs when the fetal presenting part does not completely fill the lower uterine segment during labor or when there is unusual mobility of the cord.[4] Cord prolapse is frequently encountered with breech presentation, multiple pregnancies, prematurity, and premature rupture of the membranes.

The management of cord prolapse is directed at sustaining fetal life until delivery is accomplished. Unless immediate delivery is feasible or the fetus is known to be dead, preparations should be made for an emergency cesarean section. If immediate obstetric services are not available, tocolytic therapy may be instituted to decrease uterine contractions and improve fetoplacental perfusion.[10, 11] Compression of the umbilical cord should be minimized by exerting manual pressure through the vagina to lift and maintain the presenting part away from the prolapsed cord. The patient should be placed in the knee-chest or deep Trendelenburg position, and this position should be maintained until delivery is accomplished. Some physicians recommend that following manual elevation of the presenting part, 500 to 700 ml of saline be instilled into the bladder to maintain cord decompression. Once the bladder is filled, the vaginal hand may be removed.[3, 10, 11]

With cord prolapse, the fetal prognosis is dependent on presentation, gestation, and the timing of diagnosis and management. Partial cord compression for less than 5 minutes may not be harmful. Complete occlusion for the same period or partial occlusion for a longer time is likely to cause death or severe central nervous system damage to the fetus.[3]

Inhibition of Labor

Tocolytic therapy may be indicated in the emergency department to prevent the progression of labor when fetal distress, particularly that due to cord compression, is noted and to treat preterm labor.

PRETERM LABOR

Premature delivery complicates 7 to 8 per cent of all births in the United States, and prematurity continues to be the single greatest cause of neonatal morbidity and mortality.[12, 13] A wide variety of treatments for the inhibition of labor have been advocated, including bed rest, prophylactic progesterone, ethanol, prostaglandin inhibitors, magnesium sulfate, and, most recently, β-agonist agents such as terbutaline and ritodrine. Efficacy of each of these regimes is difficult to establish, because of a paucity of well-controlled clinical studies and inconsistently defined indications for the use of tocolytic therapy. Currently the cornerstones of pharmacologic management of preterm labor are the use of β-adrenergic receptor agonists and magnesium sulfate.

The criteria for defining preterm labor vary among investigators. A presumptive diagnosis of premature labor may be made in the woman who is between 20 and 37 weeks gestation when the following conditions are present: (1) the presence of regular uterine contractions occurring at intervals of 10 minutes or less and lasting at least 30 seconds, (2) progressive cervical effacement and dilation during a period of observation, or (3) a cervix that is well effaced and at least 2 cm dilated on the patient's presentation to the hospital. Because rupture of the membranes frequently means that delivery is imminent, uterine contractions accompanied by membrane rupture may also be used to establish the diagnosis. External monitoring devices, when available, are helpful by providing objective evidence of the character of uterine contractions as well as the condition of the fetus. Extended observation is undesirable because the effectiveness of tocolytic therapy diminishes as labor advances.[1, 3, 13, 14]

Ideally, when preterm labor is suspected, obstetric consultation should be obtained and the patient transferred immediately to the labor and delivery area for monitoring and determination of fetal maturity. When appropriate obstetric facilities are not available, attempts to arrest labor should be initiated in the emergency department. Indications for tocolytic therapy in the treatment of preterm labor are provided in Table 75–2.

Table 75–2. Indications for Tocolytic Therapy in Preterm Labor

Indications
Gestational age 20 to 36 weeks
An apparently healthy fetus
Regular uterine contractions
Cervical dilation of 4 cm or less

Contraindications
Gestational age of less than 20 weeks or more than 36 weeks
Known fetal lung maturity
Uncorrected fetal distress or fetal death
Obstetric complication requiring early delivery, e.g., preeclampsia-eclampsia, abruptio placenta, or placenta previa with major hemorrhage, severe fetal disease such as hydramnios or hemolytic disease
Chorioamnionitis
Severe maternal disease such as untreated hyperthyroidism, cardiac or renal disease

(From Benson RC [ed]: Current Obstetric and Gynecologic Diagnosis and Treatment. 5th ed. Los Altos, Calif, Lange Medical Publications, 1984; Huddleston JF: Preterm labor. Clin Obstet Gynecol 25:123, 1982; Rayburn WF, DeDonato DM, Rand WK: Drugs to inhibit premature labor. In Rayburn WF, Zuspan FP [eds]: Drug Therapy in Obstetrics and Gynecology. Norwalk, Conn, Appleton-Century-Crofts, 1986.)

TOCOLYTIC THERAPY

Basic maneuvers to improve uterine and fetal status should be initiated before instituting pharmacologic tocolytic therapy when either preterm labor or fetal distress is suspected. Because uterine hypoxia may induce uterine contractions, supplemental oxygen, rapid intravenous infusion of 500 to 1000 ml of crystalloid, and assumption of the left lateral decubitus position should be attempted to improve uterine perfusion.[1, 14] If contractions persist in the emergency department despite these maneuvers, pharmacologic tocolytic therapy with either the selective β_2-adrenergic agents or magnesium sulfate may be indicated.[10]

The selective β-adrenergic agents ritodrine (Yutopar) and terbutaline (Brethine, Bricanyl) are the most commonly used tocolytic agents. Although ritodrine is the only agent currently approved by the United States Food and Drug Administration for the inhibition of labor, terbutaline has been used elsewhere as a tocolytic agent, has documented efficacy in inhibiting labor, and is frequently more readily available to the emergency physician.[12]

Dosage. Ritodrine is given as an intravenous infusion, typically consisting of 150 mg ritodrine in 500 ml fluid, which yields a final concentration of 0.3 mg/ml. The initial infusion rate is 0.1 mg per minute (0.33 ml per minute), which is increased by 0.05 mg per minute every 10 minutes until uterine contractions cease, intolerable maternal side effects develop, or a maximum dose of 0.35 mg per minute is reached.[12, 14, 16]

Terbutaline may be given subcutaneously or by intravenous infusion. When given subcutaneously a 0.25-mg dose is used, which may be repeated every 1 to 6 hours; when the intravenous route is chosen, the infusion is begun at a rate of 0.01 mg per minute and may be increased by 0.005 mg per minute every 10 minutes until a maximum dose of 0.025 mg per minute is reached, uterine contractions cease, or adverse maternal side effects develop.[10, 12, 17]

The use of the β_2-adrenergic agents is limited by dose-related major cardiovascular side effects resulting from residual β_1-activity; these include fetal and maternal tachycardia, increased maternal pulse pressure, and pulmonary edema. Maternal metabolic side effects include a decrease in serum potassium and increases in blood glucose and lactic acid. Maternal medical contraindications to the use of β-adrenergic agents include cardiac disease, hyperthyroidism, asthma requiring sympathomimetic drugs, uncontrolled diabetes, and chronic hepatic or renal disease. Commonly observed minor side effects during intravenous administration are palpitations, tremors, nervousness, and restlessness.[12, 14, 17]

Magnesium sulfate ($MgSO_4$) is not approved in the United States for use as a tocolytic agent. Although apparently less effective than ritodrine or terbutaline, magnesium sulfate is less likely to cause serious side effects and is the best alternative if β-agonist agents are contraindicated or toxic. When used as a tocolytic agent, 4 to 8 gm of magnesium sulfate is given intravenously over 20 minutes, followed by a maintenance intravenous infusion of 1 to 3 gm per hour adjusted to the cessation of uterine contractions or clinical evidence of magnesium toxicity. The major side effect of magnesium therapy is impairment of the muscles of respiration with subsequent respiratory arrest, an effect usually not seen until the serum magnesium level exceeds 10 mEq/L. The first sign of magnesium toxicity, loss of the patellar reflex, typically occurs at serum magnesium levels between 7 and 10 mEq/L and precedes the development of respiratory compromise. The presence of the patellar reflex must therefore be monitored throughout therapy. Because magnesium is almost totally excreted by the kidney, mag-

nesium is contraindicated in the presence of renal failure, and urinary output and renal function should be monitored throughout therapy. If respiratory depression develops, 10 to 20 ml of a 10 per cent calcium gluconate solution is an effective antidote.[12–14]

Vaginal Bleeding During the Third Trimester

Bleeding during the third trimester should always be considered an emergency. Profound shock secondary to exsanguinating hemorrhage may occur within minutes. Although bleeding may result from local vaginal and cervical lesions, genital lacerations, circumvallate placenta, vasa previa, or rupture of the uterus, placenta previa and premature separation of the placenta account for one half to two thirds of all cases.[18] *Placenta previa* refers to implantation of the placenta in the lower uterine segment with varying degrees of encroachment upon the cervical os. Occurring in 0.1 to 1.0 per cent of all pregnancies, placenta previa is characterized clinically by vaginal bleeding with little or no abdominal or pelvic pain. Premature separation of the placenta, or *abruptio placentae*, refers to separation of the placenta from its site of implantation in the uterus before delivery of the fetus and occurs in 0.2 to 2.4 per cent of all pregnancies. In contrast to placenta previa, abruptio placentae is associated with varying degrees of abdominal pain and uterine irritability. The degree of clinical shock may be out of proportion to the amount of apparent hemorrhage. Consumptive coagulopathy occurs in 20 to 38 per cent of all cases of abruptio placentae.[18]

As noted previously, third-trimester vaginal bleeding should always be considered an emergency. Stabilization should be initiated with at least two large-bore intravenous lines. In addition to routine laboratory work-up and the taking of blood for type and cross-matching, clotting studies, including a fibrinogen level, should be drawn. Vaginal examination is *contraindicated* in the emergency department because of the possibility of tearing or dislodging a placenta previa, which may result in profuse, potentially fatal hemorrhage.[1] The patient should be immediately transferred to the care of her obstetrician for further evaluation. Definitive diagnosis via the "double set-up" examination has generally been replaced by localization of the placenta by ultrasound.[19, 20] The accuracy of placental localization and, therefore, the confirmation of placenta previa is between 93 and 98 per cent. For unknown reasons, blood separating the placenta from its attachment is difficult to detect by ultrasound. Ultrasonography, therefore, has little value in directly diagnosing abruptio placentae but is of great value in excluding the diagnosis of placenta previa.[21, 22]

DELIVERY

Full dilation of the cervix signifies the second stage of labor, heralding delivery of the infant. Typically, the patient begins to bear down and, with descent of the presenting part, develops the urge to defecate. Uterine contractions may last 1.5 minutes and recur after a myometrial resting phase of less than 1 minute.

The mechanism of labor in vertex and breech presentations consists of engagement of the presenting part, flexion, descent, internal rotation, extension, external rotation or restitution, and expulsion (Fig. 75–8). The mechanism of labor is determined by the pelvic dimensions and configuration, the size of the fetus, and the strength of uterine contractions. Essentially, the fetus will follow the path of least resistance by adaptation of the smallest achievable

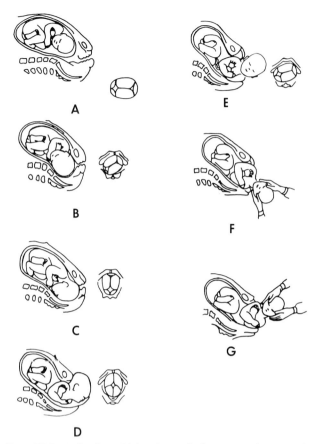

Figure 75–8. Mechanism of labor for cephalic presentation. *A,* Before labor. *B,* Engagement, flexion, and descent. *C,* Internal rotation extension. *D,* Extension to delivery of head. *E,* External rotation (restitution). *F,* Delivery of anterior shoulder. *G,* Delivery of posterior shoulder. Note that the head is being supported and guided in *F* and *G.* Traction is to be minimized. (From Romney S, Gray MK, Little AB, et al (eds): Gynecology and Obstetrics: The Health Care of Women. New York, McGraw-Hill Book Co, 1975. Reproduced by permission.)

diameters of the presenting part to the most favorable dimensions and contours of the birth canal.

The sequence of movements in vertex presentations is as follows:

1. **Engagement.** Usually occurring in the last 2 weeks of pregnancy in the primiparous patient and at the onset of labor in the multiparous patient, engagement refers to the mechanism by which the greatest transverse diameter of the head, the biparietal diameter in occiput presentations, passes through the pelvic inlet.

2. **Flexion.** Flexion of the head is necessary to minimize the presenting cross-sectional diameter of the head during passage through the smallest diameter of the bony pelvis. In most cases, flexion is necessary for both engagement and descent.

3. **Descent.** Descent is gradually progressive and is effected by uterine and abdominal contractions as well as by straightening and extension of the fetal body.

4. **Internal Rotation.** Internal rotation occurs with descent and is necessary for the head or presenting part to traverse the ischial spines. This movement is essentially a turning of the head such that the occiput gradually moves from its original, more transverse position, anteriorly toward the symphysis pubis or, less commonly, posteriorly toward the hollow of the sacrum.

5. **Extension.** Following internal rotation, the sharply flexed head reaches the anteriorly directed vulvar outlet, undergoing extension. With increasing distention of the perineum and vaginal opening, an increasingly larger portion of the occiput appears gradually. The head is born by further extensions as the occiput, bregma, forehead, nose, mouth, and finally chin pass successively over the anterior margin of the perineum.

Immediately after its birth, the head drops downward such that the chin lies over the maternal anal region.

6. **External Rotation.** External rotation or restitution follows delivery of the head as it rotates to the transverse position that it occupied at engagement. Following this movement, the shoulders descend in a path similar to that traced by the head, rotating anteroposteriorly for delivery. First, the anterior shoulder is delivered beneath the symphysis pubis, followed by the posterior shoulder across the perineum. Expulsion of the remainder of the fetal body occurs with ease.

The mechanism of the labor for breech presentations varies (Fig. 75–9). Usually the hips engage in one of the oblique diameters of the pelvic inlet. As descent occurs, the anterior hip generally descends more rapidly than the posterior hip. Internal rotation occurs as the intertrochanteric diameter assumes the anteroposterior position. Lateral flexion occurs as the anterior hip catches beneath the symphysis pubis, allowing the posterior hip to be born first. The infant's body then rotates, allowing for engagement of the shoulders in an oblique orientation. There is gradual descent, with the anterior shoulder rotating to bring the shoulders into the anteroposterior diameter of the outlet. The anterior shoulder follows lateral flexion to appear beneath the symphysis, with the posterior shoulder delivered first as the body is supported. The head tends to engage in the same diameter as the shoulders. Subsequent flexion and descent of the head occurs, following the path of the shoulders. Internal rotation occurs toward the hollow of the sacrum.

Delivery of the infant usually occurs spontaneously. The role of the physician or attendant is principally to provide control of the birth process, preventing forceful, sudden expulsion or extraction of the infant with resultant fetal and maternal injury.

Management of Delivery

EQUIPMENT (Fig. 75–10)

Obstetric pack (sterile)
   1 large basin (for placenta)
   1 pair of scissors
   2 medium Kelly clamps or umbilical tape
   1 bulb syringe or DeLee suction trap*
   1 double grip cord clamp
   3 small sterile towels
   1 package of gauze sponges
   1 baby blanket
   2 pairs of sterile gloves
   Sterile tubes for placental blood collection
Optional
   Infant resuscitation tray
   Warm blankets
   Name bands
   Heated isolette or Sterile Infant Swaddler†

---

*Argyle Manufacturing Company, St. Joseph, Missouri.
†American Hospital Supply Company, McGaw Park, Illinois.

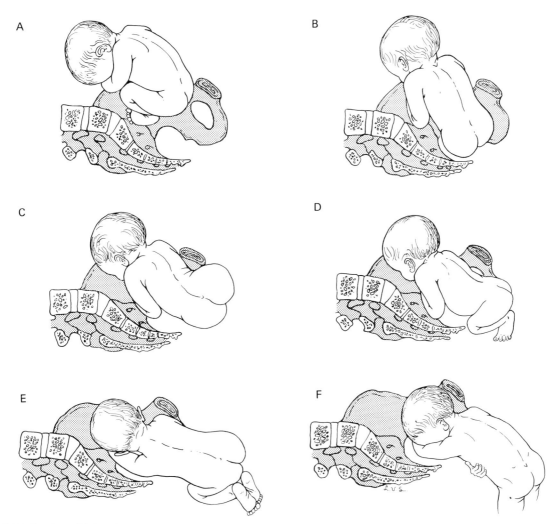

Figure 75–9. Mechanism of labor for breech presentation. *A,* Before labor. *B,* Engagement of the buttocks, internal rotation. *C,* Lateral flexion of the trunk, delivery of the buttocks. *D,* External rotation of the buttocks, engagement of the shoulders. *E,* Internal rotation of the shoulders, delivery of the posterior shoulder. *F,* Lateral flexion of the trunk, delivery of the anterior shoulder. (From Benson RC (ed): Current Obstetric and Gynecologic Diagnosis and Treatment. 3rd ed. Los Altos, Calif, Lange Medical Publications, 1980. Reproduced by permission.)

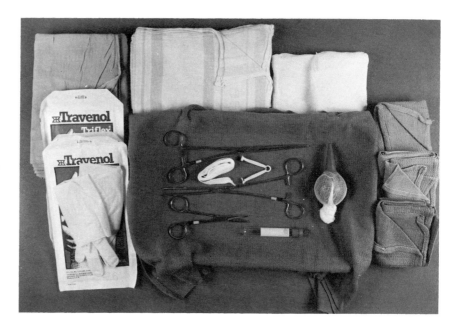

Figure 75–10. Obstetrics pack.

TECHNIQUE

Owing to the high bacterial content of the vagina and perineum, complete sterility is not a priority.[23] When time permits, however, sterile technique should be used. The hands should be cleansed and sterilely gloved. The perineum should be cleansed as described for vaginal examination and draped such that only the immediate area about the vulva is exposed. Care should be taken to avoid fecal contamination of the infant. Equipment in the obstetric pack should be sterile.

General Considerations. The patient should be positioned on a stretcher with her hips and knees partially flexed, the thighs abducted, and the soles of the feet placed firmly on the stretcher. The delivery position may be enhanced by placing the patient's buttocks on the underside of a sterile bedpan, providing up to 5 inches of additional space between the bed and the perineum.[23]

Vertex Delivery. Spontaneous delivery of the vertex-presenting infant is divided into three phases: delivery of the head, delivery of the shoulders, and delivery of the body and legs.

Delivery should be anticipated when the presenting part reaches the pelvic floor. With each contraction, the perineum bulges increasingly and the vulvovaginal opening becomes more and more dilated by the fetal head. Just before delivery, "crowning" occurs; the head is visible at the vaginal introitus, and the widest portion, or biparietal diameter, of the head distends the vulva.

Gentle, gradual, controlled delivery is desirable. As the fetal head becomes progressively more visible, one palm of the physician's hand is placed over the occipital area, providing gentle pressure to control delivery of the head. *Explosive delivery of the head should be avoided.* The other hand, preferably draped with a sterile towel to protect it from the anus, may exert forward pressure on the chin of the fetus through the perineum just in front of the coccyx in a modified Ritgen maneuver (Fig. 75–11). This maneuver extends the neck at the proper time, thereby protecting the maternal perineal musculature.

The head is gently supported during subsequent delivery of the forehead, face, chin, and neck.

After the head has been delivered, the infant's face and mouth should be quickly wiped and the oral cavity and nares should be suctioned with a bulb syringe. This minimizes the chance of aspiration of amnionic fluid, debris, and blood,

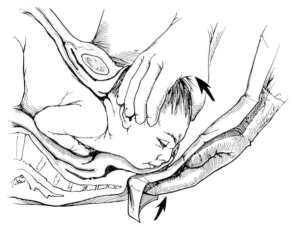

Figure 75–11. Modified Ritgen maneuver. (From Pritchard JA, MacDonald PC: William's Obstetrics. 16th ed. New York, Appleton-Century-Crofts, 1980. Reproduced by permission.)

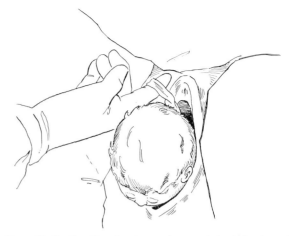

Figure 75–12. Checking for the cord around the infant's neck.

which may occur with inspiration during delivery of the thorax.

With delivery of the neck, a finger should be passed around the neck to determine whether it is encircled by one or more coils of the umbilical cord (Fig. 75–12). If a cord is felt, it should be cautiously be loosened and gently slipped over the infant's head. If this cannot be done easily, the cord should be doubly clamped and cut and the infant should be delivered *promptly*. In approximately 25 per cent of deliveries, the umbilical cord is around the infant's neck but is rarely tight enough to cause fetal hypoxia.[1]

Just before external rotation, the head usually falls posteriorly, bringing it almost into contact with the anus. As rotation occurs, the head assumes a transverse position and the transverse diameter of the thorax or bisacromial diameter rotates into the anteroposterior diameter of the pelvis. In most cases the shoulders are born spontaneously. Delivery may be aided by grasping the sides of the head and exerting *gentle* downward (posterior) traction until the anterior shoulder appears beneath the symphysis pubis. The head is then *gently* lifted upward to aid the delivery of the posterior shoulder (see Fig. 75–8). The remainder of the body usually follows without difficulty.

Delivery may be assisted by *gentle* traction on the head after the shoulders have been freed. Hooking the fingers in the axilla during delivery may result in brachial plexus injury, hematoma of the neck, or fracture of the clavicle; thus, it should be avoided. Furthermore, traction should always be exerted in the direction of the long axis of the child; if applied obliquely, traction may cause bending of the neck and excessive stretching of the brachial plexus.[1, 3, 23]

As soon as the infant is delivered, it should be held with the head lower than the body, at an angle of not greater than 15 degrees to facilitate drainage of accumulated mucus and bronchial secretions in the airway. The infant's airway should be thoroughly suctioned. Although some controversy exists as to the optimal position of the infant in relation to the mother during this stage, most authorities recommend that the infant be placed at or below the level of the vaginal introitus for 30 seconds before the cord is clamped.[1, 24] This allows up to 100 ml of blood to be transfused from the placental circulation into the infant.[1]

The umbilical cord should be cut 30 to 60 seconds after delivery. Blood samples from the placental end of the cord should be collected for determination of infant serology, including rhesus factor (Rh) studies. Two sterile clamps should be placed several inches apart, and the cord between the clamps should be cut with sterile scissors. A sterile cord clamp or cord tie of umbilical (cloth) tape is then placed around the cord, approximately 1 cm distal to the skin edge of the cord insertion site (navel).[1, 3, 23]

Immediately following the cutting of the umbilical cord, the infant should briefly be evaluated and, if necessary, resuscitation should be initiated. Because of the relatively large surface area of the neonate, attention should be directed toward maintaining body temperature by drying the neonate and placing the baby in a heated isolette, Sterile Infant Swaddler, or using warm blankets.[1, 3]

Delivery of the Placenta. Placental separation usually occurs within 5 minutes following delivery of the infant and may be recognized by the following signs:

1. The uterus becomes globular and firmer as it contracts.
2. The uterine fundus rises in the abdomen.
3. There is a sudden gush of blood.
4. The umbilical cord protrudes further out of the vagina, indicating placental descent.

Intra-abdominal pressure produced by the mother may be enough to effect complete expulsion of the placenta. If maternal force alone is insufficient to expel the placenta, it may be recovered by the Brandt-Andrews maneuver as follows (Fig. 75–13): One hand is placed on the abdomen just above the symphysis pubis. Pressure is used to elevate the uterus into the abdomen while the placenta is expressed into the vagina. The cord is kept slightly taut to help guide the placenta out of the birth canal. As the placenta passes through the introitus, fundal pressure is stopped and the placenta is gently lifted away from the introitus. Membranes that are adherent to the uterine lining should be grasped with a clamp or ring forceps and removed by *gentle* traction. Traction should never be used to pull the placenta out of the uterus, because traction may result in uterine inversion. The placenta should be examined for completeness and saved for later evaluation by the obstetrician.[1]

The uterus should be palpated and elevated when the third stage of labor has been completed. Firm compression of the uterus may express clots and stimulate the uterus to contract, reducing total blood loss. If there is persistent bleeding from a flaccid uterus, gentle massage and oxytocics may be used as necessary.[1, 3] Oxytocics should not be used before placental delivery during the third stage of delivery, because the resultant uterine contraction may entrap the placenta within the uterus. Use of oxytocics before delivery of an undiagnosed second twin may prove fatal to the entrapped fetus.

Oxytocin (Pitocin, Syntocinon) is the most commonly used oxytocic and is usually given by intravenous infusion. Twenty units of oxytocin are added to 1 liter of normal saline and are given at a rate of 10 ml per minute for several minutes until the uterus remains firmly contracted and bleeding is controlled. The infusion rate is then reduced to 1 to 2 ml per minute. If an intravenous line is not available, 5 to 10 IU (0.5 to 1.0 ml) of oxytocin may be given intramuscularly. An injection of 0.2 mg methylergonovine maleate (Methergine) may be given intramuscularly as an alternative. Because methylergonovine may cause serious hypertension and seizures, it is contraindicated in patients with hypertension and preeclampsia.[1]

Occasionally, the placenta may fail to separate completely, resulting in a retained placenta or placental fragments, with persistent uterine bleeding. Manual removal of the placenta, exploration of the uterine cavity for retained products, and, occasionally, hysterectomy are indicated. These procedures are beyond the scope of emergency department care and should be left to the obstetrician. The patient should be supported with intravenous fluid, blood, and fresh frozen plasma as indicated until definitive therapy is available. Constant firm *uterine massage* can lessen hemorrhage and may be life saving.

SHOULDER DYSTOCIA

The term *shoulder dystocia* refers to impaction of the fetal shoulders in the pelvic outlet occurring after delivery of the head in vertex presentations. Occurring more commonly with large infants, shoulder dystocia is a serious and at times fatal complication. Swartz sites an overall incidence of 0.15 per cent, increasing to 1.7 per cent in infants weighing more than 4000 g.[25] Impaction of the fetal shoulders and thorax

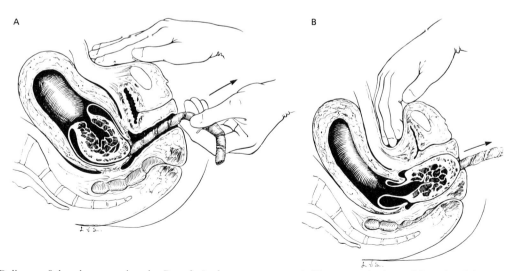

Figure 75–13. Delivery of the placenta using the Brandt-Andrews maneuver. *A,* The uterus is elevated into the abdomen as gentle traction is exerted on the cord. *B,* Pressure is exerted between the uterine fundus and the symphysis, forcing the uterus upward and the placenta outward. (From Benson RC (ed): Current Obstetric and Gynecologic Diagnosis and Treatment. 3rd ed. Los Altos, Calif, Lange Medical Publications, 1980. Reproduced by permission.)

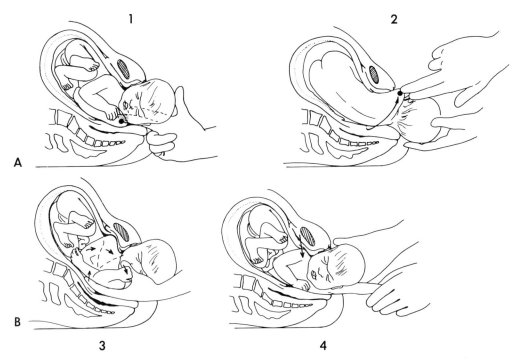

Figure 75–14. Maneuvers for shoulder dystocia. *A,* Rotation: *1.* Rotation of the posterior shoulder. *2.* Delivery of the rotated shoulder. *B,* Delivery of the posterior arm: *3.* Flexion of the posterior arm. *4.* Delivery of the posterior arm to permit delivery of the anterior shoulder. (From Romney S, Gray MK, Little AB, et al (eds): Gynecology and Obstetrics: The Health Care of Women. New York, McGraw-Hill Book Co, 1975. Reproduced by permission.)

in the maternal pelvis prohibits adequate respiration; compression of the umbilical cord frequently compromises fetal circulation.

Management. General anesthesia is desirable but is seldom available in the emergency department. A wide episiotomy reduces the incidence of major perineal lacerations and provides additional space for manipulation. Frequently, placing the mother in the extreme lithotomy position with her hips completely flexed, allowing the knees to rest upon her chest, causes the fetal shoulders to engage appropriately and enables delivery to progress.[26–28] If this simple change in maternal position fails to effect delivery, the infant should immediately be examined. The examiner's hand is inserted as far within the birth canal as possible to rule out the possibility of a fetal tumor or anomaly as the cause of obstruction. If no anomaly is found, two maneuvers are commonly used to effect delivery (Fig. 75–14). In the first maneuver, rotation of the shoulder girdle into one of the oblique pelvic diameters may be accomplished by applying pressure to the infant's posterior scapula, rotating it upward and anteriorly. When the bisacromial diameter has been dislodged from the anteroposterior diameter of the pelvis, fundal pressure alone may result in advancement of the anterior shoulder. If advancement does not occur, Wood's "screw principle" may be used. Rotation of the shoulders is continued anteriorly in a screw-like motion until the posterior shoulder passes beneath the symphysis pubis and is delivered as an anterior shoulder.[1, 25, 28, 29]

If rotation is unsuccessful, delivery of the infant's posterior arm may be used to effect delivery. The physician's hand is passed into the uterus along the hollow of the sacrum, bringing down the entire posterior arm by flexing the elbow, looping a finger around the forearm, and delivering it. Frequently, the anterior shoulder usually follows without difficulty. If the anterior shoulder cannot be delivered, rotation of the shoulder girdle into one of the oblique

diameters of the pelvis aids delivery.[1, 28, 30] This maneuver is highly effective but may result in uterine rupture and other serious lacerations of the maternal perineum.[3]

Cleidotomy, division of the clavicles to reduce the bulk of the shoulder girdle, is the ultimate solution for cases of shoulder dystocia but should be done only under the direct supervision of the obstetrician.

BREECH DELIVERY

When compared with cephalic presentations, the breech delivery is associated with a greater incidence of prematurity, prolapsed cord, low implantation of the placenta, uterine and congenital abnormalities, multiple pregnancies, and increased perinatal morbidity and mortality rates.[1, 3, 19, 31, 32] The incidence of breech presentation varies inversely with gestational age and weight. At term, the incidence of breech presentation 3 to 4 per cent; from 28 to 38 weeks, 17 per cent; and at less than 28 weeks gestation, 40 per cent.[33]

Although increased rates of prematurity and congenital anomalies associated with breech presentation account for much of the perinatal loss, when these factors are excluded, the perinatal mortality rate for breech remains three to four times that for vertex presentations.[32, 34, 35] Fetal distress also occurs more frequently. Whereas umbilical cord prolapse occurs in only 0.3 to 0.5 per cent of vertex presentations, the incidence rate increases to 3.8 to 5.2 per cent in breech presentations.[33] Prolapse occurs more commonly with footling and incomplete presentations than with frank breech. Frank breech is the most frequent type of breech presentation, occurring in approximately 65 per cent of the cases; complete breech occurs in about 10 per cent of the cases and footling or incomplete breech occurs in about 25 per cent.[3]

The increased use of cesarean section has greatly decreased the morbidity and mortality associated with breech delivery. Although cesarean section is now recognized as the standard of care, vaginal delivery may be the method of choice in carefully selected cases.[32, 35, 36] The emergency physician seldom, if ever, is called on to make the decision as to the most appropriate means of delivery but, rather, could be faced with the imminent vaginal delivery of the breech infant. Breech delivery is most appropriately performed with both a physician and an assistant present.

Types. There are three types of vaginal breech delivery.

Spontaneous Breech. This type of delivery is that in which the infant is delivered spontaneously without any manipulation or traction other than supporting the infant. Although this form of delivery is rare with term infants, there is little associated traumatic morbidity.

Partial Breech Extraction. In this type of delivery, the infant is delivered spontaneously as far as the umbilicus; the remainder of the body is extracted.

Total Breech Extraction. The entire body of the infant is extracted by the physician in total breech extraction.

Delivery is easier and perinatal morbidity and mortality are reduced when the breech is born spontaneously to the level of the umbilicus.[1, 37] If fetal distress develops before this time, however, a decision must be made whether to perform a total breech extraction or prepare for cesarean section. Total breech extraction is indicated only if there is a definite diagnosis of fetal distress unresponsive to routine maneuvers and cesarean section cannot be performed promptly. To perform any vaginal breech delivery, the birth canal must be sufficiently large to allow passage of the fetus without trauma and the cervix must be completely effaced and dilated. If these conditions do not exist, a cesarean section is indicated. To ensure full cervical dilation in the footling or complete breech, it is important that the feet, legs, and buttocks advance through the introitus to the level of the fetal umbilicus before the physician intervenes in delivery and further extraction is attempted. *The mere appearance of the feet through the vulva is not in itself an indication to proceed with delivery.*

Technique. If fetal distress is documented and total

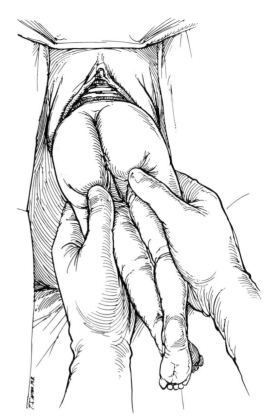

Figure 75–16. Breech extraction. Traction of the legs and thighs. (From Taylor ES: Obstetrics and Fetal Medicine. 2nd ed. Baltimore, Williams & Wilkins, 1977. Reproduced by permission.)

extraction is deemed necessary, the following procedures are carried out. The physician's hand is introduced into the vagina, and both feet of the fetus are grasped, with the index finger placed between the fetal ankles. Gentle traction is applied until the feet are pulled through the vulva (Fig. 75–15). At this point, a wide episiotomy is usually made. Because the legs are slippery and difficult to hold owing to vernix caseosa, they should be wrapped in a sterile towel as they emerge through the vulva. Downward gentle traction is continued as successively higher portions of the legs and thighs are grasped (Fig. 75–16). When the breech appears at the vulva, gentle traction is applied until the hips are delivered. As the buttocks emerge, the fetal back usually rotates anteriorly. The thumbs of the physician are then placed over the sacrum while the fingers are placed over the hips, and gentle downward traction is continued (Fig. 75–17). As the scapulas emerge, the infant usually rotates back to its original position, with the back directed laterally.

If spontaneous rotation does not occur, slight rotation should be added to the traction to bring the bisacromial diameter of the fetus into the anteroposterior diameter of the pelvis (Fig. 75–18). Delivery of the shoulders should not be attempted until the lower halves of the scapula are delivered outside the vulva and the axilla becomes visible at the introitus. Two methods of shoulder delivery are commonly used. In this first method, with the scapulas visible, the trunk is rotated such that the anterior arm and shoulder appear at the vulva and can be easily released and delivered. The body of the fetus is then rotated in the reverse direction to deliver the other shoulder and arm beneath the symphysis pubis. In the second method, if trunk rotation is unsuccessful, the posterior shoulder must be delivered first. The feet are grasped in one hand and drawn upward over the

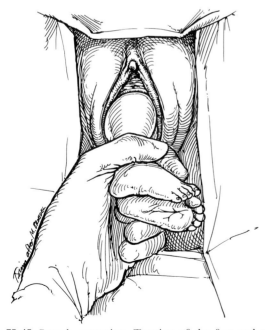

Figure 75–15. Breech extraction. Traction of the feet and ankles. Note that the index finger is placed between the ankles. (From Pritchard JA, MacDonald PC: William's Obstetrics. 16th ed. New York, Appleton-Century-Crofts, 1980. Reproduced by permission.)

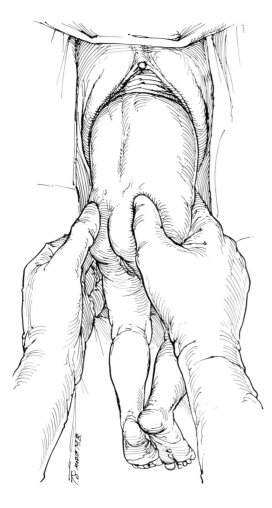

Figure 75–17. Breech extraction. The physician's hands are placed over the infant's sacrum to deliver the body. (From Taylor ES: Obstetrics and Fetal Medicine. 2nd ed. Baltimore, Williams & Wilkins, 1977. Reproduced by permission.)

mother's groin. In this manner, leverage is exerted on the posterior shoulder, which slides out over the perineal margin, usually followed by the arm and hand. The anterior shoulder, arm, and hand are then delivered beneath the symphysis pubis by downward traction on the fetal body (Fig. 75–19).

Occasionally, spontaneous delivery of the arm and hand do not follow delivery of the shoulder. If this occurs, upward traction of the fetal body should be continued after delivery of the posterior shoulder. Two fingers of the physician are then passed along the fetal humerus until the fetal elbow is reached. The fingers are used to splint the fetal arm, which

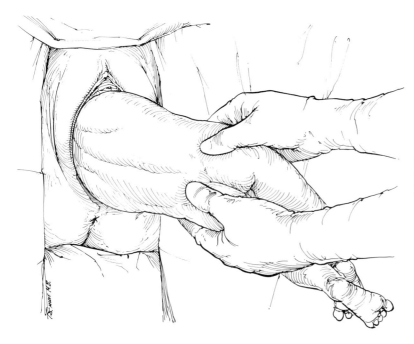

Figure 75–18. Breech extraction. Rotation occurs as the scapulae emerge. (From Taylor ES: Obstetrics and Fetal Medicine. 2nd ed. Baltimore, Williams & Wilkins, 1977. Reproduced by permission.)

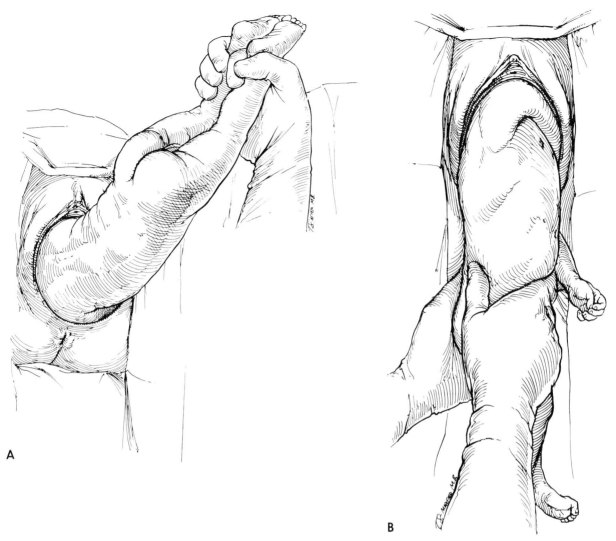

Figure 75–19. Breech extraction. *A*, Delivery of the posterior shoulder by upward traction on the fetal body. *B*, Delivery of the anterior shoulder beneath the symphysis by downward traction. (From Taylor ES: Obstetrics and Fetal Medicine. 2nd ed. Baltimore, Williams & Wilkins, 1977. Reproduced by permission.)

is then swept downward and delivered. The anterior arm may then be delivered by depression of the fetal body alone. In some cases it may be necessary to sweep the anterior arm down over the thorax using two fingers as a splint.

After the shoulders appear, the head usually occupies one of the oblique diameters of the pelvis, with the chin directed posteriorly. The head may then be extracted using the Mauriceau maneuver. With the fetal body resting upon the physician's palm and forearm, the index and middle finger of the hand are placed over the infant's maxilla, flexing the fetal head. Two fingers of the other hand are hooked over the fetal neck, and, grasping the shoulders, downward traction is applied until the suboccipital region appears under the symphysis pubis (Fig. 75–20). As the body of the fetus is then elevated toward the mother's abdomen, the fetal mouth, nose, brow, and eventually occiput successively emerge over the perineum. Suprapubic pressure applied by an assistant is helpful in delivery of the head. If delivery of the head is not effected by the Mauriceau maneuver, forceps delivery may be necessary. Forceps application is beyond the scope of this text.

At times, delivery of a frank breech may be necessary. Facilitated by an episiotomy, the breech should be allowed to deliver spontaneously as far as possible. Moderate traction

may be exerted by a finger placed in each fetal groin (Fig. 75–21). Once the knees appear outside the birth canal, the legs may be slowly flexed to assist delivery, which usually occurs without trauma.

Complications. Traumatic morbidity associated with breech presentations is approximately 12 times that of vertex presentations and is directly related to the manipulations used to effect delivery and the relationship of fetal size to that of the maternal pelvis.[38] One of the most significant features of breech delivery is that progressively increasing diameters and less distensible fetal parts must traverse the maternal pelvis.

If cephalopelvic disproportion is not diagnosed until the fetal body has been delivered and if the fetal head will not descend, the prognosis is grave. In addition, whereas in vertex presentations, in which moulding the fetal head is gradual, occurring over the course of hours, in breech presentation, moulding is abrupt, subjecting the delicate supporting tissues of the aftercoming head to sudden and often violent stresses. Intracranial hemorrhage is the most frequent cause of death in breech delivery, with injury to the spinal cord, liver, adrenal glands, and spleen occurring in decreasing order of frequency.[1, 39]

Both assisted breech delivery and breech extraction

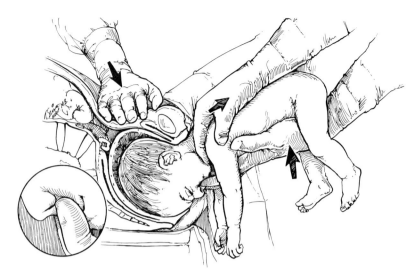

Figure 75–20. Mauriceau maneuver: delivery of the aftercoming head. While suprapubic pressure is applied by an assistant, the head is gently flexed by pressure on the mandible. (From Taylor ES: Obstetrics and Fetal Medicine. 2nd ed. Baltimore, Williams & Wilkins, 1977. Reproduced by permission.)

involve a change in motive powers for delivery, substituting traction from below for pressure from above and increasing the probability of occurrence of unilateral or bilateral nuchal arms or hyperextension of the fetal head. Decomposition and extraction of a frank breech infant carry significantly increased fetal risks and impose additional maternal risks because of intrauterine manipulation. The fact that manipulation does indeed correlate with traumatic morbidity was illustrated by Ravinsky and coworkers, who found that, whereas spontaneous breech delivery was associated with no traumatic complications, increasing degrees of obstetric manipulation corresponded to progressive elevations of the traumatic morbidity rate.[38] The highest traumatic maternal morbidity rate, 8.3 per cent, which is ten times the rate for assisted breech delivery and four times the rate for breech extraction, occurred with breech decomposition and extraction.

EPISIOTOMY

An episiotomy is an incision of the posterior vaginal wall and a portion of the pudenda, which is made to enlarge the vaginal introitus to permit easier passage of the fetus and theoretically to prevent perineal lacerations of the mother, preserving the structure and function of the vaginal introitus. Although about 60 per cent of women receive an episiotomy during childbirth, the routine use of the procedure has been questioned. Until further data are available this discussion will present the traditional viewpoint. An episiotomy helps to mimimize compression and trauma of the fetal head; facilitates the second stage of labor by removing the resistance of the pudendal musculature; substitutes a straight surgical incision for the ragged laceration that may result from tearing of the musculature; and may reduce the incidence of subsequent symptomatic cystocele, rectocele, and uterine prolapse. It is generally recommended that an episiotomy be performed for most breech deliveries; for deliveries in primiparous patients when possible; to facilitate delivery of premature infants; and when a perineal tear is imminent.[3]

Although both the median and mediolateral episiotomy are commonly described (Fig. 75–22), the median episiotomy is usually preferred.[4, 40–42] A median incision is the easiest type of episiotomy to perform and repair, results in the least amount of blood loss, and heals rapidly with minimal discomfort. The major disadvantage to the median incision is occasional accidental extension of the incision into the anal sphincter or through the sphincter into the rectum, resulting in third- and fourth-degree lacerations, respectively. There is minimal morbidity if laceration of the rectal sphincter is recognized early and is properly repaired. Failure to repair

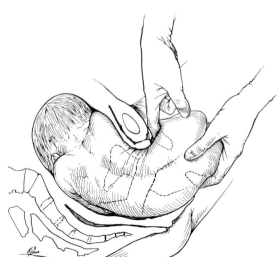

Figure 75–21. Extraction of a frank breech by moderate traction exerted with a finger in each groin. (From Pritchard JA, MacDonald PC: William's Obstetrics. 16th ed. New York, Appleton-Century-Crofts, 1980. Reproduced by permission.)

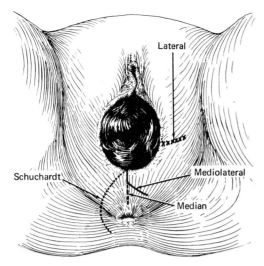

Figure 75–22. Types of episiotomy. Median and mediolateral are those most commonly performed. (From Benson RC (ed): Current Obstetric and Gynecologic Diagnosis and Treatment. 3rd ed. Los Altos, Calif, Lange Medical Publications, 1980. Reproduced by permission.)

the sphincter, however, often leads to incontinence and a rectovaginal fistula. Although a mediolateral episiotomy seldom results in extension through the anal sphincter, with this type of episiotomy blood loss is generally greater, it is more difficult to repair, and painful healing and postpartum dyspareunia often result. Of note is one large retrospective analysis showing a several fold *lower* frequency of severe perineal lacerations with the mediolateral episiotomy.[42a] The authors of that report advocate reevaluating the current use of a midline episiotomy as usual practice.

Procedure

EQUIPMENT

> Tissue scissors or scalpel (with tongue blade)
> 3–0 or 2–0 absorbable suture on atraumatic needle (e.g., chromic catgut or polyglycolic acid)
> Needle holder
> Suture scissors
> Gauze pack

TECHNIQUE

The episiotomy should be timed so that it precedes trauma to the maternal tissues and fetus but avoids excessive maternal blood loss before delivery. With vertex presentations, the episiotomy should be performed when the fetal head begins to distend the perineum and the caput becomes visible to a diameter of 3 to 4 cm during a contraction.[1, 41, 42] With breech delivery, the episiotomy is usually performed as the fetal buttocks distend the vulva but occasionally may not be necessary until delivery of the head.[4] Anesthesia for episiotomy in the emergency department is usually limited to local infiltration of the perineum with 1 or 2 per cent lidocaine.

The episiotomy is a simple incision that extends through the skin and subcutaneous tissues, the vaginal mucosa, the urogenital septum, the superior fascia of the pelvic diaphragm, and, if the episiotomy is mediolateral and deep, through the lowermost fibers of the puborectalis portion of the levator ani muscles. The incision may be made with either a scissors or a scalpel. When using a scalpel, a tongue

blade is placed between the infant's head and the maternal perineum as the perineum is incised. For the median episiotomy, the incision is made through the median raphe of the perineum almost to the anal sphincter (Fig. 75–23). For the mediolateral episiotomy, the incision is directed downward and outward in the direction of the lateral margin of the anal sphincter and may be either to the right or to the left (see Fig. 75–22).

Following delivery of the infant and placenta, the episiotomy is repaired. The goals of episiotomy repair are to restore anatomy and achieve adequate hemostasis with a minimum of suture material. It is preferable to perform the closure after delivery of the placenta and following inspection and repair of the cervix and upper vaginal canal. The same principles of repair are followed for both the median (Fig. 75–24) and mediolateral (Fig. 75–25) episiotomy.

Because there is minimal tension on the closed wound, most authorities recommend the use of 3–0 or 2–0 chromic catgut or polyglycolic acid on a large, atraumatic needle. The first step is to close the vaginal mucosa using a continuous suture from the apex of the incision to the mucocutaneous junction, reapproximating the margins of the hymenal ring. Burying the closing knot in the incision, not at the hymenal ring, minimizes the amount of scar tissue and prevents tenderness and dyspareunia. All large actively bleeding vessels should be separately ligated during closure with separate absorbable suture ligatures. Next, the perineal musculature is reapproximated with three or four interrupted sutures. Closure of the superficial layers may be accomplished by one of two methods. In the first method, a continuous suture is used to close the superficial fascia from the mucocutaneous junction outward and is then continued upward as a subcuticular skin closure, returning to and ending at the mucocutaneous junction. Alternatively, several interrupted sutures may be placed through the skin and subcutaneous fascia and loosely tied. This last method of skin closure avoids burying two layers of suture in the more superficial layers of the perineum.

Alternatively, one continuous suture may be used to close the entire episiotomy in three layers. First, the vaginal mucosa is sutured as previously described. The suture is then inverted below the hymenal ring and continued out-

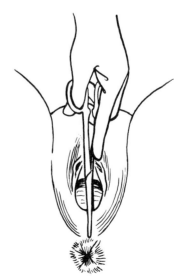

Figure 75–23. Midline (median) episiotomy. (From Romney S, Gray MK, Little AB, et al (eds): Gynecology and Obstetrics: The Health Care of Women. New York, McGraw-Hill Book Co, 1975. Reproduced by permission.)

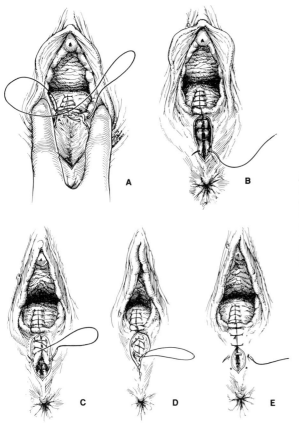

Figure 75–24. Closure of median episiotomy. *A,* Closure of mucosa and hymenal ring with continuous suture. *B,* Approximation of perineal musculature with interrupted sutures. *C,* Continuous suture to unite superficial fascia. *D,* Completion of repair by carrying continuous suture upward as a subcuticular stitch. *E,* Alternatively, closure of the superficial fascia and skin (*C* and *D*) may be accomplished by a series of loosely tied interrupted sutures. (From Pritchard JA, MacDonald PC: William's Obstetrics. 16th ed. New York, Appleton-Century-Crofts, 1980. Reproduced by permission.)

wardly, reapproximating the deep tissue. The skin and subcutaneous fascia are closed with a continuous subcuticular stitch carried upward and ending at the hymenal ring.

During episiotomy closure, it is helpful to maintain a dry field by inserting a large gauze pack in the vagina, leaving a tail or portion of the pack outside the vagina to aid in removal after the repair.

The most common complication of episiotomy is hematoma formation owing to inadequate hemostasis; a hematoma is treated by evacuation and drainage. Occasionally, large bleeding vessels will require delayed ligation. Postpartum episiotomy pain can usually be controlled by analgesics and local heat or sitz baths. Infection is a rare complication and responds readily to adequate drainage and appropriate antibiotic therapy.

IMMEDIATE POSTPARTUM HEMORRHAGE

Postpartum hemorrhage, defined as maternal blood loss greater than 500 ml during the 24 hours following delivery, is the most common cause of serious obstetric hemorrhage and accounts for up to 25 per cent of obstetric deaths caused by hemorrhage (see also Chapter 76).[1] Postpartum hemor-

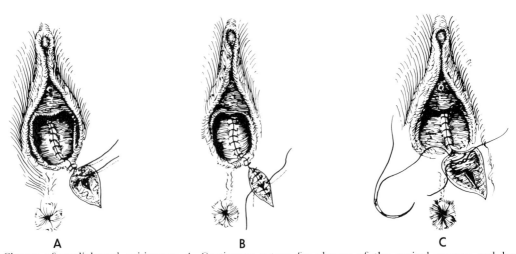

Figure 75–25. Closure of mediolateral episiotomy. *A,* Continuous suture for closure of the vaginal mucosa and hymenal ring. *B,* Approximation of the levator ani and perineal musculature. *C,* Closure of the skin. (From Benson RC (ed): Current Obstetric and Gynecologic Diagnosis and Treatment. 3rd ed. Los Altos, Calif, Lange Medical Publications, 1980. Reproduced by permission.)

rhage is conventionally divided into immediate hemorrhage occurring within 12 to 24 hours of delivery and delayed hemorrhage occurring more than 24 hours after delivery.

Postpartum hemorrhage is frequently characterized by steady moderate bleeding that persists until serious hypovolemia develops rather than by sudden massive hemorrhage. Because of the relative hypervolemia that occurs during normal pregnancy, blood loss may exceed 1500 ml before significant clinical changes in pulse and blood pressure become manifest.[43] Careful observation for blood loss, including evaluation of uterine size and consistency, is therefore mandatory during the early postpartum period.

The most common causes of immediate postpartum hemorrhage, in order of frequency, are uterine atony, lacerations of the vagina and cervix, and retained placenta or placental fragments. Less commonly, coagulation disorders, uterine rupture, uterine inversion, and paravaginal vessel laceration result in postpartum blood loss.[3, 44, 45]

Management

Management of postpartum hemorrhage consists of replacement of intravascular volume with crystalloid and blood products as needed, as well as therapy directed toward the cause of hemorrhage. The diagnosis of uterine atony, the most common cause of bleeding, is made when uterine palpation reveals a soft "boggy" uterine corpus. Although the diagnosis may be suspected on the basis of abdominal examination alone, bimanual pelvic examination is frequently necessary to confirm the diagnosis.

Uterine atony is managed by manual massage of the uterine fundus (Fig. 75–26). One hand of the physician is used to compress and massage the posterior aspect of the uterus through the abdominal wall while the knuckles of the other sterile gloved hand are used to gently massage the anterior aspect of the uterus through the vaginal wall. Oxytocics should be administered in conjunction with massage.

OXYTOCICS

Oxytocin is ideally administered as an intravenous infusion, which is prepared by adding 20 to 40 units of oxytocin

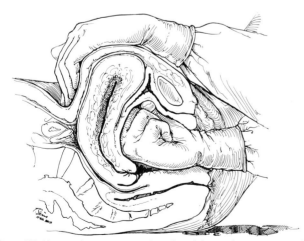

Figure 75–26. Uterine massage. One hand is used to massage the posterior aspect of the uterus through the abdominal wall. The other hand, inserted in the vagina, compresses the anterior uterus. (From Pritchard JA, MacDonald PC: William's Obstetrics. 16th ed. New York, Appleton-Century-Crofts, 1980. Reproduced by permission.)

to 1 liter of crystalloid and infused at a rate of 200 to 500 ml per hour. If intravenous access is unavailable, 10 units of oxytocin may be given intramuscularly. Because the onset of action of intravenously administered oxytocin is rapid, uterine contractions and therefore slowing of hemorrhage should be observed within minutes of administration. If bleeding persists and the uterus remains boggy despite oxytocin therapy, 0.2 mg of *methylergonovine (Methergine)* or *ergonovine (Ergotrate)* should be given intramuscularly to help stimulate uterine contractions. Typically, uterine contractions occur within minutes of ergot administration and last for several hours. Because of their tendency to cause vasoconstriction and severe hypertension in some patients, ergot preparations should be avoided in women who are known to be hypertensive or have preeclampsia.[1] If the uterus remains boggy and the bleeding persists despite uterine massage and the administration of oxytocin and an ergotamine, the use of prostaglandin therapy should be considered. An intramuscular injection of 0.25 mg of 15-methyl prostaglandin $F_2\alpha$ (Carboprost tromethamine) or, alternatively, 0.5 to 1 mg of prostaglandin $F_2\alpha$ (Dinoprost tromethamine) injected transabdominally or transvaginally into the myometrium has been reported to control postpartum hemorrhage refractory to other therapy. The use of prostaglandin compounds for the purpose of arresting postpartum hemorrhage due to uterine atony has not yet been approved by the United States Food and Drug Administration. Their use as a last resort, however, may help to control life-threatening hemorrhage unresponsive to more traditional therapies.[45, 46]

PROCEDURES

If vaginal bleeding persists despite uterine massage and a firmly contracted uterus, a cause other than uterine atony should be suspected. The labia, vagina, and cervix should be carefully inspected for lacerations. Bleeding from lacerations may be controlled by direct pressure or, in the case of cervical lacerations, by gentle application of the ring forceps to the bleeding point. Absorbable sutures may be used to control bleeding from easily accessible lacerations. Because adequate visualization of the cervix and upper vagina is difficult and repair of extensive lacerations frequently requires general anesthesia, repair of these lacerations is often better left to the obstetrician.

Although rare, occurring in approximately 1 in 4000 to 5000 deliveries, *uterine inversion* usually manifests with dramatic hemorrhage and shock occurring in 27 to 39 per cent of the patients.[41] Diagnosis is made by visualization and palpation of the soft, pear-shaped fundal wall near the cervical os or extending through it. On abdominal examination, no mass representing the uterine corpus can be palpated above the symphysis pubis. Treatment is aimed at maintaining cardiovascular stability through the use of intravenous fluids and immediate repositioning of the uterine corpus. General anesthesia is often necessary, especially if the cervix has contracted. Oxytocics should not be given until after the uterus is repositioned. If the placenta has become partially detached before replacement, the remainder should be removed immediately before further manipulation.[1, 41, 45]

Repositioning may be accomplished by inserting one hand into the vagina and extending the fingers to identify the margins of the cervix; the uterine corpus is allowed to rest in the palm of the hand. Gentle pressure exerted with the fingers on the edges of the uterus closest to the cervix in the direction of the umbilicus is followed by gradual replacement of the corpus (Figs. 75–27 and 75–28). Pressure should not initially be exerted centrally on the fundus, because this will cause the uterus to be compressed, forcing

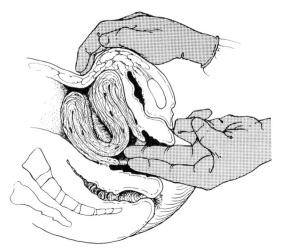

Figure 75–27. Replacement of a partially inverted uterus. (From Benson RC (ed): Current Obstetric and Gynecologic Diagnosis and Treatment. 3rd ed. Los Altos, Calif, Lange Medical Publications, 1980. Reproduced by permission.)

more "layers" of the uterus to simultaneously lie within the relatively tight cervical ring. Once the uterus has been repositioned, the placenta may be removed. Because traction on the cord of an adherent placenta is one of the principal causes of uterine inversion, this procedure may be deferred until the obstetrician arrives. Although replacement of the inverted uterus can usually be accomplished by vaginal manipulation, occasionally a dense cervical contraction ring is present, preventing repositioning. General anesthesia and laparotomy may be necessary for uterine repositioning.

Management of refractory postpartum hemorrhage requires specialized care and should be left to the obstetrician. Fluid replacement and the application of the pneumatic anti-shock garment are used to stabilize the patient in the interim.[44]

POSTMORTEM CESAREAN SECTION

Introduction

Postmortem cesarean section, one of oldest and most dramatic surgical procedures known, has long been used as an attempt to preserve the life of the unborn child.[47, 48] Earliest records trace its origin back to 715 B.C. when the legendary king of Rome Numa Pompilious decreed that the child be excised from the womb of any woman who died late in pregnancy. Under the emperors of Rome, the Caesars, this law became known as the "lex caesarea," and hence the name "cesarean operation."[49]

Pliny the Elder described the first successful postmortem cesarean delivery in 237 B.C., that of Scipio Africanus who would later become one of Rome's greatest generals. In A.D. 1280 the Catholic Church at the Council of Cologne decreed that postmortem cesarean section must be performed to permit the unborn child to be baptized and undergo a proper burial. In 1500 a Swiss sow gelder, Jacob Nufer, performed the first reported successful cesarean section with maternal survival delivering his wife of a live born infant. His wife lived to bear six more children through vaginal delivery.[49–51]

Since 1879 there have been more than 188 reports of postmortem cesarean section resulting in the delivery of a live infant.[52] Because most of the literature on postmortem cesarean section involves only small numbers of cases with emphasis on those that are successful, accurate survival statistics are difficult to ascertain. When reported, infant survival rates range from 11 to 40 per cent.[50] Because the potential for survival of a normal infant exists, cesarean delivery must be considered in any woman who suffers irreversible

cardiopulmonary arrest during the third trimester of pregnancy.[52] Although the procedure is rare, the decision and its performance may fall to the emergency physician.

Indications

Survival of the infant is directly related to the maturity of the fetus, the elapsed time from maternal death to delivery, the performance of cardiopulmonary resuscitation on the mother, and, in certain circumstances, the availability of neonatal intensive care facilities.[51, 52] Under the best circumstances the probability of infant survival is directly related to the neonatal birth weight and gestational age of the fetus. Although the lower limit of fetal viability varies among institutions, in general, survival of the fetus is unlikely if gestational age is less than 28 weeks or fetal weight is less

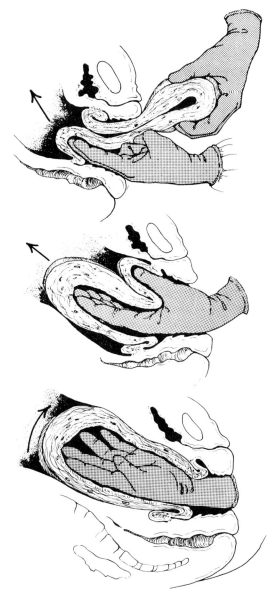

Figure 75–28. Replacement of an inverted uterus. (From Benson RC (ed): Current Obstetric and Gynecologic Diagnosis and Treatment. 3rd ed. Los Altos, Calif, Lange Medical Publications, 1980. Reproduced by permission.)

Table 75–3. Outcome of 61 Infants Who Survived Postmortem Cesarean Section from 1900 to 1985 as a Function of Time from Death to Delivery

Time (min)	Number of Patients	Normal	Neurologic Sequelae
0–5	42 (69%)	42	0
6–10	8 (13%)	7	1 (mild)
11–15	7 (11%)	6	1 (severe)
16–20	1 (2%)	0	1 (severe)
21–25	3 (5%)	1	2 (severe)

(From Katz VL, Dotters DJ, Droegemueller W: Perimortem cesarean delivery. Obstet Gynecol 68:571, 1986.)

than 1000 gm.[50, 53] If the duration of gestation is not known from the history, fetal maturity may be quickly estimated by measuring the height of the uterine fundus. At 28 weeks gestation the fundus is approximately 28 cm above the symphysis pubis or halfway between the umbilicus and the costal margin. In some institutions with advanced neonatal capabilities, infant survival may be considered possible at 26 weeks gestation or less.[54] Criteria for intervention should be established prospectively at each institution and be in accordance with the institution's general neonatal policies.[48]

The frequency of infant survival decreases and the chance of neurologic damage increases as the time from maternal death (cessation of circulation) to cesarean section rises (Table 75–3). When cesarean section is performed within 5 minutes of maternal death neonatal outcome is generally considered excellent, from 5 to 10 minutes good, from 10 to 15 minutes fair, and from 15 to 20 minutes poor. There have been no reported cases of fetal survival when cesarean delivery has been performed more than 25 minutes after maternal death.[47, 55] Because even under optimal conditions cardiopulmonary resuscitation results in a cardiac output of 30 to 40 per cent of normal and placental perfusion may be severely compromised, every attempt should be made to begin cesarean delivery within 4 minutes of the cardiopulmonary arrest, completing the procedure within 5 minutes of arrest.[48, 52] Fetal prognosis is generally better following the sudden death of a previously healthy mother than after the death of a woman with a prolonged and debilitating illness.[47, 50, 52]

Cardiopulmonary resuscitation should, of course, be initiated immediately on arrest of the mother and continued until *after* delivery of the infant. Because dextroversion of the uterus may impede venous return and further reduce maternal cardiac output in the supine patient, manual displacement of the uterus away from the inferior vena cava may be attempted by an assistant. In rare cases removal of the infant and relief of uterine compression on the vena cava has resulted in improved maternal cardiac output with subsequent survival of the mother.[48, 51]

Legal Considerations

No physician has ever been found liable for performing a postmortem cesarean section. Indeed, it is felt that the physician has the legal right and responsibility to provide the unborn fetus with every possible chance of survival when there is no hope of maternal survival.[47, 52, 55] Permission for the operation should be obtained from the family when possible but not at the expense of delaying the procedure. Failure to obtain permission should not preclude cesarean section.[50, 52, 54, 55]

Procedure

EQUIPMENT

Scalpel with a number 10 blade
Bandage scissors
Bladder retractor
Large retractors (two)
Forceps
Lap or gauze sponges
Hemostats (curved and straight)
Suction
Obstetric pack (as described earlier for vaginal delivery)

Because of the rarity of this procedure in the emergency department, it is unlikely that a specific instrument pack will be available. Minimally, a scalpel with a large blade and an obstetric pack are necessary.

TECHNIQUE

Postmortem cesarean section should be performed by the most experienced person present, preferably an obstetrician, and when possible a neonatologist should be in attendance. Cardiopulmonary resuscitation should be initiated on the mother at the time of cardiac arrest and continued throughout the procedure. Although it is helpful if fetal heart tones are present premortem, time should not be wasted searching for them.

Rapid extraction of the infant while avoiding fetal injury is the goal of the procedure. Using a large (e.g., number 10) scalpel, a classic midline vertical incision is made through the abdominal wall extending from the level of the fundus to the symphysis pubis and carried through all abdominal layers to the peritoneal cavity (Fig. 75–29). If available, retractors are placed in the abdominal wound and drawn laterally to expose the anterior surface of the uterus. The bladder is reflected inferiorly; if full it may be aspirated to evacuate it and permit better access to the uterus (Fig. 75–30). While avoiding injury to fetal parts, a small, approximately 5-cm, vertical incision is made through the lower uterine segment until amniotic fluid is obtained or until the uterine cavity is clearly entered (Fig. 75–31A). The index and long fingers are then inserted into the incision and used to lift the uterine wall away from the fetus. A bandage scissors is used to extend the incision vertically to the fundus until a wide exposure is obtained (Fig. 75–31B). The infant

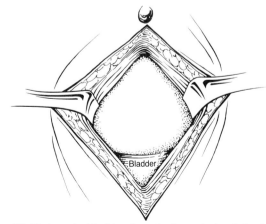

Figure 75–29. A vertical incision is made through the abdominal wall from the level of the uterine fundus to the symphysis pubis.

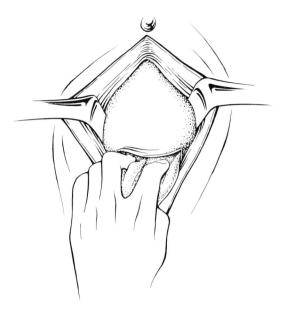

Figure 75–30. If available, retractors are used to expose the anterior surface of the uterus, and the bladder is retracted inferiorly.

is then gently delivered, the mouth and nares suctioned, and the cord clamped and cut (Fig. 75–32). Because the incision is relatively high in the uterus, the infant's head may not be readily accessible to the physician, in which case the infant's feet are grasped and the baby delivered through maneuvers similar to those of a breech delivery. Neonatal resuscitation should be carried out as necessary.

Because in rare instances relief of vena caval compression by the uterus improves maternal hemodynamics such that maternal survival is possible, maternal pulses should be checked and cardiopulmonary resuscitation continued after delivery of the infant.[54, 56, 57]

Conclusion

Postmortem cesarean section is a rarely performed but potentially life-saving procedure, which should be considered in any women in the third trimester of pregnancy who suffer irreversible cardiopulmonary arrest. Because neonatal survival is enhanced as the time from maternal death to delivery decreases while the irreversible nature of maternal cardiac arrest becomes more apparent as resuscitative efforts progress, the decision and timing of this procedure may be one of the most difficult that the emergency physician makes. Once the decision is made to perform a cesarean section, it should be done as quickly as possible by the most experienced person present. Cardiopulmonary resuscitation should be continued until after delivery of the infant. Although rare, maternal survival has been reported after "postmortem" cesarean section.

THE NEONATE

Evaluation of the neonate begins before delivery with assessment of maternal well-being, gestational age, ease and type of previous deliveries, and the recognition of fetal distress as evidenced by meconium staining of the amniotic fluid, fetal bradycardia, or evidence of cord prolapse. Care of the newborn begins with delivery of the head while the mouth and nares are suctioned. Following delivery and cutting of the umbilical cord, the infant should immediately

be placed in a supine position with the head lowered and turned to the side to prevent aspiration. Because of the relatively large surface area of the infant, temperature drops rapidly immediately after birth, with subsequent chilling, which produces shivering and increased oxygen demand. Care must be taken, therefore, to maintain body temperature by drying the baby and placing it in warm blankets, a Sterile Infant Swaddler, or a heated isolette, or if resuscitation is necessary, under a radiant warmer.

Evaluation

Traditionally, the *Apgar Scoring System*, applied at 1 and 5 minutes after birth, is the standard of neonatal evaluation (Table 75–4).[1, 3, 58] In general, the higher the score, the better the condition of the infant. The 1-minute Apgar Score reflects the need for immediate resuscitation. A score of 7 to 10 indicates that the infant is in excellent condition,

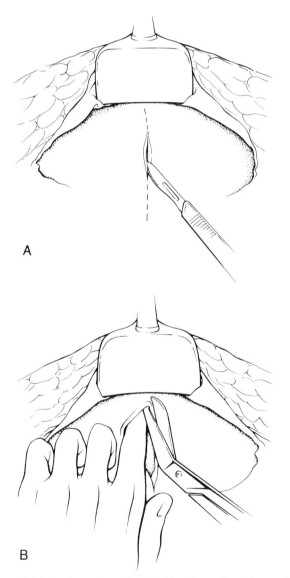

A

B

Figure 75–31. *A,* A small vertical incision is made with a scalpel through the lower uterine segment. *B,* A bandage scissors is used to extend the incision vertically to the fundus.

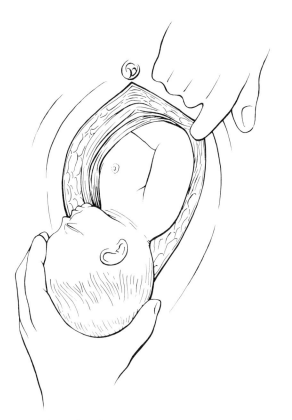

Figure 75–32. The infant is then delivered, the nares and mouth suctioned, and the cord clamped and cut.

requiring no aid other than nasopharyngeal suctioning. A moderately depressed infant with depressed respirations, flaccidity, and pallor or cyanosis usually scores 4 to 7 and may require resuscitation. A score of 0 to 4, indicating a severely depressed infant, mandates immediate resuscitation. The 5-minute Apgar Score is an indicator of neonatal and long-term prognosis; a low score suggests increased risk of subsequent infant morbidity and mortality.[1, 3, 58]

Although the Apgar Score is the traditional standard for neonatal evaluation, the decision to resuscitate and the infant's response to resuscitation can be more accurately assessed by evaluating the heart rate, respiratory activity, and neuromuscular tone of the infant.[58]

Normally, the newborn takes its first breath within a few seconds of birth and cries within 30 seconds.[1] Apnea is the most common initial manifestation of depression in the neonate and unless reversed may lead to progressive hypoxemia, hypercarbia, and acidosis. Hypoventilation quickly leads to cardiovascular depression with subsequent slowing of the heart rate, the most sensitive indication of infant distress. A heart rate of less than 100 beats per minute is considered abnormal.[58, 59]

Stabilization

EQUIPMENT

Bulb syringe or DeLee suction trap*
Oral airways (size 0, 00, and 000)
Suction catheters (size 5, 6, 8, and 10 French)
Endotracheal tubes (size 2.5 mm, 3.0 mm, and 3.5 mm)
Endotracheal tube stylet (optional)
Laryngoscope
Laryngoscope blade (straight; sizes 0 and 1)
Resuscitation bag
Face masks (sizes 0 and 1)
Wall suction
Wall oxygen
Radiant warmer

TECHNIQUE

If neonatal respirations are infrequent or absent, suctioning the mouth and pharynx with a bulb syringe or DeLee suction trap and stimulating the infant by lightly slapping the soles of the feet and rubbing the back may serve to stimulate breathing. If necessary, the airway should be gently suctioned with an 8 or 10 French suction catheter. Because deep suctioning of the oropharynx may produce a vagal response causing bradycardia or apnea, suctioning should continue for no longer than 10 seconds at a time and heart rate should be continuously monitored.[58] Because the neonate is an obligate nose breather, it is advisable to suction once through each nostril to ensure patency of the upper airway. Failure to establish effective respirations indicates either marked central nervous system depression, mechanical obstruction, or an intrinsic lung abnormality and demands active resuscitation.

If signs of airway obstruction, that is, decreased chest expansion and sternal and intercostal retractions are present and persist after suctioning, the larynx should be directly visualized with a laryngoscope. Suctioning of the larynx should be done under direct vision. For obstruction distal to the glottic opening, it is advisable to intubate the infant and suction through the endotracheal tube. Appropriate size of the endotracheal tube varies with the size of the neonate from 2.5 mm for those weighing 1000 gm or less to 3.5 mm for the term infant.

Because *meconium aspiration* is a major cause of neonatal morbidity and mortality, its prevention deserves special mention. Up to 60 per cent of neonates with meconium staining of the amniotic fluid aspirate; approximately 20 per cent of these neonates later develop pulmonary complications.[58] To prevent aspiration, neonates born with meconium staining of the amniotic fluid require thorough suctioning of the hypopharynx before the initiation of respiration, that

_____

*Vygon, East Rutherford, New Jersey.

Table 75–4. Apgar Scoring System

Sign	0	1	2
Heart rate	Absent	Slow (<100)	>100
Respiratory effort	Absent	Slow, irregular	Good, crying
Muscle tone	Flaccid	Some flexion of extremities	Active motion
Reflex irritability	No response	Grimace	Vigorous cry
Color	Blue, pale	Body pink, extremities blue	Completely pink

Table 75–5. Medications Commonly Used in Neonatal Resuscitations

Drug	Dose	Indications	Comments
Epinephrine*	0.01 mg/kg; (0.1 ml/kg of 1:10,000 solution)	Bradycardia, asystole, EMD	May be repeated every 5 minutes as required.
Sodium bicarbonate	1–2 mEq/kg	Correction of acidosis persisting after adequate ventilation	(1) Should not be used for brief episodes of arrest or to correct respiratory acidosis; (2) Because rapid infusion of hypertonic solutions may predispose to intracranial hemorrhage, each dose should be infused over 5–10 minutes in concentrations not to exceed 0.5 mEq/ml.
Atropine*	0.01–0.02 mg/kg	Bradycardia, 2- and 3-degree atrioventricular block, perhaps asystole unresponsive to epinephrine	(1) Minimum initial dose is 0.1 mg; (2) May repeat mg/kg dose every 2–5 minutes to a total dose of 0.1 mg/kg; (3) Not recommended by current ACLS guidelines for acute phase of neonatal resuscitation.
Dextrose	0.5–1.0 gm/kg	Serum glucose < 40 mg/dl	(1) Monitor serum glucose (Dextrostix) frequently; (2) Administer as dilute solution, e.g. 10% dextrose solution; (3) Follow initial bolus with continuous infusion of 5–8 mg/kg/minute.
Naloxone*	0.01 mg/kg IV or IM	Narcotic reversal as indicated	Duration of narcotic may be greater than that of naloxone; subsequent monitoring of infant required.
Calcium chloride	5–20 mg/kg	Controversial, hypocalcemia and possibly for compromised myocardial dysfunction or cardiac arrest	Not recommended by current ACLS guidelines for acute phase of neonatal resuscitation.
Cardiovascular Drips			
Epinephrine	0.1–1 μg/kg/minute	α-adrenergic agent required to maintain systemic arterial pressure	Myocardial stimulation may cause pathologic arrhythmias; excessive dose may impair renal, splanchnic, or peripheral perfusion.
Isoproterenol	0.1–1.5 μg/kg/minute titrated to desired heart rate	Bradycardia, 2- and 3-degree atrioventricular block, asystole	May cause hypotension due to β$_2$-adrenergic stimulation.
Other			
Defibrillation	1–2 watt-sec/kg	Ventricular fibrillation, ventricular tachycardia	Rarely indicated or effective.
Fluid (normal saline, lactated Ringer solution)	10–20 ml/kg	Hypovolemia	Rarely indicated. Hypovolemia most commonly occurs with placenta previa, abruption, twin-twin or feto-maternal transfusion. May require O-negative blood cross-matched with mother's blood or 5% albumin solution or other plasma substitute.

*May also be given via endotracheal tube.
ACLS, advanced cardiac life support; EMD, electrical mechanical dissociation.

is immediately after delivery of the head and before delivery of the thorax. Immediately after delivery, and if possible, before the infant has taken its first breath, laryngoscopy with intubation and tracheal suctioning is generally recommended.[58, 59]

Bag and mask ventilation should be initiated as soon as it is recognized that tactile stimulation is not sufficient to establish spontaneous ventilation or that ventilation is not adequate to maintain a heart rate of greater than 100 beats per minute.

The heart rate should be monitored during the course of neonatal evaluation and stabilization with either direct auscultation over the chest or by palpating the pulse at the base of the umbilical cord. A readily discernible heart beat of 100 or more beats per minute is acceptable. If the heart rate drops to less than 80 beats per minute and does not immediately respond to effective ventilation and oxygenation, chest compression should be instituted while ventilation is continued. The two-handed method of chest compression is preferred. The hands encircle the chest with the fingers placed over the back, and the thumbs are placed over the midportion of the sternum to provide compression. The sternum is compressed 1/2 to 3/4 inches at a rate of 120 compressions per minute. Positive-pressure ventilation should be continued with 100 per cent oxygen at a rate of 40 to 60 per minute. If there is no response in heart rate, an intravenous or umbilical line should be placed and appropriate drug therapy should be instituted. Myocardial dysfunction and shock in the neonatal period are most commonly due to profound hypoxia. If these conditions persist despite adquate ventilation, an umbilical, intravenous, or interosseous line should be established and appropriate drug therapy instituted.[58-61] The medications most commonly used in neonatal resuscitation are found in Table 75–5.

REFERENCES

1. Pritchard JA, MacDonald PC, Gant NF (eds): William's Obstetrics. 17th ed. Norwalk, Conn, Appleton-Century-Crofts, 1985.
2. Communication from the National Center for Health Statistics.
3. Benson RC (ed): Current Obstetric and Gynecologic Diagnosis and Treatment. 5th ed. Los Altos, Calif, Lange Medical Publications, 1984.
4. Romney SL, Gray MK, Little AB, et al (eds): Gynecology and Obstetrics: The Health Care of Women. New York, McGraw-Hill Book Co, 1975.
5. Abe T: The detection of the rupture of fetal membranes with nitrazine indicator. Am J Obstet Gynecol 39:400, 1940.
6. Baptisti A: Chemical test for the determination of ruptured membranes. Am J Obstet Gynecol 35:688, 1938.
7. Iannetta O: A new simple test for detecting rupture of the fetal membranes. Obstet Gynecol 63:575, 1984.
8. Friedman EA: The graphic analysis of labor. Am J Obstet Gynecol 68:1568, 1954.
9. Higgins SD: Emergency delivery: Prehospital care, emergency department delivery, perimortem salvage. Emerg Med Clin North Am 5:529, 1987.
10. Sacchetti A: Emergencies of delivery. In Farrell RG (ed): Ob/Gyn Emergencies, the First 60 Minutes. Rockville, MD, Aspen Publishers, 1986.
11. Katz Z, Lancet M, Borenstein R: Management of labor with umbilical cord prolapse. Am J Obstet Gynecol 142:239, 1982.
12. Caritis SN, Carby MJ, Chan L: Pharmacologic treatment of preterm labor. Clin Obstet Gynecol 31:635, 1988.
13. Gonik B, Creasy RK: Preterm labor: Its diagnosis and management. Am J Obstet Gynecol 154:3, 1986.
14. Huddleston JF: Preterm labor. Clin Obstet Gynecol 25:123, 1982.
15. Rayburn WF, DeDonato DM, Rand WK: Drugs to inhibit premature labor. In Rayburn WF, Zuspan FP (eds): Drug Therapy in Obstetrics and Gynecology. Norwalk, Conn, Appleton-Century-Crofts, 1986.
16. Barden TP, Peter JB, Merkatz IR: Ritodrine hydrochloride: A betamimetic agent for use in preterm labor. Obstet Gynecol 56:1, 1980.
17. Stubblefield PG, Heyl PS: Treatment of premature labor with subcutaneous terbutaline. Obstet Gynecol 59:457, 1982.
18. Abdul-Karim RW, Chevil RN: Antepartum hemorrhage and shock. Clin Obstet Gynecol 10:533, 1976.
19. Wheeler AS, Francis MJ: Anesthesia for complicated obstetrics. J Am Assoc Nurse Anesth 47:300, 1979.
20. Booher D, Little B: Vaginal hemorrhage in pregnancy. N Engl J Med 290:611, 1974.
21. Trott A: Diagnostic modalities in gynecologic and obstetric emergencies. Emerg Med Clin North Am 5:405, 1987.
22. Chinn DH, Callen PW: Ultrasound of the acutely ill obstetrics and gynecology patient. Radiol Clin North Am 21:585, 1983.
23. Jennings B: Emergency delivery: How to attend one safely. Maternal Child Nursing 4:148, 1979.
24. Yao AC, Lind J: Placental transfusion. Am J Dis Child 127:128, 1974.
25. Swartz DP: Shoulder girdle dystocia in vertex delivery: Clinical study and review. Obstet Gynecol 15:194, 1960.
26. Gonik G, Stringer CA, Held B: An alternative maneuver for management of shoulder dystocia. Am J Obstet Gynecol 145:882, 1983.
27. Hunt AB: Problems of delivery of the oversized infant. Am J Obstet Gynecol 64:559, 1952.
28. Smeltzer JS: Prevention and management of shoulder dystocia. Clin Obstet Gynecol 29:299, 1986.
29. Woods CE: A principle of physics as applicable to shoulder delivery. Am J Obstet Gynecol 45:796, 1943.
30. Mazzanti GA: Delivery of the anterior shoulder. Obstet Gynecol 13:603, 1959.
31. Brenner WE, Bruce RD, Hendricks CH: The characteristics and perils of breech presentation. Am J Obstet Gynecol 118:700, 1974.
32. Cruikshank DP: Breech presentation. Clin Obstet Gynecol 29:255, 1986.
33. James FM: Anesthetic considerations for breech or twin delivery. Clin Perinatol 9:77, 1982.
34. Morely GW: Breech presentation: A 15 year review. Obstet Gynecol 30:745, 1967.
35. Collea JV, Rabin SC, Weghorst GR, et al: The randomized management of term frank breech presentation: Vaginal delivery vs. cesarean section. Am J Obstet Gynecol 131:186, 1978.
36. Johnson CE: Breech presentation at term. Am J Obstet Gynecol 106:865, 1970.
37. Hall JE, Kohl SG, O'Brien F, et al: Breech presentation and perinatal mortality. Am J Obstet Gynecol 91:665, 1965.
38. Rovinsky JJ, Miller JA, Kaplan S: Management of breech presentation at term. Am J Obstet Gynecol 115:497, 1973.
39. Tank ES, Davis R, Holt JF, et al: Mechanisms of trauma during breech delivery. Obstet Gynecol 38:761, 1971.
40. Beynon CL: Midline episiotomy as a routine procedure. J Obstet Gynaecol Br Commonwealth 81:126, 1974.
41. Herbert WNP: Complications of the immediate puerperium. Clin Obstet Gynecol 25:219, 1982.
42. Varner MW: Episiotomy: Techniques and indications. Clin Obstet Gynecol 29:309, 1986.
42a. Shiono P, Klebanoff MA, Carey JC: Midline episiotomies: More harm than good? Obstet Gynecol 75:765, 1990.
43. Watson P: Postpartum hemorrhage and shock. Clin Obstet Gynecol 23:985, 1980.
44. Kelly JV: Postpartum hemorrhage. Clin Obstet Gynecol 19:595, 1976.
45. Herbert WN, Cefalo RC: Management of postpartum hemorrhage. Clin Obstet Gynecol 27:139, 1984.
46. Rayburn WF, Russ JS: Uterine stimulants. In Rayburn WF, Zuspan FP (eds): Drug Therapy in Obstetrics and Gynecology. Norwalk, Conn, Appleton-Century-Crofts, 1986.
47. Lattuada HP: Postmortem cesarean section: Surgical and legal aspects. Am J Surg 84:212, 1952.
48. Phelan JP: Fetal considerations in the critically ill obstetric patient. In Clark SL, Phelan JP, Cotton DB (eds): Critical Care Obstetrics. Oradell, NJ, Medical Economics Books, 1987, pp 436–460.
49. Speert H: Historical highlights. In Danforth DN (ed): Obstetrics and Gynecology. 4th ed. Philadelphia, Harper & Row, 1982, pp 2–22.
50. Arthur RK: Postmortem cesarean section. Am J Obstet Gynecol 132:175, 1978.
51. DePace NL, Betesh JS, Kotler MN: Postmortem cesarean section with recovery of both mother and offspring. JAMA 248:971, 1982.
52. Katz VL, Dotters DJ, Droegemueller W: Perimortem cesarean delivery. Obstet Gynecol 68:571, 1986.
53. Morkovin V: Trauma in pregnancy. In Farrell RG (ed): Ob/Gyn Emergencies: The First 60 Minutes. Rockville, Md, Aspen Publishers, 1986, pp 71–86.
54. Neufeld JDG, Moore EE, Marx JA, Rosen P: Trauma in pregnancy. Emerg Med Clin North Am 5:623, 1987.
55. Weber CE: Postmortem cesarean section: Review of the literature and case reports. Am J Obstet Gynecol 110:158, 1971.
56. Farrell RG: Useful ob/gyn procedures in the emergency department. In Farrell RG (ed): Ob/Gyn Emergencies: The First 60 Minutes. Rockville, Md, Aspen Publishers, 1986, pp 317–330.
57. Danforth DN: Operative delivery. In Benson RC (ed): Current Obstetric & Gynecologic Diagnosis and Treatment. Los Altos, Calif., Lange Medical Publications, 1984, pp 946–991.
58. Neonatal resuscitation. In Textbook of Advanced Cardiac Life Support. Dallas, Tex, American Heart Association, Dallas, Tex, 1987.
59. McKlveen RE, Ostheimer GW: Resuscitation of the newborn. Clin Obstet Gynecol 30:611, 1987.
60. Benitz WE, Frankel LR, Stevenson DK: The pharmacology of neonatal resuscitation and cardiopulmonary intensive care. Part 1—immediate resuscitation. West J Med 144:704, 1986.
61. Lamb FS, Rosner JS: Neonatal resuscitation. Emerg Med Clin North Am 5:541, 1987.

Chapter 76

Abnormal Vaginal Bleeding, Spontaneous Abortion, and Postpartum Hemorrhage

Roy G. Farrell

INTRODUCTION

Vaginal bleeding is a common presenting complaint in the emergency department. The sections that follow emphasize procedures that are performed in the emergency department to diagnose and treat the various causes of vaginal bleeding. These sections focus on three broad diagnostic categories: dysfunctional and perimenopausal uterine bleeding, postpartum and other life-threatening uterine bleeding, and bleeding during the first trimester of pregnancy. Specific procedures to be discussed in order of appearance are paracervical block and endometrial biopsy, tamponade of life-threatening uterine bleeding with a 30-ml Foley catheter balloon, and suction curettage for first-trimester spontaneous abortion. Pharmacologic therapy of postpartum hemorrhage is addressed in Chapter 75, and culdocentesis for evaluation of ectopic pregnancy is discussed in Chapter 77.

DYSFUNCTIONAL AND PERIMENOPAUSAL UTERINE BLEEDING

Introduction

Initial evaluation of abnormal bleeding requires establishing that a pregnancy is not present, either by an absolutely convincing history (keeping in mind that "immaculate conceptions" seem to occur with surprising frequency) or, more reliably, by an immediate pregnancy test on urine or blood that is based on monoclonal antibody detection of human chorionic gonadotropin. Anatomic causes of vaginal and cervical bleeding can usually be ruled out by a thorough pelvic examination. Systemic causes, such as thrombocytopenia, anticoagulant therapy, and hypothyroidism must be considered. Only after excluding anatomic and systemic causes of bleeding can a diagnosis of dysfunctional uterine bleeding be made definitively. Bleeding from an inflamed, friable cervix or a cervical mass must be evaluated with chlamydia and gonorrhea cultures and with a Papanicolaou test to evaluate for atypical cervical cells that are consistent with cervical carcinoma. Bleeding from inside the uterus can be evaluated for anatomic lesions (polyps, endometrial carcinoma) and for the presence of adequate estrogen stimulation (proliferative or anovulatory endometrium) and progesterone stimulation (secretory or ovulatory endometrium) by one of three procedures: endometrial biopsy, cervical dilation and endometrial curettage, or hysteroscopy, using a fiberoptic scope. A thorough endometrial biopsy can be performed easily by the emergency physician in the emergency department. It should be preceded by a paracervical block for patient comfort. The entire procedure takes about 15 minutes. It is the procedure of choice in the emergency setting and has been shown equal in diagnostic accuracy to dilatation and curettage.[1–3] Hysteroscopy has generally been reserved for those cases in which uterine bleeding persists after an endometrial biopsy or a dilation and curettage and appropriate hormone therapy to look for previously undetected anatomic lesions, such as polyps.[4] Hysteroscopy has been advocated by several researchers as superior to dilation and curettage for initial evaluation of abnormal uterine bleeding.[5–7] Hysteroscopy with directed biopsies can be performed easily in an outpatient setting and may replace blind endometrial biopsy in the future as the recommended initial procedure for evaluation of dysfunctional uterine bleeding.[8]

Hormonal Therapy versus Endometrial Biopsy

Hormonal therapy of dysfunctional bleeding can be initiated presumptively after a normal pelvic examination without endometrial biopsy in women under 30 years of age. In women older than 30 years, an attempt to rule out endometrial carcinoma and other anatomic lesions within the uterus with endometrial biopsy is recommended.[8, 9] Hormonal therapy may then be instituted if significant bleeding persists. Heavy vaginal bleeding is usually slowed considerably by endometrial biopsy. Continued heavy bleeding usually can be controlled with intravenous conjugated estrogen (Premarin), 25 mg every 30 minutes for one to three doses. Heavy bleeding not controlled by conjugated estrogen suggests an anatomic lesion and requires gynecologic consultation. Approximately 20 per cent of all postmenopausal women with uterine bleeding have endometrial carcinoma.[10] Outpatient therapy for mild to moderate uterine bleeding is best accomplished with combination estrogen-progesterone birth control preparations (Ortho-Novum 1/50 or Norinyl 1–50), two tablets twice a day for 4 days, then one tablet twice a day for 4 days, then one tablet daily for the remainder of a 21-day cycle. Close outpatient follow-up to evaluate the results of the endometrial biopsy, any continued bleeding, or both is recommended.[1]

Paracervical Block

Paracervical block is a simple and safe anesthestic technique that can be performed by the emergency physician to increase patient comfort before endometrial biopsy and suction curettage. Introduced in 1945, it has become widely accepted as the technique of choice for outpatient cervical and uterine procedures. Sensory fibers to the cervix, uterus, and upper vagina travel with the uterine blood vessels through the uterosacral ligaments and enter the uterus at the level of the internal cervical os. The ability to block these nerves through the vagina is greatly facilitated by the rich lymph and vascular anastomoses in the region. Precise placement of the anesthetic solution is therefore not important.[11]

EQUIPMENT

Paracervical block is simplified and safer to perform if a paracervical anesthesia tray is used (Fig. 76–1). This tray

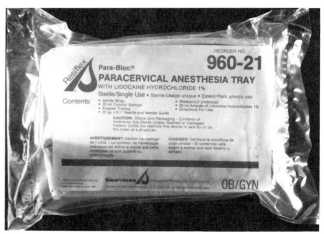

Figure 76–1. Paracervical anesthesia tray.

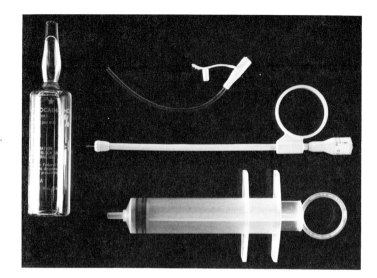

Figure 76–2. Paracervical anesthesia equipment.

provides 1 per cent lidocaine (20 ml), a trumpet-shaped plastic needle guard, and a 19-gauge needle that protrudes from the guard approximately 9 mm (Fig. 76–2).

PROCEDURE

The 20 ml of lidocaine is aspirated into the syringe, and the needle is attached with the needle guard in place. The inferior lip of the cervix is anesthetized with 1 to 2 ml of 1 per cent lidocaine solution, and then a cervical tenaculum is placed on the cervix. The cervix is elevated, and 4 to 5 ml of 1 per cent lidocaine are injected at each of four sites (the 3, 5, 7, and 9 o'clock positions) in the vaginal mucosa at its reflection onto the cervix (Fig. 76–3). Injection into the muscle of the cervix itself prevents the spread of anesthetic

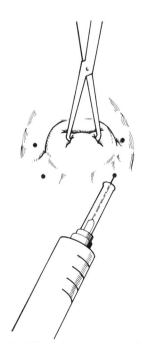

Figure 76–3. Paracervical block injection sites (the 3-, 5-, 7-, and 9-o'clock positions). The cervix is elevated with a cervical tenaculum. Then 3 to 5 ml of 1 per cent lidocaine are deposited at a depth of 6 to 12 mm at each injection site. (From Farrell RG: OB/GYN Emergencies: The First 60 Minutes. Rockville, Md, Aspen Publishers, Inc, 1986, p 323. With permission from Aspen Publishers, Inc, © 1986.)

and leads to an unsuccessful block. A period of 5 minutes is allowed for the block to take effect before an attempt is made to insert instruments into the cervix.[1]

CONCLUSION

Use of the trumpet-shaped needle guard prevents deep penetration of the needle and intravascular injection of the lidocaine, which is the only significant complication noted in the literature. In my experience and in that of my emergency physician colleagues, no complications have occurred in more than 500 cases, except an occasional lack of adequate anesthesia. In these cases, cervical block anesthesia may be supplemented by intravenous fentanyl, inhaled nitrous oxide, or both. True allergy to amide-linked local anesthetics such as lidocaine is extremely rare. Most "allergies" are reactions to preservatives in multiple-dose vials or are adverse reactions to epinephrine. Use of plain lidocaine without preservatives should minimize adverse reactions. The use of a paracervical block is not an absolute necessity for endometrial biopsy but is recommended, because patient comfort during the procedure varies considerably. Comfort during suction curettage is greatly facilitated by the paracervical block and the use of intravenous fentanyl.

Endometrial Biopsy

INDICATIONS AND CONTRAINDICATIONS

Emergency department endometrial biopsies are indicated in any woman older than 30 years of age with abnormal uterine bleeding after the physician has ruled out pregnancy and other anatomic lesions with a thorough pelvic examination and a negative pregnancy test, and after coagulation disorders are ruled out with a complete blood count and coagulation studies. Alternatives to endometrial biopsy are dilation and curettage or office hysteroscopy-guided biopsy. These last two techniques are beyond the training of most emergency physicians, however, and are often not readily available by consultation at the time one is confronted in the emergency department with a patient who needs an endometrial tissue sample before institution of hormonal therapy for her abnormal uterine bleeding.

EQUIPMENT

The Karman cannula device is disposable and is composed of a plastic suction curette (4-, 5-, and 6-mm sizes) with a plastic stylet and a separately packaged 50-ml syringe with a self-locking plunger (Fig. 76–4). Other necessary

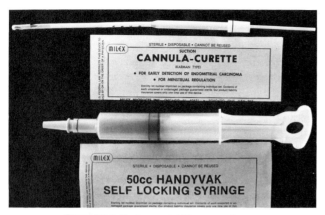

Figure 76–4. Endometrial biopsy equipment.

equipment includes a vaginal speculum, a cervical tenaculum, and a pathology specimen container with 10 per cent formalin.

PROCEDURE

Careful attention to technique is necessary to obtain a thorough scraping of the endometrial lining and high diagnostic accuracy. Before performing the biopsy, the practitioner should describe the indications and technique for endometrial biopsy to the patient and obtain verbal or written consent. The anterior (inferior) lip of the cervix is anesthetized to prevent cramping pain on application of the tenaculum, and the cervical tenaculum is applied. After administration of a paracervical block (see earlier description) and a 5-minute wait for the block to take effect, traction is placed on the cervix with the tenaculum to straighten the uterine axis and to provide countertraction while inserting the suction cannula.

While maintaining traction on the cervix in the axis of the vagina, a cannula with stylet in place is inserted into the cervical canal with slow, controlled pressure. A 5-mm cannula is adequate for most procedures, although moderate cervical stenosis may require use of a 4-mm cannula. A slight twisting motion may help the cannula pass the internal os and move into the uterine cavity. The uterine cavity is gently sounded to determine its depth, and the stylet is removed from the cannula. The 50-ml self-locking syringe is firmly attached to the cannula, and a vacuum is produced by slowly withdrawing the plunger until it locks in place at the 30-ml mark. A thorough endometrial curettage is performed by slowly scraping the lateral wall of the uterus while withdrawing the cannula and the attached syringe back to the level of the internal os. The cannula is reinserted until the posterior wall of the uterus is felt again, and the procedure is repeated approximately seven to eight times per uterine quadrant until the entire 360 degrees of the uterine cavity has been thoroughly aspirated. The cannula with the syringe attached is then removed from the uterus. Usually no more than 5 ml of tissue is aspirated. The tissue is placed in a pathology specimen jar, labeled, and sent for pathologic analysis. The patient is observed for 30 to 60 minutes to see if the bleeding has slowed considerably or has stopped. In the majority of cases, endometrial biopsy alone stops or significantly slows dysfunctional uterine bleeding enough to allow the patient to return home from the emergency department. Persistent bleeding may require hormonal therapy to achieve control.

COMPLICATIONS

Complications of endometrial biopsy are rare and are fewer than those of dilation and curettage. Complication rates for endometrial biopsy in several series representing a total of 5851 cases were 0 to 4 per 1000 for perforations, 0 to 4 per 1000 for infections, no major hemorrhage, and no unanticipated major operations.[3] Pregnancy should be ruled out with a stat human chorionic gonadotropin–β subunit test, even in those patients with a history of tubal ligation. Perforation of the uterus may occur if undue force is used and if traction is not applied through the cervical tenaculum to straighten the cervical canal. If endometrial biopsy is necessary in the presence of infection, intravenous antibiotics should be given 30 minutes before the procedure. Endometritis may occasionally develop following the procedure. Prophylactic antibiotics are indicated only in the presence of valvular heart disease or severe compromise of the immune system. On rare occasions, increased bleeding may follow an endometrial biopsy. If rapid bleeding continues, especially in an older woman, carcinoma is a more likely diagnosis. In this case, consider sending the specimen to pathology for immediate frozen section and admitting the patient. Severe cervical stenosis may prevent passage of the cannula and warrant a dilation and curettage in the operating room.

INTERPRETATION

Adequate tissue for histologic diagnosis is almost always obtained. Localized lesions, especially polyps, are occasionally missed, particularly if a thorough, four-quadrant technique is not performed. Continued bleeding indicates the need for referral for hysteroscopy with guided biopsy or dilation and curettage, or both, to identify a localized anatomic lesion.

CONCLUSION

Endometrial biopsy gives the emergency physician a very useful tool in the diagnosis of abnormal uterine bleeding. The procedure screens for intrauterine anatomic lesions and obtains a tissue sample for hormonal staging of the endometrium before instituting hormonal therapy. It is simple to perform and its diagnostic accuracy approaches that of dilation and curettage.[3] Close outpatient follow-up for evaluation of the results and need for further work-up is essential.

INTRAUTERINE TAMPONADE OF LIFE-THREATENING UTERINE BLEEDING WITH A FOLEY CATHETER BALLOON

INTRODUCTION

Rapid or exsanguinating vaginal bleeding is uncommon and is most often due to one of three problems:

1. Complications of pregnancy: postpartum bleeding, incomplete abortion, placenta previa
2. Reproductive tract neoplasia
3. Blood dyscrasia

A patient in shock from vaginal bleeding with grossly abnormal postural vital signs needs immediate fluid resuscitation, limited laboratory studies (including a complete blood count, clotting studies, pregnancy test [where indicated], and type and crossmatch for blood), rapid evaluation for the cause of the bleeding, and institution of measures to control the bleeding as soon as possible. Immediate efforts to correct any blood dyscrasias are vital. When postpartum bleeding, pregnancy, and blood dyscrasia have been ruled out, endometrial biopsy followed by conjugated estrogens (Premarin),

25 mg intravenously every 30 minutes for 1 to 3 doses, usually controls the hemorrhage.

In certain circumstances, intrauterine tamponade with a 30-ml Foley catheter balloon may facilitate control of exsanguinating uterine bleeding when endometrial biopsy and hormonal therapy fail to control severe menorrhagia. It has also proved useful in emergency control of postpartum hemorrhage.

Balloon tamponade is an excellent technique to control uterine bleeding until blood dyscrasias and clotting abnormalities can be corrected. The procedure is simple to perform and buys the emergency physician the time needed to stabilize the patient and obtain appropriate consultation.

Other commonly accepted techniques for controlling life-threatening uterine hemorrhage include surgical ligation of the uterine arteries, emergency hysterectomy, regional intra-arterial infusion of vasoconstrictive agents, and selective arterial embolization.[12, 13] Foley catheter balloon tamponade offers both an alternative to these techniques and an opportunity to stabilize the patient and to mobilize the personnel needed to provide more invasive techniques if they are still necessary.

BACKGROUND

Uterine tamponade using a Foley catheter was described by Goldrath in a series of 20 patients in 1983.[14] The procedure was successful in 17 cases, partially successful in two cases, and unsuccessful in one case. It was used in a wide variety of cases of severe uterine hemorrhage, including delayed postpartum bleeding, blood dyscrasias, severe menorrhagia with fibroids, following therapeutic abortion, and 6 weeks after undergoing a caesarean section. The two partially successful cases involved patients with an incompetent cervix who spontaneously passed the Foley balloon after 24 hours and then continued bleeding. The unsuccessful case followed a therapeutic abortion at 12 weeks. It was surmised that the uterine cavity was too large for a 30-ml balloon to affect tamponade and that a larger balloon might have been successful.

INDICATIONS

Uterine tamponade with a Foley catheter is appropriate in any case of severe uterine bleeding that does not involve pregnancy. In the first trimester, spontaneous abortion with heavy bleeding requires evacuation of the uterine contents with suction curettage. Continued heavy bleeding following suction curettage can be treated with Foley catheter tamponade, although the uterine cavity after 10 to 12 weeks of gestation may be too large for a 30-ml balloon to be effective in a tamponade. In the third trimester, placenta previa, which often requires emergency caesarean section, must be ruled out, and any insertion of instruments into the cervix is contraindicated.

During the first 1 to 2 weeks after childbirth, the technique may be unsuccessful because of uterine size and cervical dilation. Postpartum bleeding in the first week or two may require a larger balloon, although an attempt with a 30-ml Foley catheter balloon is not contraindicated. Other techniques to control postpartum hemorrhage are discussed in Chapter 75.

Foley catheter tamponade is very useful in controlling hemorrhage from the uterus of a woman who is not pregnant, including bleeding that is secondary to blood dyscrasias. If no blood dyscrasia exists, an attempt at endometrial biopsy, administration of conjugated estrogens (Premarin, 25 mg given intravenously), or both, may be considered if the patient is stable. In the unstable patient with ongoing uterine hemorrhage, Foley catheter balloon tamponade is the initial treatment of choice.

EQUIPMENT

The necessary equipment is commonly found in the emergency department: a wide selection of Foley catheter sizes with a 30-ml balloon, a syringe for inflation of the balloon, tap water or saline for balloon inflation, and a clamp to occlude the lumen of the catheter.

PROCEDURE

Anesthesia is not required for this procedure. The tip of the catheter beyond the attachment of the balloon is amputated to provide a spherical object within the uterus. The balloon is tested to ensure its integrity after cutting off the tip of the catheter. The largest caliber of Foley catheter that can be inserted through the cervix, either dilated or undilated, is placed. Usually, a uterus that has been bleeding excessively has a somewhat dilated cervix.

The balloon is distended with saline until the bleeding stops. The normal uterus has a capacity of between 5 and 10 ml. Occasionally, patients who have been bleeding excessively have a larger uterus, and up to 15 to 30 ml of saline have been required for balloon inflation. Patients with fibroids may need 30 to 40 ml. Blood sometimes drips through the Foley catheter lumen if it is of large caliber. In this case, clamping the Foley catheter provides further tamponade. The balloon is left in place for variable periods of time. Usually 12 to 24 hours is sufficient for control of the bleeding.[14] Prophylactic antibiotic coverage with ceftriaxone, 500 mg daily given intravenously, is recommended for patients whose catheters are left in place for more than a few hours or for patients who are at risk for infection (e.g., postpartum patients, patients previously exposed to instrumentation).

COMPLICATIONS

An endometritis from stasis may occur, although none of the 20 patients in the original Goldrath series developed a fever or endometritis.[14] The inflated catheter occasionally causes discomfort, which can be treated with oral analgesics. Control of bleeding from the uterus with an incompetent cervix may require a stitch around the cervix (cerclage) to retain the balloon inside the cervix. Before performing cerclage, cervical trauma is first ruled out by history and physical examination. A 0- or 00-gauge chromic or nylon suture is placed circumferentially as high as possible around the neck of the cervix. The needle is passed shallowly through the cervical muscle and around the cervix until a 360-degree suture has been placed. The suture is cinched up firmly to establish cervical competence and then is tied securely.

Retrograde bleeding through the fallopian tubes has not been reported. It is assumed that the tubal orifices are probably occluded during tamponade. In none of the cases in the original series was there clinical evidence of blood in the abdominal cavity. Two case reports describe successful use of Foley catheter balloon tamponade. One reported a case of cervical pregnancy in the late first trimester in which hysterectomy was avoided[15] and another reported two cases of postpartum hemorrhage that resulted from placental implantation in the noncontractile cervical segment of the uterus.[16]

CONCLUSION

The tamponade of severe uterine hemorrhage using a Foley catheter with a 30-ml balloon is simple, readily available, and inexpensive. Use of this technique in the emergency department may occasionally be life saving and may obviate the need for emergency surgery or arterial catheterization for vasoconstrictive infusions or selective embolectomy. This procedure, although rarely needed and only recently described, is an essential skill for any physician who treats women with acute uterine hemorrhage.

BLEEDING IN THE FIRST TRIMESTER

Overview

First-trimester bleeding may be associated with a threatened or actual miscarriage, an ectopic pregnancy, a blighted ovum, or trophoblastic disease.[17] To confirm the presence of a pregnancy, an immediate pregnancy test can be performed. Ectopic pregnancy must be ruled out. The history may reveal risk factors for ectopic pregnancy. Pain, rather than vaginal bleeding, is usually the main presenting complaint in ectopic pregnancy, although presentations vary. Pelvic examination can confirm the presence of an incomplete or inevitable abortion. Simultaneous intrauterine and ectopic pregnancies occur rarely and can present a diagnostic challenge. Ultrasound is extremely useful in localizing the pregnancy as being within the uterus. A gestational sac can be visualized by about 5 weeks of gestation, and cardiac motion within 6 to 7 weeks.[18] Quantitative serum human chorionic gonadotropin-β subunit testing is useful before 6 weeks or if the gestational sac is not visualized. Levels of human chorionic gonadotropin-β subunit that are significantly high for gestational sac size indicate the presence of trophoblastic disease. Culdocentesis (see Chapter 77) can document the presence of intraabdominal blood suggestive of ectopic pregnancy or purulent material suggestive of pelvic inflammatory disease or other infection.

Threatened abortion is defined as uterine bleeding in a patient with an intrauterine pregnancy of less than 20 weeks of gestation with a closed cervical os. With an inevitable abortion, the os is open, but no products of conception have been passed. With an incomplete abortion, products of conception have been passed, and the cervical os generally remains open; bleeding and uterine cramping continue as well. With a complete spontaneous abortion, all products of conception have been passed and cramping ceases, although mild vaginal bleeding (spotting) may continue for several days. This section describes the treatment of incomplete and inevitable abortion with the suction curettage procedure.

Suction Curettage

INTRODUCTION

Inevitable and incomplete abortion are definitively treated by evacuation of the products of conception from the uterus by suction curettage. This technique was developed in the late 1960s for therapeutic abortion and rapidly became the procedure of choice over instrument curettage for spontaneous abortion as well as for therapeutic abortion.[19] Several physicians recommended outpatient treatment of spontaneous abortion with suction curettage in the early 1970s and reported on large series of patients who had incomplete or inevitable abortions and were treated as outpatients.[19, 20] In 1982, my emergency physician group published a report on the first large series of these patients who were treated with suction curettage in the emergency department by emergency physicians and described its experience with the procedure over a 7-year period.[21] More recently, a thorough protocol for the procedure has been described in another emergency department setting.[22] The procedure takes only about 10 to 15 minutes to perform and is followed by an observation period of 2 hours, during which an oxytocin drip is infused.

Several advantages of performing the procedure in the emergency department at the time of initial presentation have been cited: rapid control of significant vaginal bleeding and elimination of painful cramping, rapid and definitive treatment of cases involving endometritis, and increased convenience and comfort for the patient through elimination of repeated examinations and inevitable delays while waiting for another physician to arrive and for an operating room to become available. Finally, the cost savings to the patient and to society in general are significant in having the procedure performed in the emergency department instead of in the operating room because of the additional services of an anesthesiologist and an operating room staff that would be required.[1]

INDICATIONS AND CONTRAINDICATIONS

Suction curettage is indicated for all cases of first-trimester incomplete and inevitable spontaneous abortion.

The diagnosis of incomplete and inevitable abortion is usually obvious from physical findings alone. If a coagulopathy is present, the procedure is contraindicated until it can be corrected, because an increased rate of hemorrhage may result. Unless the history or physical examination suggests a coagulopathy, screening patients is of low yield and generally is not indicated. Patients with evidence of endometritis, sepsis, or both should receive a dose of intravenous antibiotic (e.g., ceftriaxone, 2 gm intravenously) 30 minutes before the procedure. If the patient is allergic to cephalosporins or has a history of true anaphylaxis to penicillin, gentamycin, 2 mg/kg, plus clindamycin, 600 mg given intravenously, may be substituted. In patients with signs of hypovolemia or peritonitis, the presence of a ruptured ectopic pregnancy should be considered, and ultrasound, culdocentesis, or both should be performed. An attempt should never be made to force a suction catheter through a closed cervical os. The cervical os should admit an 8-mm suction curette if the patient has an inevitable or incomplete abortion. A closed os suggests a threatened abortion or an ectopic pregnancy. Because 50 per cent of patients who have threatened abortions go on to a normal delivery,[23] patients with a closed cervical os should be treated with bed rest and observation unless an ultrasound confirms fetal demise.

EQUIPMENT

The equipment needed for suction curettage is relatively inexpensive and easy to use. It includes an instrument tray with gauze sponges, a vaginal speculum, ring forceps, a cervical tenaculum, and a sharp uterine curette (Fig. 76–5); a paracervical anesthesia tray (Figs. 76–1 and 76–2); plastic suction curettes, sizes 8 to 11 mm (Fig. 76–6); and a vacuum curette pump and collecting apparatus (Fig. 76–7).

PROCEDURE

Patient Preparation and Anesthesia. The procedure is explained to the patient, and an informed consent form is signed. Potential complications as noted subsequently should be mentioned. Preexisting endometritis is treated with parenteral antibiotics as noted earlier. An intravenous line of 1000 ml of normal saline or lactated Ringer solution with 20 units of oxytocin is run over 2 to 3 hours.

Sedation and anesthesia are best obtained with a combination of paracervical block (see the description in this

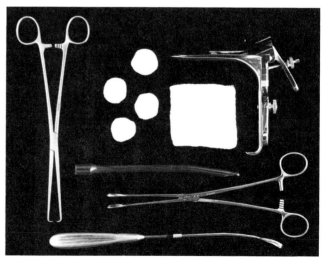

Figure 76–5. Suction curettage equipment.

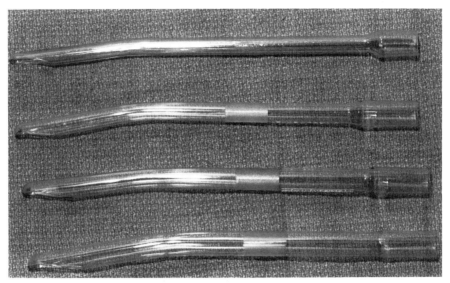

Figure 76–6. Plastic suction curettes, 8 to 11 mm.

chapter) and intravenously administered short-acting narcotics. Fentanyl (0.1 to 0.2 mg given intravenously) is an excellent short-acting narcotic; its effect is essentially gone in 45 minutes, and it can easily and quickly be reversed by naloxone if the need arises. A patient-administered nitrous oxide–oxygen mixture is also an excellent adjunct, and it gives the patient some measure of control over her experience.[1]

Technique. After allowing a paracervical block to take effect, the largest suction cannula that will pass easily through the partially dilated cervix is introduced. The tenaculum is used for traction to straighten the uterine axis if the fundus is anteflexed or retroflexed and to provide countertraction while inserting the suction cannula. The curette is inserted so that the curve of the instrument follows the axis of flexion of the uterine fundus. A gently rotating motion helps the curette pass through the internal os. Note that most perforations occur at the internal os, where the uterus is flexed on the cervical canal. The curette should *not* be forced through the os but rather rotated gently through the os with controlled pressure. The distal wall of the uterus is sounded with the curette, and the vacuum line is attached to the curette. The vacuum pump is turned to 50 to 75 mm Hg vacuum pressure, and the plastic curette is rotated 180 degrees in each direction in the uterine cavity. The suction is released by means of a slip ring on the vacuum line connector, and the curette is withdrawn. The vacuum line is removed, and the curette is reinserted gently while countertraction is applied with the tenaculum. The procedure is repeated two to three times until no more tissue is obtained. Care should be taken not to apply suction in the cervical canal because it is often painful.

Gentle manual curettage with a metal uterine curette is recommended at this point. The curette is used as an extension of the finger tips to feel for any retained tissue. It slides smoothly over retained tissue and scrapes in a grating sensation over normal uterine wall. Retained tissue can be resuctioned with a plastic curette or gently curetted with the sharp curette. Vigorous scraping with a metal curette should be avoided because it may damage the germinal layer of the uterine endometrium.

After all the instruments have been removed from the vaginal vault, the uterus is massaged firmly with bimanual pressure to stimulate uterine contraction. All pathology specimens are sent to the laboratory in an appropriate container with fixative (10 per cent formalin). The patient is observed for 2 hours while the oxytocin infusion is completed. Criteria for home discharge include the absence of significant cramping, bleeding limited to minimal spotting only, and stable postural vital signs. A repeat pelvic examination before discharge is not required in most cases.[1]

Prevention of Rh Sensitization. Many pregnant patients who have received prenatal care or who have been pregnant before already know their Rh type. If a good history of an Rh-positive blood type from a reliable patient is available,

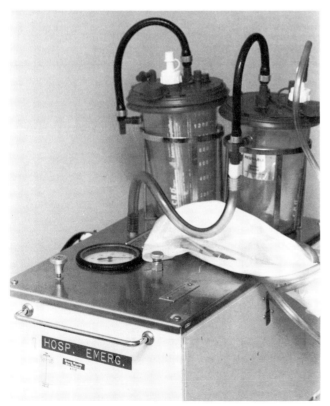

Figure 76–7. Vacuum pump and collecting apparatus.

recording of this information in the emergency department record is sufficient. Rh type can also be confirmed from old hospital charts or the patient's outpatient medical record, when available. Patients whose Rh type cannot be confirmed with reasonable certainty must be assumed to be Rh negative and to be carrying an Rh-positive fetus. Blood for Rh typing and Rh antibody titer must be sent to the laboratory. (One exception is when the biologic father is known with certainly to be Rh negative.) If the patient is confirmed to be Rh negative and if she may have been sensitized to the Rh antigen from a previous pregnancy or transfusion, an Rh antibody titer is needed (Fig. 76–8). If she is found to be Rh negative and has no antibodies, the patient must be contacted to return to the emergency department or her doctor's office for Rh immune globulin within 72 hours. Unsensitized Rh-negative patients who aborted 12 weeks or earlier may be given Rh immune globulin microdose (MicRhoGAM) within 72 hours of the miscarriage. In pregnancies of 13 weeks' duration or more, the inoculum of Rh-positive fetal cells may be too great for the microdose. Rh immune globulin (RhoGAM), which must be cross-matched with the patient's blood, is necessary in this situation.

Emotional Support and Reproductive Counseling. A vital and often neglected aspect of the care of a woman having a spontaneous abortion is the anxiety inherent in the experience of having a miscarriage and the emotional impact of unexpectedly losing a desired pregnancy. The patient's anxiety may be significant and may have several components, all of which can be addressed in the emergency department to the benefit of the patient. The patient is often frightened by the pain and bleeding and may imagine that her condition is life threatening or that the suction curettage procedure will be extremely painful. By directly addressing these concerns and reassuring the patient when appropriate, the physician can do much to allay anxiety. The physician should describe suction curettage to the patient, explaining that the procedure itself takes only 5 to 10 minutes and that she will be given medication (usually in the form of a paracervical block as well as an intravenous narcotic) to minimize any discomfort. She should also be prepared for the noise of the vacuum and the site of blood in the tubing or vacuum receptacle.

The patient often feels guilt for having done something that may have caused the miscarriage. The patient should be told that a miscarriage (the word *abortion* should be avoided because it connotes an induced pregnancy termination to most patients) is a natural process and is the body's way of getting rid of a pregnancy that was not developing properly. One out of every 4 to 5 women have a miscarriage at some time during their reproductive life. The patient should be reassured that she did nothing to cause the miscarriage. Miscarriages are rarely related to minor falls, general activity, or diet.

The patient often feels grief over the sudden loss of a fetus. This response is often present even in patients who have been planning to have a therapeutic abortion. This grief response can be especially acute in the patient who had conceived after trying to become pregnant for some time and who especially desired the pregnancy. The patient should be told that a period of mourning is normal and to be expected. It may take her several weeks before the acute sense of loss begins to dissipate. The spouse or significant other should be included in these discussions when possible, and the patient should be encouraged to seek the support of family and friends during this time. It is appropriate to take time off from work during this process, if the patient desires. Such counseling by the physician, which gives the patient permission to mourn her loss acutely, can help prevent delayed or pathologic grief reactions that can include (1) somatic distress, (2) preoccupation with thoughts of the unborn child, (3) guilt feelings, (4) feelings of anger and hostility, and (5) change in normal behavior. The patient with a history of infertility can be reassured that this pregnancy is proof of her ability to become pregnant and that, in spite of the sense of loss she feels, this pregnancy can be interpreted as a good sign that she has the potential to become pregnant again.

In addition, the patient may be concerned about the reproductive consequences of this miscarriage and curettage. Women are also concerned about what the fetus looks like and what abnormalities it has. Often the fetus has been passed already or has degenerated in utero. Little can be told by looking at an aborted fetus grossly. Show the patient the fetus if you find it *and* if she requests to see it, explaining that it will be sent to the pathology laboratory for examination and that a report will be sent to her physician. The patient should be counseled regarding future pregnancies with the following information:[24]

1. If there is *no* history of spontaneous abortion before the current one, the risk of miscarriage with the next pregnancy is unchanged (15 to 20 per cent).

2. If the patient has had at least one previous miscarriage as well as previous live births, the risk rises to 30 per cent.

3. If the patient has had at least one previous miscarriage but no live births, the risk is 45 per cent.

Other questions the patient may have include the following:

When may I try to get pregnant again? Wait three normal menstrual cycles to allow the uterine lining to build up again and be receptive for another pregnancy.

When may I have intercourse? Wait 1 week or until all bleeding has stopped to allow the cervix to close, thus minimizing any risk of inducing infection.

When should I start taking birth control pills? If the patient wishes to start birth control pills, she should wait 5 days, then begin with one pill per day, whether or not she is still bleeding.

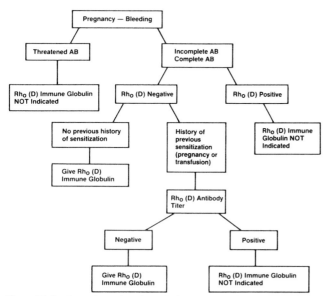

Figure 76–8. Flow chart for the administration of Rh$_0$ (D) immune globulin. (Adapted with permission from Annals of Emergency Medicine 1:41, 1975. Copyright © January/February 1975, American College of Emergency Physicians.)

Table 76–1. Patient Discharge Instructions after a Miscarriage

1. In general, you should restrict your physical activity for 24 hours after you leave the emergency department.
2. Take your temperature three times a day for 5 days after the miscarriage.
3. If your temperature is higher than 100°, call your doctor's office. If no communication can be made to his/her office, call the emergency department.
4. You may have some *bleeding* following the miscarriage. It should be no heavier than a normal period and may last as long as 2 weeks. If at any point you bleed more heavily than the heaviest day of a normal period, call your doctor's office.
5. You may have some slight cramping for the first day or two following the miscarriage. Any severe *pain or cramping* that persists after the first day or two should be brought to your doctor's attention.
6. To help prevent *infection*, you should not have intercourse or douch until the bleeding has completely stopped or until 1 week has passed. Use pads, not tampons, for the first 3 days after your miscarriage.
7. You should have a check-up in your doctor's office in about 1 month.
8. If you plan to use birth control pills for contraception after your miscarriage, you may begin the pills 5 days afterward, whether or not you are still bleeding. Take 1 pill daily.
9. Take iron pills if prescribed.
10. Take Methergine as directed
11. Return for Rh immune globulin if indicated.

Danger Signs: Pain, heavy bleeding, and fever.

If you have any questions or problems call your doctor's office

(From Farrell RG: OB/GYN Emergencies: The First 60 Minutes. Rockville, Md, Aspen Publishers, Inc, 1986. With permission from Aspen Publishers, Inc, © 1986.)

Discharge Medications and Instructions

To provide continued stimulus for uterine contraction, patients are given an ergotrate such as methylergonovine maleate (Methergine), 0.2 mg to be taken orally four times a day for 2 days. If bleeding and cramping have continued, a repeat examination and possible repeat suctioning of the uterus may be needed to remove retained products of conception. Abnormal postural vital signs indicate a need for additional isotonic saline infusion or blood transfusion. A hematocrit may be necessary after intravenous fluid replacement to assess the need for transfusion. If bleeding has stopped, postural vital signs are stable, and the hematocrit is 26 per cent or more, transfusion can usually be avoided. All patients with blood loss of more than 500 ml or a drop in hematocrit level of 4 per cent or more should be given iron supplementation (ferrous sulfate, 250 mg twice a day) on discharge for 1 month. Discharge instructions should cover recommended physical and sexual activity; danger signs of fever, bleeding, and cramping; and use of birth control, if desired by the patient (Table 76–1).

Complications

Complications of suction curettage include retained products of conception with continued bleeding, endometritis, or both. These complications occur in less than 5 per cent of cases. Serious complications, such as uterine perforation, are rare.[19]

Conclusion

Definitive treatment of incomplete and inevitable abortion by suction curettage in the emergency department or outpatient setting is a simple, straightforward procedure with minimal complications. Immediate availability of this procedure in the emergency department provides significant advantages for the patient in terms of rapid treatment of blood loss, pain, and infection and minimized anxiety and expense. A large published series of cases has demonstrated that this procedure can be safely and effectively performed by emergency physicians in the emergency department setting.[21]

References

1. Farrell RG: OB/Gyn Emergencies: The First 60 Minutes. Rockville, Md, Aspen Publishers, Inc, 1986.
2. Suarez RA, Grimes DA, Majmirdar B, et al: Endometrial aspiration with Karman cannula. Reprod Med 28:41, 1983.
3. Grimes DA: Diagnostic dilatation and curettage: A reappraisal. Am J Obstet Gynecol 142:1, 1982.
4. Zimmerman R: Dysfunctional uterine bleeding. Obstet Gynecol Clin North Am 15:107, 1988.
5. Loffer FD: Hysteroscopy with selective endometrial samples compared with D&C for abnormal uterine bleeding: The value of negative hysteroscopic view. Obstet Gynecol 73:16, 1989.
6. Gimpelson RJ, Rappold HO: A comparative study between panoramic hysteroscopy with directed biopsies and dilatation and curettage. Am J Obstet Gynecol 158:489, 1988.
7. Mencaglia L, Perino A, Hammon J: Hysteroscopy in perimenopausal and postmenopausal women with abnormal uterine bleeding. J Reprod Med 32:577, 1987.
8. Smith CB: Dysfunctional uterine bleeding. Am Fam Physician 36:161, 1987.
9. Worley RJ: Dysfunctional uterine bleeding, clarifying its definition, mechanisms, and management. Postgrad Med 79:101, 1986.
10. Fortier KJ: Postmenopausal bleeding and the endometrium. Clin Obstet Gynecol 29:440, 1986.
11. Quilligan E, Zuspan F: Operative Obstetrics. 4th ed. New York, Appleton-Century-Crofts, 1982, pp 140–143.
12. Fehrman H: Surgical management of life-threatening obstetric and gynecologic hemorrhage. Acta Obstet Gynecol Scand 67:125, 1988.
13. Mud HJ, Schattenkerk ME, Johannes ED, et al: Nonsurgical treatment of pelvic hemorrhage in obstetric and gynecologic patients. Crit Care Med 15:534, 1987.
14. Goldrath MH: Uterine tamponade for the control of acute uterine bleeding. Am J Obstet Gynecol 147:869, 1983.
15. Hurley VA, Birscher NA: Cervical pregnancy: Hysterectomy avoided with the use of a large Foley catheter balloon. Aust N Z J Obstet Gynecol Aug; 28:230, 1988.
16. Bowen LW, Beson JH: Use of a Foley catheter balloon to control postpartum hemorrhage resulting from a low placental implantation. A report of two cases. J Reprod Med 30:623, 1985.
17. Deutchman M: The problematic first-trimester pregnancy. Am Fam Physician 39:185, 1989.
18. Stabile I, Campbell S, Grudzinskas JG: Ultrasonic assessment of complications during first trimester pregnancy. Lancet 2:1237, 1987.
19. Hill DL: Management of incomplete abortion with vacuum curettage. Minn Med 54:225, 1971.
20. Filshie GM, Sanders RR, O'Brien PM, et al: Evacuation of retained products of conception in a treatment room with and without general anesthesia. Br J Obstet Gynecol 84:514, 1977.
21. Farrell RG, Stonington DT, Ridgeway RA: Incomplete and inevitable abortion: Treatment by suction curettage in the emergency department. Ann Emerg Med 11:652, 1982.
22. Brennan DB, Caldwell M: Dilatation and evacuation performed in the emergency department for miscarriage. J Emerg Nursing 13:144, 1987.
23. Funderburk SJ, Guthrie D, Medlum D: Outcome of pregnancies complicated by early vaginal bleeding. Br J Obstet Gynecol 87:100, 1980.
24. Polland FJ, Miller JR, Jones DC, et al: Reproductive counseling in patients who have had a spontaneous abortion. Am J Obstet Gynecol 127:685 1977.

Chapter 77

Culdocentesis

G. Richard Braen

INTRODUCTION

There are a number of conditions in which the clinician must sample the intraperitoneal fluid for confirming a diagnosis or for microbial culturing. This fluid can be obtained from the peritoneal cavity in a number of ways. Culdocentesis involves the introduction of a hollow needle through the vaginal wall into the peritoneal space. Culdocentesis is a simple, rapid, and safe procedure. The technique has several indications, but it is used primarily for diagnosing ruptured ectopic pregnancies and ruptured ovarian cysts and for obtaining fluid to aid in the culture diagnosis of pelvic inflammatory disease (PID).

ANATOMY

Before a culdocentesis is attempted, the clinician must be familiar with the anatomy of the rectouterine pouch (pouch of Douglas) and the vagina. In the adult female, the vagina is approximately 9 cm long. From its inferior to its superior aspect, the posterior wall of the vagina is related to the anal canal by way of the perineal body, the rectum, and the peritoneum of the rectouterine pouch.[1] The rectouterine pouch and the posterior wall of the vagina are adjacent only at the upper quarter (approximately 2 cm) of the posterior vaginal wall. The vaginal wall in this area is less than 5 mm thick. The uterus lies nearly at a right angle to the vagina.

The blood supply of the upper vagina comes from the uterine and vaginal arteries, which are branches of the internal iliac artery. The area is drained by a vaginal venous plexus that communicates with the uterine and vesical plexuses. The vagina has its greatest sensation near the introitus and little sensation in the area adjacent to the rectouterine pouch.

The rectouterine pouch is formed by reflections of the peritoneum, and it is the most dependent intraperitoneal space in both the upright and the supine positions. Blood, pus, and other free fluids in the peritoneal cavity pool in the pouch because of its dependent location. This pouch separates the upper portion of the rectum from the uterus and the upper part of the vagina. The pouch often contains small intestine and normally a small amount of peritoneal fluid.

INDICATIONS

Culdocentesis is indicated in any adult female when fluid aspirated from the rectouterine pouch will help confirm a clinical diagnosis. If ultrasound examination is not readily available, culdocentesis may be the most accurate way for the emergency physician to confirm the diagnosis of ectopic pregnancy. Analysis of peritoneal fluid is a reliable method of differentiating inflammatory from hemorrhagic pelvic pathologic conditions. Conditions in which a culdocentesis may be of diagnostic value include a ruptured viscus (particularly an ectopic pregnancy or a corpus luteum cyst), PID,

and other intra-abdominal infections (particularly appendicitis with rupture or diverticulitis with perforation), intra-abdominal injuries to the liver or the spleen, and ruptured aortic aneurysms.[3]

Ectopic Pregnancy. Ectopic pregnancy is often one of the most difficult gynecologic lesions to diagnose.[4] In a series of 300 consecutive cases of ectopic pregnancy, 50 per cent of patients received medical consultation at least two times before the correct diagnosis was made.[5] In 11 per cent of the patients in this series, the diagnosis was not made until the third medical visit. Because of the severe consequences of a ruptured ectopic pregnancy, an early, accurate diagnosis is essential. Ectopic pregnancy is the leading cause of maternal death in the first trimester of pregnancy.[6]

The clinical picture of ectopic pregnancy may include vascular collapse, pelvic pain, amenorrhea or abnormal menses, shoulder pain, syncope, cervical or adnexal tenderness, and adnexal mass, and anemia and leukocytosis. There is often a history of salpingitis, use of an intrauterine contraceptive device, or tubal ligation. No combination of these signs, symptoms, or historical data is diagnostic for an ectopic pregnancy. To confuse the diagnosis further, a normal menstrual history and a negative urine pregnancy test are found in approximately 50 per cent of patients with ectopic pregnancy.[7] The greater sensitivity of the serum human chorionic gonadotropin β subunit (β-hCG) radioreceptor assay and urine hemagglutination inhibition tests, coupled with the development of pelvic ultrasound and laparoscopy, has increased the chances for early diagnosis of *unruptured* ectopic pregnancy.[8] A sensitive and specific β-hCG test must be used. The newer urinary β-hCG tube tests provide this sensitivity.[9] One study of patients suspected of having an ectopic pregnancy had a pregnancy test rate using the urinary slide test of 80 per cent with the β-hCG latex tube test and 86 per cent with the serum hCG radioimmunoassay (RIA) test.[10] β-hCG has a serum half-life of about 2 days when there is no residual trophoblastic tissue and can be detectable in serum using β-hCG RIA for 16 to 90 days after an induced abortion (median:30), 9 to 35 days after spontaneous abortion (median:19), and 1 to 35 days after a laparotomy with the removal of an ectopic pregnancy via salpingectomy.[9]

In patients with β-hCG titres under 6000 mIU/ml (about 900 ng/mL), the presence of a noncystic mass on adnexal ultrasonography has a predictive value for ectopic pregnancy of 83 per cent, and the presence of a cystic mass has a positive predictive value of 35 per cent. The combination of a noncystic mass and fluid in the cul-de-sac (found in 22 per cent of all patients with ectopic gestations) is the best predictor of an ectopic pregnancy with a 94 per cent positive predictive value.[11] If sonographic evaluation is planned, culdocentesis ideally should be delayed to avoid iatrogenic introduction of blood into the cul-de-sac.

Culdocentesis continues to play an important role in the diagnosis of ectopic pregnancy, with an accuracy rate of 85 to 95 per cent.[5, 12, 13] Although a culdocentesis is most often positive in the presence of a frankly ruptured ectopic pregnancy, it may be diagnostic even in the nonruptured case when bleeding has been slow or intermittent. It is useful to note that many ectopic pregnancies will leak varying amounts of blood for days or weeks before rupture. Importantly, hemoperitoneum has been noted to occur in 45 to 60 per cent of cases of *unruptured* ectopic pregnancy proven at surgery.[14-16]

Pelvic Infection. Acute PID has a polymicrobial etiology.[17-19] It has been common practice to define the etiology of PID by isolation of pathogens from the endocervix. The etiology is probably better defined by examination of the tubal flora. In fact, there is little correlation between cul-de-

Table 77–1. Correlation Between the Results of Culdocenteses Performed on 77 Patients with Ectopic Gestation and Various Clinical Parameters

| | Classic Triad | | | Peritoneal Signs | Pulse ≥100 | Blood Pressure <90/40 | Mean Hematocrit | Hemoperi- toneum ≥100 ml | Ruptured Tube | Total |
	Bleeding	Pain	Adnexal Mass							
Postive	37	54	10	26	19	9	35	52	30	54
Negative	8	8	3	1	1	0	39	0	0	8
Inadequate	13	15	6	5	4	1	38	13	7	15
Total patients	58	77	19	32	24	10		65	37	77

Note: There is a *lack of correlation* between a positive culdocentesis and peritoneal signs and changes in vital signs.
(From Cartwright PS, Vaughn B, Tuttle D: Culdocentesis and ectopic pregnancy. J Reprod Med 29:88, 1984. Reproduced by permission.)

sac cultures and cervical cultures in PID.[20] Some medical centers routinely use aspirates obtained through culdocentesis to aid in determining the microbial agents causing the PID.[21] As the microbiology of PID becomes more complex and as the causative organisms develop resistance to antimicrobial agents, culdocentesis may evolve as one of the prime methods of obtaining meaningful microbiological cultures that will dictate appropriate therapy.

Blunt Abdominal Trauma. Although diagnostic peritoneal lavage remains a popular and valuable technique, the use of culdocentesis to detect hemoperitoneum has been advocated.[3, 22] Because small amounts of blood tend to collect in the rectouterine pouch, the aspiration of clear peritoneal fluid is of great potential value in *excluding* hemoperitoneum. The procedure may be more advantageous than peritoneal lavage in some instances, because there is less risk of urinary bladder perforation or bowel injury. In addition, previous abdominal surgery is not a contraindication to culdocentesis, as it is with peritoneal lavage.[23]

CONTRAINDICATIONS

The contraindications to culdocentesis are relatively few and include a pelvic mass detected on bimanual pelvic examination, a nonmobile retroverted uterus, and coagulopathies. Pelvic masses may include tubo-ovarian abscesses, appendiceal abscesses, ovarian masses, and pelvic kidneys. It has been suggested that "the only major risk with the procedure is that of rupturing an unsuspected tubo-ovarian abscess into the peritoneal cavity. This can be avoided by careful bimanual pelvic examination to exclude patients with large masses not affixed to the cul-de-sac.[20] Although there are no data to guide the age at which culdocentesis may be safely performed, the procedure is generally limited to patients who are beyond puberty. This limitation is suggested on the basis of anatomy and with the consideration that the procedure is difficult to perform through a small, prepubertal vagina.

One should not rule out a culdocentesis in the absence of classic signs of ectopic pregnancy. It is important to note that a positive culdocentesis does not consistently correlate with peritoneal irritation, blood pressure, pulse rate, or the actual volume of hemoperitoeum.[14] In fact, bradycardia in the presence of significant intraperitoneal bleeding from a ruptured ectopic pregnancy is not unusual (Tables 77–1 and 77–2).

EQUIPMENT

The equipment required for culdocentesis is listed in Table 77–3. Either an 18-gauge spinal needle or a 19-gauge butterfly needle held by ring forceps is acceptable. It is also acceptable to anesthetize the posterior vaginal wall at the site of the puncture using 1 to 2 per cent lidocaine with epinephrine through a 25-gauge needle. Some physicians use a cocaine-soaked cotton ball to anesthetize the mucosa before infiltration with a local anesthetic. Although local anesthesia is often unnecessary (because the puncture of the posterior vaginal wall at the upper one fourth of the vagina is relatively painless), there may be some advantage to its use, because multiple attempts at culdocentesis are occasionally required. In addition, the epinephrine may produce vasoconstriction and may reduce bleeding associated with the needle puncture. Although culdocentesis is not usually very painful, it may be stressful to the patient, and all attempts should be made to render the procedure as painless as possible. Consideration of parenteral analgesia and sedation (see Chapter 41) should also be made when the patient is uncomfortable or anxious.

TECHNIQUE

A culdocentesis is an invasive procedure that, in some hospitals, requires a written, witnessed, and signed consent form from the patient, parent, or guardian when the pa-

Table 77–2. Correlation Between Tubal Status and Hypotension, Tachycardia, Hematocrit, Signs of Peritoneal Irritation, and Hemoperitoneum in 77 Patients with Ectopic Gestation

	Culdocentesis- Positive	Peritoneal Signs	Blood Pressure <90/40	Pulse ≥100	Hemoperi- toneum ≥100 ml	Average Hematocrit
Ruptured (n = 37)	30	25	8	19	37	33.6
Intact (n = 40)	24	7	2	5	28	37.3
Total patients	54	32	10	24	65	

Note: The culdocentesis is frequently positive in the absence of rupture.
(From Cartwright PS, Vaughn B, Tuttle D: Culdocentesis and ectopic pregnancy. J Reprod Med 29:88, 1984. Reproduced by permission.)

Table 77–3. Equipment for Culdocentesis
Adjustable examination table with stirrups
Bivalve vaginal speculum
Uterine cervical tenaculum
19-gauge butterfly needle or 18-gauge spinal needle
25-gauge needle (for local anesthetic infiltration)
Ring sponge forceps
Syringes (20 ml)
Surgical preparation (iodinated, such as Betadine)
Sterile water, cotton balls, 4 × 4 gauze sponges
Cocaine (10% solution) or lidocaine (1%) with epinephrine
Culture media or test tube without anticoagulant

tient's condition permits. If verbal consent is obtained, this action should be witnessed and a notation in the medical record made documenting that the procedure was described, complications discussed, and any alternatives (e.g., sonography or immediate laparoscopy) offered.

Once written or verbal consent is obtained, the patient is placed in a lithotomy position with the head of the table slightly elevated (reverse Trendelenburg position) so that intraperitoneal fluid gravitates into the rectouterine pouch. The patient's feet are placed in stirrups. In selected patients, some physicians premedicate with intravenous narcotics or sedatives. The administration of nitrous oxide analgesia is also an accepted practice. Although pain may not be an overriding aspect of culdocentesis, *the judicious use of analgesia and sedation will make the procedure easier for both physician and patient.*

Radiographs when indicated in the *stable* patient are taken *prior* to culdocentesis to avoid possible confusion if a pneumoperitoneum is detected following the procedure.

A bimanual pelvic examination must be performed before culdocentesis to rule out a fixed pelvic mass and to assess the position of the uterus. The examiner then inserts the bivalve vaginal speculum and opens it widely by adjusting both the height and the angle thumbscrews. The *posterior* lip of the cervix is grasped with the toothed uterine cervical tenaculum, and the cervix is elevated (Fig. 77–1). This maneuver elevates a retroverted uterus from the pouch, exposes the puncture site, and stabilizes the posterior wall during the needle puncture. Some physicians prefer to use longitudinal traction on the cervix to produce the same result. Pain is often felt by the patient when the cervix is grasped with the tenaculum, and the patient should be forewarned of a possible sharp pain during this part of the examination. The vaginal wall adjacent to the rectouterine pouch will be tightened somewhat between the inferior blade of the bivalve speculum and the elevated posterior lip of the cervix. This tightening of the vaginal wall exposes the puncture site and keeps it from moving away from the needle when the wall is punctured.

After the tenaculum is applied and the posterior lip of the cervix is elevated or traction is applied, the vaginal wall in the area of the rectouterine pouch should be swabbed with surgical preparation followed by a small amount of sterile water. Local anesthesia may be administered at this point. Anesthesia may be injected with a separate 25-gauge needle or by the spinal needle to be used for the culdocentesis. A cotton ball soaked in cocaine solution can also be used for topical anesthesia of the posterior vaginal wall before infiltration with a local anesthetic. The needles used for both the local anesthetic and the puncture should be attached to a 20-ml syringe. A smaller syringe may not be long enough to allow adequate control of the needle, and the physician's hand may block the view of the puncture site if a smaller syringe is used.

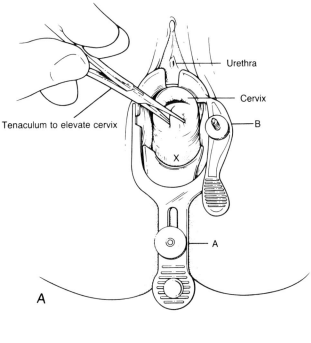

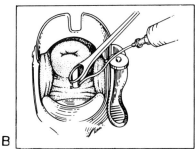

Figure 77–1. *A,* Preparation for culdocentesis. Note that one opens the speculum widely by using both the height *(A)* and the angle adjustments *(B).* The cervix is grasped on the posterior lip with a toothed tenaculum. *X* marks the site for puncture of the vaginal wall. (From Vander Salm TJ, Cutler BS, Wheeler HB: Atlas of Bedside Procedures. Boston, Little, Brown & Co., 1979.) *B,* The use of a butterfly needle for culdocentesis. The needle is inserted 1 cm posterior to the point at which the vaginal wall joins the cervix. (From Webb MJ: Culdocentesis. JACEP 7:452, 1978.)

Following local anesthesia, the syringe and the spinal needle to be used for the culdocentesis are advanced parallel to the lower blade of the speculum. It is helpful to fill the syringe with 2 to 3 ml of saline (nonbacteriostatic) before puncture. Following needle puncture, the free flow of the fluid from the syringe expels tissue that may have clogged the needle and confirms that the needle tip is in the proper position and is not lodged in the uterine wall or the intestinal wall. Saline (rather than air) is preferred, because if air is used, one must be careful in interpreting the presence of free peritoneal air on subsequent radiographs. To avoid the need to change the syringe during the procedure, lidocaine (Xylocaine) may be used for both anesthesia and confirmation of proper needle placement, but the bacteriostatic property of this agent precludes its use if the procedure is performed to obtain fluid for culture.

The vaginal wall should be penetrated in the midline 1 to 1.5 cm posteriorly (inferiorly) to the point at which the vaginal wall joins the cervix (Fig. 77–2).[24] The needle should penetrate a total of 2 to 2.5 cm.[24, 25] Suction is then applied with the syringe while the needle is slowly withdrawn. It is

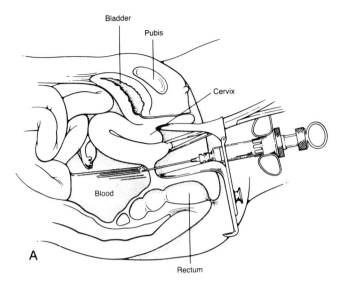

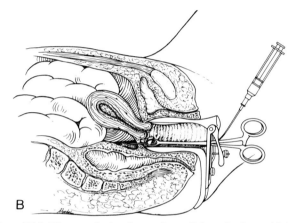

Figure 77–2. The needle is advanced parallel to the lower blade of the speculum. Aspiration is continued throughout the gradual withdrawal of the needle. *A,* The use of a spinal needle. (From Vander Salm TJ, Cutler BS, Wheeler HB: Atlas of Bedside Procedures. Boston, Little, Brown & Co, 1979.) *B,* The use of a butterfly needle and ringed forceps. (From Webb MJ: Culdocentesis. JACEP 7:452, 1978. Reproduced by permission.)

important for the physician to avoid aspirating any blood that has accumulated in the vagina from previous needle punctures or from cervical bleeding, because this may give the false impression of a positive tap. Bleeding from the puncture site in the vaginal wall is minimized if epinephrine is added to the local anesthetic.

Blood or fluid may be obtained immediately but may also be obtained just before the needle is withdrawn from the peritoneal cavity. Therefore, it is important to aspirate throughout the gradual withdrawal procedure. Because small clots may clog an 18-gauge needle, some physicians prefer using a larger gauge needle (e.g., 15 or 16 gauge), which permits easier aspiration of small clots.[4] These needles are rarely required, however. If no fluid is aspirated, the needle should be reintroduced and directed only slightly to the left or right of the midline. Directing the needle too far laterally may result in puncture of mesenteric or pelvic vessels. It is important to note that if no fluid is obtained on the first attempt, the procedure should be repeated.

Some physicians prefer the use of a 19-gauge butterfly needle held with a ring forceps (Fig. 77–3).[2] This technique offers a built-in guide to needle depth and allows for good control of the needle during puncture. An assistant must aspirate the tubing while the physician controls positioning and withdrawal of the needle.

Fluid that is aspirated may be old, nonclotting blood, bright red blood, pus, exudate, or a straw-colored and serous liquid. Any fluid that is not blood should be submitted for Gram staining, aerobic and anaerobic culture, and cell counts. Blood should be observed for clotting. Blood should also be sent for a hematocrit determination.

INTERPRETATION OF RESULTS

An interpretation of the results of a culdocentesis depends primarily on whether any fluid was obtained. In the absence of a pathologic condition, one will often aspirate a few milliliters of clear, yellowish peritoneal fluid. When there is no return of fluid of any type (a so-called dry tap), the procedure has *no diagnostic value.* Because a dry tap is nondiagnostic, it should not be equated with normal peritoneal fluid. In addition, when less than 2 ml of clotting blood is obtained, this is also considered to be a nondiagnos-

Figure 77–3. Culdocentesis may be performed with a 19-gauge butterfly needle held with ring forceps. (From Webb MJ: Culdocentesis. JACEP 7:451, 1978. Reproduced by permission.)

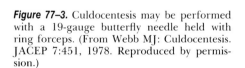

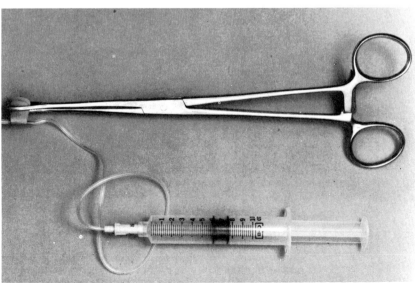

tic tap, because the source of this small amount of blood may be the puncture site on the vaginal wall. Such blood will usually clot. Over 2 ml of *nonclotting blood* is certainly suggestive of a hemoperitoneum. However, some researchers interpret as little as 0.3 ml of *nonclotting* blood as a positive tap.[14] There is no particular significance to larger amounts of blood, because absolute volume may be related to the needle position or the rate of bleeding. Brenner and coworkers reported no blood from culdocentesis in 5 per cent of patients with proven ectopic pregnancies, even when rupture had occurred.[5] In the series of 77 patients with surgically proven ectopic pregnancy reported by Cartwright and associates, a culdocentesis performed within 4 hours of surgery was positive in 70 per cent, negative in 10 per cent, and inadequate in 20 per cent.[14] "Positive" in their series was defined as obtaining at least 0.3 ml of nonclotting blood with a hematocrit of more than 3 per cent. "Negative" was defined as obtaining at least 0.3 ml of fluid with a hematocrit of less than 3 per cent, and an "inadequate" tap was one in which no fluid was obtained. In the 252 surgically proven ectopic pregnancy patients having a culdocentesis reported by Vermesh and colleagues, 83 per cent had a positive tap.[16] They defined a positive tap as nonclotting blood with a hematocrit greater than 15 per cent.

Because culdocentesis is usually used to diagnose an ectopic pregnancy, a "negative tap" is one that yields pus or clear, straw-colored peritoneal or cystic fluid. A large amount of clear fluid (greater than 10 ml) indicates a probable ruptured ovarian cyst, aspiration of an intact corpus luteal cyst, ascites, or possibly carcinoma. The significance of these fluids is outlined in Table 77–4. Elliot and colleagues[26] caution that obtaining greater than 10 ml of clear fluid should not automatically rule out an ectopic pregnancy since the latter may co-exist with other pathology.

A "positive tap" is one in which nonclotting blood is obtained. Blood remains unclotted for days in the syringe as a result of the defibrination activity of the peritoneum.

This finding is indicative of hemoperitoneum caused by conditions such as a ruptured ectopic pregnancy, a hemorrhagic ovarian cyst, or a ruptured spleen. The return of a serosanguineous fluid also suggests a ruptured ovarian cyst. The hematocrit of blood from active intraperitoneal bleeding is greater than 10 per cent. In one series, the hematocrit of blood from a ruptured ectopic pregnancy was at least 15 per cent in 97 per cent of cases.[5]

It should be emphasized that a positve culdocentesis in the presence of a positive pregnancy test does not always prove an ectopic pregnancy.[16] A ruptured corpus luteum cyst in the presence of an intrauterine pregnancy test is probably the most common cause of a "false-positive" scenario. When possible, ultrasound may help corroborate the culdocentesis findings. One study estimated a false-positive rate of 9 per cent.

COMPLICATIONS

Culdocentesis is one of the safest procedures performed in the emergency setting, and there are probably fewer complications with this technique than with peripheral venous cannulation. Complications have been reported, however, and include the rupture of an unsuspected tubo-ovarian abscess.[24] This is the most common of the serious complications. Others include perforation of the bowel, perforation of a pelvic kidney, and bleeding from the puncture site in patients with clotting disorders. Because the most common complications result from the puncture of a pelvic mass, careful bimanual examination of the patient should help prevent this problem. Puncture of the bowel and the uterine wall occurs relatively frequently, but this occurrence does not generally result in serious morbidity. Obviously, penetration of the gravid uterus has greater potential for harm. Occasionally, one will aspirate air or fecal matter,

Table 77–4. Interpretation of Culdocentesis Fluid	
Aspirated Fluid	**Condition and Suggested Differential Diagnosis**
Clear, serous, straw-colored (usually only a few milliliters)	Normal peritoneal fluid
Large amount of clear fluid	Ruptured or large ovarian cyst (fluid may be serosanguineous). Pregnancy may be coexistent.
	Ascites
	Carcinoma
Exudate with polymorphonuclear leukocytes	Pelvic inflammatory disease
	Gonococcal salpingitis
	Chronic salpingitis
Purulent fluid	Bacterial infection
	Tubo-ovarian abscess with rupture
	Appendicitis with rupture
	Diverticulitis with perforation
Bright red blood*	Ruptured viscus or vascular injury
	Recently bleeding ectopic pregnancy* (ruptured or unruptured)
	Bleeding corpus luteum
	Intra-abdominal injury
	Liver
	Spleen
	Other organs
	Ruptured aortic aneurysm
Old, brown, nonclotting blood	Ruptured viscus
	Ectopic pregnancy with intraperitoneal bleeding over a few days or weeks
	Old (days) intra-abdominal injury (e.g., delayed splenic rupture)

Note: The hematocrit of blood from a ruptured ectopic pregnancy is usually greater than 15 per cent (97.5 per cent of cases),[5] but some authors use greater than 3 percent as positive.[14]

confirming inadvertent puncture of the rectum. Although this may be disconcerting, it is seldom of serious clinical concern and requires no immediate change in therapy.

CONCLUSION

In the emergency setting, culdocentesis is a very helpful diagnostic procedure. It is used mainly in the evaluation of ectopic pregnancy but should also be considered as a diagnostic aid in the evaluation of PID and in abdominal trauma. This is a safe, simple procedure that every physician who deals with the emergency evaluation of women, *particularly women of the childbearing age*, should know and use. It is the most reliable, and certainly the most rapid, way to perform a definitive evaluation of the unstable patient with suspected ectopic pregnancy.

REFERENCES

1. Ellis H: Clinical Anatomy, A Revision and Applied Anatomy for Clinical Students. 5th ed. Oxford, Blackwell Scientific Publications, 1972, pp 129–131.
2. Webb MJ: Culdocentesis. JACEP 7:451, 1978.
3. Clarke JM: Culdocentesis in the evaluation of blunt abdominal trauma. Surg Gynecol Obstet 129:809, 1969.
4. Capraro VJ, Chuang JT, Randall CL: Cul-de-sac aspiration and other diagnostic aids for ectopic pregnancy. Int Surg 53:4, 1970.
5. Brenner PF, Roys S, Mishell DR: Ectopic pregnancy. A study of 300 consecutive surgically treated cases. JAMA 243:673, 1980.
6. National Center for Health Statistics: Final Mortality Statistics, 1975. Washington, DC, US Government Printing Office, 1977.
7. Kistner RW: The oviduct-tubal ectopic pregnancy. In Kistner RW (ed): Gynecology: Principles and Practice. 2nd ed. Chicago, Year Book Medical Publishers, 1971, pp 304–308.
8. Chung SJ: Review of pregnancy tests. South Med J 74:11, 1981.
9. Batzer FR, Corson SL: Diagnostic techniques used for ectopic pregnancy. J Reprod Med 31:86–93, 1986.
10. Braunstein GD, Asch RH: Predictive value analysis of measurements of human chorionic gonadotropin, pregnancy specific B-1 glycoprotein, placental lactogen, and cystine aminopeptidase for the diagnosis of ectopic pregnancy. Fertil Steril 39:62, 1983.
11. Romero R, Kadar N, Castro D, et al: The value of adnexal sonographic findings in the diagnosis of ectopic pregnancy. Am J Obstet Gynecol 158:52, 1988.
12. Hall RE, Tod WD: The suspected ectopic pregnancy. Am J Obstet Gynecol 81:1220, 1969.
13. Webster HD, Barclay DL, Fischer CK: Ectopic pregnancy: A seventeen-year review. Am J Obstet Gynecol 92:23, 1965.
14. Cartwright PS, Vaughn B, Tuttle D: Culdocentesis and ectopic pregnancy. J Reprod Med 29:88, 1984.
15. Romero R, Copel JA, Kadar N, et al: Value of culdocentesis in the diagnosis of ectopic pregnancy. Obstet Gynecol 65:519, 1985.
16. Vermesh M, Graczykowsk JW, Sauer MV: Reevaluation of the role of culdocentesis in the management of ectopic pregnancy. Am J Obstet Gynecol 162:411, 1990.
17. Thompson SE III, Hager WD: Acute pelvic inflammatory disease. Sex Transm Dis 4:105, 1977.
18. Eschenbach DA: Epidemiology and diagnosis of acute pelvic inflammatory disease. Obstet Gynecol 55:142S, 1980.
19. Monif GRG: Significance of polymicrobial bacterial superinfection in the therapy of gonococcal endometritis-salpingitis-peritonitis. Obstet Gynecol 55:154S, 1980.
20. Chow AW, Malkasian KL, Marchall JR, et al: The bacteriology of acute pelvic inflammatory disease, value of cul-de-sac cultures and relative importance of gonococci and other aerobic or anaerobic bacteria. Am J Obstet Gynecol 122:876, 1975.
21. Eschenbach DA, Buchanan TM, Pollock HM, et al: Polymicrobial etiology of acute pelvic inflammatory disease. N Engl J Med 293:166, 1975.
22. Generelly P, Moore TA, LeMay JT: Delayed splenic rupture: Diagnosed by culdocentesis. JACEP 6:369, 1977.
23. Olsen WR: Peritoneal lavage in blunt abdominal trauma. JACEP 2:271, 1973.
24. Webb MJ: Culdocentesis. JACEP 7:12, 1978.
25. Lucas C, Hassim AM: Place of culdocentesis in the diagnosis of ectopic pregnancy. Br Med J 1:200, 1970.
26. Elliot M, Riccio J, Abbott J: Serous culdocentesis in ectopic pregnancy; a report of two cases caused by co-existent corpus luteum cysts. Ann Emerg Med 19:407, 1990.

Chapter **78**

Examination of the Sexual Assault Victim

G. Richard Braen

INTRODUCTION

Rape is reported to be the fastest growing violent crime in the United States,[1] and it has been estimated that one of six women will be the victim of a rape or an attempted rape in her lifetime.[2] The victims of rape can experience extensive trauma (both physical and psychologic), can be exposed to disease, and can become pregnant. The physicians and nurses dealing with an alleged sexual assault victim have a professional, ethical, and moral responsibility to provide the best medical and psychologic care possible while simultaneously collecting and preserving the proper medicolegal evidence that is unique to the evaluation of alleged sexual assault cases.

The emergency department is the most common place to which victims are brought by police. This occurs for several reasons but is mainly a matter of logistics—the peak hours for this crime are from 8:00 P.M. to 2:00 A.M.,[3] and the most common days on which it occurs are weekends. In many localities, the only available physician at these times is the emergency physician, and it is often his or her responsibility to perform the evaluation and treatment. Emergency personnel can help change the psychologic and physical impact of sexual assault. Through proper care of the victim, careful and thorough acquisition of evidence, and cooperation with the law and the legal process, emergency department staff can help the victim toward recovery from the assault and can aid society in improving the prosecution and conviction rates.[4]

MANAGEMENT OF THE ADULT FEMALE SEXUAL ASSAULT VICTIM

An important aspect of performing a sexual assault evaluation is preparation. This includes the establishment of a protocol and the assembly of appropriate forms and equipment. All of this must be accomplished through a cooperative effort with the police, the crime laboratory, the hospital laboratory, crisis volunteers, and the emergency department clerical, social service, nursing, and physician staffs. Careful step-by-step planning concerning the way in which a victim is handled in the emergency department and in follow-up helps both to ensure the best care for the victim and to aid in the prosecution and conviction of assailants.

Major provisions in the emergency department protocol should include patient privacy and the designation of a separate area for the care of the victims. Emergency personnel should know the appropriate steps for evaluation and treatment of the victim, follow-up care, and maintenance of evidence. Examination kits should be available in the emergency department, and the staff should be familiar with them. A list of the contents of the kits should be kept in the department (Table 78–1). The kits save a tremendous

Table 78–1. Basic Sexual Assault Examination Kit

Contents	Purpose
Paper bags	Clothing collection
Two urine containers	Urine for pregnancy test and drug screen
Fingernail file and envelope	Fingernail scrapings
Forceps, scissors, envelope	Pubic hair trimming
Plastic comb, large paper towel, envelope	Pubic hair combing
Vaginal speculum, aspiration pipette, red-topped test tube and stopper	Aspiration of vaginal contents
Two glass slides (one frosted at one end), two cotton-tipped swabs, red-topped test tube and stopper, pencil for marking slide	Swabbing of vagina
10 ml of saline, aspiration pipette and bulb, test tube	Vaginal washing
Cervical scraper, slides, Pap smear fixative	Pap smear
Thayer-Martin plates or Transgrow media, cotton-tipped swabs	Gonorrhea culture
Three cotton-tipped swabs and a test tube or an envelope	Saliva for secretor status
Three red-topped test tubes, tourniquet, nonalcohol swab to prepare skin, syringe and needle	Blood samples
Appropriate laboratory forms, rape examination forms, labels for samples, camera and film (optional)	
5 ml of toluidine blue dye	Vaginal laceration examination

(From Braen GR: Sexual assault. In Rosen P, Baker FJ, Barkin RM, et al (eds): Emergency Medicine, Concepts and Clinical Practice. St. Louis, CV Mosby Co, 1983. Reproduced by permission.)

amount of nursing and physician time when a victim comes to the department. A "check list for sexual assault examinations" (Table 78–2) should be included in the kits. This serves as a reminder of all of the medicolegal procedures to be completed.

Even though this chapter is primarily devoted to the evaluation of the adult *female* sexual assault victim, a guideline to the evaluation of the adult male sexual assault victim, the female child victim, the male child victim, and the accused assailant is provided in Table 78–3. Each of these individuals has special needs, and separate protocols should be developed in the emergency department for them.

Consent

Consent for treatment of a victim of sexual assault is mandatory. The victim has undergone an experience in which her right to grant or deny consent was taken from her,[5] and obtaining consent for medical treatment and for the gathering of evidence has important psychologic and legal implications. The victim has the right to refuse medicolegal examination and even medical treatment. She should, however, be encouraged to have physical evidence collected in the event that she later decides to seek prosecution. Witnessed, written, informed consent therefore should be obtained before evaluation and treatment are begun. If the victim refuses any part of the examination, her wishes should be honored, and the refusal should be noted in the hospital record.

When the court orders an examination but the victim does not want to be examined, the physician must realize that an uncooperative victim (who indeed has the right to refuse examination) can make a thorough examination impossible. Pursuing an examination unwanted by the victim adds additional trauma to the victim's psychologic state, and the examining physician should discuss the situation with the authority that issued the court order and resolve the conflict before proceeding.

History

It should be emphasized that the sexual assault victim is actually a patient whose physical stability takes priority over all else (e.g., if she is in physical danger from hemorrhage, shock, or respiratory insufficiency, treatment of these conditions takes precedence).

The history appropriate to a sexual assault case basically is divided into three categories: history of the event, gynecologic history, and medical history. The history of the event should include only those elements necessary for the physician to complete a thorough physical examination and collection of evidence. Questions beyond this, such as a description of the assailant, should be left to the police investigators. Limiting the history not only shortens the evaluation in the emergency department but also helps prevent discrepancies between the emergency department history and the official police investigation report. Discrepancies could weaken the case if it comes to trial. For the sake of time, the medical history may be obtained by a nurse and expedited by the use of a checklist, which is then reviewed by the physician.

The history of the event should include the time, date, and place of the alleged assault and a description of the use of force or threats of force and the type of assault. Elements of force include the type of violence used, threats of violence, the use of restraints, the number of assailants, the use of alcohol or drugs (forcedly or willingly) by the victim, and any loss of consciousness experienced by the victim. Elements

Table 78–2. Check List for Sexual Assault Examinations

	General
_____	Photographs
	Urine
_____	Pregnancy test
_____	Urine drug screen
	Blood
_____	Serologic test for syphilis
_____	hCG-β subunit
_____	Ethanol or complete drug screen, or both
_____	Red-topped test tube for blood typing
	Pelvic Examination Specimens
_____	Pap smear
_____	Three vaginal swabs
_____	Potassium hydroxide slide
_____	Normal saline slide
_____	Dry mount slide
_____	Thayer-Martin plates (gonococcal culture)
_____	*Chlamydia* screening test
	Buccal Specimens
_____	Three buccal swabs
	Pubic Hair
_____	Combed hair
_____	Cut or plucked hair
	Fingernails
_____	Scrapings from under nails
	Clothes
_____	Panties and any other articles requested by police

of the type of assault include fondling; vaginal, oral, or anal penetration or attempted penetration; ejaculation on or in the body; the use of a condom; and the insertion of foreign bodies into the vagina or the anus. The use of force or violence is partly a police matter, but from a medical standpoint it is desirable to correlate the physical examination with a description of any force, restraint, or violence.

A basic gynecologic history should be obtained in preparation for treatment plans regarding venereal disease and pregnancy. For example, it might be important from a medicolegal standpoint to know of any recent gynecologic surgical procedure that could be misinterpreted as local trauma. The gynecologic history therefore includes the use of birth control before the attack (with information regarding any missed birth control pills), last normal menstrual period, last voluntary intercourse, gravidity and parity, recent gynecologic surgery, and recent venereal disease.

The medical history should include current medications, tetanus immunization status, and allergies. One should note whether the victim douched, bathed, urinated, defecated, used a mouthwash, or brushed her teeth following the rape. Each of these can alter the recovery of seminal specimens and other sexual assault evidence. In addition, any nonperineal or nonoral trauma should be reassessed when the medical history is taken.

Several elements of the history taken together can help the physician decide which samples to obtain. For example, sperm remain motile in the cervix for up to 5 days and remain motile in the vagina for 6 to 12 hours.[6] If the victim had voluntary intercourse 48 hours before examination and was raped 3 hours before examination, the physician should obtain samples from both the vagina and the cervix, keeping the two separate.[7] By taking a careful history, the physician is able to perform an appropriate examination given these two events.

While taking the history, the examiner should observe the patient's ability to understand and respond appropriately to questions. Some victims of sexual assault are not capable of consenting to intercourse because of mental retardation, immaturity, or intoxication with drugs or alcohol. If intoxication is suspected, appropriate testing should be undertaken. If mental retardation is suspected, formal examination of the patient's mental status should be planned for a later date.

Physical Examination

The physical examination of the sexual assault victim is an extension of the history. The purpose of the examination is twofold: to aid in the proper medical evaluation of the patient and to gather samples and observations that might serve as evidence. The findings on physical examination help the physician and the court to answer the following questions: (1) Is or was the victim capable of consenting to intercourse? (2) Was force used? (3) Did vulvar, oral, or anal penetration occur? (4) Is there collectable physical evidence from the assailant in or on the victim's body? A number of standardized examination kits have been developed to assist the physician in gathering evidence in a systematic fashion. Each kit should be reviewed for completeness as it applies to the local legal protocol.

Photographs should be considered, particularly if the victim is still wearing the clothing worn during the attack. Some institutions take their own photographs; others use police photographers. Patient consent should be obtained for photographs taken by hospital personnel, and a chain of evidence should be maintained. Self-developing film that can be permanently labeled (subject, date, details of pictured injury, and so forth) should be used. The photographs should be labeled immediately and may be added to the legal evidence. These photographs may serve as evidence or may simply refresh the examiner's memory at the time of the trial. After the victim has been photographed, she should remove her own clothing, piece by piece, placing each item in a separate *paper* bag. If semen, blood, or other foreign material is present, it will dry in a paper bag, whereas it could become moldy if placed in a plastic bag.

At this time the entirety of the patient's body, excepting the pelvic, anal, and oral areas, should be examined for signs of trauma and foreign bodies. Important areas for evaluation are the back, the thighs, the breasts, the wrists, and the ankles (particularly if restraints were used). Even in the absence of ecchymoses, tender contusions should be reported. Leaves, grass, sand, and so forth can occasionally be found in the hair or on the skin and should be retained as evidence. Areas of trauma should be documented and further evaluated (e.g., with radiographs) as indicated by the type and extent of injury. Up to 30 per cent of rape victims show external evidence of trauma.[3] This evidence may range from abrasions to multiple major blunt and penetrating trauma. In addition, dried semen stains may be visible on the hair or the skin of the victim. These appear as lightly crusted, flaking areas that can be removed by saline-moistened swabs; the swabs are then air-dried and preserved as evidence. Not only the skin but also the fingernails can contain hidden bits of evidence. Rape victims may have bits of the assailant's skin, blood, or facial hair or other foreign material from the rape site beneath their fingernails; fingernail scrapings thus should be routinely obtained.

Following this initial examination, the patient should be placed in a lithotomy position for the pelvic examination. The thighs and the perineum should be inspected for signs of trauma and for foreign materials, such as seminal stains. An ultraviolet light used in a darkened room can aid in the search for external seminal stains. Any such stains should be removed and preserved as previously described. The pubic hair should then be combed for foreign material, particularly pubic hairs from the assailant. These combings can be placed directly into a large paper envelope; the samples are submitted along with the comb. Foreign pubic hairs can help identify race and hair color, but generally there are not enough individual characteristics in hair to enable one to state positively that a hair of unknown source came from a particular person to the exclusion of all others.[8] In the future, crime laboratories may be able to perform enzyme typing of hair roots. Currently, sufficient phosphoglucomutase activity can be found in plucked hair roots to enable typing of individual roots by starch-gel electrophoresis.[9] This capability may some day be extended to hair roots collected by brushing.

The pelvic examination includes careful evaluation of the vulva and the introitus for signs of trauma, foreign material, and degree of maturity or senility. The internal examination should be done with a water-lubricated speculum.[10] The hymen should be inspected and one of the four following conditions noted: (1) that the hymen is present, intact, and free of evidence of trauma; (2) that the hymen is present and intact and shows old scarring; (3) that the hymen is present and recently ruptured; or (4) that the hymen is absent. A recently ruptured hymen is associated with bleeding or fresh clots.

The vaginal wall should be inspected for lacerations. These appear near the introitus in younger, sexually inexperienced females; in older, sexually active females they appear higher, particularly in the right fornix.[11, 12] The cervix should be inspected for signs of pregnancy, menstruation, trauma, and preexisting infection.

Table 78–3. Sexual Assault Examination Protocol for Medical Personnel

	Female Adult Victim	Female Child Victim (Prepubertal)	Male Adult Victim	Male Child Victim	Male Suspect
I. History					
A. History of the event	*	*	*	*	
1. Time, date, place	*	*	*	*	
2. Use of force, threats of force	*	*	*	*	
a. Type of violence	*	*	*	*	
b. Threats of violence	*	*	*	*	
c. Use of restraints	*	*	*	*	
d. Number of assailants	*	*	*	*	
e. Use of alcohol or drugs	*	*	*	*	*
f. Loss of consciousness	*	*	*	*	
3. Type of assault	*	*	*	*	
a. Fondling	*	*	*	*	
b. Vaginal penetration (or attempt)	*	*			
c. Oral penetration (or attempt)	*	*	*	*	
d. Anal penetration (or attempt)	*	*	*	*	
e. Ejaculation—where on or in body	*	*	*	*	
f. Was condom used?	*	*	*	*	
g. Use of lubricant	*	*	*	*	
B. Sexual history					
1. Use of birth control	*	I.A.			
2. Last voluntary intercourse or sexual activity	*	I.A.	I.A.	I.A.	*
3. Gravidity, parity	*				
4. Recent gynecologic surgery	*	I.A.			
5. Recent venereal disease	*	I.A.	*	I.A.	*
C. Medical history					
1. Current medications	*	*	*	*	*
2. Tetanus immunization status	*	*	*	*	*
3. Allergies	*	*	*	*	*
D. History of douching, bathing, urination, defecation, or enema use following the assault	*	*	*	*	
II. Physical Examination					
A. Rapid survey for airway, breathing, circulation	*	*	*	*	*
B. Inspection of clothing for signs of violence or other evidence, such as feces, semen, blood (retain appropriate evidence, consider photographs)	*	*	*	*	*
C. Examination of all areas of skin for signs of violence, foreign material (retain appropriate evidence, consider photographs)	*	*	*	*	*
D. Examination of extremities for fractures, sprains, and so forth	*	*	*	*	*
E. Examination of oral cavity for signs of trauma, infection	*	*	*	*	*
F. Examination of breasts for trauma	*	*	*	*	
G. Genital/rectal examination			*	*	*
1. Male genitalia			*	*	*
a. Examination for signs of trauma to penis, dried semen, infection, and so forth			*	*	*
b. Examination of shaft of penis for lubricant, feces, blood					*
c. Examination for signs of trauma to testicles, scrotum			*	*	*
d. Examination for vasectomy scars					*
2. Female genitalia					
a. Wood's light (filtered ultraviolet) to detect seminal stains on perineum	*	*			
b. Inspection of vulva for signs of trauma or semen	*	*			
c. Inspection of introitus	*	*			
d. Inspection of hymen	*				
i. By speculum examination	*	I.A.			
ii. By separating vulva manually	I.A.	*			
e. Inspection of vaginal vault for trauma and foreign bodies	*	I.A.			
f. Inspection of cervix	*	I.A.			
i. For parity	*				
ii. For signs of pregnancy	*	I.A.			
iii. For menstruation	*				
iv. For trauma	*	I.A.			
v. For signs of infection	*	I.A.			
g. Refer to Section III: H, I, J, K, L of this protocol	*	*			
h. Bimanual pelvic examination	*				
i. Palpation of uterus per rectum	*	*			
3. Anal and perianal area	*	*	*	*	
a. Inspection for signs of trauma	*	*	*	*	
b. Inspection for signs of lubricant, semen, blood, foreign material, pre-established infection	*	*	*	*	
c. Digital rectal examination for trauma, foreign bodies	*	*	*	*	
d. Refer to Section III: L, M, N of this protocol	*	*	*	*	

Table 78–3. Sexual Assault Examination Protocol for Medical Personnel Continued

	Female Adult Victim	Female Child Victim (Prepubertal)	Male Adult Victim	Male Child Victim	Male Suspect
III. Laboratory					
A. Photography (optional)	*	*	*	*	*
1. Signs of trauma (patient clothed)	*	*	*	*	*
2. Signs of restraint (patient clothed)	*	*	*	*	
3. Signs of trauma (patient unclothed)	*	*	*	*	*
4. Signs of restraint (patient unclothed)	*	*	*	*	
B. Clothing collection (for secretions, blood, semen, signs of violence, and so forth)	*	*	*	*	*
C. Removal of dried seminal or blood stains from skin	*	*	*	*	*
D. Fingernail scrapings for foreign material	*	*	*	*	*
E. Combings from pubic hair	*	I.A.	*	I.A.	*
F. Plucked or trimmed pubic hair	*	I.A.	*	I.A.	*
G. Plucked or trimmed head hair	*	*	*	*	*
H. Vaginal pool aspiration	*	I.A.			
1. Sperm motility and morphology	*	I.A.			
2. Acid phosphatase	*	I.A.			
3. Blood group antigens	*	I.A.			
4. Sperm precipitin test	Optional	Optional			
I. Swab of posterior vaginal fornix (same tests as previously described if vaginal aspirate not available)	*	I.A.			
J. Vaginal washing with 10 ml saline solution (same tests as described previously if vaginal aspirate not available)	*	I.A.			
K. Pap smear from cervix and vaginal wall	*	I.A.			
L. Gonorrhea cultures†	*	*	*	*	*
1. Cervix	*	I.A.			
2. Rectum	*	*	*	*	I.A.
3. Oropharynx	*	*	*	*	I.A.
M. Collection of foreign material from perianal area (especially lubricant)	*	*	*	*	I.A.
N. Rectal washing	I.A.	I.A.	I.A.	I.A.	
1. Sperm motility and morphology	I.A.	I.A.	I.A.	I.A.	
2. Acid phosphatase	I.A.	I.A.	I.A.	I.A.	
O. Saliva for secretor status	See Note 1	See Note 1	See Note 1	See Note 1	See Note 1
P. Blood samples	*	*	*	*	*
1. Serologic test for syphilis	*	*	*	*	*
2. Drug and alcohol screen	I.A.	I.A.	I.A.	I.A.	I.A.
3. Blood typing	*	*	*	*	*
4. Pregnancy test (β subunit of hCG)	See Note 2				
Q. Urine samples	I.A.	I.A.	I.A.	I.A.	I.A.
1. Pregnancy test (serum test preferred)	See Note 2				
2. Drug screen	I.A.	I.A.	I.A.	I.A.	I.A.
R. Penile shaft swabs					*
1. For vaginal epithelium					*
2. For fecal stains					*
S. Penile urethral swab			I.A.	I.A.	*
1. Gram stain for gonorrhea			I.A.	I.A.	*
2. Culture for gonorrhea			I.A.	I.A.	*
T. Radiographs for trauma	I.A.	I.A.	I.A.	I.A.	I.A.
IV. Consolidation of Evidence	*	*	*	*	*
V. Initiation of "Chain of Evidence"	*	*	*	*	*

I.A., If appropriate.

*, Indicated.

†*Chlamydia* screening tests may also be used.

Note 1: Collection of saliva for secretor status is appropriate only if samples from the body, clothing, or crime scene potentially containing antigens that could link the victim with the suspect or suspects have been or will be obtained.

Note 2: The β-hCG serum pregnancy test is more sensitive and quantitative but is not readily available in some hospitals.

After the inspection of the introitus, the vagina, and the cervix, the following samples should be obtained:

1. Any vaginal tampon that may have been inserted before or after the assault.

2. Any foreign body (I have found condoms, a bar of soap, and a handkerchief).

3. Vaginal swabs from pooled secretions in the posterior fornix (these may contain acid phosphatase or sperm).[6, 13, 14] A wet mount of one swab may reveal motile sperm if the examiner has ready access to a microscope. One swab can be used to make a dry mount for the crime laboratory, and one or two swabs can be air-dried for submission to the crime laboratory. If there are no pooled secretions, a vaginal washing using 5 ml of sterile (but not bacteriostatic) water can be obtained with a syringe. The washing can be examined for sperm and acid phosphatase.

4. A Papanicolaou (Pap) smear to determine sperm and cervical mucosa morphology. Occasionally, the Pap smear may detect sperm when other tests do not.

5. A separate swab from the cervix for sperm and acid phosphatase. Dried specimens for acid phosphatase need not be refrigerated, but liquid specimens require refrigeration.

6. A cervical culture for gonorrhea.

Each sample should be separately labeled; the label should include the area from which the specimen was collected. Some physicians also obtain cervical chlamydial cultures.

After these samples have been obtained, a bimanual pelvic examination should be performed to assess uterine size and to identify adnexal masses and tenderness.

Another test that can be performed for sexual assault victims is the toluidine blue dye test for traumatic intercourse. Genital lacerations are corroborating evidence that rape has occurred, but without specialized staining techniques the majority of small lacerations go undetected. Toluidine blue greatly increases the detection of genital lacerations by highlighting lacerations with clear, linear marks easily distinguishable from episiotomy scars, rugae,

and vulvitis. This test is highly sensitive, however, and small toluidine blue–highlighted lacerations may occur in vigorous nonrape intercourse, especially in adolescents.[15] This test involves the application of toluidine blue to the vaginal mucosa. Tears in the mucosa expose superficial nuclei of underlying cells. These nuclei have an affinity for the toluidine blue, and lacerations (small and large) become stained. In one study, 70 per cent of nulliparas and 40 per cent of the total number of patients examined within 48 hours after complaint of sexual assault demonstrated toluidine blue–positive lacerations.[16] McCauley and associates demonstrated that the use of toluidine blue increased the detection of vaginal lacerations in reported rape victims from one in 24 to 14 in 24. Toluidine blue is primarily used in gynecology for outlining cervical neoplasia.[17]

The dye is applied with cotton-tipped applicators; all excess is wiped off with cotton balls until no further dye can be removed. Lacerations retain the dye (Fig. 78–1). Toluidine blue should be applied to the external genitalia before the insertion of a speculum, because the speculum itself may cause small lacerations.[16] Because of the potential spermicidal activity of toluidine blue, the examiner must decide on a case-by-case basis when to perform this test. The dye is not absorbed systemically so it is considered safe in pregnant women. Note that the dye is not used intravaginally but only on the external areas. If seminal stains are noted on the perineum, samples should be collected before toluidine blue application.

The anorectal area should be examined for traces of foreign material (particularly lubricants) and trauma. Because of a reluctance of some victims to admit to anal or oral sodomy, an examination of these areas should be performed in all cases. Anorectal swabs should be obtained for gonorrhea culturing and sperm and acid phosphatase testing. If the patient admits to anal penetration, one can perform a rectal washing by injecting 5 to 10 ml of normal saline with a syringe and a small plastic intravenous catheter, aspirating and preserving the fluid as evidence. This washing can be examined for sperm and acid phosphatase, even

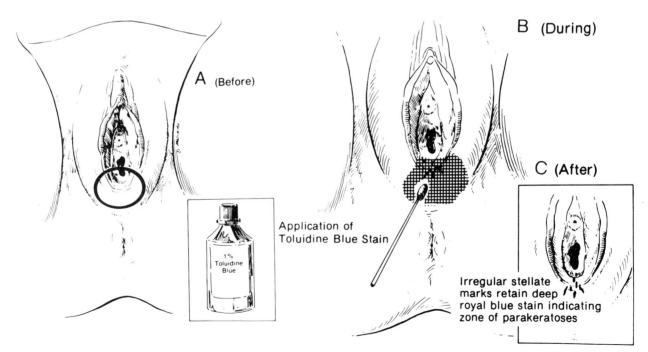

Figure 78–1. Toluidine blue application procedure. (From McCauley J, Guzinski G, Welch R, et al: Toluidine blue in the corroboration of rape in the adult victim. Am J Emerg Med 5(2):106, 1987.)

though acid phosphatase determination has been of little value from samples taken from the anal canal and the rectum.[18]

The mouth, particularly if oral sodomy is reported, should be inspected for signs of trauma. These can include bruises about the mouth, a torn frenulum of the lower lip, a torn frenulum beneath the tongue, and contusions or lacerations of the tonsillar pillars or the posterior pharyngeal wall. The examiner tests for acid phosphatase and sperm in the oral cavity by swabbing between the teeth with cotton-tipped applicators. The acid phosphatase test is seldom positive, but spermatozoa have been identified in oral smears up to 6 hours after the attack despite tooth brushing, using mouthwash, and drinking various fluids.[18] In addition, saliva samples (two to three saliva-soaked swabs) should be obtained so that one can assess the victim's secretor status of blood group antigens if foreign blood group antigens are found in the vagina. Eighty per cent of people secrete blood group antigens in saliva, semen, and so forth. Culturing of the pharynx for gonorrhea should also be performed.

Blood tests in sexual assault victims may include the following: drug and alcohol testing, blood typing, a serologic test for syphilis, and, if appropriate, a pregnancy test using the β subunit of human chorionic gonadotropin (hCG).[19, 20] If a serum pregnancy test is positive within a few hours or days of the assault, the victim was probably already pregnant at the time of the assault. If the test is negative at the initial examination but positive at a 2-week follow-up visit, it can be assumed that the victim became pregnant at or near the time of the assault.[7]

Motile and immotile sperm may be found microscopically in wet mounts of vaginal aspirates and in vaginal, oral, and rectal swabs. The samples should be examined microscopically immediately after the physical examination. The forensic pathologist may not be able to examine the samples for several hours, days, weeks, or months after they are collected, when sperm motility (a very good sign of recent intercourse) has been lost. The absence of sperm does not rule out sexual assault. The assault may have been without penetration, there may have been coitus interruptus, and the assailant may have used a condom or have had a vasectomy.

Samples and other evidence must be given to the police, a crime laboratory, or a forensic pathologist. Each sample must be labeled with the patient's name, the hospital number, the date and time of collection, the area from which the specimen was collected, and the collector's name. These specimens should then be packaged and transferred to the next appropriate official (police officer, pathologist, or other individual) along with a written "chain of evidence" that includes a list of the specimens, the signature of each person who provided them, and the signature of each person who received them. If this chain is broken, important evidence may be considered worthless in the courtroom.

Treatment

The factors of venereal disease, pregnancy, psychologic distress, and follow-up should be considered in the treatment of a sexual assault victim. Victims are reported to have a 1 in 30 chance of developing gonorrhea and a 1 in 1000 chance of developing syphilis.[3] The chance of developing a human immunodeficiency virus infection, herpes, or chlamydia from being raped has not been determined. Depending on patient reliability and other factors, a physician may choose to treat a victim as if she had been exposed to a known case of gonorrhea or may choose to rely on cultures. (When cultures are obtained from the cervix, the pharynx,

and the rectum, 90 per cent of established gonorrhea cases can be diagnosed at a single visit.[21]) Gonorrhea resulting from a rape may possibly be culturable within hours of the attack but should be almost always culturable at a 2-week follow-up visit.

Because victims tend to have a relatively low compliance with keeping follow-up visits, many physicians offer gonorrhea and chlamydia prophylaxis at the time of the initial examination. If this course of treatment is chosen, the patient is essentially treated as if she had been exposed to a male known to have gonorrhea. With the increasing prevalence of *Neiserria gonorrhoeae* strains resistant to penicillin and tetracycline, ceftriaxone has become the antibiotic of choice. Ceftriaxone also treats incubating syphilis. Intramuscular spectinomycin and oral ciprofloxacin are single-dose alternatives for penicillin- and cephalosporin-allergic patients, but neither of these has been shown to be effective against incubating syphilis. No single-dose regimen for gonorrhea is effective against coexisting *Chlamydia trachomatis* infection, and patients should also receive a 7-day course of doxycycline or tetracycline (a negative pregnancy test is a prerequisite for using either of these two antibiotics).[22] Erythromycin is an alternative agent for chlamydia prophylaxis in the pregnant patient.

Pregnancy occurs in approximately 1 per cent of victims. The examiner must be very careful to determine that pregnancy did not exist before the attack, and pregnancy tests should be obtained before any postcoital therapy is offered. The greater sensitivity of the serum pregnancy test using hCG-β subunit makes it the preferred test. This test is sensitive at 5 days after implantation of the products of conception. Newer urine tests are being developed that have a greater sensitivity than the old tests. These may be acceptable in the future. Sexual assault victims should be offered pregnancy prevention as outlined in Table 78–4. Diethylstilbestrol was once approved by the United States Food and Drug Administration (FDA) but currently is not approved as a morning-after contraceptive. Ovral is also not officially approved for this use by the FDA but is recommended by some physicians.[23] Ovral (50 µg of ethinyl estradiol and 0.5 mg of norgestral) has an unknown mechanism of action as a morning-after contraceptive. Ovral works best if begun within 12 to 24 hours following the deposit of semen in the vagina but no later than 72 hours. A total of four tablets are taken orally, two tablets at a time, 12 hours apart. Adverse effects are nausea, vomiting, and breast tenderness. If the patient vomits within 1 hour of taking a dose, the dose should be repeated. Antiemetic therapy should be offered if vomiting occurs. The failure rate of this regimen is reported to be 1.8 per cent or less.[23, 24]

Sexual assault precipitates a psychologic crisis for the patient, and psychologic care should begin when the patient

---

Table 78–4. *Alternative Drug Regimens for Pregnancy Prevention in Female Sexual Assault Victims**

Oral diethylstilbestrol in a dose of 25 mg twice daily for 5 days
Intravenous conjugated estrogen (Premarin) in a dose of 50 mg once daily for 2 days
Oral conjugated estrogen (Premarin) in a dose of 30 mg once daily for 5 days
Oral ethinyl estradiol in a dose of 5 mg once daily for 5 days
Oral ethinyl estradiol and norgestral (Ovral), 4 tablets (two at a time taken 12 hours apart)

*All should be begun within 24 hours of the sexual assault. All of these preparations may cause nausea and vomiting. Note that treatment is started only after pregnancy has been ruled out.

Table 78–5. Steps for Initial Psychologic Care by the Physician

Introduction of self
Reassurance that patient is safe
Empathetic listening to the patient about the ordeal
Informing the patient of his/her current physical condition in a
    supportive way
Involvement of the patient in procedures and decision making
    Allowing patient to determine rate of questioning
    Obtaining permission from patient for steps in examination
        and informing her of what is being done and why
    Involving patient in decisions regarding treatment (e.g., use of
        prophylactic antibiotics or pregnancy prevention)
    Involving patient in decisions regarding medical and
        psychological follow-up
    Involving patient in decisions regarding contacting and giving
        information to significant others
Brief discussion of the psychologic sequelae of sexual assault with
    the patient or contact with someone trained in crisis intervention
Arrangements for supportive follow-up

(From Martin CA, Warfield MC, Braen GR: Physician's management of the psychological aspects of rape. JAMA 249:501, 1983. Reproduced by permission. Copyright 1983, American Medical Association.)

first arrives in the emergency department.[25, 26] The victim often develops a posttraumatic stress disorder, manifested by numbed responsiveness to the external world, sleep disturbances, guilt feelings, memory impairment, avoidance of activities, and other symptoms.[27] The victim is particularly vulnerable to this stress disorder because of the following characteristics of sexual assault: (1) it is sudden, and the victim is unable to develop adequate defenses; (2) it involves intentional cruelty or inhumanity; (3) it makes the victim feel trapped and unable to fight back; and (4) it often involves physical injury.[28] The initial psychologic care of the rape victim in the emergency department is fundamental (Table 78–5). One can learn the methods for proper psychologic care with a minimum of training.

Follow-up for rape victims is essential. A 2-week follow-up examination conducted by a physician should be arranged; medical (venereal disease and pregnancy) and psychologic reevaluation is performed at this time. Further evaluations can be performed at 4 and 6 weeks at the discretion of the physician following the patient. In addition, local volunteer support groups can be of immense assistance to a rape victim, and contact with such a group should be offered to each victim of sexual assault.

It is uncommon to be called to court to testify in cases of sexual assault, but when called it is best to work with the prosecuting attorney when preparing your testimony. In some jurisdictions it is possible to minimize the time spent away from work by arranging to be called to the courtroom just before the time of testimony. Once on the witness stand, remember that one is called as the examining physician and not necessarily as an expert witness. The law requires that one testify only to one's best recollection and to what is indicated in the charting. Factual information in answer to questions should be given only if one knows the facts, and assumptions should be avoided. One should not be afraid to acknowledge the limits of one's knowledge or expertise.

Statements such as "There were marks on the body that were consistent with bite marks" are preferable to statements such as "There were bite marks." It is the court's decision whether or not a person was raped, and the clinician is there to give information on the patient's presentation, her statements, what was found, and what was done for treatment. One should stick to the facts and avoid interpretations.

REFERENCES

1. Hicks DJ: Rape: Sexual assault. Obstet Gynecol Annu 7:447, 1978.
2. Nelson C: Victims of rape: Who are they? In Warner CG (ed): Rape and Sexual Assault: Management and Intervention. Rockville, MD, Aspen Publications, 1980.
3. Schiff AF: A statistical evaluation of rape. Forensic Sci 2:339, 1973.
4. Braen GR: Sexual assault. In Rosen P, Baker FJ, Barkin RM, et al (eds): Emergency Medicine, Concepts and Clinical Practice. St. Louis, CV Mosby Co, 1983.
5. Burgess AW, Holstrom LL: The rape victim in the emergency department. Am J Nurs 73:1741, 1973.
6. Gomez RR, Wunsch CD, Davis JH, et al: Qualitative and quantitative determinations of acid phosphatase activity in vaginal washings. Am J Clin Pathol 64:423, 1975.
7. Braen GR: Physical assessment and emergency medical management for adult victims of sexual assault. In Warner CG (ed): Rape and Sexual Assault: Management and Intervention. Rockville, MD, Aspen Publications, 1980.
8. Don't miss a hair. F.B.I. Law Enforcement Bulletin 9, May 1976.
9. Twibell J, Whitehead PH: Enzyme typing of human hair roots. J Forensic Sci 23:356, 1978.
10. Togatz GE, Okagaki T, Sciarra JJ: The effect of vaginal lubricants on sperm motility in vitro. Am J Obstet Gynecol 113:88, 1972.
11. Fish SA: Vaginal injury due to coitus. Am J Obstet Gynecol 72:544, 1956.
12. Rush R, Milton PJD: Injuries of the vagina. S Afr Med J 47(Suppl):1325, 1973.
13. McCloskey KL, Muscillo GC, Noordervier B: Prostatic acid phosphatase activity in the postcoital vagina. J Forensic Sci 21:630, 1975.
14. Rupp JC: Sperm survival and prostatic acid phosphatase activity in victims of sexual assault. J Forensic Sci 14:177, 1968.
15. McCauley J, Guzinski G, Welch R, et al: Toluidine blue in the corroboration of rape in the adult victim. Am J Emerg Med 5:105, 1987.
16. Lauber AA, Souma ML: Use of toluidine blue for documentation of traumatic intercourse. Obstet Gynecol 60:644, 1982.
17. Richart RM: A clinical staining test for the in vivo delineation of dysplasia and carcinoma in situ. Am J Obstet Gynecol 86:703, 1963.
18. Enos WF, Beyer JC: Spermatozoa in the anal canal and rectum and in the oral cavity in female rape victims. J Forensic Sci 23:231, 1978.
19. Hayman CR: Serologic tests for syphilis in rape cases. JAMA 228:1227, 1974.
20. Saxena BB, Hasan SH, Haour F, et al: Radio-receptorassay of human gonadotropin: Detection of early pregnancy. Science 184:793, 1974.
21. US Department of Health, Education and Welfare: VD Fact Sheet 1975 (32nd ed). DHEW Pub. No. (CDC) 76–8195. Atlanta, Centers for Disease Control, 1975.
22. Treatment of sexually transmitted diseases. The Med Letter on Drugs and Therapeutics, 32 (issue 810):5–10, Jan, 1990.
23. Ovral as a morning-after contraceptive. The Med Letter on Drugs and Therapeutics, 31 (issue 803):93–94, Oct, 1989.
24. Bagshaw SN, Edwards D, Tucker AK: Ethinyl diestradiol and d-norgestrel is an effective emergency postcoital contraceptive: A report of its use in 1,200 patients in a family planning clinic. Aust NZ J Obstet Gynaecol 28:137, 1988.
25. Burgess AW, Holstrom LL: Rape trauma syndrome. Am J Psychiatry 131:981, 1974.
26. Martin CA, Warfield MC, Braen GR: Physician's management of the psychological aspects of rape. JAMA 249:501, 1983.
27. American Psychiatric Association Committee on Nomenclature and Statistics: Diagnostic and Statistical Manual of Mental Disorders. 3rd ed. Washington, DC, American Psychiatric Association, 1980.
28. Andreasen NC: Post-traumatic stress disorder. In Kaplan HI, Freedman AM, Sadock BJ (eds): Comprehensive Textbook of Psychiatry III. Vol. 2. Baltimore, Williams & Wilkins, 1980, pp 1517–1525.

Chapter 79

Removal of an Intrauterine Device

Samuel Timothy Coleridge

INTRODUCTION

Intrauterine contraceptive devices (IUDs) remain the third most popular method of temporary contraception used by married couples in the United States and are second only to oral contraceptives in effectiveness in preventing pregnancy.[1, 2] An estimated 60 million women use IUDs (80 per cent live in China, 6 per cent in developed countries, and 0.5 per cent in sub-Saharan Africa).[3] It is generally accepted that the mechanism of action of the IUD is the production of a local sterile inflammatory reaction caused by the presence of a foreign body in the uterus. The addition of copper increases this inflammatory reaction. Copper ions as well as the locally released high levels of progesterone probably also act to prevent the normal process of implantation.[4-7] On removal of an IUD, the inflammatory process rapidly disappears, although controversy exists as to whether the mechanism of resumption of fertility is the same as that following discontinuation of mechanical methods, such as the condom or the diaphragm.[8]

In general, with IUDs the pregnancy rate is less than 2 per cent, the rate of expulsion is as high as 5 to 15 per cent, and the rate of removal for medical reasons is 15 per cent. The major reasons for removal are uterine bleeding and lower abdominal pain during the first 3 to 6 months of use. The incidence of each complication diminishes in subsequent years.[3, 5, 9-12] The complications of IUDs include an increased odds ratio of 1.0 to 12.3 of developing pelvic inflammatory disease (PID),[5, 8, 13-27] a 1.1 to 13.7 per cent increased risk of extrauterine pregnancy if the patient with an IUD should get pregnant,[5, 7, 11, 22-24, 28-39] and an increased incidence of uterine perforation and uterine bleeding.[3, 10, 40, 41] In pregnant patients who fail to remove the IUD, there is an increased risk of spontaneous and septic abortion with both increased mortality and increased morbidity,[1, 5, 19, 22, 29, 42-45] a higher incidence of abruptio placenta and placenta previa,[17] and a possible increased risk of prematurity with IUDs containing copper.[5] A disproportionate number of cases of actinomycosis-like organisms have been identified in Papanicolaou (Pap) smears of patients with IUDs, but the rarity of pelvic actinomycosis rules against the routine removal of IUDs for asymptomatic IUD users with smears that are positive for actinomycosis-like organisms.[7, 22, 46, 47] However, a few investigators have noted an association between intrauterine fungal contamination and neonatal death in two case reports.[48, 49] There is no evidence to suggest that IUDs are associated with an increased incidence of congenital anomalies.[5, 22]

Several long-term studies have indicated that IUDs are not associated with an increased incidence of carcinoma of the cervix or the endometrium.[5] It is estimated, however, that among IUD users mortality is 3 to 5 deaths per million females annually, mainly as a result of infection. The IUD is as safe as or safer than other methods of contraception, including sterilization, and safer than no contraception, regardless of age group. However, in nonmonogamous relationships, contraceptive use of the IUD or oral contraceptive pill alone can no longer be advised owing to the lack of protection against sexually transmitted diseases.

In the United States, IUD usage peaked in 1972 with nearly 10 per cent of married women using the IUD. Then in 1986 the major United States distributors of IUDs announced that they were withdrawing them from the market. This was attributable more to the rising costs of liability insurance associated with one particular IUD (the Dalkon Shield) than to medical or safety considerations. Two

years later, in 1988, the Copper T 380A was released by Gyno-Pharma Inc. (Somerville, N.J.), with described design improvements and, more significantly, a detailed informed consent procedure.[50, 51] In February 1989, the Diagnostic and Therapeutic Technology Assessments (DATTA) panel of obstetrician-gynecologist consultants from the American Medical Association overwhelmingly considered both the copper-containing and progesterone-releasing IUDs as safe and effective. They went on to conclude that when IUDs are used in women in monogamous relationships, these devices were reliable in reducing pregnancy with relatively few side effects.[3, 7, 16, 52] This issue continues to be debated primarily because of differences in methodology used for reporting the complications of salpingitis (clinical versus pathologic diagnosis) and unwanted pregnancy (control group of non-IUD users).[11, 13-15, 17, 18, 37, 39, 53-57]

Pelvic inflammatory disease associated with IUD usage is related to insertion.[16] In one study, transient bacteremia resulting from vaginal organisms was found in 13 per cent of women 4 to 6 minutes after insertion of new devices.[54] Some data suggest that PID occurring more than a few months after insertion of copper-bearing devices is due to infections by STD and is not related to IUDs.[16] It has been speculated that IUDs may facilitate the ascension of lower tract infections due to organisms such as *Neisseria gonorrhea* or *Chlamydia trachomatis* but have no effect on the ascension of non-STD organisms.[14] The suggestion that bacteria penetrate the cervical mucus along the IUD string has been refuted by Jacques and associates, but the theory of bacteria attaching to spermatozoa entering the cervix remains plausible.[3, 58]

IUD users do not have any higher incidence of chlamydial infection.[47, 53, 55] Several studies challenge the high incidence of PID associated with IUD users (relative risks ranging from 1.0 to 120.6) and assert that women in stable monogamous relationships have no increased risk of primary tubal infertility associated with IUD usage.[13, 14, 16-18, 37, 39, 54, 56, 57]

Intrauterine devices and all contraceptive methods protect against ectopic pregnancy. The risk of ectopic pregnancy in IUD users is 40 per cent of that among women not using contraception, but 3 to 4 per cent of pregnancies in IUD users are ectopic.[7, 11, 38]

Several researchers have found that women with an IUD in place at the estimated time of conception are three to eight times more likely to experience second trimester fetal loss than are women who conceive without an IUD in place.[42, 44, 45] If the IUD is removed during the first trimester, there is little increase in the risk of second trimester fetal loss over patients who conceive without an IUD in place. The observed 20.3 per cent incidence of second trimester fetal loss is similar to the 17 per cent incidence of spontaneous abortion among nonusers of IUDs. In contrast, the estimated relative risk of fetal loss for women with an IUD in place at conception that was not removed in the first trimester is 10.3 per cent higher than the risk in nonusers.[7, 28, 29, 42]

The relative risk for septic second trimester fetal loss in patients with IUDs versus nonseptic losses in this group ranges from twofold to thirteenfold.[10, 11] There is no association between IUD use in the recent past (less than 1 year) or in the remote past (greater than 1 year) and second or third trimester fetal loss, provided there is no IUD in situ at conception. The type of IUD does not affect the risk of fetal loss.[19, 21, 42] The clinical features of the febrile spontaneous abortion in IUD users and in nonusers are similar; both groups of patients experience mainly localized symptoms, such as pelvic pain, uterine cramping, and vaginal hemorrhage.[44] This differs from the generalized symptoms that have been reported with maternal deaths. The clinical course of an IUD-associated maternal death from spontaneous abortion begins with generalized symptoms of septicemia, which precede the abortion. Fever was the presenting sign in 13 of 17 women who died with IUDs in place in Cates's study. No maternal deaths from an IUD in situ occurred during the first trimester; however, the risk of maternal death was 50 times greater in women who continued their pregnancy with an IUD in situ than in those who did not.[29]

Uterine perforation, although not common, is a potentially serious complication. *Perforation usually occurs initially at insertion* and is related to the shape of the IUD and the amount of force needed during insertion.[10, 59] During the months following insertion, continued uterine contractions may be responsible for either partial or complete perforation through the uterine musculature. The "widened Lippe's loop" on plain anteroposterior roentgenograms of the pelvis has been described as diagnostic for perforations of this type

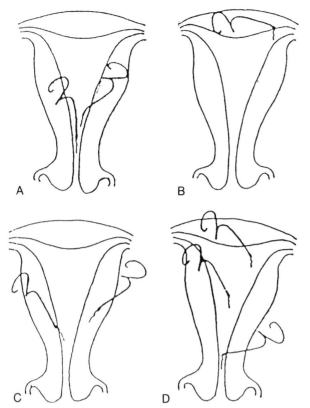

Figure 79–1. Types of partially perforated intrauterine devices (IUDs). For schematic purposes, the underlined number indicates the preponderant compartment involved; however, all degrees of perforation are possible. Uterine perforation has occurred with all types of IUDs; the IUD represented here is a stylized version. The string of the IUD is shown as missing at the external os because this is most often the case. *a*, Type 1–2; type 1–2. IUD present in compartments 1 (uterine cavity) and 2 (myometrium). *b*, Type 2. IUD present in compartment 2. *c*, Type 2–3; type 2–3. IUD present in compartments 2 and 3 (peritoneal cavity). *d*, Type 1–2–3; type 1–2–3; type 1–2–3. IUD present in compartments 1, 2, and 3. (From Zakin D, Stern WZ, Rosenblatt R: Complete and partial uterine perforation and embedding following insertion of intrauterine devices 1. Classification, complications, mechanism, incidence, and missing string. Obstet Gynecol Surv 36:335, 1981. Reproduced by permission. © Williams & Wilkins, 1981.)

of IUD. Eisenberg describes the distance from the bullous tip at the end of the loop to the second loop as approximately 1 cm in every case (normal controls were usually 2 or 3 mm and never greater than 5 mm).[60] Contiguous organs can become involved, particularly the rectosigmoid colon, the small bowel, and the bladder. In addition, problems can occur in more esoteric locations (e.g., fistulas to the abdominal wall).[10, 61] The detailed description and classification of uterine perforations by Zakin and associates is recommended for a discussion of the multiple possibilities involved and for an explanation of why gentle traction for removal with or without sonography, radiography, or hysterography is indicated rather than repeated forceful attempts at removal (Fig. 79–1).[10, 40, 62]

INDICATIONS FOR IUD REMOVAL

Bleeding and pain are the most common causes for termination of the IUD. Removal is usually requested within the first 6 months after insertion when these features are present. If a woman with an IUD in situ becomes pregnant, it is advisable to remove her IUD as soon as the pregnancy is recognized to give her pregnancy the optimal chance of progressing to term and to eliminate the possibility of

maternal death in the second or third trimester from sepsis. The IUD can usually be easily withdrawn by the physician if the string is visible. If the IUD cannot be removed, interruption of the pregnancy should be offered as an option. If the patient elects to maintain her pregnancy with the IUD in place, she should be warned of the increased risk of sepsis and should be closely followed for signs of septicemia.[1, 5, 28, 42, 44]

Likewise, the shortened or invisible IUD string suggests either (1) tail retraction within the cervical canal or uterine cavity (e.g., from uterine enlargement due to tumor or pregnancy or from rotation of the device within the uterine cavity), (2) unnoticed expulsion, or (3) uterine perforation and misplacement within the uterine wall, broad ligament, or abdominal cavity.[41, 63] Any of these conditions merits attempted IUD removal.[10, 22] The presence of endometritis in a patient with an IUD in place is also an indication for IUD removal. Although the issue is controversial, the consensus is that the IUD may act as a foreign body and may prohibit eradication of the bacterial infection with antibiotics alone.[26, 27, 64] It is generally advised that broad-spectrum antibiotics be given for 7 to 14 days after IUD removal if PID is diagnosed. Antibiotics are not required if IUD removal is accomplished in the absence of infection.

The two IUDs currently in use in the United States require replacement at different intervals. The Progestasert ($84 each) is replaced annually, and the Paragard TCu-380A ($140 each) is normally replaced every 4 years. It has been recommended that prophylactic antibiotics be given to patients at risk for complications from bacteremia (e.g., those who may be immunocompromised and those with valvular disease or a prosthetic valve).[54]

EQUIPMENT

Equipment useful for simple IUD removal is depicted in Figure 79–2. A tray containing the uterine sound, a tenaculum, and Bozman forceps (numbers 1, 6, and 5) is often adequate. Included on the tray should be a Novak curette, sponge forceps, and, possibly, the IUD extractor device (numbers 4, 3, and 2).

PROCEDURE

Prior to removal of the IUD, a consent form should be signed by all patients, particularly the pregnant patient. The patient should be given instructions regarding the procedure, the probable side effects of mild uterine cramping and spotting for a few days, and the possible complications of uterine perforation and induced abortion if she is pregnant. The patient should be cautioned to return immediately if fever develops.

Removal of the IUD during menses is somewhat easier, although this is not always possible. Swabbing the cervix with a povidone-iodine or soap solution is recommended before the insertion of any instrument in the uterine cavity. Slow removal of the IUD by gentle, constant traction with the Bozman forceps is usually successful. A sudden jerking movement may cause the string to break. If the IUD does not dislodge easily, sounding the uterus and gently probing the device may facilitate removal. If this is not adequate, then progressive dilation of the cervix is appropriate. Placement of a Lamicel sponge into the cervical canal allows for painless, reversible softening and dilation of the cervix, which proves particularly valuable for removal of retracted IUDs in nulliparas but requires a delay of 5 hours or more for full effect.[64-69] A tenaculum to steady the cervix or to

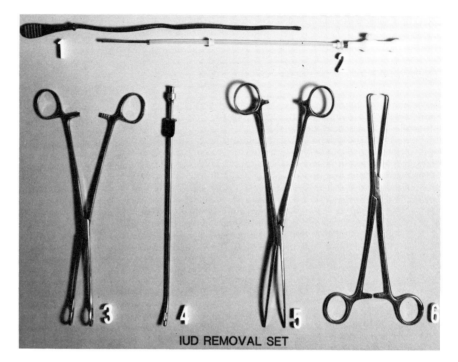

Figure 79–2. Implements for removal of an intrauterine (IUD) device. *1,* Uterine sound. *2,* IUD extractor device. *3,* Sponge (ring) forceps. *4,* Novak curette. *5,* Bozman forceps. *6,* Tenaculum.

straighten the ante- or retroverted uterus may be useful. A paracervical block of anesthesia is indicated when significant patient discomfort exists.[10, 30]

When the string is not visible at the cervical os, pregnancy must be excluded before the uterine cavity can be explored. After pregnancy has been ruled out, the cervix is grasped with a tenaculum, and the uterine cavity is explored with a sound to locate the IUD. After the presence and the position of the device have been noted, an IUD extractor, as described by Landesman (number 4; Fig. 79–2),[70] or a Novak curette is passed beyond the IUD and is withdrawn. Likewise, Husemeyer and Gordon advocate use of a plastic endometrial curette, the Mi-Mark Helix (Simpson/Basye Inc.) device, originally designed to obtain endometrial mucus, as an IUD extractor similar to the Landesman device.[63, 71] The Retrievette is a similar instrument used in Europe to retrieve retracted IUD threads.[72] Another useful device is the Rocket retrieval forceps from London.[73] With repeated gentle passes of any such extractor, the string becomes visible or the device itself is visible at the external cervical os. Once visualization is assured, a Bozman or sponge (ring) forceps can be used to grasp the IUD and complete the extraction. Avoidance of winding or angulating the thread about the jaws of the instrument is important.[41]

If the device is not felt, a radiograph can be obtained. The uterine sound should be inside the uterine cavity to demonstrate the cavity position in both posteroanterior and lateral films.[10, 30, 40] Practitioners in some institutions prefer to use sonography to determine location.[5, 10, 74–77] Magnetic resonance imaging has also been used and found to be safe (i.e., the IUD does not move under the influence of the magnetic field, does not heat up, and does not produce artifacts on the image screen.[78] If the IUD is outside the uterus, referral in a routine but timely manner to a gynecologist for laparoscopy and removal is indicated to prevent potential adhesions and bowel obstruction. Similarly, the Majzlin Spring IUD (which was withdrawn from the market in 1973) is extremely likely to be embedded, and the patient with this device should be referred to a gynecologist for removal.[79] An intratubal (P-block, Mark 9) device is marketed. This device must be inserted and removed hysteroscopically.[80]

If the patient is pregnant and wishes to maintain her pregnancy, she should be thoroughly counseled that removal statistically improves the chances for a successful outcome but that a spontaneous abortion may also occur. Removal of the IUD with a visible string should be accomplished with gentle traction. The patient should be told to return if bleeding, cramping, or signs of infection occur.

COMPLICATIONS

As previously stressed, removal of IUDs from the uterine cavity—whether diagnosed as free, embedded, or partially perforated (see Fig. 79–1)—should be accomplished cautiously and in a tentative fashion. It should be predetermined that attempts at removal will be stopped if undue resistance to instrumental traction is encountered. Complications of severe continuous or delayed bleeding, uterine cramping, or signs of sepsis suggest uterine perforation, and no further attempts at extraction in the emergency department are appropriate if these are present.[10, 40] Urgent referral to a gynecologist after telephone consultation is necessary. If uterine perforation occurs, the patient should be started on broad-spectrum antibiotics and typed for possible blood transfusion if hemorrhage is present.

Intravenous or oral antibiotics for 1 to 2 weeks in the symptomatic patient with PID are mandatory *with* IUD removal to prevent bacteremia or septicemia. Some physicians recommend antibiotic therapy be initiated *prior* to IUD removal. Although extended therapy before removal has been recommended by some, a 30-minute delay following intravenous antibiotic administration in the noncompromised patient (without valvular heart disease) should be adequate in the patient *without* uterine perforation. If the device is removed because of persistent cramping or uterine bleeding in the absence of infection, prophylactic antibiotics are not routinely given. It must be stressed, however, that low-grade endometritis is often difficult to exclude in the presence of pain and bleeding in the IUD user, and a course of antibiotics is justified in borderline cases.

Generally, only mild analgesia, if any, need be prescribed following the extraction. Alternative means for future birth control should be advocated for the patient who experiences an IUD-related complication.

CONCLUSION

Voluntary removal of the IUD is generally a simple procedure when the device is indeed intrauterine. In the pregnant patient, removal is both recommended and generally safe in the first trimester. When the IUD string of a nonpregnant patient cannot be seen, appropriate investigation for its location by radiographs with an intrauterine sound in place or by sonography is indicated if cervical dilation with gentle, unhurried, and careful endocervical and intrauterine probing is unsuccessful. If the IUD is not easily found or if gentle, constant traction is ineffective in removing the IUD, then one should consider uterine perforation. Referral to a gynecologist is appropriate for further investigation; hysteroscopy, laparoscopy, or laparotomy may be required. Removal can be difficult and even hazardous, depending on the degree of myometrial penetration or the extrauterine location.

REFERENCES

1. Cates W, Jr, Ory HW, Tyler CW: Publicity and the public health: The elimination of IUD-related abortion deaths. Fam Plann Perspect 9:138, 1977.
2. Gairola GA, Hockstrasser DL, Garkovich LE: Modern contraceptive practice in rural Appalachia. Am J Public Health 76:1004, 1986.
3. Diagnostic and therapeutic technology assessment (DATTA). Intrauterine device. JAMA 261:2127, 1989.
4. Beerthuizen RJ, Van Wijck JA, Eskes TK, et al: IUD and salpingitis: A prospective study of pathomorphological changes in the oviducts in IUD-users. Eur J Obstet Gynecol Reprod Biol 13:31, 1982.
5. Mischell D: Intrauterine devices. Clin Obstet Gynecol 6(1):27, 1979.
6. Ortiz ME, Croxatto HB: The mode of action of IUDs. Contraception 36:37, 1987.
7. Grimes DA: Reversible contraception for the 1980's. JAMA 255:69, 1986.
8. Eschenbach DA: Do IUDs increase relative risk of infection? Contemporary OB/GYN 14:93, 1979.
9. Chaudhury RR: Current status of research on intrauterine devices. Obstet Gynecol 34:333, 1980.
10. Zakin D, Stern WZ, Rosenblatt R: Complete and partial uterine perforation and embedding following insertion of intrauterine devices I. Classification, complications, mechanism, incidence, and missing string. Obstet Gynecol 36:335, 1981.
11. Sivin I, Stern J: Long-action, most effective copper T IUDs: A summary of U. S. experience, 1970–75. Studies in Fam Planning 10:263, 1979.
12. Sivin I, Schmidt R: Effectiveness of IUD's: A review. 36:55, 1987.
13. Kirsnon B, Poindexter AN, Spitz MR: Pelvic adhesions in intrauterine device users. Obstet Gynecol 71:251, 1988.
14. Lee NC, Rubin GL, Borucki R: The intrauterine device and pelvic inflammatory disease revisited: New results from the Women's Health Study. Obstet Gynecol 72:1, 1988.
15. Rioux J-E, Cloutier D, Dupont P, Lamonde D: Long-term study of the safety of the Dalkon Shield and Gyne-T 200 intrauterine device. CMAJ 134:747, 1986.
16. Mishell DR: Contraception. N Engl J Med 320:777, 1989.
17. Lee NC, Rubin GL, Ory HW, Burkman RT: Type of intrauterine device and the risk of pelvic inflammatory disease. Obstet Gynecol 62:1, 1983.
18. Cramer DW, Schiff I, Schoenbaum SC, et al: Tubal infertility and the intrauterine device. N Engl J Med 312:941, 1985.
19. Burkman RT: Association between intrauterine device and pelvic inflammatory disease. Obstet Gynecol 57:269, 1981.
20. Edelman DA: Pelvic inflammatory disease and the intrauterine device: A causal relationship. Int J Gynecol Obstet 17:504, 1980.
21. Eschenbach DA, Harnisch JP, Holmes KK: Pathogenesis of acute pelvic inflammatory disease: Role of contraception and other risk factors. Am J Obstet Gynecol 8:838, 1977.
22. Keith LG, Berger GS, Edelman DA: Clinician's guide to using IUD's—safely. Contemporary OB/GYN 19:159, 1982.
23. Malhotra N, Chaudhury RR: Current status of intrauterine devices II. Intrauterine devices and pelvic inflammatory disease and ectopic pregnancy. Obstet Gynecol Surv 37:1, 1982.
24. Oser S, Liedholm P, Gullberg B, Sjoberg NO: Risk of pelvic inflammatory disease among intrauterine device users irrespective of previous pregnancy. Lancet 1:386, 1980.
25. Vessey MP, Yeates D, Flavel M, McPherson K: Pelvic inflammatory disease and the intrauterine device: Findings in a large cohort study. Br Med J 282:855, 1981.
26. Westrom L, Bengtsson LP, Mardh PA: The risk of pelvic inflammatory disease in women using intrauterine contraceptive devices as compared to non-users. Lancet 2:161, 1976.
27. Westrom L: The risk of pelvic inflammatory disease in women using intrauterine contraceptive devices as compared to non-users. Lancet 2:221, 1974.
28. Alvior G: Pregnancy outcome with removal of intrauterine device. Obstet Gynecol 41:894, 1973.
29. Cates W, Jr, Ory HW, Rochat RW, Tyler CW: The intrauterine device and deaths from spontaneous abortion. N Engl J Med 295:1155, 1976.
30. Hatcher RA, Stewart GK: Contraceptive Technology. Irvington Publishing, New York, NY, 1981, pp 72–97.
31. McMorries KE, Lofton RH, Stinson JC, Cummings RV: Is the IUD increasing the number of ovarian pregnancies? Contemporary OB/GYN 13:165, 1979.
32. Ory HW: Ectopic pregnancy and intrauterine contraceptive devices: New perspectives. Obstet Gynecol 57:137, 1981.
33. Pagano R: Ectopic pregnancy: A seven-year survey. Med J Aust 2:526, 1981.
34. Progestasert IUD and ectopic pregnancy in patients using IUDs. FDA Drug Bulletin 8:37, 1978.
35. Tatum HJ, Schmidt FH: Contraceptive and sterilization practices and extrauterine pregnancy: A realistic perspective. Fertil Steril 28:407, 1977.
36. Vessey MP, Yeates D, Flavel R: Risk of ectopic pregnancy and duration of use in an intrauterine device. Lancet 2:501, 1979.
37. Marchbanks PA, Annegers JF, Coulam CB, et al: Risk factors for ectopic pregnancy: A population based study. JAMA 259:1823, 1988.
38. Kulig JW: Adolescent contraception: Nonhormonal methods. Pediatr Clin North Am 36:717, 1989.
39. Chow W-H, Daling JR, Weiss NS, et al: IUD use and subsequent tubal ectopic pregnancy. Am J Public Health 76:536, 1986.
40. Zakin G, Lindgren S: Influence of an intrauterine device on the course of an acute salpingitis. Contraception 24:199, 1981.
41. Ansari AH: Diagnosis and management of intrauterine device with missing tail. Obstet Gynecol 44:727, 1974.
42. Foreman H, Stadel BV, Schlesselman S: Intrauterine device usage and fetal loss. Obstet Gynecol 58:669, 1981.
43. Kelaghan J, Rubin GL, Ory HW, Layde PM: Barrier-method contraceptives and pelvic inflammatory disease. JAMA 248:184, 1982.
44. Kim-Farley RJ, Cates W, Jr, Ory HW, Hatcher RA: Febrile spontaneous abortion and the IUD. Contraception 18:561, 1978.
45. Shine RM, Thompson JF: The in-situ IUD and pregnancy outcome. Am J Obstet Gynecol 119:124, 1974.
46. O'Connor KF, Bagg MN, Croley MR, Schabel SI: Pelvic actinomycosis associated with intrauterine devices. Radiology 170:559, 1989.
47. Edelman DA: IUD complications in perspective. Contraception 36:159, 1987.
48. Smith CV, Horenstein J, Platt LD: Intraamniotic infection with *Candida albicans* associated with a retained intrauterine contraceptive device: A case report. Am J Obstet Gynecol 159:123, 1988.
49. Misenhimer HR, Garcia-Bunuel R: Failure of intrauterine contraceptive device and fungal infection in the fetus. Obstet Gynecol 34:368, 1969.
50. Pitkin M: The return of the IUD (editorial). Obstet Gynecol 72:119, 1988.
51. Amstey MS: The return of the IUD (letter). Obstet Gynecol 73:137, 1989.
52. Sweet RL, Gibbs RS: Pelvic inflammatory disease. In Infectious Diseases of the Female Genital Tract. Baltimore, Williams & Wilkins, 1985, p. 54.
53. Guderian AM, Trobough GE: Residues of pelvic inflammatory disease in intrauterine device users: A result of the intrauterine device or *Chlamydia trachomatis* infection? Am J Obstet Gynecol 154:497, 1986.
54. Murray S, Hickey JB, Houang E: Significant bacteremia associated with replacement of intrauterine contraceptive device. Am J Obstet Gynecol 156:698, 1987.
55. Edelman DA: The use of intrauterine contraceptive devices, pelvic inflammatory disease, and *Chlamydia trachomatis* infection. Am J Obstet Gynecol 158:956, 1988.
56. Kramer RL: The intrauterine device and pelvic inflammatory disease revisited: New results from the Women's Health Study. Obstet Gynecol 73:300, 1989.
57. Tatum HJ, Connell EB: A decade of intrauterine contraception: 1976 to 1986. Fertil Steril 46:1, 1981.
58. Jacques M, Olson ME, Costerton JM: Microbial colonization of tailed and tailless intrauterine contraceptive devices: Influence of the mode of insertion in the rabbit. Am J Obstet Gynecol 154:648, 1986.
59. Vessey MP, Johnson B, Doll R, Peto R: Outcome of pregnancy in women using an intrauterine device. Lancet 1:495, 1974.
60. Eisenberg RL: The widened loop sign of Lippe's loop perforations. AJR 116:847, 1972.
61. Schwartzwald D, Mooppan M, Tancer ML, et al: Vesicouterine fistula with menouria: A complication from an intrauterine contraceptive device. J Urol 136:1066, 1986.
62. Reinbach D, Carr ND: Strangulating small bowel obstruction due to an intrauterine contraceptive device. Br J Surg 74:112, 1987.
63. Ansari AH, Hoffman D: Retrieval of intrauterine contraceptive device with missing tail by means of a plastic curette (Mi-Mark). Am J Obstet Gynecol 142:1061, 1982.
64. Soderberg G, Lindgren S: Influence of an intrauterine device on the course of an acute salpingitis. Contraception 24:199, 1981.
65. Wheeler RG, Schneider K: Properties and safety of cervical dilators. Am J Obstet Gynecol 146:597, 1983.

66. Nicolaides KH, Welsh CC, MacPherson MBA, et al: Lamicel: A new technique for cervical dilatation before first trimester abortion. Br J Obstet Gynecol 90:475, 1983.
67. Johnson IR, MacPherson MBA, Welch CC, Filshie GM: A comparison of Lamicel and prostaglandin E$_2$ vaginal gel for cervical ripening before induction of labor. Am J Obstet Gynecol 151:604, 1985.
68. Hale RW, Pion RJ: Laminaria: An underutilized clinical adjunct. Clin Obstet Gynecol 15:829, 1972.
69. Johnson N, Moodley J: Retrieval of intrauterine contraceptive devices with missing tails, using Lamicel. Br J Obstet Gynecol 95:97, 1988.
70. Landesman R: An intrauterine device. Obstet Gynecol 37:618, 1971.
71. Husemeyer RP, Gordon H: Retrieval of contraceptive-device threads from within the uterine cavity. Lancet 1:807, 1979.
72. Akerlund M: Retrieval of intrauterine devices with missing tails, using Lamicel. Br J Obstet Gynecol 95:254, 1988.
73. Stubbelfield PG, Fuller AF, Foster SC: Ultrasound-guided intrauterine removal of intrauterine contraceptive devices in pregnancy. Obstet Gynecol 72:961, 1988.
74. McArdle CR: Ultrasonic localization of missing intrauterine contraceptive devices. Obstet Gynecol 51:330, 1978.
75. Carroll R, Gombergh R: Empty-bladder (hysterographic) view on US for evaluation of intrauterine devices. Radiology 163:822, 1987.
76. Ron-El R, Weinraub Z, Langer R, et al: The importance of ultrasonography in infertile women with "forgotten" intrauterine contraceptive devices. Am J Obstet Gynecol 161:211, 1989.
77. Parsons J, McEwan JA: Transvaginal ultrasonography to ascertain the position of an IUD. N Engl J Med 321:546, 1989.
78. Mark AS, Hricak H: Intrauterine contraceptive devices: MR imaging. Radiology 162:311, 1987.
79. Weiss BD: The Majzlin spring revisited. Am Fam Phys 26:123, 1982.
80. Brundin J: Observations on the mode of action of an intratubal device, the P-block. Am J Obstet Gynecol 156:997, 1987.

Neurologic Procedures

Chapter 80

Insertion of Cervical Traction Devices

Robert G. R. Lang

INTRODUCTION

Caliper traction devices or "skull tongs" are important not only to immobilize the cervical spine and prevent further injury but also to reduce a fracture-dislocation. Return of vertebral elements to their anatomic position can be associated with marked improvement of a neurologic deficit if spinal cord transection has not occurred. Cervical traction can also give dramatic symptomatic relief in undisplaced fractures associated with severe neck pain.

Skull tongs are inserted to provide steady traction by means of weights attached to the tongs by a cord. The weight of the body provides counter traction. Insertion of skull tongs can be easily carried out in the emergency department using only local anesthetic.

Cervical immobilization should begin in the prehospital care phase of trauma management. In-line axial manual stabilization in the neutral position is often required while awaiting radiographs if an unstable cervical fracture is suggested by clinical and historical (mechanism of injury) findings. Caliper traction should complement the more rapidly introduced techniques of cervical immobilization discussed in Chapter 62.

BACKGROUND

Until the early 1930s, skeletal traction was accomplished by halter, casts, or rings with turnbuckles.[1] These devices were often unsatisfactory because the patient was in a recumbent position and had adjacent injuries, encroachment of the anterior surface of the neck, pain, and pressure sores.

Skeletal skull traction was first described by Crutchfield in 1933.[1] His first case was a woman severely injured in an automobile accident. In addition to a complete fracture-dislocation of the axis, she had multiple facial lacerations and a compound fracture of the mandible. Ordinary methods for reduction of the cervical fracture could not be used; so, on the suggestion of Dr. Coleman, burr holes were drilled through the outer table in the parietal eminences, Edmonton extension tongs were inserted, and traction was applied.

In the same year, Neubeiser described the use of number 8

I would like to thank Edean Berglund, Medical Librarian at St. Peter Hospital, for her assistance in obtaining the reference material; Teresa Edwards, for typing the second edition original manuscript; Elaine Dunn, for typing the revisions; and my wife, Nancy, for her assistance. I would also like to thank Dr. James Stone, Chairman, Division of Neurosurgery, Cook County Hospital, for his critical review of the neurosurgical chapters in the first edition. Many of his recommendations have been incorporated into the second edition.

Kirby fishhooks, with the barbs removed, inserted under the zygomatic processes.[2] A device with blunt hooks was later developed by Selmo, but it resulted in disfiguring incisions for insertion under the zygomatic processes.[3] In 1940, Peyton used number 5 fishhooks, with the barbs removed, inserted under the zygomatic arches percutaneously.[4] This traction device left minimal, if any, scars after removal, and the hooks could be easily maintained while in place.

In 1935, Crutchfield developed small skull tongs,[5] but an unfortunate error in construction made many of the initial instruments almost worthless.[6] For proper application, the maximum spread of the tongs had to be at least 10 cm, whereas many of the defective tongs had spreads of less than 7 cm.

Over the years, a variety of skull traction devices were developed, each bearing the name of its developer. Barton, Blackburn, and Vinke are among the better known types. The correctly constructed small tongs of Crutchfield were perhaps the most popular of their time and indeed are still in use in many institutions.

In 1973, Gardner described spring-loaded points for cervical traction.[7] His "skull traction tong" gained popularity very quickly and is now the principal device in use. The spring-loaded points require no skin incision for insertion and can be inserted in minutes. When properly inserted, they rarely pull out and can be left in place for prolonged periods of time. They will readily tolerate up to 65 lb of traction.

Low profile skull tongs developed at the University of Virginia have the positive features of both the Crutchfield and Gardner-Wells tongs. The University of Virginia tongs allow increased head mobility while tolerating up to 90 lb of traction without pulling free.[8] Unfortunately, the ideal skull tongs have yet to be developed. Minns and Sutton studied the mechanics of various skull traction calipers. They suggest that the ideal skull tongs would be a cone type of caliper with the Stratford modification (3-cm elliptical support) using a spring-loaded system above the swivel pin, parallel to the compressing turnbuckle, with pin tips angled 67 degrees.[9]

In recent years, there has been a tendency toward more aggressive early surgical stabilization of cervical fracture dislocations. The development of the Halo brace has allowed earlier ambulation of patients with unstable cervical spine injuries.[10] Patients who previously remained in tongs on spinal frames for 16 to 20 weeks are now frequently up within 1 to 2 weeks after injury.

INDICATIONS

Skull tongs should be inserted in all patients with unstable cervical spine injuries and in those with stable subluxations that need to be reduced prior to immobilization, including fracture-dislocations, subluxations, unilateral and bilateral locked facets in the lower cervical region (C3 to C7), hangman's fracture (C2 pedicles) with and without subluxation, fractures of the odontoid process, and possibly Jefferson's fracture (ring of the atlas). A pure, severe ligamentous injury, often associated with a teardrop fracture, may also be unstable and require traction. Cervical burst fractures with neurologic deficit or pain and spasm should be immobilized in skull tongs.

Insertion of skull tongs should be carried out as soon as technically possible in patients who have obvious fracture-dislocations and neurologic deficits when on-site neurosurgical consultation is not rapidly available. Early reduction can sometimes result in a dramatic reversal of neurologic deficit. While the early application of appropriate traction can be beneficial, the merit of cervical traction with tongs over simple conventional cervical immobilization during interhospital transfer to a tertiary trauma facility is controversial.

Skull tongs are *not* indicated for stable compression fractures of the vertebral bodies or fractures of cervical spinous processes (clay-shovelers' fracture) unless they are associated with severe ligamentous disruption. Skull tongs are also not indicated for thoracic or lumbar fracture-dislocations. Placement of tongs directly over skull fractures is to be avoided. Skull tongs generally should not be used in preadolescent children. Skull tongs must be used with great care and under constant supervision in the case of an agitated, confused, and restless patient. When clinically indicated, computed tomography (CT) of the head should be performed prior to insertion of skull tongs.

If instability or the extent of injury is uncertain despite quality cervical radiographs, the patient's neck should be immobilized in a Philadelphia collar and the patient should be admitted to the hospital and kept at bed rest until muscle spasm resolves. Flexion-extension views, with the physician in attendance, can then be carried out under fluoroscopy to determine whether instability is present. Tomography (both standard and computed) should also be considered.

EQUIPMENT

INSERTION OF GARDNER-WELLS TONGS

Disposable safety razor
Povidone-iodine (Betadine) soap and solution
One per cent lidocaine (Xylocaine) with 1 per
    100,000 epinephrine
12-ml syringe
19-gauge 1½-inch needle
27-gauge 1½-inch needle
Gardner-Wells skull tongs
Suitable bed or frame with pulleys and weights
    for establishing cervical traction

INSERTION OF CRUTCHFIELD TONGS

Disposable safety razor
Povidone-iodine (Betadine) soap and solution
One per cent lidocaine (Xylocaine) with 1 per
    100,000 epinephrine
12-ml syringe
19-gauge 1½-inch needle
27-gauge 1½ inch needle
Scalpel handle with number 11 blade
Sterile metal ruler
Blue marking pen
Twist drill
Twist drill bit with 4-mm point-fixed guard
Crutchfield tongs with minimum spread of
    10 mm point to point
Suitable bed or frame with pulleys and weights
    for establishing cervical traction

INSERTION OF UNIVERSITY OF VIRGINIA TONGS

Disposable safety razor
Povidone-iodine (Betadine) soap and solution
One per cent lidocaine (Xylocaine) with 1 per 100,000
    epinephrine
12-ml syringe
19-gauge 1½-inch needle
27-gauge 1½-inch needle
University of Virginia skull tongs
Suitable bed or frame with pulleys and weights for
    establishing cervical traction

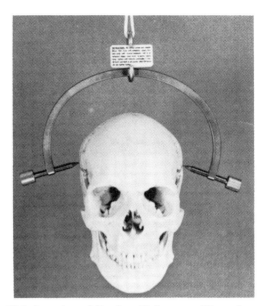

Figure 80–1. Insertion of Gardner-Wells tongs. The points are applied above the ears and below the "equator." Flexion or extension of the head is determined by height of the pulley. Note that the instructions attached to the tong always face anteriorly. (From Gardner WJ: The principle of spring-loaded points for cervical traction. Technical note. J Neurosurg 39:543, 1973. Reproduced by permission.)

TECHNIQUE

Insertion of Gardner-Wells Tongs

The scalp is shaved above both ears for a diameter of about 5 cm. The skin is then scrubbed with povidone-iodine soap and painted with povidone-iodine solution.

The tongs are inserted above and slightly behind the ears and below the "equator" of the skull. The points should be located just below the temporal ridges, about 5 cm above the mastoid bone (Figs. 80–1 and 80–2). Placing the tongs directly above the external canals distributes the pulling force too far anterior.

Infiltration of 1 per cent lidocaine with epinephrine is least painful when carried out with a 27-gauge 1½-inch needle. It is important to raise a large wheal in the skin and then infiltrate subcutaneous tissue, muscle, and especially the sensitive pericranium. Approximately 4 ml of local anesthetic should be infiltrated on each side.

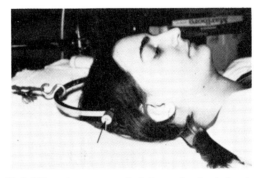

Figure 80–2. When the outer end of the spring-loaded point barely protrudes beyond the flat surface, the spring is fully compressed. (From Gardner WJ: The principle of spring-loaded points for cervical traction. Technical note. J Neurosurg 39:543, 1973. Reproduced by permission.)

One side of the tongs has a spring-loaded point to indicate when proper "squeeze pressure" has been achieved. As pressure increases, the indicator begins to emerge. The tongs are inserted by simply applying the points to the infiltrated skin and then tightening each side alternately until the spring indicator on the spring-loaded point barely protrudes from the flat surface of the knurled end (see Fig. 80–2). A protrusion of 1 mm or a distance equal to the thickness of the associated lock washer is generally recommended. This indicates that the spring is fully compressed and is exerting 30 lb of "squeeze" between the points. The tong is tilted (rocked) back and forth to ensure proper seating and is then retightened if the indicator has recessed. Traction is now applied. The tightness of the tongs should be checked after 24 hours to ensure that the indicator is flush with the outer flat surface of the screw assembly. The depth of penetration is self-limited by a gradual lessening of spring tension accompanied by an exponential increase in the surface area of contact between the tapered points and the bone.

The skin should be cleaned daily with peroxide around the pin sites. Povidone-iodine solution for cleaning is avoided, because it can cause corrosion of the pins.

Insertion of Crutchfield Tongs

The scalp is shaved for 6 cm on each side of the sagittal midline in line with the mastoid tips. The Crutchfield tongs are opened so that the distance between the tips is 11 cm. The sagittal midline is marked with a sterile blue marking pen, and the tips of the opened tongs are applied to the skin equidistant from the midline (Fig. 80–3). The point at which the tips touch the skin is marked with the pen and then infiltrated with 1 per cent lidocaine with 1 per 100,000

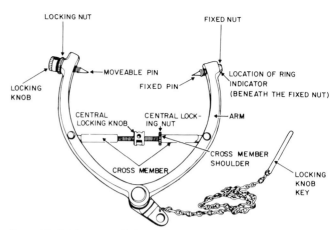

Figure 80–4. Diagram of the University of Virginia tongs. (From Rimel RW, et al: Modified skull tongs for cervical traction: Technical note. J Neurosurg 55:848, 1981. Reproduced by permission.)

epinephrine. A skin wheal is raised, and approximately 3 ml should be infiltrated at each site down to and including the pain-sensitive pericranium. Stab wounds, just large enough to permit entry of the drill bit so that the pins will fit snugly and limit bleeding, are then made in the skin with a number 11 blade. A 4-mm point with a fixed guard is used to drill the holes on each side of the skull to a depth of 4 mm. The skull must be drilled to the full depth of the guard or else the points of the tongs may later slip out. After each hole has been drilled, its depth should be checked by slipping the drill point from the edge to the depth of the hole and observing the distance through which it passes.

When drilling is completed, the points of the tongs are slipped into the holes and the instrument is tightened and locked. The tongs should be checked every 2 or 3 days and tightened only when necessary. Pin sites are cleaned with peroxide daily.

Insertion of University of Virginia Tongs

The scalp is shaved above both ears for a diameter of about 5 cm. The skin is then scrubbed with povidone-iodine soap and painted with povidone-iodine solution. The inter-pin distance for the tongs is first approximated to the appropriate skull size by turning the central locking knob on the cross member (Fig. 80–4). The central locking nut should be turned away from the cross member shoulder to allow free adjustment. The moveable pin is adjusted until it is protruding slightly less than the fixed pin.

The tongs are inserted just below the equator of the skull about 5 cm superior to the mastoid bone. The fit is approximated by turning the central knob of the cross member to close the tongs. The central locking knob is turned until the pressure on the pins first begins to move the fixed nut slightly away from the arm shoulder. The moveable pin is then tightened until the ring indicator located beneath the nut of the fixed pin is in view. The nut will then be protruding 2 mm. The pins are then exerting 30 lb of pressure between the points. The central locking knob is then tightened against the central locking nut with the locking knob key. This will prevent inadvertent loosening of the device.

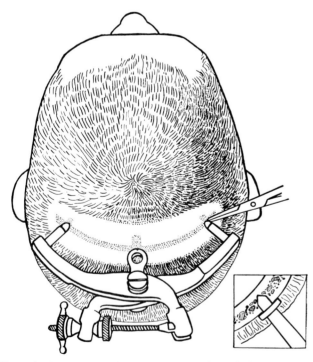

Figure 80–3. Procedure for correct application of the skull tongs developed by Crutchfield. Lines are painted on the scalp to indicate the midline of the skull and the approximate plane of the cervical articulations (through mastoid tip). (From Crutchfield WG: Skeleton traction in treatment of injuries to the cervical spine. JAMA 155:29, 1954. Copyright 1954, American Medical Association.)

Application of Traction

Traction should be applied in the plane of the articulating facets to eliminate an uneven pull on muscles and

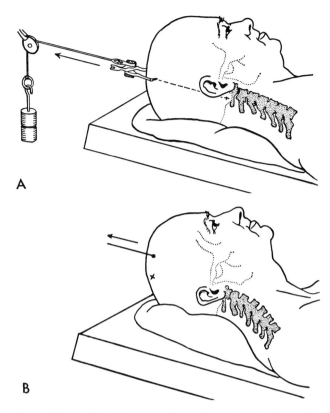

A

B

Figure 80–5. *A,* Traction correctly applied in the plane of the articulating facets. *B,* Ineffective traction applied in a plane anterior to that of the articulating facets, which may even increase the deformity in cases of anterior displacement of the upper segment. (From Crutchfield WG: Skeletal traction in treatment of injuries to the cervical spine. JAMA 155:29, 1954. Reproduced by permission. Copyright 1954, American Medical Association.)

tendons (Fig. 80–5*A*). Tongs are frequently applied too far forward on the skull (Fig. 80–5*B*). The tips of the traction device should be directly perpendicular to the mastoid tips. The minimal corrective pull varies according to the level of injury and the position of the patient while in traction. Weights listed in Table 80–1 are only an approximation for various levels of cervical spine injury with the head of the patient's bed elevated no more than 20 degrees. No effort should be made to bring about a rapid reduction. Force sufficient to accomplish this may injure soft tissues and endanger the spinal cord. A minimal corrective pull that provides immediate protection for the spinal cord and begins

Table 80–1. Suggested Weights for the Treatment of Fractures and Dislocations at Various Levels in the Cervical Spine

Level	Minimum Weight (lb)	Maximum Weight (lb)
1st	5	10
2nd	6	10–12
3rd	8	10–15
4th	10	15–20
5th	12	20–25
6th	15	20–30
7th	18	25–35

(From Crutchfield WG: Skeletal traction in treatment of injuries to the cervical spine. JAMA 155:31, 1954. Reproduced by permission. Copyright 1954, American Medical Association.)

the reduction that may be complete within 1 hour should be applied. When a very strong pull is used, portable radiographs should be carried out every 15 minutes until it is shown that the force is not too strong. Overdistraction must be avoided at all cost. Beware of lytic spinal lesions. A pathologic fracture may be present. Neoplastic destructive spinal lesions can be especially prone to separation and spinal injury with overdistraction. Also, in some cases of trauma the spinal ligaments are so badly torn that traction considerably widens the intervertebral space and additional serious injury may occur to the spinal cord or cervical nerves. If follow-up radiographic examination does not show complete reduction and if there is no wide gap between the bodies of the affected vertebrae, additional weight is added gradually. After the vertebrae have been pulled sufficiently apart for them to slip back into position, no additional weight should be added, even though some deformity is present. The same amount of pull or even less pull usually brings about complete and satisfactory reduction within a few days. Analgesia and sedatives may be required to keep the patient comfortable while traction is being applied. As soon as satisfactory alignment has been obtained, the pull for holding the corrected position is reduced to a minimum (5 to 7 lb).

COMPLICATIONS

The potentially most serious complication with application of skull tongs for cervical traction is overdistraction and worsening of the patient's neurologic condition. This complication has been reported in several cases.[11] Simple traction on the patient's shoulders for visualization of lower cervical vertebrae during a portable cervical radiograph has also resulted in distraction.[12] Immediate follow-up radiographs are needed after application of tongs, after the addition of any weight, and at regular intervals while the patient is in traction. Muscle relaxants such as diazepam (Valium) and analgesics will significantly reduce the amount of weight required for reduction and maintenance of position; overdistraction is likely to occur with a general anesthetic if the amount of weight is not adequately reduced during the procedure.

Skull tongs may pull out if they are not checked periodically for tightness, and perforation of the inner table has been reported with Gardner and Crutchfield tongs.[1, 13] Inner-table penetration can be prevented by correctly applying the tongs and by not overtightening them. Periodic tangential views of the skull will provide early identification of inner-table perforation and may prevent secondary complications, such as intracranial bleeding or brain abscess. Infection around the pin sites is another frequent problem. Most infections are localized cellulitis and can be prevented by regular cleaning with hydrogen peroxide and shaving of the pin sites. Osteomyelitis and brain abscess have been reported infrequently.[14] Frank psychosis can develop while patients are in tongs. Psychotic patients will require adequate sedation and constant supervision.

CONCLUSION

Skull traction devices are an effective way to reduce fracture-dislocations and stabilize the cervical spine.

Ease of application of Gardner-Wells tongs makes them preferable for use in the emergency department, but Crutchfield tongs are better tolerated by the patient when prolonged traction is anticipated.

Application of skull tongs for cervical traction to reduce a fracture-dislocation is best done under the care of a neurosurgeon or orthopedic surgeon who has had training in spinal injuries. In circumstances in which these specialists are not immediately available, early reduction of a fracture-dislocation prior to transfer may improve a patient's neurologic deficit by relieving pressure on the spinal cord and its vascular supply. When circumstances permit, discussion with the receiving specialist is preferred prior to tong placement and initiation of traction. Adequate precautions against overdistraction must always be taken.

Finally, the use of high dose methylprednisolone therapy may be beneficial in cord injuries up to 8 hours post-trauma.[15] An initial bolus of 30 mg/kg, followed by an infusion of 5.4 mg/kg/hr for the next 23 hours has been recommended.

REFERENCES

1. Crutchfield WG: Skeletal traction for dislocation of the cervical spine. South Surg 2:156, 1933.
2. Neubeiser BL: A method of skeletal traction for neck extension. J Missouri Med Assoc 30:495, 1933.
3. Selmo JD: Traction on the zygomatic process for cervicovertebral injuries. Am J Surg 46:405, 1939.
4. Peyton WT, Hall HB, French LA: Hook traction under zygomatic arch in cervical spine injuries. Surg Gynecol Obstet 79:311, 1944.
5. Crutchfield WG: Further observations on treatment of fracture dislocations of cervical spine with skeletal traction. Surg Gynecol Obstet 63:513, 1936.
6. Crutchfield WG: Skeletal traction in treatment of injuries to the cervical spine. JAMA 155:29, 1954.
7. Gardner WJ: The principle of spring-loaded points for cervical traction. Technical note. J Neurosurg 39:543, 1973.
8. Rimel RW, Butler AB, Winn R, et al: Modified skull tongs for cervical traction. J Neurosurg 55:848, 1981.
9. Minns RJ, Sutton RA: The mechanics of skull traction calipers. Injury 16:464, 1985.
10. Nickel VL, Perry J, Garrett A, et al: The Halo. A spinal skeletal traction fixation device. J Bone Joint Surg 50:1400, 1968.
11. Fried LC: Cervical spinal cord injury during skeletal traction. JAMA 229:181, 1974.
12. Kaufman HH, Harris JH, Jr, Spencer JA, Kopanisky DR: Danger of traction during radiography for cervical trauma (letter). JAMA 247:2369, 1982.
13. Feldman RA, Khayyat GF: Perforation of the skull by a Gardner-Wells tong. J Neurosurg 44:119, 1976.
14. Weisl H: Unusual complications of skull caliper traction. J Bone Joint Surg 54B:143, 1972.
15. Bracken MB, Shepard MJ, Collins WF, et al: A randomized controlled trial of methylprednisolone or naloxone in the treatment of acute spinal cord injury. N Engl J Med 322:1405, 1990.

Chapter 81

Emergency Drainage of Traumatic Intracranial Hematomas

Robert G. R. Lang

INTRODUCTION

Head injury, termed the *silent epidemic* by the National Head Injury Foundation, disables 30,000 to 50,000 people a year in the United States,[1] and in most published trauma series it accounts for approximately half the fatalities.[2] Although up to 60 per cent of deaths from head injury occur before people are admitted to the hospital,[3] an intracranial hematoma will be present in about 40 per cent of unconscious patients with head injuries who arrive in the emergency department.[4] The mortality rate of these patients has been quoted at a staggering 45 to 90 per cent.[4]

If we assume that brain shift leading to tentorial herniation is an emergency condition that becomes more profound with time, early decompression should result in better survival with less neurologic deficit. Indeed, few medical conditions require more urgent care. Seelig and coworkers reported 30 per cent mortality in patients with acute subdural hematoma who underwent surgery within the first 4 hours following injury and a 90 per cent mortality in those who had surgery later.[5] Bricolo and Pasut had an overall mortality

I would like to thank Edean Berglund, Medical Librarian at St. Peter Hospital, for her assistance in obtaining the reference material; Teresa Edwards, for typing the second edition original manuscript; Elaine Dunn, for typing the revisions; and my wife, Nancy, for her assistance. I would also like to thank Dr. James Stone, Chairman, Division of Neurosurgery, Cook County Hospital, for his critical review of the neurosurgical chapters in the first edition. Many of his recommendations have been incorporated into the second edition.

of 5 per cent in 107 consecutive cases of extradural hematoma and based the better outcome on reducing delays in diagnosis and treatment of intracranial hematomas.[6] Clearly, there is a large group of patients who might benefit from emergency burr holes or twist drill trephination when other conservative measures for lowering intracranial pressure (ICP) have failed.

INTRACRANIAL ANATOMY AND PATHOPHYSIOLOGY

An understanding of the basic pathophysiology of brain shift and altered cerebral blood flow is important for everyone treating the head injured patient.

The cranial cavity is surrounded by a rigid nondistensible structure, the skull, and divided into compartments by the semirigid densely fibrous folds of dura mater: the falx cerebri and tentorium cerebelli (Fig. 81–1). There are three primary components within the cranial cavity: cerebrospinal fluid (CSF), blood, and semigelatinous brain. If there is any addition to the volume of one of the cranial components by hematoma, pus, edema, or tumor, there must be a corresponding decrease in the volume of one or more of the three primary components, otherwise pressure within the compartment rises. Compensation does indeed occur when CSF is expressed from the ventricles and subarachnoid cisterns, when blood is expressed from the collapsible veins, and, in cases of slow growing tumors, when a certain amount of interstitial fluid is squeezed from the brain itself. Once the volume of the mass exceeds the compensating capacity of the compartmental components, pressure rises very rapidly, often within minutes, and brain shift occurs from one compartment toward another. Because of the attachment of cranial nerves and delicate blood vessels the brain tolerates shift very poorly. Ropper correlated progressive lateral displacement of the pineal gland on computed tomography (CT) scan with progressive impairment of consciousness from drowsiness (3 to 4 mm) to coma (8 to 13 mm).[7] In the case of an expanding temporal epidural hematoma, the most medial part of the brain, the uncus, will begin to pass into the tentorial notch (uncal herniation) and the cingulate gyrus will pass under the falx (subfalcine herniation) (Fig. 81–2). The herniating uncus commonly exerts pressure on the oculomotor nerve in the tentorial notch, resulting in pupillary dilation on the side of the hematoma (Fig. 81–3). Pupillary dilation is the most reliable sign for determining

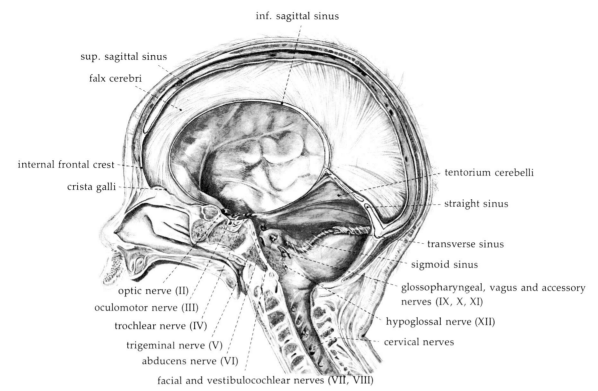

Figure 81–1. Folds of the dura mater. (From Grant JCB: An Atlas of Anatomy. 5th ed. Baltimore, Williams & Wilkins, 1962. Reproduced by permission. © Williams & Wilkins, 1962.)

the side of the hematoma but is correct in only 80 per cent of the cases.[8] When pupillary dysfunction does occur contralateral to the mass lesion, it is often due to direct pressure of the tentorium cerebelli on the displaced oculomotor nerve contralateral to the mass. As brain shift continues, the opposite cerebral peduncle can also be forced against the free edge of the tentorium, producing extremity paralysis on the same side of the hematoma (Kernohan's notch) (see Fig. 81–2). Direct pressure on the ipsilateral cerebral peduncle or, in the case of a posterior frontal hematoma, the motor cortex itself can produce a contralateral paralysis. Thus, paralysis is not as accurate a localizing sign as is pupillary dilation and can be present on the same or opposite

side of the hematoma. Further herniation and shift of the midbrain will result in tearing of delicate perforating vessels and the characteristic midbrain hemorrhages of Duret (Fig. 81–4). At this point, irreversible damage has occurred. Damage to the midbrain reticular formation results in deep unconsciousness and cessation of eye movements, and the pupils become fixed at midposition.

The infratentorial compartment is much smaller than the two supratentorial compartments; compensatory mechanisms are exhausted much more quickly, and volumes tolerated are much smaller. Patients with initial symptoms of drowsiness, incoordination, ataxia, and nystagmus may suddenly become deeply unconscious and apneic. Bradycardia and wide pulse pressure from direct brain stem pressure are more common with infratentorial masses. There can be

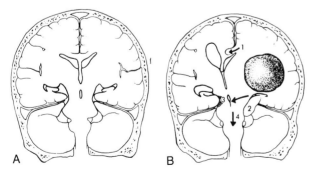

Figure 81–2. Intracranial shifts from supratentorial lesions. *A,* Relationships of the various supratentorial compartments as seen in a coronal section. *B,* Herniation of the cingulate gyrus under the falx *(1),* herniation of the temporal lobe into the tentorial notch *(2),* compression of the opposite cerebral peduncle against the unyielding tentorium, producing Kernohan's notch *(3),* and downward displacement of the brain stem through the tentorial notch *(4).* (From Plum F, Posner JB: The Diagnosis of Stupor and Coma. 2nd ed. Philadelphia, FA Davis Co, 1972. Reproduced by permission.)

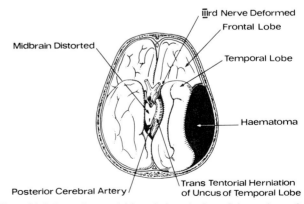

Figure 81–3. Lateral tentorial herniation. A view of the undersurface of the cerebrum shows the distortion produced by a hematoma in the right temporal region. (From Jennett B, Teasdale G: Management of Head Injuries. Philadelphia, FA Davis Co, 1980. Reproduced by permission.)

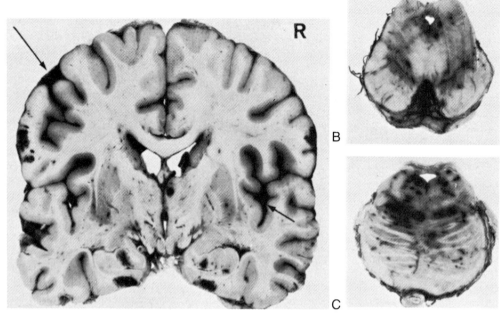

Figure 81–4. Multiple fractures of both sides of the skull in a 47-year-old man. *A,* Coronal section of the brain. Note the contusions in the right and left parietal regions and in the parahippocampal gyri (related to the edge of the tentorium cerebelli). Hemorrhages are present in the hippocampi and in the right thalamus. Subarachnoid blood *(arrows)* and a little intraventricular blood are also seen. *B,* Midbrain. There are several hemorrhages. *C,* Pons. Numerous hemorrhages are present in the floor of the fourth ventricle and in the tegmental region. (From Blackwood W, Corsellis JAN, McMenemy WH: Greenfield's Neuropathology. 3rd ed. London, Edward Arnold, 1976. Reproduced by permission.)

upward herniation through the tentorial notch or downward herniation of cerebellar tonsils through the foramen magnum (tonsillar herniation) (Fig. 81–5). Infratentorial hematomas are difficult to diagnose without CT. If a fracture is seen extending through the occipital bone to the foramen magnum, one should suspect an infratentorial hematoma.

While the relationship between increased ICP and brain shift is one mechanism for impairment of brain function,

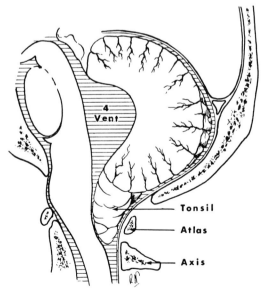

Figure 81–5. Cerebellar tonsils driven between the posterior arch of the atlas and the medulla, which is compressed. (From Jennett B: An Introduction to Neurosurgery. 3rd ed. Chicago, Year Book Medical Publishers, 1977. Reproduced by permission.)

Miller also implicates the influence of ICP on cerebral blood flow.[9] A constant blood flow to the brain is normally maintained by automatic changes in cerebrovascular resistance at the arteriole level, despite fluctuations in the systemic blood pressure. This is known as cerebral autoregulation and will function in the presence of moderate elevations of ICP. Repeated elevations of ICP, however, are believed to damage cerebral autoregulation.[9] When autoregulation is lost, increased ICP reduces cerebral blood flow. As intracranial pressure approaches mean arterial blood pressure, blood flow ceases. This quickly leads to cerebral ischemia and infarction.

BACKGROUND

Successful evacuation of traumatic intracranial hematomas has been carried out since ancient times. Neolithic skulls more than 4000 years old have been found with fractures and man-made defects that suggest surgical removal of bone (Fig. 81–6). Bony proliferation around the edges suggests that the patients survived not only their injury but also the surgery.[10] Implements made of stone (flint), obsidian, shell, and even sharks' teeth were used in various parts of the world,[11] and techniques for trephination included scraping, sawing, and boring. The ancient Egyptians may have used trephining for the treatment of migraine and epilepsy,[12] but it is not mentioned as a treatment for head injuries in Breasted's translation of the Edwin Smith papyrus.[13]

Greek and Roman surgeons were more concerned with the skull fracture itself than with intracranial hematomas. Trephination was practiced by the Hippocratic school, but its rationale was not clearly stated by Hippocrates. It seems that the elimination of blood was not a primary consideration, because the operator often left a thin shell of bone intact.[10] It appears that trephination was practiced more as a prophylactic measure to allow the products of suppuration to escape than as a method of relieving pressure. Later, in approximately 30 B.C., Celsus recommended trephining for meningeal hemorrhage.[14] The important conclusion that pressure on the brain rather than the skull fracture itself was the most significant factor

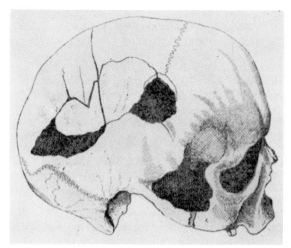

Figure 81–6. Skull from Prunieres' collection, showing a large fracture with defects suggesting the surgical removal of bone. (From Walker AE: Clinical Neurosurgery. Baltimore, Williams & Wilkins, 1959. Reproduced by permission. © Williams & Wilkins, 1959.)

in head injury was not reached, however, until the time of Rhazes, an Arabic physician, who lived about A.D. 900.[15] Unfortunately, Arabic surgeons of Rhazes' era apparently had lost the art of trephination.[16]

Gradually, a better understanding of the pathophysiology of head injury evolved. The significance of the dilated pupil cannot be attributed to any one author, but Jean Louis Petit, in the mid-eighteenth century, recognized that a history of unconsciousness after head injury, followed by a lucid period and then progressive lethargy, was indicative of an extradural hemorrhage. He recommended trephination in all cases of scalp wound with fracture—"Not only to elevate the bone and remove splinters but to give exit of blood effused between the dura and the bone."[16] Hill and Petit operated on subdural hematomas to allow extravasated blood to escape.[10]

Trephination became unpopular during the early nineteenth century because of the high incidence of sepsis, but, after the introduction of the antiseptic technique by Lister in 1867, this rapidly changed. Diagnostic burr holes became so popular in the early twentieth century that they were often done without clear indications; thus, the term *woodpecker surgery* was coined.

Despite the more liberal use of burr holes, extradural hemorrhage remained in most circumstances a lethal condition. One reported series of 99 patients in 1927 had a mortality rate of 86 per cent.[17] With the development of neurosurgery as a subspecialty, one might have expected a progressive decline in mortality throughout the mid-twentieth century. A review of the literature on epidural hemorrhage by Hooper (1959), however, revealed a disparity in mortality statistics. Nine separate studies between 1938 and 1958 had a mortality rate in excess of 30 per cent, whereas another eight studies were under 30 per cent. This led to a review of his own 83 cases in which there were 19 deaths (23 per cent). He stated "That between all these causes of death lies the major factor—delay in operative intervention."[17] The importance of immediate decompression when rapid neurologic deterioration occurred was becoming increasingly recognized in the neurosurgical literature. Although cerebral angiography had reduced the need for diagnostic burr holes, Jamieson and Yeland (1968) reported that epidural hematomas were usually found under the most prominent fractures and that angiography was an unnecessary delay.[18] They had a mortality rate of only 8 per cent with early evacuation. Other more recent studies have clearly established the relationship between early surgical decompression in a patient with an intracranial mass lesion and a better outcome.[5, 6, 19–21]

There have been, however, infrequent reports of trephination in the emergency department. Burton and Blacker (1965) reported on the use of a compact hand drill for emergency decompression.[22] They found this to be most useful for chronic subdural hematomas

that were liquefied and that could easily be evacuated by subsequent needle puncture through the trephine hole. The use of the compact hand drill for trephination was only of occasional assistance in the management of acute head injuries in which epidural or subdural hematomas often consisted of clotted blood, which made aspiration through a needle difficult. Mahoney and associates (1981) reported better results with emergency twist drill trephination.[23] Twist drill trephinations were performed in patients with signs of brain herniation and in whom there was no time for diagnostic studies. Although twist drill holes are easier to place than burr holes, the problem of inadequate decompression remains.

At Cook County Hospital, an emergency burr hole tray is kept ready for use in the emergency department. If a trauma patient with a dilated pupil does not respond to mannitol within 10 to 15 minutes, a low temporal burr hole is placed on the side of the large pupil (or first pupil to dilate) and is enlarged to a small craniectomy.[24] If extradural or subdural hematoma is present, it exudes under pressure. The last pupil to dilate often becomes smaller. When a hematoma is not found on the side of the dilated pupil, the patient's head is turned and a burr hole is placed on the opposite side. The patient is then taken to the operating room for a large fronto-temporo-parietal craniotomy. A CT scan is then performed in the immediate postoperative period to rule out additional hematomas elsewhere in the brain.[25]

The advent of CT has made diagnosis much more rapid. CT scanners are frequently located in close proximity to emergency departments, and an accurate diagnosis can be established in a matter of minutes. Interestingly, Bricolo and Pasut (1984) have linked the increasing availability of CT scanners in small community hospitals to delays in transfer for definitive neurosurgical care.[6] Precious minutes can be wasted in the CT scanner; however, a study by Andrews and colleagues (1986) failed to show improved outcome with burr hole exploration over early CT scanning in severely head injured patients.[26]

Even though experiences in the Korean and Vietnamese wars have led to the development of efficient civilian transport systems for critically injured patients, delay in transfer time still results in significant morbidity and mortality. Studies in the British Isles, where regional medical care has been developed to a very sophisticated degree, have shown that one third of avoidable deaths from head injury were a result of delay in evacuation of an intracranial hematoma.[27] Studies carried out at neurosurgical centers in the United States have shown delays of 1 to 3 hours for treatment of severely head injured patients who are transferred from outlying hospitals.[28] A study by Stone and coworkers (1986) at Cook County Hospital confirmed, over a 12 1/2-year period, decreased morbidity and mortality in patients taken directly to a regional trauma center compared with those patients transferred from outlying hospitals.[20] Fortunately, helicopters and mobile intensive care units are becoming more widely available and should increase the efficiency of transfer to a regional neurosurgical center.

The literature now contains isolated reports of surgical decompression by nonsurgeons in the emergency department[29] and, indeed, by a nonphysician (dentist)[30] that resulted in rapid reversal of neurologic signs of tentorial herniation and full recovery of their respective patients. A review of 50 head injured patients treated with diagnostic burr holes by general surgeons in American Samoa demonstrated an overall mortality rate of 18 per cent. Twenty-three out of the 27 unconscious or obtunded patients had an intracranial hematoma, which was then surgically decompressed. Three of the nine deaths were attributable to a delay in burr hole placement of 24 to 48 hours for evacuation of an intracranial hematoma. The only complication directly attributable to burr hole placement was one superficial wound infection. The nearest neurosurgical center was in Hawaii, 3000 miles away.[31]

INITIAL NONOPERATIVE TREATMENT

The importance of early correct management of the head injured patient from the scene of the accident to the emergency department cannot be overemphasized. The first priority is to get oxygen to the brain. All unconscious patients should be intubated to provide an unobstructed airway, to facilitate ventilatory support, and to prevent aspiration. Lidocaine (10 mg/ml) 1.5 mg/kg is given intravenously 1 minute prior to intubation to blunt the rise in ICP associated with intubation.[32, 33] One should avoid securing the tube with constricting circumferential tapes about the neck, because they can impede venous return. A cricothyroidotomy may be necessary if severe facial fractures are present or if an unstable cervical spine injury is likely. Hyperventilation to a Pco₂ of 30 mm Hg should be routine because excessive hyperventilation will promote vasoconstriction of intracranial vessels.[34] End-tidal CO_2 measurements may provide a useful means of monitoring ventilation.[35]

The blood pressure must be sufficient to perfuse the brain. Hypotension is not a characteristically early feature of severe head injuries and usually indicates an overlooked extracranial injury or severe bleeding from scalp lacerations. Approximately 5 per cent of severe head injuries have associated cervical spine fractures,[36] so great care must be taken to immobilize the spine until adequate radiographs can be obtained. If no cervical fracture is found, the head should be elevated 20 degrees in the neutral position to promote venous drainage and to lower ICP while mean arterial blood pressure is maintained.[37]

Mannitol, 1 gm/kg, should be administered intravenously only when signs of tentorial herniation have developed. The drug can be lifesaving and will often rapidly reverse neurologic deterioration. Indiscriminate use of mannitol may mask signs of impending herniation and give a false sense of security. Hyperosmolar agents work by extracting fluid from normal brain tissue, thereby decreasing ICP. As the pressure decreases, the tamponade effect of the blood clot may be lost and further bleeding may occur. Additional improvement, with repeated doses of mannitol, is less likely with acute bleeding. Some centers also routinely administer furosemide (Lasix), 0.5 mg/kg, in addition to mannitol to further dehydrate the brain while preparing for surgery.

A CT scan or an angiogram must be promptly carried out on all patients who receive mannitol. These studies provide useful diagnostic and anatomic information in patients who do not have progressive herniation. Optimally, hematomas will be discovered prior to the development of brain herniation. CT scan is the procedure of choice for patients with head injuries. Angiography is now used only when a scanner is not available.

INDICATIONS FOR EMERGENCY CRANIAL DECOMPRESSION

Emergency decompression should be performed on any patient who demonstrates or has a history of *progressive neurologic deterioration* and signs of brain herniation. Serial neurologic examinations by the emergency physician are the most reliable indicators of deterioration, but properly trained paramedical personnel can also provide this vital information. Patients who are *immediately* rendered unconscious, who have fixed dilated pupils, and who show absence of eye movements, abnormal posturing (decerebrate) or no extremity response to pain, and irregular or absence of breathing from the time of the accident are likely to have sustained a severe generalized brain contusion. The critical damage occurred at the time of injury, and burr holes will generally *not* be of value. A CT scan or an angiogram must nonetheless be performed to confirm this clinical impression, as nearly 50 per cent of acute subdural hematomas present with the history "unconscious from the time of injury."[24]

A history of head trauma in an unconscious patient with a fixed dilated pupil, hemiplegia, and a skull fracture on the side of the dilated pupil strongly suggests *but does not guarantee* an intracranial hematoma on the same side as the dilated pupil. If the pupil remains dilated after initial nonoperative treatment has been completed, one should immediately create a burr hole. There is usually only a brief period of time before the other pupil dilates and irreversible brain damage occurs.

In the absence of other mitigating information, the first burr hole should be made in the temporal area. Frontal and parietal burr holes should be carried out only if the temporal burr hole is negative and if there is a high level of suspicion of a clot in these areas, i.e., a fracture line there. Epidural hematomas are almost always located under the fracture or area of scalp contusion,[17] whereas subdural hematomas are usually much more extensive and may even develop opposite the site of initial injury. The reduction in ICP is directly proportional to the amount of blood removed. A large fronto-temporo-parietal craniotomy is the preferred treatment for acute subdural hematomas, but this may not be feasible until the patient is transferred to a larger medical center. For similar reasons the burr hole should be expanded to a limited craniectomy approximately 3 cm in diameter if the burr hole is positive for either an epidural or subdural hematoma.

When it is not known which pupil was the first to dilate, emergency *bilateral* burr holes may be necessary as a last resort in the trauma patient who has progressively deteriorated and developed bilateral fixed dilated pupils. In all situations, if burr holes result in negative findings on one side, the other side should always be explored.

Suboccipital burr holes should be considered in any patient who has an occipital skull fracture that extends into the foramen magnum and shows signs of brain stem compression. The burr hole should be placed on the side of the fracture.

There are no absolute contraindications to performing emergency burr holes; however, one subgroup of patients deserves special mention. Prothrombin time (protime) and partial thromboplastin time should be performed with an unconscious patient, and fresh frozen plasma should be administered if a coagulopathy is discovered. Those patients who are on anticoagulants or who are known hemophiliacs are especially susceptible to intracranial hematomas following head injury. If it is known that the patient has been taking anticoagulants, 20 mg of vitamin K should be given promptly along with fresh frozen plasma after the blood samples for coagulation times have been drawn. Additional doses should be given as needed. Uncontrollable bleeding during the procedure is a definite risk if the patient's coagulopathy has not been reversed completely. In a life-threatening emergency, coumadin-induced bleeding may be immediately reversed with prothrombin complex (konyne or Proplex), but this results in almost a 100 per cent incidence of hepatitis.

Patients who have intracranial hematomas but show no sign of tentorial herniation should *not* be subjected to emergency burr holes. These patients should be taken promptly to the operating room by a neurosurgeon. If a neurosurgeon is not available, arrangements should be made for the patient to be immediately transferred to a medical center with a neurosurgeon on staff. Mannitol should be available to the patient during transfer but should be given only if lateralizing signs of tentorial herniation develop. The neurosurgical team at the receiving hospital should be alerted by radiotelephone about any change in the patient's condition. After arrival, the patient can then be taken directly to the operating room or to the CT scanner if no prior significant lesion has been detected.

EQUIPMENT

STANDARD EMERGENCY BURR HOLE TRAY

Essential Equipment
  Number 4 scalpel handle
  Number 12 blade
  Cushing periosteal elevator
  Number 3 Penfield elevator
  2 self-retaining retractors (standard 14.8-cm Wullstein)
  2 hemostats
  Hudson brace
  Cushing perforator and burr attachments for Hudson brace
  Dural hook
  Number 6 scalpel handle and number 11 blade
  Small cottonoids (1 to 2 cm² gauze)
Suture Material
  3–0 silk on spool
  2–0 Vicryl (atraumatic needle)
  2–0 nylon (cutting needle)
Hemostatic Agents
  Topical thrombin
  Gelfoam
  Bone wax
Available with Tray but Separately Wrapped
  Kerrison rongeurs (upbiting 5 mm)
  Leksell rongeurs (full curve wide jaw)
  Small perforator and burr attachments for infants and small children
  Dural suction catheter and sterile tubing for attachment to suction
  Number 19 needle
  Number 22 needle
  6-ml syringe

TWIST DRILL TREPHINATION TRAY

Scalpel with number 11 blade
15/64-inch-diameter Matthews hand drill

TECHNIQUES

Temporal Burr Hole

The patient is first placed in a supine position with a sandbag or folded towel under one shoulder, and the head is rotated so that the side with the dilated pupil is uppermost. The sandbag prevents kinking of the neck and obstruction of venous return (Fig. 81–7). It is often helpful to have a gloved assistant hold the head. The hair is shaved from the temporal scalp, and the head is then scrubbed with povidone-iodine scrub. These procedures can be carried out during other resuscitative measures so that critical minutes are not wasted. The area is then painted with povidone-iodine solution and draped with sterile towels.

A 4-cm vertical skin incision is made, two fingerbreadths anterior and three fingerbreadths above the anterior tragus of the ear (Fig. 81–8). The superficial temporal artery palpable just anterior to the ear should be avoided, and the incision should not extend below the zygoma to prevent injury to the superior branch of the facial nerve. The zygoma is palpable as a ridge of bone that extends toward the outer canthus of the eye from a point just superior and anterior to the external ear canal.

The incision should first be made through skin and subcutaneous tissues so that bleeding from any branches of the superficial temporal artery can be clamped and ligated. The self-retaining retractor is inserted, and the superficial

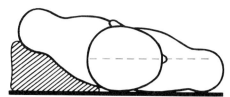

Figure 81–7. The head is turned to the side, and a sandbag is placed under the opposite shoulder. (From Kempe LG: Operative Neurosurgery. Vol 1. Berlin, Springer-Verlag, 1968. Reproduced by permission.)

fascia of the temporalis muscle is exposed. This is divided vertically with a scalpel, and a Cushing periosteal elevator is then scraped back and forth to free the attachments of muscle from the squamosal temporal bone. There is usually some bleeding from the muscle, but this can be controlled by inserting the self-retaining retractor deeper into the wound or by placing another retractor at right angles to the first. The outer surface of the temporal bone should now be visible, and a fracture line can sometimes be identified.

The perforator is connected to the Hudson brace and drilling is begun (Fig. 81–9). A perforating hole is first drilled and then enlarged with a burr. Inserting the tip of the perforator into the fracture line may prevent slippage on the initial turns. It is important to hold the brace perpendicular to the skull so that a clean direct hole is drilled. Firm steady pressure should be used, and frequent checks should be made to assess the depth of the hole. Perforation of the inner table will not be obvious unless an epidural clot is present. The white dura is of a similar color as the surrounding bone. The bone dust must be carefully cleared away with saline irrigation or with the curette to enable one to see the fine line between the inner table and the dura. The soft dura will "give" slightly if gentle pressure is applied with the rounded end of the curette. It is very

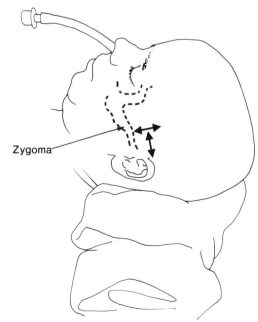

Zygoma

Figure 81–8. The temporal burr hole is placed just above the midpoint of the zygomatic arch and two fingerbreadths anterior to the external auditory canal. (From Simon R, Brenner B: Procedures and Techniques in Emergency Medicine. Baltimore, Williams & Wilkins, 1983. Reproduced by permission. © Williams & Wilkins, 1983.)

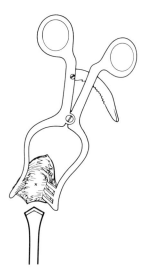

Figure 81–9. The standard hand-held drill introduced through an incision is shown. The drill is centered along the periosteal surface of the outer table. (From Simon R, Brenner B: Procedures and Techniques in Emergency Medicine. Baltimore, Williams & Wilkins, 1983. Reproduced by permission. © Williams & Wilkins, 1983.)

important not to overdrill with the perforator, because the dura can be torn, or worse, the instrument may plunge into the brain. As soon as the tip of the perforator penetrates the inner table, the perforator bit should be switched to the burr. Drilling is then completed, but it is advisable to leave a thin rim of bone to prevent plunging with the burr.

The rim can be scooped out more safely with a curette. This can be done by using the edge of the hole as a fulcrum and directing pressure upward while the curette is turned on its axis. Any bleeding from bone is controlled by application of bone wax. The dark clotted blood of an epidural hematoma or the dura should now be clearly visible. If a subdural hematoma is present, the dura will have a dark-bluish tinge. If the burr hole is to be enlarged, a Penfield number 3 elevator should be inserted between the inner table and the dura all around the burr hole to prevent attached dura from being caught in the jaws of the rongeur. Either a Kerrison or Leksell rongeur can be used (Fig. 81–10). The bone is always removed with upward pressure as the jaws are being closed. An epidural clot should be suc-

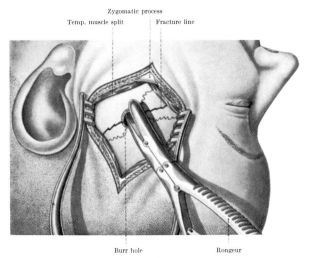

Figure 81–10. Enlarging the burr hole for a left temporal craniectomy. (From Kempe LG: Operative Neurosurgery. Vol 1. Berlin, Springer-Verlag, 1968. Reproduced by permission.)

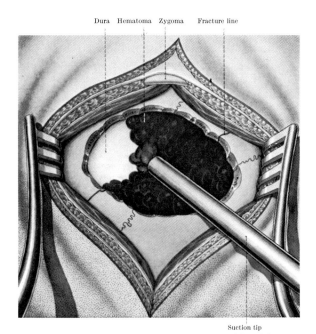

Figure 81–11. A temporal craniectomy for an epidural hematoma. Note that the craniectomy reached down to the level of the zygoma. (From Kempe LG: Operative Neurosurgery. Vol 1. Berlin, Springer-Verlag, 1968. Reproduced by permission.)

tioned cautiously with the dural suction catheter (Fig. 81–11). In an epidural hematoma, the blood is usually thick and clotted. If liquid, it implies continued bleeding. The middle meningeal artery lies deep in relation to the clot, its branches being stripped from the inner surface of the bone by the expanding hematoma. Frequently, because of its arterial origin, the bleeding may be profuse. Blood loss must be replaced with adequate transfusion of crystalloid solutions and blood to maintain normal arterial pressure.

Optimally, the patient will soon be taken to the operating room where adequate exposure can be obtained. The bleeding can then be controlled with bipolar cauterization of the vessel. If the patient is to be transferred and if specialist care is not immediately available, an attempt should be made to find the bleeding point. If suctioning provides clear visualization, bleeding can be controlled with a silk stitch.[38] A 4–0 silk suture on a tapered needle is passed around the vessel proximal to the bleeding point and tied. Great care must be taken not to injure a pial vessel on the brain surface, which would lead to a subdural hematoma. Meningeal bleeders are difficult to control without cautery, because the vessel is enclosed within the layers of the dura and is not amenable to clipping or clamping unless the dura is incised. Alternatively, in the presence of uncontrollable bleeding, the wound should be packed lightly with gauze and left open. The head is then elevated 30 degrees to slow bleeding. If bleeding is from the base of the skull where the artery enters through the foramen spinosum, bone must be removed inferiorly toward the zygoma and the opening must be plugged with bone wax. Further bleeding between the dura and the bone can be controlled by inserting thin strips of thrombin-soaked Gelfoam or muscle stamps around the bony edges. Thin strips or stamps of muscle can be obtained from the temporalis muscle and placed between dura and bone.

In the case of a subdural hematoma, the dura is opened by first inserting the dural hook through the outer layer of the dura and pulling upward. The dura is then opened with a number 11 blade, using gentle stroking motions rather than plunging with the tip of the blade. When the dura is first penetrated, there will often be a sudden gush of bloody fluid if a subdural hematoma is present. When the opening is large enough, a small cottonoid should be inserted to protect the brain beneath and a cruciate opening should be completed. Suctioning a subdural clot is hazardous because of the unprotected brain beneath the clot. The suction should be turned down, and the finger hole on the dural suction catheter should be kept open. The amount of blood that should be removed in an emergency setting is difficult to quantify. Suffice it to say that the object of the procedure is partial decompression; removal of large amounts of clots, particularly in the case of a subdural hematoma, can unleash hemorrhage from large dural veins which may not be controllable. Bleeding points on the surface of the brain can usually be controlled by applying a small piece of thrombin-soaked Gelfoam or muscle stamps and holding them in place with moist cottonoids.

Prior to closure, a pocket should be created around the burr hole by using the periosteal elevator under the temporalis muscle. This will allow further bleeding to accumulate outside the cranial cavity while arrangements are made for more definitive neurosurgical treatment. Under ideal circumstances, the muscle fascia is closed with running 0–0 Vicryl suture and the skin is closed with a running 2–0 nylon interlocking suture. A quick temporary closure can be performed with a running 2–0 nylon interlocking suture catching skin, subcutaneous tissue, and muscle.

Needling the brain for intracerebral clots is extremely hazardous and should not be carried out in the emergency department. If the brain is bulging out of the initial burr hole, it is likely that a clot is present at some other location, perhaps on the other side. Frontal and parietal burr holes should then be considered, and contralateral burr holes should be contemplated if the initial holes result in negative findings.

Frontal and Parietal Burr Holes

Frontal (anterior) burr holes are made through a 4-cm incision located three fingerbreadths from the midline and three fingerbreadths from the hairline (Fig. 81–12). Parietal (posterior) burr holes are placed four fingerbreadths directly behind the frontal burr hole. The parietal incision should be curved inferiorly so that it may later be incorporated in a skin flap if necessary.

There is no muscle, so skin incisions are made through all layers to the skull. The pericranium is freed by blunt dissection using the scalpel handle. After the self-retaining retractor is inserted, additional cuts may be necessary in the pericranium to create a free surface for the perforator. The convexity of the skull in the frontal and parietal regions makes it more difficult to determine when the brace is perpendicular to the surface, and there is often a tendency to cut the burr hole on a bevel. It is most important that the perforator not bevel toward the midline because of the superior sagittal sinus and large perforating veins in the midline. Arachnoid villi tend to be evident toward the midline, and when a hole is drilled over them, they often bleed profusely. Such hemorrhaging can be controlled by application of thrombin-soaked Gelfoam and a moist cottonoid. If bleeding persists and is uncontrollable, the hole can be plugged with bone wax and another hole can be drilled. Closure of the frontal and parietal burr holes in the emergency department should involve use of one layer of 2–0 nylon through skin and galea if the patient is being taken to the operating room. If not, a two-layer closure with 2–0 inverted Vicryl in the galea and 2–0 nylon in the skin is the preferred technique.

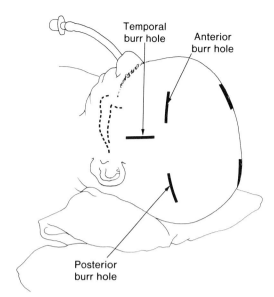

Figure 81–12. The sites of incision and burr hole placement. (From Simon R, Brenner B: Procedures and Techniques in Emergency Medicine. Baltimore, Williams & Wilkins, 1983. Reproduced by permission. © Williams & Wilkins, 1983.)

Suboccipital Burr Holes

A patient with posterior clots will usually need assisted ventilation. In addition, positioning of the patient will require maximal neck flexion. Such a patient should therefore have been intubated and undergone cervical spine x-rays prior to positioning. The patient is then turned on his side with the head supported on folded towels and the neck maximally flexed by an assistant. The side on which the clot is suspected should be in the uppermost position. The occipital and upper cervical regions must be shaved and scrubbed with povidone-iodine. After infiltration with lidocaine and epinephrine (to control surface bleeding), an incision is made midway between the external occipital protuberance and the mastoid and is extended 4 cm into the upper cervical region. The posterior fossa is located below the superior nuchal line. The skin and subcutaneous tissues are densely adherent to the underlying tissues and can be undermined with lateral cuts just above the muscle layer. This will allow insertion of the self-retaining retractor. The muscles are then divided vertically. The occipital artery may cause troublesome bleeding and should be ligated. The attachments of the muscles below the superior nuchal line are separated from the occipital bone with a periosteal elevator, and, if necessary for better exposure, the attachments along the superior nuchal line may also be divided.

Laterally, it is important to stop at the emissary veins from the proximal sigmoid sinus, which penetrate the occipital bone just behind the mastoid. Very profuse venous bleeding may occur if these veins are damaged. If this occurs, bleeding from the bone should be controlled with bone wax and the head should be elevated to collapse the veins. Suture ligature in the muscle may be necessary, and muscle stamps applied with moist cottonoids can be used to control dural sinus bleeding.

The burr hole should be drilled over the fracture site, if it is evident, and must be either above or below the superior nuchal line to avoid the transverse sinus (Fig. 81–13). If the burr hole is too far lateral, mastoid air cells can be penetrated. If the mastoid air cells are entered, they

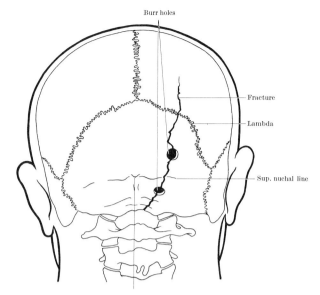

Figure 81–13. The placement of burr holes in extradural hematoma over the occipital and suboccipital areas. (From Kempe LG: Operative Neurosurgery. Vol 1. Berlin, Springer-Verlag, 1968. Reproduced by permission.)

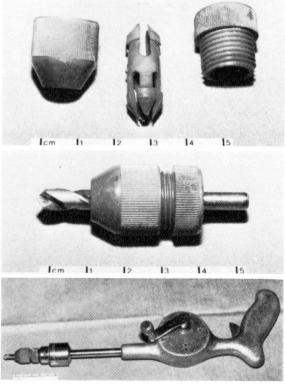

A

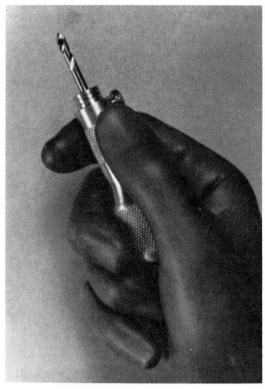

B

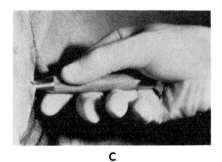

C

Figure 81–14. *A: Top,* Twist drill stop, unassembled. From left to right are the end cap, the central sleeve, and the front cap. *Center,* The twist drill stop in place on the drill bit. *Bottom,* The twist drill with the bit and fully assembled. (From Grode ML, Carton CA: Drill stop for twist drill. Technical note. J Neurosurg 52:599, 1980. Reproduced by permission.) *B,* Method of grasping a compact hand drill. The bit length can be varied by using a set screw. (From Burton C, Blacker HM: A compact hand drill for emergency brain decompression. J Trauma 5:643, 1965. Reproduced by permission. © Williams & Wilkins, 1965.) *C,* Trephining the skull. (From Mahoney BD, Rockswold GL, Ruiz E, et al: Emergency twist drill trephination. Neurosurgery 8:552, 1981. Reproduced by permission. © Williams & Wilkins, 1981.)

should be plugged with bacitracin- or neomycin-impregnated bone wax. Also, the transverse sinus curves laterally as the sigmoid sinus and passes deep to the mastoid. The sigmoid sinus must also be avoided. Thus, it is important that the burr hole be drilled in the center, midway between the mastoid and external occipital protuberance and midway between the superior nuchal line and ring of foramen magnum. If an epidural hematoma is not encountered, the dura should be opened. Following the procedure the muscle fascia is closed with 0–0 Vicryl suture and the skin is closed with 2–0 nylon interlocking suture.

Temporal Twist Drill Trephination

Twist drill trephination uses a 15/64-inch drill bit secured to either a standard surgical drill (Fig. 81–14*A*) or a hand twist drill (Fig. 81–14*B*). The equipment for this technique and the technique itself are simpler than those for burr holes, and twist drill trephination can be performed more quickly. The hole, however, is very small, and further decompression by craniectomy is not possible. The procedure is carried out through a small incision rather than by direct vision as in the case of burr holes. Damage to underlying brain by an inadvertent plunge might be less severe with a twist drill than with the perforator or burr. Unfortunately, only a limited amount of clotted blood can be removed, and there is no exposure to control meningeal or surface bleeding.

Mahoney and associates[23] have used twist drill trephination for emergency decompression in patients with uncal herniation.[23] Their technique is as follows. After suitable cervical radiographs have been obtained, the patient can be positioned nose up or turned to the side with a sandbag under the shoulder. The hair on the side of the dilated pupil is shaved, and the head is scrubbed with povidone-iodine while other resuscitative measures are being taken. A 2.5-cm vertical incision is made two fingerbreadths anterior and two to three fingerbreadths superior to the tragus of the ear after infiltrating the skin with lidocaine and epinephrine (Fig. 81–15). A 15/64-inch-diameter Matthews hand drill (Codman Surgical Instruments, Randolph, MA) is used to trephine the skull (see Fig. 81–14*C*). Binding of the drill bit can be felt at the diploë and inner table. On penetrating the inner table, the drill is withdrawn and the wound is observed for return of blood. The source of bright red bleeding is likely to be the skin margin or the diploë. Dark clotted blood indicates an epidural hematoma if the dura was not lacerated. If no blood returns, the dura is elevated with a dural hook and a nick is carefully made in the dura with a number 11 blade. Once again, the wound is observed for the return of dark blood, this time from a

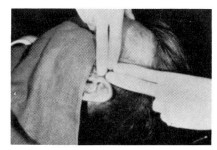

Figure 81–15. Measuring the location of the incision. (From Mahoney BD, Rockswold GL, Ruiz E, et al: Emergency twist drill trephination. Neurosurgery 8:552, 1981. Reproduced by permission. © Williams & Wilkins, 1981.)

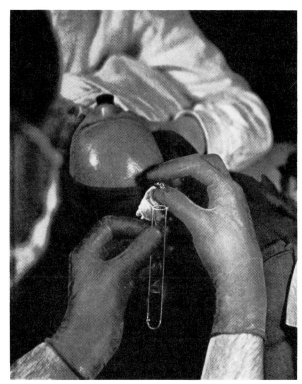

Figure 81–16. Note that the subdural needle is placed away from the midline. The shaft of the needle is held firmly against the scalp so that it will not wiggle. (From Ingraham FD, Matson DD: Neurosurgery of Infancy and Childhood. Springfield, Ill, Charles C Thomas, 1954. Reproduced by permission.)

subdural hematoma. If dark red blood is obtained, it can sometimes be further evacuated by careful suctioning with a sterile catheter.

Infant Subdural Tap

The infant is placed supine in the nose-up position, and excessive flexion of the neck is avoided. The scalp is then shaved over the lateral margins of the anterior fontanelle. The skin is scrubbed with povidone-iodine for 10 minutes, then draped with sterile towels; local anesthetic is not used. A subdural needle is inserted through the skin at the extreme lateral limit of the anterior fontanelle where it meets the coronal suture (Fig. 81–16). A zig-zag puncture is used to prevent later leakage of subdural fluid. The needle is first inserted through the skin, then the skin is moved with the needle in place before the pericranium is penetrated. The needle is then pushed through the pericranium into the subdural space. The subdural fluid is allowed to drain spontaneously, and specimens are collected for Gram stain, culture, cells, sugar, and protein. The fluid is never aspirated for fear of drawing pial vessels into the point of the needle. If a pial vessel is punctured, bleeding will usually cease spontaneously. The procedure is then repeated on the opposite side. A firm sterile occlusive dressing should then be applied. If continued leakage occurs from the puncture site, colodium-impregnated cotton fluff applied over the puncture wound and elevation of the head 20–30 degrees will usually stop it.

Ventricular Puncture

Acute obstruction to the flow of CSF can produce severe headaches, vomiting, unconsciousness, and death from cen-

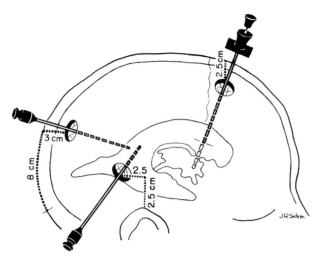

Figure 81–17. The three standard trephination sites used to gain access to the lateral ventricles. The anterior site, or Kocher point, is 3 cm posterior to the normal hairline and 2.5 cm lateral to the midline. The Keen point or lateral trephine opening permits tapping of the trigone of the lateral ventricle. The Keen point is 2.5 cm behind and 2.5 cm above the top of the ear. The posterior aspect of the lateral ventricle is approached through a posterior parietal trephine opening that is 8 cm above the inion and 2.5 to 3 cm lateral to the midline. (From Zingesser LH, Schechter MM: Encephalography. *In* Youmans JR: Neurological Surgery. 2nd ed. Vol 1. Philadelphia, WB Saunders Co, 1982. Reproduced by permission.)

tral brain herniation. There are multiple causes for acute hydrocephalus. Most patients with this disorder seen in the emergency department have an obstructed shunt. In certain cases, a small cyst (colloid cyst) acts like a ball valve at the foramen of Monro. Subarachnoid hemorrhage, infection, and various congenital conditions can all cause hydrocephalus. Most often, symptoms progress gradually, and the majority of shunt obstructions can be relieved by tapping the shunt through its reservoir. In certain cases, direct ventricular puncture will be lifesaving.

A needle can be inserted into the lateral ventricle through either a frontal or parietal burr hole (Fig. 81–17). The point of reference for a frontal approach is the inner canthus of the ipsilateral eye, whereas for a parietal approach, the pupil of the ipsilateral eye is the reference point. A maximum of three attempts should be made. The ventricles are usually encountered at a depth of 5.5 cm from the burr hole, but in hydrocephalic patients, they can be encountered at much shallower depths.

Possible complications include ventriculitis, intraventricular hemorrhage, and porencephaly. The needle must be held steady while it is in the brain.

COMPLICATIONS

The most serious complication of emergency burr hole placement would be an inadvertent plunge with the perforator or burr. Frequent checks of the depth of the hole and controlled pressure are most important to prevent this catastrophe. A plastic drill stop has been designed for twist drills to prevent inadvertent plunge with this instrument (see Fig. 81–14C).[39] If the brain is penetrated, bleeding is usually from superficial vessels in the pial arachnoid. Such bleeding can be controlled with pieces of thrombin-soaked Gelfoam. The head should be elevated to slow the bleeding

and the patient transferred to a neurosurgical center as soon as possible.

Infection is a possible complication. Mahoney and associates reported one death from Pseudomonas meningitis in a patient who had an emergency twist drill trephination.[23] The patient had multiple injuries, including basal skull fractures, and a direct causal relationship to the trephination could not be established. Patients who receive emergency burr holes should be covered with a broad-spectrum antibiotic such as ceftriaxone.

Perforation of major sinuses or other vessels can occur if the burr holes are placed in an improper location.

CONCLUSION

Emergency trephination was performed by Mahoney and colleagues[23] on 41 patients.[23] Ten patients had bilateral procedures, resulting in a total of 51 trephinations. Twenty-three of these patients had significant extracerebral hematoma, and 18 others had cerebral contusions and intraparenchymal or extraventricular hematomas. Thirty-two of the patients died (78 per cent) and nine survived. Of the 23 patients with extracerebral hematomas, 6 of them showed therapeutic efficiency with a rapid decrease in the size of the previously dilated pupil shortly after release of the clotted blood (estimated range 10 to 50 ml; average about 20 ml). Of the six patients who showed a therapeutic response, three of them later died because of their injuries and three recovered to an independent functional state.

Hoff and associates[40] performed exploratory burr holes on 100 patients who had signs of tentorial herniation.[37] In one third of the patients, extracerebral hematomas were shown on the initial burr hole examination. Forty-seven of the patients survived, and, of these patients, 22 had removal of a significant hematoma. In four of these patients, the burr holes were nondiagnostic and the hematomas were removed after angiography or CT scanning. In the remaining 25 survivors, no further operations for removal of intracranial clot were required. Hoff and coworkers believe that early burr hole exploration was beneficial to one third of their patients.

There is an understandable hesitancy for personnel who do not have formal neurosurgical training to drill holes in the skull and attempt to evacuate intracranial blood. Certain skills are required, but the degree of difficulty should be no greater than insertion of a chest tube. The techniques described should be optional procedures in the emergency physician's management of patients with multiple trauma.

Early diagnosis and immediate surgical decompression of significant intracranial hematomas are now the accepted neurosurgical standards of care for patients with severe head injuries. Optimally these patients are taken from the scene of the accident directly to a regional trauma center where subspecialty support including neurosurgery is available. Cranial burr hole decompression in the emergency department should only be performed on the preterminal patient who is developing clinical signs of brain herniation and is unresponsive to conservative measures and in whom there is a high index of suspicion for an intracranial hematoma.

REFERENCES

1. Clifton GC: Head injury incidence and organization of prehospital care. Neurol Clin IV:3, 1982.
2. Pitts LH, Martin N: Head injuries. Surg Clin North Am 62:47, 1982.
3. Field JH: Epidemiology of Head Injuries in England and Wales. London, Department of Health and Social Security, Her Majesty's Stationery Office, 1976.
4. Becker DP, Miller JD, Ward JD, et al: The outcome from severe head injury with early diagnosis and intensive management. J Neurosurg 47:491, 1977.
5. Seelig JM, Becker DP, Miller JD, et al: Traumatic acute subdural hematoma: Major mortality reduction in comatose patients treated within four hours. N Engl J Med 304:1511, 1981.
6. Bricolo AP, Pasut LM: Epidural hematoma: Toward zero mortality. A prospective study. Neurosurgery 14:8, 1984.
7. Ropper AW: Lateral displacement of the brain and level of consciousness in patients with an acute hemispheral mass. N Engl J Med 314:953, 1986.

8. Bruce DA, Gennarelli TA, Langfitt TW: Resuscitation from coma due to head injury. Crit Care Med 6:254, 1978.
9. Miller JD: Volume and pressure in the craniospinal axis. Clin Neurosurg 22:76, 1975.
10. Walker AE: The dawn of neurosurgery. Clin Neurosurg 6:3, 16, 1959.
11. Parry TW: Trephination of the living human skull in prehistoric times. Br Med J March 17, 1923.
12. Mumford JG: Narrative of surgery; a historic sketch. In Keen's Surgery. Philadelphia, WB Saunders Company, 1907.
13. Breasted JH: The Edwin Smith Papyrus. Chicago, University of Chicago Press, 1930.
14. Celsus AC: DeMedicina, trans. WG Spencer, Vol. 3. London, W Heineman Ltd., 1938, pp 294–649.
15. Mettler CC: History of Medicine. York, PA, Maple Press Co., 1947, p 826.
16. Horrax H: Neurosurgery: A Historical Sketch. Springfield, Charles C Thomas, Publisher, 1952, p 135.
17. Hooper R: Observations on extradural hemorrhage. Br J Surg 47:71, 1959.
18. Jamieson KG, Yelland JON: Extradural hematoma. Report of 167 cases. J Neurosurg 29:13, 1968.
19. Soloniuk D, Pitts LH, Lovely M, Bartkowski H: Traumatic intracerebral hematomas: Timing of appearance and indications for operative removal. J Trauma 26:787, 1986.
20. Stone JL, Lowe RJ, Jonasson O, et al: Acute subdural hematoma: Direct admission to a trauma center yields improved results. J Trauma 26:445, 1986.
21. Rockswold GL, Leonard PR, Nagib MG: Analysis of management in thirty three closed head injury patients who talked and deteriorated. Neurosurgery 21:51, 1987.
22. Burton C, Blacker HM: A compact hand drill for emergency brain decompression. J Trauma 5:643, 1965.
23. Mahoney BD, Rockswold GL, Ruiz E, Clinton JE: Emergency twist drill trephination. Neurosurgery 8:551, 1981.
24. Stone JL, Rifai MHS, Sugar O, et al: Subdural hematomas: Part I acute subdural hematoma. Progress in definition of clinical pathology and therapy. Surg Neurol 19:216, 1983.
25. Stone JL: Personal communication, September 3, 1983.
26. Andrews BT, Pitts LH, Lovely MP, Bartkowski H: Is computed tomo-

graphic scanning necessary in patients with tentorial herniation? Results of immediate surgical exploration without computed tomography in 100 patients. Neurosurgery 19:408, 1986.
27. Jeffreys RV, Jones JJ: Avoidable factors contributing to the death of head injury patients in general hospitals in Mersey region. Lancet 2:459, 1981.
28. Rimel RW, Jane JA, Edlich RF: An educational training program for the care at the site of injury of trauma to the central nervous system. Resuscitation 9:23, 1981.
29. Springer MFB, Baker FJ: Cranial burr hole decompression in the emergency department. Am J Emerg Med 6:640, 1988.
30. Reyna TM, Madauss WC: Emergency treatment of epidural hematoma: Case report. Mil Med 146:504, 1981.
31. Schecter WP, Peper E, Tuatoo V: Can general surgery improve the outcome of head injury victim in rural america? A review of experience in American Samoa. Arch Surg 120:1163, 1985.
32. Hamil SF, Bedford RF, Weaver DC, Coloham AR: Lidocaine before endotracheal intubation: Intravenous or laryngotracheal? Anaesthesiology SS:578, 1981.
33. Ampel L, Hott KA, Sielaff GW, Sloan TB: An approach to airway management in the acutely head-injured patient. J Emerg Med 6:1, 1988.
34. Cold GE: Does acute hyperventilation provoke cerebral oligaemia in comatose patients after head injury? Acta Neurochir (Wien) 96:100, 1989.
35. Mackersie RC, Karagianes TG, York J, et al: End-tidal PCO2 monitoring during resuscitation of severe head injuries. (abstract) Crit Care Med 17:S45, 1989.
36. Saul TG, Ducker TB: Management of severe head injuries. Mo State Med J 45, 1981.
37. Davenport A, Will EJ, Davison AM: Effect of posture on intracranial pressure and cerebral perfusion pressure in patients with fulminant hepatic and renal failure after acetaminophen self-poisoning. Crit Care Med 18:286, 1990.
38. Rosenfeld JV: The emergency burr hole: Indication and technique. Papua New Guinea Med J 25:189, 1982.
39. Grode ML, Carton CA: Drill stop for twist drill—technical note. J Neurosurg 52:599, 1980.
40. Hoff JT, Spetzler R, Winestock D: Head injury and early signs of tentorial herniation—a management dilemma. West J Med 128:112, 1978.

Chapter 82

Spinal Puncture and Cerebrospinal Fluid Examination

Jon C. Kooiker

INTRODUCTION

Spinal fluid examination is performed in an emergency setting for the purpose of obtaining information that will be relevant to the diagnosis and treatment of specific disease entities. Many urgent and life-threatening conditions require immediate and accurate knowledge of the nature of the cerebrospinal fluid (CSF). Certain harmful consequences may result from a spinal puncture, however, and this procedure should follow a careful neurologic examination with thought given to the risks and merits of the procedure in each given situation.

In 1885, Corning punctured the subarachnoid space to introduce cocaine into a living patient.[1] Quincke (1891) first removed CSF in a diagnostic study and introduced the use of a stylet.[2] He studied cellular contents and measured protein and glucose levels. Quincke was also the first to record pressure with a manometer. Subsequently, increasingly sophisticated bacteriologic, biochemical,

cytologic, and serologic techniques were introduced. In 1918, Dandy replaced spinal fluid with air to determine normal brain anatomy and changes that would indicate disease.[3] Iodinized oil and, more recently, water-soluble contrast media have been used to delineate the spinal subarachnoid space and cerebral cisterns.[4] Other uses of the spinal puncture include injection of anesthetic agents, chemotherapeutic agents, and antibiotics and drainage of fluids.

ANATOMY OF SPINAL FLUID FORMATION AND CIRCULATION

In the adult, approximately 140 ml of the spinal and cranial cavities is occupied by CSF. This volume is the result of a balance between continuous secretion (primarily by the ventricular choroid plexus) and absorption into the venous system (chiefly by way of the arachnoid villi). After formation, the fluid passes out of the ventricles by way of the foramina of Luschka and Magendie. The fluid then flows into the spinal subarachnoid space, the basilar cisterns, and the cerebral subarachnoid space. Production is approximately 0.35 ml per minute, and CSF ventricular production is such that there is a net flow out of the ventricles of 50 to 100 ml per day.

Spinal fluid may have an embryologic nutritive function; at maturity the CSF most likely acts as a mechanical barrier between the soft brain and the rigid fibrous-osseous dura, skull, and vertebral column. It also appears to support the weight of the brain.[5] Contraction and expansion of the CSF may accommodate changes in brain volume. Additional functions, including intracerebral transport and maintenance of a stable chemical environment of the central nervous system (CNS), have been reviewed by Fishman.[6]

INDICATIONS FOR SPINAL PUNCTURE

In recent years, the indications for spinal puncture have been reduced with the introduction of new noninvasive diagnostic procedures—primarily computed transaxial tomography (CT). A few clinical situations require an early, or even an emergent, spinal puncture. The primary indication for an emergent spinal tap is the possibility of CNS infection. CSF should be examined in patients with a fever of unknown origin, especially if an alteration of consciousness is present, even in the absence of meningeal irritation. Meningeal signs need not be present in patients who are old, debilitated, immunosuppressed, or receiving anti-inflammatory drugs or who have had partial treatment with antibiotics. In a newborn, even a fever is not a dependable sign; temperatures may be normal or even subnormal. A tense and bulging fontanelle is somewhat more reliable, although this sign may be absent in a dehydrated child. In a child between the ages of 1 month and 3 years, fever, irritability, and vomiting are the most common symptoms of meningitis. Typically, handling is painful for the child, and the child cannot be comforted. In addition, the older child may complain of a headache. In all ages, the patient looks unusually ill and appears drowsy with a dulled sensorium.[7-9] Physical signs become more useful in diagnosing meningitis in children past 3 years of age. These include nuchal rigidity, Kernig's sign (efforts to extend the knee are resisted), and Brudzinski's sign (passive flexion of one hip causes the other leg to rise, and efforts to flex the neck make the knees come up). A useful aid in distinguishing neck rigidity of meningeal origin from that caused by primary pain in the cervical muscles and the soft tissues is the usual preservation of lateral movement in meningeal irritation. A petechial skin rash in a febrile child should also raise the possibility of *Neisseria* meningitis.[10]

The second indication for an emergent spinal puncture is a suspected spontaneous subarachnoid hemorrhage. The diagnosis will usually be made by CT or by the finding of blood in the spinal fluid. A small "warning bleed" from a subarachnoid hemorrhage may not be diagnosed with either a CT scan or lumbar puncture. If CT is available, then this noninvasive radiologic procedure, which has the potential to distinguish between aneurysmal and primary intracerebral bleeding, is preferred over spinal puncture.[11] A normal computed tomogram, however, *may not rule out a subarachnoid hemorrhage, and an appropriate clinical setting requires a confirmatory spinal puncture.*[12] Failure to detect blood radiographically may indicate a small bleed or a predominant basal accumulation of blood. If a patient is seen several days after the hemorrhage, the blood may have become isodense with brain and may no longer be visible.[13, 14] The proper diagnosis would then require spinal puncture. Since 5 to 8 per cent of acute subarachnoid hemorrhages will not be detected by the initial CT scan, some authors maintain that a lumbar puncture is mandatory to rule out the diagnosis with certainty.[14a, 14b]

The usual clinical picture of a subarachnoid hemorrhage is a severe and sudden excruciating headache. The location of the headache is variable and does not give a clue as to the site of hemorrhage. Nausea, vomiting, and prostration are common symptoms, with approximately one third of patients becoming unconscious at the onset. Examination shows an acutely ill patient with an altered mental status. Meningeal signs are commonly present at the time of the initial examination and usually develop in all cases within 2 to 3 days. Meningeal signs may become more severe during the first week after hemorrhage and correspond to the breakdown of blood in the spinal fluid. During the first week, many patients are febrile, reflecting a chemical hemic

meningitis.[15, 16] In theory, a small subarachnoid hemorrhage may take several hours to reach the lumbar region. Thus, it is possible that such a patient might have normal lumbar CSF if examined soon after rupture. A second, delayed lumbar puncture may occasionally be required for diagnosis in such a situation. If the neurologic picture demonstrates localizing findings, the presence of a large intracranial hematoma should be suspected, and spinal puncture is contraindicated until CT (or arteriography) delineates the nature of the lesion.

In a patient with suspected cerebral embolus or evolving infarct, either a computed tomogram or clear spinal fluid should be obtained prior to the use of anticoagulants. This seems particularly applicable if neurologic deficits or an altered mental state persists.[17]

Other nonemergent reasons for CSF examination include evaluation of CNS syphilis, instillation of chemotherapy and positive contrast agents, evaluation of suspected multiple sclerosis, and treatment of headache from subarachnoid hemorrhage or benign intracranial hypertension.[18] Carcinomatous meningitis and suspected spinal cord compression from metastatic disease may require spinal puncture for myelography. The availability of magnetic resonance imaging (MRI) is a suitable alternative for identifying compressive myelopathies.

CONTRAINDICATIONS

Spinal puncture is absolutely contraindicated in the presence of infection in the tissues near the puncture site.[5, 6] Spinal puncture is relatively contraindicated in the presence of increased intracranial pressure from a space-occupying lesion. Caution is particularly advised when lateralizing signs (hemiparesis) or signs of uncal herniation (unilateral third nerve palsy with altered level of consciousness) are present. In such cases, a tentorial or cerebellar pressure cone may be precipitated or aggravated by the spinal puncture. Cardiorespiratory collapse, stupor, seizures, and sudden death may occur when pressure is reduced in the spinal canal.[18] The risk seems to be particularly pronounced in patients with brain abscess.[19, 20] Brain abscesses frequently occur as expanding intracranial lesions with headache, mental disturbances, and focal neurologic signs rather than as infectious processes with signs of meningeal irritation. In 75 per cent of cases, a primary source of chronic suppuration is present.[19] Metastatic hematogenous spread of bacterial infection (from sepsis, intrathoracic infection, or congenital cardiac malformations with endocarditis) and prior otolaryngologic infection are of major importance in the genesis of cerebral abscesses. Although the CSF is usually abnormal (elevated pressure, elevated white blood cell count, and elevated protein concentration), spinal puncture in patients with possible brain abscess should be discouraged. Five of Samson and Clark's 22 patients exhibited signs of midbrain compression within 2 hours of lumbar puncture.[20] Evidence of herniation markedly reduces the patient's chances for survival.

Patients with ruptured brain abscesses, unfortunately, may present with an associated purulent meningitis. If the history suggests possible brain abscess, CT can rapidly diagnose and localize the lesion.[21-23] Kaufman and Leeds reported rapid and accurate demonstration in nine cases of brain abscesses and in six cases of subdural and epidural empyema with no false-negative studies.[21] Since the appearance of brain abscesses on computed tomograms is similar to that of neoplastic and vascular lesions, however, false-positive reports of brain abscess may be encountered.

Trauma to the dural or arachnoid vessels may result in

blood contaminating the spinal fluid. This generally is of little consequence. Spinal epidural hematomas may occur but are rare complications of lumbar puncture in individuals receiving anticoagulant therapy or in patients with disease associated with abnormal clotting mechanisms, especially thrombocytopenia. Edelson and colleagues found over 100 cases of spinal epidural hematoma, approximately one third associated with anticoagulant therapy.[24] Most articles describe isolated cases.[17, 24–26] Spinal subdural hematomas following lumbar puncture are even more rare than epidural hematomas. When a patient is anticoagulated or has a coagulopathy, the tap should be performed by experienced physicians, who are less likely to traumatize the dura. The patient should be carefully followed for progressive back pain, lower extremity motor and sensory deficits, and sphincter impairment after the procedure. *Complaints of motor weakness, sensory loss, or incontinence following lumbar puncture should be thoroughly investigated.* Lumbar puncture may be performed in the presence of a coagulation defect if it is confined to situations in which it may provide essential information, such as in the diagnosis of meningitis. In cases of severe thrombocytopenia, the infusion of platelets prior to the lumbar puncture may be desirable. Similarly, the infusion of clotting factors in the hemophiliac patient and normalization of the prothrombin time with fresh frozen plasma in the anticoagulated patient are desirable if the clinical situation permits such delay.

If the history and physical examination suggest a treatable illness, such as meningitis, then the physician may perform a spinal puncture after careful consideration of the entire clinical picture. In all cases, the study should be undertaken after careful thought regarding how the results will assist in patient evaluation and treatment. It is unlikely that the spinal puncture will alter management in the presence of a neoplasm, a hematoma, a completed nonembolic infarct, or cranial trauma.

TECHNIQUE

Lumbar puncture is carried out with the patient in the lateral recumbent position. A line connecting the posterior superior iliac crests will intersect the midline at approximately the L4 spinous process (Fig. 82–1).[27, 28] The adjacent interspace above or below may be used, depending upon which area appears to be most open to palpation. The space between lumbar vertebrae is relatively wide. In the thoracic region, the spinous processes overlap and are directed caudally, and therefore there is no midline area free of overlying bone. In the adult, the spinal cord extends to the lower level of L1 or the body of L2, thus eliminating higher levels as sites for puncture. The puncture in adults and in older children may be performed from the L2 to L3 interspace to the L5 to S1 interspace. Developmentally, the spinal canal and the spinal cord are of equal length in the fetus. Growth of the cord does not keep pace with longitudinal growth of the spinal canal. At birth, the cord ends at the level of the L3 vertebra. The needle in infants should be placed at the L4 to L5 or L5 to S1 interspaces. The subarachnoid space extends to an S2 vertebral level; however, the overlying bony mass prevents entry into this lower-most portion of the subarachnoid space.[27]

Almost all patients are afraid of a spinal puncture because they have heard stories of severe complications. Explaining the procedure in advance and discussing each step during the course of the test aids in reducing patient tension and helps the physician. The physician should inquire about history of allergies to local anesthetic agents and topical antiseptics. A standard informed consent form is available in hospitals. In view of the transient nature of physician-patient relations in emergency departments, this should be used when spinal punctures are performed, providing the patient is competent and of legal majority or an appropriate guardian is present.

The next important step is positioning of the patient. The patient is given a pillow to keep his head in the same plane as the vertebral axis. The shoulders and the hips are positioned perpendicular with the table. A firm table or bed is desirable whenever possible. Flexion of the neck does *not* facilitate the procedure to any great extent, and since severe flexion may add to the patient's discomfort, this step may be omitted. The patient's lower back should be arched toward the physician. Some physicians place the patient in a sitting position, because the midline is more easily identified when the patient is sitting. The higher CSF hydrostatic pressure in a sitting, dehydrated patient may aid CSF flow. Caution regarding orthostatic blood pressure changes and airway maintenance must be observed when the patient is sitting for the procedure. An assistant must also help support the patient during the procedure.

Sterile gloves must be used. The examiner should wash the patient's back with an antiseptic solution applied in a circular motion and should increase the circumference of the pattern with each motion. A povidone-iodine solution will decrease skin flora to a bacterial count of zero to two bacteria per square inch. Friction during skin preparation helps remove loose debris.[28] The patient should be warned that the solution will be cold. The excess fluid is removed with a dry sterile gauze pad. A sterile towel is placed between the patient's hip and the bed. Commercial trays have a

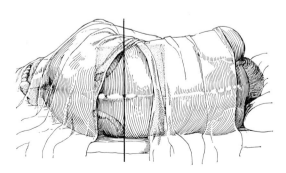
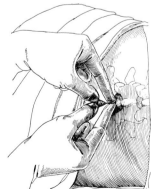

Figure 82–1. When the patient has been correctly positioned for the lumbar tap *(left),* an imaginary line connecting the iliac crests will be exactly perpendicular to the bed. Insertion sites are marked by "x"; the operative field is draped. The needle should be inserted perpendicularly (or nearly so) to the plane of the back, with the forefingers of both hands guiding it in *(right).* (From Cole M: Pitfalls in cerebrospinal fluid examination. Hosp Pract 47, 1969. Illustration by Carol Donner. Reproduced by permission.)

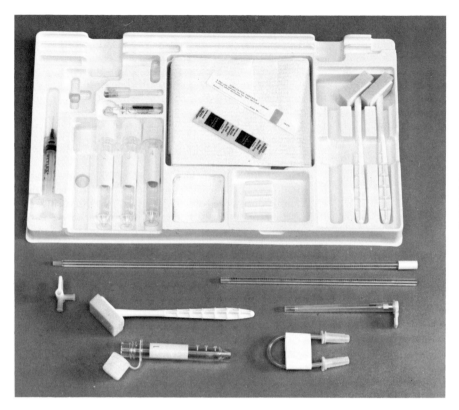

Figure 82–2. Standard lumbar puncture tray. Separate equipment is available for infants, children, and adults. (Courtesy of the American Pharmaseal Company, Glendale, Calif.)

second sterile drape with a hole that may be centered over the site selected for the tap (Fig. 82–2).

The skin and deeper subcutaneous tissue are infiltrated with local anesthetic (1 per cent lidocaine). The patient should be warned about transient discomfort from the anesthetic. Anesthetizing the deeper subcutaneous tissue renders the procedure almost painless. Merely raising a skin wheal is insufficient anesthesia. While waiting for the anesthetic to take effect, the physician should attach the stopcock and manometer and see that the valve is working. A 3½-inch, 20-gauge needle should be used in adults, and a 2½-inch, 22-gauge needle should be used in children. (A 1½-inch, 22-gauge needle is available for infants.) A needle of this size has enough rigidity to allow the procedure to be accomplished easily but makes less of a dural tear than do larger instruments. The patient should be told to report any pain and should be informed that he will feel some pressure.

The needle is placed into the skin in the midline parallel to the table. The needle is held between both thumbs and index fingers. After the subcutaneous tissue has been penetrated, the needle is angled toward the umbilicus. The bevel of the needle should be facing laterally. It has been speculated that pointing the bevel laterally may allow the needle to penetrate the transverse fibers of the dura rather than cut through them, allowing for less spinal fluid leakage after the needle has been withdrawn.

The supraspinal ligament connects the spinous process; the interspinal ligaments join the inferior and superior borders of adjacent spinous processes. The ligamentum flavum is a strong, elastic, yellow membrane that may reach a thickness of 1 cm in the lumbar region. The ligamentum flavum covers the interlaminary space between the vertebrae and functions to assist the paraspinous muscles in maintaining an upright posture (Fig. 82–3). The ligaments are stretched in a flexed position and are more easily crossed by

the needle. The ligaments offer resistance to the needle, and a "pop" is often felt as they are penetrated. One should remove the stylet frequently to see if the subarachnoid space has been reached. The "pop" is occasionally not felt with the very sharp needles in disposable trays.

If bone is encountered, the needle must be partially withdrawn to the subcutaneous tissue. The physician should

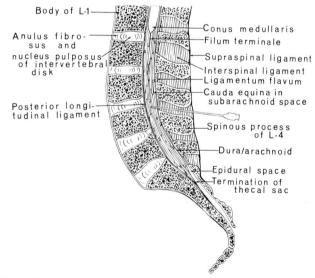

Figure 82–3. Midsagittal section through lumbar spinal column with spinal puncture needle in place between spinous processes of L-3 and L-4. Note the slightly ascending direction of the needle. The needle has pierced three ligaments and the dura/arachnoid and is in the subarachnoid space. (From Lachman E: Anatomy as applied to clinical medicine. New Physician 145, 1968. Reproduced by permission.)

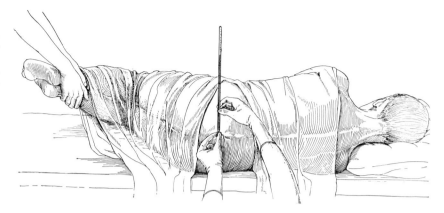

Figure 82–4. Opening pressure should be measured, not estimated, by means of an air-water manometer affixed to the needle by a three-way stopcock, thus allowing pressure to be taken and fluid withdrawn through a single needle. If the manometric reading is elevated initially, the assistant or nurse gently extends the patient to see if elevation will subside to normal limits (80 to 180 mm H_2O). (From Cole M: Pitfalls in cerebrospinal fluid examination. Hosp Pract 47, 1969. Illustration by Carol Donner. Reproduced by permission.)

repalpate the back and ascertain that the needle is in the midline. If bone is again encountered, the needle should be slightly withdrawn and reangled, with the point placed so it angles more sharply cephalad. This should avoid hitting the inferior spinous process.

Clear fluid will flow from the needle when the subarachnoid space has been penetrated. The physician should attach the manometer and record the opening pressure. A three-way stopcock is supplied in disposable trays; this allows both collection and pressure to be measured by a single needle (Fig. 82–4). The patient is then asked to relax and to extend his legs to decrease intra-abdominal pressure. The fluid column is observed for phasic changes with respirations and arterial pulsations. This ensures placement in the subarachnoid space. If the needle is against a nerve root or is only partially within the dura, the pressure may be falsely low, and respiratory excursions will not be seen in the manometer.[29] Minor rotation of the needle may solve these problems. Hyperventilation to relax the patient should not be attempted, since this will reduce the pressure readings owing to hypocapnia and resultant cerebral vasoconstriction.

After measuring the pressure, the physician should turn the stopcock and collect enough fluid to perform all desired studies. Even if the pressure is elevated, sufficient fluid should be removed for performance of all indicated studies, since the risk of the procedure involves the dural rent and not the amount of fluid removed. Presumably, more fluid will be lost subsequently through the hole in the dura. A dressing is placed over the puncture site. Commercial trays supply four specimen tubes. Tube 1 is used for determining protein and glucose levels and for electrophoretic studies; tube 2 is used for microbiologic and cytologic studies; tube 3 is for cell counts and serologic tests for syphilis. In the presence of bloody CSF, cell counts should be performed in tubes 1 and 3 to help differentiate traumatic taps. One may compare water placed in tube 4 with CSF in tube 3 to detect cloudiness or discoloration.

Traumatic taps can be avoided by proper patient and needle positioning. A traumatic tap most commonly occurs when the subarachnoid space is transfixed at the extrance of the ventral epidural space, where the venous plexus is heavier. A plexus of veins forms a ring around the cord, and these veins may be entered if the needle is advanced too far ventrally or is directed laterally (Fig. 82–5). If blood is encountered and fluid does not clear, the procedure should be repeated at a higher interspace with a fresh needle. A traumatic tap, per se, is not a particularly dangerous problem, and no specific precautions are needed if blood-tinged fluid is obtained. Observation for signs of cord or spinal nerve compression from a developing hematoma should be routine for these patients.

Lateral Approach in Lumbar Puncture

The supraspinal ligament may be calcified in older people, making a midline perforation difficult. A calcified ligament may deflect the needle. In this case, a slightly lateral approach may be used. As the lower lamina rises upward from the midline, the needle is directed slightly cephalad to miss the lamina and slightly medially to compensate for the lateral approach.[27] The needle passes through the skin, superficial fascia, fat, the dense posterior layer of thoracolumbar fascia, and the erector spinae muscles. The needle then penetrates the ligamentum flavum (bypassing the supraspinal and interspinal ligaments), the epidural space, and the dura before CSF is obtained (Fig. 82–6).

Cisternal Puncture. In situations in which lumbar puncture is contraindicated (such as local infection or acute trauma to the lumbar spine), cisternal, or suboccipital, punc-

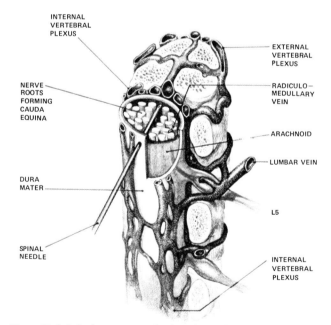

Figure 82–5. Spinal contents at the fourth and fifth lumbar vertebrae to show the relationship of a lumbar puncture needle to the major vessels at this level. The major radiculomedullary vein, shown accompanying the L-5 nerve root, is situated far laterally to a needle correctly positioned in the midline of the dural sac. Note the avascular subdural space. (From Edelson RN, Chernik IVL, Rosner JB: Spinal subdural hematomas. Arch Neurol 31:134–137, 1974. Illustration by Lynn McDowell. Reproduced by permission. Copyright 1974, American Medical Association.)

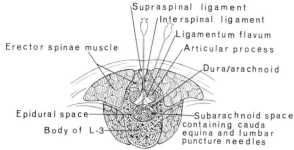

Figure 82–6. Horizontal section through the body of L-3. Note the two puncture needles in the subarachnoid space. The medial one is in the midline corresponding to the position in Figure 82–3. The lateral one exemplifies the lateral approach, which avoids the occasionally calcified supraspinal ligament. Note the lateral needle piercing the intrinsic musculature of the back and only one ligament, the ligamentum flavum. (From Lachman E: Anatomy as applied to clinical medicine. New Physician 145, 1968. Reproduced by permission.)

ture is the usual alternative. Technical problems, such as morbid obesity, cord tumor, arachnoiditis, bony deformities, or prior spinal surgery (fusion), may make lumbar puncture impossible. Contrast material may be injected into the cisterna magna to identify the rostral extent of the lesion when lumbar myelography has shown a complete block.

The patient is cleaned and anesthetized in a manner similar to that for a lumbar puncture after the neck has been shaved from the external occipital protuberance to the mastoid process laterally. The patient is preferably placed in a lateral decubitus position, but a sitting position can be used. A pillow is placed under the head to keep the neck and the vertebral axis in the same plane. The patient's neck is flexed to his chest. The spinal needle is placed in the midline halfway between the spinous process of C 2 and the inferior occiput. The needle is angled cephalad through the subcutaneous tissue until it comes in contact with the bony occiput. The needle is then withdrawn and subsequently advanced at a less acute angle with the horizontal plane of the cervical spine. This is repeated until the dural "pop" is felt. As in the lumbar region, the stylet should be removed frequently so the dura is not punctured unknowingly. Fluid is removed in the usual manner. Dural veins are less extensive, and bloody taps are less common. Low-pressure headaches are less common, presumably because the subarachnoid pressure is lower and the dural tear can heal faster.

Lateral Cervical Puncture

The patient is placed in a supine position and fully sterilized and anesthetized. A 20-gauge lumbar puncture needle is inserted perpendicular to the neck and parallel to the bed. The landmark for insertion is a point 1 cm inferior and 1 cm dorsal to the mastoid process. The physician frequently removes the stylet to check for fluid return and, as at other sites, advances the needle slowly. If the needle goes too deeply and encounters paraspinous muscles, it is probably too deep posteriorly and should be repositioned more anteriorly. If bone is encountered, more dorsal placement is needed. Pressure and fluid samples are collected, as in other sites.[30]

The contraindications to cisternal and cervical punctures are the same as those to lumbar puncture. Both techniques are easily mastered, but prior demonstration of the procedure by an experienced neurologist or neurosurgeon is advised. When lumbar puncture cannot be performed for

technical reasons and meningitis is suspected, then placement of the needle under fluoroscopy may help obtain spinal fluid.

Lumbar Puncture in Infants

Lumbar puncture in infants is usually performed to exclude meningitis. The sitting position may allow the midline to be more easily identified. Some authors use a nonstyleted needle in small infants, because this device allows the pressure to be estimated as the needle punctures the dura.[31] The failure to use a stylet may be the source of later development of an interspinal epidermoid tumor.[32, 33] A technique of lumbar puncture in the neonate using a butterfly infusion set needle has been described as a simplified procedure that may be useful in the squirming or hyperactive patient.[31]

If the child's neck is very tightly flexed, CSF may not be obtained. If the head is held in midflexion, however, CSF usually flows briskly. Prolonged severe flexion of the neck in an infant may produce dangerous airway obstruction; the airway should be checked if the infant suddenly stops crying. Incorrect positioning usually results in multiple punctures and a bloody tap. If CSF fails to flow, gentle suction with a 1.0-ml syringe may be used to exclude a low-pressure syndrome. Local anesthesia is seldom administered to the neonate, and pressure readings are of little clinical value in the struggling child. Positioning is very important in the infant and is best accomplished by an assistant, who maintains the spine maximally flexed by partially overlying the child and holding him behind the shoulders and the knees. The infant has poor neck control; hence, the assistant must also ensure that the child maintains an open airway.

Studies have shown that hypoxemia may occur from extrathoracic compression of the chest by abdominal contents, and a sitting position is suggested by some authors.[32] This is a problem primarily in neonates. However, all infants with serious cardiopulmonary disease should be closely monitored during the procedure. Particular attention should be given to avoiding neck and trunk flexion.

COMPLICATIONS

Implantation of Epidermoid Tumors

An epidermoid tumor or cyst is a mass of desquamated cells containing keratin within a capsule of well-differentiated stratified squamous epithelium. Congenital lesions are rare and arise from epithelial tissue that becomes sequestrated at the time of closure of the neural groove between the third and fifth weeks of embryonic life. Acquired intraspinal epidermoid tumors result from implantation of epidermoid tissue into the spinal canal at the time of lumbar puncture performed with needles without stylets or with illfitting needles.[33, 34] The clinical syndrome consists of pain in the back and the lower extremities developing years after spinal puncture. Myelography is required for diagnosis and surgery for treatment. Failure to use a stylet may also result in aspiration of a nerve root into the epidural space.

Postspinal Headache

A number of complications from lumbar puncture have been reported. By far the most common is the "postspinal headache." This occurs after 5 to 30 per cent of spinal taps.[6, 35, 36] The syndrome starts up to 48 hours after the procedure and usually lasts for 1 to 2 days and occasionally up to 14 days. Exceptional cases lasting months have been described. The headache usually begins within minutes after the patient arises and characteristically ceases as soon as he assumes a recumbent position. The pain is usually cervical and suboccipital in location but may involve the shoulders and the entire cranium. Exceptional cases include autonomic symptoms of nausea, vomiting, and vertigo. The syndrome is caused by leakage of fluid through the dural puncture site. This results in an absolute reduction of CSF volume below the cisterna magna and a downward movement of the brain with displacement and stretching of pain-sensitive structures, such as meninges and vessels, which, in turn, causes a traction headache. In the recumbent position there is relief, since the weight of the brain is shifted cephalad. Dural leakage has been confirmed at surgery for disc disease and by at least one isotope myelographic study.[37] The size of the dural rent seems to correlate with the frequency of post–lumbar puncture headaches.[38]

Using normal volunteers, Tourtellotte and coworkers found the incidence of postural headache to be one case per nine subjects with the use of a 26-gauge needle and one case per three subjects with a 22-gauge needle.[38] The headache was reported to be milder when the smaller needle was used. Practically speaking, a 26-gauge needle is difficult to place and to manipulate into a position in which it does not become intermittently obstructed by nerve roots. In addition, a syringe is needed to withdraw fluid, and pressure cannot be easily recorded. Theoretically, the incidence of headache is greater with an 18-gauge needle.

Other factors claimed to influence the incidence of postspinal headache have been reviewed by Fishman.[6] The incidence is higher in young patients than in older patients and is also increased in females. Psychologic factors, quantity of CSF removed, forced bed rest, post–lumbar puncture hydration, and position during lumbar puncture have not been found to be relevant in the incidence of headache. Some reports suggest a lower incidence with the lateral approach resulting from the production of holes in the dura and the arachnoid that do not overlap.

The influence of activity on post–spinal puncture headache has been studied with contradicting results, including worsening of, improvement in, and no effect on the incidence of headaches when patients were mobilized.[6, 29, 36, 39, 40] Brocker studied 1094 patients and reported a reduction of headache from 36.5 to 0.5 per cent by having the patients lie prone instead of supine for 3 hours after puncture with an 18-gauge needle.[39] He concluded that the prone position caused hyperextension of the spine and disrupted alignment of the holes in the dura and the arachnoid, making a leak less likely. Others have failed to show a decrease in duration, severity, or incidence of spinal headache with 24 hours of bed rest.[40] Interestingly, Vilming and colleagues noted a slight reduction in post–lumbar puncture headache if immediate mobilization was undertaken.[41]

Many medications have been advocated for treatment of post–spinal puncture headache: barbiturates, codeine, neostigmine, ergots, diphenhydramine hydrochloride (Benadryl), dimenhydrinate (Dramamine), amphetamine sulfate (Benzedrine), caffeine, ephedrine, intravenous fluids, magnesium sulfate, and vitamins.[6] Sechzer and Abel[41a] in a double-blind demand method found caffeine sodium benzoate (500 mg in 2 ml normal saline given IV push) to be effective in 75 per cent of patients. Additional patients responded to a second injection one to two hours later. Other clinicians prefer to put 500 mg of caffeine sodium benzoate in a liter of saline and infuse the fluid over one hour.[41b] This approach is contraindicated in the patient at risk for xanthine toxicity (e.g., supratherapeutic theophylline level, history of cardiac dysrhythmias).

Most clinicians generally follow the practice of using a styleted needle that is as small as possible. A 20- to 22-gauge needle is often used for adults because of its stiffness and ease of fluid flow. Multiple punctures should be avoided. There is no certainty about activity and position immediately after the procedure, although Brocker's results with the prone position are impressive.[39] Most postspinal headaches can be managed with bed rest with the head in the horizontal position. Dehydration should be avoided, since it lowers CSF pressure and might aggravate the headache. While simple analgesics are commonly prescribed, they have no apparent advantage over bed rest and fluid intake. In the absence of a postural headache it is not necessary to stress immobilization or bed rest after lumbar puncture.[42] A patient with a prolonged headache after spinal puncture should be reassessed to rule out other structural causes of headaches. If the headache is not postural, other causes should be sought.

In cases in which a prolonged low-pressure headache exists, the placing of an epidural blood patch by experienced anesthesiologists is highly successful.[43, 44] An epidural tap is performed at the level of the prior lumbar puncture. Ten to 20 ml of autologous blood is drawn aseptically into a syringe and slowly injected (1 to 2 ml every 10 seconds) into the epidural space at the site of the dural puncture. The injection is slowed or discontinued if back pain or paresthesias develop. The patient is kept supine for 1 hour while receiving intravenous hydration. Relief usually occurs at the time of the procedure. Pain relief is due to the blood patch forming a gelatinous tamponade, hence stopping the spinal fluid leak and providing an immediate elevation of CSF pressure. Patch failures (15 to 20 per cent) are believed to be due to improper needle placement, injection of an inadequate quantity of blood, or an incorrect diagnosis. A second patch will often be successful.

Complications reported after an epidural patch include back stiffness (15 per cent), paresthesias, radicular pain, subdural hematoma, adhesive arachnoiditis, and bacterial meningitis.[43, 44] The procedure should be used in patients with refractory headaches who fail to respond to conservative therapy and should be performed by physicians trained in the procedure.

Infection

Spinal puncture is absolutely contraindicated in the presence of local infection at the puncture site (cellulitis, epidural abscess, or furunculosis) because of the danger of inducing meningitis.

The postulation that an association exists between performance of a lumbar puncture during bacteremia and later development of meningitis has been examined by several laboratory and clinical investigators.[45, 46] The meningitis could be coincidental ("spontaneous meningitis") or could result from leakage of blood containing bacteria into the subarachnoid space after lumbar puncture ("lumbar puncture–induced meningitis"). Eng and Seligman reported that 14 per cent of 165 cases of bacteremia caused by *Streptococcus pneumoniae*, *Haemophilus influenzae*, and *Neisseria meningitidis* had evidence of meningitis at the time of initial lumbar puncture.[47] They argue that one cannot easily differentiate spontaneous meningitis from lumbar puncture–induced meningitis with these organisms because of their ability to invade the meninges spontaneously. Eng and Seligman identified a spontaneous meningitis in 0.8 per cent of patients (7 of 924) with sepsis due to other organisms, and 2.1 per cent of these patients (3 of 140) had a clinical course consistent with a lumbar puncture–induced meningitis. These differences were not statistically significant, and the investigators concluded that the occurrence was "rare enough to be clinically insignificant."

Teele and coworkers, however, reported that 7 of 46 children developed meningitis after an initial normal lumbar puncture in the presence of bacteremia.[46] *S. pneumoniae, H. influenzae,* and *N. meningitidis* were recovered in all cases. All cases of "lumbar puncture–induced meningitis" occurred in children under 1 year of age who received no antimicrobial therapy at the time of initial cultures. Teele and associates advise that, for children less than 1 year of age, the presence of a high fever and leukocytosis should prompt hospitalization and treatment for bacteremia and meningitis pending culture results suggestive of infection or development of clinical infection at other sites, such as otitis media or pneumonia. Positive blood cultures would then require a second lumbar puncture to exclude the development of meningitis and to determine the length of antibiotic therapy.

Other studies suggest that the development of meningitis in children with occult bacteremia is more strongly associated with *S. pneumoniae, H. influenzae* type B, or *N. meningitidis* species of bacteria and *not* with the performance of lumbar puncture.[48] Suspected bacteremia is not a contraindication for performing a lumbar puncture; delay in diagnosis because of concern regarding the risks of a lumbar puncture is more serious than the risk of causing meningitis with the procedure.[49, 50]

Herniation Syndromes Following Lumbar Puncture

Lumbar puncture is of value in confirming a diagnosis of meningitis and subarachnoid hemorrhage. Lumbar puncture can be dangerous in patients with intracranial mass lesions, however. Particularly with supratentorial mass lesions, there may be large pressure gradients between the cranial and lumbar compartments. When brain volume is increased because of a mass lesion or edema, rostrocaudal displacement may occur following lumbar puncture if the skull is intact. Lowering the lumbar pressure by removing CSF may increase the gradient, promoting both transtentorial and foramen magnum herniation. The frequency with which a lumbar puncture causes or accelerates transtentorial herniation is difficult to determine, because a patient might have developed herniation spontaneously without the procedure. Conflicting data are present in the literature. Korein and coworkers, in a personal series and literature review of 418 cases, concluded that the risk of an unfavorable response following lumbar puncture is less than 1.2 per cent.[51] Zisfein and Tuchman[51a] in another retrospective analysis of 38 patients with intracranial mass lesions found only one that died after lumbar puncture. That patient was comatose with fixed dilated pupils and absent caloric response prior to the tap.

Duffy encountered 30 cases referred to a neurosurgical service over a 1-year period because of complications of lumbar puncture.[18] Thirteen patients lost consciousness immediately following lumbar puncture, and another 15 showed a decreased level of consciousness within 12 hours following lumbar puncture. Three patients stopped breathing during the procedure. Twelve died within 10 days of the lumbar puncture. Only 10 of the 30 had papilledema, and in half the lumbar pressure was normal. In each case, clinical deterioration occurred within 12 hours of the lumbar puncture. The use of a small needle and the removal of limited volumes of CSF may not prevent herniation in the presence of increased intracranial pressure, because fluid seepage through the dura may be considerable. This may explain a progressive and worsening herniation syndrome.

A careful neurologic examination should precede all spinal punctures. When there is a history of headache with progressive mental changes and the development of localizing neurologic signs, then spinal puncture should *not* be performed as the initial diagnostic procedure unless there is a suspicion of infection. When these findings are present and meningitis is still clinically suspected, an initial dose of antibiotic should be administered empirically while awaiting computed cranial tomography and subsequent lumbar puncture. Appropriate cultures of blood and other body fluid should be obtained prior to antibiotic administration. Papilledema is not a constant feature, even when the history suggests a protracted course.

A computed tomogram should identify hemorrhagic lesions and most neoplasms and should aid in the decision regarding the need for and the risk involved with spinal puncture. Computed cranial tomography may help recognize patients with unequal pressures between intracranial compartments who are at risk for cerebral herniation. It has been shown that a small dural puncture site allows less spinal fluid to leak into surrounding tissues after the procedure.[52] CT findings that suggest unequal pressure between intracranial compartments include: lateral shift of midline structures, loss of suprachiasmatic and circum-mesencephalic cisterns, shift or obliteration of the fourth ventricle, and failure to visualize the superior cerebellar and quadrigeminal plate cisterns with sparing of the ambient cisterns.[52] The presence of a posterior fossa mass would be a strong contraindication to a lumbar puncture. Because of bone and motion artifact, the posterior fossa unfortunately may be a difficult area to visualize.

Recognition of Herniation Syndromes

Herniation syndromes are the result of downward displacement of the hemispheres and the basal ganglia, which compress and displace the diencephalon and the midbrain rostrocaudally through the tentorial notch. Etiologic features and pathogenesis are detailed in the monograph by Plum and Posner.[53] Herniations have the potential to initiate vascular and obstructive complications that aggravate the original expanding lesion and can create an irreversible pathologic process. The anterior cerebral artery may be compressed against the falx and may increase ischemia and edema of the herniating hemisphere. Midline displacement posteriorly compresses the deep great cerebral vein and raises pressure in its area of drainage. Compression of the posterior cerebral artery at the tentorial notch can produce occipital infarction and swelling. In addition, kinking of the aqueduct may interfere with CSF circulation. This blockage may produce a normal spinal CSF pressure. Transtentorial herniation displaces the brain stem downward, stretching medial perforating branches of the basilar artery, as the artery is tethered to the circle of Willis. This produces brain stem ischemia and hemorrhages.

In general, pathologic changes with supratentorial mass lesions spread through the hemisphere and move rostrally and caudally in a progressive manner, with progressive dysfunction of the hemisphere and, subsequently, succeeding levels of the brain stem. The infrequent exceptions are seen in patients with acute cerebral-intraventricular hemorrhage and in patients with hemispheral mass lesions with incipient herniation who undergo lumbar puncture. Such conditions may rapidly progress from hemispheral dysfunction to sudden medullary failure.

Central, or *transtentorial,* herniation occurs in response to lesions of the frontal, parietal, and occipital lobes and the extracerebral lesions lying toward the vertex or the fronto-occipital lobes (Fig. 82–7). Frequently, patients are subacutely or chronically ill with bilateral disease, and the diagnosis may be uncertain. Initially, subjects exhibit a change in alertness or behavior. If the supratentorial lesion enlarges, compressing the diencephalon, stupor and then coma develop. At this point, monitoring of respiratory, ocular, and motor signs helps in diagnosing a supratentorial lesion and in determining the rostrocaudal direction of the disease process. Respirations at this time may be interrupted

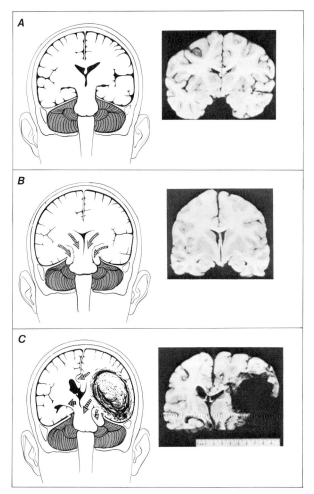

Figure 82–7. Intracranial shifts from supratentorial lesions. *A,* The relationships of the various supratentorial and infratentorial compartments as seen in a coronal section. *B,* Central transtentorial herniation. The photograph is taken of a patient with carcinoma of the lung and multiple cerebral metastases (none is apparent in this section) who died after developing signs and symptoms of the central syndrome of rostral-caudal deterioration. The brain is swollen: The diencephalon is compressed and elongated, and the mammillary bodies lie far caudal to those in the normal brain. Neither the cingulate gyrus nor the uncus is herniated. *C,* Uncal and transtentorial herniation. The photograph is of a patient who developed a massive hemorrhagic infarct and died after developing the syndrome of uncal herniation. The cingulate gyrus is herniated after the falx; there is hemorrhagic infarction of the opposite cerebral peduncle and marked swelling and grooving of the uncus on the side of the lesion. Central downward displacement is also present but is less marked than in *B* above. (From Plum F, Posner J: The Diagnosis of Stupor and Coma. Philadelphia, FA Davis Co, 1980. Reproduced by permission.)

by deep sighs or yawns and periodic breathing of the Cheyne-Stokes type (periods of hyperpnea regularly alternating with apnea). Pupils are small but react briskly. Eye movements may be conjugate or slightly divergent with roving eye movements. Caloric testing with cold water produces a conjugate slow tonic movement to the side of irrigation. Many individuals have a hemiparesis prior to herniation. As the diencephalic stage of the central syndrome evolves, the contralateral hemiplegia may worsen, with the homolateral limbs developing a paratonic resistance to movement, but the individual continues to respond to noxious stimuli appropriately. At this stage both plantar responses are extensor. Decorticate responses appear and consist of flexor muscle hypertonus in the upper extremity with predominantly extensor hypertonus in the leg. Recognition of a diencephalic stage of herniation is important in that it gives warning that a potentially reversible lesion may become irreversible.

Once midbrain signs develop, they will probably reflect infarction rather than reversible ischemia and compression. The chances of successfully removing or alleviating a supratentorial mass are small once the midbrain stage is reached.

Patients who develop midbrain and upper pons failure exhibit a sustained tachypnea; pupils dilate to a fixed midposition (3 to 5 mm), and oculovestibular reflexes become difficult to obtain, requiring side-to-side head movements and cold caloric irrigation. Dysconjugate eye movements appear with failure to adduct (internuclear ophthalmoplegia). Motor responses give way to extensor hypertonus in all limbs (decerebrate rigidity). Midbrain damage results from ischemia and infarction, and few patients recover.

As the brain stem becomes more ischemic, the pupils maintain a fixed position, eye movements are lost, and decerebration gives way to flaccidity. The medullary stage consists of irregular respirations with long periods of apnea. The pupils dilate and the blood pressure falls, with death being inevitable.

Uncal herniation occurs when expanding lesions in the temporal fossa shift the medial temporal lobe (uncus) and the hippocampal gyrus medially over the incisural edge of the tentorium. This flattens the midbrain, pushing it against the contralateral incisura. The third nerve and the posterior cerebral artery on the side of the lesion are caught between the swollen uncus and the free edge of the tentorium (Figs. 82–8 and 82–9). The earliest sign is a unilaterally sluggish or slightly dilated pupil. Because the diencephalon may not be the first structure encroached upon, impaired consciousness is not consistently present as an early sign of uncal herniation. Other respiratory, ocular, and motor findings may not be appreciably changed from earlier examinations. Pupillary dilation may persist for several hours, but once the patient progresses beyond this stage there is a tendency for midbrain dysfunction to occur rapidly. Ipsilateral external ophthalmoplegia soon follows pupillary dilation along with stupor and coma. Oculovestibular reflexes disappear as ischemia spreads to the midbrain. As the opposite cerebral peduncle is compressed against the tentorial edge, hemiplegia may appear ipsilaterally to the expanding supratentorial lesion (Kernohan's notch). Decerebrate posturing develops, with the opposite pupil becoming dilated and fixed. Progression then proceeds as described for the central syndrome. As with transtentorial herniation, once midbrain failure occurs, survival is much less likely.

Backache and Radicular Symptoms

Minor backache commonly results from the trauma of the spinal needle. Frank disk herniation has been reported

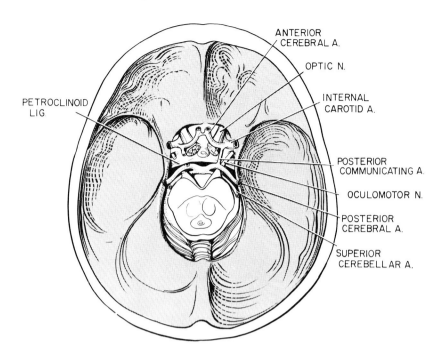

ANTERIOR
CEREBRAL A.

OPTIC N.

INTERNAL
CAROTID A.

PETROCLINOID
LIG.

POSTERIOR
COMMUNICATING A.

OCULOMOTOR N.

POSTERIOR
CEREBRAL A.

SUPERIOR
CEREBELLAR A.

Figure 82–8. The floor of the anterior and middle fossae, illustrating the tentorial notch and the way in which the third nerve passes between the posterior cerebral and superior cerebellar arteries over the petroclinoid ligaments. (From Plum F, Posner J: The Diagnosis of Stupor and Coma. Philadelphia, FA Davis Co, 1980. Reproduced by permission.)

from the passing of the needle beyond the subarachnoid space into the annulus fibrosis. Transient sensory symptoms from irritation of the cauda equina are also quite common.

Other reported complications include transient unilateral or bilateral sixth nerve palsies caused by stretching or displacement of the abducens nerve as it crosses the petrous

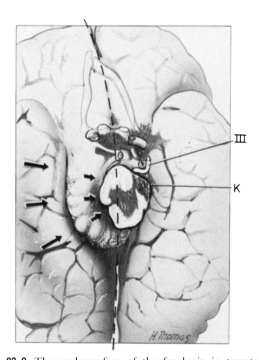

III

K

Figure 82–9. The undersurface of the forebrain in transtentorial herniation. Compare the positioning of cranial nerve III and the adjacent posterior cerebral artery as well as the shape of the midbrain with those in Figure 82–8. Large arrows point to the edge where the hippocampus herniated through the tentorium. Small arrows and the dotted line indicate the lateral shift of the mesencephalon, which produces a hemorrhagic Kernohan notch at point K. (From Plum F, Posner J: The Diagnosis of Stupor and Coma. Philadelphia, FA Davis Co, 1980. Reproduced by permission.)

ridge of the temporal bone, subarachnoid hemorrhage, epidural hematoma, anaphylactoid reactions to local anesthetics, settling of cord tumors, and retroperitoneal abscess produced by dural laceration in patients with meningitis.[54] Most of these are rare and seldom encountered.[6, 24, 26]

Most of the complications of lateral cervical and cisternal puncture are similar to those encountered with a lumbar puncture. In addition, perforation of a large vessel with resultant cisterna magna hematoma or obstruction of vertebral artery flow has been described. Puncture of the medulla oblongata may cause vomiting or apnea, and puncture of the cord may be associated with pain.[30] Long-lasting side effects of cord puncture are probably minor. In addition, traumatic tap and postspinal headache may occur with lateral cervical and cisternal puncture.

INTERPRETATION

Pressure

The pressure of the spinal fluid is of great clinical importance. It should be accurately measured whenever possible. Accurate measurement is dependent upon patient cooperation. Normal pressure is between 70 and 180 mm H_2O. In the sitting position, lumbar pressure should not rise above the foramen magnum. Increased intracranial pressure can result from expansion of the brain (edema, hemorrhage, or neoplasm), overproduction of CSF (choroid plexus papilloma), a defect in absorption, or obstruction of flow of CSF through the ventricles. Cerebral edema may be associated with meningitis, carbon dioxide retention, subarachnoid hemorrhage, anoxia, congestive heart failure, or superior vena cava obstruction. Pressure may be falsely elevated in a tense patient, when the head is elevated above the plane of the needle, and, possibly, with marked obesity or muscle contraction.[5] Pressure is not usually measured in the neonate, since a struggling or crying child will have a falsely elevated pressure.

Low pressure should suggest obstruction of the needle by meninges. Low pressure can also be seen with spinal block. Rarely, a primary low-pressure syndrome occurs in a setting of trauma, following neurosurgical procedures, secondary to subdural hematomas in elderly patients, with barbiturate intoxication, and in cases of CSF leakage through holes in the arachnoid.[55, 56]

The Queckenstedt test is useful for demonstrating the presence of obstruction in the spinal subarachnoid space.[5, 6, 35] The test is seldom performed today, because myelographic techniques have been refined. This test may be of use in the management of a patient with a myelopathy whose general medical state makes the examiner reluctant to perform a myelogram or in whom the need for myelography is uncertain. With the patient in the lateral recumbent position, jugular vein compression causes decreased venous return to the heart. This distends cerebral veins and causes a rise of intracranial pressure, which is transmitted throughout the system and is measured in the manometer. After 10 seconds of bilateral compression, CSF pressure usually rises to 150 mm H_2O over the initial reading and returns to the baseline in 10 to 20 seconds after release. If there is no change in the lumbar pressure or if the rise and fall are delayed, it should be concluded that the spinal subarachnoid space does not communicate with the cranial subarachnoid space. In this situation, Pantopaque should be injected before removal to facilitate subsequent performance of a myelogram. This is necessary because the lumbar dural sac may collapse, making it impossible to re-enter the canal. If cervical cord disease is suspected, the test should be repeated with the neck in the neutral position, hyperextended, and flexed. When lateral sinus obstruction is suspected, unilateral jugular venous compression may be used (Tobey-Ayer test).

Appearance

If the spinal fluid is not crystal clear, a pathologic condition of the CNS should be suspected. The examiner should compare the fluid with water, viewing down the long axis of the tube or holding both tubes against a white background. A glass tube is preferred, because plastic tubes are frequently not clear. The fluid may be clear with as many as 400 cells/mm³.[6]

Xanthochromia is a yellow-orange discoloration of the supernate of centrifuged spinal fluid. Xanthrochromia is produced by red cell lysis and is caused by one or more of the following pigments: oxyhemoglobin, bilirubin, and methemoglobin. Oxyhemoglobin causes a red color, bilirubin a yellow color, and methemoglobin a brown color. Oxyhemoglobin is seen within 2 hours of subarachnoid bleeding and red cell lysis. Formation reaches a maximum in 24 to 48 hours after hemorrhage and disappears in 3 to 30 days.[5, 35, 57] The appearance of bilirubin in the CSF involves the conversion of oxyhemoglobin by the enzyme hemeoxygenase. The enzyme is found in the choroid plexus, the arachnoid, and the meninges. Enzyme activity appears approximately 12 hours after the bleed.[5, 57] Bilirubin may persist for 2 to 4 weeks. Bilirubin in CSF caused by hepatic or hemolytic disease does not appear until a serum level of 10 to 15 mg total bilirubin per 100 ml is reached, unless underlying disease associated with a high CSF protein is present.

Oxyhemoglobin and bilirubin may be measured chemically or by spectrophotometric analysis. Demonstration of these compounds in CSF may help in the distinction between recent intracranial hemorrhage and a traumatic tap. Oxyhemoglobin may form as a result of red cell lysis if the tube has been allowed to stand for more than 1 hour before testing, however.

Methemoglobin is a reduction product of oxyhemoglobin characteristically found in encapsulated subdural hematomas or in old intracerebral hematomas.

Cells

The technique involved in cell counts is reviewed in several sources.[5, 6, 35, 57] Cell counts above 5 per mm³ should be taken to indicate the presence of a pathologic condition. In a study of 135 normal university students, Tourtellotte and Shorr reported almost exclusively lymphocytes and monocytes, and the presence of one to five lymphocytes in the CSF may be normal.[5] It has been stated that polymorphonuclear leukocytes are never seen in normal individuals. With the use of the cytocentrifuge, however, an occasional specimen may show a neutrophil in an otherwise normal individual.[6] Such a finding should routinely prompt culture of the spinal fluid, since the presence of a neutrophilic pleocytosis is commonly associated with bacterial infections or the early stages of viral infections, tuberculosis, meningitis, hematogenous meningitis, and chemical meningitis due to foreign bodies. The fluid from a traumatic tap should contain about 1 white blood cell per 700 red cells if the complete blood count (CBC) is normal, but this is highly variable. Formulas to assess the contribution of total CSF cell count and protein values from traumatic taps have been proposed but do not have uniform support.[57, 58] All blood-contaminated CSF should be cultured, especially that from uncooperative infants and children being evaluated for sepsis.[59, 60] One study suggests that one to two polymorphonuclear leukocytes are normal and correlate with CSF blood contamination.[61]

As many as 30 per cent of patients may exhibit CSF pleocytosis after a generalized or focal seizure. In a review of 102 patients without CNS infection who had lumbar puncture within 48 hours of a seizure, Prokesch reported an average of 72 cells per mm³, noting the presence of both polymorphonuclear and mononuclear cells.[62] Although these patients did not have CNS infection, many did have serious intracranial pathology (subdural hematoma, subarachnoid hemorrhage, or stroke).

Small lymphocytes may be seen in normal individuals. Small and large immunocompetent cells are found with a variety of bacterial, fungal, viral, granulomatous, and spirochetal diseases as well as the presence of foreign substances.

Eosinophils are always abnormal and most commonly represent a parasitic infestation of the CNS. They may also be seen after myelography and pneumoencephalography and, to a minor degree, in other inflammatory diseases, including tuberculous meningitis and neurosyphilis; CSF eosinophilia has also been reported in cases of subarachnoid hemorrhage, lymphoma, and Hodgkin's disease.[63]

Glucose

The normal range of CSF glucose is between 50 and 80 mg/dl, which is between 60 and 70 per cent of the glucose concentration in the blood. Values below 40 mg/dl are invariably abnormal. Hyperglycemia may mask a depressed CSF glucose level, and the CSF to blood glucose ratio should be measured routinely. Between 90 and 120 minutes are required before the CSF glucose reaches the steady state with blood glucose changes, such as after the intravenous injection of glucose. When CSF glucose is of diagnostic importance, CSF and blood samples should be obtained after a 4-hour fast.

Glucose enters the CSF by way of the choroid plexus as well as by transcapillary movement into the extracellular space of the brain and the cord by carrier-mediated transport. It then equilibrates freely with the CSF subarachnoid

Table 82–1. Low CSF Glucose Syndromes	
Bacterial meningitis	Syphilis
Tuberculous meningitis	Chemical meningitis
Fungal meningitis	Subarachnoid hemorrhage
Sarcoidosis	Mumps meningitis
Meningeal carcinomatosis	Herpes simplex encephalitis
Amebic meningitis	Hypoglycemia
Cysticercosis	Trichinosis

space. Fishman concludes that a low CSF glucose concentration indicates increased glucose utilization in the brain and the spinal cord and, to a lesser degree, by polymorphonuclear leukocytes and inhibition of membrane carrier systems.[6] Once in the CSF, glucose undergoes glycolysis and there is an invariable rise in CSF lactate levels. Glucose levels remain subnormal for 1 to 2 weeks following the effective treatment of meningitis.

Low CSF glucose levels may be found in several diseases of the nervous system, as noted in Table 82–1. Only low concentrations of glucose are of diagnostic value, and elevated CSF glucose levels generally have no significance; elevation usually reflects hyperglycemia.

Protein

The normal range of the lumbar CSF protein level is 15 to 45 mg/dl. Infants normally have a lower level than adults, and protein levels may drop after a lumbar puncture. The concentration is lower in the ventricles (5 to 15 mg/dl) and the basilar cisterns (10 to 25 mg/dl), reflecting a gradient in the permeability of capillary endothelial cells to proteins in the blood, to the so-called blood-brain barrier. Most of the proteins in CSF normally come from the blood, which normally has a protein concentration of up to 8000 mg/dl. Protein entry is determined by molecular size and relative impermeability of the blood-CSF barrier. Faulty reabsorption of protein by arachnoid villi may also elevate protein levels. Increases in CSF total protein levels suggest that a disease state may be present. Levels greater than 500 mg/dl are uncommon and are seen mainly in meningitis, in subarachnoid bleeding, and with spinal tumors. The high levels seen with cord tumors result from an increase in local capillary permeability. With high levels (generally 1000 mg/dl), CSF may clot (Froin's syndrome).

Hemorrhage into the CSF or the introduction of blood by a traumatic tap increases CSF protein levels. If the serum protein is normal, the CSF protein should theoretically rise by 1 mg for every 1000 red cells, but this is quite variable. The inflammatory effect of hemolyzed erythrocytes may also significantly increase CSF protein.

Selective measurement of gamma globulin fractions in CSF has proved to be of diagnostic value in suspected cases of multiple sclerosis; several reviews are available.[64-66] Elevated CSF IgG has been found in many chronic inflammatory conditions, including syphilis, viral encephalitis, subacute sclerosing panencephalitis, progressive rubella encephalitis, tuberculous meningitis, sarcoidosis, cysticercosis, and acute postinfectious polyneuropathy (Guillain-Barré syndrome).

Chloride

CSF chloride was used in diagnosing tuberculous meningitis but has little current application in clinical neurology.

The Traumatic Tap

It should not be difficult to distinguish between subarachnoid bleeding and bloodshed by the spinal needle if certain steps are taken *at the time of the initial puncture*. In traumatic punctures the fluid generally clears between the first and third tubes as the needle is washed by spinal fluid. Decreasing cell counts on the first and third tubes helps confirm this. In a recent hemorrhage, however, a declining cell count may represent layering of cells in a recumbent patient. The fluid should then be centrifuged. With moderately blood-stained fluid, the supernatant should be clear if the red cells have been present for less than 2 hours (traumatic tap). Red cells undergo hemolysis in the CSF after a few hours to produce xanthochromia. Xanthochromia persists for up to 4 weeks, depending on the number of red cells that were originally present. It should be noted that an early CSF examination may show clear fluid prior to the development of hemolysis, even after spontaneous subarachnoid bleeding. Xanthochromia may be seen after a traumatic tap if the red cell count exceeds 150,000 to 200,000, however. The yellow color may appear if sufficient serum is present.[67] The presence of a clot in one of the tubes strongly favors a traumatic tap. In subarachnoid hemorrhage, clotting does not occur because blood is defibrinated at the site of the hemorrhage. Any lumbar puncture performed several days after a traumatic tap may yield stained fluid. An immediate repeat puncture at a higher interspace yielding clear CSF may also help distinguish a traumatic tap.

CSF Analysis with Infections

BACTERIAL

The CSF findings are essential in establishing the diagnosis of acute bacterial meningitis. CSF analysis establishes the diagnosis, the causative organism, and the choice of antibiotics and helps determine management. CSF must be transported to the laboratory immediately and examined at once. In cases of meningococcal infection, a delay in processing may cause the diagnosis to be missed, since the organism tends to autolyze rapidly. Speed is only slightly less important with other organisms, since early initiation of antibiotic therapy is crucial.

The Gram stain is of great importance, since this often dictates the initial choice of antibiotic therapy. It has been suggested that the physician become expert at examining Gram stains of CSF, and the editors suggest that one should spend 10 minutes personally examining each CSF specimen. Gram-negative intra- or extracellular diplococci are indicative of *N. meningitidis*. Small gram-negative bacilli may indicate *H. influenzae*, especially in children. The presence of gram-positive cocci indicates *S. pneumoniae*, *Streptococcus*, or *Staphylococcus*. Twenty per cent of Gram stains may be falsely negative because too few organisms are present.[57] The Gram stain smear is more likely to be positive in patients who have not received prior antibiotic therapy.

For culture, blood and chocolate agar are required. *N. meningitidis* and *H. influenzae* grow best on chocolate agar. The plates are incubated under 10 per cent carbon dioxide. Thioglycolate medium is used for possible anaerobic organisms. Cultures are examined at 24 and 48 hours, but plates should be kept for at least 7 days.[68]

While the culture is pending, one may suspect a bacterial infection in the presence of an elevated opening pressure and a marked pleocytosis ranging between 500 and 20,000 white cells per mm³. The differential count is usually chiefly neutrophils. A count above 1000 cells/mm³ seldom occurs in

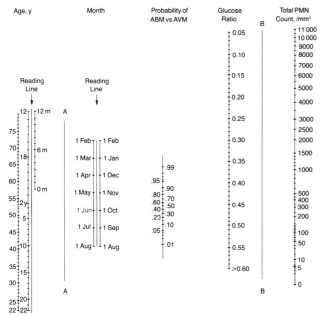

Figure 82–10. Nomogram for estimating the probability of bacterial (ABM) versus viral (AVM) meningitis. Step 1: Place the ruler on reading lines for patient's age and month of presentation, and mark the intersection with line A. Step 2: Place the ruler on the values for the glucose ratio and total polymorphonuclear leukocyte (PMN) count in cerebrospinal fluid, and mark the intersection with line B. Step 3: Use the ruler to join the marks on lines A and B; then read off the probability of ABM versus AVM. (From Spanos A, Harrell FE Jr, Durack DT: Diagnosis of acute meningitis: An analysis of the predictive value of initial observations. JAMA 262:2700, 1989. Copyright 1989, American Medical Association. Reprinted by permission.)

viral infections. Occasionally, acellular fluid may be found in the severely immunosuppressed patient or others with appropriate presentations. Repeat lumbar puncture may be required in febrile patients in whom the clinical features remain compatible with meningitis.[69, 70]

CSF glucose levels less than 40 mg/dl or less than 60 per cent of a simultaneous blood glucose level should raise the question of bacterial meningitis, even in the presence of a negative Gram stain and a low cell count. Glucose levels with bacterial meningitis are occasionally below 10 mg per dl. The CSF protein content in bacterial meningitis ranges from 500 to 1500 mg/dl and usually returns to normal by the end of therapy. Spanos and colleagues[70a] have developed a useful nomogram to help distinguish bacterial from viral infections (Fig. 82–10).

A useful test that can be performed in nearly all laboratories is the measurement of CSF lactate levels. In bacterial and fungal meningitis, levels are increased.[71] Lactic acid may be elevated even in patients who have received antibiotics for 1 or 2 days.[71] Lactic acid levels in viral infections tend to be normal, whereas values in bacterial meningitis are usually two to four times greater than the normal concentration of approximately 1.6 mEq/L.

A recent study by Durack and Spanos questions the use of repeat spinal taps as a test of meningitis cure.[72] Their review of 165 meningitis cases revealed 13 instances in which the repeat tap led to unnecessary intervention and two others in which treatment failure was *not* detected by the repeat spinal tap.

MICROBIAL ANTIGENS

Currently, several tests other than CSF culture and Gram stain are available to establish a bacterial etiology of meningitis. These include blood cultures, CSF counterimmunoelectrophoresis (CIE), CSF latex agglutination (LA), and coagglutination counterimmunoelectrophoresis (COLA). In approximately 50 per cent of bacterial meningitis cases, blood cultures are positive for the etiologic agent.[73]

CIE utilizes wells in two rows of agarose gel. A different antiserum is placed in each well. A current is passed through the gel with the reactants then moving toward each other by electrophoretic mobilization of the antigen. A line of precipitation visualized in 1 to 4 hours represents positive reaction between antiserum and antigen.[74]

Particle agglutination involves staphylococcal coagglutination and latex agglutination. Antibody on the surface of a colloid combines with antigen binding sites to cross link the colloid forming antigen bridges. A matrix forms and appears as a macroscopic agglutination. Agglutination tests can detect approximately ten times less antigen than CIE. False-positive tests can occur in the presence of rheumatoid factor, serum complement components, and possibly other serum proteins.

Another technique having some potential use is the enzyme-linked immunosorbent assay (ELISA). This technique may detect 100 to 1000 times less antigen than agglutination tests but requires 4 hours to perform.

A positive CSF antigen test may be expected in 70 to 90 per cent of patients with *Neisseria* meningitis. This compares with a positive Gram stain in approximately 70 per cent of patients. Positive latex antigen tests have been reported in approximately 60 per cent of *Streptococcus pneumoniae* meningitis cases, with a positive Gram stain in 80 per cent. A positive latex test and Gram stain are reported in approximately 85 per cent of *Haemophilus influenzae* meningitis cases.[73, 74] The Gram stain may be difficult to assess after antibiotic therapy has been initiated. Bacterial antigens may persist in the CSF for several days after antibiotic therapy. Approximately 25 to 33 per cent of positive tests are lost per day of appropriate antimicrobial therapy. A negative test, however, does not rule out bacterial meningitis.[75] In addition, blood and urine should be examined for antigen. Often antigen may be found only in the urine. Urine needs to be concentrated and may have the disadvantage of reflecting urinary tract infections. The particle agglutination test for *H. influenzae* type B may be positive for up to 10 days after children have received *H. influenzae* polysaccharide vaccine.

Antigen tests are not useful in diagnosing gram-negative bacillary, staphylococcal, and listeria meningitis. In addition, although antigen tests may identify the bacterial pathogen, they do not provide information about the antibiotic susceptibility of the organism.

EMPIRIC ANTIBIOTIC USE PRIOR TO LUMBAR PUNCTURE

Many patients are transported to a referral center after a clinical diagnosis of meningitis is made. In some instances, CSF examination cannot be performed prior to transport. The initial physician may have to decide whether to initiate empiric antibiotic therapy. Prior antibiotic administration could obscure the bacterial etiology, whereas a delay in initiating therapy may increase the morbidity and mortality of the illness. It may be difficult to identify individuals at risk for a fulminant course.

Talan and associates note that oral antibiotic treatment results in a decrease in the number of positive CSF cultures by 4 to 33 per cent and a decrease in positive CSF Gram stains of 7 to 41 per cent. After 24 hours as many as 38 per cent may have positive cultures.[73] In this situation antigen tests and blood cultures may be of help. Although there are no data to confidently address the potential advantages or disadvantages of antibiotic therapy prior to lumbar puncture, it is reasonable to initiate therapy on the premise that a delay may be deleterious. If a lumbar puncture cannot be done, consultation with physicians at the referral center would seem appropriate. If a lumbar puncture is performed, a portion of the CSF should be sent with the patient.

Approximately 75 per cent of all cases of bacterial meningitis occurring in children under 10 years of age are due to *H. influenzae*. *H. influenzae* appears to be easier to grow from early postantibiotic cultures and is more likely to be associated with positive blood cultures and antigen tests. In the pediatric population a single dose of antibiotic prior to transport is unlikely to prevent bacterial indentification. In neonates, adults, and immunosuppressed patients, the sensitivity of blood cultures and immunologic tests is less reliable. CSF examination before antibiotic administration or *early* in the course of treatment is suggested.

For immunocompromised and postneurosurgical patients, a third-generation cephalosporin (cefotaxime, ceftizoxime, ceftazidime, or ceftriaxone) and vancomycin should be used for coverage against staphylococci, *L. monocytogenes*, and gram-negative organisms.[76] Table 82–2 offers guidelines for emergency antibiotic therapy.

VIRAL STUDIES

The organisms most commonly isolated in viral meningitis are the enteroviruses (Coxsackie, ECHO) and mumps virus. Enteroviruses are most commonly seen in the summer

Table 82–2. Emergency Department Therapy of Suspected Bacterial Meningitis

Age Group	Intravenous Antibiotic Therapies
Birth to 7 days	Ampicillin 100–150 mg/kg/day, divided every 12 hours Plus Cefotaxime 100 mg/kg/day, divided every 12 hours
8 to 28 days	Ampicillin 150–200 mg/kg/day, divided every 8 hours Plus Cefotaxime 150–200 mg/kg/day, divided every 8 hours
28 days to 2 months	Ampicillin 200–300 mg/kg/day, divided every 6 hours Plus Cefotaxime 200 mg/kg/day, divided every 6 hours
2 months to 6 years	Ceftriaxone 100 mg/kg/day, divided every 12 hours
6 to 18 years	Penicillin G 250,000 U/kg/day, divided every 3 to 4 hours Or Ceftriaxone 100 mg/kg/day, divided every 12 hours (recommended for PCN allergic patients)
18 to 65 years	Penicillin G 24 million units/day, divided every 4 hours Or Ceftriaxone 4 gm/day, divided every 12 hours
65 years and older	Ampicillin 6–12 gm/day, divided every 3 to 4 hours Plus Ceftriaxone 4 gm/day, divided every 12 hours

(From Trott A: Acute meningitis. Crit Decis Emerg Med 3:1, 1988. Reproduced by permission.)

and fall, and mumps appears most frequently in the winter and spring. Viral cultures in most hospitals are not available and play little role in acute decisions regarding diagnosis and treatment. A tentative diagnosis may be based on analysis of the CSF.

The cell count in viral meningitis and encephalitis characteristically shows 10 to 1000 cells/mm^3. The differential cell count is predominantly lymphocytic and mononuclear in type. In the early stages of meningoencephalitis, however, polymorphonuclear cells may predominate, making the distinction between viral and bacterial infections difficult. In such cases, a repeat tap in 12 to 24 hours will assist in clarifying the diagnosis. Protein levels are usually mildly elevated, but normal levels may be seen. The CSF glucose is characteristically normal; however, notable exceptions include some cases of mumps meningoencephalitis and herpes simplex encephalitis. CSF pleocytosis and elevated protein levels have also been found in asymptomatic HIV-seropositive individuals.[76a]

If the CSF cannot be delivered to the viral laboratory in 24 to 48 hours, it should be refrigerated at 4° C. Members of the enterovirus group are occasionally isolated from CSF. Herpes and arboviruses are rarely found in CSF. In known viral CNS disease, the stool is more rewarding (85 per cent positive) than CSF (10 per cent positive).[68] Since CSF is normally sterile, any isolate is significant, whereas a stool isolate does not necessarily indicate that the agent is responsible for CNS disease.

NEUROSYPHILIS

The true incidence of this disease is unknown. Approximately 5000 new cases of neurosyphilis are estimated to occur in the United States each year.[77] The natural history and clinical manifestations have been modified in the antibiotic era. The widespread use of oral antibiotics has changed neurosyphilis into a chronic partially treated meningitis. Seizures were considered in the preantibiotic era to complicate general paresis only late in the course of the illness, and then only in untreated patients. Previously, seizures were reported as an early manifestation in less than 5 per cent of symptomatic neurosyphilis cases. Seizures now occur in 25 per cent of symptomatic cases and may on occasion be the sole manifestation of neurosyphilis.[77] Seizures are usually partial (focal), with one third of patients having no interictal clinical findings. A treponemal serologic test should be obtained in every adult with acquired partial seizures.

Ophthalmologic findings are frequently present in syphilis. These include a slowly progressive optic atrophy, an acute optic neuritis, cranial oculomotor neuropathy, and a chorioretinitis. A more specific sign is a dissociated pupillary response to light and convergence with loss of the light reflex (Argyll Robertson pupil). Meningovascular neurosyphilis involves infection of both the meninges and the cerebral vasculature. The clinical picture is that of a cerebral infarct or an acute meningoencephalitis. Other less common modern syndromes are reviewed in standard texts.[15]

CSF findings suggestive of neurosyphilis include more than five leukocytes per mm^3, elevated protein concentration, elevated gamma globulin concentration, and a positive serologic test for syphilis. Glucose is usually normal; the colloidal gold test has largely been replaced by electrophoretic analysis of gamma globulin.

Serologic tests for syphilis are either treponemal or nontreponemal. Nontreponemal tests detect a nonspecific globulin complex called reagin. Reagin tests, such as the Venereal Disease Research Laboratory (VDRL) flocculation test, lack sensitivity and should not be used to exclude the diagnosis of neurosyphilis. One third to one half of patients with neurosyphilis will have a negative VDRL test in the serum, and more than one third will have a negative VDRL test in the CSF.[77]

Treponemal tests provide evidence of a specific immune response to *Treponema pallidum*. Currently, the serum fluorescent treponemal antibody absorption (FTA-ABS) is the test of choice to confirm the diagnosis of neurosyphilis. The serum FTA-ABS test is reactive in 95 to 100 per cent of cases of neurosyphilis. A negative serum FTA-ABS test makes CSF examination unnecessary. Its false-positive rate is less than 1 per cent, but the incidence of biologic false-positive tests may increase in the presence of collagen vascular disorders.

A positive serum treponemal test indicates past infection with syphilis and may be reactive indefinitely, even after treatment. Therefore, CSF is used as a guide to the presence and the activity of neurosyphilis. The VDRL test is currently the test of choice in CSF and, when positive, is strong evidence for neurosyphilis. False-positive CSF-VDRL tests are rare. The FTA-ABS test is not currently used in CSF; the false-positive rate is between 4 and 6 per cent and is felt possibly to represent antibodies that have passively entered from serum.[78] The FTA-ABS test measures IgG antibody and cannot differentiate active from past infection. The CSF-VDRL either may be reactive by contamination with seropositive blood (traumatic tap, subarachnoid hemorrhage) or may occur with entry of serum reagin into CSF during meningitis.

There is some concern that today many patients with parenchymal neurosyphilis have normal CSF. A test has been developed in primates to demonstrate the presence of *T. pallidum* with normal CSF parameters. This finding leads to the recommendation that a patient with signs of progressive neurosyphilis and a positive treponemal serologic test be treated with antibiotics regardless of the CSF findings. A CSF pleocytosis may be provoked after 1 week of therapy and may supply supportive evidence for a diagnosis of neurosyphilis.

FUNGAL

The most common CNS fungal infection is cryptococcosis. Most patients are found to have elevated intracranial pressure. A lymphocytic pleocytosis with cell counts under 500 cells/mm³ is present. Glucose levels are low in 50 per cent of cases. Most CSF specimens will exhibit an elevated CSF protein. With the India ink preparation, the organisms may be seen in 50 per cent of cases. CSF cultures are positive in approximately 90 per cent of cases. Cisternal punctures for fluid analysis may be helpful in undiagnosed cases of lymphocytic meningitis in which multiple lumbar punctures have not confirmed the diagnosis.[79] Several serologic tests are available and are of value in the diagnosis and prognosis of cryptococcal meningitis and meningoencephalitis. These are based on the detection of cryptococcal polysaccharide capsular antigens in the CSF.[80] Cryptococcal antigens will be positive in more than 90 per cent of proven cases of cryptococcal meningitis. The false-positive rate is significant and is reported to be as high as 20 per cent in the CSF. Many false-positive results are caused by the presence of rheumatoid factor.[79] CNS cryptococcal infection can have a rather insidious onset (over several weeks) in the AIDS patient; headache and behavioral changes are most commonly recognized.

TUBERCULOSIS

If tuberculosis is suspected, a large volume of CSF (10 ml) is required for adequate culture. The cell count varies from 100 to 400 cells/mm³, with a lymphocytic predominance. Protein levels are elevated (100 to 500 mg/dl); CSF glucose may be depressed. Acid-fast stains must be examined by experienced observers. Fluid is inoculated onto Löwenstein-Jensen medium, and the absence of growth on the medium should not be considered negative until 8 weeks after incubation.[81]

CONCLUSION

A spinal tap should only be performed when the treating physician believes the CSF specimen(s) will be of diagnostic value. The procedure is often indicated in the diagnosis of meningitis or subarachnoid hemorrhage. Most contraindications are relative and not absolute, particularly if infection is an overriding consideration.

REFERENCES

1. Corning JL: Spinal anaesthesia and local medication of the cord. NY State Med J 42:483, 1885.
2. Quincke H: Die lumbar Punktur des Hydrocephalus. Klin Wochenschr 28:929 and 965, 1891.
3. Dandy WE: Experimental hydrocephalus. Ann Surg 70:129, 1919.
4. Sackett JF, Scruthe CM: New Techniques in Myelography. Hagerstown, MD, Harper & Row, 1979.
5. Tourtellotte WW, Shorr RJ: Cerebrospinal fluid. In Youmans JP (ed): Neurological Surgery, Vol. 1. Philadelphia, W. B. Saunders Co, 1982, pp 423–486.
6. Fishman RA: Cerebrospinal Fluid in Diseases of the Nervous System. Philadelphia, W. B. Saunders Co, 1980.
7. Smith DH: The challenge of bacterial meningitis. Hosp Pract 11:71, 1976.
8. Cramblett HG: Managing the child with bacterial meningitis. Hosp Pract 63, Dec. 1969.
9. Mattheis AW, Wehrle PF: Management of bacterial meningitis in children. Pediatr Clin North Am 15:185, 1968.
10. Greiseler PJ, Nelson KE: Bacterial meningitis without clinical signs of meningeal irritation. South Med J 75:448, 1982.
11. Hayward RD, O'Reilly G: Intracerebral hemorrhage, accuracy of computerized transverse axial scanning in predicting the underlying aetiology. Lancet 1:1, 1976.
12. Bouzarth WF, Hedges JR: Computed tomography and lumbar puncture. J Am Coll Emerg Phys 8:164, 1979.
13. Bergstrom M: Variation with time of the attenuation values of intracranial hematomas. J Comput Assist Tomogr 1:57, 1977.
14. Bergstrom M: Computed tomography of cranial subdural and epidural hematomas: Variation of attenuation related to time and clinical events such as rebleeding. J Comput Assist Tomogr 1:449, 1977.
14a. Fontanarosa PB: Recognition of subarachnoid hemorrhage. Ann Emerg Med 18:1199, 1989.
14b. Adams HP, Kassell NF, Torner JC, et al: CT and clinical correlations in recent aneurysmal subarachnoid hemorrhage. a preliminary report of the Cooperative Aneurysm Study. Neurology 33:981, 1983.
15. Vick NA: Grinker's Neurology. Springfield, IL, Charles C Thomas, 1976, pp 514–524 and 560–576.
16. Sundt TM: Intracranial aneurysms and subarachnoid hemorrhage. In Siekert RG (ed): Cerebral Vascular Survey Report. Rochester, MN, Whiting Press, 1980, pp 306–318.
17. Ruff RL, Dougherty JL: Evaluation of acute cerebral ischemia for anticoagulant therapy: Computed tomography or lumbar puncture. Neurology 31:736, 1981.
18. Duffy GP: Lumbar puncture in the presence of raised intracranial pressure. Br Med J 1:407, 1969.
19. Breuer NS, MacCarty CS, et al: Brain abscess: A review of recent experience. Ann Intern Med 82:571, 1975.
20. Samson DS, Clark K: A current review of brain abscess. Am J Med 54:201, 1973.
21. Kaufman P, Leeds N: Computed tomography (CT) in the diagnosis of intracranial abscesses. Neurology 27:1069, 1977.
22. Zimmerman RA, Bilaniuk LT, Shipkin PM, et al: Evolution of cerebral abscess: Correlation of clinical features with computed tomography. Neurology 27:14, 1977.
23. Rotheram E, Kessler L: Use of computerized tomography in nonsurgical management of brain abscess. Arch Neurol 36:25, 1979.
24. Edelson RN, Chernik NZ, Posner JB: Spinal subdural hematomas complicating lumbar puncture. Arch Neurol 31:134, 1974.
25. Laglia AG, Eisenberg RL, Weinstein PR, Mani RL: Spinal epidural hematoma after lumbar puncture. Ann Intern Med 88:515, 1978.
26. Senelick RC, Norwood CW, Cohen GH: "Painless" spinal epidural hematoma during anticoagulant therapy. Neurology 26:213, 1976.

27. Lachman E: Anatomy as applied to clinical medicine. New Phys 145, June 1968.
28. Foers CS: Skin preparation for lumbar puncture. JAMA 258:1241, 1987.
29. Cole M: Pitfalls in cerebrospinal fluid examination. Hosp Pract 47, July 1969.
30. Zivin J: Lateral cervical punctures: An alternative to lumbar puncture. Neurology 28:616, 1978.
31. Greensher J, Mofenson HC, Borofsky LG, et al: Lumbar puncture in the neonate: A simplified technique. J Pediatr 78:1034, 1971.
32. Weisman LE, Merenstein GB, Steinbarger JR: The effects of lumbar puncture position in sick neonates. Am J Dis Child 137:1077, 1983.
33. Shaywitz BD: Epidermoid spinal cord tumors and previous lumbar puncture. J Pediatr 80:638, 1972.
34. Batnitzky S, Keucher TR, Mealey J, et al: Iatrogenic intraspinal epidermoid tumors. JAMA 237:148, 1977.
35. Cole M: Examination of the cerebral spinal fluid. In Toole JF (ed): Special Techniques for Neurologic Diagnosis. Philadelphia, F. A. Davis Co, 1969, pp 29–48.
36. Petito F, Plum F: The lumbar puncture. N Engl J Med 290:225, 1981.
37. Lieberman LM, Tourtellotte WW, Newkirk TA: Prolonged post–lumbar puncture cerebral spinal fluid leakage demonstrated by radioisotope myelography. Neurology 21:925, 1971.
38. Tourtellotte WW, Henderson WG, Tucker RP, et al: A randomized double-blind clinical trial comparing the 22 versus the 26 gauge needle in the production of the post–lumbar puncture syndrome in normal individuals. Headache 12:73, 1972.
39. Brocker RJ: A technique to avoid post spinal-tap headache. JAMA 168:261, 1958.
40. Carbaat PAT, van Crevel H: Lumbar puncture headache: Controlled study on the preventive effect of 24 hours' bed rest. Lancet 2:1133, 1981.
41. Vilming ST, Schrader H, Monstad I: Post–lumbar puncture headache: The significance of body posture. A controlled study of 300 patients. Cephalagia 8:75, 1988.
41a. Sechzer PH, Abel LA: Post-spinal anesthesia headache treated with caffeine: Evaluation with demand method. Part I. Curr Ther Res 24:307, 1978.
41b. Jarvis AP, Greenawalt JW, Fagraeus L: Intravenous caffeine for postdural headache. Anesth Analg 65:316, 1986.
42. Dieterich M, Brandt T: Is obligatory bed rest after lumbar puncture obsolete? Eur Arch Psych Neurol Sci 235:71, 1985.
43. Bradsky JB: Epidural blood patch: A safe effective treatment for post lumbar puncture headaches. West J Med 129:85, 1978.
44. Olsen KS: Epidural blood patch in the treatment of post–lumbar puncture headache. Pain 30:293, 1987.
45. Petersdorf RG, Swarner DR, Garcia M: Studies on the pathogenesis of meningitis. II. Development of meningitis during pneumococcal bacteremia. J Clin Invest 41:320, 1962.
46. Teele DW, Dashefsky B, Rakusan T, Klein JO: Meningitis after lumbar puncture in children with bacteremia. N Engl J Med 305:1079, 1981.
47. Eng R, Seligman S: Lumbar puncture–induced meningitis. JAMA 245:1456, 1981.
48. Shapiro ED, Aaron NH, Wald ER, Chiponis D: Risk factors for development of bacterial meningitis among children with occult bacteria. J Pediatr 109:15, 1986.
49. Krishra V, Liu V, Singleton AF: Should lumbar puncture be routinely performed in patients with suspected bacteremia? J Nat Med Assoc 75:1153, 1983.
50. Fedor HM, Adelman AM, Pugno PA, Dallman J: Meningitis following normal lumbar punctures. J Fam Pract 20:437, 1985.
51. Korein J, Cravito H, Leicach M: Reevaluation of lumbar puncture. Neurology 9:290, 1959.
51a. Zisfein J, Tuchman AJ: Risks of lumbar puncture in the presence of intracranial mass lesions. Mt Sinai J Med 55:283, 1988.
52. Growe DJ, Baker AL, Bell WO, Ball MRet al: Contraindications to lumbar puncture as defined by computed cranial tomography. J Neurol Neurosurg Psychiatry 50:1071, 1987.
53. Plum F, Posner J: The Diagnosis of Stupor and Coma. Philadelphia, F. A. Davis Co, 1980, pp 96–112.
54. Levine JF, Hiesiger EM, Whelan MP, et al: Pneumococcal meningitis associated with retroperitoneal abscess. JAMA 248:2308, 1982.
55. Shenkin HA, Finneson BE: Clinical significance of low cerebral spinal fluid pressure. Neurology 8:157, 1958.
56. Bell WE, Joynt RJ, Sahs A: Low spinal fluid pressure syndromes. Neurology 10:512, 1960.
57. Ward P: Cerebrospinal fluid data. I. Interpretation in intracranial hemorrhage and meningitis. Postgrad Med 68:181, 1980.
58. Osborne JP, Pizer B: Effect on the white cell count of contaminating cerebrospinal fluid with blood. Arch Dis Child 56:400, 1981.
59. Novak R: Lack of validation of standard corrections for white blood cell counts of blood-contaminated cerebrospinal fluid in infants. Am J Clin Pathol 32:95, 1984.
60. Mehl AL: Interpretation of traumatic lumbar puncture. Clin Pediatr 25:523, 1986.
61. Hayward RA, Oye RK: Are polymorphonuclear leukocytes an abnormal finding in cerebrospinal fluid? Arch Intern Med 148:1623, 1988.
62. Prokesch RC: Cerebrospinal fluid pleocytosis after seizure. South Med J 76:322, 1983.
63. Kiberski T: Eosinophils in the cerebrospinal fluid. Ann Intern Med 91:70, 1979.
64. Hersey LA, Trotter JL: The use and abuse of the cerebrospinal fluid IgG profile in the adult: A practical evaluation. Ann Neurol 8:426, 1980.
65. Laurenzi M, Mavra M, Kam-Hansen S, Link H: Oligoclonal IgG and free light chains in multiple sclerosis demonstrated by thin layer polyacrylamide gel. Ann Neurol 8:241, 1980.
66. Johnson KA, Nelson BJ: Multiple sclerosis: Diagnostic usefulness of cerebrospinal fluid. Ann Neurol 2:425, 1977.
67. McNememey WH: The significance of subarachnoid bleeding. Proc R Soc Med 47:701, 1954.
68. Schaffer JG, Goldwin M: Medical microbiology. In Henry JB (ed): Todd, Sanford, and Davidson's Clinical Diagnosis and Management by Laboratory Methods. Philadelphia, W. B. Saunders Co, 1974, p 946.
69. Vorki A, Vorki AP, Puthuran P: Value of second lumbar puncture in confirming a diagnosis of aseptic meningitis. Arch Neurol 36:571, 1979.
70. Ris J, Mancebo J, Domingo P, et al: Bacterial meningitis despite "normal" CSF findings. JAMA 254:2893, 1985.
70a. Spanos A, Harrell Jr FE, Durack DT: Differential diagnosis of acute meningitis: an analysis of the predictive value of initial observations. JAMA 262:2700, 1989.
71. Beatty NH, Oppenheimer S: Cerebrospinal fluid lactic dehydrogenase and its isoenzymes in infections of the central nervous system. N Engl J Med 297:1197, 1968.
72. Durack DT, Spanos A: End-of-treatment spinal tap in bacterial meningitis: Is it worthwhile? JAMA 248:75, 1982.
73. Talan D, Hoffman JR, Yoshikawa TT, Overturf GD: Role of empiric parenteral antibiotics prior to lumbar puncture in suspected bacterial meningitis. State of the art. Rev Infect Dis 10:365, 1988.
74. Edberg SC: Conventional and molecular techniques for the laboratory diagnosis of infections of the central nervous system. Neurol Clin 4:13, 1986.
75. Klein JO, Feigin RD, McCraken GH: Report of the task force on diagnosis and management of meningitis. Pediatrics 78:959, 1986.
76. Trott A: Acute meningitis. Crit Dec Emerg Med 3:1, 1988.
76a. Chalmers AC, Aprill BS, Shepard H: Cerebrospinal fluid and human immunodeficiency virus: findings in healthy, asymptomatic, seropositive men. Arch Intern Med 150:1538, 1990.
77. Hanson JR: Modern neurosyphilis: A partially treated chronic meningitis. West J Med 135:191, 1981.
78. Jaffe HW: The laboratory diagnosis of syphilis. Ann Intern Med 83:846, 1975.
79. Yoshikawa TT: Management of central nervous system cryptococcosis. West J Med 132:123, 1980.
80. Goodman JS, Kaufman L, Koenig MG: Diagnosis of cryptococcal meningitis. N Engl J Med 285:434, 1971.
81. Kennedy DH, Fallon RJ: Tuberculous meningitis. JAMA 241:264, 1979.

Chapter *83*

Caloric Testing

Paul B. Baker

INTRODUCTION

An accurate assessment of the comatose patient requires a thorough neurologic examination, with careful evaluation of the patient's responses to a variety of external stimuli. In an individual with normal brain stem function, stimulation of the vestibular labyrinth will result in compensatory deviation of the eyes. This response is known as the vestibulo-ocular reflex and forms the physiologic basis for the caloric test of the vestibular system. During caloric testing, a thermal stimulus, usually water at a specific temperature, is delivered to the external auditory canal to activate the labyrinth and produce the characteristic ocular movements. Pathologic conditions involving either the vestibular or oculomotor reflex pathways will alter or abolish the response to caloric stimulation.

Caloric tests are performed in both conscious and unconscious patients, depending upon the diagnostic circumstances. Quantitative caloric examination is conducted in the ambulatory patient for evaluation of possible vestibular dysfunction. This type of testing requires precisely controlled irrigation temperatures and specialized recording devices and is best undertaken in a properly equipped laboratory under the supervision of an experienced neurotologist. However, the neurologist, neurosurgeon, or emergency physician may perform *qualitative* caloric testing in the comatose patient for detection of gross disruption of vestibulo-ocular reflex pathways indicative of structural lesions or metabolic abnormalities involving the brain stem. In this setting, large quantities of ice water provide maximal stimulation of the vestibular apparatus. Such testing needs no special expertise and can be done at the bedside using equipment readily available in the emergency department. This simple procedure can provide valuable diagnostic and prognostic information necessary for management of the comatose patient.

BACKGROUND

In the middle of the nineteenth century, Brown-Séquard first described the effects of introducing cold water into the ear canal.[1] The clinical importance of the phenomenon was first realized in 1906 by Bárány, who developed a caloric procedure using an ice water stimulus.[2] He postulated, correctly, that caloric stimulation of the auditory canal induced formation of convection currents within the semicircular canals of the vestibular labyrinth.

Different methods of caloric testing were later proposed by Kobrak and others, but standardization of the procedure awaited the introduction of the Fitzgerald-Hallpike technique in 1942.[3] This technique, which uses both warm and cool water stimuli under rigidly specified conditions, permits quantification of normal and abnormal caloric responses. Today, most formal caloric testing of conscious patients is based on variations of the original Fitzgerald-Hallpike procedure.

The value of caloric testing in the assessment of the comatose patient was emphasized by the work of Klingon and Bender and associates in the 1950s.[4, 5] Vaernet and Ethelberg studied the changes in caloric reactions during transtentorial herniation of the brain stem.[6, 7] Blegvad reported the effects of barbiturate intoxication upon the vestibulo-ocular reflex.[8]

More recent advances include the development of electronystagmography (ENG), which provides a graphic record of reflex eye movements and permits precise determination of the intensity of the caloric response.[9] Researchers have recently investigated the use of heated air as an alternative to traditional water caloric tests.[10]

PHYSIOLOGY AND FUNCTIONAL ANATOMY

Proper performance and interpretation of the caloric test require a basic understanding of the structure and function of both the vestibular and oculomotor systems. The anatomic pathways underlying the vestibulo-ocular reflex begin in the posterior portion of the labyrinth of the inner ear. The peripheral vestibular apparatus is located within the temporal bone and consists of the utricle, the saccule, and the lateral, anterior, and posterior semicircular canals (Fig. 83–1). Because of its proximity to the external ear canal, the lateral or horizontal canal is of principal interest in caloric testing. Note that the lateral canal is oriented at a 30-degree angle to the horizontal (Fig. 83–2). Deflections of the cupula due to movement of endolymphatic fluid within the canal result in polarization changes in the underlying hair cell, which in turn are relayed to the afferent limb of the primary vestibular neuron.

Impulses of the primary neuron travel via Scarpa's ganglion and CN VIII to the brain stem to synapse with secondary vestibular neurons in the superior and medial vestibular nuclei of the upper medulla and lower pons (Fig. 83–3). Although the connections between the vestibular and oculomotor nuclei in the brain stem are quite complex, two main pathways exist. The direct projection runs from the vestibular complex to the nuclei of CN III and CN VI via the medial longitudinal fasciculus (MLF) and involves only three neurons: the primary vestibular, secondary vestibular, and oculomotor neurons.[11] The indirect projection between these same nuclei occurs over multisynaptic circuits in the tegmental reticular formation.[12] Another brain stem structure contributing to the vestibulo-ocular interaction is the parapontine reticular formation (PPRF), a poorly characterized group of pontine neurons that coordinates both voluntary and involuntary lateral gaze. The PPRF receives multiple inputs, including projections from the vestibular system and the contralateral frontal cortex, and sends output to oculomotor neurons through both the direct and indirect pathways. Excitatory impulses originating in the lateral canal finally travel via the oculomotor and abducens nerves to the

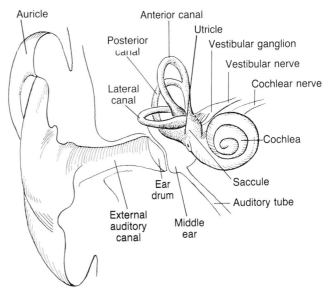

Figure 83–1. Diagram of the external, middle, and inner ear, showing the relationship of the semicircular canals to the external auditory canal. (Ossicles have been removed for clarity.) (Modified from Noback CR, Demarest RJ: The Human Nervous System. New York, McGraw-Hill Book Co, 1981, p 342.)

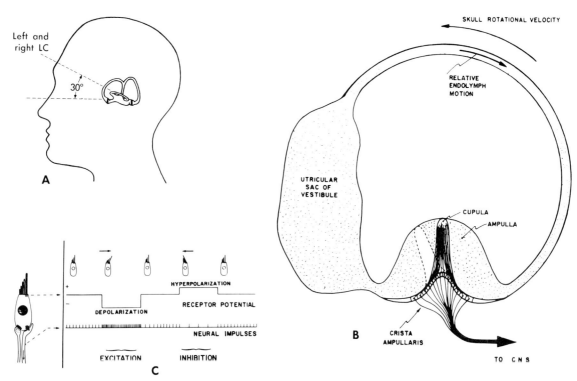

Figure 83–2. *A,* The long axis of the lateral canal forms a 30-degree angle with the horizontal plane. This alignment must be compensated for during caloric testing by proper positioning of the patient. (From Barber HO, Stockwell CW: Manual of Electronystagmography. 2nd ed. St. Louis, CV Mosby Co, 1980. Reproduced by permission.) *B,* Schematic diagram of the semicircular canal, showing the relationship between endolymphatic flow and cupular deviation. (From Jones GM, Milfum JH: Trans Biomed Eng BME-12, pp 54–64, © 1965 IEEE.) *C,* Diagram showing the effect of deflection on the underlying hair cell and its associated primary vestibular neuron. (From Flock A: In Durrant JD, Lovrinic JH: Bases of Hearing Science. 2nd ed. Baltimore, Williams & Wilkins, 1984. Reproduced by permission. © Williams & Wilkins, 1984.)

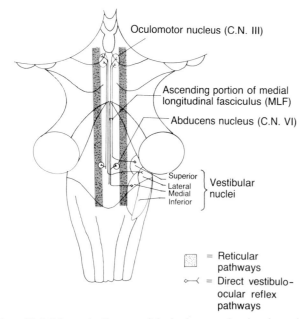

Figure 83–3. Schematic diagram of the brain stem, showing the major elements of the vestibulo-ocular reflex (VOR) pathway. The solid line indicates the direct projection between the vestibular nuclei and the third and sixth nucleus. The stippled area represents the indirect projections between the nuclei. (Modified from Barr ML, Kiernan JA: The Human Nervous System—An Anatomical Viewpoint. 5th ed. Philadelphia, JB Lippincott Co, 1988, p 330.)

ipsilateral medial rectus and contralateral lateral rectus muscles.

Rotation of the head generates flow of endolymphatic fluid within the semicircular canals. The firing rate of the primary vestibular neuron is dependent upon the direction of flow. For example, in the lateral canal, flow toward the ampulla (ampullopetal) increases the rate, whereas flow away from the ampulla (ampullofugal) decreases the rate.[13] Increased firing on one side results in conjugate deviation of the eyes toward the opposite side, whereas decreased firing causes deviation to the same side. This principle forms the physiologic basis of caloric testing. When the lateral canal is placed in the vertical position and ice water is infused into the ear, the endolymph nearest the canal will cool and sink, resulting in ampullofugal flow (Fig. 83–4). As the firing rate decreases, the eyes conjugally deviate toward the side of irrigation. Likewise, if warm water were used in the same position or if the canal were inverted 180 degrees, the opposite would occur.

Eye movements induced by caloric stimulation in conscious, neurologically normal individuals are more complex. Ice water infusions will induce a rhythmic jerking of the eyes that includes a slow deviation toward the irrigated side followed by a quick compensatory saccade toward the midline. This is known as *caloric nystagmus.* By convention, *caloric nystagmus is named for the fast component,* thus the popular mnemonic "Fast COWS" (Cold irrigation—Opposite beating nystagmus; Warm irrigation—Same-sided beating nystagmus). Most sources attribute the slow phase of nystagmus to vestibular activity transmitted over the direct pathway,

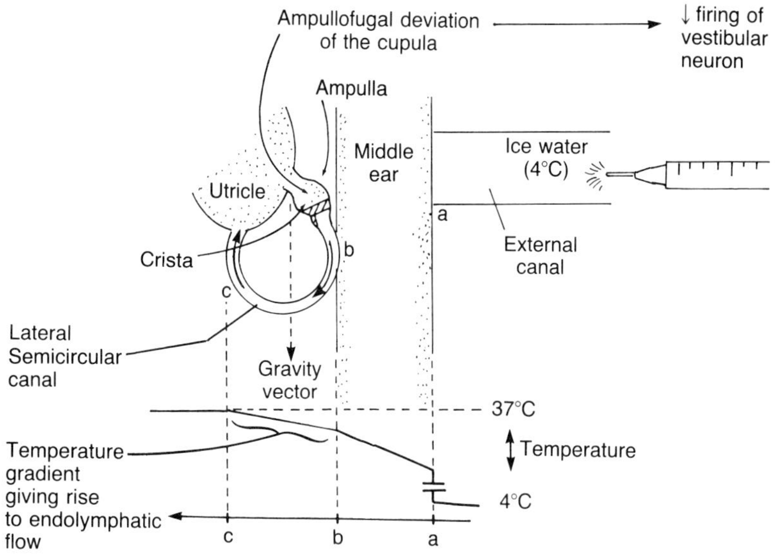

Figure 83–4. The effects of ice water irrigation on the lateral semicircular canal. The cooler endolymph sinks, resulting in ampullofugal flow and decreased neural firing of the primary vestibular neuron. Actual temperature changes within the endolymphatic fluid are on the order of 1° to 2° C. (Modified from Baloh RW, Honrubia V: Clinical Neurophysiology of the Vestibular System. Philadelphia, FA Davis Co, 1979, p 133.)

whereas the fast phase is believed to be generated by the PPRF in conjunction with cortical activity and carried over indirect pathways within the reticular formation. Numerous factors, both physiologic and pathologic, can alter caloric-induced eye movements.

EQUIPMENT

The equipment needed for performance of the caloric test is minimal and readily available in the emergency department or hospital ward. Although almost any size syringe will suffice, a 12- or 35-ml plastic syringe is ideal for irrigation. The syringe may be used as is, or a short length of soft plastic tubing may be attached. A good source of tubing is a butterfly catheter with the needle cut off. Several hundred ml of ice water should be available, although larger quantities of cool (less than 25° C) tap water can be used with similar results if ice is unavailable. Sterile or bacteriostatic saline may be used, although its advantage over tap water has not been shown. A small basin is useful to collect water as it drains from the ear canal.

Additional required equipment includes an otoscope, several sizes of ear speculums, and equipment for removal of cerumen. Towels and a thermometer that reads from 0 to 50° C are also helpful.

INDICATIONS AND CONTRAINDICATIONS

Caloric testing of the comatose patient is indicated when the physician needs information regarding the functional integrity of the brain stem. When the cause of the coma is initially unknown, caloric testing will assist in differentiation among structural, metabolic, and psychogenic causes for unresponsiveness. Even when the etiology is clearly known, caloric testing will provide an indication of the depth of coma and the prognosis for eventual recovery.

In conscious patients who complain of vertigo, caloric testing may be indicated for the nonemergency evaluation of possible vestibular disorders. Ice water produces maximal stimulation of the labyrinth and may induce nausea and vomiting in awake, susceptible individuals. These patients are best referred to a qualified neurotologist, who can conduct more accurate testing in the ENG laboratory with much less discomfort to the patient.

There are few contraindications to caloric testing. An absolute contraindication is the presence of a basilar skull fracture, either documented radiologically or suspected by clinical signs, because of the risk of introducing infection into the central nervous system (CNS) through an associated dural tear. If bilateral fracture can be readily excluded, testing of the intact ear with both warm and cold water will yield results similar to those of the standard bilateral examination.

Relative contraindications to water caloric testing include perforations of the tympanic membrane (those not due to temporal fractures), otitis media and externa, and the presence of previous otologic surgery (e.g., mastoidectomy). Although the risk of otitis media is probably small, carrying out the caloric test in the comatose patient under these conditions remains a matter of clinical judgment. When available, auditory evoked potentials provide an alternative source of information when caloric testing is contraindicated.

PROCEDURE

Caloric testing should be deferred until the patient's condition has been stabilized, including protection of the airway and evaluation of the cervical spine in trauma patients. A thorough neurologic assessment should be performed prior to caloric testing, with special attention given to the ocular examination. Pupillary responses, spontaneous ocular movements, and resting eye position should be accurately recorded. The ears should be inspected prior to insertion of the otoscope. If active bleeding or cerebrospinal fluid otorrhea/rhinorrhea is noted in the trauma victim, caloric testing and further otoscopic examination should be curtailed and the patient should be treated for a probable basilar skull fracture. If the external ear canal appears normal, the otoscopic examination should be completed. Signs of active ear infection or perforation of the tympanic membrane are contraindications to caloric testing. Tympanic rupture, hemotympanum, and step deformities of the canal may indicate fracture of the temporal bone; caloric testing in this situation is contraindicated (Fig. 83–5). Excess cerumen and foreign material must be removed, and the tympanic membrane must be clearly visualized. The ear speculum may be left in the canal as a guide for irrigation.

The patient should be placed in a supine position, with the head or upper body raised 30 degrees (two pillows will result in the appropriate angle). This angle places the lateral

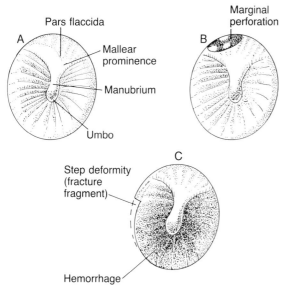

Figure 83–5. Appearance of the tympanic membrane in a normal individual *(A)*, in a patient with a superior marginal perforation and keratoma *(B)*, and in a patient with a step deformity caused by a longitudinal fracture of the temporal bone with associated hemotympanum *(C)*. (Modified from Baloh RW, Honrubia V: Clinical Neurophysiology of the Vestibular System. Philadelphia, FA Davis Co, 1979, p 105.)

canal in the vertical position and ensures a maximal response. The patient should be draped with a towel, and a small basin should be positioned below the ear to collect the water outflow. A container should be filled with several hundred ml of ice water and placed near the bedside.

The syringe and catheter system *(minus the needle)* should be filled with 10 ml of ice water, and the irrigation stream should be directed at the upper posterior portion of the tympanic membrane. Because the goal of the qualitative caloric test is to induce a maximum response, the amount and rate of infusion are not critical. As a general guide, 5 to 10 ml of ice water should be initially infused over a period of 5 to 10 seconds; amounts less than 5 ml may be advisable in suspected cases of light coma or psychogenic unresponsiveness. If no response is noted within 1 or 2 minutes, up to several hundred ml should be infused before declaring that there is no response. Testing of the contralateral ear may begin 5 or 10 minutes after the eyes have returned to their original position. At the conclusion of the testing, the otoscopic examination should be repeated to check for blanching of the tympanic membrane, a sign that the irrigation stream was properly directed.

Observation of eye deviation is easier when an assistant holds the patient's eyelids open. Movement usually occurs after a latency of 10 to 40 seconds, with persistence of the response for as long as 4 or 5 minutes. Small deviations may be detected by focusing on a small scleral vessel. Alternatively, a dermographic pencil may be used to mark the initial position of the pupil with respect to the eyelid.

Variations of the caloric technique may be useful in certain situations. Warm water caloric testing may be performed if no response to bilateral ice water caloric testing is obtained or in cases in which only one ear can be tested. Water temperature should be kept below 50° C. The response elicited will be the opposite of that obtained with ice water. In patients who fail to respond to ice water caloric testing alone, additional stimulation may be obtained by combining irrigation with repeated head turning away from

the irrigated side (the "doll's eye" maneuver). *Obviously, cervical injury must be excluded prior to using this technique.* This combination of techniques may produce eye movements in patients who do not respond to caloric testing alone.[14] Eviatar and Goodhill have described a technique for caloric testing in tympanic perforations using a small latex finger cot placed in the ear canal to prevent water from entering the middle ear.[15]

The technique of bilateral caloric testing is used to evaluate vertical gaze disorders and involves the simultaneous delivery of equal amounts of ice water to both ear canals. A large syringe can be attached to a Y-connector, or two separate syringes can be used. Two people are needed to administer the caloric challenge properly. In normal individuals, upward beating nystagmus is seen after a latency of 1 to 3 minutes (as expected, the opposite is seen with warm water). The mechanism of this phenomenon is not clear, but it may involve stimulation of the remaining two semicircular canals.

COMPLICATIONS

There are few complications with caloric testing, and they can be avoided by carefully selecting those patients who are tested and the equipment and technique used. Using needles or other sharp objects to irrigate the ear may result in laceration or perforation of the tympanic membrane or canal wall if the patient moves unexpectedly. The use of plastic syringes and soft catheter tubing will aid in reducing such occurrences.

Other potential complications of caloric testing include otitis media, meningitis, and the induction of vomiting and subsequent aspiration. Ice water irrigation in the presence of tympanic membrane perforation will increase the chance of middle ear infection; however, the incidence of this complication following caloric testing has not been reported. Meningitis may follow basilar skull fractures with meningeal tears; the additional risk of calorics in such situations is not known. Therefore, caloric testing should be omitted in the head injured patient if there is any suspicion of temporal fracture. Although ice water irrigation may produce nausea and even emesis in a few awake patients, vomiting or aspiration has not been reported as a complication of caloric testing in the comatose patient. Nevertheless, it is advisable to delay testing until the patient's airway is protected.

INTERPRETATION

The first phase of interpretation of the caloric test involves analysis of initial eye position and spontaneous eye movements prior to irrigation. Comatose patients with intact oculomotor pathways will usually have their eyes directed straight ahead or slightly divergent. Unilateral destructive lesions of the cerebral hemisphere can cause conjugate deviation of the eyes *toward* the side of the lesion, whereas irritative foci, as might be seen in status epilepticus, can cause conjugate deviation *away* from the affected side. Deviations of this type can usually be overcome by caloric stimulation, although combined irrigation and head turning may be required in the first hours following the insult. Lesions in or near the PPRF in the brain stem cause conjugate deviation *away* from the side of the lesion that usually cannot be overcome by calorics. Conjugate downward deviation can be seen with structural lesions of the brain stem or in the deeper phases of metabolic coma. Dysconjugate gaze either indicates damage at the level of the oculomotor nuclei or below or reflects disruption of the ocular muscles themselves.[16] Dysconjugate gaze may also be seen in drug-induced coma in the presence of a structurally intact brain stem pathway. In the very late stages of brain stem dysfunction, the eyes will usually return to the central position. Spontaneous roving movements of the eyes, either conjugate or dysconjugate, may be seen in supratentorial insults, but these too disappear with brain stem involvement.[14] Ocular "bobbing" is an intermittent, spontaneous downward jerking of the eyes that may occur with massive pontine lesions. There is paralysis of both voluntary and reflex lateral gaze, and caloric stimulation may increase the rate of bobbing without causing lateral deviation of the eyes.[17] Ocular "dipping" is a more prolonged, downward conjugate deviation of the eyes and has been reported in cases of severe anoxic encephalopathy (e.g., carbon monoxide poisoning).[18] The pathophysiologic basis of these eye movements is poorly understood.[19]

The second phase of interpretation involves analysis of eye movements following caloric irrigation. Reactions to ice water stimuli may be divided into four categories: normal nystagmus, conjugate deviation, dysconjugate deviation, and absent responses (Fig. 83–6). The first reaction, normal nystagmus with the fast component beating away from the side of ice water irrigation, is seen in normal, alert individuals, in cases of psychogenic unresponsiveness, and in those who have very mild organic disturbances of consciousness. The intensity of nystagmus is highly variable in conscious subjects and depends upon the degree of visual fixation and the level of mental alertness. The response is present in more than 90 per cent of children by the age of 6 months and declines in magnitude only after the seventh decade of life.[20, 21] Corneal reflexes and responses to facial pinprick may be abolished by hypnotic suggestion in susceptible individuals; however, caloric nystagmus appears to be immune to similar manipulation.[22]

Normal nystagmus is the usual result of caloric testing in cases of psychogenic unresponsiveness due to catatonia, hysterical conversion, schizophrenia, and malingering. Hyperactive caloric responses result from testing in the presence of tympanic perforation and mastoid disease. Hypoactive responses are recorded in a wide variety of vestibular and neurologic disorders.

Hypoactive responses usually require quantitative caloric testing with ENG for detection. Caloric nystagmus may be *inverted* (beating to the wrong side) or *perverted* (beating in the wrong plane); both responses are seen in brain stem lesions. *Pseudocaloric nystagmus* is a pre-existing latent nystagmus that is brought out by the general arousal of ice water irrigation and can be distinguished from true nystagmus by its failure to reverse directions with warm water irrigation.

As the level of coma deepens, the fast phase of nystagmus becomes intermittent and finally disappears, probably as a result of decreased activity in the cortex and reticular formation.

In the second type of caloric response, the eyes deviate conjugately toward the side of ice water stimulation (they "look" toward the source of irritation). When present, this reaction indicates intact brain stem function and is seen during general anesthesia, in supratentorial lesions *without brain stem compression*, and in most but not all metabolic and drug-induced comas. In such situations, bilateral simultaneous irrigation with ice water will result in conjugate downward deviation, implying that brain stem centers for vertical gaze are functional.

Dysconjugate reactions constitute the third type of caloric response to ice water stimuli. The most common dysconjugate reaction is internuclear ophthalmoplegia, in which a lesion of the MLF causes weakness or paralysis of the *adducting* eye following caloric irrigation. Internuclear

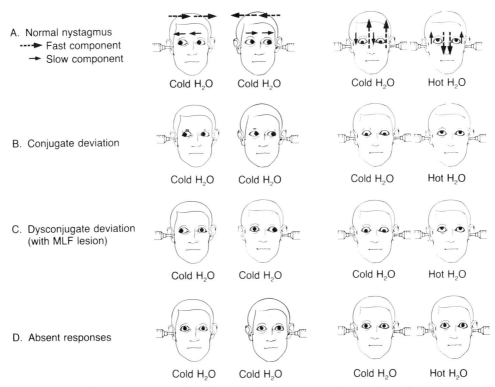

A. Normal nystagmus
- - - → Fast component
→ Slow component

Figure 83–6. The four types of caloric responses seen with unilateral and bilateral irrigations. *A*, Normal nystagmus. *B*, Conjugate deviation. *C*, Dysconjugate deviation. The most common type, internuclear ophthalmoplegia, is shown here. Vertical eye movements usually remain intact in this lesion. *D*, Absent caloric responses. MLF, Medial longitudinal fasciculus. (Modified from Plum F, Posner JB: The Diagnosis of Stupor and Coma. 3rd ed. Philadelphia, FA Davis Co, 1980, p 55.)

ophthalmoplegia may be due to acute damage to the rostral pons or may be seen as a manifestation of multiple sclerosis or previous vascular insult.

In acute supratentorial lesions, the development of dysconjugate caloric responses is a significant sign that may indicate compression of the brain stem and impending herniation. Caloric responses of this type are less common with metabolic and drug-induced coma and, when present in metabolic coma, have less ominous significance. Reversible internuclear ophthalmoplegia has been reported in hepatic coma and may occur during phenytoin, barbiturate, and amitriptyline toxicities. Forced downward deviation of the eyes, either conjugate or dysconjugate, may be seen in sedative-hypnotic–induced coma when unilateral caloric testing is performed.[23]

Palsies of the oculomotor nerves are another cause of dysconjugate reactions, although most should be apparent before irrigation. Etiologies include diabetic neuropathy (especially CN VI), increased intracranial pressure, and Wernicke's encephalopathy. Finally, Plum and Posner report that unusual and poorly characterized caloric responses may be obtained from the testing of comatose patients with long-standing, severe brain injury.[16]

Absent caloric responses are the fourth category of reactions to ice water stimuli. As a general rule, the oculo-vestibular response is preserved longer than other brain stem reflexes; however, the oculocephalic or "doll's eye" response may persist in the absence of caloric responses due to bilateral labyrinthine disease because of additional input from proprioceptive receptors in the neck. Loss of caloric responses in comatose patients with structural lesions is usually a sign of brain stem damage. In supratentorial lesions, progressive loss of caloric responses may be seen in the final stages of transtentorial herniation. The oculovestibular reflex may also be transiently absent or decreased on the side opposite massive supratentorial damage during the first hours following injury.[24] Absent caloric responses may occur in any subtentorial lesion that affects vestibular reflex pathways, including pontine hemorrhage, basilar artery occlusion, cerebellar hemorrhage or infarction with encroachment upon the brain stem, and any expanding mass lesion within the posterior fossa. Calorics may disappear in deep coma resulting from subarachnoid hemorrhage, perhaps owing to pressure upon the brain stem.

The vestibulo-ocular reflex is usually retained until the late stages of metabolic coma. When the reflex does disappear, as in the case of hepatic coma, it is frequently a preterminal event.[25] Nevertheless, caloric responses may be transiently absent in certain types of drug-induced coma, with the *eventual complete recovery of the patient*. The vestibulo-ocular reflex seems particularly sensitive to the effects of sedative-hypnotics (barbiturates, glutethimide), antidepressants (amitriptyline, doxepin), and anticonvulsants (phenytoin, carbamazepine).[8, 26, 27] Obviously, neuromuscular blocking agents (e.g., succinylcholine) will abolish caloric-induced ocular movements.

Finally, the caloric response may be absent for reasons other than those responsible for the coma. Inadequate irrigation due to excess cerumen or poor technique and unilateral or bilateral dysfunction of the peripheral vestibular apparatus must be considered. Bilateral loss of caloric response (arreflexia vestibularis) is uncommon in conscious patients, constituting 1.7 and 0.2 per cent of the ENG clinical population in two large series of patients.[28, 29] Some of the causes of unilateral and bilateral loss of oculovestibular reflexes in conscious patients are listed in Table 83–1.

The vestibulo-ocular reflex has *prognostic* as well as diagnostic significance in the comatose patient. In a study of 100 patients who were comatose from head trauma, absence

Table 83–1. Possible Causes of Absent Vestibulo-ocular Reflex In Conscious Patients

Inadequate Irrigation	**Traumatic**
Cerumen Impaction	Previous temporal fracture
Postinfectious	Previous head injury
Meningitis	Postlabyrinthectomy
Encephalitis	**Labyrinthine**
Syphilis	Vestibular neuronitis
Neoplastic	Suppurative labyrinthitis
Acoustic neuroma	**Congenital**
Other cerebellopontine	Congenital hydrocephalus
angle tumors	Hereditary spinocerebellar
Posterior fossa tumors	degeneration
Inflammatory	**Idiopathic**
Systemic lupus	**Drugs**
erythematosus	Aminoglycoside antibiotics
Cogan's Syndrome	Neuromuscular blocking
	agents
	Anticonvulsants*

*Reported rarely in conscious patients who have taken more than normal therapeutic dosage.

of calorics at 1 to 3 days following injury was associated with extremely high mortality.[30] Testing in the immediate post-traumatic period may yield inconsistent responses and is of considerably less prognostic value. Levy and coworkers studied 500 cases of nontraumatic, non–drug-induced coma in a large multicenter effort. Absence of the vestibulo-ocular reflex correlated with less than a 5 per cent chance of achieving functional recovery within 1 year when tested within 6 to 24 hours of coma onset.[31] In one study of comatose patients, the combination of absent vestibulo-ocular reflex and absent pupillary light reflex at 24 hours was associated with a 100 per cent mortality.[32] Complete loss of caloric responses is part of the criteria for the legal diagnosis of "brain death" in many localities and correlates with the irreversible cessation of cerebral function at least as well as an isoelectric electroencephalogram (EEG).[33] Excessive reliance on a single clinical sign must be avoided, and decisions regarding neurologic prognosis and future therapy should be based on complete consideration of all evidence available to the physician.

CONCLUSION

The caloric test is a simple, easily performed procedure that should be a part of the complete neurologic assessment of the comatose patient, unless contraindicated. In the emergency patient, this test should be reserved for the stable patient undergoing secondary assessment. Even when the etiology of the coma is known, the test can provide a baseline for the evaluation of future changes in the patient's status. The examination requires minimal equipment and can be conducted in a few minutes while awaiting laboratory results or during preparation for computed tomographic scanning. Complications are few if patients are properly selected and when correct technique is used. When reliably interpreted, caloric testing furnishes valuable diagnostic and prognostic information necessary for proper care of the comatose individual.

REFERENCES

1. Brown-Séquard C: Course of Lectures on the Physiology and Pathology of the Central Nervous System. Philadelphia, Collins, 1860, p 187.
2. Bárány R: Untersuchungen über den vom Vestibularapparat des Ohres reflektorisch ausgelosten rhythmischen Nystagmus und seine Begleiterscheinungen Mschr. Ohrenheilk 40:193, 1906.
3. Fitzgerald G, Hallpike CS: Studies in human vestibular function: 1. Observations of the directional preponderance ("Nystagmus bereitschaft") of caloric nystagmus resulting from cerebral lesions. Brain 65:115, 1942.

4. Klingon GH: Caloric stimulation in localization of brain stem lesions in a comatose patient. AMA Arch Neurol Psychiatr 68:233, 1952.
5. Bender MB, Bergman PS, Nathanson M: Ocular movements on passive head turning and caloric stimulation in comatose patients. Trans Am Neurol Assoc 80:184, 1955.
6. Vaernet K: Caloric vestibular reactions in transtentorial herniation of the brainstem. Neurology 7:833, 1957.
7. Ethelberg S: Vestibulo-ocular reflex disorders in a case of transtentorial herniation and foraminal impaction of the brainstem. Acta Psychiatr Scand 30:187, 1955.
8. Blegvad B: Caloric vestibular reaction in unconscious patients. Arch Otolaryngol 75:36, 1962.
9. Barber H, Stockwell C: Manual of Electronystagmography. St. Louis, The C. V. Mosby Co, 1980.
10. Zangemeister WH, Bock O: Air vs. water caloric test. Clin Otolaryngol 5:379, 1980.
11. Szentagothai J: The elementary vestibulo-ocular reflex arc. J Neurophysiol 13:395, 1950.
12. Precht W: Vestibular mechanisms. Ann Rev Neurosci 2:265, 1979.
13. Baloh RW, Honrubia V: Clinical Neurophysiology of the Vestibular System. Philadelphia, F. A. Davis Co, 1979, p 40.
14. Fischer CM: The neurological exam of the comatose patient. Acta Neurol Scand (Suppl 36)45:43, 1969.
15. Eviatar A, Goodhill V: A dry calorization method for vestibular function studies. Laryngoscope 78:1746, 1968.
16. Plum F, Posner JB: The Diagnosis of Stupor and Coma, 3rd ed. Philadelphia, F. A. Davis Co, 1980, pp 57–61.
17. Susac JO, Hoyt WF, Daroff RB, et al: Clinical spectrum of ocular bobbing. J Neurol Neurosurg Psychiatr 33:771, 1970.
18. Ropper AH: Ocular dipping in anoxic coma. Arch Neurol 38:297, 1981.
19. Rosenberg ML: Spontaneous vertical eye movements in coma. Ann Neurol 20:635, 1986.
20. Eviatar L, Miranda S, Eviatar A, et al: Development of nystagmus in response to vestibular stimulation in infants. Ann Neurol 5:508, 1979.
21. Bruner A, Norris TW: Age-related changes in caloric nystagmus. Acta Otolaryngol (Suppl) 282:1, 1971.
22. Cogan DG: Brain lesions and eye movements in man. In Bender MB (ed): The Oculomotor System. New York, Harper & Row Publishers, Inc, 1964, p 487.
23. Simon RP: Forced downward ocular deviation. Arch Neurol 35:456, 1978.
24. Posner JB, Plum F: Diagnostic significance of vestibulo-ocular responses. J Neurol Neurosurg Psychiatr 38:727, 1975.
25. Hanid MA, Silk DB, Williams R: Prognostic value of the oculovestibular reflex in fulminant hepatic failure. Br Med J 1:1029, 1978.
26. Spector RH, Schnapper R: Amitriptyline-induced ophthalmoplegia. Neurology 31:1188, 1981.
27. Spector RH, Davidoff RA, Schwartzman RJ: Phenytoin-induced ophthalmoplegia. Neurology 26:1031, 1976.
28. Simons FB: Patients with bilateral loss of caloric response. Ann Otol Rhinol Laryngol 82:175, 1973.
29. Steensen SH, Toxman J, Zilstorff K: Bilateral loss of caloric response in conscious patients (arreflexia vestibularis). Clin Otolaryngol 5:373, 1980.
30. Poulsen J, Zilstorff K: Prognostic value of the caloric vestibular test in the unconscious patient with cranial trauma. Acta Neurol Scand 48:282, 1972.
31. Levy DE, Bates D, Caronna JJ, et al: Prognosis in nontraumatic coma. Ann Intern Med 94:293, 1981.
32. Mueller-Jensen A, Neunzig HP, Emskötter T: Outcome prediction in comatose patients: Significance of reflex eye movement analysis. J Neurol Neurosurg Psychiatr 50:389, 1987.
33. Hicks RG, Torada TA: The vestibulo-ocular (caloric) reflex in the diagnosis of cerebral death. Anesth Intens Care 7:169, 1979.

Chapter **84**

Myasthenia Gravis Testing

J. Stephen Huff

INTRODUCTION

Myasthenia gravis is the most common disease of neuromuscular transmission, yet has an incidence of only 1 in 20,000 of the general population. Patients with myasthenia may be grouped into two major categories. The first group shows weakness in proximal muscles, which increases with activity and later improves with rest. The other group presents with ocular complaints of diplopia or ptosis. Patients in this group may or may not have generalized symptoms as well. Fatigue is the hallmark of the disease; symptoms seem to wax and wane. Patients frequently see a number of physicians before a correct diagnosis is made.[1–3]

Myasthenia gravis results from an immune-mediated decrease of postsynaptic acetylcholine receptors (AChRs) with variable failure of neuromuscular transmission.[1, 2, 4–6] Acetylcholine (ACh) is the transmitter at the neuromuscular junction. When the nerve terminal is stimulated, ACh is released in a quantity far in excess of that needed for effective activation of the AChR. The ACh diffuses across the synaptic cleft to transiently interact with the AChR, and an electric potential is generated at the myoneural end plate. If of sufficient magnitude, this end plate potential initiates an action potential that is propagated along the muscle membrane and leads to muscle fiber contraction. The acetylcholine is rapidly hydrolyzed by acetylcholinesterase in the synaptic cleft. Figure 84–1 summarizes neurotransmitter action at the neuromuscular junction. Of the millions of receptors at each myoneural junction, only a fraction must depolarize to stimulate muscle fiber contraction. Any factor that decreases the chance of interaction of ACh with AChR de-

creases the probability of an action potential being generated. Acetylcholinesterase inhibitors (anticholinesterases) have been the mainstay of therapy for myasthenia gravis for years but have been supplemented by aggressive immunosuppressive regimens and thymectomy. Failure of neuromuscular transmission may also occur with *excessive* acetylcholinesterase inhibition; the persistence of acetylcholine in the synaptic cleft leads to continuous depolarization of the receptor.

A patient with myasthenia gravis may present to the emergency department in one of two ways that might necessitate bedside diagnostic testing. The first presentation involves a known myasthenic patient on cholinesterase inhibitor therapy with increased weakness; pharmacologic testing in this setting is controversial and is discussed in the following section. The second presentation involves a previously undiagnosed patient in whom the diagnosis of myasthenia gravis is suspected with ptosis, diplopia, or variable muscular weakness.

Various tests are available to help with the assessment of this second presentation. Acetylcholine receptor antibody assay is now readily available and positive in more than 80 per cent of patients.[7, 8] Repetitive nerve stimulation and single-fiber electromyography tests are available in the electrophysiology laboratory.[7, 9] Several pharmacologic tests have been used, including parenteral administration of edrophonium chloride (Tensilon), neostigmine, and curare. Curare has been used systemically but can also be administered into an ischemic arm; this modification is known as the regional curare test.[9] Many of these tests are seldom used or fall in the realm of the neurologist. Edrophonium administration for diagnosis of myasthenia gravis (Tensilon test) is described in detail because of the drug's rapid onset, short duration of action, and widespread acceptance for this diagnostic challenge. The "ice pack" test also is included because of early favorable reports of its utility and the noninvasive nature of the test.[10]

EDROPHONIUM (TENSILON) TEST

Background

Edrophonium chloride (Tensilon) is an acetylcholinesterase inhibitor that has been used in the diagnosis of myasthenia gravis for more than 30 years. The short duration of action of edropho-

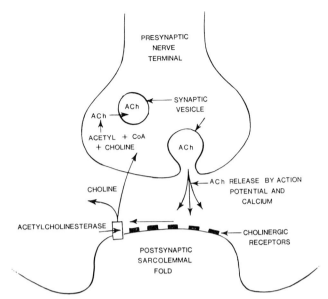

Figure 84–1. Neurotransmitter action at a neuromuscular junction. Acetylcholine *(ACh)* is formed and stored in the nerve terminal. It is released by nerve terminal depolarization in the presence of calcium and binds with receptors on the postsynaptic membrane. After producing an ionic conductance charge, it is hydrolyzed by acetylcholinesterase. (From Daube JR, Reagen TJ, Sandok BA, Westmoreland BF: Medical Neurosciences: An Approach to Anatomy, Pathology, and Physiology by Systems and Levels. Boston, Little, Brown & Co, 1986, p 278. Reproduced by permission.)

nium that made it unsatisfactory as a therapeutic agent makes it useful as a diagnostic agent.[11] The drug's onset of action is rapid, and the duration of maximal effect is short, usually less than 2 minutes. Any effect resolves within 5 to 10 minutes.[11]

Edrophonium administration in conjunction with electrophysiologic studies is frequently useful. In evaluating diplopia, many ophthalmologists use red-green filters (Lancaster test) with administration of edrophonium. Opinions vary strongly with regard to the usefulness of this procedure.[12–15]

Edrophonium administration has also been recommended in the past to monitor acetylcholinesterase inhibitor therapy.[16, 17] Currently the consensus is that edrophonium is not reliable in titrating the effect of anticholinesterase medication.[9, 18]

Myasthenic crisis may be loosely defined as respiratory distress in a myasthenic patient. Earlier concepts included "myasthenic" crisis from insufficient drug administration, "cholinergic" crisis from cholinesterase inhibitor overdosage, and the "brittle" patient with rapidly changing drug requirements,[16, 17, 19–21] but terminology in this setting remains controversial.[18, 22] Even the clinical existence of the different types of crisis has been debated.[18] Certainly in the myasthenic patient with respiratory distress, airway management and assisted ventilation are first priorities. Edrophonium administration should not be viewed as a possible alternative to intubation and ventilation. Several authorities advocate withdrawing all cholinesterase inhibitors in this setting because most patients show increased responsiveness to cholinesterase inhibitors after several days off the drug.[18, 22] Others advocate a trial of edrophonium chloride at reduced dosage (1 to 2 mg) only after respiratory support is achieved.[16, 17, 21, 23]

Indications and Contraindications

The bedside Tensilon test is indicated for diagnosis in patients suspected of having myasthenia gravis. For simple clinical use, a muscle that is clearly weak must be identified. Ptosis is a commonly monitored sign. A clinically evident extraocular muscle weakness is another example of a clinical situation that might allow direct observation of a single weak

muscle becoming stronger in response to the drug. Simple grip dynamometry does not aid in evaluation; a repetitive measure of grip strength (ergogram) is necessary. If a specific muscle cannot be isolated for objective testing, edrophonium administration should be deferred and other approaches to diagnosis pursued as discussed previously.

A history of asthma or cardiac dysrhythmias is a relative contraindication to administration of cholinesterase inhibitors. Administration of edrophonium to a patient with myasthenia gravis being treated with cholinesterase inhibitors is controversial, and many investigators consider myasthenic crisis to be a contraindication to edrophonium administration,[18, 22] though series of patients with myasthenic crisis continue to report its use.[21, 23]

Equipment

The following materials are needed for testing an adult. Intravenous access should be secured with D₅W at a keep-open rate or with a heparin lock. Ten milligrams of edrophonium chloride (Tensilon) should be drawn up in a tuberculin syringe. Edrophonium chloride is supplied in 1- and 10-ml vials at a concentration of 10 mg/ml. A second syringe of normal saline should be available to administer as a placebo, though some clinicians have recommended nicotine, calcium chloride, or atropine for this purpose.[17] Atropine and other cardiovascular drugs and resuscitative equipment should be readily available. Cardiac monitoring is generally recommended. Photographic recording equipment is desirable to objectively document improvement in motor function.

Procedure

Ideally, one person is available to administer the edrophonium or placebo and a second individual is free to observe the effect of medication on the patient. It is best if the person evaluating the response does not know which syringe contains edrophonium and which contains saline, thus creating a double-blind testing situation.

The paretic muscle to be tested is identified. Ptosis is an easily testable sign and generally used when present. The principles involved with assessing treatment of ptosis may be extended to testing other muscles. The patient is instructed to look upward for several moments in an attempt to fatigue the levators. The degree of ptosis is noted and documented by measurements or photographs. After a moment's rest, with the patient looking straight ahead, 0.2 ml of the test substance in one syringe is injected (2 mg edrophonium if active substance). If there is no response within 1 minute, another 0.3 ml is injected (3 mg edrophonium if active substance). If there is still no response, the remainder of the syringe is injected 3 minutes later. Any increase in strength reflected by an increase in palpebral fissure size is noted. The procedure may then be repeated with the other test substance.

Complications

A small percentage of individuals are hypersensitive to even the initial small dose of edrophonium and show cholinergic side effects of salivation, lacrimation, and miosis. These effects are transient. Atropine 0.5 mg may be given intravenously if necessary to counteract these symptoms. A smaller number of patients may experience symptomatic bradycardia that responds to atropine.

Interpretation

The key to the procedure is in the interpretation. If a clearly paretic muscle has been identified, objective signs of improvement in the strength of that muscle within a moment of administration of edrophonium and the fading of that improvement over the next 5 minutes are criteria for a positive test. Up to 90 per cent of patients with myasthenia have a positive test under ideal circumstances.[16, 17] False-negative results do consistently occur.

For the treatment of ptosis, a positive test consists of the patient having increased ability to elevate the eyelids after administration of 5 to 10 mg of edrophonium. The ptosis returns within 5 minutes. Subjective increases in general strength or relief of fatigue do *not* constitute a positive test. Fasciculations, brief twitches of muscles, are not usually observed in the patient with myasthenia who has received edrophonium, in contrast to normal subjects. The test may be repeated in 30 minutes if necessary.

Normal subjects have no change in muscle strength. They may transiently experience the side effects of salivation, lacrimation, and diaphoresis. Perioral, periocular, or lingual fasciculations are almost always noted in the normal patient following edrophonium administration.

The reproducible and unequivocal reversal of weakness in a specific muscle is extremely specific for myasthenia. False-positive test results have been reported in patients with Eaton-Lambert syndrome[24] and rarely in patients with intracranial lesions.[25, 26] Other rare reports of positive test results involve patients with amyotrophic lateral sclerosis. A "perverse" reaction has been noted rarely, in which a paretic extraocular muscle weak from other causes becomes even weaker with edrophonium administration.[13]

ICE PACK TEST

Background

It has been observed clinically that myasthenic patients have exacerbations of weakness with environmental heat and improvement in strength with cold temperatures. A simple bedside test uses these observations to evaluate ptosis.[10] Ice placed in a surgical glove or wrapped in a towel is placed lightly over the eyelid of a patient. Cooling of the eyelid below 29° C is accomplished within 2 minutes. The ptosis has been noted to improve in 80 per cent of the small group tested. Although the reported number of patients evaluated by this method is small, the test is included here because of its potential application in the emergency department, its lack of side effects, and its noninvasive nature.

Indications

Unilateral or bilateral ptosis of uncertain etiology in which myasthenia is a diagnostic possibility is the sole indication for this test.

Procedure

Ice and a surgical glove or towel are the only materials required. A camera to record any response is optional.

The degree of ptosis of the patient is noted and, ideally, photographed. Momentary upward gaze may be used to provoke the ptosis. If bilateral ptosis is present, the more affected eye should be tested. Eyelid cooling is accomplished by lightly holding the wrapped ice to the patient's eyelid for 2 minutes or until patient discomfort limits the application. The width of the palpebral fissure is immediately compared with the pretest width (Fig. 84–2*A* and *B*).

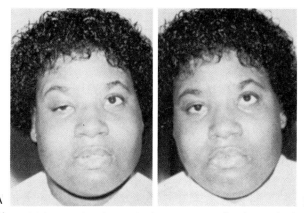

Figure 84–2. *A*, Before ice pack placement. *B*, After ice pack placement, showing improvement in ptosis of the right eye. (From Sethi KD, Rivner MH, Swift TR: Ice pack test for myasthenia gravis. Neurology 37:1383, 1987.)

Complications

Patient discomfort from the ice pack application may limit the cold exposure time to less than 2 minutes but still may allow a successful test.

Interpretation

A clear improvement of ptosis in the cooled eye is the criterion for a positive test. The effect should be reproducible. In the limited study, the ice pack test is at least as sensitive as edrophonium administration in improving ptosis in patients with ocular myasthenia. False-negative results do occur probably at about the same frequency as those in Tensilon testing. One individual has been reported with a negative ice pack test who had a positive Tensilon test. An equivocal Tensilon test was reported in another individual who had a clearly positive ice pack test. Normal individuals showed no change in palpebral fissure width after the cold exposure. There are no reports of false positives. The only reported series consists of ten myasthenic patients and seven control subjects.[10]

CONCLUSION

The bedside Tensilon test has a long history of utility in diagnosing myasthenia gravis but has been largely replaced by acetylcholinesterase receptor assay in the ambulatory setting. On occasion when rapid diagnosis is desired or myasthenia is suspected in the face of a normal acetylcholine receptor titer, a carefully performed Tensilon test is still clinically valuable. The use of the Tensilon test in the setting of myasthenic crisis is controversial and discouraged.

The ice pack test is so simple and noninvasive that it should become the initial procedure of choice in the emergency department for evaluating the possibility of ocular myasthenia. A positive ice pack test result strongly suggests ocular myasthenia gravis and alleviates any need for the Tensilon test. False-negative results do occur, and additional testing should be performed if the clinical suspicion for myasthenia gravis is strong.

REFERENCES

1. Newsom-Davis J: Diseases of the neuromuscular junction. In Asbury AK, McKhann GM, McDonald WI (eds): Diseases of the Nervous System: Clinical Neurobiology. Philadelphia, WB Saunders Co, 1986, p 269.
2. Seybold ME: Myasthenia gravis: A clinical and basic science review. JAMA 250:2516, 1983.

3. The diagnosis of myasthenia gravis (editorial). Lancet 1:658, 1986.

4. Drachman DB: Myasthenia gravis (2 parts). N Engl J Med 298:136 and 186, 1978.

5. Drachman DB: Pathophysiology of the neuromuscular junction. In Asbury AK, McKhann GM, McDonald WI (eds): Diseases of the Nervous System: Clinical Neurobiology. Philadelphia, WB Saunders Co, 1986, p 2269.

6. Engle AG: Myasthenia gravis and myasthenic syndromes. Ann Neurol 16:519, 1984.

7. Kelly JJ, Daube JR, Lennon VA, et al: The laboratory diagnosis of mild myasthenia gravis. Ann Neurol 12:238, 1982.

8. Soliven BC, Lange DJ, Penn AS, et al: Seronegative myasthenia gravis. Neurology 38:514, 1988.

9. Patten BM: Myasthenia gravis. Muscle Nerve 1:190, 1978.

10. Sethi KD, Rivner MH, Swift TR: Ice pack test for myasthenia gravis. Neurology 37:1383, 1987.

11. Osserman KE, Kaplan LI: Rapid diagnostic test for myasthenia gravis: Increased muscle strength, without fasciculations, after intravenous administration of edrophonium (Tensilone) chloride. JAMA 150:265, 1952.

12. Seybold ME: The office Tensilon test for ocular myasthenia gravis. Arch Neurol 43:842, 1986.

13. Daroff RB: The office Tensilon test for ocular myasthenia gravis. Arch Neurol 43:843, 1986.

14. Younge BR, Bartley GB: Lancaster test with Tensilon for myasthenia. Arch Neurol 44:472, 1987.

15. Daroff RB: Lancaster test with Tensilon for myasthenia. Arch Neurol 44:472, 1987.

16. Osserman KE, Genkins G: Critical reappraisal of the use of edrophonium (Tensilon) chloride tests in myasthenia gravis and significance of clinical classification. Ann NY Acad Med 135:312, 1966.

17. Osserman KE, Genkins G: Studies in myasthenia gravis: Review of a twenty-year experience in over 1200 patients. Mount Sinai J Med 38:497, 1971.

18. Rowland LP: Controversies about the treatment of myasthenia gravis. J Neurol Neurosurg Psychiatry 43:644, 1980.

19. Osserman KE, Kaplan LI: Studies in myasthenia gravis: Use of edrophonium chloride (Tensilon) in differentiating myasthenic from cholinergic weakness. Arch Neurol Psych 70:385, 1953.

20. Tether JE: Management of myasthenic and cholinergic crisis. Am J Med 19:740, 1955.

21. Gracey DR, Divertie MB, Howard FM: Mechanical ventilation for respiratory failure in myasthenia gravis: Two-year experience with 22 patients. Mayo Clin Proc 58:597, 1983.

22. Griggs RC, Donohoe KM: Emergency management of neuromuscular disease. In Henning, RJ, Jackson DL (eds): Handbook of Critical Care Neurology and Neurosurgery. New York, Praeger, 1985.

23. Sellman MS, Mayer RF: Treatment of myasthenic crisis in late life. South Med J 78:1208, 1985.

24. Oh SJ, Cho HK: Edrophonium responsiveness not necessarily diagnostic of myasthenia gravis. Neurology 38(suppl 1):124, 1988.

25. Dirr LY, Donofrio PD, Patton JF, et al: A false-positive edrophonium test in a patient with a brainstem glioma. Neurology 39:865, 1989.

26. Moorthy G, Drachman DB, Kirkham TH, et al: Ocular pseudomyasthenia or ocular myasthenia "plus": A warning to clinicians. Neurology 39:1150, 1989.

Ophthalmologic, Otolaryngologic, and Dental Procedures

Chapter 85

Ophthalmologic Procedures

David H. Barr, John R. Samples, and Jerris R. Hedges

The following sections discuss procedures commonly performed by emergency physicians during the evaluation and treatment of many eye injuries and diseases. The emphasis of these sections is on the practical application of the techniques and includes cautions to be heeded by the emergency physician.

DILATING THE EYE

Introduction

Dilating the eye is an essential step in the management of common eye emergencies. It is useful for both diagnostic and therapeutic purposes. Angle-closure glaucoma may be precipitated by dilating the pupil of the patient with a narrow angle. Systemic reactions can be produced by mucosal absorption of dilating medications. To minimize complications, the correct agent must be chosen and the proper technique used.

There are two types of dilators: sympathomimetics, which stimulate the dilator muscle of the iris, and cycloplegics, which block the parasympathetic stimulus that constricts the iris sphincter. Cycloplegics also block the contraction of the ciliary muscles, which control the focusing of the lens of the eye. This second effect of cycloplegics is of great importance in the use of dilators therapeutically for iritis.

Cycloplegics were used cosmetically as early as Galen's time. Beginning in the early 1800s, extracts from the plants *Hyoscyamus* and belladonna were used in ophthalmology. Atropine was first isolated in 1833. Epinephrine was used on eyes in 1900 as the first sympathomimetic.[1]

Indications and Contraindications

There are diagnostic and therapeutic indications for dilating the pupil. Dilation is indicated for *diagnosis* when the fundus cannot be examined adequately through an undilated pupil. Such a situation is presented by the elderly patient with miotic pupils and cataracts. Dilation is *therapeu-*

tically useful for many ophthalmic conditions, including inflammation in the eye. In the emergency setting, corneal injury with a secondary traumatic iritis is a common example. Dilation helps the inflamed eye in two ways. First, it keeps adhesions (synechiae) from forming between the iris and other ocular structures. Such adhesions eventually limit the movement of the pupil and may precipitate glaucoma. Second, cycloplegic dilating agents relax the ciliary muscle spasm that often accompanies an inflamed eye and thus reduce the pain associated with inflammation.

Whenever dilation is performed, it is important to note on the patient's chart the dose and time that agents have been given to avoid confusion during subsequent neurologic evaluation. Dilation is contraindicated in the presence of narrow angles. Patients who are predisposed to having narrow anterior chamber angles are often unaware of this condition. Patients who are using drops such as a β-blocker, a miotic, or an epinephrine compound are often those who have open-angle glaucoma and are not likely to have an intraocular pressure rise with dilation.

The depth of the anterior chamber can be estimated with a penlight by shining a light in from the side and seeing if the nasal side of the iris lights up. Normally a uniform illumination of the iris is seen. However, when there is a forward convexity of the iris, only a sector of iris is illuminated with a penlight held tangential to the eye (Fig. 85–1). With a slit lamp, the depth of the anterior chamber angle can be assessed directly. The definitive test for assessing the anterior chamber angle is gonioscopy, in which the anterior chamber angle structures are viewed directly by means of a special mirrored contact lens and the slit lamp.

Systemic effects can develop following the application of eye drops.[2] The reader should review the following sections on agents and complications before using these drugs in patients with compromised cardiovascular function.

Agents[3, 4]

Only two dilators are really needed in the emergency department. Phenylephrine (Neo-Synephrine) 2.5 per cent is used for diagnostic dilation of the pupil for visualization of the fundus. The drug is short acting, and since accommodation is not affected, the patient's vision is not altered. Phenylephrine 10 per cent should not be used routinely because it can seriously elevate the blood pressure in susceptible adults.[5, 6] For therapeutic cycloplegia in iritis, homatropine 5 per cent works well. Although Table 85–1 indicates a maximum duration of 3 days, 24 hours is a more common duration. Therefore, homatropine 5 per cent is a useful agent for traumatic iritis.

Individuals with lightly pigmented irides tend to have a greater sensitivity to the cycloplegics than do individuals

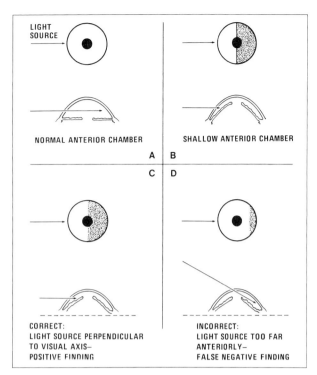

LIGHT
SOURCE

NORMAL ANTERIOR CHAMBER

SHALLOW ANTERIOR CHAMBER

A	B
C	D

CORRECT:
LIGHT SOURCE PERPENDICULAR
TO VISUAL AXIS—
POSITIVE FINDING

INCORRECT:
LIGHT SOURCE TOO FAR
ANTERIORLY—
FALSE NEGATIVE FINDING

Figure 85–1. Anterior chamber depth and transillumination test. *A,* Normal anterior chamber with negative transillumination test. *B,* Shallow anterior chamber with positive transillumination test. *C,* Shallow anterior chamber with correctly placed light source yielding a true positive test result. *D,* Shallow anterior chamber with incorrectly placed light source giving a false-negative test result. (From Bresler MJ, Hoffman RS: Prevention of iatrogenic acute narrowangle glaucoma. Ann Emerg Med 10:535, 1981. Reproduced by permission.)

with greater pigmentation; the cycloplegic effect may therefore be more prolonged in people with light eyes. Atropine should not be used for traumatic iritis because the undesirable effects of pupillary dilation and blurred vision persist for a week or longer following healing of associated corneal abrasions. Atropine drops may be prescribed as part of the therapy for nontraumatic iritis following appropriate ophthalmologic consultation.

The physician should be aware that malingerers may use mydriatics to dilate a pupil unilaterally for the purpose of feigning neurologic disease. Normally, a pupillary dilation caused by intracranial third cranial nerve compression will constrict with 2 per cent pilocarpine eye drops. The mydriatic-treated eye can be identified by full motor function of the third cranial nerve and the absence of miosis following pilocarpine instillation. It should be noted that legitimate patients may not recall the name of an eye medicine that they used but will usually recall whether the bottle had a red cap, as is found on all cycloplegic solutions. An unexpected mydriasis in a trusted patient may be the result of such an agent. Medications that constrict the pupil, such as pilocarpine, have a green cap.

Procedure

The instillation of mydriatics is similar to the administration of other eye solutions. For medicolegal purposes, visual acuity should be noted before the instillation of the medicine. This documents that any decreased vision is not the result of the mydriatic.

The patient is placed in a supine or a comfortable semirecumbent position. The patient is instructed to gaze at an object (such as a fixture on the ceiling) in the upper visual field. The physician gently depresses the lower lid using a finger on the epidermis (Fig. 85–2). A *single* drop of the solution is instilled into the lower lid fornix, and the patient is permitted to blink and to spread the medication. More than a single drop is not recommended, because it produces reflex tearing and reduces the concentration in contact with the conjunctiva. The patient should be forewarned that the medication is uncomfortable and that the closed eye can be blotted but *not* rubbed with a tissue after the medicine is used. If the desired effect is not noted in 15 to 20 minutes, a repeat dose may be used but is seldom required.

Complications

As mentioned in the section on contraindications, any dilator can precipitate an attack of angle-closure glaucoma

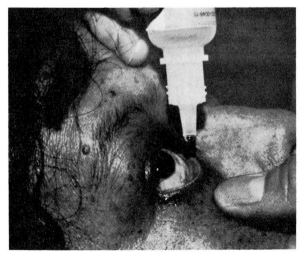

Figure 85–2. Administration of eye drops. The patient should lie in a supine position or with the head tilted back. The patient's gaze should be directed upward. A single drop of medicine is instilled in the lower conjunctival fornix. The patient should be instructed to close the eyelids for 1 minute to increase the contact of the medicine with the globe and to decrease the medication outflow down the tear duct and over the lid margin. (From Waring GO: The eye at first sight. Emerg Med November 15, 1979, p. 26. Reproduced by permission.)

Table 85–1. Mydriatic Agents

Agent	Maximum Mydriasis	Duration of Mydriasis	Common Trade Name
Sympathomimetics*			
Phenylephrine, 2.5% or 10%†	20 minutes	3 hours	Neo-Synephrine
Cocaine, 5% or 4%	20 minutes	2 hours	—
Parasympatholytics (Cycloplegics)			
Atropine, 1%	40 minutes	12 days	—
Scopolamine, 0.25%	30 minutes	7 days	—
Homatropine, 5%‡	30 minutes	1 to 3 days	—
Cyclopentolate, 1%	30 minutes	6 to 24 hours	Cyclogyl
Tropicamide, 1%	30 minutes	4 hours	Mydriacyl

*Preferred for funduscopic examination.
†A 10 per cent solution may produce cardiovascular reaction and hence should not be used.
‡Preferred for iritis or corneal abrasion therapy.

in susceptible patients.[7] In a case of angle-closure glaucoma, the patient complains of smoky vision with "halos" around lights as well as a severe, aching pain. There may be nausea and vomiting. The affected eye becomes injected in association with a hazy cornea, elevated pressure on tonometry, and an oval, fixed pupil. Immediate consultation with an ophthalmologist should be obtained. The treatment usually includes osmotic agents, carbonic anhydrase inhibitors, pilocarpine, and, later, definitive laser or surgical procedures.

The practitioner should be aware that the use of eye medications may introduce infections. Most solutions contain bactericidal ingredients, although contamination of the tips of the droppers can still occur.[8] Only newly opened bottles of eye medication should be used if the practitioner suspects a deep corneal injury or if the patient has had recent eye surgery.

Any cycloplegic (in contrast with a sympathomimetic) blurs a patient's near vision. Patients should be forewarned of this effect. Vision will be less blurred in adults over 45 years of age, who generally have a reduced ability to focus for near vision. Although most adults will be able to drive safely, even with both eyes affected, it is advisable to have someone else drive whenever feasible. Light sensitivity caused by pupillary dilation may also be bothersome; sunglasses are sufficient for this problem.

Systemic reactions can be produced by sympathomimetic and cycloplegic eye drops.[2, 9–19] Following instillation of eye drops into the conjunctival sac, systemic absorption can occur through the conjunctival capillaries as well as by way of the nasal mucosa, the oral pharynx, and the gastrointestinal tract after passage through the lacrimal drainage system. Mucosal hyperemia enhances absorption. Symptoms can often be avoided by digital pressure on the nasal canthus, thus occluding the puncta.[2]

Thirty-three cases of adverse reactions associated with 10 per cent phenylephrine have been described.[6] These include 15 myocardial infarctions (11 deaths), seven cases of precipitation of angle-closure glaucoma, and development of systemic cardiovascular or neurologic reactions.

THE FLUORESCEIN EXAMINATION

Introduction

Fluorescein staining of the eye should be part of the evaluation of all cases of eye trauma and infection. It is a quick and easy technique that is crucial for the proper diagnosis and management of common eye emergencies.

Sodium fluorescein is a water-soluble chemical that fluoresces—it absorbs light in the blue wavelengths and emits the energy in the longer green wavelengths. It fluoresces in an alkaline environment (such as in the Bowman membrane, which is located below the corneal epithelium) but not in an acidic environment (such as in the tear film over an intact corneal epithelium).[20] Thus it is very useful in revealing even minute abrasions on the cornea.

Fluorescein was first used in ophthalmology in the 1880s.[21] It was first used as a drop, but when the danger of contamination by bacteria (especially *Pseudomonas*) was recognized in the 1950s,[22] fluorescein was impregnated into paper strips. These now come in individual sterile wrappers and should be used instead of the premixed solution.

Indications and Contraindications

Fluorescein staining is indicated for evaluation of all suspected abrasions, foreign bodies, and infections of the eye.[23] This includes "simple" cases of conjunctivitis, which may actually be herpetic keratitis. In actuality, any red eye should be stained.

Fluorescein permanently stains soft contact lenses. Therefore, when fluorescein is used, soft contacts should first be removed and the patient cautioned not to put the lenses back into the eye for several hours. Topically administered fluorescein is considered nontoxic,[24] although reactions to a fluorescein-containing solution have been described. These reports of vagal reactions[25] and generalized convulsions[26] are rare and are believed to be caused by agents other than fluorescein in the solution. The practitioner who chooses to use one of the fluorescein-containing solutions rather than the fluorescein-impregnated strips should be aware of these potential idiosyncratic reactions.

The physician should also be aware that fluorescein dye may enter the anterior chamber of the eye in the presence of deep corneal defects. This form of intraocular fluorescein accumulation is also nontoxic. When the anterior chamber is viewed under the blue filter of the slit lamp, a fluorescein "flare" is visible. This flare reaction should not be confused with the flare reaction noted with iritis.

Procedure

Ideally one should not use topical anesthetics before fluorescein staining, because some patients will develop a superficial punctate keratitis from the anesthetic,[27] which can confuse the diagnosis. However, with patients who are tearing profusely and who are squeezing their eyes shut from an abrasion or a foreign body, the examination often is impossible if a topical anesthetic is not first used.

The fluorescein strip is grasped by the nonorange end, and the orange end is wetted with *one* drop of saline (most conveniently available as a small bottle of artificial tears) or dextrose solution. The wetted strip is then placed gently onto the inside of the patient's lower lid. The strip is withdrawn and the patient is instructed to blink. The patient's blinking spreads the fluorescein over the eye. The key to a good examination is a *thin* layer of fluorescein over the corneal and conjunctival surfaces. If the strip is heavily wetted before application in the lower fornix, the eye may become flooded with the solution, thus making evaluation difficult. On the other hand, use of a dry strip in the unanesthetized eye may be irritating. If too much dye accumulates, the patient can remove the excess by blotting the closed eye with a tissue. The physician uses a Wood lamp, the blue filter of a slit lamp, or simply a penlight with a blue filter to examine the eye in a darkened room, checking for areas of bright green fluorescence on the corneal and conjunctival surfaces. Following the completion of the fluorescein examination, excess dye should be irrigated from the eye to minimize damage to the patient's clothing from dye-stained tears.

A special use for fluorescein is in the *Seidel* test[28] for detection of perforation of the eye. To perform this test, the physician instills a large amount of fluorescein onto the eye by profusely wetting the strip. The eye is then examined for a small stream of fluid leaking from the globe. This stream will fluoresce blue or green in contrast with the orange color of the rest of the globe flooded with fluorescein.[29]

Interpretation

Fluorescein is mainly used for evaluation of corneal injuries. Although conjunctival abrasions pick up the stain, most of the staining on the conjunctiva represents patches of mucus rather than a real pathologic condition. Corneal staining is more specific for injury, and the pattern of injury often reflects the original insult.

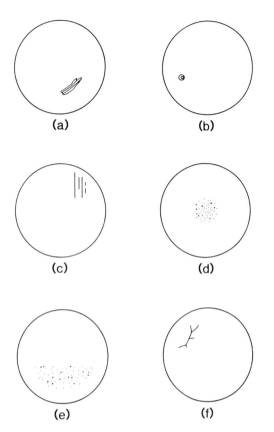

Figure 85–3. Typical corneal defect patterns for specific injuries. *A*, Typical abrasion. *B*, Abrasion around a corneal foreign body. *C*, Abrasion from a foreign body under the upper lid. *D*, Injury from excessive wearing of a contact lens. *E*, Ultraviolet exposure (resulting from sunlamp exposure, welding, or snow blindness). *F*, Herpetic dendritic keratitis.

The corneal staining shows patterns as illustrated in Figure 85–3. Abrasions usually occur in the central cornea because of the limited protection of the patient's closing eyelids. The margins of the abrasions are usually sharp and linear if seen in the first 24 hours. Circular defects are seen about embedded foreign bodies and may persist for up to 48 hours following removal of a superficial foreign object. Deeply embedded objects may be associated with defects persisting for longer than 48 hours. Objects under the upper lid (including some chalazions) produce vertical linear lesions on the upper surface of the cornea. Hard contact lens overuse diminishes the nutrient supply to the cornea. The central cornea receives the most injury and thus fluoresces brightly when stained. Ultraviolet light exposure from sunlamp abuse, snow blindness, or welding flash produces a superficial punctate keratitis, which in its mildest form may not be visible without a slit lamp. The central cornea is the least protected by the lids, and a central horizontal bandlike keratitis can result. Herpetic lesions may develop anywhere on the cornea. Classically, these lesions are dendritic, although ulcers may also be punctate or stellate.[30, 31]

Any area of corneal staining with an infiltrate or opacification beneath or around the lesion should alert the practitioner to the possibility of a viral,[30] bacterial,[32] or fungal[33] *keratitis*. Urgent ophthalmologic consultation should be obtained so that cultures of the possible etiologic agents can be procured and treatment initiated.

Frequently, practitioners are unaware that many *Pseudomonas* organisms fluoresce when exposed to ultraviolet light.[34] The presence of fluorescence before the instillation of fluorescein in the red eye should suggest the possibility of a pseudomonal infection.

Conclusion

Fluorescein staining is a quick, easy diagnostic procedure that should be part of every eye evaluation. The extra minute that the examination takes provides a wealth of diagnostic information for patients with eye trauma or infection. With the exception of the reactions noted with fluorescein solution, the potential discoloration of soft contact lenses, and the potential for infection when the solutions rather than fluorescein-impregnated paper strips are used, no complications are associated with the procedure.

EYE IRRIGATION

Introduction

Eye irrigation is the crucial first step in the treatment of chemical injuries to the eye. Irrigation should be clinically appropriate to the exposure and severity of the injury. Serious chemical injury to the eye requires irrigation at the site of injury, *before* the patient is brought to the emergency department.[35] Corneal injury can occur within seconds of contact with an alkaline substance. Eye irrigation often must be continued in the emergency department.

This section discusses methods of irrigation. Although it is best to irrigate liberally, copious irrigation is not needed when the patient has gotten a small amount of a noncaustic, nonalkaline compound in the eye.

Indications and Contraindications

Irrigation is indicated for all acute chemical injuries to the eyes. Irrigation may also be therapeutic for patients having a foreign body sensation with no visible foreign body. Small, unseen foreign material in the conjunctival tissues may be flushed out with irrigation. There is no contraindication to eye irrigation, but if there is also a possible perforating injury to the eye, the irrigation must be performed especially gently and carefully.

Equipment

The following equipment is necessary for eye irrigation:

1. Topical anesthetic, such as proparacaine 0.5 per cent.
2. Sterile irrigating solution. Usually, intravenous saline in a bag with tubing is the easiest to obtain.
3. A basin to catch the fluid.
4. Cotton-tipped applicators.
5. Gauze pads to help hold the patient's lids open.
6. Lid retractors.
7. Irrigating device (e.g., Morgan Therapeutic Lens or modified central venous catheter) for prolonged irrigation.

Procedure

BASIC TECHNIQUE

Topical anesthetic is instilled. Any particulate matter should be swept out of the conjunctival fornices with moistened cotton-tipped applicators.[36] This requires eversion of the upper lid (see the section on foreign body removal and Fig. 85–4). During actual irrigation, the lids must be held open. It is easiest to use the gauze pads to get a grip on the

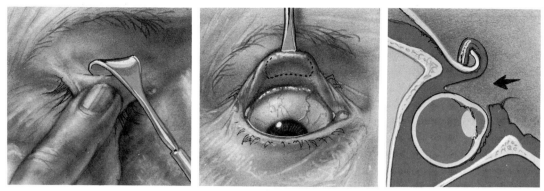

Figure 85–4. Double eversion of upper lid using a lid retractor. (From Fogle JA, Spyker DA: Management of chemical and drug injury to the eye. In Haddad LM, Winchester JF: Clinical Management of Poisoning and Drug Overdose, 2nd ed. Philadelphia, WB Saunders Co, 1990. Reproduced by permission.)

wet, slippery lids. At times the patient has blepharospasm to such a degree that lid retractors (Desmarres or paper clip retractors—Fig. 85–5) may be necessary (Fig. 85–6). When lid retractors are used, the practitioner must be certain that the eye is well anesthetized, that the retractors do not injure the globe or the lids, and that chemicals are not harbored under the retractors.

Paton and Goldberg recommend an ipsilateral facial nerve block for severe blepharospasm (Fig. 85–7).[37] To avoid swelling of the periorbital tissue, the facial nerve is blocked just anterior to the condyloid process of the ipsilateral mandible. A line of anesthesia (2 per cent lidocaine) is placed subcutaneously to temporarily paralyze the orbicularis muscle.

The saline exiting from the intravenous tubing is directed over the globe and into the upper and lower fornices. The choice of fluid is less important than the rapidity of irrigation initiation. Tap water should be readily available at the scene of the injury, and copious immediate irrigation should be encouraged before patient transport to the hospital. Prehospital care providers should be taught to irrigate all acid injuries of the eye for at least 5 minutes at the scene and to irrigate all alkali injuries for at least 15 minutes.[38, 39] Normal saline solution is preferred for eye irrigation, because it is nonirritating and isotonic without dextrose. Dextrose can be quite sticky if spilled and may serve as a nutrient for an opportunistic bacterial infection.

Care should be taken to direct the irrigating stream

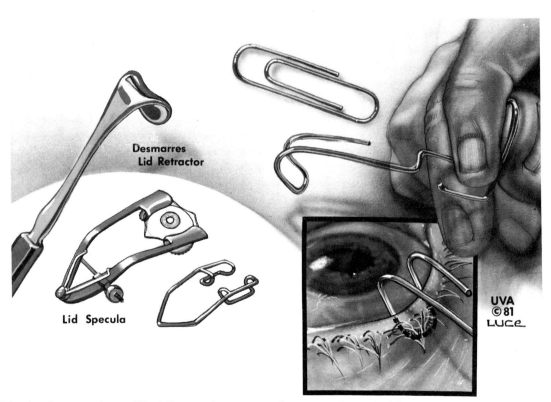

Figure 85–5. Devices for separating eyelids. A Desmarres retractor and a retractor improvised from a paper clip allow active manipulation of lids. Free-standing specula may require a seventh nerve block to reduce blepharospasm. (From Fogle JA, Spyker DA: Management of chemical and drug injury to the eye. In Haddad LM, Winchester JF: Clinical Management of Poisoning and Drug Overdose, 2nd ed. Philadelphia, WB Saunders Co, 1990. Reproduced by permission.)

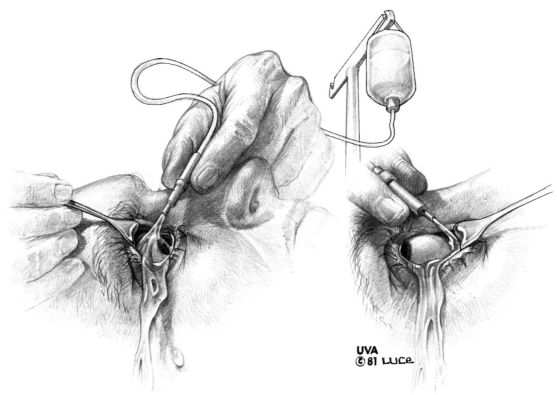

Figure 85–6. Irrigation technique using a Desmarres retractor for lid separation. (From Fogle JA, Spyker DA: Management of chemical and drug injury to the eye. In Haddad LM, Winchester JF: Clinical Management of Poisoning and Drug Overdose, 2nd ed. Philadelphia, WB Saunders Co, 1990. Reproduced by permission.)

onto the conjunctiva and then across the cornea without letting the stream splash directly onto the cornea, because the mechanical injury of the solution striking the eye can of itself be harmful. Direct irrigation of the cornea can result

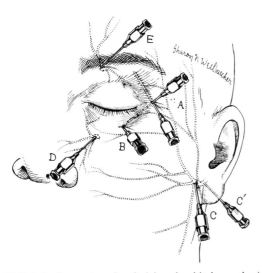

Figure 85–7. Injection points for facial and orbital anesthesia and akinesia. *A*, Van Lint technique of orbicularis infiltration. *B*, Retrobulbar injection site. *C*, O'Brien facial nerve block. *C'*, Alternative facial nerve block by tympanomastoid fissure injection. *D*, Infraorbital sensory block. *E*, Supraorbital sensory block. Injection of orbicularis *(A)* or facial nerve *(C* or *C')* permits examination and treatment of the eye in the setting of severe blepharospasm. (From Deutsch TA, Feller DB: In Paton and Goldberg's Management of Ocular Injuries. 2nd ed. Philadelphia, WB Saunders Co, 1985, p 17.)

in the development of a superficial punctate epithelial keratopathy.

DURATION OF IRRIGATION

Although Gombos recommends that a full liter of irrigating solution be used in every case of caustic injury,[10] the duration of the irrigation is best determined by the extent of exposure and the causative agent. Acids are quickly neutralized by the proteins of the eye surface tissues and, once irrigated out, cause no further damage.[41] The only exceptions are hydrofluoric and heavy metal acids, which can penetrate through the cornea. Alkalis can penetrate rapidly and if not removed (because of the slow dissociation of the cation from combination with proteins) will continue to produce damage for days.[42] Therefore, prolonged irrigation is indicated; at least 2 liters of solution should be used over 20 minutes for any significant alkaline injury.[43] If the nature of the offending agent is in doubt, prolonged irrigation should be used.

Ophthalmologic consultation should be obtained for all alkaline, hydrofluoric acid, and heavy metal acid injuries. Irrigation on an inpatient basis may be required for a period of 24 hours or more. This is especially likely when corneal hazing is present. It should be noted that the magnesium contained in sparklers combines with water from tears to produce magnesium hydroxide.[44] Such fireworks accidents should be treated as alkaline injuries rather than thermal injuries. Eye damage from hair straighteners[45] and phosphate-free detergents[46] must also be treated as alkaline injuries.

A good method of checking the effectiveness of irrigation is to measure the pH of the conjunctival fornices with a pH paper strip.[47] The pH indicator on urine multi-indicator sticks can also be used. The pH indicator on urine dipsticks is conveniently closest to the handle; all the distal indicator squares can be cut off with scissors. The normal tear film pH is 7.4. If the pH measured in the conjunctival fornices after the initial irrigation is still abnormal, irrigation is to be continued. If the pH is normal after irrigation, one should check it again in 20 minutes to make sure that it remains normal.

Delayed pH changes are usually the result of incomplete irrigation and inadequate swabbing of the fornices. In anticipation of this deficiency, one should measure the pH deep in the fornices. Often, double-lid eversion with a lid elevator is required to expose the upper fornix for swabbing, irrigation, and pH testing (see Fig. 85–4).

PROLONGED IRRIGATION

Prolonged irrigation may be required with alkali burns. Ophthalmologic consultation is essential in such situations. One technique for prolonged irrigation uses a contact lens–type irrigation device (e.g., Morgan Therapeutic Lens), which allows for continuous irrigation once the more vigorous irrigation described earlier has been used. During use, the device is set on the anesthetized eye, and the lids are allowed to close around the intravenous tubing adaptor (Fig. 85–8). Continuous flow through the device onto the cornea and into the fornices occurs. This contact lens device can become uncomfortable, because local anesthetic agents are washed out during the irrigation process; the anesthetic agent must be reapplied frequently during irrigation for patient comfort. The repeated use of the anesthetic agent may itself inhibit corneal healing.

Another irrigation device can be made for the pro-longed irrigation of the fornices by modification of a small-caliber central venous catheter. Multiple perforations are made with a scissors or a scalpel in the distal portion of the catheter. This perforated section is placed in the inferior fornix of the anesthetized eye beginning at the lateral canthus and is then looped back in the upper lid fornix (Fig. 85–9). The patient is instructed to tilt his head toward the side of the tubing to permit drainage into a laterally placed basin. After loosely applying an eye patch, one attaches the catheter to an intravenous setup for continuous irrigation. An anesthetic agent is also needed with this technique, albeit less frequently than with the contact lens–type device.

Lippas described the successful treatment of two alkaline burns using a similar but more invasive continuous irrigation technique for prolonged irrigation following immediate copious irrigation.[48] Continuous irrigation of an alkaline injury with a 10 or 20 per cent acetylcysteine (Mucomyst) solution to inhibit collagenase has been recommended,[49] although one should await ophthalmologic consultation before using this method.

Complications

The only complication from irrigation is abrasion of the cornea or the conjunctiva. This can be a mechanical injury from trying to keep the lids open in an uncooperative patient or a fine punctate keratitis from the irrigation itself.[50] If a superficial corneal defect occurs, it is treated in the usual manner by patching. Deep or penetrating corneal injuries are likely to be the result of the caustic chemical and require emergency ophthalmologic consultation.

In general, the emergency physician should not patch

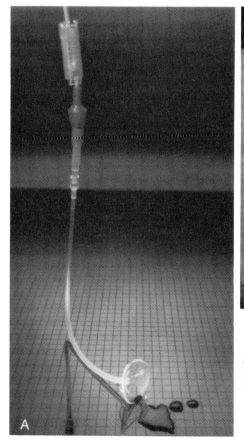
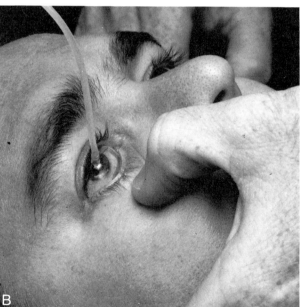

Figure 85–8. *A,* The Morgan Therapeutic Lens attached to intravenous tubing. *B,* Placement of the device into the eye for irrigation. (Courtesy of MorTan, Inc., Missoula, Mont.)

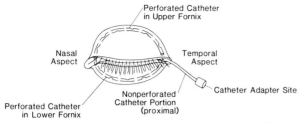

Figure 85–9. Continuous irrigation device. A perforated central venous catheter is looped in the fornices of the anesthetized eye, beginning from the temporal border of the eyelids. The eye is lightly patched after catheter placement.

these deeper injuries. They should receive continuous irrigation pending ophthalmologic consultation. Superficial injuries not associated with corneal hazing should be treated in a manner similar to that for corneal abrasions. There is some experimental evidence that massive parenteral or oral ascorbic acid supplementation may prevent the development of deep corneal injury,[51] although this treatment has not gained universal acceptance.

Conclusion

Eye irrigation is easy, and complications associated with the technique are minimal. At times, the physician may be unsure whether a chemical injury is toxic enough to warrant irrigation. One should irrigate if any doubt exists rather than omit this vital procedure and permit the progression of eye injury.

OCULAR FOREIGN BODY REMOVAL

Introduction

Patients with an external foreign body in the eye are frequently seen in emergency departments. They are often in pain and desperate for help. A high degree of suspicion for foreign body injuries and perforations of the eye is necessary, because such injuries may be occult and not readily detected. Not all foreign body injuries are associated with pain; glass embedded in the cornea may be particularly difficult to detect. This section reviews the procedures for locating and removing extraocular foreign bodies. A brief discussion covering evaluation for perforation of the globe and for an intraocular foreign body is presented. Care of the patient following removal of an extraocular foreign body is reviewed.

Indications and Contraindications

Removal of extraocular foreign bodies is always indicated. The timing of removal and the technique that is required vary according to the patient's clinical status and the type of injury received. For the most part, the emergency physician can proceed directly to removal of the object using the techniques described in this section. When the patient is extremely uncooperative (e.g., a mentally deficient individual or a young child) or when the injury is complicated (e.g., deeply embedded object, multiple foreign objects from a blast injury, or possible globe penetration), immediate ophthalmologic consultation is indicated. A penetrating injury to the cornea is particularly troublesome in that iris tissue may prolapse and may appear to represent a corneal foreign body (Fig. 85–10).

Equipment

The following equipment is necessary for extraocular foreign body removal:

1. Topical anesthetic, such as proparacaine 0.5 per cent.
2. Sterile cotton-tipped applicators.
3. Fluorescein strips.
4. Magnification: loupes plus a Wood lamp or a slit lamp.
5. Eye spud or 25-gauge needle attached to a 3-ml syringe or to the tip of a cotton-tipped applicator.
6. Dilator drops, such as Homatropine 5 per cent or Cyclopentolate 1 per cent.
7. Antibiotic ointment, such as sulfacetamide 10 per cent.
8. Eye patches.
9. Tape (nonallergenic paper tape is preferable).

Consideration of Intraocular Foreign Body

The emergency physician should always remain cognizant of the potential for an intraorbital or intraocular foreign body when examining the patient with a "foreign body" sensation. Penetrating injuries represent a greater threat of visual loss than extraocular foreign bodies and can be disastrous if overlooked.

The clinical presentation is helpful in the determination of which patients are at risk for a penetrating injury to the globe. An individual who complains of a foreign body sensation in the *absence* of trauma or one whose history is simply that something "fell" or "blew" into the eye is at *low* risk for a globe perforation. On the other hand, there is a greater probability of globe penetration in the individual who has sustained a high-velocity wound to the eye (e.g., drilling or grinding metal, blasting rock). The presence of any of the following physical findings should alert the physician to a probable *intra*ocular foreign body: irregular pupil, shallow anterior chamber on slit lamp examination, prolapsed iris, positive Seidel test (see the section on fluorescein examination), focal conjunctival swelling and hemorrhage, hyphema, lens opacification, and reduced intraocular pressure. (It should be noted that *tonometry should not be performed in the presence of other physical findings suggesting penetration of the globe*.) One should be aware that a penetrating injury may *not* be associated with eye pain. Strong historical evidence and physical findings supporting a diagnosis of penetration of the globe should prompt emergent ophthalmologic consultation.

Often, *intra*ocular foreign bodies are not visible on direct

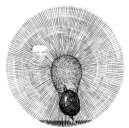

Figure 85–10. Corneal laceration with prolapse of the iris. The extruded iris is dark in appearance, mimicking a corneal foreign body. The pupil is irregular, pointing toward the laceration. Also note the presence of a small hyphema inferiorly. (From Deutsch TA, Feller DB: Paton and Goldberg's Management of Ocular Injuries. 2nd ed. Philadelphia, WB Saunders Co, 1985. Reproduced by permission.)

ophthalmoscopy. Although orbital radiographs for radiopaque objects and sonograms of the globe have been used for indirect foreign body localization,[52] computed tomography of the orbit is now considered the most useful technique.[53, 54] Patients with a suspected metallic foreign body should *not* undergo magnetic resonance imaging if the foreign body may be *intra*ocular. Therapy of intraocular and intraorbital foreign bodies must be individualized. Often, an ophthalmologist can localize an intraocular foreign body (if the vitreous is clear) using indirect ophthalmoscopy. The role of the emergency physician is to suspect the diagnosis, to protect the eye from further harm, and to obtain ophthalmologic consultation. The remainder of this section addresses the problem of extraocular foreign bodies.

Procedure

FOREIGN BODY LOCATION

The first step is to locate the foreign body. A drop of both topical anesthetic and fluorescein is applied to the inside of the lower lid (see the section on the fluorescein examination). Vertical corneal abrasions from foreign bodies under the lids are helpful for localizing these hidden foreign objects (see Fig. 85–3*C*). One should use a penlight and loupes or a slit lamp to examine the bulbar conjunctiva by having the patient look in all directions. The physician examines the inside of the lower lid by pulling it down with the thumb while the patient looks up. One everts the upper lid by having the patient look down as the end of an applicator stick is pressed against the superior edge of the tarsal plate of the upper lid. Meanwhile, the physician grasps the lashes and pulls down and then up to flip the lid over (Fig. 85–11).

Minute foreign bodies under the lid will be missed with simple visual inspection. Ideally, the everted lid should be examined under magnification with loupes or a slit lamp. With simple lid eversion it is still not possible to see the far recesses of the upper conjunctival fornix. Although double eversion of the upper lid (see Fig. 85–4) is helpful, the best way to rule out a foreign body in the upper fornix is to sweep the anesthetized fornix with a wetted applicator as the upper lid is held everted. The applicator tip should be examined for removed foreign material. Small conjunctival foreign bodies not hidden by the lids are often best removed with a wetted nasopharyngeal swab (e.g., nasopharyngeal Calgi-Swab).

The cornea is then reexamined. Most corneal foreign

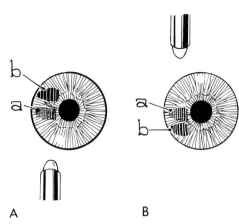

Figure 85–12. An "invisible" corneal abrasion casts an obvious shadow on the iris. The relative positions of *(a)* the corneal abrasion and *(b)* the iris shadow depend on the direction of the incident light (as in *A* and *B*). (From Paton D, Goldberg MF: Management of Ocular Injuries. Philadelphia, WB Saunders Co, 1976. Reproduced by permission.)

bodies have an area of fluorescein staining around them. A slit lamp makes the examination easy. If the physician is limited to loupes and a penlight, the light is shined diagonally on the cornea. One then finds a foreign body directly or indirectly by noting a shadow on the cornea or the iris (Fig. 85–12).[55]

With a history of a high-speed projectile hitting the eye, one must rule out an intraocular foreign body. Except in the case of a blast injury, if one foreign body is found on the surface of the globe, it is highly unlikely that there is a second foreign body inside the eye. If a foreign body cannot be found on the surface despite a suggestive history, the eye should be examined for physical evidence of penetration as discussed earlier. The pupil is dilated and the fundus is examined. If in doubt regarding an intraocular foreign body, one should consider computed tomography and ophthalmologic consultation.

FOREIGN BODY REMOVAL

Once an extraocular foreign body is located, the technique of removal depends on whether it is embedded. If the foreign body is lying on the surface, a stream of water ejected from a syringe through a plastic catheter usually washes the object onto the bulbar conjunctiva. Once the foreign body is on the conjunctiva, a wetted cotton-tipped applicator can be gently touched to the conjunctiva, and the object will adhere to the applicator tip. Overzealous use of an applicator for corneal foreign body removal can lead to extensive corneal epithelial injury. A spud device is required for removal of objects that cannot be irrigated off the cornea.

Embedded corneal foreign bodies are best removed with a commercial spud device or a 25- or 27-gauge needle on a small-diameter syringe or a cotton-tipped applicator. The applicator or the syringe serves as a handle for the attached needle. Contrary to what one might expect, it is difficult to penetrate the sclera or the cornea with a needle.[56] As with removal of conjunctival foreign bodies, the eye must be well anesthetized. The patient should be positioned such that the head is well secured (preferably in a slit lamp frame). The patient must be instructed to gaze at an object in the distance (e.g., the practitioner's ear when a slit lamp is used) to stabilize the eye further. The spud device is held *tangentially*

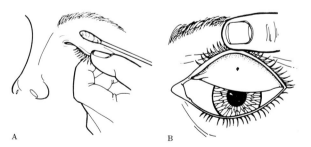

Figure 85–11. Single upper lid eversion. *A,* The end of a cotton-tipped applicator is placed above the tarsal plate while the lashes and the lid margin are pulled down and out. *B,* One everts the lid and holds it by pressing the lashes against the superior orbital rim. (From Pavan-Langston D: Manual of Ocular Diagnosis and Therapy. 3rd ed. Boston, Little, Brown, 1991. Reproduced by permission.)

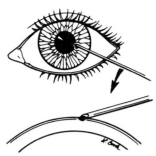

Figure 85–13. Removal of a superficial corneal foreign body. Side view illustrates the thickness of the cornea relative to the beveled needle edge. The needle or eye spud should be tangential to the cornea, and the object should be gently scraped off the cornea. (From Pavan-Langston D: Manual of Ocular Diagnosis and Therapy. 3rd ed. Boston, Little, Brown, 1991. Reproduced by permission.)

to the globe, and the foreign object is picked or scooped out (Fig. 85–13). During removal, the physician should brace his or her hand against the patient's face. It also may be helpful to brace the elbow with a pad or half-full tissue box to provide further support to the arm as the foreign body is removed. The right-handed physician should place the lower hand against the left maxillary bone when removing a foreign object from the left eye and against the bridge of the patient's nose or infranasal area when removing an object from the right eye. These positions should be reversed by the left-handed physician. The use of loupes or a slit lamp for magnification is recommended to minimize further injury during removal. In particular, corneal contact with the spud device is more readily discerned when magnification is used. Only topical anesthesia is required to remove foreign bodies from the cornea. Although the patient may feel pressure during foreign body removal, pain should not be felt after the eye is anesthetized.

RUST RINGS

A common problem with metallic foreign bodies is rust rings. These can develop within hours because of oxidation of the iron in the foreign body. There are two preferred techniques for removal of a rust ring. The most direct method is to remove it at the same time as the foreign body, either with repeated picking away with a spud device or with a rotating burr. The second approach is to let the iron of the rust ring poison and kill the surrounding epithelial cells during a 24- to 48-hour patching period. At that time, the rust ring will be soft and often comes out in one solid plug.[57] Following rust ring removal, the eye must be patched again for another 24 hours to allow the residual corneal defect time to heal. Generally, a small rust ring produces little visual difficulty unless it is directly in the line of sight. The rust ring, if large, may delay corneal healing.

MULTIPLE FOREIGN BODIES

The patient with multiple foreign bodies in the eye, such as from an explosion, should be referred to an ophthalmologist. A technique that may be chosen by the ophthalmologist is to denude the entire epithelium with alcohol and remove the superficial foreign bodies. The deeper ones gradually work their way to the surface, sometimes years later.[58]

AFTERCARE

After removing the foreign body, one should patch the eye if there is any corneal abrasion (see the section on patching). An antibiotic ointment is frequently instilled before patching, but the value of the ointment for very *superficial* corneal defects following foreign body removal is unknown. Conjunctival abrasions do not need patching. If the eye is patched, the patient should be reexamined in 24 hours. An antibiotic ointment is applied before placement of the patch. If the patient sustains a *superficial* injury from the foreign body and an eye patch is applied primarily for comfort, the physician may wish to instruct the patient to return only if the eye does *not* feel completely normal *or* if there is any blurred vision. The majority of superficial injuries heal without difficulty. The patient should be warned that the foreign body sensation may return temporarily before patch removal when the anesthetic agent has worn off.

USE OF OPHTHALMIC ANESTHETIC AGENTS

Application of topical anesthetic agents can be both diagnostic and therapeutic. Relief of discomfort with topical anesthetic use suggests a conjunctival or corneal injury. An ocular irritant may also be masked by the use of these agents. Classic teaching is that the anesthetic preparations should not be self-administered by patients. The absence of protective reflexes while the patient is under the effect of the medicine may encourage the patient to use the eye while a foreign body or a corneal infection inflicts further corneal injury.

As evident from Table 85–2, the anesthetic solutions that are commonly used have a duration of action of less than 20 minutes. The patient requiring patching may need a more extended period of pain relief. The discomfort associated with a healing corneal lesion is usually made tolerable by a pressure patch, bed rest, analgesics, and sedatives (e.g., secobarbital or chloral hydrate). Even in the absence of infection or a retained foreign body, the *repeated* use of ophthalmic anesthetic ointments may be detrimental to corneal healing. The frequent removal of a pressure patch to anesthetize the cornea may lead to disruption of migrating corneal epithelial cells and may thus prolong corneal repair.

A final word of caution should be added regarding the

Table 85–2. **Ophthalmic Anesthetic Agents**			
Generic Name	Tetracaine	Proparacaine	Benoxinate
Trade Name	Pontocaine	Ophthaine, Ophthetic	Dorsacaine
Concentration	0.5 to 1.0%	0.5%	0.4%
Onset of Anesthesia	Less than 1 minute	Less than 20 seconds	1–2 minutes
Duration of Anesthesia	15–20 minutes	10–15 minutes	10–15 minutes
Comments	Marked stinging; also available in ointment	Least irritating; no cross-sensitization with other agents	Only anesthetic compatible with fluorescein in solution

use of ophthalmic solutions. Guaiac solutions are commonly supplied in dropper bottles similar in size and appearance to those containing ophthalmic solutions. Well-intentioned emergency department personnel may store the guaiac reagent bottles with the ophthalmic bottles. One should encourage both color coding of the bottles and examination of the bottle before each use to avoid corneal injury from the guaiac reagent.

Complications

Complications associated with ocular foreign body removal are rare. The most frequent problem is incomplete removal of the foreign body. In such cases the epithelium has difficulty healing over the affected area, and thus the eye stays inflamed. Eventually, the diseased epithelium either sloughs off and heals or heals over the foreign body remnants, which are gradually absorbed. In either case, the adverse effects on the eye are minimal; a minute scar on the cornea, even directly in the center, will rarely affect the vision. Nonetheless, incomplete removal of a corneal foreign object warrants ophthalmologic follow-up.

Conjunctivitis may develop following removal of an extraocular foreign body. In most cases, the bacteria producing the infection are introduced by the patient through rubbing of the irritated eye.

Although perforation of the globe by the physician's spud device is theoretically possible, this complication is exceedingly rare. To our knowledge, only one anecdotal case occurred some 20 years ago. Treatment of such a minor corneal puncture wound would consist of antibiotics, eye shield placement, and ophthalmologic consultation. Permanent sequelae are unlikely to develop.

It should be mentioned again that much epithelial injury can occur when cotton-tipped applicators are vigorously used to remove corneal foreign bodies. Indeed, we condemn the use of cotton-tipped applicators for *corneal* foreign body removal.

Conclusion

Ocular foreign bodies are one of the most common eye emergencies. Searching for and removing the foreign body is usually straightforward. The only real trap is missing an intraocular foreign body. This must be ruled out if there is a history of a high-speed projectile hitting the eye or if physical findings suggestive of globe penetration are present.

EYE PATCHING

Introduction

Patching the lids shut is the last step in treatment of a number of common eye emergencies. Many physicians, however, have only a vague idea of what the purpose of patching is, how to do it, and how to follow up. Even this simple procedure can be performed incorrectly.

Patching may be used for several goals. A simple patch may be applied to protect the dilated eye from bright light. Pressure patching as discussed in this section is the use of a patch to hold the eyelid closed to facilitate healing of a corneal defect.

Indications and Contraindications

Patching is indicated whenever the surface of the cornea has been injured. This can occur following a mechanical

abrasion, such as a fingernail scratch, or after the removal of a foreign body. Chemical damage, damage from prolonged contact lens use, and ultraviolet light injuries, which are commonly seen in the emergency department, also require patching. With each of these forms of injury, the purpose of the patch is to keep the lids from moving over the cornea and to keep light out. After patching, the patient immediately experiences less pain and tearing and the epithelium heals faster.

Patching is contraindicated when the corneal epithelial loss results from an active infection—such as a corneal ulcer—rather than from an abrasion. The first consideration in the differentiation between ulcer and abrasion is the history of the injury (how recently it occurred and how clean the offending object was). The second determining factor is the appearance of the cornea (that is, an ulcer will have an infiltrate of white cells beneath the area of epithelial loss and will be accompanied by a purulent discharge). A pressure patch should never be applied to an eye with a penetrating injury. A protective cup is the preferred covering pending ophthalmologic consultation.

Equipment

The following equipment is necessary for patching the eye: two gauze eye patches, tape (e.g., 1-inch paper tape, preferably nonallergenic), an antibiotic ointment (e.g., sulfacetamide 10 per cent), and a dilator drop (cyclopentolate [Cyclogel] 1 per cent or homatropine 5 per cent). The tape should be precut into 4-inch strips and should be kept within reach. Commercial patching products are also available and are discussed below.

Procedure

Before patching a corneal abrasion, one should apply both a dilator drop and an antibiotic ointment.[59] The dilator must be a cycloplegic to relax the ciliary muscle spasm that accompanies corneal abrasions. Both cyclopentolate 1 per cent and homatropine 5 per cent last approximately 24 hours. The patient should be checked for a narrow anterior chamber before the drop is instilled (see Fig. 85–1). Antibiotic ointment is used prophylactically, although it is rare for abrasions to become infected.[60] In the past it was thought that the ointment vehicle would slow epithelial healing, but the vehicles that are currently used do not have this effect.[61–63]

An effective patch must be put on tightly enough to keep the lids shut. The physician should have the patient shut both eyes and should remind him to keep them shut throughout the entire procedure. Two patches are used. The vertically positioned first patch is doubly folded and placed over the closed lids. The unfolded second patch is then put horizontally over the first (Fig. 85–14). The tape strips are stretched diagonally from the center of the forehead to the cheekbone. The physician can pull up the skin of the cheek; when he lets go, the tape will be even tighter. If the tape completely covers the patch, slippage of the patch and resultant eye movement are avoided (Fig. 85–15). The tape should not extend onto the angle of the mandible, because mastication loosens the tape in such a situation. Some physicians paint the skin about the eye with tincture of benzoin to help secure the tape. Care must be taken not to introduce the benzoin into the eye. The presence of extensive facial hairs may prevent tight taping of the patch. An adjustable elastic strap pressure patch (e.g., Presspatch II, Precision Therapeutics, Inc., Las Vegas, Nev.) may be useful in this setting (Fig. 85–16).

It is imprudent to leave a pressure patch on for more

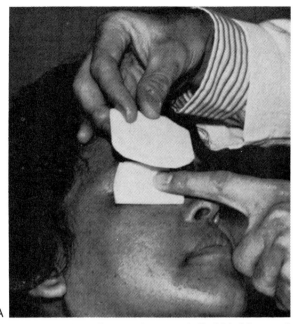
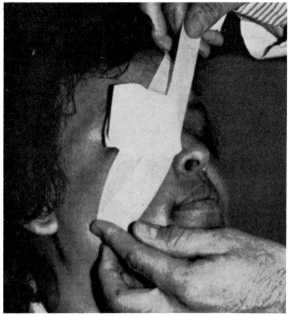

A   B

Figure 85–14. Application of eye patch. *A,* Vertically folded first patch in orbital recess. *B,* Horizontally oriented second patch with forehead to cheek taping. (From of Waring GO: Emerg Med, November 15, 1979, p 39.)

than 24 hours. When repatching to promote healing is required, a clean patch should be applied within each 24 hours. Repatching prevents a patch from becoming moist and serving as a nidus for the development of infection.

The Donaldson Eyepatch (Keeler Instruments, Inc., Broomall, Pa.) is a commercial product used for enforced eyelid closure that avoids the bulkiness of pressure patching (Fig. 85–17). The device has two components: one adheres to the upper lid, and the other is a circle that adheres to the ipsilateral cheek. A tab on the upper component connects by Velcro to the lower component. This patch may be advantageous in some settings, but its design may encourage some individuals to release the lid closure prematurely.

Complications

There are few complications involved in patching. It is possible to patch the patient's lashes in between the lids so that they abrade the cornea. This can occur if the patient partially opens his eye during the procedure. You can avoid this by insisting that both eyes stay closed during the entire patching.

Most problems develop when the eye is not securely patched and excessive lid motion occurs. In this situation the corneal epithelial cells are not permitted to migrate over and close the epithelial defect. This leads to increased pain

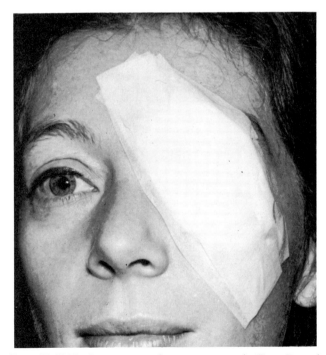

Figure 85–15. Final appearance of pressure eye patch. (From Deutsch TA, Feller DB: Paton and Goldberg's Management of Ocular Injuries. 2nd ed. Philadelphia, WB Saunders Co, 1985. Reproduced by permission.)

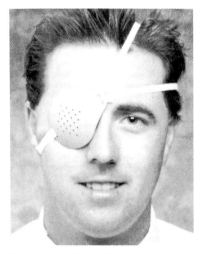

Figure 85–16. Use of the adjustable elastic strap pressure patch, Presspatch II. (Courtesy of Precision Therapeutics, Inc., Las Vegas, Nev.)

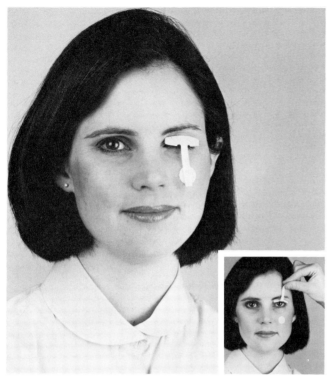

Figure 85–17. Donaldson Eyepatch (Keeler Instruments, Inc.). Inset shows the means by which the patch can be released for eye inspection or medication administration.

and delayed healing. Some corneal defects are extensive and may require 3 to 5 days for healing. Patients with extensive injuries should be followed frequently and treated with cycloplegics, pain medication, and (if clinically indicated) sedatives for sleep. The practitioner should document the size of the corneal defect at each visit. If healing does not occur in a progressive fasion, ophthalmologic consultation should be obtained. As mentioned earlier, patching when a corneal ulcer is present is contraindicated. A corneal "abrasion" that does not heal could very well be a herpetic ulcer.

All patients whose eyes have been patched for a corneal abrasion should be warned about possible *recurrent erosions* that might occur in the future as a complication of the original injury. The original abrasion may appear to have healed perfectly, but days, weeks, or even months later a small area of corneal epithelium can come off, re-creating the symptoms of the original abrasion. This usually occurs in the mornings as the patient opens his eyes. These erosions may heal before the patient is reexamined and can be very puzzling. The cause is a failure of bonding of the corneal epithelium to its basement membrane.[64] Patients who develop this syndrome are given 5 per cent sodium chloride ointment to use nightly to prevent the erosions; some require bandage-soft contact lenses.[65]

Conclusion

Patching should be an easy, straightforward procedure. A common problem is the lack of follow-up instructions given to the patient after the patching. Too often, the patient is given a bottle of antibiotic to be used every 4 hours and only vague recommendations for a follow-up check. When patients remove the patch to put in an antibiotic drop, they are never able to replace the patch properly again. Instead, they should be told to keep the patch on for 24 hours and to return to have their abrasion checked by a

physician after that time. This is the only safe way of ensuring that the abrasion has healed properly. As discussed earlier, trustworthy patients with very *superficial* corneal injuries may be given more responsibility (and instruction) for their own subsequent care. The physician should, however, make a follow-up telephone call to these individuals if they choose not to return to ascertain their compliance with the instructions.

The patient with an eye patch should be instructed to rest the uninjured eye. Reading should be discouraged, because involuntary movement of the patched eye will result. Watching television from a distance of 10 feet or more promotes eye fixation and is acceptable. Distant vision is unaffected by patching, although a small degree of peripheral vision is lost on the patched side. Driving after a patch is placed is generally safe, although not advisable. The patient should be driven home from the hospital to minimize the medicolegal risk to both patient and physician if the patient becomes involved in an accident. An elderly patient may require assistance with routine ambulation after eye patching.

CONTACT LENS PROCEDURES

Introduction

An estimated 15 million Americans wear a form of contact lenses.[66] Removal of these lenses in the emergency department may be required to permit further evaluation of the eye or to prevent injury from prolonged wear. Emergency physicians also evaluate patients for "lost" contacts, which may be trapped under the upper lid. At times, the patient may request that the physician remove a lens that he has failed to extract from the cornea. This section on contact lens procedures addresses these concerns and discusses injuries associated with removal attempts, the mechanism of injury from prolonged wear, and instructions to be given to patients at discharge.

The first "contact" lenses were scleral lenses made of glass. These lenses, covering the cornea as well as much of the surrounding sclera, are reported to have been in use from 1888 to 1948.[67] Glass corneal lenses (sitting entirely on the cornea) made by the Carl Zeiss Optical Works of Jena were first described in 1912. A practical synthetic scleral lens using methyl methacrylate rather than glass was discussed by Mullen and Obrig in 1938.[68, 69] In 1947, Tuohy redeveloped the corneal lens using methyl methacrylate. This was the forerunner of the current hard contact lens.[70] The development in Czechoslovakia of lenses made of soft gas-permeable polymers was reported in 1960.[71] These hydrogel (hydrophilic gelatinous-like) lenses have evolved into today's soft contact lenses.

Mechanism of Corneal Injury from Contact Lens Wear

HARD CONTACT[72]

The oxygenation of the cornea is dependent on movement of oxygen-rich tears under the hard contact lens during blinking. During the "adaptation" phase of early wear, the wearer of hard contacts produces hypotonic tears as a result of mechanical irritation from the lens. This results in corneal edema, which reduces subsequent tear flow under the lens during blinking. Extended wear at this time leads to corneal ischemia with superficial epithelial defects predominantly in the central corneal area (see Fig. 85–3D), where the least tear flow occurs. With adaptation, the tears become isotonic and the blinking rate normalizes, permitting extended wear. It should be noted that during early adaptation blinking is more rapid than normal and then slows to a subnormal rate during late adaptation. Mucus delivery to the cornea in the tear film may also play an important role in maintaining corneal lubrication. Tight-fitting contacts may never permit good tear flow despite an adaptation phase; individuals with tightly fitted lenses may never be able to wear their original contacts for longer than 6 to 8 hours. Lenses that are excessively loose can also cause corneal injury by moving during blinking. Rough or cracked edges can compound these injuries.

In the emergency department, the patient who presents with irritation caused by prolonged wear may be either a new or an "adapted" wearer. The adapted wearer may have been exposed to chemical irritants (e.g., smoke), which reduce the tonicity of tears and lead to corneal edema and decreased tear flow. Alternatively, the adapted wearer with irritation may have ingested sedatives (e.g., alcohol) or may have fallen asleep wearing the contacts, thus decreasing blinking and tear flow. Another possibility is that the patient may actually be wearing tight-fitting contacts that have never allowed true adaptation despite many months of wear.

The patient with the overwear syndrome usually awakens 3 hours after removing the lenses. The patient experiences intense pain and tearing similar to that caused by a foreign body. The delay in the onset of symptoms until after removal of the lenses is caused by a temporary corneal anesthesia produced by the anoxic metabolic by-products that build up during extended lens wear.[73] A second factor is the slow passage of microcysts of edema, which are pushed up to the corneal surface by mitosis of the underlying cells. When the cysts break open on the surface, the corneal nerve endings are exposed.[74]

Most patients with the overwear syndrome can be managed with reassurance, frequent administration of artificial tears, oral analgesics, and advice to "wait it out" in a darkened room. Some patients require patching for comfort. A patient who has experienced no problems with contact lenses before an overwear episode can return to using the lenses after 2 or 3 days of wearing glasses but should be advised to build up wearing time gradually. A patient who was having chronic problems with lens comfort before the episode should check with an ophthalmologist before using the contacts again.

SOFT CONTACT[75]

Although there is also oxygenation of the cornea by way of the tear film with soft contact lenses, only approximately one tenth of the flow behind the lens that occurs with a hard lens is present during soft contact wear. The high degree of lens gas permeability permits the majority of oxygenation to occur directly through the lens. The hydrogel lens is more comfortable than the hard contact because lid motion over the lens is smooth. The minimization of lid and corneal irritation allows a more rapid adaptation phase because the initial reflex-induced tearing and blinking changes are reduced. Nonetheless, the lenses may still lead to corneal edema and secondary hypoxic epithelial changes if worn for an excessive period when blinking is inhibited. Some individuals can tolerate the lenses for extended periods and may on occasion sleep with the contacts in place, although this practice is not encouraged. Newer extended-wear hydrogel lenses (e.g., Permalenses) permit wear for several weeks without injury. These lenses are not discernible from standard soft lenses on examination.

Although the acute overwear syndrome that occurs with hard contacts can also occur with soft lenses, it is very infrequent. More commonly, ocular damage from soft contact lenses falls into one of the three following categories:

1. Corneal neovascularization. Often the patient is asymptomatic, but on slit lamp examination fine vessels are seen invading the peripheral cornea. The treatment is to have an ophthalmologist refit the patient with looser or thinner lenses or with contacts that are more gas permeable.

2. Giant papillary conjunctivitis.[76] The patient notes decreased lens tolerance and increased mucus production. On examination of the tarsal conjunctiva (best seen on eversion of the upper lid), large papillae are seen. These grossly appear as a cobblestoned surface. The treatment is to discontinue wearing the lenses until the process reverses and then have the lenses refitted.

3. A sensitivity reaction to the contact lens solutions (usually Thimerosol or Chlorhexidine).[77, 78] There is diffuse conjunctival injection and sometimes a superficial keratitis. The treatment is to switch to preservative-free saline with the use of heat sterilization.

All three of the aforementioned problems with soft lenses have bilateral, subacute onsets and do not require emergency treatment. The only form of ocular damage associated with soft contact lenses that is a true emergency is a bacterial or fungal corneal ulcer.[79-81] Because the nature of soft contact lenses is to absorb water, they can also absorb pathogens, which then can invade the cornea. This is especially true if the soft lens is worn continuously during both day and night. The patient presents with a painful, red eye associated with discharge and a white infiltrate on the cornea. Immediate ophthalmologic consultation is required for appropriate culturing and antimicrobial treatment.

Indications for Removal

Removal of a contact lens is recommended in the following situations:

1. Contact lens wearer with an altered state of consciousness. The emergency physician should always be aware that the patient with a depressed or acutely agitated sensorium may be unable to express the need to have his contact lenses removed. Furthermore, it is likely that patients with a depressed sensorium will have decreased lid motion. During the secondary survey of these patients, the emergency physician should identify the presence of the lenses and should arrange for their removal and storage to prevent harm from excessive wear or possible accidental dislodgment at a later time. Without magnification, soft contacts may be difficult to see. Examination with an obliquely directed penlight should reveal the edge of the soft lens a few millimeters from the limbus on the bulbar conjunctiva.

2. Eye trauma with lens in place. Following measurement of visual acuity with the patient's lenses in place, the contacts should be removed to permit more detailed examination of the cornea. It should be noted that fluorescein may discolor hydrogel lenses; when possible, extended-wear lenses should be removed before the use of this chemical. After the dye is instilled, the eyes should be flushed with normal saline; at least 1 hour should pass before reinsertion.[82] The recent availability of single-use droppers of 0.35 per cent fluorexon (Fluresoft) has permitted the safe staining of eyes when soft lenses are to be worn immediately following the examination. A limited eye irrigation following the use of fluorexon drops is still recommended before the reinsertion of soft contacts.

3. Inability of the patient to remove the contact lens. A patient may present with a hard contact that cannot be removed because of corneal edema from prolonged wear. Alternatively, the patient may present with a "lost contact" that is believed to be behind the upper lid. It should be noted that there is no urgency for contact removal in the prehospital setting; hence, removal can wait until the patient has been evaluated by a physician.

Contraindication to Removal

The only major problem with contact lens removal occurs when the cornea may have been perforated. In this case, the suction cup technique of removal described later is preferred.

Procedure

HARD CONTACT LENS REMOVAL

A number of maneuvers have been devised for removal of the corneal lens. One technique is to first lean the patient's face over a table or a collecting cloth. The physician pulls the lids temporally from the lateral palpebral margin to lock the lids against the contact lens edges. The patient should look toward his nose and then downward toward his chin. This movement works the lower eyelid under the lower lens edge and flips the lens off the eye. The technique requires a cooperative patient, because the physician must pull the patient's lids tightly against the edge of the contact lens. The movement of the patient's eye then flips the contact free.

In the unresponsive patient, a modification of the technique can be used while the patient is supine. The physician takes a more active role in lid movement using the following procedure: One thumb is placed on the upper eyelid and the other on the lower eyelid near the margin of each lid. With the lens centered over the cornea, the eyelids are opened until the lid margins are beyond the edges of the lens (Fig. 85–18A). The physician then presses both eyelids gently but firmly on the globe of the eye and moves the lids so that they are barely touching the edges of the lens (Fig.

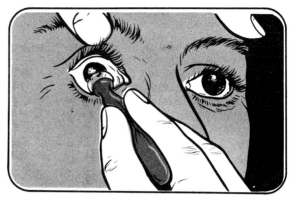

Figure 85–19. Use of a moistened suction cup to remove a hard contact lens. (From Grant HD, Murray RH, Bergeron JF: Brady Emergency Care. 5th ed, © 1990, pp 338–339. Reprinted by permission of Prentice Hall, Englewood Cliffs, New Jersey.)

85–18B). One presses slightly harder on the lower lid to move it under the bottom edge of the lens. As the lower edge of the lens begins to tip away from the eye, the lids are moved together, allowing the lens to slide out to where it can be grasped (Fig. 85–18C). The physician should remember to use clean hands when removing the lens.

Alternatively, one can move the lens gently off the cornea using a cotton-tipped applicator to guide the lens onto the sclera, where the applicator tip can be forced under an edge of the lens to flip the contact loose. Topical anesthesia is indicated when using an applicator and the patient is awake. Care must be taken with this technique to avoid contact of the applicator with the cornea when the lens is moved off the eye. Perhaps the easiest technique is to use a moistened suction-tipped device and simply lift the lens off the cornea (Fig. 85–19). A drop of honey on the fingertip can be used by the patient or the physician to remove a hard contact lens if a suction-tipped device is not available. The honey is easily washed off a hard lens.

Scleral lenses (those hard contact lenses that cover both the cornea and an amount of the sclera) can be removed by an exaggeration of the manual technique described earlier (Fig. 85–20). Elevation of the lens with a cotton-tipped applicator or a suction-tipped device is also an effective technique.

SOFT CONTACT LENS REMOVAL

With clean hands, the physician pulls down the lower eyelid using the middle finger. The tip of the index finger is placed on the lower edge of the lens. The lens is slid down onto the sclera and is compressed slightly between the thumb and the index finger. This pinching motion folds the lens and allows removal from the eye (Fig. 85–21).

Lens Storage

After a contact lens has been removed, it should be stored in sterile normal saline solution. It is best to use the patient's own storage container and, if available, a buffer solution. A variety of alternative sterile containers are available for use in the emergency department. One should be certain that right and left lenses are kept separate and in appropriately labeled containers. The containers should be kept with the patient until a friend or family member can procure them or should be locked with the patient's valuables.

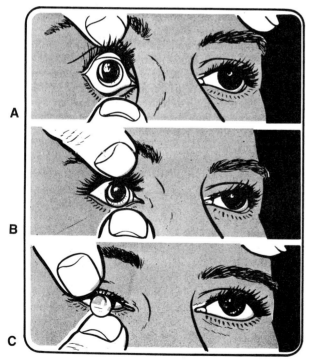

Figure 85–18. Manual technique for removing a hard contact lens. *A,* Separation of lids. *B,* Entrapment of lens edges with lids. *C,* Expulsion of lens by forcing of lower lid under inferior edge of lens. (From Grant HD, Murray RH, Bergeron JF: Brady Emergency Care. 5th ed, © 1990, pp 338–339. Reprinted by permission of Prentice Hall, Englewood Cliffs, New Jersey.)

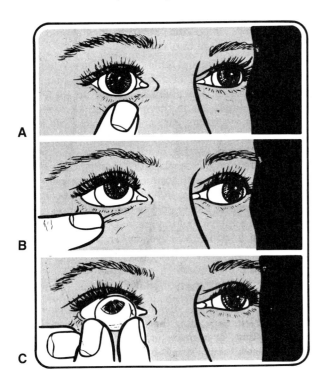

Figure 85–20. Removal of a hard scleral lens. *A,* Separation of lids. *B,* Forcing of lower lid beneath edge of scleral lens by temporal traction on lower lid. *C,* Lifting of lens off eye. (From Grant HD, Murray RH, Bergeron JF: Brady Emergency Care. 5th ed, © 1990, pp 338–339. Reprinted by permission of Prentice Hall, Englewood Cliffs, New Jersey.)

Evaluation of the "Lost Contact"

A patient may present with a request to be examined for a "lost" contact lens. The patient may be unsure if the lens is hidden under a lid, remains on the cornea, or is truly outside the eye.

The evaluation of the patient with a "lost" contact should begin, as should all eye examinations, with the measurement of visual acuity. Visual acuity is preferably measured using a 20-foot eye chart. A diminished visual acuity in the eye in which a patient "just can't seem to take out" a soft contact lens may be the most convincing evidence that the lens is missing. Although transparent, soft contacts in proper position are usually seen easily when viewed closely with loupes or on slit lamp examination. The lens forms a fine line where it ends on the sclera several millimeters peripherally

to the limbus. Hard contact lenses are even more evident as they change in position on the cornea. (Hard scleral lenses appear similar to the soft contacts when in proper location and in general are too large to be lost in the upper fornix.)

If the contact is not evident on initial inspection, the lids are everted as discussed in the section on foreign body removal (double eversion of the upper lid). If the lens is still not visible, a drop of topical anesthetic is placed in the eye. The upper fornix is gently swept with a wetted cotton-tipped applicator while the patient looks toward his chin. If the lens is still not evident although the patient remains insistent that it is in the eye, one may perform a fluorescein examination after explaining that the dye will color the lens (permanently). The upper lid should again be doubly everted and visualized using an ultraviolet light source.

If the lens remains elusive, the patient should be re-

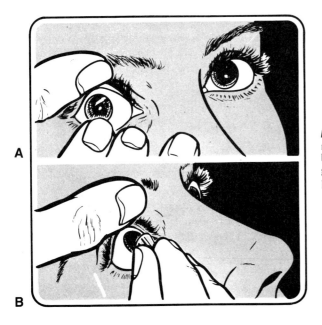

Figure 85–21. Removal of a soft contact lens. *A,* Separation of lids and movement of contact onto sclera using index finger. *B,* Pinching of lens between thumb and index finger. (From Grant HD, Murray RH, Bergeron JF: Brady Emergency Care. 5th ed, © 1990, pp 338–339. Reprinted by permission of Prentice Hall, Englewood Cliffs, New Jersey.)

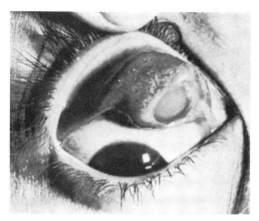

Figure 85–22. Hard contact lens embedded in conjunctival tissue of upper lid. (From Mandell RB: Contact Lens Practice. 3rd ed. Springfield, Ill, Charles C Thomas, 1981. Reproduced by permission.)

assured that a thorough examination has been performed and that no object has been located under the eyelids or on the cornea. The cornea should then be examined for defects that warrant antibiotic ointment and a pressure patch (as discussed in the section on patching). Follow-up with the patient's eye specialist for a replacement lens and further reassurance is encouraged. One should also ask the patient to retrace movements at the time the contact began to give trouble or was missed and to check the clothing being worn for the presence of the lens. A final possibility is that the patient may have accidentally placed the two lenses together in the same side of the carrying case, causing them to stick together. In fact, patients have inadvertently placed one contact over the other—both in the same eye! One should note that hard contacts have been found embedded in conjunctival tissue under the upper lid (Fig. 85–22), at times for more than a year.[83, 84]

Complications of Lens Removal

Unless care is used during lens removal, a corneal abrasion can occur. It may be difficult at times to determine whether the injury was produced by the patient or was a result of the physician's technique. Fortunately, the corneal injury is usually of a superficial nature and responds well to eye patching.

Conclusion

Contact lens removal is seldom a difficult task. More challenging situations are the identification of emergency patients at risk of overuse corneal injury, the evaluation of patients who cannot locate a soft lens, and the instruction of patients with contact lens–related problems concerning aftercare.

TONOMETRY

Introduction

Tonometry is the estimation of intraocular pressure obtained by measurement of the resistance of the eyeball to indentation of an applied force. Elevated intraocular pressure is associated with visual field loss and blindness. Sudden elevation of intraocular pressure can follow trauma or occur with primary angle-closure glaucoma. Often, patients with primary angle-closure glaucoma

come to the emergency department with systemic complaints that include nausea, vomiting, and headache; the emergency physician must determine the intraocular pressure and its relationship to the systemic symptoms. Occasionally, such patients are surprisingly free of pain in or about the eye.

Patients with an elevated intraocular pressure are at risk for retinal hypoperfusion when their systemic blood pressure is suddenly lowered. The emergency physician who treats patients in shock or uses potent antihypertensive agents needs to remain vigilant for the development of decreased retinal perfusion. Monitoring such patients for retinal artery perfusion with the direct ophthalmoscope is helpful.

Background

Ophthalmologists depended on tactile estimation of eye pressure until the 1860s, when von Graefe developed the first mechanical tonometer.[85] Applanation tonometry was introduced in 1885 by Maklakoff[86] but was not popularized until Goldmann improved the instrument in the 1930s.[87] Schiötz developed an impression tonometer in 1905 and modified it in the 1920s; this form is still in use today.[88] Aside from modifications in configuration, current tonometers closely resemble the devices popularized by Schiötz and Goldmann. The most dramatic variations are the Mackay-Marg tonometer,[89] which permits a continuous tonographic recording, and the noncontact tonometer, which is a pneumatic applanation tonometer.[90] Pocket-sized tonometers using the MacKay-Marg tonometer principle are now in use. One such device is the Tono-Pen XL (Bio-Rad, Ophthalmic Division, Santa Ana, Calif.).[91] These devices are portable, lightweight, and relatively accurate, with built-in provisions for calibration.

Tonometric Techniques

There are three tonometric techniques that are reliable and clinically useful for estimating intraocular pressure:

1. The impression method, whereby a plunger 3 mm in diameter deforms the cornea and the "indentation" is measured. This technique was popularized by Schiötz and commonly bears his name.

2. The MacKay-Marg method, a refined version of the impression technique, whereby smaller amounts of cornea are indented.

3. The applanation method, whereby a plane surface is pressed against the cornea.

One can either measure the pressure necessary to flatten a defined area or determine the size of a flattened area produced by the defined pressure. These tonometric techniques are based on the Imbert-Fick law, which states: If a plane surface is applied with force (F) to a thin, spheric membrane within which a pressure (P_t) exists, at equilibrium the expression $P_t = F/A$ is valid if A is the area of the applied surface (Fig. 85–23). It should be noted that the

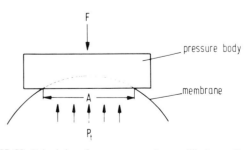

Figure 85–23. Principle of tonometry. At equilibrium: $P_t = F/A$. (From Draeger J, Jessen K: Tonometry and tonography. In Bellows JG: Glaucoma: Contemporary International Concepts. New York, Masson Publishing USA, 1979. Reproduced by permission.)

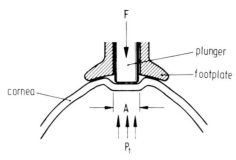

Figure 85–24. Principle of impression tonometry. In reality, P_t is increased slightly by the weight of the instrument. (From Draeger J, Jessen K: Tonometry and tonography. In Bellows JG: Glaucoma: Contemporary International Concepts. New York, Masson Publishing USA, 1979. Reproduced by permission.)

Schiötz tonometer (Fig. 85–24) actually measures the total intraocular pressure (initial pressure plus the pressure added by the weight of the tonometer and the plunger). Friedenwald[92] empirically found that a "rigidity coefficient" could be introduced to allow an estimation of the true intraocular eye pressure. One must be aware, however, that calculated conversion tables for Schiötz tonometers use an average estimate of the rigidity coefficient and hence are not accurate when eye rigidity is altered (e.g., after scleral buckle procedures for retinal detachment or with extreme myopia). Although the applanation tonometer (Fig. 85–25) also increases the intraocular pressure during measurement, the applied pressure is much smaller and is partially countered by the surface tension of the eye tear film. Studies have shown the applanation tonometer measurements to be within 2 per cent of the true intraocular pressure.[93]

The noncontact tonometer is a pneumatic applanation tonometer that permits intraocular pressure measurement without eye contact. A pulsed air jet is used to deform the cornea. The technique is also dependent on ocular rigidity. Although readings taken by different examiners correlate well, the measurements are altered by the use of local anesthetics and show a wide standard deviation of measurement in patients with pathologic elevation of ocular pressure (when standard applanation tonometry is used as a reference).[94] Furthermore, the technique is not useful with corneal surface irregularities (e.g., corneal edema, keratoconus, corneal perforation) or when medications in viscous preparations have been used.

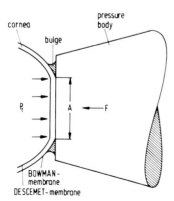

Figure 85–25. Principle of applanation tonometry. The effect of surface tension counters the pressure rise produced by application of the instrument. (From Draeger J, Jessen K: Tonometry and tonography: In Bellows JG: Glaucoma: Contemporary International Concepts. New York, Masson Publishing USA, 1979. Reproduced by permission.)

Indications for Tonometry

Measurement of intraocular pressure in the emergency department is part of any complete eye examination. Special situations in which tonometry is required are as follows:

1. *Confirmation of a clinical diagnosis of acute angle-closure glaucoma.* The middle-aged or elderly patient who presents with acute aching pain in one eye, blurred vision (including "halos" around lights), and a red eye with a smoky cornea and a fixed midposition pupil obviously needs a pressure reading. Sometimes the findings are less dramatic, and sometimes the patient complains mostly of nausea and vomiting that suggest a "flu" rather than an eye disorder.

2. *Determination of a baseline ocular pressure following blunt ocular injury.* Patients with hyphema often have acute rises in intraocular pressure because of blood obstructing the trabecular meshwork.[95] Later, angle recession can cause a permanent form of open-angle glaucoma. Arts and coworkers suggest that an intraocular pressure greater than 22 mm Hg or a difference of 3 mm Hg or greater between eyes is a good marker for ocular "injury" in the setting of an orbital fracture.[96]

3. *Determination of a baseline ocular pressure in a patient with iritis.* Patients with iritis can develop both open- and closed-angle glaucoma as well as steroid-induced glaucoma.

4. *Documentation of ocular pressure in the patient at risk for open-angle glaucoma.* All patients over the age of 40 with a familial history of open-angle glaucoma, optic disk changes, visual field defects, and pressures over 21 mm Hg should be referred to an ophthalmologist for further work-up. Referral should also be made for those patients with suspiciously cupped disks who have normal pressures; some of these patients may have "low-pressure" glaucoma associated with visual field defects.

5. *Measurement of ocular pressure in patients with glaucoma and hypertension.* There is conflicting evidence[97–104] concerning the relationship between acute reductions in systemic blood pressure and further visual field loss in glaucoma patients. Progressive or rapid visual field loss is a rare but reported phenomenon in association with systemic blood pressure reduction. The prudent physician measures the intraocular pressure and consults with the glaucoma patient's ophthalmologist before instigating treatment for systemic hypertension. Consideration should also be given to the use of a β-blocking agent to lower intraocular and systemic pressures simultaneously.

Contraindications to Tonometry

Tonometry is relatively contraindicated in eyes that are infected.[105] One should sterilize a tonometer before and after applying it to a potentially infected eye. Infected eyes are preferably measured with either a noncontact tonometer or a device with a covered tip (e.g., Tono-Pen). The contact portions of any device should be swabbed with alcohol and allowed to dry prior to use on another eye. Not all viruses may be destroyed by alcohol cleansing. Hydrogen peroxide is effective for deactivating the human immunodeficiency virus responsible for the acquired immunodeficiency syndrome (AIDS). Ultraviolet sterilization, cold-sterilizer bathing of the footplate and plunger, and ethylene oxide sterilization have been advocated as alternatives to sterilize the Schiötz tonometer tip. The Schiötz tonometer may also be used with sterile disposable coverings (marketed as Tonofilm). Nonetheless, measurement of intraocular pressure in an obviously infected eye can be deferred until a subsequent visit to the emergency department or private physician unless the red eye demands an immediate determination of intraocular pressure. Examples of a need for immediate tonometry in the setting of a red eye are suspected angle-closure glaucoma (acute onset of redness and pain in the eye with smoky vision, a cloudy cornea, and a fixed pupil in mid-dilation) and iritis (ciliary injection with photophobia), in which secondary angle-closure or steroid-induced pressure changes may occur. Reported cases of conjunctivitis spread by tonometry predominantly tend to be viral infections. Particular efforts should be made to avoid use of the instrument on patients with active facial or ocular herpetic lesions or on patients with AIDS.

The presence of corneal defects also represents a relative contraindication to tonometry.[21] The use of a tonometer on an abraded cornea may lead to further injury and is commonly deferred until a subsequent visit. Patients who cannot maintain a relaxed position (e.g., because of significant apprehension, blepharospasm, uncontrolled coughing, nystagmus, or uncontrolled singultus) are unlikely to permit an adequate examination and can receive corneal injury when sudden movements occur during an examination. Furthermore, tonometric examination, with the exception of the palpation technique (through the lids) and the noncontact method, should not be performed on a cornea without complete anesthesia.

Tonometry should *not* be performed with a suspected penetrating ocular injury.[105] Globe perforation may be exacerbated by pressure on the globe with resultant extrusion of intraocular contents. Slit lamp examination can be used for detection of a possible perforation.

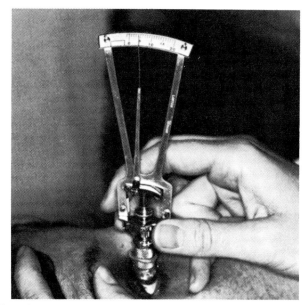

Figure 85-26. One technique of lid separation and Schiötz tonometer placement. Lid separation pressure is applied to the bony orbital rims. The tonometer is held vertically during use, and the physician's hand is established against the patient's facial bones. (From Keeney AH: Ocular Examination, 2nd ed. St. Louis, CV Mosby Co, 1976. Reproduced by permission.)

Procedure

PALPATION TECHNIQUE

All forms of tonometry are essentially ways of determining the ease of deforming the eye; an eye that can easily be deformed has a low pressure. The most direct way to do this is simply to press on the sclera through the lids and grossly compare one eye with the other. One can easily distinguish the rock-hard eye of acute glaucoma from the normal opposite eye by this method. Another method is to anesthetize the eyes topically and press a wetted applicator on the sclera of each eye. Again, eye deformation is inversely related to ocular pressure. Rigidity of the globe also is a factor in this crude method of tonometry.

IMPRESSION (SCHIÖTZ) TECHNIQUE

Use of the Schiötz tonometer requires relaxation on the part of the patient and steadiness on the part of the physician. The patient is placed in either a supine or a semirecumbent position and is instructed to gaze at a spot directly above the eyes. A spot on the ceiling should suffice; alternatively, the patient can stretch the arm up over the head and gaze at the thumb. A drop of topical anesthetic is placed in each eye. The patient is allowed to blink while the physician blots the tears away with a tissue. Rubbing the eyes lowers intraocular pressure.

The patient *keeps both eyes wide open and fixed on an object*, and the physician separates the eyelids on the side to which he or she is standing. Care must be taken to direct pressure onto the orbital rims rather than into the orbit, because pressure directed into the orbit falsely raises the reading (Fig. 85–26). The tonometer is momentarily held over the open eye, and the patient is informed that the instrument will block vision in the one eye. The patient is instructed to continue to gaze at the fixation point as though the instrument were not there. After the patient relaxes the involun-

tary muscle contraction that occurs when the instrument is first placed in the line of sight, the instrument is gently lowered onto the middle portion of the cornea. The instrument should be vertically aligned with the footplate resting on the cornea; the reading should be in midscale. Should the reading be on the low end of the scale (less than 5 units), additional weight should be added to the plunger after the instrument has been removed. The process should be repeated as before with the additional weight.

The opposite eye should be measured in the same fashion. A converted scale reading giving an intraocular pressure of greater than 21 mm Hg requires ophthalmologic consultation (Table 85–3). Associated symptoms or signs of angle-closure glaucoma (primary or secondary) represent an ophthalmologic emergency.[106]

Errors with Impression Tonometry. Inaccurate readings can occur with the Schiötz tonometer for a variety of reasons. If the plunger is sticky, falsely low readings may be obtained. Plunger motion and the zero point of the tonometer should be checked on a firm test button before use. A sticky plunger can be cleaned with isopropyl alcohol and dried with a tissue. When the lids are held open, pressure directed into the orbit elevates the intraocular pressure and provides a falsely elevated reading. The following eye movements have been found to elevate the intraocular pressure: closure of the lids (increase by 5 mm Hg), blinking (increase by 5 to 10 mm Hg), accommodation (increase by 2 mm Hg), and looking toward the nose (increase by 5 to 10 mm Hg).[107] Repeated measurements or prolonged measurements have been found to lower the intraocular pressure approximately 2 mm Hg and may also lower the pressure in the opposite eye.[108] As mentioned in the introduction to this section, the calibration of the Schiötz tonometer is based on a mean rigidity coefficient. Factors that produce a reduction in ocular rigidity falsely lower the measured pressure. These factors include high myopia, anticholinesterase drugs, overhydration (4 cups of coffee or 6 cans of beer), and scleral buckle operations.[107, 109]

Table 85–3. Schiötz Tonometry

Tonometer Scale Reading (units)	Tonometer Weights (grams)		
	5.5 (mm Hg)	7.5 (mm Hg)	10 (mm Hg)
2.50	27	39	55
3.00	24	36	51
3.50	22	33	47
4.00	21	30	43
4.50	19	28	40
5.00	17	26	37
5.50	16	24	34
6.00	15	22	32
6.50	13	20	29
7.00	12	18	27
7.50	11	17	25
8.00	10	16	23
8.50	9	14	21
9.00	8	13	20
9.50	8	12	18
10.00	7	11	16

The table provides estimates of the intraocular pressure to the nearest mm Hg for the different weight of the Schiötz tonometer. Accuracy is most dependable with scale readings larger than 5. If the scale reading is less than 5, use the next highest weight that will give a reading of 5 or more.

Ocular pressure measurements can vary with ocular perfusion. When measured after a premature ventricular contraction, the intraocular pressure may be reduced as much as 8 mm Hg.[110] Similarly, decreased venous return as produced by breath holding, the Valsalva maneuver, or a tight collar can increase the intraocular pressure.[107]

APPLANATION TECHNIQUE[111, 112]

One can perform this technique using a slit lamp attachment for an applanation tonometer with the patient's head stabilized in the headrest of the slit lamp (see the following section on the slit lamp examination) (Fig. 85–27). A portable device is also available and is similar in principle. The portable device is not discussed specifically.

The patient must be comfortable and relaxed. The physician should anesthetize the eye as discussed previously, avoiding ocular pressure, which can lower the subsequent measurements. Fluorescein should be applied to each eye. Excess fluorescein should be blotted from the eye. The patient's head should be in the slit lamp with the forehead firmly against the headrest, and the physician should direct the patient to gaze straight ahead. One can use a light for fixation or can ask the patient to focus on the physician's ear on the side opposite the eye being examined.

The cobalt blue light filter is placed in the light beam, and the slit diaphragm is opened fully. The light arm is angulated to shine on the applanation prism in the region of the encircling black line near the anterior prism tip at an angle of 45 to 60 degrees to the line of observation. The voltage is turned to the maximum setting, and the low-power microscopic system is focused through the plastic prism so that the front face is clearly seen through the chosen eyepiece. The pressure knob of the tonometer is turned to 1 gm (10 mm Hg), bringing the prism arm to its forward stop. Thus, when corneal contact is made, the prism will be exerting only light pressure. The room lights are dimmed.

The patient's eye that is being examined and the applanation prism are watched from the side (or with the eye not sighting through the microscope) as the instrument is brought forward by the "joy stick" control until gentle contact is made between the prism face and the corneal center. Contact is evidenced by an immediate bluish glow throughout the limbus. The patient's lids must be wide open and unblinking. Contact with the lid margins produces reflex blinking, and the lids may require separation by the physician's fingers. Pressure during lid separation must be exerted only against the orbital rims. Through the microscope, the physician sees two blue semicircles (surrounding the flattened area of cornea). Each semicircle is bordered by an arc of green light and pulses synchronously with the cardiac rate (Fig. 85–28).

The semicircles should be of equal size; their width should be approximately one tenth the diameter of the flattened surface contained within each arc. If the semicircles are grossly widened, either excessive tears are present or the prism was probably wet before contact. A wet prism must be withdrawn, dried, and reapplied. If the semicircles are grossly narrowed, the tear film has dried excessively. In this case, the prism must be withdrawn and the patient instructed to blink several times before contact with the cornea is attempted again. If the semicircles are so broad that they extend beyond the illuminate field, there is excessive flattening, and the slit lamp must be drawn back. If the semicircles suddenly shrink, either the patient has moved back or the instrument has been backed away from the eye. The semicircles should be of equal extent above and below a horizontal dividing line. If the dividing line is not horizontal, the applanation prism assembly should be rotated on its holder until the line is horizontal. If the semicircles are not equally divided above and below the line, vertical adjustments of the slit lamp should be made.

Readings should be taken at approximately the midpoint between systole and diastole, when the inner (concave) boundaries of each semicircle rhythmically glide past each other through excursions of equal distance (see Fig. 85–28C). One finalizes adjustments to the end point of properly located and sized semicircles by rotating the pressure knob back and forth. When applanation pressure exceeds intraocular pressure, the semicircles are too small to intersect.

At the end point is a flattened disk area 3.06 mm in diameter within the 7-mm diameter of the prism face. Here

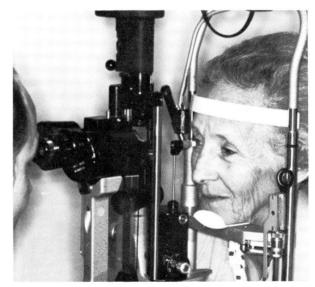

Figure 85–27. Goldmann applanation tonometer with the biprism in contact with the patient's right cornea. (From Keeney AH: Ocular Examination, 2nd ed. St. Louis, CV Mosby Co, 1976. Reproduced by permission.)

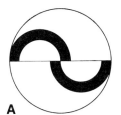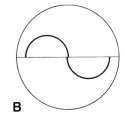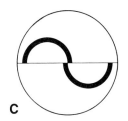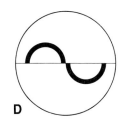

A   B   C   D

Figure 85–28. Schematic representation of semicircles seen through the contact applanation prism of the Goldmann tonometer. *A,* Semicircles are too wide, suggesting excessive moistening of the prism or cornea. The prism must be withdrawn and dried. *B,* Semicircles are too narrow, suggesting that the lacrimal fluid has dried out, as during a prolonged measurement. The prism must be withdrawn so that the patient may blink a few times. The measurement is then repeated. *C,* Semicircles are of appropriate width, and their inner borders just touch. Cardiac pulsations transmitted through the globe cause rhythmic or pulsating movement of the semicircles over each other through a small amplitude. *D,* Semicircles are slightly separated, indicating applied pressure below that of the eye. The measuring drum must be turned to increase applanation pressure until the end point is reached. (From Keeney AH: Ocular Examination, 2nd ed. St. Louis, CV Mosby Co, 1976. Reproduced by permission.)

the attractive surface tension of the tears toward the prism is counterbalanced by the elasticity, or springiness, of the cornea; at this point the grams of force applied through the prism (indicated on the pressure knob) are directly convertible (when multiplied by 10 into millimeters of mercury) to express intraocular pressure. With an applanation tonometer, the average intraocular pressure in a seated adult is 14 to 17 mm Hg.

After use, the tonometer should be wiped dry and removed for storage if used infrequently in the emergency department. One should verify the pressure adjustment periodically using the test weight or metal balance bar supplied with the instrument.

Potential sources of error with the applanation tonometer are similar to those mentioned for the impression tonometer, with the exception that ocular rigidity is not a factor. Inaccuracies primarily result from ocular motion or tensing of the lids.

Complications

When tonometric instruments are used properly and reasonable precautions are taken, complications are unusual. The eye with preexisting corneal injury should be spared the additional trauma of tonometer placement. Corneal abrasions can be produced by ocular movement during testing. In particular, patients with uncontrollable nystagmus, singultus, or coughing or those who are extremely apprehensive should not be subjected to tonometry. Infection can be transmitted by the use of the instrument. Careful cleansing of the device and avoidance of tonometry in patients with obvious conjunctivitis, corneal ulcers, or active herpetic lesions should minimize the risk of spreading the infection to the unaffected eye or to subsequent patients. Although protective coverings can be placed over the tonometer contact, tonometry can usually be postponed in the aforementioned individuals until the risk of infection is minimal. Extrusion of ocular contents with penetrating injuries is a potential but rare complication.

Conclusion

Tonometry is an easily learned technique that should be used by the emergency physician for the detection of elevated intraocular pressure. An elevated intraocular pressure in conjunction with physical findings suggestive of acute angle-closure glaucoma is an indication for therapy and consultation with an ophthalmologist. The baseline measurement of intraocular pressure will aid the ophthalmologist in subsequent evaluation of a referred patient. In addition, the emergency physician can serve as a referral source for patients with elevated intraocular pressure who are suspected of having open-angle glaucoma. In particular, future drug therapy for systemic hypertension may be altered by the presence of concomitant intraocular hypertension. The emergency physician who aggressively manages patients with hypertensive crises must also be aware of potential visual field defects when systemic blood pressure is vigorously lowered without concurrent lowering of intraocular pressure.

SLIT LAMP EXAMINATION

Introduction

The slit lamp is an extremely useful instrument; it makes the examination of the anterior segment of the eye a pleasure. The instrument can reveal pathologic conditions that would otherwise be invisible. The slit lamp permits detailed evaluation of external eye injury and is the definitive tool for diagnosing anterior chamber hemorrhage and inflammation. The emergency physician should not attempt to diagnose any but the simplest of eye problems without the aid of a slit lamp.

Background[113]

Since the 1800s, physicians have searched for a better way both to magnify and to illuminate the anterior segment of the eye. In 1891, Aubert developed the first true binocular stereoscopic microscope. Then, in 1911, Gullstrand introduced a slit illuminator device. The microscope and the illuminator were combined by Henker in 1916; the result was the first true slit lamp. Goldmann improved the mechanical supports for the microscope and the illuminator and in 1937 marketed a slit lamp that resembles closely the device that is used today.

Indications and Contraindications

The slit lamp can be used in every eye examination. It is especially useful in the emergency department for the diagnosis of corneal abrasions, foreign bodies, and iritis.[114] The slit lamp facilitates foreign body removal and is also used in conjunction with most applanation tonometers. Although portable slit lamp instruments exist, emergency physicians generally have access only to a stationary, upright device. Therefore, in the absence of a portable device, a slit lamp examination is contraindicated in patients who cannot tolerate an upright sitting position (e.g., those with orthostatic syncope).

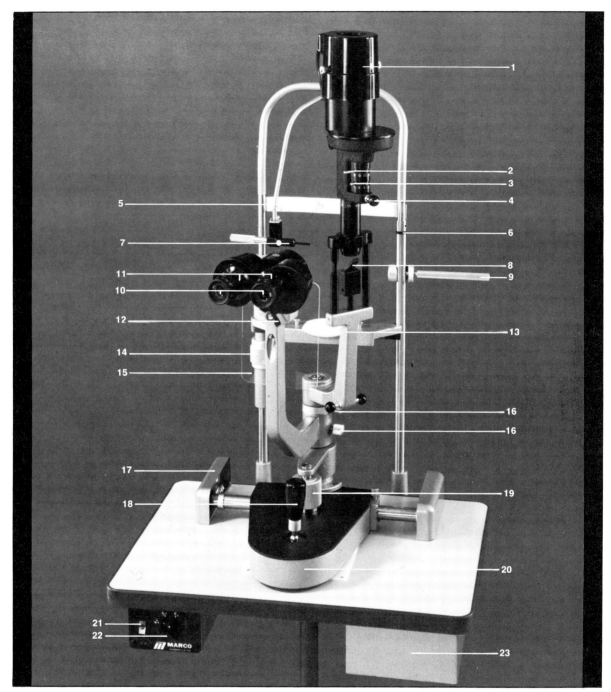

MARCO I PRIMARY CARE SLIT LAMP

NOMENCLATURE

1. Cover for Lamp Bulb
2. Slit Width Controls (Red-Free Filter)
3. Slit Height Control (Cobalt Blue Filter)
4. Control of the Rotation of Slit
5. Headrest
6. Eye Level Marker
7. Fixation Lighthead
8. Mirror
9. Examiner's Handrest
10. Eyepieces
11. Knurled Rings for Refractive Error Adjustment
12. High-Low Magnification Lever
13. Patient's Chinrest
14. Headrest Elevation Control
15. Breath Shield
16. Fixing Screws for Arm
17. Rail Covers
18. Joystick
19. Elevation Control
20. Slit Lamp Base
21. On-Off Switch
22. Intensity Control
23. Accessory Storage Drawer

Figure 85–29. Slit lamp controls. (From Marco Equipment, Inc.: Operating Instructions for Slit Lamp Microscopes. Jacksonville, Fla, Marco Equipment, Inc.)

Equipment

The slit lamp has three essential components: a binocular microscope mounted horizontally, a light source that can create a beam of variable width, and a mechanical assembly to immobilize the patient's head and to manipulate the microscope and the light source. The location and arrangement of the knobs that control these components vary in devices made by different manufacturers. Usually, by simply turning each knob and watching the results, one can quickly master a new machine. Figure 85–29 illustrates the location of the functional controls on one particular instrument.

The first knob that one should locate is the on/off switch for the entire machine. Often this switch incorporates or is adjacent to a rheostat that provides two or three different power settings. The lowest setting is adequate for routine examination and will preserve bulb life. One can use a high-intensity setting when examining the anterior chamber with a narrow slit beam. Often, these controls are located on a transformer placed beneath the table to which the slit lamp has been attached. The second knob that one should find is the locking nut for the mechanical assembly. This must be loosened in order for the assembly to be moved.

The patient should be comfortable while sitting with the head in the device. The patient's forehead should be firmly against the headrest, and the chin should be in the chin rest. By varying the table height and height of the chin rest, one should be able to maximize the comfort of the patient's neck and back. The chin rest should be adjusted to align the patient's eye level with the mark on the headrest support rods.

The binocular microscope has a control for varying the magnification. Usually low powers, such as $10\times$ or $16\times$, are the most useful. A higher power is helpful when the anterior chamber is examined for cells and flare and when the cornea is examined in minute detail. The binocular interpupillary distance should be adjusted to match that of the examiner. One can focus the eyepieces by moving the instrument forward and backward until the narrowed vertical beam is sharpest on the patient's cornea when viewed with the unaided eye. Then, while viewing through each eyepiece individually, the physician adjusts the focus of each to produce a sharp image of the anterior cornea.

The light source is mounted on a swinging arm. There are knobs to vary the width and the height of the light beam. There are also filters that can be "clicked" in; only white and blue are usually needed. The angle of the slit beam can be varied from vertical to horizontal. The vertical alignment is preferred for routine examinations in the emergency department.

Both the microscope and the light source are mounted on swivel arms, linked at their base to a movable table. One can change the position of this table by pushing on any part of it. For finer movements, the physician uses a "joy stick." One can vary the height of the microscope and the light source by twisting either the joy stick or a separate knob at the base, depending on the design of the instrument.

Procedure[115, 116]

There are three setups that every slit lamp operator must know. The first is for an overall screening of the anterior segment of the eye. For examination of the patient's right eye, the light source is swung to the examiner's left at a 45-degree angle while the microscope is directly in front of the eye. The slit beam is set at the maximum height and the minimum width using the white light. To scan across the patient's cornea, one first focuses the beam on the cornea by moving the entire base of the slit lamp forward and backward. One then moves the whole base left and right to scan across. The 45-degree angle between the microscope and the light source should not be varied. The most common mistake is to try to scan by swinging the arm of the light source in an arc; this does not work because the light beam will remain centered on the same point of the patient's eye. The examiner scans across at the level of the conjunctiva and the cornea and then pushes slightly forward on the base and scans at the level of the iris. The depth of the anterior chamber is determined by this low magnification set-up. When the depth of the anterior chamber is reduced, one should suspect a corneal perforation or a predisposition to angle-closure glaucoma.

This basic set-up can also be used to examine the conjunctiva for traumatic lesions, inflammation, and foreign bodies. The lids can be examined for hordeolum, blepharitis, or trichiasis. Complete lid eversion (as described in the section on foreign body removal) can be performed in conjunction with the slit lamp examination to permit evaluation of the undersurface of the upper lid for foreign body retention.

Corneal foreign body removal can be enhanced by use of the slit lamp. In particular, the instrument allows stabilization of the patient's head. Magnification also minimizes corneal injury during foreign body or rust ring removal. The upper eyelid may be immobilized by a cotton-tipped applicator, as discussed previously. The physician's hand can be steadied against the patient's nose, cheek, or forehead or against the support rods of the headrest. The patient should be instructed to stare straight ahead at a fixed light or at the physician's ear during removal of the foreign body.

The second set-up is essentially the same as the first but uses the blue filter. The purpose is to identify any areas of fluorescein staining. After fluorescein is applied, the blue filter is "clicked" into position, and the beam is widened to 3 or 4 mm. It should be noted that a patient can tolerate a wider beam without photophobia if it is blue. Corneal defects (as discussed in the section on the fluorescein examination) are sought with this set-up. The blue filter is also used with applanation tonometry, as discussed in the section on tonometry.

The purpose of the third set-up is to search for cells in the anterior chamber—either the white cells of iritis or the red cells of a microscopic hyphema. The height of the beam should be shortened to 3 or 4 mm and should be as narrow as possible. The microscope should be switched to high

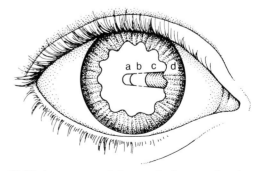

Figure 85–30. Appearance of the eye during anterior chamber examination: *a,* corneal reflection; *b,* anterior chamber (potential location of cells or flare); *c,* lens reflection; *d,* iris. The slit of light shines in the temporal to nasal direction at 45 degrees to the anterior surface of the cornea.

power. The beam is first focused on the center of the cornea and is then pushed forward slightly so that it is focused on the anterior surface of the lens. When the joy stick is again pulled back to a focus point midway between the cornea and the lens, it will be focused on the anterior chamber (Fig. 85–30). One should keep the beam centered over the pupil so that there is a black background. Normally, the aqueous humor of the anterior chamber is totally clear. If small particles are visible floating up or down through the beam, these are usually circulating cells. If the beam lights up the aqueous like a searchlight in the fog, then the examiner has found the protein flare that accompanies iritis. Note should be made of the fact that fluorescein can penetrate an abraded cornea, producing a fluorescein flare on slit-lamp evaluation. To avoid confusion, some physicians prefer to examine for anterior chamber flare before the stain is used.

Conclusion

In practice, the three set-ups described here take only 1 minute per eye. Experience with the instrument enhances the ability of the user. The device is helpful for the evaluation of ocular infections and corneal lesions, the removal of corneal foreign bodies, the measurement of intraocular pressure by applanation tonometry, and the diagnosis of iritis.

REFERENCES

Dilating the Eye

1. Duke-Elder S: System of Ophthalmology. Vol III. St. Louis, CV Mosby Co, 1962, pp 542, 571.
2. Adler AG, McElwain GE, Merli GJ, et al: Systemic effects of eye drops. Arch Intern Med 142:2293, 1982.
3. American Academy of Ophthalmology: Ophthalmology Basic and Clinical Science Course. Rochester, Minn, American Academy of Ophthalmology, 1977, p 127.
4. Physicians' Desk Reference for Ophthalmology. Oradell NJ, Medical Economics Co, 1982, p 2.
5. Lanscke RK: Systemic reactions to topical epinephrine and phenylephrine. Am J Ophthalmol 61:95, 1966.
6. Fraunfelder FT, Scafidi AF: Possible adverse effects from topical ocular 10% phenylephrine. Am J Ophthalmol 85:447, 1978.
7. Bresler MJ, Hoffman TLS: Prevention of iatrogenic acute narrow-angle glaucoma. Ann Emerg Med 10:535, 1981.
8. Hovding G, et al: Bacterial contamination of drops and dropper tips of in-use multidose bottles. Acta Ophthalmol 60:213, 1982.
9. Solosko D, Smith RB: Hypertension following 10% phenylephrine ophthalmic. Anesthesiology 36:187, 1972.
10. McReynolds WV, Havener WH, Henderson JW: Hazards of the use of sympathomimetic drugs in ophthalmology. Arch Ophthalmol 56:176, 1956.
11. Kim MK, Stevenson CE, Mathewson MD: Hypertensive reactions to phenylephrine eye drops in patients with sympathetic denervation. Am J Ophthalmol 85:862, 1978.
12. Adler AG, McElwain GE, Martin JH, et al: Coronary artery spasm induced by phenylephrine eye drops. Arch Intern Med 141:1384, 1981.
13. Fraunfelder FT: Interim report: National registry of possible drug induced ocular side effects. Ophthalmology 86:126, 1979.
14. Hoefnagel D: Toxic effects of atropine and homatropine eye drops in children. N Engl J Med 264:168, 1961.
15. Heath WE: Death from atropine poisoning. Br Med J 2:608, 1950.
16. Freund M, Meun S: Toxic effects of scopolamine eye drops. Am J Ophthalmol 70:637, 1970.
17. Beswick JA: Psychosis from cyclopentolate. Am J Ophthalmol 53:879, 1962.
18. Binkharst RD, Weinstein GW, Borety RM, et al: Psychotic reaction induced by cyclopentolate: Results of pilot study and double-blind study. Am J Ophthalmol 55:1243, 1963.
19. Carpenter WT Jr: Precipitous mental deterioration following cycloplegia with 0.2% cyclopentolate HC1. Arch Ophthalmol 18:445, 1967.

The Fluorescein Examination

20. Havener WA: Ocular Pharmacology. St. Louis, CV Mosby Co, 1978 p 413.
21. Duke-Elder S: System of Ophthalmology. Vol. VII. St. Louis, CV Mosby Co, 1962, p 243.

22. Vaughn DG: The contamination of fluorescein solutions. Am J Ophthalmol 39:55, 1955.
23. Paton D, Goldberg MF: Management of Ocular Injuries. Philadelphia, WB Saunders Co, 1976, p 194.
24. Grant MW: Toxicology of the Eye. Springfield, Ill, Charles C Thomas, 1974, p 495.
25. National Registry of Drug Induced Ocular Side Effects, Case Reports 404a, 404b, 421. Portland, Ore, University of Oregon Health Sciences Center, 1979.
26. Cohn HC, Jocson VL: A unique case of grand mal seizures after Fluress. Ann Ophthalmol 13:1379, 1981.
27. Havener WA: op. cit., pp 70–74.
28. Cain W Jr, Sinskey RM: Detection of anterior chamber leakage with Seidel's test. Arch Ophthalmol 99:2013, 1981.
29. Havener WA: op. cit., p 419.
30. Sexton RR: Herpes simplex keratitis. In Wilson LA (ed): External Diseases of the Eye. Hagerstown, Md, Harper & Row, 1979, pp 235–260.
31. Sexton RR: Superficial keratitis. In Wilson LA (ed): External Diseases of the Eye. Hagerstown, Md, Harper & Row, 1979, pp 203–213.
32. Wilson LA: Bacterial corneal ulcers. In Wilson LA (ed): External Diseases of the Eye. Hagerstown, Md, Harper & Row, 1979, pp 215–233.
33. Jones DB: Fungal keratitis. In Wilson LA (ed): External Diseases of the Eye. Hagerstown, Md, Harper & Row, 1979, pp 265–277.
34. Weiss JN, Kreter JK, Dalton HP, et al: Detection of *Pseudomonas aeruginosa* eye infections by ultraviolet light. Ann Ophthalmol 14:242, 1982.

Eye Irrigation

35. Paton D, Goldberg MF: op. cit., p 166.
36. Ibid., p 167.
37. Ibid., p 168.
38. American Academy of Orthopedic Surgeons: Emergency Care and Transportation of the Sick and Injured. 3rd ed. Menasha, Wis, George Banta Co, Inc, 1981, p 298.
39. Grant HD, Murray RH, Bergeron JF: Emergency Care. 3rd ed. Bowie, Md, RJ Brady Co, 1982, pp 166–167.
40. Gombos GM: Handbook of Ophthalmologic Emergencies. Flushing, NY, Medical Examination Publishing Co, 1973, p 90.
41. Paton D, Goldberg MF: op. cit., p 163.
42. Ibid., p 164.
43. Pavan-Langston D: Manual of Ocular Diagnosis and Therapy. Boston, Little, Brown & Co, 1980, p 32.
44. Harris LS, Cohn K, Galin MA: Alkali injury from fireworks. Ann Ophthalmol 3:849, 1971.
45. Smith RS, Shear G: Corneal alkali burns arising from accidental instillation of a hair straightener. Am J Ophthalmol 79:602, 1975.
46. Scharpf LG Jr, Hill ID, Kelly RE: Relative eye-injury potential of heavy-duty phosphate and non-phosphate laundry detergents. Food Cosmet Toxicol 10:829, 1972.
47. Havener WA: op. cit., p 573.
48. Lippas J: Continuous irrigation in the treatment of external ocular diseases. Am J Ophthalmol 57:298, 1964.
49. Vaugn D, Asbury J: General Ophthalmology. 8th ed. Los Altos, Calif, Lange Medical Publishers, 1977, p 40.
50. Rost KM, Jaeger RW, deCastro FJ: Eye contamination: A poison center protocol for management. Clin Toxicol 14:295, 1979.
51. Levinson RA: Ascorbic acid prevents corneal ulceration and perforation following experimental alkali burns. Invest Ophthalmol 15:992, 1976.

Ocular Foreign Body Removal

52. Paton D, Goldberg MF: op. cit., pp 111–129.
53. Grove AS, New PFJ, Momose KJ: Computerized tomographic (CT) scanning for orbital evaluation. Trans Am Acad Ophthalmol Otolaryngol 79:137, 1975.
54. Lobes LA Jr, Grand MG, Reece J, et al: Computerized axial tomography in the detection of intraocular foreign bodies. Ophthalmology 88:26, 1981.
55. Paton D, Goldberg MF: op. cit., p 195.
56. Pavan-Langston D: op. cit., p 37.
57. Newell FW: Ophthalmology Principles and Concepts. St. Louis, C. V. Mosby, 1978, p 186.
58. Paton D, Goldberg MF: op. cit., pp 200, 203.

Eye Patching

59. Paton D, Goldberg MF: op. cit., p 202.
60. King JWR, Brison RJ: Emergency department management of traumatic corneal epithelial injuries without topical antibiotic prophylaxis. (abstract) J Emerg Med 8:373, 1990.
61. Havener WA: op. cit., p 119.

62. Hanna C, Fraunfelder FT, Cable M, et al: The effect of ophthalmic ointment on corneal wound healing. Am J Ophthalmol 76:193, 1973.
63. Fraunfelder FT, Hanna C, Cable M, et al: Entrapment of ophthalmic ointment in the cornea. Am J Ophthalmol 76:475, 1973.
64. Sexton RR: Superficial keratitis, op. cit., pp 208–210.
65. Laibson PR: Epithelial basement membrane dystrophy and recurrent corneal erosion. In Fraunfelder FT, Roy FH (eds): Current Ocular Therapy. Philadelphia, WB Saunders Co, 1980, pp 362–363.

Contact Lens Procedures

66. Forstot SL, Ellis PP: Identifying and managing contact lens emergencies. E R Reports 3:35, 1982.
67. Mandell RB: Contact Lens Practice. Springfield, Ill, Charles C Thomas, 1981, p 11.
68. Obrig T, Salvatori P: Contact Lenses. 3rd ed. New York, Obrig Laboratories, 1957, p 188.
69. Mullen JE: Contact Lens. US Patent 2,237,744.
70. Nugent MW: The corneal lens, a preliminary report. Ann West Med Surg 2:241, 1948.
71. Dreifus M, Wichtenle O, Lim D: Intercameral lenses of hydrocolloid acrylates. Cesk Oftalmol 16:154, 1960.
72. Mandell RB: op. cit., pp 142–168.
73. Krezanoski JZ: Physiology and biochemistry of contact lens wearing, In Encyclopedia of Contact Lens Practice. Vol 4. South Bend, Ind, International Optic, 1959, pp 18–26.
74. Cogger TJ: Correction with hard contact lenses, In Duane TD (ed): Clinical Ophthalmology. New York, Harper & Row, 1982, p 17.
75. Mandell RB: op. cit., pp 496–513.
76. Fowler SA, Allansmith MR: Evolution of soft contact lens coatings. Arch Ophthalmol 98:95, 1980.
77. Mondino BJ, Gorden LR: Conjunctival hyperemia and corneal infiltrates with chemically disinfected soft contact lenses. Arch Ophthalmol 98:1767, 1980.
78. Shaw EL: Allergies induced by contact lens solutions. Contact Intraocular Lens Med J 6:273, 1980.
79. Krachmer JH, Purcell JJ Jr: Bacterial corneal ulcers in cosmetic soft contact lens wearers. Arch Ophthalmol 96:57, 1978.
80. Bohigian GM: Management of infections associated with soft contact lenses. Ophthalmology 86:1138, 1979.
81. Binder PS: Complications associated with extended wear of soft contact lenses. Ophthalmology 86:1093, 1979.
82. Mandell RB: op. cit., p 574.
83. Long JC: Retention of contact lens in upper fornix. Am J Ophthalmol 56:309, 1963.
84. Michaels DD, Zugsmith GS: An unusual contact lens complication. Am J Ophthalmol 55:1057, 1963.

Tonometry

85. Duke-Elder S: System of Ophthalmology. Vol VII. St. Louis, CV Mosby Co, 1962, pp 349–350.
86. Maklakoff C: L'ophthalmotonometrie. Arch Ophthalmol (Paris) 5:159, 1885.
87. Goldmann H: Un nouveau tonometre à applanation. Bull Soc Franc Ophthalmol 67:474, 1955.
88. Schiötz H: Tonometry. Br J Ophthalmol 4:201, 1920.
89. Mackay RS, Marg E: Fast automatic electronic tonometers based on an exact theory. Acta Ophthalmol 37:495, 1959.

90. Grolman B: A new tonometer system. Am J Ophthalmol 49:646, 1972.
91. Boothe WA, Lee DA, Panek WC, et al: The Tono-Pen: A manometric and clinical study. Arch Ophthalmol 106:1214, 1988.
92. Friedenwald JS: Tonometer calibration: An attempt to remove discrepancies found in the 1954 calibration used for the Schiötz tonometers. Trans Am Acad Ophthalmol Otolaryngol 61:108, 1957.
93. Goldmann H, Schmidt TH: Über Applanation stonometrie. Ophthalmologica 134:221, 1957.
94. Longham ME, McCarthy E: A rapid pneumatic applanation tonometer. Arch Ophthalmol 79:389, 1968.
95. Wilensky JT: Blood induced secondary glaucomas. Ann Ophthalmol 11:1659, 1979.
96. Arts HA, Eisele DW, Duckert LG: Intraocular pressure as an index of ocular injury in orbital fractures. Arch Otolaryngol Head Neck Surg 115:213, 1989.
97. Krakan CET: Intraocular pressure elevation—cause or effect in chronic glaucoma? Ophthalmologica 182:141, 1981.
98. Bouzas A, Kampitospoulos G, Kalliterakis E: La decoloration paillaire dans les hemorragies gastrointestinales. Bull Soc Ophthalmol Fr 87:296, 1975.
99. Jampol LM, Board RJ, Manmenu AE: Systemic hypotension and glaucomatous changes. Am J Ophthalmol 85:154, 1978.
100. Drance SM, Sweeney VP, Morgan RW, et al: Factors involved in the production of low tension glaucoma. Can J Ophthalmol 9:399, 1974.
101. Harrington DO: The pathogenesis of the glaucoma field. Clinical evidence that circulatory insufficiency in the optic nerve is the primary cause of visual field loss in glaucoma. Am J Ophthalmol 47:177, 1959.
102. Francois J, Neetans A: The deterioration of the visual fields in glaucoma and the blood pressure. Doc Ophthalmol 28:70, 1970.
103. Jonasson F: Dangerous antihypertensive treatment. Br Med J 2:1218, 1979.
104. Phelps GK, Phelps CD: Blood pressure and pressure amaurosis. Invest Ophthalmol 14:237, 1975.
105. Keeney AH: Ocular Examination. St. Louis, CV Mosby Co, 1970, pp 120–123.
106. Hillman JS: Acute closed-angle glaucoma: An investigation into the effect of delay in treatment. Br J Ophthalmol 63:817, 1979.
107. Gorin G: Clinical Glaucoma. New York, Marcel Dekker, 1977, p 76.
108. Wilke K: Effects of repeated tonometry. Genuine and sham measurements. Acta Ophthalmol 50:574, 1972.
109. Harbin TS, Laikam SE, Lipsitt K, et al: Applanation—Schiötz disparity after retinal detachment surgery utilizing cryopexy. Ophth AAO 86:1609, 1979.
110. Lichter PR, Bergstrom TJ: Premature ventricular systole detection by applanation tonometry. Am J Ophthalmol 81:797, 1976.
111. Keeney AH: Ocular Examination, Basis and Technique. St. Louis, CV Mosby Co, 1976, pp 141–147.
112. Chandler PA, Grant WM: Glaucoma. 2nd ed. Philadelphia, Lea & Febiger, 1979, p 11.

Slit Lamp Examination

113. Tate GW, Safir A: The slit lamp: History, principles, and practice. In Duane TD (ed): Clinical Ophthalmology. Vol I. New York, Harper & Row, 1981, Chapter 59.
114. Pavan-Langston D: op. cit., p 9.
115. Cogger TJ: Correction with hard contact lenses. In Duane TD (ed): Clinical Ophthalmology. Vol I. New York, Harper & Row, 1981, Chapter 54.
116. Keeney AH: op. cit., pp 85–90.

Chapter 86

Otolaryngologic Procedures

Tom I. Abelson and William J. Witt

PHYSICAL EXAMINATION OF THE LARYNX

All physicians have the ability to visually examine the larynx. To do so requires only a knowledge of several techniques, including indirect laryngoscopy, telescopic examination of the larynx, and flexible laryngoscopy, and practice in their use.

Indications

In an emergency department setting, laryngoscopy is indicated when visualization of the hypopharynx and larynx might enhance the ability to diagnose and treat the patient's problem. Unexplained hoarseness, dysphagia, odynophagia, recurrent aspiration, and a feeling of a lump or foreign body in the throat are all indications for laryngoscopy.

There are some situations in which laryngoscopy should be avoided or should be performed only under very controlled circumstances. In children with epiglottitis, in patients with foreign bodies that are partially obstructing the airway, and in patients with severe neck trauma (including possible laryngotracheal separation or crush injuries of the larynx), all examinations should be performed in an operating room or in a specially prepared room in the emergency department. In these situations, the examining physician and team must be prepared to perform *any* procedure necessary to secure an airway under *any* circumstance. The team must be able to immediately intubate the patient, even under difficult circumstances. If attempts at intubation are unsuccessful, the ability to pass a rigid bronchoscope and to perform an emergency tracheotomy or cricothyrotomy is critical. Any manipulation or examination of the larynx in these situations may precipitate complete airway obstruction.

It should also be stressed that patients who have laryngeal symptoms but normal results from emergency department laryngoscopic examination should have close otolaryngologic follow-up and repeat examination. When laryngeal findings are evident on examination, repeat examination to document complete resolution of these findings is indicated.

Indirect Laryngoscopy

The oldest technique for examination of the larynx and the one used most commonly by otolaryngologists is indirect laryngoscopy, using a headlight or head mirror with an angled laryngeal mirror. Using this technique, most larynges are visualized with the excellent and undistorted optics of a flat reflecting mirror. The few cooperative patients who cannot be examined with the indirect mirror technique include those with severe psychologic gag reflex that cannot be overcome with topical anesthesia; those with uncontrollable coughing; and those with cervical spine, pharyngeal, or oral conditions that prevent appropriate positioning or visualization.

Procedure. The patient is seated in an upright position with the legs uncrossed, the upper torso leaning slightly forward, and the head slightly extended in the "sniffing" position. If the head mirror is placed over the physician's left eye, the light bulb is placed to the patient's right or vice versa. It does not matter which side is used. The light bulb is placed just behind and to the side of the patient's head at a slightly higher level than the patient's eyes. This placement prevents the physician's hands from interfering with the light shining on the head mirror. An unfrosted 150-watt light bulb provides excellent illumination. Some otolaryngologists place this light in a silver or white reflector. Use of a headlight precludes the need for the reflecting light. The examination can be performed with the physician either sitting or standing.

The keys to satisfactory examination of the larynx are practice, a reassured patient, and avoidance of contact with the *posterior pharyngeal wall* and the *posterior tongue*. Touching either of these areas elicits a gag reflex, but contact with the soft palate or uvula usually is tolerated. During the examination, the patient is advised to relax and to breathe continuously in and out through the mouth. It is important that patients not hold their breath, because in doing so, they often constrict the pharyngeal inlet, initiating contact with the mirror and precipitating a gag reflex. The patient is asked to protrude the tongue, which is grasped with a gauze sponge between the thumb and forefinger, pulling it outward and downward. This movement tends to raise the larynx and pull the epiglottis forward, opening the laryngeal inlet. The patient is instructed to keep the eyes open and to gaze at an object over the physician's shoulder. This maneuver minimizes supratentorial input to the gag reflex. The laryngeal mirror is slightly warmed, either in a flame or other type of warmer, and is tested for excess heat on the physician's hand or cheek before introduction into the patient's mouth. Warming the mirror inhibits fogging. Commercial solutions (Clear-dip) may also be used. While encouraging the patient to relax and to continue inhalation and exhalation, the mirror is passed into the mouth and over the back of the tongue where it can be gently placed against the soft palate and uvula if necessary (Fig. 86–1).

By reflecting the light off the mirror and by rotating the mirror, the base of the tongue, vallecula, epiglottis, pyriform sinus, postcricoid area, arytenoids, aryepiglottic folds, false vocal cords, ventricles, true vocal cords, supraglottic area, and the upper part of the trachea can be examined. The anterior commissure of the vocal cords is the most difficult area to examine, because the epiglottis tends to overhang it. By asking the patient to phonate a high-pitched sound such as "Eeeeee," the larynx is further raised and tilted to permit more complete examination of the anterior larynx. Vocal cord mobility can also be observed through this maneuver.

In patients who are unable to control their gag reflex or in those in whom it is difficult to avoid touching sensitive areas, a topical anesthetic, gargle, or spray can be used. Those agents containing benzocaine (Cetacaine or Hurricaine) are most commonly used. If, despite adequate anesthesia, the patient is still unable to be examined, one of the two techniques described below can be used.

The authors would like to thank Kathy Jung, medical illustrator, and Jeri Kay, typist.

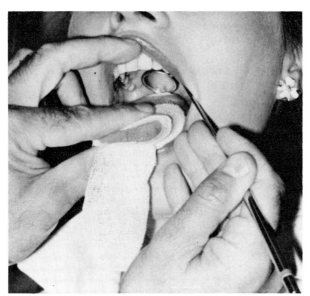

Figure 86–1. To insert the laryngeal mirror, the patient's tongue is grasped between the thumb and first or second finger with a gauze pad. The other finger is used to retract the upper lip. The indirect laryngeal mirror is passed into the mouth, avoiding contact with the tongue. It can touch the palate and uvula without creating a gag reflex. Contact with the posterior pharynx should also be avoided. Contrary to the illustration, the wearing of latex gloves is recommended.

Laryngoscopy by Angled Telescopes

In the second method for visually examining the larynx, one of several 90-degree or 70-degree telescopes is used. One popular telescope is the LarynxVue II (Fig. 86–2*A*). This type of telescope obtains its energy from a wall plug or lightweight battery pack that can be carried on the physician's belt. Many other telescopes with external light sources are also available. These endoscopes are frequently used by otolaryngologists for video and stroboscopic laryngoscopy.

Procedure. The patient is positioned in a manner identical to that used for indirect laryngoscopy (Fig. 86–2*B*). Topical anesthesia is used, if necessary. As the instrument is passed into the oral cavity, it is rested on either a guide attached to the hand that is holding the tongue or rested on the fingers of that hand. It is important to place the instrument in a position very close to that needed for examination of the larynx under direct vision before beginning to look through the eyepiece. Again, by asking the patient to breathe quietly, to phonate, to take a deep breath, or to cough gently, the larynx can be examined for mucosal lesions and for function.

Flexible Fiberoptic Laryngoscopy

In patients who have a psychologic gag reflex that cannot be controlled by reassurance or topical anesthesia or in those with anatomic abnormalities that preclude examination of the larynx via the oral cavity, a flexible fiberoptic laryngoscope or bronchoscope passed through the nose permits examination of the larynx. Several companies, including Machida and Olympus, manufacture flexible scopes specifically designed for examination of the nasopharynx and larynx. These scopes are very small and do not have suction channels. They are shorter than bronchoscopes and can be attached to lightweight, portable light sources.

Procedure. The physician must carry out a thorough examination of the nose to determine the side of the nasal cavity through which he or she will pass the instrument. After this decision has been made, topical anesthetic and vasoconstrictor medications are applied to the nasal mucosa. This step greatly enhances the patient's comfort and cooperation during the procedure and permits a more leisurely evaluation. Four per cent topical lidocaine can be applied by spray or on cotton pledgets as described in the section on epistaxis in this chapter. An alternative is to use several drops of topical epinephrine mixed with a few ml of 4 per cent lidocaine. This mixture is applied to self-made rolled pledgets of cotton, which are placed in the floor of the nose and along the inferior turbinate on the side to be examined (see Fig. 86–19). After waiting several minutes, the nose is reexamined. It is often useful to place another larger pledget farther into the nose to anesthetize the nasal cavity posteriorly. After the nose is adequately vasoconstricted, a small amount of 10 per cent lidocaine is sprayed through that nostril to partially anesthetize the nasopharynx and posterior pharyngeal wall. To prevent unnecessary concern or even panic, the patient must be told that when the pharynx is numb it feels swollen *even though it is not*, and that it may seem hard to swallow *even though it is not!*

The patient is again positioned in the "sniffing" position. The scope is warmed to prevent fogging and is placed into the anterior nares under direct vision. Once it is passed into the nasal vestibule, vision through the scope demonstrates the clearest path. This may be below or above the inferior turbinate. As the nasal choana is approached, the eustachian tube orifice is seen. The scope can be turned sideways and flexed to see the eustachian tube on the other side (it curves around the posterior margin of the septum to accomplish this). One turns the scope inferiorly to see the posterior

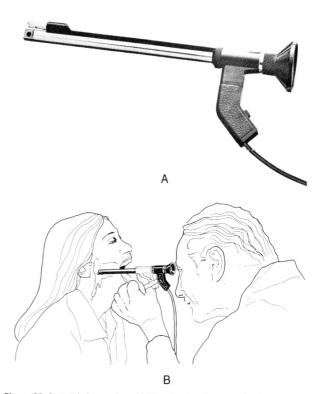

Figure 86–2. *A*, Right-angle self-illuminating laryngeal telescope. The one pictured is called the LarynxVue II. It can be used as presented or with a guide strapped to the examiner's thumb. (Courtesy of Astralite Corp., 4378 East LaPalma Avenue, Anaheim, Calif 92807). *B*, The laryngeal telescope is held in the same hand that holds the patient's tongue, leaving the other hand free to use instruments.

surface of the palate and uvula. If the scope fogs or becomes covered by mucus, the patient can be asked to swallow and the palate will clean the lens. The tonsils, base of tongue, and posterior pharyngeal wall can now be seen, and the larynx will appear in the distance. The scope is advanced to bring the larynx into closer view, but it should not be passed below the level of the tip of the epiglottis unless the larynx itself has been anesthetized. The valleculae, epiglottis, pyriform sinuses, arytenoids, false vocal cords, true vocal cords, and subglottis should be visualized systematically so as not to miss unexpected abnormalities. Phonation and deep breathing as well as gentle coughing can demonstrate vocal cord function or dysfunction.

Which Procedure Should be Used?

Indirect laryngoscopy using an angled mirror requires the least expensive equipment and provides the best optics, because there is minimal distortion from a good mirror. This technique requires practice to become proficient. Therefore, it is valuable to practice indirect laryngoscopy on normal patients to gain confidence in the technique and to become familiar with normal anatomy. Many physicians who infrequently examine the larynx find the right-angle telescope easier to use. Although the optics in these telescopes are not as good as those provided by a mirror, they *are* excellent and the laryngeal view may be better. The fiberoptic flexible laryngoscope is generally reserved for use when the other techniques are not successful. It must be stressed that no examination yields adequate results unless the physician has experience using the technique and is thoroughly comfortable with the normal anatomy and variations thereof that will be observed.

Use of the Head Lamp

Direct "through the eye" illumination is necessary to accomplish many of the procedures required for treatment of head and neck diseases. Many physicians find that a headlight is more convenient to use and provides more flexibility than the head mirror. The light source of a headlight must emanate from directly between the eyes rather than from the forehead or the side in order to provide enough direct light into the depths of the nasal or oral cavities.

Procedure. The key to success is to line up the direction of the light beam with a comfortable head position. First, the headgear is placed in position and tightened enough to prevent slippage but not so tight as to cause pressure or pain over the length of a procedure. Next, the clinician gazes comfortably at a spot on the patient or on the clinician's outstretched hand at a comfortable working distance. Finally, without moving his or her eyes or head, the physician moves the headlight into position, so that the light beam is focused on the spot where he or she would like to work while not obstructing the view of either eye. If it is necessary to turn constantly to bring the light into the appropriate position, these steps must be repeated. With the equipment in the appropriate position, the light automatically shines where the operator is directly looking.

PROCEDURES IN THE EXTERNAL AUDITORY CANAL

Anatomy

The external auditory canal, or meatus, is S shaped and is approximately 2.5 cm long. The lateral one third is

cartilaginous, and the medial two thirds is bony. The medial margin of the canal is the tympanic membrane, which lies in an oblique position with its anterior edge deeper than its posterior edge. (This oblique position permits a larger tympanic membrane to fit into the restricted size of the ear canal, resulting in greater mechanical advantage for carrying sound energy to the inner ear.) The bony canal is directed slightly downward and forward in relation to the cartilaginous canal; thus, pulling the pinna upward, backward, and outward tends to straighten the canal and permits a better view of the tympanic membrane. The external canal is intimately related to the temporomandibular joint, the parotid gland, and the mastoid air cells.

The skin of the osseous canal is very thin, with few cutaneous organs. The skin of the cartilaginous canal is thicker, with hair follicles, sebaceous glands, and apocrine glands. Cerumen is formed by these glands and from exfoliated cells of the skin. Cerumen is bacteriostatic and water-repellent, not waterproof. Under positive pressure or after repeated douching with water or after mild trauma (e.g., by cotton-tipped applicators), the protection offered the skin by the cerumen may be breached. Water, debris, and bacteria can then enter the follicular space and precipitate an infection.[1]

Examination

A thorough examination with good illumination and a gentle but effective touch is required to evaluate the external ear canal. Illumination can be provided in several ways. The hand-held otoscope can be equipped with fiberoptic heads, which provide excellent illumination. The operating head otoscope may not be quite as bright as the fiberoptic otoscope but permits the passage of instruments through the earpiece for the removal of debris while still providing magnification (Fig. 86–3).

The headlight or head mirror and light bulb can serve to illuminate the ear canal through a separate metal or plastic speculum. This method maximizes the ability to use

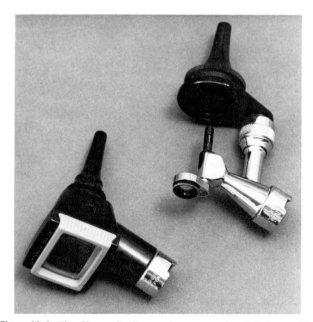

Figure 86–3. The fiberoptic diagnostic otoscope head *(left)* provides the best lighting for examination of the ear canal but is more difficult to use with instruments. The operating head *(right)* provides both magnification and access for instruments to the ear canal.

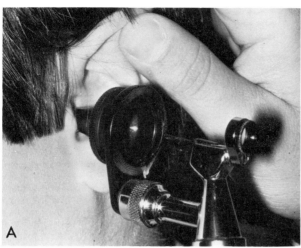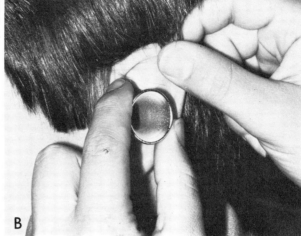

Figure 86–4. *A,* Patient being examined using an otoscope with an operating head. Note that the pinna is pulled upward and backward. *B,* Patient being examined using a metal speculum. Light is supplied with a head mirror or a headlight. This method of examination provides the most flexibility when instruments must be used.

instruments but provides no magnification unless loupes are used (Fig. 86–4). The best illumination is provided by the operating microscope, which also permits binocular vision and frees both hands for manipulation.

Cerumen Impaction

Cerumen and squamous debris normally migrate out of the healthy ear canal, but impaction of cerumen may occur for various reasons. An unusually tortuous canal, a small meatus, or a large number of vibrissae may impede removal of cerum. Cotton-tipped applicators are frequently used by patients for self-cleaning. Although some earwax may be removed by the sides of an applicator, the tip often pushes the wax deeper into the canal. It is not unusual to find a deep cerumen impaction with a concavity the size and shape of the tip of a cotton-tipped applicator. Earwax is frequently brown or black in color.

The most common complaint of the patient with cerumen occlusion is of a blocked ear. Slight unsteadiness and even dizziness and mild pain are often reported. A superimposed external otitis may be present from the patient's attempts to remove the cerumen. Hearing loss frequently occurs suddenly. Hearing is not affected by cerumen as long as a tiny air passage exists through it. If water or manipulation blocks that passageway, a significant conductive hearing loss results. Removal of the impaction results in a most grateful and relieved patient.

REMOVAL OF CERUMEN

Procedure. Cerumen can be removed by irrigation, suction, or metal probe curettage. Irrigation is simple and usually effective and hence often the initial procedure of choice if there is no history of a perforated tympanic membrane. Irrigation may be accomplished with a DeVillbiss irrigator activated by compressed air (Fig. 86–5). Alternatively, a metal ear syringe or Waterpik can be used. One can also use a 20-ml syringe and a butterfly infusion catheter (Fig. 86–6). The metal tip and plastic butterfly are cut off,

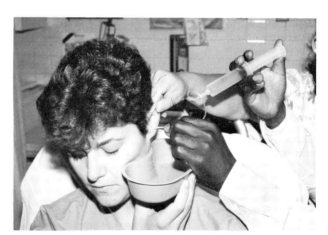

Figure 86–6. Irrigation is a simple, painless, and usually successful way to remove cerumen. After a wax-softening agent has been instilled for 15 to 20 minutes, an assistant applies traction on the ear to straighten the canal, and the plastic tubing of a 19-gauge butterfly device (needle and wings removed) is inserted 1 cm into the canal. A basin is held by the patient, and warm water is introduced with a 20-ml syringe. A number of irrigations may be required, and the procedure may be supplemented with careful removal of large cerumen pieces with a curette.

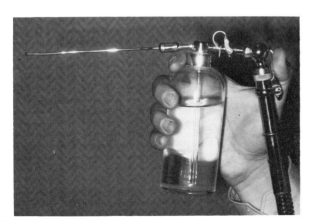

Figure 86–5. This DeVillbiss irrigator uses compressed air to eject the irrigant, which should be at or near body temperature to avoid caloric stimulation of the inner ear. The more conventional metal ear syringe can be equally effective and does not require a source of compressed air to function.

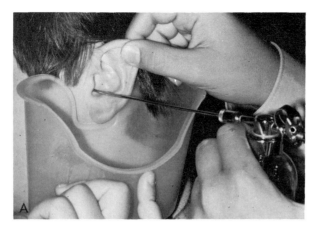

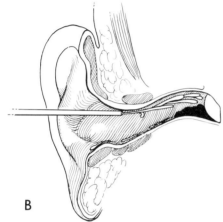

Figure 86–7. *A,* The patient is positioned for irrigation of the external auditory canal. The patient is holding a specially shaped ear basin to catch the irrigating fluid. The auricle is pulled upward, backward, and outward to straighten the ear canal, and the irrigation is directed along the posterior superior canal wall. Water warmed to approximately body temperature should be used to avoid caloric stimulation of the semicircular canals. *B,* The tip of the irrigator is passed only into the cartilaginous section of the external ear canal.

and the plastic catheter is placed in the external canal. Irrigation fluid is then inserted through the syringe. An 18-gauge Teflon intravenous catheter can likewise be used with a 20-ml syringe for irrigation. The patient or an assistant holds a kidney basin or an ear basin to catch the irrigating fluid. The irrigator is *inserted only into the cartilaginous canal and is directed along the superior canal wall* (Fig. 86–7). The irrigant is tap water, at or near body temperature, to prevent caloric stimulation of the inner ear and resultant pain or vertigo. There is no advantage to irrigating with peroxide or other solutions. Most cerumen can be removed with persistent irrigation, although it may require numerous attempts. Irrigation is a safe and easy method that rarely fails if one is persistent. Tympanic membrane perforation is a theoretic complication but occurs very rarely when the previously discussed methods have been used properly. Irrigation, however, should not be performed if there is a history of a perforated tympanic membrane, because water within the middle ear space inevitably results in infection and pain.

Occasionally, irrigation loosens but does not remove debris, and it may be necessary to alternate between irrigation and manual removal. After irrigation, the ear canal should be dried with a cotton-tipped applicator or a few drops of 70 per cent alcohol. If irrigation is not successful

and if external otitis is not present, a cerumen-softening solution such as Cerumenex may be placed in the ear for 15 to 30 minutes, and the irrigation should be repeated. One in vitro study of ceruminolytics found 5 per cent sodium bicarbonate more effective than commercial products.[1] Occasionally, 2 to 3 days of softening at home is required. The disadvantage of this procedure is that some patients develop a contact dermatitis to the softening agent.

The consistency of cerumen varies. A soft, semiliquid wax is best removed with irrigation. More firm cerumen can be removed mechanically. A wire loop or blunt right-angle hook is introduced under direct vision along, but not touching, the skin of the ear canal. Flexible plastic cerumen loops may also be used to remove soft wax less traumatically (e.g., Flex-Loop, Bionix Development Partners, Toledo, Ohio). Cerumen is gently teased away from the skin into the center of the canal (Fig. 86–8). The instrument is then passed just beyond the bolus, turned 90 degrees to engage the cerumen, and withdrawn. At all times, both hands should be supported against the head of the patient so that they move with the head, preventing aural injury. *A confident, gentle touch is critical,* because a loop or hook improperly used may be very painful and traumatic to the patient. It is not uncommon to precipitate bleeding of the canal, because the skin is quite fragile. It is imprudent to persist in removal techniques if the pain or bleeding caused by the procedure is significant. Patients can be prepared by warning them and then deliberately but gently touching the canal skin so they are less startled when manipulation begins. An anxious patient may not tolerate the procedure after the first perception of pain. *It is difficult to safely remove cerumen from a screaming or agitated child;* hence, irrigation often is the method of choice for pediatric patients.

External Otitis

The symptoms of external otitis or swimmer's ear are varied and include itching, fullness, hearing loss, drainage, burning, and pain. These symptoms may occur in any combination and range from mild to severe. As previously suggested, humidity, high temperatures, local trauma, and introduction of an exogenous material are the conditions

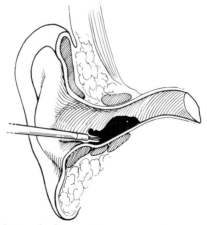

Figure 86–8. Removal of impacted cerumen using a small wire loop or cerumen spoon. This procedure is done under direct vision generally through a speculum or otoscope (not pictured in the drawing). The key is to separate the cerumen from the skin of the ear canal and to move it toward the center of the canal before attempting to extract it.

most often associated with external otitis. Senturia and colleagues divide the disease into three stages.[1a]

1. Preinflammatory
2. Acute inflammatory
    Mild
    Moderate
    Severe
3. Chronic inflammatory

The preinflammatory stage manifests with mild edema and itching and can easily lead to the mild-acute stage, with erythema, edema, and some debris. In the moderate-acute stage, pain and edema are more severe with partial blockage of the ear canal with debris. In the severe stage, pain is intense. Manipulation of the pinna and tragus causes pain. The ear canal may be completely occluded by tissue edema and debris. Pain may radiate to the jaw or neck. Infraauricular or cervical lymph adenopathy is often evident. *Pseudomonas* is most often identified in cultures, but the associated cellulitis is usually caused by gram-positive organisms. The chronic stage is identical to any chronic dermatitis with exfoliative debris, scaling, and gram-negative or fungal contamination.

TREATMENT

Procedure. The techniques used in the treatment of external otitis are designed (1) to remove debris from the canal so that medication can come in contact with the skin, (2) to provide antimicrobial or antifungal action, and (3) to decrease the inflammatory response.

Treatment of the preinflammatory stage involves removal of debris and the use of ear drops. Debris may be removed by irrigation with 3 per cent hypertonic saline, by suction, or by swabbing the canal under otoscopic vision with self-made cotton-tipped applicators (Figs. 86–9 and 86–10). Note that commercial *flexible* urethral or nasopharyngeal swabs (Calgi-Swab) can be used for this purpose. The cotton of the applicator is soaked with the medicated solution that the patient will use as drops for several days. Solutions with polymyxin, neomycin, and hydrocortisone (Cortisporin Otic Suspension or Solution, Coly-Mycin S Otic) are most commonly used. Note that Cortisporin Otic Solution contains preservatives that can irritate the middle ear if the tympanic membrane is perforated. Therefore, the cloudy *suspension* and not the clear *solution* should be used if a tympanic membrane defect is suspected. Solutions that acidify the ear canal are also effective microbials. Acetic acid and hydrocortisone (VoSol HC) or a saturated solution of boric acid in alcohol (made by the pharmacist) may be useful. Allergy to neomycin is common. However, if medication is changed because of sensitivity and the reaction persists, it should be remembered that propylene glycol may also cause skin reactions and is a carrier in many of these medications.

If the ear canal is patent, it is easy for the patient to apply the ear drops at home. The patient is instructed to place four to six drops of medication in the affected ear while lying down with the affected ear up. The tragus and pinna are manipulated to work the drops into the canal. The patient should remain in that position for about 5 minutes. A wad of cotton is placed in the concha to catch the extra medication that will drain out when the patient sits up. The drops are placed two to four times per day, depending upon the severity of the disease. When eczema of the skin of the concha or pinna is present, a corticosteroid cream is also used.

The mild acute inflammatory stage is treated in a similar manner; however, *irrigation is avoided* because the irritation

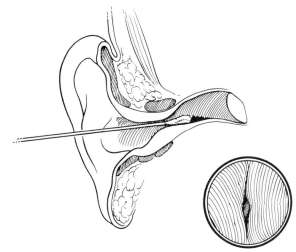

Figure 86–9. Diagram showing a severe stage of external otitis with edema almost closing the external canal. A self-made cotton-tipped applicator is represented cleaning debris from the ear canal to permit medicated ear drops to come in contact with the skin. This applicator is used under direct vision generally through an otoscope (not pictured here).

may cause increased swelling of the canal. The moderate acute inflammatory stage may be associated with significant edema of soft tissue and debris; hence antibiotic drops may be impeded from entering the canal easily. The canal must first be cleared of debris using cotton-tipped applicators and suction if necessary. Occasionally, a short-acting intravenous narcotic may be helpful with this painful procedure. Bleeding may be easily precipitated, and one should not be overzealous in attempting to remove every bit of debris. If the pain is intolerable, one should treat for 24 to 48 hours before proceeding with further débridement of the canal. A wick is then inserted into the ear canal to draw the medication drops into the ear. This can be done in many ways. One-quarter-inch Nu-Gauze (Johnson & Johnson) impregnated with an antibiotic and corticosteroid cream (Cortisporin Cream) can be packed into the ear canal. This is done through the otoscope using a small alligator forceps, and the leading edge of the gauze is placed as deeply into the canal as possible. The deeper parts of the canal are carefully packed through the otoscope. The otoscope is removed, and the rest of the lateral part of the external canal is packed.

A second method is to place just one thickness of Nu-Gauze into the ear canal without packing it tightly. The patient can then apply ear drops, which will be drawn into the canal by the gauze. A cotton wick may be fashioned by wrapping cotton around a forceps. The cotton is dipped into the antibiotic solution and gently placed into the canal. If the wick is thin enough, it will reach deeply into the canal. The cotton is then kept moist with repeated antibiotic drops.

Commercially made wicks are available as well. These wicks, such as the Pope Ear Wick (Merocel brand surgical sponge) are compacted and firm and are easily introduced into the ear canal (Fig. 86–11). Ear drops are absorbed into the sponge, which expands gently and softens. Thus the drops are brought into contact with the skin, and the pressure helps to diminish swelling, often dramatically. With any method, the patient keeps the wick moistened with applications of ear drops, which are allowed to soak in. The patient or physician removes the wick or pack 24 to 36 hours later and continues using the drops as previously indicated.

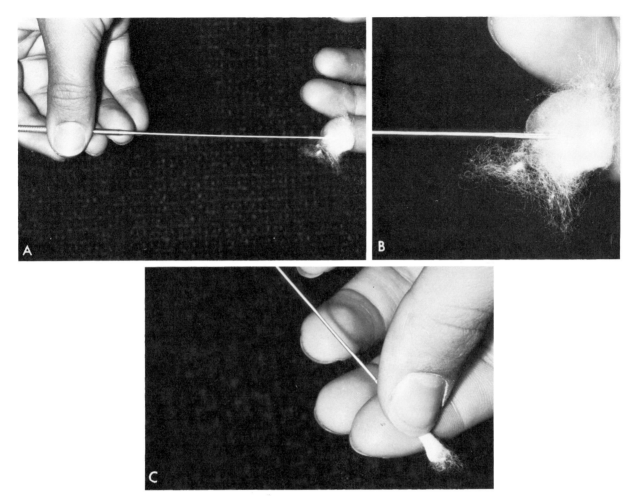

Figure 86–10. *A–C*, Individual applicators are made by applying a small tuft of cotton to a wire applicator and rotating it. The size of the tuft of cotton can be varied as needed. These applicators are used to clean the external ear canal and to apply topical medications.

In most cases, it is desirable to see the patient 24 to 36 hours later to ensure that a reaccumulation of debris has not occurred. Patients with this amount of edema are placed on an oral antibiotic as well. Reasonable choices are erythromycin, amoxicillin/clavulinic acid, and cephalosporins. Oral analgesics are frequently required for this painful condition.

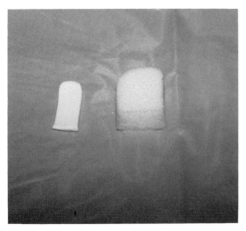

Figure 86–11. The Merocel nasal tampon (or external ear canal wick) is available in various sizes. The dehydrated material *(left)* quickly expands *(right)* on contact with blood or when irrigated with saline to compress a nose bleed or to function as an ear wick.

In the severe acute inflammatory state of external otitis, pain and diffuse inflammation are most prominent. Temporomandibular motion may be quite painful, resulting in poor oral intake. Nausea and vomiting secondary to pain may complicate the syndrome. Strong pain medication is indicated, as well as some sedation to permit sleep. A gauze wick is again used; however, because of severe edema and pain, the wick can be inserted only a short distance. The patient should be started on a broad-spectrum oral antibiotic. The patient is seen again in 24 hours, at which time the gauze wick can be changed and most likely can be more deeply inserted. Within 48 hours, marked improvement is generally seen.

During the entire course of treatment for any stage of external otitis, the patient must be advised to keep the ears dry. When bathing, cotton impregnated with Vaseline can be placed in the concha, and care should be taken to prevent water from seeping into the ear canal. If the canal does get wet, drops should be applied immediately. Following resolution of the infection, the canal is kept dry after swimming or bathing with a few drops of isopropyl (rubbing) alcohol or by drying the canal with a hair dryer.

It should be noted that although cultures are not routinely taken for uncomplicated otitis externa, *Pseudomonas* or *Proteus* may frequently be isolated. The cellulitis, however, may be due to other organisms. Therefore, the local antibiotic drops are sufficient for gram-negative organisms, whereas the previously mentioned antibiotics seem to hasten the resolution of the surrounding cellulitis. Patients do not need to be admitted to the hospital for intravenous antibiotics to treat *Pseudomonas* or *Proteus* infections unless they fail to respond to the previous course of therapy.[1] The only time when this advice does not hold true is in the case of malignant external otitis, which is also discussed in this chapter.

Otomycosis

Fungi can cause external otitis of any degree. The mycelia and spores are visible as a fuzzy coating on the skin of the ear canal. The most common fungus to cause this type of infection is *Aspergillus niger*. If fungi are observed, corticosteroids are avoided. Effective antifungal agents to use in this situation are M-Cresyl Acetate, a saturated solution of boric acid in alcohol, or a 1 per cent solution of clotrimazole (Lotrimin).

TREATMENT

The critical aspect of treatment is complete manual removal of the organism. This is accomplished using cotton-tipped applicators impregnated with the treatment solution. Care must be taken to avoid depositing the medication, which can be quite irritating, on the external skin. A complete swabbing of the ear canal and removal of all debris is usually sufficient to control this disease.

A follow-up visit in 3 to 7 days is indicated to permit reapplication of medication and recleaning of the canal if the infection recurs. Otomycosis can also complicate chronic bacterial external otitis and may not be obvious. In recurrent cases, it is useful to culture for fungus. Because special media are required, the bacteriology laboratory should be consulted about the techniques of culturing the specimen. In chronic cases, any one of several antimycotic agents can be used, including Halotex, Lotrimin, Micatin, Tinactin, and Nilstat. These agents can be used as drops in the ear canal or applied to the ear canal using cotton-tipped applicators. It must be stressed that cleansing of the ear canal is the most critical aspect of the treatment of fungal disease.

Malignant External Otitis

Malignant external otitis is misnamed, because it does not represent a neoplastic process. However, it certainly is malignant in relation to its progressive and often life-threatening characteristics. The disease presents in diabetics, in immunosuppressed patients, or in patients who are taking systemic steroids. It manifests as an external otitis due to *Pseudomonas*, resulting in extensive necrosis and osteomyelitis that may progress to the base of the skull, resulting in cranial nerve deficits and potentially death.

The disease is recognized by its severity and poor response to usual treatment. Granulation tissue is often seen in the ear canal. A severe external otitis in such patients warrants immediate otolaryngologic evaluation. Treatment requires hospitalization, varying degrees of débridement and long-term, high-dose intravenous antibiotics, although reports support treatment with some oral agents, such as ciprofloxacin once a positive response to treatment is seen. It is presumed that the severity of the disease is related to compromised local defense mechanisms.

Foreign Body of the Ear

The presence of a foreign body is a challenge to the emergency physician, although many of the techniques for removal of a foreign body are similar to those used for the removal of cerumen. The junction of the cartilaginous and bony sections of the external auditory canal is both the narrowest point of the canal and the location of a curve in the canal. Thus most foreign bodies lodge in the outer two thirds of the canal and are relatively easy to remove. Those lying more medial are in a more sensitive portion of the canal and may be lying on the tympanic membrane. The nature of the foreign body is determined by history and direct examination. Efforts at removal in the emergency department should not be persistent when removal is difficult. Timely referral to a specialist is generally preferred for complicated cases.

Procedure. The first attempt at removal is the best chance for success. The ear canal may be irrigated with water to remove small, hard objects in the same manner in which cerumen is removed (see Figs. 86–6 and 86–7). Irrigation should not be used when the foreign body is a seed or bean, because these organic objects may swell, rendering removal more difficult.

Illumination for the removal of foreign bodies of the ear canal is critical. An operating microscope should be used, if available. Binocular vision provides depth of field perception and permits more accurate placement of instruments. An operating head on an otoscope or a head mirror with separate speculum can be used. Wire loops, blunt hooks of various sizes, suction heads (numbers 3 and 5), and alligator forceps should be available (Fig. 86–12).

A frequent foreign body found in children is a bead or the eye from a stuffed toy. These polished, smooth materials can be exceedingly difficult to grasp. If there is a space between the object and the skin of the ear canal, a right-angle hook can be passed beyond it, turned 90 degrees, and withdrawn with the bead (Fig. 86–13). The Richards Manufacturing Company manufactures a plastic suction catheter with a soft funnel tip. The suction catheter can often grasp and easily withdraw a smooth foreign body, making a difficult task both easy and safe (Fig. 86–14). A Fogarty catheter may be passed beyond the foreign body, the balloon inflated, and the catheter withdrawn to force the object from the canal. Care must be taken in this situation, however, to avoid puncturing the eardrum.

Living insects present a special challenge when lodged in the ear. Their movement can be exceedingly irritating, and the insect itself or the patient's attempts to remove the insect may excoriate the canal skin. The insect is first

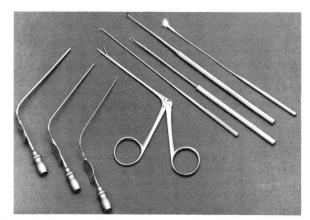

Figure 86–12. *Left to right*: suction tips (numbers 7, 5, and 3), alligator forceps, right-angle blunt hook, wire loop, ear curette, and self-made cotton-tipped applicators. All these instruments are used when working within the ear canal. All can cause damage unless managed in a controlled manner under direct vision.

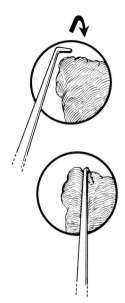

Figure 86–13. This technique may be used to remove hard, smooth foreign bodies or firm concretions of cerumen. A small, blunt, right-angle hook (available in various sizes) is passed between the foreign body and canal skin under direct vision. After its tip is medial to the foreign body, it is rotated 90 degrees and withdrawn.

suffocated by filling the ear canal with mineral oil, ether, or alcohol. The insect can then be removed by irrigation or other mechanical means. An insect often fragments, making irrigation the most useful technique.

Alligator forceps are useful when the object has an easily grasped edge or protrusion. When not using binocular vision, special care must be taken to prevent the open jaws from touching the canal skin.

The keys to successful removal of a foreign body in the ear are good lighting and equipment and a cooperative patient. Even the most cooperative patient may become difficult after the first inadvertent twinge of pain. It is impossible for anyone to lie still while someone touches an unanesthetized tympanic membrane. It is also impossible for an assistant to hold the head of an uncooperative patient still enough for delicate instrumentation of the ear canal. Instrumentation of the ear canal may also produce a reflex cough in older children and adults.

The removal of foreign bodies can be facilitated by local anesthesia or the judicious use of sedation (see Chapter 41), but very young or mentally impaired children may require general anesthesia. The injection of local anesthetic in the ear canal is quite painful and should not be given to compensate for poor illumination or faulty techniques. The hand-held speculum, with either an operating microscope, headlight, or head mirror, permits the mobility necessary to give these injections. A 3 to 5-cm needle (25 or 27 gauge) is used, and a three-finger syringe provides the best control. One per cent lidocaine, with or without epinephrine (1:100,000), is used.

The subcutaneous injections are made in four quadrants to encircle the ear canal. This field block is placed laterally, near the opening of the meatus. The largest speculum permitting a good view of the canal is used. The speculum is then withdrawn slightly, and the injection is made just under the skin. Less than 0.5 ml is used in each quadrant, just enough to slightly bulge the skin forward (Fig. 86–15). After waiting 2 to 3 minutes, the speculum can be reintroduced. If more anesthesia is necessary, a very small injection can be made in the anterior and posterior canal walls, just

under the skin at the junction of the bony and cartilaginous canals. The skin is very thin in this area; thus, care must be taken to avoid lacerations. If placed correctly, a small bleb of anesthesia dissects down toward the tympanic membrane. As mentioned previously, the placement of local anesthetic should not change the care with which objects are removed, because lacerations of the canal, skin, or tympanic membrane are to be avoided.

Perforation of the Ear Drum

Traumatic perforation of the tympanic membrane most commonly follows a slap to the ear or an uncontrolled dive into a swimming pool. Trapped air in the external ear canal is pressurized and implodes the eardrum to the point of rupture. Other trauma can also cause perforation, and temporal bone or base of the skull fracture, facial paralysis, and cochlear or vestibular injury must be ruled out. If there is no history of loss of consciousness, facial weakness, nystagmus, or vertigo, and if any hearing loss is conductive and not sensorineural (based on an audiogram or tuning fork testing with Weber lateralizing to the injured side and bone conduction being greater than air conduction), then a simple perforation can be suspected. Insufflation of the external ear canal should be performed to assess the possibility of round window damage and endolymph loss. The production of vertigo with insufflation warrants an immediate otolar-

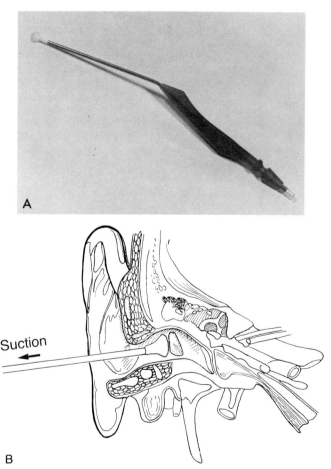

Figure 86–14. *A* and *B*, This suction catheter has a soft, flexible funnel-shaped tip, which is able to grasp some foreign bodies of the ear or nose and provide a mechanism for easy removal. (Courtesy of Richards Manufacturing Co.)

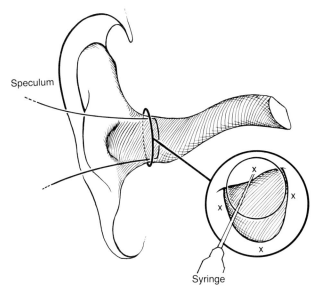

Figure 86–15. Four-quadrant field block anesthesia of the external auditory canal. Local anesthetic is injected subcutaneously in the four quadrants of the lateral portion of the ear canal. The largest speculum that will fit is used to guide the injections. The speculum is withdrawn slightly, tilted toward each of the four quadrants, and the needle is inserted subcutaneously *(x)*. A very small amount of anesthetic (0.25 to 0.50 ml) is injected to produce a slight bulge in the soft tissue. A total of 1.5 to 2.0 ml of anesthetic is usually sufficient to anesthetize the ear canal and permit painless removal of a foreign body.

yngologic referral. Often blood or swelling of the ear canal prevents clear observation of the perforation. If there is any question as to the diagnosis, perforation should be suspected and the patient instructed and treated as follows.

Foreign material is cleaned from the ear canal if possible, but one should *never irrigate an ear that may have a ruptured tympanic membrane.* A loop or suction can be used under direct vision through the operating head of an otoscope or a microscope, if available. The patient is advised to keep all water out of the ear, because water entering the middle ear inevitably results in infection. Cotton with Vaseline or silicone ear plugs can be used to protect the middle ear during showering but should not be relied on completely.

The need for antibiotics, ear drops, or both is not clear. We prefer to use Cortisporin Otic Suspension (the Solution will burn) in cases that are contaminated by water or foreign material, and to prescribe broad-spectrum antibiotics. In clean, dry perforations secondary to a slap no medication is necessary. The patient is advised to report any drainage (bloody or purulent), and is seen in follow-up in 5 to 7 days. The vast majority of traumatic perforations heal without sequelae.

EPISTAXIS

Nasal hemorrhage is one of the most common otolaryngologic emergencies confronting the emergency physician. Most episodes of epistaxis are controlled by patients outside the hospital setting, despite the fact that many commonly used methods of control are based on folk remedies. Lying with the head hanging over the edge of a bed allows the blood to run posteriorly to be swallowed but increases venous pressure and can prolong bleeding. Although holding ice behind the neck is innocuous, it is also ineffective in controlling bleeding. Epistaxis is frequently terrifying to the

patient and to the physician who is not comfortable with all aspects of treatment. An anterior septal bleed is a minor inconvenience, whereas massive posterior bleeding may be disastrous.

Anatomy and Physiology

The nasal mucosa serves to warm and humidify inspired air. To this end, it is supplied with freely anastomosing blood vessels from the internal and external carotid systems. The external carotid provides the major blood supply via the internal maxillary artery (leading to the greater palatine and sphenopalatine arteries) and the facial artery. The internal carotid artery supplies the nose via the ophthalmic artery (leading to the anterior ethmoid artery) and the posterior ethmoid artery. The sphenopalatine artery is the site of bleeding in most posterior bleeds. Bleeding from the upper recesses of the nasal chamber originates mainly from the ethmoid arteries. Terminal branches of the internal and external carotid systems supply the nasal septum. Knowledge about the detailed anatomy of these vessels becomes critically important when dealing with the surgical ligation of vessels for uncontrolled nasal hemorrhage. In the usual emergency department situation, the important distinctions are knowing which side is bleeding and whether it is anterior or posterior.

Most nose bleeds occur in the anterior or caudal septum in an area of anastomosing vessels called *Little's area* (Fig. 86–16). The relatively exposed position of this area accounts for the most common cause of bleeding, mucosal disruption. It is common for bleeding to occur spontaneously, without identifying precipitating factors. Although local mucosal trauma is most often involved, patients are reluctant to admit to nose picking or the use of cocaine.

Mucosal problems can be caused by digital or external trauma, simple drying of the mucosa, upper respiratory infection, irritants (over-the-counter medications such as nose sprays and chemicals such as cocaine), or foreign bodies. The use of aspirin can prolong any minor bleed. Vascular abnormalities, including superficial vasculature, varices, and hereditary hemorrhagic telangiectasia, account for a small percentage of epistaxis cases. Platelet and coagulation disorders are also uncommon but cause a significant percentage of severe and difficult-to-control episodes of bleeding. Benign and malignant tumors are always included in the differential diagnosis, especially in patients with recurrent posterior bleeds and increasing nasal obstruction. Hypertension is frequently encountered in the patient with epistaxis.

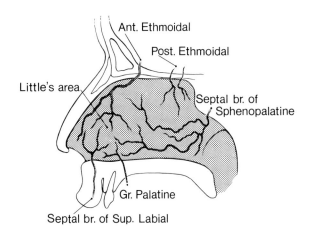

Figure 86–16. Little's area contains the Kiesselbach plexus of arterioles and is the most common site of epistaxis.

In the past, it has been thought to be a major cause of epistaxis, but hypertension is probably more often the result of fear or a reflection of arteriosclerosis, rather than a cause of bleeding.

History

One should always inquire about the following specifics: What is the past medical history? What medications (including over-the-counter medications) are taken? From which nostril did the bleeding start? Did it run out of the nose or drain posteriorly? Is there a past history of similar bleeding? If so, how was it controlled? If the patient attempted to squeeze the nostrils closed, did the bleeding stop or drain into the pharynx? Was there an inciting incident or was the bleed spontaneous? Did the blood clot? Is the patient taking anticoagulants or aspirin? Is there bleeding in the bowels, urine, or gums? Are there skin ecchymoses? The answers to many of these questions will help indicate the anterior or posterior location of the bleeding. In anterior epistaxis, blood tends to flow out of the nostril and tends to stop with external pressure. When external pressure causes the bleeding to flow into the nasopharynx, it is apparent that the source of bleeding may be more posterior. Trauma results in anterior epistaxis more often than posterior epistaxis.

It is not uncommon to encounter patients who have stopped bleeding by the time they reach the emergency department. In such cases, one is tempted to do nothing, because the problem appears to have been solved. Once the patient returns home, however, the bleeding often recurs. *It is prudent to attempt to identify the bleeding site in all patients*, and one should not be reticent to provoke bleeding by stroking the septum with a cotton-tipped applicator or by having the patient blow the nose, so that definitive steps may be taken to prevent rebleeding.

Treatment

Because physical examination and treatment are so intertwined, they will be discussed together. Throughout the entire encounter, the physician must provide reassurance. As mentioned previously, many epistaxis patients are terrified. They have blood coming from within their head, and they may have heard that epistaxis precedes stroke or that it serves to prevent a stroke. Although epistaxis is messy and scary, it is rarely life threatening.

The patient should be told that every step in the treatment will be explained before it is carried out and that the bleeding *will* be controlled. A hospital gown or other cover is provided for both the patient and the doctor, but the patient should be asked not to worry about or be embarrassed by soiling of clothes or instruments with blood. After the bleeding has been stopped, everything can be cleaned up. An emesis basin is kept handy, because swallowed blood often induces nausea, and the patient may vomit large quantities of clot or coffee-ground material.

General Approach

If the patient has been bleeding for a few days or orthostatic changes have occurred, a complete blood count and coagulation studies are ordered. *If the patient is taking anticoagulants, clotting studies are mandatory*, even in cases of the most minor bleeding. The persistence of epistaxis in the patient on aspirin should also suggest a possible von Willebrand disease associated with a prolonged partial thromboplastin time. If the patient is hypotensive, an intravenous infusion should be started for volume replacement and blood should be sent for typing and possible cross-matching. *Simply treating hypertension will not stop most nose bleeds.* Moderate hypertension is best left untreated, because it usually subsides following successful treatment of the bleeding. Most physicians prefer to sedate hypertensive and extremely anxious patients with diazepam or morphine intramuscularly before attempting to manipulate the nose. Patients who remain hypertensive after bleeding has been controlled may require medication to control the blood pressure. Laboratory studies are not required for most nose bleeds, but it should be noted that significant blood loss may occur in patients with chronic epistaxis.

Equipment

Chair with headrest
Headlight, or head mirror and light bulb
Suction and several suction tips (8 to 10 French catheter)
Clothing protection
Nasal speculum
Bayonet forceps
Topical anesthetic and vasoconstrictor
Cotton
Kidney basin
Cautery material (silver nitrate or heat cautery)
1.25-cm (½ inch) × 180-cm (72 inch) Vaseline gauze packing
Tongue depressors
2 small red rubber catheters
Number 2 silk surgical thread
Gauze pads
Tonsil clamp or hemostat
Balloon tampons (pediatric Foley catheters are adequate) for posterior bleeds

Examination

The patient is seated in an upright position, leaning slightly forward in the "sniffing" position. Remember that the floor of the nose is parallel to the palate and only a small part of the nasal cavity can be seen with the patient's head tilted backward (Fig. 86–17). The physician may either sit or stand. *A nasal speculum is always used to properly visualize the anterior nasal mucosa* (Fig. 86–18). The head mirror and light are the simplest way to provide direct "from the eye" illumination; however, for those not experienced in the use of the mirror, a headlight may be easier to use. A hand-held flashlight or other light source does *not* provide an adequately directed light beam, does not permit visualization of the nasal cavities, and makes treatment difficult.

With all the necessary or potentially necessary equipment available, with the patient reassured and positioned, and with an assistant standing by, the examination can begin. *Blood clots must be expelled from the nasal cavities before the nose can be properly examined.* This can be accomplished with suction or by asking the patient to vigorously blow the nose. Often, the expulsion of clots results in a marked diminution of the rate of bleeding. Before medications are placed in the nose, a careful search for the bleeding site is made. After an initial inspection, one may instill topical anesthetic and vasoconstrictors in the side from which there was bleeding. Four per cent cocaine provides the optimal combination of local anesthesia and vasoconstriction. Because of cocaine's low therapeutic-to-toxicity ratio and its strictly controlled status, it is often simpler, safer, and more convenient to use a combination of 4 per cent lidocaine and topical epinephrine. Twenty milliliters of 4 per cent lidocaine mixed with 0.25 ml of 1:1000 topical epinephrine gives an appropriate

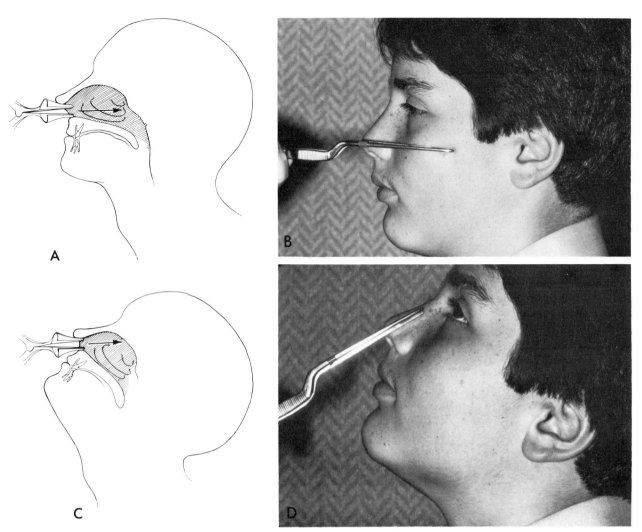

Figure 86–17. *A* and *B*, Photograph showing the correct position for examining and treating disease of the nasal cavity. The patient is in the "sniffing position," sitting upright or leaning slightly forward with the head only slightly extended. When the nasal tip is raised with the nasal speculum, the view is parallel to the floor of the nose and allows visualization of the entire nasal cavity. *C* and *D*, When told that their nose will be examined, most patients extend the neck and look toward the ceiling. In this position, only the most anterior portions of the nasal cavity are visible.

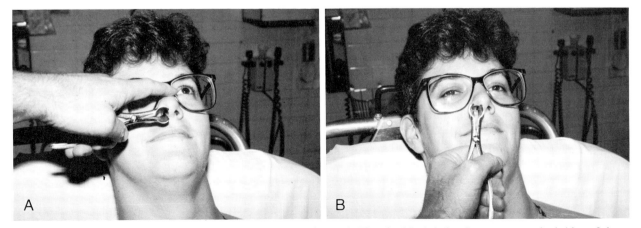

Figure 86–18. To examine a nose properly, a nasal speculum must be used. The physician's index finger rests on the bridge of the nose, and the speculum is spread in an inferior to superior direction *(A)*. It is incorrect to spread laterally with the speculum unsupported *(B)*.

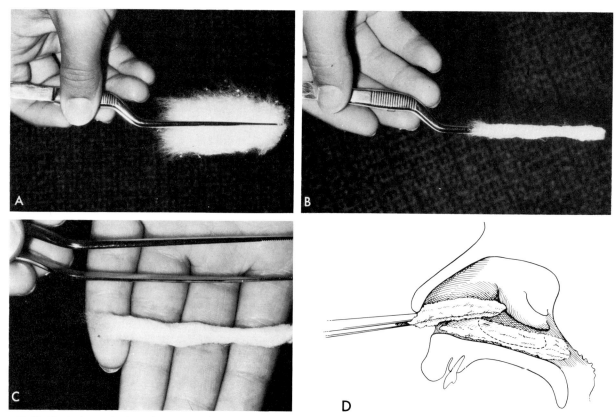

Figure 86–19. Topical anesthetic and vasoconstrictors are applied on individually made cotton pledgets. The size of the pledget may be changed according to the extent of the nasal cavity to be anesthetized and the size of the patient. *A,* An appropriately sized cotton pledget is grasped in a bayonet forceps. *B,* The cotton is then grasped with the opposite hand, and the forceps is rotated. *C,* The pledget is removed and is ready for insertion. *D,* To completely anesthetize the nasal cavity, three pledgets are necessary. The first is placed on the floor of the nose, the second in the middle meatus between the inferior and middle turbinates, and the third in the roof of the nasal cavity and the anterior nasal vestibule. *Note:* This pledget technique can be used to make a cotton wick for the treatment of otitis externa.

concentration of the vasoconstrictor. Another option is to alternate between plain 4 per cent lidocaine and 1/2 per cent or 1 per cent Neo-Synephrine. One can inadvertently cause a patient to be cocaine toxic if the 10 per cent cocaine solution is used or if the nose is repeatedly packed. A maximum of 4 ml of 4 per cent cocaine solution or 2 ml of 10 per cent solution should be used in adults or 3 mg/kg in a child (*Note*: 4 per cent cocaine contains 40 mg/ml). It should be noted that cocaine toxicity is poorly understood, and reactions have occurred with lower doses, although other reports describe safe use of much higher doses.[2] Cocaine should be avoided in the elderly or in those with known coronary artery disease.

If an anterior bleeding site is easily seen, one may simply place a ball of cotton soaked with anesthetic in the nasal cavity and have the patient squeeze the nostrils together. Often, cotton pledgets are required for adequate anesthesia or vasoconstriction.

The technique for placing local anesthesia pledgets is illustrated in Figure 86–19. The cotton pledgets are left in place for 5 minutes. After they are removed, if bleeding has not significantly diminished, new cotton pledgets can be placed for another 5 minutes to ensure adequate vasoconstriction and anesthetic effect (some of the anesthetic may have been washed away with the bleeding). The patient is told that the topical anesthetic may drain into the throat and produce a sensation of not being able to swallow. Reassurance of the temporary nature of this condition and of the fact that they actually can swallow when they make the attempt will calm most patients. The pledgets are then

removed, and the nose is examined. With the nasal speculum in one hand and the 8 or 10 French suction tip in the other, the nose can be examined while gently suctioning blood away to see the spot that is bleeding. *The key to successful treatment of epistaxis is identification of the site of bleeding!*

ANTERIOR EPISTAXIS

As mentioned previously, the most common site of bleeding is from the easily visualized part of the nasal septum. The exact spot of bleeding can be identified using gentle suction if the bleeding is brisk or diffuse. If the hemorrhage has stopped with vasoconstriction but the bleeding site is not apparent, bleeding may be provoked by gentle stroking with a cotton-tipped applicator. If a prominent blood vessel or excoriated area is visible, cauterization can be used. Silver nitrate sticks are most commonly used to control this type of bleeding when a definite bleeding site has been identified. The mucosa is cauterized by firmly touching the area around the bleeding site for 10 to 15 seconds and turning the end of the silver nitrate stick. Cautery should begin in concentric circles, starting away from the bleeding site itself so as to cauterize the vessels feeding the site of injury. When silver nitrate is applied, the mucosa turns a gray to black color. When approaching the site itself, it is often helpful to begin just above it and come down on it so that the silver nitrate does not become coated with blood before touching the area that is bleeding. One cannot cauterize an actively bleeding vessel with silver nitrate; hemostasis before cautery is required. Frequently repeated, overly aggressive, or bilateral cautery with silver nitrate can produce septal perforation.

The patient should be informed that some pressure might be felt during cauterization but that pain will not be a problem if the mucosa is anesthetized properly. If any burning results, the nose should be reanesthetized. At times, mucus draining over the cauterized area can carry silver nitrate into the floor of the nose and unanesthetized areas. Therefore, after controlling bleeding, it helps to wipe the area with a cotton pledget impregnated with local anesthetic. There should be no concern about causing bleeding while wiping the area, because this would indicate inadequate cauterization. It is common for patients to sneeze soon after the silver nitrate is applied.

Nasal packing is not usually necessary for a first time bleed, especially if the bleeding site is small and easily cauterized. Patients should be advised not to place anything inside the nose and to be careful not to insert fingers into the nostrils when wiping the nose with tissues. They should be advised not to blow the nose and to open the mouth to relieve pressure when sneezing. The patient should be observed for 30 minutes in the emergency department to be certain that bleeding does not recur.

Aspirin should not be used for the next 3 to 4 days. Antibiotics or decongestants are not required. Patients are advised to avoid strenuous activity for a few days. Minor rebleeding should be treated at home with rest and by pinching the nose continuously for 20 minutes. Vaseline or antibiotic ointment may be applied to the cauterized area to prevent dryness; however, this should not be done for more than several days. A crust usually forms and should be permitted to release itself.

Should bleeding recur from the same spot within several days, the procedure should be repeated and the nose packed according to the following directions. The purpose of the packing is not only to control bleeding with pressure but also to protect the cauterized area from drying and trauma and to permit healing. Generally, packing alone without cautery should not be used for control of anterior epistaxis, especially if it is done as a blind procedure without identifying the bleeding point. Movement of the packing may continue to abrade the mucosa and actually prolong bleeding or permit it to recur as soon as the packing is removed. The physician should note that nasal packing is quite uncomfortable and sometimes painful and try to avoid packing the nose unless the bleeding cannot be controlled with cautery alone. Bilateral anterior packs should also be avoided when possible.

The technique for placing an anterior pack is critical. A poorly placed pack does not control bleeding, may fall out sooner than is desired, or may fall backward into the nasopharynx, causing discomfort and a feeling of choking in an already fearful patient. Blind packing with large amounts of loose gauze should not be attempted. The key to placement of packing is adequate visualization and the placement of packing in an "accordion" manner, so that part of each layer of packing is near the front of the nose (Fig. 86–20). As each layer is placed, the nasal speculum is removed and replaced above it and the packing is gently pushed down to the floor of the nose. It should not be necessary to force the packing tightly into the nose. In a difficult-to-control nose bleed, 180 cm of 1.25 cm (½ inch) Vaseline gauze packing can be placed fairly easily and gently, if done correctly. When just covering a cauterized area, it is not necessary to place this much packing, but it should be remembered that a very small amount may easily become dislodged. For a simple anterior pack, an alternative to Vaseline gauze is the Merocel nasal tampon (see Fig. 86–11). The anterior pack is removed in 2 to 4 days.

An anterior pack is an intranasal foreign body. As such, it stimulates nasal mucus production and may block normal drainage of the paranasal sinuses. Occasionally, one will see blood from the ocular puncta, because blood may be forced back through the lacrimal duct. If mucus production is excessive, a decongestant or antihistamine may be given orally. Antibiotics should be routinely used, and coating the packing gauze with antibiotic ointment is suggested.

POSTERIOR EPISTAXIS

Posterior epistaxis is identified by nasal hemorrhage that tends to flow posteriorly into the nasopharynx and pharynx. Posterior bleeding is also suggested when an anterior bleed appears to be bilateral. If an anterior pack has already been placed, hemorrhage continues posteriorly. Anterior nasal packing is unsuccessful in controlling posterior epistaxis, because the packing material cannot exert direct pressure on a posterior bleeding site. Although humidification and vasoconstrictor sprays may be effective for controlling many cases of posterior epistaxis, recalcitrant cases may require placement of a posterior pack. The purpose of the posterior pack is twofold. The pack may actually compress the bleeding point and stop hemorrhage. More often, it simply forms a buttress against which an anterior pack is placed to tamponade the bleeding sites, while preventing the packing from falling into the nasopharynx.

There are two major types of postnasal packs. The classic posterior nasal pack (Fig. 86–21) consists of a gauze tampon placed transorally into the nasopharynx and held in place by silk strings or umbilical tape brought out through the nostril. The second type of posterior pack consists of an inflatable balloon, which is placed transnasally, blown up in the nasopharynx, and retracted into the posterior nasal cavity. Because they are more convenient to use and less uncomfortable to the patient during placement, balloon devices have become more popular. Both methods are described here.

The classic gauze nasal pack is formed of rolled gauze or a cotton-filled gauze pad (see Fig. 86–21B). The end of the pack or the middle of the gauze roll is tied twice with number 2 silk ties or umbilical tapes. All strands are left long. After anesthetizing the patient's nose and posterior pharyngeal wall, a small number 10 French red rubber catheter is placed through the bleeding nostril and brought out through the mouth. A catheter placed in the nonbleeding side can be used to retract the palate anteriorly while positioning the pack (see Fig. 86–21C). Two of the silk ties secure the pack to the end of the catheter. This catheter is then pulled back through the nose, bringing the ties out with it. The sutures themselves are then grasped, and the pack is pulled into the nasopharynx.

Placement of the pack is facilitated by directing the pack into the patient's oral cavity and nasopharynx with a finger (see Fig. 86–21D). This uncomfortable step must be accomplished as smoothly and efficiently as possible. A silk tie is left protruding from the mouth and can be used later for removal of the pack. The string can be taped to the patient's cheek. An assistant then holds mild tension on the ties to hold the posterior pack in position *while anterior nasal packing is placed* as previously described.

The silk sutures are tied over a large gauze pad or a dental roll to hold the posterior pack in position. This pad can cause alar or columellar necrosis if it is too small or too tight. The postnasal pack is left in place for 3 to 5 days, and

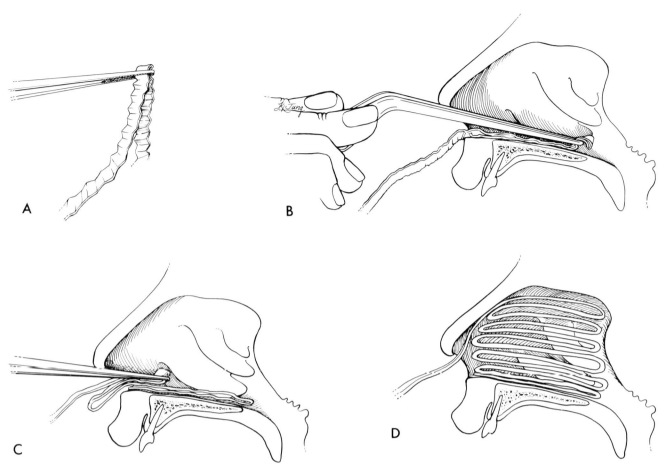

Figure 86–20. The key to placement of an anterior nasal pack that will control epistaxis adequately and stay in place is to lay the packing into the nasal cavity in an "accordion" manner, so that part of each layer of packing lies anteriorly, preventing the gauze from falling posteriorly into the nasopharynx. *A*, The first layer of ¼-inch Vaseline gauze strip is grasped approximately 2 to 3 cm from its end. *B*, This first layer is then placed on the floor of the nose through the nasal speculum (not pictured here). The bayonet forceps and nasal speculum are then withdrawn. *C*, The nasal speculum is reintroduced on top of the first layer of packing, and a second layer is placed in an identical manner. After several layers have been placed, it is often useful to reintroduce the bayonet forceps to push the previously placed packing down onto the floor of the nose, making it tighter and more secure. *D*, A complete anterior nasal pack can tamponade a bleeding point anywhere in the anterior nasal cavities and will stay in place until removed by the physician or patient.

the patient is hospitalized and carefully observed as described below. The entire procedure is obviously uncomfortable for the patient; however, if it is explained in advance and accomplished rapidly, a very effective, custom-made tampon can be placed.

As previously mentioned, inflatable balloon packs are the most convenient packs to use and are successful in controlling most cases of posterior epistaxis. There are two general types of balloon tampons. The first is a Foley catheter with a 30-ml balloon (Fig. 86–22). Some physicians prefer to use a 10 French pediatric Foley catheter with a smaller balloon. The tip of the catheter is cut off so that it does not push against the posterior pharyngeal wall and cause necrosis or gagging. After clearing the nose of clots, determining the site of bleeding, and applying topical anesthesia, a 12 to 16 French Foley catheter is placed along the floor of the nose until the balloon is seen in the nasopharynx. The balloon is then slowly filled with 5 to 15 ml of water, and the Foley catheter is retracted anteriorly to wedge the balloon snugly in the posterior nasal cavity. If the soft palate is grossly displaced inferiorly or if there is significant pain, the balloon is slightly deflated. An anterior pack is then placed as previously described. The catheter is held in position with slight tension by padding the alar and nasal columella with

gauze and applying a nasogastric tube clamp or plastic umbilical clamp.

Several companies manufacture balloon tamponade devices specifically designed for the temporary control of epistaxis. These devices are often effective for the control of bleeding in the emergency department and are more easily placed than the conventional posterior gauze packs.

A balloon tamponade device is a double balloon system that serves as both an anterior and posterior pack, eliminating the need to place an additional pack after the posterior pack has been positioned. Two such devices are the Gottschalk Nasostat (Sparta Surgical Corp., Hayward, Calif.) balloon and the Exomed Epistat (Exomed Inc., Jacksonville, Fla.).

The device resembles a nasal airway with a double-lumened, independently inflatable, low-pressure double balloon system (Fig. 86–23). To use the balloon, the nose is cleared of clots, the device is lubricated with an anesthetic ointment, and the deflated system is slowly passed along the floor of the nose. The device is fully advanced so that the posterior balloon extends into the nasopharynx. The posterior balloon is inflated with 4 to 8 ml of water, and slight forward traction is applied. The anterior balloon is then *slowly* inflated with 10 to 25 ml of air or saline, securing the

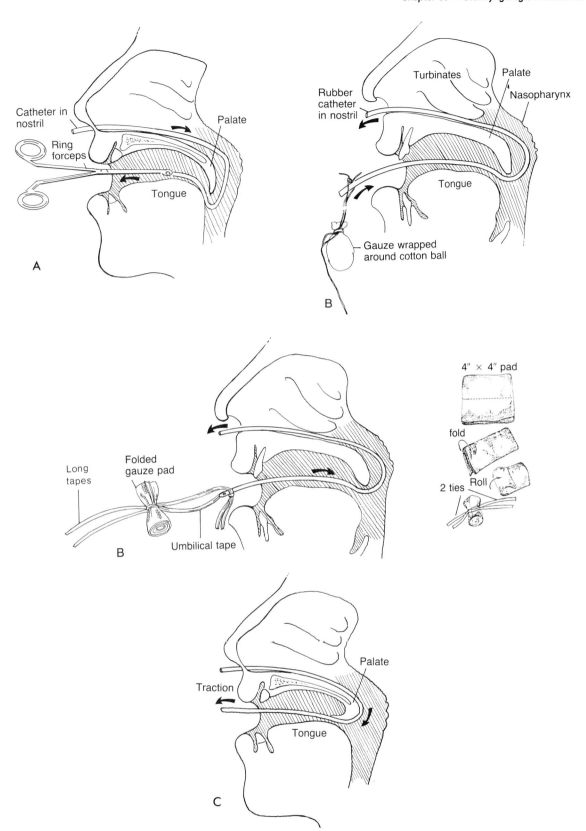

Figure 86–21. Posterior nasal pack. *A*, Following topical anesthesia, a red rubber catheter is passed through the nose and carefully grasped in the oral pharynx with ringed forceps and brought out through the mouth. *B, Upper*, A posterior nasal pack made by wrapping a cotton ball in a 4-inch by 4-inch gauze pad and tying two long silk sutures or umbilical tapes around the neck of the pack. *Lower*, Alternatively, a gauze pad can be folded and rolled into a cylinder and tied with two strings. Two of the strings are used to tie the pack to the tip of the catheter. *C*, As an option, a second catheter, which has been passed through the nonbleeding side and brought out the mouth, can be used to retract the palate forward to aid in the placement of the pack (not shown). The optional catheter is removed after the pack is in the proper position.

Illustration continued on following page

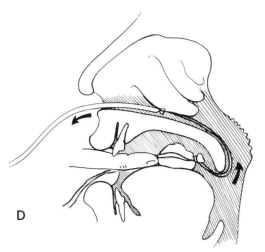

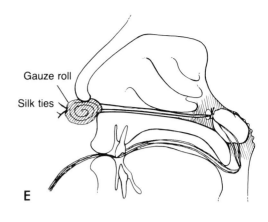

Figure 86–21 *Continued D,* The finger is used to guide the pack through the mouth and into the proper position as traction on the catheter pulls the pack from above. This uncomfortable step is the most difficult of the procedure and must be performed deliberately and smoothly. If the patient has teeth, a dental roll or bite block is placed to prevent the patient from biting the physician's finger. *E,* Proper position of the posterior pack, wedged in the posterior portion of the nose. A long strand attached to the pack exits from the mouth and is taped to the cheek. If the pack slips posteriorly, the mouth string is pulled to prevent suffocation. A large gauze pad or roll is used to keep slight tension on the pack (after the anterior pack has been placed). A large roll is used to prevent pressure necrosis on the nasal ala and columella.

anterior pack. Even minimal balloon inflation may be painful. *Inflation should be done slowly and should be stopped if pain is severe.*

The device is constructed of soft, pliable silicone rubber, which allows atraumatic expansion of the balloon into the entire nasal cavity. If the patient complains of excessive pain, the anterior balloon is slightly deflated.

If the balloon tampons are unsuccessful in controlling epistaxis, they should be replaced with conventional packs before more complicated techniques are attempted. Patients with the balloon devices are treated similarly to those with conventional posterior packs.

As an alternative to a nasal balloon or traditional packing, both anterior and limited posterior nose bleeds may be treated with the Merocel nasal tampon (Merocel Corp., Mystic, Conn.). This material is also used as a wick for otitis externa. The tampon is a fiberless, absorbent, radiopaque, synthetic material that is inserted in a dehydrated, slightly rigid, compact form. Upon exposure to blood or saline the sponge quickly expands to form a soft compressive tampon (see Fig. 86–11). Some prefer to cover the dry tampon with Gelfoam powder to promote hemostasis or to place Gelfoam or Surgicel sponge between the septum and the Merocel. After proper evaluation, anesthesia, and shrinkage of the nasal mucosa, the desired length (anterior or posterior size) of Merocel sponge is quickly inserted into the nose with a few millimeters remaining just outside the nostril. Coating the stiff sponge with antibiotic ointment will facilitate passage and later removal of the tampon. The speed of insertion is important and should take only a few seconds, because the tampon expands almost immediately on exposure to moisture. Once it is in place, irrigation with saline fully expands the tampon. The device remains in the nose for 24 to 48 hours and is usually more comfortable than a balloon or gauze packing. Before removal, the sponge is rehydrated and should be easily withdrawn in a single quick motion.

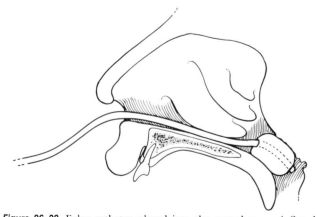

Figure 86–22. Foley catheter placed into the nasopharynx, inflated with water, and retracted into position. The distal tip of the catheter has been cut off. An anterior pack (not shown) is then placed around the catheter. The ala and columella are protected with gauze padding, and a plastic umbilical clamp or nasogastric clamp is applied to the catheter to maintain slight tension on the balloon.

Care of the Patient with a Posterior Nasal Pack

All patients with formal posterior nasal packs should be admitted to the hospital. Selected patients who have access to close follow-up may be treated as outpatients with the Merocel nasal tampon. Posterior packs are uncomfortable when being placed and annoying when in place. Mild sedation is often required for packs to be tolerated. Posterior nasal packs are associated with a significant incidence of morbidity and even mortality. Complications include hypoventilation with hypoxia and hypercarbia, infection, pain, and dysphagia.

Because many patients with severe posterior epistaxis are elderly and have some manifestations of arteriosclerosis or chronic lung disease, they are susceptible to life-threatening complications from even mild hypoxia. Cook and Komorn noted a statistically significant decrease in P_{O_2} (average 7.5 to 11 mm Hg) and an increase in P_{CO_2} (average 7 to 13 mm Hg) in patients with anterior and posterior nasal packs who were treated with sedation and bed rest.[3] The changes were most pronounced in patients with preexisting

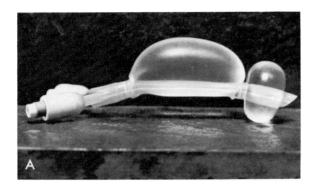

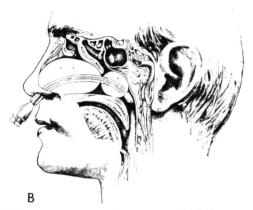

Figure 86–23. *A* and *B,* The balloon tamponade device serves as both an anterior and posterior pack. It is easily inserted and is often successful for the temporary control of posterior epistaxis in the emergency department. The balloon shown here is the Epistat balloon. (Courtesy of Exomed Inc., Jacksonville, Fla.)

chronic obstructive pulmonary disease. The presence of a previously reported reflex increase in pulmonary vascular resistance (the so-called *nasopulmonary reflex*),[4] has not been confirmed. There is, however, no question that hypoxia, hypercarbia, and death can follow the placement of these packs. Therefore, patients with posterior packs must be closely monitored, preferably in an intensive care setting, for at least the first night.

The accidental dislodgment of a posterior pack into the airway could be disastrous. The emergency removal of the classic pack by pulling the mouth string should be familiar to all nursing personnel. Patients should be routinely provided with humidification and oxygen as indicated by blood gas determinations. Sedation should be used with extreme caution. Broad-spectrum antibiotics are given routinely to help prevent complications of bacterial nasopharyngitis and sinusitis caused by blockage of the sinus ostea and poor drainage. Oral intake may be compromised because of discomfort, and fluid balance must be carefully monitored. Other complications include necrosis of the nasal ala or columella from improper padding, necrosis of the palate, or nasal mucosa. Complications increase with the length of packing, and the posterior pack should be removed within 3 to 5 days.

Uncontrolled Epistaxis

There are a few patients whose epistaxis cannot be controlled by the methods previously described. In some, the bleeding site can be identified and cauterized by exami-

nation under anesthesia. In others, ligation of vessels is necessary. The anterior and posterior ethmoid arteries can be ligated through an external incision medial to the medial canthus of the eye. The sphenopalatine artery and other branches from the external carotid system are approached through the maxillary sinus and lie just posterior to its posterior wall.

More recently, epistaxis has been controlled by embolization of the internal maxillary artery (usually with Gelfoam) after catheterization under radiologic control. Each of these methods of treating epistaxis has risks and potential complications, but the details are beyond the scope of this book; a complete discussion can be found in the otolaryngology literature.[2]

Nasal Packing and Toxic Shock Syndrome

In 1982 Tag and colleagues described two cases of toxic shock syndrome related to nasal packing.[5] Toxic shock syndrome is a severe illness characterized by sudden onset of high fever with vomiting, diarrhea, and myalgia, followed by development of hypotension and, in severe cases, shock. The diagnosis is further supported by the presence of multiple organ system dysfunction. About 10 days after onset, there is desquamation of the skin, particularly of the palms and soles. The syndrome had been described 2 years earlier and was felt to be related to tampon use and associated with a toxin-producing *Staphylococcus aureus.*

Subsequent articles have substantiated that toxic shock syndrome can occur following many surgical procedures including nasal surgery, and is thought to be related to rapid growth of toxin-producing staphylococcal organisms in susceptible hosts.[6–8] Most cases have involved patients with postoperative nasal packing. These articles have led many surgeons to use antistaphylococcal antibiotics as long as packing is in place. The effectiveness of this measure has not been established. However, *an awareness of the syndrome, and the need for a high level of suspicion in early postoperative patients who develop fever, nausea, and vomiting cannot be stressed enough.* Rapid recognition of the problem, removal of packing, intravenous hydration, antibiotics, and steroids can prevent a catastrophe.

Conclusion

Most cases of epistaxis can be readily controlled in the emergency department with a minimum of complications. One should not, however, underestimate the amount of blood that can be lost in chronic epistaxis. Significant hemorrhage may not be appreciated until the patient faints in the waiting room during his third visit within 1 week for seemingly minor bleeding. Elderly patients are especially prone to complications and require thorough investigation and definitive measures to stop the bleeding. Finally, persistent bleeding should always raise the possibility of a bleeding disorder or an occult nasopharyngeal carcinoma. All but the most straightforward cases of epistaxis require follow-up evaluation.

SEPTAL HEMATOMA

The portion of the nasal septum that provides support to the tip of the nose consists of a thin section of cartilage enveloped by a layer of mucoperichondrium on each side. When nasal trauma occurs, with or without fracture, the bending and shearing forces can cause separation of the perichondrium from the cartilage. The resultant potential space may fill with blood, resulting in a septal hematoma. Failure to recognize and appropriately treat a septal hema-

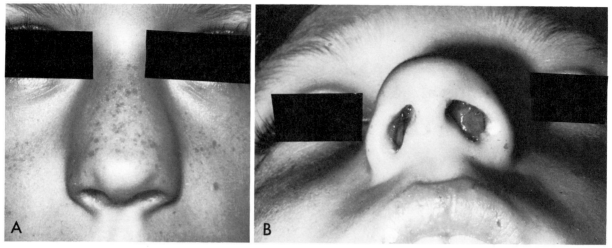

Figure 86–24. Photograph of a left septal abscess in a 7-year-old boy who sustained blunt nasal trauma 1 week previously. He had immediate nasal obstruction that persisted, and he presented with fever, widening of the nasal dorsum *(A)*, and a visible mass in the nose *(B)*. Early diagnosis and treatment of septal hematoma would have prevented this complication.

toma can have disastrous cosmetic and even life-threatening consequences. If the hematoma becomes infected, cartilage destruction with a saddle nose deformity can result. Meningitis or cavernous sinus thrombosis can complicate inadequately treated septal abscess. Posterior septal hematomas also occur and may be more difficult to recognize.

Diagnosis

A thorough nasal examination is indicated after any degree of nasal trauma. Suspicion of septal hematoma is heightened if nasal obstruction has resulted, but an adequate nasal airway does not rule out hematoma. As discussed in the section entitled "Epistaxis," good "from the eye" illumination is required. The nasal mucosa is anesthetized and vasoconstricted as previously described. A fresh septal hematoma is often the same color as the nasal mucosa and may not be ecchymotic. Therefore, it may easily be missed unless the septum is palpated with a blunt instrument. On palpation one finds a boggy, fluctuant septum that may be tender to the touch. A septal hematoma can occur on one or both sides (Fig. 86–24). The patient with a septal hematoma or abscess may complain of nasal pain out of proportion to other findings.

Treatment

Because the cartilage receives its nutrient supply via the perichondrium and because devitalized septal cartilage will inevitably become infected and "melt away," the key to treatment is to reestablish close approximation of the perichondrium and cartilage. A long vertical incision is made through the mucosa overlying the hematoma (Fig. 86–25). A small cup forceps or punch forceps is used to remove a small area of mucosa to allow constant drainage. All clots are removed with suction or irrigation (normal saline). A small drain such as a sterile rubber band is placed, and the nose is packed with an anterior pack as described in the section entitled "Epistaxis." Broad-spectrum antibiotics are used. The packing is removed daily, and recurrent hematoma is reaspirated. When no recurrence is seen, the drain is removed. The following day the packing is discontinued. The patient is advised to avoid blowing the nose and to

open the mouth when sneezing to avoid large intranasal pressure changes. Continued observation is indicated until healing is completed.

Bilateral hematomas can be handled in one of two ways. After one side has been incised and drained as previously described, a piece of septal cartilage can be removed to permit drainage through the septum from the opposite side. Extreme care must be taken to avoid a mucosal laceration on the second side; otherwise, a septal perforation is likely to occur. The second method is to incise the mucosa on each side, leaving the cartilage intact. Here, it is critical that the two incisions be staggered so that they are not directly

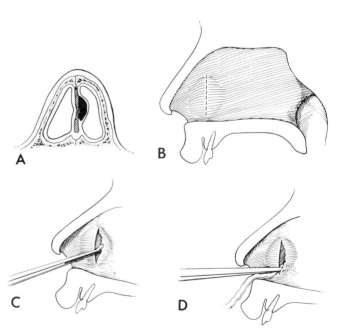

Figure 86–25. *A*, A small left-sided septal hematoma. *B*, After applying appropriate topical anesthesia, supplemented with local infiltrative anesthesia if necessary, an incision is made through the mucosa and the perichondrium covering the hematoma. *C*, A small cup forceps or scissor is used to remove enough mucosa to help prevent premature closure of the wound and reaccumulation of hematoma. *D*, A sterile rubber band is then placed as a drain, and the nares is packed as described in the section entitled "Epistaxis."

opposite one another; otherwise, septal perforation is likely to occur. Septal perforation often results in recurrent epistaxis and nasal stuffiness or even saddle deformity.

At the first sign of suppuration, hospital admission, wide drainage, irrigation, and intravenous antibiotics are indicated to avoid both saddle deformity and infectious complications such as meningitis or cavernous sinus thrombosis.

NASAL FRACTURES

Nasal fractures are one of the most common facial injuries seen in the emergency department. Epistaxis, swelling, periorbital ecchymosis, and obvious deformity suggest a displaced nasal fracture. Radiographs can demonstrate the presence or absence of fracture in some cases but do not always correlate with the clinical picture.

It should be remembered that one of the functions of the facial bone structure is to protect the brain from trauma. Patients with suspected facial fractures must be evaluated for intracranial and neck injury prior to dealing with the fracture. As discussed earlier, the next most serious associated injury is septal hematoma, which must be ruled in or out.

Most cases of nasal fracture are accompanied by enough soft tissue swelling that definitive treatment is impossible immediately. The patient is advised to take measures to minimize swelling (ice packs for the first 24 hours, and head elevation) and to be reevaluated by an appropriate specialist in 3 to 5 days, unless that specialist prefers to see the patient immediately. After the swelling has gone down, the extent of deformity can be accurately assessed, and the success of intervention can be confirmed. Simple fractures can be treated by closed reduction under local or topical anesthesia, as described subsequently. More extensive or difficult-to-evaluate injuries might require sedation or general anesthesia and more extensive manipulation to be reduced.

Procedure. In the unusual circumstance where the deformity is a simple (unilateral) depressed lateral nasal bone and swelling is minimal, closed reduction can be attempted in the emergency department. Informed consent must be obtained and includes a description of the procedure, and the reasons that guarantees cannot be made. Impacted bones may be difficult to manipulate. Green-stick fractures may not reduce at all, or may reduce, only to return to an abnormal position. Pre- and postoperative photographs are important in our present medicolegal climate.

The nose is carefully and patiently topically anesthetized as described in the section on epistaxis or as shown in Figure 86–26. Special care is taken to anesthetize the high anterior area under the nasal bones. We do not use local anesthesia for most simple fractures (which are the only ones that can be treated in the emergency department), because the injections are more uncomfortable than the procedure itself. However, 1 per cent lidocaine with or without 1:100,000 epinephrine can be used intranasally deep to the nasal bone and externally as well. A scalpel handle is coated with lidocaine jelly and is introduced into the nose and moved anterior under the depressed nasal bone (Fig. 86–27). With firm constant (not sudden) pressure the displaced bone is moved back into its normal position. If this occurs with a "pop" and the nose looks perfect, an excellent result will usually be obtained. If the bone does not move or if it immediately begins to return to a depressed position, a green-stick fracture or impaction is suspected, and the patient must be referred.

There is controversy concerning the use of an external

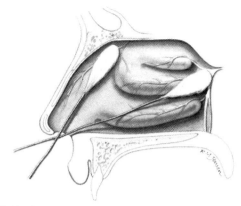

Figure 86–26. Placement of local anesthetic in the nose for anesthesia before reduction of nasal fracture by blockage of the anterior ethmoidal nerve superiorly and the sphenopalatine ganglion at the posterior end of the middle turbinate. (From DeWeese DD, Saunders WH, Schuller DE, Schleuning AJ II (eds): Otolaryngology: Head and Neck Surgery. 7th ed. St. Louis, CV Mosby Co, 1988.)

dressing or splint after closed reduction. We do not cover the nose after simple reductions, for fear that a dressing can depress the fracture again during placement, or can cover incomplete reduction. Other clinicians believe that the dressing protects the nose and reminds the patient and others not to bump it again. If a dressing is applied it is removed in 5 to 10 days. Antibiotics are not routinely prescribed for nasal fractures but should be considered if an open fracture exists.

NASAL FOREIGN BODIES

Nasal foreign bodies are most commonly found in children and include objects such as buttons, beads, cotton, beans, and other appropriately sized objects. Vegetable foreign bodies will absorb water from the nasal mucosa and swell with time, making removal much more difficult than insertion. A child with a retained nasal foreign body often

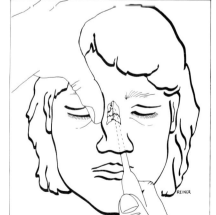
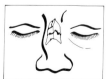

Figure 86–27. Reduction of a depressed and dislocated nasal bone fracture. This reduction is accomplished in two steps following anesthesia by first elevating the depressed nasal bone as illustrated and then manually displacing the pyramid to the midline. The handle of a scalpel may be used if an elevator is unavailable. (From Adams GL, Boies LR Jr, Hilger PA (eds): Boies Fundamentals of Otolaryngology. 6th ed. Philadelphia, WB Saunders Co, 1989.)

presents with a foul odor, unilateral purulent rhinorrhea, or persistent epistaxis.

Procedure. The key to removal of a nasal foreign body is reassurance and immobilization of the child, good lighting, and appropriate instrumentation.[9] As for removal of foreign bodies of the ear, prolonged attempts at removal should be avoided in the emergency department. In a very young or uncooperative patient, general anesthesia is indicated. In selected cases, sedation (see Chapter 41) is appropriate. Topical anesthesia and vasoconstriction can be applied as a spray or by drops, using 4 per cent topical lidocaine and 0.25 per cent phenylephrine hydrochloride or 1 ml of 4 per cent cocaine solution (maximum dose: 3 mg/kg). The nose is then carefully examined, and a determination is made as to which instrument provides the best chance for removal of the foreign body. A smooth, round object can be removed using the suction instrument pictured in Figure 86–14 or using right-angle hooks as described in Figure 86–13. An alligator forceps or bayonet forceps can be used to grasp an object that has a small leading edge. Unlike foreign bodies of the ear, foreign bodies in the nasal cavity cannot be removed by irrigation, because the nasal cavity is open posteriorly. One should not push a nasal foreign body back into the pharynx hoping that the object will be swallowed, because aspiration may occur.

Fox describes the successful use of a number 4 Fogarty vascular catheter for the removal of blunt nasal foreign bodies in children.[9] The catheter is passed beyond the foreign body, and the balloon is inflated. Slow, gentle traction is maintained on the catheter while the object is carefully extricated. This technique may be less traumatic than manual removal with forceps.

The Fogarty catheter balloon may also be used to stabilize the foreign body from behind while it is removed with forceps, because attempts to remove a foreign body may result in the object being forced into the oral pharynx, with subsequent aspiration. Aspiration is especially likely in the struggling child. A balloon inflated behind the foreign body helps to prevent this.

AURICULAR HEMATOMA

The anatomy of the pinna of the ear correlates in many ways with that of the nasal septum. It consists of cartilage enveloped on each side by perichondrium covered closely by skin. As previously noted, cartilage is avascular and receives its nutrients and oxygenation through the perichondrium. Any process that disrupts the close approximation of perichondrium to cartilage can threaten its integrity.

Auricular hematoma may occur after any blunt trauma, but it occurs most commonly in wrestlers as a result of a shearing force that separates the perichondrium from the cartilage. If left untreated, such a hematoma tends to become infected and the resultant chondritis produces a cosmetic auricular deformity called *cauliflower ear* (Fig. 86–28).

Procedure. The first step in treatment of an auricular hematoma consists of sterile needle aspiration of the hematoma (Fig. 86–29).[10] If aspiration is successful, a pressure dressing is applied as described in Figure 86–30.

The ear must be reexamined daily for reaccumulation of the hematoma, because recurrence is common. The ear must be examined sooner if pain increases or if there is fever, because these findings indicate possible infection.

Reaspiration may be required at the patient's return visit, but if the hematoma recurs after reaspiration, it should be incised and drained, using strict sterile technique. A sterile rubber band or small Penrose drain can be used as a drain (Fig. 86–31) and a pressure dressing is reapplied. The ear should be reexamined in 2 to 3 days, and the patient should be kept on a broad-spectrum antibiotic. If the hematoma does not reform, the drain can be removed in 2 to 3 days and a pressure dressing is left in place for one more day.

An alternative technique for applying a pressure dressing consists of a tie-over stent (Fig. 86–32).[11] A sterile dental roll is cut to the size of the hematoma and placed over it. A second dental roll is placed in the postauricular sulcus. A 3–0 or 4–0 monofilament suture on a straight needle is placed through the center of one dental roll, through the ear, back

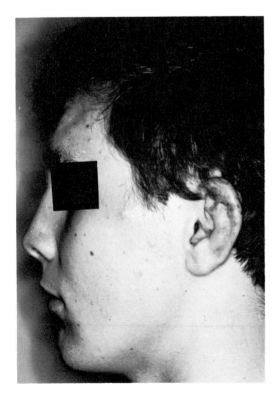

Figure 86–28. High-school wrestler with a cosmetic auricular deformity known as *cauliflower ear*, resulting from inadequate removal of blood from an auricular hematoma.

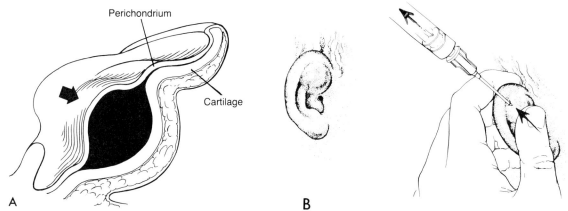

Figure 86–29. *A,* Subperichondrial hematoma within the concha of the ear. *B,* Needle aspiration of an auricular hematoma. A topical antiseptic is used to clean the ear, but local anesthesia is seldom required. While stabilizing the pinna with the thumb and fingers, the most fluctuant part of the hematoma is punctured with a 20-gauge needle. The thumb "milks" the hematoma into the syringe until the entire hematoma has been evacuated. The thumb maintains continued pressure on the ear for 3 minutes after the needle has been withdrawn. A pressure dressing is then applied, and the ear is checked for reaccumulation of blood in 24 hours. Reaspiration may be required, and persistent accumulations require incision and drainage. (*B* redrawn from Fleisher Gr, Ludwig S, Henretig FM, et al: Textbook of Pediatric Emergency Medicine. Baltimore, Williams & Wilkins, 1983. © Williams & Wilkins, 1983.)

through the posterior dental roll, and through the ear again, where the two ends are tied. Additional tie-over sutures are used as necessary. Care must be taken to ensure that the vascular supply to the auricle is not compromised by sutures tied too tightly. The patient and family are advised to observe the auricle frequently and to return to the doctor if discoloration occurs. Again, the ear is examined daily and if there is no reaccumulation of hematoma and no compromise of the skin, this type of pressure dressing is left in place for 3 to 5 days, with the patient on a broad-spectrum antibiotic. As in the case of septal hematoma, any sign of abscess or chondritis is treated with aggressive surgical drainage and intravenous antibiotics in the hospital.

PERITONSILLAR ABSCESS

Peritonsillar abscess, also called *quinsy,* is the most common head and neck abscess in adults. It most frequently occurs in teen-agers and young adults and rarely occurs in children younger than 10 years old. Over the past decade, the treatment for peritonsillar abscess has undergone controversial changes.

Anatomy

The palatine tonsils are aggregations of lymphatic tissue covered by mucous membrane. They are located in the tonsillar fossa, between the glossopalatine arch (anterior tonsillar pillar) and the pharyngopalatine arch (posterior tonsillar pillar). The lateral or deep surface of the tonsil is adherent to a fibrous capsule, which is separated from the inner surface of the superior pharyngeal constrictor muscle by loose connective tissue. This muscle lies between the tonsil and the external maxillary artery. The internal carotid artery lies 2.0 to 2.5 cm behind and lateral to the tonsil.

Pathophysiology

A peritonsillar abscess begins as a tonsil infection that extends through the capsule into the soft connective tissue between the tonsil and the superior constrictor muscle. Here

the infection suppurates and extends superiorly into the soft palate, where the median raphe limits its medial extent. Usually, the abscess will form over the superior lateral aspect of the tonsil, but it can form in the mid-posterior portion, and more uncommonly, along the inferior tonsillar pole.

The abscess can spontaneously rupture into the oropharynx, followed by resolution of the process. If rupture occurs during sleep, pyogenic aspiration may occur. A breakthrough can also occur through the superior pharyngeal constrictor muscle into the parapharyngeal space, resulting in a deep neck space infection and its potential complications. Occasionally, edema of the larynx may follow if the abscess extends down the lateral pharyngeal wall. Deep cervical vessel thrombosis and septicemia are also possible complications.

The bacteria most commonly associated with peritonsillar abscess is group A streptococcus. However, gram-negative and mixed anaerobic infections are common. Because of the frequency of prior antibiotic coverage, cultures taken during incision and drainage may be sterile.

Although peritonsillar abscess usually follows untreated or inappropriately treated tonsillitis, we have seen several cases that followed treatment of tonsillitis with intramuscular long-acting penicillin or other, appropriate oral antibiotics.

Diagnosis

The typical patient with a peritonsillar abscess gives a history of a generalized sore throat in the recent past (2 days to 2 weeks), which was either not treated or partially treated with antibiotics. Before seeking medical attention, the pain localizes to one side, frequently with ipsilateral otalgia. The patient becomes toxic with temperature elevations between 101° and 103° F. Trismus develops because of pterygoid muscle irritation, making intraoral examination difficult. As the abscess expands, swallowing becomes more painful, eventually resulting in drooling and possibly dehydration if the process lasts long enough. The patient develops so-called hot potato muffled speech, and halitosis may be severe. Tender ipsilateral cervical lymph adenopathy is usual, and secondary torticollis may develop, with the head tilted toward the affected side.

Physical examination is difficult, secondary to trismus;

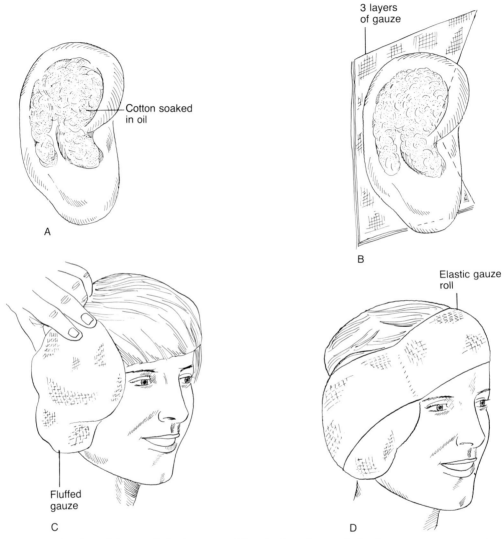

Figure 86–30. Compression dressing of the ear. Following successful aspiration of an auricular hematoma, a compression dressing is used to prevent reaccumulation of the hematoma or fluid. *A,* Dry cotton is first placed into the ear canal. A conforming material is then carefully molded into all the convolutions of the auricle. One may use Vaseline gauze or cotton soaked in mineral oil or saline. *B,* When the convolutions are fully packed, a posterior gauze pack is placed behind the ear. A V-shaped section has been cut from the gauze to allow it to fit easily behind the ear. *C,* Multiple layers of fluffed gauze are placed over the packed ear, and the entire dressing is held in place with Kling or an elastic gauze roll *(D).* The ear is thus compressed between two layers of gauze, and the packing ensures even distribution of pressure to all parts of the auricle.

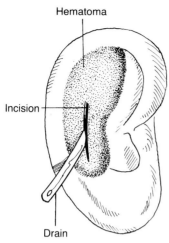

Figure 86–31. If repeated aspiration of an auricular hematoma is unsuccessful, the hematoma is incised and drained, as shown. The drainage incision must go through the perichondrium to be successful. Following placement of the drain beneath the perichondrium, a compression ear dressing is placed, as shown in Figure 86–30.

however, an accurate assessment and treatment can usually be accomplished. It is important to reassure the patient and to encourage the patient to relax and open the mouth as wide as possible. Depress the tongue with a tongue depressor, preferably the L-shaped metal depressor, which gives greater leverage and keeps the examiner's hand out of the field of vision. Placing the depressor at the level of the tonsil gives the best visualization. Positioning the depressor too far posteriorly causes reflex gagging, whereas positioning it too far anteriorly results in inadequate exposure.

The affected tonsil usually appears larger than its counterpart, is hyperemic, and may be covered with exudate (Fig.

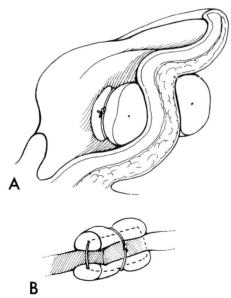

Figure 86–32. *A,* After aspiration by needle or incision and drainage, sterile dental rolls are used as a tie-over stent. *B,* One suture has been placed through the center of each roll, and the other is perpendicular to it and surrounds both dental rolls. The sutures are tied firmly but must not be so tight that pressure necrosis is risked.

86–33). The tonsil is displaced downward, forward, and medially by the inflamed and edematous palate. The uvula is usually edematous and may seem to point toward the unaffected side. A useful sign is that the normally sharp cuff-like border of the anterior tonsillar pillar is obliterated by bulging edema.

Digital palpation is not recommended unless carotid aneurysm is suspected, as secondary spasm may cause injury to the examining finger. Fluctuation is not needed to make the diagnosis or to initiate treatment, because the abscess may not yet have "headed."

The differential diagnosis includes severe unilateral tonsillitis, acute leukemia, chancre, gumma, carcinoma, carotid artery aneurysm, and tumor of the parapharyngeal space. These diagnoses can usually be ruled out because the peritonsillar abscess is an acute process, associated with toxicity and surrounding tissue edema, especially of the uvula. It is often more difficult to rule out peritonsillar cellulitis, because the history and physical findings can be almost identical to those of an abscess. Differentiation between peritonsillar abscess and cellulitis can be made during the course of treatment.

Treatment

The treatment for peritonsillar abscess has undergone change over the past 10 years. If a true abscess has formed, some type of drainage is necessary to prevent the complications previously described.

If the suspected diagnosis is peritonsillar *cellulitis,* the patient is treated with high-dose amoxicillin/clavulinic acid, clindamycin, or late generation cephalosporins, and analgesics. Cellulitis may be differentiated from abscess by clinical response to therapy or more definitively by needle aspiration. Most patients with cellulitis do not have severe trismus and do respond to antibiotics. With a responsible nontoxic patient who can maintain close contact with the physician, this treatment can be done on an outpatient basis, provided that the patient is advised to call the physician if the symptoms become more severe with increasing fever, trismus, or pain. The patient should be seen again within 24 hours unless there is marked improvement in the symptoms. If there is any question about being able to maintain close follow-up or if the patient is unable to adequately take oral antibiotics and fluids, hospitalization with intravenous antibiotics and fluids is indicated. Penicillin has been the mainstay of treatment in the past, pending cultures from the abscess fluid; however, broad-spectrum antistaphylococcal antibiotics such as the new cephalosporins, clindamycin, and amoxicillin/clavulinic acid are probably more commonly used today. If symptoms worsen and if the situation does not improve in 24 hours, the diagnosis of peritonsillar abscess becomes evident.

The classic treatment of a peritonsillar *abscess* is incision and drainage, followed by an interval tonsillectomy in 4 to 8 weeks. Tonsillectomy was suggested to prevent recurrence of peritonsillar abscess, and the time period of 4 to 8 weeks was decided on so that inflammation would have subsided but dense scarring would not yet have occurred.

During the mid to late 1970s, emergency tonsillectomy gained some popularity for the treatment of peritonsillar abscess.[12] Removing the tonsil completely unroofs the abscess cavity and serves to prevent future infections. The fear of operative bleeding and septicemia is unfounded, because all these patients are treated with preoperative intravenous antibiotics, and the surgery is performed under endotracheal anesthesia to control the airway. It is now apparent that this procedure is safe; however, emergency tonsillectomy is based

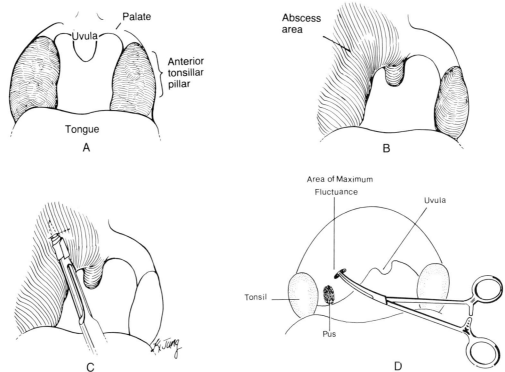

Figure 86–33. *A,* In tonsillitis, the tonsils are enlarged. They may be covered by white exudate. The margin between the tonsil and the anterior tonsillar pillar and palate is well defined. *B,* In peritonsillar abscess, the tonsil, palate, and anterior tonsillar pillar may be bulging medially in one unit. The margin between the tonsil, palate, and anterior tonsillar pillar is somewhat effaced. The uvula is usually edematous and may be pointing toward the opposite tonsil. *C,* The safest area to incise and drain a peritonsillar abscess is usually just above the tonsil in the soft palate. This location, with tape wrapped around the knife blade to prevent deep penetration, will serve to guard the deep vessels of the neck from inadvertent injury. *D,* Following mucosa incision, a hemostat is placed in the incision and gently spread to break up loculations and enhance drainage.

on the premise that peritonsillar abscesses are recurrent and that tonsillectomy will eventually be necessary.

Studies indicate that this premise may be incorrect. Retrospective studies indicate that recurrence rates for abscesses may be as low as 7 per cent in children, suggesting that the need for tonsillectomy is doubtful.[13] Tonsillectomy is probably only indicated for patients with recurrent abscesses; those who have complications of an abscess, such as airway compromise or parapharyngeal space infection; or those who have other indications for tonsillectomy, notwithstanding the present abscess.

While generally used for diagnostic purposes, in some patients needle aspiration is curative treatment, along with antibiotics for peritonsillar abscess. Spires compared needle aspiration with incision and drainage and concluded that the advantages of needle aspiration alone as the primary drainage procedure outweigh the acceptably low failure rate, making it the initial procedure of choice.[14] One approach is to use aspiration to confirm the presence of an abscess in questionable cases. However, since both procedures are best tolerated and are most accurate in a patient locally anesthetized, one can then proceed with incision and drainage after a positive tap. *A negative needle aspiration does not completely rule out abscess.*

Needle aspiration in the emergency department is not appropriate for the uncooperative patient or the patient with severe trismus. Such patients should have aspiration and/or incision and drainage under general anesthesia. For the cooperative patient, aspiration or incision and drainage as outlined below is generally possible.

Once peritonsillar abscess has been diagnosed by the patient's history and physical examination, a lack of response to oral or intravenous antibiotics, or a positive tap, an incision and drainage is indicated. Toxic or unreliable patients should be admitted to the hospital. With appropriate reassurance and encouragement and with the prospect of both immediate and great relief of the worst of their symptoms, most patients are able to cooperate with an incision and drainage carried out under local anesthesia in an outpatient setting.

Procedure. Preparation is the same for aspiration and incision and drainage. Again, good "through the eye" lighting with a head mirror or headlight is necessary. The patient is seated upright with his head supported by a headrest. The mouth is anesthetized with topical anesthesia such as 4 to 10 per cent lidocaine or Cetacaine spray. The area in which the incision will be made is then infiltrated with approximately 1 ml of 1 to 2 per cent lidocaine combined with epinephrine in a concentration of 1:100,000, using a fine needle (25 or 27 gauge). In the presence of trismus, this is best accomplished with either a spinal needle and a 3–5 ml syringe, a 3.75 cm 27-gauge needle on a tuberculin syringe or a dental injection set-up (see Chapter 87). Lidocaine is used to anesthetize the overlying oropharyngeal mucosa where the incision is made, not the underlying abscess wall. It is our impression that, with careful infiltration, there is much less discomfort during the actual incision and drainage.

The incision or aspiration is made in the soft palate in the area that is bulging most prominently. This is usually just superior and lateral to the tonsil. As mentioned, some physicians prefer to localize the incision site with a 20-gauge needle on a syringe. A needle guard can be made by amputating the distal 0.5 cm of the plastic needle cover provided with individually packaged needles. With the needle cover (guard) over the needle and taped to the syringe to avoid displacement of the guard, the needle protrudes only a short distance past the tip of the cylindrical guard. This minimizes the risk of major vessel injury when aspirating for purulence. If purulence is not found at the first site, a second aspiration is attempted 1 cm caudad; a third attempt may be made if needed 1 cm below the second site, at the lower tonsillar pole.

Once purulence is found, as much pus as possible is aspirated. Alternatively incision and drainage can be made at this site. The incision is 1 to 2 cm long and can be made with a number 15 or 11 blade. It is useful to place tape around the blade as pictured in Figure 86–32*C*, leaving approximately 0.5 cm of the blade exposed to prevent an uncontrolled deeper incision. It must be remembered that the major vessels of the neck travel within the parapharyngeal space lateral to the tonsil. The patient is advised to expectorate the pus after abscess incision. Suctioning with a tonsil suction tip or a number 9 to 10 Frazier suction tip will aid in the removal of pus. A closed Kelly clamp is then cautiously placed through the incision and gently opened to open up loculated abscess spaces (see Fig. 86–32*D*). A culture of the abscess wall, preferably for aerobic and anaerobic bacteria, is taken at this time. The patient's mouth can then be rinsed with hydrogen peroxide. The small amount of bleeding that invariably occurs with this procedure will spontaneously stop. Drains are never placed in peritonsillar abscesses.

After incision and drainage, antibiotics are continued for a total of 3 weeks. The lengthy postoperative course of antibiotics empirically seems to decrease the incidence of recurrence. The postoperative treatment may be performed on an outpatient basis or started while the patient is still in the hospital if there is a question of the ability for adequate oral intake and follow-up. The patient is seen routinely midway through the course of treatment, as well as 1 week after the cessation of all antibiotics. Recurrence of symptoms always requires *prompt* reevaluation.

REFERENCES

1. Robinson AC, Hawke M: The efficacy of ceruminolytics: Everything old is new again. J Otolaryngol 18:263, 1989.
1a. Senturia BH, Marcus MD, Lucente FE: Diseases of the External Ear. An Otologic-Dermatologic Manual. 2nd ed. New York, Grune & Stratton, Inc, 1980.
2. Abelson TA, Gluckman J: Epistaxis. In Paparella MM, Shumrick DA, Meyerhoff WL, et al (eds): Otolaryngology. 3rd ed. Philadelphia, WB Saunders Co, 1991.
3. Cook TA, Komorn RM: Statistical analysis of the alterations of blood gases produced by nasal packing. Laryngoscope 83:1802, 1973.
4. Larsen K: Arterial blood gases and pneumatic nasal packing in epistaxis. Laryngoscope 92:586, 1982.
5. Tag AR, Mitchell FB, Harell M, Morrison WV: Toxic shock syndrome: Otolaryngologic presentations. Laryngoscope 92:1070, 1982.
6. Jacobson JA, Kasworm EM: Toxic shock syndrome after nasal surgery. Arch Otolaryngol Head Neck Surg 112:329, 1986.
7. Barbour SD, Shlaes DM, Guertin SR: Toxic-shock syndrome associated with nasal packing: Analogy to tampon-associated illness. Pediatrics 73:163, 1984.
8. Wagner R, Toback JM: Toxic shock syndrome following septoplasty using plastic septal splints. Laryngoscope 96:609, 1986.
9. Fox JR: Fogarty catheter removal of nasal foreign bodies. Ann Emerg Med 9:37, 1980.
10. Potsic WP: Management of trauma of the external ear. In English GM (ed): Otolaryngology: A Textbook. New York, Harper & Row, 1981, Chapter 14.
11. Scarcella JV: Tie-over dressing to prevent recurrence of a hematoma of the ear. Plast Reconstr Surg 61(4):610, 1978.
12. Templer JW, Holinger LD, Wood RP 2nd, et al: Immediate tonsillectomy for the treatment of peritonsillar abscess. Am J Surg 134:596, 1977.
13. Holt GR, Tinsley P: Peritonsillar abscess in children. Laryngoscope 91:1226, 1981.
14. Spires JR, Owens JJ, Woodson GE, Miller RH: Treatment of peritonsillar abscess: A prospective study of aspiration vs incision and drainage. Arch Otolaryngol Head Neck Surg 113:984, 1987.

Chapter **87**

Emergency Dental Procedures

James T. Amsterdam

INTRODUCTION

Patients with a variety of general dental, oral, and maxillofacial emergencies may present to any emergency unit. Emergencies may range from an agonizing toothache to massive maxillofacial trauma or infection. Most general dental emergencies can be evaluated and managed initially by the emergency physician; however, pediatric dental emergencies and dentoalveolar trauma may require immediate dental consultation and early follow-up. In addition, consultation is essential in maxillofacial trauma or in certain dental infections in which a seemingly minor problem may have potential life-threatening implications, including airway compromise, septi-

cemia, and dehydration. The management of oral and facial pain, dentoalveolar trauma, dental infection, and maxillofacial trauma requires an understanding of the anatomy of the stomatognathic system; the relevant anatomy is therefore discussed. This chapter concludes with an overview of the oral manifestations of systemic disease that are of particular importance to the emergency physician. Intraoral and extraoral local anesthesia can be very useful in the diagnosis and management of dental emergencies. This topic is covered in Chapter 39.

ANATOMY

Stomatognathic System

The muscles of mastication are divided into two groups: the supramandibular muscles, or elevators of the mandible, and the inframandibular muscles, or depressors. The most important elevating muscles are the masseters, the medial pterygoids, and the temporalis. The bilateral simultaneous function of this group is to move the condyle of the mandible superiorly and posteriorly. The muscles involved in the depressor function of the mandible are the lateral pterygoids, the digastric muscles, the geniohyoid, and the mylohyoid. The unilateral contraction of the lateral pterygoid muscle causes movement of the mandible to the opposite side. If both lateral pterygoids contract simultaneously, the mandible is depressed, causing the jaw to open in a downward and forward movement.

The original contributions by both Barry Hendler, D.D.S., M.D., and Louis F. Rose, D.D.S., M.D., to this material are greatly appreciated.

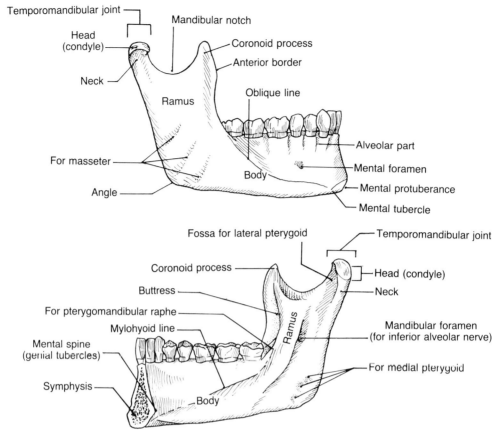

Figure 87–1. Anatomy of the mandible. (Redrawn from Grant JC: Grant's Atlas of Anatomy. 5th ed. Baltimore, Williams & Wilkins, 1962. © Williams & Wilkins, 1962.)

The mandible is essentially formed bilaterally by two rami—the horizontal portion and the ascending portion (Fig. 87–1). The ascending ramus of the mandible extends up to form two processes: the coronoid process, which extends anteriorly, and the more important condylar process, which extends posteriorly. The temporomandibular articulation is a diarthrosis joining the mandibular fossa and the articular tubercle of the temporal bone with the condyle of the mandible. A fibrous connective-tissue articular disk or meniscus intervenes between the articulating bones. A joint capsule surrounds the temporomandibular joint. The capsule consists of an outer fibrous layer, which is strengthened on its lateral surface to form the temporomandibular joint and the capsular ligaments. The capsular ligaments reinforce the capsule and function to limit mandibular movement. A small amount of synovial fluid may be found in the articular spaces. Frequently, trauma to the mandibular condyle produces pain resulting from extension or torquing of these ligaments, which should be distinguished from pain caused by a fracture in this area.

Teeth

A tooth has been described as a homogeneous body of dentin surrounding a central pulp—the neurovascular supply—from which the microporous dentin is nourished and was initially derived. The pulp continuously lays down additional dentin throughout life. The tooth may also be divided into coronal and root portions. The enamel-covered coronal portion is the part that is normally seen in the mouth. The root portion of the tooth, which serves to anchor

it, is covered with cementum, a substance that is much softer than enamel (Fig. 87–2).

There are numerous classifications for the teeth. The permanent dentition generally consists of 32 teeth, which comprise four types—incisors, canines, premolars, and molars (Fig. 87–3). If one begins from the midline and counts backward one will find one central incisor, one lateral incisor, one canine, two premolars, and three permanent molars in the normal dental anatomy. The third molar is commonly referred to as the wisdom tooth. Agenesis, or absence, of any of these teeth can occur occasionally. In addition, a patient can have extra, or supernumerary, teeth, which are somewhat small and unusually shaped. There are many methods of notation in the literature for numbering or

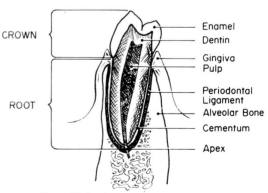

Figure 87–2. The dental anatomic unit.

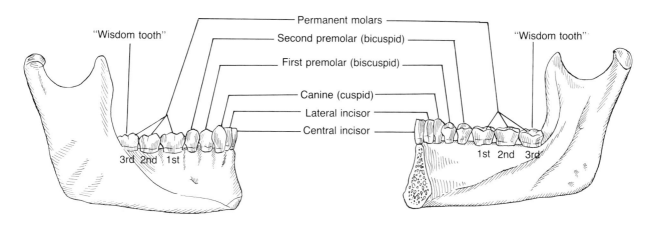

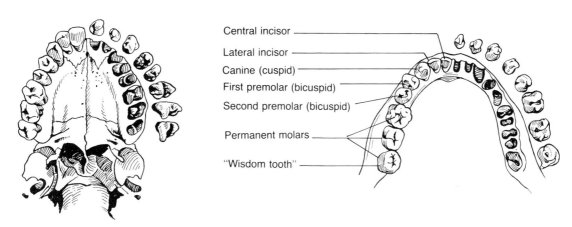

Figure 87–3. Classification of teeth. (Redrawn from Grant J, Basmajian J: Grant's Method of Anatomy. 7th ed. Baltimore, Williams & Wilkins, 1965. © Williams & Wilkins, 1965.)

classifying teeth. Although some systems are more universal than others, it is perhaps best for the emergency physician simply to describe the type of tooth and the location involved in a particular emergency, for example, an upper right second premolar or a lower left canine. Dental nomenclature that may be of use to the emergency physician includes the following terms:

Facial: That part of a tooth that faces the oral vestibule, or the cheek and the lips. In the area of incisors to canines this surface is called the *labial* surface; for premolars and molars it is referred to as the *buccal* surface.

Oral: That part of a tooth that faces the tongue or the palate, usually referred to as the *lingual* surface of the tooth.

Approximal: The contacting areas of adjacent teeth. The area closest to the midline is called the *mesial* surface, and the area toward the posterior aspect of the mouth is referred to as the *distal* surface.

Occlusal: Biting surfaces of the premolars and the molars.

Incisal: Biting surface of the canines and incisors.

Apical: The tip of the root.

Coronal: Toward the biting surface of the tooth.

Periodontium

The normal periodontium can be divided into two major components, the gingival unit and the attachment apparatus. The *gingival unit* is composed of the soft tissues investing the teeth and the alveolar bone. The *gingiva* is covered by a keratinized, stratified squamous epithelium. It extends from the free gingival margin to the mucogingival junction. In a position apical to the mucogingival junction is the *alveolar mucosa*, which is covered by a nonkeratinized, stratified squamous epithelium and is continuous with the mucosa of the lip and the cheek.

In healthy individuals, the gingiva is attached tightly to the tooth. From a level that is coronal to the margin of the alveolar bone to the level of the cementoenamel junction, connective tissue fibers from the gingiva insert into the cementum of the root.

Coronally to the epithelial attachment is a space bounded on one side by enamel and on the other by a continuation of the gingival epithelium. This space is called the *gingival sulcus*. It is the cuff that is formed around the necks of the teeth by the gingival tissues. The gingiva lining this space is not attached to the tooth and is therefore called *free gingiva*. The gingiva apical to the base of the gingival sulcus is called *attached gingiva*. In the healthy periodontium, the gingival sulcus is rarely greater than 2 to 3 mm in depth.

The *attachment apparatus* is, as the name implies, the group of structures that attach the teeth to the jaws. It consists of the cementum covering the root, the alveolar bone surrounding the root, and the periodontal ligament. The periodontal ligament is composed of collagen fibers that insert on one end in the alveolar bone and on the other end in the cementum. It is important to note that the union of the tooth to the alveolar bone is not a direct calcific union but a fibrous attachment. The anatomy of the dental unit (crown and root) and the periodontium is illustrated in cross section in Figure 87–2.

DENTAL ALVEOLAR TRAUMA

Fractures of Teeth

The simplest type of dental trauma involves the fracture of anterior teeth. The management of dental fractures is based on (1) the extent of the fracture in relation to the pulp of the tooth and (2) the age of the patient. A classification system, the Ellis system, was developed to describe the anatomy of fractures of teeth. The emergency physician may alternatively use a descriptive classification of traumatic injuries to teeth and supporting structures, as advocated by Johnson.[1]

The Ellis class I fracture involves only the enamel portion of the tooth (Fig. 87–4). This is generally a minor problem and requires immediate intervention only if a sharp piece of tooth is causing trauma to soft tissues. In such situations, the rough edge may be smoothed with something as simple as an emery board, or the patient may be referred at his convenience to a general dentist for more definitive management. What is perhaps most important is that the emergency physician can reassure anxious parents that with plastic enamel bonding materials, a cosmetic restoration of the tooth is possible. It would be inappropriate for the emergency physician to attempt the immediate restoration of these teeth; however, no irreversible damage would occur from the smoothing of rough edges. These fractures are not painful and do not result in sensitivity to heat or cold.

The Ellis class II fracture is a more complicated fracture in that it involves not only the enamel but also the exposure of dentin. On inspection, dentin is identified by its pinkish or yellow appearance as opposed to the white hue of enamel. The patient with exposed dentin may frequently complain of sensitivity to hot or cold or even air. The immediate treatment of the Ellis class II fracture is dictated by the age

	Eruption (Months)	Root Completed (Years)
Deciduous Teeth		
Central incisor	6–9	½–2
Lateral incisor	7–10	1½–2
Cuspid	16–20	2½–3
	Eruption (Years)	**Root Completed (Years)**
Permanent Teeth		
Maxillary central incisor	7–8	10
Maxillary lateral incisor	8–9	11
Maxillary cuspid	11–12	13–15
Mandibular central incisor	6–7	9
Mandibular lateral incisor	7–8	10
Mandibular cuspid	9–11	12–14

Table 87–1. *Eruption of Deciduous and Permanent Anterior Teeth*

(Adapted from Wheeler R: Dental Anatomy and Physiology. Philadelphia, WB Saunders Co, 1969, p 30.)

of the patient (Table 87–1). Because as the tooth matures the pulp continues to produce a larger amount of dentin and the pulp itself shrinks in size, the dentin that is exposed in the Ellis class II fractures in patients less than 12 years of age is closer to pulpal tissue.

Because dentin is a microtubular structure that can permit the passage of microorganisms from the oral environment directly to the pulp, contamination and resulting inflammation to the pulp can be anticipated in affected patients if dentin is exposed to the oral environment for more than 24 hours. Therefore, because of the possibility of damage to the pulp, the management of Ellis class II fractures in younger patients (under 12 years of age) requires the immediate placement of a dressing on the exposed dentin. The dressing not only provides pain relief but also helps prevent infection.

A simple dressing that the emergency physician can apply consists of a calcium hydroxide resin paste (Dycal), which is available from dental supply companies (Fig. 87–5). One prepares calcium hydroxide paste by mixing a small amount of base and accelerator from two tubes with an applicator. The exposed dentin is dried with a piece of

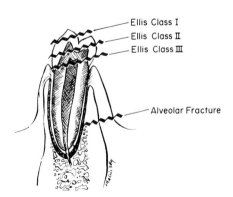

Figure 87–4. The Ellis classification for fractured alveolar teeth.

Ellis Class I
Ellis Class II
Ellis Class III

Alveolar Fracture

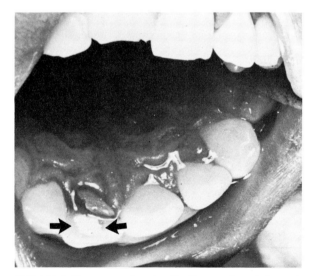

Figure 87–5. Temporary dressing for fractured tooth *(arrows)*.

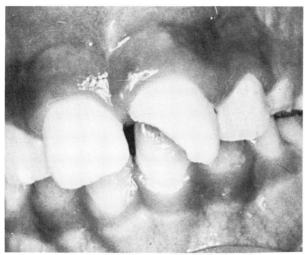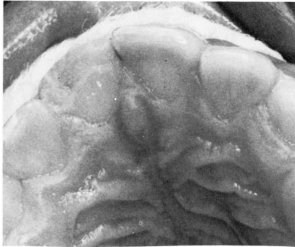

Figure 87–6. Recognition of the Ellis III fracture. (From Johnson R: The treatment of the child patient. In University of Pennsylvania School of Dental Medicine: Continuing Dental Education. Vol 2, no. 2. Philadelphia, University of Pennsylvania, 1978. Reproduced by permission.)

gauze, and a small amount of calcium hydroxide is placed on the exposed area with a cleansed applicator instrument; the tooth surface must be perfectly dry or the Dycal will not adhere. The tooth is then covered with a small piece of aluminum foil or preferably dental "dry" foil. Dycal will set in approximately 2 minutes and will set more quickly if exposed to humidity. Dycal is easily removed by the dentist. Patients are advised not to eat solid foods to prevent dislodging of the Dycal dressing.

More sophisticated techniques involve covering the tooth with the plastic bonding materials described previously; an aesthetic restoration will then result. The patient treated by the emergency physician requires referral within 24 hours. In simple class II fractures, older patients (12 to 14 years), who have a greater dentin-to-pulp ratio, may be advised to avoid extremes in temperature and to seek dental care the following day. A protective dressing need not be routinely applied. Patients with severe Ellis class II fractures (which may usually be recognized because of their larger exposed areas of pinkish- or yellowish-tinged dentin) should be treated with a dressing in a manner similar to that for younger patients. Analgesics may also be required, depending on the degree of sensitivity of the patient. It should be noted that the correct management of Ellis class II fractures may obviate the need for root canal therapy. The emergency physician, however, should warn any patient who has sustained trauma to the anterior teeth, no matter how minor, that disruption of the neurovascular supply to the tooth may have occurred. The long-term complication of the initial trauma may be necrosis of the pulp or resorption (dissolving) of the root.

Ellis class III fractures of the teeth involve, in addition to fracture of enamel and exposure of dentin, the actual exposure of the pulp. One may differentiate the Ellis class III fracture from the Ellis class II fracture by gently wiping a tooth clean with a piece of gauze to remove any blood that may be present from soft tissue trauma. The tooth is then examined for any red blush of dentin or frank drops of blood that may be extruded from the pulp. A patient may complain of exquisite pain; however, on occasion the tooth may be in "shock," in which case the patient feels little sensitivity in the tooth.

Ellis class III fractures are true dental emergencies and require immediate attention from a general dentist or en-

dodontist (root canal specialist) (Fig. 87–6). Ultimate treatment will consist of the total removal of pulpal tissue (pulpectomy). Alternatively, in the case of primary teeth, partial amputation of pulpal tissue (pulpotomy) may be performed. Delaying either of these procedures will result in significant pain and, probably, abscess formation. Some reports have recommended the use of the endodontic barbed broach for the removal of exposed pulp in the emergency department. A barbed broach, when twisted in the root canal, engages the remaining pulp; when the broach is removed, the pulp is generally attached. Even in the hands of an endodontist, the use of this instrument is difficult, and it is prone to breakage in the root canal. A broken instrument in a root canal is difficult to remove and may necessitate the extraction of the tooth. Therefore, emergency physicians and other nondentists generally should not attempt to use this instrument. If a dentist is not immediately available, the tooth may be temporarily covered with aluminum or preferably dental dry foil so as to minimize pulpal irritation and pain. Because of bleeding or other sources of moisture, it may be difficult to apply Dycal to these fractures effectively. Analgesics should be prescribed, and the patient should be told to see a dentist as soon as possible. It should be noted that one should neither prescribe nor apply any of the over-the-counter topical dental analgesic preparations. Although these agents may give the patient temporary relief from pulpal pain, they often cause severe soft tissue damage because of their irritant effects, and they are caustic to the tooth. Use of these agents has been known to result in sterile abscesses. In all cases of tooth fracture, the soft tissue should be palpated for tooth fragments and radiographed if swelling limits the examination and if one has not accounted for tooth fragments.

Subluxation and Avulsed Teeth

The same force that may have resulted in the fracture of anterior teeth may also result in actual loosening of the tooth in its socket. This is called *subluxation*. Traumatized teeth should always be examined for subluxation by pressure applied with the fingers or with two tongue blades on each side of the tooth. The tooth is wiggled in a back-and-forth motion. A more subtle indication that teeth have been traumatized is the appearance of blood in the gingival crevice of the tooth. Teeth that are minimally mobile usually heal well if the patient is kept on a soft diet for 1 to 2 weeks. Teeth that appear grossly mobile to the eye require stabilization as soon as possible. The techniques for stabilization are described later. Although stabilization procedures are usually performed by the general dentist or the oral and maxillofacial surgeon, the techniques that are described can be used by the emergency physician who is trained in such procedures. As a temporary measure for teeth that are very loose, it is often useful to have the patient bite gently on a piece of gauze to keep the tooth in place pending examination by a dentist or an oral surgeon.

AVULSED AND INTRUDED TEETH

Teeth that have been completely avulsed from the socket constitute a true dental emergency. If the patient is unaware of the location of the missing tooth, a complete *intrusion* of the tooth below the level of the gingiva must be ruled out with a radiograph (Fig. 87–7). An intruded tooth has been forced back into the alveolar bone, implying disruption of the supporting structures and possible fracture of the alveolar bone. Intrusion may be missed by a superficial examination, and one should not automatically conclude that all spaces in dentition following trauma represent avulsed teeth. Dice and coworkers[9] have reported a case in which an intruded tooth was initially thought to be a fractured tooth; a facial cellulitis and subsequent periodontal infection developed as a result of the misdiagnosis. Intruded primary teeth ("baby teeth") in the absence of infection are allowed to erupt for 6 weeks before considering repositioning. Intruded permanent teeth are surgically repositioned with a forceps and are then stabilized. Failure to diagnose intruded teeth may also result in cosmetic deformity.

As in other cases of dental alveolar trauma, the management of an avulsed tooth depends on the age of the patient and the length of time that the tooth has been absent from the oral cavity. Avulsed primary anterior teeth in the pediatric patient (aged 6 months to 5 years) *are not replaced into their sockets.* Loss of these primary anterior teeth poses no threat to normal development and alignment of permanent teeth. Reimplanted primary teeth have a high tendency to ankylose, or fuse to the bone itself. The most serious consequence of an ankylosed primary tooth is facial deformity in the child. As growth continues, it may hinder the eruption of the permanent tooth, and as time progresses

ankylosed teeth are surgically more difficult to remove. Temporary prosthetic replacement of avulsed primary teeth is easily accomplished if a cosmetic effect is desired.

In general, *permanent* teeth should be replaced in their sockets as soon as possible. Care must be taken that the tooth not become dehydrated and that the remaining periodontal ligament fibers are disturbed as little as possible. The transport medium is also important in terms of pH and osmolarity to preserve the cells of the periodontal ligament fibers.[3] A percentage point for successful reimplantation is lost every minute that the tooth is absent from the oral cavity. This time interval can be extended from 4 to 12 hours if the tooth is placed in a medium consisting of a pH-balanced cell culture fluid such as Hanks solution. A system called the Emergency Tooth Preserving System (Biological Rescue Producers, Inc., Pottstown, Pa.) is now available, which contains the cell-preserving fluid in a break-resistant, sterilized container, that does not need to be refrigerated. An avulsed tooth is simply dropped in the system's basket, which sits in the fluid, and the cap is replaced. When the tooth is needed, the basket is lifted out of the container. Teeth that have been absent from the oral cavity for more than 20 minutes should also be placed in this fluid for at least 30 minutes to rehydrate the periodontal ligament cells.

Therefore, when a call is received about an avulsed tooth, the first question that should be asked is the age of the patient. If it has been determined that the tooth is permanent, the parent or patient should be instructed to rinse the tooth under running tap water only if there is gross debris and to reimplant the tooth in its socket immediately. If actual reimplantation is not possible, the patient should be advised to bring the tooth to the emergency unit as quickly as possible, preferably in a cup of milk. Alternatively, the patient may be allowed to place the tooth in his or her own mouth to bathe in saliva, but care should be taken that the tooth is not swallowed. In all cases, one should attempt to prevent dehydration of the avulsed tooth, because teeth that become dehydrated have the poorest prognosis for healing.

The procedure for the reimplantation of permanent teeth in the emergency unit is illustrated in Figure 87–8. The avulsed tooth is held by the crown at all times. It is rinsed under saline or under running water to remove gross debris but is *not* scrubbed to conserve as much of the remaining periodontal ligament fibers as possible, because these fibers ultimately play a role in reattachment. Ideally, if the Emergency Tooth Preserving System (ETPS) is avail-

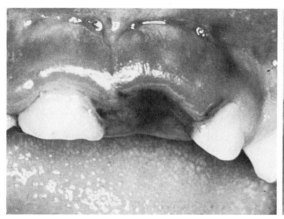
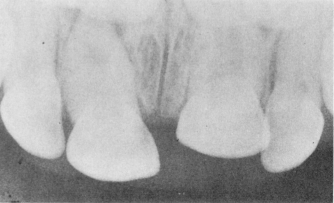

Figure 87–7. Intruded tooth secondary to trauma. A dental radiograph is necessary to determine intrusion or avulsion. (From Johnson R: The treatment of the traumatized incisor in the child patient. In University of Pennsylvania School of Dental Medicine: Continuing Dental Education. Vol 2, no. 2. Philadelphia, University of Pennsylvania, 1978. Reproduced by permission.)

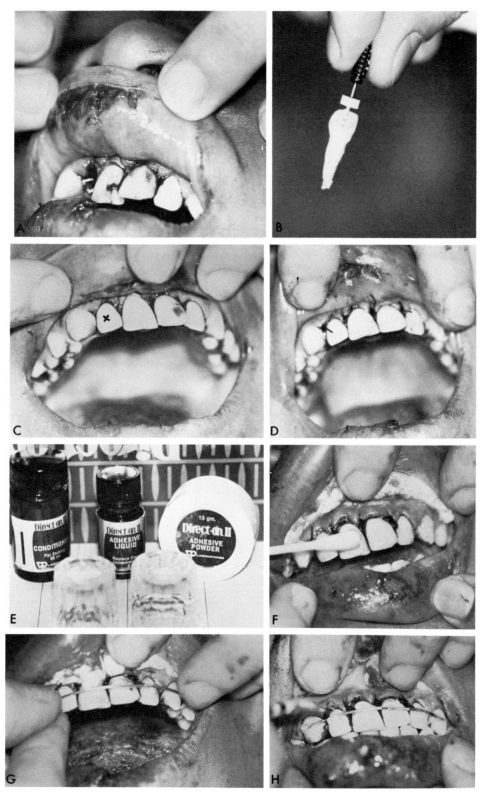

Figure 87–8. Procedure for reimplantation and stabilization of avulsed permanent teeth. *A* and *B*, The tooth is held in gauze and rinsed; root canal therapy is performed, if indicated. *C*, The tooth is reimplanted (marked with an *x*). *D*, Gingival lacerations are closed. The tooth is then acid etched and bonded to the arch wire. *E*, Direct-on system. *F*, Acid etching. *G*, Wire application. *H*, Wire bonding.

able in the emergency department, the avulsed tooth can be cleansed by soaking in this system. Indeed, if the tooth has been avulsed for longer than 20 minutes, it should be soaked in the preserving solution for 30 minutes. If the patient has other more serious injuries, the tooth can remain in the ETPS until reimplantation can be accomplished. The socket is then inspected. Blood clots or bone fragments, which may prevent reimplantation, should be irrigated or removed by gentle suction. When reimplantation is delayed (one-half hour or more), local anesthesia is suggested (see later). The socket is suctioned and débrided of foreign matter, and the tooth is immediately reimplanted. The socket should not be sharply scraped, because this may damage the periodontal ligament or the attachment fibers. If the tooth does not fully sit in the socket as compared with the alignment of the adjacent teeth or if there is confusion as to the position of the tooth after reimplantation, the procedure should stop at this point. The patient should then gently bite on a piece of gauze until seen by a general dentist or an oral and maxillofacial surgeon or the tooth can be transported in the ETPS medium to the dentist.

Prognosis of Avulsed Teeth. When a tooth is avulsed, the neurovascular supply to the tooth is completely disrupted. If the tooth is reimplanted within a few minutes, there may be some restoration of the neurovascular supply, but most avulsions result in hypoxia and ultimate necrosis of the pulp. Therefore, almost all reimplanted teeth require subsequent root canal therapy within a short period (i.e., within 7 days). The purpose of root canal therapy is to débride the pulp, to render the tooth insensitive to pain, and to fill and seal the pulp chamber with an inert material. This inert material prevents infection or chronic inflammation, which may discolor the tooth or interfere with stabilization of the tooth by the periodontal ligament.

The object of immediate reimplantation is not to keep the tooth alive but to keep the periodontal ligament alive, thus ensuring a retained functional tooth. Healing of the periodontal ligament is variable following reimplantation. In addition, some resorption of the root surface always follows replantation. The degree of resorption varies and may even result in ankylosis of the tooth with surrounding bone. Although the long-term prognosis favors retaining an avulsed tooth if timely treatment is available, the patient should always be advised of the possibility of losing the tooth in a few months to a number of years following reimplantation. In general, immature permanent teeth have a better prognosis for survival than do older teeth.

Stabilization Techniques. Avulsed teeth require immediate stabilization so that they will not exfoliate. Although stabilization is normally performed by the general dentist or the oral and maxillofacial surgeon, there are situations in which it may be performed by the emergency physician. Stabilization is indicated in the case of a single avulsed tooth that has been placed back into the socket with satisfactory alignment. Satisfactory alignment of the tooth is judged both by visual inspection and by a report from the patient that there is no prematurity of occlusion when the jaw is closed. Even a millimeter of extrusion of a reimplanted tooth may cause occlusal disharmony in some patients, and we believe that finite occlusal adjustment should not be performed by the emergency physician.

Any tooth stabilized by the emergency physician should be evaluated by the general dentist or the oral and maxillofacial surgeon within 24 hours. Several techniques are available to the emergency physician for the stabilization of a single avulsed tooth. The application of Erich arch bars is perhaps the oldest technique used for stabilization of avulsed teeth. These arch bars are also used for the stabilization of mandibular and maxillofacial fractures. Figure 87–9 shows

the application of the Erich-type arch bar. The application of the arch bar is not a simple technique and consequently is not recommended for application by the nondentist. A temporary and readily available measure to stabilize avulsed or subluxated teeth in the emergency unit by nondentists has been described by Medford.[4] A temporary splint that has been accepted by the Council on Dental Therapeutics of the American Dental Association[5] is the commercially available Coe-Pak (Coe Laboratories, Inc., Chicago, Ill.). Coe-Pak is a zinc oxide preparation that sets to semihardness. It is prepared from tubes that contain a base and a catalyst (Fig. 87–10). Following reimplantation of the tooth, the splint material is applied in a soft, clay-like consistency and is molded over the gingival line and into the spaces between the teeth. A liquid diet is possible with the splint in place, and the patient should be directed to see a dentist within 24 hours.

Another system is available for stabilization of teeth. The avulsed teeth are first stabilized with light ligature wire (Fig. 87–11). Light ligature wire is approximately 28 gauge. A band of wire is looped circumferentially around the avulsed tooth. The area encompassed by the wire should also include at least one to two teeth adjacent to the avulsed tooth. For example, in the case of an avulsed upper left central incisor, the wire would include the upper right lateral incisor and the upper left lateral incisor or canine tooth. The wire is gently wrapped at the area of the canine tooth. This wire is further stabilized interdentally with small sections of wire. These are passed labially above the light ligature wire and interdentally over both sections of it in a lingual direction. They are then brought anteriorly under both sections of the wire and are finally tied on the anterior side. The interdental sections are secured, and the initial wire is tightened at the area of the canine. Care must be taken at this point not to break the wire; if this occurs, the entire procedure must be redone. Light ligature wire has poor tensile strength and loosens rapidly. Therefore, this wire is secured with bonding material made of beads of acid-etched resin. In addition to the acid etching, a material called "Direct-on," consisting of a powder and liquid, is used with a brush. Small beads of material are placed on the wire, bonding it to each individual tooth. This procedure may be performed in a matter of minutes.

Avulsed teeth are stabilized for approximately 10 days to 2 weeks and are then brought back into function. However, if teeth are reimplanted by an emergency department physician, the patient should be seen by the dentist in 24 to 48 hours. General precautions to be taken to avoid long-term complications are explained to the patient, as in any type of dentoalveolar trauma. When there are concomitant alveolar fractures, the stabilization of avulsed or subluxated teeth serves to stabilize not only the teeth but also their alveolar bone. In this situation, therapy is directed toward the conservation and healing of bone, and therefore stabilization is left for a minimum of 6 weeks, recognizing the risk of possible ankylosis of the teeth. The indiscriminate loss of alveolar bone leads to much more difficult prosthetic restoration of this area than with the removal of an ankylosed tooth. Generally, prophylactic antibiotics (phenoxymethyl penicillin, 250 to 500 mg four times a day) are used when avulsed teeth are reimplanted in the oral cavity. Tetanus prophylaxis should also be instituted when needed.

Lacerations Associated with Dentoalveolar Trauma

Subluxated or avulsed teeth are frequently accompanied by associated lacerations of the gingiva, the mucosa, the lips,

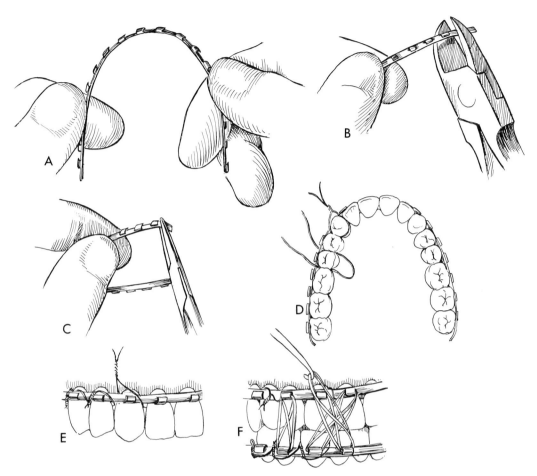

Figure 87–9. Application of Erich arch bars. *A, B,* and *C,* A commercially available arch bar is shaped to fit the maxillary and mandibular arches. *D* and *E,* Stainless steel wire secures the bar to the necks of the teeth. *F,* The maxilla and the mandible are brought into occlusion and are held in place with rubber bands. (From Converse JM: Reconstructive Plastic Surgery. 2nd ed. Vol 2. Philadelphia, WB Saunders Co, 1977. Reproduced by permission.)

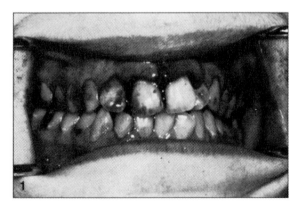

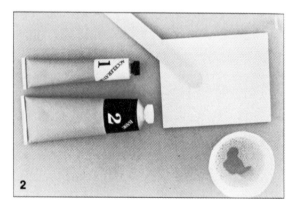

Figure 87–10. Stabilization of teeth with Coe-Pak. *1,* Dental trauma on examination. *2,* Armamentarium.

Illustration continued on following page

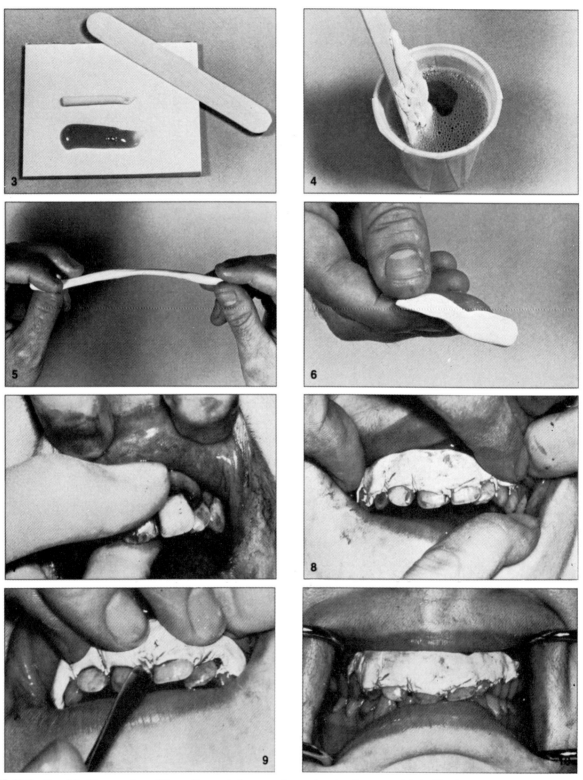

Figure 87-10 *Continued 3*, Dispensation of ingredients. *4*, Storage of spatulated splint material. *5*, Shaping the splint material into rope form. *6*, The splint material ready for application. *7*, Repositioning the traumatized teeth. *8*, Applying the splint to the cervical line and embrasures. *9*, Adapting the splint to the embrasures with a blunt instrument. *10*, The patient in full closure to check for interferences. (From Medford HM: Temporary stabilization of avulsed or luxated teeth. Ann Emerg Med 11:490, 1982. Reproduced by permission.)

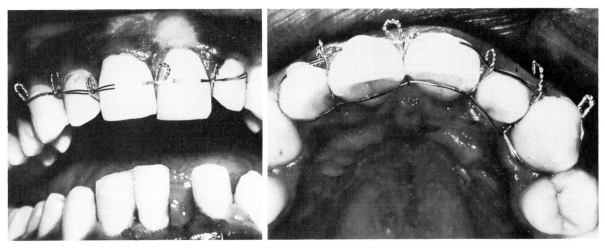

Figure 87–11. Stabilization of teeth with ligature wire.

and other facial soft tissues. Emergency physicians must remember that the stabilization procedures described previously should always precede the definitive closure of any soft tissue laceration. The lips and the oral mucosa undergo constant manipulation during the stabilization procedures for teeth; therefore, carefully placed sutures may be torn and may increase the existing soft tissue injury, making aesthetic closure more difficult. Plastic closure, once dental stabilization has been first performed, may then be left undisturbed.

Gingival avulsions should be placed in approximately their original position with fine silk sutures. Gingiva is very friable, and suturing may be difficult. The suture may be passed between teeth and may be anchored to the mucosa on the other side of the teeth. When appropriate, patients with large gingival avulsions should be referred to the oral surgeon.

A frequently encountered problem is that of the through-and-through laceration resulting in an open communication between the skin and the oral cavity. This may result from a tooth being forced through the upper or lower lip. Occasionally, pieces of a fractured tooth are found imbedded in the soft tissue. Devitalized tissue should be removed by sharp débridement, and the area should be irrigated under pressure. After appropriate débridement and irrigation, it is best to close mucosal lacerations larger than 0.5 cm with sutures. Mucosal lacerations can be closed with 4–0 Dexon or Vicryl or 3–0 to 4–0 black silk sutures; gingival lacerations are closed with 4–0 black silk. The cut ends of nylon sutures are very irritating and should not be used. Large, open intraoral mucosal lacerations result in much discomfort for the patient and frequently become infected from the accumulation of debris.

Patients with sutured intraoral lacerations are advised to keep the area clean by rinsing with warm saline and swabbing locally with hydrogen peroxide. Lip sutures may be covered with a thick coating of petrolatum jelly or antibiotic ointment. Patients are given the usual wound precautions and are checked within 24 to 48 hours. A certain amount of edema may be found when the wound is checked; in addition, a whitish granulation tissue, resembling pus, may have developed. The emergency physician should not immediately assume that this means that the area is infected. Significant pain usually signifies infection, however. If there is any suspicion of infection, the patient should be rechecked at 24-hour intervals until the edema has resolved. Frank infection should be treated with penicillin and hot com-

presses. Occasionally, sutures may need to be removed to promote drainage. Like patients with reimplanted avulsed teeth, individuals with through-and-through lacerations should be given tetanus prophylaxis; antibiotic coverage is often prescribed. Penicillin or erythromycin is advocated by many. It should be noted that there are few clinical studies to support the routine use of prophylactic antibiotics in intraoral lacerations. Skin sutures are frequently removed in 3 to 5 days to minimize scar formation. Intraoral sutures are removed in 5 to 7 days.

HEMORRHAGE

Oral hemorrhage may be spontaneous from the gingiva or, more commonly, may be the result of dental treatment, especially the surgical extraction of teeth. Patients with this complaint frequently present at night, when their dentist or oral surgeon is not immediately available. A patient presenting with a bleeding gingiva should be questioned about any recent dental scaling, curettage, or other procedures. Such bleeding usually responds to peroxide mouth rinses and local pressure with gauze. In patients with advanced periodontal disease, small remnants of missed granulation tissue may ooze continuously for hours. Spontaneous gingival hemorrhage without a history of recent dental therapy may be the initial presentation of a systemic process, for example, leukemia or coagulopathy. A decision to investigate such hemorrhage with laboratory testing is based on the extent of the hemorrhage, the age of the patient, and other information obtained from the history and physical examination.

Most commonly, patients present with bleeding following dental extraction. Postextraction bleeding most often responds to sustained pressure, which can be produced by having the patient bite on gauze. Patients frequently report that they have already been doing this for hours. One should then ask whether the patient has been spitting excessively, smoking cigarettes, or using straws, each of which may create a negative intraoral pressure. A negative intraoral pressure removes blood clots from sockets and aggravates postextraction bleeding.

The procedure for the management of postextraction bleeding is a very systematic one. If clots are present, they should be removed with suction or wiped with gauze. Patients are then instructed to bite on gauze for 15 to 20 minutes. If bleeding continues after 15 to 20 minutes, local anesthesia consisting of 2 per cent lidocaine (Xylocaine) with 1:100,000 or 1:50,000 epinephrine is infiltrated in the area of the socket to a point at which the tissue blanches (turns white). Gauze pressure is then reapplied. The epinephrine reduces bleeding, and the lidocaine allows the patient to bite without pain. Continued bleeding after 20 minutes may respond to the placement of a small piece of Surgicel or Gelfoam in the socket. This is then secured with a 3–0 black silk suture.

Sustained vigorous oozing after all the aforementioned procedures have been performed warrants a screening co-agulation profile, consisting of a complete blood count with differential, prothrombin time and partial thromboplastin time, and a platelet count. Postextraction bleeding is often caused by aspirin use. The patient must be questioned about all medication that may contain aspirin. Postextraction bleeding may also be the initial manifestation of a coagulopathy, such as hemophilia, especially in younger individuals. In some instances, postextraction bleeding results from improper surgical technique or flap design or lack of a sufficient number of sutures. Such flaps may need to be revised and resutured.

Following treatment, the emergency physician should warn the patient to avoid all liquids and solid foods for 2 hours and to avoid extremes in temperature, excessive spitting, smoking, or the use of straws or aspirin. If bleeding occurs at home, gauze pressure should be used.

The patient should be advised of the possibility that a *dry socket* will develop in 2 to 3 days. The patient becomes aware of a dry socket when excruciating pain develops in the area of the socket and a foul odor or taste occurs in the mouth after a day or two of no pain. Patients should know that the pain of a dry socket is easily managed by their dentist or an emergency physician. Application of local anesthesia to the area of the involved tooth, gentle irrigation of the socket, and application of an iodoform pack dipped in eugenol or Campho-Phenique or a commercial sedative dressing relieves the pain. The packing is placed gently in the socket while avoiding manipulation of the walls of the socket. A dry socket is a localized alveolar osteitis. Because of the high incidence of osteomyelitis secondary to scraping of a dry socket to initiate bleeding, aggressive débridement of the dry socket is contraindicated.

Patients with dry sockets are frequently given oral antibiotics (penicillin or erythromycin is preferred). The use of topically applied antibiotics is not indicated because of the increased incidence of sensitivity reactions. The dressing is replaced at 24-hour intervals until the patient is pain-free.

In addition to dental extractions, bleeding is frequently seen after periodontal (gingival) surgery. The tissue involved in the surgical site is usually covered with a surgical dressing, which may be dislodged by bleeding. Bleeding following periodontal surgery will generally respond to gauze pressure. It should be noted, however, that the periodontal surgical dressings are extremely important for wound healing, and the incorrect placement of the pack can result in treatment failure. Therefore, the periodontist should be informed immediately that bleeding has occurred and should see the patient as soon as possible.

DRAINAGE OF AN INFECTION OF DENTAL ORIGIN

Acute infection of the oral cavity and the jaws can be minor or life-threatening. The most common dental infection is the periapical abscess, or the acute alveolar abscess, which usually begins in the periapical region of the tooth as a result of nonvitality or degeneration of the pulp. One can usually easily manage these infections by treating the tooth with endodontics or extraction.

Periodontal and pericoronal infections are generally more difficult to manage. Most intraoral infection forms an abscess and drains intraorally. When the infection is well contained, drainage of these areas is generally easy. Extension of this same infection to the fascial planes of the head and neck, however, may result in much more serious infection in the parapharyngeal space or may track exteriorly to drain at the surface of the skin (Fig. 87–12). Drainage of an infection of dental origin by the emergency physician should be limited to well-confined intraoral abscesses requiring intraoral drainage and fluctuant extraoral swellings that require drainage externally by an incision on the face.

Pulpal Infection (Abscessed Tooth)

Although physical and chemical injuries to teeth result in pulpal necrosis and infection, dental infection most frequently is the result of a carious (decay) exposure of the pulp. Destruction of the enamel and the dentin by caries opens a portal to the pulp for oral microorganisms. Before invasion of the pulp by microorganisms, the affected tooth usually becomes sensitive. Invasion of the pulp produces either a localized or a generalized pulpal infection. If the portal of entry into the pulp is adequate to allow spontaneous drainage, the patient may be asymptomatic. If drainage is obstructed, rapid involvement of the entire pulp results in pulpal necrosis. The patient can experience moderate to severe pain that has been ranked second only to that of renal colic. Untreated inflammation progresses through the teeth and extends into the periapical region; irritation in this area by inflammatory products in the necrotic pulp may result in the formation of periapical granuloma. This process may be asymptomatic and persists as long as drainage through the tooth continues.

Treatment consists of removing the infected pulp and obliterating the pulp chamber, allowing the tooth to remain (root canal therapy), or extracting the infected tooth and draining the periapical region. Antibiotic therapy is indicated if drainage cannot be established when the infection has perforated the cortex and has spread into the surrounding soft tissue. Frequently, physical examination reveals a grossly decayed tooth. Alternatively, no apparent pathologic condition may be seen, or many teeth may appear decayed. One may localize the offending tooth by percussing individual teeth with a tongue blade; in most cases, tapping the involved tooth elicits a sharp pain.

In most minor dental infections, oral phenoxymethyl penicillin in doses of 250 to 500 mg four times a day is the drug of choice. Erythromycin, 250 to 500 mg four times a day; clindamycin (Cleocin), 150 to 300 mg four times a day; and cephalexin (Keflex), 250 to 500 mg four times a day, are alternatives. Analgesics can be prescribed. If the infection has broken through the cortex and there is subperiosteal extension of the infection with swelling, incision and drainage is the treatment of choice, as in any abscess.

Periodontal Infection

Periodontal disease is a progressively destructive bacterial process involving the supporting structures of the teeth, which include the gingiva, the periodontal ligament, and the alveolar bone. Unlike the relatively confined pulp chamber, inflammatory exudate produced in periodontal infection usually drains freely, and the patient experiences little, if

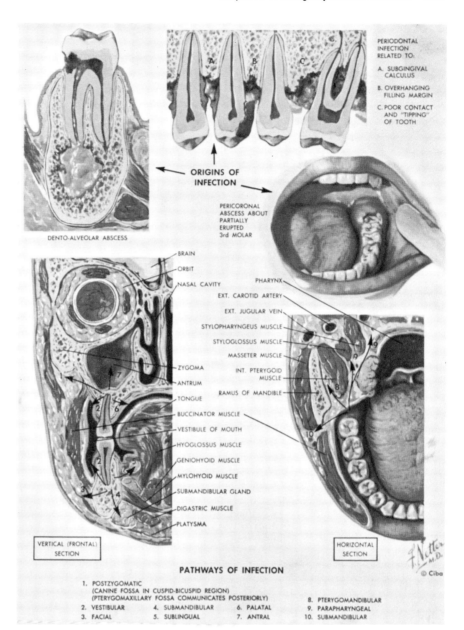

Figure 87–12. Origin and pathways of dental infection. (From Netter F: CIBA collection of medical illustrations. Vol 3: Digestive System, part I, section V, plate no 6. Reproduced by permission.)

any, discomfort. Significant symptoms may not be apparent for many years. If for any reason drainage from the infected area is interrupted, the inflammation becomes acute and is similar to an acute periapical infection that spreads to the soft tissue. The lack of a carious lesion in the involved tooth and a dental radiograph helps in distinguishing between these two processes. In most cases, acute periodontal infections tend to remain in the intraoral soft tissues rather than spread to the face and the neck.

Immediate treatment of periodontal infections includes drainage of the infected tissue (see later discussion), which may require removal of the involved tooth. Antibiotic therapy is usually instituted only if drainage cannot be achieved or if spread to tissues of the face and the neck has occurred. Follow-up periodontal therapy is needed to prevent recurrence. Warm saline rinses frequently promote drainage in periodontal areas, and antibiotics are prescribed if there are systemic manifestations. The condition usually does not require urgent referral. Frequently, a scaling and curettage of the area relieves the abscess. In the emergency unit,

however, incision and drainage of the abscess is generally preferred.

Pericoronal Infection

Pericoronitis occurs when debris and microorganisms become trapped under soft tissues that partially overlie the crown of a tooth, usually in an erupting or partially impacted third molar (wisdom tooth). A localized infection that drains from under the tissue becomes established. If drainage is interrupted by sudden swelling of the overlying tissue, caused either by trauma from an impacted third molar or by the inflammatory process itself, the entrapped exudate will spread through other pathways, usually into the pterygomandibular or submasseteric spaces (see Fig. 87–12). The underlying bone is generally not involved. Clinically, marked trismus secondary to irritation of the masseter or the medial pterygoid muscles predominates. The pericoronal tissues are erythematous and swollen. Digital pressure in the area often

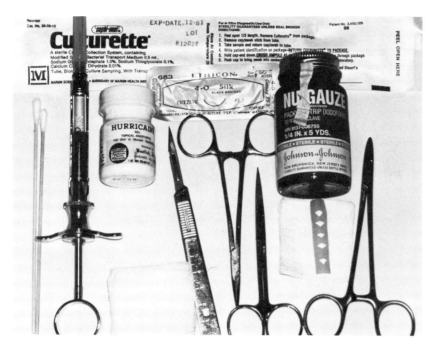

Figure 87–13. Equipment for incision and drainage of dental infection.

elicits pain and produces a small amount of exudate under the infected flap.

Treatment includes antibiotics in virtually all cases. Removal of the impacted tooth or the infected tissue ensures good drainage. Frequent irrigations with warm saline during this period are beneficial and should be instituted immediately. An oral and maxillofacial surgeon should be consulted in 24 to 48 hours. Fluctuant swelling is amenable to incision and drainage. Soft tissue dissection should be performed with caution, because the space extends posteriorly in the retropharyngeal area. Incisions are made with great care in this region because of the proximity of the internal carotid artery, which may have been moved anteriorly with tissue swelling.

In many instances, progression of oral infection may cause acute facial cellulitis. The extent of the cellulitis, of course, is dependent upon the virulence of the organism and the resistance of the host. In general, cellulitis from odontogenic infections arising from the maxillary teeth involves the lower half of the face and the neck. This pertains only to the earlier stages of infection, because in many instances the entire side of the face may be involved, regardless of the origin of infection. In the nondebilitated host, most untreated odontogenic infections tend to localize and drain spontaneously (usually extraorally).

Technique of Incision and Drainage

INTRAORAL TECHNIQUE

Before attempting incision and drainage of an intraoral abscess, the emergency physician should first determine whether the infection or abscess is a simple one. The patient should have minimal trismus and should be able to open the mouth widely to allow inspection of the pharynx. The area of maximal fluctuance is anesthetized superficially with either a topical anesthetic spray, such as Cetacaine, or (better) 2 per cent lidocaine (Xylocaine) with 1:50,000 epinephrine by injection until tissue blanching occurs. One should always remember that attainment of profound anesthesia in an infected site is often difficult. Superficial anesthetic techniques are used so as not to track infection more distally

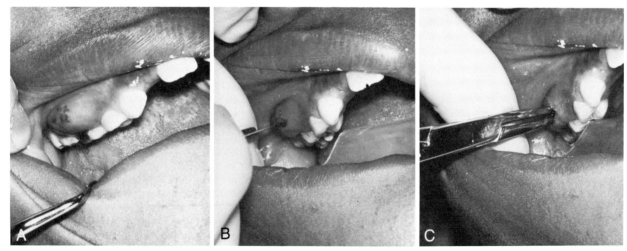

Figure 87–14. *A,* Drainage of localized dental infection. *B,* Incision. *C,* Blunt dissection.

with a long needle. When regional nerve blocks distant to the area of infection are possible, they should be considered (see Chapter 39).

The required equipment for incision and drainage consists of the instruments found in a standard incision and drainage tray (Fig. 87–13). A number 11 scalpel blade is recommended, as are a mosquito hemostat and drain material (such as one-fourth-inch iodoform gauze or a small 3-cm fenestrated Penrose drain). Antiseptic cleansing of the area to be drained is generally not necessary. A small 1-cm incision is made superficially over the area of fluctuance, with the point of the scalpel blade always facing toward the alveolar bone (Fig. 87–14). Blunt dissection is then carried out with a mosquito hemostat to avoid any vascular structures. Cultures of draining pus may be obtained at the discretion of the clinician. Cultures are recommended for complicated abscesses and when the patient is immunocompromised. The drained area is copiously irrigated. If possible, one places the iodoform or the Penrose drain by packing the site and securing one end of the drain with a black silk suture (4–0) to prevent aspiration of the drain. The patient is instructed to continue warm salt water rinses hourly for the next 24 to 48 hours and to rinse several times during the night. The drain is removed in 24 to 48 hours, and intraoral rinsing is continued every 4 hours for another day. Patients generally begin taking oral antibiotics during the course of this therapy. Although the emergency physician may manage the initial phase of the dental infection, referral to a dentist or an oral and maxillofacial surgeon is required for definitive therapy of the infection.

EXTRAORAL TECHNIQUE

If the dental infections described in the preceding section do not drain intraorally, they may spread to the face. Again, the emergency physician must determine that the infection, although it has an extraoral spread, is a simple one. The patient should have no trismus, and the retropharynx should be adequately visualized. Drainage of an infection of dental origin on the face requires more attention and care because of the cosmetic consequences of the procedure (Fig. 87–15). The patient is placed in a reclining position and is externally draped well so as to prevent drainage of purulence on the patient's clothing, the stretcher, and other materials in the treatment area. The skin is cleansed with a scrub, prepared with povidone-iodine solution, and draped in an appropriate manner. The skin is anesthetized superficially with 2 per cent lidocaine (Xylocaine) and 1:100,000 epinephrine.

It is important to note that the incision in this case will not be made over the area of maximal fluctuance but inferiorly to the area of infection in a zone of *healthy* skin. A 1.0- to 1.5-cm incision that follows the natural tissue line as closely as possible is made through skin and subcutaneous tissue; blunt dissection with a mosquito hemostat is then carried out toward the area of infection to establish drainage. A culture should be taken, and the area should be gently irrigated with saline. Again, a Penrose drain should be placed. The area is covered with a gauze dressing, and the patient is instructed to remove the dressing four times a day and to apply heat in order to promote drainage in this zone. It is important to note that this is one of the few indications for the application of warm compresses to the face in the presence of dental infection. In general, all attempts should be made to establish drainage intraorally, but this procedure is used when extraoral drainage is inevitable. Any facial infection of dental origin that requires 24 hours of heat to obtain maximal fluctuance for drainage extraorally can probably be managed at that time with intraoral drainage. Ob-

viously, scarring results from any extraoral drainage. Therefore, the procedure should be avoided if possible, but if it is necessary, the incision is made over healthy tissue.

COMPLICATED HEAD AND NECK INFECTIONS

The emergency physician is often responsible for the actual incision and drainage of simple dental infections. When the infections described previously extend to the fascial compartments of the head and the neck, they immediately fall into the serious and complicated category (Fig. 87–16). The spread of dental infection through fascial planes of the head and the neck is particularly serious. Toxic febrile patients with marked trismus require immediate attention to airway and the early institution of intravenous antibiotics. The patient should immediately be referred to the oral and maxillofacial service for admission.

A common complicated infection of dental origin seen by the emergency physician is Ludwig angina. This infection is a bilateral, board-like swelling involving the submandibular, submental, and sublingual spaces with elevation of the tongue. Emergency physicians frequently see affected patients before elevation of the tongue, during the initial manifestations of the infection. In the early stages, Ludwig angina may appear deceptively benign (Fig. 87–17A). Brawny induration is characteristic, and there is no fluctuance present for incision and drainage. Infection is commonly caused by hemolytic *Streptococcus* organisms, although it may be a *Staphylococcus/Streptococcus* mixed infection or a combination of aerobic or anaerobic organisms. The presence of anaerobes commonly accounts for the presence of gas in the tissues. Chills, fever, difficulty in swallowing, stiffness of tongue movements, and trismus are common presenting signs. Respiration becomes increasingly difficult as the tongue is elevated, and the oral pharynx becomes edematous (Fig. 87–17B). Progression to airway obstruction may be rapid—over only a few hours.

Treatment consists of high-dose intravenous antibiotic therapy. Intubation or tracheostomy should be considered in the acute stage to maintain the airway if respiration becomes embarrassed. Constant observation is important, since the airway may become obstructed without much warning. Although hospital admission (preferably in a surgical intensive care setting) is mandatory, surgical intervention may be required only if antibiotic therapy is not successful. The most common locations of dental infection in this condition are the lower second and third molar teeth; pus formation usually occurs medially or on the lingual aspect of the mandible. In Ludwig angina, as in any parapharyngeal space infection, mediastinal descent can occur because of the communication of the parapharyngeal space with the visceral space.

Therapeutic Considerations

The most important therapeutic modality for pyogenic orofacial infections of odontogenic origin is surgical drainage and removal of necrotic tissue. The need for definitive restoration or extraction of the infected teeth, the primary source of infection, is readily apparent. Antibiotic therapy, although important in halting local spread of infection and preventing hematogenous dissemination, cannot substitute for evacuation of pus.

Penicillin remains the antibiotic of choice for treating orofacial infections of odontogenic origin. *Bacteroides fragilis*, which is highly resistant to penicillin, is not normally a resident in the oral cavity; however, this organism has been

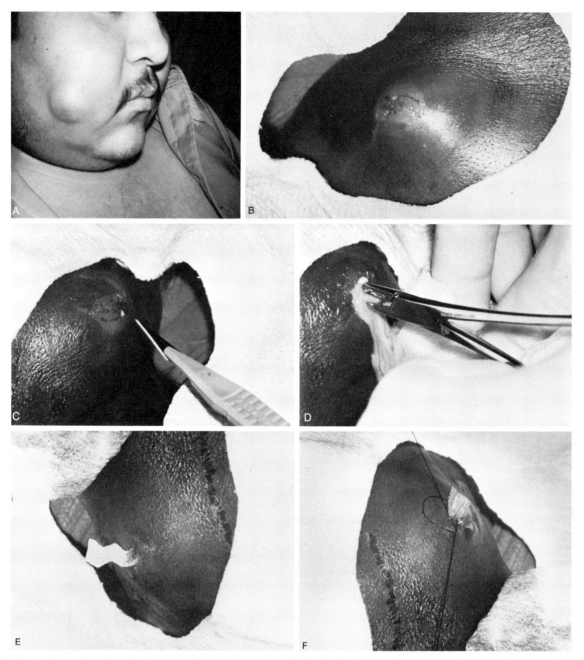

Figure 87–15. *A*, Illustration of a facial abscess that points extraorally. *B–F*, Technique of cutaneous drainage in a second patient. *B*, Anesthetic infiltrated below abscessed area. *C*, Incision. *D*, Drainage with blunt dissection. *E*, Gauze packing. *F*, Gauze sutured in place.

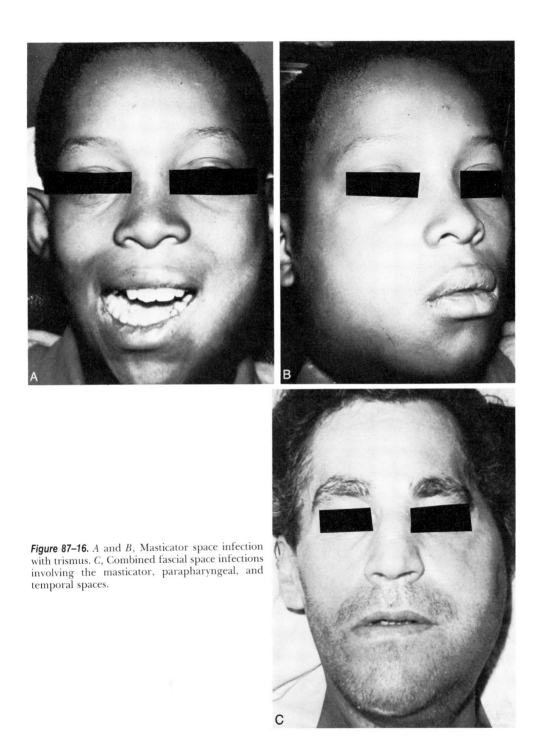

Figure 87–16. *A* and *B*, Masticator space infection with trismus. *C*, Combined fascial space infections involving the masticator, parapharyngeal, and temporal spaces.

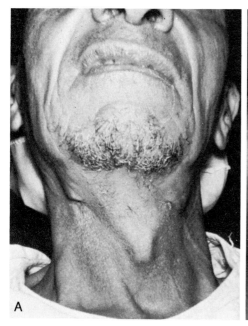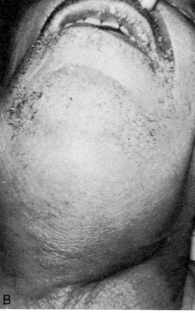

Figure 87–17. *A*, Ludwig angina may initially appear benign. *B*, In Ludwig angina, rapid progression may compromise the airway in a few hours.

recovered in 15 to 20 per cent of anaerobic pleuropulmonary infections and is presumably related to aspiration of oropharyngeal flora. It is interesting to note that penicillin has remained effective in such cases despite recovery of this organism as part of the mixed flora.

Cephalosporins, particularly cefoxitin (Mefoxin), may be excellent alternatives for penicillin-allergic patients, because the action of these agents against oral-obligate anaerobes is comparable with that of penicillin and they also are effective against certain aerobic bacteria. The usual dosage of a cephalosporin is 1 to 2 gm intramuscularly or intravenously every 6 hours. Clindamycin (600 mg intramuscularly or intravenously every 8 hours) is also highly effective, especially against anaerobes, when used in a controlled fashion and when possible side effects are monitored. Erythromycin is generally active against most indigenous oral bacteria but is comparatively less active against anaerobic and microaerophilic streptococci, *Fusobacterium*, and anaerobic gram-negative cocci. Chloramphenicol, although highly active against obligate anaerobes, is potentially toxic and should be reserved for situations in which the pathogenic role of *B. fragilis* is of prime importance or for use as an alternative agent in patients allergic to penicillin, cephalosporins, or clindamycin.

DISORDERS OF THE TEMPOROMANDIBULAR JOINT AND RELATED STRUCTURES

Mandibular Dislocation

In acute dislocation of the mandible, the condyle moves too far anteriorly in relation to the eminence and becomes locked (Fig. 87–18). Subsequent muscular trismus prevents the condyle from moving back into the temporal fossa. The spasm of the external pterygoid, masseter, and internal pterygoid muscles as well as associated edema result in extreme discomfort and anxiety for the patient. It is difficult for the patient to verbalize a complaint because he cannot close the mouth. Predisposing factors include anatomic disharmonies between the fossa and the interior articular eminence, weakness of the capsule forming the temporomandibular ligaments, and torn ligaments. Dislocation is likely to occur during maximum opening, such as occurs during yawning, laughing, or "popping" of the mandible in an open

position. Although the temporomandibular joint is a double joint, dislocation may occur bilaterally or unilaterally. The jaw may be locked open symmetrically or may deviate to the side opposite the side of dislocation. Palpation of the temporomandibular joints may reveal them to be anterior to the articular eminence. In the face of trauma, radiographs should be taken to rule out fracture, since the clinical picture of both these conditions is similar and similar occlusal disturbances are produced. Radiographs may not be necessary on an emergency basis if there is no history of trauma or if the condition is recurrent.

TECHNIQUE FOR REDUCTION

If one appreciates the anatomy of the temporomandibular joint, the proper sequence for manual manipulation to reduce the dislocation is clear (see Fig. 87–18*D*). Following dislocation, the powerful masseter muscles may be in tremendous spasm. For a smooth reduction, it is mandatory to relieve the patient's pain and tense muscle spasm with diazepam or a narcotic by slow intravenous injection. Some advocate direct injection of the condylar area with a local anesthetic. When the patient is sufficiently relaxed and analgesia is obtained, the physician faces the patient and grasps the mandible with both hands—one on each side with the thumbs (which have been wrapped with gauze or tongue blades) facing the occlusal surfaces of the posterior teeth. The finger tips are placed around the inferior border of the mandible in the region of the angles. Some prefer to have the patient seated in a chair or on the floor with the patient's back against the wall. Downward pressure is slowly and steadily applied to free the condyles from their anterior position to the eminence. The chin is then pressed backward after the jaw has been forced downward, and the mouth is closed while the condyle returns to its position in the fossa. In cases of severe muscle spasm, the jaw may snap back quickly. Therefore, protection of the thumbs is essential.

Following the procedure, the patient should be instructed to stay on a soft diet for 1 week, to avoid wide opening of the mandible, and to take analgesics and muscle relaxants. Local heat may also provide relief. Chronic dislocators or patients who suffer acute recurrences may be helped by a bandage applied around the head holding the mandible to the maxilla for 2 weeks to prevent maximum opening, but this is rarely used. Very severe cases may

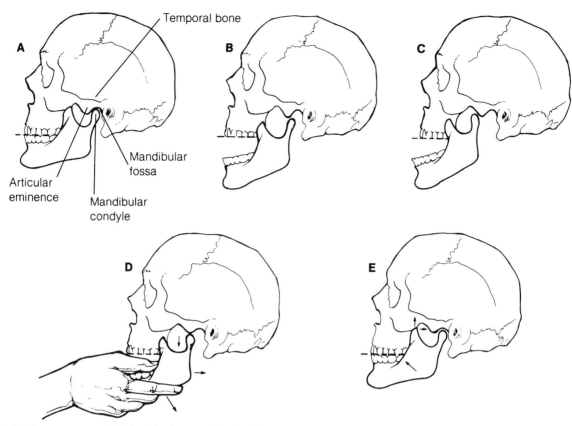

Figure 87–18. The temporomandibular joint in normal and dislocated positions. *A,* Closed position, with the mandibular condyle resting in the mandibular fossa, behind the articular eminence. *B,* In maximally open position, the condyle is just under and slightly behind the eminence. *C,* The dislocated jaw traps the condyle forward of and slightly above the eminence. *D,* To reduce the dislocation, pressure is applied to the lower molars near the jaw angle in a downward and backward direction (with well-padded thumbs!). As soon as the condyle is past the articular eminence, the muscles will cause the jaw to return to the normal closed position *(E),* usually with a swift snap. (From Amsterdam JT, Hendler BH, Rose LF: Temporomandibular joint dislocation. Consultant 23:151, 1982. Reproduced by permission.)

require intermaxillary wiring and fixation for complete control with the use of Erich arch bars (described in the section on dentoalveolar trauma). Patients who have suffered dislocation of the temporomandibular joint should be referred to an oral and maxillofacial surgeon for follow-up, since chronic dislocation may require a surgical alteration of the eminence for relief.

Temporomandibular Myofascial Pain Dysfunction Syndrome

The temporomandibular myofascial pain dysfunction syndrome, or simply the TMJ syndrome, is a complex neuromuscular disturbance possibly resulting from and definitely aggravated by occlusal disturbances and disharmonies between occlusal relations and the anatomy of the temporomandibular joint. Other entities, such as trauma, psychologic tension, and neuromuscular habits (e.g., bruxism and clenching), contribute to the problem. Patients who present to the emergency unit frequently complain of unilateral facial pain. The pain is fairly nonspecific and is generalized to the region of the temporomandibular joint. The pain is of a dull nature in most patients and increases throughout the day with continued jaw motion. Clinical examination frequently reveals spasm of the masseter muscle externally and the internal pterygoid muscle intraorally. There is usually limitation of opening. Radiographs of the temporomandibular joint are usually normal unless there is an associated temporomandibular joint degenerative disease.

When the diagnosis of TMJ syndrome is suspected, it is important for the emergency physician to rule out acute otalgia or pain of odontogenic origin.

TREATMENT

Severe trismus associated with TMJ syndrome may be treated by the emergency physician locally with the application of a refrigerant anesthetic spray, such as ethyl chloride. The skin of the patient's face around the masseter muscle at the angle of the mandible is covered with a light coating of petrolatum jelly. A towel is placed over the midline of the face to protect the region of the eye, and ethyl chloride is gently sprayed at the angle of the mandible in a rotary fashion from a distance of approximately 10 inches. The physician should take care not to produce frostbite of the tissues. The patient is instructed to open and close the mouth gently as the refrigerant spray is being applied. Frequently, this breaks the muscle spasm. Diazepam may also be of use. Physiotherapy is continued at home and consists of the application of moist heat for 15 minutes four times a day. The patient should stay on a soft diet for approximately 2 weeks. Analgesics, such as aspirin or aspirin-codeine combinations, are effective, as are muscle relaxants and tranquilizers.

Patients should be referred to a general dentist, a periodontist, or a periodontal prosthodontist for follow-up and a course of therapy consisting of occlusal adjustment, if indicated. It is possible that some patients may have to be referred to an oral and maxillofacial surgeon for an intra-articular injection of cortisone or, rarely (in the most intractable cases), surgery (high intracapsular condylectomy). The various methods described here should always be attempted by a dentist before intra-articular injection of steroids is considered. Although useful, the intra-articular injection of steroids in the temporomandibular joint is associated with a high incidence of subsequent fibrosis.

CONCLUSION

Although patients having dental complaints do not represent a high percentage of emergency visits, individuals with dental emergencies frequently do present to the emergency unit. The most common procedures available to the emergency physician in the management of general dental emergencies have been described in detail in this chapter. Although many procedures, such as the stabilization of a reimplanted avulsed tooth, are more easily and perhaps better performed by a dentist or an oral and maxillofacial surgeon, in some cases this type of consultation may not be readily available for several days. Emergency physicians can render a great service to the patient in these cases by performing whatever stabilization is possible for the reimplanted tooth. The majority of procedures described in this chapter are useful for the emergency physician and should be performed whenever indicated. The emergency physician should feel free to call on dental colleagues for further demonstration and explanation when necessary.

REFERENCES

1. Johnson R: Descriptive classification of trauma—the injuries to the teeth and supporting structures. J Am Dent Assoc 102:195, 1981.
2. Dice WH, Pryor GJ, Kilpatrick WR: Facial cellulitis following dental injury in a child. Ann Emerg Med 11:541, 1982.
3. Lindskog S, Blomlof L: Influence of osmolality and composition of some storage media on human periodontal ligament cells. Acta Odontol Scand 40:435, 1982.
4. Medford HM: Temporary stabilization of avulsed or luxated teeth. Ann Emerg Med 11:490, 1982.
5. American Dental Association Council on Dental Therapeutics: Accepted Dental Therapeutics. 38th ed. Chicago, American Dental Association, 1979.

General References

6. Alderman M: Disorders of the temporomandibular joint and related structures. In Lynch M (ed): Burket's Oral Medicine. Philadelphia, JB Lippincott Co, 1977, pp 235–274.
7. Akamine RN: Diagnosis of traumatic injuries of the face and jaws. Oral Surgery 8:349, 1955.
8. Amsterdam J: General dental emergencies. In Tintinalli J, et al (eds): Emergency Medicine: A Comprehensive Study Guide. 2nd ed. New York, McGraw-Hill Book Co, 1988, pp 612–617.
9. Amsterdam J: Dental emergencies. In Rosen P, Baker FJ, Barkin RM, et al (eds): Emergency Medicine: Concepts and Clinical Practice. 2nd ed. St. Louis, CV Mosby Co, 1988, pp 1051–1067.
10. Amsterdam J, Rose LF: Dental alveolar trauma. Curr Top Emerg Med II, Vol 2(9):1, 1981.
11. Amsterdam J, Hendler B: Approach to oral and facial pain. Curr Top Emerg Med II, Vol 2(10):1, 1981.
12. Andreason JO: Traumatic injuries of the teeth. St. Louis, CV Mosby Co, 1972.
13. Brightman VJ: Chronic oral sensory disorders—pain and dysgeusia. In

Lynch M (ed): Burket's Oral Medicine. Philadelphia, JB Lippincott Co, 1977, pp 302–342.
14. Buzzard EM, Smith HC, Hayton-Williams DS: Symposium: Medical and surgical considerations in the treatment of maxillofacial injuries. Br Dent J 116:63, 1964.
15. Braham R, Roberts M, Morris M: Management of dental trauma in children and adolescents. J Trauma 17:857, 1977.
16. Committee on Trauma, American College of Surgeons: The Management of Fractures and Soft Tissue Injuries. 2nd ed. Philadelphia, WB Saunders Co, 1965, pp 16–20, 247–264.
17. Converse JM, Smith B: Blowout fractures of the floor of the orbit. In Converse JM (ed): Reconstructive Plastic Surgery. 2nd ed. Vol 2. Philadelphia, WB Saunders Co, 1977, pp 752–775.
18. Dingman RO, Natvig P: Surgery of Facial Fractures. Philadelphia, WB Saunders Co, 1964.
19. Gibson DE, Verono AA: Dentistry in the emergency department. JEM 5:35, 1987.
20. Hagan EH, Huelke DF: An analysis of 319 case reports of mandibular fractures. J Oral Surg 19:93, 1961.
21. Hendler BH: Maxillofacial fractures—spread of infection of odontogenic origin. In Tintinalli J, et al (eds): Emergency Medicine: A Comprehensive Study Guide. 2nd ed. New York, McGraw-Hill Book Co, 1988.
22. Hendler BH, Quinn PD: Fatal mediastinitis secondary to odontogenic infection. J Oral Surg 36:308, 1978.
23. Hendler B, Amsterdam J: Infection of dental origin. Curr Top Emerg Med II 2(8):1, 1981.
24. Hendler BH, Wagner D: Problem—blow to the jaw, Trauma Rounds. Emerg Med 5:60, 1973.
25. Hendler BH, Wagner D: Injury to the lip and oral mucosa, Trauma Rounds. Emerg Med 6:278, 1974.
26. Huelke DF, Harger JH: Maxillofacial injuries: Their nature and mechanisms of productions. J Oral Surg 27:451, 1969
27. Kruger GO: Textbook of Oral and Maxillofacial Surgery. 5th ed. St. Louis, CV Mosby Co, 1979.
28. Laskin D: The role of the dentist in the emergency room. Dent Clin North Am 19:675, 1975.
29. LeFort R: Etude expérimentale sur les fractures de la machoire supérieure. Rev Chir (Paris) 23:360, 1901.
30. Lind GL, Spiegel EH, Muson ES: Treatment of traumatic tooth avulsion. Anesth Analg 61:469, 1982.
31. Lynch M (ed): Burket's Oral Medicine. 8th ed. Philadelphia, JB Lippincott Co, 1984.
32. McCarthy F: Emergencies in Dental Practice: Prevention and Treatment. Philadelphia, WB Saunders Co, 1979.
33. Osbon DB: Facial trauma. In Irby WB (ed): Current Advances in Oral Surgery. Vol 1. St. Louis, CV Mosby Co, 1974, pp 214–241.
34. Rose LF: General health affecting periodontal disease and therapeutic response. In Goldman HM, Cohen DW: Periodontal Therapy. 6th ed. St. Louis, CV Mosby Co, 1979.
35. Shafer WG, Hine MK, Levy BM: Oral Pathology. 3rd ed. Philadelphia, WB Saunders Co, 1974, pp 308–365.
36. Ship I, Lynch M: General health status affecting periodontal disease and therapeutic response. In Goldman HM, Cohen DW (eds): Periodontal Therapy. 5th ed. St. Louis, CV Mosby Co, 1973.
37. Sicher H: Structural and functional basis for disorders of the temporomandibular articulation. J Oral Surg 13:275, 1955.
38. Sicher H: The Propagation of Dental Infections in Oral Anatomy. St. Louis, CV Mosby Co, 1965, pp 470–482.
39. Solinitzky O: The fascial compartments of the head and neck in relation to dental infections. Bull Georgetown U Med Ctr 7:86, 1954.
40. Smith B, Converse JM: Early treatment of orbital floor fractures. Trans Am Acad Ophthalmol Otolaryngol 61:602, 1957.
41. Thoma KH: Oral Surgery. 5th ed. St. Louis, CV Mosby Co, 1969.
42. Thompson CW: Primary care of the acute trauma patient. In Irby WB (ed): Current Advances in Oral Surgery. St. Louis, CV Mosby Co, 1977.
43. Weisgold A, Baumgarten H, Rose L, Amsterdam J, Brown S: Dental medicine. In Kaye D, Rose L (eds): Fundamentals of Internal Medicine. St. Louis, CV Mosby Co, 1983, pp 1228–1251.
44. Wise RA, Baker HW: Surgery of the Head and Neck. 3rd ed. Chicago, Year Book Medical Publishers, 1968, pp 80–122.

Microbiologic Procedures

Chapter **88**

Direct Preparation of Stained and Unstained Clinical Materials*

Frank P. Brancato and Jon Jui

INTRODUCTION

Histologists have used organic dyes to stain tissues since 1856. In 1869, Hoffman used these dyes to stain bacteria. In 1875, Weigert stained cocciform bacteria in tissue with methyl violet. Three years later, Koch introduced dried bacterial films on glass and stained these films with various dyes. Early in the next decade, Ehrlich (1882) developed a method for acid-fast staining of bacteria, followed 2 years later by Gram's accidental discovery of a differential staining technique that now bears his name. One of the numerous modifications of the Gram stain is in use in clinical laboratories over most of the world.

Interest in the physiology and method of disease production by bacteria, however, took precedence over the microscopic examination of these organisms in clinical materials. For the first half of the twentieth century, there was scant attention in the literature regarding the direct microscopic examination of clinical material either as a wet mount or as a Gram-stained film on a glass slide. This is not to imply that microscopic examinations of Gram-stained smears were not being done. These smears were being done in all medical bacteriology courses; however, they were of colonies from cultures or of growth in broth.

In 1958, Newman[1] and, in 1959, Blenden[2] emphasized the importance of the initial microscopic examination in selecting the proper culture medium and in evaluating the culture results. Brancato and Parker,[3] in 1966, provided their direct smear data based on experience compiled from 1954 to 1964 at the Seattle U.S. Public Health Service Hospital. Their data documented the benefit of this tool to the patient, to the physician, and to the microbiologist. Path Capsule 26, published and copyrighted in 1965 by the College of American Pathologists,[4] very succinctly pointed out the value of direct smear results. In the 1970s Provine and Gardner[5] and, a few years later, others[6–12] reaffirmed their conclusions. As Washington[13] wrote about the Gram-stained smear in 1979: "Curiously this test is *vastly* underused, sometimes misused, and *often* misinterpreted" (my emphasis).

INDICATIONS

A direct preparation is indicated when the practitioner concludes after physical examination of the patient that an

*A photomicrograph atlas is provided on page 1076.

infection may be present or must, at least, be ruled out. This conclusion can be supported rapidly and accurately, in most instances, by microscopic examination of a direct smear of appropriate clinical material. The direct smear can also aid in the choice of antibiotic therapy, provided the bacterial morphology and staining properties are correlated with the associated cellular reaction and clinical picture to suggest a specific infecting organism or category of organisms.

The importance of the collection of the clinical material, which forms the base from which an accurate smear and, if necessary, a culture can be prepared, has been emphasized but never often enough. In the following section, primary attention is directed toward the collection of clinical material from various body areas.

COLLECTION TECHNIQUE (General Principles)

Body Fluids and Transudates

The vascular network is accessed via venipuncture and the central nervous system via lumbar tap. Body cavities are accessed via pleural, peritoneal, or joint tap.

Collection

1. Sterilize the skin surface selected for penetration (alcohol rub, povidone-iodine rub followed by alcohol rub; allow to dry).
2. Administer local anesthetic when clinically indicated, using sterile technique.
3. Penetrate with a sterile needle and syringe.
4. After aspiration of specimen, remove trapped air from syringe and replace needle guard.

Direct Examinations

1. Gram-stained smear (except blood).
2. India ink mount (spinal fluid).
3. Wright-Giemsa–stained smear (blood when blood parasites are a consideration).
4. Acid-fast–stained smear.
5. Acridine orange–stained smear (if fluorescent microscope is available).

Discussion

These fluids and transudates are sterile and, other than blood, normally are free of host-reactive cells, such as leukocytes. The presence of a host reaction strongly points to a microbial infection. Organisms are also uncommonly seen in direct smears from these body fluids. To see at least one organism per oil immersion field, there must be at least 100,000 organisms per ml (conservatively). Rarely are organisms seen when the count is under 10,000 per ml.[14–16] Consequently, materials should be forwarded to the laboratory for culture when a host reaction is present, even though no organisms are seen on the smear.

Exudates from Sites with Resident Flora

Primary sites with resident flora include the upper respiratory tract, the female urogenital tract, draining cutaneous lesions, and anorectal lesions.

Collection

1. Rinse and gently cleanse the site free of contamination from earlier exudation.
2. Touch two sterile swabs (cotton, calcium alginate) to fresh exudate.
3. Make thin smear by rolling one swab over a 1-sq cm area of a clean glass slide. Several slides may be made.
4. Insert the other swab into sterile tube (dry or with suitable carrying fluid, such as 1 to 2 ml of physiologic saline or broth).

Direct Examinations

1. Gram-stained smear.
2. Acid-fast–stained smear.

Discussion

The existence of a resident flora presents two problems. First, because collection is affected, the lowest possible level of contamination by the resident flora must be sought. Second, interpretation of the smear microscopically and, if cultured, of the culture findings in the presence of resident flora may be difficult.

It is immediately obvious that a knowledge of the resident flora and their levels at the aforementioned body sites is necessary.[17] Not as obvious is the need for knowledge about the host reaction in the form of inflammation and phagocytic cells at these sites. In normal individuals or in immunosuppressed individuals, such host reactions are generally reduced or lacking.

Sterile Fluids Generally Collected by Passage Through the Area Having Resident Flora

LOWER RESPIRATORY TRACT

Collection

1. The patient rinses the oral cavity and throat by gargling with tap water; then the patient expectorates a *deep* cough sputum into a sterile container (quality, not quantity, of the specimen is the goal).

Alternatives

2. Nasotracheal aspiration. Sterile tubing is passed through the nasal passage into the trachea.
3. Transtracheal aspiration (as per needle cricothyroidotomy discussed in Chapter 7).

Direct Examinations

1. Gram-stained smear.
2. Acid-fast–stained smear.
3. Wright-Giemsa–stained smear (for quantitation of eosinophils).
4. Acridine orange–stained smear (if fluorescent microscope is available).

UPPER URINARY TRACT

Collection

1. The patient voids a clean catch (midstream) specimen. The external genitalia are first cleansed front to back, and the patient is encouraged to void approximately 20 ml of urine before collecting 1 to 2 ml in a sterile container for smear and culture (if indicated).

Alternatives

2. An in-and-out catheterized specimen collected in a sterile container.
3. Patients with indwelling catheters should have a new sterile catheter placed before collection of the specimen.
4. Suprapubic tap, best obtained from hyperdistended bladder. Cleanse and anesthetize the skin; then aspirate (see Chapter 73).

Direct Examinations

1. Gram-stained smear.
2. Acridine orange–stained smear (if fluorescent microscope is available).

MALE UROGENITAL TRACT

Collection

1. If penile discharge is present, the external genitalia are washed and the discharge is expressed by gentle massage, and collected with a sterile swab. Place discharge in plugged or capped tube.
2. If no penile discharge is present, the external genitalia are washed and a thin alginate swab (may or may not be moistened with sterile water) is inserted approximately 2 cm into the distal urethra and rotated gently. The swab is then placed in a plugged or capped tube.[18]

Direct Examination

1. Gram-stained smear.

CLOSED CUTANEOUS LESIONS SUCH AS FURUNCLES AND VESICLES

Collection

1. Swollen lesion (pooled exudate). Sterilize the surface (e.g., povidone-iodine rub followed by alcohol rub) and aspirate exudate with a sterile needle and syringe. Alternatively, one can incise and drain the lesion, collecting a sample with a sterile swab from the inner wall of the lesion.
2. Inflammation with no obvious exudate accumulating. After sterilizing the surface, insert and withdraw approximately 0.5 ml of sterile physiologic saline from the margin of the lesion with a sterile needle and syringe (see Chapter 48).

Direct Examinations

1. Gram-stained smear.
2. Wright-Giemsa–stained smear (for herpetic infection–associated multinuclear giant cells).

Discussion

Exudates derived from closed lesions represent a significant proportion of the clinical materials submitted to the laboratory, and, if the specimen has been properly collected, a direct smear evaluation can result in highly accurate and rapid guidance to the requestor.

Excretion with Resident Flora (Feces)

Collection

1. Fluid feces. Have the patient defecate directly into a waterproof container with secure lid.
2. Formed feces. Have the patient provide a sample as discussed earlier. Examine the entire surface for adhering helminths or parts thereof; then take small portions from different specimen areas, especially those with mucus or

blood, using a disposable wood spatula (tongue blade), and place them in a waterproof container.

Direct Examinations

1. Place a drop of freshly passed (warm) fluid feces on a slightly warmed slide. Immediately seal it with a petrolatum-rimmed coverslip.

2. Gram-stained smear of thin film of fluid feces or of mucus or blood adhering to formed feces.

3. Wright-Giemsa–stained smear of thin film of fluid feces or of mucus or blood adhering to formed feces.

PRIMARY STAINING METHODS

Procedural steps for popular staining methods are listed in Table 88–1. Additional comments regarding the methods are provided in the following sections.

Gram Stain

The Gram stain allows one to see the morphologic differences among bacteria and separates bacteria into two broad groups. The ability of bacteria to retain the primary crystal violet dye and to resist decolorization is termed *gram-positive*. *Gram-negative* denotes that the primary dye stain taken up by the organism is susceptible to decolorization.

Although gram-positive bacterial cell walls resist decolorization, some decolorization is possible with errors in technique,[19] and gram-positive organisms may be incorrectly perceived as gram-negative. The following procedural points, which may influence the degree of decolorization, should be noted. A thick smear is more resistant to decolorization than a thin smear; thus it is important to spread the specimen evenly over the slide so that individual cells may be separated from one another. Air drying a smear may be

---

Table 88–1. *Common Staining Methods*

Gram Stain

Fixation

Prepare a thin smear by spreading material from swab (or 0.01 ml calibrated loop in the case of unspun urine) evenly onto a glass slide over a 2-cm² area. Allow the slide to air dry, then *briefly* heat fix.

Primary Stain

Flood the slide with crystal violet, or methyl violet, 6B for several seconds. Rinse the slide with tap water immediately, and drain off the water. During drainage, the slide should be held vertically with the frosted end up and the unfrosted end resting on blotting paper.

Mordant

Flood the slide with Gram's iodine for at least 10 seconds. Rinse with tap water and drain again, as previously.

Decolorization

Flood the slide with acetone-alcohol (1:1), drain, and repeat the acetone-alcohol flood. Rinse the slide with tap water, and drain. Note that at the end of this step the slide should be similar in appearance to the original unstained smear. Some authors recommend either 95 per cent ethanol or acetone alone rather than the combination (1:1) used here.

Counterstain

Flood the slide with 0.1 per cent aqueous basic fuchsin, and rinse with tap water. Drain the slide, and allow it to air dry.

Note that many laboratories use safranin rather than basic fuchsin for counterstaining. Basic fuchsin tends to produce a darker counterstain.

Kinyoun-Tergitol Acid-Fast Stain

Fixation

A thin smear is prepared on a glass slide. The smear is air dried and briefly heat fixed.

Primary Stain

Flood the slide with carbol-fuchsin, and allow the slide to stand for at least 1 minute.

Decolorization

Decolorize the slide with acid alcohol until the washing is no longer red.

Counterstain

Counterstain the slide with methylene blue for 30 seconds. Rinse the slide with tap water, and allow it to air dry. Acid-fast organisms retain the carbol-fuchsin red stain.

Wright-Giemsa Stain

Fixation

A thin smear is fixed by flooding the slide with methanol for 1 minute. A thick smear, if blood is studied, is allowed to dry for at least 1 hour but less than 8 hours. The thick smear is subsequently immersed in distilled water for 5 minutes.

Primary Stain

The smear is flooded with filtered Wright-Giemsa stain for 10 to 30 minutes.

Rinse

The stain is washed off with buffered water. The slide is held vertically over blotting paper and allowed to drain, then it is allowed to air dry.

Methylene Blue Wet Mount

Preparation

A drop of specimen is placed beside a drop of methylene blue on a glass slide. The drops are allowed to mix.

Coverslip and Seal

A coverslip is placed over the specimen stain mixture. Vaseline is used to seal the edges of the coverslip. The specimen is allowed to stand 5 to 10 minutes to permit complete staining prior to examination. Overstaining can occur after 30 minutes.

Acridine Orange Stain

Fixation

A thin smear is prepared in the standard manner. The smear is allowed to air dry and is then briefly heat fixed.

Stain

The slide is flooded with 0.5 per cent acridine orange solution (0.15 M acetate buffer, pH 4.0) for 2 minutes.

Rinse

The slide is rinsed with tap water and allowed to air dry. The slide is examined under high-dry and oil immersion magnification with a fluorescent microscope. Microbes will stain orange against a faint green background with this method.

an inadequate method for fixation of the specimen. Gentle heating of the slide with an alcohol lamp or Bunsen burner allows for better fixation. Heat fixation should not be excessive and, optimally, when time permits, should be done *after* the specimen has been allowed to air dry. A few quick passes over an open flame is usually sufficient for heat fixation. The flame should not be used to dry the specimen. Excessive heating may damage cell walls and may cause a gram-positive organism to stain negatively. Some authorities prefer to fix the specimen with methanol.[19]

The leukocytes may serve as a guide to decolorization. Normally, the crystal violet is completely removed from the leukocyte with the decolorizer, and the leukocyte assumes the red color of the counterstain. Retention of the violet stain by the leukocyte is presumptive evidence of insufficient decolorization. As a general guide to the use of the decolorizer, one should use the decolorizer until the solution flows colorlessly from the edge of the slide.

Gram iodine, a mordant composed of aqueous iodine with potassium iodide (I_2-KI), forms a stable complex with the crystal violet, which limits the degree of decolorization of the organism. The solution has a relatively short half-life. Gram iodine may be somewhat unstable if it is stored for long periods of time, and the iodine may be lost from the solution. The available iodine concentration of an open bottle stored at 25° C decreases to 10 per cent of its original concentration at 30 days. As the concentration of iodine decreases, the smear may become more susceptible to decolorization. The problem of iodine loss may be remedied by using iodophor as the mordant.

Host cells, epithelial and reactive, thin organisms (spirochetes), and protozoan appendages (flagella of the Mastigophora) are distinctly stained by the use of basic fuchsin as the counterstain.

Acid-Fast Stain

The Kinyoun-tergitol modification is a rapid, cold method for staining those organisms with cell walls resistant to decolorization with a dilute acid solution. With careful timing, the acid-fastness of all mycobacteria and nocardias can be demonstrated. The acid-fast stain can be modified to detect *Pneumocystis carinii*, cytomegalovirus inclusion bodies, and *Legionella*.[20] Rather than decolorizing as in step 3 of the procedure (see Table 88–1), the slide is washed with tap water. The counterstain (methylene blue) is allowed to sit a full 5 minutes before again being rinsed with tap water.

Wright-Giemsa Stain

This commonly used hematologic tool is effective in differentially staining leukocytes, multinuclear giant cells, blood parasites, and some fecal protozoa.

Methylene Blue Wet Mount

This stain provides a rapid demonstration of the presence of fecal leukocytes and also emphasizes nuclear details of intestinal protozoa.[21] The technique is also helpful in the rapid analysis of cerebral spinal fluid.

Acridine Orange Stain

This stain is useful in staining certain body fluids in which there may be a paucity of microbes, making them difficult to discern among the host cells and debris.[22, 23] The disadvantage of this staining method is that a fluorescent microscope must be available.

DIRECT SMEAR EVALUATION

General

The routine evaluation of a direct smear can be done at all hospitals, and the equipment should be available in the emergency department for use by the physician when time allows. The stained specimens are best evaluated with the low-dry and the high-power oil immersion lenses without a coverslip. The most frequent errors are improper collection and improper preparation of the material and a hasty evaluation of the slide under the microscope. At least 5 minutes of uninterrupted examination of a slide is necessary for optimal evaluation. Although it is time consuming to look at all smears and although most laboratories have personnel with these skills, in such critical illnesses as suspected meningitis, all smears should be viewed personally by the physician in charge.

Individuals not completely at ease with the microscopic examination of direct smears of clinical materials will find Charts 88–1 through 88–5, Microbiology Algorithms, of help. Some of the algorithms have corresponding illustrations of a diagnostic field to further aid the neophyte. Because an infecting organism and the host-reactive cells do not differ markedly from one clinical material to another, repetition is avoided by presenting descriptive algorithms and illustrations of their presence in only one clinical material.

Upper Respiratory Tract

Various anatomic areas of the upper respiratory tract may manifest signs of infection (e.g., pharynx, tonsils, sinuses, gingiva, and epiglottis). Because these areas can be visualized relatively easily, a thin smear made from a swab of the inflamed site or the purulent area quickly reveals the presence and type of host reaction and the associated probable etiologic agent.

Keitel,[24] Provine and Gardner,[5] and Bannatyne and associates[25] stated that the abundant upper respiratory mixed flora, including numerous streptococci, rendered the Gram-stained pharyngeal smear difficult to interpret and generally worthless in diagnosing the cause of pharyngitis. In these publications, there was no mention of attention being given to the host's cellular reaction in interpreting the significance of the organisms present. The data in Table 88–2 reveal the considerable degree of accuracy of the direct Gram-stained smear in the presumptive diagnosis of streptococcal pharyngitis. These data have been affirmed elsewhere.[7, 10–12]

Chart 88–1 (Microbiology Algorithm for Upper Respiratory Tract Infections) presents the evaluation of Gram-stained smears for upper respiratory infections. The importance of correlating the bacterial and host cell reaction is emphasized in this chart. Illustrative examples are shown in Figures 88–1 through 88–5.

The emergency physician can use the Gram-stained smear as a screening tool to limit the number of throat cultures or fluorescent antibody studies carried out in his practice. A positive direct smear is strong, presumptive evidence of a group A β-hemolytic streptococcal pharyngitis.[7, 10–12] Because of a small but definite number of false-negative pharyngeal direct smears for group A β-hemolytic streptococcal pharyngitis, the physician must use clinical

Table 88–2. Incidence of Group A Beta-Hemolytic Pharyngitis with Smear-Culture Correlation (Seattle U.S. Public Health Service Hospital, 1964–1979)

	Number	Percentage
Positive smear with positive culture	3,610	91.4
Negative smear with positive culture	338	8.6
Total streptococcal isolates with smears	3,948	
Total pharyngeal cultures with smears	42,035*	100

*Most cultures had a negative smear and a negative culture for streptococci. Unfortunately no count was kept of the very small number of cases with positive smears with negative cultures, which were considered culture failures.

judgment in determining how to work up symptomatic patients with a negative smear.[26]

Other infections with characteristic Gram-stained direct smears that require antibiotic therapy include *Corynebacterium diphtheriae* or *Corynebacterium hemolyticum* pharyngitis (see Fig. 88–5), and Vincent infection (see Fig. 88–4). The presence of several species of *Neisseria (N. sicca, N. subflava, N. flavescens,* and *N. lactamica)* and *Branhamella catarrhalis* (formerly *N. catarrhalis)* as endogenous flora minimizes the usefulness of the direct smear in diagnosing *Neisseria gonorrhoeae* pharyngitis.[27] Nonetheless, the presence of gram-negative intracellular diplococci (see Fig. 88–20) together with a suggestive case history should prompt culture for *N. gonorrhoeae.*

Lower Respiratory Tract

Expectorated sputum often containing varying amounts of cellular and microbial contamination from the upper respiratory tract is the most common sputum specimen submitted to the laboratory. Endotracheal tube collections are the second most often submitted. Specimens from endotracheal tubes generally reveal upper respiratory contamination but often to a lesser degree than that found in deep cough specimens. Less often received are transtracheal specimens.

The quality of the material submitted as sputum should be ascertained by careful macroscopic and microscopic scrutiny. Macroscopic examination not only reveals the presence of food, tobacco, or other contamination, which would render the specimen less than satisfactory, but also may disclose the presence of mucopurulent patches, which would reverse the earlier opinion.

In addition to the rapid Gram stain, a wet mount of sputum has been advocated by Epstein[28] as a faster method by which structures such as eosinophils, Charcot-Leyden crystals (see Fig. 88–27), Curschmann spirals (see Fig. 88–10), and alveolar macrophages would be revealed, which are likely to be missed or inadequately distinguished by the Gram stain. The addition of buffered crystal violet to a wet sputum mount has also been proposed as a method of enhancing cellular differentiation.[29] Although it takes more time, a Wright-Giemsa–stained thin sputum film is helpful in differentiating and quantifying eosinophils and polymorphonuclear leukocytes. A 10 per cent sodium hydroxide, wet mount of expectorated sputum can establish the diagnosis of *Coccidioides immitis* pneumonitis (see Fig. 88–9).

Bartlett[30] and Heinemann and coworkers[8] found smear and culture correlation more than 50 per cent of the time. Yet, in a survey by Heinemann and associates,[8] only 13 of 38 hospitals in the Philadelphia area included a Gram stain routinely in the evaluation of sputum.

Interestingly, the microbiologic significance of clinical material from the lower respiratory tract, specifically expectorated sputum, has been under adverse criticism in recent years.[31] What may appear to be a good collection of sputum as evidenced by the direct Gram-stained smear, revealing many neutrophils, numerous bacteria of one morphologic type, and only rare or no squamous epithelial cells, may sometimes be at odds with physical and radiologic findings. Although a positive Gram stain for gram-positive diplococci will correlate with a positive sputum growth of *Streptococcus*

Chart 88–1. Microbiology Algorithm: Upper Respiratory Tract Infections Gram-Stained Smear Evaluation*

1. No inflammatory cells, only squamous epithelial cells (SEC) and mixed resident flora (see Fig. 88–1).
   Impression: no pathology evident; normal.
2. Intact mixed leukocytes. Foamy macrophages may be present; ciliocytophthoria (disrupted ciliated columnar epithelial cells) may be present. Mixed resident flora (see Fig. 88–2).
   Impression: presumptive viral infection.
3. Host reaction as in No. 2, but mixed resident flora is present in overwhelming numbers.
   Impression: presumptive viral infection, with abundant microbial overgrowth (bacterial component).
4. Host reaction as in No. 2, but elongated, encapsulated, gram-positive diplococci are very prominent and associated with leukocytes.
   Impression: presumptive viral infection, with presumptive *Streptococcus pneumoniae* (bacterial component) infection.
5. Host reaction as in No. 2, but small, gram-negative coccobacilli are very prominent and associated with leukocytes.
   Impression: presumptive viral infection, with presumptive *Haemophilus* (bacterial component) infection.
6. Host reaction as in No. 2, with neutrophils prominent and numerous gram-negative diplococci, often phagocytized.
   Impression: presumptive viral infections with presumptive *Neisseria* (bacterial component) infection.
7. Host reaction as in No. 2, but large, plump, gram-negative diplobacilli *(Moraxella)* are very numerous.
   Impression: presumptive viral infection, with postnasal drainage.
8. Host reaction as in No. 2, but with marked numbers of spherical, gram-positive cocci in clusters with diphtheroids.
   Impression: presumptive viral infection; pharyngeal aspiration from "runny" nose *(Staphylococcus* and *Corynebacterium).*
9. Many leukocytes generally disrupted; spherical, single, and paired. Gram-positive cocci associated with leukocytic remnants (see Fig. 88–3).
   Impression: presumptive group A β-hemolytic streptococcus infection.
10. Many neutrophils generally disrupted; numerous fusobacteria and treponemes (see Fig. 88–4).
    Impression: Vincent infection.
11. Many leukocytes, generally neutrophils, intact and disrupted; slender pleomorphic, gram-positive bacilli are prominent and associated with the leukocytes (see Fig. 88–5).
    Impression: presumptive *Corynebacterium diphtheriae* vs. *C. haemolyticum* infection.

*At least five different portions of the smear must be examined with lower-power and oil immersion lens.

Chart 88–2. Microbiology Algorithm: Lower Respiratory Tract Infections Gram-Stained Smear Evaluation*

1. 25 or more squamous epithelial cells (SEC) per low-power field (LPF); resident flora of upper respiratory tract (URT).
   Impression: gross URT contamination; poor collection.
2. 11–25 SEC/LPF; resident flora of URT; few scattered leukocytes.
   Impression: moderate URT contamination; fair collection.
3. 4–10 SEC/LPF; scant resident flora of URT; leukocytes present.
   Impression: slight URT contamination; good collection.
4. 0–3 SEC/LPF; many leukocytes present, generally neutrophils.
   Impression: good collection, most microbial pneumonias; etiologic agent generally abundant and associated with neutrophils
   (*Streptococcus pneumoniae* (see Fig. 88–7), *Haemophilus influenzae* (see Fig. 88–6), *Staphylococcus aureus, Klebsiella*).
5. 0–3 SEC/LPF; mixed intact leukocytes; foamy macrophages often abundant; some URT flora may be present with minimal cellular association.
   Impression: good collection; presumptive viral or mycoplasma pneumonia.†
6. 0–3 SEC/LPF; few to many intact, mixed leukocytes; ciliated columnar epithelial cells may be prominent (if fragmented, they are called *ciliocytophthoria*).
   Impression: Good collection; presumptive viral bronchial entity (see Fig. 88–2).

*At least five different portions of the smear must be examined with low-power and oil immersion lens.
†Mycoplasma pneumonias generally present with a nonproductive cough.

---

pneumoniae (pneumococcus) in 60 to 90 per cent of cases of community-acquired pneumonias, a Gram stain may miss up to 38 per cent of specimens ultimately growing pneumococcus.

Exudative upper respiratory tract infection must be ruled out, because aspiration of upper respiratory exudate may be coughed up and, mistakenly, assumed to be sputum. Aspiration of potential pathogens into the lower respiratory tract may or may not produce tracheitis, bronchitis, bronchiolitis, or pneumonitis. Without the direct microscopic examination, the value of the sputum culture has been questioned, and rightly so, by various investigators.[8, 9, 32] It appears that in the clinical analysis of materials from the respiratory tract, both upper and lower, the Gram-stained smear and other direct microscopic procedures should be guides to culture interpretation and arbiters of the accuracy and quantification of the culture.

The emergency physician can best use the direct sputum smear (wet mount as discussed by Epstein[28] or Gram stain) to support a clinical and radiologic diagnosis of pneumonia. The absence of a chest film abnormality in a normally hydrated patient should make one suspicious of the diagnosis of pneumonitis even in the presence of a productive cough. The examination of such a patient's sputum should suggest whether the illness is allergic, viral, bacterial, or a combination of pathogens (see Chart 88–2: Microbiology Algorithm for Lower Respiratory Tract Infections) (Figs. 88–6 through 88–10). The Kinyoun-tergitol acid-fast stain can be used to identify presumptive *Mycobacterium tuberculosis* in expectorated sputum (see Fig. 88–8). This rapid stain is relatively easy to perform and should be considered by the emergency physician for high-risk patients with pulmonary symptoms.

Microscopic examination of sputum should also suggest the origin of the specimen, whether it be upper or lower respiratory tract, because more than 25 squamous epithelial cells per low-power field[33] are indicative of gross upper respiratory tract contamination and culture is not warranted. Wong and colleagues[34] compared six different criteria, including the one just mentioned,[33] in determining the quality of sputum. The other criteria included a complicated scoring system of pluses for leukocytes and minuses for epithelial cells;[35, 36] averaging the number of epithelial cells per low-power field, with 10 being the cutoff point for an acceptable sample;[37] averaging the number of leukocytes per low-power field, with 25 being the cutoff point;[38] and averaging the ratio of leukocytes to epithelial cells, with 10 being the cutoff point.[39] These different screening criteria yielded similar results.

Urinary Tract

Urinary tract excretions represent a large proportion of the clinical materials submitted for microbiologic analysis. Urine is sterile and practically acellular unless an infection is present. Most specimens are ordered as clean catch (midstream) voided urine for culture, however, and all voided specimens must pass through the urogenital tract. Only a scrupulous collection technique will prevent contamination of the urine with resident flora or with infectious organisms and host-reactive cells of the urogenital tract (especially in the female). The difficulty in securing a suitable collection is greatly magnified in debilitated, obese, aged, very young, or certain types of handicapped individuals. Catheterization may be resorted to in some female patients, with the knowledge that there is a risk of an infection being initiated where there was none initially.[40, 41] Kaye[42] estimates the incidence of infection after single catheterization in the female under the following circumstances: if the patient is ambulatory-nonpregnant (1 per cent), hospitalized-nonpregnant (4 per cent), bedridden-nonpregnant (13 per cent), or pregnant and catheterized at delivery (20 per cent).

The data in Table 88–3 illustrate the smear-culture correlation of urines submitted to the laboratory of the Seattle U.S. Public Health Service Hospital over an 11-year period. These data are slightly more accurate than those of Barbin and associates,[43] who had an 8 per cent negative microscopy culture result. They used a technique developed

Table 88–3. Urine Smear-Culture Correlation (Seattle U.S. Public Health Service Hospital, 1969–1979)

	Number	Percentage
Positive smear-culture agreement Either positive smear with positive culture or negative smear with negative culture	64,279	98.9
Negative smear culture agreement Either positive smear with negative culture or negative smear with positive culture	761	1.2
Total urine specimens	65,079	100

by Kunin[44] in which a drop of manually agitated, uncentrifuged urine was used for a wet reading under a coverslip using oil immersion. The sample was considered positive if there was at least one bacterium per oil field in each of the five fields *and* if the bacteria had smooth surfaces without adherent material.

The Gram-stained direct smear of properly handled, uncentrifuged voided or catheterized urines has a value that cannot be overstated. The following features of the specimen are immediately revealed: contamination or lack of contamination; if contamination is present, its degree and origin; presence or absence of inflammatory cells; and suggestion of a particular etiologic agent. It is important to emphasize that the unspun urine sample is the sample of choice.

The number of leukocytes and bacteria in the centrifuged specimen varies greatly, depending on the force and length of centrifugation. In an obviously infected urine, spinning down a sample may concentrate pathogens and facilitate identification but the sediment should not be quantitated for purposes of determining or ruling out infection. The Gram-stained direct smear provides useful clinical information and avoids needless cultures (see Chart 88–3: Microbiology Algorithm for Urinary Tract Infections) (see also Figs. 88–21 and 88–22). The emergency physician may prefer the wet mount technique described previously[43] to the technique of reading the Gram-stained smear. Certainly, the speed with which the wet mount technique can be performed lends itself well to emergency care. The practitioner should be aware, however, that the wet mount technique has a 4 per cent false-positive and a 4 per cent false-negative potential when compared with the standard urine culture (positive culture: colony count greater than 10^5 per ml).

Urogenital Tract

The normal male urogenital tract mucosa and secretions are considered sterile, whereas in the normal female (approximately 12 to 45 years of age), the presence of a resident flora of acidophilic, facultative to anaerobic microbes (essentially lactobacilli) results in a varying degree of protection from pathogens.

Wald[48] found that a 10-minute examination of a cervical Gram-stained smear for at least eight or more pairs of gram-negative, kidney bean–shaped diplococci in polymorphonuclear leukocytes was specific for gonorrhea in the female adolescent (see Fig. 88–20). He found that when the smear was positive, the culture was positive in 96 per cent of the cases. The test is faulty primarily in its sensitivity; if the culture was positive, the smear was positive 63 per cent of the time. This correlates with the 38 to 69 per cent sensitivity rate reported elsewhere in the literature for older women.[49–52]

Lossick and colleagues[53] found the cervical Gram stain to be 97 per cent specific. Use of the Gram stain, combined with epidemiologic treatment of potentially exposed patients, permitted treatment of 91 per cent of the infected women at the initial clinic visit. Of patients with positive cultures who were not treated initially, 7.3 per cent developed salpingitis between visits. This stresses the value of the cervical smear Gram stain in the evaluation and treatment of gonorrhea. The presence of a vaginal discharge in the preadolescent female should alert the practitioner to the possibilities of a vaginal foreign body or sexual abuse.[54] Smear and culture evaluation of the vaginal discharge is warranted.[55, 56]

In the symptomatic male with a urethral discharge, the finding of typical gram-negative, intracellular diplococci within pus cells has a 93 to 99 per cent sensitivity rate.[49] The smear has also been found to detect 70 per cent of the subsequently culture-proven cases of gonorrhea in asymptomatic males.[37] Chart 88–4 (Microbiology Algorithm for Male Urogenital Tract Infections) describes an approach to evaluating the urethral Gram-stained smear of male patients. One should be aware that in the male, the distal portion of the urethral meatus harbors a "skin" flora that consists of micrococci and diphtheroids that could conceivably contaminate a deeper collection. The long urethra prevents contamination by anorectal flora.

In Chart 88–5 (Microbiology Algorithm for Female Urogenital Tract Infections), the author's approach to evaluating vaginal smears is described (see also Figs. 88–17 through 88–19). Note that in the female, the proximity of the anorectal opening to the vulva is an ever-present source of contamination. *Gardnerella vaginalis* (formerly *Haemophilus vaginalis* and *Corynebacterium vaginale*) vaginitis is suggested on Gram stain by the large numbers of gram-variable, small coccobacilli (salt and pepper appearance) and "clue" cells

---

Chart 88–3. Microbiology Algorithm: Urinary Tract Infections Gram-Stained Smear Evaluation*

1. No inflammatory cells; no organisms.
   Impression: normal (no infection).
2. No inflammatory cells; squamous epithelial cells (SEC); resident urogenital flora (varies with gender).
   Impression: poor collection.
3. Male: 1–3 WBC/LPF†; no organisms, or there may be urogenital meatal flora such as diphtheroids and staphylococci.
   Impression: not an infection of the urinary tract.
4. Female: 5–10 WBC/LPF; varying numbers of SEC; no organisms, or there may be urogenital flora such as lactobacilli, streptococci, etc.
   Impression: not an infection of the urinary tract.
5. Male: 4 or more WBC/LPF; female: 10 or more WBC/LPF; no organisms seen (bacterial count may be under 10,000/ml).
   Impression: should be cultured; may represent a urethral syndrome patient.[45–47]
6. Rare–many WBC/LPF, gram-negative bacilli generally plump.‡
   Impression: presumptive acute infection; obtain culture (see Fig. 88–21).
7. Rare–many WBC/LPF, and SEC often present; mixed gram-negative bacilli; chaining or clumping gram-positive cocci may also be present.
   Impression: presumptive chronic infection often precipitated by instrumentation; obtain culture.
8. Male: generally older than 45 years; WBC and Gardnerella-type bacilli (often in clumps).
   Impression: prostatism with a microbial component and not a cystitis.

*Entire film (0.01 ml of unspun urine) screened under low-power magnification and at least 10 oil immersion fields examined.
†WBC (white blood cells)/LPF (low-power field): rare, 1–3; few, 4–10; moderate, 11–25; many, more than 25.
‡Organisms/OIF (oil immersion field): 10^5/ml, averages 1/OIF for 10 OIF; 6×10^4/ml to 9×10^4/ml, 5–9 in 10 OIF; 10^4/ml to 5×10^4/ml, 1–5 in 10 OIF.

Chart 88–4. Microbiology Algorithm: Male Urogenital Tract Infections Gram-Stained Smear Evaluation*

---

1. Many neutrophils; gram-negative diplococci; "key" cells (at least three pairs of cocci intracellular and no other organisms).
   Impression: neisserial, presumptive *Neisseria gonorrhoeae* infection (see Fig. 88–20).
2. Many leukocytes and squamous epithelial cells (SEC) may be present; many phagocytized microbes.
   Impression: microbial (could be *Gardnerella, Escherichia, Streptococcus, Candida, Haemophilus*); may be secondary to viral or chlamydial urethritis.
3. At least 10 WBC/high-power field (HPF); scattered round-to-cuboidal epithelial cells; no organisms or meatal "skin" flora (diphtheroids, micrococci).
   Impression: nongonococcal urethritis.
4. Many intact mixed WBCs; foamy macrophages; no specific microbial agent seen in Gram stain.
   Impression: nongonococcal urethritis; possible viral or chlamydial urethritis.
5. Many WBCs; no specific microbial agent seen in Gram stain.
   Impression: nongonococcal urethritis; rule out trichomoniasis.
6. Chancres
   soft: chancroid—*Haemophilus ducreyi*: Gram stain of chancre exudate not of much value because of microbial contamination.
   hard: syphilis—*Treponema pallidum*: darkfield microscopic examination and/or serologic tests necessary as organism does not take the Gram stain as does *Treponema genitalis*.

---

*At least five different portions of the smear must be examined with low-power and oil immersion lens.

Chart 88–5. Microbiology Algorithm: Female Urogenital Tract Infections Gram-Stained Smear Evaluation*

General Statement:
Normal vaginal-cervical secretions vary among women and in each throughout the menstrual cycle. Lactobacilli are the normal resident flora, but occasionally other acidophilic organisms such as *Escherichia* and streptococci may be present.
Leukocytes (WBC) and erythrocytes (RBC) are also found periodically, often in large numbers.
1. Many squamous epithelial cells (SEC); WBCs, few to many, may be present; normal flora are numerous.
   Impression: normal flora (Fig. 88–17).
2. Cellular aspect as in No. 1: lactobacilli and yeast-type fungal elements are prominent.
   Impression: if pseudomycelium and budding yeast cells are present, candidiasis; specific diagnosis of *Candida albicans* if germ tube is seen in the smear (see Fig. 88–18).
   Impression: if only budding yeast cells are seen, may be *Torulopsis glabrata (Candida glabrata)*.
3. Many WBCs; SECs may or may not be present; abnormal bacterial flora are generally abundant and mixed.
   Impression: *Trichomonas vaginalis* may be present; discernible with low-power scanning (see Fig. 88–19).
   Impression: *Neisseria gonorrhoeae* may be present; diagnosis is established if "key" cell (at least three pairs of intracellular gram-negative diplococci and no other organisms are seen) is present.
4. Many WBCs and SECs; many small, gram-variable, pleomorphic bacilli; these may be phagocytized and/or the SECs may be completely covered by adhering organisms ("clue" cells).
   Impression: *Gardnerella vaginalis*.†
5. Many WBCs; SECs may or may not be prominent; many small, slightly curved, slender, gram-negative bacilli with pointed ends.
   Impression: *Mobiluncus* sp.
6. Mixed WBCs and SECs in variable numbers; one of the following organisms may be predominant in a mixed flora (*Escherichia, Clostridium, Bacillus, Staphylococcus*).
   Impression: Some strains of these organisms produce enzymes, such as lecithinase, which may act as a mucosal irritant.
7. Many cervical epithelial cells; sometimes their nuclei are naked; few other cellular components are present; resident flora are generally few in number.
   Impression: chronic cervicitis; postmenopausal.

---

*At least five different portions of the smear must be examined with low-power and oil immersion lens.
†Special stains, serologic tests, and possibly cultural procedures are necessary to rule out chlamydia, viruses, mycoplasma, etc.[45–47]

(vaginal epithelial cells stippled with small coccobacilli).[58] The wet preparation will reveal many coccobacilli, often in clumps, floating between the epithelial cells and, at times, the "clue" cells.[59] This form of vaginitis is susceptible to metronidazole.[59, 60] Action against symbiotic anaerobic bacteria may be the mechanism of response.[61]

The wet preparation (a drop of vaginal secretion mixed with a drop of saline) examined under high-dry power is also useful for diagnosing trichomoniasis.[62, 63] The motile, pear-shaped organisms are slightly larger than polymorphonuclear leukocytes (see Fig. 88–19). Because the organisms "round up" when they die and are difficult to differentiate from white blood cells, the wet preparation should be examined immediately. The sensitivity of the wet preparation has been estimated at approximately 76 per cent.[62, 63]

Candidiasis can also be diagnosed by wet mount with a sensitivity ranging from 40 to 80 per cent.[59, 61] Mixing the discharge with 10 per cent potassium hydroxide (KOH) or sodium hydroxide (NaOH) solution and briefly heating the slide will lyse the other cellular elements, thus aiding in the visualization of the fungi. The hydroxide wet mount is not suitable for determining the presence of trichomonads. The sensitivity of the Gram stain for candidiasis (see Fig. 88–18) has been estimated to approach 100 per cent.[64]

Exudates (Other Than Respiratory or Urogenital)

Cutaneous exudates represent a significant portion of the clinical materials submitted to the microbiology laboratory (Figs. 88–11 through 88–15). Smear correlation with culture result is rarely a problem, but this information does not always contribute to the immediate care of the patient. Unopened abscesses, furuncles, and vesicles are excellent sources of diagnostic smears when sampled immediately upon incision and drainage, and yield approximately 100 per cent accuracy. Spontaneously draining abscesses, abrasions, ulcers, and wounds, however, are not adequate sources of smears.

After gentle cleansing with saline-soaked gauze, the extending edge of shallow ulcers generally supplies stained films accurately portraying host-reactive cells with probable specific etiologic associated microbes. In Fig. 88–16, a 10 per cent NaOH or KOH wet mount of skin scrapings from a shallow, slightly raised, discolored lesion confirms the clinical diagnosis of tinea versicolor due to *Pityrosporum orbiculare*. The acid-fast stain of an ulcer-like lesion may reveal acid-fast organisms that could be *Mycobacterium marinum*, *M. ulcerans*, or *M. leprae*.

In deep lesions, such as osteomyelitis, it is necessary to penetrate more deeply to obtain exudate. Too often, surface exudate will yield a potentially pathogenic microbe mistakenly considered the causative agent, which is located much deeper in the lesion.

A knowledge of the location of the lesion is essential to the microscopist. Proximity to the various body apertures increases the risk of transposed resident flora contaminating lesions or aggravating infections initiated by another microbe.

One special technique, the *Tzanck smear*, is an important tool in the rapid diagnosis of viral infections.[65] The Tzanck smear offers several advantages to the emergency physician. It is inexpensive; simple to perform; and provides timely, reliable, diagnostic information.[66]

The Tzanck smear is most reliable in the diagnosis of herpes simplex and varicella-zoster infections. The sensitivity of the smear in the vesicular, pustular, and crusted stages is 67 per cent, 55 per cent and 17 per cent, respectively.[67, 68] In expert hands, sensitivity, specificity, and positive and nega-

tive predictive values are 80 per cent, 90 per cent, 88 per cent, and 82 per cent, respectively.[66] The Tzanck smear may actually be superior to direct immunofluorescence assay and culture results.[69] One disadvantage should be mentioned. The microscopic cytomorphology of varicella-zoster and herpes simplex infections is identical. Therefore the Tzanck smear is not able to differentiate between these types of infections.[66]

Although the technique is relatively simple, care needs to be taken to optimize results. Sampling early vesicular and multiple lesions maximizes the possibility of a positive preparation.[70] The Tzanck test is insensitive on lesions that have spontaneously ruptured to become shallow ulcers.[71] A number 15 scalpel is used to unroof the vesicle, and the fluid is blotted away with a cotton swab. The blade is then used to scrape the base of the lesions to collect a sample of cells. Care should be taken not to cause bleeding, since blood cells will make interpretation difficult. Once an adequate sample has been collected, the cells should be transferred gently to the glass slide by touching the blade to the surface of the slide in a series of small rapid blots.[72] This will minimize smearing and crushing of cells. The slide is then air dried and stained with Wright-Giemsa or methylene blue stain. The slide is examined under low (100×) and high power (400×) for the presence of multinucleated giant cells diagnostic of infection with a herpes group virus.

Intestinal Tract

Commonly, a smear of a freshly passed portion of feces and, less commonly, smears of fecal exudate secured by proctoscopy or sigmoidoscopy may be subjected to microscopic examination. In recent years, swabs of the distal 2 to 3 cm of the anal mucosa with attendant stained smears have been studied with promising results (see Figs. 88–23 through 88–27). Multiple smears should be prepared so that a Gram stain and a Wright-Giemsa stain can be done. Methylene blue staining of wet mounts for leukocytes and microbes may be desired.[21]

Exudate from the anorectal or sigmoid mucosa has been important in various instances, reducing the problem of determining the etiologic agent from the abundant resident flora. A report of a *Streptococcus pyogenes* epidemic due to an anal mucosa carrier was published by McIntyre.[73] Schroeter and Reynolds[74] reported that 30 per cent of the failures in the treatment of gonorrhea in 908 female patients would have been missed if rectal mucosa cultures had not been done concurrently with cultures of the cervical site. Unfortunately, direct smears were not done in either of the aforementioned studies. Other studies have reported a 30 to 48 per cent sensitivity rate of the rectal smear in detecting the presence of gonorrhea.[49, 75]

In another report, direct Gram-stained smears of anal mucosa exudate from a homosexual male revealed the presence of numerous treponemes.[76] Therapeutic clearing of the organisms and exudate with antibiotics occurred, suggesting a treponemal etiology. Microscopic examination of exudate from numerous bleeding petechiae in another patient undergoing sigmoidoscopy revealed an overwhelming number of treponemes, accounting in all probability for the positive fecal occult blood. Using the Gram stain, Quinn and associates[77] reported the presence of anorectal leukocytic exudate in 42 of 52 male homosexuals. In 28 of these men and in 2 of 10 men without an exudate, one or more probable etiologic agents were identified. Despite the purulent exudates, the etiologic agents, including *N. gonorrhoeae* in 7 men, were not always seen by Gram stain.

Gram-stained and Wright-Giemsa–stained thin smears

of fluid feces can aid in the diagnosis of giardiasis, cryptosporidiosis, and other diarrhea-causing agents.[78, 79] Ho and colleagues[80] found that the Gram stain of stool was greater than 43 per cent sensitive and greater than 99 per cent specific for *Campylobacter* enteritis. An S-shaped (equivalent sign) or "seagull"-shaped gram-negative curved rod was found to be diagnostic of *Campylobacter jejuni*. False-positive smears were rare. Direct wet mount smears of fluid feces that are examined when they are freshly passed and warm may be more rapid aids in establishing an early diagnosis of strongyloidiasis (larva), of amebiasis (trophozoite), giardiasis (trophozoite), cryptosporidiosis (oocyst), and other parasitic infections. Immunocompromised patients are at high risk for superinfection with various protozoan parasites and with the helminth *Strongyloides stercoralis*.[78–82]

The macroscopic examination of formed feces may frequently reveal the clearly visible (2 × 1 cm or larger) proglottids of Taenia, especially *Taenia saginata*, the beef tapeworm, or the less visible (about 1 cm × 0.5 mm) female gravid *Enterobius vermicularis*, the pinworm.[83] Even when the macroscopic examination is negative, the modified Graham cellulose tape technique, in which the adhesive side of the tape is first applied to the perianal folds and then placed adhesive side down on a glass slide,[84, 85] is a microscopic examination that can be easily and rapidly carried out and is very effective.[86] The characteristic spherical ova of Taenia (35 micron diameter), containing a hexacanth embryo (six hooklets), or the characteristic egg-shaped ova of *Enterobius* (about 60 × 26 microns), containing a motile embryo, are easily recognized and identified using the low-power (100×) and the high-dry power (450×) microscope lens. A single negative examination does not rule out either of these parasites because of variables that can alter the findings, such as bathing just before the examination, the time of the day that the collection is made, and so on. Consequently, multiple examinations may be necessary. One text suggests that seven examinations be carried out on different days before a negative diagnosis is reported.[87] Brugmans and coworkers[88] pointed out that analysis of a placebo treatment group yielded a false-negative rate (13 per cent [children] to 24 per cent [adults]) with either one or two examinations in the group that was negative before receiving the placebo but positive afterwards. The rate was 6 per cent (adults) to 14 per cent (children) in the group that was positive before receiving the placebo but negative afterwards.

CONCLUSION

In the last few years, there has been increased emphasis on the value of the direct analysis of clinical materials. This direct analysis may vary from an unstained wet mount (in saline or 10 per cent hydroxide) to variously stained wet mounts and dried thin smears. The microscope used may be compound, phase, darkfield, or fluorescent. The Gram-stained thin smear viewed through the compound microscope is the most familiar approach.

The expression that "An immediate Gram stain of a specimen often provides proof of goodwill; . . ."[89] is woefully inadequate. Although the patient is the primary beneficiary of this rapid and accurate tool, it must be stressed that the requestor is the recipient of the confidence factor. This may be defined as the laboratory-physical examination correlation. Moreover, the microbiologist also benefits because the direct analysis provides a very basic type of quality control by delineating the quality of the submitted specimen, the degree and type of host reaction, if any, and the probable etiologic agent. With this information, the microbiologist can determine whether to proceed with culture of the specimen, what substrates to use in culturing it, and what results to expect.

In this text, special emphasis is placed on the fact that the same value can be obtained from direct analysis of materials from the upper respiratory tract as from other areas or tracts of the body.

In any area in which there is an abundant resident flora, knowledge of the components of such a flora and a careful collection technique will eliminate any hesitancy in "reading" such smears and producing a rapid, highly accurate smear report.

REFERENCES

1. Newman JP: Diagnostic bacteriological procedures and the practitioner. MSU Veterinarian, Fall 1958, p11.
2. Blenden DC: Bacteriology in the veterinarian's office. Vet Scope 9:7, 1959.
3. Brancato FP, Parker MJ: The stained direct smear of clinical material. Health Lab Sci 3:69, 1966.
4. Path Capsule 26. The routine throat culture. College of American Pathologists, 1965.
5. Provine H, Gardner P: The Gram-stained smear and its interpretation. Hosp Prac 85, 1974.
6. Baker LH, Hodges GR: Examination of pharyngeal secretions to determine the etiology of pharyngitis. Am J Med Sci 272:89, 1976.
7. Hedges JR, Wagner DK: Pharyngeal gram stains in the treatment of sore throats. JACEP 7:229, 1978.
8. Heinemann HS, Chawla JK, Lofton WM: Misinformation from sputum cultures without microscopic examination. J Clin Microbiol 6:518, 1977.
9. Bartlett RC, Tetreault J, Evers J, et al: Quality assurance of Gram-stained direct smears. Am J Clin Pathol 72:984, 1979.
10. Crawford G, Brancato F, Holmes K: Streptococcal pharyngitis: Diagnosis by Gram stain. Ann Int Med 90:293, 1979.
11. Sharma SC, Subbukrishnan P: Streptococcal pharyngitis—rapid diagnosis by Gram stain. Postgrad Med J 57:13, 1981.
12. Jui J, Norton R, Edminster S, et al. Gram stain for streptococcal pharyngitis. Ann Emerg Med 14:191, 1985.
13. Washington JA II: Use and abuse of the Gram-stained smear. Clin Microbiol Newsletter 1:4, 1979.
14. Willis HH, Cummings MM: Diagnostic and Experimental Methods in Tuberculosis. 2nd ed. Springfield, Ill, Charles C Thomas Publishing Co, 1952, p 95.
15. Barry AL, Smith PB, Turck M: Laboratory diagnosis of urinary tract infections. Cumitech 2. American Society of Microbiologists, Washington, DC, April, 1975.
16. Isenberg HD, Schoenknecht FD, von Graenitz A: Collection and processing of bacteriological specimens. Cumitech 9. American Society of Microbiologists, Washington, DC, August 1979.
17. Rosebury T: Life on Man. New York, Berkley Publishing Group, 1952.
18. Kellogg DS Jr, Holmes KK, Hill GA: Laboratory diagnosis of gonorrhea. Cumitech 4. American Society of Microbiologists, Washington, DC, October 1976.
19. Magee CM, Rodehaever GT, Edgerton MT, et al: A more reliable gram staining technique for diagnosis of surgical infections. Am J Surg 130:341, 1975.
20. Macher AM: Presented at 22nd Interscience Conference on Antimicrobial Agents and Chemotherapy. 1982.
21. Nair CP: Rapid staining of intestinal amoeba on wet mounts. Nature 172:1051, 1953.
22. Kronvall G, Myhre E: Differential staining of bacteria in clinical specimens using acridine orange buffered at low pH. Acta Pathol Microbiol Scand (B) 85:249, 1977.
23. Murray PR: Principles and uses of bacterial stains. API Species 6:1, 1982.
24. Keitel HG: Pitfalls in laboratory tests. Pediatr Clin North Am 12:17, 1965.
25. Bannatyne RM, Clausen C, McCarthy LR: Laboratory diagnosis of upper respiratory tract infections. Cumitech 10. American Society of Microbiologists, Washington, DC, December 1979.
26. Wood RW, Tomkins RK, Wolcott BW: An efficient strategy for managing acute respiratory illness in adults. Ann Intern Med 93:757, 1980.
27. Rein MF: Gonorrhea. In Practice of Medicine, Vol III. New York, Harper & Row, Publishers, 1975, pp 1–18.
28. Epstein RL: Constituent of sputum: A simple method. Ann Intern Med 77:259, 1972.
29. Chodosh S: Examination of sputum cells. N Engl J Med 282:854, 1970.
30. Bartlett RC: How fast to go—how far to go. In Lorian V (ed): Significance of Medical Microbiology in the Care of Patients. Baltimore, Williams & Wilkins, 1977, pp 15–35.
31. Quintiliani R: Complete abandonment urged for expectorated sputum tests. Clinical Lab Forum: July, 1971.
32. Barrett-Connor E: Nonvalue of sputum culture in the diagnosis of pneumococcal pneumonia. Am Rev Respir Dis 103:845, 1971.
33. Geckler RW, Gremillion DH, McAllister CK, et al: Microscopic and bacteriological comparison of paired sputa and transtracheal aspirates. J Clin Microbiol 6:396, 1977.
34. Wong LK, Barry AL, Horgan SM: Comparison of six different criteria for judging the acceptability of sputum specimens. J Clin Microbiol 16:627, 1982.
35. Bartlett RC: Medical Microbiology: Quality, Cost, and Clinical Relevance. New York, John Wiley & Sons, 1974, pp 24–31.

36. Barry AL: Clinical specimens for microbiologic examination. In Hoeprich PD (ed): Infectious Diseases. 2nd ed. New York, Harper & Row, 1978, pp 92–96.
37. Murray PR, Washington JA II: Microscopic and bacteriologic analysis of expectorated sputum. Mayo Clin Proc 50:339, 1975.
38. Van Scoy RE: Bacterial sputum cultures: A clinician's viewpoint. Mayo Clin Proc 52:39, 1977.
39. Heinemann HS, Radano RR: Acceptability and cost savings of selective sputum microbiology in a community teaching hospital. J Clin Microbiol 10:567, 1979.
40. Beeson PB: Editorial: The case against the catheter. Am J Med 24:1, 1958.
41. Kimmelstiel P, Kim OJ, Beres J, et al: Chronic pyelonephritis. Am J Med 30:589, 1961.
42. Kaye D: Host defense mechanisms in the urinary tract. Urol Clin North Am 2:407, 1975.
43. Barbin GK, Thorley JD, Reinarz JA: Simplified microscopy for rapid detection of significant bacteriuria in random urine specimens. J Clin Microbiol 7:286, 1978.
44. Kunin CM: The quantitative significance of bacteria visualized in the unstained urinary sediment. N Engl J Med 265:589, 1961.
45. Paavonen J: Chlamydia trachomatis-induced urethritis in female partners of men with nongonococcal urethritis. Sex Transm Dis 6:69, 1979.
46. Stamm WE, Wagner KF, Amsel R, et al: Etiology of acute urethral syndrome (abstract). Clin Res 1:79, 1980.
47. Greenberg RN, Rein MF, Sanders CV, et al: Urethral syndrome in women. JAMA 245:923, 1981.
48. Wald ER: Gonorrhea: Diagnosis by Gram stain in the female adolescent. Am J Dis Child 131:1094, 1977.
49. Rothenberg RB, Simon R, Chipperfield E, et al: Efficacy of selected diagnostic tests for sexually transmitted disease. JAMA 235:49, 1976.
50. Caldwell JG, Price EU, Pagin GJ, et al: Sensitivity and reproductivity of Thayer-Martin culture medium in diagnosing gonorrhea in women. Am J Obstet Gynecol 109:463, 1971.
51. Parisen H, Farmer AD: Diagnosis of gonorrhea in the asymptomatic female. South Med J 61:505, 1968.
52. Thin RNT, Williams IA, Nicol CS: Direct and delayed methods of immunofluorescent diagnosis of gonorrhea in women. Br J Vener Dis 47:27, 1970.
53. Lossick JG, Smeltzer MP, Curran JW: The value of the cervical Gram stain in the diagnosis and treatment of gonorrhea in women in a venereal disease clinic. Sex Transm Dis 9:124, 1982.
54. Tokarski PA: Sexual abuse of the child. Top Emerg Med 3:15–21, 1982.
55. Folland DS, Burke RE, Hinman AR, et al: Gonorrhea in preadolescent children: An inquiry into source of infection and mode of transmission. Pediatrics 60:153, 1977.
56. Farrell MK, Billmire ME, Shamroy JA, et al: Prepubertal gonorrhea: A multidisciplinary approach. Pediatrics 67:151, 1981.
57. Handsfield HH, Lipman TD, Harnish JP, et al: Asymptomatic gonorrhea in men: Diagnosis, natural course, prevalence, and significance. N Engl J Med 209:117, 1974.
58. Smith RF, Rodgers HA, Hines PA, et al: Comparisons between direct microscopic and cultural methods for recognition of Corynebacterium vaginale in women with vaginitis. J Clin Microbiol 5:268, 1977.
59. Balsdon MJ, Taylor GE, Pead L, et al: Corynebacterium vaginale and vaginitis: A controlled trial of treatment. Lancet 1:501, 1980.
60. Pheifer TA, Forsyth PS, Durfee MA, et al: Nonspecific vaginitis role of Haemophilus vaginalis and treatment with metronidazole. N Engl J Med 298:1429, 1978.
61. Spiegal CA, Amsel R, Eschenbach D, et al: Anaerobic bacteria in nonspecific vaginitis. N Engl J Med 303:601, 1980.
62. McClennon MT, Smith JM, McClennon CE: Diagnosis of vaginal mycosis and trichomoniasis. Reliability of cytologic smear, wet smear, and culture. Obstet Gynecol 40:231, 1972.
63. Nagesha CN, Ananthakrishna WL, Sulochana P: Clinical and laboratory studies on vaginal trichomoniasis. Am J Obstet Gynecol 106:933, 1970.
64. Eddie DAS: The laboratory diagnosis of vaginal infection caused by Trichomonas and Candida (Monilia) species. J Med Microbiol 1:153, 1968.
65. Tzanck A: Le cytodiagnostic immédiat en dermatologie. Ann Dermatol Syph 8:205, 1948.
66. Oranje AP, Elzo Folkers: The Tzanck smear: Old, but still inestimable value. Pediatr Dermatol 5:127, 1988.
67. Solomon AR, Rasmussen JE, Weiss JS: A comparison of the Tzanck smear and viral isolation in varicella and herpes zoster. Arch Dermatol 122:282, 1986.
68. Folkers E, Poranje A, Duivenvoorden JN, et al: Tzanck smear in diagnosing genital herpes. Genitourin Med 64:249, 1988.
69. Sadick NS, Swenson PD, Kaufman RL, Kaplan MH: Comparison of detection of varicella-zoster virus by the Tzanck smear, direct immunofluorescence with a monoclonal antibody, and virus isolation. J Am Acad Dermatol 17:64, 1987.
70. Solomon AR, Rasmussen JE, Varani J, et al: The Tzanck smear in the diagnosis of cutaneous herpes simplex. JAMA 251:633, 1984.
71. Brown ST, Jaffe HW, Zaidi A, et al: Sensitivity and specificity of diagnostic tests for genital infection with Herpes hominis. Sex Transm Dis 6:10, 1979.
72. Solomon AR: The Tzanck smear: Viable and valuable in the diagnosis of herpes simplex, zoster, and varicella. Int J Dermatol 25:169, 1986.
73. McIntyre DM: An epidemic of Streptococcus pyogenes puerperal and postoperative sepsis with an unusual carrier site—the anus. Am J Obstet Gynecol 101:308, 1968.
74. Schroeter AL, Reynolds G: The rectal culture as a test of cure of gonorrhea in the female. J Infect Dis 125:499, 1972.
75. Bhattacharyya MN, Jephcott AE: Diagnosis of gonorrhoea in women. Role of the rectal sample. Br J Vener Dis 50:109, 1974.
76. Kaplan LR, Takeuchi A: Purulent rectal discharge associated with a nontreponemal spirochete. JAMA 241:52, 1979.
77. Quinn TC, Corey L, Chaffee RG, et al: The etiology of anorectal infections in homosexual men. Am J Med 71:395, 1981.
78. Tzipori S, Angus KW, Gray EW, et al: Vomiting and diarrhea associated with cryptosporidial infection (letter). N Engl J Med 303:818, 1980.
79. Garcia LS, et al: Clinical laboratory diagnosis of Cryptosporidium from human fecal specimens. Clin Microbiol Newsletter 4:136, 1982.
80. Ho DD, Ault MJ, Ault MA, et al: Campylobacter enteritis: Early diagnosis with Gram's stain. Arch Int Med 142:1858, 1982.
81. Parasite causes death in immunodeficient patients. JAMA (Medical News) 224:581, 1973.
82. Bradley SL, Dines DE, Brewer NS: Disseminated Strongyloides stercoralis in an immunosuppressed host. Mayo Clin Proc 53:332, 1978.
83. Markell EK, Voge M: Medical Parasitology. 5th ed. Philadelphia, W. B. Saunders Company, 1981.
84. Graham CF: A device for the diagnosis of Enterobius vermicularis. Am J Trop Med 21:159, 1941.
85. Brooke MM, Donaldson AW, Mitchell RB: A method of supplying cellulose tape to physicians for diagnosis of enterobiasis. Public Health Rep 64:897, 1949.
86. Mazzotti L, Osorio MT: The diagnosis of enterobiasis. Comparative study of the Graham and Hall techniques in the diagnosis of enterobiasis. J Lab Clin Med 30:1046, 1945.
87. Kolmer JA, Boerner F: Approved Laboratory Technic. 4th ed. East Norwalk, Conn, D Appleton-Century Co, 1945, p 571.
88. Brugmans JP, Thienpont DC, van Wijngaarden I, et al: Mebendazole in enterobiasis: Radiochemical and pilot clinical study in 1,278 subjects. JAMA 217:313, 1971.
89. Isenberg HD: The role of clinical microbiology in health care. American Society of Microbiologists Newsletter 48:101, 1982.

Description of Photomicrographs in Figures 88–1 Through 88–6

Figure Number	Source	Preparation	Chart Index	Description	Interpretation	Comment
88–1	Throat	Gram	Chart 88–1 (#1)	Squamous epithelial cells; resident flora	Normal	
88–2	Throat	Gram	Chart 88–1 (#2)	*Ciliocytophthoria* (cough cells); resident flora	Viral	Coughing is a primary symptom of viral upper respiratory tract infection
88–3	Throat	Gram	Chart 88–1 (#9)	Disrupted leukocytes; associated spherical gram-positive cocci	Streptococcal (*Streptococcus pyogenes*)	Generally in pairs or singly; rarely very short chains
88–4	Throat	Gram	Chart 88–1 (#10)	Disrupted leukocytes; gram-negative bacilli (slightly curved and pointed ends) and undulating fine filaments	Vincent disease (*Fusobacterium* and *Treponema*)	Anaerobic entity; generally secondary infection; other bacteria often present
88–5	Throat	Gram	Chart 88–1 (#11)	Leukocytes generally intact; associated slender, pleomorphic, gram-positive bacilli	Arcanobacterium (*Corynebacterium haemolyticum*)	Often mimic streptococcal infection, even including rash
88–6	Sputum	Gram	Chart 88–2 (#4)	Leukocytes; "foamy" macrophages; many small gram-negative coccobacilli	Viral with *Haemophilus*	Part of resident flora; this bacillus is often very numerous in viral infections

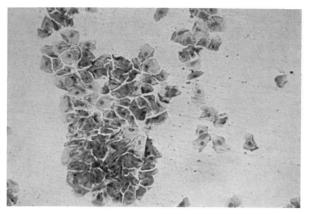

Figure 88–1.

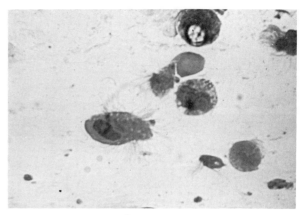

Figure 88–2.

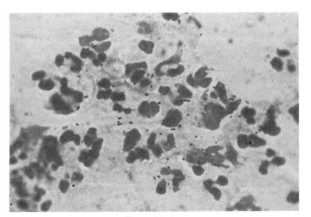

Figure 88–3.

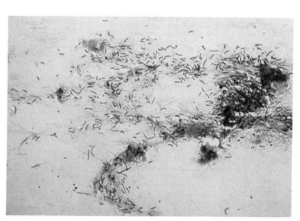

Figure 88–4.

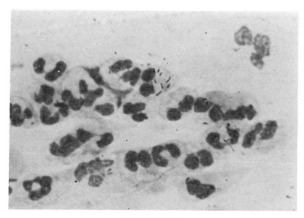

Figure 88–5.

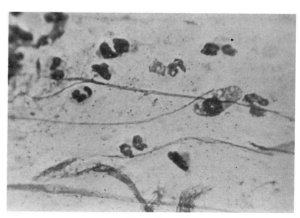

Figure 88–6.

Description of Photomicrographs in Figures 88–7 through 88–12

Figure Number	Source	Preparation	Chart Index	Description	Interpretation	Comment
88–7	Sputum	Gram	Chart 88–2 (#4)	Leukocytes; macrophages; numerous encapsulated elongated, gram-positive diplococci (short chains)	Viral with *Streptococcus pneumoniae*	As with *Haemophilus*
88–8	Sputum	Kinyoun		Slender, beaded, acid-fast bacilli	*Mycobacterium tuberculosis*	Specimen digested and concentrated
88–9	Sputum	Sodium hydroxide (10 per cent)		Two thick-walled spherules; squamous epithelial debris; resident flora	*Coccidioides immitis*	Easily seen on low power (100 ×) with controlled lighting
88–10	Sputum	Gram		Coiled, snake-like mucus strands	Curschmann spirals characteristic of bronchial asthma but may be encountered in other catarrhal conditions	Sometimes eosinophils and Charcot-Leyden crystals enveloped
88–11	Eye drainage	Gram		Fibrinoleukocytic debris; plump gram-negative diplobacilli	*Moraxella*	Resident flora of nasopharyngeal mucosa; reflects eye contamination by nasal discharge
88–12	Ear discharge	Gram		Cellular debris (leukocytes and epithelial cells); conidia and gram-variable fungal hypha	*Aspergillus* most likely	Slender gram-negative bacilli; pleomorphic gram-positive bacilli; gram-positive cocci also present

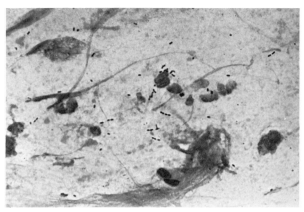

Figure 88–7.

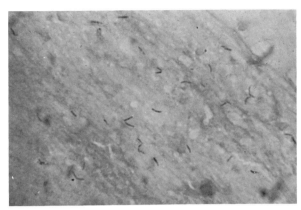

Figure 88–8.

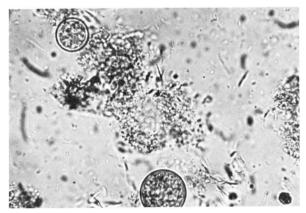

Figure 88–9.

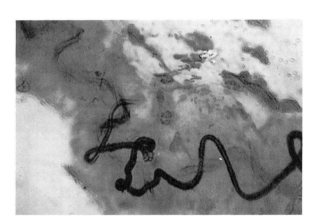

Figure 88–10.

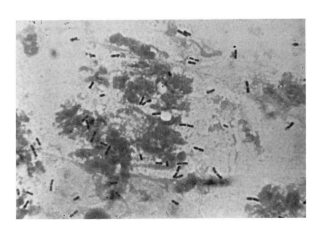

Figure 88–11.

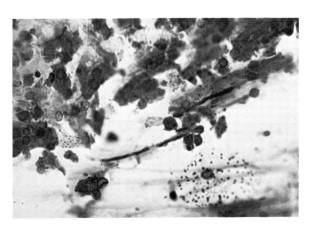

Figure 88–12.

Description of Photomicrographs in Figures 88–13 Through 88–18

Figure Number	Source	Preparation	Chart Index	Description	Interpretation	Comment
88–13	Cheek abscess	Gram		Many neutrophils; fragmented slender gram-positive filaments	Actinomycosis *(Actinomyces israelii)*	Resident flora of dentiginous crevices and tonsillar crypts—"sulfur" granule
88–14	Foot lesion	Gram		Many neutrophils; associated spherical gram-positive cocci in clumps	Staphylococcal *(Staphylococcus aureus)*	Often resident flora of skin and mucosa
88–15	Gangrene ankle	Gram		Large gram-positive bacilli in seroerythrocytic matrix; rare neutrophils	Gas gangrene *(Clostridium perfringens)*	Host reaction appears mild relative to the dangerous nature of the lesion
88–16	Skin scrapings from chest	Sodium hydroxide (10 per cent)		Squamous epithelial cells; clusters of spherules and short filaments	*Pityrosporum furfur* (formally *Malassezia furfur*)	Easily seen on low power; diagnostic of tinea versicolor
88–17	Vagina	Gram	Chart 88–5 (#1)	Squamous epithelial cells; uniform, moderately thick gram-positive bacilli; spermatozoa	Normal *(Lactobacillus)*	
88–18	Vagina	Gram	Chart 88–5 (#2)	Squamous epithelial cells and leukocytes; budding yeast cells and filaments; germ tube present	*Candida albicans*	The presence of germ tube is diagnostic

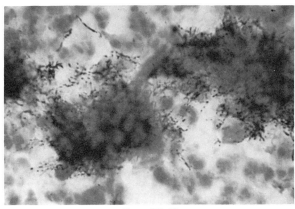

Figure 88–13.

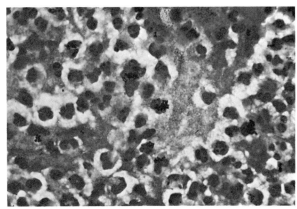

Figure 88–14.

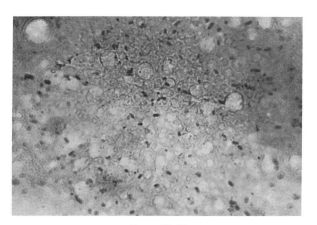

Figure 88–15.

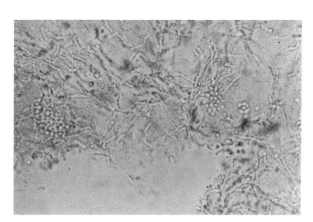

Figure 88–16.

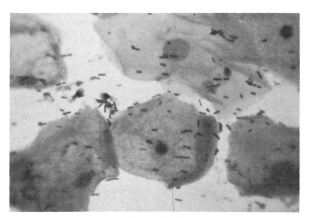

Figure 88–17.

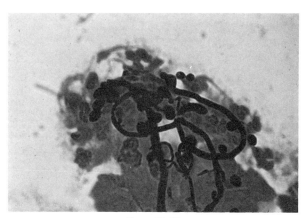

Figure 88–18.

Description of Photomicrographs in Figures 88–19 Through 88–24

Figure Number	Source	Preparation	Chart Index	Description	Interpretation	Comment
88–19	Vagina	Gram	Chart 88–5 (#3)	Neutrophils; four trichomonads	*Trichomonas vaginalis*	Flagella seen in two lenticular nuclei; small relative to cell size
88–20	Urethra	Gram	Chart 88–4 (#1)	Neutrophils; associated gram-negative diplococci (often intracellular)	Neisserial (*Neisseria gonorrhoeae*)	"Key" cells = only gram-negative diplococci within neutrophils
88–21	Urine	Gram	Chart 88–3 (#6)	Neutrophils; associated plump gram-negative bacilli	Coliforms (*Escherichia coli*)	Most common cause of acute bacterial urinary tract infection
88–22	Urine	Gram		Neutrophils; associated slender gram-negative bacilli	Pseudomonad (*Pseudomonas aeruginosa*)	Generally in chronic infections, especially after instrumentation
88–23	Fluid feces	Wright-Giemsa		Mucus shreds; leukocytes; fecal flora; protozoa	*Cryptosporidium* (approximately 4 microns in diameter)	Internal content took stain, but electron microscopy used for detail
88–24	Mucoid feces	Wright-Giemsa		Pear-shaped, binucleated protozoa; some fecal flora	*Giardia lamblia* trophozoites	

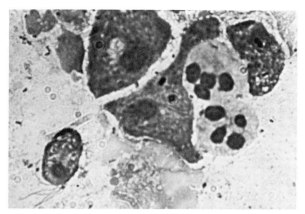

Figure 88–19.

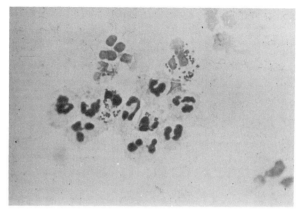

Figure 88–20.

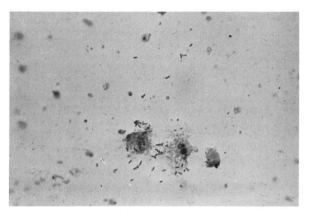

Figure 88–21.

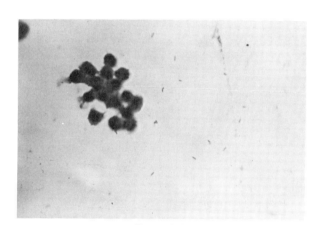

Figure 88–22.

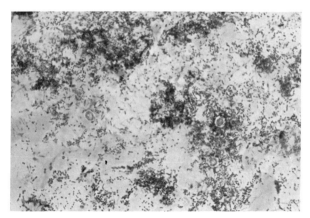

Figure 88–23.

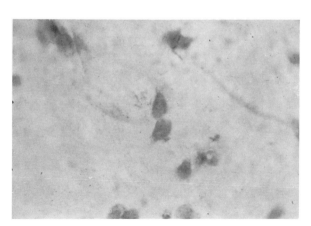

Figure 88–24.

Description of Photomicrographs in Figures 88–25 Through 88–27

Figure Number	Source	Preparation	Chart Index	Description	Interpretation	Comment
88–25	Anal folds	Cellulose tape		Multiple ovoid bodies	Ova of *Enterobius vermicularis*	Easily seen on low power
88–26	Fluid feces	Direct		*Amoeba* trophozoite with ingested yeast cells	Presumptive *Entamoeba histolytica*	Rapid directional mobility on warm mount
88–27	Fluid feces	Direct		Elongated, diamond-shaped crystals	Charcot-Leyden crystals in mucosal secretions following foreign body irritation; associated with elevated eosinophil levels	Exact nature unknown; generally in bronchial asthma and in amebic colitis

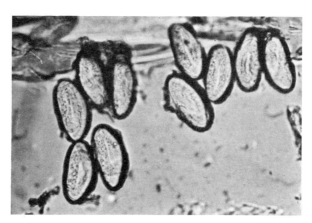

Figure 88–25.

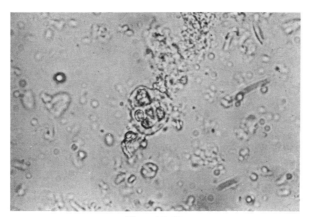

Figure 88–26.

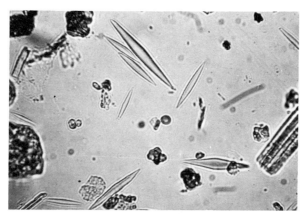

Figure 88–27.

Chapter 89

Rapid Microbial Detection Systems

A. Roy Magnusson and Jon Jui

INTRODUCTION

Evolving molecular biologic technologies have made rapid antigen or antibody detection a reality in everyday clinical practice. These techniques have enabled the clinician to make an earlier diagnosis, initiate earlier appropriate specific therapy, eliminate additional costly tests, shorten hospitalization time, and improve diagnostic accuracy. Commercial rapid antigen assay kits are available for the detection of group A streptococcal pharyngitis, *Neisseria gonorrhoeae*, and *Chlamydia trachomatis* endocervicitis or urethritis. In addition, rapid detection assays for the common organisms causing meningitis (*Haemophilus influenzae* type B, *Streptococcus pneumoniae*, group B streptococcus, *Neisseria meningitidis* [types A, B, C]) have been developed. Viable methods have also been developed for the rapid detection of pyuria, bacteriuria, and human immunodeficiency virus (HIV-1) antibody.[1-4]

Several different techniques have been used for detection of antigen or antibody. All techniques exploit the high degree of sensitivity and specificity of antigen-antibody interactions. The assays may contain either antigen to detect antibodies or antibodies to detect antigens. A variety of techniques have been used to amplify these reactions. These include such techniques as fluorescent staining, latex particle agglutination, enzyme-linked immunosorbent assay, countercurrent immunoelectrophoresis, radioimmunoassay, and staphylococcal coagglutination.

Immunofluorescent Staining. The immunofluorescent staining technique incubates the patient's fixed smears with a monoclonal antibody specific for an organism or group of organisms. Specific fluorescein-conjugated antiserum directed against the initial antibody is added to the monoclonal antibody attached smears. Finally, the prepared smears are examined by fluorescence microscopy. Fluorescence techniques, although sensitive, are not useful in quantification of antigens or antibodies. In addition, immunofluorescent staining requires the laboratory to maintain special diagnostic equipment and to train its personnel for proper interpretation of the smears.[5-7]

Latex Particle Agglutination and Coagglutination. Latex particle agglutination uses latex particles coated with antibody. A lattice forms in the presence of antigen; the resultant latex particle agglutination is visible to the observer. Nonspecific agglutination, detected by using control reagents, is the most common pitfall of this assay.

Coagglutination tests operate in a similar fashion, except coated inactivated staphylococci replace the latex beads. Staphylococci have a surface protein (protein A) that binds antibody via its Fc portion; the active site is then free to react with antigen. The agglutination of the staphylococcal cells makes the antigen-antibody reaction visible. The presence of specific antibodies to staphylococcal cell wall in the patient's specimen that cross react with the staphylococcal proteins of the assay can cause occasional false-positive reactions. Both agglutination techniques do not require special equipment and results are available in less than 15 minutes.[8, 9]

Enzyme-Linked Immunosorbent Assay. The classic enzyme-linked immunosorbent assay (ELISA) application uses test wells coated with antibody (or antigen). A monoclonal antihuman IgG specific to the antigen-antibody complex is linked to an enzyme such as peroxidase or alkaline phosphatase. This enzyme is used as an indicator, turning positive in the presence of an antigen-antibody complex.

Radioimmunoassay. A radioactive marker (such as I[125]) is linked to monoclonal human anti-IgG antibody. The emitted radiation indicates the presence of the antibody; the test is performed in a manner similar to ELISA.

Countercurrent Immunoelectrophoresis. In countercurrent immunoelectrophoresis, antigen is placed in a well on the cathode side of an agarose slide and electrophoresed toward the anode. Antibody is placed in the well on the anode side and migrates toward the cathode by endo-osmotic flow. A precipitin line forms at antibody-antigen equivalence. Because the majority of antigens of bacteria that cause meningitis are anions, the method is useful in the rapid diagnosis of central nervous system infection.[10-13]

CLINICAL APPLICATION OF IMMUNOCHEMICAL TECHNIQUES

Sexually Transmitted Diseases

CHLAMYDIA TRACHOMATIS

Genital infections with *C. trachomatis* are now recognized as a major public health problem in the United States. *C. trachomatis* may be responsible for as many as 50 per cent of the cases of nongonococcal urethritis in men and mucopurulent cervicitis in women. These infections, if left untreated, often produce serious sequelae such as epididymitis, endometritis, pelvic inflammatory disease, perihepatitis, and cervical dysplasia.[14] The clinical manifestations of *C. trachomatis* infections are often subtle and nonspecific, with many patients being asymptomatic. Effective diagnosis and identification of *Chlamydia* in clinical specimens have been difficult. *Chlamydia*, an obligate intracellular microorganism, requires cell culture systems to grow in vitro. These culture systems have several disadvantages. They are expensive, require a high level of quality control, are not readily available, and take 2 to 7 days to identify the presence of the organism.[15-17]

Two commercial kits that identify *Chlamydia* directly from smears of clinical specimens are available, making the diagnosis of chlamydial infections possible at medical facilities without tissue culture capabilities.

Fluorescent Antibody Technique (MicroTrak by SYVA). This method uses monoclonal antibodies that have been prepared against the major outer membrane protein of all 15 known human serovariants of *C. trachomatis*, for both forms of the organism: the infectious elementary body, and the metabolically active replicating reticulate body.[16] These antibodies are labeled with fluorescein isothiocyanate. When the specimen is applied directly to a slide well and stained, the antibody conjugate binds specifically to *C. trachomatis* present in the smear. Unbound antibody is rinsed away and the slide is viewed under a fluorescence microscope. Positive smears demonstrate apple green elementary or reticulate bodies contrasted by the reddish brown background of the counterstained cells.[16]

Collection Techniques. Specimen collection is a critical step in performing an accurate fluorescent antibody study. Even samples collected under study conditions result in inadequate specimens 12 per cent of the time.[15]

Recommended methods of attaining urethral samples in males require that a Dacron swab be inserted 2 to 4 cm into the urethra, then rotated gently and withdrawn. Cervical samples may be collected with either a brush or a small swab. The brush is recommended in women who are not pregnant. The cervical swabs may be used in pregnant women or if the cervical os is too small to admit the brush.

The exocervix is first wiped with a cotton or Dacron swab to remove excess mucus. The brush or swab is gently inserted into the os. The brush is left in place for 2 to 3 seconds, then rotated one full turn (360 degrees). The swab is simply rotated for 5 to 10 seconds. The brush or swab should be withdrawn without touching any vaginal surfaces.[15, 16, 18]

Methods for collecting rectal, conjunctival, and nasopharyngeal samples are outlined in the kit directions.[18]

Slides should be prepared immediately from the collected specimen. The swab or brush is rolled over the slide in an effort to cover the well evenly. After the slide is allowed to air dry, it is flooded with 0.5 ml of methanol provided in the kit. Again the slide is air dried and transported to the lab where specimens should be stored at room temperature and stained as soon as possible.[16, 18]

Wiping the cervix to clear debris deserves special mention. Embil and coworkers found that when multiple samples are taken, the first or second samples taken yielded 67 per cent positive results, while the fourth or fifth swabs yielded 82 per cent results. They suggest that the cervix must be cleared of debris to obtain cells that contain *Chlamydia*.[19]

Fluorescent Antibody Staining and Interpretation. The staining and interpretation of the slides require a certain amount of expertise as well as special equipment. Technicians require a minimum of 4 hours of microscope training time to read the slides accurately.[20]

Thirty microliters of reagent containing the fluorescent antibody is added to the slide and incubated for 15 minutes. The slide is then rinsed and mounting reagent added before coverslip placement. A fluorescent microscope is required to read the slide. At least 10 elementary bodies should be identifiable at a magnification of $400\times$ on the 8-mm slide for a test to be considered positive.[18, 20]

Several studies have reported sensitivity and specificity data for this method.[15, 16, 20–25] Sensitivity varies from 70 to 96 per cent. Specificity has been consistently high, ranging from 94 to 99 per cent. Although some investigators have suggested that decreasing the criteria for a positive test from 10 to 5 particles per slide would increase the sensitivity to 92 per cent, the recommended standard remains 10 stained particles per slide.[16, 18, 20]

ELISA Technique (Chlamydiazyme). The other commercial kit available involves the use of antibodies to *Chlamydia* and anti-IgG antibodies that are enzyme linked. Specimens are collected and then placed in specimen storage reagent for transport to the lab. Specimen buffer reagent is added and the solutions are incubated for 10 minutes. Samples are centrifuged for three 15-second cycles. They are then placed in plastic wells with one polystyrene bead each and incubated for 45 minutes. The beads are washed, and rabbit antibody to *Chlamydia* is added to the wells and incubated for 45 minutes. After a washing, peroxidase conjugated antibody to rabbit immunoglobulin is added and incubated for 45 minutes. Finally, the specimens are then placed in a spectrophotometer for analysis of color change. If antigen is present in the specimen, the rabbit antibody will attach to it. Subsequently the peroxidase-conjugated antibody to rabbit antibody will attach to the complex, thus fixing the enzyme to the antigen and producing a color change.[26]

When compared with culture results, the sensitivity of this method is 82 to 86 per cent and specificity is 90 to 98 per cent.[27, 28]

Neisseria Gonorrhoeae

Gonozyme. Rapid diagnosis of gonococcal infections would be clinically advantageous and commercial kits have been developed for this purpose. To date, no commercially available test has proven optimal for direct detection of gonococcal antigen in patient specimens.

Two commercial tests show promise. Gonodecten (Gd; U.S. Packaging Corp., LaPorte, Ind.) is a 3-minute test that detects cytochrome oxidase enzymes produced by *N. gonorrhoeae* in urethral discharge.[29] This test in symptomatic males is sensitive and a useful screening method.

The Gonozyme test (Abbott Laboratories, North Chicago, Ill.) detects gonococcal antigen, and results are available within 1 hour. The Gonozyme test has a sensitivity of 95 to 100 per cent and a specificity of 97 to 100 per cent when used in male patients seen in a high-risk setting.[30, 31] However, the predictive value of this test in patient populations with low prevalence of disease is questionable.[32, 33] In addition, the specificity of this test is low enough in women to require a confirmation culture to eliminate the possibility of a false-positive test.[32–36] Finally, the Gonozyme test is unable to detect the presence of antibiotic-resistant strains of *N. gonorrhoeae*, a significant clinical problem in many areas of the country.[30]

Thus the combination of Gram stain and culture remains the mainstay for the diagnosis of *N. gonorrhoeae* infections.

Meningitis

Rapid antigen tests have been commercially available to detect the capsular polysaccharide antigens of the commonly diagnosed meningeal pathogens. However, Gram stain and culture of the cerebrospinal fluid (CSF) remain the standard method of determining the etiologic diagnosis of bacterial meningitis.

Wilson and Smith noted that 78 per cent (70 of 89) of positive patient specimens detected by the latex particle agglutination (LPA) Bactigen tests had the appropriate organism detected on Gram-stained smears of CSF. False-positive results are uncommon with CSF LPA tests, although false-positive reactions have occurred in urine samples even with preboiling.[37] These tests are of particular use in the setting of a patient with negative blood cultures, CSF cultures, and Gram stains.

CIE, LPA, and CoA are currently the CSF antigen detection techniques available in most clinical laboratories. The majority of investigations have found LPA to detect lower amounts of antigen than CIE or CoA.[37, 38–41] The capsular polysaccharide of *H. influenzae* type B is the most reliably detected of the four most commonly seen organisms.[37]

Haemophilus Influenzae *Type B*

The sensitivity of immunochemical tests in detection of *H. influenzae* is greater than with other similar bacterial antigens.[37] This has been explained by the need to develop antisera against only one strain of one organism. Both LPA and CoA were similar in sensitivity and both were superior to CIE.[38, 42–44] The percentage of positive tests compared to culture-positive CSF samples ranges from 54 to 92 per cent for CIE to 94 to 100 per cent for LPA and CoA.[45–49, 50] Gram-stained smears were more sensitive than CIE and nearly as sensitive as LPA.[48] Both CIE and LPA detected antigen in some samples of negative Gram-stained smears.[48–50] False-positive results were uncommon with all techniques and ranged from 0.1 to 0.5 per cent.[37]

Concentrated urine specimens have also been used to detect *H. influenzae* antigen. In culture-positive CSF samples, both CIE and LPA detected *H. influenzae* antigen in the concentrated urine in 91 per cent of cases.[51] In a few culture-negative samples, both CIE and LPA techniques detected antigen.[52] Certain investigators have found the indirect enzyme-linked immunosorbent assay to be highly sensitive and specific in detecting *H. influenzae* type B antigen.[41, 53, 54]

However, the commercial application of this technology is currently not available.

NEISSERIA MENINGITIDIS

Detection of bacterial antigen of *N. meningitidis* depends on the serogroup of *N. meningitidis* encountered. The combination of patients from multiple studies suggests the most sensitive of the techniques is LPA detecting 78 per cent of meningococcal antigen.[37] In contrast, the CIE method detects 60 per cent and CoA 39 per cent of patients with meningococcal meningitis.[9, 13, 37, 48, 55–59] The majority of the clinical trials have been performed on patients with group A and C meningococcal infections, which account for only 25 per cent of the meningococcal infections in the United States.

Only limited data are available with group B meningococcal infections. Several investigators have noted the difficulty in detecting *N. meningitidis* group B polysaccharide antigen by LPA with the sensitivity of LPA ranging from 60 to 80 per cent.[9, 37, 50, 53, 60] CIE has not proven to be of value with this antigen.[50, 53] Williams and Hart report the use of the LPA preparations using monoclonal meningococcal group B antibody (Wellcome Diagnostics). Seven of the eight CSF (87 per cent) specimens of *N. meningitidis* were positive by LPA.[61]

Antigen tests were more often positive in Gram-stained negative meningococcal samples than with other pathogens. CoA is relatively insensitive. False-positive results were distinctly uncommon but have been noted in patients with *Escherichia coli* infections.[38]

STREPTOCOCCUS PNEUMONIAE

Detection of *S. pneumoniae* by CIE, CoA, and LPA ranges from 67 to 100 per cent.[37] LPA is the most promising technique. A number of investigators report 65 to 100 per cent sensitivity using this technique.[37, 39, 40, 61] False-positive results have been rare and have occurred in patients with *E. coli, Klebsiella,* or meningococcal infections.[38, 39, 62]

GROUP B STREPTOCOCCUS

LPA is superior to CIE and CoA and is the preferred method of rapid detection of group B streptococcus antigen.[63–71] Many investigators have reported positive predictive values approaching 100 per cent in small numbers of patients.[37] False-positive tests with the latex agglutination assay have been noted with group G streptococcus[65] and *S. pneumoniae.*[63] Researchers have developed an extremely sensitive enzyme immunoassay for the rapid detection of streptococcal antigen in cerebrospinal fluid that is more sensitive and specific than the currently available immunodiagnostic tests. However, this test has remained a research tool.[72]

Human Immunodeficiency Virus

A new 5-minute latex agglutination test for HIV antibodies has been approved by the United States Food and Drug Administration. The test, *Recombingen HIV-1 LA* (Baxter Healthcare Corporation, Deerfield, Ill.), is based on highly purified recombinant HIV envelope (gp120 and gp41) antigen harvested from genetically engineered *E. coli.* These antigens are attached to polystyrene beads, which in the presence of specific antibodies form visible aggregates. Riggin and coworkers found the Recombingen test to possess 100 per cent sensitivity and 99.6 per cent specificity when compared with Western blot and ELISA.[73] Clinical trials in Africa suggest this test possesses both sensitivity and specificity approaching 99 per cent.[74, 75] The assay can detect HIV-1 antibodies within 5 minutes in whole blood, serum, or plasma. The cost for an individual test is approximately ten dollars.

Potential applications of this test include its use as a rapid screening test for determining the risk of exposure and need for prophylaxis in health care workers exposed to the blood products. This assay would enable developing world laboratories to test for the HIV virus antibody without the costly training and equipment currently required for the ELISA antibody screening tests.

Acute Pharyngitis

GROUP A STREPTOCOCCUS

Pharyngitis is a common presenting complaint in the office and emergency department. Numerous etiologic agents have been identified. Viral agents associated with pharyngitis include adenovirus, influenza A and B, parainfluenza, enterovirus, respiratory syncytial virus, herpes simplex type I virus, and Epstein-Barr virus. Bacterial causes include group A streptococcus, group C,G, and F streptococcus, *C. trachomatis* and TWAR, *Mycoplasma pneumoniae,* and *N. gonorrhoeae.*[76] *H. influenzae* and *Neisseria meningitidis* may cause sore throat but usually in the setting of systemic disease.

The diagnostic approach and medical treatment of pharyngitis has focused on the identification and eradication of group A streptococcus from the throat for several reasons. Antibiotic therapy has well-documented efficacy in the prevention of the long-term complications of streptococcal infections such as rheumatic heart disease.[77, 78] In addition, there is evidence that an early course of antibiotics will shorten the course of streptococcal pharyngitis.[79, 80] Finally, antibiotics have not been demonstrated to be effective in nonstreptococcal pharyngitis.[81]

Throat Culture—The Gold Standard. With the emphasis on early treatment, methods of rapid identification of group A streptococcus became important. Although the throat culture is considered the gold standard in the diagnosis of streptococcal pharyngitis, it is not without its limitations. First, reading throat cultures is a sophisticated skill requiring practice and training. Several studies have demonstrated that interpretation of throat culture results is fraught with error.[82–85] Glass and Bottone compared results interpreted by pediatric housestaff with the interpretations of trained lab technicians and found that physicians in training did not identify 60 per cent of the positive cultures.[83] Although the specificity of throat cultures approaches 99 per cent, the sensitivity of a single throat culture compared with that of many throat cultures ranges from 76 to 90 per cent.[86–89] This varies with the collection technique, the culture medium, and identification techniques used. To make matters worse, office cultures are less accurate than those done in the lab. Merenstein and Rogers noted only an 80 per cent agreement between throat cultures processed in both office and laboratory. They also noted that there was clinical improvement in patients with negative cultures, suggesting that some patients may have had undetected clinical streptococcal infections.[90] Other studies have demonstrated difficulties with office-based cultures.[79, 81, 84] Office-based throat culture sensitivity may be as low as 29 to 60 per cent with specificity in the 76 to 99 per cent range. Another major drawback is the 24 to 48 hours required to incubate throat cultures. Because early treatment is more effective in reducing symptoms, the physician is faced with the decision of whether to empirically treat the undiagnosed pharyngitis. Finally, both the physician and patient spend considerable time and effort in follow-up of culture results.

Immunoassays for Group A Streptococcus. The shortcomings of throat cultures have prompted the development of newer methods of detecting group A streptococcus in pharyngeal specimens. These rapid screens have several advantages. They provide an immediate diagnosis, thus eliminating both delays in therapy and the need for follow-up contact for culture results. Early institution of antibiotic treatment will possibly shorten the clinical course of the pharyngitis.[79, 81, 90–94]

Rapid strep tests involve a two-step process based on the immunologic differences in the "C carbohydrate," a molecule within the cell wall of various subgroups of streptococcus species. The first step is to extract the antigen from the cell wall. Commercial kits contain the reagents necessary for the extraction process. These reagents are one of two types. Nitrous acid extraction is the quickest method, requiring 5 to 10 minutes. Enzyme extraction, another commonly used method, requires 60 minutes. The second step involves the use of antibodies to the C carbohydrate attached to something that will result in a measurable end point. Kits vary in the type of visual end point used. Examples of commonly used end points include the agglutination of latex particles, color changes, or the release of a fluorescent component visible under ultraviolet light.

Latex Agglutination. These test kits use latex particles (covered with antibody) that are added to the extracted specimen. If the group A antigen is present, crosslinking occurs, resulting in visible agglutination.

ELISA Technique. This method involves the use of monoclonal antibodies in an enzyme-linked immunosorbent assay. The extraction process is followed as above. The extracted specimen is poured onto a plate coated with rabbit antistreptococcal A antibody. If bacterial antigen is present, it binds to the antibody on the plate. Then rabbit antistreptococcal A antibody conjugated with alkaline phosphatase is added, which in turn binds to the now fixed specimen antigen-antibody complex. After a washing step to remove unfixed enzyme-conjugated antibody, a substrate is added, which in the presence of bound enzyme changes color.

Sensitivity and Specificity. Several studies have compared rapid strep screens to the throat culture standard.[95–105] The specificity of most kits approaches 98 per cent. The sensitivity, however, has been the source of some concern. A number of studies have estimated the sensitivities to range from 80 to 95 per cent when compared to throat culture techniques. Reported sensitivities based on performance of the test by nonlaboratory personnel have been even lower. Slifkin and Gil found the latex agglutination test to be 99 per cent specific and 95 per cent sensitive.[100] Despite the potentially high sensitivity, the possibility exists that 1 patient in every 20 with streptococcus pharyngitis could go untreated owing to a false-negative streptococcal screen. This has led some clinicians to recommend the use of "backup" cultures in patients with significant pharyngitis and negative rapid strep screens.[104] Another approach is to empirically treat patients with classic clinical features and to use the streptococcal screen on patients with low probability of bacterial infection who might not be available for "call-back" if the throat culture is positive.

How to Choose a Test Kit. There are several kits available on the market and the final choice will depend on the individual needs of a particular lab or office. There are several criteria that are useful in deciding which kit best fits your needs.

1. The reported sensitivity should exceed 90 to 95 per cent. Specificity should be close to 100 per cent.

2. The actual hands-on time required by the nurse or technician should be less than 5 minutes. Nitrous acid extraction techniques are considerably quicker than enzyme extraction kits (5 minutes compared to 60 minutes).

3. The latex agglutination tests have an average cost of less than two dollars not including controls (ELISA kits cost twice as much).

4. An end point should be easy to define for even inexperienced staff. Kits vary in the end point reaction used to determine positive from negative. The ELISA test is easier to read for the beginner than latex agglutination methods.

5. The kits should also contain clear instructional material as well as both positive and negative control specimens.

6. The kit should not require elaborate storage procedures. Some kits require refrigeration of reagents at specific temperatures with a warm-up period required before use.

Performance of the Rapid Strep Test. Because there are so many variations and kits on the market, it is important to read instructions carefully when buying a new kit or changing to another brand. The sales representative should review the instructions during a hands-on inservice. There should be sufficient practice by those using controls contained in the kit to demonstrate proficiency. Initially, parallel testing with throat cultures is recommended to document the personnel's accuracy in performing the rapid assay. Daily positive controls should be used to test the quality of the reagents. Negative controls should be run with each test or batch. This often makes comparison and identification of a positive test easier.

Urinary Tract Infections

URINE LEUKOCYTE ESTERASE AND NITRITE ASSAY

The need for a rapid, accurate indicator of urinary tract infections and the emphasis for cost containment has led to the use of urinary dipstick analysis as a screening aid for patients with urinary tract complaints.[106–109] In 1979, Banauch reported the first trial with the use of the leukocyte esterase (LE) test as a marker for white blood cells in urine.[110] Since then, numerous investigators have published statistical data either in support of[111–127] or against[128–135] the use of LE and nitrite dipstick screening.

Both the nitrite and LE tests are colorometric methods. The nitrite dipstick test detects nitrites, which are the byproducts of nitrate-reducing bacteria in the bladder. These bacteria convert dietary nitrates to nitrites. An amine impregnated on the dipstick pad forms a diazomium compound in the presence of nitrites. This results in a pink color reaction within 60 seconds. Leukocyte esterase is an enzyme found in azurophilic or primary neutrophilic granules of polymorphic leukocytes. This enzyme is not normally found in serum, urine, or kidney tissue. Leukocyte esterase reacts with a chloracetate stain impregnated in the dipstick pad resulting in an indoxyl moiety that is oxidized by room air. A blue color develops in 1 to 2 minutes. Tables 89–1 and 89–2 show the common causes for false-positive tests.[136, 137]

The sensitivity and specificity of the nitrite dipstick, LE dipstick, and their combined use is shown in Table 89–3. The nitrite dipstick compared with the LE dipstick is more specific (92 to 100 per cent vs. 64 to 82 per cent) but not as sensitive (35 to 85 per cent vs. 72 to 97 per cent).[136] Studies using both the nitrite and LE dipsticks to detect bacteriuria report sensitivities ranging from 72 to 100 per cent and specificities ranging from 50 to 90 per cent. Positive predictive values range from 24 to 94 per cent and negative

Table 89–1. Causes of Inaccurate Nitrite Dipstick Tests

False positives
  Specimen contamination
  Prolonged exposure to room air
False negatives
  Presence of nonnitrate reducing organisms (e.g., many non-
    Enterobacteriaceae species)
  Presence of organisms that further reduce nitrate to ammonia
  Not performed on first morning-voided specimen
  Frequent voiding
  Dilute urine
  High specific gravity
  Urine pH <6
  Presence of urobilinogen
  Large dietary intake of vitamin C

Table 89–3. Sensitivity and Specificity of Nitrite and Leukocyte Esterase Dipsticks for Detecting Bacteriuria

Dipstick Test	Range of Reported Sensitivity (%)	Range of Reported Specificity (%)
Nitrite	35–85	92–100
Leukocyte esterase (LE)	72–97	64–82
LE and nitrite	70–100	60–98

Twenty-five of these 81 patients had *C. trachomatis* on culture. Twenty-four of the 25 (96 per cent) specimens were LE positive. This was contrasted with only 11/25 (44 per cent) specimens being gram-positive. All controls were LE negative.[139] Sadof and coworkers had similar results in a study of 54 sexually active adolescent males testing the reliability of LE in first-catch urine specimens to detect urethritis caused by *N. gonorrhoeae* and *C. trachomatis*. In these patients with urinary symptoms, the LE dipstick had a 94 per cent sensitivity, 89 per cent specificity, 81 per cent positive predictive value, and a 97 per cent negative predictive value.[140]

predictive values from 92 to 100 per cent using a positive urine culture at greater than 10^5 colony count as a gold standard.[136] Requiring both components to be positive greatly improved the specificity from 72 to 99.5 per cent at the expense of decreasing sensitivity from 100 to 35 per cent.[114]

The characteristics of the emergency department population must be considered, since predictive value analysis depends on disease prevalence. Ideally, a test should have both a high sensitivity and specificity. Tests that minimize both false-negative and false-positive results are preferred. Gallagher and colleagues[138] have found the nitrite reagent to give false-positive results with prolonged exposure to air. By 5 days, the reagent strips display 20 per cent false-positive results with air exposure.

Chernow and colleagues in a study of fresh urine specimens from 203 patients found that the LE test was 100 per cent sensitive and 76 per cent specific.[121] Gutman and Solomon prospectively evaluated 1079 clean-catch, midstream samples from male veteran patients. Using positive dipstick readings for LE, nitrite, and protein, the sensitivity, specificity, positive predictive value, and negative predictive value for specimens containing more than or 10^3 CFU s/ml were 80 per cent, 71 per cent, 48 per cent, and 91 per cent. Clinical data were reviewed in 38 patients with one or more dipstick-negative, culture-positive urines. Most of these patients were neurologically compromised patients who lacked clinical or other laboratory evidence suggesting urinary tract infection. They concluded that in their predominately male patient population clinically significant bacteriuria is an unlikely finding in a dipstick-negative urine.[122]

Dipstick-negative, culture-positive urine specimens may result from unusual patterns of infection. Wu and colleagues in a study of immunosuppressed patients reported a low sensitivity (66 per cent) and a very low negative predictive value (46 per cent) of the LE-nitrite screening test.[131]

Finally, some investigators have found the LE test to be useful as a rapid screen for nongonococcal urethritis. Perera and colleagues studied 81 men with urethral syndrome.

CONCLUSION

The integration of rapid microbiologic assays for antigen and antibody detection in practice of emergency medicine has been swift. Rapid assays have numerous intrinsic benefits to the practice of emergency medicine. These benefits include increased speed, decreased cost, earlier appropriate therapy, and decreased need for repeated visits. In addition, the decreased dependence on expensive laboratory facilities makes these tests attractive to the physician practicing in a rural or third world setting.

The key question is the extent to which rapid methodology will become a culture substitute versus a culture supplement. The physician needs to evaluate the impact of both false-positive and false-negative results before adopting a rapid screen methodology as a substitute for culture. In addition, the physician needs to recognize the population or settings where prior trials of the rapid test have been conducted. These settings may not be similar to his or her practice. Finally, before choosing a test, the physician must consider the reliability, ease of use, quality assurance, and medicolegal issues related to the test.

Major technologic advances such as monoclonal antibodies and molecular probes have the potential to increase the sensitivity and specificity of these rapid tests. The availability of this technology will have a significant impact on the practice of emergency medicine in the future.

REFERENCES

General

1. Brooks GF, York MK: Cost-effective clinical microbiology and newer test of importance to the practitioner. In Remington JS, Swartz MN (eds): Current Clinical Topics in Infectious Disease 7. New York, McGraw-Hill Book Co, 1987, pp 157–193.
2. Todd JK: Test selection for the pediatric office laboratory. In Aronoff SC, Hughes WT, Kohl S, et al (eds): Advances in Pediatric Infectious Disease. Chicago, Year Book Medical Publishers, 1988, 3, pp 111–124.
3. Saglio SD, Henley CE: Rapid assay kits for common microbiologic agents. AFP 36:169, 1987.
4. Spector SA, Dankner WM: Rapid viral diagnostic techniques. In Aronoff SC, Hughes WT, Kohl S, et al (eds): Advances in Pediatric Infectious Disease. Chicago, Year Book Medical Publishers, 1986, 1, pp 37–59.

Immunofluorescent Staining

5. Clausen CR: Detection of bacterial pathogens in purulent clinical specimens by immunofluorescence techniques. J Clin Microbiol 13:1119, 1981.
6. Fox HA, Hagen PA, Turner DJ, et al: Immunofluorescence in the

Table 89–2. Causes of Inaccurate Leukocyte Esterase Dipstick Tests

False positives
  Contamination during collection
False negatives
  Increased specific gravity
  Glycosuria
  Presence of urobilinogen
  Therapy with phenazopyridine hydrochloride, nitrofurantoin, or rifampin
  Large dietary intake of vitamin C

diagnosis of acute bacterial meningitis: A cooperative evaluation of the technique in a clinical laboratory setting. Pediatrics 43:44, 1969.

7. Biegeleisen JZ, Mitchell MS, Marcus BB, et al: Immunofluorescence techniques for demonstrating bacterial pathogens associated with cerebrospinal meningitis. I. Clinical evaluation of conjugates on smears prepared directly from cerebrospinal fluid sediments. J Lab Clin Med 65:976, 1965.

Latex Particle Agglutination and Coagulation

8. Dajani AS: Agglutination test for the diagnosis of meningitis. In Coonrod JD, Kunz LJ, Ferraro MJ (eds): The Direct Detection of Microorganisms by Counterimmunoelectrophoresis in Clinical Samples. Orlando, Fla, Academic Press, 1983, p 87.
9. Dirks-Go SI, Zanen HC: Latex agglutination, counterimmunoelectrophoresis, and protein A coagglutination in diagnosis of bacterial meningitis. J Clin Pathol 31:1167, 1978.

Countercurrent Immunoelectrophoresis

10. Estela LA, Heinrichs TF: Evaluation of the counterimmunoelectrophoretic (CIE) procedure in the clinical laboratory setting. Am J Clin Pathol 70:239, 1978.
11. Finch CA, Wilkinson HW: Practical considerations in using counterimmunoelectrophoresis to identify the principal causative agents of bacterial meningitis. J Clin Microbiol 10:519, 1979.
12. Naiman HL, Albritton WL: Counterimmunoelectrophoresis in the diagnosis of acute infection. J Infect Dis 142:524, 1980.
13. Higashi GI, Sippel JE, Girgis NI, et al: Counterimmunoelectrophoresis: An adjunct to bacterial culture in the diagnosis of meningococcal meningitis. Scand J Infect Dis 6:233, 1974.

Chlamydia Trachomatis

14. Holmes KK: The Chlamydia epidemic. JAMA 245:1718, 1981.
15. Shafer MA, Vaughan E, Lipkin ES, et al: Evaluation of fluorescein-conjugated monoclonal antibody test to detect *Chlamydia trachomatis* endocervical infections in adolescent girls. J Pediatr 108:779, 1986.
16. Tam MR, Stamm WE, Handsfield HH, et al: Culture independent diagnosis of *Chlamydia trachomatis* using monoclonal antibodies. N Engl J Med 310:1146, 1984.
17. Ripa KT, Mardh PA: New simplified culture technique for *Chlamydia trachomatis*. In Hobson D, Holmes KK (eds): Nongonococcal Urethritis and Related Infections. Washington DC, American Association of Microbiology, 1977, pp 323–327.
18. Syva MicroTrak, *Chlamydia trachomatis* Direct Specimen Test. Package insert, Syva Co., 1987.
19. Embil JA, Thiebaux HJ, Manuel FR, et al: Sequential cervical specimens and the isolation of *Chlamydia trachomatis*: Factors affecting detection. Sex Transm Dis 10:62, 1983.
20. Stamm WE, Harrison HR, Alexander ER, et al: Diagnosis of *Chlamydia trachomatis* infections by direct immunofluorescence staining of genital secretions. Ann Intern Med 101:638, 1984.
21. Lipkin ES, Moncada JV, Shafer MA, et al: Comparison of monoclonal antibody staining and culture in diagnosing cervical chlamydial infection. J Clin Microbiol 23:114, 1986.
22. Forbes BA, Bartholoma N, McMillan J, et al: Evaluation of a monoclonal antibody test to detect *Chlamydia* in the cervical and urethral specimens. J Clin Microbiol 23:1136, 1986.
23. Uyeda CT, Welborn P, Ellison-Birang N, et al: Rapid diagnosis of chlamydial infections with the MicroTrak direct test. J Clin Microbiol 20:948, 1984.
24. Quinn TC, Warfield P, Kappus E, Barbacci M, et al: Screening for *Chlamydia trachomatis* infection in an inner-city population: A comparison of diagnostic methods. J Infect Dis 152:419, 1985.
25. Lindner FE, Geerling S, Nettum JA, Miller SL, et al: Identification of *Chlamydia* in cervical smears by immunofluorescence: Technic, sensitivity, and specificity. Am J Clin Pathol 85:180, 1986.
26. Chlamydiazyme (TM) Diagnostic Kit. Package insert. Abbott Laboratories, Diagnostis Division, 1985.
27. Amortegui AJ, Meyer MP: Enzyme immunoassay for detection of *Chlamydia trachomatis* from the cervix. Obstet Gynecol 65:523, 1985.
28. Jones MF, Smith TF, Houglum AJ, et al: Detection of Chlamydia trachomatis in genital specimens by the Chlamydiazyme test. J Clin Microbiol 20:465, 1984.

Neisseria Gonorrhoeae

29. Janda WM, Jackson T: Evaluation of Gonodecten for the presumptive diagnosis of gonococcal urethritis in men. J Clin Microbiol 21:143, 1985.
30. Burns M, Rossi PH, Cox DW, et al: A preliminary evaluation of the gonozyme test. Sex Transm Dis 10:180, 1983.
31. Hossain A, Bakir TM, Siddiqui M, et al: Enzyme immunoassay (EIA) in

the rapid diagnosis of gonorrhoea. J Hyg Epidemiol Microbiol Immunol 32(4):425, 1988.
32. Demetriou E, Sackett R, Welch DF: Evaluation of an enzyme immunoassay for detection of *Neisseria gonorrhoeae* in an adolescent population. JAMA 252:247, 1984.
33. Martin R, Coopes S, Neagle P, et al: Comparison of Thayer-Martin, Transgrow, and Gonozyme for detection of *Neisseria gonorrhoeae* in a low risk population. Sex Transm Dis 13:108, 1986.
34. Martin R, Wentworth BB, Coopes S, et al: Comparison of Transgrow and Gonozyme for detection of *Neisseria gonorrhoeae* in mailed specimens. J Clin Microbiol 19:893, 1984.
35. Danielsson D, Moi H, Forslin L: Diagnosis of urogenital gonorrhoea by detecting gonococcal antigen with a solid phase enzyme immunoassay (Gonozyme). J Clin Pathol 36:674, 1983.
36. Aardoom HA, DeHoop D, Iserief CA, et al: Detection of *Neisseria gonorrhoeae* antigen by a solid-phase enzyme assay. Br J Vener Dis 58:359, 1982.

Meningitis

37. Wilson CB, Smith AL: Rapid tests for the diagnosis of bacterial meningitis. In Remington JS, Swartz MN (eds): Current Clinical Topics in Infectious Disease 7. New York, McGraw-Hill Book Co, 1987, pp 134–156.
38. Thirumoorthi MC, Dajani AS: Comparison of staphylococcal coagglutination, latex agglutination, and counterimmunoelectrophoresis for bacterial antigen detection. J Clin Microbiol 9:28, 1979.
39. Tilton RC, Dias F, Ryan RW: Comparative evaluation of three commercial products and counterimmunoelectrophoresis for the detection of antigens in cerebrospinal fluid. J Clin Microbiol 20:231, 1984.
40. Habte-Gabr E, Muhe L, Olcen P: Rapid etiological diagnosis of pyogenic meningitis by coagglutination, latex agglutination and immunoosmophoresis of cerebrospinal fluid, serum and urine. Trop Geogr Med 39:137, 1987.
41. Pepple J, Moxon ER, Yolken RH: Indirect enzyme-linked immunosorbent assay for the quantitation of the type-specific antigen of *Haemophilus influenzae B*: A preliminary report. J Pediatr 97:233, 1980.
42. Shaw ED, Darker RJ, Feldman WE, et al: Clinical studies of a new latex particle agglutination test for detection of *Haemophilus influenzae* type B polyribose phosphate antigen in serum, cerebrospinal fluid, and urine. J Clin Microbiol 15:1153, 1982.
43. McGraw TP, Bruckner DA: Sensitivity of commercial agglutination and counterimmunoelectrophoresis methods for the detection of *Haemophilus influenzae* type B capsular polysaccharide. Am J Clin Pathol 80:703, 1983.
44. Ward JI, Siber GR, Scheifele DW, et al: Rapid diagnosis of *Haemophilus influenzae* type B infections by latex particle agglutination and counterimmunoelectrophoresis. J Pediatr 93:37, 1978.
45. Granoff DM, Congeni B, Baker R, et al: Countercurrent immunoelectrophoresis in the diagnosis of *Haemophilus influenzae* type B infection. Am J Dis Child 131:1357, 1977.
46. Belmaaza A, Hamel J, Mousseau S, et al: Rapid diagnosis of severe *Haemophilus influenzae* serotype B infections by monoclonal antibody enzyme immunoassay for outer membrane proteins. J Clin Microbiol 24:440, 1986.
47. Daum RS, Siber GR, Kamon JS, et al: Evaluation of a commercial latex particle agglutination test for rapid diagnosis of *Haemophilus influenzae* type B infection. Pediatrics 69:466, 1982.
48. Colding H, Lind I: Counterimmunoelectrophoresis in the diagnosis of bacterial meningitis. J Clin Microbiol 5:405, 1977.
49. Shackelford PG, Campbell J, Feigin RD: Countercurrent immunoelectrophoresis in the evaluation of childhood infections. J Pediatr 85:478, 1974.
50. Bortolussi R, Wort AJ, Casey S: The latex agglutination test versus counterimmunoelectrophoresis for rapid diagnosis of bacterial meningitis. CMA 127:489, 1982.
51. Feigin RD, Wong M, Shackelford PG, et al: Countercurrent immunoelectrophoresis of urine as well as CSF and blood for diagnosis of bacterial meningitis. J Pediatr 93:773, 1976.
52. Leinonen M, Kayhty H: Comparison of counter-current immunoelectrophoresis, latex agglutination, and radioimmunoassay in detection of soluble capsular polysaccharide antigens of *Haemophilus influenzae* type B and *Neisseria meningitidis* of groups A or C. J Clin Pathol 31:1172, 1978.
53. Sippel JE, Prato CM, Girgis NI, et al: Detection of *Neisseria meningitidis* group A, *Haemophilus influenzae* type B, and *Streptococcus pneumoniae* antigens in cerebrospinal fluid specimens by antigen capture enzyme-linked immunosorbent assays. J Clin Microbiol 20:259, 1984.
54. Wetherall BL, Hallsworth PG, McDonald PJ: Enzyme-linked immunosorbent assay for detection of *Haemophilus influenzae* type B antigen. J Clin Microbiol 11:573, 1980.
55. Olcen P: Serological methods for rapid diagnosis of *Haemophilus influenzae*, *Neisseria meningitidis*, and *Streptococcus pneumoniae* in cerebrospinal fluid: A comparison of co-agglutination, immunofluorescence and immunoelectroosmophoresis. Scand J Infect Dis 10:283, 1978.
56. Greenwood BM, Whittle HC, Dominic-Rajkovic O: Countercurrent

immunoelectrophoresis in the diagnosis of meningococcal meningitis. Lancet 2:519, 1971.

57. Whittle HC, Greenwood BM, Davidson NM, et al: Meningococcal antigen in diagnosis and treatment of group A meningococcal infections. Am J Med 58:823, 1975.

58. Edwards EA, Muehl PM, Peckinpaugh RD: Diagnosis of bacterial meningitis by counterimmunoelectrophoresis. J Lab Clin Med 80:449, 1972.

59. Hoffman TA, Edwards EA: Group-specific polysaccharide antigen and humoral antibody response in disease due to *Neisseria meningitidis*. J Infect Dis 126:336, 1972.

60. Leinonen M, Herva E: The latex agglutination test for the diagnosis of meningococcal and *Haemophilus influenzae* meningitis. Scand J Infect Dis 9:187, 1977.

61. Williams RG, Hart WC: Rapid identification of bacterial antigen in blood cultures and cerebrospinal fluid. J Clin Pathol 41:691, 1988.

62. Wasilauskas BL, Hampton KD: Determination of bacterial meningitis: A retrospective study of 80 cerebrospinal fluid specimens evaluated by four in vitro methods. J Clin Microbiol 16:531, 1982.

63. Edwards MS, Kasper DL, Baker CJ: Rapid diagnosis of type III group B streptococcal meningitis by latex particle agglutination. J Pediatr 95:202, 1979.

64. Bromberger PI, Chandler B, Gezon H, et al: Brief clinical and laboratory observations: Rapid detections of neonatal group B streptococcal infections by latex agglutination. J Pediatr 96:104, 1980.

65. Friedman CA, Wender DF, Rawson JE: Rapid diagnosis of group B streptococcal infections utilizing a commercially available latex agglutination assay. Pediatrics 73:27, 1984.

66. Baker CJ, Webb BJ, Jackson CV, et al: Countercurrent immunoelectrophoresis in the evaluation of infants with group B streptococcal disease. Pediatrics 65:1110, 1980.

67. Siegel JD, McCracken GH: Detection of group B streptococcal antigens in body fluids of neonates. J Pediatr 93:491, 1978.

68. Typlin BL, Koranyi K, Azimi P, et al: Counterimmunoelectrophoresis for the rapid diagnosis of group B streptococcal infections. Clin Pediatr 18:366, 1979.

69. Strechenberg BW, Schreiner RL, Grass SM, et al: Countercurrent immunoelectrophoresis in group B streptococcal disease. Pediatrics 64:632, 1970.

70. Webb BJ, Edwards MS, Baker CJ: Comparison of slide coagglutination test and countercurrent immunoelectrophoresis for detection of group B streptococcal antigen in cerebrospinal fluid from infants with meningitis. J Clin Microbiol 11:263, 1980.

71. Webb BJ, Baker CJ: Commercial latex agglutination test for rapid diagnosis of group B streptococcal infection in infants. J Clin Microbiol 12:442, 1980.

72. Polin RA, Kennett R: Use of monoclonal antibodies in an enzyme-linked inhibition assay for rapid detection of streptococcal antigen. J Pediatr 97:540, 1980.

Human Immunodeficiency Virus

73. Riggin CH, Beltz GA, Hung CH, et al: Detection of antibodies to human immunodeficiency virus by latex agglutination with recombinant antigen. J Clin Microbiol 25:1772, 1987.

74. Quinn TC, Riggin CH, Kline RL, et al: Rapid latex agglutination assay using recombinant envelope polypeptide for the detection of antibody to the HIV. JAMA 260:510, 1988.

75. Van DePerre P, Nzaramba D, Allen S, et al: Comparison of six serological assays for human immunodeficiency virus antibody detection in developing countries. J Clin Microbiol 26:552, 1988.

Acute Pharyngitis

76. Komaroff AL, Aronson MD, Pass TM, et al: Serologic evidence of chlamydial and mycoplasmal pharyngitis in adults. Science 222:927, 1983.

77. Denny FW: Effect of treatment on streptococcal pharyngitis: Is the issue really settled? Pediatr Infect Dis 4:352, 1985.

78. Wannamaker LW, Rammelkamp CH Jr, Denny FW, et al: Prophylaxis of acute rheumatic fever by treatment of the preceding streptococcal infection with various amounts of depot penicillin. Am J Med 10:673, 1951.

79. Krober MS, Bass JW, Michels GN: Streptococcal pharyngitis: Placebo controlled double blind evaluation of clinical response to penicillin therapy. JAMA 253:1271, 1985.

80. Randolph MF, Gerber MA, DeMeo KK, et al: Effect of antibiotic therapy on the clinical course of streptococcal pharyngitis. J Pediatr 106:870, 1985.

81. McDonald CJ, Tierney WM, Hui SL, et al: A controlled trial of erythromycin in adults with nonstreptococcal pharyngitis. J Infect Dis 152:1093, 1985.

82. Mandzac AM: Throat culture processing in the office: A warning. JAMA 200:208, 1967.

83. Glass R, Bottone EJ: Inaccuracy of house staff in reading throat cultures. JAMA 240:2651, 1978.

84. Battle CV, Glasgow LA: Reliability of bacteriologic identification of beta-hemolytic streptococci in private offices. Am J Dis Child 122:134, 1971.

85. Crawley R, Belsey R, Brock D, et al: Regulation of physician's office laboratories: The Idaho experience. JAMA 255:374, 1986.

86. Laatsch LJ: Pharyngeal carriage of beta-hemolytic streptococci and the effect of laboratory exposure in medical technology students. J Med Tech 2:106, 1985.

87. Centor RM, Meier FA, Dalton HP: Throat cultures and rapid tests for diagnosis of group A streptococcal pharyngitis. Ann Intern Med 105:892, 1986.

88. Halfon ST, Davies AM, Kaplan O, et al: Primary prevention of rheumatic fever in Jerusalem schoolchildren. II. Identification of beta-hemolytic streptococci. Isr J Med Sci 4:809, 1968.

89. Dingle JH, Abernethy TJ, Badger GF, et al: Endemic exudative pharyngitis and tonsillitis. JAMA 125:1163, 1944.

90. Merenstein JH, Rogers KD: Streptococcal pharyngitis: Early treatment and management by nurse practitioners. JAMA 227:1278, 1974.

91. Roenstien BJ, Markowitz M, Gordis L: Accuracy of throat cultures processed in physician's offices. J Pediatr 76:606, 1970.

92. Brink WR, Rammelkamp CH, Denny FW, et al: Effect of penicillin and aureomycin on the natural course of streptococcal tonsillitis and pharyngitis. Am J Med 10:300, 1951.

93. Brumfitt W, Slater JDM: Treatment of acute sore throat with penicillin. Lancet 1:8, 1957.

94. White CB, Lieberman MM, Morales E: An in vitro comparison of eight rapid streptococcal antigen detection tests. J Pediatr 113:691, 1988.

95. Dobkin D, Shulman ST: Evaluation of an ELISA for group A streptococcal antigen for the diagnosis of pharyngitis. J Pediatr 110:566, 1987.

96. Chang MJ, Mohla C: Ten-minute detection of group A streptococci in pediatric throat swabs. J Clin Microbiol 21:258, 1985.

97. Miceika BG, Vitous AS, Thompson KD: Detection of group A streptococcal antigen directly from throat swabs with a ten minute latex agglutination test. J Clin Microbiol 21:467, 1985.

98. White CB, Bass JW, Yamada SM: Rapid latex agglutination compared with the throat culture for the detection of group A streptococcal infection. Pediatr Infect Dis 5:208, 1986.

99. Roddey OF, Clegg HW, Clardy LT, et al: Comparison of a latex agglutination test and four culture methods for identification of group A streptococci in a pediatric office laboratory. J Pediatr 108:347, 1986.

100. Slifkin M, Gil GM: Evaluation of the Culturette brand ten minute group A strep ID technique. J Clin Microbiol 20:12, 1984.

101. Polin RA, Kennett R: Use of monoclonal antibodies in an enzyme linked inhibition assay for rapid detection of streptococcal antigen. J Pediatr 97:540, 1980.

102. Gerber MA, Randolph MF, Tilton RC: Enzyme fluorescence procedure for rapid diagnosis of streptococcal pharyngitis. J Pediatr 108:421, 1986.

103. Gerber MA, Randolph MF, Chanatry J, et al: Antigen detection test for streptococcal pharyngitis: Evaluation of sensitivity with respect to true infections. J Pediatr 108:654, 1986.

104. Radetsky M, Wheeler RC, Roe MH, et al: Comparison evaluation of kits for rapid diagnosis of group A streptococcal disease. Pediatr Infect Dis 4:274, 1985.

105. Fischer PM: Rapid testing of streptococcal pharyngitis. Primary Care 13:657, 1986.

Urinary Tract Infections

106. Kunin CM, DeGroot JE: Self-screening for significant bacteriuria. JAMA 231:1349, 1975.

107. Finnerty FA, Johnson AC: A simplified accurate method for detecting bacteriuria. Am J Obstet Gynecol 101:238, 1968.

108. Czerwinski AW, Wilkerson RG, Merrill JA, et al: Further evaluation of the Griess test to detect significant bacteriuria. Am J Obstet Gynecol 110:677, 1971.

109. Sleigh JD: Detection of bacteriuria by a modification of the nitrite test. Br Med J 1:765, 1965.

110. Banauch D: Detection of leukocytes in urine by means of a test strip: A cooperative study at eleven centers. Dtsch Med Wochenschr 104:1236, 1979.

111. Loo SYT, Scottolini AG, Luangphinith S, et al: Urine screening strategy employing dipstick analysis and selective culture: An evaluation. Am J Clin Pathol 81:634, 1984.

112. Loo SYT, Scottolini AG, Luangphinith S, et al: Performance of a urine screening protocol. Am J Clin Pathol 85:479, 1986.

113. Males BM, Bartholomew WR, Amsterdam D: Leukocyte esterase-nitrite and bioluminescence assays as urine screens. J Clin Microbiol 22:531, 1985.

114. Oneson R, Groschel DH: Leukocyte esterase activity and nitrite test as a rapid screen for significant bacteriuria. Am J Clin Pathol 83:84, 1985.

115. Perry JL, Mathews JS, Weesner DE: Evaluation of leukocyte esterase activity as a rapid screening technique for bacteriuria. J Clin Microbiol 15:852, 1982.

116. Pezzlo MT, Wetkowski MA, Peterson EM, et al: Detection of bacteriuria and pyuria within two minutes. J Clin Microbiol 21:578, 1985.

117. Pfaller MA, Koontz FP: Laboratory evaluation of leukocyte esterase and

nitrite tests for the detection of bacteriuria. J Clin Microbiol 21:840, 1985.

118. Sawyer KP, Stone LL: Evaluation of a leukocyte dipstick test used for screening urine cultures. J Clin Microbiol 20:820, 1984.

119. Smalley DL, Dittmann AN: Use of leukocyte esterase-nitrite activity as predictive assays of significant bacteriuria. J Clin Microbiol 18:1256, 1983.

120. Wenk RE, Dutta D, Rudert J, et al: Sediment microscopy, nitrituria, and leukocyte esteraseuria as predictors of significant bacteriuria. J Clin Lab Automation 2:117, 1982.

121. Chernow B, Zaloga GP, Solano S, et al: Measurement of urinary leukocyte esterase activity: A screening test for urinary tract infections. Ann Emerg Med 13:150, 1984.

122. Gutman SI, Solomon RR: The clinical significance of dipstick-negative, culture-positive urines in a veterans population. Am J Clin Pathol 88:204, 1987.

123. Leighton PM, Little JA: Leucocyte esterase determination as a secondary procedure for urine screening. J Clin Pathol 38:229, 1985.

124. Shaw ST, Poon SY, Wong ET: "Routine urinalysis." Is the dipstick enough? JAMA 253:1596, 1985.

125. Hughes JG, Snyder RJ, Washington JA II: An evaluation of a leukocyte esterase/nitrite test strip and a bioluminescence assay for detection of bacteriuria. Diagn Microbiol Infect Dis 3:139, 1985.

126. Kincaid-Smith P, Bullen M, Mills J, et al: The reliability of screening tests for bacteriuria in pregnancy. Lancet 2:61, 1964.

127. Takagi LR, Mruz RM, Vanderplow MG: Screening obstetric outpatients for bacteriuria. J Reprod Med 15:229, 1975.

128. Jones C, MacPherson DW, Stevens DL: Inability of the chemstrip LN compared with quantitative urine culture to predict significant bacteriuria. J Clin Microbiol 23:160, 1986.

129. Sewell DL, Burt SP, Gabbert NJ, et al: Evaluation of the Chemstrip 9™ as a screening test for urinalysis and urine culture in men. Am J Clin Pathol 83:740, 1985.

130. Wilkins EGL, Ratcliffe JG, Roberts C: Leukocyte esterase-nitrite screening method for pyuria and bacteriuria. J Clin Pathol 38:1342, 1985.

131. Wu TC, Williams EC, Koo SY, et al: Evaluation of three bacteriuria screening methods in a clinical research hospital. J Clin Microbiol 21:796, 1985.

132. McNeely SG, Baselski VS, Ryan GM: An evaluation of two rapid bacteriuria screening procedures. Obstet Gynecol 69:550, 1987.

133. Murray PR, Smith TB, McKinney TC: Clinical evaluation of three urine screening tests. J Clin Microbiol 25:467, 1987.

134. Damato JJ, Garis J, Hawley RJ, et al: Comparative leukocyte esterase-nitrite and Bact-T-Screen studies using single and multiple urine volumes. Arch Pathol Lab Med 112:533, 1988.

135. Archbald FJ, Verma U, Tajani NA: Screening for asymptomatic bacteriuria with microstix. J Reprod Med 29:272, 1984.

136. Pels RJ, Bor DH, Woolhandler S, et al: Dipstick urinalysis screening of asymptomatic adults for urinary tract disorders. JAMA 262:1221, 1989.

137. Alwall N, Lohi A: Factors affecting the reliability of screening tests for bacteriuria I. Acta Med Scand 193:499, 1973.

138. Gallagher EJ, Schwartz E, Weinstein RS: Performance characteristics of urine dipsticks stored in open containers. Am J Emerg Med 8:121, 1990.

139. Perera SAB, Jones C, Srikantha V, et al: Leucocyte esterase test as rapid screen for non-gonococcal urethritis. Genitourin Med 63:380, 1987.

140. Sadof MD, Woods ER, Emans SJ: Dipstick leukocyte esterase activity in first-catch urine specimens. JAMA 258:1932, 1987.

Chapter **90**

Blood Cultures and Anaerobic Culture Techniques

Jon Jui and Frank P. Brancato

BLOOD CULTURES

Introduction

Hippocrates considered blood one of four humors in the body, the proper balance of which results in the body's good health. Today, it is recognized that blood plays an essential role in infectious disease. As Bennett and Beeson[1] state, "Of all tissues which display defensive powers, the blood stands at the top." In addition to the importance of blood as a carrier of antibodies and phagocytic cells, it is also important as a disseminator of disease-causing microbes and toxins throughout the body. Detection and identification of microorganisms in the blood are two of the most important functions of a clinical microbiology laboratory.

Studies have shown that blood is rarely directly invaded by microorganisms.[1] Bacteria usually enter the circulation through the lymphatic system, and bacteremias follow increased lymph flow from infected foci. Exceptions to this are intravascular infections, such as endocarditis, suppurative thrombophlebitis, and mycotic aneurysm or uncontrolled infections such as typhoid fever and brucellosis. Although entrance into the blood stream by microbes or microbial toxins is considered by some investigators to be a relatively benign event in itself compared with focal tissue invasion, systemic manifestations such as fever, chills, and malaise can be important causes of clinical concern, especially when no tissue foci are immediately obvious. The likelihood of bacteremia is related to

local conditions that favor drainage of lymph from infected areas. Nodes throughout the body usually function as microbial filters as lymph enters the blood stream. Nonetheless, nodes may malfunction and hence increase the likelihood of bacteremia in the following situations: when an extensive number of microbes reach the node, early in the infection when there may be a deficiency of phagocytic cells in the nodes, when the perfusion pressure of the lymph is high, when the microbes are unusually virulent or survive ingestion to be ingested later in the blood stream, or when the node is manipulated.[1]

Clinically, bacteremia may be transient, intermittent, or continuous. Transient bacteremia is common and may occur from manipulation of infected or contaminated tissues, such as gastrointestinal procedures, dental procedures, instrumentation of the genitourinary tract, or surgical incision of an abscess. Sigmoidoscopy-associated bacteremia has been reported to occur in as many as 9.5 per cent of patients, and the rate associated with barium enema has ranged as high as 40 per cent.[2] Also, transient bacteremia may occur in the early phases of other infections such as pneumococcal pneumonia. The significance of a transient bacteremia varies with host resistance and the recurrence of the precipitating cause.

Bacteremia and septicemia are not synonymous. Bacteremia represents the presence of bacteria in the blood stream, whereas septicemia refers to the presence of bacterial toxins in the blood stream. Bacteremia usually results in chills and fever, but bacteremias can be present without detectable systemic symptoms.[3] Septicemia, on the other hand, can result from bacterial toxins disseminating into the blood stream from an infected focus (toxemia). Furthermore, a bacteremia of low order of magnitude may lead to septicemia with negative cultures because of the paucity of organisms.

The importance of early detection and early institution of appropriate antibiotic and therapeutic modalities in the bacteremic patient have been the subject of many investigations. Weinstein and colleagues[4, 5] reviewed the laboratory, epidemiology, and clinical significance of 500 patients with bacteremia and fungemia. Total mortality in this population was 42 per cent with half of all deaths directly due to infections. The immunocompromised and the elderly had markedly greater mortality. The risk of death was particularly high in patients with enterococcal, facultative gram-negative, fungal, polymicrobial, or hospital-acquired sepsis. The use of appropriate antibiotics and additional therapeutic maneuvers such as surgical drainage increased survival.[4, 5]

Indications for Blood Culture

The culturing of blood has become a major component of the clinical microbiology laboratory. A patient with a fever of unknown origin is a prime candidate for blood culture because bacteremia with sepsis is a likely possibility. The blood culture may provide the only positive isolation of an organism that is causing a hidden focal infection somewhere in the body. Indications for blood culturing in the emergency department include the following: (1) evaluation of a toxic-appearing patient with normal immune defenses and a fever, (2) evaluation of a toxic-appearing patient with immune dysfunction with or without fever (immunosuppressed, elderly, neonate), and (3) documentation of infection and determination of the sensitivity of the organism in the patient with suspected endocarditis or other infectious focus with bacteremia. Special issues are relevant to the culturing of different age groups.

FEBRILE ADULT

The proper management of the febrile adult emergency department patient and the role of blood cultures have received limited investigation. Several cited potential advantages include fewer admissions with outpatient assessment of blood culture results, identification of bacteria not accessible via other culture techniques, and earlier identification of organisms. Potential disadvantages include the cost of blood cultures, false-positive results that require follow-up, and increased responsibility and liability for the health care provider.[6] In 1976, Eisenberg and coworkers prospectively studied the course of febrile patients who presented to an emergency department. The determination of which patient received blood cultures was left to the discretion of the treating physician. They found bacteremia in nine of the 86 patients admitted but in only one of the 124 not admitted. In addition, contamination caused ten other additional positive cultures. These investigators concluded that the frequency of bacteremia among febrile adult outpatients was about 5 per cent, with the physician identifying most of these patients clinically. They concluded that the routine use of blood cultures in febrile adult patients discharged from the emergency department resulted in a high cost for a minimal return.[7] In a similar study in 1984, Stair and Lenhart conducted both a prospective and retrospective study of the use of blood cultures at the Georgetown University Hospital emergency department. The retrospective portion of the study spanned over one year. During that period, the emergency department discharged 17 patients with positive blood cultures. Clinical correlation revealed that contamination caused 15 of the 17 positive blood cultures in discharged patients. Prospectively, investigators found ten positive cultures from 100 consecutive blood cultures obtained from the emergency department. Only four of the ten were judged to be "true positives" with the remainder believed to be the result of contamination. In only one of the ten, did the culture affect the clinical course. This was a young woman with *Escherichia coli* bacteremia secondary to a urinary tract infection with an antibiotic-resistant organism.[6]

A number of developments have occurred since the publication of this study. Pressure for effective use of scarce hospital resources, increased cost for hospitalization, and the advent of broad-spectrum, long-acting, effective antibiotics with central nervous system penetration have been the nidus for the development of other management options.

Sklar and Rusnak, in a study of 86 emergency department patients discharged home from whom blood cultures were obtained, concluded that the selective use of blood cultures on patients with risk factors for endocarditis, pneumonia, and urosepsis may be beneficial. Five of these 86 (5.8 per cent) patients had positive blood cultures. Three of the five patients were subsequently diagnosed to have endocarditis. All patients with a diagnosis of endocarditis had identifiable risk factors. No obvious morbidity occurred in the three endocarditis patients between culturing and admission to the hospital. In addition, the study suggested that the rate of bacteremia of patients hospitalized versus those discharged home was not statistically different (7.4 per cent versus 5.8 per cent).[8]

Multiple investigators support the concept of selective culturing of the adult with low risk factors for bacteremia.[6, 8, 9] Some recommendations to the treating physician are notable:

1. The physician's clinical impression of the adult patient at low risk for outpatient evaluation should guide the decision to obtain blood cultures.

2. The adult at high risk for septicemia should be hospitalized. Three blood cultures should almost always suffice to establish or rule out bacteremia.[10, 11]

3. Patients released from the emergency department who have had blood cultures obtained must have strict follow-up evaluations and procedures. Close follow-up within 12 to 24 hours or sooner after the initial visit is strongly recommended.

4. Special discharge precautions including verification of telephone numbers or designation of a close relative of the patient whom the physician can contact are vital.

5. Explicit return instructions regarding the circumstances warranting return to the emergency department with verification of patient understanding of the discharge instructions are required. These factors must be documented in the patient record.

6. Close coordination and communication with the physician who will see the patient in follow-up are essential.[5, 9]

7. The use of presumptive antibiotic therapy before receiving laboratory results is a rational and cost-effective plan of management at the discretion of the treating physician. The antibiotic chosen should have (1) appropriate antimicrobial coverage, (2) demonstrated therapeutic efficacy for the clinical illness, and (3) a long therapeutic half-life (12 to 24 hours).

FEBRILE CHILD

The pediatric literature has established the concept of "occult bacteremia." The definition of occult bacteremia is a "condition in which bacteremia is present and confirmed by laboratory study, and in which clinical signs and symptoms are minimal."[9] For this reason, the utility of blood culturing in children is quite different from adults. Attempts to ascertain the incidence and proper management of the febrile child have been the source of multiple studies. The incidence of bacteremia in the emergency or outpatient setting is estimated to be 5 per cent in febrile children (range 2.8 to 13 per cent).[12–20] Risk factors of occult bacteremia in children include young age (6 to 24 months), high fever (>38.9° C), and high white blood cell (WBC) count (>15,000 to 20,000 WBC/mm³).[12–15, 18, 19, 21–25] Other investigators suggest the use of the sedimentation rate or C-reactive protein to be useful in the identification of the febrile child with bacteremia.[22, 26, 27] Interestingly, most children with occult bacteremia discharged to home improve with oral antimicrobial therapy.[27–29] However, a small number of the children not treated with antibiotics will continue to be ill, develop new or progressive focal disease, and have persistent bacteremia.[12, 13, 24, 27–29]

The management of children with low risk for bacteremia during their first visit raises the issue of whether presumptive therapy with antimicrobial agents for the child with risk factors will decrease the morbidity of bacteremia. Only limited data exist, and often the numbers in the studies are too small to make any definite conclusion. Investigations by both Bratton and colleagues and Marshall and associates suggest that the outcome of children with unsuspected bacteremia whose treatment was initiated on the first visit was better than the outcome of those untreated.[28, 29] However, in both studies, the two groups were not comparable. In a prospective randomized clinical trial, Carroll and co-workers studied 96 children whose treatment was randomized to either penicillin or placebo. Cultures revealed ten children to be bacteremic. Four of the five treated children showed improvement. All five untreated children were unimproved and two developed meningitis.[27] However, this study's methodology and statistical evaluation have received wide criticism. Jaffe and colleagues studied a total of 955 febrile children ages 3 to 36 months with no focal bacterial infection. Their investigation was a prospective, double-blind, clinical treatment trial of febrile children with no focal evidence of infection. Randomization of treatment occurred to either ampicillin or placebo. Twenty-seven children (2.8 per cent) had bacteremia with pathogenic organisms. Although the numbers were small, there were no significant differences in the incidence of major infectious morbidity associated with bacteremia between the antibiotic treated (2 out of 19) and placebo groups (1 out of 8).[19]

In conclusion, there is no adequate trial to definitively determine the efficacy of presumptive antimicrobial therapy in preventing either morbidity or mortality in the febrile child with occult bacteremia. More important, a trial using an effective, long-acting antimicrobial with excellent central nervous system penetration such as ceftriaxone has not been published. Nonetheless, a number of recommendations can be made for blood culture use in the "febrile child":

1. Physicians should obtain at least one blood culture in the patient younger than 3 months of age who is suspected to be bacteremic. Because "occult bacteremia" is not a recognized entity in this age group, these patients should receive a septic workup as for admitted patients to determine the source of the fever or infection.

2. The physician should consider the diagnosis of occult bacteremia in a child between the ages of 3 months and 24 months presenting with a temperature higher than 39° C, a leukocyte count greater than or equal to 15,000/mm³, or an erythrocyte sedimentation rate of greater than or equal to 30 mm/hour. At least one blood culture should be obtained.

3. Many investigators believe that if the physician decides to manage the patient as an outpatient, initiation of presumptive therapy is advisable pending culture results.[9, 20, 30] The choice should be a long-acting antibiotic with the proper antimicrobial spectrum and with documented efficacy for patients with bacteremia and meningitis. In this age group (3 months to 24 months), antimicrobial activity against *Streptococcus pneumoniae, Neisseria meningitidis,* and *Haemophilus influenzae* is mandatory.[31]

Collection Technique

Venous blood is usually drawn for culture. Collection of venous blood is less hazardous than that of arterial blood and it has been shown, at least in patients with subacute bacterial endocarditis, that arterial blood is no more likely to contain organisms than is venous blood.[32] In fact, indwelling arterial lines may be contaminated and yield false-positive culture results.[33] To minimize contamination with skin flora, antisepsis must be obtained at the site of proposed venipuncture. Because it may be difficult to disinfect the skin of the groin, it is best to avoid femoral vein puncture when obtaining blood for culture.

Many reports cite iodine as superior to other materials for producing skin antisepsis.[34–39] Story[40] and Lee and associates,[41] however, reported studies that indicate that two washes with 70 per cent isopropyl alcohol compare favorably with an iodine wash followed by an alcohol wash. Coulthard and Sykes[42] found isopropyl alcohol to be more effective than ethyl alcohol.

The optimal method may be a three-step procedure.[43, 44] First, the site is cleansed with 70 per cent isopropyl alcohol. Second, a 2 per cent tincture of iodine or 10 per cent povidone-iodine is applied concentrically. Many authorities advise using a soaked sponge to keep the puncture site wet with the solution for a full 2 minutes before venipuncture. Third, after venipuncture, the residual iodine is removed with an alcohol sponge to prevent burns or sensitization. Eisenberg and colleagues[7] reversed the order, using tincture of iodine first and then scrubbing with alcohol prior to venipuncture, without increasing the rate of contamination. A common procedural error is to contaminate the skin with a finger, which is used to palpate a vein before venipuncture.

Scott[45] found that the use of two needles significantly reduced the number of contaminated cultures. This is supported by the work of Eisenberg and coworkers,[7] who had a low contamination rate using two needles. The first needle is used to draw the sample; it is then discarded, and a second sterile needle is used to inject the collected blood into the culture media. While confirming the lower contamination rate with the two-needle technique (0.6 versus 2.2 per cent), Leisure and colleagues recommend using a single needle and caution that recapping of needles may increase the risk of needle stick injury to the clinician.[45a] Needles should be directly placed in a sharps container without recapping whenever possible.

Today, many commercially packaged blood culture kits provide a two needle setup in which the needles are joined by sterile tubing. One needle is for the venipuncture, and the other side punctures the culture bottle or collection container, thereby allowing the blood to flow directly from the patient's vein into the culture media. If two collection bottles (broth media) are used with the double needle and tubing apparatus, the anaerobic bottle is filled first (5 to 10 ml blood added). The aerobic bottle is then "filled" and allowed to vent by removing the venipuncture needle from the arm. If a single collection bottle is used, the bottle is "filled" as for an anaerobic culture and the specimen is subsequently split in the laboratory, with venting of the aerobic portion at that time. Hoffman and associates[46] warn that if blood is drawn for multiple purposes in a single syringe, the blood culture bottles should be inoculated before entering other collection tubes. They reported that reflux of blood introduced into EDTA (ethylenediamine tetraacetic acid)-containing tubes resulted in false-positive blood cultures with *Serratia marcescens.*

Tonnesen and colleagues[47] reported obtaining promising results using blood drawn from indwelling venous catheters compared with venipuncture. Handsfield[48] pointed out that the false-positive rate of 37 per cent in the data of Tonnesen and coworkers[47] was not acceptable. Although it is tempting to aspirate blood from indwelling venous catheters such as a central venous pressure line, such practice results in a higher level of contamination and should not be used when venipuncture sites are available. Wormser and coworkers used a variety of indwelling catheters and found catheter blood cultures to be 96 per cent sensitive and

98 per cent specific.[48a] These results are somewhat better than those of earlier reports and may in part be due to a brief duration of catheter placement (92 per cent drawn within 4 days of placement).

It should be noted that clotted blood or citrated blood is generally unsuitable for culture, because the isolation rate from these samples is substantially decreased.[49]

Smears

Unless the bacteremia is overwhelming, direct Wright-Giemsa or Gram-stained blood smears or buffy-coat smears are generally of no value.[50, 51] This opinion may be reversed if an acridine orange stain is done as early as 6 hours after incubation of the blood culture.[52] Mirrett and associates demonstrated that this stain was more sensitive than methylene blue or Gram stains when small numbers of organisms are involved.[52]

Cultures

It is standard practice to vent one bottle of culture medium, thus replacing the partial vacuum in the bottle with air to enhance the growth of aerobes. This is done by puncturing the diaphragm of the collection bottle with a cotton-plugged needle to allow equilibration. One bottle is left unvented to facilitate recovery of anaerobes. This may be done in the laboratory or at the patient's bedside.

In recent years, many substrates for culturing blood have been devised. These have varied from fluid to fluid-agar slant bottles with additives, which not only serve as anticoagulants but also are capable of neutralizing some antibiotics, complement, lysozyme activity, and phagocytosis. If a patient has previously been treated with penicillin, for example, one may add penicillinase directly to the culture to inactivate the antibiotic remaining in the blood sample. Although this practice is controversial, it may be of value in some instances. If a patient is currently taking antibiotics, the laboratory should be informed so that appropriate steps may be taken to maximize the culture yield. It has become obvious that no specific substrate will suffice to isolate all microbes that might be found in the blood stream. Most laboratories use a two-bottle system to cover aerobic and anaerobic flora and incubate these at 37° C for 7 days. The time period may be extended to 14 days if the patient has been partially treated. Approximately two thirds of blood cultures from bacteremic patients who have not been treated with antibiotics will be positive within 24 hours, and 90 per cent will be positive within 3 days.

VOLUME

The volume of blood cultured is important. Various investigators have shown that increasing the inoculum from 2 ml to as high as 40 ml yielded corresponding increased numbers of positive cultures.[53–55] Most commercial and laboratory-prepared systems are suitable only for between 2 and 10 ml of inocula. The 10-ml inoculum, which is preferable for adults, is not suitable for children. Generally, in children, 1 to 5 ml of blood is recommended for culture, and the younger the child, the smaller the amount.[56] A minimum ratio of blood to broth, 1:10, will usually suffice if one is in doubt as to the volume of blood required. Because fresh human serum has inherent bactericidal properties, it is important to quickly dilute or neutralize this effect with culture media.

TIMING

The timing of the blood culture is important, especially in instances in which the bacteremia may be transient (occurring after insult to infected tissues) or intermittent (undrained abscesses sporadically seeding). The classic teaching method suggests that blood for culture should be drawn just before a chill or febrile episode, but in practice, the onset of such episodes results in blood cultures being initiated after the chill or temperature spikes. Musher and coworkers[57] reported on fever patterns in 102 patients and concluded that in most infectious states, the release of pyrogenic substances into the blood stream is continuous. Exaggeration of the normal variation probably results because of reactivity of the hypothalamus to these stimuli and varies in accordance with circadian rhythm. These findings do not support the recommendation to draw blood cultures just before fever spikes in infected patients unless one were to presume that bacteremia also has a diurnal variation.

The timing of blood culture is even more complicated when one considers the fact that the influx of bacteria into the blood stream will produce a shaking chill or fever only when following a lag period of 30 to 90 minutes. If the host's defenses are active, bacteria may be rapidly removed from the blood by phagocytosis and the blood culture taken at the time of the rigor may be negative. The ideal time for obtaining a blood culture may be determined only retrospectively.

In most adult infections, 2 or 3 cultures, taken at 1-hour intervals, are recommended, but if immediate antimicrobial therapy is planned, the interval should be reduced appropriately.[56] In critically ill patients, it is best to draw all blood samples simultaneously from different anatomic sites and to begin antibiotic therapy promptly. If three separate blood cultures are taken over 24 hours in the nontoxic bacteremic patient, the cumulative yield has been shown to be 99 per cent in the bacteremic adult. A single blood culture has been shown to be frequently satisfactory in the bacteremic neonate.[58]

CONTAMINATION AND FALSE-POSITIVE CULTURES

Gross contamination of blood cultures may occur, resulting in pseudobacteremia.[59] Contamination with skin bacteria often produces blood cultures that are positive for diphtheroids, micrococcus species, bacillus, and staphylococcus epidermidis. It should be noted that these organisms can occasionally be true pathogens, especially in immunosuppressed patients.

Contamination can be kept to a minimum if proper attention is focused on technique. Generally "false-positive" blood cultures can be identified by the clinical course of the patient and the failure of repeat cultures to grow the same organism. In contaminated specimens, growth in the broth generally does not appear earlier than the third or fourth day of incubation and the organism will often not grow in more than one sample.

Ideally, contamination should occur in less than 3 per cent of all blood cultures performed.[60] To attain this goal, it is preferable to have blood drawn directly from the patient into the blood culture media using a double-ended needle. After the needle has been withdrawn, the culture is a closed system, and it should not be reopened unless it is necessary to check growth. A diphasic or triphasic fluid-agar slant or similar modification[61] would eliminate the need for blind subcultures (required when broth type substrates are used). Even the proposed use of acridine orange–stained smears as an alternative to early routine subcultures[56] would require entry into a closed system. Consequently, to reduce the risk of contamination, these procedures should be performed in laminar air-flow facilities, with aseptic technique.

Most of the additives in blood culturing have potential disadvantages that must be considered.[62–65] There have been false-positive diagnoses of bacteremias with *Escherichia*[66] and with *Moraxella*[67] owing to the addition of contaminated penicillinase when the blood cultures were initiated. There is no definitive evidence that penicillinase enhances isolation of bacteria from blood, but its use does enhance the risk of contamination.

Various radiometric methods of assaying blood for bacteria are available commercially.[68] The degree of information produced by these instruments must be weighed against their high initial cost, continuing operating costs, and performance efficiency. Results of controlled evaluation studies of radiometric methods are not encouraging.[59]

FUNGAL CULTURES

Generally, fungi are difficult to isolate in blood cultures, and it may take 4 to 6 weeks to obtain a positive yield. If a fungemia is suspected, it is best to discuss culture media and technique with the laboratory before cultures are taken. Cultures of bone marrow are occasionally positive in deep mycoses when blood cultures are negative.

Occasionally, blood cultures are positive in cases of disseminated histoplasmosis or candidiasis, but other fungi, such as Cryptococcus and Aspergillus or fungi-like bacteria such as Nocardia and Actinomycosis, are rarely isolated from the blood.

ANAEROBIC CULTURE TECHNIQUES

Introduction

Pure anaerobic infections are rarely encountered. The presence of anaerobes, as a microbial component of an infection in which facultative microbes are also prominent, however, is not rare. Unfortunately, the presence of the anaerobes in such an infection may often be overlooked. Because anaerobic infections are often polymicrobic in nature, it is common to find numerous different strains of anaerobic bacteria associated with a single localized necrotic infection, such as an abscess. Anaerobes are the predominant normal flora of the skin and mucous membranes. The resident flora of the various mucosal tracts and epithelial glandular areas of the body consist of a mixed microbial population, including surface aerobes and deep anaerobes with facultative organisms throughout. Often the synergistic interaction of the organisms is required for pathogenicity. Given a suitable environment in an immunocompromised or otherwise weakened host or when local tissue redox potentials are reduced by ischemia, necrosis, or infection, the anaerobes can cause an infection or compound the seriousness of an existing infection. A relatively common example of such an anaerobic disease entity is Vincent's oral mucosal disease (fusospirochetal necrotizing lesions). Anaerobes indigenous to the tonsillar crypts (actinomycetes, fusobacteria, spirochetes, peptostreptococci) that are introduced into other anatomic sites (Table 90–1) such as the lungs can cause life-threatening, often slowly resolving disease in the form of an aspiration pneumonia or a lung abscess.

Certain clinical findings are often associated with the presence of anaerobic bacterial disease. The presence of a foul-smelling discharge, infection located in or adjacent to a mucous membrane, or the presence of crepitus (subcutaneous emphysema) or gangrene suggest infection by anaerobes. Some common primary anaerobic infections include dental abscess, infected human bites, infections developing in patients with malignancies where necrotic tissue is seen, septic thrombophlebitis, pelvic inflammatory disease, perirectal abscess, lung abscess, and those developing in patients who are on aminoglycoside antibiotics.

Table 90–1. Anaerobes Isolated from Selected Clinical Materials (Seattle U.S. Public Health Service Hospital)	
Throat Cultures 1967–1979: 34,856	
Vincent angina	357
Vincent angina and *Streptococcus pyogenes*	2
Vincent angina and *Corynebacterium hemolyticum*	1
Peptostreptococcus	2
Peptostreptococcus and *Haemophilus influenzae*	1
Bacteroides	1
Blood Cultures 1962–1979: 18,912	
Clostridium	2(2)*
C. perfringens	4(3)
C. histolyticum	2(1)
C. lentoputrescens	1(1)
C. cochlearum	1(1)
Propionibacterium acnes	125(125)
Peptococcus	4(4)
Peptostreptococcus	23(17)
Bacteroides	29(22)
Fusobacterium	1(1)
Bacteroides and *Peptostreptococcus*	9(2)
Bacteroides and enteric *Streptococcus*	2(2)
Mixed anaerobes	2(2)
Pleural Fluid	
C. difficile	1

*Isolates (patients).

Indications for Anaerobic Culture

The isolation and identification of anaerobic bacteria are often expensive and time consuming. Not all infections require highly specialized anaerobic culture techniques, and only certain specimens should be cultured for anaerobic bacteria. Potential specimens for anaerobic culture include all cutaneous lesions and fluid aseptically aspirated from sites that are sterile under normal conditions. Such fluids include blood, spinal fluid, pleural fluid, transtracheal aspirate, and pus obtained directly from an abscess cavity or by culdocentesis. Upper respiratory tract collections, expectorated sputum, feces, urogenital collections, and voided urine are generally cultured only aerobically or under increased carbon dioxide–reduced oxygen tensions. Certainly, when there has been suspected or obvious soil and/or foreign body contamination of wounds, direct smears (generally Gram-stained) and anaerobic cultures should be performed. Likewise, when there has been penetration through a mucosal area harboring anaerobes or a suspected pulmonary aspiration of fluids from similar mucosal areas, direct smears and anaerobic cultures should be done.

It is common to obtain a report of "no growth" in foul-smelling abscess cultures. Such cultures are often anaerobic strains that would have been positive if careful anaerobic cultures had been performed.

Collection Technique

Classically, collection and culture techniques stress speed as an essential element. It has been shown that this process may not be that urgent.[69] Thirty-seven strains of anaerobes previously considered to be oxygen-sensitive were actually aerotolerant, surviving in purulent exudate exposed to air at room temperature up to 24 hours before processing.[69] Not all clinical materials are as dense as purulent exudate, however, so that a careful collection technique and expeditious transport to the laboratory are essential for maximum yield.[70]

Generally, ordinary cotton swabs or applicators are unsatisfactory for collecting anaerobic organisms. If the specimen is fluid, it is best to collect the specimen with a sterile needle and syringe. Once the fluid is aspirated, air should be expelled from the syringe and the needle capped to minimize exposure to atmospheric oxygen. If an abscess is to be cultured, percutaneous aspiration of pus for culture and Gram stain before incision and drainage is preferred. When a swab is used to make the collection, the swab should be inserted deeply in a thioglycolate (without indicator) or other suitable reduced broth tube immediately. Oxygen-free tubes that contain swabs are available for obtaining anaerobic cultures. Such tubes should not be opened until the culture is taken. The tube is then sealed promptly, and the specimen is quickly transported to the laboratory.

Smears

In the hands of an experienced clinical microscopist, direct smears of clinical material often will be interpreted as consisting of anaerobic bacteria with a significant host-cell relationship and may establish the microbiologic diagnosis. The direct smear of a possible clostridial-caused gangrenous infection is essential and can be lifesaving, because time is extremely important.

Because the initial incubation period for anaerobes is usually 48 hours, the immediate examination of a Gram-stained smear of clinical material for anaerobes is more urgent than when aerobes or facultative organisms are suspected to be the etiologic agent. Note that the highly toxic *Clostridium perfringens* organism is present in approximately 50 per cent of gangrenous lesions.[71]

Cultures

The same nutritionally enriched broths that are available commercially for the isolation of aerobic and facultative microbes can be used for the isolation of anaerobic microbes. *Unvented* vacuum bottles of commercially produced media have a sufficiently low redox potential to support the growth of anaerobic bacteria.[72] Therefore, thioglycolate broths and other specially prepared anaerobic broths are not needed initially.

Conclusion

Because such a large proportion of the resident flora of the upper respiratory mucosa, the female urogenital mucosa, cutaneous glands, and the colon are anaerobes (reported as 10:1 for the first three cited areas and at least 1000:1 for the colon),[71] smears and cultures of drainage from these areas or from lesions near these areas must be interpreted very cautiously. Certainly, clinical findings have an even more important role in these instances. The foul odor of expectorated sputum from a patient with aspiration pneumonia and probable lung abscess, fetid breath of persons with sore throats or sinusitis, and stench or crepitation at a wound site[73] suggest the presence and significance of anaerobes such as species of *Bacteroides*, *Peptostreptococcus*, *Actinomyces*, and *Clostridium*.

REFERENCES

Bacteremia and Blood Culture

1. Bennett IL Jr, Beeson PB: Bacteremia: Consideration of some experimental and clinical aspects. Yale J Biol Med 26:241, 1954.

2. Everett ED, Hirschmann JV: Transient bacteremia and endocarditis prophylaxis. A review. Medicine 56:61, 1977.
3. Gleckman R, Hibert D: A febrile bacteremia: A phenomenon in geriatric patients. JAMA 248:1478, 1982.
4. Weinstein MP, Reller LB, Murphy JR, et al: The clinical significance of positive blood cultures: A comprehensive analysis of 500 episodes of bacteremia and fungemia in adults. I. Laboratory and epidemiologic observations. Rev Infect Dis 5:35, 1983.
5. Weinstein MP, Reller LB, Murphy JR, et al: The clinical significance of positive blood cultures: A comprehensive analysis of 500 episodes of bacteremia and fungemia in adults. II. Clinical observations, with special reference to factors influencing prognosis. Rev Infect Dis 5:54, 1983.
6. Stair TO, Lenhart M: Outpatient blood cultures: Retrospective and prospective. Audits in one emergency department (letter). Ann Emerg Med 13:986, 1984.
7. Eisenberg JM, Rose JD, Weistein A: Routine blood cultures from febrile outpatients. JAMA 236:2863, 1976.
8. Sklar DP, Rusnak R: The value of outpatient blood cultures in the emergency department. Am J Emerg Med 5:95, 1987.
9. Lyman JL: Use of blood cultures in the emergency department. Ann Emerg Med 15:308, 1986.
10. Aronson MD, Bor DH: Blood cultures. Ann Intern Med 106:246, 1987.
11. Washington JA, Ilstrup DM: Blood cultures: Issues and controversies. Rev Infect Dis 8:792, 1986.
12. McGowan JE, Bratton L, Klein JO, et al: Bacteremia in febrile children seen in a "walk-in" pediatric clinic. N Engl J Med 25:1309, 1973.
13. Teele DW, Pelton SI, Grant MJA, et al: Bacteremia in febrile children under 2 years of age: Results of cultures of blood of 600 consecutive febrile children seen in a walk in clinic. J Pediatr 87:227, 1975.
14. McCarthy PL, Grundy GW, Spiesel SZ, et al: Bacteremia in children: An outpatient clinical review. Pediatrics 57:861, 1976.
15. McCarthy PL, Dolan TF: Hyperpyrexia in children. Am J Dis Child 130:849, 1976.
16. Hoekelman R, Lewin EB, Shapira MB, et al: Potential bacteremia in pediatric practice. Am J Dis Child 133:1017, 1979.
17. Kline MW, Lorin MI: Bacteremia in children afebrile at presentation to an emergency room. Pediatr Infect Dis J 6:197, 1987.
18. Dagan R, Powell KR, Hall CB, et al: Identification of infants unlikely to have serious bacterial infection although hospitalized for suspected sepsis. J Pediatr 107:855, 1985.
19. Jaffe DM, Tanz RR, Davis AT, et al: Antibiotic administration to treat possible occult bacteremia in febrile children. N Engl J Med 317:1175, 1987.
20. Crocker PJ: Occult bacteremia in the emergency department. Ann Emerg Med 13:45, 1984.
21. Baron MA, Fink HD: Bacteremia in private pediatric practice. Pediatrics 66:171, 1980.
22. Crain EF, Shelov SP: Febrile infants: Predictors of bacteremia. J Pediatr 101:686, 1982.
23. Brook I, Gruenwald LD: Occurrence of bacteremia in febrile children seen in a hospital outpatient department and pediatric practice. South Med J 77:1240, 1984.
24. Dashefsky B, Teele DW, Klein JO: Unsuspected meningoccemia. J Pediatr 102:69, 1983.
25. Todd J: Childhood infections: Diagnostic value of peripheral white blood cell and differential cell counts. Am J Dis Child 127:810, 1974.
26. McCarthy PL, Jekel JF, Dolan TF: Temperature greater than or equal to 40° C in children less than 24 months of age: A prospective study. Pediatrics 59:663, 1977.
27. Carroll WL, Farrell MK, Singer JI, et al: Treatment of occult bacteremia: A prospective randomized clinical trial. Pediatrics 72:608, 1983.
28. Bratton L, Teele DW, Klein JO: Outcome of unsuspected pneumococcemia in children not initially admitted to the hospital. J Pediatr 90:703, 1977.
29. Marshall R, Teele DW, Klein JO: Unsuspected bacteremia due to haemophilus influenzae: Outcome in children not initially admitted to hospital. J Pediatr 95:690, 1979.
30. Klein JO: Bacteremia in febrile children managed out of hospital. In Remington JS, Swartz MN (eds): Current Clinical Topics of Infectious Disease, Volume 6. New York, McGraw-Hill, 1975, pp 184–195.
31. Cherry JD: Selection of antimicrobial agents for initial treatment of suspected septicemia in infants and children. Rev Infect Dis 5(Suppl):s32–s39, 1983.
32. Mallen MS, Hube EL, Brenes M: Comparative study of blood cultures made from artery, vein, and bone marrow in patients with subacute bacterial endocarditis. Am Heart J 33:692, 1947.
33. Vaisanen IT, Michelsen T, Valtonen V, et al: Comparison of arterial and venous blood samples for the diagnosis of bacteremia in critically ill patients. Crit Care Med 13:664, 1985.
34. Braude AI, Sanford JP, Bartlett JE, Mallery OT: Effects and clinical significance of bacterial contaminants in transfused blood. J Lab Clin Med 39:902, 1952.
35. Gardner AD: Rapid disinfection of clean unwashed skin. Lancet 255:760, 1952.
36. Gershenfeld L: Iodine. In Reddish GF (ed): Antiseptics, Disinfectants, Fungicides, and Chemical and Physical Sterilization. Philadelphia, Lea & Febiger, 1954.

37. Lovell DL: Preoperative skin preparation with reference to surface bacteria contaminants and resident flora. Surg Clin North Am 26:1053, 1946.

38. Scurr CF: Emergencies in general practice: Accidents with injections. Br Med J 1:1289, 1956.

39. Zintel HA: Asepsis and antisepsis. Surg Clin North Am 36:257, 1956.

40. Story P: Testing of skin disinfectants. Br Med J 2:1128, 1952.

41. Lee S, Schoen I, Malkin A: Comparison of use of alcohol with that of iodine for skin antisepsis in obtaining blood cultures. Am J Clin Pathol 47:646, 1967.

42. Coulthard CE, Sykes G: Germicidal effect of alcohol. Pharm J 137:79, 1936.

43. Washington JA II: Blood cultures: Principles and techniques. Mayo Clin Proc 50:91, 1975.

44. Tandberg D, Reed WP: Blood cultures following rectal examination. JAMA 239:1789, 1978.

45. Scott AC: Blood-culture technique: Two needles or one (letter). Lancet 1:1414, 1979.

45a. Leisure MK, Moore DM, Schwartzman JD, et al: Changing the needle when inoculating blood cultures: A no-benefit and high-risk procedure. JAMA 264:2111, 1990.

46. Hoffman PC, Arnow PM, Goldman DA, et al: False-positive blood cultures: Association with nonsterile blood collection tubes. JAMA 236:2073, 1976.

47. Tonnesen A, Peuler M, Lockwood WR: Cultures of blood drawn by catheters vs venipuncture. JAMA 235:1877, 1976.

48. Handsfield HH: Blood cultures drawn through catheters (letter). JAMA 236:2944, 1976.

48a. Wormser GP, Onorato IM, Preminger TJ, et al: Sensitivity and specificity of blood cultures obtained through intravascular catheters. Crit Care Med 18:152, 1990.

49. Ellner PD, Stoessel CJ: The role of temperature and anticoagulant on the in vitro survival of bacteria in blood. J Infect Dis 116:238, 1966.

50. Bartlett RC, McCarthy L: Edited transcript, Pfizer Diagnostics "Dialogue." (Annual Meeting) American Society of Microbiologist, Chicago, Illinois, 1974.

51. Reik H, Rubin SJ: Evaluation of the buffy-coat smear for rapid detection of bacteremia. JAMA 245:357, 1981.

52. Mirrett S, Lauer BA, Miller GA, et al: Comparison of acridine orange, methylene blue, and Gram stains for blood culture. J Clin Microbiol 15:562, 1982.

53. Hall MM, Ilstrup DM, Washington JA 2d: Effect of volume of blood cultured on detection of bacteremia. J Clin Microbiol 3:643, 1976.

54. Tenney JH, Reller LB, Mirrett S, et al: Controlled evaluation of the volume of blood cultured in detection of bacteremia and fungemia. J Clin Microbiol 15:558, 1982.

55. Washington JA 2d: Conventional approaches to blood culture. In The Detection of Septicemia. Boca Raton, Fla, CRC Press, Inc, 1978, pp 41–88.

56. Reller LB, Murray PR, MacLowry JD: Blood cultures II. Cumitech 1. Washington JA 2d (coordinating ed). Washington, DC, American Society of Microbiologists, June 1982.

57. Musher DM, Fainstein V, Young EJ, et al: Fever patterns: Their lack of clinical significance. Arch Intern Med 139:1225, 1979.

58. Franciosi RA, Favara BE: A single blood culture for confirmation of the diagnosis of neonatal sepsis. Am J Clin Pathol 57:215, 1972.

59. Griffin MR, Miller AD, Davis AC: Blood culture cross contamination associated with a radiometric analyzer. J Clin Microbiol 15:567, 1982.

60. Wilson WR, Van Scoy RE, Washington JA 2d: Incidence of bacteremia in adults without infection. J Clin Microbiol 2:94, 1975.

61. Pfaller MA, Sibley TK, Westfall LM, et al: Clinical laboratory comparison of a slide-blood culture system with a conventional broth system. J Clin Microbiol 16:525, 1982.

62. Rosner R: Effect of various anticoagulants and no anticoagulant on ability to isolate bacteria directly from parallel clinical blood specimens. Am J Clin Pathol 49:216, 1968.

63. Evans GL, Cekoric T Jr, Searcy RL: Comparative effects of anticoagulants on bacterial growth in experimental blood cultures. Am J Med Tech 34:1, 1968.

64. Pai CH, Sorger S: Enhancement of recovery of Neisseria meningitidis by gelatin in blood culture media. J Clin Microbiol 14:20, 1981.

65. Hall MM, Warren E, Ilstrup DM, Washington JA 2nd: Comparison of sodium amylosulfate and sodium polyanetholsulfonate in blood culture media. J Clin Microbiol 3:212, 1976.

66. Norden CW: Pseudo-septicemia. Ann Intern Med 71:789, 1969.

67. Faris HM, Sparling FF: Mima polymorpha bacteremia. JAMA 219:76, 1972.

68. Carlson LG, Plorde JJ: Influence of a blood culture inoculation technique on detection of bacteremia by the BACTEC system. J Clin Microbiol 16:590, 1982.

Anaerobic Culture Techniques

69. Bartlett JG, Sullivan-Sigler N, et al: Anaerobes survive in clinical specimens despite delayed processing. J Clin Microbiol 3:133, 1976.

70. Holdeman LV, Cato EP, Moore WEC (eds): Anaerobe Laboratory Manual, 4th ed. Blacksburg, Va, Virginia Polytechnic Institute and State University, 1977.

71. Finegold SM, Shepherd WE, Spaulding EH: Practical anaerobic bacteriology. Cumitech 5. Washington, DC, American Society of Microbiologists, April, 1977.

72. Reller LB, Murray PR, MacLowry JD: Blood cultures II. Cumitech 1. Washington JA 2d (coordinating ed). Washington, DC, American Society of Microbiologists, June 1982.

73. Pulaski EJ: Common Bacterial Infections. Philadelphia and London, WB Saunders Co, 1964, pp 76–80.

Chapter **91**

Procedures Pertaining to Hypothermia

David P. Sklar and David Doezema

INTRODUCTION

The spectacular reports of survival after up to 66 minutes of cold water immersion fuel our fascination with hypothermia.[1, 2] The severely hypothermic patient appears at times to lie suspended somewhere between life and death, and physicians continue cardiopulmonary resuscitation (CPR) long past the time other patients would be declared dead, occasionally succeeding in resuscitating a hypothermic patient who leaves the hospital neurologically intact.[3-6] The medical literature discussing treatment for the patient presenting with a subnormal core temperature has been characterized by anecdotal reports, patient selection bias, and uncontrolled studies.[7-10] However, since the condition is relatively rare, most physicians cannot rely upon their own experience to help them evaluate treatment recommendations.

We provide a critical review of approaches and procedures appropriate to the management of several categories of hypothermic patients. Our recommendations combine treatment efficacy with safety. Before describing procedures and making recommendations, we will define essential terms and briefly review the pathophysiology of hypothermia.

DEFINITIONS

Accidental hypothermia (AH) has been defined as an unintentionally induced decrease in the core (vital organ) temperature below 35° C.[11] Victims of hypothermia can be separated into the following categories: *mild* hypothermia 35 to 33° C (95.0 to 91.4° F), *moderate* hypothermia 32 to 28° C (89.1 to 82.4° F), and *severe* hypothermia 27 to 9° C (80.6 to 48.2° F).[11] Other factors that may be useful in separating groups of AH patients include the presence of underlying illness,[12-16] altered neurologic state on arrival, hypotension, and the need for prehospital CPR.[17] A hypothermia outcome score has been developed that incorporates some of these factors.[17]

Mild to moderate hypothermia may easily be overlooked in the emergency department, because the signs and symptoms may be misleading. A common error is failure to routinely obtain a core temperature on all patients. Presenting symptoms such as confusion in the elderly and combat-

iveness in the intoxicated patient may not initially be recognized as symptoms of hypothermia. *Hypothermic patients frequently will not feel cold* or shiver, and a "paradoxical undressing" has been described in confused patients who apparently have the sensation of heat at lowered body temperatures.

CORE TEMPERATURE MEASUREMENT

Accurate temperature measurement is important to guide diagnostic and therapeutic decisions. A core temperature can be estimated with a rectal probe, although rectal temperature often lags behind core temperature.[11] Esophageal probes may be used, although they may be affected by warm humidified air therapy, which is commonly used in severe hypothermia. Oral temperatures are not reliable if the patient is uncooperative or tachypneic[18] or if the thermometer does not record temperatures in the hypothermic range and are *inappropriate* for evaluating significant hypothermia. Other possible sites for temperature measurement include the tympanic membrane and the urinary bladder.[19] Fresh urine temperature can closely approximate core temperature.[20] Standard glass/mercury thermometers generally cannot record temperatures of less than 34° C, although some models are available to record temperatures as low as 24° C (Dynamed, Inc., Carlsbad, CA). For monitoring purposes we recommend rectal or bladder probes and tympanic membrane temperature measurement to guide therapy (Fig. 91–1). The rectal probe should be inserted at least 10 cm beyond the anal sphincter and its position frequently verified. One should remember that temperature gradients exist in the human body and consistency of monitoring at one or more sites is mandatory. A chart that converts Centigrade to Fahrenheit temperatures will assist the clinician in assessing the severity of hypothermia (Fig. 91–2).

PATHOPHYSIOLOGY

Accidental hypothermia occurs when the body's heat producing mechanisms cannot keep up with heat loss. Heat production occurs through basal metabolic functions and muscular activity. Heat production can be increased from the basal rate of 100 kcal/hr to 500 kcal/hr by shivering.[21, 22] Heat loss occurs through radiation, conduction, evaporation, and convection. Vasoconstriction and shunting of blood can preserve core temperature at the expense of a further temperature decrease of the skin. As the core body temperature drops below 33° C, the patient becomes confused and ataxic.[22] Shivering stops at about 32° C. Atrial fibrillation occurs frequently as the temperature continues to drop,[23] and the patient loses consciousness.[22] A J-wave in the electrocardiogram (ECG) often appears prior to ventricular fibrillation (Fig. 91–3). Ventricular fibrillation may occur below 29° C and becomes common as the core drops to

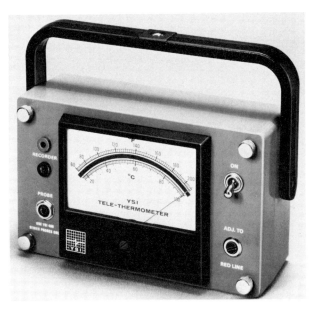

Figure 91–1. Electric thermometer (without probe). This is model 43TA with Fahrenheit and Celsius scales. Infrared tympanic membrane thermometers are acceptable alternatives, but the rectal probe has the advantage of providing a continuous readout. (Courtesy of Yellow Springs Instrument Company, Yellow Springs, Ohio.)

25° C.[22] The electroencephalogram (EEG) flattens at 19 to 20° C,[24] and asystole commonly occurs at 18° C but has been seen at higher temperatures. The lowest recorded temperature for a survivor of AH is 16° C.[25]

INITIAL EVALUATION AND STABILIZATION OF THE HYPOTHERMIC PATIENT

Overall, one must realize that with the reduction of core and cellular temperatures, it is not surprising to find a parallel reduction in all parameters of vital activity, because the enzymatic rate of metabolism itself decreases two to three times with each 10° C drop and cerebral blood flow decreases 6 to 7 per cent per 1° C drop. Profound hypothermia results in coma, hyporeflexia, fixed and dilated pupils, severe bradycardia, and often unobtainable blood pressure. In severe hypothermia, a pulse may not be palpable and blood pressure measurement may require the use of a Doppler device.[16] ECG monitoring provides rate and rhythm status. All patients who have more than minimal impairment require frequent determination of their oxygenation, ventilation, and acid/base status via arterial blood gases.

All patients should have an adequate-bore intravenous (IV) line established for fluid, glucose, and possible drug administration. Most hypothermic patients are *dehydrated*, because fluid intake is reduced and cold causes a diuresis; maintenance IV fluids should be given routinely. Warming of all IV fluids to 40 to 42° C is reasonable, but the usual volumes administered will not contribute many calories of heat.

With a mild to moderate reduction in core temperature, the level of mentation correlates with the severity of the AH or associated illness or both. In alcoholics or diabetics, coma at higher core temperatures may be due to unsuspected hypoglycemia, and a trial of glucose by bolus infusion is justified. In the 22 cases of AH reviewed by Fitzgerald, all except two were alcoholics.[26] The serum glucose was less than 50 mg/dl in 41 per cent (nine patients). This study noted glycosuria in two patients, even when low serum glucose values were evident, and described a renal tubular

glycosuria in AH. Such glycosuria may worsen or cause hypoglycemia; *glycosuria in AH is no guarantee of adequate serum glucose*. This supports the routine use of supplemental IV glucose unless a normal serum glucose can be quickly assured. IV thiamine (100 mg) and a trial dose of 2 mg IV naloxone (Narcan) should also be given to *all obtunded victims* to treat potential thiamine deficiency and narcotic overdose, respectively. Although failure to rewarm spontaneously has been noted in victims with hypothyroidism and other endocrine deficiencies, the use of thyroid hormones and steroids is reserved for those patients with suspected thyroid and adrenal insufficiency, respectively.

Antibiotics are not routinely indicated in uncomplicated mild hypothermia. Although there is no consensus on the value of routine antibiotic therapy in severe AH, the inaccuracy of historical, laboratory, and clinical data in distinguishing the infected from the noninfected hypothermic patient has prompted some authors to advocate the routine initiation of broad-spectrum antibiotic therapy upon admission of severely hypothermic patients.

TREATMENT OVERVIEW

The treatment of AH involves support of basic bodily functions, i.e., airway, breathing, and circulation, while preventing further heat loss and augmenting heat production. Although AH may be lethal, the speed and manner of warming the patient may also be harmful by causing or worsening hypotension, a paradoxical decrease in core temperature,[9, 27, 28] and cardiac dysrhythmias.[29, 30] Other complications may include bleeding[8, 31] and infection of surgical incisions. Invasive therapy should be carefully considered and individualized to the severity of the hypothermia and the condition of the patient, and one should avoid the temptation to *overtreat and overmonitor with invasive techniques the otherwise stable hypothermic patient*.

As opposed to the need for rapid temperature correction with *hyperthermia*, a condition in which it is essential to lower the core temperature as rapidly as possible, a more gradual and conservative approach is generally advocated

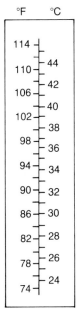

Figure 91–2. Temperature conversion scale. To change Celsius (centigrade) to Fahrenheit, multiply the Celsius temperature by 9/5 and add 32. To change Fahrenheit to Celsius, subtract 32 from the Fahrenheit number and multiply by 5/9.

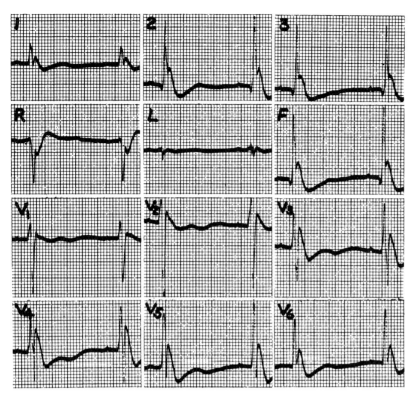

Figure 91–3. In severe hypothermia, the electrocardiogram (ECG) exhibits marked elevation of the "J deflection," so-called Osborne waves. The height of the J wave is proportionate to the degree of hypothermia, and this finding is usually most marked in the midprecordial leads. The ECG is of a patient with sinus bradycardia, but approximately half of patients with a temperature below 32° C will develop slow atrial fibrillation, a rhythm that usually converts spontaneously with rewarming. (From Marriott HJ: Practical Electrocardiology. 8th ed. Baltimore, Williams & Wilkins, 1988. © Williams & Wilkins, 1988.)

for rewarming the moderately *hypothermic* patient. Although the ideal rewarming rate is unknown and clearly varies with each case, it is logical to be content with a 0.5 to 2.0° C per hour rise in temperature *in the otherwise stable patient* (Table 91–1). Patients who slowly become hypothermic over hours or days may not tolerate nor require invasive procedures or aggressive therapy.

The patient with severe underlying problems such as hypoglycemia, sepsis, adrenal crisis, drug overdose, or hypothyroidism should be treated appropriately for those conditions as well as for hypothermia, as long-term outcome may depend more on treatment of the underlying illness than the hypothermia.[32, 33]

For patients with AH that is mild, removal of wet clothing followed by passive external rewarming with blankets will generally suffice. Passive external warming results following the addition of increased insulation, preventing further heat loss so that the body's own mechanisms for heat production can restore normal temperature. The technique is simple; however, the patient must be capable of generating enough body heat for this method to be successful. Patients who cannot shiver, patients who are hypotensive, or patients who are intoxicated or malnourished may not have this capability; however, most patients with mild hypothermia can be warmed gradually with passive rewarming techniques (Fig. 91–4). Survival rates using passive external rewarming have ranged from 55 to 100 per cent.[7, 8, 32–35]

For patients in the moderate or severe category of hypothermia, a more aggressive approach may be warranted. The options available are active external rewarming and active core rewarming. Active core rewarming techniques can be further divided into less invasive and more invasive techniques.

Active External Rewarming

The application of heat to the skin of the hypothermic patient has been termed *active external rewarming*.

INDICATIONS

Although there is some suggestion that active external rewarming may be associated with an increase in mortality over other treatments,[9, 17] we will describe it briefly because it may have a place in the adjunctive care of moderately hypothermic, otherwise healthy individuals. Furthermore, in settings where more aggressive warming techniques are precluded owing to lack of equipment or personnel, active external rewarming may be the only option available to the rescuer, paramedic, or physician.

PROCEDURE

The techniques most commonly used include immersion of the hypothermic patient (except the extremities and head) into a warm (40° C) bath (Fig. 91–5) and the use of warm water–filled heat exchange blankets, e.g., "heating blankets," electrical heating blankets, or a sheet cradle.[36] A warm

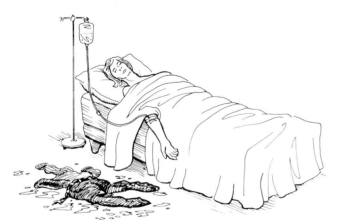

Figure 91–4. Passive external rewarming features: Further heat loss must be stopped through insulation and environmental manipulation. Internal heat generation is required for rewarming. Rewarming rates are relatively slow.

Table 91–1. *Warming Rates (°C/hr)*

	Passive External	Active External	Inhalation of Warm Air	Peritoneal Lavage	Colon/Gastric/ Bladder Lavage	Cardiac Bypass
1st Hour	1.4	1.5	1.5	1.5	1.3	1.0
2nd Hour	1.4	2.4	2.0	2.5	1.7	2.7
3rd Hour	1.8	2.0	1.9	3.2	1.8	3.2

(From Danzl D, Pozos RS: Multicenter Hypothermia Study. Ann Emerg Med 16:1042, 1987. Reproduced by permission.)

immersion tank of the type present in most burn units can be used. The patient should receive supplemental IV fluid[36] that has been warmed to 40° C, given at a rate sufficient to generate a urinary output of 30 to 40 ml per hour. An initial fluid bolus of 500 ml of 5 per cent dextrose and normal saline may be beneficial. (Note that blood pressure is not an accurate way to gauge fluid resuscitation, since serious hypothermia is always accompanied by "physiologic" hypotension.) Close monitoring of the patient's acid-base status should accompany immersion into the tank. Since patients requiring mechanical ventilation have rarely been subjected to tank immersion, it cannot be recommended for hypothermic patients who require intubation. Rewarming rates ranging from 0.90 to 8.8° C per hour have been reported.[9, 10]

If a heating blanket is used, the patient can be placed on the warm heat source while receiving other treatments that may be difficult or impossible to carry out in a tub, such as defibrillation, CPR, or more invasive warming techniques.

COMPLICATIONS

The concern with this treatment is that surface vasodilation may produce a relative hypovolemia in the hypothermic patient. A further decrease in the core temperature may occur as the blood courses through still cold extremities and returns to the heart. In the study by Miller and coworkers, mortality with this method was 64.43 per cent.[9] However, others have described a 95 per cent survival rate.[10] One study with human volunteers with mild to moderate hypothermia comparing external rewarming with inhalation with warm air demonstrated superior warming rates using external rewarming without adverse effect.[37] Importantly, CPR and other advanced cardiac therapy and/or monitoring are impossible with immersion rewarming.

Fluid resuscitation may account for some of the survival variability reported. Until adequately studied, passive external rewarming should only be considered in a clinically monitored setting for moderately hypothermic or mildly

hypothermic patients who can protect their airway. When using a heating device, the potential for burns to the areas in greatest contact with the heating source should also be monitored.

Active Core Rewarming

There is accumulating evidence that active core rewarming may decrease mortality from severe hypothermia exposure compared with other techniques.[17] Several methods have been described including the use of warm humidified air through an endotracheal tube or mask (Fig. 91–6), peritoneal lavage (see Fig. 91–6), gastric or bladder lavage with warm fluid, cardiopulmonary bypass (Fig. 91–7), hemodialysis, and thoracotomy with mediastinal lavage (Fig. 91–8). These techniques transfer heat actively to the body core, achieving varying rewarming rates. The specific techniques as well as some of the advantages and disadvantages for each procedure will be described.

LESS INVASIVE TECHNIQUES

Inhalation of Heated Humidified Oxygen or Air
Background. The use of warm humidified oxygen to treat hypothermia was described by Lloyd in 1973,[38] and it has been used successfully since then.[8] Miller and colleagues reported average rates of rewarming of 0.74° C per hour via mask and 1.22° C per hour via endotracheal tube with heated aerosol at 40° C.[9] Faster rewarming rates may be accomplished using a maximum safe aerosol temperature of 45° C. The Multicenter Hypothermia Study showed an average first and second hour rewarming rate of 1.5 to 2° C for mask and endotracheal tube inhalation in severe hypothermia.[39] This rate was somewhat less in moderate hypothermia. There was also a trend toward a better outcome using this method.[17]

The core rewarming occurs through the following mechanisms. The warmed alveolar blood returns to the heart, thereby warming the myocardium. The warmed humidified air delivered to the alveoli also warms contiguous structures in the mediastinum by conduction. Finally, warming the inhaled air or oxygen eliminates a major source of heat loss.

Indications and Contraindications. The use of heated humidified air or oxygen is a simple technique that should be used routinely, either by itself or in combination with other methods, in all patients with hypothermia, regardless of severity. If the correct equipment is available, it can be used in the field as well as the hospital.[38, 40] Mouth-to-tube ventilation in the intubated hypothermic prehospital patient has the theoretical advantage of providing warm humidified air without special equipment. The ventilating rescuer can inhale oxygen prior to expiring into the patient's endotracheal tube to provide air with increased oxygen content.

There are no contraindications for or reported complications from the use of warm humidified air for hypothermia, and there is no "afterdrop."[11, 27, 28]

Procedure. A heated cascade nebulizer can be used with

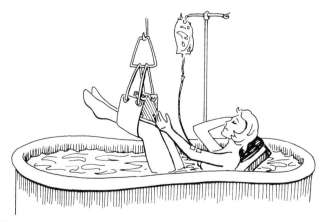

Figure 91–5. Active external rewarming features: A heat source warms the skin. Rates of rewarming are very rapid in some series. There have been suggestions of increased mortality with this method when used for patients with moderate to severe hypothermia.

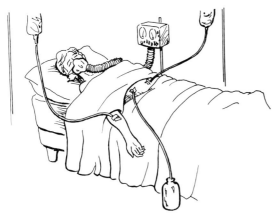

Figure 91–6. Active core rewarming methods: Inhalation of warm, humidified air or oxygen causes gradual core rewarming. This method can be combined with other methods such as heated intravenous fluids. Peritoneal lavage is a more rapid method of core rewarming that requires placement of one or more intraperitoneal catheters.

a mask for patients with spontaneous respirations or with a volume ventilator for intubated patients. It is important to monitor the inspired air to maintain a temperature of approximately 45° C.[41] Temperatures greater than 50° C may burn the mucosa, and temperatures less than 45° C do not deliver maximum heat. The air or oxygen must be humidified,[11] and the heater module may need modification, as many units have feedback mechanisms that shut off at a given temperature. In our institution, we found that without modification, we were delivering humidified air at no greater than 40° C using all available ventilators. In many cases the air temperature was only 30° C.

One can calculate the amount of heat in kilocalories delivered, but it is sufficient to monitor the patient's rectal or tympanic temperature to determine effectiveness.[42] If the warming rate is acceptable, inhalation therapy may be sufficient by itself to treat the hypothermic patient.

Conclusions. Recent studies have suggested that the rewarming rate of inhalation therapy is inferior to that of peritoneal lavage, thoracic lavage, and bath rewarming.[43] However, since inhalation therapy can be combined with any and all other methods of rewarming and because it is relatively noninvasive and inexpensive, it should be considered as the initial treatment of choice for hypothermic patients.

Peritoneal Dialysis

Background. Peritoneal dialysis (lavage) is an ideal treatment for severe hypothermia because it is available in most hospitals and does not require any unusual equipment or training. Rewarming rates of 1 to 3° C per hour, depending on the dialysis rate, can be achieved without sophisticated equipment that may delay therapy or require transfer of the patient to a tertiary care facility.[39, 44]

Peritoneal dialysis rewarming was first used successfully in a patient in ventricular fibrillation with a temperature of 21° C.[45] Since that time, there have been reports of successful rewarming with peritoneal lavage in stable, severely hypothermic patients and unstable hypothermic patients in cardiac arrest.[27, 44, 46] Peritoneal lavage works through heat transfer from lavage fluid to the peritoneal cavity. The peritoneal great vessels and abdominal organs provide a large surface area for heat exchange. As in other rewarming methods, there are proponents and detractors;[47] however, there are few controlled comparisons with other methods,[43] and failures are probably not reported.

Indications and Contraindications. Peritoneal dialysis is indicated in any severely hypothermic patient (temperature less than 28° C), especially patients in cardiac arrest. It is particularly useful in hypothermic patients who have overdosed with a dialyzable toxin. Other less invasive methods, such as gastric or bladder lavage or warm nebulized air or oxygen inhalation, may be preferred in stable patients with temperatures greater than 26 to 28° C. Peritoneal dialysis should not be performed on patients with previous abdominal surgery.

Equipment. Minimal equipment is needed. We recommend using the Seldinger technique, as described by Lazarus and Nelson,[48] with a commercially available disposable kit (Arrow Peritoneal Lavage Kit, Product No. AK-09000, Arrow International, Inc., Reading, PA) because of the minimal morbidity associated with this procedure (see Chapter 56).

Procedure. The patient should be supine with a Foley catheter in place. After infiltration with lidocaine, an infraumbilical stab incision is made with a number 11 blade, and an 18-gauge needle is placed into the peritoneal cavity directed toward the pelvis at a 45-degree angle. A standard flexible J-wire is inserted through the needle, and the needle is removed. The 8 French dialysis catheter is passed over the wire with a twisting motion, and the wire is removed.

Lavage rates of 4 to 12 liters per hour can be achieved with two catheters. Fluid is warmed with a standard blood warmer to 40 to 45° C. We recommend standard 1.5 per cent dextrose dialysate solution, adding potassium (4 mEq/L) if the patient becomes hypokalemic. Ringer's solution and normal saline have also been used successfully.[49] The rate should be at least 6 liters per hour and preferably 10 liters per hour.[49]

Complications. The method we describe has a complication rate of less than 1 per cent[48, 50] and, in our hospital, has had no morbidity. A "mini-lap" using direct dissection may also be used but may have a higher complication rate.[50]

Conclusions. Peritoneal dialysis is a useful method because it uses readily available fluid and can be done with a self-contained disposable kit. If a hospital also treats trauma victims, the same lavage kit can be used for evaluation of abdominal trauma. If combined with warm nebulized inhalation, warming rates of 4° C per hour can be achieved.[39]

Gastrointestinal/Bladder Rewarming

Background. Gastric or bladder irrigation offers some of the same advantages as peritoneal dialysis without invading the peritoneal cavity. Heat is delivered to structures in close proximity to the core. In the Multicenter Hypothermia Study, gastric/bladder/colon lavage had a first hour rewarming rate of 1 to 1.5° C for severe hypothermia and a second hour rewarming rate of 1.5 to 2° C for severe hypothermia.[39] In a multifactorial analysis of the Multicenter Hypothermia

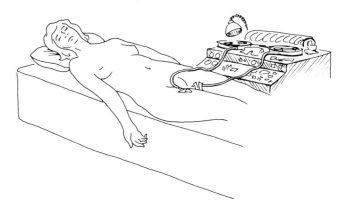

Figure 91–7. Active core rewarming cardiac bypass features: Bypass technology and a surgical team are needed. The rewarming rates are rapid. This method is useful in a patient with cardiac arrest; the technique is invasive and expensive.

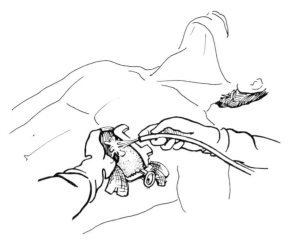

Figure 91–8. Active core rewarming open thoracic lavage features: The heart is warmed directly. This method requires surgical backup and is relatively invasive. The rewarming rates are rapid.

Study, there was a trend toward improved survival in patients on whom this method was used.[17]

Although the amount of heat delivered with gastric lavage is much less than that delivered with peritoneal dialysis, it is somewhat easier to use and less invasive. When combined with other methods, gastric or bladder lavage provides significant warming.[6, 39] Serum electrolytes should be monitored if large volumes of tap water are used, as dilutional electrolyte disturbances may occur. Children may be more susceptible to electrolyte changes with tap water irrigation.[31]

Indications. Warmed gastric or bladder lavage is indicated in moderate or severe hypothermia. It can be combined with other warming techniques when rapid rewarming is needed.

Contraindications. Patients who are obtunded and lack protective airway reflexes should have endotracheal intubation prior to gastric lavage to prevent aspiration of gastric contents. The reader is referred to the appropriate chapters concerning nasogastric tube placement (Chapter 51), gastric lavage (Chapter 53), and urethral catheterization (Chapter 73) for specific contraindications to these procedures.

Equipment. We recommend using large diameter 39 to 40 French lavage tubes with normal saline warmed to 40 to 45° C and a Y connector and clamp as described in Chapter 53. Although smaller tubes are easily passed nasally, we recommend oral placement of the large lavage tubes. A modified Sengstaken tube with gastric and esophageal balloons may also be used.[52]

Procedure. Two hundred to 300 ml aliquots of fluid may be instilled into the stomach before removal and gravity drainage. For bladder irrigation the optimal volume is not known but bladder distension should be avoided. One hundred to 200 ml aliquots should be sufficient. The amount of time that the irrigant should be left before removal is not known, but we recommend rapid exchanges with a dwell time of 1 to 2 minutes to limit the cooling of the irrigant fluid.

Complications. Complications include trauma to the nasal turbinates (especially if a large tube is passed nasally), gastric and esophageal perforation, dilutional hyponatremia, inadvertent placement of the tube in the lungs, and pulmonary aspiration. All of these can be minimized by careful, proper technique.

Conclusions. Gastrointestinal and bladder lavage with heated fluids is easily performed using equipment and solutions available in any hospital. Because of its ease and availability, it can be started early in the resuscitation and combined with any other rewarming method to give a significant added increment of heat.

MORE INVASIVE TECHNIQUES

Thoracic Cavity Lavage

Background. Thoracic cavity lavage can be performed either *closed,* through chest tubes placed in the one hemithorax,[43, 53–55] or *open,* after resuscitative thoracotomy.[36, 56, 57] The former approach offers the advantages of being less invasive and being based upon procedures more commonly used by the emergency physician. Further, closed-chest cardiopulmonary resuscitation can be continued while this technique is used. The open thorax approach offers the theoretic advantage of direct heart warming and the option of open-chest cardiac massage.

Indications. Thoracic cavity lavage should be considered for patients requiring rapid core rewarming in the setting of inadequate perfusion (e.g., shock or during cardiopulmonary resuscitation) when cardiac bypass is not available. Open thoracic lavage should be considered in those patients who will receive open chest massage or thoracotomy for other reasons, e.g., hypothermic arrest with penetrating trauma. Generally, thoracic lavage is contraindicated for patients with mild or moderate hypothermia who can be rewarmed by other less invasive methods. The technique should be avoided in the patient with a coagulopathy unless needed as a life-saving measure.

Procedure

Closed thoracic lavage: Two large bore thoracostomy tubes (e.g., 36 Fr in 70-kg adults) are placed in one hemithorax (see Chapter 9). Iversen and colleagues[55] recommend one placed in the fourth intercostal space in the posterior axillary line and the other in the third intercostal space in the midclavicular line. A nonrecycled system has been described for thoracic lavage.[55] One chest tube is infused with 3-liter bags of heated normal saline (40 to 41° C) using a high-flow fluid infuser (e.g., Level-1 Fluid Warmer, Technologies Inc., Marshfield, Mass.). The effluent is collected with an autotransfusion thoracostomy drainage set (e.g., Pleurevac, Deknatel A-5000-ATS, Fall River, Mass.) and the removable reservoir repeatedly emptied as needed. Iversen and associates[55] were able to deliver fluid at an average rate of 180 ml/min for 2.5 hours using this system. Brunette and colleagues[54] used a continuous-flow recycled fluid system with a roller pump and external heat exchanger to circulate thoracic fluid at a rate of 300 ml/min. The use of a single chest tube system using a Y-connector arrangement similar to gastric lavage (see Chapter 53) is also effective. Aliquots of 200 to 300 ml with a 2-minute dwell time followed by suction drainage (at 20 cm H_2O) are recommended.

Closed-chest massage is used until adequate spontaneous perfusion occurs. Closed-chest defibrillation may be required in the patient warmed to 30° C with persistent ventricular defibrillation. Thoracic lavage generally is continued until the patient's temperature approaches 35° C.

Open thoracic lavage: A left thoracotomy is performed as described in Chapter 18. Saline warmed to 40 to 41° C can then be continuously poured into the thoracic cavity, bathing the heart while an assistant suctions the excess fluid from the lateral edge of the thoracotomy. Alternatively, fluid may be added to the thorax and mediastinum intermittently and suctioned after several minutes, and more warm saline may be added (see Fig. 91–8). This technique also allows for direct myocardial temperature monitoring. Direct cardiac massage is used until adequate spontaneous perfusion occurs. Direct cardiac defibrillation may be required in the patient warmed to 30° C with persistent ventricular defibrillation. When defibrillation is successful, direct myocardial warming should continue until the patient's temperature approaches 35° C.

Conclusions. While thoracic lavage clinically has not been investigated in a controlled fashion, it has been anecdotally successful in hypothermic arrest patients.[54-57] Animal studies of closed thoracic lavage suggest that it is an effective rewarming technique.[43, 53] Nonetheless, thoracic lavage should be restricted to those patients with inadequate spontaneous perfusion to permit less aggressive techniques and in the setting where more definitive therapy (e.g., cardiac bypass) is not rapidly available.

Cardiac Bypass. The use of cardiac bypass through either the femoral artery–femoral vein or aorta-caval procedure can result in rapid rewarming but requires surgical expertise, availability of appropriate equipment, and technical support.[2, 3, 29] This procedure has not been compared with other rewarming methods in a controlled fashion. Its main advantages would appear to be the rapid rate of warming it produces and the elimination of the need for CPR in the arrested patient. Warming rates of 2 to 3° C per hour can be reliably achieved with this technique.[39] Drawbacks include potential delays in assembling the appropriate team and equipment, delays due to the time necessary to complete the operation, complications from the operation, the expense of the procedure and bypass equipment, and the potential for infection. Also, it has not been shown that more rapid warming rates improve survival. Until clear advantages to this procedure in the hypothermic patient are shown, it cannot be recommended for routine use in severely hypothermic patients. Its use in extreme situations that may include cardiac arrest should be based upon individual characteristics of the patient, physician team, and hospital resources, with the full knowledge that no consensus concerning its use presently exists.

Hemodialysis. Hemodialysis has also been utilized to achieve core rewarming after placement of a shunt. Some of the potential advantages and drawbacks of cardiac bypass also apply to this procedure, although slower warming rates have been reported. For patients who have ingested a dialyzable toxin, hemodialysis can be used to both remove the toxin and rewarm the blood.[58] In such cases its use may be appropriate.

Experimental Techniques. Radiowave rewarming is one experimental rewarming technique that has shown promise, although it has not yet been described in human hypothermic victims. Radiowave rewarming appears to be a rapid, safe, noninvasive technique.[57] However, if proven effective and safe in human trials, the technology for performing this procedure may not be readily available to the victim when needed.

ADJUNCTIVE THERAPY FOR HYPOTHERMIC PATIENTS

Cardiac Arrest

Rapid rewarming and restoration of cardiac rhythm is essential for patients in cardiopulmonary arrest and can best be achieved by a combination of passive and multiple active core rewarming techniques. Since numerous cases of survival from hypothermic cardiac arrest with prolonged external cardiac compression exist,[6, 39] thoracotomy is not mandatory but does offer some theoretical advantages, such as increased cardiac output with open-chest massage,[60] direct observation of cardiac activity, and direct warming of cardiac tissue with thoracic cavity lavage of warm fluid. The optimal rate of cardiac compression in hypothermia is not known, but be-

cause of decreased oxygen consumption of vital organs, the rate required in hypothermic cardiac arrest may be less than that recommended in normothermic cardiac arrest. However, there is no evidence that standard CPR is harmful in the hypothermic patient; therefore, we recommend standard CPR for nonperfusing hypothermic patients. The duration of CPR depends upon the time required to raise the core temperature to a level at which defibrillation should be successful (above 30° C), but other factors that may occur in individual cases make any specific temperature recommendation for cessation of CPR efforts impossible. Certainly survival is highly unlikely in patients with a core temperature below 10° C, and patients who persist in asystole or go from ventricular fibrillation to asystole as they are warmed past 32° C are unlikely to respond. Elevated potassium and BUN levels may portend an irreversible process[17, 29] and should be measured in the early stages of resuscitation. However, the unusual reports of survival with prolonged CPR in hypothermic patients make extended efforts to resuscitate such patients reasonable. Under favorable conditions, hypothermic cardiac arrest patients may reasonably be admitted to an intensive care unit for a 4- to 5-hour trial of rewarming with CPR in progress.

Airway Management

A secure functioning airway must be maintained for the hypothermic patient, just as in any critically ill patient. In mild hypothermia, heated humidified oxygen can be delivered effectively by a face mask. The hypothermic patient can be combative and uncooperative and may require arm restraints if a mask is used. For the patient with decreased sensorium who cannot reliably maintain his airway or the hypothermic patient who may be hypoxic, endotracheal intubation may be performed safely without the added risk of ventricular dysrhythmias.[9, 39] The technique for endotracheal intubation depends on the specific presenting circumstances and the expertise of the operator. Once an endotracheal tube has been placed and secured, it may be used for treatment of the patient with warm humidified oxygen.

Acid-Base Disturbances

The interpretation of arterial blood gases in the hypothermic patient has been reviewed.[61, 62] Although correction of reported results to reflect the hypothermic state has been described, the use of *uncorrected* pH to guide therapy with bicarbonate or hyperventilation has more recently been advocated.[61, 62] The appropriate use of bicarbonate in the acidotic, critically ill patient is currently controversial.[63, 64] Similar controversy surrounds the use of bicarbonate in the hypothermic patient. Even though alkalosis is protective for ventricular fibrillation,[61] it is probably better to modify pH by ventilatory adjustment. Arterial pH did not correlate with patient death in the Multicenter Hypothermia Study.[39] If the clinician attempts to treat the acidosis, the pH uncorrected for temperature appears preferred.

ADJUNCTIVE PHARMACOTHERAPY AND MONITORING

Cardiac irritability, particularly refractory ventricular fibrillation, may be present on the patient's initial arrival or may occur during rewarming. Bretylium tosylate is an antidysrhythmic agent[65] that has been used successfully to treat two hypothermic patients in ventricular fibrillation[30, 66] and may prevent ventricular fibrillation in patients at risk for this dysrhythmia.[67] However, routine administration of this medication to hypothermic patients has not been studied on humans in a controlled fashion. Other pharmacologic agents, including lidocaine, have limited value in hypothermia.[68] Even though digitalis may be less dysrhythmogenic in hypothermia for a given blood level, there is no clear indication for its use.[69] Most supraventricular dysrhythmias, including atrial fibrillation, convert spontaneously as the patient is warmed and therefore do not necessarily require treatment in the hypothermic state. Magnesium has been used successfully to defibrillate hypothermic ventricular fibrillation.[70] Dopamine has been used in reports of successful resuscitation of hypotensive hypothermic patients, and there is some theoretical support for its occasional use.[68]

Intravenous fluid should be given early because most hypothermic patients have intravascular volume depletion. Dextrose 5 per cent with normal saline has been advocated as the ideal initial resuscitation fluid.[11] Potassium should be avoided until electrolytes are measured and normal renal function confirmed.

Placement of a Swan-Ganz catheter and close monitoring of urinary output may assist in the fluid management of severely hypothermic patients. The risks of precipitating ventricular fibrillation should be weighed against the potential benefits of the Swan-Ganz catheter.

Elevation of creatine phosphokinase (CPK) in hypothermic patients may indicate rhabdomyolysis, and careful monitoring of renal function with aggressive fluid replacement may prevent the development of renal failure.

FROSTBITE

Hypothermic patients frequently suffer from frostbite in addition to their systemic hypothermia. Frostbite usually involves the hands, feet, ears, and nose, and the exposed skin goes through a number of progressively deleterious physiologic changes upon exposure to the cold. Mild cold injury is termed *frostnip*, a condition that involves only the skin, sparing the subcutaneous tissues. The skin is blanched and numb but the injury is immediately reversible with no permanent sequelae if the area is quickly rewarmed. Nonfreezing temperatures also produce *trenchfoot*, an intermediate in the progression to true frostbite.

In frostbite the skin and subcutaneous tissue are actually frozen. The affected extremity is hard, solid, and blanched. Clear or hemorrhagic bullae may be present. Initially there is no pain or feeling in the frostbitten extremity. After rewarming, the affected area develops severe edema and blistering, eventually exhibiting dry gangrene and mummification leading to tissue sloughing.

Physiologically, frostbite involves the initial extracellular formation of ice crystals followed by delayed but progressive ischemia in the affected area. Interstitial ice crystal formation is a hypertonic state that leads to cellular dehydration and cell death. Cellular water loss enhances extracellular ice formation, leading to further damage from increased pressure on blood vessels and cells. Cold also increases blood viscosity, promotes vasospasm, and precipitates microthrombus formation. The cascade of injurious events in frostbite may be mediated by prostaglandins.

Rapid rewarming is the treatment of choice for frostbite.[71] The aim is to limit the length of time the tissue remains in the frozen state. The most practical way to rewarm an extremity is to totally immerse the area in warm water at 104 to 108° F (40 to 42° C) for 15 to 30 minutes. The affected area should be carefully protected to assure

that the tissue is not additionally injured through contact with the sides or rim of the container. After thawing, the area should be meticulously protected from injury. An extremity should be elevated and cotton or gauze placed between the toes/fingers to limit maceration. The use of topical aloe vera (a thromboxane inhibitor) and systemic antiprostaglandins (such as ibuprofen) may be helpful. There is no proven benefit to the use of heparin or low molecular weight dextran, vasodilators, steroids, or immediate surgical sympathectomy. The use of antibiotics is controversial, although some authors advocate penicillin prophylactically. Débridement of tissue should be avoided in the emergency department.

CONCLUSION

As a general guideline, one should take a conservative approach to rewarming the stable hypothermic patient, with avoidance of overtreatment and the selective and careful use of invasive monitoring. In moderate hypothermia, underlying problems should be sought, passive rewarming and basic support started, and less invasive core rewarming begun. This approach should include mask ventilation with warm humidified air or oxygen in the conscious patient and intubation and ventilation in the unconscious patient. In selected patients, gastric or peritoneal lavage with warm fluid may be considered. For severely hypothermic, *unstable* patients, cardiac bypass and thoracic lavage may offer additional benefits including rapid warming rates and direct heart warming. The benefits should be weighed against the time, expense, and danger of complications these procedures entail.

It is ironic that as we consider costly procedures for resuscitating hypothermic patients, many of whom are elderly and alcoholic, we have not considered preventive measures. In fact, many of the same patients who become interesting hypothermic cases visit emergency departments as part of a daily quest for shelter. We often take pride in sending these emergency department "abusers," without obvious acute medical problems, back out into the streets to make room for "real" sick patients whom we can help. However, it may well be that the most effective emergency department procedure to combat hypothermia is a chair in the waiting room on a cold winter night.

REFERENCES

1. Siebke H, Breivik H, Rod T, et al: Survival after 40 minute submersion without cerebral sequelae. Lancet 1:1275, 1975.
2. Bolte RG, Black PG, Bowers RS: The use of extracorporeal rewarming in a child submerged for 66 minutes. JAMA 266;377, 1988.
3. Maresca L, Vasko JS: Treatment of hypothermia by extracorporeal circulation and internal rewarming. J Trauma 27:89, 1987.
4. Althaus U, Aeberhard P, Schupbach P: Management of profound accidental hypothermia with cardiorespiratory arrest. Ann Surg 195:492, 1982.
5. Towne WD, Geiss WP, Yanes HO: Intractable ventricular fibrillation associated with profound accidental hypothermia—Successful treatment with partial cardiopulmonary bypass. N Engl J Med 287:1135, 1972.
6. Schissler P, Parker MA, Scott SJ, Jr: Profound hypothermia: Value of prolonged cardiopulmonary resuscitation. South Med J 74:474, 1981.
7. White JD: Hypothermia: The Bellvue experience. Ann Emerg Med 11:417, 1982.
8. O'Keefe KM: Accidental hypothermia: A review of 62 cases. JACEP 6:491, 1977.
9. Miller JW, Danzl DF, Thomas DM: Urban accidental hypothermia: 135 cases. Ann Emerg Med 9:456, 1980.
10. Zachary L, Kucan JO, Robson MC, et al: Accidental hypothermia treated with rapid rewarming by immersion. Ann Plast Surg 9:238, 1982.
11. Danzl DF: Accidental hypothermia. In Rosen P, et al (eds): Emergency Medicine: Concepts and Clinical Procedures. 2nd ed. St. Louis, C. V. Mosby Co, 1988, pp 663–692.
12. Lewin S, Brettman LR, Holzman RS: Infections in hypothermic patients. Arch Intern Med 141:920, 1981.
13. Bryant RE: Factors affecting mortality in gram negative rod bacteremia. Arch Intern Med 127:120, 1971.
14. Forester CF: Coma in myxedema. Arch Intern Med 111:734, 1963.
15. Strauch BS, Felig P, Baxter JD, et al: Hypothermia in hypoglycemia. JAMA 210:345, 1969.
16. Morris DL, Chambers HF, Morris MG, et al: Hemodynamic characteristics

of patients with hypothermia due to occult infection and other causes. Ann Intern Med 102:153, 1985.

17. Danzl DF, Hedges JR, Pozos RS, et al: Hypothermia outcome score: Development and implications. Crit Care Med 17:227, 1989.

18. Tandberg D, Sklar D: The effect of tachypnea on the estimation of body temperature by an oral thermometer. N Engl J Med 308:945, 1983.

19. Lilly JK, Beland JP, Zekan S: Urinary bladder temperature monitoring: A new index of body core temperature. Crit Care Med 8:742, 1980.

20. Fox RH, Woodward PM, Exton-Smith AN, et al: Body temperature in the elderly: A national study of physiological, social and environmental conditions. Br Med J 1:200, 1973.

21. Bangs CC: Hypothermia and frostbite. Emerg Clin North Am 2:475, 1984.

22. Moss J: Accidental severe hypothermia. Surg Gynecol Obstet 162:501, 1986.

23. Schwab RH, Lewis DW, Killough JH, et al: Electrocardiographic changes occurring in rapidly induced deep hypothermia. Am J Med Sci 248:290, 1964.

24. Bering EA, Jr: Effects of profound hypothermia and circulatory arrest on cerebral oxygen metabolism and cerebrospinal fluid electrolyte composition in dogs. J Neurosurg 39:199, 1974.

25. DaVee TS, Reineberg EJ: Extreme hypothermia and ventricular fibrillation. Ann Emerg Med 9:100, 1980.

26. Fitzgerald FT: Hypoglycemia and accidental hypothermia in an alcoholic population. West J Med 133:105, 1981.

27. Harnett RM, O'Brien EM, Sias FR, et al: Initial treatment of profound accidental hypothermia. Aviat Space Environ Med 51:680, 1980.

28. Hayward JS, Eckerson JD, Kemna D: Thermal and cardiovascular changes during three methods of resuscitation from mild hypothermia. Resuscitation 11:21, 1984.

29. Hauty MG, Esrig BC, Hill JG: Prognostic factors in severe accidental hypothermia in experience from the Mt. Hood tragedy. J Trauma 27:1107, 1987.

30. Danzl D, Sowers MD, Vicerio SJ: Chemical ventricular defibrillation in severe accidental hypothermia. Ann Emerg Med 11:698, 1982.

31. Fruehan AE: Accidental hypothermia: Report of eight cases of subnormal body temperature due to exposure. Arch Intern Med 106:218, 1960.

32. Hudson LD, Conn RD: Accidental hypothermia: Associated diagnoses and prognosis in a common problem. JAMA 227:37, 1974.

33. Weyman AE, Greenbaum PM, Grace WJ: Accidental hypothermia in an alcoholic population. Am J Med 56:13, 1974.

34. Fitzgerald FT, Jessup C: Accidental hypothermia: A report of 22 cases and review of the literature. Adv Intern Med 27:127, 1982.

35. Gregory RT, Doolittle WH: Accidental hypothermia. Part II, Clinical implications of experimental studies. Alaska Med 15:48, 1973.

36. Leddingham I McA, Mone JG: Treatment of accidental hypothermia: A prospective clinical study. Br Med J 280:1102, 1980.

37. Romet TT, Hoskin RW: Temperature and metabolic responses to inhalation and bath rewarming protocols. Aviat Space Environ Med 59(7):630, 1988.

38. Lloyd ELL: Accidental hypothermia treated by central rewarming through the airway. Br J Anaesth 45:41, 1973.

39. Danzl D, Pozos RS: Multicenter Hypothermia Study. Ann Emerg Med 16:1042, 1987.

40. Lloyd ELL, Conliffe NA, Orgel H, Walker PN: Accidental hypothermia: An apparatus for central re-warming as a first aid measure. Scot Med J 17:83, 1972.

41. Shanks CA, Sara CA: Temperature monitoring of the humidifier during the treatment of hypothermia. Med J Aust 2:1351, 1972.

42. Myers RA, Britten JS, Cowley RA: Hypothermia: Quantitative aspects of therapy. JACEP 8:523, 1979.

43. Otto RJ, Metzler MH: Rewarming from experimental hypothermia, comparison of heated aerosol inhalation, peritoneal lavage and pleural lavage. Crit Care Med 16:869, 1988.

44. Troelson S, Rybro L, Knudsen F: Profound accidental hypothermia treated with peritoneal dialysis. Scand J Urol Nephrol 20:221, 1986.

45. Lash RF, Burdett JA, Ozil T: Accidental profound hypothermia and barbiturate intoxication—Report of rapid "core" rewarming by peritoneal dialysis. JAMA 201:269, 1967.

46. Pickering BG, Bristow GK, Craig DB: Case history number 97: Core rewarming by peritoneal irrigation in accidental hypothermia with cardiac arrest. Anesth Analg 4:574, 1977.

47. O'Connor JP: Use of peritoneal dialysis in severely hypothermic patients (Letter to the Editor). Ann Emerg Med 15:104, 1986.

48. Lazarus HM, Nelson JA: The surgeon at work. A technique for peritoneal lavage without risk or complication. Surg Gynecol Obstet 162:501, 1986.

49. Lonning PE, Skulberg A, Abyholm F: Accidental hypothermia. Acta Anaesth Scand 30:601, 1986.

50. Howdieshell TR, Osler TH, Demarest GB: Open versus closed peritoneal lavage with particular attention to time, accuracy and cost. Am J Emerg Med 7:367, 1989.

51. Peterson LD: Electrolyte depletion following emergency stomach evacuation. Am J Hosp Pharm 36:1366, 1979.

52. Ledingham IM, Douglas IH, Routh GS, et al: Central rewarming system for treatment of hypothermia. Lancet 1:1168, 1980.

53. Brunette DD, Sterner S, Robinson EP, et al: Comparison of gastric lavage and thoracotomy cavity lavage. Ann Emerg Med 16:1222, 1987.

54. Brunette DD, Sterner SP, Ruiz E: Closed thoracic cavity lavage for the treatment of severe environmental hypothermia. (abstract). Ann Emerg Med 19:492, 1990.

55. Iversen RJ, Atkin SH, Jaker MA, et al: Successful CPR in a severely hypothermic patient using continuous thoracostomy lavage. Ann Emerg Med 19:1335, 1990.

56. Coughlin F: Heart warming procedure. N Engl J Med 326:288, 1973.

57. Linton AL, Ledingham IM: Severe hypothermia with barbiturate intoxication. Lancet 1:24–26, 1966.

58. Lee HA, Ames AC: Hemodialysis in severe barbiturate poisoning. Br Med J 1:1217, 1965.

59. White JD, Butterfield AB, Nucci RC, et al: Rewarming in accidental hypothermia. Radio wave vs. inhalation therapy. Ann Emerg Med 16:50, 1987.

60. Del Guercio LRM, Feins NR, Cohn JD, et al: Comparison of blood flow during external and internal cardiac massage in man. Circulation 31(Suppl):171, 1965.

61. Delaney KA, Howland MA, Vassallo S, et al: Assessment of acid base disturbances in hypothermia and their physiological consequences. Ann Emerg Med 18:72, 1988.

62. Swain JA: Hypothermia and blood pH: A review. Arch Intern Med 148:1643, 1988.

63. Sacpoule PW: Lactic acidosis: The case against bicarbonate therapy. Ann Intern Med 105:276, 1986.

64. Maring RG, Cohen JJ: Bicarbonate therapy for organic acidosis: The case for its continued use. Ann Intern Med 106:615, 1987.

65. Koch-Weser J: Drug therapy: Bretylium. N Engl J Med 300(9):473, 1979.

66. Kochar G, Kahn SE, Kotler MN, et al: Bretylium tosylate and ventricular fibrillation in hypothermia. Ann Intern Med 105:624, 1986.

67. Murphy K, Nowak RM, Tomlanovich MC: Use of bretylium tosylate as prophylaxis and treatment in hypothermic ventricular fibrillation in the canine model. Ann Emerg Med 15:1160, 1986.

68. Nicodemus EF, Chaney RD, Herold R: Hemodynamic effects of inotropes during hypothermia and rapid rewarming. Crit Care Med 9:325, 1981.

69. Szekely P, Wynne NA: The effects of digitalis on the hypothermic heart. Br Heart J 22:647, 1960.

70. Buky B: Effect of magnesium on ventricular fibrillation due to hypothermia. Br J Anaesth 42:886, 1970.

71. McCauley RL, Hing DN, Martin RC, et al: Frostbite injuries: A rational approach based on the pathophysiology. J Trauma 23:143, 1983.

Chapter 92

Procedures Pertaining to Hyperthermia

Dwight E. Helmrich and Scott A. Syverud

INTRODUCTION

The ravages of heatstroke have long been recognized. A Roman army was decimated by heat in 24 B.C. King Edward's heavily armored crusaders were defeated by "heat and fever" during the final battle of the Holy Land. Eleven thousand Peking residents died during a heat wave in 1743. In contrast, malignant hyperthermia and neuroleptic malignant syndrome have only been recognized and described in the last 30 years.[8, 9] These latter conditions are largely iatrogenic, most commonly triggered by modern pharmacologic therapy.

Heatstroke remains a common clinical problem with significant morbidity and mortality.[1] As is the case with accidental hypothermia, published clinical studies of heatstroke treatment techniques have largely been limited to retrospective case series without concurrent control or comparison groups.[2–7] A variety of cooling techniques have been advocated during the last 50 years. Although some cooling techniques have been compared in controlled models of heatstroke, when choosing a cooling technique to use in clinical practice, the reader must weigh several factors including speed of cooling, ease of use, and safety.

Before considering the various cooling techniques, it is essential that the underlying disorder of hyperthermia be clearly understood. Heat illness presents a spectrum of disease from mild heat exhaustion (primarily a volume loss disorder) to severe heatstroke (with thermal-related end-organ injury). The latter includes the skeletal muscle disorder known as malignant hyperthermia. Treatment of this spectrum of disease requires a discriminating approach, including supportive care only for heat exhaustion and rapid cooling for heatstroke. Malignant hyperthermia requires specific pharmacologic therapy (e.g., dantrolene) in addition to cooling measures. A brief discussion of hyperthermic disorders is therefore necessary before describing cooling techniques.

NORMAL THERMOREGULATION

Heat is a by-product of metabolism in all living organisms. In the resting adult, basal metabolism produces approximately 75 kcal/hr of heat load.[10] Physical activity increases this basal heat production significantly.[11] Moderate exercise generates about 300 kcal/hr of heat for brief periods of time.[12] Under normal circumstances, metabolic heat load is transferred from the core to the skin by increasing cutaneous blood flow.[13] Heat can then be dissipated from the body by convection, radiation, conduction, and evaporation. However, convection, radiation, and conduction require a thermal gradient to be effective. At ambient temperatures approaching body temperature, evaporation becomes the only functioning heat loss mechanism. The vaporization of 1.7 ml of sweat can liberate 1 kcal of body heat when the relative humidity is low.[14] When the relative humidity is high, evaporative heat loss is rendered ineffective. Therefore, high ambient temperature and high humidity retard heat dissipation. Heat storage and rising core temperature result.[15, 16]

In the ensuing discussion, temperatures will be given in degrees Celsius (centigrade). A temperature conversion scale is provided in the previous chapter (see Fig. 91–2).

TYPES OF HYPERTHERMIA

Mild Heat Illness

Heat cramps and heat exhaustion are induced by a hot environment. The body's heat dissipation mechanisms are able to keep up with heat production and absorption in these disorders, albeit at a price. Symptoms of these disorders are largely due to the mechanisms used by the body to dissipate heat. In spite of these symptoms, the body temperature remains at or near normal. Rapid cooling techniques are *not* required, and supportive care and hydration in a cool environment are usually adequate therapy.

Heat cramps are severe muscle cramps of large muscle groups (usually in the lower extremities). This disorder occurs after heavy exercise in a hot environment. Heavy sweating with inadequate hypotonic fluid replacement (water) is a common historical point. Rest in a cool environment and vigorous fluid replacement with isotonic solutions (normal saline) are usually adequate therapies. *Heat exhaustion* is a poorly defined syndrome with a spectrum of nonspecific symptoms that occur after heat exposure. Malaise, flu-like symptoms, orthostasis, dehydration, nausea, and headache may all occur. As distinct from the more severe heat disorders, mental status is normal and body temperature is normal or only mildly elevated. As with heat cramps, rehydration, rest, and supportive care in a cool environment are adequate therapy for heat exhaustion. Rapid cooling techniques are not required.

Heatstroke

When the body's normal heat dissipation mechanisms are overwhelmed, core temperature elevation and heatstroke rapidly ensue. Two forms of heatstroke are described in the literature. *Classic* (nonexertional) *heatstroke* usually occurs during summer heat waves. The poor, urban elderly are at greatest risk.[7] Lack of air conditioning, marginal cardiovascular status, and medications that interfere with heat dissipation predispose this population to heatstroke. The similarity between adults with nonexertional heatstroke and children with hemorrhagic shock and encephalopathy syndrome has been emphasized.[16a, 16b] These children are generally overdressed or wrapped in blankets and suffering from a viral infection. *Exertional heatstroke*, a consequence of strenuous physical activity even in temperate climates, usually afflicts a younger segment of the population. Highly motivated, poorly acclimatized athletes and military recruits are common victims, as are individuals who perform heavy physical labor in a hot, humid environment.[17]

The degree of hyperthermia necessary to produce heatstroke in man is unknown. In tissue culture cells, thermal injury is observed in the range of 40 to 45° C.[18] Studies with hyperthermia in cancer therapy reveal that tissue sensitivity to heat is increased by relative hypoxia, ischemia, and acidosis.[19] The duration of thermal insult measured as degree-minutes is also an important variable.[20]

The key clinical findings in the diagnosis of heatstroke are (1) a history of heat stress or exposure, (2) a rectal temperature greater than 40° C, and (3) central nervous system (CNS) dysfunction, i.e., altered mental status, disorientation, stupor, seizures, or coma.

The sequelae of heatstroke are caused by thermal damage to multiple organ systems.[3, 23] Stupor, seizures, and coma can result as direct effects of heat on the CNS. Cardiovascular collapse results from dehydration, maximal cutaneous vasodilation, and direct heat–induced myocardial depression.[21] Coagulopathies and liver dysfunction occur as consequences of thermal breakdown and consumption of serum proteins as well as direct heat damage to hepatic cells.[22] Renal failure can result from myoglobinuria (related to rhabdomyolysis) and acute tubular necrosis.[1]

The treatment of these sequelae in acute heatstroke does not differ from that in other disorders, with the sole exception that rapid cooling is necessary to prevent further damage and reverse heat stress.

Malignant Hyperthermia

Malignant hyperthermia is an inherited abnormality of the skeletal muscle membrane.[9] In response to certain stresses or drugs (Table 92–1), patients with this disorder sustain a massive efflux of calcium from skeletal muscle sarcoplasmic reticulum, resulting in contraction of the sarcomeres, skeletal muscle rigidity, increased skeletal muscle metabolism and heat production, and, finally, systemic hyperthermia. Hyperthermia is a late development occurring after rigidity has been present for some time and the body's normal heat dissipation mechanisms have been overwhelmed. The earliest signs of malignant hyperthermia are increased carbon dioxide production, muscle rigidity, and tachycardia. Cardiac output and cutaneous blood flow also increase to maximize heat loss. Malignant hyperthermia is diagnosed based on the clinical triad of (1) exposure to an agent or stress known to trigger the condition (see Table 92–1), (2) skeletal muscle rigidity, and (3) hyperthermia. High levels of expired carbon dioxide (from increased skeletal muscle metabolism) may also indicate this diagnosis.

Malignant hyperthermia is usually encountered in the operating room while patients are undergoing general anesthesia. However, cases of malignant hyperthermia may be encountered anywhere general anesthetics or neuromuscular blocking agents are used. Patients with malignant hyperthermia triggered by environmental or emotional stress may present de novo to the emergency department.[24]

As with heatstroke, treatment of malignant hyperthermia requires rapid cooling and supportive care for the sequelae described previously. Unlike heatstroke, malignant hyperthermia requires specific pharmacologic therapy to stop excess heat production by skeletal muscle. Dantrolene sodium induces muscle relaxation in malignant hyperthermia by blocking calcium release from muscle cell sarcoplasmic reticulum.[25] In all cases of malignant hyperthermia, the inciting stimulus (see Table 92–1) should be discontinued immediately and dantrolene therapy administered. Rapid

Table 92–1. Triggers for Malignant Hyperthermia

Drugs	Conditions
Halothane	Heat stress
Methoxyflurane	Vigorous exercise
Enflurane	(?) Emotional stress
Diethyl ether	
Cyclopropane	
Succinylcholine	
Tubocurarine	
Lidocaine	
Mepivicaine	
(?) Nitrous oxide	
(?) Isoflurane	
(?) Gallamine	

cooling, although an important part of treatment, takes second priority to these measures.

Neuroleptic Malignant Syndrome

Neuroleptic malignant syndrome (NMS) was first described in the late 1960s and is characterized by fever, muscle rigidity, altered level of consciousness, and autonomic instability.[8] This uncommon disorder follows the therapeutic use of neuroleptic drugs including phenothiazines, butyrophenones, thioxanthenes, lithium, and tricyclic antidepressants. Muscle rigidity can manifest as oculogyric crisis, dyskinesia, akinesia, dysphagia, dysarthria, or opisthotonos. Temperatures can exceed 42° C. Initial agitation often progresses to stupor and coma. Catatonia and mutism may also be present. Autonomic instability is manifested as tachycardia, hypotension or hypertension, sweating, and incontinence. Ventilations may be impaired by chest wall rigidity.

This syndrome is more likely to occur at the initiation of or after an increase in neuroleptic dosage. It may occur if antiparkinsonian drugs are suddenly discontinued. NMS resembles malignant hyperthermia but usually takes considerably longer to develop (2 to 3 days) and lasts longer (5 to 10 days) after the inciting drug is discontinued. Mortality is high (30 per cent) and is usually caused by respiratory failure, renal failure, cardiovascular collapse, or thromboembolic disease. Unlike malignant hyperthermia, NMS is thought to be caused by a central disorder of thermoregulation.

Treatment of severe NMS (i.e., hypotension, hyperthermia, marked rigidity) closely follows that of malignant hyperthermia except that therapy must be maintained for several days until symptoms resolve. Discontinuation of the triggering neuroleptic, rapid cooling, and supportive treatment for ensuing organ failure remain the cornerstones of therapy.

COOLING TECHNIQUES

General Considerations

Heatstroke mortality is proportional to the magnitude and duration of thermal stress measured in degree-minutes.[26, 27] Given that rapid cooling is accepted as the cornerstone of effective heatstroke therapy, the clinician must choose which cooling technique to use. Studies in animal models have been based on the assumption that the fastest cooling technique is the best. In clinical patient care, other factors will also influence the choice of technique. Patient access, monitoring, safety, ease of use, and availability are all considerations in addition to speed of cooling. A technique that may not be the most rapid but allows easy patient access and is readily available may be preferable to more cumbersome (albeit more rapid) cooling techniques in some clinical settings.

The cooling rates achieved in various human and animal studies of heatstroke are summarized in Table 92–2. The relative advantages and disadvantages of various cooling techniques are outlined in Table 92–3.

Indications for Rapid Cooling

Rapid cooling should be instituted as soon as the diagnosis of heatstroke (rectal temperature > 40° C, altered mental status, history of heat stress or exposure) is made. Rapid cooling is also indicated for the treatment of malignant

Table 92–2. Cooling Rates Achieved with Various Cooling Techniques

Technique	Author/Year	Reference	Species	Rate (° C/min)
Evaporative	Weiner/1980	28	Human	0.31
	Barner/1984	29	Human	0.04
	Al-Aska/1987	30	Human	0.09
	Kielblock/1986	31	Human	0.034
	Wyndam/1959	32	Human	0.23
	White/1987	33	Dog	0.14
	Daily/1948	34	Rat	0.93
Immersion (ice water)	Weiner/1980	28	Human	0.14
	Wyndam/1959	32	Human	0.14
	Magazanik/1980	35	Dog	0.27
	Daily/1948	34	Rat	1.86
Ice packing (whole body)	Kielblock/1986	31	Human	0.034
	Bynum/1978	36	Dog	0.11
Strategic ice packs	Kielblock/1986	31	Human	0.028
Evaporative and strategic ice packs	Kielblock/1986	31	Human	0.036
Cold gastric lavage	Syverud/1985	37	Dog	0.15
	White/1987	33	Dog	0.06
Cold peritoneal lavage	Bynum/1978	36	Dog	0.56

Note: The obvious variation in cooling rates reported using the same technique can be explained by several factors. Animals studies usually produce faster cooling rates than those observed with the same technique in humans, probably owing to a higher body surface area to mass ratio in animals. Human volunteers with elevated body temperature but not heatstroke (i.e., Kielblock, 1986) may not cool as fast as actual heatstroke patients (Al-Aska, 1987). Air flow rates, water temperature, and lavage rates also affect cooling rate.

hyperthermia but should be instituted concurrently with the discontinuation of the triggering agent or drug and the administration of dantrolene. In NMS, cooling measures should be used if the rectal temperature exceeds 40° C. Since studies show that the degree of organ damage correlates with the degree and duration of temperature elevation above 40° C, a reasonable clinical goal is to reduce the temperature to below 40° C within 1 hour of the start of therapy.[26, 27]

Contraindications for Rapid Cooling

Rapid cooling, per se, is never contraindicated in the presence of heatstroke. Immersion cooling is relatively contraindicated when cardiac monitoring of an unstable patient is required or when limited personnel make constant patient supervision impossible. Iced gastric lavage is contraindicated in patients with depressed airway reflexes unless the airway is protected by endotracheal intubation.[37] This technique is also contraindicated by conditions that preclude placement of an oro- or nasogastric tube. Iced peritoneal lavage is contraindicated when multiple previous abdominal surgeries make placement of a lavage catheter risky owing to potential bowel perforation (see also Chapter 56).

Evaporative Cooling

INTRODUCTION

Evaporating water is thermodynamically a much more effective cooling medium than melting ice. Evaporating 1 gm of water

Table 92–3. Advantages and Disadvantages of Various Cooling Techniques

Technique	Advantages	Disadvantages
Evaporative	Simple, readily available Noninvasive Easy monitoring and patient access Relatively more rapid	Constant moistening of skin surface required to maximize heat loss
Immersion	Noninvasive Relatively more rapid	Cumbersome Patient monitoring and access difficult Shivering Poorly tolerated by conscious patients
Ice packing	Noninvasive Readily available	Shivering Poorly tolerated by conscious patients
Strategic ice packs	Noninvasive Readily available Can be combined with other techniques	Relatively slower Shivering Poorly tolerated by conscious patients
Cold gastric lavage	Can be combined with other techniques	Relatively slower Invasive May require airway protection Human experience limited
Cold peritoneal lavage	Very rapid	Invasive Human experience limited

requires 540 kcal. Melting 1 gm of ice requires only 80 kcal. In theory, therefore, evaporative cooling should be approximately seven times more efficient than ice packing. In practice, evaporative cooling is more efficient, but not nearly to the degree thermodynamics would predict.[32] In separate human studies, Wyndam and colleagues and Weiner and Khogali found evaporative cooling to be 1.5 to 2.2 times faster than ice water immersion.[28, 32] In human volunteers with mild, exercise-induced hyperthermia, Kielblock and associates found evaporative cooling no faster than whole body ice packing.[31] In clinical practice, ice water immersion or ice packing causes heat loss by conduction as well as by heat consumption by the phase change of melting ice.

Despite the continued enthusiasm of some clinicians for ice water immersion, evaporative cooling is the fastest noninvasive cooling technique in human studies.[28, 31, 32] To maximize evaporative cooling rates, several factors must be optimized.[38] Air flow rates must be high (large fans are required). The temperature of the air must be warm, as evaporation is decreased at lower temperatures. The entire body surface must be exposed to air flow and continuously moistened with water (ideally the patient is suspended in a mesh sling to expose the back to air flow and moisture). Finally, the temperature of the water used to moisten the skin must be tepid (15° C). If the water is ice cold, evaporation will be slow. Conversely, if it is hot, conductive heat gain may occur.

Weiner and Khogali have constructed a sophisticated "body cooling unit" (BCU) to maximize evaporative cooling.[28] Patients in the BCU are suspended in a mesh net. High air flow rates (30 m/min) at temperatures of 45° C are maintained both anterior and posterior to the mesh net. Atomized water at 15° C is continuously sprayed on all body surfaces. Using this device, Weiner and Khogali achieved rapid cooling rates under laboratory conditions.[28]

The realities of clinical practice make these conditions hard to reproduce. Half the body surface (the back) will usually be unavailable for evaporative cooling. Air flow rates and temperatures are usually limited by the ambient temperature in the treatment facility and the size and power of the fan available. These realities are reflected by the slower cooling rates Al-Aska and coworkers achieved when treating heatstroke victims with evaporative cooling in a clinical setting[30] (see Table 92–2).

PROCEDURE

Evaporative cooling is accomplished by undressing the patient completely, positioning a fan or fans (usually at the foot of the bed or stretcher) as close to the patient as possible, and then sponging the skin continuously with tepid 15° C water. A single care provider can continue the technique and monitor the patient once cooling has been initiated. It is important to keep as much body surface as possible moist and exposed to the air flow. Covering sheets or clothing will impede skin evaporation and cooling.

COMPLICATIONS

Complications of evaporative cooling are rare and are more often attributable to the underlying disorder than to the cooling technique. Wet skin may interfere with electro-cardiogram (ECG) monitoring, but this can usually be avoided by using electrodes on the patient's back. Shivering occurs infrequently with this technique when compared with other cooling techniques because the water is relatively warm (15° C).[30] If significant shivering does occur, it can be reduced with phenothiazine administration (chlorproma-zine, 25 to 50 mg intravenously for adults), although this treatment is not necessary unless shivering causes significant cooling delays. Evaporative cooling should be discontinued when the rectal temperature reaches 39° C. Continued cooling beyond this temperature may lead to subsequent "overshoot hypothermia" due to continued core temperature drops after active evaporative cooling is discontinued.

Immersion Cooling

INTRODUCTION

It would seem obvious that the fastest way to cool a heatstroke patient would be immersion in ice water. In one of the first studies of heatstroke cooling techniques, Daily and Harrison demonstrated that rats with hyperthermia cooled faster with ice water immersion than with evaporative cooling.[34] Some contemporary sources continue to recommend ice water immersion as the cooling technique of choice for heatstroke, usually citing Daily and Harrison's work as a reference.[39, 40]

Intuition, in this case, has proven to be incorrect. Studies in humans comparing ice water immersion with evaporative cooling have demonstrated evaporative cooling to be considerably faster.[28, 31, 32] An explanation of the discrepancy between Daily and Harrison's results and subsequent human studies can be inferred. Daily and Harrison studied rats with intact coats of fur who were heated until they collapsed in a hot, humid environment. They then compared the cooling rate observed with ice water immersion with that observed when the rat was dunked in ice water, then held in front of a fan.[34]

Clearly, cooling a rat with an intact coat of fur is not the same as cooling a human heatstroke victim. The higher body surface area to mass ratio of the rat would make conductive heat loss in ice water relatively more efficient than in humans. Fur impedes evaporative heat loss and is not a factor in humans. Finally, a single dunking in 0° C water is not the optimal technique for evaporative cooling.

Nonetheless, in clinical trials, cold water immersion remains the second fastest noninvasive cooling technique available (see Table 92–2). In situations where evaporative cooling is not available, immersion may be the cooling technique of choice.

Several factors are important in maximizing the rate of immersion cooling. Conductive heat loss is dependent on cutaneous blood flow to maintain a heat gradient from skin to water. Intense cutaneous vasoconstriction will impede conductive heat loss. Maga-zanik and associates, in a canine study, have suggested that warmer water (15° C) may actually cool faster than ice water (0° C) owing to this factor.[35] The optimal water temperature for cooling human heatstroke patients has not been defined.

Regardless of the water temperature, it is clear that increasing surface area increases conductive heat loss. Maximizing the body surface area in contact with the water will increase cooling rates with immersion cooling. In clinical practice, this means that complete immersion of the trunk and extremities will cool faster than partial immersion of the trunk (back only) with the extremities extended out of the bath.

PROCEDURE

Immersion cooling is accomplished by undressing the patient completely prior to transfer to a tub of water of a depth sufficient to cover the torso and extremities. Various water containers have been used. A regular bathtub, if available, can be used. Most clinical reports have described tubs that can be moved to the emergency treatment area when needed. A plastic child's wading pool and a decontam-ination tub or stretcher with waterproof sides and drainage capability are examples of the latter approach. The patient's head must be continuously supported out of the bath. Temperature and ECG leads must be securely attached to the patient if monitoring is to be continued during immersion. The patient should be removed from the bath when rectal temperature reaches 39° C because core temperature will continue to drop for a short period even after the patient is removed. An electronic temperature monitor with a long flexible rectal probe is useful for continuous temperature monitoring during immersion.

COMPLICATIONS

The common complications of immersion cooling are shivering and the loss of monitoring capability. Phenothia-zines (chlorpromazine, 25 to 50 mg intravenously for adults) can be used to decrease shivering, but blood pressure must be monitored closely after use of this α-blocking agent. Magazanik and coworkers have suggested that warmer water temperatures (15 ° C) will minimize shivering and increase cutaneous blood flow, thereby increasing cooling rates. Shivering and cutaneous vasoconstriction in particular are concerns with this technique. Shivering generates considerable heat through muscle metabolism. Cutaneous vasoconstriction impedes conductive heat loss. Advocates of ice water immersion have recommended continuous massage of the skin to stimulate cutaneous blood flow.[40] The efficacy of this approach has not been proven.

Patient monitoring is a problem under water. Electrodes on the nonimmersed upper shoulders can be used. ECG artifact often becomes a major problem during vigorous shivering. This cooling technique is not recommended for patients with unstable cardiac rhythms or patients who are at risk for developing these rhythms. A significant change in cardiac rhythm might go undetected during the labor-intensive process of immersion cooling.

Patient access for resuscitative procedures is also a major problem with this technique. Should the patient develop ventricular fibrillation, he must be removed from the bath and dried prior to defibrillation. Invasive and diagnostic procedures, e.g., intravenous (IV) access and radiography, cannot be performed during the cooling period. Care must be taken to avoid displacement of IV lines during placement in and removal from the bath.

As body temperature drops, mental status will improve in many heatstroke victims. When awake, most people find ice water immersion difficult to tolerate. IV sedation may be required.

Finally, this technique is labor intensive. Several care givers must be present throughout the process. The head must be maintained out of the bath. If massage is used, one or more individuals will need to immerse their own hands in water to continuously massage the patient. IV medications and constant attention to temperature and ECG monitors are also necessary. This cooling technique should only be used if adequate personnel are available.

Whole Body Ice Packing

INTRODUCTION

Packing the heatstroke victim in ice may maximize conductive heat loss without the attendant logistical problems caused by water immersion. Constant attendance, as required for skin moistening for evaporative cooling and as described for immersion cooling, may not be necessary with ice packing. Kielblock and colleagues demonstrated in a human study of mild, exercise-induced hyperthermia that whole body ice packing cooled just as fast as evaporative cooling (see Table 92–2).[31] Whether these results will also be observed in heatstroke victims with much higher body temperatures remains to be determined. Further study of this technique is required before making a clear recommendation regarding its use in heatstroke.

PROCEDURE

Whole body ice packing is accomplished by undressing the patient completely, then covering the extremities and torso with crushed ice. As with any cooling technique, constant temperature monitoring using an electric thermometer and a long flexible rectal probe is recommended.

The ice should be removed and the patient should be dried off when the rectal temperature reaches 39° C. A large supply of crushed ice will be needed whenever this technique is used. Whole body ice packing can usually be performed on the emergency department stretcher without additional equipment. As with immersion cooling, ECG monitoring can potentially be difficult owing to shivering artifact and displacement of electrodes.

Conscious patients usually do not tolerate ice packing well. IV sedation or restraint may be required. Excessive shivering can be treated with phenothiazines (chlorpromazine, 25 to 50 mg IV for adults) if the rate of cooling is decreased.

Strategic Ice Packs

INTRODUCTION

Some authorities have suggested that selective placement of ice packs over areas of the body where large blood vessels run close to the skin may be an effective cooling technique.[41] Cooling in these areas would occur despite cutaneous vasoconstriction owing to direct conductive heat loss from the blood within the vessel, across the vessel wall, subcutaneous tissue, and skin, to the ice. The most common areas used for strategic ice packing are the anterior neck (carotid and jugular vessels), the axilla (axillary artery and vein), and the groin (femoral vessels). Kielblock and associates' study of this technique reported a cooling rate slightly slower than that seen with evaporative or whole body ice pack cooling (see Table 92–2).[31] A combination of strategic ice packs with evaporative cooling resulted in faster cooling than either technique alone, although the relative increase achieved by adding ice packs to evaporative cooling was small.[31]

In unconscious patients or in awake patients who can tolerate ice packs without excessive shivering, this technique could be added to evaporative cooling. A definite conclusion as to the efficacy of strategic ice packs alone or in combination with other techniques will require further study.

PROCEDURE

This technique is best accomplished by placing large plastic bags filled with crushed ice or an ice water mixture in both axilla and over both femoral triangles. If the neck is used, the packs must be placed laterally, with care taken not to compress the trachea or apply excessive weight over the carotid arteries. The neck area should probably not be packed in the presence of carotid bruits or a history of cerebrovascular disease.

COMPLICATIONS

Complications of strategic ice packing are limited to shivering and patient discomfort as described for whole body ice packing previously. The ice packs should be removed when the rectal temperature reaches 39° C to avoid excessive core temperature drop.

External Versus Core Cooling

All of the external cooling techniques described previously are noninvasive and use heat loss by evaporation or conduction across the skin as the primary cooling mechanism. With each of these techniques, dropping of the central temperature will continue even after the technique is discontinued and the skin is dried. This is due to a delay in the establishment of an equilibrium between the cold skin and the core. The amount of "core afterdrop" can exceed 2° C. For this reason, cooling should usually be discontinued when the core temperature reaches 39° C.

Since the sites of significant cell damage with heatstroke are centrally located (liver, kidney, heart, and so on), central cooling techniques theoretically are preferable to external techniques. Iced gastric lavage and peritoneal lavage are the two central techniques that have been studied in both animal models and human heatstroke.[36, 37, 42, 43] Cooling via the respiratory tract has been studied in animals but not investigated clinically.[44] Central cooling techniques are necessarily more invasive than external techniques and therefore have the potential for more significant complications.

Cold Gastric Lavage

INTRODUCTION

The stomach lies in close proximity to the liver, great vessels, kidneys, and heart. The gastric mucosa is not subject to the intense vasoconstriction observed on skin exposure to ice water.[45] For these reasons, lavage of the stomach might be expected to be an effective central cooling method. In a canine model, lavage with ice water at a rate of 200 ml/min produced cooling rates that were slower than those seen with evaporative cooling.[33] Human heatstroke victims have been successfully cooled with gastric lavage, but only in combination with external techniques.[42] Cold gastric lavage seems best suited for use in patients with severe hyperthermia who are cooling at a slow rate with external techniques alone. The presence of an endotracheal tube and the passage of a large-bore gastric tube make rapid lavage without aspiration possible. This technique should be reserved for patients whose airway is protected by endotracheal intubation and who do not have a contraindication to gastric tube placement (see Chapters 51 and 53).

PROCEDURE

Cold gastric lavage is best accomplished by instilling 10 ml/kg of iced tap water into the stomach as rapidly as possible (usually over 30 to 60 seconds). After a 30- to 60-second dwell time, the water is removed by suction or gravity.[37] Cooling will theoretically be faster if a high temperature gradient is maintained in the stomach. To this end, the lavage should proceed quickly. A faster lavage rate is usually maintained if suction is used to withdraw instilled fluid. A large container of ice water maintained 3 to 4 feet above the patient will facilitate instillation of fluid. This container should be directly connected to the lavage tubing and should ideally allow passage of water but not ice, which may occlude the tube. Since large volumes of water are needed, it is helpful if additional water and ice can be added to the container without interrupting the lavage. A large syringe can be used as an alternative to gravity instillation, but this is usually slower.

A simple system that accomplishes this procedure can be devised from readily available equipment in most emergency departments. A standard lavage set-up (for use in drug overdoses) and a large-bore gastric tube are used. The lavage bag is cut open at the top to allow water and ice to be added. It is then suspended above the patient and connected to the orogastric tube by Y tubing with clamps. The other arm of the Y tubing is connected to suction. Using the clamps, ice water can intermittently be instilled by gravity and withdrawn by suction.

COMPLICATIONS

A major potential complication of cold gastric lavage is pulmonary aspiration. The use of a cuffed endotracheal tube should minimize the incidence of this complication. Owing to the large volume of water used and the frequent depression of airway reflexes seen with severe heatstroke, this technique should not be used in a patient who is not endotracheally intubated.

If tap water is used, water intoxication, hyponatremia, and other electrolyte disturbances are *potential* complications. Water is absorbed from the stomach and with large-volume lavage may pass the pylorus into the small intestine. In canine studies, large-volume gastric lavage with tap water did not cause electrolyte abnormalities.[37] The actual incidence of these potential complications in human heatstroke has not been determined. The use of normal saline instead of tap water would eliminate this potential problem.

Theoretically, the passage of cold water through the esophagus directly behind the heart has the potential to induce cardiac dysrhythmias. Dysrhythmias have not been observed in canine studies or in case reports of human heatstroke victims cooled with this technique.[37, 42]

Cold Peritoneal Lavage

INTRODUCTION

The surface area and blood flow of the peritoneum greatly exceed those of the stomach. Peritoneal lavage would therefore be expected to exchange heat much faster than gastric lavage. Bynum and coworkers' study of peritoneal lavage (6° C fluid) in dogs demonstrated the fastest cooling rate ever reported in large animal or human studies (see Table 99–2).[36] A case report of peritoneal lavage cooling in human heatstroke also demonstrated rapid cooling.[43] As with gastric lavage, this central cooling technique offers the advantage of directly cooling the core organs that are most susceptible to thermal damage. Unlike gastric lavage, endotracheal intubation is not required.

Peritoneal lavage is also the most invasive cooling technique. Surgical placement of the lavage catheter is necessary. Since heat exchange is more efficient across the peritoneum, smaller volumes of fluid can be used. This cooling technique is contraindicated by conditions that preclude placement of a lavage catheter (i.e., multiple abdominal surgical scars) (see Chapter 56).

Peritoneal lavage is the most rapid central cooling technique. It can theoretically be combined with other techniques to speed cooling of the heatstroke patient with refractory hyperthermia. Being the most invasive cooling technique, it requires time, proper equipment, and surgical expertise to institute. Its use is probably best suited to situations in which heatstroke patients are not responding to external cooling and adequate equipment and personnel are readily available.

PROCEDURE

To institute peritoneal lavage cooling, several (2 to 8) liters of sterile saline should be immersed in an ice water bath to cool them while the catheter is being placed. A standard peritoneal lavage catheter (as for diagnostic use in trauma patients) is placed using any of the techniques described in Chapter 56.[43] Use of a larger peritoneal dialysis catheter may speed fluid instillation and withdrawal. Actual lavage volumes and rates have not been established. One approach is to instill and withdraw 500 to 1000 ml every 10 minutes until adequate cooling has been achieved. Rectal temperature may be falsely low during the lavage owing to the presence of cold water about the rectum at the level of the rectal temperature probe.[36] It may be preferable to monitor tympanic membrane esophageal temperature when using this technique. The lavage should be discontinued when core temperature reaches 39° C to avoid excessive core afterdrop.

COMPLICATIONS

The potential complications of peritoneal lavage cooling are primarily related to placement of the catheter and include bowel or bladder perforation and placement into the rectus sheath rather than the peritoneum. Please see

Chapter 56 for a more in-depth discussion of these complications.

Other Cooling Techniques

The respiratory tract is commonly used to rewarm hypothermic patients (see Chapter 91).[46] Efforts to use the respiratory tract to cool heatstroke victims have thus far been unsuccessful. High-frequency jet ventilation (HFJV) causes core cooling in critically ill patients.[47, 48] The use of HFJV in a canine model of heatstroke has shown it to be a relatively ineffective cooling technique.[44] Heat loss by convection (air transfer) is relatively inefficient compared with the conductive heat loss mechanism used by other cooling techniques. The use of dry, hot air to maximize evaporative heat loss from the lungs might cause respiratory complications.[48]

Ice water lavage of the bladder and colon have not been investigated as cooling techniques. Obvious logistical problems decrease the potential effectiveness of these techniques. In addition, the central cooling rate achieved would probably not be faster than the relatively slow rate seen with gastric lavage.

Dantrolene sodium administration is key to the effective treatment of malignant hyperthermia.[49] This drug induces skeletal muscle relaxation by blocking the release of calcium within muscle cells. It has been suggested that dantrolene administration might speed cooling of heatstroke victims by reducing skeletal muscle heat production.[24, 50] In a canine study of externally induced hyperthermia, dantrolene administration did not result in faster cooling rates than those seen with spontaneous room air cooling alone.[51] A small human study of exercise-induced heatstroke during a religious pilgrimage has suggested that dantrolene may speed cooling rates in exertional heatstroke.[52] Dantrolene administration is best reserved for patients with clinical muscle rigidity or suspected malignant hyperthermia. The routine use of this drug in heatstroke patients is not recommended.

Hemodialysis or partial cardiopulmonary bypass could theoretically be used to cool heatstroke patients. There are no animal or clinical data in the literature evaluating these invasive central cooling techniques. The downdraft of a hovering helicopter has been used as an evaporative cooling adjunct at one center.[53]

CONCLUSION

Rapid cooling is the key step in the emergency management of heatstroke patients. Evaporative cooling is clearly the technique of choice. It combines the advantages of simplicity and noninvasiveness with the most rapid cooling rates achieved with any external technique. It is also logistically easier to institute, maintain, and monitor evaporative cooling than any other cooling technique. If a patient is not cooling rapidly with evaporative cooling, other techniques can be added. Strategic ice packs can be used. If the patient is endotracheally intubated, gastric lavage can be used. If facilities and personnel are available, peritoneal lavage cooling can be instituted as a rapid central cooling technique. If muscle rigidity is present or if malignant hyperthermia is suspected, dantrolene sodium should be administered. A reasonable clinical goal is to reduce the rectal temperature to 40° C or below within 60 minutes of instituting therapy.

Immersion cooling should be limited to situations in which electric power for evaporative cooling is unavailable (e.g., in wilderness settings where bodies of cool water are available nearby and the victim is far from more sophisticated medical care). Other cooling techniques require further study before a clear recommendation as to their efficacy can be made.

REFERENCES

1. Clowes GHA, Jr, O'Donnell TF, Jr: Heat stroke. N Engl J Med 12:564, 1974.
2. Ferris EB, Jr, Blankenhorn MA, Robinson HW, Cullen GE: Heat stroke: Clinical and chemical observation on 44 cases. J Clin Invest 17:249, 1938.
3. Shibolet S, Coll R, Gilat T, Sohar E: Heatstroke: Its clinical picture and mechanism in 36 cases. Q J Med New Series 36(144):525, 1967.
4. Yaqub BA, Al-Harthi SS, Al-Orainey IO, et al: Heatstroke at the Mekkah pilgrimage: Clinical characteristics and course of 30 patients. Q J Med New Series 59(229):523, 1986.
5. Graham BS, Lichtenstein MJ, Hinson JM, Theil GB: Nonexertional heatstroke: Physiologic management and cooling in 14 patients. Arch Intern Med 146:87, 1986.
6. Tucker LE, Stanford J, Graves B, et al: Classical heatstroke: Clinical and laboratory assessment. South Med J 78(1):20, 1985.
7. Sprung CL: Hemodynamic alterations in heat stroke in the elderly. Chest 75(3):362, 1979.
8. Martin ML, Lucid EJ, Walker RW: Neuropletic malignant syndrome. Ann Emerg Med 14(4):354, 1985.
9. Symposium on malignant hyperthermia. Br J Anaesth 60:251, 1988.
10. Bradbury PA, Fox RH, Goldsmith R, et al: Resting metabolism in man at elevated body temperatures. Physiol Soc Jan 14, 61P, 1967.
11. Hanson PG, Zimmerman SW: Exertional heatstroke in novice runners. JAMA 242(2):154, 1979.
12. Hensel H: Neural processes in thermoregulation. Physiol Rev 53(4):948, 1973.
13. Rowell LB: Cardiovascular aspects of human thermoregulation. Circ Res 52(4):367, 1983.
14. Kew MC: Temperature regulation in heatstroke in man. Israel J Med Sci 12(8):759, 1976.
15. Shibolet S, Lancaster MC, Danon Y: Heat stroke: A review. Aviat Space Environ Med 5:280, 1976.
16. O'Donnell TF, Jr, Clowes GHA, Jr: Circulatory abnormalities of heat stroke. N E J Med 12:734, 1973.
16a. Sofer S, Phillip M, Hershkowits J, et al: Hemorrhagic shock and encephalopathy syndrome: Its association with hyperthermia. Am J Dis Child 140:1252, 1986.
16b. Weibley RE, Pimentel B, Ackerman NB: Hemorrhagic shock and encephalopathy syndrome of infants and children. Crit Care Med 17:335, 1989.
17. Spaul WA, Greenleaf JE: Heat stress field study. US Navy Med Mar-Apr, 25, 1984.
18. Overgaard K, Overgaard J: Investigations on the possibility of a thermic tumour therapy—I. Europ J Cancer 8:65, 1972.
19. Gerweck LE: Hyperthermia in cancer therapy: The biological basis and unresolved questions. Cancer Res 45:3408, 1985.
20. Oleson JR, Calderwood SK, Coughlin CT, et al: Biological and clinical aspects of hyperthermia in cancer therapy. Am J Clin Oncol 11(3):368, 1988.
21. Costrini AM, Pitt HA, Gustafson AB, Uddin DE: Cardiovascular and metabolic manifestations of heat stroke and severe heat exhaustion. Am J Med 66:296, 1979.
22. Sohal RS, Sun SC, Colcolough L, Burch GE: Heat stroke: Electron microscopic study of endothelial cell damage and disseminated intravascular coagulation. Arch Intern Med 122:43, 1968.
23. Hubbard RW, Matthew CB, Durkot MJ, Francesconi RP: Novel approaches to the pathophysiology of heatstroke: The energy depletion model. Ann Emerg Med 16(9):1066, 1987.
24. Jardon OM: Physiologic stress, heat stroke, malignant hyperthermia—a perspective. Milit Med 147:8, 1982.
25. Ward A, Chaffman MO, Sorkin EM: Dantrolene: A review of its pharmacodynamic and pharmacokinetic properties and therapeutic use in malignant hyperthermia, the neuroleptic malignant syndrome and an update of its use in muscle spasticity. Drugs 32:130, 1986.
26. Vicario SJ, Okabajue R, Haltom T: Rapid cooling in classic heatstroke: Effect on mortality rates. Am J Emerg Med 4(5):394, 1986.
27. Hubbard RW, Bowers WD, Matthew WT, et al: Rat model of acute heatstroke mortality. J Appl Physiol 42(6):809, 1977.
28. Weiner JS, Khogali M: A physiological body-cooling unit for treatment of heat stroke. Lancet Mar 8, 507, 1980.
29. Barner HB, Masar M: Field evaluation of a new simplified method for cooling of heat casualties in the desert. Mili Med 149:95, 1984.
30. Al-Aska AK, Abu-Aisha H, Yaqub B, et al: Simplified cooling bed for heatstroke (letter). Lancet Feb 14, 381, 1987.
31. Kielblock AJ, Van Rensburg JP, Franz RM: Body cooling as a method for reducing hyperthermia. S Afr Med J 69:378, 1986.
32. Wyndham CH, Strydom NB, Cooke HM, et al: Methods of cooling subjects with hyperpyrexia. J Appl Physiol 14(5):771, 1959.
33. White JD, Riccobene E, Nucci R, et al: Evaporation versus iced gastric lavage treatment of heatstroke: Comparative efficacy in a canine model. Crit Care Med 15(8):748, 1987.
34. Daily WM, Harrison TR: A study of the mechanism and treatment of experimental heat pyrexia. Am J Med Sci 215:42, 1948.
35. Magazanik A, Epstein Y, Udassin R, et al: Tap water, an efficient method for cooling heatstroke victims—a model in dogs. Aviat Space Environ Med 51(9):864, 1980.

36. Bynum G, Patton J, Bowers W, et al: Peritoneal lavage cooling in an anesthetized dog heatstroke model. Aviat Space Environ Med 49(6):779, 1978.
37. Syverud SA, Barker WJ, Amsterdam JT, et al: Iced gastric lavage for treatment of heatstroke: Efficacy in a canine model. Ann Emerg Med 14:424, 1985.
38. Khogali M, Weiner JS: Heat stroke: Report on 18 cases. Lancet Aug 9, 276, 1980.
39. Treatment of heat injury. Med Lett Drugs Ther 32(822):66, 1990.
40. Cummings P: Felled by the heat. Emerg Med June 30, 95, 1983.
41. Noakes TD: Heatstroke during the 1981 National Cross-Country Running Championships. S Afr Med J 61:145, 1982.
42. Slovis CM, Anderson GF, Casolaro A: Survival in a heatstroke victim with a core temperature in excess of 46.5°. Ann Emerg Med 11:269, 1982.
43. Horowitz BZ: The golden hour in heat stroke: Use of iced peritoneal lavage. Am J Emerg Med 7(6):616, 1989.
44. Barker WJ, Amsterdam JT, Syverud SA, et al: High-frequency jet ventilation cooling in a canine hyperthermia model. Ann Emerg Med 15:680, 1986.
45. Carlson LD, Hsieh ACL, Fullington F, Elsner RW: Immersion in cold water and body tissue insulation. Aviat Med Feb, 145, 1958.
46. Lloyd EL: Airway warming in the treatment of accidental hypothermia: A review. J Wilderness Med 1:65, 1990.
47. Smith RB, Cutaia F, Hoff BH, et al: Long term transtracheal high frequency ventilation in dogs. Crit Care Med 9:311, 1981.
48. Keszler M, Klein R, McClellan L, et al: Effects of conventional and high frequency jet ventilation on lung parenchyma. Crit Care Med 10:514, 1982.
49. Harrison GG: Control of the malignant hyperpyrexic syndrome in MHS swine by dantrolene sodium. Br J Anaesth 47:62, 1975.
50. Lydiatt JD, Hill GE: Treatment of heatstroke by dantrolene. JAMA 246:41, 1981.
51. Amsterdam JT, Syverud SA, Barker WJ, et al: Dantrolene sodium for treatment of heatstroke victims: Lack of efficacy in a canine model. Am J Emerg Med 4:399, 1986.
52. Channa AB, Seraj MA, Saddique AA, et al: Is dantrolene effective in heat stroke patients? Crit Care Med 18:290, 1990.
53. Poulton TJ, Walker RA: Helicopter cooling of heatstroke victims. Aviat Space Environ Med 58:358, 1987.

Chapter 93

The Amobarbital Interview

Kenneth V. Iserson

INTRODUCTION

Emergency physicians occasionally encounter patients presenting with complaints of sudden, nontraumatic paresis or paralysis of the extremities, as well as those presenting in catatonia-like states.[1] Although an underlying primary psychiatric etiology is usually suspected by the experienced emergency physician, nagging questions about the presence of exotic or rare organic etiologies usually remain.[2] This dilemma, as well as the physician's frequent inability to alleviate acute symptoms, often causes difficulty and confusion in the patient's initial disposition and treatment. The use of sodium amobarbital (Amytal) interviews in these patients quickly resolves such problems.[3, 4] The procedure can be easily accomplished in either the emergency department or the physician's office in about 20 minutes.

BACKGROUND

Amobarbital (sodium iso-amyl ethyl barbiturate) was first synthesized by the Lilly Company in the late 1920s. It is a moderately long-acting barbiturate with a moderately rapid induction time.[5] In 1930, W. J. Bleckwenn began using amobarbital to produce a drug-induced narcosis for the treatment of neuropsychiatric disorders.[6-8] The technique was quickly picked up and expanded by much of the psychiatric community under the general term narcoanalysis.[9, 10] It was generally used in institutionalized or long-term patients. World War II brought a resurgent interest in the amobarbital interview. At this time, it was introduced for use in acute paralysis, amnesia, aphonia, or pseudocatatonic states on the front lines. Grinker and Spiegel used the technique successfully for both diagnostic and therapeutic purposes.[11, 12] Since World War II, however, the psychiatric community has lost interest in narcoanalysis. Current textbooks of psychiatry give little space to narcoanalysis, and many practicing psychiatrists have little familiarity with the technique.[13]

Recently, the emergency medicine community has developed an interest in narcoanalysis for symptoms similar to the "war neuroses."[14] A series of actual emergency department cases of catatonic-like symptoms and conversion reactions has also been reported.[15]

INDICATIONS

The amobarbital interview is a rapid and safe method for distinguishing and treating the functional factors that contribute to several types of symptom complexes presenting to the emergency department.

Over the years, a variety of indications have been developed for acute outpatient use of the amobarbital interview. These indications include the following:

1. Resolve conversion symptoms so that their crystallization and permanence may be avoided.
2. Treat acute panic states following such traumatic events as rape, catastrophic loss, or disaster.
3. Diagnose and treat mute and unresponsive patients (benign stupor) or patients with acute hysterical amnesia.
4. Diagnose malingering.
5. Reveal suicidal ideations.
6. Gain information in criminal cases (of dubious merit or legal worth).[16]
7. Differentiate between organic illness or organic psychosis and functional psychosis.
8. Differentiate functional psychiatric disorders, such as multiple personality disorders or pseudodementia, from other psychiatric disorders.[17-19]

The use of the test to differentiate an organic from a functional illness can be of considerable concern and of life-threatening importance to those involved with the care of catatonic-like patients. Because many patients choose the emergency department as their first access into the medical system, an organic etiology for such complaints must be considered by the emergency physician. Many psychiatrists have lost sight of this possibility[1] or have come to rely heavily on "medical clearance," which is, at times done hastily in a busy emergency department by psychiatrically inexperienced physicians. Patients who appear to be catatonic or in benign stupor have been reported to have such conditions as intracranial infections[20, 21] and hemorrhage,[22] endocrine abnormalities,[23] liver failure,[24] atrioventricular (AV) malformations, tumors, and drug ingestions.[25] Delay in diagnosis and therapy has led to deaths in patients with these conditions as well as in those with acute lethal catatonia.[26] Either an admission protocol (vital signs, history, and physical examination) or the amobarbital interview should suggest an organic etiology for these patients.[1]

Most emergency department experience with the amobarbital interview has been with adults presenting with one of two specific syndromes, either hysterical conversion reactions that significantly impair the patient's functions or a catatonia-like state. The catatonia-like state is different from the common condition that Plum and Posner describe as psychogenic unresponsiveness.[27] Patients with psychogenic unresponsiveness are usually hysterical, with symptoms lasting for several minutes. They lie with their eyes closed and actively resist opening the lids. When opened, the eyelids flutter or close rapidly rather than with the smooth motion seen in coma. These patients normally will respond quickly to noxious stimuli and a firm approach by the emergency department staff.

Patients in a catatonia-like state, however, often present either in a state of mute wakefulness without response to verbal or tactile stimuli or in a mildly stuporous condition. Patients in a state of mute wakefulness will often track the observer with their eyes (coma vigil, akinetic mutism) and may show a waxy flexibility of the extremities.[25] Those in stupor are sometimes mistakenly assumed to have either a neurologic condition or drug ingestion.

CONTRAINDICATIONS

Contraindications to the amobarbital interview fall into two categories: psychiatric and medical (Table 93–1). From the psychiatric standpoint, most contraindications are relative ones. That is, potential benefit from the procedure must be weighed against the potential harm under the circumstances. Patients presenting with an overt paranoid reaction or those patients unwilling to passively submit to the procedure are unlikely to gain maximum benefit and may incur additional psychiatric trauma by undergoing the interview. Likewise, the patient who is overeager may be describing a condition from which secondary gain is involved in having the procedure performed. Using this technique on such patients may be both dangerous and unnecessary.

Medical contraindications are both absolute (i.e., porphyria and barbiturate allergy) and relative. Relative contraindications include already being under the influence of depressant drugs and having a history of barbiturate addiction, although the interview can also be used as a test of current addiction. However, even when there is concomitant drug ingestion, the interview may still be performed if the dose of amobarbital is very carefully titrated. Relative contraindications also include the presence of severe liver, cardiac, or renal disease. Severe hyper- or hypotension may suggest an organic cause, but use of the drug in these states poses a medical risk only if more than the maximum safe

dose (500 mg amobarbital sodium intravenously) is given. The presence of mild pulmonary infection, pulmonary edema, or laryngitis poses only the theoretical risk of increasing the chance of laryngospasm. Generally, in the presence of significant concomitant medical diseases, it is best to forego the amobarbital interview and concentrate on stabilizing the patient in the emergency department. The interview may be performed later in the hospital stay.

EQUIPMENT

One should never attempt the amobarbital interview unless one has the proper time, space, equipment, and ancillary personnel available. A relatively quiet room, a stretcher or table with side rails up, and basic resuscitation equipment (airway, intubation equipment, Ambu bag) are the primary requirements. Intravenous equipment (generally 0.9 NS or D_5NS) with an injection port should be used. Amobarbital sodium (Amytal sodium, Lilly) is supplied as a dry powder, which must be reconstituted with sterile water. In reconstituting the amobarbital, it is important to rotate, not shake, the ampule. Five hundred milligrams of amobarbital sodium should be prepared as a 5 per cent by weight solution by diluting 500 mg of the powder in 10 ml of sterile water.

Sodium amobarbital is not the only drug that has been used in this manner. Some psychiatrists now use thiopental and mixtures of thiopental and amobarbital.[28] Others have used chloroform, cannabis indica, paraldehyde, scopolamine, chloral hydrate, and most modern barbiturates for the same purpose.[29] Amobarbital, however, seems to be the best choice for emergency department use. (The editors recommend that the procedure be done only with amobarbital.) Aside from the wealth of clinical experience with amobarbital in this setting and its theoretical superiority over thiopental for interviewing,[30] it is already familiar to most emergency physicians and is stocked as a second-line anticonvulsant in some departments.

PROCEDURE

A medical history emphasizing prior psychiatric problems, drug overdose and abuse, allergies, medications, and contraindications to the procedure must be obtained from the patient, relatives, or friends. A complete physical examination must be performed to identify any obvious organic problems. Glucose, blood urea nitrogen (BUN), electrolytes, and a complete blood count (CBC) are obtained in cases of stupor. Samples for toxicology should be obtained, and glucose, naloxone, and thiamine should be administered. Prior records, when obtainable, should be reviewed. If a proper history, physical examination, or laboratory analysis is not possible, the procedure should not be performed. *The physician's zeal to try the procedure should not tempt her or him to take short cuts or to hastily examine the patient.*

After deciding that the symptoms are possibly of a nonorganic psychiatric etiology, the procedure of the amobarbital interview is explained to the patient and/or his relatives. Reassurance should be given that Amytal is not, in fact, "truth serum." The patient should be placed in a relatively quiet room with the patient's relative or a chaperone in attendance. It may be extremely helpful for relatives to observe the interview, because it is often difficult for them to comprehend that certain symptoms, such as paralysis, have a psychogenic basis. Successful results may further reinforce the need for the family to arrange for follow-up psychiatric care.

Table 93–1. Contraindications to Use of Amobarbital Interview

	Medical Contraindications	Psychiatric Contraindications
Absolute	Porphyria Allergy to barbiturates	None
Relative	History of barbiturate addiction Under influence of depressant drugs Severe liver, cardiac, or renal disease Severe hyper- or hypotension (only if more than 500 mg is used) Pulmonary infection or edema	Paranoid reaction Unwilling patient Overeager patient

An intravenous line should be secured in a large peripheral vein. Sodium amobarbital (5 per cent solution) is administered at a rate of 50 mg (0.5 ml) per minute. A conversation (or monologue in the stupor cases) about benign, nonthreatening topics should be held with the patient during induction. A calm, reassuring attitude and suggestions similar to those given during hypnotic inductions are useful, because the effect of the interview may be as great as that of the medication.[31, 32]

There is a close similarity between the state produced with Amytal and the light stages of hypnosis.[33] Some investigators have, in fact, considered it just another hypnotic medium that allows simple, direct psychotherapy with little or no analysis.[34] If a psychiatrist is present during the interview, some of the information obtained can be beneficial in future analysis. We suggest that whenever possible, the interview should be performed in consultation with a psychiatrist who will be involved in the subsequent care of the patient.

The levels of narcosis are staged using the criteria developed by Lorenz and associates.[35] The interview is conducted during stage II narcosis. Stage I narcosis is reached when the responsive patient describes his first symptoms: fatigue, light headedness or dizziness, or blurring or double vision. Stage II occurs when the responsive patient becomes euphoric or drowsy and when the unresponsive patient begins answering questions. Stage III, absence of corneal reflexes, should be avoided.

When stage II is reached, the actual interview is begun. It usually requires 250 to 500 mg of amobarbital to reach this stage, although some investigators report success with as little as 100 mg.[14] The patient is initially questioned regarding such nonthreatening topics as identification data, his current personal situation, predisposing factors, and further medical history (including drug ingestion).

The next stage of the interview is tailored to the specific problem. For example, if the patient has paralysis of an arm or leg, the interviewer suggests that the patient try to move and use the affected part. Once the paralysis is overcome, the interviewer reinforces the fact that the extremity is now back to normal and that it will continue to be normal after the patient leaves the hospital. It is not advisable to confront the patient with a psychiatric diagnosis at this time, even though such a diagnosis is now obvious to the family. If the patient is catatonic or unresponsive, spontaneous speech or movement will return, and it is emphasized to the patient that such a responsive state is normal and desirable. Patients with organic/toxic psychoses will not respond verbally and will merely fall asleep or become more sedated during the interview. If this occurs during the interview process, the interview can be terminated with the knowledge that the patient should be presumed to have an organic etiology. Patients who have an organic basis for paresis or paralysis will still show this deficit during the interview.

Near the end of the interview, it is suggested to the patient that he remember a pleasant occurrence. This helps to improve the patient's emergence from the interview. A few patients may become slightly upset during the interview. They can be given an extra 50 to 100 mg of amobarbital at the conclusion of the interview to obtain a slightly longer sleep period.[36] Respirations are the only vital sign monitored after the procedure begins. As long as sodium amobarbital is given by this protocol, there are no significant effects on blood pressure, pulse, or respiratory rate.[35] A cardiac monitor is not required routinely but is advised in any patient with cardiovascular disease and in the elderly. Patients who are not hospitalized should be observed for 2 to 4 hours after the interview has been completed. Patients usually fall asleep for 2 to 3 hours following the conclusion of the

interview, and when the patient is awakened, the proper disposition should be made.

Catatonic and pseudocatatonic patients who now have established psychiatric diagnoses should be admitted to a psychiatric service. Patients with resolved conversion reactions can be discharged with follow-up. When a psychiatric basis cannot be proven, the patient requires further evaluation for a presumed organic etiology.

COMPLICATIONS

Many thousands of amobarbital interviews have been conducted, usually in settings that are not conducive to advanced life support, with few complications.[9, 35, 37, 38] Nevertheless, resuscitation facilities must be readily available if this procedure is undertaken. The few complications reported have been primarily respiratory depression or apnea and were associated with too rapid administration (greater than 50 mg per minute) or occasionally too much (greater than 500 mg) of the drug.[38] Vasomotor collapse and laryngospasm have also been reported on rare occasions. The latter complications are reported to occur only in stage III (usually greater than 700 mg) or anesthetic levels of narcosis, and they are not reported at all in most series. Most complications are probably related to physician error or inaccurate calculation of drug doses.

INTERPRETATION

The patient with a supposed psychiatric symptom who does not initially respond to the amobarbital interview warrants intensive investigation for an anatomic/physiologic basis for the deficit. Failure to alleviate symptoms with the amobarbital interview is often due to the failure of the physician to make the proper pre-interview diagnosis. This is usually the result of an inadequate physical examination or incomplete laboratory or radiographic evaluation prior to the technique being used. If the patient has a firm belief or delusion, such as a feeling that he is God or that he is from outer space, the amobarbital interview will not abolish that belief. Likewise, it obviously will not render a schizophrenic normal while under the influence of the drug.[39]

Some cases of catatonia may not respond to this technique. It must be emphasized, however, that if a psychiatric diagnosis is not firmly made from the results of the interview, it is mandatory that the patient receive intensive medical care and evaluation before he is referred to a psychiatric facility.

CONCLUSION

The amobarbital interview has been shown to be a rapid and safe technique that can be readily performed by the emergency physician. It is useful for the confirmation of the psychiatric basis of stupor in catatonic-like patients and for diagnosis and resolution of similarly based nontraumatic paresis and paralysis. When possible, we suggest that the procedure be carried out in conjunction with a psychiatric evaluation to obtain the maximum clinical benefit.

References

1. Belfer ML, d'Autremont CC: Catatonia-like symptomatology: An interesting case. Arch Gen Psychiatry 24:119, 1971.
2. Slater E: Diagnosis of "hysteria." Br Med J 1:827, 1922.
3. Mann J: The use of sodium amobarbital in psychiatry. Ohio State Med J 65:700, 1969.
4. Stevens H: Conversion hysteria: A neurologic emergency. Mayo Clin Proc 43:54, 1968.

5. Churchill-Davidson HC: A Practice of Anaesthesia. Philadelphia, WB Saunders Co, 1978.
6. Bleckwenn WJ: Narcosis as therapy in neuropsychiatric conditions. JAMA 95:1168, 1930.
7. Bleckwenn WJ: Sodium amytal in certain nervous and mental conditions. Wis Med J 29:693, 1930.
8. Bleckwenn WJ: The use of sodium amytal in catatonia. Association for Research in Mental Diseases 10:224, 1931.
9. Horsley JS: Narco-analysis. J Ment Sci 82:416, 1936.
10. Lindemann E: Psychological changes in normal and abnormal individuals under the influence of sodium amytal. Am J Psychiatry 88:1038, 1932.
11. Grinker RR, Spiegel JP: War Neuroses. Philadelphia, Blakiston, 1945.
12. Grinker RR, Spiegel JP: Men Under Stress. Philadelphia, Blakiston, 1945.
13. Cole JO, Davis JM, Freedman AM, et al: Comprehensive Textbook of Psychiatry, 2nd ed. Baltimore, Williams & Wilkins, 1975, pp 1968–1969.
14. Wettstein RM, Fauman BJ: The amobarbital interview. JACEP 8:272, 1979.
15. Iserson KV: The emergency amobarbital interview. Ann Emerg Med 9:513, 1980.
16. Redlich FC, Ravitz LJ, Dession GH: Narcoanalysis and truth. Am J Psychiatry 107:586, 1951.
17. Marcum JM, Wright K, Bissell WG: Chance discovery of multiple personality disorder in a depressed patient by amobarbital interview. J Nerv Ment Dis 174:489, 1986.
18. Markowitz J, Viederman M: A case report of dissociative pseudodementia. Gen Hosp Psychiatry 8:87, 1986.
19. Ross CA, Anderson G: Phenomenological overlap of multiple personality disorder and obsessive-compulsive disorder. J Nerv Ment Dis 176:295, 1988.
20. Raskin DE, Frank SW: Herpes encephalitis with catatonic stupor. Arch Gen Psychiatry 31:544, 1974.
21. Penn H, Racy J, Lapham L, et al: Catatonic behavior, viral encephalopathy, and death. Arch Gen Psychiatry 27:758, 1972.
22. Michaels LJ: Catatonic syndrome in a case of subdural hematoma. J Nerv Ment Dis 117:123, 1953.
23. Hockaday TDR, Keynes WM, McKenzie JK: Catatonic stupor in elderly woman with hyperparathyroidism. Br Med J 1:85, 1966.
24. Jaffe N: Catatonia and hepatic dysfunction. Dis Nerv Syst 28:606, 1976.
25. Morrison JR: Catatonia: Diagnosis and management. Hosp Commun Psychiatry 26:91, 1975.
26. Regestein QR, Alpert JS, Reich P: Sudden catatonic stupor with disastrous outcome. JAMA 238:618, 1977.
27. Plum F, Posner JB: The Diagnosis of Stupor and Coma. Philadelphia, FA Davis Co, 1972, pp 217–221.
28. Smith JW, Lemere F, Dunn RB: Pentothal interviews in the treatment of alcoholism. Psychosomatics 12:330, 1971.
29. Hart WL, Ebaugh FG, Morgan DW: The amytal interview. Am J Med Sci 210:125, 1945.
30. Naples M, Hackett TP: The amytal interview: history and current uses. Psychosomatics 19:98, 1978.
31. Stevenson I, Buckman J, Smith BM, et al: The use of drugs in psychiatric interviews: Some interpretations based on controlled experiments. Am J Psychiatry 131:707, 1974.
32. Smith BM, Hain JD, Stevenson I: Controlled interviews using drugs. Arch Gen Psychiatry 22:2, 1970.
33. Burnett WE: A critique of intravenous barbiturate usage in psychiatric practice. Psychiatr Q 22:45, 1948.
34. Morris DP: Intravenous barbiturates: An aid in the diagnosis and treatment of conversion hysteria and malingering. Milit Surg 96:509, 1945.
35. Lorenz WF, Reese HH, Washburne AC: Physiological observations during intravenous sodium amytal medications. Am J Psychiatry 13:1205, 1934.
36. Marcos LR, Goldberg E, Feazell D, et al: The use of sodium amytal interviews in a short-term community-oriented inpatient unit. Dis Nerv Ssyt 38:283, 1977.
37. Kameneva EN, Yagodka PK: Sodium amytal: Its therapeutic and diagnostic uses. Neuropathologiya Psykhatriya 12:44, 1943.
38. Lambert C, and Rees WL: Intravenous barbiturates in the treatment of hysteria. Br Med J 2:70, 1944.
39. Sullivan DJ: Psychiatric uses of intravenous sodium amytal. Am J Psychiatry 99:411, 1942.

Appendix

Commonly Used Infusion Rates

*Mary Ann Howland and
Elaena Quattrocchi*

AMINOPHYLLINE

Dosage

Aminophylline is given as a loading dose of 5.6 mg/kg, followed by a continuous infusion to maintain the serum theophylline level between 10 and 20 µg/ml. There is considerable variation in theophylline metabolism, and serum levels must be monitored carefully. Aminophylline is 80 per cent theophylline. Note that the dose given is expressed in aminophylline units, but serum levels measure theophylline.

Note: Premature infants and some neonates have decreased theophylline elimination that may result in toxicity if the infusion rates for children or adults are used for calculations. Elderly patients with chronic obstructive pulmonary disease; patients with liver disease or concomitant respiratory infections; or patients who are taking medications (e.g., erythromycin, cimetidine, contraceptives, allopurinol) have decreased theophylline clearance.

Available Preparations

Each 10-ml ampule contains 250 mg of aminophylline; each 20-ml ampule contains 500 mg aminophylline. The concentration of aminophylline in each ampule is 25 mg/ml.

Aminophylline—Loading Dose
(5.6 mg/kg,* based on a zero theophylline level to start)†

				Weight					
10 kg	*20 kg*	*30 kg*	*40 kg*	*50 kg*	*60 kg*	*70 kg*	*80 kg*	*90 kg*	*100 kg*
56 mg	112 mg	168 mg	224 mg	280 mg	336 mg	392 mg	448 mg	504 mg	560 mg

*Diluted in 50 to 100 ml and infused over a period of 20–30 minutes; frequent monitoring of serum theophylline levels is required.
†*Note:* In adults and children, 1 mg/kg of theophylline raises the serum theophylline level by approximately 2 µg/ml.

Aminophylline—Maintenance Dose*
(250 mg diluted in 250 ml; concentration of 1 mg/ml)

	Infusion Rate (microdrops/min or ml/hr)									
Age Group and Dose	*10 kg*	*20 kg*	*30 kg*	*40 kg*	*50 kg*	*60 kg*	*70 kg*	*80 kg*	*90 kg*	*100 kg*
Children, ages 1–9 years 1 mg/kg/hr	10	20	30	40	—	—	—	—	—	—
Children, older than 9 years, healthy adult smokers 0.75 mg/kg/hr					37	45	52	60	67	75
Healthy adults, nonsmokers 0.5 mg/kg/hr					25	30	35	40	45	50
Adults with cardiac failure or liver disease 0.25 mg/kg/hr					12	15	17	20	22	25

*Frequent monitoring of serum theophylline levels is required.

INTRAVENOUS NITROGLYCERIN

Note: Filters and plastic bottles and tubing (especially polyvinyl chloride tubing) may absorb nitroglycerin. Glass infusion bottles, special tubing (supplied by manufacturer), and the avoidance of in-line filters are recommended.

Dosage

There is no fixed optimum dose. The usual starting dose is 3 to 5 µg/minute, with increases of 5 to 10 µg/minute every 5 minutes depending on the clinical response.

Available Preparations

Several preparations, which differ in concentration, volume per ampule, and solvents are available.

NITRO-BID (Marion Laboratories)

Each 1-ml ampule contains 5 mg nitroglycerin.
Each 5-ml ampule contains 25 mg nitroglycerin.
Each 10-ml ampule contains 50 mg nitroglycerin.

NITROSTAT (Parke-Davis)

Each 10-ml ampule contains 8 mg nitroglycerin.

TRIDIL (American Critical Care)

Each 10-ml ampule contains either 5 or 50 mg nitroglycerin.
Each 5-ml ampule contains 25 mg nitroglycerin.

Nitro-Bid or Tridil (50 mg diluted in 1000 ml; concentration 50 µg/ml)	
2.5	3
5	6
10	12
15	18
20	24
30	36
40	48
50	60
60	72
80	96
100	120

Note: This is *not* a dose/weight calculation.
For 25 mg/500 ml (50 µg/ml), use same infusion rate as in chart.
For 50 mg/500 ml (100 µg/ml), divided the infusion rate by 2 for desired microdrops/min.
For 25 mg/1000 ml (25 µg/ml), multiply the infusion rate by 2 for desired microdrops/min.

Nitrostat (8 mg diluted in 250 ml; concentration of 32 µg/ml)*	
Dose (µg/min)*	**Infusion Rate** (microdrops/min or ml/hr)
5	9
10	18
15	27
20	36
30	54
40	72
50	90†
60	108†
80	144†
100	180†

Note: This is *not* a dose/weight calculation.
†It may be more reasonable to increase concentration to limit volume.
For 16 mg/250 ml (64µg/ml), divide the infusion rate by 2 for desired microdrops/min.
For 24 mg/250 ml (96 µg/ml), divide the infusion rate by 3 for desired microdrops/min.
For 16 mg/500 ml (32 µg/ml), use same infusion rate.

DOBUTAMINE (DOBUTREX)

Dosage

There is no fixed optimum dose. The infusion rate may be started at 2.5 µg/kg/minute and increased every 5 to 10 minutes based on the clinical response. Doses up to 40 µg/kg/minute have been used.

Available Preparation

DOBUTREX (Lilly Pharmaceutical Company)

Each 20-ml ampule contains 250 mg dobutamine.

Dobutamine (250 mg diluted in 250 ml; concentration of 1000 μg/ml)			
Dose (μg/kg/min)	**Infusion Rate** (microdrops/min or ml/hr for various weights)		
	50 kg	*70 kg*	*100 kg*
2.5	7.5	10.5	15
5	15	21	30
10	30	42	60
15	45	63	90
20	60	84	120*
30	90	126*	180*
40	120	168*	240*

*It may be more reasonable to double the concentration to reduce the volume.
For 250 mg/500 ml (500 μg/ml), multiply the infusion rate by 2 for desired microdrops/min.
For 250 mg/1000 ml (250 μg/ml), multiply the infusion rate by 4 for desired microdrops/min.
For 500 mg/250 ml (2000 μg/ml), divide the infusion rate by 2 for desired microdrops/min.
For 500 mg/500 ml (1000 μg/ml), use same dose schedule as in the chart.
For 500 mg/1000 ml (500 μg/ml), multiply the infusion rate by 2 for desired microdrops/min.
For 1000 mg/250 ml (4000 μg/ml), divide the infusion rate by 4 for desired microdrops/min.

DOPAMINE

Dosage

There is no fixed optimum dose. An infusion rate of 2 to 5 μg/kg/minute is considered to be low and is a reasonable starting dose. Rates of 5 to 10 μg/kg/minute are moderate, and rates of 10 to 20 μg/kg/minute are large. Doses up to 50 μg/kg/minute have been used.

Available Preparations

INTROPIN (American Critical Care)

Each 5-ml vial, ampule, or syringe may contain *either* 200 mg, 400 mg, or 800 mg of dopamine HCl.

DOPAMINE HCl (Elkins-Sinn)

Each 5-ml ampule may contain *either* 200 mg or 400 mg of dopamine HCl.

DOPASTAT (Parke-Davis)

Each 5-ml ampule contains 200 mg of dopamine HCl.

Dopamine (800 mg diluted in 500 ml; concentration of 1600 μg/ml)			
Dose (μg/kg/min)	**Infusion Rate** (microdrops/min or ml/hr for various weights)		
	50 kg	*70 kg*	*100 kg*
5	9.4	13	19
10	19	26	37.5
15	28	39	56
20	37.5	52.5	75
30	56	79	112.5

For 800 mg/250 ml (3200 μg/ml), divide the infusion rate by 2 for desired microdrops/min.
For 800 mg/1000 ml (800 μg/ml), multiply the infusion rate by 2 for desired microdrops/min.
For 400 mg/250 ml (1600 μg/ml), use the same dose schedule as in the chart.
For 200 mg/250 ml (800 μg/ml), multiply the infusion rate by 2 for desired microdrops/min.
For 200 mg/500 ml (400 μg/ml), multiply the infusion rate by 4 for desired microdrops/min.

ISOPROTERENOL (ISUPREL)

Dosage

There is no fixed optimum dose. The usual starting dose is 1 to 2 μg/minute, with increases of 1 to 2 μg/minute every 5 to 10 minutes depending on the clinical response.

Available Preparations

Each 5-ml ampule contains 1 mg isoproterenol. The concentration is 0.2 mg/ml as a 1:5000 solution. It is also available as 1-ml ampules containing 0.2 mg of isoproterenol.

Isoproterenol (Isuprel) (2 mg diluted in 250 ml; concentration of 8 μg/ml)	
Dose* (μg/min)	**Infusion Rate** (microdrops/min or ml/hr)
1	7.5
2	15
4	30
6	45
8	60
10	75
12	90
14	105†
16	120†
20	150†

*Note that this is *not* a dose/weight calculation.
†It may be more reasonable to increase concentration to limit volume.
For 2 mg/500 ml (4 μg/ml), multiply the infusion rate by 2 to obtain desired microdrops/min.
For 1 mg/250 ml (4 μg/ml), multiply the infusion rate by 2 to obtain desired microdrops/min.
For 1 mg/500 ml (2 μg/ml), multiply the infusion rate by 4 to obtain desired mcirodrops/min.
For 4 mg/250 ml (16 μg/ml), divide the infusion rate by 2 to obtain desired microdrops/min.

NOREPINEPHRINE (LEVOPHED)

Note: Norepinephrine should be administered with a solution containing dextrose as opposed to a plain saline solution to protect the drug from loss of potency owing to oxidation.

Dosage

There is no fixed optimum dose. The usual starting dose is 2 to 4 μg/minute, with increases of 2 to 4 μg/minute every 5 to 10 minutes depending on the clinical response.

Available Preparations

Each 4-ml ampule contains 4 mg norepinephrine, at a concentration of 1 mg/ml.

Norepinephrine (Levophed) (8 mg diluted in 500 ml; concentration of 16 μg/ml)	
Dose (μg/min)*	**Infusion Rate** (Microdrops/min or ml/hr)
1	3.75
2	7.5
4	15
6	22.5
8	30
10	37.5
12	45
16	60
20	75

*Note that this is *not* a dose/weight calculation.
For 16 mg/500 ml (32 μg/ml), divide the infusion rate by 2 to obtain desired microdrops/min.
For 4 mg/500 ml (8 μg/ml), multiply the infusion rate by 2 to obtain desired microdrops/min.

PROCAINAMIDE (PRONESTYL)

Dosage

A loading dose may be given by intermittent intravenous injection (slow push not to exceed 50 mg/minute) at a dose of 100 mg every 5 minutes or as a continuous intravenous infusion at 20 mg/minute. The loading dose should not exceed 1 gm. A constant maintenance infusion of 1 to 4 mg/minute may be started following the loading dose.

Available Preparations

Each 10-ml ampule provides 1 gm of procainamide at a concentration of 100 mg/ml. It is also available as 2-ml ampules providing 500 mg/ml.

Procainamide Maintenance Dose (Pronestyl) (2 gm diluted in 500 ml; concentration of 4 mg/ml)		
Dose (mg/min)*		**Infusion Rate** (microdrops/min or ml/hr)
Low	1	15
	2	30
	3	45
High	4	60

*Note that this is *not* a dose/weight calculation (see following table).

Procainamide Maintenance Dose (Pronestyl) (2 gm diluted in 500 ml)			
Maintenance Dose (calculated by weight)	**Infusion Rate** (microdrops/min or ml/hr for various weights)		
	50 kg	*70 kg*	*100 kg*
1.4 mg/kg/hr (low)	17.5	24.5	35
2.8 mg/kg/hr (average)	35	49	70

LIDOCAINE HCl

Note: Lidocaine should be administered as a loading dose followed by a continuous infusion.

Dosage

The average loading dose over the first 20 minutes is 150 to 225 mg, *in divided doses*. The first bolus should not exceed 100 mg. Immediately following the first bolus, an infusion of 1 to 4 mg/minute is begun, depending on the clinical condition and the response to therapy. A reasonable regimen for lidocaine loading is to give an initial 75 to 100 mg bolus, followed by 50 mg every 5 minutes to a total of 200 to 225 mg. The infusion rate should not exceed 300 mg/hr.

Available Preparations

Although many preparations for intravenous infusion are available, it is most reasonable to use 1 gm/5 ml-vial or 2 gm/10 ml-vial (such as the Inject-all syringe safety vial by Bristol).

Lidocaine HCl (2 gm diluted in 500 ml; concentration of 4 mg/ml)		
Dose (mg/min)*		**Infusion Rate** (microdrops/min or ml/hr for average 70-kg adult)
Low	1	15
	2	30
	3	45
High	4	60

*Note: This is *not* a dose/weight calculation (see following table).
For 1 gm/500 ml (2 mg/ml), multiply the infusion rate by 2 to obtain desired microdrops/min.

Lidocaine HCl (2 gm diluted in 500 ml; concentration of 4 mg/ml)			
Dose	**Infusion Rate** (microdrops/min or ml/hr for various weights)		
	50 kg	*70 kg*	*100 kg*
10 μg/kg/min (hepatic insufficiency or older than 70 years)	7.5	10.5	15
20 μg/kg/min (hepatic insufficiency or older than 70 years)	15	21	30
30 μg/kg/min	22.5	31.5	45
40 μg/kg/min	30	42	60
50 μg/kg/min (high dose)	37.5	52.5	75

For 1 gm/500 ml (2 mg/ml), multiply the infusion rate by 2 to obtain desired microdrops/min.

METARAMINOL (ARAMINE)

Dosage

There is no fixed optimum dose. An intravenous infusion is titrated according to the clinical response.

Available Preparation

ARAMINE (Merck Sharp and Dome)

Each 10-ml ampule contains 100 mg metaraminol (10 mg/ml).

Infusion

Mix 1 to 4 vials in 250 to 1000 ml and begin as a slow infusion, changing the rate every 5 to 10 minutes, depending on the clinical response.

Suggested starting dose: dilute 100 mg/250 ml and begin at 10 microdrops/minute. Wait at least 5 minutes before increasing the dose.

INTRAVENOUS ETHANOL (in the treatment of poisoning by methanol or ethylene glycol)

Note: Concentrations higher than 10 per cent are not recommended for intravenous administration. Concentrations higher than 30 per cent are not recommended for oral administration.

The dose schedule is based on the premise that the patient initially has a *zero* ethanol level. The aim of therapy is to maintain a serum ethanol level of 100 to 150 mg/dl, but constant monitoring of the ethanol level is required because of wide variations in endogenous metabolic capacity. Activated charcoal adsorbs oral ethanol. Ethanol is removed by dialysis, and the infusion rate of ethanol must be increased during dialysis.

Prolonged ethanol administration may lead to *hypoglycemia*.

Note: 10 per cent ethanol for infusion may be difficult to find in the hospital pharmacy. To formulate 10 per cent ethanol for infusion, (1) remove 50 ml from a 1-liter bottle of 5 per cent ethanol/D5W and replace it with 50 ml of 100 per cent ethanol, or (2) remove 100 ml from a 1-liter bottle of D5W and replace it with 100 ml of 100 per cent ethanol.

Intravenous Ethanol: Loading Dose
(A 10% volume/volume concentration yields approximately 100 mg/ml)

	Volume of Loading Dose (given over 1–2 hours as tolerated)					
	10 kg	*15 kg*	*30 kg*	*50 kg*	*70 kg*	*100 kg*
Loading dose of 1000 mg/kg of 10% ethanol (infused over 1–2 hours as tolerated). *Assumes a zero ethanol level to start.* Aim is to produce a serum ethanol level of 100–150 mg/dl.	100 ml	150 ml	300 ml	500 ml	700 ml	1000 ml

Oral Ethanol: Loading Dose
(A 20% volume/volume concentration yields approximately 200 mg/ml)

	Volume of Loading Dose					
	10 kg	*15 kg*	*30 kg*	*50 kg*	*70 kg*	*100 kg*
Loading dose of 1000 mg/kg of 20% ethanol, diluted in juice. May be administered orally or via nasogastric tube. *Assumes a zero ethanol level to start.* Aim is to produce a serum ethanol level of 100–150 mg/dl.	50 ml	75 ml	150 ml	250 ml	350 ml	500 ml

Intravenous Ethanol: Maintenance Dose

(A 10% volume/volume concentration yields approximately 100 mg/ml. Infusion to be started immediately following the loading dose. Aim is to maintain serum ethanol level of 100–150 mg/dl*)

Normal Maintenance Range	Infusion Rate (microdrops/min or ml/hr for various weights)†					
	10 kg	15 kg	30 kg	50 kg	70 kg	100 kg
80 mg/kg/hr	8	12	24	40	56	80
110 mg/kg/hr	11	16	33	55	77	110
130 mg/kg hr	13	19	39	65	91	130
Approximate maintenance dose for chronic alcoholic						
150 mg/kg/hr‡	15	22	45	75	105	150
Range required during hemodialysis						
250 mg/kg/hr‡	25	38	75	125	175	250
300 mg/kg/hr‡	30	45	90	150	210	300
350 mg/kg/hr‡	35	53	105	175	245	350

*Serum ethanol levels should be monitored closely.

†Rounded off to nearest drop.

‡At higher infusion rates, it may be necessary to administer by volume rather than by microdrops/min. Because microdrops/min equal ml/hr, the infusion rate in the chart may be used to calculate both microdrops/min and ml/hr.

Oral Ethanol: Maintenance Dose

(A 20% volume/volume concentration yields approximately 200 mg/ml. Infusion to be given each hour immediately following a loading dose. Aim is to maintain serum ethanol level of 100–150 mg/dl.*
Each dose may be diluted in juice and given orally or via nasogastric tube.)

Normal Maintenance Range	Infusion Rate (ml/hr† for various weights‡)					
	10 kg	15 kg	30 kg	50 kg	70 kg	100 kg
80 mg/kg/hr	4	6	12	20	28	40
110 mg/kg/hr	6	8	17	27	39	55
130 mg/kg/hr	7	10	20	33	46	66
Approximate range for chronic alcoholic or for patient receiving continuous oral activated charcoal						
150 mg/kg/hr	8	11	22	38	53	75
Range required during hemodialysis						
250 mg/kg/hr	13	19	38	63	88	125
300 mg/kg/hr	15	23	46	75	105	150
350 mg/kg/hr	18	26	52	88	123	175

*Serum ethanol levels should be monitored closely.

†For a 30% concentration, divide the amount by 1.5.

‡Rounded off to nearest ml.

SODIUM NITROPRUSSIDE

Dosage

There is no fixed optimum dose. Infusion rates range from 0.5 to 10 µg/kg/minute. The dose is titrated to the clinical response. An infusion pump should be used.

Available Preparations

NIPRIDE (Roche)

NITROPRESS (Abbott)

SODIUM NITROPRUSSIDE (Elkins-Sinn)

Each 5 ml vial contains 50 mg sodium nitroprusside.

Mix only in D5W, and wrap bottle in aluminum foil. Monitor for cyanide toxicity and methemoglobinemia at the higher doses.

Sodium Nitroprusside
(50 mg diluted in 250 ml; concentration of 200 µg/ml)

Dose* (µg/kg/min)	Infusion Rate (microdrops/min or ml/hr for various weights)		
	50 kg	*70 kg*	*100 kg*
0.5	7.5	10.5	15
3	45	63	90
6	90	126*	180*
8	120*	168*	240*
10	150*	210*	300*

*It may be more reasonable to increase concentration to limit volume.
For 50 mg in 500 ml (100 µg/ml), multiply the infusion rate by 2 for desired microdrops/min.
For 100 mg in 250 ml (400 µg/ml), divide the infusion rate by 2 for desired microdrops/min.
For 100 mg in 500 ml (200 µg/ml), use same dose schedule as in chart.
For 200 mg in 250 ml (800 µg/ml), divide the infusion rate by 4 for desired microdrops/min.

TISSUE PLASMINOGEN ACTIVATOR/ALTEPLASE (ACTIVASE)

Dosage

A total dose of either 100 mg in patients over 65 kg or 1.25 mg/kg in patients less than 65 kg should be administered in the following fashion: 60 per cent of the total dose in the first hour with 6 per cent to 10 per cent of the total as a loading dose over 1 to 2 minutes; the remaining 40 per cent of the total dose administered in two equal amounts over the second and third hour.

Available Preparation

Activase

Each vial contains 20 mg or 50 mg of lyophilized powder, which needs to be reconstituted with sterile water for injection without preservatives (provided with vial). It then may be further diluted with normal saline or dextrose.

Tissue Plasminogen Activator/Alteplase (Activase)
(Based on a reconstituted strength of 1 mg/ml*)

	Patient Weight				
	45 kg	*50 kg*	*55 kg*	*60 kg*	*65 kg or greater*
Total dose† (1.25 mg/kg) (Some calculations are rounded off)	56 ml	62.5 ml	70 ml	75 ml	100 ml
Initial bolus‡ Administer over 1–2 minutes (10% of total dose)	5.6 ml	6.25 ml	7 ml	7.5 ml	10 ml
Followed immediately by First hour (50% of total dose)	28 ml	31 ml	35 ml	37.5 ml	50 ml
Second hour (20% of total dose)	11.2 ml	12.5 ml	14 ml	15 ml	20 ml
Third hour (20% of total dose)	11.2 ml	12.5 ml	14 ml	15 ml	20 ml

*If the drug is further diluted to a concentration of 0.5 mg/ml, *double* the volume.
†Note that mg equals ml if reconstituted and infused without further dilution.
‡Withdraw bolus dose with a syringe from reconstituted vial, place remaining drug into *empty* intravenous bag.
Note: Additional therapy includes: oxygen, intravenous nitroglycerin, lidocaine for reperfusion arrhythmias, aspirin therapy when not contraindicated, and routine systemic heparinization.
Cautions: Avoid use of central venous lines, intramuscular injections, and arterial blood gas sampling in noncompressible arteries. Hold venipuncture sites for 20 minutes and monitor intravenous sites for bleeding.
Relative contraindications include: bleeding disorders, trauma, recent stroke (<6 months), recent surgery (<2 weeks but <2 months if neurosurgery), gastrointestinal or genitourinary bleeding (<4 weeks), prolonged cardiopulmonary resuscitation, ? menstruation, ? pregnancy, uncontrolled hypertension, known central nervous system aneurysm, neoplasm, or arteriovenous malformation.

HEPARIN SODIUM: LOADING DOSE/CONTINUOUS INFUSION

Dosage

An intravenous loading dose of 5000 to 10,000 units (50 units/kg in children) for deep vein thrombosis, coronary occlusion, or pulmonary embolism, followed by a continuous infusion of 1000 units/hr (15 to 25 units/kg/hr in children).* In preparing the solution, the heparin should be diluted in D5W or 0.9 per cent sodium chloride and inverted six times to avoid pooling. Aim for activated partial thromboplastin (PTT) of 1.5 to 2 times control.†

Available Preparations

There are many different concentrations available in vials, ampules, and syringes. Some preparations contain parabens or benzyl alcohol.

Example Concentrations

1000 units/ml, 5000 units/ml, 10,000 units/ml, 20,000 units/ml, and 40,000 units/ml.

Clinical Use

For 1000 units/hr infusion, add 25,000 units of heparin to 1000 ml of saline (concentration of 25 units/ml) and infuse at a rate of 40 ml/hr over 24 hours. Alternatively, add 25,000 units of heparin to 500 ml of saline (concentration of 50 units/ml) and infuse at a rate of 20 ml/hr.

VASOPRESSIN INFUSION (8-Arginine—Vasopressin, Antidiuretic Hormone)

Injection

Dosage

As adjunctive therapy for hemorrhage from esophageal varices,‡ dilute in 0.9 per cent sodium chloride or D5W to 0.1 to 1.0 unit/ml. Initial intravenous infusion of 0.2 to 0.4 units/minute may be increased gradually to 0.9 units/minute if necessary.§ Tapering is usually attempted after 24 hours but may be delayed for 3 days to 2 weeks. Always use with infusion pump. Extravasation may lead to severe tissue necrosis.

Available Preparations

Each 0.5-ml ampule provides 10 units. Vasopressin is also available in 1-ml ampules at a concentration of 20 units/ml (Lypho Med, Quad, Parke-Davis). Do *not* use preparation in oil.

Intravenous Vasopressin Continuous Infusion (100 units diluted in 200 ml 0.9% NaCl or D5W: concentration of 0.5 units/ml)		
Dose* (units/min)		**Infusion Rate** (microdrops/min or ml/hour)
Starting	0.1	12
	0.2	24
	0.4	48
	0.6	72
High	0.9	108

Note: This is *not* a dose/weight calculation.

---

*Assumes normal coagulation profile.

†Neutralization of heparin effect: infuse no more than 25 to 50 mg of protamine sulfate slowly over 10 minutes. Each mg of protamine neutralizes 100 units of heparin, but heparin is rapidly metabolized. Assume the half-life of heparin to be 1½ hours following intravenous injection. Hypotension and anaphylactoid reactions may be seen with protamine injection.

‡Not in FDA approved labeling.

§Monitor carefully. Side effects include hypertension, cardiac arrhythmias, myocardial/splanchnic ischemia, decreased cardiac output.

RITODRINE HYDROCHLORIDE (YUTOPAR) INFUSION

Note: Maternal pulmonary edema has been reported with this drug.

Dosage

To inhibit premature labor, dilute in D5W and begin continuous infusion at a rate of 50 to 100 µg/minute. *Note:* This is *not* a dose/weight regimen. Gradually titrate in 50 µg/minute increments at 10- to 15-minute intervals until the desired effect is achieved. The usual dose is 150 to 350 µg/minute. This is generally continued for 12 hours after cessation of uterine contractions. An infusion pump or controlled infusion device is required.

Available Preparations

As a concentrate that must be diluted before use. Each 5-ml vial or ampule provides a total of 50 mg of ritodrine at a concentration of 10 mg/ml (DuPont, Lyphomed, Astra, Quad). Also available at a concentration of 15 mg/ml in a 10-ml vial and syringe containing 150 mg total (DuPont, Lyphomed, Astra, Quad).

Ritodrine Hydrochloride: Continuous Infusion
(150 mg diluted in 500 ml of D5W; concentration of 300 µg/ml)

Dose* (µg/min)		Infusion Rate (microdrops/min† or ml/hr)
50	initial	10
100	dose	20
150		30
200		40
250		50
300		60
350		70‡

*Note: This is *not* a dose/weight calculation.
†Standard microdrop chamber.
‡If fluid restriction is necessary, the concentration can be increased.

NALOXONE HYDROCHLORIDE (NARCAN)

Dosage

Start with a loading dose of 0.4 to 2.0 mg intravenous push. Consider lower dose for a pregnant or a suspected opioid-dependent individual to prevent vomiting from opioid withdrawal. Always be prepared to protect the airway. In children, administer 0.01 mg/kg. If no response and opioids are suspected, consider 10 to 20 mg intravenous push (0.1 to 0.2 mg/kg in children).* If a clinical response is noted, continue with a maintenance dose titrated to keep the patient stable and not in overt withdrawal. The hourly maintenance dose is approximately two thirds of the effective loading dose, given as a constant infusion.

Available Preparations

Each 2-ml ampule contains 2 mg at a concentration of 1 mg/ml. Also available in 10-ml vials and 1- and 2-ml syringes at the same concentration. Also available in a concentration of 0.4 mg/ml in a 1-ml ampule or syringe and a 10-ml vial and at 0.02 mg/ml in 2-ml ampules. Various manufacturers.

---

*There is no set maximum limit to the bolus. However, if no response occurs at 20 mg, an effect from a larger dose is unlikely. Overdose of naloxone has not been reported.

Continuous Infusion

Dilute 10 mg in 500 ml of D5W or 0.9% sodium chloride; final concentration of 0.02 mg/ml. May also use 20 mg in 500 ml for a concentration of 0.04 mg/ml.

Maintenance Dose

Depends on the loading dose. If the loading dose was appropriate, then give the maintenance dose listed below and titrate for the desired clinical effect. If withdrawal occurred with the loading dose, use the lesser maintenance dose (highly variable) and titrate to respiratory function and clinical response.

Naloxone		
Effective Loading Dose (mg)	**Infusion Rate (ml/hr)**	
	0.02 mg/ml	*0.04 mg/ml*
0.4	13	6
1.0	33	16
2	66	33
5	165	82
10	330	165

PHENYTOIN SODIUM (DILANTIN)

Dosage

An intravenous loading dose of 15 to 20 mg/kg, infused at a maximum rate of 40 to 50 mg/minute (1 mg/kg/minute in the neonate). The therapeutic serum level is 10 to 20 μg/ml, but higher levels may be required for patients with status epilepticus. In the elderly or in the presence of cardiovascular instability, a slower infusion rate is recommended. Infuse with electrocardiogram, blood pressure, and pulse monitoring. Infuse by direct intravenous infusion into a large vein to avoid extravasation or dilute* in 0.9 per cent sodium chloride to a concentration of less than 6.7 mg/ml and infuse with an infusion pump or a volume control device.

Available Preparations

Each 5-ml vial provides 250 mg (50 mg/ml). Also available at a concentration of 50 mg/ml in 2-ml and 5-ml ampules, vials, and prefilled syringes. Various manufacturers.

Intravenous Phenytoin: Loading Dose (Add 1 gm of phenytoin to 200 ml of saline* [concentration 5 mg/ml] and infuse at a maximum rate of 8 ml/min (40 mg/min).† In children, the maximum infusion rate is 1 mg/kg/min.)				
Loading Dose (mg/kg)	**Total Volume (ml) of 5 mg/ml Concentration Administered**			
	30 kg	*60 kg*	*70 kg*	*80 kg*
10	60	120	140	160
15	90	180	210	240
18	108	216	252	288
20	120	240	280	320

*Incompatible with any glucose-containing solution. Do not use unless solution is clear. May also use 500 mg per 100 ml saline for the same final concentration.

†Main complications are pain at infusion site and hypotension. Both may be avoided with slower infusion rates and piggybacking the infusion into a concurrent saline infusion.

---

*Not in FDA approved labeling.

ESMOLOL HYDROCHLORIDE (BREVIBLOC)

Dosage

For supraventricular tachycardia, a loading dose of 500 µg/kg is given over 1 minute, followed by a maintenance infusion of 50 µg/kg/minute for 4 minutes. A second loading dose of 500 µg/kg may be infused over 1 minute if the response is not optimal, followed by a maintenance infusion of 100 µg/kg/minute (range 50 to 200 µg/kg/minute)* Monitor heart rate and blood pressure carefully. Maintenance infusion may be continued for 24 hours. Concentrations exceeding 10 mg/ml are irritating. Use infusion pump. Elimination half-life is approximately 9 minutes.

Available Preparations

As a concentrate that must be diluted before use, each 10-ml ampule contains 2.5 g of esmolol (with 25 per cent alcohol and 25 per cent propylene glycol additives). Also available in a single-dose 10-ml vial containing 100 mg.

Esmolol Hydrochloride Injection: Loading Dose
(2.5 g diluted in 250 ml of D5W or D5NS: final concentration of 10 mg/ml. Sequence of loading dose given over 1 minute followed by maintenance dose for 4 minutes. If the response is inadequate, repeat the loading dose followed by 4 minutes of increased maintenance dose to assess the response. Must use infusion pump. Because the pump is controlled with ml/hr rates, the following doses are expressed in ml/hr.)

Infusion Rate (Over First Minute Only)
(set infusion pump at the following ml/hr for various weights: 10 mg/ml concentration)

Dose (µg/kg/min)	50 kg	60 kg	70 kg	80 kg	90 kg	100 kg
500	150	180	210	240	270	300

Esmolol Hydrochloride Injection: Maintenance Dose

Infusion Rate by Pump
(ml/hr for various weights: 10 mg/ml concentration)

Dose (µg/kg/min)	50 kg	60 kg	70 kg	80 kg	90 kg
50	15	18	21	24	27
100	30	36	42	48	54
150	45	54	63	72	81
200	60	72	84	96	108

*Repeat loading doses of 500 µg/kg may be given over 1 minute, and the maintenance dose may be increased by increments of 50 µg/kg/minute for 4 minutes to assess response.

Index

Note: Numbers in *italics* refer to illustrations; numbers followed by (t) indicate tables.